Algorithms in PEDIATRICS

Algorithms in PEDIATRICS

Second Edition

Editors

Anand S Vasudev
DNB D (Ped) DCP MNAMS MICP (USA) FIAP FIMSA
Visiting Consultant Pediatric Nephrologist
Indraprastha Apollo, Max, and Holy Family Hospital
New Delhi, India

Nitin K Shah
MD DCH DNB
Section Head
Department of Pediatrics
PD Hinduja National Hospital, Mumbai
Visiting Pediatric Hematologist Oncologist
BJ Wadia Hospital for Children, Mumbai
Apollo Hospitals
Navi Mumbai, Maharashtra, India
President, Indian Academy of Pediatrics, 2006

Foreword

Vasant Khalatkar

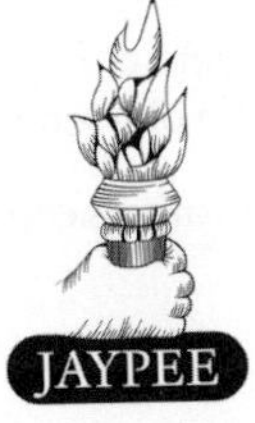

JAYPEE BROTHERS MEDICAL PUBLISHERS
The Health Sciences Publisher
New Delhi | London

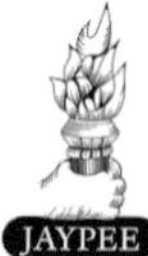

Jaypee Brothers Medical Publishers (P) Ltd

Headquarters
EMCA House, 23/23-B
Ansari Road, Daryaganj
New Delhi 110 002, India
Landline: +91-11-23272143, +91-11-23272703
+91-11-23282021, +91-11-23245672
e-mail: jaypee@jaypeebrothers.com

Corporate Office
4838/24, Ansari Road, Daryaganj
New Delhi 110 002, India
Phone: +91-11-43574357
Fax: +91-11-43574314
e-mail: jaypee@jaypeebrothers.com

Overseas Office
JP Medical Ltd.
83, Victoria Street, London
SW1H 0HW (UK)
Phone: +44-20 3170 8910
e-mail: info@jpmedpub.com

EU GPSR Authorised Representative
Logos Europe, 9 rue Nicolas Poussin
17000, La Rochelle, France
Phone: +33 (0) 6 67 93 73 78
e-mail: contact@logoseurope.eu

Website: www.jaypeebrothers.com
Website: www.jaypeedigital.com

Inquiries for bulk sales may be solicited at: jaypee@jaypeebrothers.com

Algorithms in Pediatrics

First Edition: 2017

Second Edition: **2026**

ISBN: 978-93-5696-476-1

Printed in India at Sterling Graphics Pvt. Ltd.

Contributors

Aakanksha Raghuvanshi
MBBS DOMS DNB
Assistant Professor
Department of Ophthalmology
ESIC Medical College and Hospital
Faridabad, Haryana, India

Aaqib Zaffar Banday MD DM
Lecturer
Department of Pediatrics
Government Medical College
Srinagar, Jammu and Kashmir, India

Aathira Ravindranath MD DM
Consultant
Department of Pediatric Gastroenterology
Apollo BGS Hospitals
Mysuru, Karnataka, India

Abhaya Gupta
MBBS DNB MCh MRCS
Professor (Additional)
Lokmanya Tilak Municipal Medical College (LTMMC) and General Hospital (LTMGH)
Mumbai, Maharashtra, India

Abheet Gupta BS (Psychology)
Psychosocial Rehabilitation Practitioner
Department of Psychosocial Rehabilitation
Behavioral Health Services North
Plattsburgh, New York, USA

Abhijeet Saha
MBBS MD FISPN FIPNA FISPD FRCPCH
Director Professor
Division of Pediatric Nephrology
Department of Pediatrics
Lady Hardinge Medical College
New Delhi, India

Abhishek S Aradhya MD DM
Consultant Neonatologist
Department of Pediatrics
Ovum Woman and Child Speciality Hospital
Bengaluru, Karnataka, India

Aditya P Modak
MBBS DNB (Pediatrics) FIAP (IDPCCM)
Junior Consultant
Department of PICU/NICU
Jupiter Lifeline Hospital
Thane, Maharashtra, India

Ajai Kumar Prithvi
DNB (Pediatrics) DM (Neonatology) DrNB (Neonatology)
Associate Consultant
Department of Neonatology
KIMSHealth
Thiruvananthapuram, Kerala, India

Ajit Gajendragadkar MD DCH
Consultant Pediatrician
Department of Pediatrics
PD Hinduja Hospital and Medical Research Centre (MRC)
Mumbai, Maharashtra, India

Akash Bihari Pati
MS (Gen. Surg) MCh (Ped. Surg)
Additional Professor
Department of Pediatric Surgery
All India Institute of Medical Sciences
Bhubaneswar, Odisha, India

Alapan Mahapatra
MBBS MD (Pediatrics)
Fellow in Pediatric Endocrinology
Department of Endocrinology
Regency Center for Diabetes, Endocrinology and Research (CDER)
Medinipur, West Bengal, India

Alaric J Aroojis
MBBS Diploma (Orthopedics) MS (Orthopedics) DNB (Orthopedics)
Honorary Consultant
Bai Jerbai Wadia Hospital for Children, Mumbai
Consultant
Department of Pediatric Orthopedics
Lilavati and Hinduja Hospital
Mumbai, Maharashtra, India

Alpana A Utture
MD (Pediatrics) DM (Neonatology) Fellowship RNSH (Australia)
Head of Unit and Senior Consultant
Bai Jerbai Wadia Hospital for Children
Mumbai, Maharashtra, India

Amar Jeet Chitkara
MD DNB FIAP
Senior Director
Max Superspeciality Hospital
Shalimar Bagh, New Delhi, India

Amar Shah
MB MS MAMS MCh (Pediatric Surgery) FRCS (Pediatric Surgery, England)
Director
Department of Neonatal and Pediatric Surgery
Amardeep Multispeciality Children Hospital and Research Centre
Ahmedabad, Gujarat, India

Ameet Kishore
MBBS (AFMC) FRCS (Glas) FRCS (Edin) FRCS-ORL (UK)
Senior Consultant
Department of ENT, Head and Neck Surgery
Indraprastha Apollo Hospital
New Delhi, India

Amit Kumar Meena
MD (Dermatology) DNB (Dermatology) MRCP (SCE)
Senior Resident
Department of Dermatology and STD
Lady Hardinge Medical College
New Delhi, India

Amrit Tuteja
DrNB (Neonatology) DNB (Pediatrics) MBBS
Consultant
Department of Neonatology
Max Superspeciality Hospital
New Delhi, India

Anand Alladi MS MCh (Pediatric Surgery)
Professor
Department of Pediatric Surgery
Bangalore Medical College and Research Institute
Bengaluru, Karnataka, India

Anand P Rao MD DNB
Consultant
Department of Pediatric Rheumatology
Manipal Hospital
Bengaluru, Karnataka, India

Anand S Vasudev
DNB D (Ped) DCP MNAMS MICP (USA) FIAP FIMSA
Visiting Consultant Pediatric Nephrologist
Indraprastha Apollo, Max, and Holy Family Hospital
New Delhi, India

Anant Bangar
MBBS DNB (Pediatric Surgery)
Consultant Pediatric Surgeon
Department of Pediatric Surgery
Lilavati Hospital and Research Centre
Mumbai, Maharashtra, India

Anirban Chatterjee MS DNB MNAMS
Senior Consultant
Department of Orthopedics
Medica Superspecialty Hospital
Kolkata, West Bengal, India

Aniruddha Ghosh MD DNB MNAMS
Assistant Professor
Department of Pediatric Medicine
Institute of Child Health
Kolkata, West Bengal, India

Anirudh Shah
MS FRCS (England) FRCS (Edinburgh)
Director
Department of Pediatric Surgery
Amardeep Multispeciality Children Hospital and Research Centre
Ahmedabad, Gujarat, India

Anjali Kulkarni
MD FRCPCH Fellowship in Neonatology (Au)
Consultant
Pediatrician and Neonatologist
Doorstep Health Services
Pune, Maharashtra, India

Anju Aggarwal MD (Pediatrics) FIAP
Director Professor and Head
Department of Pediatrics
University College of Medical Sciences and Guru Teg Bahadur Hospital
New Delhi, India

Anju Gupta MD
Professor
Department of Pediatrics
Postgraduate Institute of Medical Education and Research
Chandigarh, India

Anju Virmani
MBBS MD (Pediatrics) DNB (Endocrinology)
Director
Department of Pediatric Endocrinology
Max Smart Super Specialty Hospital
Senior Consultant Endocrinologist/ Diabetologist
Madhukar Rainbow Children's Hospital
New Delhi, India

Ankit Parakh MD (Pediatrics)
Associate Director
Department of Pediatrics
BLK-Max Hospital
New Delhi, India

Anoop K Verma MBBS MD FIAP
Director
Department of Pediatrics
Swapnil Nursing Home and Research Centre
Raipur, Chhattisgarh, India

Anshu Srivastava
MD (Pediatrics) DM (Gastroenterology)
Professor
Department of Pediatric Gastroenterology
Sanjay Gandhi Postgraduate Institute of Medical Sciences
Lucknow, Uttar Pradesh, India

Anupam Sachdeva MD
Chairman
Division of Pediatric Hematology-Oncology and Bone Marrow Transplantation
Co-Director
Institute of Child Health
Sir Ganga Ram Hospital
New Delhi, India

Anupam Sibal
MD FIMSA FIAP FRCP (Glasgow) FRCP (London) FRCPCH FAAP
Group Medical Director
Senior Pediatric Gastroenterologist and Hepatologist
Department of Pediatric Gastroenterology
Apollo Hospitals
New Delhi, India

Anurag Bajpai MD FRACP SCE (UK)
Consultant Pediatric and Adolescent Endocrinologist
Director
MedEClasses
Department of Pediatric Endocrinology,
Regency Hospital Limited
Kanpur, Uttar Pradesh, India

Anurag Krishna MCh FAMS
Chairman
Department of Pediatrics and Pediatric Surgery
Max Healthcare Institute
New Delhi, India

Apaopa Thekho MD (Dermatology)
Senior Resident
Department of Dermatology, Venereology, and Leprosy
ESIC Medical College and Hospital
Faridabad, Haryana, India

Arjun A Dhawale MS DNB MRCSEd
Surgeon
Department of Orthopedics and Spine Surgery
Sir HN Reliance Foundation Hospital and BJ Wadia Hospital for Children
Mumbai, Maharashtra, India

Arun G Roy MD DM
Senior Consultant and Head
Department of Neurology
Apollo Adlux Hospital
Kochi, Kerala, India

Arvind S Bais MS (ENT) FIMSA
Retired Director Professor and Head, ENT, and Former Principal
Department of ENT and Head Neck Surgery
Lady Hardinge Medical College
New Delhi, India

Ashish Jain
MBBS MD (Pediatrics) DNB (Pediatrics) DM (Neonatology)
Professor and Head
Department of Neonatology
Maulana Azad Medical College and Lok Nayak Hospital
New Delhi, India

Ashish Mehta
MD (Pediatrics) Fellowship in Neonatology (College of Pediatrics, Australia)
Director and Consultant Neonatologist
Arpan Newborn Care Centre
Ahmedabad, Gujarat, India

Ashwani Kumar MBBS DNB MNAMS
Consultant
Department of ENT and Head and Neck Surgery
Indraprastha Apollo Hospital
New Delhi, India

Aspi J Irani MD DCH
Pediatrician
Nanavati Super Speciality Hospital
Mumbai, Maharashtra, India

ATK Rau MD DipHA FAMS
Senior Professor
Department of Pediatrics
Shridevi Trust Institute of Medical Sciences
Tumkur, Karnataka, India

Avantika Tiwari
MBBS DrNB (Pediatric Surgery)
Senior Resident
Department of Pediatric Surgery
Narayana Health Hospitals
Bengaluru, Karnataka, India

Ayesha Mariam
MBBS DCH DNB (Pediatrics) PDF Neurology (IAP)
Registrar (Pediatric Neurology)
Department of Pediatrics
Apollo Children's Hospital
Chennai, Tamil Nadu, India

Baldev S Prajapati
MD (Pediatrics) DPed FIAP MHAMS
Professor and Head
Department of Pediatrics
GCS Medical College, Hospital and Research Centre
Ahmedabad, Gujarat, India

Barath Jagadisan MBBS MD PDCC
Consultant
Department of Pediatric Hepatology
King's College Hospital, NHS Foundation Trust
Denmark Hill, London, UK

Bharat Agarwal
MD DCH DNB MNAMS FIAP
Professor Emeritus and Former Head
Department of Pediatric Hematology and Oncology
BJ Wadia Hospital for Children
Mumbai, Maharashtra, India

Bharati MD (Dermatology)
Senior Resident
Department of Dermatology and STD
Lady Hardinge Medical College
New Delhi, India

Bhaskar Saikia MD IDPCCM
Senior Consultant—Pediatric Intensivist
Department of Pediatrics
Max Superspeciality Hospital
New Delhi, India

Bikrant Bihari Lal MD DM
Associate Professor
Department of Pediatric Hepatology
Institute of Liver and Biliary Sciences
New Delhi, India

Chandan S
MBBS MD (Pediatrics)
Senior Resident
Department of Neonatology
Maulana Azad Medical College and Lok Nayak Hospital
New Delhi, India

D Venkata Umesh Reddy
MBBS MD DM (Pediatric Gastroenterology)
Consultant Pediatric Gastroenterologist, Hepatologist and Interventional Endoscopist
Department of Pediatric Gastroenterology
Ankura Hospital for Women and Children
Hyderabad, Telangana and Vijayawada, Andhra Pradesh, India

Deepa Sharma
MBBS DNB Fellowship in Vitreoretina
Chief Medical Officer
Department of Ophthalmology
Atal Bihari Vajpayee Institute of Medical Sciences (ABVIMS) and Dr RML Hospital
New Delhi, India

Deepak Chawla
MD DM (Neonatology)
Professor
Department of Neonatology
Government Medical College and Hospital
Chandigarh, India

Deepti Suri MD DNB
Professor of Pediatric Allergy and Immunology
Department of Advanced Pediatric Center
Postgraduate Institute of Medical Education and Research
Chandigarh, India

Devinder Rai
MBBS MS (ENT)
Senior Consultant
Department of ENT
Sir Ganga Ram Hospital
New Delhi, India

Dhulika Dhingra MBBS MD (Pediatrics)
Specialist
Department of Pediatrics
National Institute of TB and Respiratory Diseases
New Delhi, India

Digvijay Singh MD FAICO
Director
Department of Ophthalmology
Noble Eye Care
Gurugram, Haryana, India

Dimple Jain
MBBS MD (Pediatrics) MRCPCH PDCC (Pediatric Gastroenterology)
Consultant Pediatric Gastroenterologist, Hepatologist, Liver Transplant Physician
Department of Pediatrics
Jupiter Hospital
Thane, Maharashtra, India

Dinesh K Chirla
MD DM (Neonatology) FRCPCH (UK)
Neonatal Fellow (Australia) Fellow in PICU (UK)
Director
Department of Neonatology and Pediatric Intensive Care
Rainbow Children's Hospital
Hyderabad, Telangana, India

Divij Sachdeva MD
Associate Consultant
Pediatrics, Hematology, Oncology and BMP Unit
Institute of Child Health
Sir Ganga Ram Hospital
New Delhi, India

Divya Arun Kondgekar
MBBS MD FPCS (MUHS)
Senior Resident
Department of Pediatric Surgery
Bai Jerbai Wadia Hospital for Children
Mumbai, Maharashtra, India

Ganesh S Jevalikar MD PDCC
Principal Consultant
Department of Endocrinology and Diabetes
Max Healthcare
New Delhi, India

Gaurav Mandhan
DM (Neonatology) MD (Pediatrics)
MRCPCH FIAP (Neonatology)
Director and Consultant
Department of Neonatology and Pediatrics
Miracles Apollo Cradle Hospital
Gurugram, Haryana, India

Gauri Kapoor
MD (Pediatrics) PhD (Molecular Oncology)
Director and Head
Department of Pediatric Hematology and Oncology
Rajiv Gandhi Cancer Institute and Research Centre
New Delhi, India

Gautam S Agarwal MS MCh
Senior Consultant
Department of Pediatric Surgery
Kokilaben Dhirubhai Ambani Hospital
Mumbai, Maharashtra, India

Geminiganesan Sangeetha
MD MRCPCH PhD
Assistant Professor
Department of Pediatrics
(Pediatric Nephrology Division)
Sri Ramachandra Institute of Higher Education and Research
Chennai, Tamil Nadu, India

Gurleen Sikka
MBBS MD RCPCH Fellowship (Neonatology)
Consultant
Department of Neonatology and Pediatrics
CK Birla Hospital
New Delhi, Delhi, India

Harshika Chawla
MBBS MS (Ophth) FICO FRCOpth
Clinical Fellow Oculoplastics
Department of Oculoplasty
Royal Victoria Infirmary
Newcastle Upon Tyne, UK

Himanshu Acharya MBBS MS MCh DNB
Associate Professor
Department of Pediatric Surgery
Netaji Subhash Chandra Bose Medical College
Jabalpur, Madhya Pradesh, India

Himanshu Garkoti
MS DNB (Ophthalmology)
Senior Resident (Vitreo-retina, Uvea, Neuro-ophthalmology)
Department of Ophthalmology
Atal Bihari Vajpayee Institute of Medical Sciences
New Delhi, India

Hina Kauser MBBS MS
Professor
Department of Ophthalmology
Hamdard Institute of Medical Sciences and Research
New Delhi, India

Hitesh B Chauhan MS
Pediatric Orthopedic Surgeon
Department of Pediatric Orthopedics
Rainbow Superspeciality Hospital and Children's Orthopedic Centre
Ahmedabad, Gujarat, India

Ira J Holla MBBS FAAP
Assistant Professor
Division of Newborn Medicine
University of Mississippi Medical Center
Madison, Mississippi, USA

Ira Shah
MD (Pediatrics) DCH (Gold Medalist) FCPS
Diploma in Pediatric Infectious Diseases (UK)
Professor and Head
Department of Pediatric Infectious Diseases and Pediatric Gastroenterology and Hepatology
BJ Wadia Hospital for Children
Mumbai, Maharashtra, India

Jasodhara Chaudhuri
MD MRCPCH (UK) FRCPCH (UK) DM (Neurology)
Assistant Professor
Department of Neuromedicine
Nil Ratan Sircar (NRS) Medical College
Kolkata, West Bengal, India

Jaswinder Kaur
MD Fellowship in Pediatric Gastroenterology, Hepatology and Nutrition (ISPGHAN)
FNB Trainee
Department of Pediatric Gastroenterology, Hepatology and Liver Transplantation
Indraprastha Apollo Hospital
New Delhi, India

Jayakumar Vaikundam
MD (Ped) DCH DM (Neuro)
Chairman and Senior Consultant Neurologist
Department of Neurology
JK Institute of Neurology
Madurai, Tamil Nadu, India

Jayanth S Sampath
MBBS FRCSEd MSc
Consultant Pediatric Orthopedic Surgeon
Department of Pediatric Orthopedics
Rainbow Children's Hospital
Bengaluru, Karnataka, India

Jayashree A Mondkar MD DCH
Professor Emeritus
Lokmanya Tilak Municipal General Hospital and Medical College
Mumbai, Maharashtra, India

Jaydeep Choudhury
DNB (Pediatrics) MNAMS FIAP
Professor
Department of Pediatrics
Institute of Child Health
Kolkata, West Bengal, India

John Matthai
DCH MD FAB (Pediatric Gastroenterology) FRCPCH
Consultant
Pediatric Gastroenterologist
Masonic Children's Hospital
Coimbatore, Tamil Nadu, India

Jyoti Sharma
MD (Pediatrics) DNB (Pediatrics) Fellow IPNA, Fellow ISN (Pediatric Nephrology)
Senior Consultant (Pediatric Nephrology)
Renal Unit
Department of Medicine
King Edward Memorial Hospital
Pune, Maharashtra, India

Kana R Jat MD (Pediatrics)
Additional Professor
Department of Pediatrics
All India Institute of Medical Sciences
New Delhi, India

Kanishka Das
MS DNB (Gen. Surg) MCh DNB MNAMS (Ped. Surg)
Professor
Department of Pediatric Surgery
All India Institute of Medical Sciences
Bhubaneswar, Odisha, India

Karunesh Kumar MD FNB
Consultant (Pediatric Gastroenterology)
Department of Pediatric Gastroenterology, Hepatology, and Liver Transplantation
Indraprastha Apollo Hospital
New Delhi, India

Kaustubh Mohite
MD (Pediatrics) Diplomat (European Pediatric Respiratory Society)
Consultant (Pediatric Pulmonology, Interventional Pulmonology and Sleep Medicine)
Department of Pediatrics
Sai Child Care Hospital, Jupiter Hospital, Apollo Hospital, SRCC Hospital, Hinduja Hospital, Kokilaben Dhirubhai Ambani Hospital
Mumbai, Maharashtra, India

Kochurani Abraham
DCH DNB (Pediatrics) Fellowship in Pediatric Endocrinology
Consultant
Department of Pediatric Endocrinology
Ankura Hospital
Pune, Maharashtra, India

Lokesh Lingappa
MD DM (Neuro) MRCPCH (UK)
Clinical Lead and Consultant Child and Adolescent Neurologist
Division of Pediatric Neurosciences
Rainbow Children's Hospital
Hyderabad, Telangana, India

M Zulfikar Ahamed
MBBS DCH DM (Cardiology) FIAP
Senior Consultant
Department of Pediatric Cardiology
KIMSHealth
Consultant, Pediatric Cardiologist
Lifeline Heart Institute
Clinical Professor
Department of Pediatric and Adolescent Cardiology
Child Development Centre (CDC)
Adjunct Professor
Department of Cardiology
KMC Manipal
Adjunct Professor
Department of Cardiology
Gokulam Medical College
Thiruvananthapuram, Kerala, India

Madhava Vijayakumar
MD DCH DNB FRCP
Professor and Head
Department of Pediatrics
Institute of Maternal and Child Health (IMCH)
Government Medical College
Kozhikode, Kerala, India

Mahesh A Mohite MD DCH
Chief Pediatrician
Sai Children's Hospital
Panvel, Maharashtra, India

Mahrukh Bhat
MBBS MS (Ophthalmology)
Assistant Professor
Department of Ophthalmology
ESIC Medical College and Hospital
Faridabad, Haryana, India

Malathi Sathiyasekaran
MD DCH MNAMS DM (Gastro)
Senior Consultant
Department of Pediatric Gastroenterology
MGM Healthcare and Rainbow Hospitals
Chennai, Tamil Nadu, India

Manas Kalra MD
Senior Consultant
Pediatrics, Hematology, Oncology and BMP Unit
Institute of Child Health
Sir Ganga Ram Hospital
New Delhi, India

Manav Deep Singh MS
Professor
Department of Ophthalmology
ABVIMS and Dr RML Hospital
New Delhi, India

Mandar Agashe MS
Consultant
Centre for Pediatric Orthopedic Care
Dr Agashe's Hospital
Mumbai, Maharashtra, India

Manika Boipai MCh (Pediatric Surgery)
Junior Pediatric Surgeon
Department of Pediatric Surgery
SRCC Children's Hospital Managed by Narayana Health
Mumbai, Maharashtra, India

Manjari Agarwal MD (Pediatrics)
Consultant
Department of Pediatric Rheumatology
Sir Ganga Ram Hospital
New Delhi, India

Manoj G Matnani
MD (Pediatrics) IPNA Fellowship (India)
Fellowship Pediatric Nephrology (UK)
Consultant Pediatric Nephrologist
Department of Pediatrics
Jehangir Hospital and Dr DY Patil Medical College
Pune, Maharashtra, India

Mehul A Shah
MD (Pediatrics) DCH (Bom) MD (USA) DABPN (USA)
Consultant Pediatric Nephrologist
Apollo Hospital and Little Stars and She Hospital
Hyderabad, Telangana, India

MKC Nair
DSc PhD MD MBA MA PG Diploma in Counseling and Ultrasonography
Director, Developmental Medicine
NIMS-Spectrum-Child Development Research Centre (CDRC)
Thiruvananthapuram, Kerala, India

Moinak S Sarma MBBS MD DM
Additional Professor
Department of Pediatric Gastroenterology
Sanjay Gandhi Postgraduate Institute of Medical Sciences
Lucknow, Uttar Pradesh, India

Monika Chhajed
MBBS DCH DNB (Pediatrics)
Consultant
Department of Pediatric Neurology
Motherhood Chaitanya Hospital
Chandigarh, India

Monjori Mitra
MBBS DCH DNB FIAP
Professor
Institute of Child Health
Kolkata, West Bengal, India

Mukesh Sanklecha MD DNB DCH
Senior Consultant
Department of Pediatrics
Bombay Hospital Institute of Medical Sciences and Saifee Hospital
Mumbai, Maharashtra, India

Mukta Mantan
MD DNB (Pediatrics) Fellowship in Pediatric Nephrology
Director-Professor
Department of Pediatrics
Maulana Azad Medical College
New Delhi, India

Murchana Khound
MBBS MD (Pediatrics) IAP Neonatology Fellowship PGDDN
Assistant Professor
Department of Pediatrics
All India Institute of Medical Sciences
Guwahati, Assam, India

Nameet Jerath
MD (Pediatrics) Fellowship Pediatric Critical Care (Hospital for Sick Kids, Toronto)
Senior Consultant
Department of Pediatric Critical Care and Pulmonology
Indraprastha Apollo Hospital
New Delhi, India

Nandkishor S Kabra
DM MD DNB MSc
Director
Neonatal Intensive Care Unit (NICU)
Department of Neonatology
Surya Hospitals
Mumbai, Maharashtra, India

Narendra R Nanivadekar
MD DCH DNB
Consultant Pediatrician and Neonatologist
Niramay Pediatric Nursing Home and Eye Care Centre
Kolhapur, Maharashtra, India

Naushin Ahmad
MBBS (Pursuing MS)
Junior Resident 3
Department of Ophthalmology
Hamdard Institute of Medical Sciences and Research
New Delhi, India

Naveen Bajaj
MD (Pediatrics) DM (Neonatology) Fellowship in Neonatal Perinatal Medicine (Canada)
Director
Department of Neonatology
Sapling Hospital
Ludhiana, Punjab, India

Naveen Jain DM (Neonatology)
Senior Consultant
Department of Neonatology
KIMSHEALTH
Thiruvananthapuram, Kerala, India

Naveen Sankhyan MD DM
Professor
Department of Pediatrics
Advanced Pediatrics Centre
Postgraduate Institute of Medical Education and Research (PGIMER)
Chandigarh, India

Neelu Desai MD DNB
Consultant
Department of Child Neurology
PD Hinduja Hospital
Mumbai, Maharashtra, India

Neevita Narayan
BSc (Speech and Hearing) MSc (Audiology) AuD (USA)
Director
SpHear Speech and Hearing Clinics
New Delhi, India

Nihaal Reddy MD
Consultant Pediatric Neuroradiologist
Rainbow Children's Hospital, Tenet Diagnostics
Hyderabad, Telangana, India

Nikita Gandhi Sethi
MD DNB (Dermatology)
Senior Consultant
Department of Dermatology, Venereology and Leprosy
DERMHealth Skin and Hair Clinic
New Delhi, India

Nitin K Shah
MD DCH DNB
Section Head
Department of Pediatrics
PD Hinduja National Hospital, Mumbai
Visiting Pediatric Hematologist Oncologist
BJ Wadia Hospital for Children
Mumbai
Apollo Hospitals
Navi Mumbai, Maharashtra, India
President, Indian Academy of Pediatrics, 2006

Noella Maria Delia Pereira
DNB (Pediatrics) DCH MRCPCH (UK) PG Diploma in Pediatric Infectious Diseases (Oxford)
Consultant (Pediatric HIV and Telemedicine)
Pediatric Centre of Excellence for HIV Care
Lokmanya Tilak Municipal General Hospital and Medical College
Mumbai, Maharashtra, India

Omkar P Hajirnis
DNB (Pediatrics) MRCPCH (UK)
Consultant Pediatric Neurologist
Department of Pediatrics
Jupiter Hospital
Thane, Maharashtra, India

PAM Kunju
MD (Pediatrics) DCH DM (Neurology) WHO Fellowship in Pediatric Neurology (USA)
Professor
Department of Pediatric Neurology
KIMSHEALTH
Thiruvananthapuram, Kerala, India

Pankaj V Deshpande
MRCP (UK) MD (Pediatrics) FCPS (Child Health) DCH
Consultant
Department of Pediatric Nephrology
Hinduja Hospital, Mahim and
Apollo Hospital, Belapur
Mumbai, Maharashtra, India

Paramanand G Andankar
MBBS DCH DNB
Chief Pediatric Intensivist and Pediatrician
Pediatric Intensive Care Unit (PICU)/ Neonatal Intensive Care Unit (NICU)
Jupiter Lifeline Hospital
Thane, Maharashtra, India

Parmarth Chandane
MD DAA Diplomate ERS
Professor (Additional)
Department of Pediatrics
Head (Pediatric Respiratory Medicine)
Bai Jerbai Wadia Children's Hospital
Mumbai, Maharashtra, India

Paula Goel MD (Pediatrics)
Consultant Pediatrician and Adolescent Specialist
Department of Pediatrics
Fayth Clinic
Mumbai, Maharashtra, India

Piyali Bhattacharya
DCH MD (Pediatrics) FIAP FRCP (London)
Senior Pediatrician
General Hospital
Sanjay Gandhi Postgraduate Institute of Medical Sciences
Lucknow, Uttar Pradesh, India

PK Pruthi MBBS DCH MD MAMS
Chairman and Senior Consultant
Division of Pediatric Nephrology and Renal Transplantation
Sir Ganga Ram Hospital
New Delhi, India

Poonam Sidana
MD (Peds) Neonatal Fellowship (Australia)
Director
Department of Pediatrics and Neonatology
CK Birla Hospital
New Delhi, India

Pradeep K Sharma MBBS MD IDPCCM
Senior Consultant and Unit Head
Department of Pediatrics
Shree Aggarsain International Hospital
New Delhi, India

Pratap Kumar Patra
MBBS MD (Pediatrics) DM (Pediatric Clinical Immunology and Rheumatology)
Additional Professor
Department of Pediatrics
All India Institute of Medical Sciences
Patna, Bihar, India

Pratibha D Singhi
MBBS MD FIAP FNAMS
Professor, Senior Consultant, and Head
Department of Pediatric Neurology
Amrita Institute of Medical Sciences
Faridabad, Haryana, India

Pratiksha Khatua MBBS MD (Pediatrics)
Fellow in Infectious Disease (IAP)
Institute of Child Health
Kolkata, West Bengal, India

Praveen Khilnani
MD FICCM FAAP (USA) FCCM (USA) MCCM (USA)
Chairman
Department of Pediatrics, Pediatric Critical Care and Pulmonology
Medanta—The Medicity
Gurugram, Haryana, India

Pravesh Yadav MD (Dermatology)
Assistant Professor
Department of Dermatology
Dr Baba Saheb Ambedkar Hospital
New Delhi, India

Preetham K Poddutoor
DCH DNB Fellow Neonatology
Head
Department of Pediatrics
Rainbow Children's Hospital
Secunderabad, Telangana, India

Preeti Singh MBBS MD
Professor
Department of Pediatrics
Kalawati Saran Children's Hospital
Lady Hardinge Medical College
New Delhi, India

Prema Raghunathan
MBBS DNB (Pediatrics) PGDAP FIAP ACME
Professor
Department of Pediatrics
Rajarajeswari Medical College and Hospital
Bengaluru, Karnataka, India

Premal Naik MS DNB
Honorary Orthopedic Surgeon
Smt. Nathiba Hargovandas
Lakhmichand (NHL) Municipal Medical
College, Ahmedabad
Director, Rainbow Superspeciality Hospital
Ahmedabad, Gujarat, India

Priya Tomar
MBBS MD Fellowship in Pediatric Cardiology
Pediatric Cardiologist
Department of Pediatric Cardiology
Child Heart Foundation
New Delhi, India

Priyanka Arora MBBS MS FPOS
Associate Professor
Department of Ophthalmology
Dayanand Medical College and Hospital
Ludhiana, Punjab, India

Priyankar Pal
MD (Pediatrics) MNAMS FIAP FRCPCH (UK)
Professor and Head
Department of Pediatric Medicine
Institute of Child Health
Kolkata, West Bengal, India

PSN Menon MBBS MD MNAMS
Former Professor
Department of Pediatrics
All India Institute of Medical Sciences
New Delhi, India

Purva Kanvinde
MBBS MD (Pediatrics) FIAP FNB
Consultant
Department of Pediatric Hematology-Oncology
Bai Jerbai Wadia Hospital for Children
Mumbai, Maharashtra, India

Purvaja Kubde MBBS MD (Pediatrics)
FNB Fellow
Department of Pediatric
Hematology-Oncology
Bai Jerbai Wadia Hospital for Children
Mumbai, Maharashtra, India

Raghupathy Palany MD DCH FRCP
Senior Consultant
Department of Pediatric and
Adolescent Endocrinology
Sagar Hospital
Bengaluru, Karnataka, India

Rajal B Prajapati MD (Pediatrics) DPed
Professor
Department of Pediatrics
GCS Medical College, Hospital and
Research Centre
Ahmedabad, Gujarat, India

Rajeev Redkar
MCh FRCS (Peds) DNB FRCS Ed FRCSG MS
FCPS IAS
Consultant
Department of Pediatric Surgery
Lilavati Hospital and Research Centre
Mumbai, Maharashtra, India

Rajesh R Chokhani MD DCH FRCPCH (UK)
Consultant Pediatrician
Department of General Pediatrics
PD Hinduja Hospital and Research Centre
Mumbai, Maharashtra, India

Rajiv Chadha MS MCh (Pediatric Surgery)
Retired Director-Professor
Department of Pediatric Surgery
Lady Hardinge Medical College and
Kalawati Saran Children's Hospital
New Delhi, India

Raju C Shah MD DPed FIAP FRCPCH (UK)
Former Professor and Head
GCS Medical College
Ankur Institute of Child Health
Ahmedabad, Gujarat, India

Ram G Holla
MBBS MD (Pediatrics) DM (Neonatology)
Senior Consultant
Department of Pediatrics and
Neonatology
Rosewalk Hospital
New Delhi, India

Ramesh Babu
MS MCh FRCS (Glas) FRCS (Edin) FRCS (Ped) PhD
Professor and Senior Consultant
Department of Pediatric Urology
Sri Ramachandra Institute of Higher
Education and Research
Chennai, Tamil Nadu, India

Ramya Bandi
MD DNB (Pediatrics) Fellowship
(Pediatric Neurology)
Consultant Pediatric Neurologist
Department of Pediatrics
Ankura Hospital for Women and
Children
Hyderabad, Telangana, India

Rashmi Kumar MD FNASc FAMS
Retired Professor and Head
Department of Pediatrics
King George's Medical University
Lucknow, Uttar Pradesh, India

Rashna D Hazarika
MBBS MD (Pediatrics) (PGIMER, Chandigarh)
Professor and Medical Superintendent
PA Sangma International Medical
College and Hospital
Ri Bhoi, Meghalaya, India

Rasiklal S Shah
MBBS MCh (Pediatric Surgeon)
Professor and Head
Department of Surgery and
Pediatric Surgery
SRCC Children's Hospital Managed
by Narayana Health
Mumbai, Maharashtra, India

Rhishikesh P Thakre
DM (Neonatology) MD DNB DCH FCPS FIAP FNNF
Senior Consultant
Neo Clinic
Chhatrapati Sambhajinagar,
Maharashtra, India

Ridhima Aggarwal MBBS MD (Pediatrics)
Senior Resident
Pediatric Clinical Immunology and
Rheumatology
Department of Pediatrics
Postgraduate Institute of Medical
Education and Research
Chandigarh, India

Ritabrata Kundu
MD (Pediatrics) FIAP
Professor (Pediatrics)
Department of Pediatric Medicine
Institute of Child Health
Kolkata, West Bengal, India

Ritika Khurana MD FNB
Junior Consultant
Department of Pediatric
Hematology-Oncology
BJ Wadia Hospital for Children
Mumbai, Maharashtra, India

Ritu Gupta MBBS DCH
Senior Consultant Pediatrician
Adolescent Health Specialist, Certified
Parenting and Youth Life Coach
Friends Eye and Childcare Centre
Noida, Uttar Pradesh, India

Rohit Vohra
MBBS MD (Pediatrics) IFPCCM Fellowship in
Pulmonology
Consultant
Department of Pediatric Intensive Care
and Pulmonology
Indraprastha Apollo Hospital
New Delhi, India

Roli M Srivastava
MBBS DCH PGDAP (Adolescent Pediatrics) MD
Consultant
SKIN MIRACLE Aesthetics, Anti-aging,
Laser and Wellness Centers
Retired Scientist
Reproductive and Child Health Division
Indian Council of Medical Research
(ICMR)
Kanpur, Uttar Pradesh, India

Ruchi Nimish Nanavati
MBBS MD (Pediatrics) IBCLC FNNF
Professor and Ex-Head
Department of Neonatology
Seth Gordhandas Sunderdas (GS)
Medical College and
King Edward Memorial (KEM) Hospital
Mumbai, Maharashtra, India

Rujuta Mehta
MBBS MS (Orthopedics) DNB (Orthopedics)
Honorary Consultant and Head
Department of Pediatric Orthopedics
Bai Jerbai Wadia Hospital for Children,
Mumbai
Consultant
Nanavati, Jaslok, Shushrusha, and
Surya Hospital
Mumbai, Maharashtra, India

Rupal Gupta MBBS MD
Senior Resident
Division of Pediatric Nephrology
Department of Pediatrics
Lady Hardinge Medical College
New Delhi, India

Rupesh Wod
MBBS MS (Orthopedics and Trauma)
Consultant Pediatric Orthopedic
Surgeon
Department of Pediatric Orthopedics
National Academy of Medical Sciences
(NAMS)
Kanti Children's Hospital
Kathmandu, Nepal

S Balasubramanian
MD DCH FRCPCH (UK)
Senior Consultant
Department of Pediatrics
Kanchi Kamakoti CHILDS Trust Hospital
Chennai, Tamil Nadu, India

S Thangavelu
MD DCH DNB MRCP
Pediatric Consultant and Director
Department of Pediatrics
Mehta Multispeciality Hospital Pvt Ltd
Chennai, Tamil Nadu, India

Sabharitha G
MBBS MD (Pediatrics)
Registrar
Department of Pediatrics
Dr Mehta's Multispeciality Hospital
Chennai, Tamil Nadu, India

Sagar Bhattad
MBBS MD (Ped) DM (Ped Clinical Immunology
and Rheumatology) Fellowship in BMT
Consultant
Pediatric Immunology, Rheumatology,
and Bone Marrow Transplant (BMT)
Department of Pediatrics
Aster CMI Hospital
Bengaluru, Karnataka, India

Sandeep A Patwardhan
MS (Orth) DOrth
Professor
Department of Pediatric Orthopedics
Sancheti Institute
Pune, Maharashtra, India

Sangeeta Mudaliar DNB (Pediatrics)
Head and Consultant
Department of Pediatric Hematology-
Oncology
Bai Jerbai Wadia Hospital for Children
Mumbai, Maharashtra, India

Sangeetha Shenoy MD (Pediatrics)
Professor
Department of Pediatrics
MS Ramaiah Medical College
Bengaluru, Karnataka, India

Sanjay M Bafna
MBBS MD (Pediatrics) European Diploma in
Pediatric Respiratory Medicine, Diploma in
Pediatric Sleep Medicine
Consultant Pediatrician, Pediatric
Pulmonologist, and Critical Care
Specialist
Department of Pediatrics
Jehangir Hospital and Bharati
Vidyapeeth Medical College and
Hospital
Pune, Maharashtra, India

Sanjay Rao
MBBS MS (Surgery) MCh (Pediatric Surgery) DNB
(Pediatric Surgery) FRCS Ed (Pediatric Surgery)
Senior Consultant and Head
Department of Pediatric Surgery
Narayana Health Hospitals
Bengaluru, Karnataka, India

Sanjay Wazir
DM (Neonatology)
Director
Department of Neonatology
Motherhood Hospital
Gurugram, Haryana, India

Sarah Paul DCH MD (Peds)
Professor (Retd.)
Department of Pediatrics
PSG Medical College
Coimbatore, Tamil Nadu, India

Sarbani S Raha MD (Peds)
Consultant Pediatric Neurologist
KGP Children Hospital and Child
Neurology and Epilepsy Clinic (CNEC)
Vadodara, Gujarat, India

Sarita Sanke MD DNB MRCP (SCE)
Senior Consultant
Department of Dermatology,
Venereology, and Leprosy
Yashoda Superspecialty Hospital
New Delhi, India

Savneet Kaur MD (Pediatrics)
Assistant Professor
Department of Pediatrics
Lady Hardinge Medical College
New Delhi, India

Seema Alam MD
Professor and Head
Department of Pediatric Hepatology
Institute of Liver and Biliary Sciences
New Delhi, India

Shachi Srivastava
MS DNB (Ophthalmology)
Assistant Professor
Department of Ophthalmology
ESIC Medical College and Hospital
Faridabad, Haryana, India

Shakuntala Prabhu
MD FRCPCH (UK)
Professor
Department of Pediatrics and Pediatric
Cardiology
Bai Jerbai Wadia Hospital for Children
Mumbai, Maharashtra, India

Shalu Gupta MD DM
Director-Professor
Department of Pediatrics
Lady Hardinge Medical College and
Kalawati Saran Children's Hospital
New Delhi, India

Sharad Nair
MBBS MS (ENT) Fellowship in Head Neck Oral
Onco Reconstructive and Microvascular Surgery
Consultant
Department of ENT, Head Neck and
Oral Cancer Surgery
Indraprastha Apollo Hospital
New Delhi, India

Shashi Vashisht MBBS MS
Retired Professor and Head
Department of Ophthalmology
ESIC Medical College
Faridabad, Haryana, India

Shekhar Patil MBBS MD DM
Consultant
Department of Neurology
Apollo Hospital
Navi Mumbai, Maharashtra, India

Shikha Jain MBBS MS
Chief Medical Officer
Department of Ophthalmology
ABVIMS and Dr RML Hospital
New Delhi, India

Shiv Sajan Saini MD DM
Associate Professor
Newborn Unit
Department of Pediatrics
Postgraduate Institute of Medical
Education and Research (PGIMER)
Chandigarh, India

Shoham Majumder
MBBS MD (Pediatrics) DM (Neonatology)
Assistant Professor
Department of Neonatology
Himalayan Institute of Medical Sciences
Dehradun, Uttarakhand, India

Shreepal Jain MBBS MD FNB FPICS
Consultant Interventional Pediatric and
Fetal Cardiologist
Bai Jerbai Wadia Hospital for Children
Mumbai, Maharashtra, India

Shyam Kukreja MBBS DCH MD (Pediatrics)
Director and Head
Department of Pediatrics
Max Super Speciality Hospital
New Delhi, India

Sikha Agarwal MD (Pediatrics)
Consultant
Department of Pediatrics and
Pediatric Rheumatology
PREP Clinic, PD Hinduja Hospital
Mumbai, Maharashtra, India

Sneha Shinde MD
FNB Fellow
Department of Pediatric Hematology-
Oncology
BJ Wadia Hospital for Children
Mumbai, Maharashtra, India

Somashekhar M Nimbalkar
MD (Ped) PGDPH CPH FIAP FNNF
Head
Department of Neonatology
Pramukhswami Medical College
Anand, Gujarat, India

Soonu Udani MD
Medical Director and Head
Department of Critical Care and
Emergency Services
SRCC Children's Hospital
Mumbai, Maharashtra, India

Soumya Tiwari MBBS MD
Professor
Department of Pediatrics
Kalawati Saran Children's Hospital
Lady Hardinge Medical College
New Delhi, India

Srijib Mukherjee
DNB FNB (Pediatric Hematology Oncology
Fellow in BMT
Children's Hospital, Westmead
Sydney, Australia

Subhasis Roy Choudhury
MS DNB MCh (Pediatric Surgery)
Director-Professor
Department of Pediatric Surgery
Lady Hardinge Medical College and
Kalawati Saran Children's Hospital
New Delhi, India

Sudha R Chandrashekhar MD ESPE
Professor
Department of Pediatrics
Bai Jerbai Wadia Hospital for Children and Seth GS Medical College
Mumbai, Maharashtra, India

Suhas V Prabhu MD DCH MNAMS
Consultant Pediatrician
Department of Pediatrics
PD Hinduja Hospital
Mumbai, Maharashtra, India

Suma Balan
MBBS MD (Pediatrics) MRCP (Pediatrics) CCT (UK)
Professor and Head
Department of Rheumatology and Clinical Immunology
Amrita Institute of Medical Sciences
Kochi, Kerala, India

Supriya Phanse Gupte
MD (Pediatrics) Fellowship in Pediatric Endocrinology
Consultant
Department of Pediatrics
Dr DY Patil Medical College, Hospital and Research Centre
Pune, Maharashtra, India

Surender K Yachha MD DM
Director and Head
Department of Pediatric Gastroenterology, Hepatology, and Liver Transplantation
Sakra World Hospital
Bengaluru, Karnataka, India

Surpreet BS Nagi DCH
Consultant
Department of Pediatrics
Dr Anand's Hospital for Children
Mumbai, Maharashtra, India

Sushma P Desai
MD (Pediatrics) DCH PGD (Adolescent Pediatrics)
Consultant Pediatrician, Adolescent Physician and Counselor
Department of Pediatrics and Adolescent Health Care
Gopi Children Hospital and "Tarun" Adolescent Health Care Center
Surat, Gujarat, India

Sushmita Banerjee
MBBS DCH MRCPI MSc (Clinical Pediatrics) FRCPCH FIAP
Consultant
Department of Pediatrics
Calcutta Medical Research Institute (CMRI)
Kolkata, West Bengal, India

Suyodhan A Reddy
MCh (Pediatric Surgery)
Senior Pediatric Surgeon and Head
Department of Pediatric Surgery
Sir JJ Group of Hospitals
Mumbai, Maharashtra, India

T Sathish Kumar MBBS MD DCH
Professor
Department of Pediatrics
Christian Medical College
Vellore, Tamil Nadu, India

Tanu Singhal MD (Pediatrics) MSc
Consultant
Department of Pediatrics and Infectious Disease
Kokilaben Dhirubhai Ambani Hospital and Medical Research Institute
Mumbai, Maharashtra, India

Tapas K Sabui MD
Professor
Department of Pediatric Medicine
Santiniketan Medical College
Bolpur, West Bengal, India

Taral V Nagda MS DNB
Pediatric Orthopedic Surgeon
Department of Pediatric Orthopedics
SRCC Children's Hospital
Mumbai, Maharashtra, India

Taru Dewan MS (Ophthalmology) FRCSEd
Professor and Head
Department of Ophthalmology
Atal Bihari Vajpayee Institute of Medical Sciences
New Delhi, India

Tulika Seth MD ABP
Additional Professor
Department of Hematology
All India Institute of Medical Sciences
New Delhi, India

Tushar Idhate
MBBS MD (Pediatrics)
Associate Professor
MGM Medical College and Hospital
Chhatrapati Sambhajinagar, Maharashtra, India

V Viswanathan
MBBS DCH MRCP PhD
Consultant Pediatric Neurologist
Department of Pediatrics
Apollo Children's Hospital
Chennai, Tamil Nadu, India

Vaishali R Deshmukh
MBBS DCH DNB (Peds) PGD-AP
Consultant, Adolescent Clinic
Deenanath Mangeshkar Hospital and Research Center and Bharati Hospital Medical College
Pune, Maharashtra, India

Vaman V Khadilkar
MD DNB FIAP MRCP (UK) DCH (London)
Consultant Pediatric Endocrinologist
Department of Peditaric Endocrinology
Jehangir Hospital
Professor
Bharati Vidyapeeth Medical College
Pune, Maharashtra, India

Varinder Singh
MD (Pediatrics)
Professor
Hamdard Institute of Medical Science and Research
New Delhi, India

Veena Kalra MBBS MD
Senior Consultant
Department of Pediatric Neurology
Indraprastha Apollo Hospital
New Delhi, India

Venkatadass K
MS (Ortho) DNB (Ortho)
Consultant and Head of Pediatric Orthopedics
Department of Orthopedics
Ganga Hospital
Coimbatore, Tamil Nadu, India

Vibhor Borkar
MBBS MD PDCC DM (Pediatric Gastroenterology)
Director
Department of Pediatric Gastroenterology, Hepatology, and Liver Transplantation
Nanavati Max Super Speciality Hospital
Mumbai, Maharashtra, India

Vibhu Mendiratta
MD (Dermatology)
Head and Director-Professor
Department of Dermatology and STD
Lady Hardinge Medical College
New Delhi, India

Vidya Yadav MD (Dermatology)
Senior Resident
Department of Dermatology
Lady Hardinge Medical College
New Delhi, India

Vignesh V
MD (Pediatrics) DM (Pediatric Gastroenterology)
Consultant
Department of Pediatric Gastroenterology
Travancore Medical College and Hospital
Kollam, Kerala, India

Vijay Viswanathan DNB DCH
Consultant Pediatric Rheumatologist
Department of Pediatrics
Pediatric Rheumatology Unit
Jupiter Hospital, Thane
Apollo Children's Hospital
Navi Mumbai, Maharashtra, India

Vijaya Sarathi
MD (Pediatrics) DM (Endocrinology)
Professor and Head
Department of Endocrinology
Vydehi Institute of Medical Sciences and Research Centre
Bengaluru, Karnataka, India

Vikas Kohli
MBBS MD (USA) American Board Certified
Director
Department of Pediatric Cardiology
Delhi Child Heart Center
New Delhi, India

Vikesh Agrawal
MBBS MS MCh FSPU FIAGS PhD Scholar
Professor and Head
Department of Pediatric Surgery
Netaji Subhash Chandra Bose Medical College
Jabalpur, Madhya Pradesh, India

Vikram Gagneja MD IDPCCM
Head
Department of Pediatrics and PICU
Manipal Hospital
New Delhi, India

Vinayan KP MD DCH DNB DM (Neurology)
Professor and Head
Department of Pediatric Neurology
Amrita Institute of Medical Sciences
Kochi, Kerala, India

Viraj Shingade MS DNB
Director
Children Orthopedic Care Institute
Pravira Hospital
Nagpur, Maharashtra, India

Vrajesh Udani MD
Consultant
Department of Child Neurology and Epilepsy
PD Hinduja Hospital and Medical Research Centre
Mumbai, Maharashtra, India

Zameer MM
MBBS MS (Surgery) MCh (Pediatric Surgery) MRCS
Consultant
Department of Pediatric Surgery
Narayana Health Hospitals
Bengaluru, Karnataka, India

Foreword

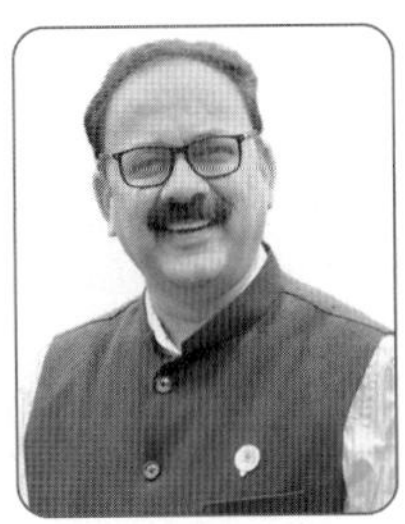

It is with immense pride and admiration that I present this latest edition of *Algorithms in Pediatrics.* This book is a testament to the evolving field of pediatrics and the relentless pursuit of excellence by its contributors. It serves as a guiding light for clinicians, providing structured algorithms that simplify complex clinical scenarios and enable timely, evidence-based decision-making.

The field of pediatrics is both challenging and rewarding, requiring precision, adaptability, and a compassionate approach. This book meets those demands by offering practical, step-by-step pathways to diagnose and manage pediatric conditions. It emphasizes the importance of a thorough history, focused examination, and rational use of investigations to ensure resource-effective and patient-centered care.

Henry David Thoreau once said, *"Our lives are frittered away by detail; simplify, simplify."* This quote captures the essence of this book, which aims to distill the vast expanse of pediatric knowledge into concise and accessible algorithms. By doing so, it equips pediatricians to navigate complex clinical challenges with clarity and confidence.

In the diverse and resource-constrained healthcare landscape of India, this book is particularly relevant. It bridges the gap between academic knowledge and real-world application, providing solutions tailored to the unique challenges faced by clinicians here. For practicing pediatricians, trainees, and even postgraduate students, this book offers invaluable insights that are not only academically enriching but also practically indispensable.

The comprehensive coverage of pediatric subspecialties, combined with its focus on logical and efficient problem-solving, makes this book a cornerstone for pediatric practice. It empowers clinicians to provide better care, optimize the use of available resources, and ultimately improve the health outcomes of our children.

I extend my heartfelt congratulations to the editors, Drs Anand S Vasudev and Nitin K Shah, for their exceptional work in creating this invaluable resource. Their dedication to advancing pediatric care through this book is truly commendable.

May this book continue to inspire and guide pediatricians as they strive to bring quality care to every child.

Warm regards

Vasant Khalatkar
MD (Ped) FIAP FICMCH
PG Diploma in Pediatric Infectious Diseases (UNSW)
Fellow Guide Diploma Child Health (DCH)
Director
Colours Children Hospital for Pediatric Intensive Care
Nagpur, Maharashtra, India
National President
Indian Academy of Pediatrics (IAP), 2025

Preface to the Second Edition

It gives us immense pleasure to present to you the second edition of *Algorithms in Pediatrics*. Pediatrics is rapidly advancing with the growth of its subspecialties. At times, it becomes difficult for busy pediatricians, whether in practice, in teaching institutions, or pursuing their postgraduation, to read through lengthy texts of different subspecialties. Keeping this in mind, we thought of bringing forth this concise book on algorithms, which deals with common and practical topics of everyday requirements in different pediatric specialties.

The book has been designed with a practical approach in mind, with an algorithm for each topic, along with a concise text to use the algorithms. The text has been kept simple and easily comprehensible. The book can be consulted rapidly in the emergency room, wards, outpatient departments, or busy clinics.

The book contains 19 subspecialty sections, a total of 166 chapters. This was an immense work, which could not have been possible without the help and coordination of the section editors. We are very thankful to all the section editors.

A large number of luminaries and experts in the field of pediatrics and its subspecialties have contributed their mind and might in bringing out this second edition of the book. We are thankful to all these contributors.

We are also thankful to M/s Jaypee Brothers Medical Publishers (P) Ltd, New Delhi, India, for publishing this book.

We are also grateful to our respective spouses for being tolerant and supportive of us in this endeavor.

Anand S Vasudev
Nitin K Shah

Preface to the First Edition

It gives us immense pleasure to present to you the 1st edition of *"Algorithms in Pediatrics"*. Pediatrics is rapidly advancing with the growth of its subspecialties. At times, it becomes difficult for busy pediatricians, whether in practice, in teaching institutions, or pursuing their postgraduation, to read through lengthy texts of different subspecialties. Keeping this in mind, we thought of bringing forth this concise book on algorithms, which deals with common and practical topics of everyday requirements in different pediatric specialties.

The book has been designed with a practical approach in mind, with an algorithm for each topic, along with a concise text to use the algorithms. The text has been kept simple and easily comprehendible. The book can be consulted rapidly in the emergency room, wards, outpatient departments, or in busy clinics.

The book contains 19 subspecialty sections, with 8–10 chapters in each, a total of 156 chapters. This was an immense work, which could not have been possible without the help and coordination of the section editors. We are very thankful to all the section editors.

A large number of luminaries and experts in the field of pediatrics and its subspecialties have contributed their mind and might in bringing out this book. We are thankful to all these contributors.

We are also thankful to Jaypee Brothers Medical Publishers (P) Ltd. for publishing this book.

We are also grateful to our respective spouses for being tolerant and supportive of us in this endeavor.

Anand S Vasudev
Nitin K Shah

Contents

SECTION 1 NEONATOLOGY

Section Editors: **Anjali Kulkarni, Ashish Mehta**

SECTION 2 ADOLESCENCE

Section Editors: **MKC Nair, Piyali Bhattacharya**

SECTION 3 IMMUNIZATION

Section Editors: **Amar Jeet Chitkara, Jaydeep Choudhury**

SECTION 4 OFFICE EMERGENCIES

Section Editors: **Ajit Gajendragadkar, Rajesh R Chokhani**

SECTION 5 INTENSIVE CARE UNIT

Section Editor: **Praveen Khilnani**

SECTION 10 GASTROENTEROLOGY

Section Editors: **Aathira Ravindranath, Anupam Sibal**

SECTION 11 NEUROLOGY

Section Editors: **Shekhar Patil, Vrajesh Udani**

SECTION 12 NEPHROLOGY

Section Editors: **Anand S Vasudev, Pankaj V Deshpande**

SECTION 13 ENDOCRINOLOGY

Section Editors: **Vaman V Khadilkar, Anju Virmani**

SECTION 14 RHEUMATOLOGY

Section Editor: **Priyankar Pal**

SECTION 15 PEDIATRIC SURGERY

Section Editors: **Anurag Krishna, Rasiklal S Shah**

SECTION 16 DERMATOLOGY

Section Editor: **Vibhu Mendiratta**

SECTION 17 OPHTHALMOLOGY

Section Editor: **Shashi Vashisht**

SECTION 18 EAR, NOSE, AND THROAT

Section Editor: **Ameet Kishore**

SECTION 19 ORTHOPEDICS

Section Editor: **Rujuta Mehta**

PLATE 1

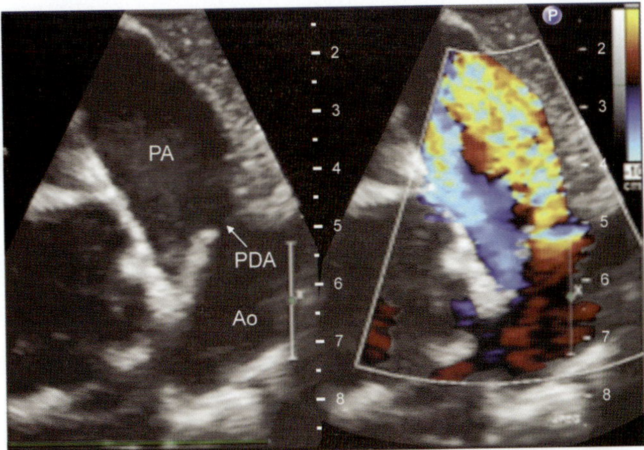

Fig. 2: Ductal view showing PDA with left to right shunt. (Ao: aorta; PA: pulmonary artery; PDA: patent ductus arteriosus) ***(Chapter 7)***.

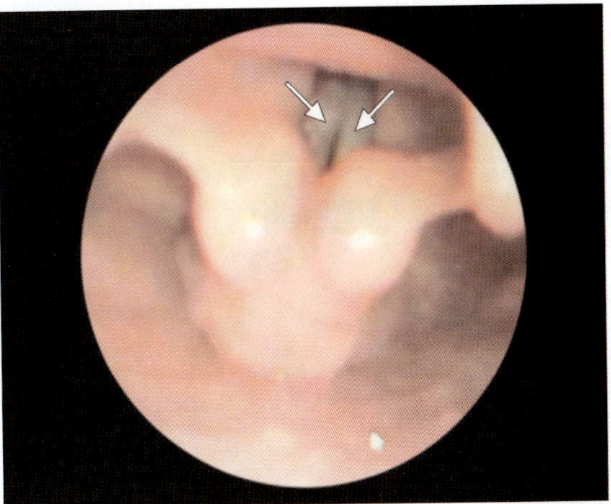

Fig. 1A: The vocal cords (VC) are swollen with marked subglottic swelling (arrow), narrowing the opening of subglottic airway ***(Chapter 33)***.

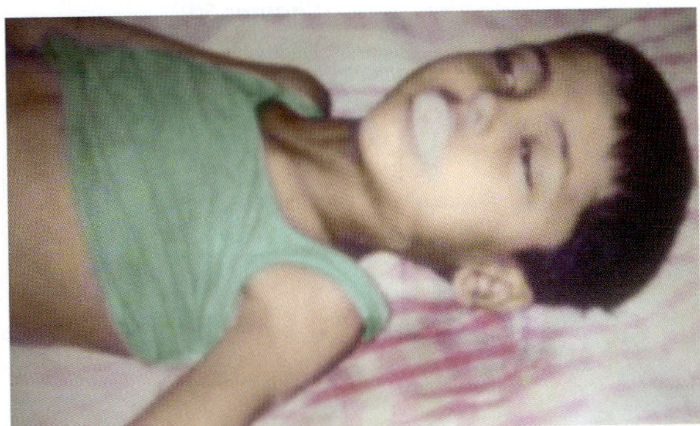

Fig. 1: Pulmonary edema ***(Chapter 40)***.

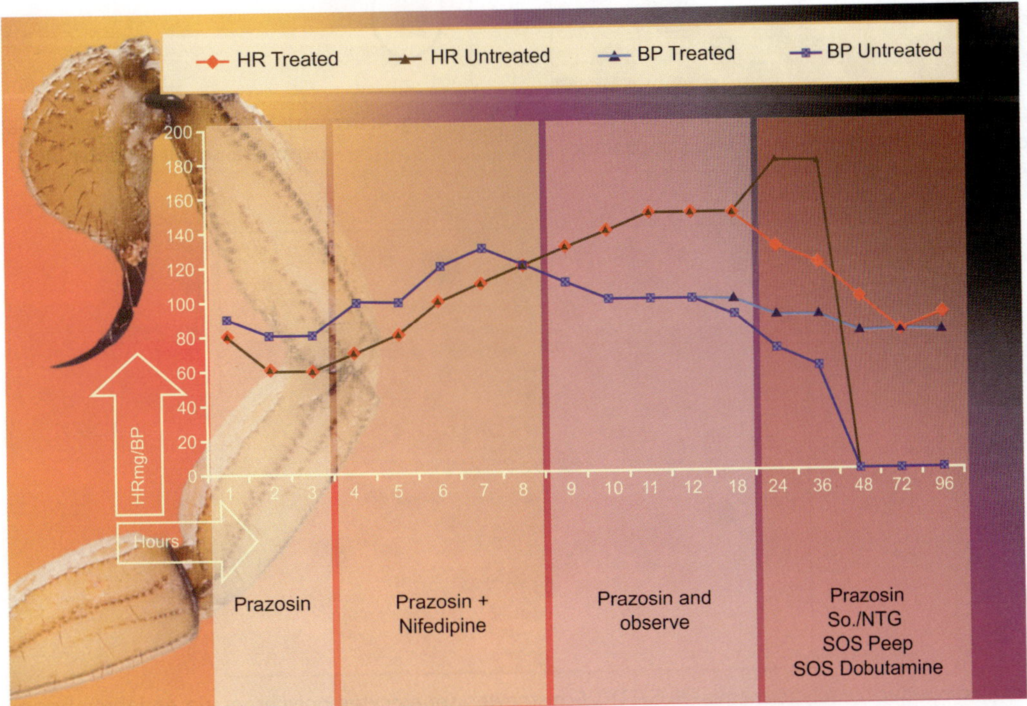

Fig. 5: Pathophysiology-guided management ***(Chapter 40)***.

PLATE 2

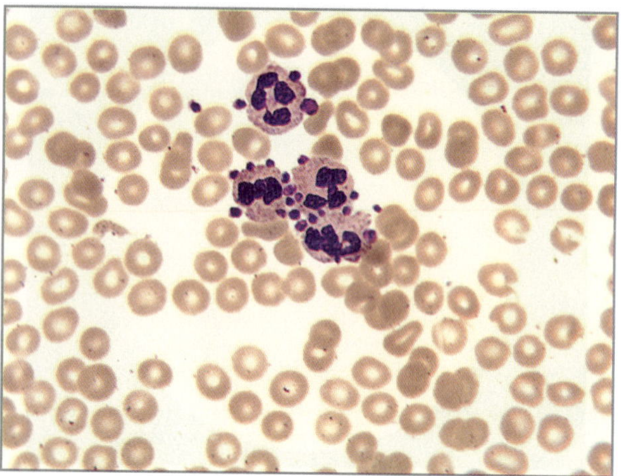

Fig. 1: Pseudothrombocytopenia due to platelet satellitism ***(Chapter 60)***.

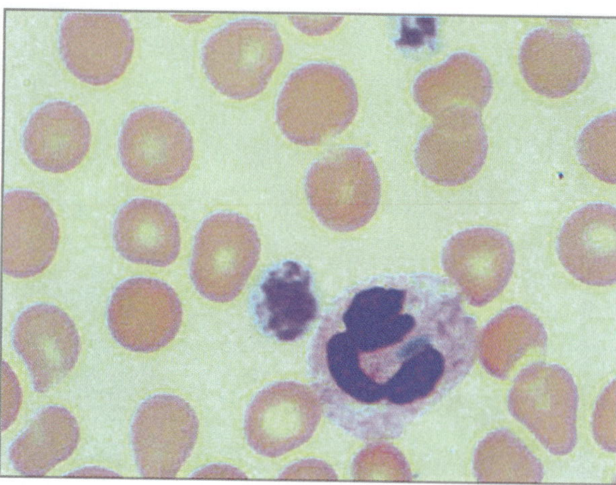

Fig. 3: May–Hegglin anomaly: Neutrophil contains multiple prominent, light blue, and round Dohle bodies, which are intracytoplasmic inclusions that consist of RNA and giant platelets ***(Chapter 60)***.

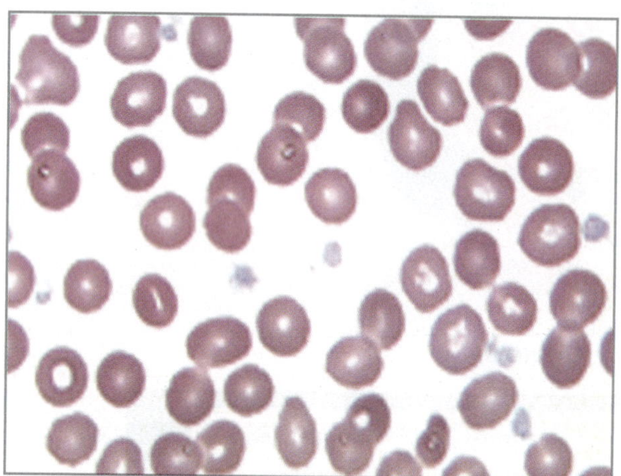

Fig. 2: Gray platelet syndrome: Large platelets which look colorless (due to absence of alpha granules), giving it a grey appearance on peripheral smear ***(Chapter 60)***.

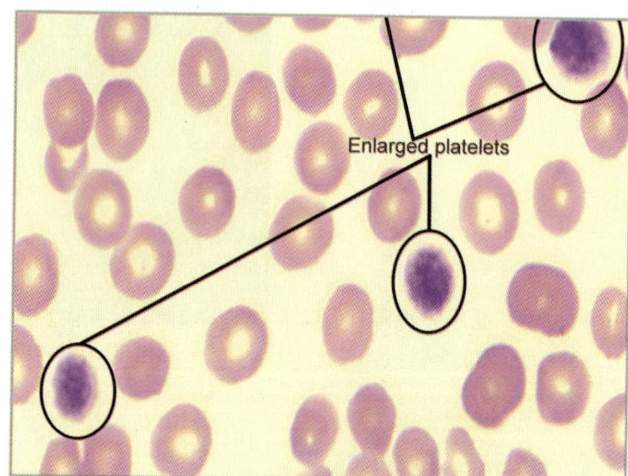

Fig. 4: Bernard–Soulier syndrome: Large platelets on peripheral smear ***(Chapter 60)***.

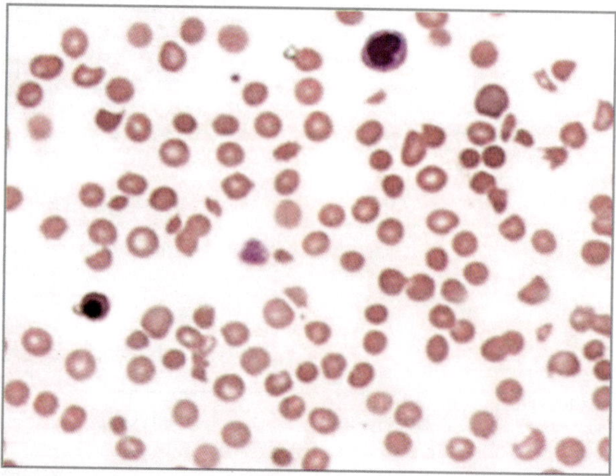

Fig. 5: Microangiopathic hemolytic anemia (HUS/TTP): Schistocytes, spherocytes, polychromasia, and thrombocytopenia on peripheral smear. (HUS: hemolytic uremic syndrome; TTP: thrombotic thrombocytopenic purpura) ***(Chapter 60)***.

PLATE 3

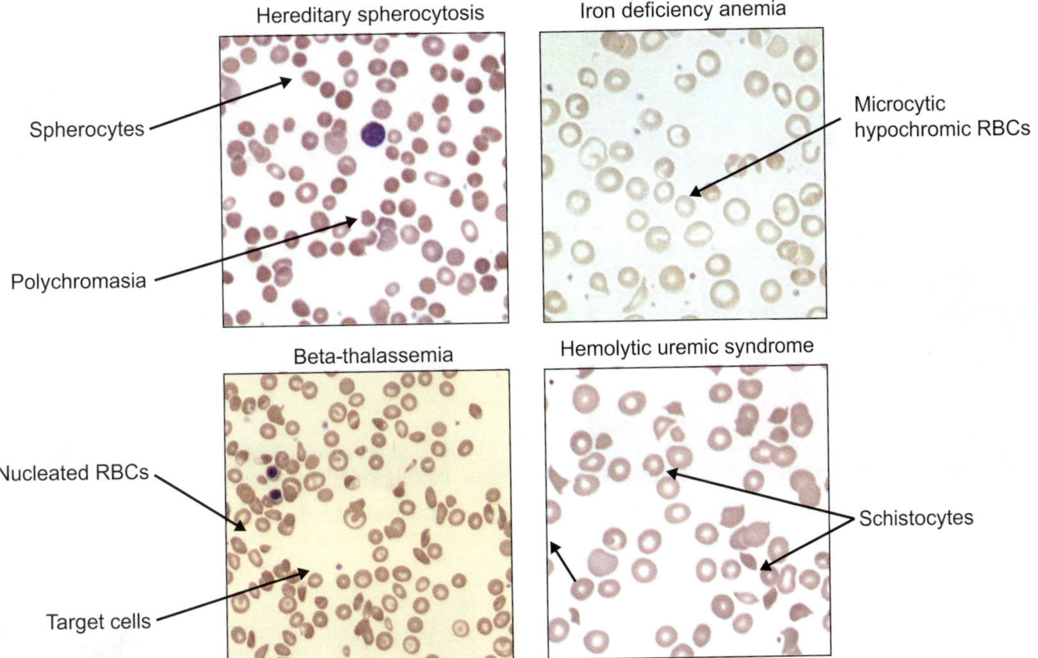

Fig. 1: Peripheral smear examination in common disorders with anemia ***(Chapter 61)***.

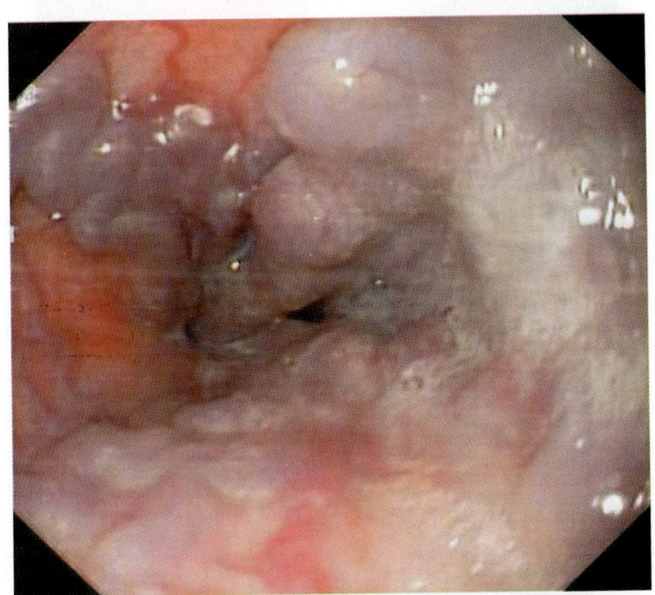

Fig. 1: Upper gastrointestinal endoscopy showing large esophageal varices ***(Chapter 79)***.

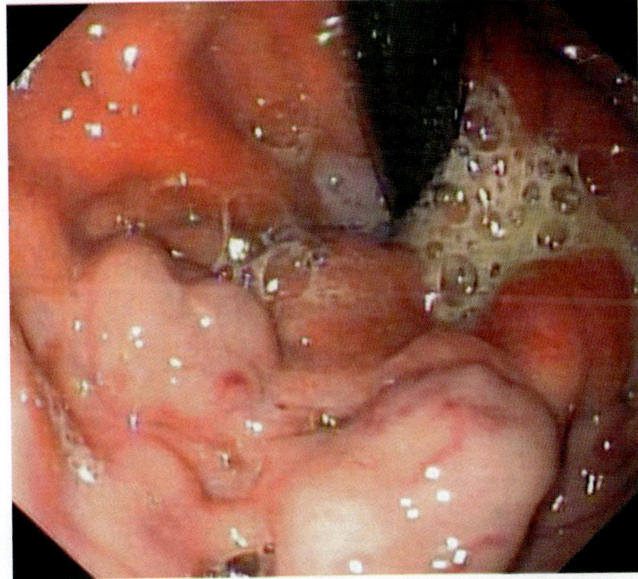

Fig. 2: Upper gastrointestinal endoscopy showing gastric varices with red color signs on retroversion ***(Chapter 79)***.

PLATE 4

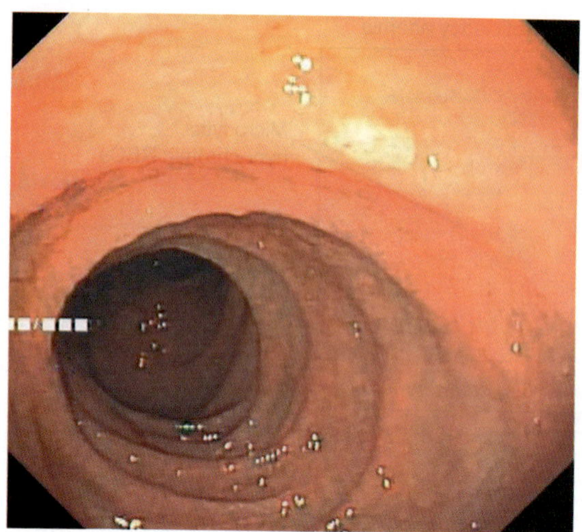

Fig. 3: Upper gastrointestinal endoscopy showing duodenal ulcer without signs of active bleeding ***(Chapter 79)***.

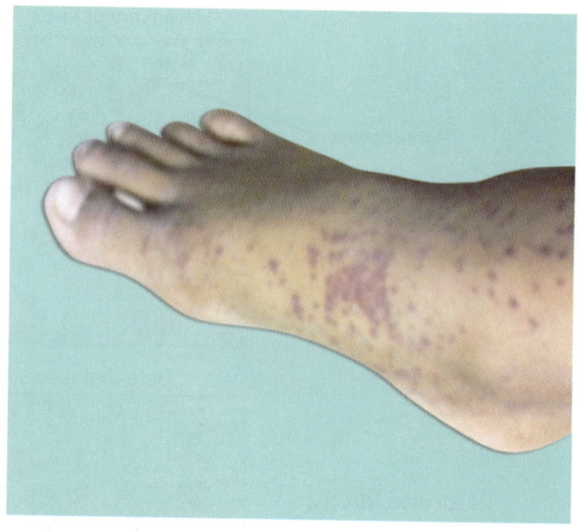

Fig. 3: Palpable Henoch–Schönlein purpura ***(Chapter 80)***.

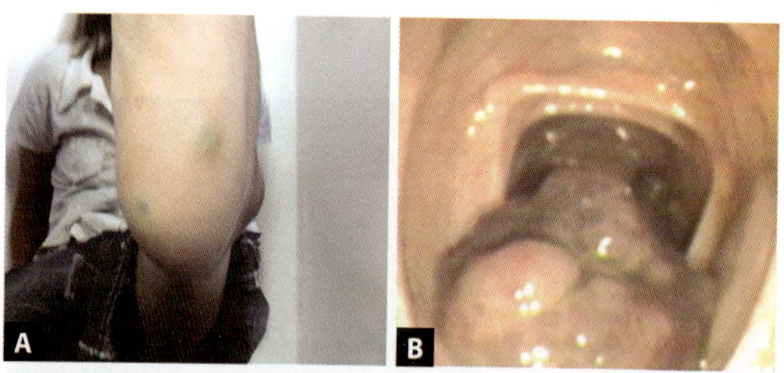

Figs. 1A and B: Bluish black hemangiomas on the sole and hemangiomas on colonoscopy (Blue rubber bleb nevus syndrome) ***(Chapter 80)***.

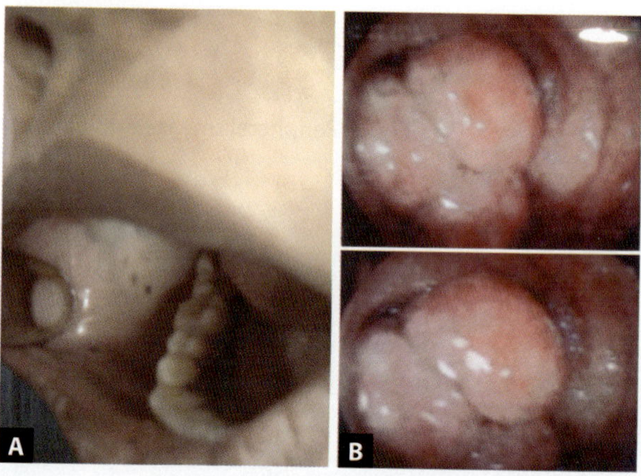

Figs. 4A and B: Oral buccal mucosal pigmentation and colonic polyps (Peutz–Jeghers syndrome) ***(Chapter 80)***.

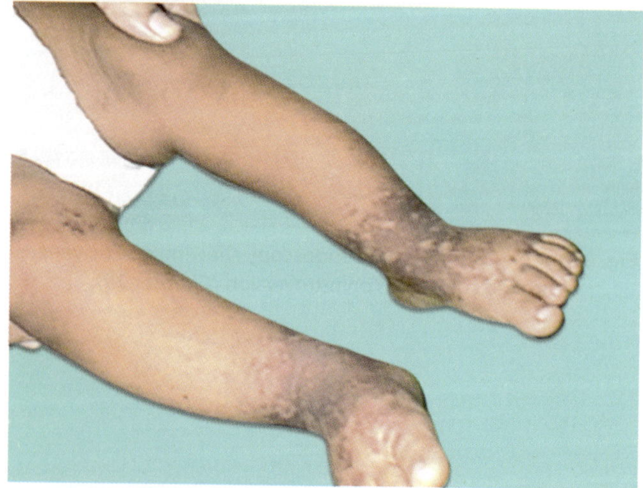

Fig. 2: Infant with dengue and thrombocytopenia with ecchymosis both ankles ***(Chapter 80)***.

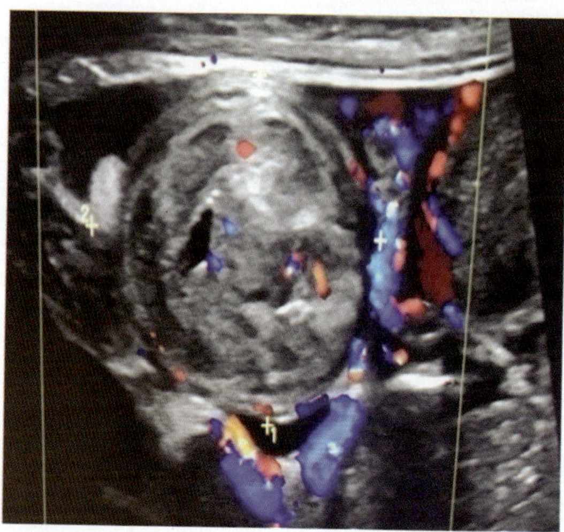

Fig. 6B: Ultrasound and Doppler study showing target sign of intussusception ***(Chapter 80)***.

PLATE 5

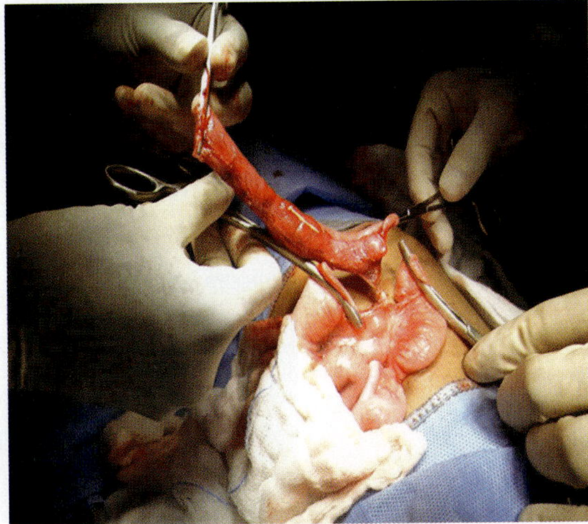

Fig. 7B: Contrast-enhanced computed tomography (CECT) abdomen demonstrating the ileal duplication confirmed on surgery ***(Chapter 80)***.

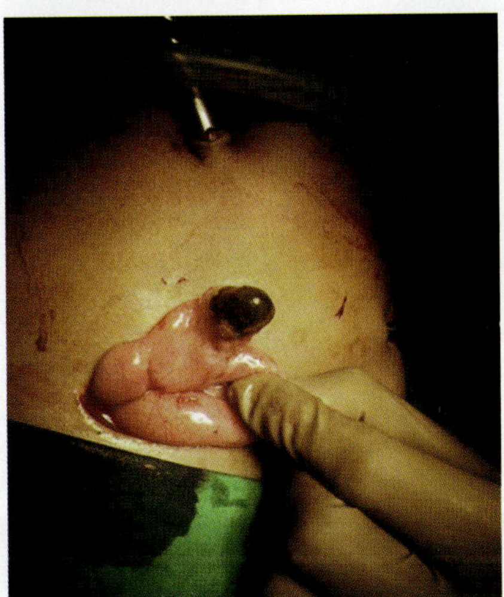

Fig. 8B: Radionuclide study technetium-99m pertechnetate scan demonstrating the Meckel's diverticulum confirmed on surgery ***(Chapter 80)***.

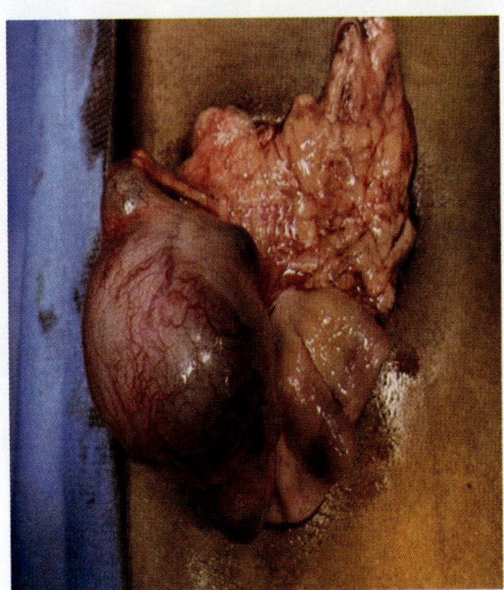

Fig. 9B: Radionuclide technetium-99m pertechnetate scan showing uptake of ileal duplication cyst confirmed on surgery ***(Chapter 80)***.

PLATE 6

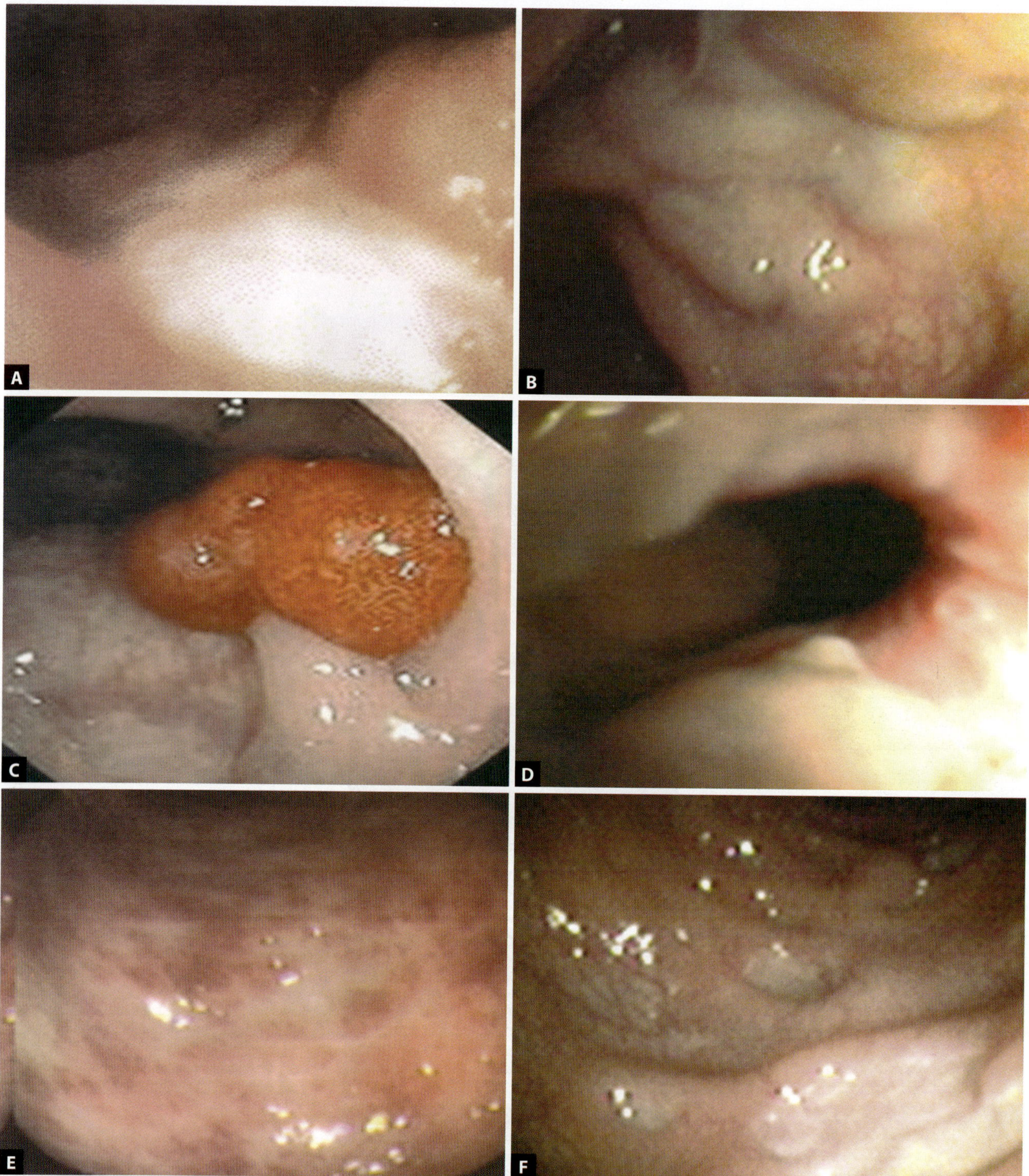

Figs. 10A to F: Colonoscopy images seen in lower gastrointestinal bleed (LGIB). (A) Solitary rectal ulcer; (B) Rectal varices; (C) Pedunculated cherry red rectal polyp; (D) Fissure-in-ano; (E) Severe ulcerative colitis; (F) Irregular ulcers seen in Crohn's disease ***(Chapter 80)***.

PLATE 7

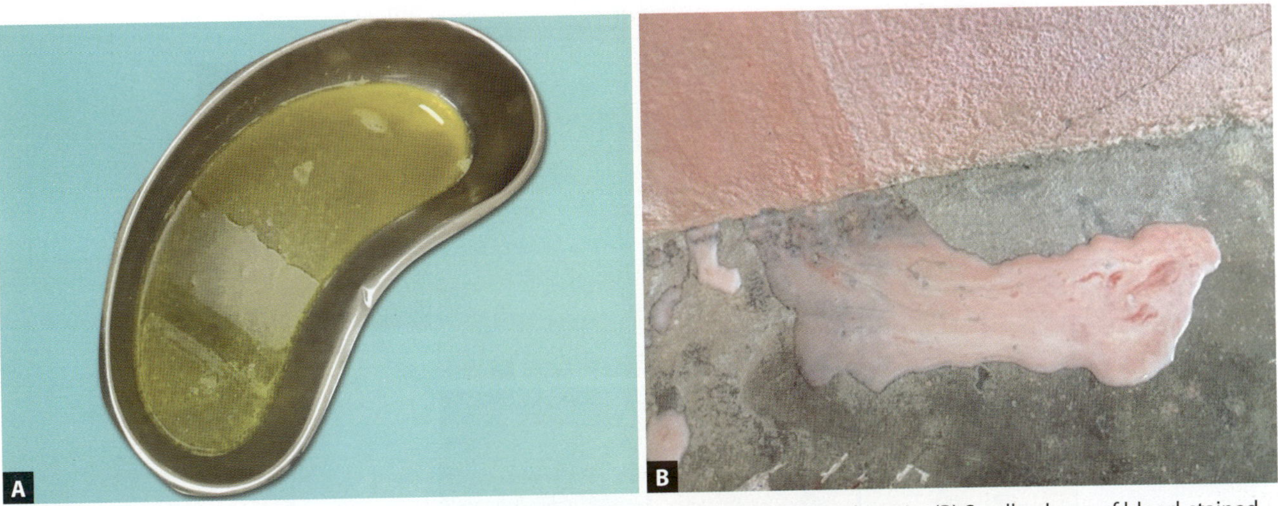

Figs. 2A and B: (A) Image showing bilious (greenish) vomiting in a 3-year-old with malrotatio; (B) Small volume of blood-stained (hematemesis) vomitus in an infant with cow milk protein allergy ***(Chapter 84)***.

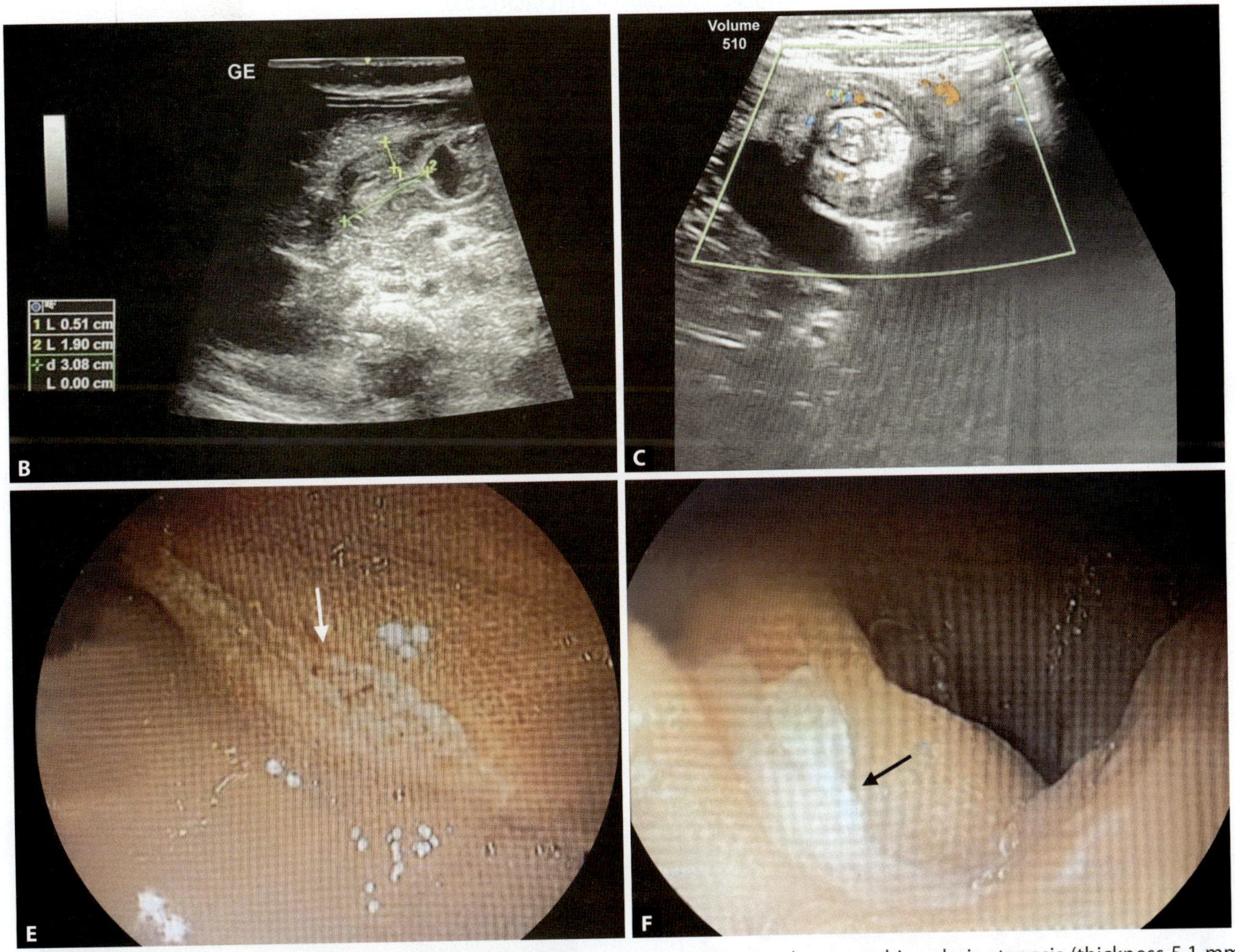

Figs. 3B, C, E and F: (B) A 3-month-old infant with ultrasound abdomen showing hypertrophic pyloric stenosis (thickness 5.1 mm, length 19 mm); (C) Target sign of intussusception in an 18 month old child; (E) A 10-year-old with a large linear gastric ulcer (white arrow; *Helicobacter pylori* positive); (F) A 6-year-old with peptic duodenal (D1 part) clean based ulcer (black arrow; *H. pylori* negative) ***(Chapter 84)***.

PLATE 8

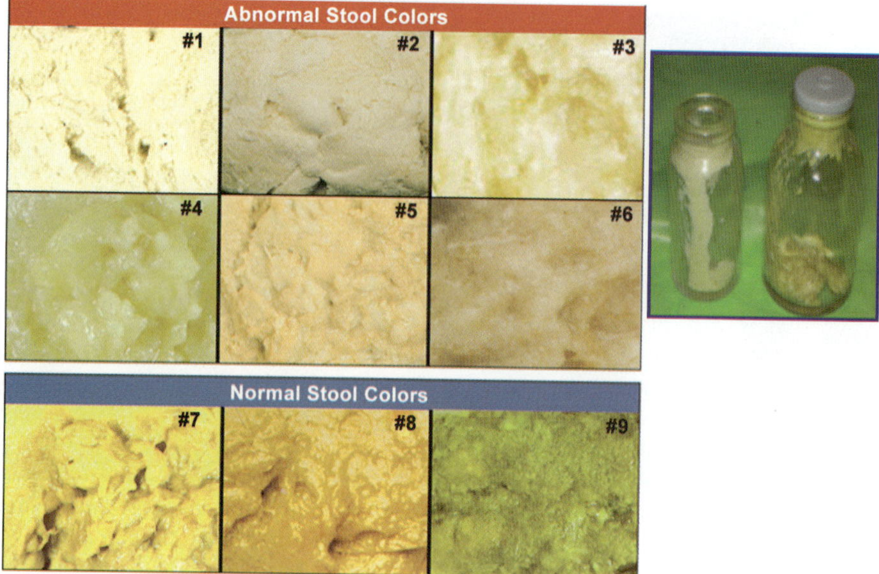

Fig. 2: Stool color chart ***(Chapter 85)***.

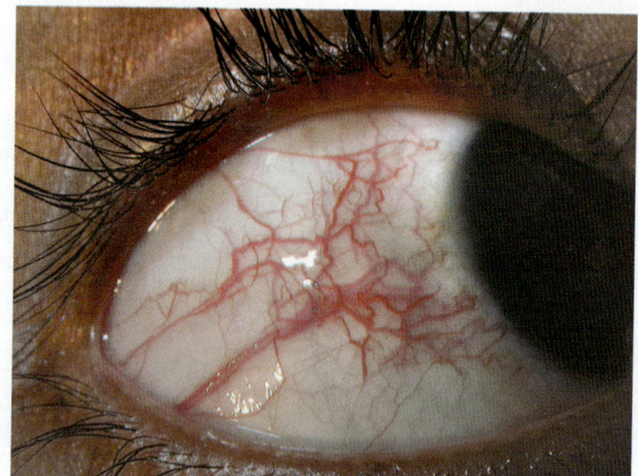

Fig. 1: Bulbar conjunctival telangiectasia ***(Chapter 93)***.

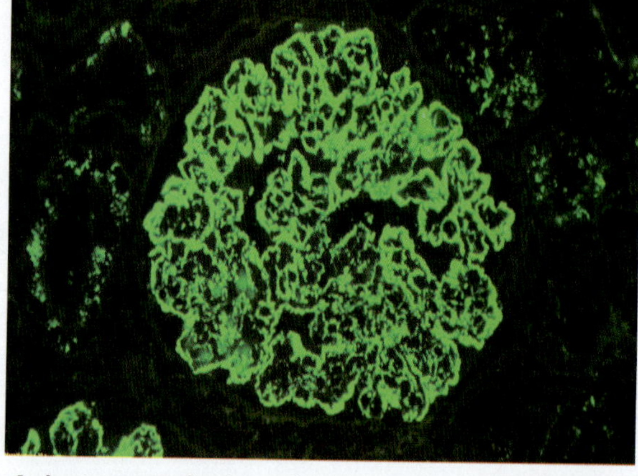

Fig. 4: Acute postinfectious glomerulonephritis. Immunofluorescence for immunoglobulin G showing smaller and spaced parietal granular deposits giving a "starry sky" appearance ***(Chapter 101)***.

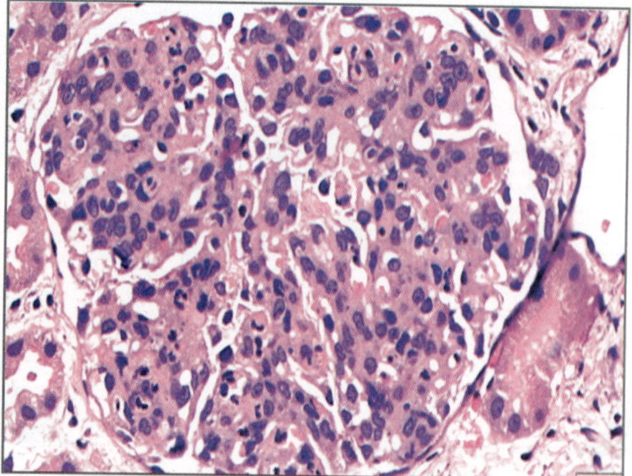

Fig. 3: Acute postinfectious glomerulonephritis. Glomerulus showing cellular proliferation obstructing capillaries and there are abundant polymorphs (hematoxylin and eosin) ***(Chapter 101)***.

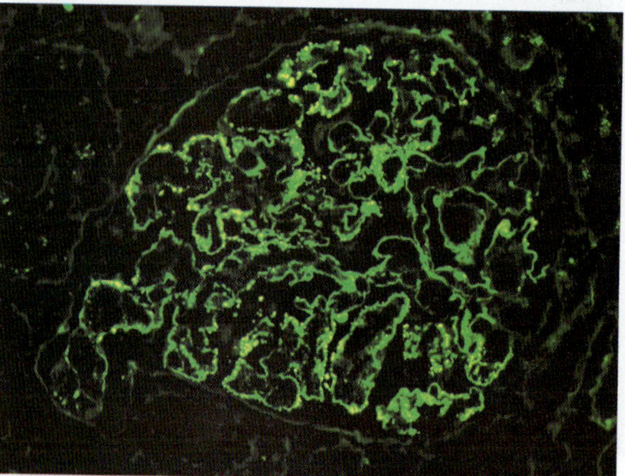

Fig. 5: Acute postinfectious glomerulonephritis. Immunofluorescence for C3 showing extensive granular deposits in the capillary walls giving it a garland appearance ***(Chapter 101)***.

PLATE 9

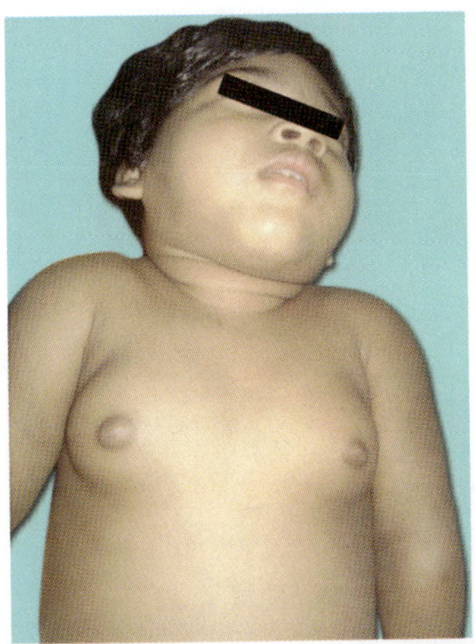

Fig. 1: Premature thelarche due to gonadotropin-dependent precocious puberty in a 4-year-old girl with spastic quadriplegia with seizures on anticonvulsant therapy ***(Chapter 113)***.

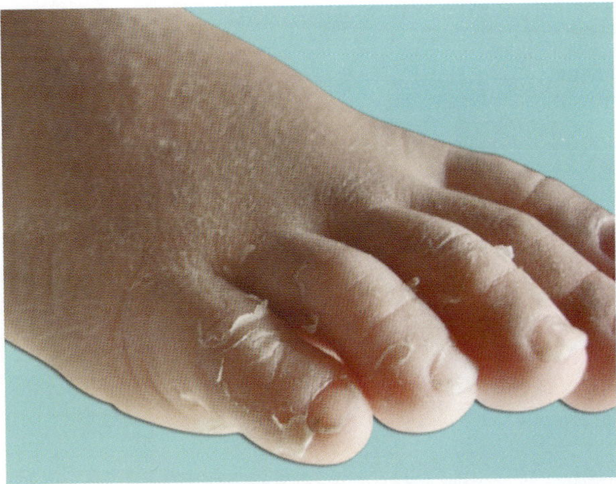

Fig. 2: Periungual desquamation in feet, which usually follows similar findings in hands ***(Chapter 122)***.

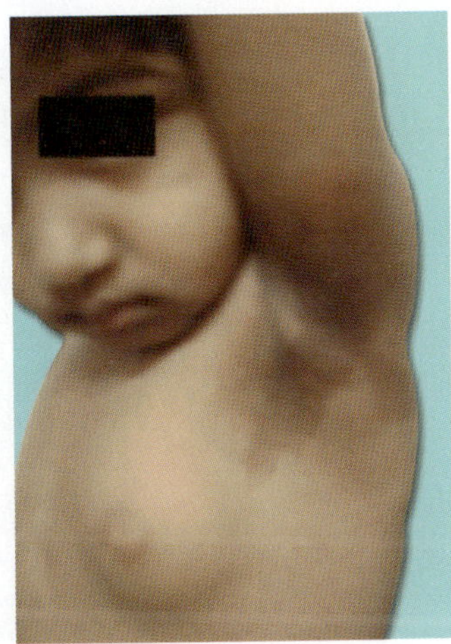

Fig. 2: McCune–Albright syndrome in a 4-year-old girl. Note the premature thelarche and the large cafe-au-lait pigmented macule in the axilla ***(Chapter 113)***.

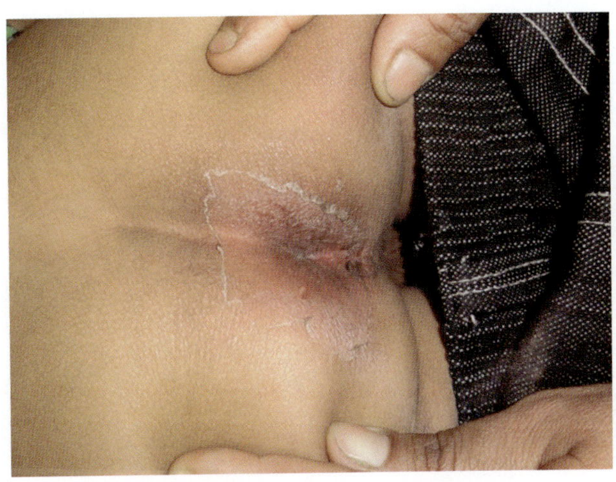

Fig. 3: Perianal desquamation ***(Chapter 122)***.

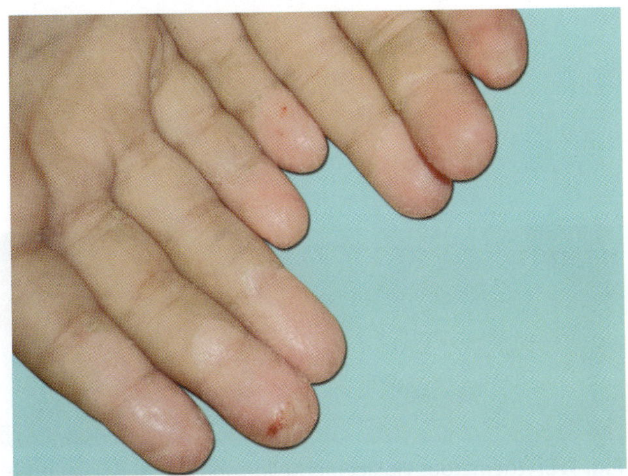

Fig. 1: Periungual desquamation in hands ***(Chapter 122)***.

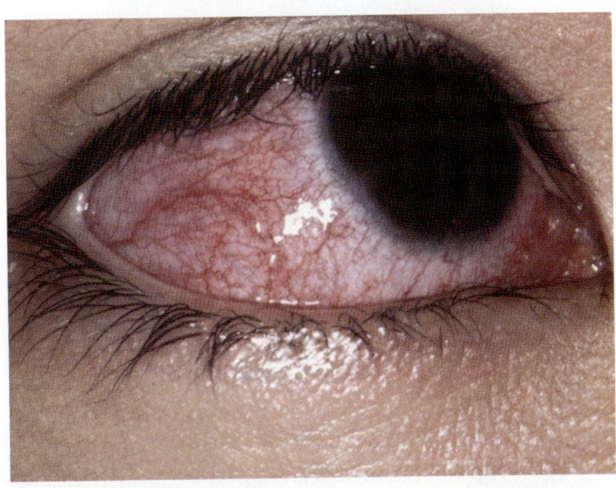

Fig. 4: Nonexudative conjunctivitis ***(Chapter 122)***.

PLATE 10

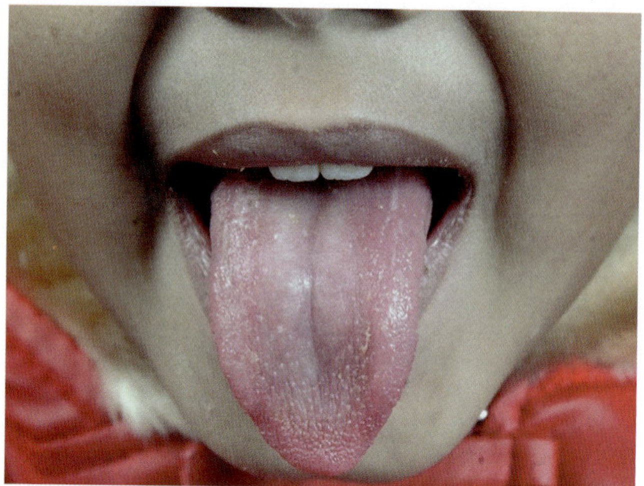

Fig. 5: Strawberry tongue ***(Chapter 122)***.

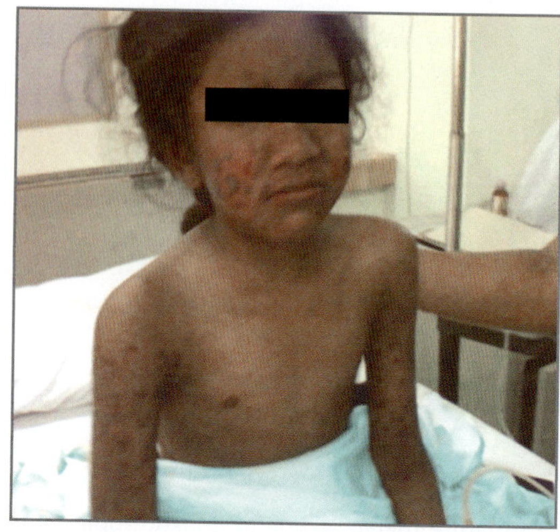

Fig. 1: Extensive rash malar and on extremities in a child with systemic lupus erythematosus ***(Chapter 124)***.

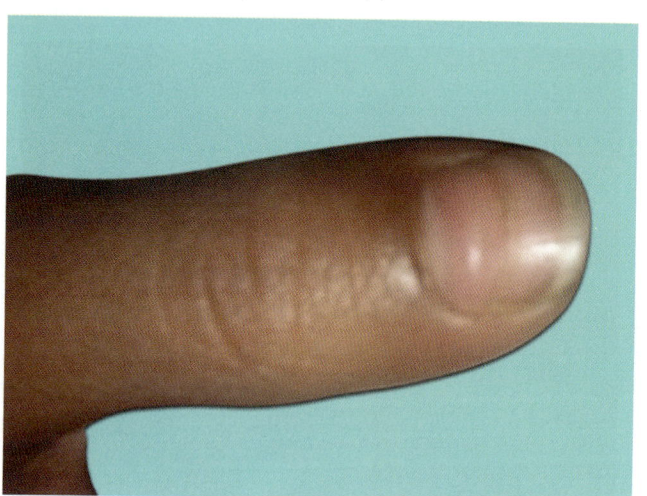

Fig. 7: Prominent Beau's lines ***(Chapter 122)***.

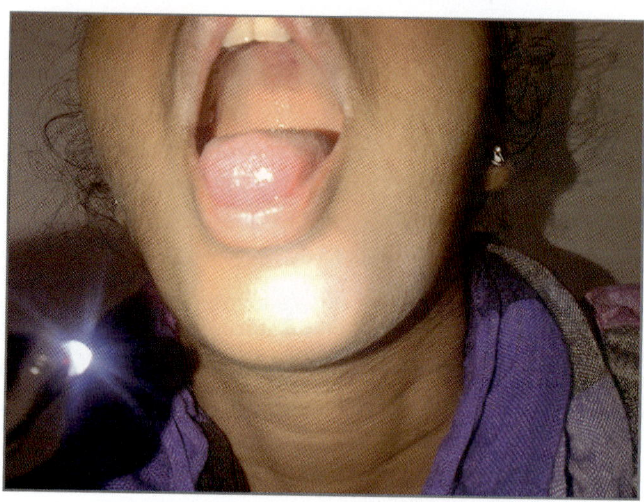

Fig. 2: Oral ulcer on hard palate in systemic lupus erythematosus ***(Chapter 124)***.

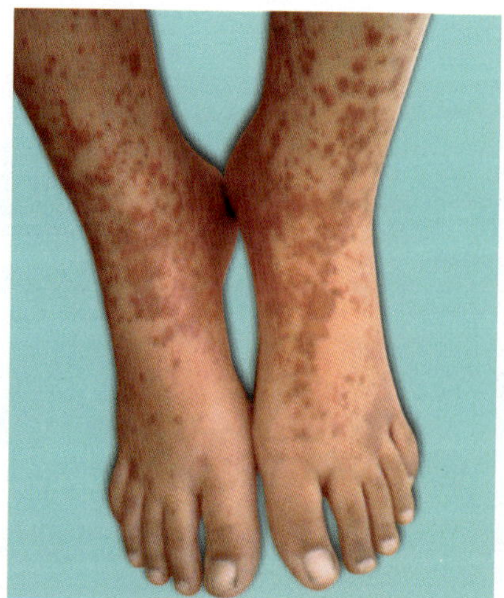

Fig. 1: Predominant lower purpura in an adolescent girl ***(Chapter 123)***.

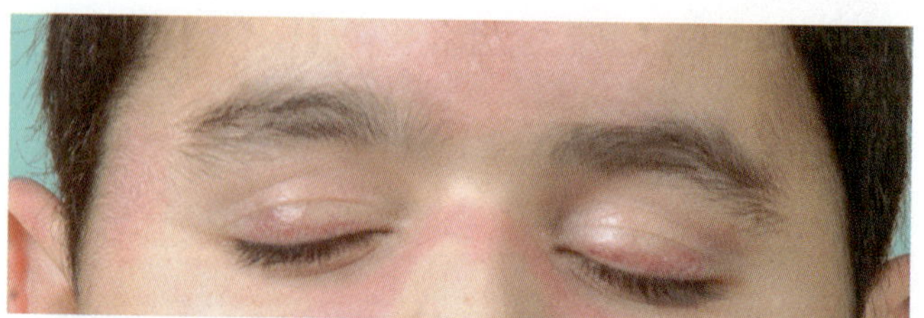

Fig. 1: Erythematous violaceous heliotrope rash seen over the upper eyelids ***(Chapter 125)***.

PLATE 11

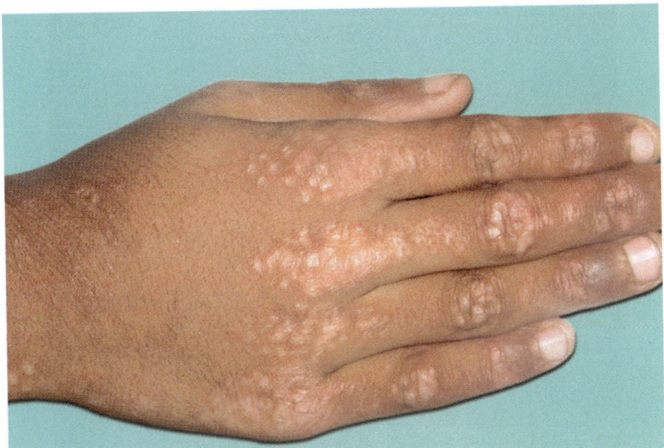

Fig. 2: Juvenile dermatomyositis. Erythematous, scaly papules noted over extensor surfaces of small joints, and wrist and elbows ***(Chapter 125)***.

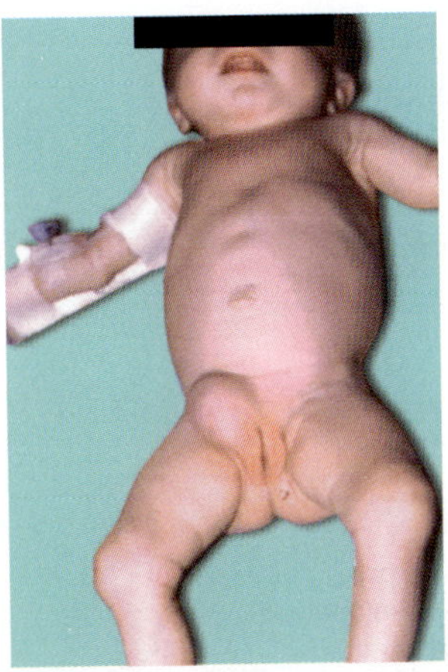

Fig. 5: Incarcerated right inguinal hernia causing intestinal obstruction ***(Chapter 129)***.

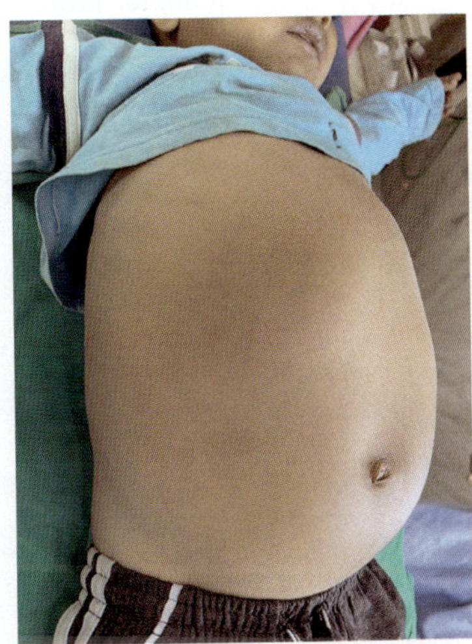

Fig. 3: Generalized abdominal distention with visible dilated bowel loops—intestinal obstruction ***(Chapter 129)***.

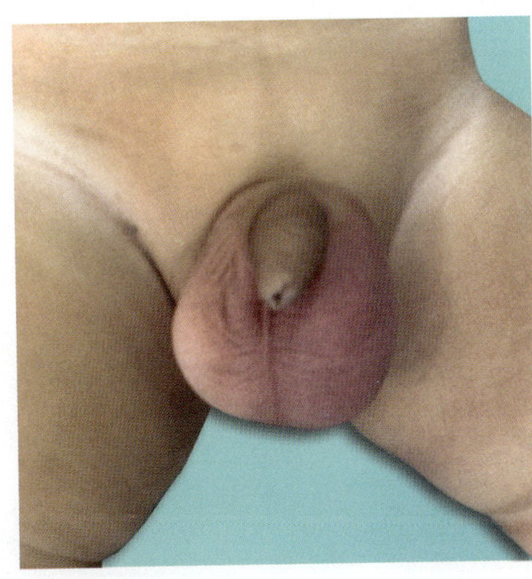

Fig. 6: Acute left scrotum (tender and red scrotum on the left)—left testicular torsion ***(Chapter 129)***.

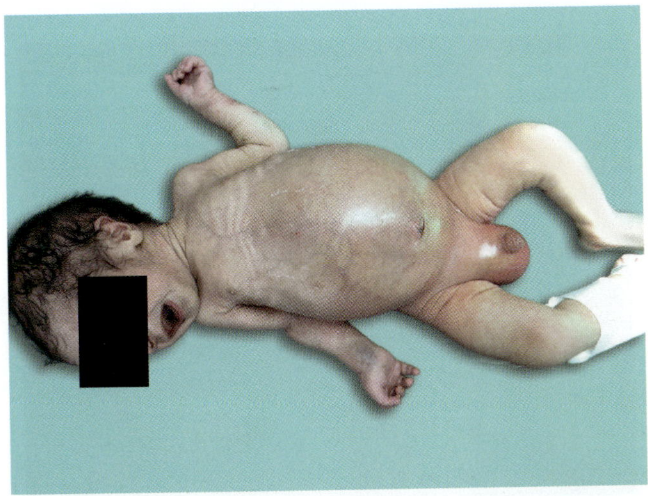

Fig. 4: Distended shiny abdomen—peritonitis ***(Chapter 129)***.

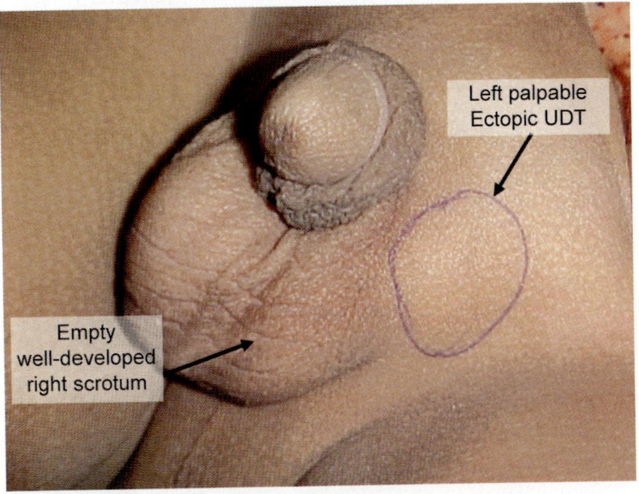

Fig. 1: Left ectopic testis—testis noted to be in ectopic site, different from the normal path of testicular descent ***(Chapter 130)***.

PLATE 12

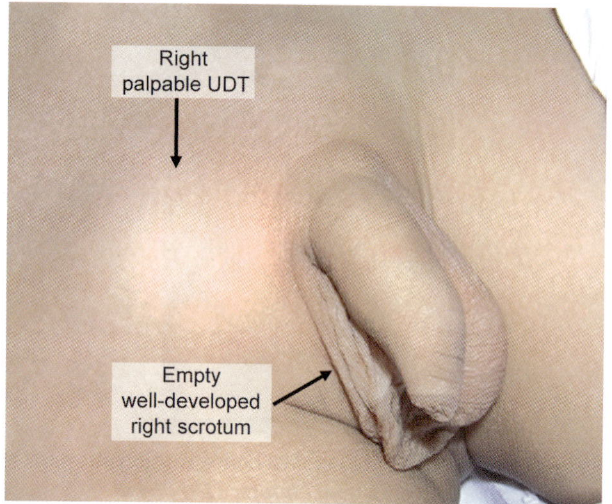

Fig. 2: Right palpable undescended testis—testis palpable in inguinal region and scrotal sac is empty but well developed ***(Chapter 130)***.

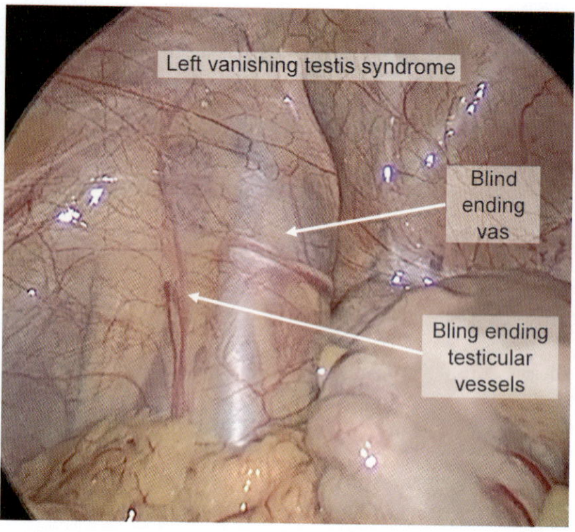

Fig. 5: Blind ending vas and vessels in left vanishing testis syndrome ***(Chapter 130)***.

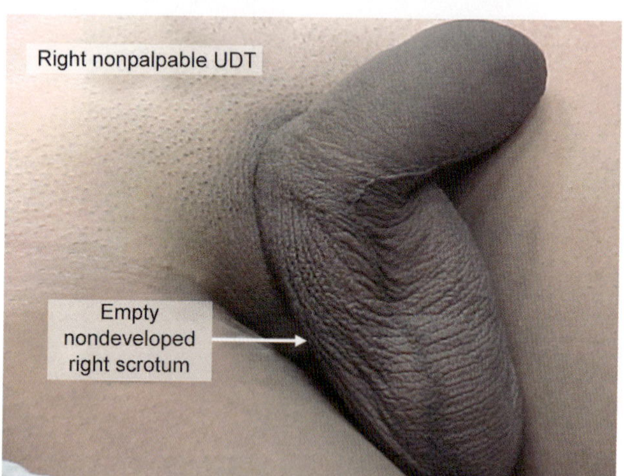

Fig. 3: Right nonpalpable undescended testis—scrotal sac is empty and underdeveloped. Further evaluation is needed to rule out intra-abdominal position, atrophy, or absence of testis ***(Chapter 130)***.

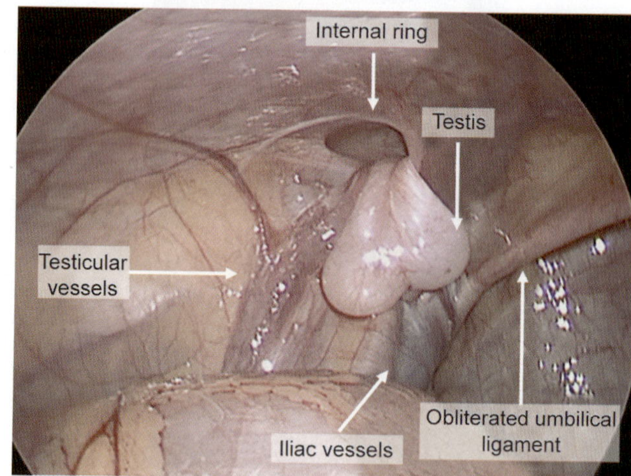

Fig. 6: Laparoscopic findings in the low abdominal testis near the internal ring ***(Chapter 130)***.

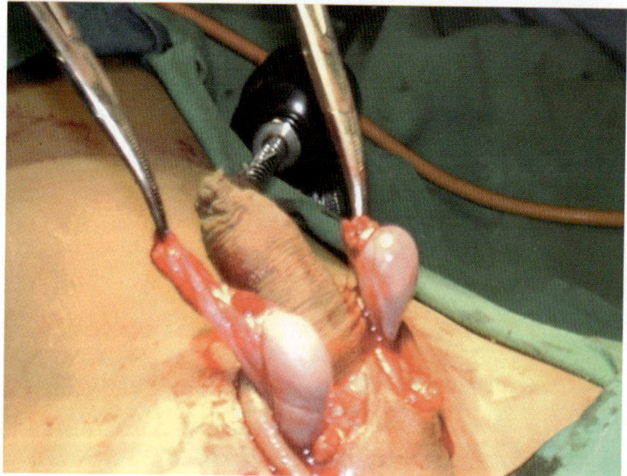

Fig. 4: Laparoscopic bilateral orchidopexy ***(Chapter 130)***.

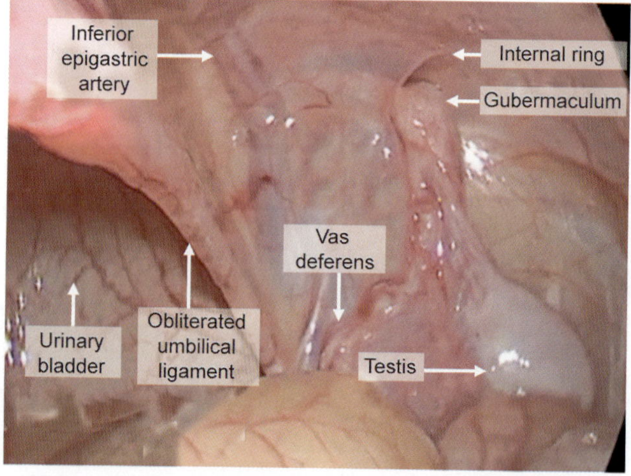

Fig. 7: Laparoscopic findings in the high abdominal testis—usually need two-stage orchidopexy ***(Chapter 130)***.

PLATE 13

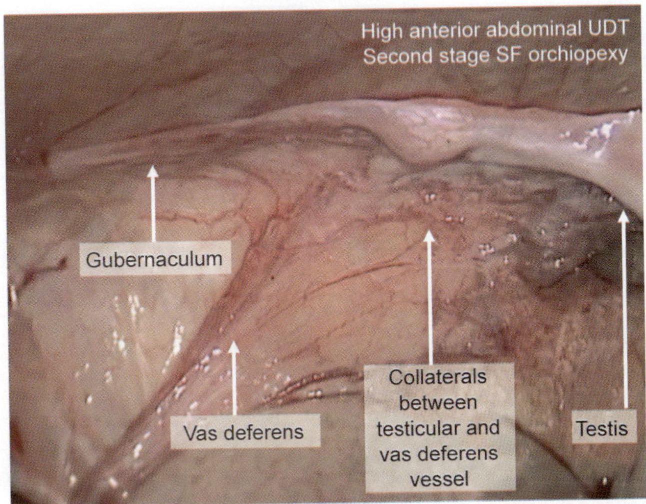

Fig. 8: Laparoscopic findings during second stage of Stephen–Fowler orchidopexy showing collaterals between artery to vas deferens and testicular artery ***(Chapter 130)***.

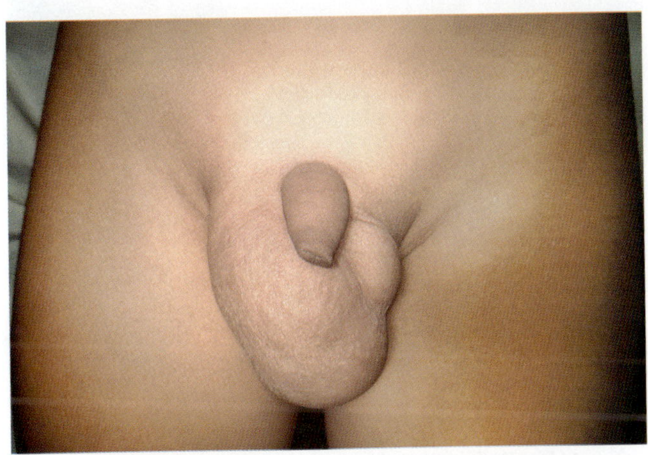

Fig. 1: Clinical picture of inguinal hernia ***(Chapter 132)***.

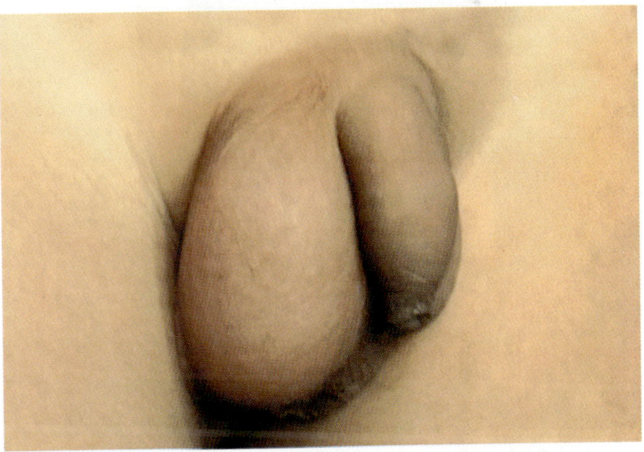

Fig. 2: Clinical picture of hydrocele ***(Chapter 132)***.

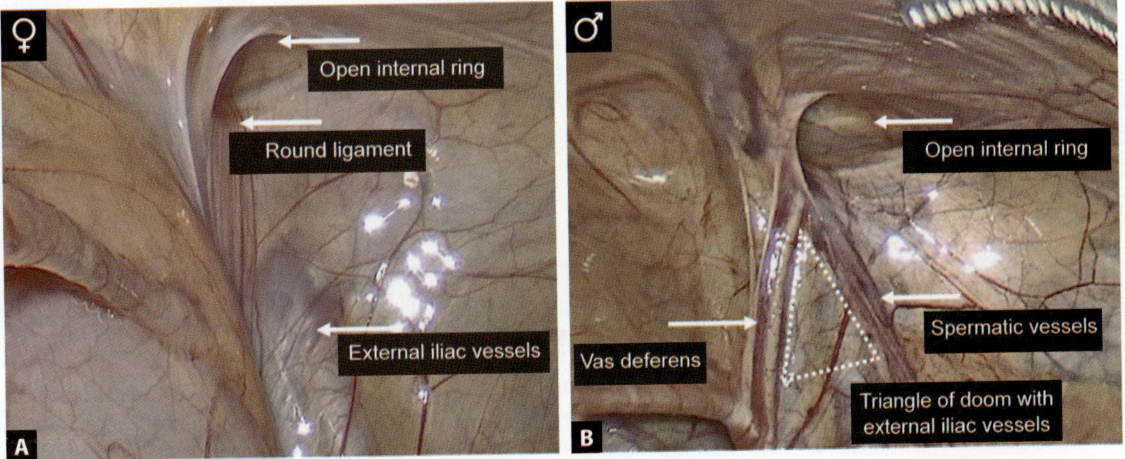

Figs. 3A and B: Laparoscopic internal view of inguinal hernia in a girl (A) and a boy (B) ***(Chapter 132)***.

PLATE 14

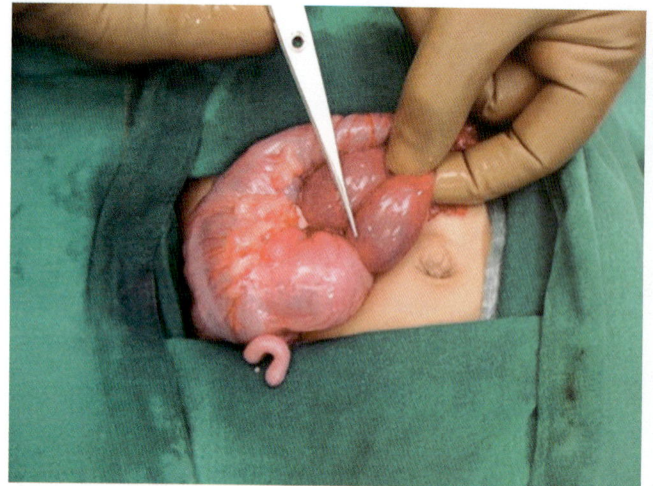

Fig. 2: Operative photograph showing the intussusception ***(Chapter 135)***.

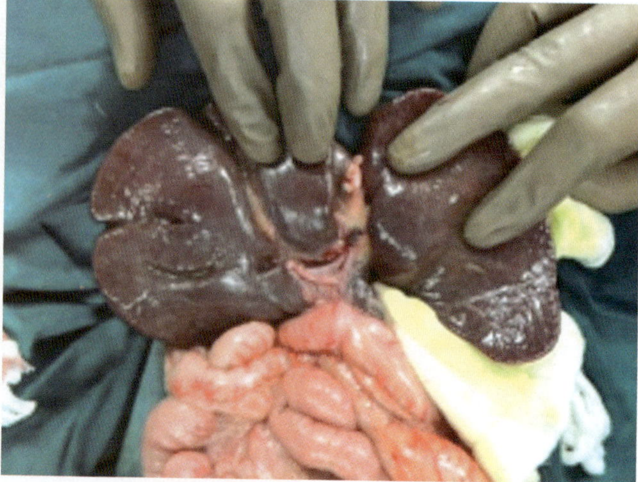

Fig. 2: Dissection of porta hepatis ***(Chapter 136)***.

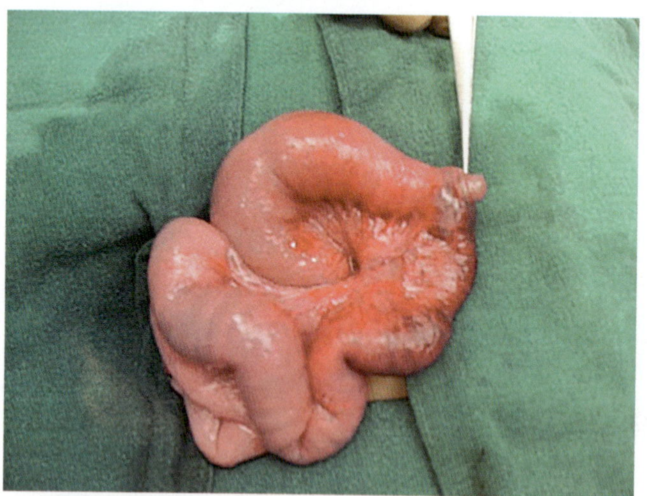

Fig. 5: Operative photograph showing a small Meckel's diverticulum as the lead point ***(Chapter 135)***.

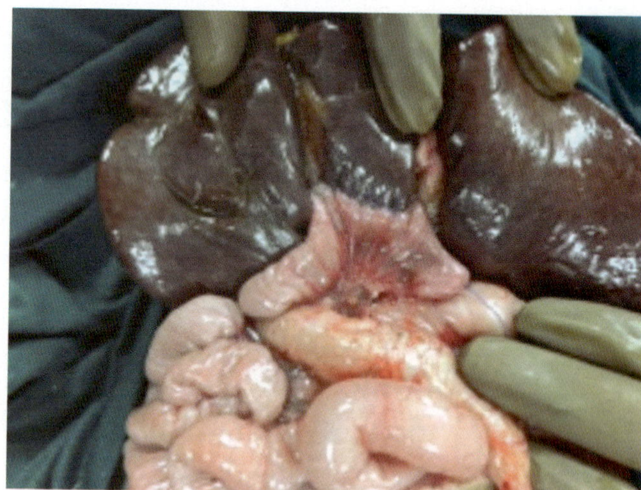

Fig. 3: Completed anastomosis ***(Chapter 136)***.

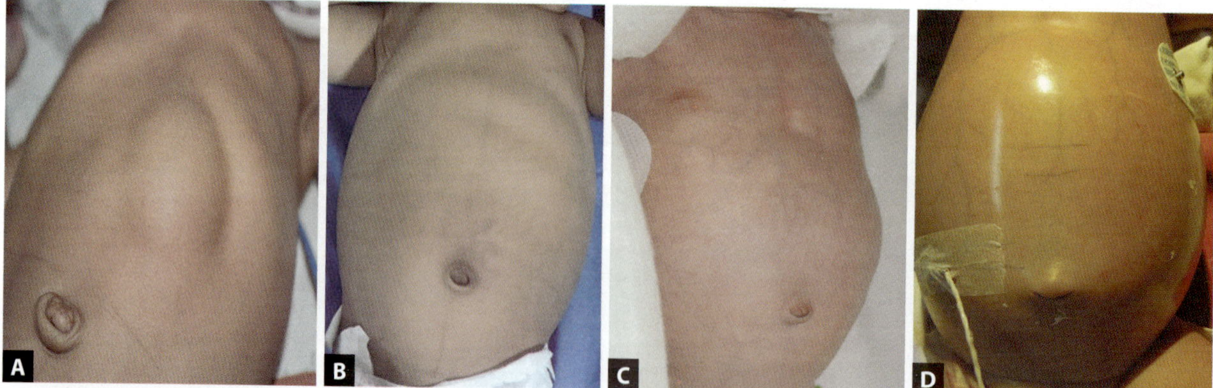

Figs. 1A to D: Spectrum of abdominal distension in neonatal intestinal obstruction. (A) Variably distended, peristaltic stomach/bowel in pyloroduodenal/upper jejunal obstruction; (B) Step-ladder bowel pattern in ileal obstruction; (C) Moderate, generalized distension and visible abdominal veins in necrotizing enterocolitis; (D) Shiny, grossly distended abdomen in Hirschsprung-associated enterocolitis ***(Chapter 137)***.

PLATE 15

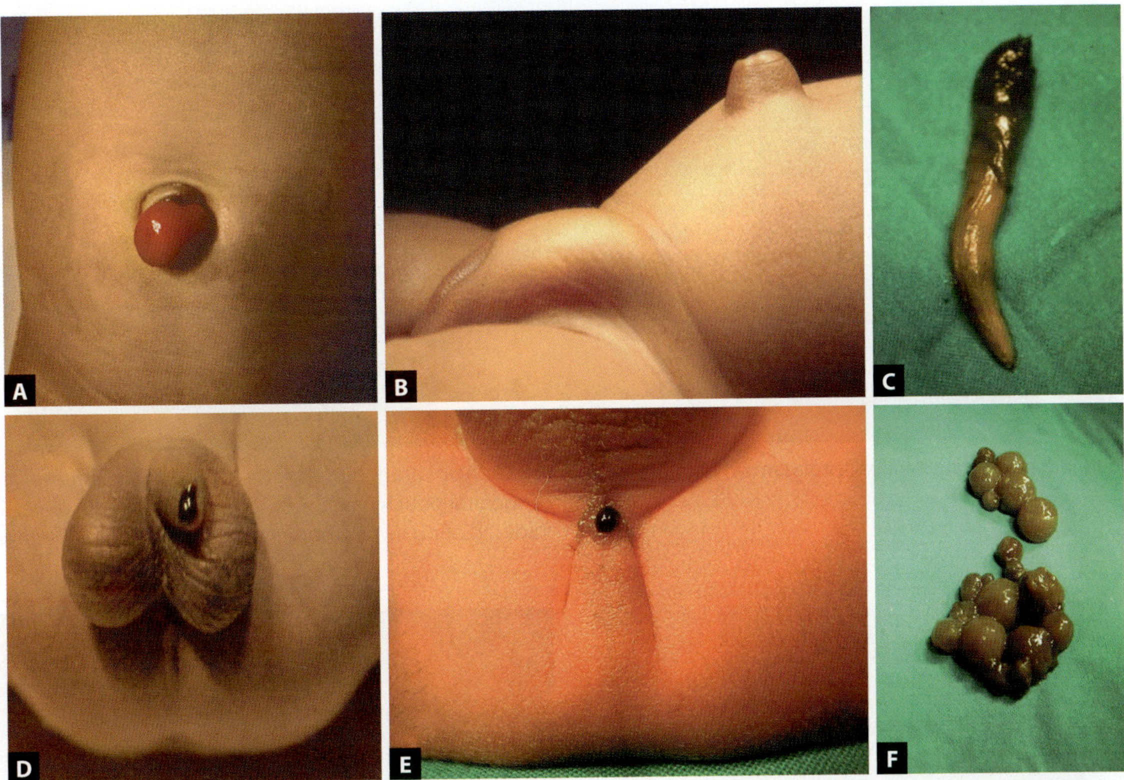

Figs. 2A to F: Typical physical signs lead to a diagnosis in neonatal intestinal obstruction. (A) Umbilical polyp in a PVID; (B) Umbilical and inguinal hernia in a neonate; (C) Meconium plug expelled by an infant of a diabetic mother; (D) Meconuria in a male, imperforate anus with high anorectal malformation; (E) Meconium extruding through perineal fistula in a male, low anorectal malformation; (F) Pale meconium pellets in distal ileal atresia. (PVID: persistent vitellointestinal duct) ***(Chapter 137)***.

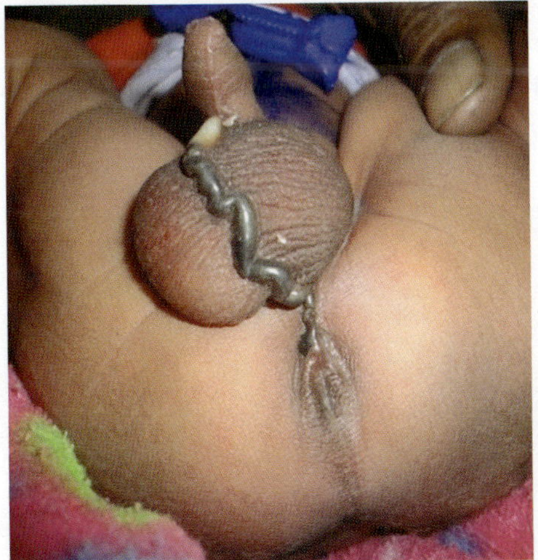

Fig. 3: Perineal fistula with meconium-filled tract along median raphé ***(Chapter 138)***.

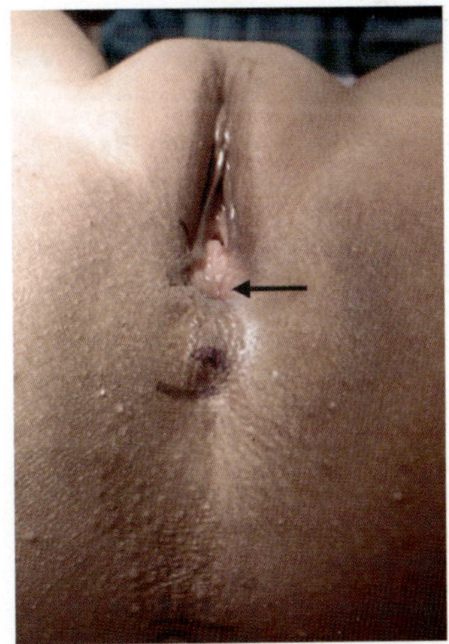

Fig. 6: Girl with vestibular fistula (arrow) ***(Chapter 138)***.

PLATE 16

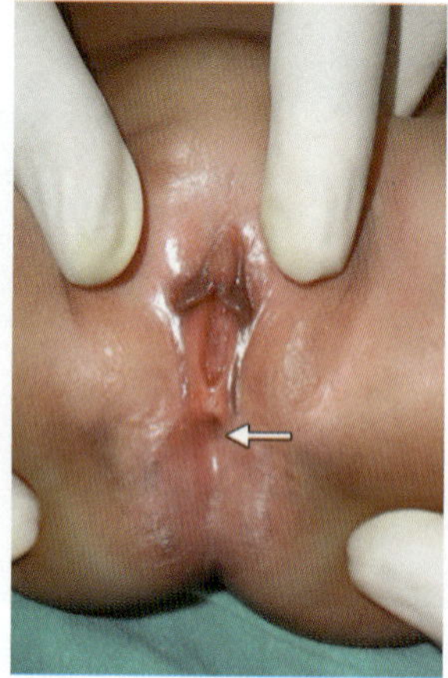

Fig. 7: Perineum of a girl with a perineal fistula (arrow) ***(Chapter 138)***.

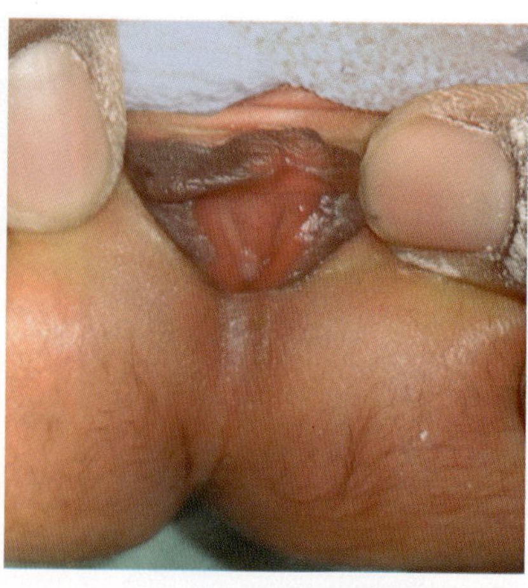

Fig. 9: Appearance of external genitalia in newborn girl with congenital pouch colon (CPC). Note wide margin of vestibule and folds radiating inward from margins of vestibule ***(Chapter 138)***.

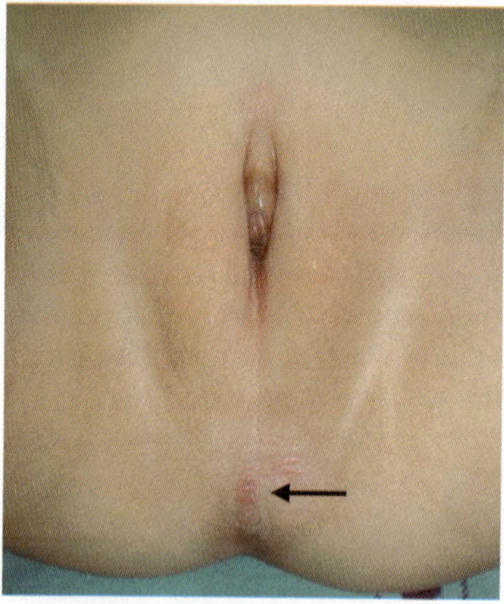

Fig. 8: Case of "persistent cloaca". Note small-looking external genitalia with a flat-bottom perineum (arrow) ***(Chapter 138)***.

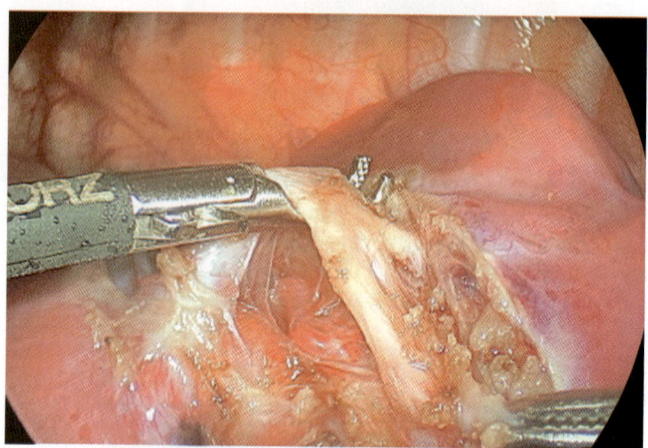

Fig. 2: Isolation of the lobar vessels prior to clamping and resection ***(Chapter 139)***.

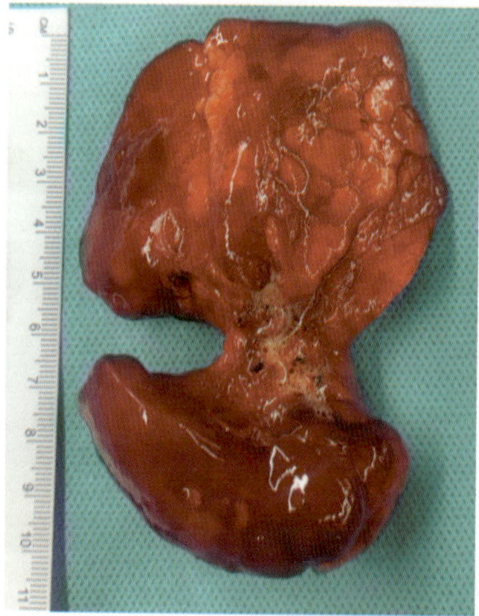

Fig. 3: Specimen of the lobe with multiple congenital pulmonary airway malformation lesions within ***(Chapter 139)***.

PLATE 17

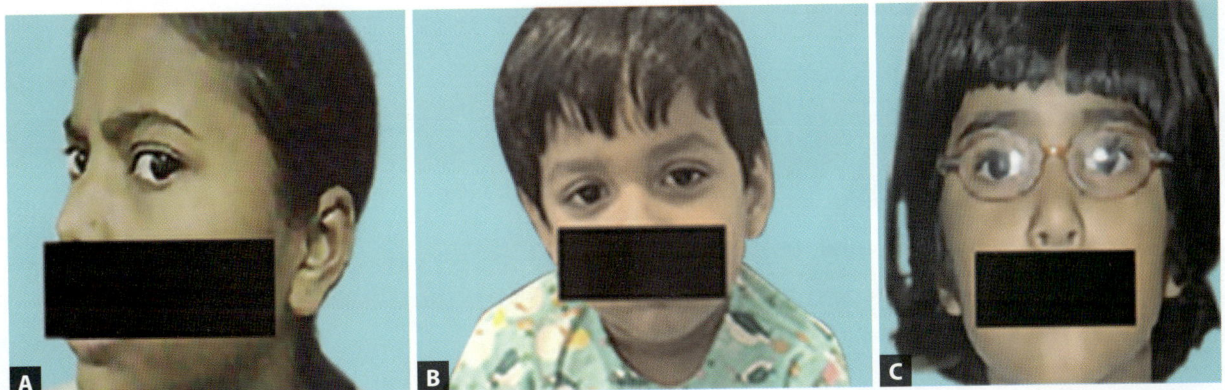

Figs. 1A to C: Various forms of ocular abnormal head posture. (A) Infantile nystagmus with null point in levoversion showing face turn to right; (B) A case of left superior oblique palsy showing a head tilt to right side; (C) A case of V pattern intermittent exotropia keeping a slight chin up posture ***(Chapter 146)***.

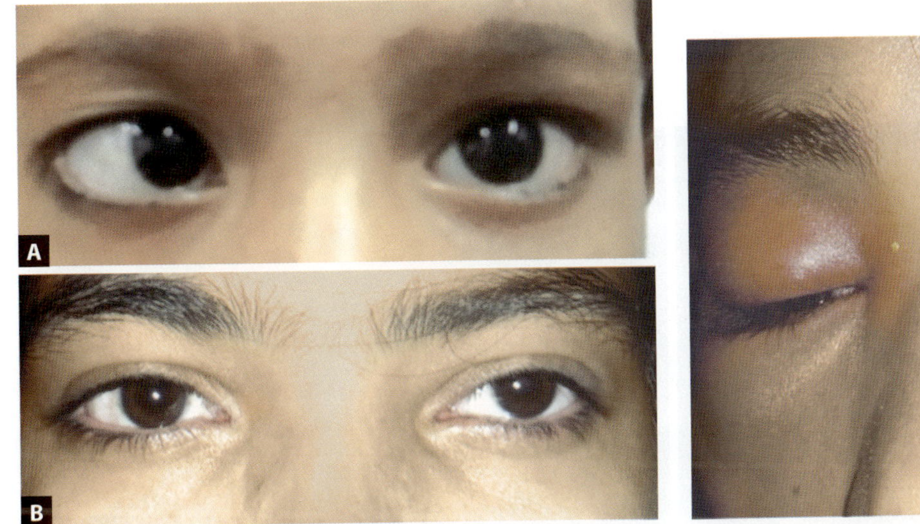

Figs. 1A and B: Horizontal deviations in strabismus. (A) Esodeviation; (B) Exodeviation ***(Chapter 148)***.

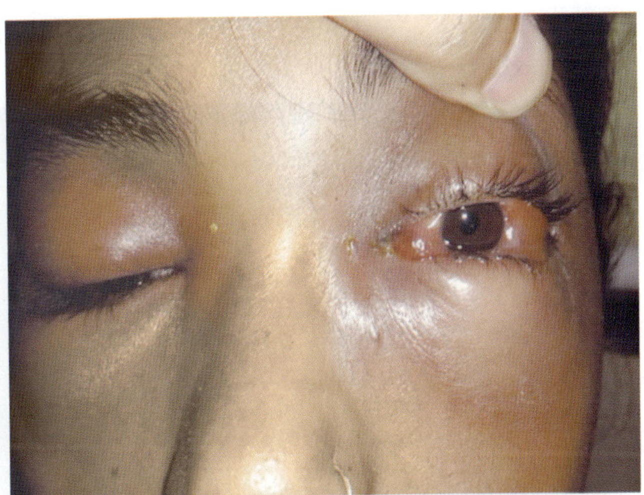

Fig. 1: Orbital cellulitis ***(Chapter 153)***.

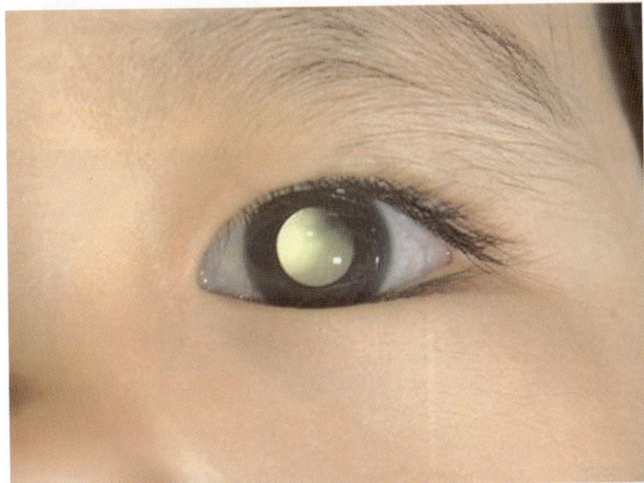

Fig. 1: White reflex in the pupillary area ***(Chapter 152)***.

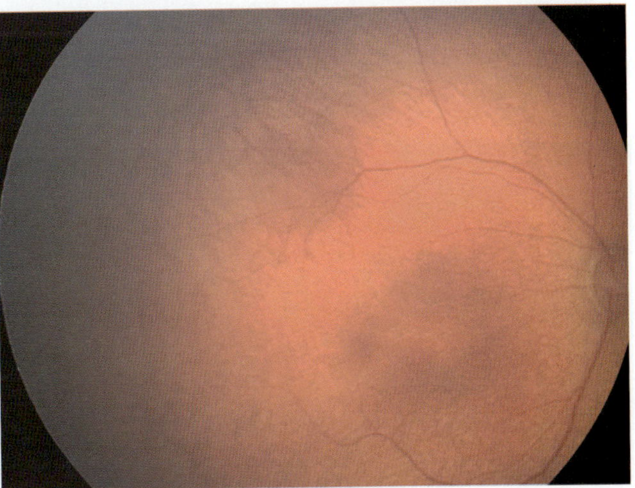

Fig. 4: Immature vascularization with peripheral avascular retina ***(Chapter 154)***.

PLATE 18

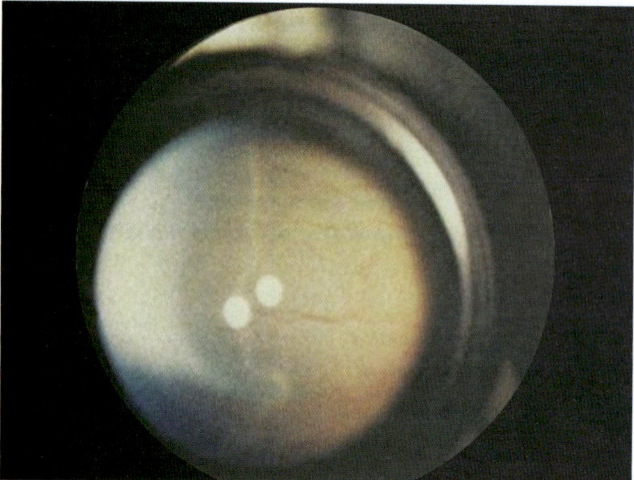

Fig. 6A: A thin flat line separates vascular from avascular retina with abnormal branching of vessels posteriorly (indicates earliest sign of abnormal vessel development) ***(Chapter 154)***.

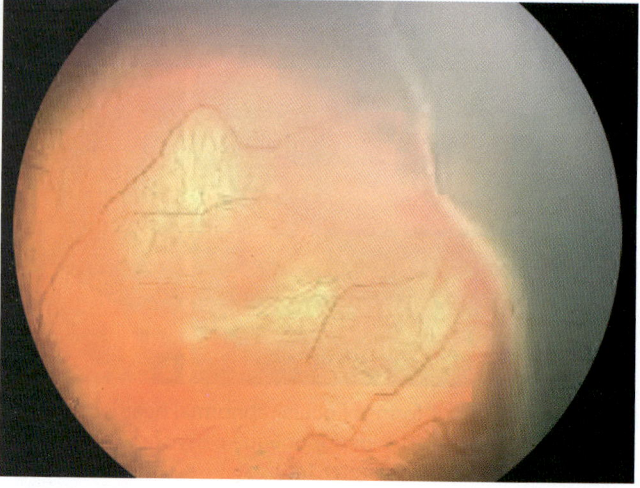

Fig. 7: *Stage II:* The Ridge—this is the hallmark of the stage 2 disease. It arises from the demarcation line and has length and width. It extends above the plane of the retina ***(Chapter 154)***.

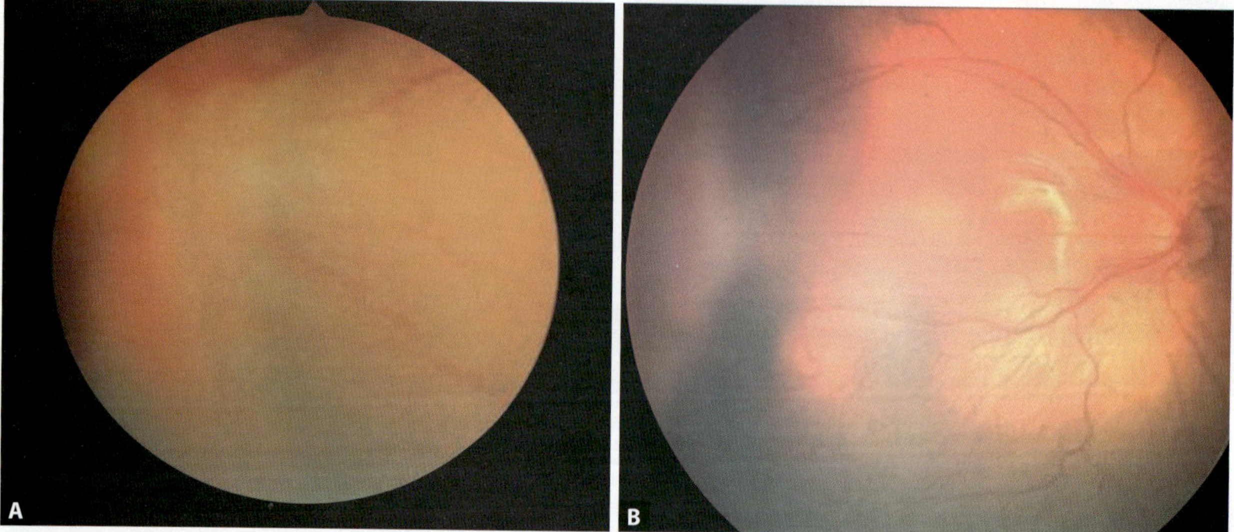

Figs. 9A and B: Partial retinal detachment (A) Stage IVa: Macula not involved; (B) Stage IVb: Macula involved ***(Chapter 154)***.

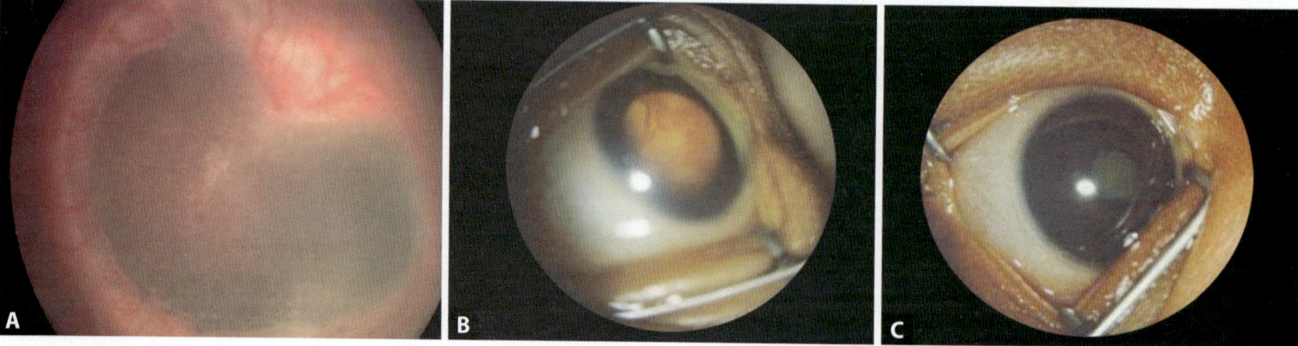

Figs. 10A to C: Plus disease ***(Chapter 154)***.

PLATE 19

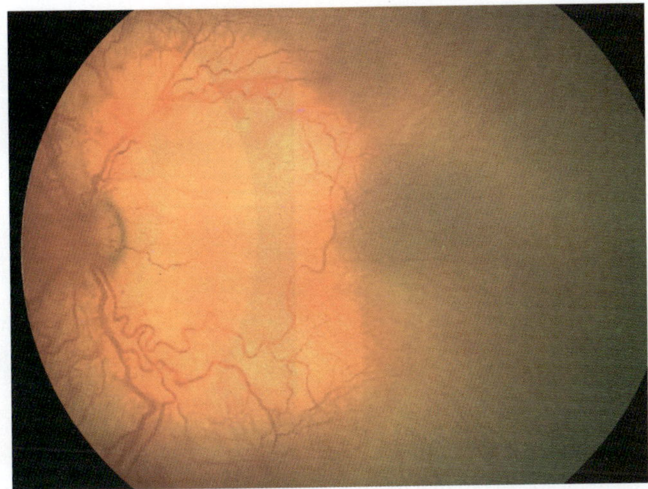

Fig. 11: Left eye of a preterm infant with aggressive posterior retinopathy of prematurity (APROP) ***(Chapter 154)***.

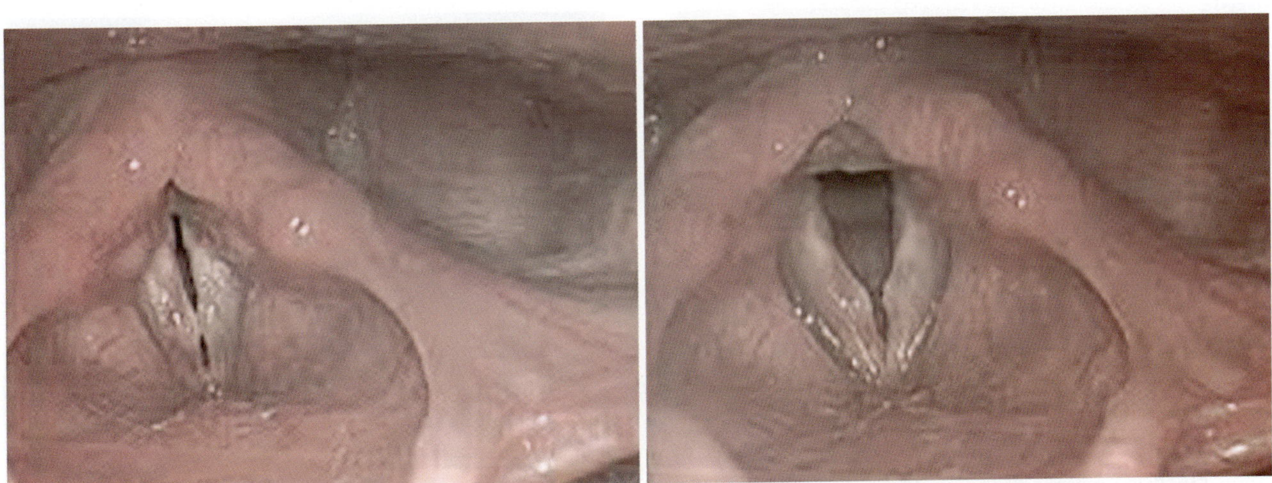

Fig. 1: Laryngoscopic image of a 7-year-old boy with bilateral vocal cord nodule ***(Chapter 156)***.

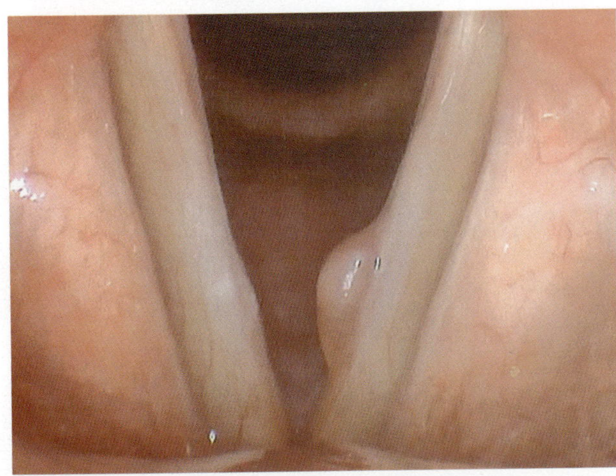

Fig. 2: Laryngoscopic image of 9-year-old girl with left vocal cord polyp ***(Chapter 156)***.

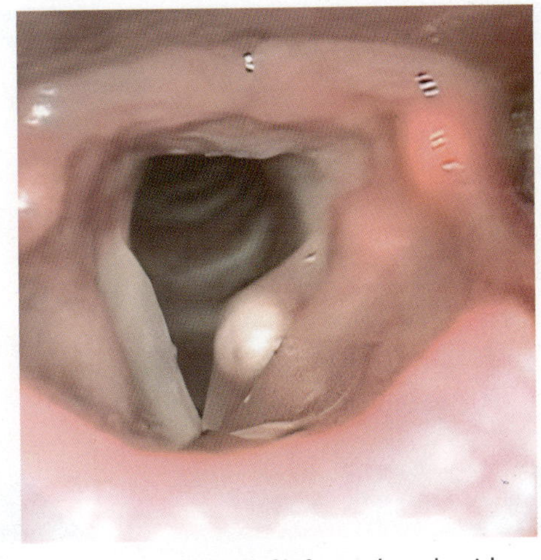

Fig. 3: Laryngoscopic image of left vocal cord epidermoid cyst ***(Chapter 156)***.

PLATE 20

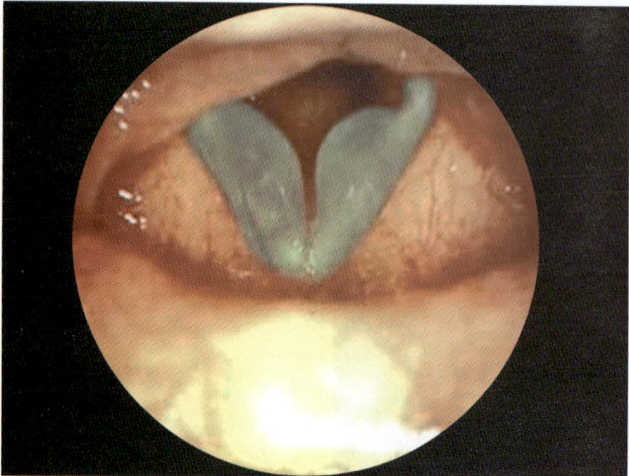

Fig. 4: Laryngoscopic image of bilateral vocal cord mucus retention cyst ***(Chapter 156)***.

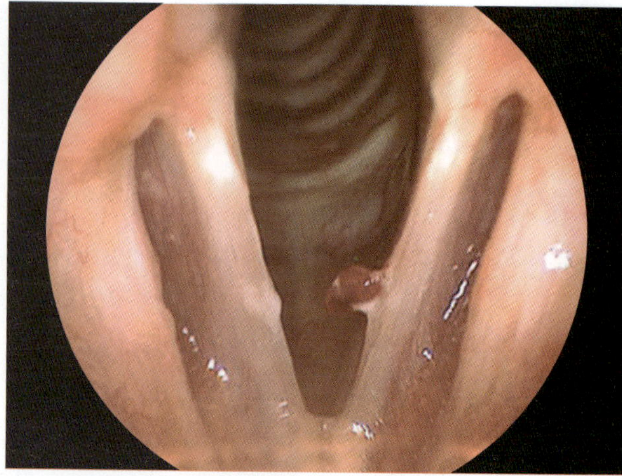

Fig. 7: Laryngoscopic image of hemorrhagic polyp ***(Chapter 156)***.

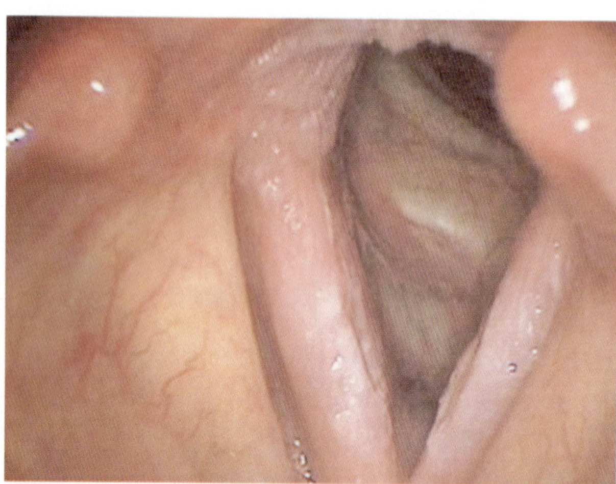

Fig. 5: Laryngoscopic image of linear grooves on bilateral vocal cords ***(Chapter 156)***.

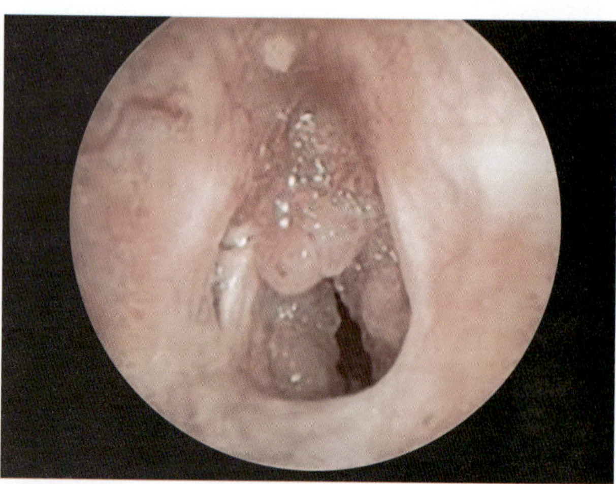

Fig. 8: Laryngoscopic image of juvenile onset juvenile onset recurrent respiratory papillomatosis (JORRP) of larynx ***(Chapter 156)***.

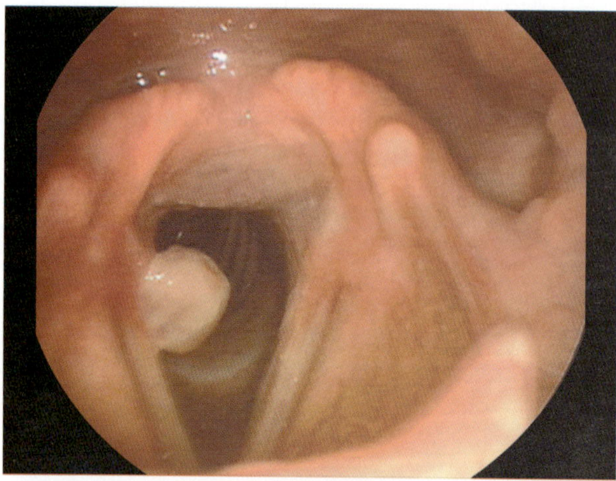

Fig. 6: Laryngoscopic image of right vocal cord granuloma ***(Chapter 156)***.

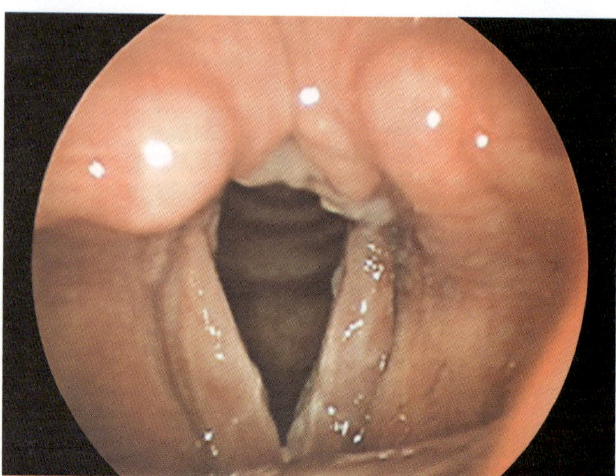

Fig. 9: Laryngoscopic image of chronic laryngitis owing to laryngopharyngeal reflux (LPR) with interarytenoid edema ***(Chapter 156)***.

PLATE 21

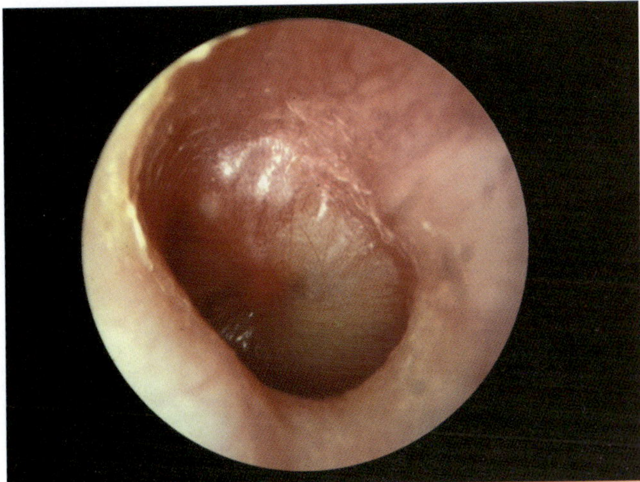

Fig. 1: Acute otitis media—bulging of tympanic membrane ***(Chapter 157)***.

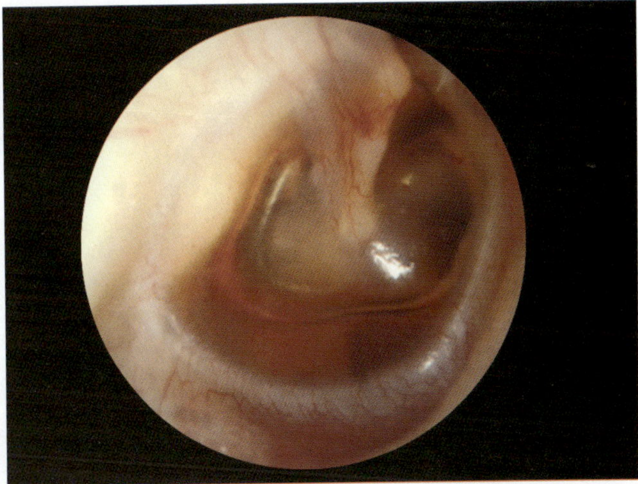

Fig. 3: Otitis media with effusion (OME)—Air fluid level ***(Chapter 157)***.

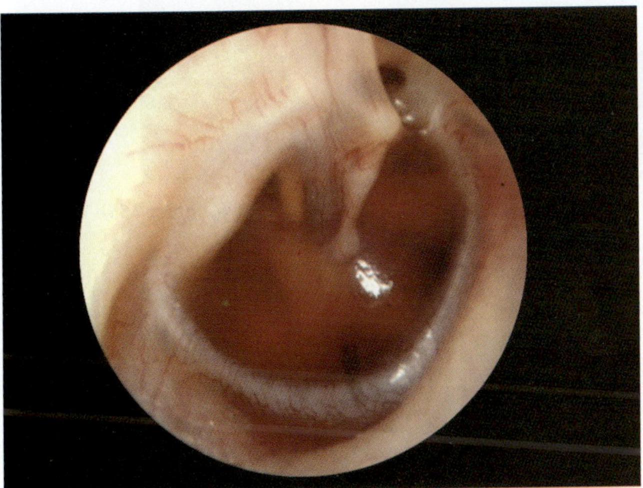

Fig. 2: Otitis media with effusion (OME)—Amber colored fluid in middle ear ***(Chapter 157)***.

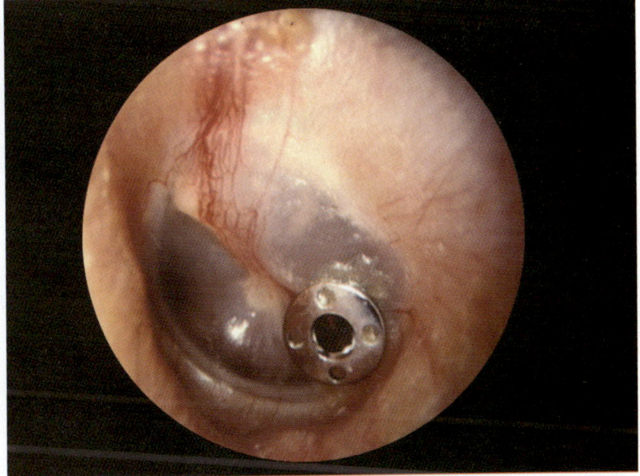

Fig. 4: Grommet in place ***(Chapter 157)***.

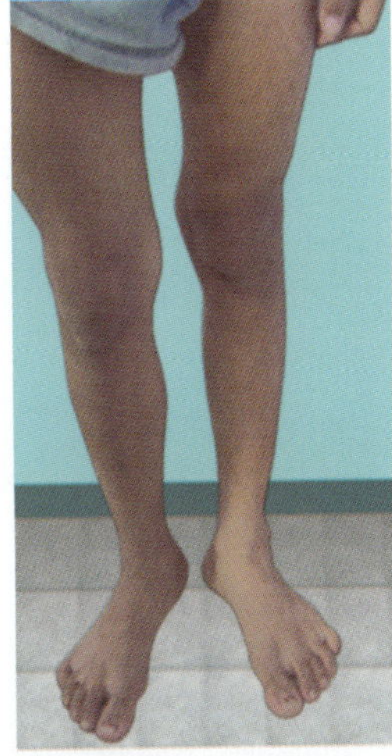

Fig. 2: Clinical photograph of the same child whose X-ray is shown in Figure 1A suggesting gross shortening of left lower limb ***(Chapter 161)***.

PLATE 22

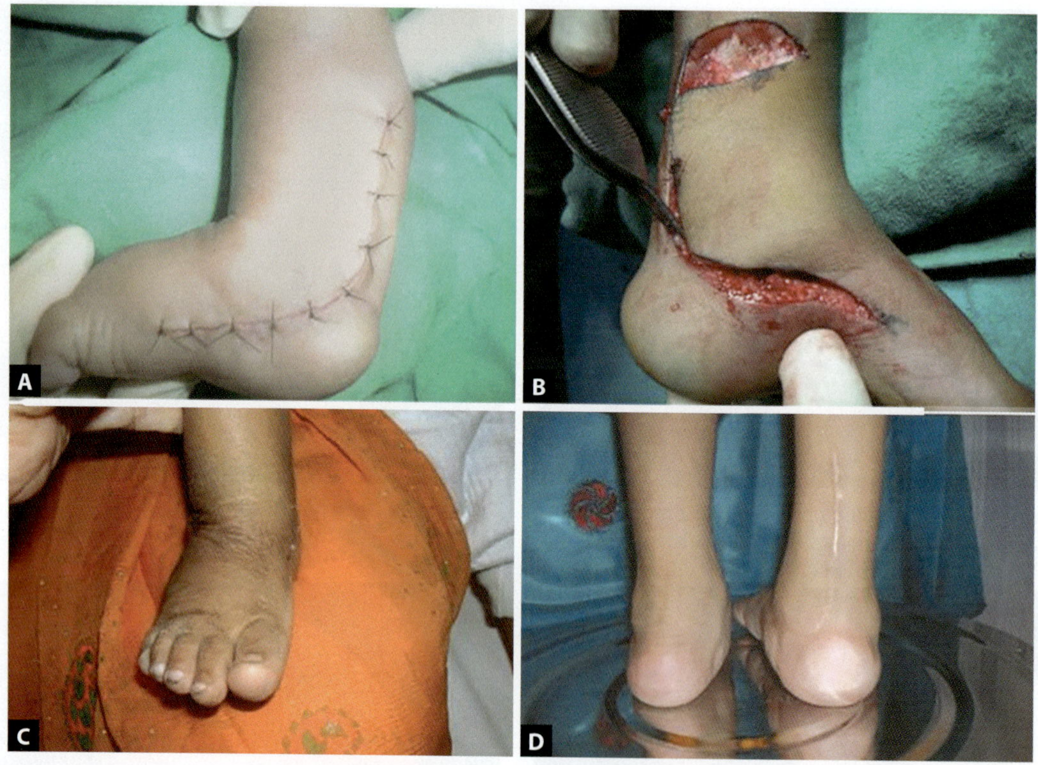

Figs. 5A to D: Steps and result of posteromedial release surgical open release for a 17-month-old boy ***(Chapter 165)***.

Neonatology

Section Editors: *Anjali Kulkarni, Ashish Mehta*

CHAPTER 1

Neonatal Resuscitation

Rhishikesh P Thakre

INTRODUCTION

The arrival of a new baby holds the potential for a medical emergency. It is noteworthy that almost half of the newborns necessitating resuscitation have no identifiable risk factors prior to birth. The essential factors here are anticipation and preparation. It is imperative to evaluate all infants for resuscitation requirements upon birth. Roughly 10% of newborns may require some form of resuscitation, with the proportion needing extensive intervention being <1%.

STANDARD PRECAUTIONS

- Every resuscitative procedure must adhere to rigorous aseptic standards.
- All resuscitation equipment must be maintained in a clean and sterile condition, with a preference for disposability where appropriate.
- Items such as suction catheters, mucus extractors, umbilical catheters, syringes, needles, and endotracheal (ET) tubes should be single-use, sterile, and disposed after use.

PREPARATION PRIOR TO BIRTH

Equipment Check

- Diverse sizes of equipment should be on hand to accommodate varying gestational needs.
- Utilization of a checklist is advisable to verify the operational status of the equipment.
- *The following equipment is considered "preferred" for resuscitation:* Compressed air, blender, pulse oximeter with neonatal probe, electrocardiogram (ECG) with chest leads, laryngeal mask airway, and plastic wrap.

Personnel

- During each delivery, there must be at least one individual designated primarily for the newborn's care, possessing the ability to initiate positive pressure ventilation (PPV) and chest compression (CC), if necessary.
- Proficient personnel for comprehensive resuscitation should be easily accessible in case the need arises.
- In situations classified as "high risk" deliveries, a minimum of two or more individuals are essential. A team leader should be identified and clear roles and responsibilities should be designated.
- Anticipated problems should be defined and plan of action be discussed.
- If time permits, parental counseling should be done.

Identifying High-risk Delivery

Focused questions (help prepare and anticipate problems during resuscitation) include: (1) What is the gestational age? (2) Is the amniotic fluid clear? (3) Are there any additional risk factors? (4) What is the umbilical cord plan?

ASSESSMENT AT BIRTH

- Need for resuscitation is identified following birth by assessment of whether the infant is "breathing or crying?"
- If breathing, the newborn does not require any further resuscitation. Early skin-to-skin contact with mother and delayed cord clamping is practiced and newborn monitored for breathing, color, and activity.
- If the baby is not breathing or crying, a series of steps may be needed to establish breathing sequentially, viz. initial steps, ventilation, CC, intubation, and/or administration of drugs.

Assessing the breathing is by observing the baby's chest movements. Breathing is adequate if a baby is vigorously crying or has good regular chest movements with no pauses or indrawing with associated good tone. Gasping or labored breathing is abnormal.

CORD CLAMPING

- All babies who establish spontaneous breathing at birth should have cord clamping delayed for at least 1 minute. The baby is placed on mother's abdomen.

- It is a safe procedure in term, preterm, and low birth weight (LBW) babies and leads to improved iron status, higher blood pressures during stabilization, lessens risk of intraventricular hemorrhage (IVH), fewer blood transfusions, and improved survival in preterm.
- Prior to arrival of the baby cord plan should include who will hold the baby, where the baby will be placed, how the babies temperature shall be maintained, how the cord will be clamped and who will time the procedure.
- Cord clamping should be done immediately if newborn is depressed, mother is hemodynamically unstable, fetal hydrops, disrupted uteroplacental circulation (e.g., bleeding vasa previa), and known twin-to-twin transfusion syndrome.

STEPS IN NEONATAL RESUSCITATION

A baby who is not breathing or crying at birth should undergo following steps of resuscitation with ongoing assessment and reassessment at every step **(Flowchart 1)**.

Initial Steps

- A baby who is not breathing or crying should be received in dry, prewarmed cloth with immediate cord clamping, and placed under a heat source.
- The head, trunk, and the limbs should be dried firmly and quickly.
- Suction of mouth followed by nose may be done if there is obvious obstruction to airway.
- Stimulation is done by rubbing the back or tapping the soles.
- The newborn is repositioned and simultaneous assessment of respiration and heart rate (HR) is done.

Response to resuscitation is best judged by increasing HR and later by establishment of spontaneous breathing. The HR is easiest and quickly assessed by palpating at the base of umbilical cord but is not reliable; hence auscultation of precordium is preferred.

Positive Pressure Ventilation

- PPV is indicated if the newborn has apnea or gasping respiration, HR < 100 beats per minute or oxygen saturation (SpO_2) below target values despite supplemental oxygen being increased to 100%.
- PPV, if indicated, should begin within first minute of birth following initial steps—first golden minute.
- A flow-inflating bag, a self-inflating bag, or a pressure-limited T-piece resuscitator can be used for PPV.
- Call for help and ask assistant to apply pulse oximeter, if available, to right hand/wrist of the newborn.
- In all newborns (term or preterm ≥32 weeks), PPV should be started with room air. If the infant is <32 weeks of gestation, 21–30% oxygen is recommended.
- Provide breaths at a rate of 40–60 per minute using pneumonic "breathe-two-three" where you squeeze the bag during "breathe" and release as you say "two three".
- You should provide breaths up to 15 seconds and check for HR. A rising HR indicates efficacy of PPV. You should then continue to provide another 15 seconds of PPV and check HR every 30 seconds thereafter.
- If there is no HR rise, check for air entry and chest movement. If not, take corrective measures for ventilation. HR is assessed every 30 seconds. Consider inserting orogastric tube if ventilation is prolonged.
- PPV is discontinued if there is rise in HR > 100 beats per minute and onset of spontaneous respiration.
- If despite adequate PPV, there is no desired response after ventilation corrective measures, one may consider intubation or initiate CC if HR is <60 beats per minute.

Intubation

- Intubation is considered if ventilation is ineffective or prolonged, CC is anticipated, administration of drugs, or suspected congenital diaphragmatic hernia.
- Intubation is performed in time limit of 30 seconds.
- There is no role of cuffed ET tubes.
- Two common and serious errors of ET intubation are malplacement of the ET tube and the use of the wrong sized tubes.

Chest Compression

- HR < 60 beats per minute despite adequate ventilation and ventilation corrective measures is an indication to start CC.
- One should ensure that assisted ventilation is being delivered optimally before starting CCs. Consider intubation if CC is to begin.
- The two-thumb encircling hands technique generates higher peak systolic and coronary perfusion pressure and is recommended for performing CCs.
- A ratio of three CCs to one ventilation is delivered in 2 seconds for uninterrupted 60 seconds compressing the one-third anteroposterior diameter of the chest over the lower thirds of the sternum below the inter nipple line.
- HR is checked every 60 seconds. Use of ECG monitor is preferred.

Flowchart 1: Indian Academy of Pediatrics Neonatal Resuscitation Program first golden minute algorithm for neonatal resuscitation.

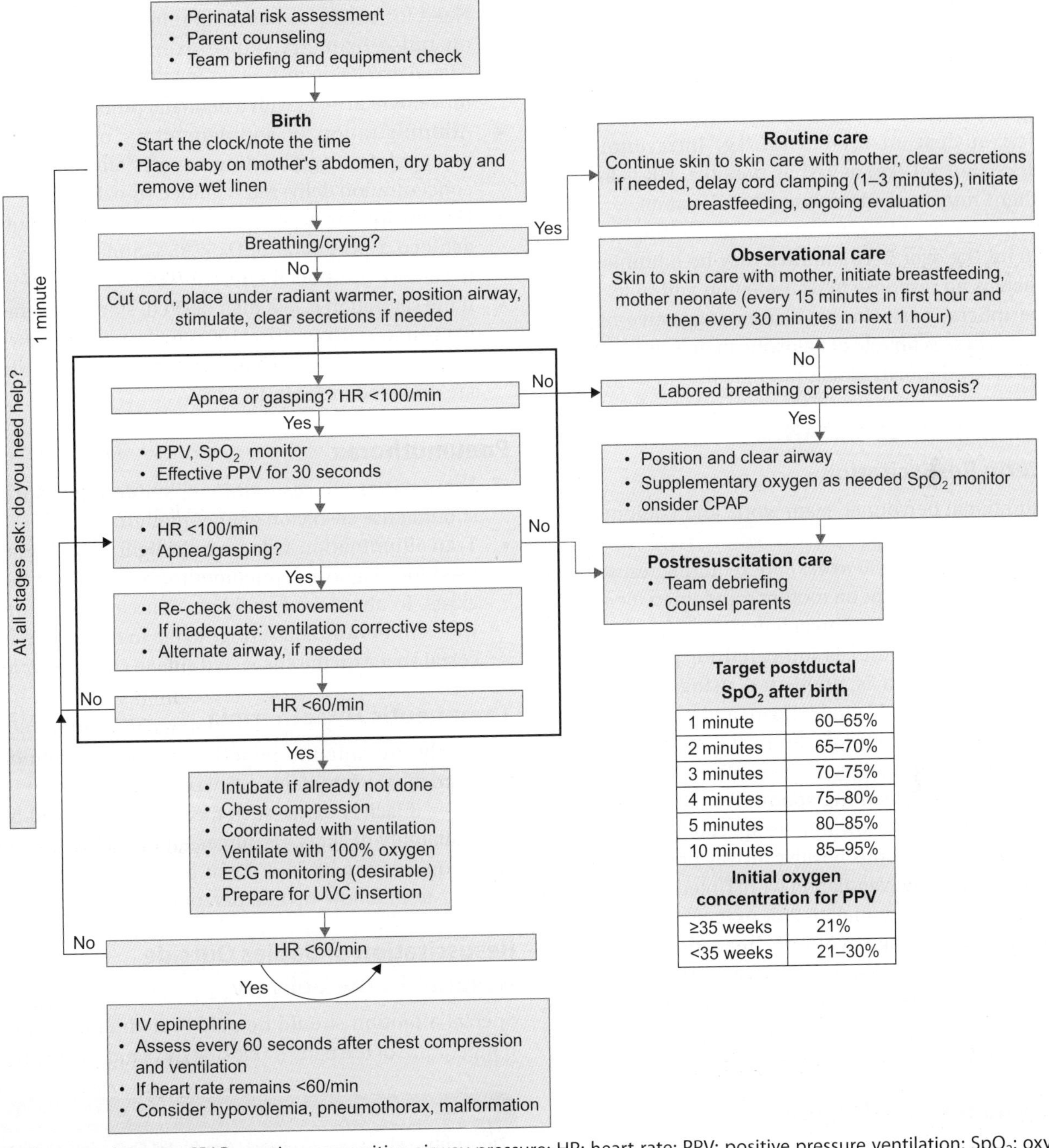

Target postductal SpO_2 after birth	
1 minute	60–65%
2 minutes	65–70%
3 minutes	70–75%
4 minutes	75–80%
5 minutes	80–85%
10 minutes	85–95%
Initial oxygen concentration for PPV	
≥35 weeks	21%
<35 weeks	21–30%

(ECG: electrocardiogram; CPAP: continuous positive airway pressure; HR: heart rate; PPV: positive pressure ventilation; SpO_2: oxygen saturation; UVC: umbilical vein catheter)

Source: Gupta P. IAP-NNF Textbook of Neonatal Resuscitation, 1st edition. New Delhi: Jaypee Brothers Medical Publishers (P) Ltd.; 2023.

If the HR is <60 beats per minute, CC with intubation is continued with administration of adrenaline; if the HR is 60–100 beats per minute, CC is stopped and ventilation continued and if the HR is >100 beats per minute with spontaneous breathing, PPV is discontinued.

Medications

- Bradycardia in the newborn infant is usually the result of inadequate lung inflation or profound hypoxemia, and establishing adequate ventilation is the most important step to correct it.

- Medications are indicated if the HR is <60 beats per minute despite 60 seconds of adequate CC and ventilation.
- The preferred mode of drug delivery is umbilical venous route.
- Epinephrine is administered in 1:10,000 concentration at dose of 0.1–0.3 mL/kg, intravenous (IV) (ET: 0.5–1 mL/kg) as fast as possible. HR is assessed after 1 minute of adrenaline administration.
- Volume expanders, normal saline or Ringer lactate, 10 mL/kg over 5–10 minutes may be administered if there is no response to resuscitation and signs of poor peripheral perfusion or history suggestive of blood loss. There is no role of naloxone in delivery room.
- ET drug administration is not reliable.

SPECIAL CIRCUMSTANCES

Preterm Resuscitation

- Additional personnel, team work, and equipment are required.
- Preterm babies (>30 weeks) not requiring resuscitation at birth can be kept on mother's abdomen for skin-to-skin contact for thermoregulation.
- A "thermal bundle" is indicated for preterm birth. Ensure the area is preheated using a warmer or portable pad. Food grade, clean, and plastic wrapping may be done skipping the initial steps for infants <32 weeks of gestation.
- If preterm is breathing spontaneously with labored respiration or has low minute specific SpO_2, consider initiating continuous positive airway pressure (CPAP). If not breathing, ventilation with T piece resuscitation is preferred with initial 21–30% oxygen.
- Gentle handling, avoiding head-down position, avoiding excess pressures of PPV or CPAP, administering surfactant after stabilization, using pulse oximeter as a guide to oxygenation and avoiding rapid infusions are good resuscitation practices.

Meconium-stained Liquor

- The resuscitation is no longer different and same steps of resuscitation are performed as for nonbreathing baby.
- A depressed infant needs initial steps with oral suction if visible secretions, ventilation with bag and mask, intubation during ventilation corrective measures, under vision tracheal suction and considering further steps based on response.
- There is no role for stomach aspiration following resuscitation.

Role of Oxygen

- Need for oxygen is based on minute specific reading on pulse oximetry. Pulse oximeter working on a "signal extraction technique" that is designed to reduce movement artifact with a neonatal probe is ideal.
- Administration of supplementary oxygen should be regulated by blending oxygen and air, and the concentration delivered is guided by oximetry.
- Healthy infants born at term may take >10 minutes to achieve a preductal SpO_2 < 95% and nearly 1 hour to achieve postductal saturation >95%.
- If the saturation is less than desired, start supplemental oxygen and titrate. Use 100% oxygen if the newborn needs CC. Minute specific SpO_2 targets for newborns are provided in **Table 1**.

Pneumothorax

- Nonresponse to resuscitation, sudden deterioration should raise suspicion of pneumothorax.
- Transillumination using a cold light source may be used for diagnosing pneumothorax bedside, if facility exists. In absence of cold light source, use a butterfly with a three-way and syringe to tap in the second intercostal space on the suspected side to confirm air leak.

Therapeutic Hypothermia

Currently, therapeutic hypothermia is not defined as standard of care for infants ≥35 weeks of gestation in India. However, if facility exists, such therapy may be used based on availability of skills, resources, multidisciplinary team care, consistent with laid down protocols with facilities for long-term follow-up and parental consent.

Resuscitation of Babies Outside Hospital/Home Delivery

Special attention should be paid to maintaining normal temperature of the baby by closing the windows to prevent

TABLE 1: Target oxygen saturation (for term and preterm).

Time (minute)	*Preductal SpO_2 after birth*
1	60–65%
2	65–70%
3	70–75%
4	75–80%
5	80–85%
10	85–95%

(SpO_2: oxygen saturation)

TABLE 2: Postresuscitation care.

	Routine care	*Observational care*	*Advanced care*
When?	For all spontaneous breathing newborns not requiring resuscitation	Postinitial steps or brief positive pressure ventilation (<1 minute)	Postpositive pressure ventilation (>1 minute), need for chest compressions, intubation or drugs or very preterm (<32 weeks)
Where?	Mother	Supervised in nursery	Neonatal intensive care unit
Care?	Counsel parents, initiate breastfeeding, assess for color, activity, and breathing	Counsel parents, observe for temperature, respiration, heart rate, and blood sugar	Team debriefing, counsel parents, sick newborn care, and monitoring

draughts, use dry warm cloth, baby cap, and skin-to-skin contact. Resuscitation can also be performed keeping baby on mother's abdomen. Baby should be transferred to facility in skin-to-skin contact with mother or using thermocol box.

To Resuscitate or Not

Such decisions should not be made based on gestational age or birth weight alone but are made with best interest of the newborn, availability of skills, expertise and resources and parental preferences. When in doubt, resuscitation should be initiated. Noninitiation is considered in anencephaly, confirmed trisomy 13 or 18, multiple complex congenital anomalies not compatible with life. Discontinuation may be considered if chances of survival are extremely poor or survival without medical support is not possible. Such decisions must be taken objectively.

Quality Improvement

To reduce the gap between what we know and what we do in delivery room series of indicators may be identified for every step of resuscitation with respect to availability, effectiveness, safety, timeliness, efficiency, equity, and accessibility. For every identified problem, policy, place, personnel, and equipment issues need to be addressed looking at all the steps involved taking every team member into confidence. Such plan-do-study-act sessions will streamline deficiencies in resuscitation.

POSTRESUSCITATION CARE

The postresuscitation care has been described in **Table 2**.

HARMFUL PRACTICES IN NEWBORN RESUSCITATION

- Routine suction of mouth and nose
- Unrestricted oxygen use without pulse oximeter
- Vigorous and prolonged tactile stimulation in a depressed baby
- Putting the baby upside down for postural drainage

CLINICAL PEARLS

- Discontinuation of resuscitative efforts may be appropriate if resuscitation in a depressed infant does not result in spontaneous circulation (no HR or breathing) despite 20 minutes of resuscitation.
- Use of pulse oximetry is desirable in following conditions: anticipated need for resuscitation, PPV, supplemental oxygen, CPAP, evaluation of cyanosis.
- Free-flow oxygen can be delivered by holding tube near the nostrils, using face mask and flow-inflating bag. It cannot be delivered by self-inflating bag.

KEY POINTS

- Preparation, anticipation, and teamwork is essential.
- All well newborns not requiring resuscitation should be offered early skin-to-skin contact and delayed cord clamping.
- Rapid assessment for need for resuscitation and initial steps should be performed within 30 seconds and PPV initiated not later than 60 seconds of birth constitutes the "first golden minute".
- The most sensitive measure of response to resuscitation is prompt improvement in HR.
- The most important and effective step in resuscitation is ventilation.
- Initiate resuscitation with room air for all newborns.

SUGGESTED READING

1. Aziz K, Lee CHC, Escobedo MB, Hoover AV, Kamath-Rayne BD, Kapadia VS, et al. Part 5: Neonatal Resuscitation 2020 American Heart Association Guidelines for Cardiopulmonary Resuscitation and Emergency Cardiovascular Care. Pediatrics. 2021;147(Suppl 1):e2020038505E.
2. Gupta P. IAP-NNF Textbook of Neonatal Resuscitation, 1st edition. New Delhi: Jaypee Brothers Medical Publishers (P) Ltd.; 2023.

CHAPTER 2

Apnea

Naveen Jain, Ajai Kumar Prithvi

INTRODUCTION

Apnea is a common problem in clinical practice of pediatricians managing preterm babies. It is a symptom of serious concern as timely intervention may be necessary to prevent death/serious hypoxia and associated morbidities. Many apnea events or a single serious apnea event may lead the clinician to investigate extensively and initiate empirical therapies ranging from antibiotics to treatment for reflux. A clinical/algorithmic approach may optimize interventions.

DEFINITION

Cessation of breathing lasting long enough* to cause hypoxia (saturation <80%), bradycardia [heart rate (HR) <100 beats per minute] or poor perfusion or poor tone.

Intermittent hypoxia (IH) describes brief, self-resolving episodes of decrease in oxygen saturation (SpO_2), without bradycardia or loss of tone.

CLINICAL EVALUATION

Apnea is always a life-threatening emergency; treatment (resuscitation) precedes evaluation. In practice, good observation is possible only after resuscitation. Classical description of apnea has been central, obstructive, and mixed based on whether baby is breathing or not at the time of apnea.

However, it is probably more useful/practical to classify babies as:

- *Well preterm baby with apnea:* Possibly apnea of prematurity (AOP)
- *Symptomatic apnea (has to be ruled out before diagnosing as AOP):* A baby with low saturations and needing oxygen to saturate even after effective breathing is established or a sick baby [any parameter of STOPS has either poor Sensorium or tone, Temperature instability, Oxygenation problems or respiratory distress, poor Perfusion, abnormalities of Sugars], or feed intolerance. Apnea in the setting of abnormal STOPS is usually secondary to a cause and needs specific investigation and treatment.

Apnea of prematurity and symptomatic apnea may benefit by stimulation of respiratory center with xanthines, high-flow nasal cannula/continuous positive airway pressure (CPAP)/nasal intermittent mandatory ventilation (NIMV); but treatment of primary cause is more important. Recurrent and severe apnea may require intubation and ventilation in both situations.

CLINICAL PEARLS

- Is the baby completely well after the apnea (AOP likely)? Or
- Does the baby still need oxygen to saturate, has poor sensorium or activity, hypo- and hyperthermia, poor perfusion, and abnormal sugars—look for a cause and treat?

COMMON CAUSES OF APNEA

- AOP
- Respiratory distress syndrome
- Sepsis
- Hypoglycemia
- *Dyselectrolytemia:* Hyponatremia, hypocalcemia, and hypokalemia
- Hypo- and hyperthermia
- Airway obstruction by secretions and poor neck position
- Anemia
- *Cardiac causes:* Patent ductus arteriosus (PDA) and pulmonary hypertension

*Usually defined as >20 seconds, but time is never measured in clinical practice!

- *Central causes:* Perinatal asphyxia, seizures, birth trauma, meningitis, intracranial hemorrhage [intraventricular hemorrhage (IVH) and subdural hemorrhage], periventricular leukomalacia (PVL), and hydrocephalus
- Necrotizing enterocolitis
- Bronchopulmonary dysplasia (BPD)
- Drug toxicity, e.g., phenobarbitone

DIFFERENTIAL DIAGNOSIS

- Periodic breathing (cessation of breathing with no cyanosis or bradycardia)
- Subtle seizures
- Gastroesophageal reflux disease (GERD)

INVESTIGATIONS

Investigations should be planned, based on the expected cause; clues may be obtained from clinical setting and physical examination.

- *First line:*
  - Blood sugar, serum electrolytes, Na, K, and Ca
  - Blood gas analysis
  - Sepsis screen including blood culture
  - Hemoglobin for anemia
  - Ultrasonography head to rule out IVH, PVL, and ventriculomegaly
  - Chest X-ray for pneumonia
- *Second line:*
  - Echocardiography to rule out PDA
  - Electroencephalogram (EEG)
  - Metabolic screen
  - Cerebrospinal fluid (CSF) study
  - Serum phenobarbitone level

MANAGEMENT

Management of newborn with apnea has been depicted in **Flowchart 1**.

Emergency

- Warmth, airway is positioned to semi extend the neck and careful suction of oronasopharynx
- Gentle stimulation of sole or by rubbing back followed by positive pressure ventilation (PPV) if no respiration after stimulation (as in Neonatal Resuscitation Program)
- Oxygen, if baby is hypoxic, to maintain SpO_2 in the range of 90–95%
- Temporarily postpone feeds
- *Methylxanthines (caffeine or aminophylline):* These are adenosine receptor antagonists and are primarily used in AOP:
  - Caffeine (standard dose regime) 10 mg/kg of caffeine base as loading dose over 30 minutes followed by 5 mg/kg/day of caffeine base in once-a-day dose regimen reduces apnea. To be continued till baby is apnea free for 7 days or >34 weeks postconceptional age. Caffeine may also be used in periextubation period to reduce the need for reintubation in very low birth weight babies. High dose up to 20 mg/kg/day has not been reported to have any adverse effects on neurodevelopment.
  - Aminophylline (loading dose) 8 mg/kg intravenous infusion over 30 minutes followed by 1.5–3 mg/kg per dose every 8–12 hourly. Caffeine is the preferred drug because of higher therapeutic safety, more reliable enteral absorption, less fluctuation of plasma levels owing to its long half-life, ease of administration (once daily), and few side effects such as tachycardia and feed intolerance as compared to aminophylline.
  - Caffeine may have action for days after stopping, and babies must be monitored in hospital for recurrence of apnea for 5–7 days after stopping caffeine.
  - Use of caffeine in babies <1,250 g or <28 weeks of gestation has been shown to decrease bronchopulmonary dysplasia and survival with better neurodevelopmental outcome at 18 months of corrected age. Prophylactic use of either aminophylline or caffeine in the prevention of AOP has been recommended by the World Health Organization (WHO), and may be considered as per local resources.

CLINICAL PEARLS

- Caffeine/aminophylline may decrease incidence and severity of apnea episodes; this *must not delay* investigating for a cause or planning for CPAP/ventilation.
- Aminophylline is similar in effectiveness (but narrow therapeutic index); close monitoring for tachycardia and feed intolerance may be required (most centers are not monitoring drug levels in India); has almost been replaced by caffeine.

Flowchart 1: Management of newborn with apnea.

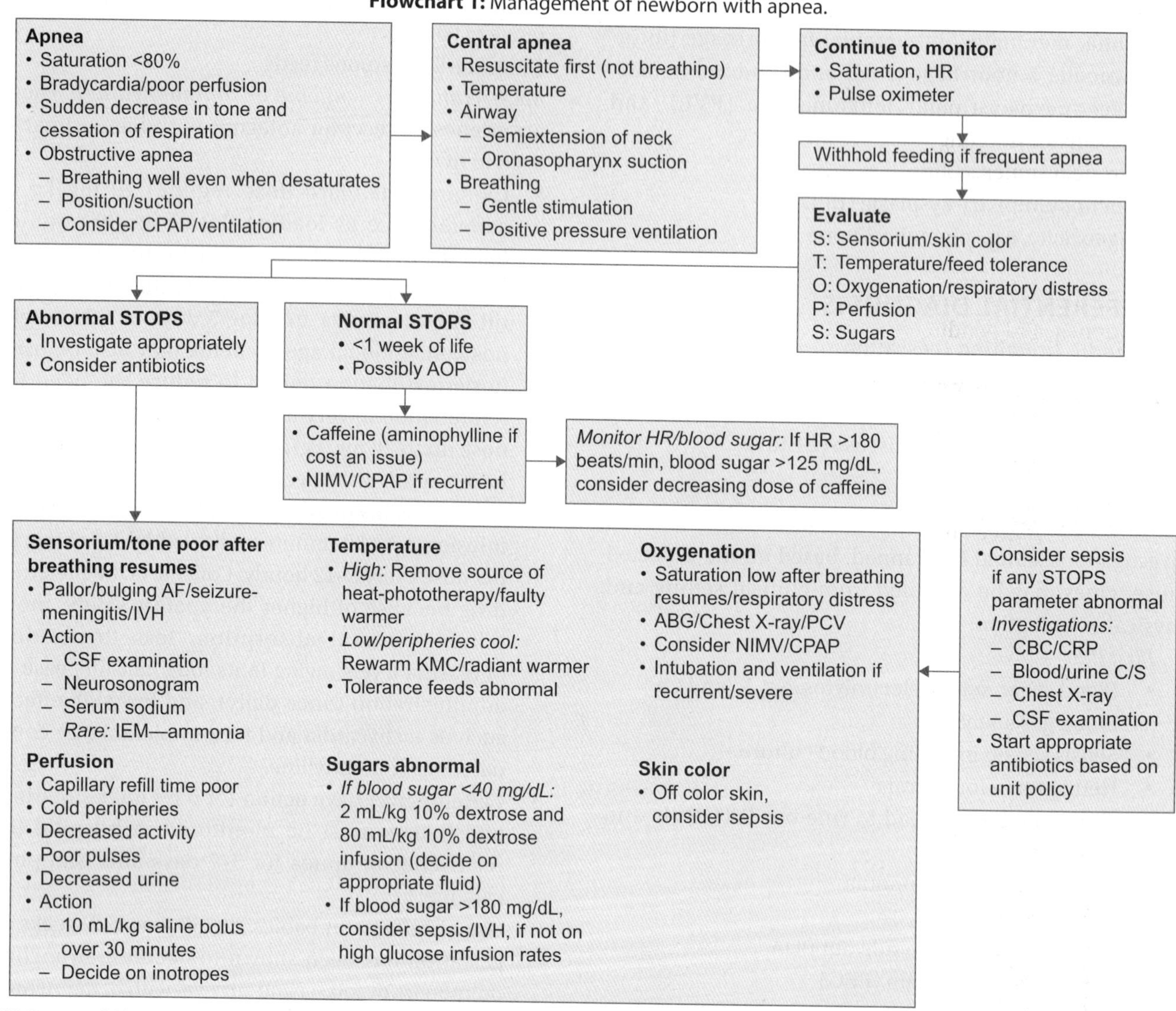

(ABG: arterial blood gas; AF: anterior fontanelle; AOP: apnea of prematurity; CBC: complete blood count; CPAP: continuous positive airway pressure; CRP: C-reactive protein; HR: heart rate; IEM: inborn error of metabolism; IVH: intraventricular hemorrhage; KMC: kangaroo mother care; NIMV: nasal intermittent mandatory ventilation; PCV: packed cell volume)

- *Oxygen:* Oxygen tubing placed close to nose with a flow rate of 3–4 L/min (infranasal oxygen) can be used in frequent IH. The risk of high fraction of inspired oxygen (FiO_2) is unlikely; however, supplemental oxygen therapy should be adjusted to maintain SpO_2 values in the targeted range (90–95%).
- *CPAP:* CPAP can be used in apnea if xanthines fail. CPAP is the preferred mode of treatment if baby has retractions or higher need for oxygen in addition to apnea. Postextubation CPAP reduces extubation failure due to apnea.
- *Heated humidified high-flow nasal cannula (HFNC):* Flow of gases >3 L/min is equally effective, especially in babies without many retractions. Post-extubation HFNC reduces extubation failure due to apnea.
- Noninvasive ventilation with nasal prongs in the form of NIMV or synchronized NIMV
- *Intubation and ventilation:* If the baby has frequent apnea on CPAP and NIMV, intubation, and mechanical ventilation should be considered without much delay.

- *Supportive care:*
  - *Avoid triggers:* Vigorous suctioning of the pharynx; oral feedings can increase the risk of apnea; tube feeds may be necessary if apnea are frequent. Prone positioning stabilizes the chest wall and may reduce apnea.
  - *Transfusion of packed red blood cells:* If packed cell volume less than thresholds for gestation age and no other evident cause of apnea.
  - Antibiotics should be initiated in sick babies with apnea, and pending reports of blood culture.

AREAS OF UNCERTAINTY IN CLINICAL PRACTICE

- The duration and frequency of apneas that can be safely tolerated
- Effect of treated and untreated apneas on neuro-development

KEY POINTS

- It is important to differentiate if the baby looks well or not.
- A well-baby is likely to have AOP, it is a diagnosis of exclusion.
- Investigations may be required in a sick baby to find causes of apnea.

SUGGESTED READING

1. Bruschettini M, Brattström P, Russo C, Onland W, Davis PG, Soll R. Caffeine dosing regimens in preterm infants with or at risk for apnea of prematurity. Cochrane Database Syst Rev. 2023;4(4):CD013873.
2. Chavez L, Bancalari E. Caffeine: Some of the Evidence behind Its Use and Abuse in the Preterm Infant. Neonatology. 2022;119(4):428-32.
3. Erickson G, Dobson NR, Hunt CE. Immature control of breathing and apnea of prematurity: the known and unknown. J Perinatol. 2021;41(9):2111-23.

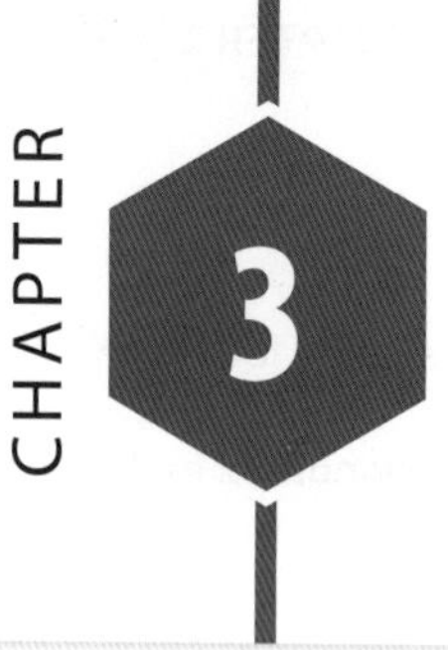

Respiratory Distress in Newborn

Murchana Khound

INTRODUCTION

Respiratory distress is a common problem in newborn and is encountered in almost 6–7% of neonates. The clinical presentation of respiratory distress in the newborn includes tachypnea (respiratory rate of >60 breaths per minute), retraction of chest (intercostals, subcostal, or supraclavicular), grunting, cyanosis, inspiratory stridor, and nasal flaring. However, conventionally, presence of any two out of retraction, grunt, and tachypnea is defined as respiratory distress. Early recognition and management is necessary to prevent mortality and to decrease morbidity.

COMMON CAUSES OF RESPIRATORY DISTRESS IN NEWBORN

Causes can be divided based on gestational age or age of onset:

- Based on gestational age **(Table 1)**
- Based on age of onset **(Table 2)**

TABLE 1: Causes of respiratory distress based on gestational age.

Preterm	***Term***
Pulmonary:	
• Respiratory distress syndrome (RDS) (hyaline membrane disease) • Congenital pneumonia • Aspiration pneumonia • Transient tachypnea of newborn (TTNB) • Pulmonary hemorrhage • Chronic lung disease	• Transient tachypnea of newborn (TTNB) • Meconium aspiration syndrome (MAS) • Congenital and acquired pneumonia • Persistent pulmonary hypertension • Pulmonary hemorrhage • Surfactant protein deficiency syndromes • Alveolar capillary dysplasia
Cardiac:	
• Congenital heart disease • Myocardial dysfunction	Same
Neuromuscular:	
• Asphyxia • Intraventricular hemorrhage • Muscular diseases (myasthenia gravis) • Spinal muscular atrophy • Medications (maternal sedation)	Same
Metabolic:	
• Hypoglycemia • Acidosis • Hypothermia • Polycythemia • Inborn errors of metabolism	Same
Surgical	Same

APPROACH TO A NEONATE WITH RESPIRATORY DISTRESS

History

A detailed good history is very important to come to a diagnosis. It is important to know if the baby is a term (>37 completed weeks of gestational age) or a preterm baby (<37 weeks of gestation). If preterm, the exact gestational age helps us to assess the risk of respiratory distress syndrome (RDS) or hyaline membrane disease. It is important to know in case of preterm baby whether antenatal steroid has been received or not. The importance of determining the time of onset of distress needs to be emphasized, as this may vary depending upon the etiology. RDS, transient tachypnea of newborn (TTNB), and meconium aspiration syndrome (MAS) are some conditions which would present in a neonate soon after birth. If feeding problems are present, such as choking or aspiration during a feed, and distress occurred after some duration after birth, aspiration pneumonia may be thought of as a cause. Congenital heart disease usually manifests with symptoms like respiratory distress after some duration after birth; acquired pneumonias will also manifest later than 48 hours after birth. Important clues for diagnosis are given in **Table 3**.

TABLE 2: Causes of respiratory distress based on age of onset.

Before 6 hours of life	*After 6 hours of life*
RDS/TTNB	Congenital heart disease
Birth asphyxia	Sepsis
Pneumothorax	Shock
MAS	Aspiration pneumonia
Congenital malformations	

(MAS: meconium aspiration syndrome; RDS: respiratory distress syndrome; TTNB: transient tachypnea of the newborn)

TABLE 3: Important clues for diagnosis.

History	*Suggestive cause*
Prolong/difficult labor, assisted delivery, fetal distress, and MSAF	Asphyxial lung disease and MAS
PPV in delivery room	Air leak
Prolonged rupture of membrane	Congenital pneumonia
Polyhydramnios	CDH and TEF
Oligohydramnios	Pulmonary hypoplasia
Maternal HTN and preeclampsia	Asphyxia and MAS
Placenta previa and abruption	Shock
Diabetes in mother	RDS and polycythemia
Family history of unexplained neonatal deaths	RDS, CHD, and IEM
Postfeed worsening	GERD, cleft palate, TEF, and IEM
Relation with crying	Worsens with crying in CHD, relieves on crying in choanal atresia
Chronic course/oxygen dependency	BPD, CHD, osteopenia of prematurity, and recurrent aspiration

(BPD: bronchopulmonary dysplasia; CDH: congenital diaphragmatic hernia; GERD: gastroesophageal reflux disease; HTN: hypertension; IEM: inborn errors of metabolism; MAS: meconium aspiration syndrome; MSAF: meconium-stained amniotic fluid; PPV: positive pressure ventilation; RDS: respiratory distress syndrome; TEF: tracheo-esophageal fistula)

Clinical Examination

The neonate should then be assessed for severity of respiratory distress and any associated neurological signs such as level of alertness, bulged fontanelle, and tone anomaly. One should also look for any signs suggestive of cardiac problem such as prolonged capillary refill time, poor pulse volume, a hepatomegaly, presence of any murmur, and any abnormality in blood pressure. Any signs indicating presence of sepsis should be looked for. If malformations are present in any part of body, it may indicate a surgical cause or a cardiac cause as the possibility for respiratory distress. Excessive frothing with inability to pass a feeding tube may indicate presence of tracheoesophageal fistula while deterioration of a baby on bag and mask ventilation and associated scaphoid shape of abdomen would indicate presence of diaphragmatic hernia. In a dehydrated baby, metabolic acidosis may be the cause. History of meconium stained liquor, and on clinical examination, meconium staining of nails, skin, umbilicus, etc. with a hyperinflated chest would indicate MAS.

CLINICAL PEARL

- A detailed history and clinical examination is very important to find the cause of respiratory distress in a newborn.

Assessment of Severity

For assessment of severity Downes score **(Table 4)** is used in both term and preterm babies and Silverman–Anderson score in preterm babies **(Fig. 1)**.

The Downes score is commonly used for assessing severity of respiratory distress objectively in a newborn as well as to assess whether baby is improving or deteriorating later on **(Table 4)**.

A score of 6 or more indicates severe respiratory distress and impending failure with need for respiratory support. A score of <6 indicates respiratory distress and

TABLE 4: Score for respiratory distress (Downes score).

Score	*0*	*1*	*2*
Respiratory rate	<60	60–80	>80
Central cyanosis	None	None with 40% fraction of inspired oxygen (FiO_2)	Need >40% FiO_2
Retractions	None	Mild	Severe
Grunting	None	Minimal	Obvious
Air entry	Good	Decreased	Very poor

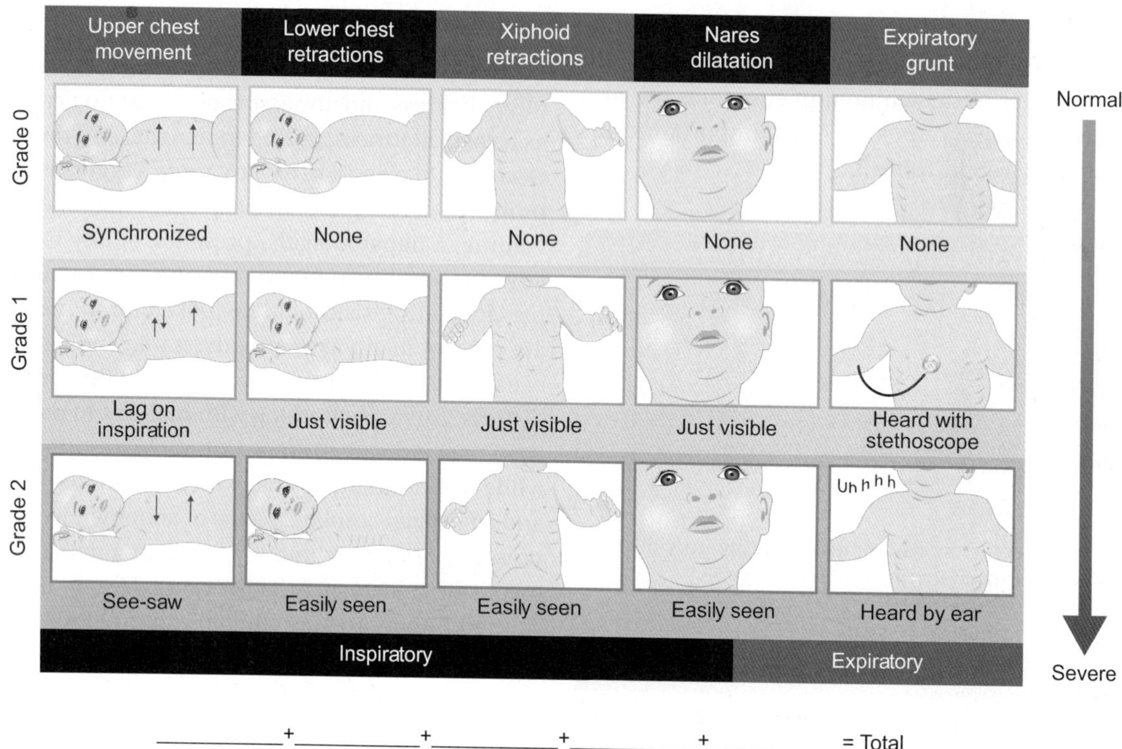

________+________+________+________+________ = Total

Fig. 1: Silverman–Anderson score in preterm babies.

may indicate oxygen supplementation with a hood if the score is <4 and a score of 4–6 indicates moderate respiratory distress with need for support with continuous positive airway pressure (CPAP).

Investigations

Based on probable diagnosis reached after thorough history and clinical examination, investigations need to be planned to confirm diagnosis. If history of prolonged rupture of membrane is present in a neonate with respiratory distress, sepsis screen which includes estimation of total leukocyte count, absolute neutrophil count, estimation of C-reactive protein level, band cell count and microerythrocyte sedimentation rate, and blood culture needs to be done. Shake test should be done if RDS is suspected. Shake test is a simple bedside test and should be done in preterm babies with respiratory distress, especially if there is no history of administration of antenatal steroid. The gastric aspirate (0.5 mL) is mixed with 0.5 mL of absolute alcohol in test tube. This is shaken for 15 seconds and allowed to stand for 15 minutes. A negative shake test, i.e., no bubbles or bubbles covering less than one-third of the rim indicates a high risk of developing RDS and the presence of bubbles more than two-thirds of the rim indicates lung maturity and decreased risk of developing RDS. A chest X-ray helps to differentiate different conditions such as RDS, TTNB, MAS, pneumonia, and different surgical conditions such as tracheoesophageal fistula and diaphragmatic hernia **(Figs. 1 to 5)**. Cardiomegaly in chest X-ray may indicate cardiac abnormality as a cause of respiratory distress. An arterial blood gas (ABG) helps further in establishing diagnosis. Other investigations are echocardiography, ultrasonography (USG) of brain, inborn errors of metabolism (IEM) screening, etc., based on suspected etiology. Lung ultrasound is an upcoming modality in diagnosis of respiratory distress in newborn as it is easy to learn, point-of-care, radiation free, quick, and repeatable. Point-of-care lung ultrasound can assist clinician in guiding respiratory support, assessing response to surfactant therapy and need of possible repeat surfactant treatment, monitoring progress of respiratory illness, assessing the therapeutic effect of thoracocentesis (i.e., pleural effusion or pneumothorax), early identification of respiratory diseases such as RDS, TTNB, and pleural effusion before getting the X-ray film, cause of sudden deterioration in respiratory status like pneumothorax, and enable prompt intervention. Classical findings in pneumothorax are

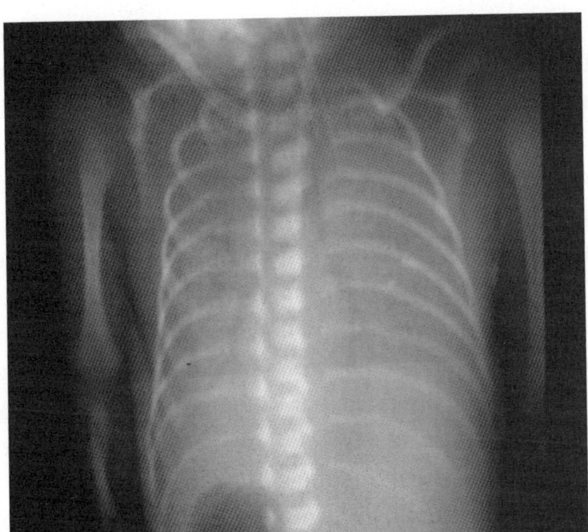

Fig. 2: Chest X-ray anteroposterior view of a premature baby showing respiratory distress syndrome (RDS), with bilateral lung fields showing ground-glass appearance with air bronchogram. If a preterm baby has respiratory distress within the first 6 hours of birth and is cyanosed or needs oxygen to maintain oxygen saturation, the diagnosis is RDS unless proved otherwise. X-ray findings would be a reticulogranular pattern in mild disease, uniform ground-glass opacity with profound under aeration in moderate disease and a "white out" picture in severe disease.

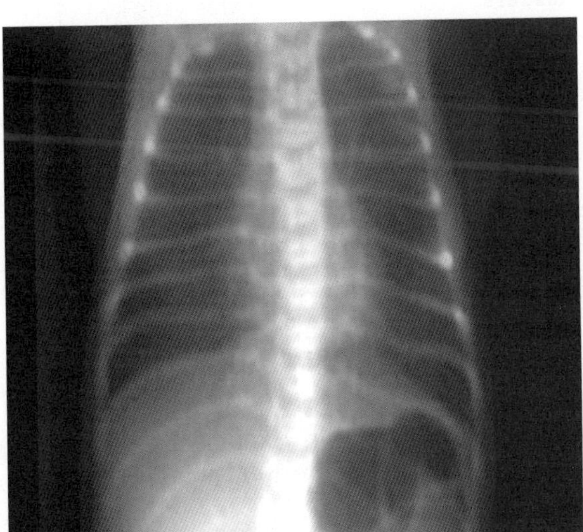

Fig. 3: Chest X-ray showing hyperinflation of lung fields, bilateral perihilar streaky opacities (sunburst), fluid in the horizontal fissure of right lung and mild to borderline cardiomegaly suggestive of transient tachypnea of newborn. Transient tachypnea of the newborn is a benign condition usually seen in term babies born by cesarean section. These babies are well and have only tachypnea with rates as high as 80–100 breaths per minute. The breathing is shallow and rapid without any significant chest retractions. It occurs because of delayed clearance of lung fluid. Management is supportive and prognosis is excellent.

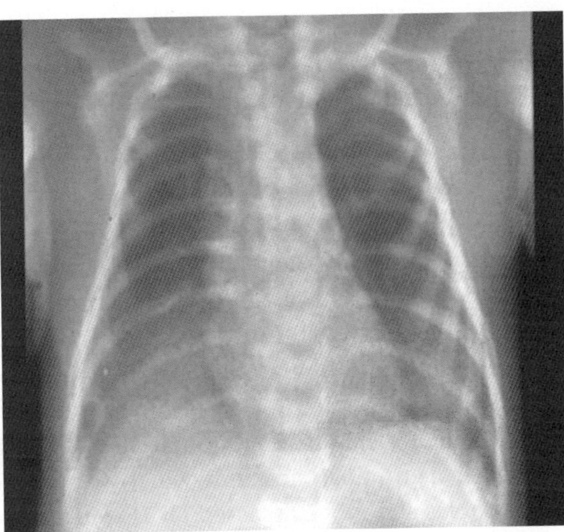

Fig. 4: Chest X-ray showing infiltrates in right lower lung which is asymmetrical bilaterally with history of prolonged rupture of membrane, suggesting congenital pneumonia. In developing countries, pneumonias account for >50% cases of respiratory distress in newborn. In congenital pneumonia, respiratory distress is noticed soon after birth or during first 24 hours. Auscultatory signs may be nonspecific. The newborn may die from pneumonia without manifesting distress. Neonates may develop pneumonia postnatally as a consequence of septicemia, aspiration of feeds, and ventilation for respiratory failure.

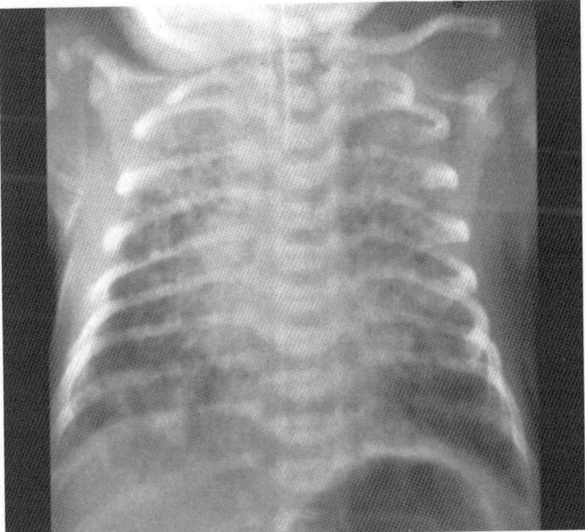

Fig. 5: Patchy opacities with intermittent hyperlucent areas suggestive of air entrapment are seen in meconium aspiration syndrome (MAS). Babies born through meconium stained liquor could have MAS and aspiration may occur in utero, during delivery or immediately after birth. Thick meconium could block air passages and cause atelectasis and air-leak syndromes.

presence of lung point, absence of lung sliding, presence of pathological A lines, absence of B lines, absence of pleural line, and bar code sign on M-mode.

MANAGEMENT (FLOWCHART 1)

General Management

Irrespective of cause, the principles of supportive therapy for respiratory distress in newborn is same and crucial in all. All babies with respiratory distress would need constant monitoring. The parameters to be monitored to find whether baby is improving or deteriorating with any indication for respiratory support are the respiratory rate, presence of grunting, chest indrawing, or any episode of apnea. Babies should be assessed for Downes score at intervals to access improvement or deterioration. Monitoring should be continued till baby no longer requires oxygen for at least a minimum period of 24 hours.

Based on severity of respiratory distress, baby would require oxygen (Downes score 1–3), continuous positive pressure ventilation (Downes score 4–6), or mechanical ventilation (Downes score >6). Oxygen can be provided with oxygen hood or nasal cannula for achieving appropriate oxygen saturation (90–95% range). Oxygen when given therapeutically should always be warmed and humidified. When oxygen hood is used for administering oxygen, oxygen flow rate should be 5–6 L/min (2–3 L/kg/min). Flow rate <3 L/min is not appropriate as may lead to carbon dioxide rebreathing. If an oxygen hood is used with all side ports closed and flow rate of 5 L/min, the baby would receive around 80% oxygen, if one side port is kept open with same flow rate, baby would receive 60% oxygen while baby would receive 40% oxygen if both side ports are kept open. The percentage of oxygen needed by baby can be determined by oxygen saturation reading shown in pulse oximeter. The aim should be to maintain oxygen saturation in the range of 90–94%. Another useful method of providing oxygen is nasal prongs. Appropriate sized prongs which fit into neonate's nostrils should be used. If baby's oxygen saturation is acceptable, we can slowly wean off oxygen.

Flowchart 1: Management of neonatal respiratory distress.

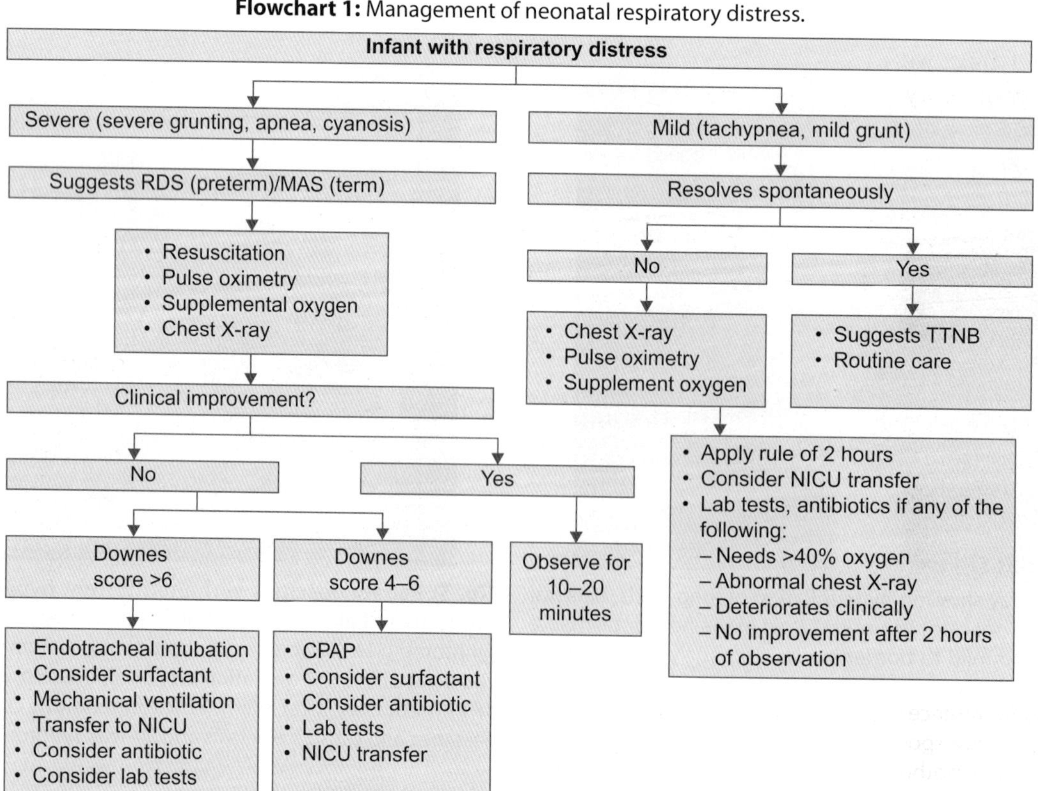

(CPAP: continuous positive airway pressure; MAS: meconium aspiration syndrome; NICU: neonatal intensive care unit; RDS: respiratory distress syndrome; TTNB: transient tachypnea of newborn)

> **CLINICAL PEARL**
>
> - During oxygen therapy, percentage of oxygen needed should be determined in a neonate by oxygen saturation reading in a pulse oximeter and ABG. Oxygen is a drug and overdose should be avoided. Target oxygen saturation should be 90–94% in neonates.

The body temperature of the neonate should be maintained in normal range (36.5–37.5°C). Fluid and electrolyte balance should be maintained. If baby is having moderate-to-severe respiratory distress, baby can be maintained on intravenous fluid. If mild respiratory distress is there, as assessed by Downes score, baby can be fed expressed breast milk by tube feeding. Blood sugar should be monitored and kept in normal range (40–125 mg/dL). Associated polycythemia or anemia should be corrected. If baby has apnea, baby should be stimulated by providing tactile stimulation or positive pressure ventilation by bag and mask. Repeated episodes might indicate need for CPAP or mechanical ventilation, if severe. Such babies would need transfer to centers with facility for CPAP or mechanical ventilation if these are not available locally **(Figs. 6A and B)**.

All babies with respiratory distress do not need antibiotics. Babies with TTNB do not need antibiotics. However, if respiratory distress is persistent or risk factors for sepsis are present, antibiotics should be started after taking cultures. If cultures come negative and clinically baby does not seem to have infection, antibiotics can be stopped.

Continuous positive airway pressure is indicated for neonates with respiratory distress if Downes score is 4–6. Experience is required for the successful application of CPAP, especially with short binasal prongs. Single prong method may be beneficial for nurseries who have less experience with short binasal prongs or when application of short binasal prongs is problematic. While commencing CPAP, it can be given at a pressure of 6–8 cm of water with sufficient oxygen to maintain target saturation. An orogastric tube needs to be passed to decompress the stomach. While baby is on CPAP, continuous monitoring of saturation, heart rate, and respiratory rate are indicated. Blood gases are indicated when pressures or oxygen percentage are changed or patient's condition shows some change. The circuit integrity should be checked periodically.

> **CLINICAL PEARL**
>
> - Downes score of 4–6 is an indication for CPAP. A score of >6 is an indication for mechanical ventilation.

Baby's improvement would be indicated by reduction in respiratory rate, stabilization or reduction of oxygen requirement to maintain saturation of 92–95%, reduction

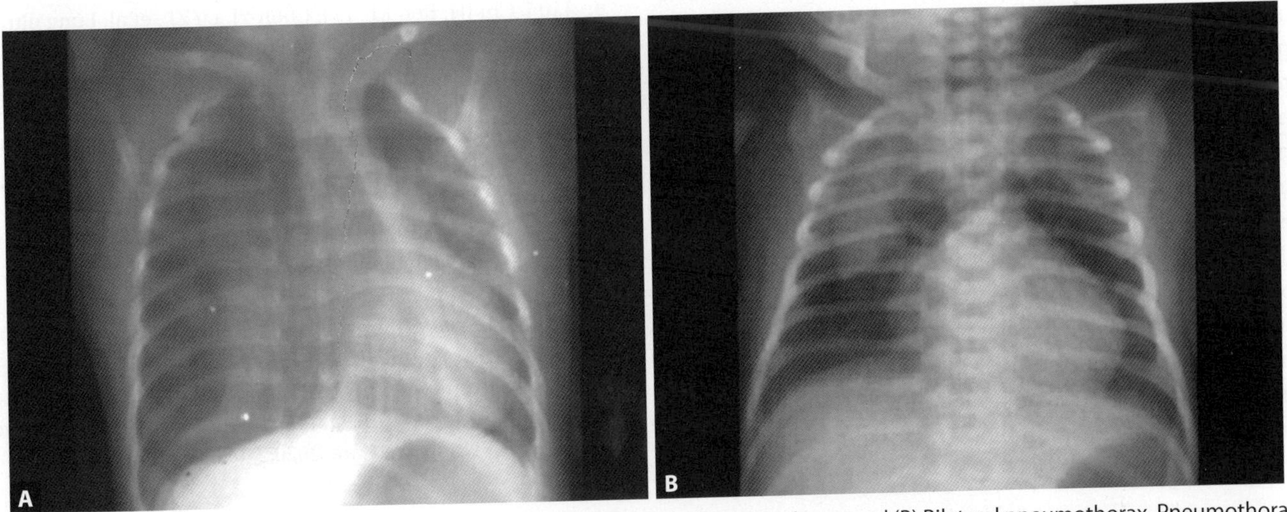

Figs. 6A and B: Presence of pneumothorax on chest X-ray, (A) Right-sided pneumothorax and (B) Bilateral pneumothorax. Pneumothorax in neonates could be spontaneous but is more often due to meconium aspiration syndrome or staphylococcal pneumonia. It is important to recognize pneumothorax because quick recognition and prompt treatment could be life-saving. The distress is usually sudden in onset and heart sounds become less distinct. Immediate management in hemodynamically unstable neonate is by emergency needle aspiration in ipsilateral second intercostal space in mid clavicular line and later chest tube drainage in ipsilateral fourth intercostal space in anterior axillary line.

in sternal and intercostal retraction, reduction in grunt, and improved ABG reports. The need for CPAP for acute lung conditions usually lasts for 1–3 days.

Weaning is commenced when saturation is >96%, retraction, grunt disappears, and respiratory rate stabilizes with normal blood gas reports. While weaning, initially fraction of inspired oxygen (FiO_2) is brought down and then pressure is reduced by 1–2 cm/h until a pressure of 5 cm is reached. When neonate is stabilized in 21% oxygen and 5 cmH_2O, ceasing CPAP is considered. However, recommencing CPAP may be needed at times if work of breathing is increased or oxygen requirement increases. Complications of CPAP, like pneumothorax, must be excluded in such babies.

Continuous positive airway pressure is said to be failed if there is rapid rise for oxygen requirement, respiratory acidosis or partial pressure of carbon dioxide >60 mm Hg, recurrent apnea and increased work of breathing indicated by excessive retraction grunt and retraction, or if agitation is not relieved.

There can be at times complications of CPAP such as pneumothorax, nasal trauma, or CPAP belly, i.e., distension of abdomen.

If CPAP fails or Downes score is >6, there is need for mechanical ventilation.

Specific Management

In case of pneumonia, antibiotic is indicated. Antibiotic of choice should be based on local antibiotic sensitivity pattern. In case of hyaline membrane disease, surfactant replacement therapy is indicated. If pneumothorax occurs, needle decompression or chest tube drainage may be required. Small pneumothoraces can be treated in term infants without invasive management through nitrogen washout. Administration of 100% oxygen can accelerate the resolution of the pneumothorax as readily absorbed oxygen replaces nitrogen in the extrapulmonary space. If the neonate is polycythemic then partial exchange transfusion is required and if anemic then packed red blood cell (PRBC) transfusion should be given according to standard transfusion policy. Ductus-dependent cardiac lesion will require initiation of prostaglandin therapy. Neonates with respiratory distress due to surgical conditions, such as tracheoesophageal fistula and diaphragmatic hernia, would need surgical intervention. Respiratory distress due to cardiac failure would need management of cardiac failure. Refractory hypoxia would indicate the need of high frequency ventilation, inhaled nitrous oxide or extracorporeal membrane oxygenation (ECMO).

KEY POINTS

- Respiratory distress occurs in 6–7% of all neonates.
- Early identification and appropriate and timely management is the key to success in management.
- Oxygen saturation in pulse oximeter should be maintained at 90–94%.
- Oxygen should be used judiciously and overdose should be avoided.
- Antibiotic use is not indicated in all patients with respiratory distress.

SUGGESTED READING

1. Frey B, Shan F. Oxygen administration in infants. Arch Dis Child Fetal Neonatal Ed. 2003;88:F84-8.
2. Hein HH, Ely JW, Lofgren MA. Neonatal respiratory distress in the community hospital: when to transport, when to keep. J Fam Pract. 1998;46:284-9.
3. Hermansen CL, Lorah KM. Respiratory distress in newborn. Am Fam Physician. 2007;76:987-94.
4. Liu J, Chi JH, Ren XL, Li J, Chen YJ, Lu ZL, et al. Lung ultrasonography to diagnose pneumothorax of the newborn. Am J Emerg Med. 2017;35(9):1298-302.
5. National Neonatology Forum. (2008). Facility based care of sick neonate at referral health facility. [online] Available from https://cghealth.nic.in/ehealth/2013/Training_Portal/pdf/FBNC/FACILITY%20BASED%20CARE%20OF%20SICK%20NEONATE%20AT%20REFERRAL.pdf. [Last accessed September, 2024].
6. Singh Y. Tissot C, Fraga MV, Yousef N, Cortes RG, Lopez J, et al. International evidence-based guidelines on point of care ultrasound (POCUS) for critically ill neonates and children issued by the POCUS Working Group of the European Society of Paediatric and Neonatal Intensive Care (ESPNIC). Crit Care. 2020;24(1):65.

Respiratory Support in Newborns

Jayashree A Mondkar, Alpana A Utture

INTRODUCTION

Respiratory disorders are one of the most common reasons for admission to the neonatal unit. Advances in neonatal respiratory care with the availability of a number of noninvasive and invasive modalities of therapy have revolutionized the management of babies with respiratory disorders, especially the extremely preterm (<28 weeks gestation at birth) and very preterm (<32 weeks gestation) group.

The aims of respiratory support are to maintain adequate oxygenation and ventilation, to reduce work of breathing and to prevent lung injury. The modalities of respiratory support commonly available in our neonatal intensive care units (NICUs) include:

Noninvasive modes of respiratory support:

- Continuous positive airway pressure (CPAP)
- Heated, humidified high-flow nasal cannula (HH-HFNC)
- Nasal intermittent positive pressure ventilation (NIPPV)/nasal intermittent mandatory ventilation (NIMV)
- Nasal high-frequency oscillatory ventilation (nasal HFOV).

Invasive ventilation:

- Conventional ventilation using a variety of modes
- High-frequency ventilation

Oxygen therapy:

- As a standalone therapy is rarely used in the acute stage of respiratory illness
- Used as part of all respiratory support modalities mentioned above

Respiratory adjuncts: The following respiratory adjuncts may be needed for management of respiratory distress along with respiratory support modalities.

- Surfactant therapy
- Adjuncts for persistent pulmonary hypertension of the newborn (PPHN): Nitric oxide, sildenafil

COMMON CLINICAL INDICATIONS FOR RESPIRATORY SUPPORT IN NEONATAL INTENSIVE CARE UNIT

Pulmonary Disorders

- Respiratory distress syndrome (RDS)
- Meconium aspiration syndrome (MAS)
- Transient tachypnea of the newborn
- Congenital pneumonia
- Community-acquired pneumonia
- Persistent pulmonary hypertension of the newborn
- Air leak syndromes
- Bronchopulmonary dysplasia (BPD)
- Pleural effusion
- Pulmonary hypoplasia
- Upper airway disorders

Surgical Disorders

- Esophageal atresia with tracheoesophageal fistula
- Congenital diaphragmatic hernia (CDH)
- Congenital pulmonary airway malformation (CPAM)
- Congenital lung cysts, bronchogenic cysts

Cardiopulmonary Disorders

- Neonatal septic shock
- Shock associated with structural cardiac defects

Central Nervous System Disorders

- Perinatal asphyxia and hypoxic ischemic encephalopathy
- Apnea of prematurity
- Neonatal encephalopathy
- Neuromuscular disorders

OXYGEN THERAPY

Indications

Oxygen therapy is indicated for hypoxemia resulting from reduced alveolar oxygen content, low ventilation–perfusion ratio, reduced diffusion capacity, or extrapulmonary right-to-left shunts. The aim of therapy is to achieve adequate tissue oxygenation without creating oxygen toxicity and oxidative stress. Strategies to "normalize" oxygenation with use of high FiO_2 result in high rates of retinopathy of prematurity, chronic lung disease, brain, and other organ injury, especially in the premature infant.

CLINICAL PEARL

- Oxygen therapy should be used judiciously and blended air–oxygen mixture using a blender preferably with an oxygen analyzer should be used at all times to target oxygen saturation between 91 and 95%.

Oxygen is usually administered:

- By means of a head box, mask, and nasal cannula. An external air–oxygen blender should be used to titrate the fraction of oxygen delivered. It may be used for mild-to-moderately severe respiratory disorders in term babies without evidence of respiratory failure.
- *As part of assisted therapy:* CPAP or mechanical ventilation wherein supplemental oxygen is administered by the mixture of air and oxygen in the CPAP device or ventilator.

CLINICAL PEARLS

- Gas warming and humidification is essential to avoid drying of the airways and secretions as well as to avoid convective heat losses when using head box, nasal cannulas, or assisted ventilation.
- No role for standalone oxygen therapy in preterm with RDS as alveolar recruitment is the key to management.

Flowchart 1: Algorithm for management of respiratory distress syndrome.

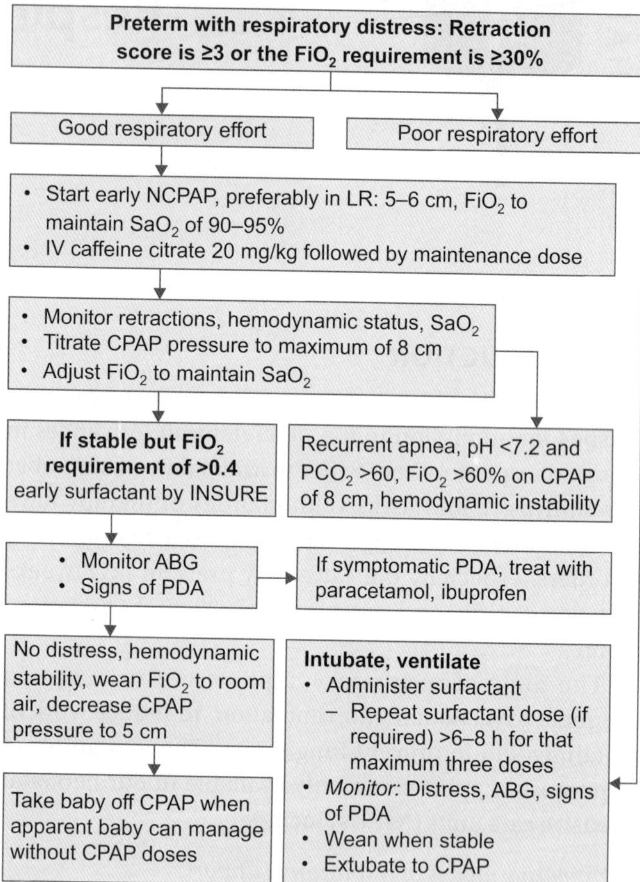

(ABG: arterial blood gas; FiO_2: fraction of inspired oxygen; INSURE: INtubatio-SURfactant-Extubation; LR: labor room; NCPAP: nasal continuous positive airway pressure; $PaCO_2$: partial pressure of arterial carbon dioxide; PDA: patent ductus arteriosus; RDS: respiratory distress syndrome; SaO_2: arterial oxygen saturation)

NONINVASIVE RESPIRATORY SUPPORT (FLOWCHART 1)

Noninvasive respiratory support has become the mainstay of respiratory therapy in the NICU so as to reduce complications of invasive mechanical ventilation like ventilator-associated pneumonias and bronchopulmonary dysplasia.

Types of Noninvasive Ventilation

Continuous Positive Airway Pressure

Continuous positive airway pressure is the application of continuous distending pressure to the airways of a spontaneously breathing baby. Current evidence strongly supports the role of early use of CPAP to reduce the need for intubation, invasive ventilation, and surfactant therapy for extremely low birth weight (ELBW) babies by 50%.

Mechanism of action:

- Alveolar stabilization and maintenance of functional residual capacity (FRC)
- Facilitates gas exchange by preventing collapse of the alveoli at end expiration
- Decreases the work of breathing as the pressure required to overcome the collapsing forces generated by surface tension is reduced when the alveolus remains inflated at end expiration
- Conserves surfactant
- Decreased ventilation–perfusion mismatch

- Helps maintain upper airway stability by stenting the airway and decreasing obstruction
- Lowers airway resistance to gas flow in patients with obstructive lung disease and apnea
- Augments stretch receptors and decreases diaphragmatic fatigue
- Reduces intracardiac left-to-right shunt

Contraindications:

- Pneumothorax
- Choanal atresia
- Cleft lip or palate
- Congenital diaphragmatic hernia
- Tracheoesophageal fistula
- Cardiac failure or hemodynamic instability

Continuous positive airway pressure delivery systems:

- *Continuous flow CPAP system:* Continuous flow CPAP consists of gas flow generated at a source and directed against the resistance of the expiratory limb of the circuit. Ventilator-derived CPAP and bubble CPAP are examples of continuous flow devices.
- *Ventilator-based CPAP:* Ease of use, pressure stability, and an effective alarm system. Ventilator CPAP is typically used for infant extubated from mechanical ventilator.
- *Bubble CPAP:* In this system of delivery, the nasal interface is attached to a circuit with a gas source providing blended, warm, humidified gas at flow rate of 5–8 L/min; the expiratory limb is partly submerged under water. The height of the submerged water column in centimeters represents CPAP pressure in centimeters. The benefits of bubble CPAP are ease of setup and low cost. However, as there is no audible pressure disconnect alarm, no warning occurs even when there are leaks in the system. Visual alarm of "no bubbling" and clinical observations of the patient are essential to maintaining patient safety.
- *Variable flow CPAP:* Variable flow CPAP represents a sophisticated technology of CPAP delivery with visual and audible alarms. The major benefit is a decrease in the work of breathing due to the variable flow. However, it requires specific equipment such as flow drivers, generators, nasal interface, and circuits that are expensive. Although data suggests that some of these systems are superior to others, in clinical practice, the stability of the nasal interface is probably the most important factor determining the success or failure of this form of respiratory support.

CLINICAL PEARL

Endotracheal CPAP should never be used as it significantly increases the work of breathing. It is like breathing through a straw.

Interface used for delivery of continuous positive airway pressure: Nasal mask or short binasal prongs are used as interface. Studies suggest that nasal masks may reduce treatment failure and also nasal injury.

Initiating continuous positive airway pressure:

- Continuous positive airway pressure should be initiated in the labor room, in infants who have sufficient respiratory drive and evidence of respiratory distress, especially in ELBW babies. >50% of ELBW infants who are not depressed at birth can be managed successfully with nasal continuous positive airway pressure (NCPAP), avoiding the use of invasive ventilation. For any preterm with RDS, CPAP should be promptly instituted if the Silverman Anderson retraction score is ≥3.
- Place the baby supine with a slight head extension
- Choose the appropriate sized nasal mask or short binasal prongs size 0 or 1. Avoid pressure of the prongs against the nasal septum.
- Start with a CPAP of 5–6 cmH_2O, flow of 5–7 L/min of blended, warm, humidified gas.
- Use appropriate FiO_2 to maintain SaO_2 between 91 and 95%.
- Titrate CPAP pressure till the grunting and retractions are relieved or till a maximum of 8 cmH_2O.
- If FiO_2 requirement is >0.3 with need for CPAP pressure ≥6, administer surfactant as early rescue therapy (within 2 hours of birth) should be administered by less invasive surfactant administration (LISA) if adequate expertise available or by INtubation-SURfactant-Extubation (INSURE) technique. LISA is preferable as it lowers the need for invasive ventilation as well as risk of BPD compared to INSURE.
- A second and rarely a third dose of surfactant is indicated by 6–12 hours if the mean airway pressure (MAP)/CPAP pressure remains ≥7 and FiO_2 >0.4.
- All preterm babies <32 weeks with RDS needing respiratory support, especially those receiving surfactant should be monitored by point of care echocardiography at 24 hours (and repeated 12–24 hourly) for the presence of a hemodynamically significant

symptomatic PDA. Symptomatic hsPDA should be managed appropriately with ibuprofen or paracetamol as needed.

CLINICAL PEARLS

- Any kind of noninvasive support demands same vigilance as invasive support.
- Adequacy of flow is decided by bubbling at expiratory limb both during inspiration and expiration.
- Adequacy of oxygenation is decided by SpO_2 on pulse oximeter.
- Adequacy of pressure is decided by reduction in chest retractions.

Failure of continuous positive airway pressure:

- Oxygen requirement >60% to maintain saturation 91–95% at CPAP pressure of 8 cmH_2O
- Arterial blood gas (ABG) showing respiratory acidosis with pH <7.20 with partial pressure of carbon dioxide >60 mm Hg
- Recurrent apneic episodes
- Increased work of breathing (sternal and intercostal recession/grunt/tachypnea)

CLINICAL PEARL

- Before using alternative mode of ventilation for continuous positive airway pressure failure, quickly go through checklist to ensure adequate flow delivery, adequate pressure, and position of interface.

Complications of CPAP:

- *Pneumothorax:* Incidence varies between 0.5 and 2% though the Continuous Positive Airway Pressure or Intubation at Birth (COIN) study showed a higher incidence of 9%. In this trial, CPAP pressure of 8 cmH_2O was used compared to conventional 5–6 cm of NCPAP.
- *CPAP belly:* Benign gaseous abdominal distention that can be minimized by evacuating the gas in the stomach routinely by maintaining an open-to-air orogastric tube while on CPAP.
- *Nasal injury:* This occurs due to care-related problems and is preventable with proper nasal mask/prong size and position, minimizing tubing torque, gentle intermittent cleansing, and proper heating and humidification of inspired gases.

CLINICAL PEARL

- Advantage of noninvasive respiratory support outweighs complications related to it.

Heated Humidified High-flow Nasal Cannula

The heated and humidified high-flow nasal cannula (HH-HFNC) is a simple method of providing noninvasive respiratory support. The system consists of heated and humidified, blended air–oxygen gas delivered to the baby by nasal cannula with short binasal prongs. Generally, flow rates of 3–6 L/min are used. Care should be taken to ensure that the nasal prongs do not fit the nares tightly (the external diameter of the prongs should occupy not more than 50% of the diameter of the nares) as very high distending pressure can be generated.

The mechanism of action of HH-HFNC includes "washout" of the exhaled carbon dioxide in the nasopharyngeal dead space and reduction of inspiratory resistance thereby work of breathing. Blended gas administered at flow rates of more than 1 L/min produces some amount of distending airway pressure. The distending pressure generated by HH-HFNC is variable, depending on the size of the nasal cannula, and the flow rate.

The HH-HFNC may be used as a primary respiratory support for RDS as an alternative to nasal CPAP in more mature preterm infants, postextubation from invasive ventilation or to transition a baby off CPAP. The benefits of HH-HFNC are the simplicity of application of the cannula, less risk of damage to the nares and nasal septum, comfort for more mature babies with RDS, and ease of handling and feeding the baby on this therapy.

Noninvasive Positive Pressure Ventilation/ Noninvasive Mechanical Ventilation

This is a method of assisted mechanical ventilation without an endotracheal (ET) tube in the trachea, and using either nasal mask or nasal prongs as the interface. The ventilator delivers peak inspiratory pressure (PIP), positive end-expiratory pressure (PEEP) at the set inspiratory time, rate, and FiO_2.

Noninvasive mechanical ventilation (NIMV) may be delivered as:

- Synchronized nasal intermittent positive pressure ventilation (SNIPPV)
- Nonsynchronized nasal intermittent positive pressure ventilation.

  The NIMV should preferably be synchronized.

Mechanism of action: Like CPAP, NIMV expands the lung, increases FRC, prevents alveolar collapse, and improves ventilation–perfusion mismatch.

Synchronized noninvasive positive pressure ventilation (NIPPV) results in a higher tidal volume compared to NCPAP breaths and nonsynchronized NIMV. Whether synchronized or not, NIPPV improves thoracoabdominal asynchrony and chest wall stabilization, resulting in a decreased work of breathing.

Nasal High-frequency Ventilation

In this modality, nasal interface is used along with the high-frequency mode of ventilation. Nasal HFOV is also being studied for use as a primary modality and for post-extubation to reduce extubation failure. More studies are required before this modality can be considered as standard of care.

MECHANICAL VENTILATION (TABLES 1 AND 2 AND FLOWCHARTS 1 AND 2)

Conventional Ventilation

Indications

- Apnea
- Respiratory failure characterized by:
  - PaO_2 <50 mm Hg on FiO_2 >0.6
  - $PaCO_2$ >55–60 mm Hg with pH <7.25
- Continuous positive airway pressure failure
- Shock

TABLE 1: Suggested initial settings on ventilator.

Settings	*Normal lung*	*RDS*	*MAS*
PIP (cmH_2O)	12–14	16–18	16–18
PEEP (cmH_2O)	3–4	5–8	4–5
FiO_2	10% higher than head box or CPAP FiO_2		
Rates (per min)	25–30	40–60	40–60
Flow (L/min)	8–10	8–10	8–10
Inspiratory time (s)	0.36–0.40	0.36–0.40	0.36–0.38

(CPAP: continuous positive airway pressure; MAS: meconium aspiration syndrome; PEEP: positive end-expiratory pressure; PIP: peak inspiratory pressure; RDS: respiratory distress syndrome)

TABLE 2: Target blood gases.

	Preterm	*Term*
pH	7.25–7.35	7.35–7.40
PaO_2	50–70	60–80
$PaCO_2$	40–50	35–45

($PaCO_2$: partial pressure of arterial carbon dioxide; PaO_2: partial pressure of arterial oxygen)

CLINICAL PEARL

Decision to provide ventilatory support should not be exclusively based on blood gas.

Modes of Ventilation

Conventional ventilation is time-cycled pressure-limited. Currently, patient triggered modes of ventilation like synchronized intermittent mandatory ventilation (SIMV) and assist control with volume guarantee are preferred. Pressure support ventilation (PSV) is a mode of ventilation in which patient's spontaneous breaths are augmented by supplemental inspiratory pressure. This may be used along with SIMV or CPAP. It is particularly useful

Flowchart 2: Management of meconium aspiration syndrome.

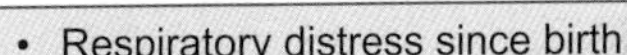

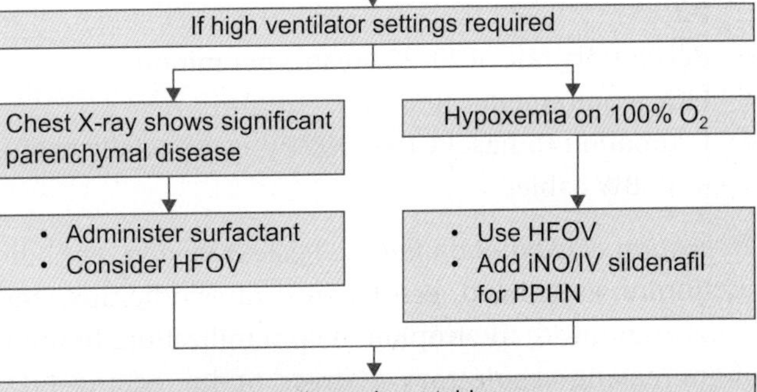

(ABG: arterial blood gas; HFOV: high-frequency oscillatory ventilation; MAS: meconium aspiration syndrome MSAF: meconium-stained amniotic fluid)

in weaning off ventilation. Flow cycling is increasingly being used wherein the breath is terminated not at a set inspiratory time but when inspiratory flow is reduced to 30% of the peak flow. Flow cycling gives inspiratory as well as expiratory synchrony.

Weaning

- In volume guarantee mode, there is auto weaning of pressure once lung compliance improves. In other modes, gradually decrease the most damaging parameters, i.e., FiO_2 and PIP first based on clinical and ABG improvement.
- Improvement of lung compliance on the pressure volume loops and tidal volume scalers is a good indicator while considering weaning.
- Diuresis in preterm is also a good indicator of improving lung function.
- Changes are accomplished in small decrements (PIP 1–2 cmH_2O, FiO_2 5%, rate 5 breaths per min).
- Repeated assessment should be done to determine readiness for extubation at the earliest to minimize ventilator-induced lung injury and chronic lung disease.
- Once the patient is clinically stable, blood gases have normalized, and X-ray shows improvement and the ventilator settings are minimum baby should be extubated. Preterm should be extubated to CPAP/NIPPV to avoid extubation failure and need for reventilation.

Extubation Criteria

- 12–14 cmH_2O (larger babies may be extubated with PIP 14)
- Respiratory rate of 20–25 breaths per minute
- FiO_2 requirement <40%
- Extubation to nasal CPAP/NIPPV is especially useful in VLBW babies

Prevention of extubation failure: Postextubation, periodic suctioning as needed, gentle chest physiotherapy, and nebulization with ipratropium help stabilization. In event of increasing respiratory distress or increasing FiO_2 requirement postextubation, consider increasing CPAP pressure/NIPPV, nursing the baby in prone position and do oronasal suctioning. Consider treatment with injection dexamethasone, 3 doses 0.15 mg/kg/dose 12 hourly to treat airway inflammation related to intubation especially when the infant has been on invasive ventilation for over a week.

High-frequency Oscillatory Ventilation

High-frequency oscillatory ventilation (HFOV) is a type of mechanical ventilation that uses a constant distending pressure (MAP) with pressure variations (ΔP) oscillating around the MAP at very high rates (up to 900 cycles per min). This creates small tidal volume, often less than the dead space.

Indications

At present, HFOV is generally used as a rescue therapy.

- *Failure of conventional ventilation in the term infant:* Persistent pulmonary hypertension of the newborn, MAS
- Air leak syndromes [pneumothorax, pulmonary interstitial emphysema (PIE)]
- *Congenital diaphragmatic hernia:* Certain centers use HFOV as a primary modality of respiratory therapy for CDH, however, HFOV has not been proved superior to conventional ventilation.
- Failure of conventional ventilation in the preterm infant (severe RDS, PIE, pulmonary hypoplasia) or to reduce barotrauma when conventional ventilator settings are high.

Initial Settings on High-frequency Oscillatory Ventilation

On an HFOV ventilator, the oxygenation is controlled by changing the MAP also called Paw or by the FiO_2.

Ventilation is controlled by the amplitude (ΔP) and the frequency.

In contrast to conventional ventilation, decreasing the frequency increases the tidal volume delivered, thereby increasing the carbon dioxide washout.

Initial settings: Aim is to maximize recruitment of alveoli—

- Set MAP 2–3 cmH_2O above the MAP on conventional ventilation
- Set frequency to 8–10 Hz for term babies and 10–12 Hz for preterms
- Generally, the frequency is set at 10 Hz, inspiratory time at 33%, and rarely require change throughout the course of ventilation
- Set amplitude to get good vibrations (wobble) of chest, abdomen, and upper thighs.

Ventilator Setting Adjustments on High-frequency Oscillatory Ventilation

Table 3 describes ventilator adjustments on high-frequency oscillatory ventilation.

Chest X-ray: Follow-up chest radiograph in 4–6 hours is recommended to assess the expansion.

Thereafter, repeat chest radiography with acute changes in patient condition.

Suctioning:

- Suction is indicated for diminished chest wall movement (chest wobble), elevated carbon dioxide, and/or worsening oxygenation suggesting airway or ET tube obstruction, or if there are visible/audible secretions in the airway
- Avoid in the first 24 hours of HFOV unless clinically indicated
- Press the "stop" button briefly while quickly inserting and withdrawing suction catheter (PEEP is maintained). Indwelling suction catheter is required.

Weaning:

- Reduce FiO_2 to <40% gradually
- Reduce MAP when chest radiograph shows evidence of overinflation (>9 ribs) or hyperoxemia on ABG.
- Reduce MAP by 1-2 cmH_2O to 8–10 cmH_2O
- In air leak syndromes, reducing MAP takes priority over weaning the FiO_2
- Wean the amplitude in 2–4 cmH_2O decrements based on $PaCO_2$
- Discontinue HFOV when MAP 8–10 cmH_2O and amplitude 20–25
- If infant is stable, oxygenating well and blood gases are satisfactory, then infant could be extubated to CPAP or switched to conventional ventilation.

TABLE 3: Ventilator adjustments on high-frequency oscillatory ventilation.

Poor oxygenation	*Over-oxygenation*	*Under-ventilation*	*Over-ventilation*
Increase FiO_2	Decrease FiO_2	Increase amplitude	Decrease amplitude
Increase MAP (Paw)* (1–2 cmH_2O)	Decrease MAP (1–2 cmH_2O)	Decrease frequency by 1–2 Hz	Increase frequency by 1–2 Hz

Note: *Pressure airway.
(FiO_2: fraction of inspired oxygen; MAP: mean airway pressure)

KEY POINTS

- Decision to provide respiratory support to neonate is never solely based on blood gas.
- Noninvasive support is a preferable modality to avoid lung injury.
- Irrespective of the mode being used, always adjust ventilator settings, keeping in mind pathophysiology of the disease state.
- High-frequency ventilation has a proven role as a rescue therapy. It is not a panacea of all respiratory problems of neonate.

SUGGESTED READING

1. Bhandari V, Black R, Gandhi B, Hogue S, Kakkilaya V, Mikhael M,. et al. RDS-NExT workshop: consensus statements for the use of surfactant in preterm neonates with RDS. J Perinatol. 2023;43:982-90. https://doi.org/10.1038/s41372-023-01690-9
2. Boost II collaborative groups. Oxygen saturation and outcomes in preterm infants. N Engl J Med. 2013;368:2094-104.
3. Collaborative CCDH, Puligandla P, Skarsgard E, Offringa M, Adatia I, Baird R, et al. Diagnosis and management of congenital diaphragmatic hernia: a clinical practice guideline. CMAJ. 2018;190(4):E103-12.
4. Donn SM, Sinha SK. Assisted ventilation and its complications. In: Martin RJ, Fanaroff AA, Walsh MC (Eds). Fanaroff and Martin's Neonatal-perinatal Medicine: Diseases of the Fetus and Infant, 9th edition. Philadelphia: Mosby/Elsevier; 2011.
5. Goldsmith J, Karotkin E. Assisted Ventilation of the Neonate, 7th edition. Amsterdam: Elsevier Publication; 2022.
6. Lemyre B, Deguise M-O, Benson P, Kirpalani H, Ekhaguere OA, Davis PG. Early nasal intermittent positive pressure ventilation (NIPPV) versus early nasal continuous positive airway pressure (NCPAP) for preterm infants. Cochrane Database Syst Rev. 2023;(7):CD005384.
7. Morley CJ, Davis PG, Doyle LW, Brion LP, Hascoet JM, Carlin JB. COIN Trial Investigators. Nasal CPAP or intubation at birth for very preterm infants. N Engl J Med. 2008;358(7):700-8.
8. Prakash R, De Paoli AG, Oddie SJ, Davis PG, McGuire W. Masks versus prongs as interfaces for nasal continuous positive airway pressure in preterm infants. Cochrane Database Syst Rev. 2022;(11):CD015129.
9. Sweet DG, Carnielli VP, Greisen G, Hallman M, Klebermass-Schrehof K, Ozek E, et al. European Consensus Guidelines on the Management of Respiratory Distress Syndrome: 2022 Update. Neonatology. 2023;120(1):3-23.

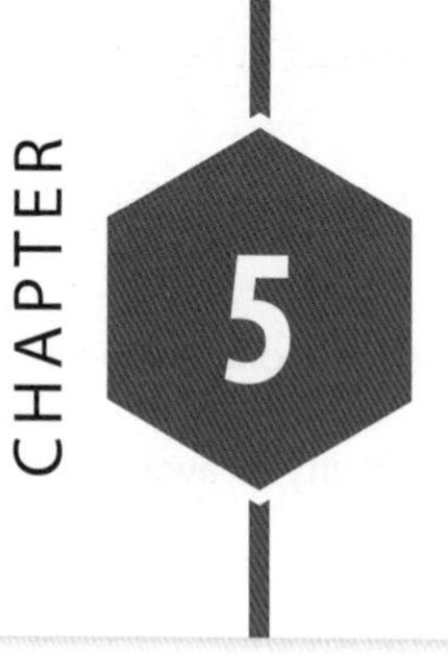
CHAPTER 5

Persistent Pulmonary Hypertension of the Newborn

Ira J Holla, Ram G Holla

INTRODUCTION

Fetal circulation is characterized by the systemic and pulmonary circulations functioning in series, with high pulmonary vascular resistance (PVR) and right to left shunting at the levels of the ductus arteriosus and foramen ovale. In the fetus, only about 10–15% of right ventricular (RV) output perfuses the lungs, with the rest of the RV outflow being shunted through the ductus arteriosus into the aorta. At birth, there is a fall in the PVR due to lung expansion and increasing partial pressure of oxygen, and a simultaneous rise in systemic vascular resistance (SVR) due to clamping of the umbilical cord. This causes reversal of the direction of shunting through the foramen ovale and ductus arteriosus (from higher pressure systemic circulation to lower pressure pulmonary circulation). Humoral mediators such as prostaglandins and prostacyclins released in response to elevated arterial oxygen content and pH further constrict the ductus and cause smooth muscle relaxation of pulmonary vasculature. This transforms the fetal circulation which is characterized by pulmonary and systemic circuits in series, to the adult circulation, in which the two circuits function in parallel.

Failure to achieve or sustain the normal decrease in PVR at birth results in persistent shunting of blood to the path of least resistance, which in this case would be from the high pressure pulmonary circulation to relatively lower pressure systemic circulation leading to cyanosis, also known as persistent pulmonary hypertension of the newborn (PPHN).

ETIOPATHOGENESIS OF PERSISTENT PULMONARY HYPERTENSION OF THE NEWBORN

Normal pulmonary vascular development in infancy requires maintenance of low PVR after birth and is necessary for normal lung function and growth. The developing lung is subject to multiple genetic, pathological, and/or environmental influences that can adversely affect lung adaptation, development, and growth, leading to pulmonary hypertension.

Persistent pulmonary hypertension of the newborn can be classified based on etiology into two distinct categories, i.e., primary (or idiopathic) and secondary.

Primary idiopathic PPHN accounts for only 10–20% of cases of PPHN and is characterized by absence of parenchymal or pulmonary vascular disease in the presence of severe pulmonary hypertension.

Secondary PPHN accounts for the vast majority (80–90%) of PPHN cases and can be secondary to one of the following:

- *Parenchymal disease* [e.g., meconium aspiration syndrome (MAS), respiratory distress syndrome (RDS), and congenital pneumonia/sepsis]
- *Pulmonary hypoplasia* [secondary to oligohydramnios from prolonged rupture of membranes, renal agenesis, and congenital diaphragmatic hernia (CDH)]
- *Abnormal or delayed transition* at birth (secondary to perinatal asphyxia and alveolar capillary dysplasia).

The top five causes of PPHN are sepsis (30%), MAS (24%), idiopathic (20%), RDS (7%), and CDH (6%). About 15–20% of cases of MAS may develop PPHN.

> **CLINICAL PEARL**
>
> - PPHN is caused by failure of pulmonary pressures to fall after birth leading to right-to-left shunting, hypoxemia, acidosis, and shock.

CLINICAL MANIFESTATIONS OF PERSISTENT PULMONARY HYPERTENSION OF THE NEWBORN

- The outstanding feature of PPHN is central cyanosis. Hypoxemia out of proportion to the degree of

TABLE 1: Mechanisms leading to pulmonary hypertension in the newborn.

Abnormally constricted blood vessels	*Structurally abnormal pulmonary vasculature*	*Hypoplastic pulmonary vasculature*	*Functional obstruction to pulmonary flow*
• Acute perinatal hypoxia • Meconium aspiration • Sepsis or pneumonia • Respiratory distress syndrome • Hypoventilation • Central nervous system depression • Hypothermia	• Placental insufficiency • Prolonged gestation • In utero closure of ductus arteriosus: Aspirin, nonsteroidal anti-inflammatory drugs • Idiopathic	• Diaphragmatic hernia • Lung dysgenesis • Pleural effusion • Congenital lung hypoplasia • Potter sequence • Thoracic dystrophies • Alveolar capillary dysplasia	• Polycythemia • Hyperfibrinogenemia

parenchymal lung disease can be seen in idiopathic pulmonary hypertension.

- Labile hypoxemia which is defined as a marked change in oxygen saturation (SpO_2) with little to no change in ventilatory or fraction of inspired oxygen (FiO_2) settings is caused by shift in direction of shunt with subtle change in PVR–SVR balance.
- Symptoms generally begin at birth, but definitely before 12 hours.
- *Differential saturation:* Preductal SpO_2 may be 10% higher (or more) than postductal saturation. Arterial blood gas may show similar findings [partial pressure of arterial oxygen (PaO_2) >20 mm, higher in the preductal sample). A subset of infants may have right to left shunting only at the level of the foramen ovale and not at the ductus, and may fail to show differential cyanosis **(Table 1)**.

Respiratory symptoms are related to the underlying disease, distress being the most severe in MAS, diaphragmatic hernia, RDS, pneumonia, etc.

DIFFERENTIAL DIAGNOSIS

Primary pulmonary disease without elevated PVR and structural heart disease associated with right to left shunting should be excluded before a diagnosis of PPHN can be made.

> **CLINICAL PEARL**
>
> *Differential oxygenation:* SpO_2 10% higher, PaO_2 20 mm Hg higher in preductal than postductal samples.

Clinical signs favoring cyanotic congenital cardiac disease over persistent pulmonary hypertension of the newborn are as follows:

- Cardiomegaly
- Weak pulses
- Active precordium
- Pulse differential between upper and lower extremities
- Pulmonary edema
- Grade 3+ murmur
- Persistent pre- and postductal arterial oxygen tension (PaO_2) at or <40 mm Hg.

INVESTIGATIONS AND DIAGNOSIS

- Chest X-ray usually shows the underlying pulmonary disease or may be normal. The cardiac silhouette is usually normal. Pulmonary blood flow may be diminished leading to a "black lung" appearance.
- The electrocardiogram is usually normal for age.
- An echocardiography must be performed in every baby with PPHN for diagnosis and exclusion of cardiac disease, and is the gold standard for diagnosis of pulmonary hypertension. The size, direction, and location of the shunt should be assessed. Echocardiographic signs of pulmonary hypertension include flattening or leftward deviation of interventricular septum, right-to-left or bidirectional shunt at the level of the ductus arteriosus and/or at the level of the foramen ovale, and tricuspid valve regurgitation. Tricuspid regurgitant (TR) jet velocity on continuous wave Doppler along with simultaneous systemic pressure measurement can estimate degree of pulmonary hypertension. ECHO also helps guide choice of pulmonary vasodilator by assessing presence and degree of ventricular dysfunction. In all cases, response to treatment, particularly changes in cardiac output and direction of ductal shunting, should be assessed by repeated echocardiographic assessments.
- *Hyperoxia test:* Hyperoxia with or without hyperventilation can help to predict the presence and

reversibility of pulmonary hypertension. However, with the wide availability of bedside stat ECHO, this test has fallen out of practice due to the potential adverse effects of hyperoxia and alkalosis.

MANAGEMENT

Management of a neonate with PPHN **(Flowchart 1)** constitutes a medical emergency in which correction of hypoxia is important for reversal of pulmonary hypertension, limitation of shunting, establishment of systemic perfusion, and prevention of end organ damage.

- *General measures:*
  - Correct underlying metabolic/hematological derangements:
    - Correct acidosis, hypoglycemia, hypocalcemia, polycythemia, and hypothermia
    - Treatment directed at the specific disorder causing PPHN, e.g., CDH
  - *Monitoring:*
    - Blood pressure—preferably intra-arterial
    - Pulse oximetry (both pre- and postductal)
    - Transcutaneous oxygen/carbon dioxide or end-tidal CO_2
    - End organ perfusion—urine output, lactate, and capillary refill time
    - Postductal blood gas assessments

Flowchart 1: Management of a neonate with PPHN.

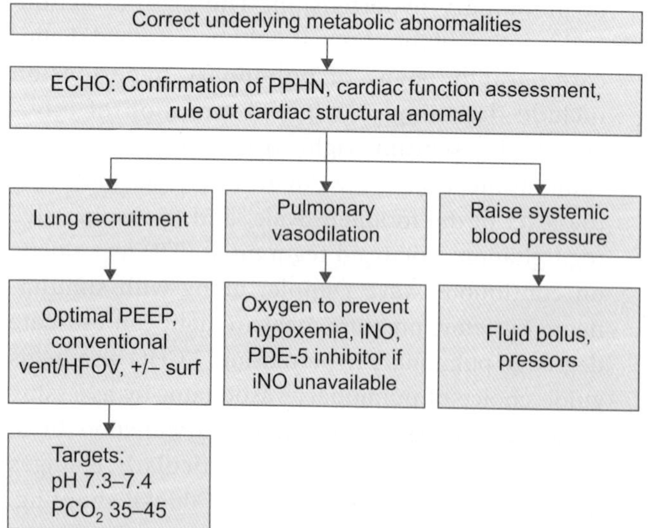

(HFOV: high-frequency oscillatory ventilation; iNO: inhaled nitric oxide; PCO_2: partial pressure of carbon dioxide; PDE-5: phosphodiesterase-5; PEEP: positive end-expiratory pressure; PPHN: persistent pulmonary hypertension of the newborn)

    - Monitoring of blood gas should be accompanied by charting of trends in PaO_2, partial pressure of arterial carbon dioxide ($PaCO_2$), alveolar-arterial oxygen gradient ($AaDO_2$), and oxygenation index **(Appendix)**

Functional ECHO in monitoring the course of PPHN:

- Parameters assessed include TR jet velocity, TR pressure gradient, septal curve (infra/iso/suprasystemic pressure), RV or right atrial dilation, and direction of shunt.
- The presence of persistent right to left shunt at the ductal level after therapeutic optimization is associated with increased risk of death prior to 28 days of life.
- With improvement in clinical picture (decreasing FiO_2 requirement, improving PaO_2) repeat ECHO may show iso- or subsystemic RV pressure and bidirectional or left to right shunt at the ductal and atrial levels.
  - Minimize stress/stimulation: The hyper-reactive pulmonary circulation is highly sensitive to catecholamines leading to increased PVR. Stress should be blocked by silence, avoidance of disturbance, gentle handling, eye covers/ear muffs, and sedation.
    - Fentanyl (2–5 μg/kg/h) as a continuous infusion
    - Morphine (5–10 μg/kg/h) as a continuous infusion
    - Midazolam (10–60 μg/kg/h) as a continuous infusion
    - PRN doses of fentanyl/midazolam prior to care times/interventions
    - Very agitated or unstable neonates, particularly if breathing out of phase, may be paralyzed with pancuronium (0.1 mg/kg/dose; every 1–4 h PRN) or vecuronium, but only after adequate sedation/analgesia has been given
  - Maintain hematocrit above 45%
- *Ventilation:* Optimize lung recruitment and reduce ventilation-perfusion mismatch. Specific approaches to respiratory support and mechanical ventilation vary. A gentle approach that maintains adequate oxygenation and mild hyperventilation ($PaCO_2$ 35–45 mm Hg, and pH at 7.3–7.4), generally lowers the PVR to the extent of abolishing right to left shunting. The state of the underlying lung should dictate the specific respiratory management strategy, always keeping in mind that high intrathoracic pressure may worsen the situation by impeding cardiac output and elevating PVR. High-frequency oscillatory ventilation (HFOV) is often useful

in treating infants whose PPHN is associated with severe pulmonary parenchymal disease. Neonates with PPHN have cardiopulmonary instability, and weaning from ventilation should be done very gradually to prevent reversal. Surfactant may be beneficial in cases of parenchymal lung disease such as MAS which can lead to surfactant inactivation.

- *Optimize cardiac output and left ventricular function, maintain systemic blood pressure:* The aim of cardiovascular management is to optimize systemic blood pressure to levels above the pulmonary pressure in order to minimize or eliminate right to left shunt. Target mean blood pressure levels would be 45–55 mm Hg. Low blood pressure may be normalized using:
  - *Volume expansion:* Especially in hypovolemic conditions (e.g., hemorrhage, hydrops, and capillary leak) or decreased SVR (e.g., septic shock) or systemic hypotension
  - *Vasopressors:* Dopamine, dobutamine, and/or adrenaline often are necessary to achieve adequate cardiac output. Dopamine in doses >10 µg/kg/min and adrenaline increase SVR through stimulation of α- and β-receptors. High doses of both may stimulate pulmonary α-receptors, leading to increased PVR. When cardiac function is poor, cardiotonic medications, such as milrinone that enhance both cardiac output and lower PVR, might be useful.
- *Decrease PVR:*
  - *Oxygen:* Being a potent vasodilator, oxygen therapy along with optimal ventilation is the cornerstone of the management of PPHN. However, excessive and prolonged exposure to oxygen can lead to paradoxical hypercontractility of the pulmonary vasculature and should be avoided. Preductal PaO_2 over 150 mm Hg should prompt cautious weaning of FiO_2.
  - *Nitric oxide:* Nitric oxide relaxes the vascular smooth muscle and causes pulmonary vasodilation. Inhaled nitric oxide (iNO) is administered by conventional or high frequency ventilation wherein it diffuses into ventilated alveoli, causes localized vasodilatation and improved oxygenation, in addition to decreasing PVR, with no effect on SVR due to its short half-life and rapid scavenging by hemoglobin in blood. iNO will be effective only once adequate lung expansion and alveolar opening has been achieved, such that it can reach the level of the alveoli and diffuse through to the pulmonary vasculature. Post hoc analysis of a study looking at early initiation of iNO suggested that use of surfactant before iNO initiation decreased the incidence of extracorporeal membrane oxygenation (ECMO) or death. iNO is started at the maximum dose of 20 ppm. Further increase in dose of iNO was not found to confer any further benefit and was associated with higher risk of methemoglobinemia. An oxygenation index (OI) >15–20 is typically used as an indication to start iNO. Response to iNO is defined as an increase in the PaO_2/FiO_2 ratio of 20 mm Hg or more and should be seen very soon after initiation of iNO. iNO can cause worsening pulmonary congestion in the presence of left ventricular (LV) dysfunction, and is contraindicated in case of certain structural cardiac anomalies such as total anomalous pulmonary venous return (TAPVR) with obstructed venous return, wherein it can worsen pulmonary venous congestion.
  - Weaning of iNO should be done in a slow, stepwise process to prevent rebound pulmonary hypertension.
  - *Phosphodiesterase inhibitors:* In cases where systemic blood pressure is normal, sildenafil, which is a phosphodiesterase-5 (PDE-5) inhibitor, may be considered. Sildenafil increases levels of cyclic-GMP (cGMP) which causes smooth muscle relaxation. However, sildenafil can cause transient systemic hypotension.
  - *Alkalinization:* Alkalosis reduces PVR. Alkalosis can be achieved by gentle hyperventilation aiming for a pH of 7.35–7.45. The use of alkali infusion to achieve higher pH (>7.5) has fallen out of favor due to impaired cerebral perfusion in the presence of high pH which was found to lead to worse neurological outcomes and profound sensorineural hearing loss.
- *ECMO:* ECMO often is lifesaving therapy for infants with PPHN who fail conventional management and/or iNO treatment. It is important to note that ECMO is not a cure for PPHN, but rather a temporizing measure in order to give the lungs a chance to rest and recover. Persistent OI >40 in the presence of optimal ventilatory and oxygenation strategies is typically used as an indication for initiation of ECMO.

Ligation or pharmacological closure of the duct is not useful and may be detrimental. There is insufficient data to justify the use of other proposed medical therapies including magnesium sulfate, calcium channel blockers, adenosine, inhaled prostacyclin, ethyl nitrite, bosentan (endothelin receptor antagonist), and inhaled or intravenous tolazoline.

OUTCOMES IN NEONATES WITH PULMONARY HYPERTENSION

Mortality from PPHN varies widely (4–33%) depending on multiple factors such as underlying etiology, severity of pulmonary hypertension, cardiac function, presence of complications such as pneumothorax, and clinical setting. According to a study done in the United States, overall mortality from PPHN was found to be 7.3%, with in hospital mortality of 6.5%, and 1-year postdischarge mortality of 0.7%. The rate of postdischarge mortality within 1 year of life, and hospital readmission was found to be nearly threefold higher in infants with PPHN as compared to infants without PPHN. Of all infants with PPHN who survived to hospital discharge, 28.6% required readmission within the first year of life as compared to 9.8% without PPHN, and approximately one-third of these readmissions were for respiratory causes. On further analysis, they found that postdischarge mortality and hospital readmission rates were highest in infants with PPHN secondary to CDH or respiratory tract anomalies as compared to PPHN secondary to MAS or sepsis. Infants who survive to discharge are at increased risk of long-term neurodevelopmental impairment, hearing abnormalities, and cognitive deficits. These infants should receive multidisciplinary follow-up which should include audiology referral, physical therapy, and occupational therapy.

APPENDIX: OXYGENATION PARAMETERS

PAO_2 = [(Barometric Pressure – Partial Pressure of water vapor) × FiO_2] – [$PaCO_2$/RQ]
= [(760 – 47) × 0.21] – [40/0.8]
= 150 – 50 = 100 mm Hg (Approximately)

Alveolar to Arterial Oxygen Gradient = $PAO_2 - PaO_2$

Where RQ is Respiratory Quotient; PAO_2 is alveolar partial pressure of oxygen; PaO_2 is arterial partial pressure of oxygen; and PCO_2 is partial pressure of CO_2.

2. Oxygenation index: $\frac{(MAP \times FiO_2 \times 100)}{PaO_2}$

KEY POINTS

- PPHN is more common in term and post-term newborns.
- Assessment of pre- and postductal saturations helps in early diagnosis.
- Congenital heart disease should always be ruled out in a patient having clinical features of PPHN.
- HFOV and iNO have revolutionized the treatment of PPHN.

SUGGESTED READING

1. Baquero H, Soliz A, Neira F, Venegas ME, Sola A. Oral sildenafil in infants with persistent pulmonary hypertension of the newborn: a pilot randomized blinded study. Pediatrics. 2006;117(4):1077-83.
2. Breinig S, Dicky O, Ehlinger V, Dulac Y, Marcoux MO, Arnaud C. Echocardiographic parameters predictive of poor outcome in persistent pulmonary hypertension of the newborn (PPHN): preliminary results. Pediatr Cardiol. 2021;42(8):1848-53.
3. Goldsmith JP, Karotkin E, Suresh G, Keszler M. Assisted Ventilation of the Neonate: An Evidence-Based Approach to Newborn Respiratory Care, 6th edition: Amsterdam, Netherlands: Elsevier; 2016.
4. Konduri GG, Sokol GM, Van Meurs KP, Singer J, Ambalavanan N, Lee T, et al. Impact of early surfactant and inhaled nitric oxide therapies on outcomes in term/late preterm neonates with moderate hypoxic respiratory failure. J Perinatol. 2013;33(12):944-9.
5. Konduri GG, Solimano A, Sokol GM, Singer J, Ehrenkranz RA, Singhal N, et al; Neonatal Inhaled Nitric Oxide Study Group. A randomized trial of early versus standard inhaled nitric oxide therapy in term and near-term newborn infants with hypoxic respiratory failure. Pediatrics. 2004;113(3):559-64.
6. Lakshminrusimha S, Keszler M. Persistent pulmonary hypertension of the newborn. Neoreviews. 2015;16(12): e680-92.
7. Lipkin PH, Davidson D, Spivak L, Straube R, Rhines J, Chang CT. Neurodevelopmental and medical outcomes of persistent pulmonary hypertension in term newborns treated with nitric oxide. J Pediatr. 2002;140(3):306-10.
8. Martinho S, Adão R, Leite-Moreira AF, Brás-Silva C. Persistent pulmonary hypertension of the newborn: pathophysiological mechanisms and novel therapeutic approaches. Front Pediatr. 2020;8:342.
9. Monfredini C, Cavallin F, Villani PE, Paterlini G, Allais B, Trevisanuto D. Meconium aspiration syndrome: a narrative review. Children (Basel). 2021;8(3):230.
10. Singh Y, Lakshminrusimha S. Pathophysiology and management of persistent pulmonary hypertension of the newborn. Clin Perinatol. 2021;48(3):595-618.
11. Steurer MA, Baer RJ, Oltman S, Ryckman KK, Feuer SK, Rogers E, et al. Morbidity of persistent pulmonary hypertension of the newborn in the first year of life. J Pediatr. 2019;213:58-65.

Bronchopulmonary Dysplasia

Naveen Bajaj, Ruchi Nimish Nanavati

INTRODUCTION

Chronic lung disease (CLD) or bronchopulmonary dysplasia (BPD) is a clinical syndrome seen in very preterm infants that results in decreased oxygenation, an increased work of breathing, and lung abnormalities that persist into childhood. In very low birthweight (VLBW) infants, overall incidence is 12–15% and is inversely related to gestational age and birth weight. Although it can occur in full-term infants, it is uncommon in infants born after 32 weeks of gestation.

> **CLINICAL PEARL**
>
> Bronchopulmonary dysplasia mainly occurs in VLBW babies.

DEFINITION (CLASSIFICATION)

The following classification systems have been described.

NICHD 2018 (Higgins et al.)

A premature infant (<32 weeks GA) with BPD has persistent parenchymal lung disease, radiographic confirmation of parenchymal lung disease, and at 36 weeks postmenstrual age (PMA) requires 1 of the following fraction of inspired oxygen (FiO_2) ranges/oxygen levels/O_2 concentrations for ∇ 3 consecutive days to maintain arterial oxygen saturation in the 90–95% range **(Table 1)**.

NICHD 2019 (Jensen et al)

Respiratory support at 36 weeks PMA regardless of prior or current O_2 therapy (FiO_2):

- *No BPD:* No support
- *Grade 1 BPD:* Nasal cannula <2 L/min
- *Grade 2 BPD:* Nasal cannula >2 L/min or noninvasive positive airway pressure
- *Grade 3 BPD:* Invasive mechanical ventilation

These criteria correctly predicted death or serious respiratory morbidity in 81% of study infants.

The more specific old term BPD instead of the more recent term CLD is preferred, because this disease is clearly distinct from the multiple CLDs of later life.

In recent years, with improved survival of extreme premature infants, the clinical and X-ray findings that define BPD have changed and a milder clinical disease called "new BPD" has emerged **(Table 2)**.

TABLE 1: Bronchopulmonary dysplasia (BPD) severity grading according to NICHD 2018.

Grades	*Invasive IPPV*	*nCPAP, NIPPV, or nasal canula flow of ≥3 L/min*	*Nasal canula flow of 1–<3 L/min*	*Hood O_2*	*Nasal canula flow of <1 L/min*
I	–	21	22–29	22–29	22–70
II	21	22–29	≥30	≥30	>70
III	>21	≥30	–	–	–
III (A)	Early death (between 14 days postnatal age and 36 weeks) owing to persistent parenchymal lung disease and respiratory failure that cannot be attributable to other neonatal morbidities (e.g., NEC, IVH, redirection of care, episodes of sepsis, etc.)				

(IPPV: intermittent positive pressure ventilation; IVH: intraventricular hemorrhage; nCPAP: Nasal continuous positive airway pressure; NIPPV: nasal intermittent positive pressure ventilation; NEC: necrotizing enterocolitis)

TABLE 2: Old versus new bronchopulmonary dysplasia (BPD).

	Old BPD (Classic BPD)	*New BPD (Atypical BPD)*
Infants at risk	Larger, more mature	Very low birth weight
Airway injury	Severe	Mild-to-none
Fibrosis	Severe	Minimal
Alveoli	Develop in regions without fibrosis	Uniform arrested development
Causes	Oxygen, ventilation	Interference with development
X-ray	Overinflation and cystic emphysema	Diffuse haziness or fine, lacy pattern

CLINICAL PEARL

(New BPD) a milder form of disease is more common than old BPD nowadays.

OLD AND NEW BRONCHOPULMONARY DYSPLASIA

Incidence

Incidence is inversely proportional to GA and birthweight (BW). Although, it can occur in full-term infants, it is uncommon in infants born after 30 weeks of GA.

- *GA <28 weeks:* 40%
- *GA <24 weeks:* 90%
- *BW <1500 g:* 12–15%
- *BW <750 g:* 80%

PATHOGENESIS

Bronchopulmonary dysplasia is caused by multiple adverse events during pre- and postnatal period **(Flowchart 1)**.

Predisposing Factors

- Fetal growth restriction
- Lack of administration of antenatal steroids
- Prematurity/low BW
- Perinatal asphyxia
- High intermittent positive pressure ventilation/oxygen requirement
- Barovolutrauma
- High initial fluid intake
- Respiratory distress syndrome (RDS), patent ductus arteriosus (PDA), and pulmonary interstitial emphysema
- *Chorioamnionitis:* Fetal inflammatory response syndrome
- Nosocomial infections
- Colonization with *Ureaplasma urealyticum*
- Genetic predisposition.

CLINICAL PEARL

Prematurity, RDS, ventilation, and infections are common predisposing factors.

CLINICAL FEATURES

Bronchopulmonary dysplasia usually develops in premature neonates being treated with oxygen and positive pressure ventilation for respiratory failure, most commonly due to RDS. It is often anticipated when mechanical ventilation or oxygen dependence extend beyond 10–14 days. Common clinical pointers are:

- Preterm on ventilator, failure to wean, and extubation failures
- Persistent or increased oxygen requirement
- Signs of respiratory distress
- Barrel-shaped chest
- Severe bronchospasm leading to frequent desaturations (BPD spells)
- Cardiomegaly, hypertension, and cor pulmonale
- Copious secretions, tracheo- and bronchomalacia
- Feed intolerance, failure to thrive

CLINICAL PEARL

Ventilatory or oxygen dependency beyond 2 weeks of life is an early suspicious sign of BPD.

Chest X-ray

Northway originally described the four stages of radiographic appearances in BPD **(Table 3)**.

The new BPD on X-ray only shows diffuse haziness, occasionally, infiltrates, or segmental atelectasis.

Flowchart 1: Bronchopulmonary dysplasia pathogenesis.

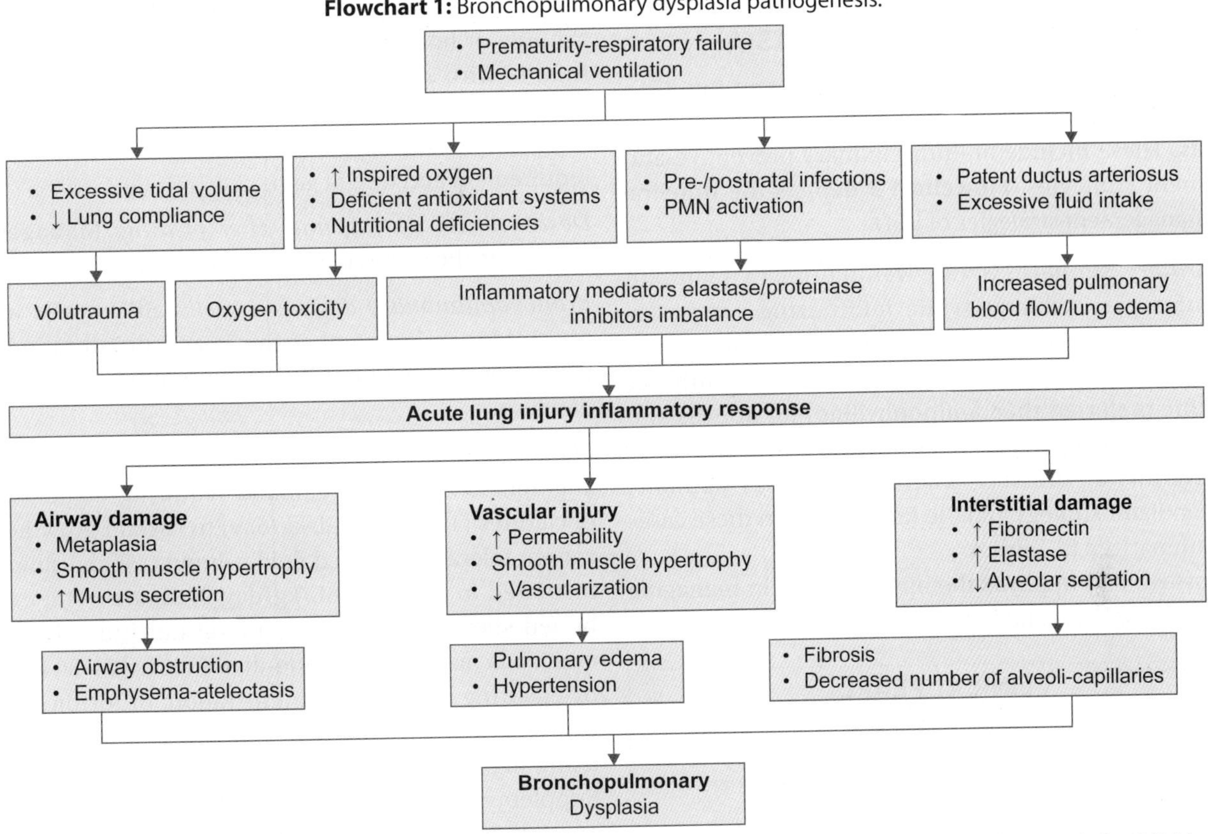

Source: Bhandari V, Bhandari A, Rajiv PK. Bronchopulmonary dysplasia. In: Rajiv PK, Vidyasagar D, Lakshminrusimha S (Eds). Essentials of Neonatal Ventilation, 1st edn. India: Elsevier, 2019. pp. 461-90.

TABLE 3: X-ray staging and appearance of bronchopulmonary dysplasia.

Stage	*Day*	*X-ray appearance*
Stage I (mild)	2–3 days	Identical to respiratory distress syndrome
Stage II (moderate)	4–10 days	Pulmonary parenchymal opacities
Stage III (severe)	10–20 days	Radiolucent cysts giving bubbly lung appearance
Stage IV (advanced)	30 days	Marked hyperinflation, emphysematous lung, fibrous streaks, and cardiomegaly

Pulmonary Functions

- Increased airway hyper-reactivity, high airway resistance, and decreased compliance results in markedly increase work of breathing, hypoventilation, and hypercapnia.
- Airway resistance increases markedly during active expiratory efforts such as in physical agitation.
- *PV loop:* High airway resistance, decreased compliance, increased work of breathing
- *Flow volume loop:* Ski slope signs suggestive of expiratory flow limitation (in severe cases)
- Functional residual capacity is initially normal or low but increases in advanced stages.

Echocardiography

Pulmonary hypertension may be seen in established BPD and reflects the severity of disease.

DIFFERENTIAL DIAGNOSIS

- Bacterial or viral pneumonia
- Pulmonary lymphangiectasia
- Recurrent aspirations
- Total anomalous pulmonary venous connections.

TREATMENT STRATEGIES FOR SUSPECTED BRONCHOPULMONARY DYSPLASIA

Though there is no single magical therapy for BPD, multiple "best practices" result in better outcome of these infants. These include multidisciplinary preventive and treatment strategies. **Flowchart 2** depicts the timeline and management strategies of BPD.

Respiratory support: Gentle ventilation to maintain adequate gas exchange while minimizing ventilator-induced lung injury. The aim is to ventilate for the shortest possible time, wean gradually, use methylxanthines (caffeine preferred than aminophylline) for apneas and in periextubation period, and extubate to nasal continuous positive airway pressure (CPAP) as early as possible. The ventilator strategy and the targets used in these cases are summarized in **Table 4**.

Postextubation physiotherapy is helpful in managing segmental collapse and increased airway secretions.

CLINICAL PEARL

- Gentle ventilation, early extubation, and use of noninvasive ventilation are the goals.

Flowchart 2: Management strategies for bronchopulmonary dysplasia.

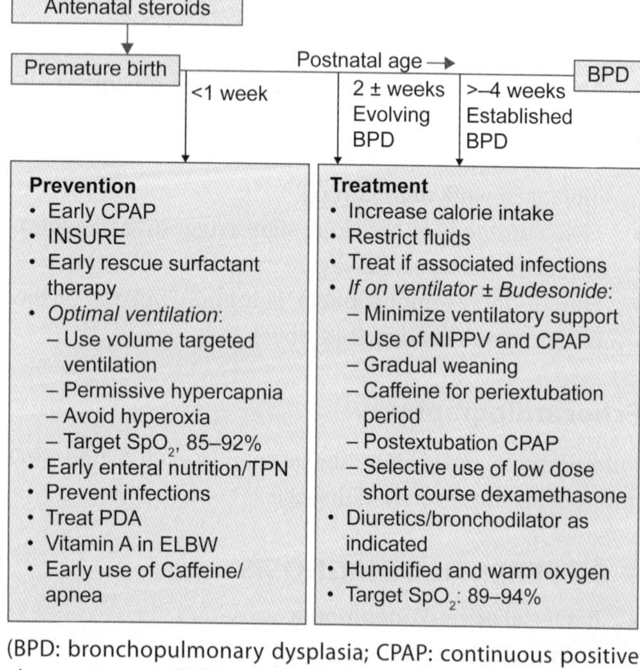

(BPD: bronchopulmonary dysplasia; CPAP: continuous positive airway pressure; ELBW: extremely low birth weight; PTV: patient triggered ventilation; PDA: patent ductus arteriosus; SpO_2: blood oxygen saturation level; TPN: total parenteral nutrition)

Delivery of oxygen: Warm humidified oxygen by nasal cannula or hood to maintain SpO_2 between 91 and 95% Infants with no other medical problem can be given home oxygen therapy by nasal cannula from a portable oxygen cylinder/oxygen concentrator. Monitor oxygen requirement and weight gain.

Desaturation during and after feeding: Managed by increasing the inspired oxygen concentration.

Bronchopulmonary dysplasia spells: BPD spells which are sudden episodes of cyanosis and desaturation due to expiratory flow limitation may require sedation and paralysis.

Fluid and nutrition: Even though these neonates have an augmented metabolic demand requiring higher intake of calories (120–160 kcal/kg/day) to sustain growth, they cannot tolerate increased fluid volumes. Hence, fluids are restricted to 120–150 mL/kg/day. Neonates who cannot be fed should be given parenteral nutrition. Those on oral feeds may be fed calorie-dense feeds (24–30 kcal/oz) by ensuring hind milk administration, or fortification of expressed breast milk with human milk fortifier or by using high calorie formula to provide 130 kcal/kg/day. Supplementation with medium chain triglyceride oil is another option. Adequate intake of calcium, phosphorus, vitamins, and iron should be ensured.

Treatment of infections: Bacterial or fungal infections are frequent in BPD infants and worsen the lung damage and should be investigated and treated.

- *Postnatal corticosteroids (See* **Table 5**)*: Drug treatment* **(Table 6)**: Before a drug is initiated in a case of BPD, one should always revisit the decision and seriously consider if that drug is required.

TABLE 4: Ventilatory strategy and arterial blood gas targets in bronchopulmonary dysplasia.

Ventilatory strategy	*Target arterial blood gas values*
Slow rates: 20–40/min	*pH:* 7.25–7.3
Lowest possible PIP: 15–20 cm H_2O	*PaO_2:* 60–80 mm Hg
Moderate PEEP: 5–6 cm H_2O	*$PaCO_2$:* 55–60 mm Hg
Inspiratory time: 0.3–0.5 s	*SpO_2:* 91–95%
Tidal volume: 5–8 mL/kg	$PaCO_2$ levels can be ignored if pH >7.25

(PIP: peak inspiratory pressure; PEEP: positive end-expiratory pressure; Ti: inspiratory time, SpO_2: blood oxygen saturation level; PaO_2: partial pressure of arterial oxygen; $PaCO_2$: partial pressure of arterial carbon dioxide)

TABLE 5: Postnatal corticosteroids.

Timing	*Dosage*	*When to use*	*Cautions*
Prophylaxis ("early" <7 days) Hydrocortisone in extremely preterm infants	• Starting at <24 hours of age • *Hydrocortisone 10-day course:* 1 mg/kg/day div BID ×7 days, 0.5 mg/kg/day QD ×3 days (PREMILOC trial)	<28 weeks if unit BPD risk is high	Do not use with NSAIDs due to risk of intestinal perforation
Early evolving BPD (7–28 days)	• *Dexamethasone 10-day course:* 0.15 mg/kg/day ×3 days, 0.10 mg/kg/day ×3 days; 0.05 mg/kg/day ×2 days; 0.02 mg/kg/day ×2 days (DART regimen) • *Hydrocortisone 22-day course:* 5 mg/kg/day div Q6 h ×7 days; 3.75 mg/kg/day div Q8 h ×5 days; 2.5 mg/kg/day div Q12 ×5 days; 1.25 mg/kg/day QD ×5 days (STOP-BPD regimen)	• <28 weeks of GA and on invasive ventilation for >7 days, consider dexamethasone at ~21 days of age • Hydrocortisone preferred if given between 7 and 21 days of age	Preference for hydrocortisone as it is safer for brain
Later evolving BPD (>28 days up to 36 weeks' PMA)	*Dexamethasone 9-day course:* • 0.2 mg/kg/day div q12 h ×3 days • mg/kg/day div q12 h ×3 days • 0.05 mg/kg/day q12 h ×3 days (Modified DART protocol)	Best to start < 50 days of age	Risk for adrenal suppression
Established BPD >36 weeks' PMA	*Prednisolone 14-day course (Bhandari et al):* • 2 mg/kg/day div BID ×5 days • 1 mg/kg/day QD ×3 days • 1 mg/kg/day QoD ×3 doses *Prednisolone 28+ day course (Linafelter et al.):* • 2 mg/kg/day ×7 days • 1 mg/kg/day QD ×7 days • 0.5 mg/kg/day QD ×7 days • 0.5 mg/kg 3×/week ×7 day	• Use Bhandari course, for NICU babies on venti, CPAP or high-flow support (more than 2L NC) • Consider longer course if escalation of respiratory support warranted when tapering steroid • Only go back to previous dose Once, then continue wean	Risk for adrenal suppression

(BPD: bronchopulmonary dysplasia; CPAP: continuous positive airway pressure; NICU: neonatal intensive care unit; PMA: postmenstrual age)

TABLE 6: Drug dosage.

Drug	*Dosage*	*Side effects*
Caffeine	• *Loading:* 20–25 mg/kg IV over 30 min or PO (equivalent to 10–12.5 mg/kg caffeine base) • *Maintenance:* 5–10 mg/kg of caffeine citrate IV or PO once daily	Restlessness, vomiting, and tachycardia
Diuretics		
Furosemide	• *IV:* 1–2 mg/kg/dose q 12–24 hourly • *Oral:* 2–6 mg/kg q 6–8 hourly	• Hypercalciuria • Nephrocalcinosis
Chlorothiazides	Oral 10–20 mg/kg q 12 hourly	Ototoxicity
Spironolactone	Oral 0.5–1.5 mg/kg q 12 hourly	Hypokalemia, alkalosis
Bronchodilators	*Inhalation*	
Salbutamol	Inhalational 0.1–0.5 mg/kg q 2–6 hourly	Tachycardia, tremors
Ipratropium	Inhalational 0.025 mg/kg q 8 hourly	
Dexamethasone		
Use minimal possible dose and for minimum duration of 3–7 days and only in infants who are >7 days old and cannot be weaned off from mechanical ventilation	*Intravenous:* • 0.15 mg/kg/day × 3 days • 0.1 mg/kg/day × 2 days • 0.05 mg/kg/day × 2 days in two divided doses	• Hyperglycemia, hypertension, gastrointestinal hemorrhage, and perforation • Poor neurodevelopment outcome

(IV: intravenous; PO: per os)

Follow these principles of drug therapy:

- All drugs have adverse effects
- Anticipate that a drug may have no therapeutic effect
- If you start a drug, be willing to stop it.

CLINICAL PEARL

- Use steroids for specific indications in the smallest possible dose and for shortest duration. Avoid using drug, especially steroids.

Preventive Strategies

Avoidance of factors that predispose to lung injury is cornerstone of management of BPD. Some of the proven strategies in the management of BPD are as follows:

- Antenatal steroids
- Resuscitation as NRP 2020 guidelines. Use of T-piece resuscitator preferable.
- *Ventilation strategies:* Aim is to minimize lungs injury by optimizing the ventilator strategies which includes:
  - Early institution of CPAP
  - *Early surfactant therapy (within 2 hours):* Use INSURE (INtubation, SURfactant administration and Extubation to CPAP)/MIST (Minimally Invasive Surfactant Therapy)/LISA (Less Invasive Surfactant Administration) technique for surfactant administration followed by CPAP/NSIMV
  - *Use of patient triggered ventilation:* More physiological

  Prefer use of volume-triggered ventilation over pressure limited ventilation:
  - *Permissive hypercapnia:* Accepting PCO_2 levels as high as 55 mm Hg with pH greater than or equal to 7.25
  - *Avoidance of hyperoxia:* Target SpO_2: 91–95% in acute phase of ventilation
  - *High-frequency oscillation:* Less injurious to lungs, but no evidence for its benefits in routine use.
- *Early use of caffeine therapy:* Within first 72 hours, preferably as early as feasible
- Prophylactic hydrocortisone ("Early"<7 days) starting at <24 hours of age in extremely preterm babies.
- Low fluid intake
- Aggressive nutrition strategies
- Prevention of nosocomial infections
- Aggressive treatment of hemodynamically significant (hs)-PDA
- *Vitamin A:* Essential for lung development and differentiation. Its use in extremely low birthweight (ELBW) babies as 5,000 IU IM three times/week for 4 weeks reduces risk of BPD
- *Inhaled nitric oxide:* Proven role yet to be established

CLINICAL PEARL

- Respiratory strategies aim to minimize lung injury and early use of caffeine reduces the chances of developing BPD.

INFANT STIMULATION AND PARENTAL SUPPORT

Infants with severe BPD may be ventilator dependent for many weeks or months and thus, deprived of normal parental stimulation. A well-organized stimulation program and parental participation help in reducing infant's neurodevelopmental delays and allaying parental anxiety.

DISCHARGE PLANNING

Usually, oxygen can be discontinued in before discharge. However, home oxygen therapy is a safe alternative to long-term hospitalization in selected cases:

- Stable babies with no other medical illness
- Stable oxygen requirement
- Parents prepared and trained
- Follow-up is ensured.

OUTCOME

The outcome has improved because of better management and milder form of the disease.

Mortality is low; however, when it occurs is usually because of respiratory failure, infections, pulmonary hypertension, and cor pulmonale. Infants with severe BPD are at higher risk of:

- Growth failure
- Feeding problems and gastroesophageal reflux
- Recurrent chest infections
- Hyper-reactive airway disease
- Long-term neurodevelopmental sequelae
- Recurrent hospitalization
- Increased mortality

KEY POINTS

- Bronchopulmonary dysplasia is mainly a disease of extreme preterm and VLBW babies, contributing to morbidities such as neurodevelopment impairment, recurrent respiratory illnesses, and growth failure.
- Prematurity, severity of respiratory disease, and ventilation are the main risk factors.
- Preventive strategies such as antenatal steroids, early use of surfactants, gentle ventilation, early and aggressive use of CPAP, and early caffeine therapy reduce the incidence of BPD.
- Early extubation should be the goal for all preterm babies requiring mechanical ventilation.
- Systemic steroids should be used only in selective cases.
- Nutrition, early stimulation, and parental anxiety should be addressed timely.
- Use of anti-inflammatory agents such as inhaled nitric oxide, late use of surfactant and antioxidants may be promising therapies in the future.

SUGGESTED READING

1. Bancalari EH, Walsh MC. Bronchopulmonary dysplasia. In: Martin RJ, Fanaroff AA, Walsh MC (Eds). Fanaroff and Martin's Neonatal-Perinatal Medicine Disease of the Fetus and Infant, 9th edn. Philadelphia: Elsevier; 2011. pp. 1179-91.
2. Davis JM, Rosenfield WN. Bronchopulmonary dysplasia. In: MacDonald MG, Seshia MMK, Mullett MD (Eds). Avery's Neonatology Pathophysiology and Management of the Newborn, 6th edn. Philadelphia: Lippincott Williams and Wilkins; 2005. pp. 568-99.
3. Htun ZT, Schulz EV, Desai RK, Marasch JL, McPherson CC, Mastrandrea LD, et al. Postnatal steroid management in preterm infants with evolving bronchopulmonary dysplasia. J Perinatol. 2021;41:1783-96.
4. Jobe AH, Bancalari E. Bronchopulmonary dysplasia. Am J Respir Crit Care Med. 2001;163:1723-9.
5. Korones Sheldon B. Complications. In: Goldsmith JP, Karotkin EH (Eds). Assisted Ventilation of the Neonate, 5th edn. Philadelphia: Saunders; 2011. pp. 389-425.
6. Patel RM, Leong T, Carlton DP, Vyas-Read S. Early caffeine therapy and clinical outcomes in extremely preterm infants. J Perinatol. 2013;33(2):134-40.

Patent Ductus Arteriosus

Divya Arun Kondgekar, Shreepal Jain, Shakuntala Prabhu

INTRODUCTION

Patent ductus arteriosus (PDA) is defined as the persistence of the ductus arteriosus (DA) after birth. During embryonic development, the DA plays a crucial role in fetal circulation; however, it becomes largely redundant after birth.

INCIDENCE AND RISK FACTORS

Patent ductus arteriosus is one of the most prevalent forms of acyanotic congenital heart disease, with an incidence ranging from approximately 1 in 5,000 to 1 in 2,000 live births, accounting for 10–12% of all congenital heart defects. It is most common cardiac condition affecting neonates. The incidence of PDA is inversely proportional to the gestational age and birth weight of the neonate. The DA is found to be patent at day 4 of life in about 80% of neonates born at 25–28 weeks compared to 10% in those born at 30–37 weeks. In neonates born at <24 weeks, the incidence is about 90%.

Maternal rubella infection during the first trimester is linked to the occurrence of PDA in neonates. Furthermore, PDA is associated with several genetic syndromes, such as trisomy 21, trisomy 18, Char syndrome, 4p deletion, Holt–Oram syndrome, and Carpenter syndrome.

ANATOMY

The DA is a vessel that connects the left pulmonary artery (LPA) near its origin to the descending aorta just distal to the left subclavian artery. During fetal life, the DA has a diameter equal to that of the descending aorta, allowing the right ventricle (RV) to eject 90% of its stroke volume into the descending aorta via the DA. Morphologically, the DA is typically funnel-shaped, being wider at the aortic end and narrower at the pulmonary end **(Table 1)**.

PATHOPHYSIOLOGY

The DA shunts oxygenated blood from the main pulmonary artery to the descending aorta, bypassing the high-resistance pulmonary circuit in the fetus **(Fig. 1)**. In fetal life, the DA remains patent due to low oxygen tension, arachidonic acid pathway metabolites (prostaglandins) in the circulating blood, and locally released nitric oxide. Functional closure of the PDA begins

TABLE 1: Determinants of ductal response and shunt volume.

Determinants of ductal response	
Factors causing the closure of PDA: • Exposure to high oxygenated blood • Cessation of prostaglandin supply from the placenta due to umbilical cord clamping • Metabolism of circulating prostaglandins by the neonatal lungs	*Factors responsible for patency of DA:* • Term neonates—abnormality in the signaling pathway of ductal smooth muscles • Preterm neonates—immaturity of the ductus and immature ductal responses to postnatal transition
Determinants of shunt volume	
• Relative changes in the systemic and pulmonary vascular resistances • Pressure gradient between aorta and pulmonary artery • *Ductal anatomy:* Size, length, and shape • Ductal tissue elastance	

(PDA: patent ductus arteriosus)

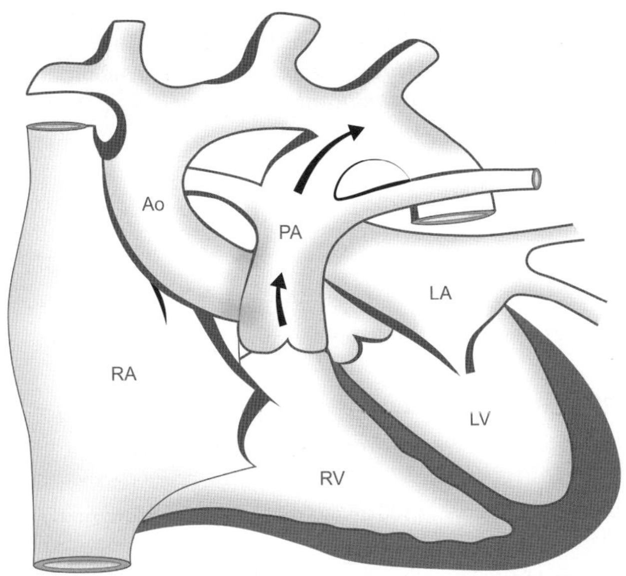

Fig. 1: Representation of fetal cardiac anatomy. Patent ductus arteriosus is the vessel connecting pulmonary artery (PA) and aorta (Ao). The arrow denotes blood flow from the right ventricle to the descending aorta in the fetal life. (LA: left atrium; LV: left ventricle; RA: right atrium; RV: right ventricle)

10–15 hours after birth and is completed in 24–48 hours. Anatomic closure begins at 48–72 hours and may take up to several weeks **(Fig. 1)**.

CLINICAL PRESENTATION (TABLE 2)

Hemodynamically insignificant PDA may be silent or present as an incidentally detected murmur. Hemodynamically significant PDA (hsPDA) results in lower systemic diastolic pressure, which may lead to end-organ damage. This phenomenon is labeled as "ductal steal". Studies have demonstrated the association of hsPDA with necrotizing enterocolitis, intraventricular hemorrhage, bronchopulmonary dysplasia, acute kidney injury, and death. However, there is insufficient evidence to determine whether systemic complications associated with hsPDA in extremely low birth weight (ELBW) neonates are due to PDA or prematurity.

CLINICAL PEARLS

- Incidentally detected and hemodynamically insignificant PDA can be managed conservatively.
- Majority of the PDAs undergo spontaneous closure by 3 months in term infants and by 1 year in preterm infants.

TABLE 2: Signs and symptoms of hemodynamically significant patent ductus arteriosus.

Clinical presentation	
Symptoms	***Signs***
• Apneic spells • Increased ventilator requirement/oxygen dependency • Difficulty to wean off ventilator support • Shock • Pulmonary/ET hemorrhage • Complicated recovery from HMD/RDS/BPD	• Persistent tachycardia • Hyperdynamic precordium • Bounding pulses with wide pulse pressure • Poor peripheral perfusion • Continuous murmur at 2nd LPSB • Low cardiac output state secondary to ductal steal

(BPD: bronchopulmonary dysplasia; HMD; hyaline membrane disease; LPSB: left parasternal border; RDS: respiratory distress syndrome)

Hemodynamically Significant Patent Ductus Arteriosus

Previously, all PDAs were considered significant and treated. Despite advances in defining PDA in neonates, there are no universally accepted guidelines for management. Transthoracic echocardiography is considered the gold standard for diagnosing neonatal PDAs and assessing their hemodynamic significance. The appearance of echocardiographic signs of hsPDA occurs, on average, 2 days before clinical signs develop. The diagnosis of hsPDA should be based on a combination of echocardiographic parameters and clinical signs, considering the presence of any other comorbidities **(Table 3)**.

Researchers have studied the role of biochemical markers in indicating the presence of hsPDA both independently and in conjunction with echocardiography. Serum markers like B-natriuretic peptide (BNP), amino-terminal pro-B-type natriuretic peptide (NT-proBNP), and cardiac troponin T (cTnT), as well as urinary markers like neutrophil gelatinase-associated lipocalin and heart-type fatty acid-binding protein, are used to predict ductal closure timing. Additionally, assessing cerebral and abdominal oxygenation using near-infrared spectroscopy might help to identify patients with compromised hemodynamic status.

CLINICAL PEARLS

- It is important to rule out duct-dependent congenital heart diseases before attempting closure of PDA.
- Decision regarding closure of PDA should depend on the both clinical findings and echocardiographic parameters.

TABLE 3: Echocardiographic indicators of hemodynamically significant patent ductus arteriosus.

Echocardiography		*Echo view*	*Hemodynamically insignificant*	*Hemodynamically significant*
Ductal dimension				
1.	Ductal size (mm) (*Note:* In preterm and low birth weight neonates this may not be applicable. Hence presence of other indices should be evaluated)	High parasternal short axis view/ ductal view	<1.5	≥1.5
2.	Direction of the shunt	High parasternal short axis view/ ductal view	Left to right	
3.	Velocity and gradient in systole and diastole (V_{max}:V_{min})	High parasternal short axis view/ ductal view (CWD)	<2	≥2
Indicators of pulmonary overcirculation				
4.	LVO (mL/kg/min)	Parasternal long axis view + apical 5 chamber view (PWD)	<300 mL/kg/min	≥300 mL/kg/min
5.	LVEDD (Z-score)	Parasternal long axis view (M-mode)	<2	≥2
6.	LA:Ao	Parasternal long axis view (M-mode)	<1.4	≥1.4
7.	Pulmonary vein d wave velocity (mean) (m/s)	High suprasternal view (PWD)	<0.3	≥0.3
8.	LPA diastolic velocity (m/s)	High parasternal view (PWD)	<0.5	≥0.5
9.	Mitral valve E:A	Apical four chamber view (PWD)	<1	≥1
Effects on systemic circulation				
10.	Flow in descending aorta	Subcostal abdominal sagittal (PWD)	Forward flow	Absent/reversal flow

(LA:Ao: left atrium to aortic valve ratio; LPA: left pulmonary artery; LVEDD: left ventricular end diastolic dimension; LVO: left ventricular output; V_{max}: maximum velocity; V_{min}: minimum velocity)

APPROACH TO NEONATAL PATENT DUCTUS ARTERIOSUS

The utility of prophylactic PDA closure in premature infants has been questioned due to the lack of any significant reduction in morbidity and mortality associated with ductal closure. Studies have indicated that closure of PDA did not improve outcomes concerning bronchopulmonary dysplasia (BPD), NEC, IVH, retinopathy of prematurity (ROP), periventricular leukomalacia, long-term neurodevelopmental status, and mortality. As a result, many neonatologists have adopted a conservative approach, which has shown a similar incidence of NEC, IVH, and BPD compared to medical treatment **(Table 4 and Flowchart 1)**.

Nonpharmacological/Conservative Management

In more mature neonates, conservative management of PDA may suffice while awaiting spontaneous closure. Preterm or LBW neonates with hemodynamically insignificant PDA can be conservatively managed. This approach includes careful fluid restriction (110–130 mL/kg/day, with monitoring of urine output) and increasing peak end-expiratory pressure (PEEP) to manage pulmonary edema. The use of diuretics is controversial, as there is a lack of evidence supporting improved outcomes in very premature infants.

Pharmacological Management

The Food and Drug Administration (FDA) has approved indomethacin and ibuprofen for medical closure of PDA. These drugs inhibit the cyclooxygenase site of the prostaglandin synthase enzyme, preventing prostaglandin synthesis and causing constriction of the PDA. Ibuprofen is associated with a lower risk of NEC and acute kidney injury compared to indomethacin. Ibuprofen is administered as 10 mg/kg for the first dose, followed by 5 mg/kg for the second and third doses, given 24 hours apart.

TABLE 4: Management strategies in neonatal PDA (based on the modality).

Management strategies in neonatal PDA					
Asymptomatic		***Symptomatic***			
			Nonpharmacological		
Conservative	***Prophylactic***	***Pharmacological***	***Conservative***	***Catheterization***	***Surgical***
• Watchful wait • Routine neonatal care	• Prophylactic closure is no longer recommended • Some centers practice prophylactic closure in extremely premature babies • Medical closure is preferred	• *Ibuprofen:* 10 mg/kg first dose followed by 5 mg/kg × 2 doses IV/orally 24 hours apart (long course for 5 days) • *Indomethacin:* 0.2 mg/kg/dose × 3 doses IV 12 hours apart • *Paracetamol:* 15 mg/kg/dose × 6 hourly IV/orally for 3 days (long course 5 days)	• *Fluid restriction:* 110–130 mL/kg/day • *Ventilatory strategies:* High positive end-expiratory pressure and lower inspiratory time • Maintaining a thermoneutral environment • Renal function test and serum electrolytes monitoring	• *Indication:* Neonates requiring high ventilatory settings with large PDA and failure of 2 courses of medical therapy. Contraindication to medical closure • Coil or device closure of PDA	• *Indication:* Neonates requiring high ventilatory settings with large PDA and failure of 2 courses of medical therapy. Contraindication to medical closure • Surgical ligation of PDA

(PDA: patent ductus arteriosus)

Flowchart 1: Algorithm for approach to neonatal PDA.

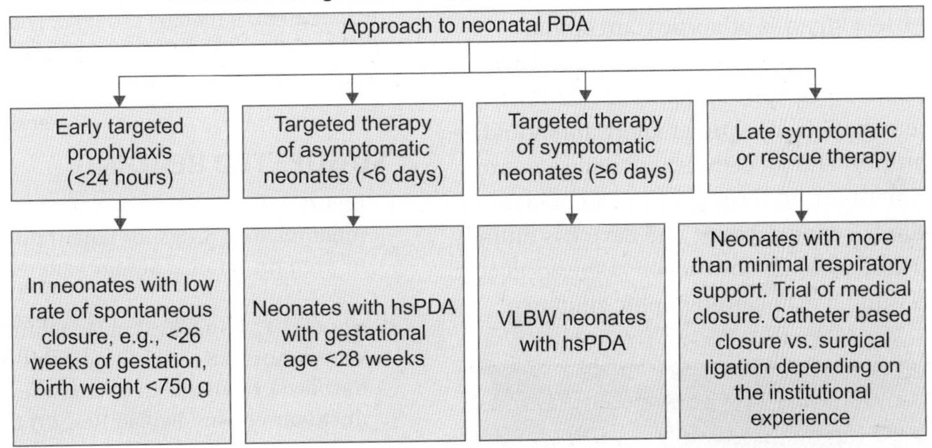

(hsPDA: hemodynamically significant PDA; PDA: patent ductus arteriosus; VLBW: very low birth weight)

A Cochrane review found that intravenous administration of ibuprofen was less effective than the oral route. Additionally, another study indicated that extremely low birth weight (ELBW) infants who received oral ibuprofen had higher rates of PDA reopening compared to those who received IV ibuprofen. Evidence also supports that oral ibuprofen is safe in low birth weight infants.

The US FDA has not approved acetaminophen for the medical treatment of PDA in neonates. Acetaminophen inhibits the peroxidase enzyme responsible for the prostaglandin synthesis, causing the narrowing of the PDA. Acetaminophen can be given orally or intravenously in the dosage of 15 mg/kg/dose every 6 hours for 3 days; can be extended up to 7 days if initial treatment fails. Due to its better safety profile and similar closure rates, acetaminophen is widely used for medical closure of PDA.

Surgical Ligation of Hemodynamically Significant Patent Ductus Arteriosus

Neonates or infants with hsPDA (>3 mm) that does not respond to medical closure are suitable candidates for surgical closure. Other indications include failure after at least two attempts of medical closure or contraindications to pharmacological management. The surgical approach involves a left thoracotomy (with operative mortality typically less than 5% in preterm infants). However, infants undergoing surgical ligation are at increased risk of developing post-ligation cardiac syndrome (PLCS), a rare but serious complication characterized by maladaptation between systemic and pulmonary vascular responses leading to a low cardiac output state. Additional complications associated with surgical closure of PDA include vocal cord paralysis, diaphragm paralysis, chylothorax, hemo-/pneumothorax, and bronchopulmonary dysplasia.

Transcatheter Closure of Hemodynamically Significant Patent Ductus Arteriosus

Transcatheter closure of hsPDA in preterm neonates is gaining popularity due to its minimally invasive nature and wide availability. In 2016, Zahn performed transcatheter closure of PDA in extremely preterm neonates (mean weight 1,249 grams) with a successful closure rate of 88% and a 12.5% adverse event rate. At the 11-month follow-up, all 24 patients were alive with no residual PDA and no left pulmonary artery stenosis or aortic coarctation.

Percutaneous PDA closure can also be performed bedside using echocardiography and portable fluoroscopy; however, a catheterization lab is preferable. Care should be taken during transport and procedure to provide a thermoneutral environment for preterm babies. Duct closure is preferred using only venous access. The device is entirely released in the PDA, avoiding obstruction at the aortic and pulmonary artery under echocardiographic guidance.

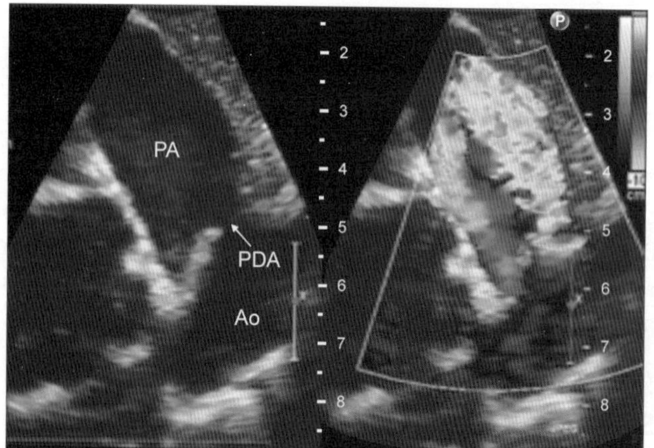

Fig. 2: Ductal view showing PDA with left to right shunt. (Ao: aorta; PA: pulmonary artery; PDA: patent ductus arteriosus) *(For color version, see Plate 1)*

The FDA has approved the use of the Amplatzer PICCOLO ductal occluder for transcatheter closure of PDAs in preterm infants weighing as little as 700 grams. In a multicenter trial of 200 patients, the implant success rate was 95.5% overall and 99% in neonates weighing 700–2,000 grams. The effective closure rate at 6 months follow-up was 100%. PLCS is less common compared to surgical ligation of PDA, although further studies are required **(Fig. 2)**.

KEY POINTS

- Ductus arteriosus plays an important role in fetal circulation, however, its patency in the postnatal period may cause hemodynamic compromise in some neonates and warrant treatment.
- Spontaneous closure of PDA may take up to 3 months in term infants and up to 1 year in preterm infants.
- Echocardiography is gold standard for early diagnosis and monitoring of neonatal PDA.
- Duct-dependent congenital heart defects should be ruled out prior to starting medical/interventional closure of PDA.
- Medical closure of PDA is widely practiced, however, transcatheter closure is becoming popular in the current era. Trial of medical therapy should only be given weighing the risk–benefit ratio and taking into consideration the adverse effects of pharmacotherapy.

SUGGESTED READING

1. Benitz WE, Bhombal S. The use of non-steroidal anti-inflammatory drugs for patent ductus arteriosus closure in preterm infants. Semin Fetal Neonatal Med. 2017;22:302-7.
2. Chock VY, Punn R, Oza A, Benitz WE, Van Meurs KP, Whittemore AS, et al. Predictors of bronchopulmonary dysplasia or death in premature infants with a patent ductus arteriosus. Pediatr Res. 2014;75:570-85.
3. Clyman RI, Couto J, Murphy GM. Patent ductus arteriosus: are current neonatal treatment options better or worse than no treatment at all? Semin Perinatol. 2012;36:123-9.
4. Clyman RI, Saha S, Jobe A, Oh W. Indomethacin prophylaxis for preterm infants: the impact of 2 multicentered randomized controlled trials on clinical practice. J Pediatr. 2007;150:46-50.
5. El-Khuffash AF, Molloy EJ. Influence of a patent ductus arteriosus on cardiac troponin T levels in preterm infants. J Pediatr. 2008;153:350-3.
6. Erdeve O, Yurttutan S, Altug N, Ozdemir R, Gokmen T, Dilmen U, et al. Oral versus intravenous ibuprofen for patent ductus arteriosus closure: a randomised controlled trial in extremely low birthweight infants. Arch Dis Child Fetal Neonatal Ed. 2012;97:F279-83.

7. Heuchan AM, Clyman RI. Managing the patent ductus arteriosus: current treatment options. Arch Dis Child Fetal Neonatal Ed. 2014;99:F431-6.
8. Jain A, Shah PS. Diagnosis, evaluation, and management of patent ductus arteriosus in preterm neonates. JAMA Pediatr. 2015;169(9):863-72.
9. Kulkarni M, Gokulakrishnan G, Price J, Fernandes CJ, Leeflang M, Pammi M. Diagnosing significant PDA using natriuretic peptides in preterm neonates: a systematic review. Pediatrics. 2015;135:e510-25.
10. Mitchell SC, Korones SB, Berendes HW. Congenital heart disease in 56,109 births: incidence and natural history. Circulation. 1971;43:323-32.
11. Noori S, McCoy M, Friedlich P, Bright B, Gottipati V, Seri I, et al. Failure of ductus arteriosus closure is associated with increased mortality in preterm infants. Pediatrics. 2009;123:e138-44.
12. Oncel MY, Yurttutan S, Erdeve O, Uras N, Altug N, Oguz SS, et al. Oral paracetamol versus oral ibuprofen in the management of patent ductus arteriosus in preterm infants: a randomized controlled trial. J Pediatr. 2014;164:510-4.e1.
13. Sathanandam SK, Gutfinger D, O'Brien L, Forbes TJ, Gillespie MJ, Berman DP, et al. Amplatzer Piccolo Occluder clinical trial for percutaneous closure of the patent ductus arteriosus in patients ≥700 grams. Catheter Cardiovasc Interv. 2020;96:1266-76.
14. Shepherd JL, Noori S. What is a hemodynamically significant PDA in preterm infants? Congenit Heart Dis. 2019; 14:21-6.
15. Skelton R, Evans N, Smythe J. A blinded comparison of clinical and echocardiographic evaluation of the preterm infant for patent ductus arteriosus. J Paediatr Child Health. 1994;30:406-11.
16. Slaughter JL, Cua CL, Notestine JL, Rivera BK, Marzec L, Hade EM, et al. Early prediction of spontaneous Patent Ductus Arteriosus (PDA) closure and PDA-associated outcomes: a prospective cohort investigation. BMC Pediatr. 2019;19:333.
17. Zahn EM, Peck D, Phillips A, Nevin P, Basaker K, Simmons C, et al. Transcatheter closure of patent ductus arteriosus in extremely premature newborns: early results and midterm follow-up. JACC Cardiovasc Interv. 2016;9:2429-37.

CHAPTER 8

Update on Neonatal Shock

Abhishek S Aradhya, Shiv Sajan Saini

INTRODUCTION AND DEFINITION

Shock is defined as a clinical syndrome of acute circulatory dysfunction, resulting in insufficient delivery of oxygen and vital nutrients to tissues relative to their metabolic demand, which leads to cell death and organ dysfunction. Shock is manifested by either hypotension and/or features of hypoperfusion such as cold extremities, poor pulse volume, prolonged capillary filling time, metabolic acidosis, etc. The case fatality rates in neonatal shock are very high. Therefore, early recognition and appropriate intervention are the key to improved survival and better neurodevelopmental outcomes.

The incidence of shock in neonatal intensive care unit (NICU) is variable and depends on the rate of preterm admissions and infection rates. The incidence increases with decreasing gestation age and is frequent in extreme preterms. The incidence varies between 3 and 10% of NICU admissions. The incidence increases to 10–28% in extreme preterms and is around 4% in <36 weeks of gestation.

PATHOPHYSIOLOGY

Shock is a pathologic state either due to reduced oxygen delivery, increased oxygen consumption or inadequate oxygen utilization. This tissue and cellular hypoxia switch the metabolism to anaerobic conditions leading to accumulation of lactic acid another and anions. Increasing levels of these metabolites result in metabolic acidosis and interferes with cellular functions, thus leading to organ dysfunction and death.

During circulatory instability, tissue perfusion is compromised. At the initial stages, circulation to vital organs (brain, heart, and adrenals) is maintained at the cost of nonvital organs (skin, muscles, gut, lungs, etc.). This phenomenon is known as the *diving reflex*. Compromised tissue perfusion in the early stages of circulatory instability clinically manifests as a change in skin color (pale or off-colored), cold peripheries, weak pulses, delayed capillary refill time (CRT), and decreased urine output. The blood pressure (BP) is maintained at this stage. This condition is also commonly referred to as *peripheral circulatory failure* or *compensated shock*. On the contrary, a new unit could have flash capillary refill, flushed skin, and a CRT <1 second. This condition is known as warm shock. Later with the involvement of vital organs, myocardial performance decreases and adrenal dysfunction sets in. Such neonates develop hypotension and progress to *decompensated shock*. Although shock and hypotension are loosely used interchangeably, however, it is important to realize that hypotension is a late manifestation of shock. As the neonate transitions from compensated to decompensated shock, the outcome worsens, and the risk of mortality increases.

In neonates, various clinical conditions cause circulatory instability. These include (but are not limited to) asphyxia, circulatory maladaptation while transitioning from fetal to neonatal life especially in extremely preterm neonates, intracardiac shunts, sepsis, fluid loss, adrenal insufficiency, arrhythmias, air leaks, and raised intrathoracic pressure. A prospective observational study done in a tertiary care set-up showed that the three most common reasons of shock in neonates include septic shock, severe birth asphyxia, and hemodynamically significant patent ductus arteriosus (HS-PDA). These conditions involve alteration in one or more domains of normal circulation, i.e., preload, myocardial contractility and afterload. Additionally, absolute or relative adrenal insufficiency contributes to hypotension. **Table 1** summarizes the main pathophysiological mechanisms in various etiologies of neonatal shock.

TABLE 1: Pathophysiology in different causes of shock in neonates.

Clinical scenario	*Preload*	*Myocardial contractility*	*Afterload*	*Main mechanism*
Hypovolemia, e.g., diarrhea, polyurea, fetomaternal bleed, intracranial bleed, etc.	Decreased as intravascular volume is reduced	Not affected	Not affected, may slightly increase initially	Predominantly decreased preload
Septic shock	Relative hypovolemia due to venodilation and capillary leak	Depressed myocardial systolic and diastolic functions	Decreased vasomotor tone	All three domains affected
Asphyxia	Increases	Depressed due to myocardial injury	Increases initially, at later stages decreases	Predominantly myocardial dysfunction
Intracardiac shunts, e.g., PDA	Increases	Hyperdynamic circulation and diastolic dysfunction initially, later systolic dysfunction	Decreased due to systemic to pulmonary shunts	Predominantly myocardial dysfunction and decreased afterload
Transitional circulation in ELBW neonates	Increases	Depressed (suddenly increased LV afterload after birth)	Increases in early stages	Predominantly myocardial dysfunction
Adrenal insufficiency	Variable	Depressed	Decreased	Combination of decreased afterload and myocardial dysfunction
Raised intrathoracic pressure, e.g., pneumothorax, high pressures on ventilator, etc.	Decreased (poor venous return)	Not affected primarily, however low output due to poor myocardial capacity to distend	Increases as intrathoracic pressure compresses vessels	Mainly decreased preload, poor cardiac filling

CLINICAL FEATURES

Hemodynamic stability is commonly assessed by heart rate (HR), pulse volume, temperature (core and peripheral temperature), BP, CRT, color, and urine output. Details of these clinical manifestations as follows:

- *Heart rate abnormalities:* Tachycardia (HR >160 beats/min) is a nonspecific finding commonly seen in shock. Tachycardia is primary compensatory mechanisms in neonates to increase cardiac output as there is limited ability to increase stroke volume. Bradycardia is a preterminal finding. There are several causes of tachycardia in newborns, especially dehydration, pain, PDA, drug effect (caffeine), sepsis, etc., making it a nonspecific hemodynamic sign. Tachycardia in isolation warrants careful evaluation and close monitoring to avoid progression to decompensated shock.
- *Hypotension:* It is defined as BP below 5th centile for gestational age. Apart from hemodynamic assessment, BP measurement helps to identify ductal-dependent systemic circulation, where BP in the lower limbs is lower than in the right upper limb. **Table 2** depicts BP thresholds at the 5th centile as per gestational age (Modified from McNamara, et al.). Traditionally, BP is used to measure the adequacy of systemic circulation. However, it is important to understand the limitations of BP during the assessment of hemodynamic stability in neonates.

TABLE 2: Blood pressure thresholds at the 5th centile as per gestational age.

Gestation (weeks)	*5th centile (mm Hg)*		
	Systolic	*MAP*	*Diastolic*
<30	42	30	20
31	45	30	20
32	46	30	21
33	47	30	22
34	48	31	23
35	49	32	24
36	50	32	25

(MAP: mean arterial pressure)

- BP by noninvasive methods directly measures mean arterial pressure (MAP). It then derives systolic BP (SBP) and diastolic BP by mathematical algorithms. Usually, BP obtained by noninvasive methods are higher than invasive methods especially at lower values. There is poor agreement between noninvasive and invasive BPs.
- It is well known that low BP is a late sign of shock.
- BP is a product of cardiac output and systemic vascular resistance (SVR). If cardiac output is decreased, the tissue perfusion also decreases. Decreased cardiac output may be masked if SVR is elevated. Thus, despite BP being stable during shock, the tissue perfusion may be seriously compromised.
- BP correlates poorly with systemic blood flow in extremely preterm neonates. These neonates can have low BP but can have adequate perfusion. Thus, in this population, BP as a number needs to be interpreted cautiously by assessing perfusion. Nevertheless, it has been shown that below a MAP of 30 mm Hg, cerebral autoregulation is lost. Thus, MAP should be targeted above 30 mm Hg even in extremely preterm neonates.

- *Delayed CRT:* Commonly, assessed over the bony surface like sternum. Flash refill indicates warm shock. Delayed CRT >3 seconds in presence of other signs of poor perfusion indicates shock.
- *Other signs of hemodynamic monitoring:* Low pulse volume or thready pulses, a core-peripheral temperature difference of >3°C (mainly for term neonates), pale color, and mottling.
- *Other organ involvement due to poor perfusion:*
  - *Neurologic signs:* Nonspecific signs such as lethargy, irritability, poor tone, and poor neonatal reflexes can be present. Decreased cerebral perfusion can also cause periodic breathing or apnea in later stages.
  - *Respiratory signs:* Tachypnea is a common finding either due to lung involvement by sepsis or as a compensatory response to metabolic acidosis.
  - *Renal signs:* There is generally decreased urine output, azotemia, and electrolyte imbalance.

Though there are many clinical signs of hemodynamic assessment, these signs have some limitations. While some of the signs of peripheral circulation are nonspecific, e.g., HR, some others are subjective, e.g., feeble pulses. Individually, CRT and core-periphery temperature differences correlate poorly with organ perfusion. Therefore, no single parameter of peripheral circulation in isolation can accurately detect shock/circulatory instability. Therefore, combined information of all parameters [HR, CRT, color, urine output, and temperature (core and peripheral temperature)] should be utilized for assessment of circulation.

Due to the subjective nature of many of the signs of hemodynamic assessment, a requirement of an objective definition of shock was felt. An objective definition of *septic shock* was proposed by the International Pediatric Sepsis Consensus Conference. Septic shock is defined as the presence of cardiovascular dysfunction in the presence of sepsis. Cardiovascular dysfunction is defined if the neonate has either of the following criteria despite administration of isotonic intravenous fluid ≥40 mL/kg in 1 hour:

- Decrease in BP (hypotension) <5th percentile for age or SBP <2SD below normal for age OR
- Need for vasoactive drug to maintain BP in normal range (dopamine >5 µg/kg/min or dobutamine, epinephrine, or norepinephrine at any dose) OR
- *Two of the following:* Unexplained metabolic acidosis—base deficit >5.0 mEq/L; increased arterial lactate > two times upper limit of normal; oliguria—urine output <0.5 mL/kg/h, prolonged capillary refill—>5 seconds; Core to peripheral temperature gap >3°C.

However, this definition is applicable only to the term neonates. Wynn and Wong proposed a modified definition for preterm neonates. The salient differences in the definition for preterm neonates (from International Pediatric Sepsis Consensus Definition) are: Fluid administration limit is >10 mL/kg in infants <32 weeks, SBP <2SD, or MAP <30 mm Hg with CRT >4 seconds. Although this definition is given for the diagnosis of neonatal septic shock, it may be used for the diagnosis of other types of shock.

However, two parameters in the above definition are laboratory variables which may not be available in all settings and they can also be increased in other clinical conditions. Later, Davis et al. gave a clinical definition of septic shock for full-term neonates. They defined neonatal septic shock in the presence of three or more of following eight features: (1) Temperature <36°C or >38°C, (2) SBP <60 mm Hg, (3) HR >205/min, (4) respiratory rate (RR) >60/min, (5) CRT ≥3 seconds, or <1 second, (6) mental status abnormality, (7) weak or bounding pulses, and (8) cool, flushed, or mottled skin. This definition is applicable to children and term neonates. For preterm neonates, a consensus definition has not been established, primarily due to the absence of normative BP and hemodynamic data across various degrees of prematurity. Nonetheless, the same criteria are often applied to preterm neonates in clinical practice.

INVESTIGATIONS

Shock is a clinical diagnosis. Laboratory investigations may aid in the diagnosis, but contribute to categorize the severity and etiology of shock. The laboratory workup includes metabolic, biochemistry, hematological, and microbiological workup.

The correctable metabolic/biochemical derangements should be screened and managed upfront in all cases, which include blood glucose levels, serum electrolytes, and serum calcium. Hypoglycemia and electrolyte disturbances should be treated aggressively.

Blood gas analysis is a useful means to get information about metabolic status as well as respiratory gas exchange. Modern blood gas machines are also capable of measuring serum electrolytes including ionized calcium levels, hematocrit, blood glucose as well as serum lactate levels. In the presence of poor perfusion, anaerobic metabolism leads to metabolic acidosis and increased lactate. Elevated lactate (>4 mmol/L as a standalone laboratory variable) and mixed venous saturation are not good markers of shock in neonates. Apart from systemic hypoperfusion states, lactate is also produced in local ischemic conditions and even in neonatal sepsis without shock. Furthermore, its levels may increase in the presence of liver dysfunction due to decreased metabolism. Importantly, lactate levels can transiently rise after improvement in circulation as the lactate from underperfused tissues shifts to central circulation with an improvement in circulatory status.

Hematological workup includes assessment of hematocrit, complete blood count (CBC), and platelet levels. In sepsis, leukocyte counts may be either elevated or low (predominantly leukopenia in neonates). In addition, absolute neutrophil count can be low and immature to total neutrophil ratio (ITR) can be elevated (>0.2).

Microbiological investigations must be performed whenever septic shock is considered. Blood culture should be obtained before giving the first dose of antibiotics. The culture of cerebrospinal fluid (CSF) should be sent in all cases of sepsis once stabilized. Site-specific infective focus (aspirates, swabs, etc.) should be cultured, wherever indicated. If viral infections (especially herpes simplex virus) are suspected, appropriate serologies/polymerase chain reaction (PCR) should be performed to identify causative organisms.

Functional echocardiography has gained importance for hemodynamic assessment in the last few years.

- For preload assessment, inferior vena cava (IVC) collapsibility is proposed. There is currently not enough literature on neonates to support its use in preload assessment. Nevertheless, the presence of collapsing IVC during inspiration, and narrower left ventricular cavity (opposite papillary muscles coming in contact with each other during systole i.e., *kissing sign*) suggests decreased intravascular volume status.
- Assessment of cardiac systolic functions (i.e., ejection fraction and fractional shortening etc.)
- Diastolic functions (e.g., early to atrial peak systolic velocity ratio, isovolumetric relaxation time, etc.) can help in diagnosing myocardial dysfunction.

There is no parameter to directly measure SVR. SVR is indirectly estimated by the formula (BP = CO × SVR). Additionally, functional echocardiography can help to exclude common mimickers of sepsis-like HS-PDA, duct-dependent systemic circulation such as hypoplastic left heart, coarctation of aorta, etc. Details of functional echocardiography are beyond the scope of the current text which is available in published reviews on this topic.

Central venous pressure, mixed venous oxygen saturation (SvO_2), and arteriovenous difference have been used to assess tissue hypoxia in older children and adults. Their widespread use in neonates is limited due to the invasive nature of the measurement and limited experience. Additionally, there is limited experience in assessing microcirculatory parameters [e.g., near-infrared spectroscopy (NIRS), the plethysmographic signal of pulse oximeter-perfusion index, and visible light technology] in the management of neonatal shock.

TREATMENT

Initial stabilization—TABC (temperature, airway, breathing, and circulation):

- As with all emergencies in neonates, the management of shock starts with the provision of a thermoneutral environment.
- The airway is stabilized followed by providing breathing support either with CPAP or mechanical ventilation depending on the severity of respiratory distress as well as hemodynamic compromise. Although CPAP can be

Flowchart 1: Algorithm for stepwise, time-sensitive management of shock.

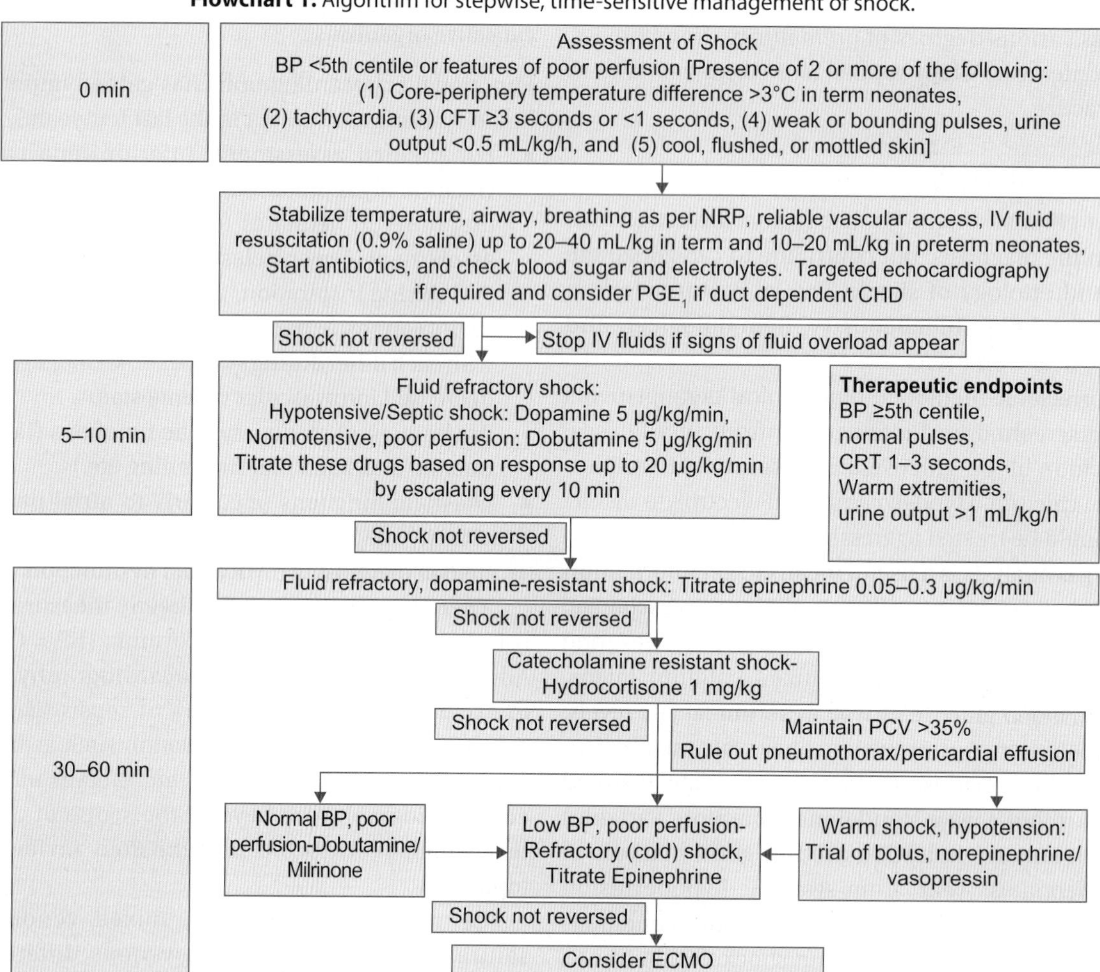

(CHD: congenital heart disease; CRT: capillary refill time; ECMO: extracorporeal membrane oxygenation; PGE: prostaglandin E1; PT: preterm)
Source: Modified from Davis et al.

tried in the early stages of shock (*compensated shock*), it may be preferable to intubate and start elective positive pressure ventilation in the presence of hypotension or requirement of more than one vasoactive agent.

- An intravenous line is required for fluid/vasoactive drug administration. With the initiation of vasoactive agents, enteral feeds should be stopped, and IV maintenance fluids should be started. Central venous access (umbilical venous on first day of life or PICC line) is preferable for reliable delivery of vasopressors **(Flowchart 1)**.

Volume Resuscitation

Volume resuscitation is the first line of therapy in neonatal shock. Crystalloids (normal saline) are preferred over 5% albumin as they are associated with a lower risk of fluid overload. Further albumin is associated with an increased risk of infection and impaired gas exchange. An initial fluid bolus of 10 mL/kg (irrespective of gestational age) is infused over 15–30 minutes (longer duration for ELBW neonates). Up to 40 mL/kg is advised for term neonates and 10–20 mL/kg for preterm neonates. The conservative fluid resuscitation in preterm neonates is advised due to increased risk of fluid overload, the opening of PDA, and intraventricular hemorrhage. Currently, there is no gold standard measure for preload optimization. Therefore, fluid resuscitation is guided by response to fluid bolus(s) and signs of fluid overload. Functional echocardiography may offer additional clues as discussed previously. It is important to realize that absolute hypovolemia is unlikely except in conditions of blood loss/GI loss. Thus, fluid should be used cautiously in the management of shock secondary to asphyxia, PDA, and transitional circulation where myocardial dysfunction is mainly implicated.

Pharmacologic Therapy

The mainstay of pharmacologic therapy is three classes of drugs based on their predominant actions: (1) Inotropes, (2) vasopressors, and (3) lusitropes. Inotropes primarily increase myocardial contractility and hence are suitable for conditions in which myocardial dysfunction is a primary problem, e.g., birth asphyxia or transitional circulation, etc. Vasopressors improve BP through an increase in vascular tone and are thus suitable for conditions with decreased afterload, e.g., septic shock and/or in the presence of hypotension. Lusitropes improve myocardial relaxation, increase systemic blood flow, and are thus useful for conditions with myocardial diastolic dysfunction. Appropriate vasoactive agents should be chosen based on underlying pathophysiology and intended effect. A single drug can have either an inotropic or vasopressor effect depending on its infusion rate. Commonly used agents in neonates, their doses, and their predominant actions are summarized in **Table 3**.

As a general rule, inotropes are advised in peripheral circulatory failure with normal BP. Vasopressors are used in hypotension. Depending on the underlying pathophysiological mechanism, the initial choice of vasoactive agents may vary. The choice of vasoactive agents in different clinical scenarios is as follows:

- *Shock in transitional circulation:* Although usually practiced, fluid resuscitation should be cautiously used as generally there is no setting of volume loss. However, at least one bolus should be given in setting of immediate cord clamping. Dobutamine should be started initially to support poor myocardial performance. If there is hypotension, vasopressors are required in addition.

TABLE 3: Vasoactive drugs, dose and important actions.

Agent	*Dose*	*Action*	*Special features*
Dopamine	*Inotrope:* 5–9 µg/kg/min, mainly on β-receptors	↑ HR and ↑ myocardial contractility	• 5% Dextrose is preferred for dilution. Preferable to change infusions every 12 hours rather than 24 hours • Acts by releasing stored norepinephrine; the stores might exhaust with continuing shock • Thyroid screening to be postponed till 12 hours after the drug is stopped
	Vasopressor: 10–20 µg/kg/min (vasopressor), mainly on α-receptors	↑ BP by increasing SVR in addition to above effects	
Dobutamine	5–20 µg/kg/min	↑ contractility, cardiac output, ↓ SVR	Direct actions on β-receptors, effective in presence of myocardial dysfunction. Increases cardiac contractility better than dopamine
Epinephrine	0.05–0.2 µg/kg/min (inotropy)	↑ contractility and HR	• Direct actions on adrenergic receptors • Caution beyond 0.5 µg/kg/min as arrhythmias may happen • Adverse effect include ↑ HR, serum lactate and hyperglycemia
	≥0.3–1.0 µg/kg/min (vasopressor)	↑ SVR	
Milrinone	• *Loading:* 50–75 µg/kg IV over 60 min; • *Maintenance:* 0.25–0.75 µg/kg/min	*Both inotropy and lusitropy;* ↓ vascular tone in pulmonary and systemic circulation	• Main role in post cardiac surgery • Useful adjunct to iNO in presence of PPHN • More effective than dobutamine in presence of diastolic dysfunction • Cautious in presence of hypotension
Vasopressin	0.01–0.12 units/kg/h	↑ SVR; releases cortisol in presence of ACTH	• Indicated in warm, vasopressor resistant shock • Caution in presence of myocardial dysfunction • Watch for oliguria as ↓ renal blood flow is known
Noradrenaline	0.02–1.0 µg/kg/min	↑ SVR	Mainly in warm shock
Levosimendan	0.1–0.4 µg/kg/min	Positive inotropy and lusitropy, ↓ SVR	Limited evidence of efficacy. Useful in postoperative care of congenital heart diseases

(ACTH: adrenocorticotropin; BP: blood pressure; HR: heart rate; SVR: systemic vascular resistance; PPHN: persistent pulmonary hypertension of the newborn)

However, vasopressors should be carefully used as they can markedly increase SVR, thereby decreasing cardiac output further. A stepwise titration of a low-to-moderate dose of epinephrine (0.05–0.3 μg/kg/min) is advised in hypotensive neonates to achieve a mean BP 3–6 mm Hg higher than gestational age.

- *Very low birth weight (VLBW) neonates with HS-PDA:* The principles of management include restoring hemodynamic stability as well as pharmacological closure of PDA. To decrease left-to-right shunt through PDA, one should use maneuvers to keep slightly higher pulmonary vascular resistance, e.g., adjusting ventilator settings to avoid hyperoxia, keeping slightly higher PCO_2 values, higher positive end-expiratory pressure, etc. No well-controlled trials are comparing different vasoactive agents in the management of shock in neonates with PDA. Bouissou et al. found that dopamine (<10 μg/kg/min) increased BP and systemic blood flow in preterm hypotensive neonates with PDA. Therefore, dopamine in inotropic doses (5 to <10 μg/kg/min) or dobutamine (10–20 μg/kg/min) should be the first line of management in such cases. Epinephrine (0.1–0.5 μg/kg/min) should be used if there is no response to dopamine and dobutamine.
- *Shock in neonates with severe birth asphyxia:* In severely asphyxiated neonates, multiple derangements such as capillary leak syndrome, myocardial dysfunction, and PPHN may occur together. Therefore, therapy must be individualized and constantly adjusted. Fluids should be given cautiously in the absence of setting of volume loss. However, one bolus can be safely given as most of these neonates receive immediate cord clamping. In normotensive patients with poor peripheral circulation, dobutamine should be used. In normotensive neonates with poor peripheral circulation and concomitant PPHN, Milrinone can be considered. In cases of hypotension, dopamine should be started and gradually titrated. Inhaled nitric oxide should be considered for neonates with PPHN.
- *Septic shock:* Fluid resuscitation (10–40 mL/kg) should be given initially as there is relative hypovolemia. The traditional initial choice of vasoactive drug is dopamine (10–20 μg/kg/min) in hypotensive neonates. Epinephrine (0.2–0.5 μg/kg/min) should be added if neonates remain hypotensive despite dopamine infusion. Use of epinephrine and norepinephrine as a first-line vasoactive drug is emerging, however, currently there is no conclusive evidence of their superiority over dopamine. In contrast, a normotensive septic neonate, with signs of peripheral circulatory failure, should be treated with dobutamine or dopamine (5–9 μg/kg/min).
- *Late-onset glucocorticoid responsive circulatory collapse:* It occurs after the first week of life in VLBW infants in the absence of other common causes such as sepsis, PDA, blood loss, or other obstructive causes of shock. Relative adrenal insufficiency is implicated in its pathophysiology. It is characterized by sudden onset hypotension and is usually resistant to fluid resuscitation and vasoactive support. Hydrocortisone is given at 0.5–1.0 mg/kg IV every 6–8 hourly for 48 hours. If responsive, hydrocortisone is continued for 3–5 days. If poor response persists vasopressin can be considered.

Steroids

Steroids are indicated as an adjunct to first-line inotrope in catecholamine-resistant shock. Steroids are initiated early, if the neonate requires >10 μg/kg/min dopamine and a directly acting drug (epinephrine >0.1 μg/kg/min or dobutamine >10 μg/kg/min). They increase BP and decrease vasopressor requirement in such neonates. Given the lack of long-term safety data of steroids on developing brain and the prolonged half-life of steroids in preterm neonates, lower doses are preferred. Hydrocortisone is given as 0.5–1.0 mg/kg q 6–8 hourly for 48 hours and 12 hourly therefore for next 3 days.

Supportive Management

Broad-spectrum antibiotics (as per the local sensitivity pattern) should be started, wherever the possibility of sepsis cannot be ruled out based on clinical risk factors and presentation. The first dose should be administered as early as possible within the first hour of shock. Enteral feeds should be withheld. However, trophic feeding can be continued if abdominal examination is normal. Parenteral nutrition may be considered. Routine sedation is not required. Avoid hyperglycemia and maintain electrolytes and calcium in their normal range. Maintain hematocrit >35%. In bleeding tendencies, vitamin K injection, platelet concentrates for platelet count <50,000/mm^3 and fresh frozen plasma (FFP) transfusions should be considered for coagulopathy. Consider venoarterial extracorporeal membrane oxygenation (ECMO) for refractory. Shock wherever facilities are available.

Other specific management such as prostaglandin E1 (PGE1) can be considered to maintain systemic circulation if duct-dependent systemic circulation is suspected.

OUTCOMES

Neonates with shock are likely to have a longer duration of hospital stay, chronic lung disease, growth failure, retinopathy of prematurity, and adverse neurodevelopmental outcomes. Mortality rates up to 40–50% are reported in VLBW in various studies from developed nations, and studies from developing countries have shown 70–80% mortality in septic shock. Poor prognostic factors in such studies are refractory shock at onset, acute renal failure, disseminated intravascular coagulation (DIC), neutropenia, metabolic acidosis, and hypothermia. Neurodevelopmental outcomes following septic shock at 18 months of age show a higher risk of impairment especially in preterm neonates. Severe sequelae either cerebral palsy, visual impairment, severe developmental delay, or short bowel syndrome have been described up to 19% at 18 months follow-up and the combined risk of death or severe sequelae in half of them.

KEY POINTS

- Shock is not just hypotension; it includes both impairment in perfusion and or blood pressure.
- Shock involves disturbances in either one or all of preload, myocardial contractility, and afterload.
- It is preferable to target MAP > 30 mm Hg in extreme preterms to maintain cerebral perfusion pressure.
- Volume resuscitation is the first line of treatment and crystalloids are preferred over colloids.
- Dopamine remains the first choice conventionally in septic shock until further evidence.
- Need close neurodevelopment follow-up as up to 20% can have varying degrees of disability.

SUGGESTED READING

1. Angus DC, van der Poll T. Severe sepsis and septic shock. N Engl J Med. 2013;369:840.
2. Barrington KJ. Hypotension and shock in the preterm infant. Semin Fetal Neonatal Med. 2008;13:16-23.
3. Baske K, Saini SS, Dutta S, Sundaram V. Epinephrine versus dopamine in neonatal septic shock: a double-blind randomized controlled trial. Eur J Pediatr. 2018;177(9): 1335-42.
4. Batton B, Li L, Newman NS, et al. Early blood pressure, antihypotensive therapy and outcomes at 18-22 months' corrected age in extremely preterm infants. Arch Dis Child Fetal Neonatal Ed. 2016;101:F201.
5. Bouissou A, Rakza T, Klosowski S, Tourneux P, Vanderborght M, Storme L. Hypotension in preterm infants with significant patent ductus arteriosus: effects of dopamine. J Pediatr. 2008;153:790-4.
6. Brierley J, Carcillo JA, Choong K, Cornell T, Decaen A, Deymann A, et al. Clinical practice parameters for hemodynamic support of pediatric and neonatal septic shock: 2007 update from the American College of Critical Care Medicine. Crit Care Med. 2009;37:666-88.
7. Burns ML, Stensvold HJ, Risnes K, Guthe HJ, Astrup H, Nordhov SM, et al. Inotropic therapy in newborns, a population-based national registry study. Pediatr Crit Care Med 2016;17:948-56.
8. Davis AL, Carcillo JA, Aneja RK, Deymann AJ, Lin JC, Nguyen TC, et al. American College of critical care medicine clinical practice parameters for hemodynamic support of pediatric and neonatal septic shock. Crit Care Med. 2017;45:1061-93.
9. Dempsey E, Rabe H. The Use of Cardiotonic Drugs in Neonates. Clin Perinatol. 2019;46(2):273-90.
10. Dionne JM, Bremner SA, Baygani SK, Batton B, Ergenekon E, Bhatt-Mehta V, et al. Method of blood pressure measurement in neonates and infants: a systematic review and analysis. J Pediatr. 2020;221:23.
11. Evans N. Which inotrope for which baby? Arch Dis Child Fetal Neonatal Ed. 2006;91:F213-20.
12. Giesinger RE, McNamara PJ. Hemodynamic instability in the critically ill neonate: an approach to cardiovascular support based on disease pathophysiology. Semin Perinatol. 2016;40:174-88.
13. Goldstein B, Giroir B, Randolph A. International pediatric sepsis consensus conference: definitions for sepsis and organ dysfunction in pediatrics. Pediatr Crit Care Med. 2005;6:2-8.
14. Higgins S, Friedlich P, Seri I. Hydrocortisone for hypotension and vasopressor dependence in preterm neonates: A meta-analysis. J Perinatol. 2010;30:373-8.
15. Iijima S. Late-onset glucocorticoid-responsive circulatory collapse in premature infants. Pediatr Neonatol. 2019; 60(6):603-10.
16. Kawai M. Late-onset circulatory collapse of prematurity. Pediatr Int. 2017;59(4):391-6.
17. Kermorvant-Duchemin E, Laborie S, Rabilloud M, Lapillonne A, Claris O. Outcome and prognostic factors in neonates with septic shock. Pediatr Crit Care Med. 2008;9:186-91.
18. Kirupakaran K, Mahoney L, Rabe H, et al. Understanding the stability of dopamine and dobutamine over 24 h in simulate neonatal ward conditions. Paediatr Drugs 2017;19(5):487-95.
19. Lasky T, Greenspan J, Ernst FR, Gonzalez L. Dopamine and dobutamine use in preterm or low birthweight neonates in the premier 2008 database. Clin Ther. 2011;33:2082-8.

20. McLean CW CR, Noori S, Seri I. Cerebral circulation and hypotension in the premature infant—diagnosis and treatment. In: JMP (Ed). Controversies in Neonatal Neurology. Philadelphia: Saunders; 2008. pp. 3-26.
21. McNamara PJ WD, Giesinger RE, Jain A. Hemodynamics. In: MacDonald MG SM, (Ed). Avery's Neonatology: Pathophysiology and Management the Newborn. Philadelphia: Wolters Kluwer; 2016. pp. 457-86.
22. Mertens L, Seri I, Marek J, Arlettaz R, Barker P, McNamara P, et al. Writing Group of the American Society of Echocardiography (ASE); European Association of Echocardiography (EAE); Association for European Pediatric Cardiologists (AEPC). Targeted neonatal echocardiography in the neonatal intensive care unit: practice guidelines and recommendations for training. Eur J Echocardiogr. 2011;12:715-36.
23. Mertens L, Seri I, Marek J, et al. Targeted neonatal echocardiography in the neonatal intensive care unit: practice guidelines and recommendations for training. Eur J Echocardiogr. 2011;12:715-36.
24. NNF Clinical Practice Guidelines development group. (2023). Diagnosis and management of shock in neonates. Online] Available from Accessed from https://www.nnfi.org/nnf-cpg-guidelines.php [Last accessed December, 2024].
25. Noori S, Seri I. Neonatal blood pressure support: the use of inotropes, lusitropes, and other vasopressor agents. Clin Perinatol. 2012;39:221-38.
26. Osborn DA, Evans N, Kluckow M. Clinical detection of low upper body blood flow in very premature infants using blood pressure, capillary refill time, and central-peripheral temperature difference. ADC Fetal Neonatal Ed. 2004;89:F168-73.
27. Saini SS, Kumar P, Kumar RM. Hemodynamic changes in preterm neonates with septic shock: a prospective observational study. Pediatr Crit Care Med. 2014;15:443-50.
28. Seri I, Noori S. Diagnosis and treatment of neonatal hypotension outside the transitional period. Early Hum Dev. 2005;81:405-11.
29. Seri I. Management of hypotension and low systemic blood flow in the very low birth weight neonate during the first postnatal week. J Perinatol. 2006;26:S8-13;discussion S22-3.
30. Shah BA, Padbury JF. Neonatal Sepsis: an old problem with new insights. Virulence. 2014;5:170-8.
31. Singh Y, Katheria AC, Vora F. Advances in Diagnosis and Management of Hemodynamic Instability in Neonatal Shock. Front Pediatr. 2018;6:2.
32. Watterberg K. Evidence-based neonatal pharmacotherapy: postnatal corticosteroids. Clin Perinatol. 2012;39:47-59.
33. Wong J, Shah P, Yoon E, Yee W, Lee S, Dow K. Inotrope use among extremely preterm infants in Canadian Neonatal Intensive Care Units: variation and outcomes. Am J Perinatol 2015;32:9-14.
34. Wynn JL, Wong HR. Pathophysiology and treatment of septic shock in neonates. Clin Perinatol. 2010;37:439-79.

Anemia in Neonate

Nandkishor S Kabra

INTRODUCTION

Anemia is one of the most common hematological abnormalities in newborn. Normal erythropoiesis in newborns is influenced by several factors, especially erythropoietin. Erythropoietin stimulates maturation of red blood cell (RBC) precursors.

It is defined as a hemoglobin or hematocrit value that is >2 standard deviations below the mean for age **(Tables 1 and 2)**.

TABLE 1: Normal hematological values in full term infants.

	Hb (g/dL)	*PCV (%)*	*Reticulocyte count (%)*
Age (days)			
1	19.0 ± 2.2	61 ± 7	3.2 ± 1.4
2	19.0 ± 1.9	60 ± 6	3.2 ± 1.3
3	18.7 ± 3.4	62 ± 9	2.8 ± 1.7
4	18.6 ± 2.1	57 ± 8	1.8 ± 1.1
5	17.6 ± 1.1	57 ± 7	1.2 ± 0.2
6	17.4 ± 2.2	54 ± 7	0.6 ± 0.2
7	17.9 ± 2.5	56 ± 9	0.5 ± 0.4
Age (weeks)			
1–2	17.3 ± 2.3	54 ± 8	0.5 ± 0.3
2–3	15.6 ± 2.6	46 ± 7	0.8 ± 0.6
3–4	14.2 ± 2.1	43 ± 6	0.6 ± 0.3
4–5	12.7 ± 1.6	36 ± 5	0.9 ± 0.8
5–6	11.9 ± 1.5	36 ± 6	1.0 ± 0.7

(Hb: hemoglobin; PCV: packed cell volume)

ETIOLOGY

Three general causes include blood loss, increased RBC destruction, and decreased RBC production.

1. *Blood loss, the most common cause of neonatal anemia, includes:*
   - *Obstetrical causes:* Placental abruption, placenta previa, trauma to placenta or umbilical cord during delivery, and rupture of anomalous placental vessels
   - *Fetomaternal transfusion:* 8% of normal pregnancies have some admixture
   - Fetoplacental transfusion due to positioning of infant above level of placenta after delivery and partial cord occlusion (e.g., with nuchal or prolapsed cord).
   - *Twin-twin transfusion:* Occurs only with monochorionic (i.e., monozygotic) twins and when there are placental vessels which allow shunting of blood from one twin to the other. Donor will have anemia of variable severity and recipient will have polycythemia of variable severity.
   - Internal hemorrhage such as intracranial hemorrhage (ICH), intraventricular periventricular hemorrhage, subgaleal hemorrhage, cephalohematoma, adrenal hemorrhage, subcapsular hematoma of liver, or ruptured viscus (e.g., spleen)
   - Iatrogenic blood loss secondary to sampling of blood for laboratory tests. This is the most common cause of anemia (and transfusion) in small premature infants.
2. *Increased RBC destruction:*
   - *Intrinsic causes:* Hereditary RBC disorders (rare), including RBC enzyme defects [e.g., glucose-6-phosphate dehydrogenase (G6PD) deficiency, hexokinase deficiency, and pyruvate kinase deficiency], RBC membrane defects (e.g., hereditary spherocytosis, elliptocytosis, and stomatocytosis), and hemoglobinopathies (e.g., α-thalassemia)
   - *Extrinsic causes:* Immune hemolysis (Rh incompatibility, ABO incompatibility, and minor blood group incompatibility, e.g., Kell and Duffy)

TABLE 2: Normal hemoglobin levels (g/dL) in preterms.

	Postnatal age (weeks)				
Birth weight (g)	*2*	*4*	*6*	*8*	*10*
800–1,000	16.0 (14.8–17.2)	10.0 (16.8–13.2)	8.7 (7.0–10.2)	8.0 (7.1–9.8)	8.0 (6.9–10.2)
1,001–1,200	16.4 (14.1–18.7)	12.8 (7.8–15.3)	10.5 (7.2–12.3)	9.1 (7.8–10.4)	8.5 (7.0–10.0)
1,201–1,400	16.2 (13.6–18.8)	13.4 (8.8–16.2)	10.9 (8.5–13.3)	9.9 (8.0–11.8)	9.8 (8.4–11.3)
1,401–1,500	15.6 (13.4–17.8)	11.7 (9.7–13.7)	10.5 (9.1–11.9)	9.8 (8.4–12.0)	9.9 (8.4–11.4)
1,501–2,000	15.6 (13.5–17.7)	11.0 (9.6–14.0)	9.6 (8.8–11.5)	9.8 (8.4–12.0)	10.1 (8.6–11.8)

- *Acquired hemolysis:* Infection, disseminated intravascular coagulation, and drugs.

3. *Decreased RBC production:*
   - Anemia of prematurity due to transient deficiency of erythropoietin
   - Aplastic or hypoplastic anemia (e.g., Diamond-Blackfan)
   - Bone marrow suppression (e.g., with rubella or parvovirus B19 infection)
   - Nutritional anemia (e.g., iron deficiency), usually after neonatal period.

CLINICAL PEARL

Anemia in neonates is the most common hematologic abnormality.

CLINICAL FINDINGS

This will vary with the severity of anemia and other associated conditions. The major physiologic impact of anemia is decreased oxygen delivery to tissues, resulting in compensatory responses and acute/chronic consequences. There may be no signs with mild anemia. With more severe anemia, examination findings include pallor, tachycardia, tachypnea, apnea, increase in oxygen requirements, lethargy, poor feeding, hepatosplenomegaly (hemolytic disease), jaundice, wide pulse pressure, hypotension, and metabolic acidosis.

CLINICAL APPROACH

History

- *Family history:* Anemia, jaundice, gallstones, splenectomy, and ethnicity
- *Maternal history:* Anemia, blood group and Rh type, blood or blood product transfusions, viral exanthematous illness during pregnancy, per vaginal bleeding, and multiple gestation: twin-to-twin transfusion, type of delivery (instrumental), and complications of labor and delivery
- *Neonatal history:* Age at onset, physical findings, and to know the cause of anemia **(Table 3)**

Physical Examination

- Look for cephalohematoma, subgaleal hemorrhage, petechiae, and overt bleeding from gastrointestinal tract and umbilical cord
- *Pallor with prolong capillary refill time:* Tachycardia, hypotension, and acute blood loss
- *Pallor without signs of decompensation:* Chronic blood loss
- *Pallor, jaundice, and hepatosplenomegaly:* Chronic hemolysis
- Failure to thrive may be a manifestation of chronic anemia
- *Examination of placenta:* For evidence of hematoma, retroplacental clots, infection, and arteriovenous anastomosis in monochorionic placenta.

CLINICAL PEARL

A systemic approach is required to identify exact cause of anemia and a protocol base management is must to correct it.

INVESTIGATIONS (FLOWCHART 1)

- Complete hemogram with peripheral smear and reticulocyte count and RBC indices
- Blood group and direct Coombs test
- *Serum bilirubin:* Increased levels of indirect bilirubin suggestive of chronic hemolysis
- *Kleihauer–Betke test of mother's blood:* Estimation of fetal blood lost into maternal circulation can be made by using the formula 2,400 × fetal/maternal cells = mL of fetal blood, e.g., 1/600 red cells in mother's

TABLE 3: Classification of anemia in the newborn.

Reticulocyte count	*Bilirubin*	*Coombs test*	*RBC morphology*	*Diagnostic possibilities*
Normal or low	Normal	Negative	Normal	Physiologic anemia of infancy or prematurity; congenital hypoplastic anemia; other causes of decreased production
Normal or high	Normal	Negative	Normal	Acute hemorrhage (fetomaternal, placental, umbilical cord, or internal hemorrhage)
High	High	Positive	• Hypochromic microcytes • Spherocytes	• Chronic fetomaternal hemorrhage • Immune hemolysis (blood group incompatibility or maternal autoantibody)
Normal or high	High	Negative	• Spherocytes • Elliptocytes • Hypochromic microcytes • Spiculated RBCs • Schistocytes and RBC fragments • Bite cells (Heinz bodies with supravital stain) • Normal	• Hereditary spherocytosis • Hereditary elliptocytosis • α- or γ-thalassemia syndrome • Pyruvate kinase deficiency • Disseminated intravascular coagulation; other microangiopathic processes • Glucose-6-phosphate dehydrogenase deficiency • Infections; enclosed hemorrhage (cephalohematoma)

(RBC: red blood cell)

Source: Christou HA. Anemia. In: Cloherty JP, Eichenwald EC, Hanson AR, Stark AR (Eds). Manual of Neonatal Care, 7th edition. (South Asian Edition). Philadelphia: Wolters Kluwer; 2012. pp. 563-71.

Flowchart 1: Approach to anemia in newborn.

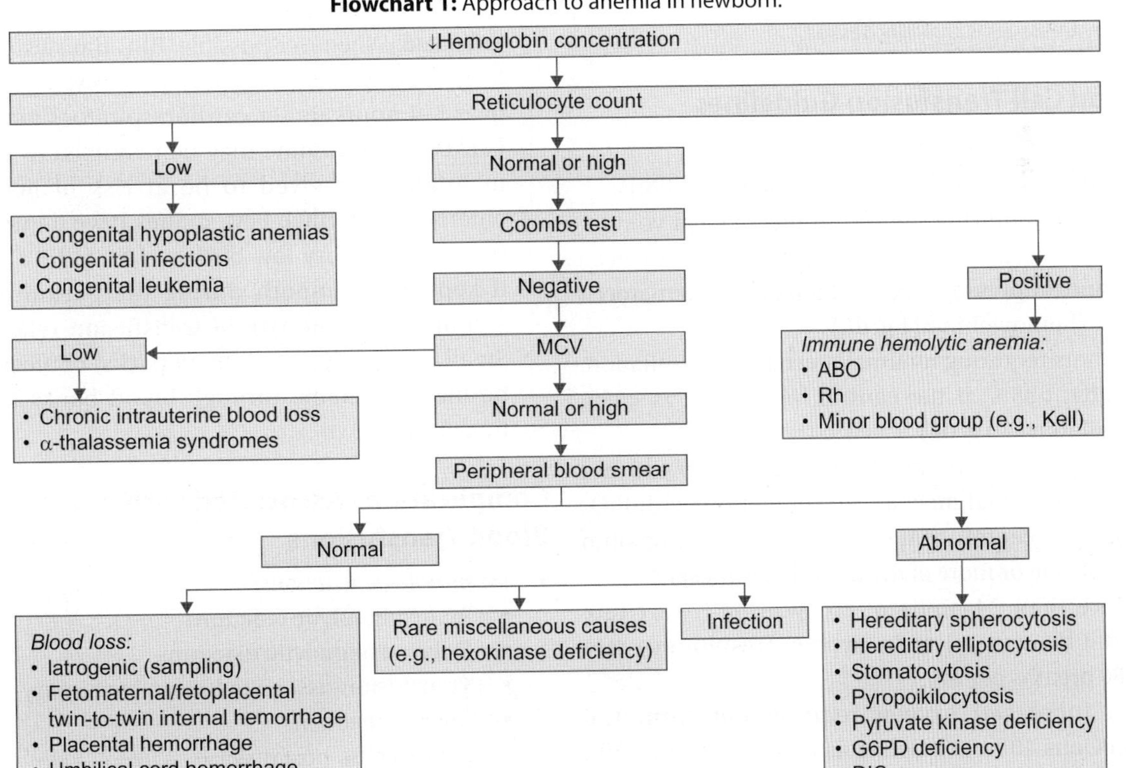

(DIC: disseminated intravascular coagulation; G6PD: glucose-6-phosphate dehydrogenase; MCV: mean corpuscular volume)

circulation is fetal, then 2,400 × 1/600 = 4 mL of fetal blood in maternal circulation

- Thick and thin peripheral smear for malarial parasites
- Urine for hematuria
- Stool for occult blood
- *TORCH screen (toxoplasma, other agents, rubella, cytomegalovirus, and herpes simplex virus,):* Baby and mother
- Ultrasound skull for evidence of ICH/intraventricular hemorrhage
- Test for G6PD deficiency
- Bone marrow examination, if indicated.

MANAGEMENT

- *Fluid resuscitation:* Normal saline push followed by packed cell transfusion: acute blood loss
- Treat the underlying cause, e.g., treatment of sepsis and toxoplasmosis
- *Iron therapy:* 6 mg/kg/day for 3 months: chronic blood loss.

CLINICAL PEARL

In preterm and term infants, packed RBCs transfusion should be considered if an immediate need for increased oxygen delivery to tissues is clinically desired.

Red Blood Cell Transfusion Guidelines for Premature Infants

Consider RBC transfusions in the following conditions:

- For infants requiring significant mechanical ventilation, defined as fraction of inspired oxygen (FiO_2) >40% and/or pressor support if the central hematocrit is <40% (hemoglobin <11 g/dL)
- For infants requiring minimal mechanical ventilation, with FiO_2 >35%, if the central hematocrit is <35% (hemoglobin <10 g/dL)
- For infants on supplemental oxygen who are not requiring minimal mechanical ventilation, with FiO_2 <25%, if the central hematocrit is >25% (hemoglobin <8 g/dL), one or more of the following is present:
  - More than 24 hours of tachycardia (heart rate >180 beats/min) or tachypnea (respiratory rate >80 breaths per min)
  - An increased oxygen requirement from the previous 48 hours, define as greater than fourfold increase in nasal cannula flow (i.e., 0.25–1 L/min) or an increase in nasal continuous positive airway pressure (CPAP) >20% from the previous 48 hours (i.e., 5–6 cmH_2O)
  - Weight gain <10 g/kg/day over the previous 4 days while receiving >100 kcal/kg/day
  - An increase in the number or severity of apnea and bradycardia (in general >10 spells or >3 spells requiring bag and mask ventilation; however, absolute number is up to individual interpretation)
  - Infant undergoing surgery
- For infants without any symptoms, if the central hematocrit is <20% hemoglobin (<7 g/dL) and the absolute reticulocyte count is <3%
- For infants with a cumulative blood loss of 10% or more of blood volume in a 72-hour period when the infant has significant cardiorespiratory illness, if further blood sampling is anticipated. Stable infants are not transfused only to replace blood lost through phlebotomy. If an erythrocyte transfusion is not given, "blood out" may be replaced mL for mL with 0.9% saline when 10–15 mL of blood per kg body weight is reached, in order to avoid hypovolemia. In addition to the saline used for the above indication, clinicians may administer additional albumin, fresh frozen plasma, platelet transfusions as they deem clinically indicated. Whenever possible, RBC transfusion should be given as 10–20 mL/kg, intravenously, infused slowly over 3–4 hours under cardiorespiratory monitoring. Packed RBCs volume may be restricted to 10 mL/kg in infants perceived to be at risk of necrotizing enterocolitis (NEC). Few studies have demonstrated that preterm very low birth weight (VLBW) infants, if kept nil by mouth during the period of transfusion reduce the risk of transfusion related NEC. Small packs (triple and penta packs) of blood should be made available through blood banks for blood transfusion.

Complications Associated with Blood Transfusions

- *Immunologic reactions:*
  - Acute hemolytic reactions
  - Delayed hemolytic reactions
  - Transfusion-associated acute lung injury
  - Allergic reactions
  - Graft-versus-host disease
- *Infections:* Human immunodeficiency virus, hepatitis B and C, cytomegalovirus, malaria, and syphilis

- Volume overload
- Transfusion-related acute gut injury in premature infants
- Hypocalcemia
- Transfusion with adult packed RBCs may theoretically increase the release of oxygen and may cause hyper-oxemia and toxicity
- Hypothermia, if large quantity of cold blood is used.

Prevention of Anemia of Prematurity

- *Maintain record of phlebotomy losses:* Transfuse the babies to replace phlebotomy losses, if exceeding 10% of blood volume in 72 hours (only in babies with significant cardiorespiratory illness)
- *Prophylactic iron therapy:*
    - Babies <1,500 g = 3–4 mg/kg/day starting at 2 weeks of life
    - Babies >1,500 g = 2–3 mg/kg/day starting at 2 weeks of life

CLINICAL PEARL

- Delay the cord clamping at birth in preterm infants to improve hemoglobin levels and reduce future transfusion needs.

- *Use of recombinant human erythropoietin (rhEPO):*
    - *Indication:* Prevention of anemia of prematurity in VLBW infants
    - *Dose:* 100–300 IU/kg/dose subcutaneously on alternate day for 6 weeks (start at 2 weeks of age)
    - Supplement with iron (6 mg/kg/day)
    - In exclusively breastfed preterm infants, vitamin E supplementation is not indicated.

AREAS OF UNCERTAINTY

- When infants are transfused at lower hemoglobin values for the gestational age, postnatal age, and the need for assisted respiratory support (oxygen, CPAP, and mechanical ventilation), it is considered as a restricted transfusion approach. The use of restrictive as compared to liberal hemoglobin thresholds in VLBW infants results in modest reductions in exposure to transfusion and in hemoglobin levels. Restrictive practice does not appear to have a significant impact on death or major morbidities at first hospital discharge or at follow-up. However, given the uncertainties of these conclusions, it would be prudent to avoid hemoglobin levels below the lower limits tested in clinical studies
- Early administration of erythropoiesis-stimulating agents (such as rhEPO) can modestly reduce the need for RBCs transfusions, the volume of RBCs transfused, and the number of donors an infant is exposed to. However, these reductions are generally considered clinically insignificant.

KEY POINTS

- Anemia in neonates is the most common hematologic abnormality.
- Causes of anemia include blood loss, increased red blood cell (RBC) destruction, and decreased RBC production.
- While investigating a newborn with anemia, a systematic approach as depicted in **Flowchart 1** is desirable.
- Delay the cord clamping at birth in preterm infants to improve hemoglobin levels and reduce future transfusion needs.
- Use laboratory tests judiciously.
- Monitor phlebotomy losses.
- Start oral iron therapy in preterm infants by 2 weeks of age as infant is established on full enteral feeds.
- Consider for erythropoietin therapy from first week of life in extremely low birth weight infants.
- In preterm and term infants, packed RBCs transfusion should be considered if an immediate need for increased oxygen delivery to tissues is clinically desired.

SUGGESTED READING

1. Aher SM, Ohlsson A. Early versus late erythropoietin for preventing red blood cell transfusion in preterm and/or low birth weight infants. Cochrane Database Syst Rev. 2020;2(2):CD004865.
2. Aher SM, Ohlsson A. Late erythropoiesis-stimulating agents to prevent red blood cell transfusion in preterm or low birth weight infants. Cochrane Database Syst Rev. 2020;1(1):CD004868.
3. Angelidou AI, Christou HA. Anemia. In: Eichenwald EC, Hanson AR, Martin CR, Stark AR (Eds). Cloherty and Stark's Manual of Neonatal Care, South Asian Edition (adaptation of 8th edition), Gurgaon: Wolters Kluwer Health (India); 2021. pp. 635-45.
4. Calberg K. Neonatal erythrocyte disorders. In: Gleason CA, Sawyer T (Eds). Avery's Diseases of the Newborn, 11th edition. Philadelphia: Elsevier; 2024. pp. 996-1024.
5. Dror Y, Chan AKC, Baker JM, Avila ML. Hematology. In: McDonald MG, Seshia MMK (Eds). Avery's Neonatology, Pathophysiology and Management of the Newborn, 7th edition. Philadelphia: Wolters Kluwer; 2016. pp. 872-930.
6. Franz AR, Engel C, Bassler D, Rüdiger M, Thome UH, Maier RF, et al; ETTNO Investigators. Effects of Liberal

vs Restrictive Transfusion Thresholds on Survival and Neurocognitive Outcomes in Extremely Low-Birth-Weight Infants: The ETTNO Randomized Clinical Trial. JAMA. 2020;324(6):560-70.

7. Houben NAM, Fustolo-Gunnink S, Fijnvandraat K, Caram-Deelder C, Carrascosa MA, Beuchée A, et al; International Neonatal Transfusion Point Prevalence Study Group. Red Blood Cell Transfusion in European Neonatal Intensive Care Units, 2022 to 2023. JAMA Netw Open. 2024;7(9): e2434077.
8. Juul SE, Vu PT, Comstock BA, Wadhawan R, Mayock DE, Courtney SE, Robinson T, et al; Preterm Erythropoietin Neuroprotection Trial Consortium. Effect of High-Dose Erythropoietin on Blood Transfusions in Extremely Low Gestational Age Neonates: Post Hoc Analysis of a Randomized Clinical Trial. JAMA Pediatr. 2020;174(10): 933-43.
9. Keir AK, Wilkinson D, Andersen C, Stark MJ. Washed versus unwashed red blood cells for transfusion for the prevention of morbidity and mortality in preterm infants. Cochrane Database Syst Rev. 2016;2016(1): CD011484.
10. Kirpalani H, Whyte RK, Andersen C, Asztalos EV, Heddle N, Blajchman MA, et al. The Premature Infants in Need of Transfusion (PINT) study: a randomized, controlled trial of a restrictive (low) versus liberal (high) transfusion threshold for extremely low birth weight infants. J Pediatr. 2006;149:301-07.
11. Kirpalani H, Bell EF, Hintz SR, Tan S, Schmidt B, Chaudhary AS, et al; Eunice Kennedy Shriver NICHD Neonatal Research Network. Higher or Lower Hemoglobin Transfusion Thresholds for Preterm Infants. N Engl J Med. 2020;383(27):2639-51.
12. Ohlsson A, Aher SM. Early erythropoiesis-stimulating agents in preterm or low birth weight infants. Cochrane Database Syst Rev. 2020;2(2):CD004863.
13. Paul DA, Leef KH, Locke RG, Stefano JL. Transfusion volume in infants with very low birth weight: a randomized trial of 10 versus 20 ml/kg. J Pediatr Hematol Oncol. 2002; 24:43-6.
14. Whyte R, Kirpalani H. Low versus high haemoglobin concentration threshold for blood transfusion for preventing morbidity and mortality in very low birth weight infants. Cochrane Database Syst Rev. 2011;(11):CD000512.

Coagulation and Bleeding Disorders in the Neonate

Deepak Chawla

INTRODUCTION

Bleeding is an alarming symptom at any age, more so in a young infant. Loss of blood from intravascular space may manifest as overt bleeding like upper or lower gastrointestinal bleeding or pulmonary hemorrhage or as covert bleeding like intracranial hemorrhage. In addition, a neonate may manifest bleeding tendency by development of facial purpura after birth, prolonged bleeding from venipuncture sites and oozing from umbilical cord. Objective of this chapter is to delineate an approach to diagnose underlying cause and plan treatment of a bleeding neonate.

HEMOSTASIS IN NEONATE

Knowledge of components of hemostatic system and their physiological variation in term and preterm neonates is essential to develop understanding of causes of bleeding and to correctly interpret results of laboratory investigations. Components of hemostatic system include procoagulant factors, inhibitors of coagulation, fibrinolytic system, platelets, and endothelium **(Flowchart 1)**. In neonates, there is decreased activity of procoagulant system which is balanced by decreased activity of coagulation inhibitors and fibrinolytic system so that a healthy term neonate does not develop bleeding or thrombosis despite passing through birth canal and undergoing postnatal extracellular fluid constriction **(Table 1)**.

CLINICAL PEARL

- Laboratory values of coagulant factors in neonates should be based on gestation- and postnatal-age-based reference values.

CAUSES OF BLEEDING IN NEONATES

Bleeding in neonates may result from decreased number or function of platelets and specific deficiencies of coagulation factors **(Table 2)**. Some systemic disorders can cause more widespread disturbance in hemostatic mechanism.

CLINICAL PEARL

- Pregnancy complications are the most common underlying cause of early-onset thrombocytopenia. Systemic infections are most common underlying cause of late-onset thrombocytopenia.

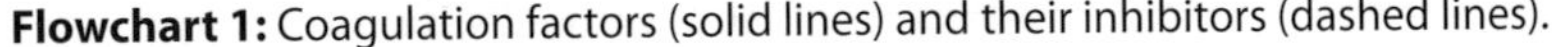

Flowchart 1: Coagulation factors (solid lines) and their inhibitors (dashed lines).

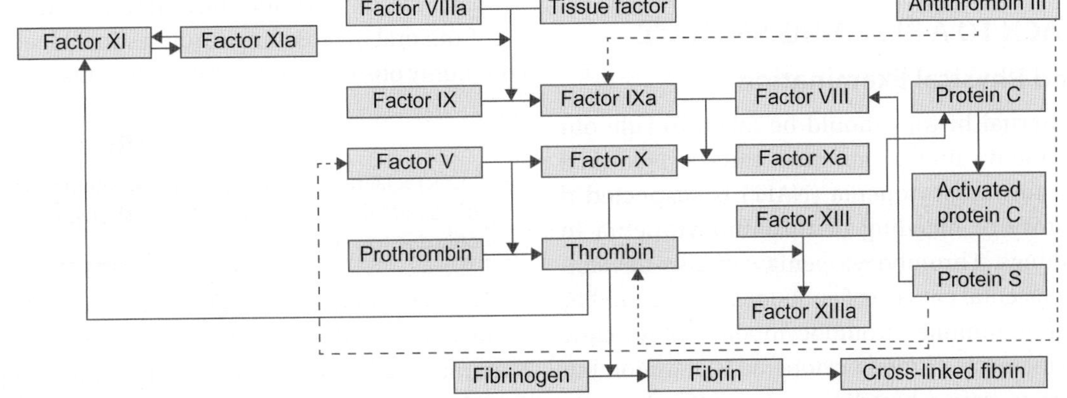

TABLE 1: Hemostatic system in a neonate in comparison to adults.

Component of hemostatic system	*Alteration*
Platelets	• Platelet count comparable to adults • Smaller and more immature megakaryocytes • Lower thrombopoietin levels in thrombocytopenic neonates
Fibrinogen, factor V and factor VIII	Comparable to adults
von Willebrand factor	Increased
Other coagulation factors	Decreased (by 50% as compared to adults)
Antithrombin III, protein C and protein S	Decreased
Plasminogen	Decreased

TABLE 2: Common causes of bleeding in neonates.

Platelets	*Coagulation factors*
Early onset (within 72 h of birth): • Pregnancy complications (gestational hypertension, intrauterine growth restriction) • Early onset sepsis • Neonatal alloimmune thrombocytopenia • Neonatal autoimmune thrombocytopenia • TORCH infections *Late onset (after 72 h of birth):* • Late-onset sepsis • Necrotizing enterocolitis • TORCH infections	• Vitamin K deficiency – Early (within 24 h) – Classical (24 h to 7 days) – Late (2–12 weeks) • Hemophilia A (classical hemophilia due to factor VIII deficiency) • Hemophilia B (factor IX deficiency) • Disseminated intra-vascular coagulation • Liver disease

[TORCH: toxoplasmosis, other (syphilis, varicella zoster, parvovirus B19), rubella, cytomegalovirus, and herpes infections]

APPROACH TO A BLEEDING NEONATE

History and Physical Examination

Detailed maternal history should be taken to rule out thrombocytopenia due to immune causes. Neonatal alloimmune thrombocytopenia (NAIT) is suspected if there is history of bleeding or thrombocytopenia in previous siblings. Thrombocytopenia can also develop due to transplacental passage of antibodies from a mother affected by autoimmune thrombocytopenia or systemic lupus erythematosus. Thrombocytopenia is common but rarely severe to cause bleeding in neonates born to pregnancies complicated by gestational hypertension, intrauterine growth restriction, or hemolysis, elevated liver enzyme levels, and a low platelet count (HELLP) syndrome. History must be sought for systemic disorders which can cause disseminated intravascular coagulation like birth asphyxia and neonatal sepsis. Inherited deficiencies of coagulation factors can be suspected if parents have a consanguineous marriage, or previous siblings are affected. Hemophilia A and B are X-linked recessive disorders while von Willebrand factor deficiency can be autosomal dominant or recessive. Presence of skeletal abnormalities like absent thumb or absent radius bone indicates Fanconi anemia or thrombocytopenia absent radius syndrome. Chromosomal disorders like trisomy 13, 18, or 21 can be associated with thrombocytopenia.

CLINICAL PEARL

- Detailed family history should be taken to rule out inherited or maternal causes of bleeding in a neonate.

Gestation at birth, age at onset of bleeding, and site of bleeding can indicate underlying cause. Bleeding in an otherwise healthy term or late preterm neonate indicates either coagulation factor deficiency or NAIT. Early-onset thrombocytopenia (within 72 h of birth) in a preterm neonate is most commonly due to maternal illness while late-onset thrombocytopenia (after 72 h of birth) is most commonly due to sepsis or necrotizing enterocolitis. Intracranial bleed without significant birth trauma indicates presence of underlying bleeding disorder. Subdural hemorrhage is more common with hemophilia while intraparenchymal bleed is more common with thrombocytopenia (e.g., NAIT). Other common sites of bleeding in coagulation factor deficiency include oozing from umbilical stump, prolonged bleeding from venipuncture or heel stick sites, large caput succedaneum, or large cephalhematoma without birth trauma. Mucosal bleeds, e.g., from oral mucosa or gastrointestinal bleeds, are more commonly observed in thrombocytopenia.

CLINICAL PEARL

- Intracranial bleed in a term neonate should raise suspicion of coagulation dysfunction. Mucosal bleed is most commonly due to platelet disorders.

History should be sought about maternal intake of medications and administration of vitamin K at birth. Maternal intake of antitubercular or antiepileptic drugs may be associated with development of early-onset vitamin K deficiency bleeding (VKDB) which presents within first 24 hours of birth. Neonates not receiving the recommended dose of vitamin K at birth may develop classical (24 h to 7 days after birth) or late onset (2–12 weeks) VKDB.

Laboratory Investigations

Essential laboratory investigations that should be done in neonates with bleeding include platelet count, prothrombin time (PT), activated partial thromboplastin time (aPTT), and fibrinogen levels **(Flowchart 2)**. Prothrombin time is prolonged in deficiency of vitamin K-dependent coagulation factors (II, VII, IX, and X). Activated partial thromboplastin time is prolonged in deficiency of vitamin K-dependent coagulation factors and deficiency of contact factors (XI, XII, prekallikrein, and high molecular weight kininogen). If PT, aPTT, and platelets counts are normal, bleeding may occur because of decreased factor XIII, α2-antiplasmin activity, or abnormal platelet functions. In a sick neonate, more widespread derangement of the laboratory markers indicates decreased synthesis due to liver disorder or consumption coagulopathy.

CLINICAL PEARL

- Initial workup in a bleeding neonate should include platelet count, prothrombin time, activated partial thromboplastin time, and fibrinogen levels.

Specific factor assay can be done on clinical suspicion. However, results need to be interpreted carefully in view of altered levels in neonates. Levels of factor VIII are comparable to adults. Therefore, classical hemophilia can be diagnosed in neonates. On the other hand, levels of factor IX are about 15% of the adult level and, therefore, hemophilia B can be diagnosed only by 6–12 months of age when levels reach the adult range. Prothrombin time and aPTT are influenced by ratio of blood and citrate in the sample; therefore, care must be taken while withdrawing the sample.

Additional laboratory investigations may be warranted as per clinical suspicion. For example, severe early onset thrombocytopenia (platelet count <50,000/μL) in a preterm neonate may be because of congenital infections for which appropriate diagnostic test should be done. Conversely, mild early onset transient thrombocytopenia in a small-for-gestation neonate may be because of gestational hypertension in mother and no further investigations are needed.

MANAGEMENT

Thrombocytopenia

Management of thrombocytopenia consists of treating underlying cause and if needed giving platelet transfusion. Due to its propensity to cause severe thrombocytopenia and serious bleeding, NAIT must be differentiated from other causes of perinatal thrombocytopenia. NAIT must be suspected if all of the following are present: (1) platelet count below 50,000/μL, (2) intracranial hemorrhage in a baby weighing >2,200 g without birth asphyxia and documented fetal or neonatal bleeding, and (3) no additional neonatal disorder. In case of NAIT, platelet transfusion is indicated if platelet counts are below 30,000/μL. In case of active bleeding, platelet transfusion can be given if platelet count is below 50,000/μL and in case of ICH below 100,000/μL. If available, single donor platelets (SDP) that are human platelet antigen compatible with

Flowchart 2: Laboratory investigations in a bleeding neonate.

Bleeding neonate → Healthy / Sick

	Healthy					Sick	
Investigations	**Immune/ congenital thrombocytopenia**	**Vitamin K deficiency**	**Hemophilia**	**Factor VII deficiency**	**Factor XIII deficiency**	**Liver disease**	**DIC**
Platelets count	↓	Normal	Normal	Normal	Normal	Normal	↓
PT	Normal	↑	Normal	↑	Normal	↑	↑
APTT	Normal	↑	↑	Normal	Normal	↑	↑
Fibrinogen	Normal	Normal	Normal	Normal	Normal	Normal/↓	↓

(PT: prothrombin time; APTT: activated partial thromboplastin time; DIC: disseminated intravascular coagulation)

the neonate are preferred. If these are not available without delay, random donor platelets can be transfused. Administration of intravenous immunoglobulin (1 g/kg for 2 days) may increase platelet count in immune thrombocytopenia. Platelet counts need to be monitored for first 2 weeks after birth. Neonatal autoimmune thrombocytopenia associated with maternal autoimmune thrombocytopenia is less severe, rarely associated with intracranial hemorrhage and can be monitored while it undergoes self-resolution. Platelet transfusion and IVIG can be considered if platelet count is below 30,000/μL.

Due to lack of demonstrable efficacy in preventing serious hemorrhages, threshold platelet count below which platelet transfusion is given has become more stringent with time. Most of neonates with platelet count above 20,000/μL will not develop a serious bleed. Therefore, this cutoff may be used in otherwise healthy neonates with thrombocytopenia. Higher cutoff of 30,000/μL may be used in neonates at higher risk of bleeding which include extremely low birthweight neonates in their 1st week after birth, unstable blood pressure records, previously existing grade 3 or 4 intraventricular hemorrhage, current minor bleeds, coexisting coagulopathy or before exchange transfusion or surgery. In case of active major bleeding, platelet count may be maintained above 50,000/μL. Platelets can be obtained by pooling from multiple donors (platelet concentrate) or by apheresis from a single donor.

CLINICAL PEARL

- Platelet count should be maintained above 50,000/μL in a neonate with active bleeding and above 30,000/μL in a neonate without active bleeding.

Coagulopathy

Vitamin K deficiency can be treated by administration of vitamin K by subcutaneous or intravenous route. Effect of parenteral vitamin K starts within 4 hours. In case of active bleeding, fresh frozen plasma (FFP) can be administered.

In case of classical hemophilia, treatment of choice is administration of factor VIII concentrate. If not available, cryoprecipitate or FFP can be given. Dose of cryoprecipitate is 2 mL/kg or 1 unit/7 kg. Fresh frozen plasma can be administered in a dose of 10–20 mL/kg. Specific deficiencies of other coagulation factors are rare and can be managed by administration of cryoprecipitate or FFP.

Fresh frozen plasma can be given in neonates with coagulopathy due to disseminated intravascular coagulation (DIC) or liver failure as multiple coagulation factors are deficient, for management of a congenital clotting factor deficiency if specific replacement is not available, to control active bleeding in vitamin K deficiency, prophylaxis of bleeding during an invasive procedure in a neonate with coexisting coagulopathy, and for reconstitution of blood for exchange transfusion. FFP should not be used for prevention of intraventricular hemorrhage, treatment of sepsis, partial exchange transfusion, or deranged coagulation profile without bleeding during therapeutic hypothermia.

Supportive and specific care for underlying systemic causes of bleeding like sepsis and NEC should be given.

KEY POINTS

- In neonates, coagulation cascade remains same as pediatric patients, while causes for bleeding differ. It involves factors related to maternal causes and intrapartum insults.
- Laboratory values of coagulation factors are different than adults.
- Platelet and component therapy should be used very judiciously. Clinical status need be considered while planning for the transfusions.

SUGGESTED READING

1. Bussel JB, Sola-Visner M. Current approaches to the evaluation and management of the fetus and neonate with immune thrombocytopenia. Semin Perinatol. 2009;33:35-42.
2. Moskowitz NP, Karpatkin M. Coagulation problems in the newborn. Curr Paediatr. 2005;15:50-6.
3. Motta M, Guaragni B. Evidence-based guidelines for administering fresh frozen plasma in the NICU. Hematology and Transfusion Medicine: Neonatology Questions and Controversies. Amsterdam: Elsevier; 2023. Chapter 14, pp. 171-84.
4. Poterjoy BS, Josephson CD. Platelets, frozen plasma, and cryoprecipitate: what is the clinical evidence for their use in the neonatal intensive care unit? Semin Perinatol. 2009;33:66-74.
5. Sola-Visner M. Platelets in the neonatal period: developmental differences in platelet production, function, and hemostasis and the potential impact of therapies. Hematology Am Soc Hematol Educ Program. 2012;2012:506-11.
6. te Pas AB, Lopriore E, van den Akker ES, Oepkes D, Kanhai HH, Brand A, et al. Postnatal management of fetal and neonatal alloimmune thrombocytopenia: the role of matched platelet transfusion and IVIG. Eur J Pediatr. 2007;166:1057-63.

Neonatal Hyperbilirubinemia (Unconjugated)

Poonam Sidana, Gaurav Mandhan, Gurleen Sikka

INTRODUCTION

Unconjugated neonatal hyperbilirubinemia (NNH) is one of the most common problems faced by pediatricians attending to neonates. Incidence is reported as 60% in term and around 80% in preterm neonates. Incidence and severity are inversely related to gestational age at birth. It is a benign condition which resolves by itself in most of the cases. Careful monitoring of all newborn infants and the application of appropriate treatments are essential, because high bilirubin concentrations can cause acute bilirubin encephalopathy and kernicterus **(Flowchart 1)**.

Flowchart 1: Flow diagram for infants during the birth hospitalization to determine postdischarge follow-up for infants who have not received phototherapy.

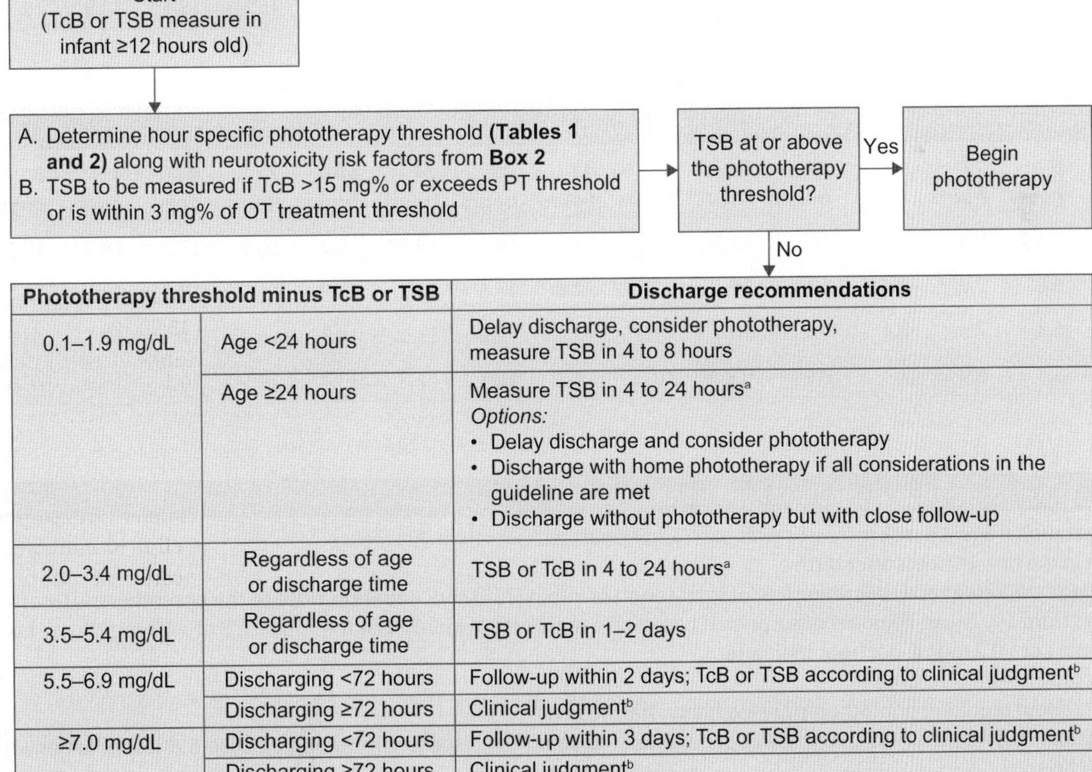

Phototherapy threshold minus TcB or TSB		Discharge recommendations
0.1–1.9 mg/dL	Age <24 hours	Delay discharge, consider phototherapy, measure TSB in 4 to 8 hours
	Age ≥24 hours	Measure TSB in 4 to 24 hours[a] *Options:* • Delay discharge and consider phototherapy • Discharge with home phototherapy if all considerations in the guideline are met • Discharge without phototherapy but with close follow-up
2.0–3.4 mg/dL	Regardless of age or discharge time	TSB or TcB in 4 to 24 hours[a]
3.5–5.4 mg/dL	Regardless of age or discharge time	TSB or TcB in 1–2 days
5.5–6.9 mg/dL	Discharging <72 hours	Follow-up within 2 days; TcB or TSB according to clinical judgment[b]
	Discharging ≥72 hours	Clinical judgment[b]
≥7.0 mg/dL	Discharging <72 hours	Follow-up within 3 days; TcB or TSB according to clinical judgment[b]
	Discharging ≥72 hours	Clinical judgment[b]

Note:

[a]Use clinical judgment and shared decision making to determine when to repeat the bilirubin measure within this 4–24-hour time window.

[b]Clinical judgment decisions should include physical examination, the presence of risk factors for the development of hyperbilirubinemia **(Box 1)** or hyperbilirubinemia neurotoxicity risk factors **(Box 2)**, feeding adequacy, weight trajectory and family support.

In 2022, the American Academy of Pediatrics (AAP) has revised its earlier guidelines for management of unconjugated hyperbilirubinemia for babies born at gestation of 35 weeks or more. It has made recommendations for primary prevention (e.g., maternal Rh typing and treatment) and secondary prevention (e.g., risk factor assessment and close monitoring for the development of hyperbilirubinemia, and, when necessary, treatment). The presence of hyperbilirubinemia neurotoxicity risk factors lowers the threshold for treatment with phototherapy and the level at which care should be escalated.

However for babies born at <35 weeks, National Institute for Health and Care Excellence (NICE) guidelines continue to be used for guiding treatment as no other guideline specifically addresses this population.

AAP guidelines have defined following risk factors for developing NNH **(Box 1)** and factors which can increase the risk of neurotoxicity **(Box 2)** as follows.

TABLE 1: Phototherapy thresholds, ≥35 weeks, without neurotoxicity risk factors (AAP, 2022).

	6 hours	*12 hours*	*18 hours*	*24 hours*	*30 hours*	*36 hours*	*42 hours*	*48 hours*	*54 hours*	*60 hours*	*72 hours*	*4 days*	*5 days*	*8 days*	*12 days*
≥40 weeks	10	11.1	12.2	13.3	14.3	15.3	16.2	17.1	17.8	18.5	19.8	21.8	21.8	21.8	21.8
39 weeks	9.5	10.6	11.8	12.8	13.8	14.8	15.7	16.6	17.4	18.1	19.5	21.5	21.7	21.7	21.7
38 weeks	9	10.1	11.2	12.3	13.3	14.2	15.1	16	16.8	17.5	18.8	20.8	20.9	21.2	21.7
37 weeks	8.4	9.5	10.7	11.8	12.6	13.6	14.5	15.4	16.2	16.9	18.1	20	20.2	20.4	20.9
36 weeks	7.9	9	10.2	11.2	12.2	13	14	14.8	15.5	16.2	17.5	19.4	19.5	19.8	20.1
35 weeks	7.3	8.5	9.7	10.6	11.5	12.5	13.4	14.2	14.9	15.6	16.8	18.5	18.8	19	19.4

TABLE 2: Phototherapy thresholds, ≥35 weeks, with neurotoxicity risk factors (AAP, 2022).

	6 hours	*12 hours*	*18 hours*	*24 hours*	*30 hours*	*36 hours*	*42 hours*	*48 hours*	*54 hours*	*60 hours*	*72 hours*	*4 days*	*5 days*	*8 days*	*12 days*
≥38 weeks	7.4	8.4	9.5	10.5	11.5	12.3	13.2	14	14.6	15.2	16.5	18.2	18.2	18.2	18.2
37 weeks	6.8	7.9	9	10	11	12	12.8	13.5	14.2	14.8	16	17.9	18	18.2	18.2
36 weeks	6.3	7.5	8.4	9.5	10.4	11.2	12	12.8	13.5	14.1	15.2	17	17.1	17.5	18
35 weeks	5.8	6.9	7.9	8.9	9.8	10.5	11.2	12.1	12.8	13.4	14.5	16.1	16.2	16.6	17.1

BOX 1: Risk factors for developing significant hyperbilirubinemia.

- Lower gestational age (i.e., risk increases with each additional week less than 40 weeks)
- Jaundice in the first 24 hours after birth
- Predischarge transcutaneous bilirubin (TcB) or total serum bilirubin (TSB) concentration close to the phototherapy threshold
- Hemolysis from any cause, if known or suspected based on a rapid rate of increase in the TSB or TcB of >0.3 mg/dL per hour in the first 24 hours or >0.2 mg/dL per hour thereafter
- Phototherapy before discharge
- Parent or sibling requiring phototherapy or exchange transfusion
- Family history or genetic ancestry suggestive of inherited red blood cell disorders, including glucose-6-phosphate dehydrogenase (G6PD) deficiency
- Exclusive breastfeeding with suboptimal intake
- Scalp hematoma or significant bruising
- Down syndrome
- Macrosomic infant of a diabetic mother

MANAGEMENT PLAN FOR A JAUNDICED NEONATE

- History and examination
- Serum bilirubin (TSB) level
- Risk assessment based on total TSB, history, and examination
- Physiological or pathological
- Investigate as needed **(Box 3)**
- Decide need to follow-up or intervene

MONITORING AND TREATMENT

In an ideal situation, treatment guidelines should be based on epidemiological data collected from a local population. In India, in view of paucity of any national database on neonatal jaundice, AAP guidelines (2022) for NNH management and NICE guidelines are being used in most centers depending upon gestation at birth. It is important to understand that use of these guidelines is primarily for deciding intervention and escalation of treatment. Monitoring frequency, stopping of phototherapy, and follow-up may have to be decided keeping in mind local factors like availability of TCB/TSB, financial issues, level and accessibility of healthcare facility.

BOX 2: Risk factors for neurotoxicity in hyperbilirubinemia.

- Gestational age <38 weeks, risk increases with decreasing gestation
- Albumin <3 g/dL
- Isoimmune hemolytic disease (positive DAT), G6PD deficiency or other hemolytic condition
- Sepsis
- Significant clinical instability in last 24 hours

BOX 3: Investigations.

The following investigations may be done, in the order of priority, depending on clinical evaluation:

- Serum bilirubin, total and conjugated, can use transcutaneous bilirubin if baby >35 weeks/>24 hours/not under phototherapy
- Blood group of the baby and the mother
- Direct Coombs test in Rh isoimmunized/ABO incompatibility
- Hemogram, reticulocyte count, peripheral smear for hemolysis/red blood cell morphology
- Glucose-6-phosphate dehydrogenase level in a male neonate in high prevalence areas
- Sepsis workup in sick neonate
- Thyroid profile
- Investigations for rare causes as applicable

Salient points of AAP guidelines 2022 are as follows:

1. For prevention of hyperbilirubinemia, effort should be made to do ABO an Rh typing of all antenatal mothers. Eligible mothers should be screened for anti-erythrocyte antibodies and managed appropriately. If mother not screened antenatally, blood group and DCT of the baby should be done on cord blood or soon after baby is born.
2. Support breastfeeding while providing treatment. There is no need to give water or dextrose to prevent jaundice. Supplementation with formula may be considered in selected cases with suboptimal breast-feeding, excessive weight loss and approaching treatment threshold.
3. Universal TcB (transcutaneous) or TSB (total serum bilirubin) is recommended between 24 and 48 hours or earlier if baby is being discharged.
4. TcB correlates well with TSB at TSB level <15 mg%
5. TSB needs to be done if TcB is within 3 mg% or higher than treatment threshold/age <24 hours/TcB >15 mg%
6. TSB is to be used for deciding the need for phototherapy, escalation of care or exchange transfusion and stopping treatment.
7. If more than one TcB or TSB levels are available, they can be used to check rate of rise and risk of requiring phototherapy.
8. Neonates requiring phototherapy should be given intensive phototherapy (*irradiance of at least 30 microwatt/cm^2/nm at a wavelength of around 475*)
9. TSB should be repeated within 12 hours of starting phototherapy based on clinical scenario.
10. Phototherapy can be stopped if TSB is 2 mg% below the hour specific threshold level at which treatment was started. Treatment could be prolonged if risk of rebound is high or postdischarge follow-up is uncertain.
11. After stopping treatment, TSB should be done between 24 and 48 hours depending upon the risk of rebound hyperbilirubinemia. TCB can be done if baby has been off phototherapy for 24 hours.
12. Care needs to be escalated if TSB is 2 mg% below exchange threshold which includes shifting the baby to neonatal intensive care unit (NICU) with facility to perform ET, intensive phototherapy, IV fluids, and get serum albumin, TSB , direct bilirubin levels and arrange blood for exchange transfusion. TSB needs to be repeated 2 hourly pending exchange transfusion till TSB is below escalation value **(Flowchart 2)**.

13. Urgent exchange transfusion should be performed if baby shows signs of acute bilirubin encephalopathy.
14. Intravenous immunoglobulin (IVIG) infusion in a dose of 0.5–1 g/kg over 2 hours may be used in babies with isoimmune hemolytic disease who reach or exceed escalation level and can be repeated after 12 hours.
15. In a neonate with TSB at exchange threshold level without any signs of bilirubin encephalopathy, if TSB drops to a level below exchange transfusion threshold while arranging for procedure, exchange transfusion may be deferred while continuing intensive phototherapy with TSB level every 2 hours till TSB reaches below escalation level **(Tables 3 to 6)**.
16. Prolonged indirect hyperbilirubinemia is suspected when TSB remains within 2 mg% of phototherapy levels after >7 days of age. This needs to be followed up and investigated further with appropriate tests as per clinical scenario.
17. For a breasted baby, if still icteric at 3–4 weeks or for a formula fed baby icteric at 2 weeks, TSB and direct bilirubin should be done to look for possible cholestasis. Review metabolic screen for any risk factors in this regard.

Flowchart 2: Approach to escalation of care. The escalation-of-care threshold is 2 mg/dL below the exchange transfusion threshold.

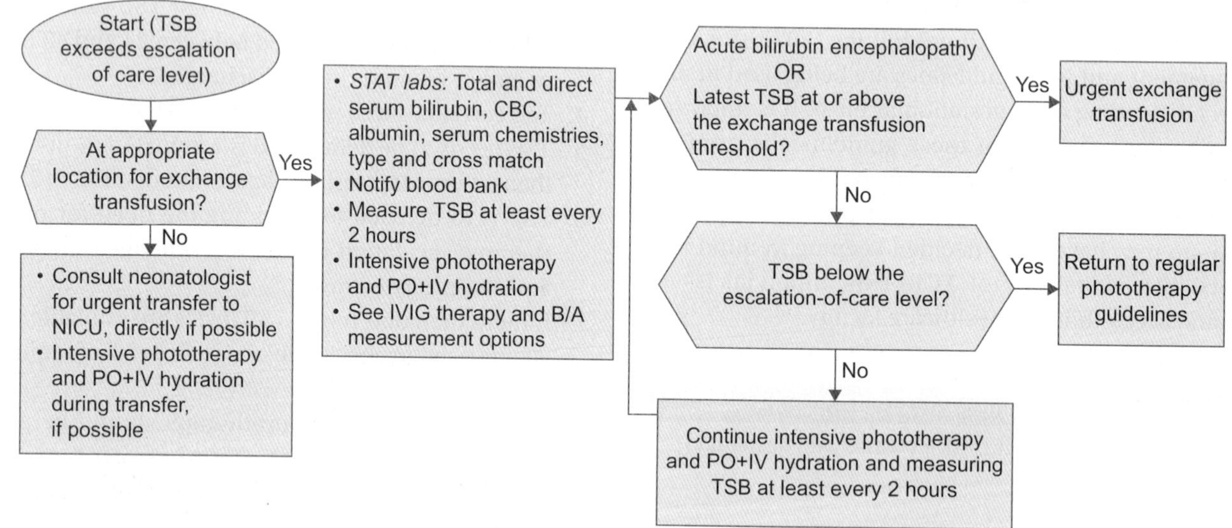

(IVIG: intravenous immunoglobulin; B/A: bilirubin to albumin ratio; NICU: neonatal intensive care unit; TSB: total serum bilirubin)

TABLE 3: Phototherapy thresholds for neonates <35 weeks (NICE, 2015).

	0 hour	*6 hours*	*12 hours*	*18 hours*	*24 hours*	*30 hours*	*36 hours*	*42 hours*	*48 hours*	*54 hours*	*60 hours*	*66 hours*	*≥72 hours*
34 weeks	2.3	3.2	4.4	5.6	6.1	7	8.2	8.8	10.2	11.1	12.3	13.2	14
33 weeks	2.3	3.2	4.1	5.3	6.1	7	7.9	8.8	9.6	10.5	11.7	12.6	13.5
32 weeks	2.3	3.2	4.1	5	5.8	6.7	7.6	8.5	9.4	10.2	11.1	12	12.9
31 weeks	2.3	3.2	4.1	4.7	5.8	6.4	7.3	8.2	9.1	9.9	10.8	11.4	12.3
30 weeks	2.3	2.9	4.1	4.7	5.6	6.1	7	7.9	8.5	9.4	10.2	11.1	11.7
29 weeks	2.3	3.2	3.8	4.4	5.3	6.1	6.7	7.6	8.2	9.1	9.9	11	11
28 weeks	2.3	2.9	3.8	4.4	5	5.8	6.4	7	7.9	8.5	9.4	9.9	11
27 weeks	2.3	2.9	3.5	4.1	4.7	5.6	6.1	6.7	7.6	8.2	8.8	9.4	9.9
26 weeks	2.3	4.9	3.5	4.1	4.7	5.3	5.8	6.4	7	7.6	8.2	8.8	9.4
25 weeks	2.3	2.9	3.4	3.9	4.5	5	5.6	6.1	6.6	7.2	7.7	8.2	8.8
24 weeks	2.3	2.8	3.3	3.8	4.3	4.8	5.3	5.8	6.2	6.7	7.2	7.7	8.2

TABLE 4: Exchange transfusion thresholds for neonates <35 weeks (NICE, 2015).

	0 hour	*6 hours*	*12 hours*	*18 hours*	*24 hours*	*30 hours*	*36 hours*	*42 hours*	*48 hours*	*54 hours*	*60 hours*	*66 hours*	*≥72 hours*
34 weeks	4.7	5.8	7	8.2	9.6	11.1	12.3	13.5	14.6	15.8	17.5	18.7	19.9
33 weeks	4.7	5.8	7	8.2	9.4	10.5	11.7	13.2	14.3	15.8	17	18.1	19.3
32 weeks	4.7	5.8	7	8.2	9.4	10.5	12.3	12.9	14	15.2	16.4	17.5	18.7
31 weeks	4.7	5.8	7	8.2	9.4	10.2	11.4	12.6	13.5	14	15.8	17	18.1
30 weeks	4.7	5.8	6.7	7.9	9.1	9.9	11.1	12.3	13.2	14.3	15.5	16.4	17.5
29 weeks	4.7	5.8	6.7	7.6	8.8	9.6	10.8	11.7	12.9	14	14.9	15.8	17
28 weeks	4.7	5.6	6.7	7.6	8.5	9.4	11	11	12	13	15	15	16
27 weeks	4.7	5.6	6.7	7.3	8.5	9.4	10	11	12	13	14	15	16
26 weeks	4.7	5.6	6.4	7.3	8.2	9.1	9.9	10.8	11.7	12.6	13.5	14.3	15.2
25 weeks	4.7	5.5	6.3	7.2	8	8.8	9.6	10.5	11.3	12.1	13	13.8	14.6
24 weeks	4.7	5.5	6.2	7	7.8	8.6	9.4	10.1	10.9	11.7	12.5	13.3	14

TABLE 5: Exchange transfusion thresholds, ≥35 weeks, without neurotoxicity risk factors (AAP, 2022).

	6 hours	*12 hours*	*18 hours*	*24 hours*	*30 hours*	*36 hours*	*42 hours*	*48 hours*	*54 hours*	*60 hours*	*72 hours*	*4 days*	*5 days*	*8 days*	*12 days*
≥38 weeks	18.8	19.8	20.5	21.3	22	22.8	23.4	24	24.6	25	25.9	27	27	27	27
37 weeks	17.8	18.8	19.4	20.3	21	21.8	22.4	23.1	23.7	24.3	25.1	26.6	26.8	27.0	27.0
36 weeks	16.5	17.5	18.2	19.1	19.8	20.5	21.2	21.9	22.4	23	24	25.5	25.8	26.2	26.9
35 weeks	15.5	16.3	17.2	17.9	18.5	19.2	20	20.8	21.2	21.9	22.9	24.5	24.8	25.2	26

TABLE 6: Exchange transfusion thresholds, ≥35 weeks, with neurotoxicity risk factors (AAP, 2022).

	6 hours	*12 hours*	*18 hours*	*24 hours*	*30 hours*	*36 hours*	*42 hours*	*48 hours*	*54 hours*	*60 hours*	*72 hours*	*4 days*	*5 days*	*8 days*	*12 days*
≥38 weeks	15.5	16.4	17	17.8	18.3	18.9	19.6	20.1	20.6	21.2	22.1	23.5	23.5	23.5	23.5
37 weeks	15	15.8	16.4	17.2	17.8	18.4	19	19.7	20.2	20.8	21.8	23.1	23.3	23.5	23.5
36 weeks	14.3	15.2	16	16.6	17.2	17.9	18.5	19.1	19.5	20	20.9	22.1	22.3	22.8	23.3
35 weeks	13.8	14.7	15.3	16.1	16.6	17.3	17.8	18.3	18.9	19.3	20.1	21.1	21.3	22	22.7

18. All healthcare facilities should have written policy for management of NNH. Families should be involved in decision making and care of the baby. Written plan with clear instructions for postdischarge follow-up should be given to the parents.
19. Prolonged indirect hyperbilirubinemia is suspected when TSB remains within 2 mg% of phototherapy levels after >7 days of age. This needs to be followed up and investigated further with appropriate tests as per clinical scenario.
20. For a breast fed baby, if still icteric at 3–4 weeks or for a formula fed baby icteric at 2 weeks, TSB and direct bilirubin should be done to look for possible cholestasis. Review metabolic screen for any risk factors in this regard.
21. All healthcare facilities should have written policy for management of NNH. Families should be involved in decision making and care of the baby. Written plan with clear instructions for postdischarge follow-up should be given to the parents.

Serum bilirubin:serum albumin ratio may be used to decide about need for exchange transfusion as follows ***(Table 7)***:

TABLE 7: Correlation of albumin levels with gestational age and neurotoxicity risk.

TSB:albumin	Gestation	Neurotoxicity risk factor
8 or more	38 weeks or more	Nil
7.2 or more	38 weeks or more	1
6.8 or more	35–37 weeks	Nil
6.2 or more	35–37 weeks	1

(TSB: serum bilirubin)

National Neonatology Forum (NNF) CPG guidelines 2020 differ from AAP guidelines as below:

Discontinuation of phototherapy can be done if TSB level is 2.9 mg% below the hour specific treatment threshold.

A single reading of TSB level below treatment threshold is sufficient to discontinue phototherapy for babies with nonhemolytic jaundice and 2 values are needed for hemolytic jaundice.

For babies nearing exchange transfusion, TSB can be measured 4–6 hourly after starting treatment and 8–12 hourly once TSB level is no longer close to exchange transfusion threshold.

IVIG is not recommended either prophylactically or therapeutically.

There is no use of albumin priming prior to exchange transfusion.

Modified bilirubin-induced neurologic dysfunction (BIND-M) score can be used in clinical practice to assess neurological status of the baby and manage plan intervention.

Clinical sign	Score	Severity	Remarks
Mental status			
• Normal	0		
• Sleepy but arousable • Decreased feeding	1		
• Lethargy • Poor suck • Irritable/ji@ery with short-term strong	2		
• Semi-coma • Apnea • Seizures • Coma	3		

Contd...

Contd...

Clinical sign	Score	Severity	Remarks
Muscle tone			
• Normal	0		
• Persistent mild hypotonia	1		
• Moderate hypotonia • Moderate hypertonia • Increasing arching of neck and trunk on slmulalon without spasms of arms and legs and without trismus	2		
• Persistent retrocollis • Opisthotonus • Crossing or scissoring of arms or legs but without spasms of arms and legs and without trismus	3		
Cry pattern			
• Normal	0		
• High pitched	1		
• Shrill cry	2		
• Inconsolable crying or • Cry weak or absent in child with previous history of high pitched or shrill cry	3		
Occulomotor or eye movements			
• Normal			
• Sun-seNng • Paralysis of upward gaze			
Total ABE score			

0–2: No or mild ABE; conlnue close monitoring and phototherapy.
3–5: Moderate ABE; increased risk of progression; consider exchange transfusion if bilirubin levels are high.
6–12: Severe ABE; immediate intervenlons are crilcal to prevent irreversible kernicterus.

KEY POINTS

- All neonates being discharged from hospital should be examined for jaundice. Based on risk assessment, a follow-up plan needs to be decided and explained to the parents clearly.
- Use total bilirubin for all decisions. Do not subtract conjugated bilirubin.
- Appropriate feeding, hydration, blood sugar level, and electrolyte balance must be maintained for babies requiring treatment.
- A neonate presenting in exchange range or suspected to be having bilirubin encephalopathy is a medical emergency. Treatment should be started without any delay.

SUGGESTED READING

1. Anand P, Bharathi M, Aparna, Gopalakrishnan S, Sachdeva A, Sahoo T, et al. (2019). Clinical Practice Guidelines Screening, Prevention and Management of Neonatal Hyperbilirubinemia National Neonatology Forum, India Screening, Prevention and Management of Neonatal Hyperbilirubinemia Guideline Development Group. [online] Available from https://www.researchgate.net/publication/340116901_Clinical_Practice_Guidelines_Screening_Prevention_and_Management_of_Neonatal_Hyperbilirubinemia_National_Neonatology_Forum_India_Screening_Prevention_and_Management_of_Neonatal_Hyperbilirubinemia_Guid. [Last accessed September, 2024]
2. Bhardwaj U, Kohli V, Thukral A. Management of Hyperbilirubinemia in Newborn Infants 35 or More Weeks of Gestation: American Academy of Pediatrics, 2022. Indian Pediatr. 2023;60(1):63-6.
3. Kemper AR, Newman TB, Slaughter JL, Maisels MJ, Watchko JF, Downs SM, et al. Clinical Practice Guideline Revision: Management of Hyperbilirubinemia in the Newborn Infant 35 or More Weeks of Gestation. Pediatrics. 2022;150(3):e2022058859.
4. Keren R, Luan X, Friedman S, Saddlemire S, Cnaan A, Bhutani VK. A comparison of alternative risk-assessment strategies for predicting significant neonatal hyperbilirubinemia in term and near-term infants. Pediatrics. 2008; 121(1):e170-9.
5. NICE. (2010). Jaundice in newborn babies under 28 days. [online] Available from www.nice.org.uk/guidance/cg98. [Last accessed September, 2024]

Neonatal Hypoglycemia

Amrit Tuteja

INTRODUCTION

Hypoglycemia is the most common metabolic disturbance occurring in the neonatal period. Hypoglycemia in neonates is a medical emergency and should be aggressively treated as severe, prolonged hypoglycemia in the neonatal period can have devastating outcomes, including long-term neurodevelopmental disabilities, cerebral palsy, and death.

PHYSIOLOGY

Once the umbilical cord is clamped, glucose supply is interrupted and neonatal glucose concentrations decrease, reaching a low point ~1–2 hours after birth. In turn, insulin secretion decreases while secretion of counter-regulatory hormones such as glucagon and catecholamines increases, stimulating gluconeogenesis and glycogenolysis, and resulting in a gradual increase in glucose concentrations. However, these do not reach adult concentrations until after 72 hours of age. Delay or interruption of this postnatal metabolic adaptation results in neonatal hypoglycemia.

DEFINITION

There is no uniform definition of neonatal hypoglycemia, and existing guidelines differ significantly in terms of when and whom to screen for hypoglycemia, and where to set interventional thresholds and treatment goals.

- *American Academy of Pediatrics (AAP):* AAP defines neonatal hypoglycemia in 1st 24 hours of age as per **Table 1** below:

TABLE 1: Definition of hypoglycemia as per the American Academy of Pediatrics (AAP).

	First 4 hours	*4–24 hours*
Lowest acceptable value	25 mg/dL	25–40 mg/dL
Actionable value	35 mg/dL	35–45 mg/dL

- *Pediatric Endocrine Society (PES):* The PES suggests the goal of treatment to maintain glucose concentration >50 mg/dL for those <48 hours and >60 mg/dL for those aged >48 hours.

Hypoglycemia can be classified as transient or permanent, but there is no consensus regarding the duration of the hypoglycemia to differentiate *one form from the other*. Transient hypoglycemia typically resolves within the first few days to weeks.

SCREENING

For whom, when, and how?

- For whom? **(Table 2)**
- When? **(Table 3)**
  The optimal frequency and duration of screening remain uncertain. Most protocols recommend screening within 1–2 hours after birth and then every 3 or 4 hours until euglycemia is maintained.
- How? **(Table 4)**

ETIOLOGY

Table 5 enlists common causes of hypoglycemia in neonates.

TABLE 2: Risk factor of neonatal hypoglycemia and duration of monitoring required.

Big Baby-LGA/IDM	*Small Baby-SGA/LBW/Preterm*
• Monitoring up to 12 hours • *Reason:* Transient hyper-insulinism	• Monitoring up to 48–72 hours • *Reason:* Low glycogen stores
• LGA (weight more than 90th centile) • IDM	• SGA (weight less than 10th centile) • LBW (weight <2.5 kg) • Preterm (gestation <37 weeks)

(IDM: infant of diabetic mother; LBW: low birth weight; LGA: large for gestational age; SGA: small for gestational age)

TABLE 3: Screening schedule for at risk neonates.

Risk factors	*Screening schedule*
LGA and IDM	1 hour or 30 minutes postfeed—3 hours-6 hours-12 hours
SGA, preterm, and LBW	1 hour or 30 minutes postfeed—3 hours-6 hours-12 hours then 6 hourly till 48–72 hours
Sick or on IV fluids	1 hour or 30 minutes postfeed—3 hours-6 hours-12 hours then 6 hourly

(IDM: infant of diabetic mother; IV: intravenous; LBW: low birth weight; LGA: large for gestational age; SGA: small for gestational age)

TABLE 4: Various methods of glucose monitoring.

Method	*Pros*	*Cons*	*Indication*
Laboratory	Most accurate	Costly, time taking, accuracy affected by quality of sample, and delay in reaching laboratory	Low glucometer value must be confirmed with laboratory value, especially when sending critical sample
Point-of-care testing (glucometer)	Quick, low cost, user friendly, and small volume of blood	Inaccurate at low glucose concentration	Most common screening method
Continuous glucose monitoring	Detailed information about glucose control	• Frequent calibration is required for better accuracy • Inaccurate at low glucose concentration	Not in practice as of now

TABLE 5: Etiology of neonatal hypoglycemia.

Transient	*Persistent*
Endocrine cause	
HI—Transient	HI (most common)
IDM	Panhypopituitarism
	Isolated GH deficiency
	Adrenal insufficiency (primary/secondary)
Nonendocrine cause	
Delayed enteral feeding	IEM—galactosemia, GSD, gluconeogenic disorder, FAO disorders, and organic aciduria
Prematurity	Hepatic dysfunction
IUGR/SGA	
Sepsis	
Polycythemia	

(FAO: fatty acid oxidation; GH: growth hormone; GSD: glycogen storage disorder; HI: hyperinsulinism; IDM: infant of diabetic mother; IEM: inborn error of metabolism; IUGR: intrauterine growth restriction; SGA: small for gestational age)

CLINICAL FEATURES

Common symptoms and signs of neonatal hypoglycemia are given in **Table 6**.

TABLE 6: Clinical features of neonatal hypoglycemia.

Neurogenic/ adrenergic	Sweating, pallor, temperature instability, irritability, hunger, tremulousness, tachycardia, and vomiting
Neuroglycopenic	Apnea, hypotonia, seizure, and coma

MANAGEMENT (FLOWCHART 1)

- Glucose infusion rate (GIR) =
$$\frac{\text{Dextrose concentration (\%)} \times \text{Intravenous fluid (IVF) (mL/kg/day)}}{144}$$
- >12.5% dextrose concentration needs central line.
- Send critical sample if GIR ≥ 12 mg/kg/min. Send when random blood sugar (RBS) < 50 mg/dL.
- Critical sample—laboratory RBS, insulin, cortisol, growth hormone (GH), B-hydroxybutyrate, lactate. Critical sample should be sent at RBS below 50 mg/dL.

Drugs used in persistent hypoglycemia are given in **Table 7**.

OUTCOME

Hypoglycemic brain injury can result in:
- Development delay—84%
- Seizure—66%

Flowchart 1: Management of neonatal hypoglycemia.

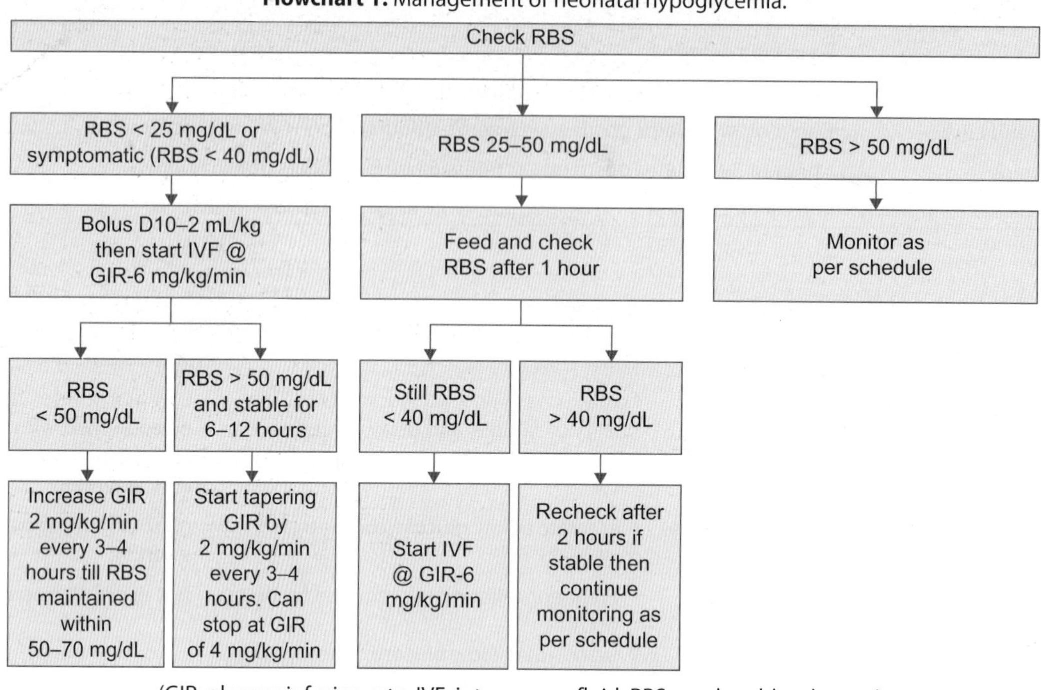

(GIR: glucose infusion rate; IVF: intravenous fluid; RBS: random blood sugar)

TABLE 7: Drugs used in persistent hypoglycemia.

Drugs	*Dose*	*Side effects*	*Comments*
Diazoxide	5–10 mg/kg/day tid to maximum of 15–20 mg/kg/day	Hypotension, fluid retention, hypertrichosis. Add chlorothiazide to reduce side effect	First-line for HI
Octreotide (long-acting somatostatin analog)	5–10 µg/kg/day up to maximum of 15–40 µg/kg/day, q 6–8 hours SC injection	Decrease in dose response after 48 hours of initiation	Second-line for HI
Hydrocortisone	5 mg/kg/day q12h	Side effects outweigh benefits	Use in adrenal insufficiency
Glucagon	1 mg/day irrespective of gestation and birth weight	Generally well tolerated	Rarely used. Only in GH deficiency or in hypopituitarism
Nifedipine	Initial—0.25–0.3 mg/kg/d to maximum of 0.5–0.8 mg/kg/d	Usually well tolerated. Hypotension reported at higher dose	Used in those unresponsive to diazoxide

(GH: growth hormone; HI: hyperinsulinism; SC: subcutaneous)

- Visual impairment—37%
- Microcephaly—32%

Table 8 shows relation between neurological outcome and neonatal neurological clinical features.

TABLE 8: Neurological outcome of neonatal hypoglycemia.

	Neurological outcome		
Clinical syndrome	*Normal (%)*	*Transient abnormality (%)*	*Abnormal (%)*
Seizure	38	12	50
No seizure	76	12	12
Asymptomatic	80	14	6

DIAGNOSIS

An MRI is a sensitive and a specific screening method for diagnosing brain injury. Diffusion-weighted imaging (DWI)

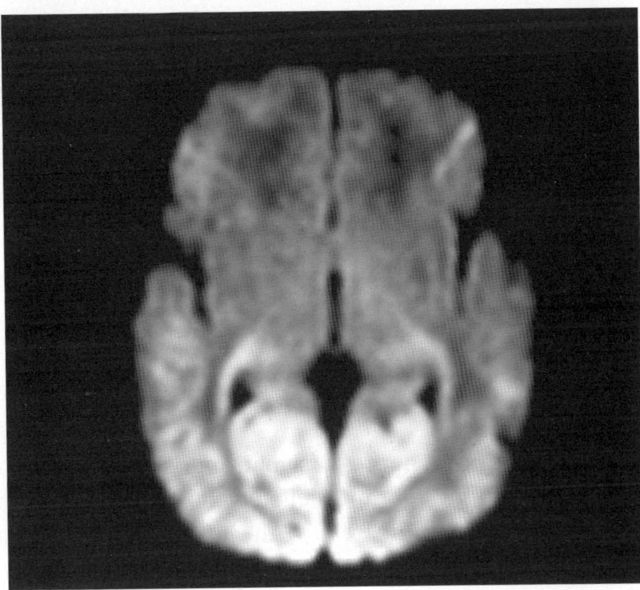

Fig. 1: Hypoglycemic brain injury.

and apparent diffusion coefficient (ADC) images can detect early brain injury, within 24 hours, latest by 5 days, while conventional MRI sequences take 5–6 days to detect them. The occipital lobes are most severely affected. The occipital lobes are most severely affected. The patterns of injury may, however, be more diverse with involvement of the basal ganglia, thalamus and the posterior limb of the internal capsule **(Fig. 1)**.

KEY POINTS

- Hypoglycemia is a medical emergency, if not properly treated can lead to a life with disability.
- Those with risk factors should be monitored for hypoglycemia.
- Early feed initiation is important to prevent hypoglycemia.
- Aim to maintain RBS at least above 40 mg/dL.
- Transient hypoglycemia usually settles by 72 hours to a week.
- Hyperinsulinism is most common cause of persistent hypoglycemia.
- GIR > 12.5 mg/kg/min needs central line.
- Symptomatic hypoglycemia can lead to brain injury and require long-term neurodevelopment follow-up. Hypoglycemic brain injury needs MRI brain imaging.

SUGGESTED READING

1. Abramowski A, Ward R, Hamdan AH. Neonatal Hypoglycemia. Treasure Island (FL): StatPearls Publishing; 2024.
2. Adamkin DH. Neonatal hypoglycemia. Semin Fetal Neonatal Med. 2017;22(1):36-41.
3. Edwards T, Harding JE. Clinical Aspects of Neonatal Hypoglycemia: A Mini Review. Front Pediatr. 2021;8:562251.
4. Garg M, Devaskar SU, Disorders of carbohydrate metabolism in the neonate. In: Martin RJ, Fanaroff AA, Walsh MC (Eds). Fanaroff and Martin's Neonatal-Perinatal Medicine: Diseases of the Fetus and Infant, 11th edition. Philadelphia: Elsevier; 2020. pp. 1584-610.
5. Harding JE, Alsweiler JM, Edwards TE, McKinlay CJ. Neonatal hypoglycaemia. BMJ Med. 2024;3(1):e000544.
6. Roeper M, Hoermann H, Kummer S, Meissner T. Neonatal hypoglycemia: lack of evidence for a safe management. Front Endocrinol. 2023;14:1179102.
7. Rozance PJ, William WH. Describing hypoglycemia—definition or operational threshold? Early Hum Dev. 2010; 86(5):275-80.
8. Stanescu A, Stoicescu SM. Neonatal hypoglycemia screening in newborns from diabetic mothers—arguments and controversies. J Med Life. 2014;7 Spec No. 3(Spec Iss 3):51-2.
9. Tas E, Garibaldi L, Muzumdar R. Glucose Homeostasis in Newborns: An Endocrinology Perspective. Neoreviews. 2020;21(1):e14-29.

Neonatal Seizures

Sanjay Wazir

INTRODUCTION

Neonatal seizures are one of the most common neurological emergencies in newborns, necessitating prompt identification and management. They often indicate underlying neurological or systemic disorders and pose a significant risk of long-term complications if not addressed effectively. This chapter provides a comprehensive guide to the evaluation and treatment of neonatal seizures, focusing on practical algorithms for clinical use.

ALGORITHM FOR MANAGEMENT OF SEIZURES

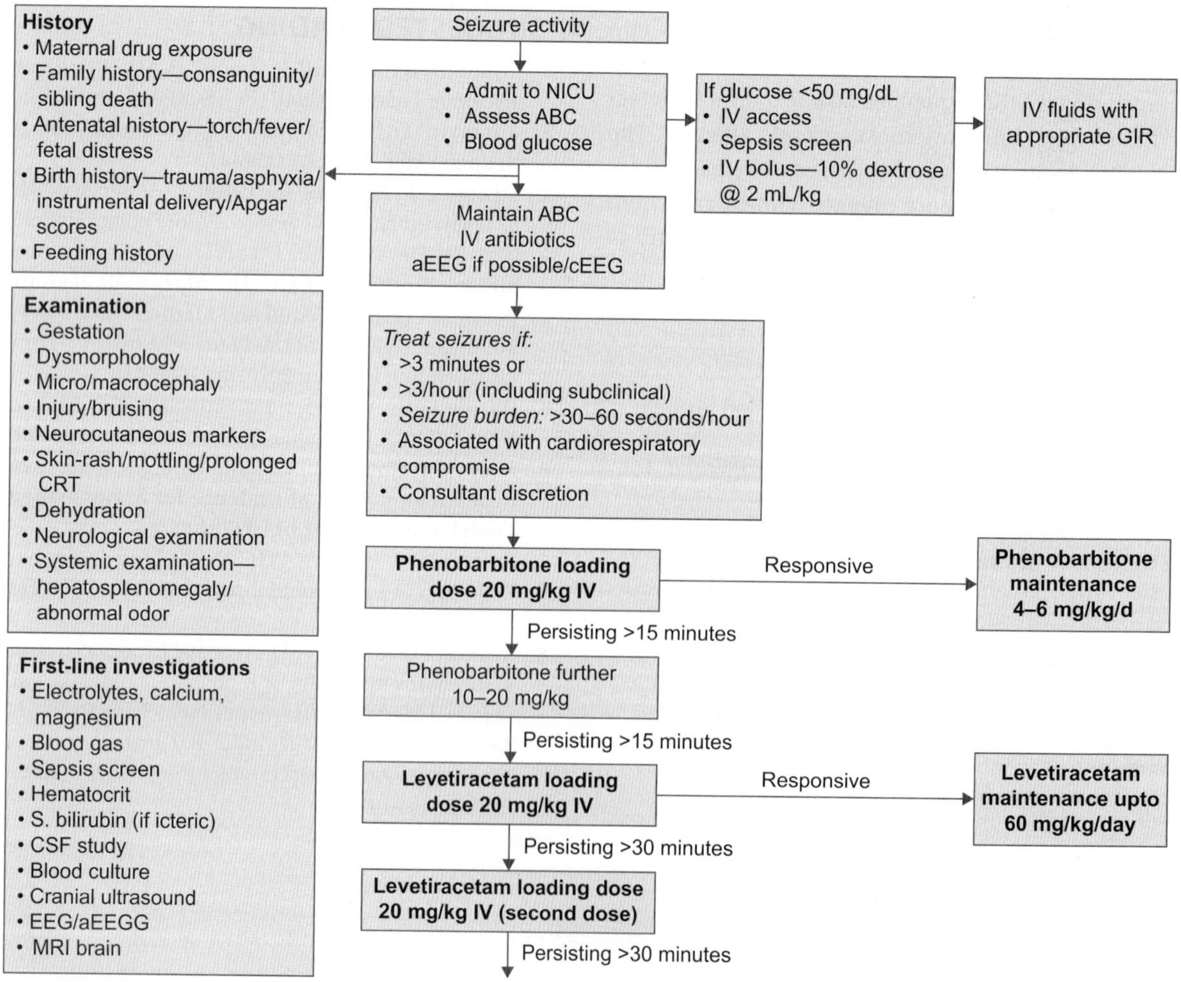

History
- Maternal drug exposure
- Family history—consanguinity/sibling death
- Antenatal history—torch/fever/fetal distress
- Birth history—trauma/asphyxia/instrumental delivery/Apgar scores
- Feeding history

Examination
- Gestation
- Dysmorphology
- Micro/macrocephaly
- Injury/bruising
- Neurocutaneous markers
- Skin-rash/mottling/prolonged CRT
- Dehydration
- Neurological examination
- Systemic examination—hepatosplenomegaly/abnormal odor

First-line investigations
- Electrolytes, calcium, magnesium
- Blood gas
- Sepsis screen
- Hematocrit
- S. bilirubin (if icteric)
- CSF study
- Blood culture
- Cranial ultrasound
- EEG/aEEGG
- MRI brain

Seizure activity
↓
- Admit to NICU
- Assess ABC
- Blood glucose

→ If glucose <50 mg/dL
- IV access
- Sepsis screen
- IV bolus—10% dextrose @ 2 mL/kg

→ IV fluids with appropriate GIR

↓ (→ History)

Maintain ABC
IV antibiotics
aEEG if possible/cEEG
↓

Treat seizures if:
- >3 minutes or
- >3/hour (including subclinical)
- *Seizure burden:* >30–60 seconds/hour
- Associated with cardiorespiratory compromise
- Consultant discretion

↓

Phenobarbitone loading dose 20 mg/kg IV — Responsive → **Phenobarbitone maintenance 4–6 mg/kg/d**

↓ Persisting >15 minutes

Phenobarbitone further 10–20 mg/kg

↓ Persisting >15 minutes

Levetiracetam loading dose 20 mg/kg IV — Responsive → **Levetiracetam maintenance upto 60 mg/kg/day**

↓ Persisting >30 minutes

Levetiracetam loading dose 20 mg/kg IV (second dose)

↓ Persisting >30 minutes

Contd...

Contd...

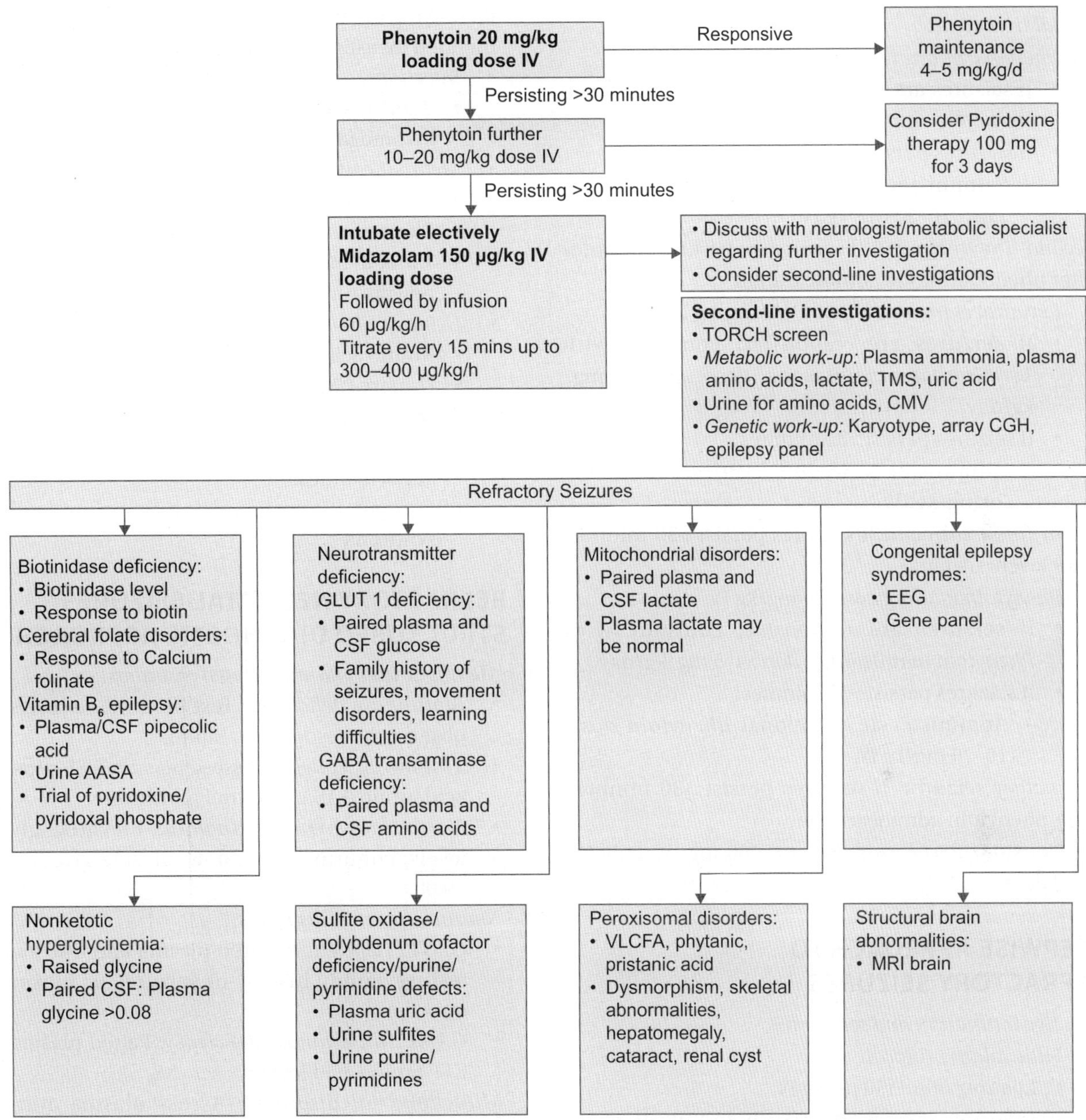

(AASA: alpha-aminoadipic semialdehyde; ABC: airway, breathing, and circulation; aEEG: amplitude-integrated electroencephalography; cEEG: continuous electroencephalography; CGH: comparative genomic hybridization; CMV: cytomegalovirus; CRT: capillary refill time; CSF: cerebrospinal fluid; EEG: electroencephalogram; GIR: glucose infusion rate; IV: intravenous; NICU: neonatal intensive care unit; TORCH: toxoplasmosis, other agents, rubella, cytomegalovirus, and herpes simplex. VLCFA: very long-chain fatty acid)

INDICATIONS TO TREAT NEONATAL SEIZURES

Neonatal seizures should be promptly treated when they meet any of the following criteria:

- Seizures lasting more than 3 minutes.
- More than 3 seizures per hour, including subclinical seizures.
- A seizure burden exceeding 30-60 seconds/hour.
- Seizures associated with cardiorespiratory compromise.
- Based on consultant discretion, particularly in cases of atypical or refractory seizures.

TREATMENT PROTOCOL

1. *Initial treatment:*
   - *Phenobarbitone loading dose:* 20 mg/kg IV.
     - If seizures are *responsive,* continue with *Phenobarbitone maintenance dose:* 4–6 mg/kg/day.
     - If seizures persist for more than 15 minutes:
       - Administer an additional *Phenobarbitone dose:* 10–20 mg/kg IV.
2. *Second-line treatment:* If seizures persist >15 minutes after phenobarbitone administration
   - *Levetiracetam loading dose:* 20 mg/kg IV.
     - If seizures are *responsive,* continue with *Levetiracetam maintenance dose:* up to 60 mg/kg/day.
     - If seizures persist >30 minutes:
       - Administer a *Second levetiracetam dose:* 20 mg/kg IV.
3. *Third-line treatment:* If seizures persist >30 minutes after levetiracetam
   - *Phenytoin loading dose:* 20 mg/kg IV.
     - If seizures are *responsive,* continue with *Phenytoin maintenance dose:* 4–5 mg/kg/day.
     - If seizures persist >30 minutes:
       - Administer an additional *Phenytoin dose:* 10–20 mg/kg IV.
4. *Refractory seizures:* If seizures persist >30 minutes after phenytoin administration
   - Consider *Pyridoxine therapy:* 100 mg IV daily for 3 days.

STEPWISE APPROACH TO REFRACTORY SEIZURES

1. *Elective intubation and sedation:*
   - *Midazolam protocol:*
     - *Loading dose:* 150 μg/kg IV.
     - *Infusion:* Start at 60 μg/kg/h and titrate every 15 minutes up to 300–400 μg/kg/h based on clinical response.
   - *Rationale:* Ensures optimal seizure control while providing sedation for mechanical ventilation, if necessary.
2. *Collaboration with specialists:*
   - Engage a *neurologist* or > to evaluate complex or atypical cases.
   - Specialists guide decisions for further investigations and advanced therapies.
3. *Second-line investigations:* For refractory seizures, identifying the underlying etiology is essential. Recommended investigations include:
   - *Infections:*
     - *TORCH screen:* Includes toxoplasmosis, rubella, cytomegalovirus (CMV), herpes.
   - *Metabolic work-up:*
     - Plasma ammonia, lactate, uric acid levels.
     - Plasma amino acid profiles.
     - Tandem mass spectrometry (TMS) for expanded newborn screening.
   - *Urine analysis:*
     - Amino acids for metabolic disorders.
     - Urinary CMV testing if infections are suspected.
   - *Genetic work-up:*
     - *Karyotype* and *array CGH* for chromosomal abnormalities.
     - *Epilepsy Gene Panel* for inherited epilepsy syndromes.

REFRACTORY NEONATAL SEIZURES: STRUCTURED DIAGNOSTIC APPROACH

1. *Metabolic and vitamin-related disorders:*
   - *Biotinidase deficiency:* Test biotinidase levels and observe the response to biotin.
   - *Vitamin B_6 epilepsy:* Assess plasma/CSF pipecolic acid, urine AASA, and trial pyridoxine.
   - *Nonketotic hyperglycinemia:* Elevated glycine levels; confirm with CSF-to-plasma glycine ratio >0.08.
2. *Neurotransmitter disorders:*
   - *GLUT1 deficiency:* Paired plasma and CSF glucose testing; family history of seizures or movement disorders.
   - *GABA transaminase deficiency:* Paired plasma and CSF amino acid levels.
3. *Mitochondrial disorders:* Assess plasma and CSF lactate levels. Note—lactate may sometimes appear normal.
4. *Peroxisomal disorders:*
   - Elevated VLCFA, phytanic acid, and pristanic acid levels.
   - *Associated features:* Dysmorphism, hepatomegaly, cataracts, skeletal abnormalities.
5. *Congenital epilepsy syndromes:* Diagnostic tools—EEG and comprehensive epilepsy gene panel testing.
6. *Structural brain abnormalities:* Brain MRI to detect malformations, structural damage, or cortical dysplasia.

KEY POINTS

- Neonatal seizures often signal underlying systemic or neurological abnormalities.
- Prompt assessment of metabolic, infectious, and structural causes is critical.
- Management should focus on stabilizing the neonate (ABC: airway, breathing, circulation) and addressing seizure activity.
- EEG remains the gold standard for diagnosis, but aEEG or clinical observation can be used where EEG is unavailable.
- A structured approach, including first-line and second-line investigations, is crucial in refractory seizures.

SUGGESTED READING

1. Spoto G, Saia MC, Amore G. Neonatal Seizures: An Overview of Genetic Causes and Treatment Options. Brain Sci. 2021.
2. Stieren ES, Rottkamp CA, Brooks-Kayal AR. Neonatal Seizures. NeoReviews. 2024.
3. Yozawitz E. Neonatal Seizures. N Engl J Med. 2023.
4. Ziobro J, Shellhaas RA. Neonatal Seizures: Diagnosis, Etiologies, and Management. Semin Neurol. 2020.

Neonatal Sepsis

Mukesh Sanklecha, Anjali Kulkarni

INTRODUCTION

Neonatal sepsis is the most common cause of mortality and morbidity in newborns in our country. Since the potential for serious adverse outcomes is high, caregivers should have a low threshold for evaluation and treatment of possible sepsis in neonates.

CLASSIFICATION BY DAY OF ONSET (TABLE 1)

Etiology-wise, sepsis can be classified as bacterial and fungal sepsis.

- *Bacterial sepsis:* Presents both as early-onset sepsis (EOS) and late-onset sepsis (LOS)
- *Fungal sepsis:* Presents commonly as LOS.

Time of onset also divides it into two categories.

RISK FACTORS FOR SEPSIS

Risk factors for sepsis are given in **Table 2**.

ORGANISMS IN NEONATAL SEPSIS

In many low- and middle-income countries, especially those in South Asia, there is no difference in the profile of organisms causing EOS and LOS. Overall, the main bacterial etiological agents reported from a large Indian study were *Acinetobacter* spp. (22%), *Klebsiella* spp. (17%), coagulase negative staphylococci (15%), *Escherichia coli* (14%), *Staphylococcus aureus* (12%), *Pseudomonas* spp. (7%), *Enterococcus* spp. (6%), and *Enterobacter* spp. (4%).

Group B *Streptococcus* does not seem common in the Indian population. *Listeria* is another organism hardly ever reported from India. The profile is different among outborn neonates admitted to Level III units with sepsis. 25% were caused by *Candida* spp. *Klebsiella pneumoniae* and *Acinetobacter baumannii* were the two most common bacterial pathogens.

TABLE 1: Classification of sepsis.

Early-onset sepsis (<72 hours)	*Late-onset sepsis (>72 hours)*
• Caused by organisms acquired before or immediately after birth (vertical infection) • Predominantly respiratory presentation	• Caused by organisms acquired from hospital or community • Varied presentation

Some experts extend the definition of EOS to 7 days and LOS to onset of symptoms beyond 7 days.

TABLE 2: Risk factors for sepsis.

Early-onset sepsis	*Late-onset sepsis*
Maternal factors: • Prolonged rupture of membranes >18 hours* • Intrapartum maternal fever >38°C within 15 days* • Foul smelling liquor* • Chorioamnionitis* • Unclean vaginal examination • Maternal leukocytosis (white blood cell >15,000) • Prolonged rupture of membrane >12 hours • Frequent (>3) per vaginal examination in labor • Vaginal positives swab for group B *Streptococcus* *Fetal factors:* • *Fetal distress:* Sustained fetal tachycardia >160/min* • Apgar <5 • Low birth weight (<1,500 g) • Prematurity <34 weeks	• Neonatal intensive care unit admission • Poor hygiene • Low and very low birth weight babies • Poor cord care • Prematurity • Bottle feeding • Invasive procedure • Superficial infection (pyoderma and umbilical sepsis) • *Fungal sepsis:* Exposure to broad-spectrum antibiotics causing alteration of normal flora

*Major risk factors

SIGNS AND SYMPTOMS ASSOCIATED WITH NEONATAL SEPSIS

Early Signs

- Respiratory distress that ranges from mild tachypnea to respiratory failure
- Increase in ventilatory support in the mechanically ventilated patient
- Lethargy or hypotonia
- Increase in apnea
- Feeding intolerance
- Temperature instability
- Hypotension or evidence of poor perfusion
- Increase in heart rate

Late Signs

- Sclerema
- Shock
- Disseminated intravascular coagulation (DIC)
- Pulmonary hemorrhage

CLINICAL PEARL

- Since the signs of neonatal sepsis are very nonspecific, any acute deterioration in a neonate should be assumed to be because of septicemia in Indian scenarios unless there are definite indications of alternative pathology.

DIAGNOSTIC WORKUP

Complete blood count (CBC) should be used after the first few hours of life in the proper clinical context. The white blood cell (WBC) and absolute neutrophil count (ANC) are most predictive of an infection when these values are low (WBC < 5,000 and ANC < 1,000]. An elevated WBC (>20,000) is neither worrisome nor reassuring in neonates. The immature to total neutrophil (I/T) ratio is the most informative if measured 1–4 hours after birth with low values (<0.15) being reassuring while elevated values (>0.3) are weakly associated with EOS. The combination of a low ANC and elevated I/T ratio is the most predictive combination of WBC indices for EOS.

- *C-reactive protein (CRP):* Rises approximately 12 hours after onset of sepsis and returns to normal within 2–7 days. Single readings have limited value and serial readings are more useful.
- *Procalcitonin:* >0.25–2 ng/L suggests sepsis and >2 ng/mL suggests strong suspicion of sepsis
- *Blood culture:* Gold standard in diagnosis till date
- Chest X-ray if respiratory distress
- *Lumber puncture:* Should be performed when index of suspicion of meningitis is high in EOS and in all cases of LOS.
- Multiplex polymerase chain reaction (PCR) of body fluids may be useful in terms of early results (2 hours turnaround time), diagnosing a nonbacterial etiology as also giving an initial clue about drug resistance.

CLINICAL PEARLS

- Blood culture should always be obtained before starting antibiotic therapy, but inability to obtain blood culture should not delay starting of treatment.
- Neutropenia in face of confirmed sepsis indicate that baby is extremely unwell.

TREATMENT

Supportive Care

- Oxygen/ventilation
- Volume expansion/maintaining blood pressure with crystalloids, colloids, and use of inotropes
- Treatment of anemia, thrombocytopenia, and DIC
- Temperature maintenance
- Treatment of hypoglycemia/hyperglycemia/hypocalcemia

Specific Treatment

All babies with presence of risk factors and/or with signs and symptoms of sepsis should be screened for sepsis and blood culture should be collected. Pending blood culture report babies should be judiciously started on antibiotics.

Antibiotics

For practical purpose, antibiotics can be classified as:

- *First-line antibiotics:* Ampicillin plus gentamicin
- *Second-line antibiotics:* Third- or fourth-generation cephalosporin/piperacillin plus tazobactam plus amikacin
- *Third-line antibiotics:* Carbapenems plus amikacin
- *Fourth-line antibiotics:* Polymyxin/colistin/vancomycin/linezolid

Choice of antibiotics should be judiciously decided **(Table 3)**. For suspected LOS, it is justified to start directly on second-line antibiotics. In EOS if high vaginal swab positive, neonate should be treated with specific antibiotics as per culture and sensitivity report. If mother is positive for group B *Streptococcus* then double dose of ampicillin should be used.

TABLE 3: Antimicrobial dosage with spectrum and schedule.

Antibiotic/antifungal	**Spectrum**	**Dose**
Ampicillin	*Listeria monocytogenes, Escherichia coli, Enterococcus,* and group B *Streptococcus*	• Mild/moderate infection: 100 mg/kg/dose • *Meningitis:* 400 mg/kg/day (interval: **Table 4**)
Cefotaxime	Gram-negative enteric bacteria and meningitis	50 mg/kg/dose (interval: **Table 4**)
Ceftriaxone*	Gram-negative bacteria and gonococcal infection	• *Sepsis:* 50 mg/kg **(Table 4)** • *Meningitis:* 80–100 mg/kg
Cefepime	Covers both gram-positive and gram-negative organism, especially *Pseudomonas aeruginosa*	• *<28 days:* 30 mg/kg/dose 12 hourly • *>28 days:* 50 mg/kg/dose 12 hourly • *Meningitis:* 50 mg/kg/dose 8 hourly
Piperacillin + tazobactam	Gram-positive and gram-negative anaerobic, e.g., *Enterococcus and Proteus*	50–100 mg/kg/dose (interval: **Table 4**)
Amikacin	Gram-negative enteric bacteria, e.g., *Serratia*	• *<29 weeks:* – *0–7 days:* 18 mg/kg/dose 48 hourly – *8–28 days:* 15 mg/kg/dose 36 hourly – *>29 days:* 15 mg/kg/dose 24 hourly • *30–34 weeks:* – *0–7days:* 18 mg/kg/dose 36 hourly – *>8 days:* 15 mg/kg/dose 24 hourly • *>35 weeks:* 15 mg/kg/dose 24 hourly
Gentamicin	Gram-negative bacteria	• *<32 weeks:* 4 mg/kg/dose 36 hourly • *>32 weeks:* 4 mg/kg/dose 24hourly
Carbapenems	Multiresistant *Klebsiella pneumoniae, Enterobacteriaceae*, and anaerobes	20–25 mg/kg/dose (interval: **Table 4**)
Colistin	*Pseudomonas aeruginosa*	50,000–75,000 units/kg/day divided 8 hourly
Vancomycin	Methicillin-resistant *S. aureus*	• *<29 weeks:* – *0–14 days:* 10–15 mg/kg/dose 18 hourly – *>14 days:* 10–15 mg/kg/dose 12 hourly • *30–42 weeks:* – *0–14 days:* 10–15 mg/kg/dose 12 hourly – *>14 days:* 10–15 mg/kg/dose 8 hourly • >42 weeks – 10–15 mg/kg/dose 6 hourly
Linezolid	Methicillin-resistant *S. aureus* refractory to vancomycin	• *<34 weeks:* 10 mg/kg/dose 12 hourly • *>34 weeks:* 10 mg/kg/dose 8 hourly
Fluconazole	*Candida* spp.	• *Prophylaxis:* 3 mg/kg/dose twice weekly • *Therapeutic:* – *<29 weeks:* - *0–14 days:* 6 mg/kg/dose 48 hourly - *>14 days:* 6 mg/kg/dose 24 hourly – *>30 weeks:* - *0–7days:* 6 mg/kg/dose 28 hourly - *>7 days:* 6 mg/kg/dose 24 hourly
Liposomal amphotericin B	Fluconazole-resistant *Candida* spp.	2.5–7 mg/kg/day as continuous infusion over 1 hour daily

*Not recommended for use in neonates with hyperbilirubinemia, concurrent administration with calcium-containing product contraindicated.

TABLE 4: Dosing interval chart.

Gestational age	*Postnatal age*	*Interval*
<29 weeks	0–28 days >28 days	12 hours 8 hours
30–36 weeks	0–14 days >14 days	12 hours 8 hours
>37 weeks	0–7 days >7 days	12 hours 8 hours

CLINICAL PEARL

- Consideration of fungal sepsis should be given for very low birth weight (VLBW) babies, especially with central lines who deteriorate on antibiotics. Fluconazole prophylaxis in such babies has shown to reduce the incidence of invasive fungal sepsis. In babies with pending culture report, it is justified to start antifungal treatment. Local antibiogram is critical in deciding use of antifungals both for prophylaxis and empiric treatment.

CLINICAL PEARL

- Irrational use of antibiotics should be avoided in neonatal intensive care unit. Clinically evaluate and consider other clinical diagnosis in the absence of positive laboratory parameters and symptomatic baby.

Management of Early-onset Sepsis

Management of EOS is represented in **Flowchart 1**. Asymptomatic neonate with minor risk factors should be observed, pending blood culture and septic screen and treatment should be started if baby becomes symptomatic or screening results are positive, whereas neonates with major risk factors should be started on antibiotics pending the sepsis screen results. All symptomatic neonates where alternative diagnosis is not possible should be started on antibiotics **(Flowchart 2)**.

Flowchart 1: Management of early-onset sepsis.

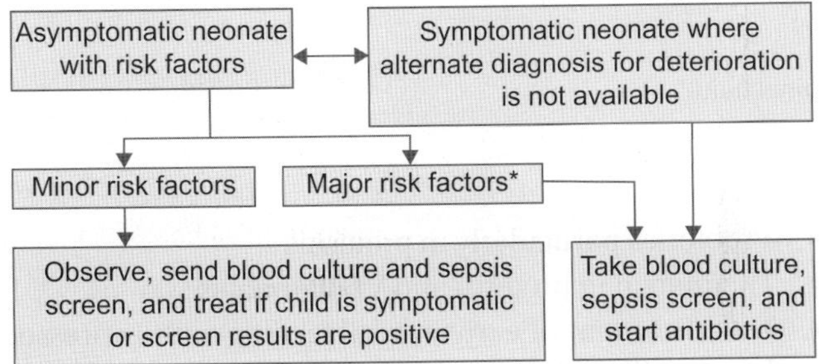

*Lumber puncture, all symptomatic infant except in premature baby with respiratory distress syndrome (RDS).

CLINICAL PEARL

- About 90% of the EOS would present with respiratory involvement.

Management of Late-onset Sepsis

Management of LOS is represented in **Flowchart 3**. All severely symptomatic infants should be started on antibiotics pending sepsis screen, blood culture, and cerebrospinal fluid examination and culture reports. Babies with minor symptoms should be started on treatment based on the sepsis screen results.

CLINICAL PEARLS

- A sepsis screen is not warranted in neonates with a high probability for sepsis. Instead, these neonates should be directly started on antibiotics pending blood culture.
- Lumbar puncture should be done in all cases of LOS.

Stopping Antibiotics

Guidelines for stopping antibiotics are illustrated in **Flowchart 4**. Duration of antibiotics depends upon clinical condition of the infant and organism identified. If septic screen and blood culture is negative and baby is asymptomatic symptoms resolved, antibiotics can be stopped after 48 hours. If blood culture is negative and clinical suspicion is high, repeat blood culture and CRP; continue antibiotics for 7–10 days till infective indices have normalized. For proven sepsis with normal cerebrospinal fluid findings, treatment should be at least 10–14 days and for meningitis, treatment should be for 21 days. For fungal sepsis, treatment duration is 3–6 weeks or 21 days after first negative blood culture.

Adjunctive Therapies in Sepsis

The following treatments have been tried with varying results but there is no evidence-based recommendation for any of these:

- Intravenous immunoglobulin (IVIG) pentoxifylline (immunomodulator)
- Granulocyte colony-stimulating factor (GCSF) with low total white blood cell (TWBC) count
- Blood exchange transfusion

Flowchart 2: Suggested algorithm for sepsis evaluation in at-risk asymptomatic infants.

Assess risk factors
- Prolonged rupture of membranes
- Preterm premature rupture of membranes
- Clinical chorioamnionitis (maternal fever, lower abdominal tenderness, leukocytosis, foul-smelling liquor)
- Frequent or unclean per vaginal examinations

Assess setting
- How premature the neonate is
- How low the birth weight is

Assess intrapartum antibiotic prophylaxis (IAP)
- Whether appropriate IAP received
- Number of hours of antibiotic coverage before delivery

↓

Estimate risk of EOS

Low risk →
- Observe carefully
- Monitor vital signs
- Consider CRP

High risk →
- Send blood culture
- Start empiric antibiotics

→ Blood culture positive, or Develops signs suggestive of EOS → Continue antibiotics, guided by sensitivity report if available

→ Blood culture sterile, clinical course not suggestive of EOS → Stop antibiotics by 24–48 hours

(CRP: C-reactive protein; EOS: early-onset sepsis)

Flowchart 3: Management of late-onset sepsis.

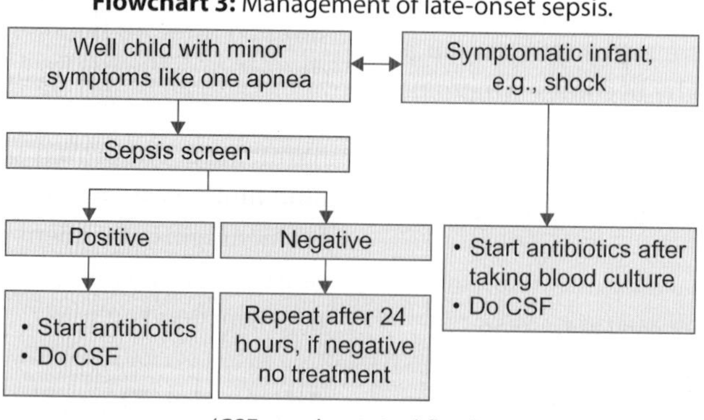

(CSF: cerebrospinal fluid)

PREVENTION

- Infection control bundles with proper perinatal asepsis
- Prophylactic vancomycin for central lines
- Probiotics particularly in preterms
- Lactoferrin in preterm and VLBW babies
- Establishment of early enteral feeding with expressed breast milk (EBM)

Flowchart 4: Stopping antibiotics.

(CRP: C-reactive protein; CSF: cerebrospinal fluid)

KEY POINTS

- Sepsis is the most common cause of mortality and morbidity in the neonatal period.
- We should have a high index of suspicion for diagnosis, and antibiotics must be used judiciously where required along with the appropriate supportive therapy.

SUGGESTED READING

1. Benitz WE, Han MY, Madan A, Ramachandra P. Serialserum C-reactive protein levels in the diagnosis of neonatal infection. Pediatrics. 1998;102:E41.
2. Hasen AR. Cloherty and Stark's Manual of Neonatal Care, 9th edition. Gurugram: Wolters Kluwer (India) Pvt. Ltd.; 2022.
3. King Edward Memorial Hospital. Neonatology Clinical Guidelines. Perth, Western Australia: King Edward Memorial Hospital; 2010.
4. Kliegman RM, Stanton BM, Geme JS, Schor NF, Behrman RE. Nelson Textbook of Pediatrics, 19th edition. Maryland Heights, Missouri: Elsevier; 2011.
5. Martin RJ, Fanaroff AA, Walsh MC. Fanaroff and Martin's Neonatal-Perinatal Medicine: Diseases of the Fetus and Infant, 9th edition. Maryland Heights, Missouri: Elsevier; 2010.
6. Remington JS, Klein JO. Infectious Diseases of the Fetus and Newborn Infant, 7th edition. Maryland Heights, Missouri: Elsevier; 2010.
7. Segar JL, Patel CA, Tierney SB. Recommended Antimicrobial Dosage Schedules for Neonates. [online] Available from https://www.uichildrens.org/uploadedFiles/UIChildrens/Health_Professionals. [Last accessed September, 2024].
8. Singh SA, Dutta S, Narang A. Predictive clinical scores for diagnosis of late-onset neonatal septicemia. J Trop Pediatr. 2003;49:235-9.
9. Young TE, Magnum B. Neofax: A Manual of Drugs Used in Neonatal Care, 23rd edition. New York: Thomson Reuters; 2010.

Approach to Congenital Heart Disease

Dinesh K Chirla, Preetham K Poddutoor

INTRODUCTION

Congenital heart disease (CHD) is as frequent as 7–8 per 100 live births. CHD can be an isolated finding or may be found in association with other malformations such as esophageal atresia, anorectal malformation, exomphalos, and skeletal defects.

About 10–15% have complex lesion with more than one cardiac abnormality and 10–15% have noncardiac abnormality **(Table 1 and Flowchart 1)**.

TABLE 1: Causes and frequency of congenital heart disease.

Causes	*Frequency (%)*	*Common cardiac abnormalities*
Chromosomal disorder		
Trisomy 21	30–40%	Atrioventricular septal defect and VSD
Trisomy 18 and 13	60–80%	Complex (VSD and PDA)
Turners (45XO)	15%	Aortic valve stenosis and coarctation of aorta
Chromosome 22q deletion	—	Aortic arch anomalies and tetralogy of Fallot
Maternal drugs		
Warfarin therapy	5%	Pulmonary valve stenosis and PDA
Fetal alcohol syndrome	25%	ASD, VSD, and tetralogy of Fallot
Maternal disorders		
Rubella infection	30–35%	Peripheral pulmonary stenosis and PDA
Systemic lupus erythematosus (SLE)	35%	Complete heart block
Diabetes mellitus	2%	Increased incidence overall (VSD, transposition, and hypertrophied septum)

(ASD: atrial septal defect; PDA: patent ductus arteriosus; VSD: ventricular septal defect)

ANTENATAL DIAGNOSIS

Checking the anatomy of fetal heart has become a routine part of the fetal anomaly scan (targeted imaging for fetal anomalies) at 18–20 weeks in most of the fetal medicine units. If an abnormality is detected, detailed fetal echocardiography is performed by pediatric cardiologists **(Flowchart 2)**. Unfortunately, these services are available only in few tertiary units or perinatal centers in India. Depending on diagnosis, some choose termination of pregnancy in complex CHD; majority can continue with pregnancy and have neonates management planned antenatally.

CLINICAL PEARL

- Neonates with duct-dependent lesion are likely to need treatment in the first 2 days.

WHEN TO SUSPECT CONGENITAL HEART DISEASE

Pathologic Murmurs

The intensity and quality of the murmur and associated findings differentiate innocent murmurs from those associated with heart disease.

The following features of murmurs are associated with structural heart disease:

- Murmur intensity grade 3 or higher
- Harsh quality
- Pansystolic duration
- Loudest at upper left, upper right sternal border, or apex
- Abnormal S2

CLINICAL PEARL

- The four S's of innocent murmur are Soft, Systolic, Asymptomatic, and left Sternal edge.

Flowchart 1: Presentation of congenital heart disease.

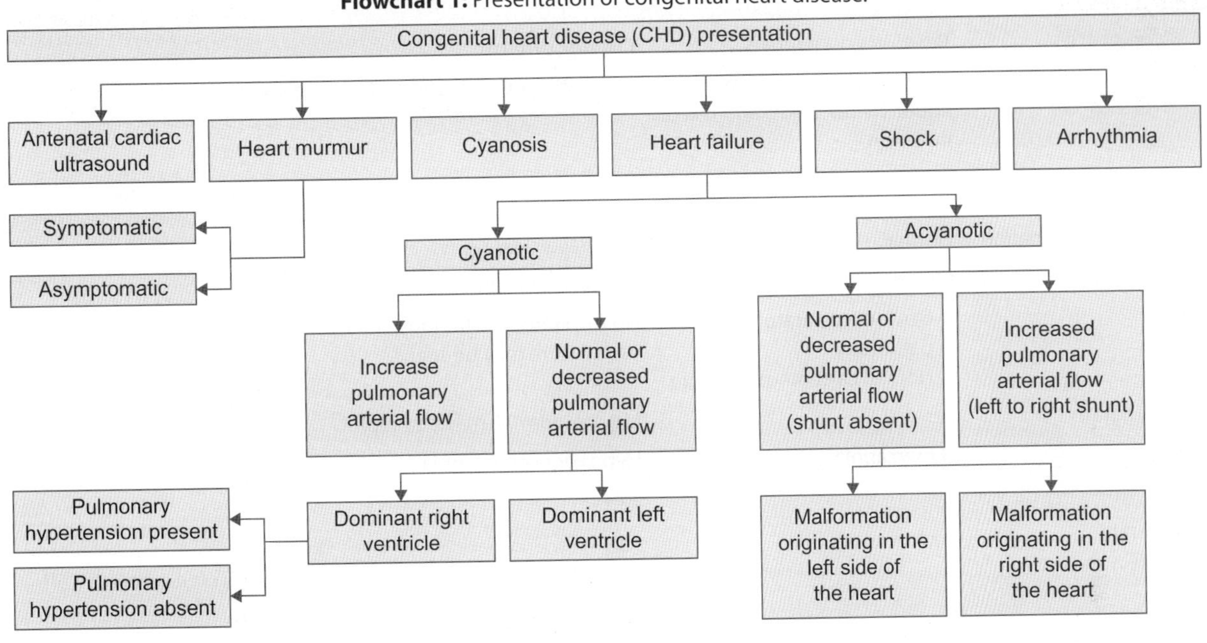

Flowchart 2: When to do fetal echocardiography.

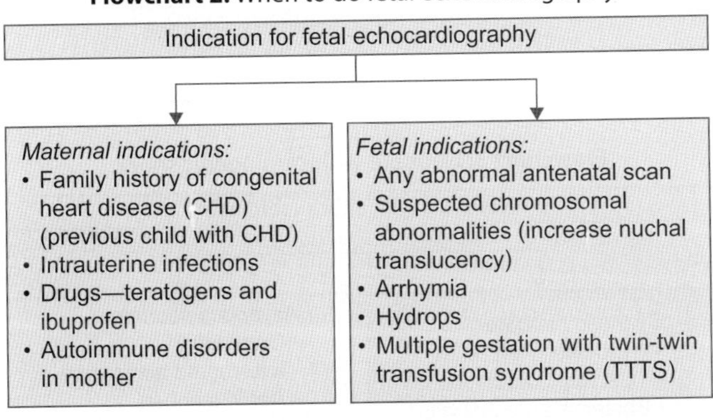

Cyanosis

Cyanosis is always suggestive of serious medical problem. Peripheral cyanosis may occur when a neonate is cold or unwell from any cause. Central cyanosis is seen on tongue. Once we rule out pulmonary disease as cause of cyanosis, we need to suspect serious cardiac abnormality. Clinically, it is sometimes difficult to identify cyanosis differentiating between cardiac and pulmonary cyanosis **(Table 2)**; always check oxygen saturation with pulse oximetry. Those with left-sided obstructive lesions present with inadequate systemic perfusion and shock, whereas those with right-sided lesions present with cyanosis because of inadequate blood reaching the lungs. In neonatal period, cardiac cyanosis may be caused by:

- *Reduced pulmonary blood flow:*
  - Critical pulmonary stenosis
  - Tetralogy of Fallot
  - Tricuspid atresia/Ebstein's
- *Poor mixing/separate parallel systemic and pulmonary circulation:* Transposition of great vessels
- *Common mixing of systemic venous and pulmonary venous blood:* Total anomalous pulmonary venous return (TAPVR), truncus arteriosus, and double outlet ventricle

Hyperoxia test can be used if echocardiography is not available.

Heart Failure

Obstruction to the outflow will lead to heart failure in neonatal period, e.g., coarctation of aorta. Based on severity of obstruction arterial perfusion is predominantly via arterial duct (right to left flow) so called duct-dependent systemic circulation.

Congenital Heart Disease

Presenting as cardiac failure: It has to be congenital heart disease presenting as cardiac failure:

- *Neonate—obstructed systemic circulation (duct-dependent): Presents with shock:*
  - Hypoplastic left heart syndrome
  - Critical aortic valve stenosis
  - Severe coarctation of aorta
  - Interruption of aortic arch

TABLE 2: Clinical features helpful in distinguishing respiratory from cardiac cyanosis.

	Respiratory cyanosis	*Cardiac cyanosis*
History	Prematurity, meconium liquor/below cords, and risk of infection	Family history of congenital heart disease
Respiration	Marked respiratory distress	Little or no respiratory distress unless shocked or metabolic disorders
Cardiovascular examination	Normal	May have clear signs
Response to oxygen	Cyanosis likely to improve	Cyanosis unlikely to improve dramatically
Chest X-ray	• Obvious respiratory pathology • Normal cardiothoracic ratio	No respiratory pathology, abnormal heart shadow, or lung vasculature may be seen
Electrocardiogram	Normal	May be normal, may be helpful
Blood gases	Hypercapnia	Hypo- or normocapnia
Heart rate	++	+++
Respiratory rate	+++	++
Grunt	++	0/+
Murmur	0	0/+/++/+++
Congestive heart failure	0	0/+/++/+++
Abnormal pulses	0	0/+
Response to O_2	+++	0/+

Note: That all categories have overlap between respiratory and cardiac causes.

- *Infants:*
  - Ventricular septal defect
  - Atrioventricular septal defect
  - Large patent ductus arteriosus

Shock

A variety of mechanisms can lead to cardiogenic shock in newborns with duct-dependent CHD when the ductus arteriosus closes **(Flowchart 3)**:

- In left heart obstructive lesions (e.g., hypoplastic left heart syndrome, critical aortic stenosis, coarctation of the aorta, and interrupted aortic arch), systemic perfusion is lost.
- In right-sided obstructive lesions (e.g., total anomalous pulmonary venous connection, tricuspid atresia, and mitral atresia), restricted pulmonary blood flow results in reduced systemic blood flow, which may result in shock.
- In lesions with parallel pulmonary and systemic circulations (e.g., transposition of the great arteries with intact ventricular septum), mixing between the two circulations is decreased, leading to hypoxia and metabolic acidosis, which results in failure and shock.

Flowchart 3: Neonate with cardiogenic shock.

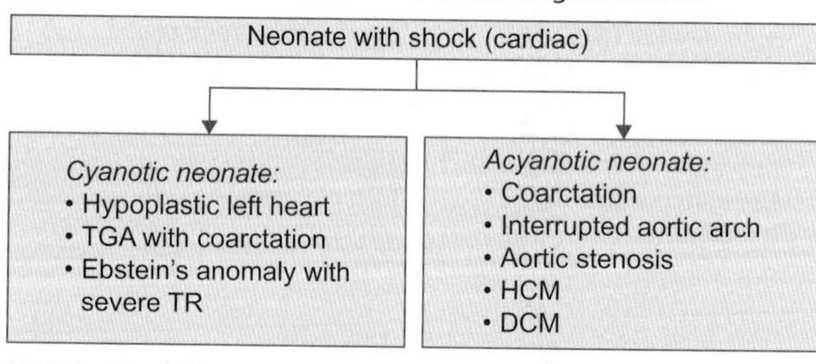

(DCM: dilated cardiomyopathy; HCM: hypertrophic cardiomyopathy; TGA: transposition of the great arteries; TR: tricuspid regurgitation)

- Cardiogenic shock must be differentiated from other causes of shock, such as sepsis. In newborns who present with shock, cardiomegaly is a helpful finding indicating a cardiac etiology.

DIAGNOSIS

If CHD is suspected, a chest X-ray and electrocardiography should be performed. Echocardiography combined with Doppler ultrasound will be able to diagnose all causes of CHD. Cardiac catheterization is seldom needed.

CLINICAL PEARL

- A normal electrocardiogram (ECG) and chest X-ray does not exclude CHD.

SPECIFIC TREATMENT

Individual treatment options for common acyanotic CHDs are given in **Table 3** and those with outflow obstruction in a well child are given in **Table 4** and for a sick child in **Table 5**. The principles of management of CHD are given in **Flowcharts 4 and 5**, and the management of heart failure is given in **Flowchart 6**.

TABLE 3: Acyanotic heart disease: Left-to-right shunts.

Lesion	*Symptoms*	*Signs*	*Management*
ASD—secundum	None	Ejection systolic murmur	Catheter device closure (3–5 years)
AVSD—partial	None, heart failure	Fixed split S2	Surgery at 3 years
VSD—small (80–90%)	None	Pansystolic murmur	None
VSD—large (10–20%)	Heart failure	Active precordium	Diuretics, captopril, surgery at 3–6 months
PDA—term	None	Continuous murmur	Coil or device closure
PDA—preterm	None, heart failure	Systolic murmur + bounding pulses	Fluid restriction, ibuprofen or indomethacin, surgical closure

(ASD: atrial septal defect; AVSD: atrioventricular septal defect; PDA: patent ductus arteriosus; VSD: ventricular septal defect)

TABLE 4: Outflow obstruction in the well child.

Lesion	*Signs*	*Management*
Aortic stenosis	Murmur, upper right sternal edge, and carotid thrill	Balloon dilatation
Pulmonary stenosis	Murmur, upper left sternal edge, and no carotid thrill	Balloon dilatation
Coarctation of aorta	Systemic hypertension, and radiofemoral delay	Surgery

TABLE 5: Left heart outflow obstruction in the sick child—duct-dependent lesion.

Lesion	*Signs*	*Management*
Coarctation of aorta and prostaglandin	Heart murmur and heart failure	Maintain ABC and immediately start prostaglandin
Interrupted aortic arch	• Weak or absent femoral pulses • Blood pressure arms > leg	
Hypoplastic left heart syndrome	• Circulatory collapse • All peripheral pulses weak or absent	• Maintain ABC and immediately start PGE • Surgery (complex) Norwood procedure.

(ABC: airway, blood, and circulation; PGE: prostaglandin E)

Flowchart 4: Cardiac conditions presenting with neonatal respiratory distress.

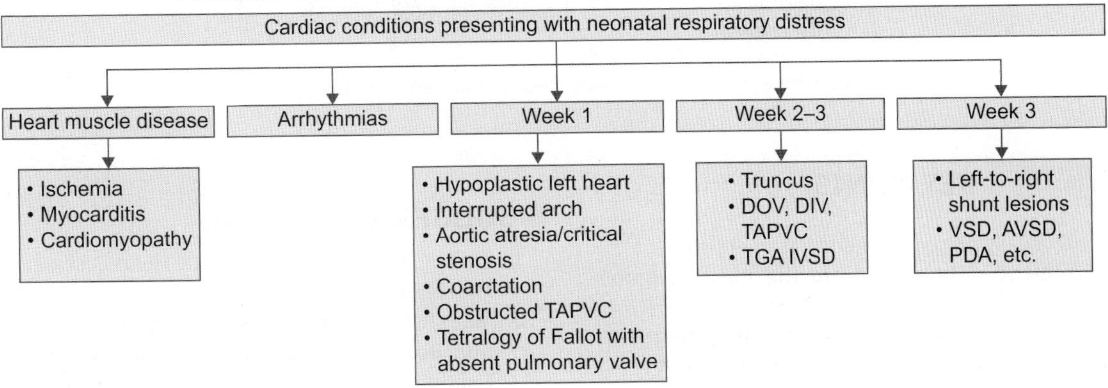

(AVSD: atrioventricular septal defect; DIV: double inlet ventricle; DOV: double outlet ventricle; IVSD: inlet ventricular septal defect; PDA: patent ductus arteriosus; TAPVC: total anomalous pulmonary venous connection; TGA: transposition of the great arteries)

Flowchart 5: Management and approach to congenital heart disease.

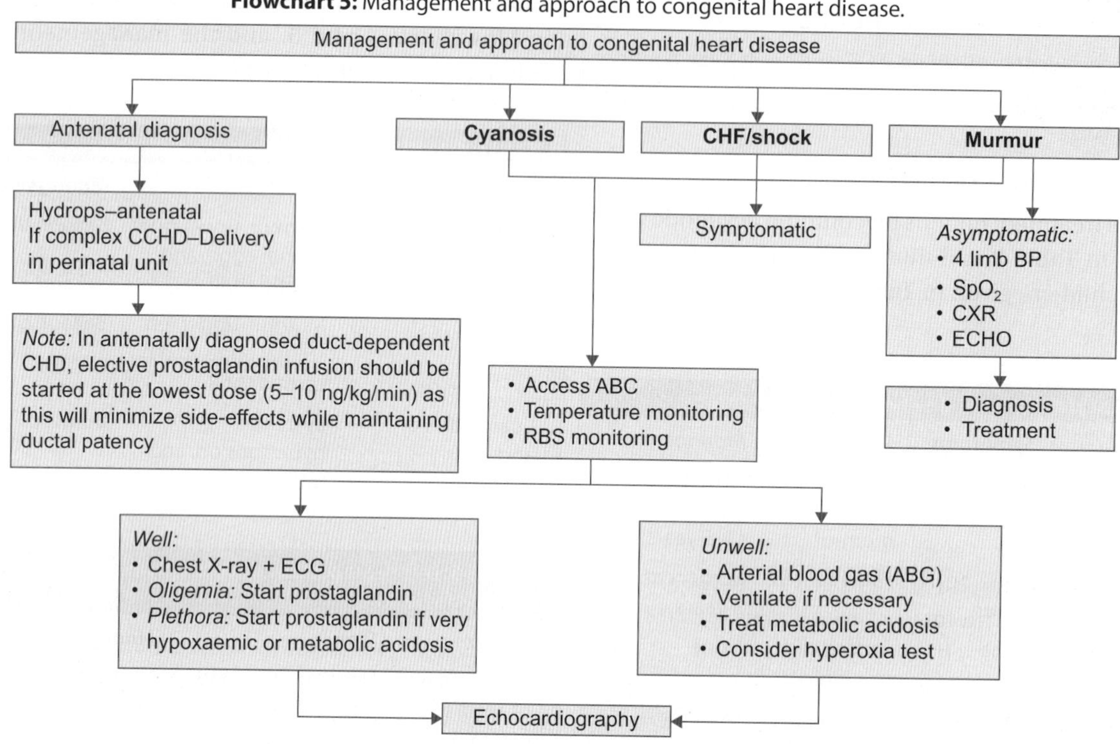

(ABC: airway, breathing, and circulation; BP: blood pressure; CCHD: critical congenital heart disease; CHF: congestive heart failure; CXR: chest X-ray; ECG: echocardiogram; ECGO: echocardiography)

Flowchart 6: Management of heart failure.

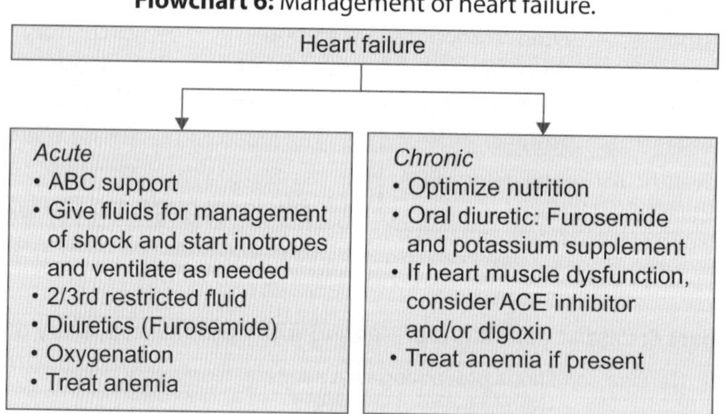

(ABC: airway, breathing, and circulation; ACE: angiotensin-converting enzyme)

KEY POINTS

- Critical CHD usually presents as neonatal emergency.
- Acyanotic left-to-right shunts are the most common anomalies.
- CHD should be considered in neonate presenting with respiratory distress once pulmonary cause is ruled out
- Check pre- and postductal oxygen saturation of all newborns before discharge or by 24 hours to screen for CHD.

SUGGESTED READING

1. Dolbec K, Mick NW. Congenital Heart Disease. Emerg Med Clin N Am. 2011;29:811-27.
2. Yates R. Cardiovascular disease. In: Rennie JM (Ed). Rennie and Roberton's Textbook of Neonatology, 5th edition. London, United Kingdom: Churchill Livingstone; 2012.
3. Yee L. Cardiac emergencies in the first year of life. Emerg Med Clin N Am. 2007;25:981-1008.

First Golden Hour Management of Preterm

Naveen Bajaj

INTRODUCTION

The "Golden Hour" is the critically important first 60 minutes of life in a preterm infant that has the potential to impact both short- and long-term outcomes. This involves many practices conducted systematically by highly specialized healthcare providers with the aim of stabilization of a preterm baby, applicable in both transport and hospital settings. Neonates especially very low birth weight (VLBW) and preterm babies ≤32 weeks of gestation are highly vulnerable to many illnesses setting up in the 1st hours of life when adaptation is critical and timing of care affects survival and long-term outcome. The prime objective of golden hour is to use evidence-based interventions and treatment for better neonatal outcome, importantly for extremely low gestational age neonates. In the golden hour, delivery room stabilization and immediate postnatal standard approach is followed with aim of practicing gentle but timely and effective interventions by an experienced and efficient team.

SPECIAL CONSIDERATIONS IN PRETERM NEONATES

- Poor thermal control
- Poor energy stores
- Poor respiratory drive
- Surfactant deficiency
- Susceptibility to intraventricular hemorrhage (IVH) and periventricular leukomalacia (PVL)
- Often born after a complication of pregnancy like antepartum hemorrhage (APH), intrauterine growth restriction (IUGR), infection, etc.
- Stressed family

AIM OF GOLDEN HOUR (FIG. 1)

- To optimize the survival free of disability in preterm infants (≤32 weeks) and VLBW by providing optimal interventions in the 1st hour of life.

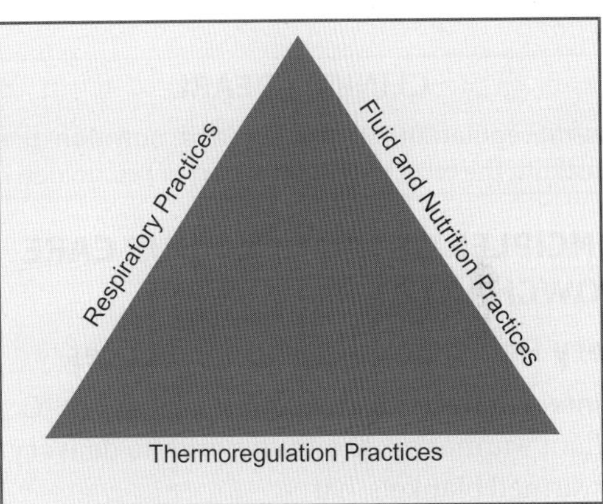

Fig. 1: The Golden Hour triad.

- To undertake all nursing and medical procedures as quickly and with as little disturbance to the infant as possible, usually within 1 hour of admission.

> **CLINICAL PEARL**
>
> Gentleness and consistencies in golden hour stabilization practices by experienced team improve neonatal outcome in preterm and VLBW babies.

BASIC PRINCIPLES

- Lung protection
- Brain protection
- Minimize damage to other organs
- Early nutrition

Techniques included in the golden hour stabilization practices are:

- Thermoregulation
- Resuscitation as per Neonatal Resuscitation Program (NRP) guidelines
- Respiratory management:
  - Oxygen targeting
  - Administering positive end-expiratory pressure (PEEP)

- Continuous positive pressure ventilation (CPAP)/ noninvasive positive pressure ventilation (NIPPV)/ heated humidified high-flow nasal cannula (HHHFNC)
- Nasal ventilator strategies to an infant in the delivery room to reduce intubations
- Identifying early those infants who need surfactant and mechanical ventilation

- Fluid and nutrition
- Treatment and prevention of infections
- Developmentally supportive care
- Family-centered care

> **CLINICAL PEARL**
>
> Thermoregulation, respiratory, and nutrition practices constitute the most important aspect of first golden hour.

PRINCIPLES OF GOLDEN HOUR CARE (FLOWCHART 1)

Delivery Room Stabilization Practices

- Maintain delivery room temperature >25–26°C
- Radiant warmer on 30 minutes prior to delivery
- Prewarmed blankets/hat
- Exothermic mattress
- Plastic wraps/bag in <29 weeks gestation
- Heated and humidified gas during resuscitation and transport (preferable)
- Delayed cord clamping for at least 60 seconds (up to 3 minutes) in stable preterms
- Stabilize spontaneously breathing preterm infants with CPAP
- Use a T-piece device rather than bag and mask if required resuscitation. If apneic, start mask ventilation/ inflations, at initial CPAP pressure of 6–8 cmH_2O and peak inspiratory pressures 20–25 cmH_2O. Use an oxygen blender and start with FiO_2 of 0.30 for babies <28 weeks, 0.21–0.30 for those 28–31 weeks, and 0.21 for 32 weeks of gestation and above. Adjust FiO_2 guided by pulse oximetry and aim for SpO_2 of 80% or more by 5 min of age. Intubation should be reserved for only for babies not responding to positive pressure ventilation via face mask or nasal prongs.
- Transport to neonatal intensive care unit (NICU) in a prewarmed incubator

Thermoregulation

Neonatal intensive care unit practices:

- Radiant warmer/incubator on 30 minutes prior to expected arrival of baby
- On admission to NICU, weigh infant in the polyethylene bag
- Use incubator in ≤28 week baby, and remove bag on admission regardless of admission temperature
- If using radiant warmer and admission temperature is <37°C leave in bag until procedures such as line insertion is completed and then remove bag. If using radiant heat source and admission temperature is ≥37°C remove bag. Place a skin temperature probe to avoid extremes in temperature.

> **CLINICAL PEARL**
>
> In extreme preterms, additional measures like use polythene bag in delivery room and transportation of infant in incubator are desired to prevent hypothermia in early hour.

Respiratory Support

Goals of treatment is to use the least amount of intervention necessary to support normal gas exchange while minimizing lung injury by early intervention, optimizing lung recruitment by using high PEEP and avoiding lung overdistention (low tidal volume 4–6 mL/kg).

- Preterm infants not needing intubation for stabilization: Initiate CPAP or NIPPV as soon as possible in all babies <30 weeks of gestational age and larger babies if they started to have signs of respiratory distress. HHHFNC can be used as an alternative, provided centers have the facility to provide CPAP or NIPPV for those falling HHHFNC. CPAP is given by short binasal prongs or mask with a starting pressure of about 6–8 cmH_2O. Give surfactant when FiO_2 > 0.3 on CPAP pressure ≥6 cmH_2O or if lung ultrasound suggests surfactant deficiency. In CPAP or NIPPV babies, use LISA technique (preferred) or INSURE for administering surfactant. Consider lower FiO_2 thresholds for very immature infants. A second and third dose of surfactant can be given if there is ongoing evidence of RDS.
- Preterm baby (especially <30 weeks of gestation) requiring intubation for stabilization: Give surfactant as early as possible. For invasive ventilation, always use patient triggered (PTV) ventilation modes. Volume targeted ventilation (VTV) or high-frequency oscillation ventilation is considered lung protective. Minimize the duration of mechanical ventilation (MV). When weaning from MV, tolerate moderate hypercarbia but maintain pH above 7.22. Try early extubation for spontaneously breathing babies and use postexubation CPAP, HHHFNC, or NIPPV immediately following surfactant.

- Use only natural surfactant.
- Oxygen saturation target should be between 91–95% with alarm limits 90–96%
- Use caffeine routinely in infants <32 weeks of gestation requiring respiratory support.

CLINICAL PEARL

- Use of prophylactic/early nasal CPAP/NIPPV and early rescue surfactant therapy is aimed to minimize lung injury.

Flowchart 1: Algorithm of golden hour management in preterm.

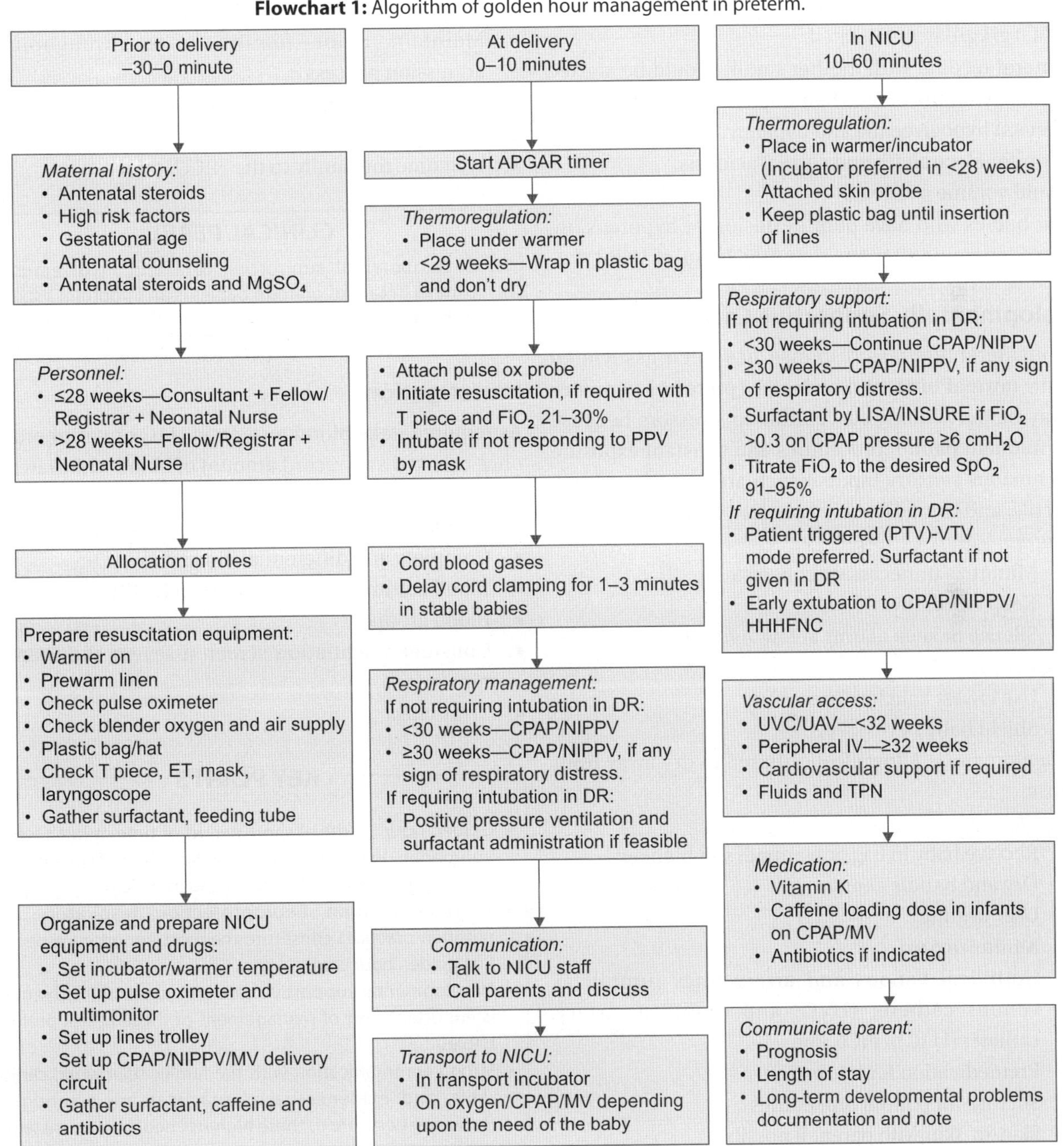

(CPAP: continuous positive airway pressure; NIPPV: nasal intermittent positive pressure ventilation; HHHFNC: heated humidified high-flow nasal cannula; MV: mechanical ventilation; PTV: patient triggered ventilation; VTV: volume targeted ventilation; UVC: umbilical venous catheter)

Fluids and Nutrition

Goal is to prevent hypoglycemia but also fluid overload:

- Start fluids 70–100 mL/kg depending upon the gestational age.
- Parenteral nutrition should be started from birth. Amino acids 1.5–2 g/kg/d should be started from day 1 and quickly built up to 2.5–3.5 g/kg/d. Lipids 1–2 g/kg/d should be started from day 1 and quickly built up to 4.0 g/kg/day as tolerated.
- Enteral feeding with mother's milk should be started from day 1 if the baby is hemodynamically stable.
- Prevent hypoglycemia and hyperglycemia.
- Monitor electrolytes and correct acidosis.
- Avoid volume overload.
- For babies who have poor perfusion or hypotension, start dopamine after one slow fluid bolus of 10 mL/kg.

Developmentally Supportive Care

- Considerable stress response has been associated with normal birth and high-risk (preterm) neonates may be particularly susceptible to stressors because of frequent painful procedures and constant exposure to noxious sensory inputs which are auditory, visual, tactile, and chemosensory in nature in NICU.
- *Sound:*
  - Minimize unnecessary conversation
  - Keep voices low
  - Silence or keep alarms at low volume
- *Light:*
  - Use lowest light level necessary
  - Shield baby's eyes
- *Chemosensory:* Allow alcohol-based to dry away from nose
- *Tactile:*
  - Receive baby in bag or warmed, soft blanket
  - Dry and handle gently
  - Use "nesting"
  - Minimize pain
  - Umbilical venous and artery lines [umbilical venous catheter (UVC) and umbilical artery catheter (UAC)]/PICC line
  - Premedication for intubation
  - Sucrose for painful procedures
  - Skin-to-skin with parent if possible

Family Involvement

Birth of a high-risk neonate is highly anxiety-provoking for families:

- Provide neonatology consultation or repeat consultation before the birth of the infant.
- Establish contact between the family and members of the NICU team and/or other support individuals before the birth of the infant.
- Maintain infant—family contact throughout the admission process.
- Ensure that the family is fully informed of their infant's condition.
- Welcome the family to the NICU.

CLINICAL PEARL

- Developmental supportive care and involvement of parents in care of preterm babies is an important aspect of management.

Investigation

As required, take blood tests from UAC or peripheral line once inserted and record amount of blood withdrawn.

- Blood glucose
- Arterial blood gas (ABG)
- Complete and differential blood counts
- Blood culture, C-reactive protein (CRP)
- Blood group
- Consider coagulation screen if severe chorioamnionitis/sepsis
- X-ray chest

KEY POINTS

- Golden hour is critical short period of time at birth where appropriate interventions (or the lack thereof) can make a difference in neonatal mortality and morbidity.
- Thermoregulation, neuroprotection, respiratory, and nutrition practices constitute the most important aspect of first golden hour care.
- Developmental supportive care and parental involvement is important part of management of these at risk preterm babies.
- Strong communication with the family, teamwork, clinical skills, and evidence-based practices are essential in delivering best care to these high-risk neonates consistently.

SUGGESTED READING

1. Davis PG, Lemyre B, De Paoli AG. Nasal intermittent positive pressure ventilation (NIPPV) versus nasal continuous positive airway pressure (NCPAP) for preterm neonates after extubation. Cochrane Database Syst Rev. 2001;(3):CD003212.
2. Rojas-Reyes MX, Morley CJ, Soll R. Prophylactic versus selective use of surfactant in preventing morbidity and mortality in preterm infants. Cochrane Database Syst Rev. 2012;(3):CD000510.
3. Stevens TP, Blennow M, Myers EH, Soll R. Early surfactant administration with brief ventilation vs. selective surfactant and continued mechanical ventilation for preterm infants with or at risk for respiratory distress syndrome. Cochrane Database Syst Rev. 2007;(4):CD003063.
4. SUPPORT Study Group of the Eunice Kennedy Shriver NICHD Neonatal Research Network. Early CPAP versus surfactant in extremely preterm infants. N Engl J Med. 2010;362(21):1970-9.
5. SUPPORT Study Group of the Eunice Kennedy Shriver NICHD Neonatal Research Network. Neurodevelopmental outcomes in the early CPAP and pulse oximetry trial. New England Journal of Medicine. 2012;367(26):2495-504.
6. SUPPORT Study Group of the Eunice Kennedy Shriver NICHD Neonatal Research Network. Target ranges of oxygen saturation in extremely preterm infants. N Engl J Med. 2010;362(21):1959-69.
7. Sweet DG, Carnielli VP, Greisen G, Hallman M, Klebermass-Schrehof K, Ozek E, et al. European Consensus Guidelines on the Management of Respiratory Distress Syndrome: 2022 Update. Neonatology. 2023;120(1):3-23.

CHAPTER 17

Perinatal Hypoxia

Ashish Jain, Chandan S

INTRODUCTION

Perinatal hypoxia/asphyxia is a common major health problem causing morbidity and mortality in neonates. According to National Neonatal-Perinatal Database (NNPD), perinatal hypoxia is the most common cause of stillbirth accounting up to 45% of cases and is one among the three leading causes of neonatal mortality. This denotes the magnitude of this serious clinical condition. Cautious monitoring and management of a neonate with perinatal hypoxia is an area of importance. Guidelines on clinical approach and management may help in improving the outcome. The management of perinatal hypoxia is evolving day by day with better understanding of its pathophysiology.

DEFINITIONS

The definitions of perinatal hypoxia vary from context to context. Thus, there is no single definition of perinatal hypoxia.

- The World Health Organization (WHO) defines perinatal asphyxia as failure to initiate and sustain breathing at birth.
- The NNPD defines perinatal hypoxia/asphyxia as moderate when there is slow/gasping breathing or an Apgar score of 4–6 at 1 minute and severe if no breathing or an Apgar score of 0–3 at 1 minute of age.
- American Academy of Pediatrics and American College of Obstetrics and Gynecology (AAP and ACOG) require presence of all of the following criteria to define perinatal asphyxia:
  - Profound metabolic or mixed acidemia (pH <7.0) in umbilical cord blood.
  - Persistence of low Apgar scores <3 for >5 minutes.
  - Signs of neonatal neurologic dysfunction (e.g., seizures, encephalopathy, and tone abnormalities)
  - Evidence of multiple organ involvement (such as that of kidneys, lungs, liver, heart, and intestine).

CLINICAL PEARLS

- No definition of perinatal asphyxia is complete, all the definitions have limitations. The definition which is feasible and sensitive and relevant for the care of the neonate should be used.
- All the definitions and grading of perinatal asphyxia are based on babies >35 weeks of gestation and preterm specific definitions are not present.

CLINICAL EVALUATION

Subsequent to the resuscitation of the baby (especially when the neonate has needed >60 seconds of positive pressure ventilation), the postasphyxiated newborn should undergo a detailed clinical evaluation, as this neonate is prone for multiorgan dysfunction as perinatal hypoxia virtually affects every organ system. Further management and outcome vary on the severity of organ dysfunction. There are several scoring systems that have being used. A scoring system that can be specifically followed for that setting should be used. Some of the scoring system would need an electroencephalography (EEG) and other investigations on the baby. The most commonly used systems are:

- Sarnat and Sarnat staging system—a descriptive staging system.
- Levene staging system—a simpler, practical staging system.
- Thompson scoring system, this offers a continuum of grading.
- Saben scoring system, which can be used very early and also delineates the mild cases.

The babies who have mild stage of the disease (Thompson score <10) are almost free of any neurodevelopmental sequelae, however, the babies with moderate and severe stage of encephalopathy (Thompson score >10 and >15) may have a neurodevelopmental impairment in 25% and 95% of cases, respectively.

A nonprogressing score is also reassuring and has a better outcome; hence the serial examination is important on day-to-day basis for the first 7 days.

CLINICAL PEARLS

- Staging/scoring system is vital in management of hypoxic-ischemic encephalopathy (HIE). Blood gas and electroencephalogram should be done wherever the facility is available.
- These systems though vital in management, a single time finding should not be used as criteria to prognosticate parents about baby. It is suggested to serially follow-up and prognosticate about the baby accordingly.

MONITORING

Neonates requiring >60 seconds of resuscitative efforts are to be shifted to neonatal intensive care unit (NICU) to monitor for encephalopathy, organ hypoxia, and initiating appropriate further management. Neonates with mild encephalopathy only require monitoring at regular intervals for signs of advanced stages of hypoxic-ischemic encephalopathy (HIE). The clinical features of HIE vary over time. The window period between these stages can be used for therapeutic intervention. Strict clinical monitoring will help in management of these neonates. Perinatal hypoxia affects virtually every organ system mainly renal, central nervous system, and cardiac. The clinical features of organ dysfunction should be looked for. Organ system dysfunction seen in perinatal hypoxia is given in **Table 1**.

DIAGNOSTICS IN BIRTH ASPHYXIA

Amplitude-integrated Electroencephalography

Amplitude-integrated electroencephalography (aEEG) is a derived simplified version of conventional EEG, a bedside tool for cerebral function monitoring, as a part of the evaluation of infants with HIE. It gives five patterns of background activity of the underlying brain. (1) Continuous normal voltage; (2) Discontinuous normal voltage; (3) Burst suppression; (4) Continuous low voltage; (5) Flat trace. Last three patterns (3), (4), and (5) suggest diffuse cortical/thalamic neuronal involvement, hence associated with poor prognosis. Additionally, the seizures persisting for >2–3 minutes can also be detected by this method. Normal sleep wake cycling is also an important prognostic pointer that can be estimated by the aEEG.

TABLE 1: Suggested monitoring in moderate-to-severe cases of perinatal asphyxia.

Organ system	*Possible dysfunctions*	*Monitoring recommended*
Temperature	Temperature dysregulation	Continuous monitoring of temperature, avoid hyperthermia of any degree
CNS	HIE, intracranial hemorrhage, seizures, long-term neurological sequelae	Staging system of HIE, aEEG monitoring where facilities are available
Cardiac	Myocardial dysfunction, valvular dysfunction, rhythm abnormalities, congestive cardiac failure	Heart rate, ECG monitoring, SpO_2 monitoring, invasive BP monitoring when required
Renal	Hematuria, acute tubular necrosis, renal vein thrombosis	Urine output measurement, urine routine examination, renal parameters, and serum electrolytes
Pulmonary	Delayed adaptation, respiratory failure, meconium aspiration, surfactant depletion, primary pulmonary hypertension, pulmonary hemorrhage	ABG monitoring, regular adjustments and monitoring of the ventilator settings
GI tract	Sluggish bowel movements, necrotizing enterocolitis, hepatic dysfunction	Abdominal girth monitoring, see for aspirates if distention present, monitor bowel sounds.
Hematological	Thrombocytopenia, coagulation abnormalities	Complete blood counts with platelets and PT, especially if bleeding
Others	Metabolic acidosis, hypoglycemia, hypocalcemia, hyponatremia, adrenal hemorrhage	Regular monitoring of the blood sugar, calcium, and electrolyte

(ABG: arterial blood gas; aEEG, amplitude-integrated electroencephalography; BP: blood pressure; CNS: central nervous system; ECG: electrocardiogram; GI: gastrointestinal; HIE: hypoxic-ischemic encephalopathy; PT: prothrombin time; SpO_2: pulse oxygen saturation)

Ultrasonography and Magnetic Resonance Imaging Brain

Early stage of perinatal asphyxia the only finding may be gross cerebral edema with obliterated ventricles later on hyperechoic basal ganglia and thalamus suggest involvement of brain. In severe cases on follow-up scans cystic encephalomalacia is apparent. Most accurate and modality of choice, conventional magnetic resonance imaging (MRI) shows abnormalities in the first 3–4 days, but generally not on the first 2 days. Diffusion-weighted imaging (DWI) sequence is not only more sensitive than conventional MRI, but also shows abnormalities earlier, often in the first 24–48 hours after birth. The patterns which are commonly seen are selective neuronal necrosis, parasagittal cerebral injury, and focal cerebral ischemic lesions.

Resistive Index in the Anterior/Middle Cerebral Artery Dopplers

The resistive index (RI) values in normal newborn are 0.74±0.08. The RI values in the early HIE (in first 24 hours) which are <0.6 (hyperemic phase) the RI in later stages of HIE >0.9 suggesting the cerebral ischemia, have a predictive role in prognosticating the neonates with HIE.

Near-infrared Spectroscopy

Measures difference in the absorption spectra of oxygenated and deoxygenated hemoglobin. Continuous noninvasive tool to assess cerebral and peripheral oxygenation and oxygen extraction. Channels applied over forehead to gauge cerebral rSO_2 and over flank to measure renal rSO_2, Normal cerebral rSO_2: 60–70% and splanchnic rSO_2: 80% useful for cerebral oxygen monitoring in term infants. Cerebral oxygenation drops in the first 4–6 hours of life following HI injury and recovers by 18–20 hours. This post HIE drop in cerebral oxygenation was less evident in infants who subsequently develop brain injury. Higher cerebral oxygenation between 24 and 36 hours of life also significantly increased the odds of having moderate-to-severe injury on MRI.

MANAGEMENT

The management is mainly supportive and comprises of cardiac, respiratory, metabolic, and neurological support in the form of maintaining optimum saturation, perfusion, blood sugar, calcium levels, and control of seizures.

Delivery Room Management

Maintain appropriate temperature, airway, and serially record Apgar score. Practicing delayed cord clamping for infants requiring resuscitation at birth is currently not recommended. However, the evidence is evolving for resuscitation with the delayed cord clamping/intact cord in the neonates with perinatal asphyxia at birth requiring resuscitation. Collect umbilical arterial cord blood after double clamping for analysis of cord arterial blood gas (ABG) that can reflect the acidemia in the perinatal period. A neonate with moderate-to-severe hypoxia is resuscitated as per the Neonatal Resuscitation Program (NRP) guidelines and transferred to NICU for further management. A neonate requiring <60 seconds of resuscitative efforts is transferred to mother's side and monitored frequently every 30 minutes–1 hour for the next 48–72 hours for development of any features of HIE **(Table 2)**.

Management in Neonatal Intensive Care Unit

Management of moderate-to-severe hypoxia consists of clinical, lab monitoring at regular intervals, and maintaining the physiology, viz., temperature, oxygenation, fluid, and electrolyte status. Any complications like seizures are promptly managed. Clinical parameters such as heart rate, respiratory rate, pulse oxygen saturation (SpO_2), temperature, blood pressure, capillary refill time, urine output, and neurological examinations for the signs of HIE should be monitored at regular intervals.

TABLE 2: Levene staging system for hypoxic-ischemic encephalopathy.

Features	*Mild*	*Moderate*	*Severe*
Consciousness	Irritable	Lethargy	Comatose
Tone	Hypotonia	Marked hypotonia	Severe hypotonia
Seizures	No	Yes	Prolonged or uncontrolled
Sucking/respiration	Poor suck	Unable to suck	Unable to sustain spontaneous respiration

Laboratory parameters to be monitored include blood sugar, blood gas, urine osmolality, serum electrolytes, and renal function tests at regular intervals. Other parameters such as electrocardiogram, and chest X-ray should be done in clinically indicated babies.

Important management guidelines for care in NICU are discussed in the following text.

Supportive Therapy

- Maintain normal temperature and avoid hyperthermia.
- Maintain adequate ventilation and oxygenation. The oxygen saturations should be targeted between 90 and 95%. Assisted ventilation should be provided in case of apnea or respiratory distress causing inadequate respiration. Permissive hypercarbia is allowed.
- Maintain fluid and electrolyte status by judicious use of fluids (need for alteration of fluids should be calculated every 12 hours initially and may be as frequent as 6–8 hourly in sick babies. Where tissue perfusion is poor, consider fluid bolus and inotrope support (dopamine and dobutamine). Dobutamine is a better choice as the peripheral vascular resistance in these babies is already high. Restricted fluid administration as a routine is not advised as it may predispose the baby to hypotension and approximately two-thirds of the cases with acute kidney injury (AKI) are nonoliguric. Restrict fluid only if there is hyponatremia (sodium <120 mg/dL) due to syndrome of inappropriate antidiuretic hormone secretion and in cases of acute renal failure. Hypoxia may cause injury to heart affecting its contractility. This can be assessed using echocardiography and managed accordingly.
- Maintain normal metabolic milieu by frequent monitoring of blood sugar. Serum calcium is monitored regularly. It is recommended to administer calcium in maintenance dose to all severely hypoxic for 2 days so as to maintain calcium in normal range.
- Seizures are serious manifestation of HIE (stage II HIE). Hypoxic seizures usually occur in the first 12–24 hours. These may be subtle or evident prominently. Electroencephalogram recording will help to identify subclinical seizures. Any metabolic disturbances such as hypoglycemia, hyponatremia, and hypocalcemia should be corrected.

Specific Therapy

Treatment of seizures: Phenobarbitone is the initial drug of choice. Loading dose of 20 mg/kg followed by two additional boluses of 10 mg/kg if seizures continue. Maintenance dose of 3–5 mg/kg/day is started after 24 hours. Monitor for respiratory depression during loading doses.

Phenytoin is added to seizures uncontrolled by phenobarbitone. Loading dose is 15–20 mg/kg and maintenance dose is 4–8 mg/kg/day.

Benzodiazepines are third-line drugs. Lorazepam is advised in doses of 0.05–0.1 mg/kg/dose intravenously. In refractory cases, consider use of investigations such as EEG, cranial ultrasonography, computed tomography scan, and MRI brain to evaluate for neural injuries.

Long-term seizure management: Following cessation of acute symptomatic seizures (electroclinical or electrographic-only seizures) without evidence for neonatal onset epilepsy, antiseizure medications should be discontinued before discharge, regardless of the MRI or EEG findings. If more than one antiseizure medication is used, the last antiseizure medication is weaned first.

- *Cardiac support:* Fluid bolus and inotrope are advised to maintain adequate perfusion.
- It is advised to withhold feeds until all parameters are stable.
- Hematologic, hepatic, and pulmonary derangements are managed accordingly.

Therapeutic Hypothermia

This is now emerging as a novel therapy in babies with perinatal asphyxia to prevent the death and neurodevelopmental impairment. This mode is used in infants of 36 weeks gestation or more with moderate-to-severe encephalopathy. It consists of moderate use of therapeutic hypothermia (33–34°C) within 6 hours of life. It has shown reduction in combined outcome of mortality or major neurodevelopmental sequelae if initiated within 6 hours of life and continued till 72 hours of age.

CLINICAL PEARLS

- Metabolic cause should be ruled out while managing seizures in a neonate with perinatal hypoxia.
- Monitoring and management of multisystem is a key factor in prognosis of the baby.

Long-term Prognosis

Thompson score **(Table 3)** of 15 or more had a high positive predictive value (PPV) of 92% and modest negative predictive value (NPV) of 82% in predicting abnormal outcome at 1 year of age. The long-term sequelae post-moderate-severe HIE vary from mild cognitive difficulties

TABLE 3: Thompson score.

Signs	*0*	*1*	*2*	*3*
Tone	Normal	Hyper	Hypo	Flaccid
LOC	Normal	Hyperalert, stare	Lethargic	Comatose
Fits	None	<3 per day	>2 per day	Refractory
Posture	Normal	Fisting, cycling	Strong distal flexion	Decerebrate
Moro	Normal	Partial	Absent	–
Grasp	Normal	Poor	Absent	–
Suck	Normal	Poor	Absent ± bites	–
Respiration	Normal	Hyperventilation	Brief apnea	IPPV
Fontanel	Normal	Full, not tense	Tense	–

(LOC: Level of consciousness; IPPV: intermittent positive pressure ventilation).

Flowchart 1: Algorithm for management of an asphyxiated baby.

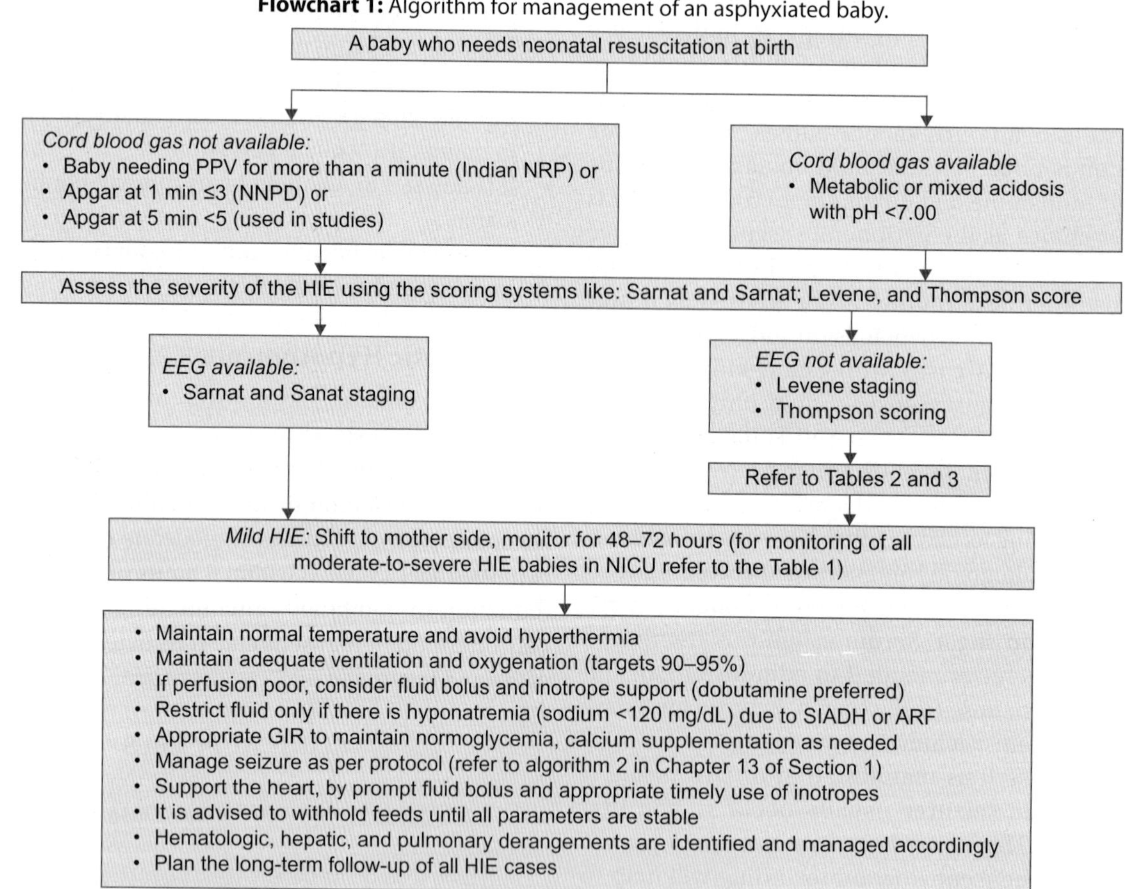

(ARF: acute renal failure; EEG: electroencephalography; GIR: glucose infusion rate; HIE: hypoxic-ischemic encephalopathy; NICU: neonatal intensive care unit; NNPD: National Neonatal-Perinatal Database; NRP: Neonatal Resuscitation Program; PPV: positive pressure ventilation; SIADH: syndrome of inappropriate antidiuretic hormone secretion)

without any motor problems to significant motor impairment affecting the quality of life. A recent systematic review which included seven studies concluded that nearly 25–60% of survivors of HIE have cognitive impairment without cerebral palsy. In another review, 30% of moderate HIE cases had cerebral palsy (CP) whilst remaining 70% without CP had significant cognitive deficits at 15–19 years.

Previously, only moderate-to-severe HIE were thought to contribute to the adverse outcomes, prospective research in mild encephalopathy (PRIME) study reported 16% of disability in mild HIE children at 18–22 months of age with 7% of them being severe, emphasizing importance of long-term follow-up needed even in mild HIE.

KEY POINTS

- Good antenatal care and prompt neonatal resuscitation are essential for prevention of perinatal hypoxia. However, in the event of a baby suffering from hypoxia at birth, adequate supportive care, and specific management can reduce the mortality and long-term morbidity provided there is least possible delay in starting the treatment.
- A system of staging like Levene staging system, a practical and easy-to-use system or others, like Thompson score, should be used in every case for better management and prognostication.
- Therapeutic hypothermia is an emerging mode of therapy in the management of an asphyxiated baby with better long-term outcome.
- The early prediction of the complications and supportive management forms the cornerstone in the management of a baby with perinatal asphyxia **(Flowchart 1)**.

SUGGESTED READING

1. Ahearne CE, Boylan GB, Murray DM. Short- and long-term prognosis in perinatal asphyxia: an update. World J Clin Pediatr. 2016;5(1):67-74.
2. Blackmon LR, Stark AR. American Academy of Pediatrics Committee on Fetus and Newborn. Hypothermia: a neuroprotective therapy for neonatal hypoxic ischemic encephalopathy. Pediatrics. 2006;117(3):942-8.
3. Goeral K, Urlesberger B, Giordano V, Kasprian G, Wagner M, Schmidt L, et al. Prediction of outcome in neonates with hypoxic-ischemic encephalopathy: role of amplitude-integrated electroencephalography and cerebral oxygen saturation measured by near-infrared spectroscopy. Neonatology. 2017;112(3):193-202.
4. Jacobs SE, Berg M, Hunt R, Tarnow-Mordi WO, Inder TE, Davis PG. Cooling for newborns with hypoxic ischaemic encephalopathy. Cochrane Database Syst Rev. 2013;1: CD003311.
5. Levene MI. The asphyxiated newborn infant. In: Levene MI, Lilford RJ (Eds). Fetal and neonatal neurology and neurosurgery. Edinburgh: Churchill Livingstone; 1995. pp. 405-25.
6. National Neonatal Perinatal Database Report (National Neonatology Forum, India); 2003. [online] Available from https://newbornwhocc.org/nnpo.aspx [Last accessed March, 2025].
7. Pressler RM, Abend NS, Auvin S, Boylan G, Brigo F, Cilio MR, et al. Treatment of Seizures in the Neonate: Guidelines and Consensus-based Recommendations: Special Report from the ILAE Task Force on Neonatal Seizures. Epilepsia. 2023;64(10):2550-70.
8. Salasa J, Tekes A, Hwang M, Northington FJ, Huisman TA. Head ultrasound in neonatal hypoxic ischemic injury and its mimickers for clinicians: a review of the patterns of injury and the evolution of findings over time. Neonatology. 2018;114:185-97.
9. Sarnat HB, Sarnat MS. Neonatal encephalopathy following fetal distress: a clinical and encephalographic study. Arch Neurol. 1976;33:696-705.
10. Thompson CM, Puterman AS, Linley LL, Hann FM, van der Elst CW, Molteno CD, et al. The value of a scoring system for hypoxic ischemic encephalopathy in predicting neurodevelopmental outcome. Acta Paediatr. 1997;86;757-61.

Calcium and Magnesium Disorders and Approach to Metabolic Bone Disease

Ashish Jain, Shoham Majumder

INTRODUCTION

Calcium is a vital mineral in the human body and plays an important role in providing structural integrity to bones and facilitating various biological processes such as energy metabolism, cell proliferation, coagulation, enzyme activity, muscle contraction, and nerve conduction. This diverse range of functions is possible due to a substantial electrochemical gradient of ionized calcium between intracellular (0.1 μmol/L) and extracellular fluid (1 mmol/L). The distribution of calcium in the body is given in **Flowchart 1**.

HYPOCALCEMIA

There is significant flux in calcium concentrations in neonatal period, especially during perinatal transition. Reference calcium ranges are given in **Table 1**. The exact definition of hypocalcemia is debatable and may depend on the gestational age, birth weight, and the clinical status of the baby. While serum calcium and ionized calcium may be linearly correlated at normal pH and albumin levels, in sick neonates the latter is a preferable marker of calcium status. Early (<72 hours) and late (>72 hours, usually after 1 week) have different etiologies and deserve separate approach for management **(Flowchart 2)**.

Flowchart 1: Distribution of calcium in the body.

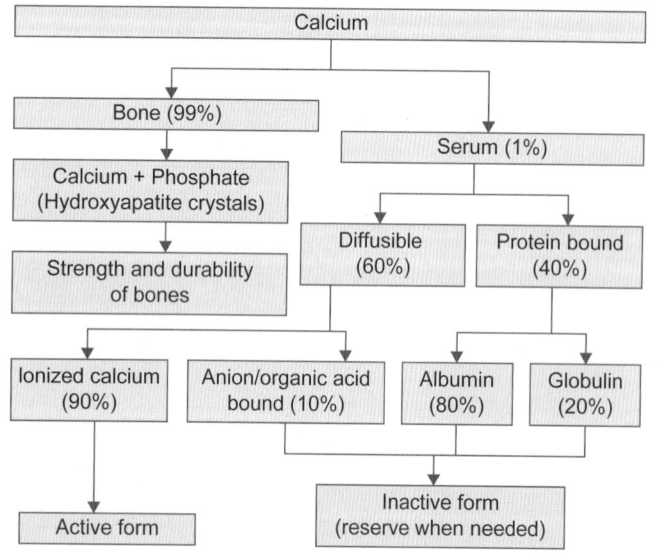

Clinical Features

Majority of hypocalcemic neonates are asymptomatic. The clinical features are variable **(Table 2)** and have no correlation with fall in calcium levels.

> **CLINICAL PEARLS**
>
> - Hypoalbuminemia can reduce total serum calcium without significant decline in ionized calcium levels.
> - Alkalosis (hyperventilation or bicarbonate infusion) or rapid buffer infusion (exchange transfusion or ECMO) reduces ionized calcium and produces clinical manifestations of hypocalcemia without reduction in serum calcium levels.

TABLE 1: Reference values of calcium.

Normocalcemia		
Total		9–10.6 mg/dL (2.25–2.65 mmol/L)
Ionized		4.84–5.0 mg/dL (1.21–1.28 mmol/L)
Hypocalcemia		
Preterm	Total	<7 mg/dL (<1.75 mmol/L)
	Ionized	<4.0 mg/dL (<1.0 mmol/L)
Term	Total	<8 mg/dL (2 mmol/L)
	Ionized	<4.4 mg/dL (<1.1 mmol/L)
Hypercalcemia		
Total		>11.0 mg/dL
Ionized		>5.0 mg/dL

Flowchart 2: Etiopathogenesis of neonatal hypocalcemia. *Black boxes:* Early-onset hypocalcemia. *Gray boxes:* Late-onset hypocalcemia.

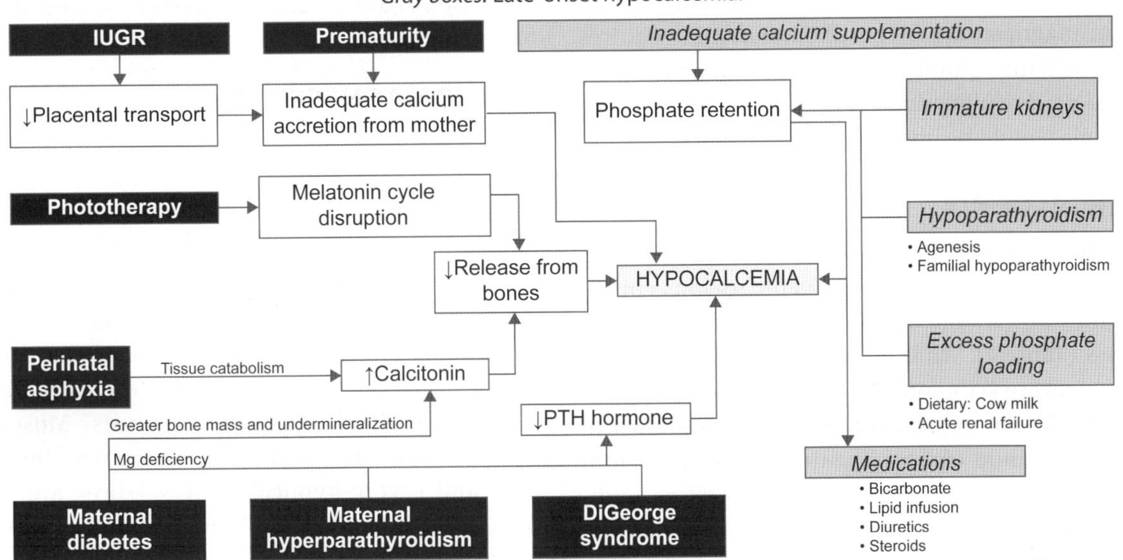

(IUGR: intrauterine growth restriction; PTH: parathyroid hormone)

TABLE 2: Clinical features of hypocalcemia.

Common	*Rare*
• Lethargy and poor feeding • Hypotonia	• Laryngospasm • Wheezing (bronchospasm)
• Apnea, tachypnea, and tachycardia	• Vomiting (pylorospasm)
• Hyperactivity • Jitteriness • Focal/generalized clonic seizures • QTc interval prolongation	• Melena

Evaluation of Neonatal Hypocalcemia

Evaluation of neonatal hypocalcemia is given in **Table 3**.

TABLE 3: Evaluation of neonatal hypocalcemia.

History	
Family history	Autosomal dominant hypercalciuric hypocalcemia, familial hypoparathyroidism
Maternal history	Diabetes mellitus, hyperpara-thyroidism, and drugs
Natal history	Prematurity, intrauterine growth restriction (IUGR), and birth asphyxia
Nutritional history	Supplementation and dosage, total parenteral nutrition (TPN), and intralipid infusion
Medication history	Diuretics and steroids
Examination	
Features of IUGR, phenotypic features of infants of diabetic mothers (IDM), dysmorphism, and skeletal dysplasias	
Investigations	
First line	Total serum calcium and ionized Ca^{2+}, phosphate, albumin, and glucose
Nonresponsive cases	Serum magnesium
Intractable cases	Parathyroid hormone, vitamin D, calcitonin, genetic studies and 24 hours urine calcium
Others	• Chest X-ray (thymic shadow and aortic arch), X-ray for skeletal dysplasias • *Electrocardiogram (ECG):* QTc interval prolongation

Management of Hypocalcemia

Emergency treatment of hypocalcemic tetany or seizures requires intravenous calcium (18 mg/kg elemental calcium commonly as 2 mL/kg of 10% calcium gluconate diluted with equal volume of dextrose over 10 minutes under cardiac monitoring). Dose can be repeated 10 minutes later in case of no response. After resolution of acute crisis, intravenous calcium can be continued as 75 mg/kg/day of elemental calcium (8 mL/kg/day of 10% calcium gluconate) till serum calcium levels stabilize. Stepwise tapering should be done (50% for 12 hours, 25% for 12 hours) before discontinuation. Supplemental calcium may be given enterally. Serum Ca^{2+} is monitored daily for 1–2 days after stopping therapy. Poor response to calcium therapy should prompt suspicions of concurrent hypomagnesemia (check section on magnesium). Hyperphosphatemia requires diet rich in calcium and low in phosphate (human milk if available or low phosphate formula feed). Persistent hypocalcemia should be investigated thoroughly.

HYPERCALCEMIA

Hypercalcemia is defined as total serum calcium >11 mg/dL (or ionized calcium >5 mg/dL). Iatrogenic reasons constitute a majority and should be ruled out before considering rarer causes **(Table 4)**. While asymptomatic in most cases, increasingly severe symptoms appear with rising calcium levels **(Table 5)**. An approach to diagnosis is shown in **Flowchart 3**. In mild cases, adjusting levels of calcium and phosphorus is adequate. In more severe cases, additional therapies include appropriate rehydration followed by furosemide to enable calcium excretion in urine. Specific therapies consist of glucocorticoids, calcitonin, bisphosphonates, parathyroidectomy, and dialysis in intractable cases.

TABLE 4: Etiology of hypercalcemia.

Iatrogenic (most common cause)	• Prematurity related hypophosphatemia • Hypervitaminosis A and D • Thiazide diuretics • Calcium salt excess	
Hyperparathyroidism	Maternal hypoparathyroidism and hypocalcemia	
	Mutation of CaSR	Neonatal severe hyperparathyroidism
		Familial hypocalciuric hypercalcemia
Hypercalcemia with skeletal dysplasia	• Infantile hypophosphatasia • Jansen metaphyseal chondrodysplasia • Williams syndrome	
Others	• Distal renal tubular acidosis • Congenital hypothyroidism • Subcutaneous fat necrosis • Blue diaper syndrome	

HYPOMAGNESEMIA

Hypomagnesemia is considered when serum magnesium levels are below 1.6 mg/dL (0.66 mmol/L) but symptoms usually appear at levels below 1.2 mg/dL (0.49 mmol/L) though there is no strict correlation. The reasons may be either due to decreased magnesium supply [intrauterine growth restriction (IUGR), maternal diabetes, and malabsorption syndromes] or increased magnesium loss (loop diuretics, high-dose aminoglycosides, exchange transfusion with citrated blood, and osmotic diuresis). Most cases are asymptomatic. In severe cases, there may hyperexcitability and severe hypocalcemic seizures unresponsive to calcium infusions. Treatment requires intravenous administration of 50% magnesium sulfate solution, 0.05–0.1 mL/kg (equivalent to 2.5–5 mg/kg of elemental magnesium) slowly over 30–60 minutes while monitoring for bradycardia and hypotension. Oral supplementation may be given at 0.2 mL/kg with at least 5–6 folds dilution to avoid osmotic diarrhea. Outcome is usually favorable.

HYPERMAGNESEMIA

Hypermagnesemia occurs when serum magnesium levels cross 2.8 mg/dL (1.15 mmol/L). It is almost always an iatrogenic event with either excessive magnesium administration to mother or neonate (antacids, enema, and total parenteral nutrition). Clinical features include bradycardia, hypotension, neuromuscular depression (lethargy, hypotonia, poor suck, and delayed passage of meconium) and respiratory failure. Calcium levels may fall due to hypermagnesemia-induced parathyroid suppression. Usually, supportive therapy is adequate as magnesium is gradually excreted by kidneys. Appropriate hydration status should be ensured. Loop diuretics may aid in excretion of magnesium. Calcium infusions may be helpful in acute

TABLE 5: Clinical features of hypercalcemia.

	Serum calcium Levels	***Clinical features***
Acute hypercalcemia	11–12 mg/dL	Asymptomatic mostly
	12–14 mg/dL	Lethargy, poor feeding, weakness, constipation, and polyuria
	>14 mg/dL	Vomiting, respiratory distress, apnea, hypotonia, lethargy, seizures, bradycardia, hypertension, and shortened QT intervals
Chronic hypercalcemia		Failure to thrive, calcifications at various organs, nephrocalcinosis, and nephrolithiasis

Flowchart 3: Evaluation of hypercalcemic neonates.

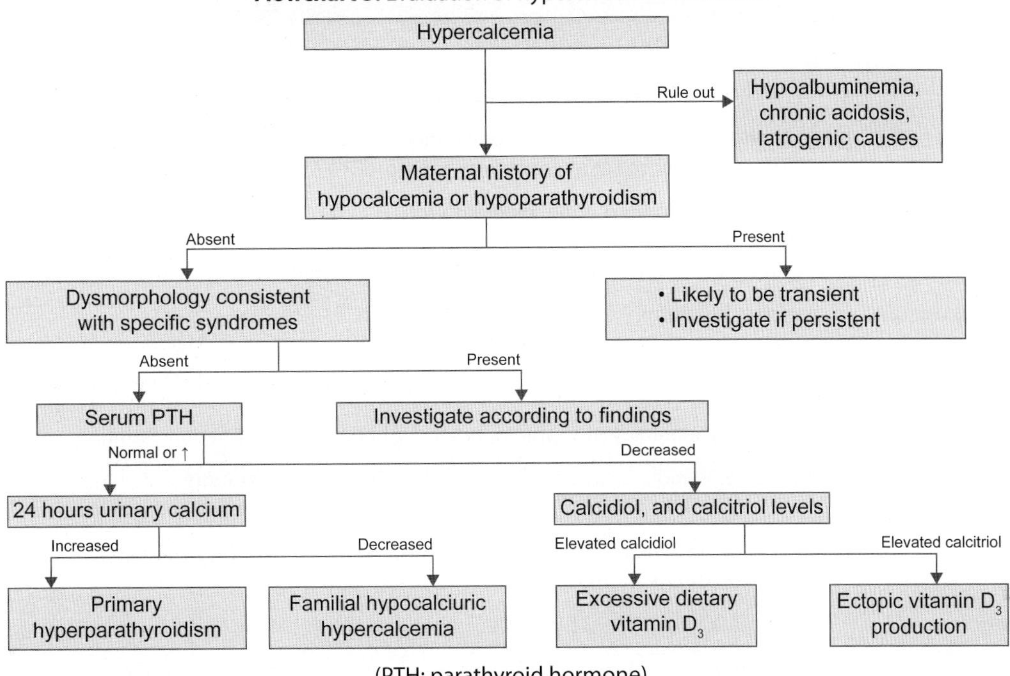

(PTH: parathyroid hormone)

symptomatic cases. For refractory cases hemodialysis may be required.

METABOLIC BONE DISEASE OF PREMATURITY

Introduction

First observed by Von Sydow in 1946, osteopenia of prematurity, now rechristened as metabolic bone disease (MBD) of prematurity, is a multifactorial disease characterized by reduced mineral content and protein matrix of bones. There is no consensus on definition at present and incidence varies according to diagnostic criteria.

Risk Factors

In fetal life, nearly 80% of bone mineral content is accrued in the third trimester. From 60 mg/day at 25 weeks, accretion rates go up to 300 mg/kg at 35 weeks onward. As a result, premature babies, especially those born at very low birth weight (VLBW) are at the highest risk. Other factors impacting placental transfer of minerals, such as preeclampsia and chorioamnionitis also increase the risks. Postnatal factors include prolonged parenteral nutrition, comorbidities, and medications which can affect bone mineralization. Neonates fed only breast milk and standard formulas are unable to meet their mineral requirements and intestinal immaturity limits absorption even in preterm neonates receiving fortified feeds. Medications such as diuretics and steroids alter mineral metabolism and predispose to MBD.

Clinical Features

Skeletal features may mimic rickets with osteopenia, craniotabes, widened anterior fontanelles and rarely pathologic long bone fractures causing pain on handling. Respiratory muscle weakness, rib softening, and fractures can cause respiratory distress, worsen pulmonary function, and result in ventilator dependence. Hypophosphatemia can affect cardiac contractility, homolysis, and leukocyte and platelet dysfunctions.

Diagnosis

Currently, there exists no single marker for screening, predicting or diagnosing MBD. Various proposed biomarkers and imaging modalities are discussed in **Table 6**. There is a lot of variation regarding screening protocol and should be customized according to unit practices and resources available **(Flowchart 4)**.

TABLE 6: Diagnostic modalities for metabolic bone disease **(MBD)**.

Serum markers			
Calcium	Not reliable as levels can remain normal at the expense of bone demineralization		
Phosphate (PO_4)	• Earliest marker of disrupted bone mineralization • Thresholds for concern vary from <5.6 mg/dL to 4 mg/dL		
Alkaline phosphatase (ALP)	• *>500 IU/L:* Impaired bone mineralization • *>700 IU/L:* Bone demineralization, even if clinically silent • ALP > 900 IU/L with PO_4 <5.6 mg/dL have 100% specificity and 70% sensitivity		
Serum parathyroid hormone (PTH)	Levels >100 pg/mL suggestive of risk for MBD		
Urine markers			
Calcium and phosphate	Can assess adequacy of supplementation. Altered by diuretic administration		
Tubular phosphorous reabsorption (TPR)	Levels >95% indicate insufficient phosphorous supplementation		
TPR + serum PTH	• *High serum PTH and low TPR:* Hypocalcemia-induced hypophosphatemia • *Normal or low PTH and high TPR:* Phosphate deficiency		
Imaging markers			
Modalities	***Significance***	***Advantages***	***Drawbacks***
Skeletal X-ray	Assesses cortical thinning of bones and fractures Not reliable in early stages as X-ray changes appear after bone mineral density reduces by 20–40%	• Cheap • Readily available	Radiation
Dual energy X-ray absorptiometry (DEXA)	• Gold standard for bone mineralization. Adaptable to preterm infants • Bone mineral density >0.068 g/cm^2 has low probability of MBD	Low ionizing radiation	Movement artifacts
Quantitative ultrasound (QUS)	Evaluates speed of sound and bone transmission time to measure both bone mineral content and organic matrix	• Cheap • No radiation	Needs further studies

Flowchart 4: Screening algorithm for **MBD**.

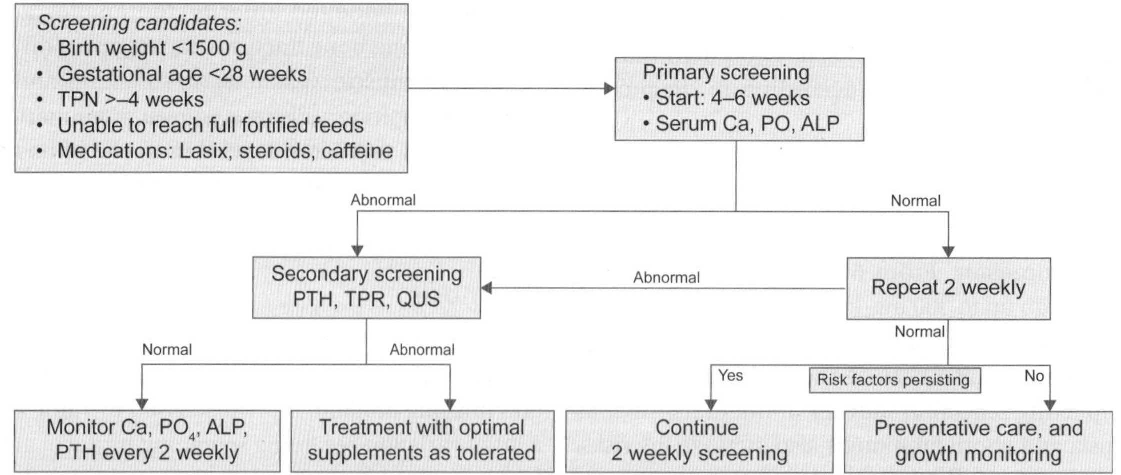

(ALP: alkaline phosphatase; MBD: metabolic bone disease; PTH: parathyroid hormone; QUS: quantitative ultrasound; TPN: total parenteral nutrition; TPR: tubular phosphorous reabsorption)

Prevention and Treatment

The goal of management is to replicate the in-utero accretion rates of third trimester while mitigating the complications.

Parenteral Nutrition

- Early initiation of mineral supplementation with adequate energy and protein to prevent catabolism.
- Adequate amount (60–120 mg/kg/day of calcium and 31–71 mg/kg/day of phosphorous) and appropriate calcium/Phosphorous (1.5:1 to 1.7:1) mass ratio is essential. Incrementally, greater doses are required in the growing phase.
- Use of organic compounds (calcium gluconate and sodium glycerophosphate), appropriate temperature and pH and order of mixing ingredients can effect supplementation.

Enteral Nutrition

- Early initiation of enteral nutrition improves endocrine adaptation and hastens gut maturity allowing better mineral absorption.
- Adequate amount (calcium of 140–160 mg/100 kcal and phosphorous of 95–108 mg/100 kcal) at appropriate mass ratios (1.5:1 to 2:1) cannot be obtained solely from unfortified breast milk even at 200 mL/kg/day.
- For persistent serum phosphorous concentration <4 mg/dL, phosphorous supplementation should be considered.
- The ideal timing of vitamin D initiation is still debatable. The dose recommendations vary from 400–1,000 IU/day.

Postdischarge Nutrition

Postdischarge calcium and phosphate supplementation may be appropriate till 40 weeks postconceptional age or till 6 months in babies with low growth velocity.

Non-nutritional Therapies

Assisted physical exercise by passive range of motion and joint compression performed 5–15 minutes for 4–8 weeks have been shown to improve bone mineralization in some studies. Medications such as steroids and furosemide should be judiciously used. Adequate counseling of caregivers and careful handling of a baby with features of MBD is essential.

Outcome

Long-term outcomes are scantily studied but most preterm babies do well with respect to bone mineralization, with bone mineral density catching up by 6 months corrected age. Some long-term associations of MBD include low peak bone mass, enamel hypoplasia, dental carries, and myopia of prematurity.

KEY POINTS

- Calcium and magnesium homeostasis is vital for physiological functioning and growth of neonate.
- Risk factors for hypocalcemia should be screened for while evaluating a neonate.
- In case of intractable neonatal seizures, hypomagnesemia should be ruled out.
- Screening for MBD is essential for at-risk neonates.
- Timely, appropriate and adequate mineral supplementation is key to prevention of MBD.

SUGGESTED READING

1. Faienza MF, D'Amato E, Natale MP, Grano M, Chiarito M, Brunetti G, et al. Metabolic bone disease of prematurity: diagnosis and management. Front Pediatr. 2019;7:143.
2. Kellar K, Pandillapalli NR, Moreira AG. Calcium and phosphorus: all you need to know but were afraid to ask. Clin Perinatol. 2023;50(3):591-606.
3. Lee B, De Beritto T. Metabolic bone disease of prematurity. Neoreviews. 2022;23(5):e311-8.

SECTION 2

Adolescence

Section Editors: *MKC Nair, Piyali Bhattacharya*

CHAPTER 19

Teen Pregnancy and Contraception

Prema Raghunathan

INTRODUCTION

Adolescents represent one-fifth of world's population. They undergo a lot of physical, emotional, behavioral, and cognitive changes along with experimentation and high-risk behavior leading to unintended pregnancy, sexually transmitted infection (STI), and unsafe abortions. The rate of birth among adolescents globally is about 11% of all births and 6.8% of women aged 15–19 years were already pregnant or mothers at the time of survey as per NFHS-5 data. Only 8% of women and 15% of men know about emergency contraception. Among this, a significant number is contributed by married adolescents in India, most other teens have sexual relationships due to peer pressure or impulsivity. Adolescents have limited education on sexuality, even if they are sexually active.

The increasing rates of teen pregnancies and abortion cause increased medical expenditure as most of these pregnancies are unplanned. They are also mostly seen in underprivileged society. Teen pregnancies push an adolescent to become school dropout, face lot of stress, and can succumb to psychological trauma. There is a higher risk of puerperal endometritis, eclampsia, and systemic infection among adolescent mothers, their babies have increased risk of low birth weight, prematurity, and severe neonatal conditions contributing to increased maternal and neonatal morbidity and mortality. Studies demonstrate that young men, like young women, have concerns about teenage pregnancy, contraceptive use, sex education, parent roles, media, and peer influence on teenager's sexual decision making. Involving young men in pregnancy prevention programs could improve understanding of the social psychology of men's development stages and perceive their sexual relationships.

Hence, clinicians caring for adolescents should step in to provide sexual education (safe sex) and contraceptive counseling as part of reproductive health. This can be imparted at school, community, and at adolescent friendly health clinics (AFHS). An assurance of confidentiality followed by systematic HEADSSS approach for psychosocial history helps adolescents to disclose sensitive issues. Life skill education and anticipatory guidance tailored to developmental stages of adolescent are cornerstone for preventing teen pregnancy. Adolescent pediatricians can help adolescents disclose pregnancy to parents in clinic itself to prevent violence and also support family in guiding further keeping legal aspects in mind.

CONTRACEPTION

Contraception counseling is an important aspect of teen care. The first step is to identify adolescent who are sexually active (maintain confidentiality) and the ones who follow abstinence. The caregivers, parents, adolescent specialist should support adolescents who follow abstinence as "abstinence is the best method of contraception". If the teen is sexually active, contraceptive counseling should be given to understand the adolescent's perception and misperception about contraceptives, risks of unprotected intercourse, educate regarding real risks, and contraindications for various methods available. Once the contraceptive method is chosen by the adolescent, the provider must discuss the common side effects, realistic expectation for failure, a contingency plan for that possibility, and strategies for close follow-up. American College of Obstetricians and Gynecologists stipulates that a routine pelvic examination with Pap smear be initiated 3 years after onset of sexual activity and annual screening for STIs.

The various contraceptive methods are broadly classified into hormonal **(Table 1)**, nonhormonal **(Table 2)**, and emergency contraception. The non-hormonal methods are barrier methods, spermicidal, and

TABLE 1: List of hormonal contraceptives.

Methods	*Available as*	*Potential side effects*	*Comments*	*Failure rates*
Commonly used methods:				
Oral contraceptive pills	• Mala D • Mala N	Breakthrough bleeding, nausea, headaches, breast tenderness	• Decreased burden: Menstrual blood loss dysmenorrhea, acne • Pelvic inflammatory disease	7%
Progestin only	Mini pills	Irregular bleeding, breast, tenderness, depression	Used among breastfeeding teens	7%
Contraceptive injections-progestin-only injection	• Depo-Provera–3 monthly • NET-EN-2 monthly	• Weight again • Acne • Depression • Irregular bleeding or amenorrhea	Not used for more than 1 year, preferred among married teens	4%
Rarely used methods:				
Vaginal ring	NuvaRing	Vaginal irritation and discharge	Decreases dysmenorrhea, acne, pelvic inflammatory disease	7%
Transdermal patch	Weekly	Allergic reaction at skin site, breast tenderness, break through bleeding	Not freely available in India	7%
Implant	Implanon	Weight gain, local insertion complications	• High efficacy • Acceptability, decreases dysmenorrhea	0.1%

TABLE 2: List of nonhormonal methods.

	Commonly used methods	
Methods	*Potential side effects*	*Comments*
Male condom	Latex allergy	• Prevents sexually transmitted diseases and human immunodeficiency virus risk • Failure rate reduced if used with other hormonal contraceptive method
Female condom	Vaginal discomfort	Not available in India, needs proper education for perfect use
Intrauterine device copper-containing	Excessive menstrual blood loss	Nonhormonal, used among parous teens
Spermicides	Urinary tract infections, allergy to ingredients	Should be used by teenage girls along with partner using condoms for maximum contraception

intrauterine devices (IUDs). The hormonal methods are combination pills or progesterone-only pills.

Nonhormonal Methods

Barrier Method

Condoms: It prevents sperms from being deposited in the vagina. The advantages are:

- There are no major side effects
- Risk of STIs reduced (acquired immunodeficiency syndrome and human papillomavirus)
- Low cost, easy availability
- Little need for advanced planning

A female condom is second choice over male condom due to its complexity of properly using device, its low typical efficacy rate, and lack of studies on effectiveness in STIs. Diaphragm and cervical caps are messy and less used by teenagers.

Spermicides

These are available as foam, cream, films, or effervescent vaginal suppositories containing nonoxynol-9. They must be placed in vaginal cavity shortly before intercourse.

Combination Methods

Use of condom by male and spermicidal foam by female adolescent is extremely effective and failure rate is 2%.

Hormonal Methods

Estrogenic substances in combination with a progestin or a progestin alone are used in these methods. The mechanism of action of both (the hormones) estrogen and progesterone combination and progesterone-only pills is to prevent luteinizing hormone (LH) surge and as a result to inhibit ovulation, they also thicken cervical mucous in such a way that prevents sperm penetration. They also cause stromal edema, regression of endometrial glands, and produce static endometrial hypoplasia. These hormones are steroidal contraceptives, can be used orally, parenterally or as devices: intrauterine and vaginal. The oral combination pills typically contain ethinyl estradiol and a progestin. The typical failure, i.e., pregnancy rates are under 1 per woman years of use. Exogenous estrogen use can cause serious side effects rarely like thrombophlebitis, myocardial infarction, hepatic adenoma, and carbohydrate intolerance. The more commonly seen adverse effects are nausea, weight gain, acne in certain progestin pills which can be reduced by using estrogen containing pills which suppresses activity of sebaceous glands. The advantages of estrogen are relief of dysmenorrhea, short menstrual cycle; estrogen containing pills have higher levels of cardioprotective high-density lipoproteins. A few extended cyclic pills are being released which can cause amenorrhea for 3 months to 1 year. However, the major disadvantages of those pills are compliance as adolescents do not take pills every day and may lead to increased failure rates and breakthrough bleeding. The recommendations for missing pills are given in **Box 1**. The most commonly used pill in India is Mala-D (norethisterone acetate + ethinyl estradiol), Mala-N (norgestrel + ethinyl estradiol) which is also supplied by Government of India. Other oral contraceptive pills (OCPs) are Ovral-L, Novelon, Femilon, and Loette.

Other combination methods are transdermal patch **(Fig. 1)** and vaginal contraceptive ring. The transdermal patch releases 20 μg ethinyl estradiol and 150 μg norelgestromin daily. This method is not popular among adolescents as patch can get partial or fully detached. The vaginal contraceptive ring (NuvaRing) is a flexible, transparent, colorless ring which is inserted into vagina by self and remains for 3 weeks where it releases 15 μg of ethinyl estradiol and 120 μg of etonogestrel/day.

In situations where estrogens are contraindicated, progestin-only pills can be used. These are called "mini pills" and are less reliable in inhibiting ovulation, compliance is poor among adolescents. The injectable progestin, medroxyprogesterone acetate, is highly effective as deep intramuscular (IM) injection 150 μg (Depo-Provera). Bone mineral density loss which is reversible side effect should be kept in mind. The progestin-only drug can also be used as subcutaneous implant.

BOX 1: Guidelines for missed OCPs.

OCP—missed pill rules:
- If the teen has missed taking OCP ask her to resume her usual pill taking schedule as early as possible (she may take two pills on the same day)
- If pills are missed in week 1 (days 1–7), emergency contraception should be considered
- If the missed pills are in week 3, she should omit the pill-free interval.
- Abstinence or condoms should be used as backup method if the following number of pills are missed:
  - Two for twenty (if two or more 20 μg ethinyl estradiol pills are missed)
  - Three for thirty (if three or more 30–35 μg ethinyl estradiol pills are missed)
- *Emergency contraception:* If you have had unprotected sex in the previous 7 days and you have missed two or more pills (i.e., more than 48 hours late) in the first week of a pack, you may need emergency contraception.

(OCP: oral contraceptive pill)

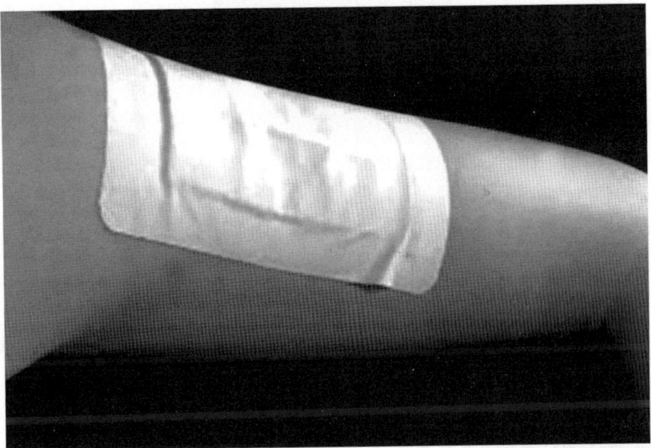

Fig. 1: Transdermal patch.

Contraindications of Combined Hormonal Contraceptives

Absolute contraindications (class 4 in the World Health Organization classification):

- Pregnancy
- Undiagnosed genital bleeding
- Breast cancer
- Past or present circulatory disease
- Thrombophilia
- Pill-induced hypertension
- Migraine with aura
- Active liver disease
- Systemic lupus erythematosus
- Hemolytic-uremic syndrome
- Thrombotic thrombocytopenic purpura

Relative contraindications (class 2 or 3 in the World Health Organization classification):

- Smoker aged over 35 years
- Hypertension (blood pressure >140/90 mm Hg)
- Diabetes
- Hyperprolactinemia
- Gallbladder disease
- Migraine without aura
- Osteosclerosis
- Sickle-cell disease

CLINICAL PEARL

Abstinence is the best contraception for teens.

EMERGENCY CONTRACEPTION

Pregnancy risk with unprotected intercourse (in midcycle) is 20–30%. The risk can be reduced if emergency contraception is used within 72 hours; these emergency contraceptive pills are combination of ethinyl estradiol and norgestrel/levonorgestrel. This helps by disrupting luteal phase and hormone pattern, makes cervix unstable, and unsuitable uterine lining for implantation. They also blunt LH surge and impair ovulation in midcycle. The important side effects are nausea and vomiting.

Potential Indications for Use of Emergency Contraception

- Lack of contraceptive use during coitus
- Mechanical failure of male condom (breakage, slippage, or leakage)
- Dislodgment, breakage, or incorrect use of diaphragm, cervical cap, or female condom
- Failure of spermicide tablet or film to melt before intercourse
- Error in practicing withdrawal (coitus interruptus)
- Missed combined oral contraceptives (any two consecutive pills)
- Missed progestin-only oral contraceptive (one or more)
- Expulsion or partial expulsion of an IUD
- Exposure to potential teratogen (such as isotretinoin or thalidomide while not using effective contraception)
- Late injection of injectable contraceptive (>2 weeks delay of a progestin-only formulation, such as depot medroxyprogesterone acetate)
- Two or more days delay in starting new vaginal ring or patch cycle
- Rape

INTRAUTERINE DEVICES (FIG. 2)

Intrauterine devices are small flexible plastic objects introduced in uterine cavity through cervix. They contain copper (Cu) or progesterone. Cu-T 380A IUD renders endometrium unsuitable for implantation, the levonorgestrel IUD acts by thickening of cervical mucosa, inhibiting sperm survival and suppresses endometrium **(Fig. 3)**. This method of contraception is used among teens who are highly sexually active but they should take measures to prevent STIs **(Flowchart 1)**.

For better understanding of contraception among adolescents, adolescent contraceptive methods can be discussed using below **Figure 3**. This is a tiered system developed by WHO. Tier 1 contraceptives are the long acting reversible contraceptives like implants and IUDs that do not rely on user and are more effective compared to Tier 2 methods which rely on consistent use like daily pill, weekly patch or vaginal ring, DMPA. The Tier 3 methods which are less effective are used during sexual activity (male and female condom, spermicide, natural family planning), or immediately after [emergency contraception (EC)].

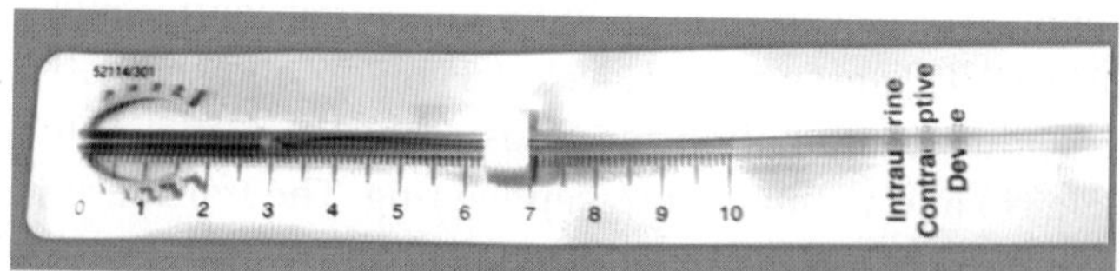

Fig. 2: Intrauterine devices.

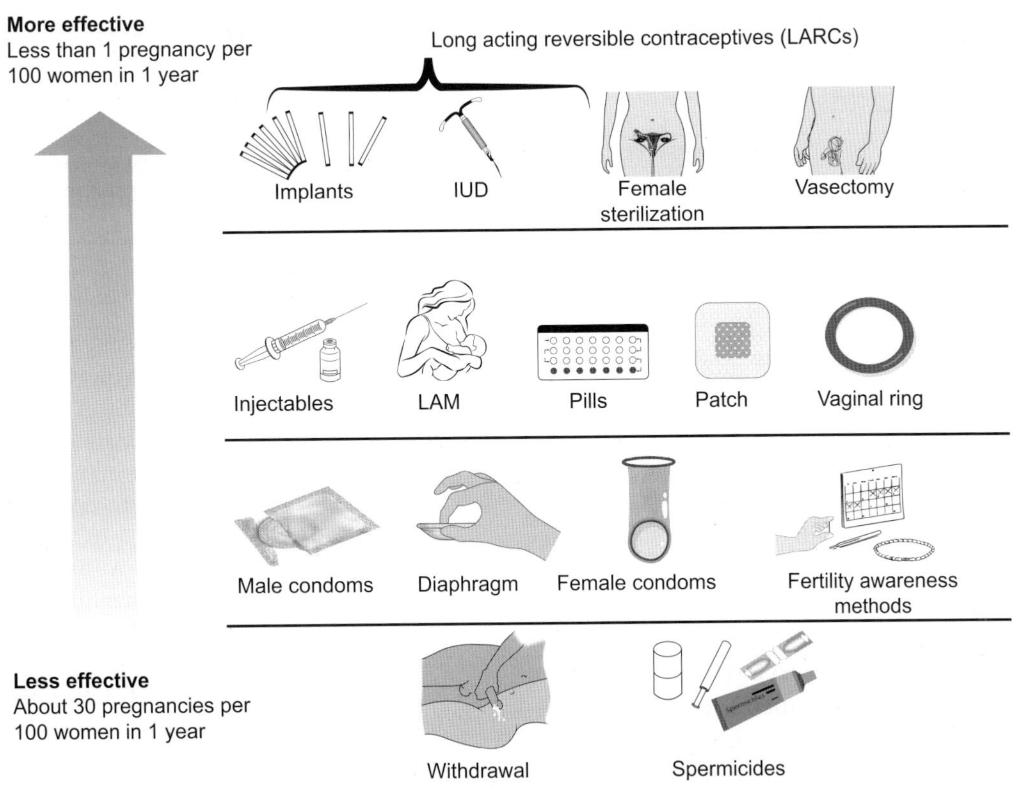

Fig. 3: World Health Organization Tiered approach to contraceptive effectiveness. (IUD: intrauterine device)
Source: Adapted from Family Planning: A Global Handbook for Providers (2018 Update).

Flowchart 1: Approach to teen contraception.

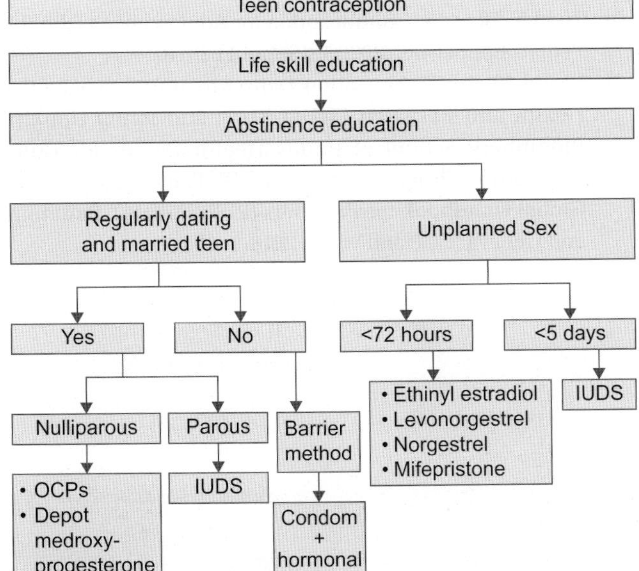

(IUDs: intrauterine device; OCPs: oral contraceptive pills)

ADOLESCENT PREGNANCY

By providing good education including sexual education to our teens, counseling them regarding abstinence, and providing life skills, teen pregnancies can be avoided. Still there are lots of pregnancies being reported. As one sector of them could be early marriages from rural population and sexual abuse. Among Indian studies, teenage pregnancy varies from 5.1% to as high as 21.12%.

The adolescent caregivers should always suspect pregnancy when there is secondary amenorrhea as most teens may be reluctant to give history of sexual activity. The methods to diagnose pregnancy are urine pregnancy test, which is sensitive by 5 days of missed cycles by 98%. Ultrasound scan detects pregnancy and can also rule out an ectopic pregnancy.

The next step after diagnosing is addressing psychosocial, emotional, and medical aspects. The options of elective termination of pregnancy or raising the child by friends/family/option of adoption can be given to family.

Flowchart 2: Teen pregnancy complications.

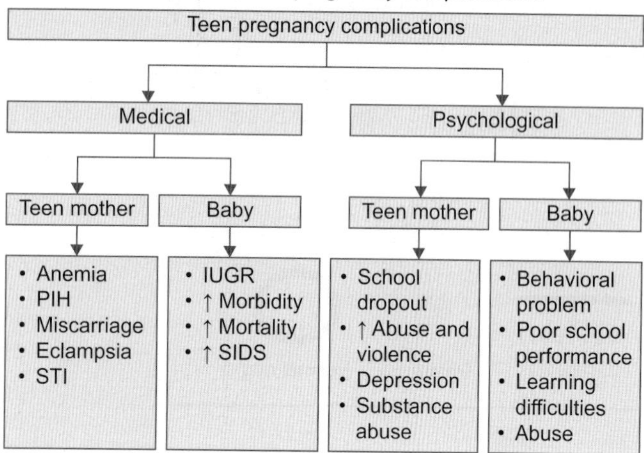

(PIH: pregnancy-induced hypertension; STI: sexually transmitted infection; IUGR: intrauterine growth retardation; SIDS: sudden infant death syndrome)

Complications due to teen pregnancy could be medical or psychosocial **(Flowchart 2)**. Most teen pregnancies do not have major medical complications. The pregnancy termination rate is about 33% in Indian statistics. Miscarriages/stillbirth rate is about 15%. Teen mothers have higher rate of anemia, pregnancy-induced hypertension, eclampsia, poor weight gain, increased STIs, increased abuse, violence, and depression. The babies of teen mothers have behavioral problems in preschool years, poor scholastic performance, learning difficulties; these could be attributed to poverty, negative parenting styles, and higher possibilities of abuse and neglect.

There are lot of educational programs for youth in various countries to educate teens about abstinence, contraception, STIs; this education and life skills training given at schools and adolescents clinics, health clinics, and/or, youth organizations have to be geared up to tackle this problem in India.

KEY POINTS

- Adolescents need sexual education.
- Encourage and support abstinence.
- Provide contraceptive counseling for sexually active teens.
- Encourage dual protection for pregnancy and sexually transmitted infections.

SUGGESTED READING

1. Adewole O, Otubanjo OM. Young Men's Perceptions of Teenage Pregnancy. The Qualitative Report. HCAS J. 2020; 25(9):3367-80.
2. Brooks RL, Shrier LA. An update on contraception for adolescents. Adolesc Med. 1999;10(2):211-9.
3. Brown RT, Braveman PK. Contraception and adolescents. Adolesc Med Clin. 2005;16(3):15-16.
4. Darroch J, Woog V, Bankole A, Ashford LS. Adding it up: Costs and benefits of meeting the contraceptive needs of adolescents. New York: Guttmacher Institute; 2016.
5. Greydanus DE, Senanayake P, Gains MJ. Reproductive health: an international perspective. Indian J Pediatr. 1999;66(3):415-24.
6. Parthasarathy A, Nair MKC, Menon PS, Bhave SY. Bhave's Textbook of Adolescent Medicine, 1st edition. New Delhi, India: Jaypee Brothers Medical Publishers; 2006.
7. Sully EA, Biddlecom A, Daroch J, Riley T, Ashford L, Lince-Deroche N, et al. Adding It Up: Investing in Sexual and Reproductive Health 2019. New York: Guttmacher Institute; 2020.
8. Todd N, Black A. Contraception for Adolescents. J Clin Res Pediatr Endocrinol. 2020;12(Suppl 1):28-40.
9. World Health Organization Department of Reproductive Health and Research (WHO/RHR) and Johns Hopkins Bloomberg School of Public Health/Center for Communication Programs (CCP) KfHP. Family Planning: A Global Handbook for Providers (2018 update). Baltimore and Geneva: CCP and WHO. 2018.

HEEADSSS Assessment of the Adolescent Child

Piyali Bhattacharya

Young people are resources to be developed, not problems to be solved.

—Pittman

INTRODUCTION

The HEEADSSS (Home, Education and employment, Eating and exercise, Activities and peer relationships, Drugs, Suicide and depression, Sexuality and Safety) assessment is a screening tool for conducting a comprehensive psychosocial history and health risk assessment of an adolescent **(Flowchart 1)**. It provides an ideal platform for a preventive health check and information about the young one's functioning in key areas of their life.

BUILD A RELATIONSHIP

- Confidently welcome the adolescent
- Respond openly to adolescent's initial reactions and feelings
- *Give clear introductions:* Yourself, your role, what you will be doing and why, e.g., "to get a better understanding of different areas of your life and how these might affect your health, I would like to ask you a few questions if it is okay with you":
    - Reassure the young person about confidentiality. However, three exceptions must be made clear to the young person and their caregivers:
        1. Harm to self
        2. Harm to others
        3. Others harming you.
    - Start with less sensitive areas of a young person's life and move towards more sensitive areas using a "third person" approach, e.g., "Some young people of your age are starting to experiment with drugs or alcohol (or sex). Have any of your friends tried these? How about yourself?"
    - Perform a risk assessment and screen for specific risk behaviors which occur in clusters.

Flowchart 1: Algorithm depicts points for interviewing and risk assessment in an adolescent child.

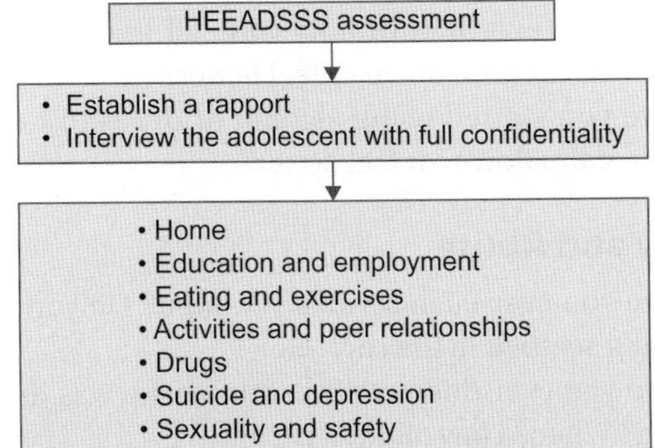

(HEEADSSS: Home, Education and employment, Eating and exercise, Activities and peer relationships, Drugs, Suicide and depression, Sexuality and Safety)

INTERVIEWING THE ADOLESCENT

Home

- How is it at home at the moment? Who lives with you? Where do you live?
- Do you have your own space? Who do you get along best with? Could you talk to them if you were worried about anything? Is there anyone new at home? Has someone left recently?
- Have you moved recently?
- Have you ever had to live away from home? (Why?)
- Have you ever run away? (Why?)
- Is there any physical violence at home?

Education and Employment

- What are your favorite subjects and least favorite subjects at school?

- How are your grades? Any recent changes? Have you changed schools in the past few years?
- Have you ever had to repeat a class? Have you ever had to repeat a grade? What are your future education/ employment plans/goals? Are you working? Where? How long?
- Tell me about your friends at school. Is your school a safe place?
- Have you ever been suspended? Expelled? Have you ever considered dropping out?
- How well do you get along with the people at school or work?
- Do you feel connected to your school? Do you feel as if you belong?
- Are there adults at school you feel you could talk to about something important? (Who?)

Eating and Exercise

- Has your weight changed recently? Are you worried about it? Have you ever dieted?
- How much exercise do you get? How much exercise do you get in an average day/week?
- What do you think would be a healthy diet? How does that compare to your current eating patterns?
- Do you worry about your weight? How often?
- Do you eat in front of the television? Computer? What would it be like if you gained/lost 10 pounds?

Activities and Hobbies

- What do you do to relax? What do you and your friends do for fun? (With whom, where, and when?)
- What do you and your family do for fun? (With whom, where, and when?)
- Do you participate in any sports or other activities?
- Do you regularly attend a club, or other organized activity?
- Do you have any hobbies?
- Do you read for fun? (What?)
- How much television do you watch in a week? How about video games? What music do you like to listen to?

Drugs, Alcohol, and Tobacco

- Lots of teenagers try smoking/alcohol, have you ever tried it?
- Have you been offered drugs? Is it hard for you to say no in this situation?
- Is there any history of alcohol or drug problems in your family? Does anyone at home use tobacco?
- Do you ever drink or use drugs when you are alone?

Sex and Relationships

- Have you ever been in a romantic relationship? Tell me about your dates
- Have any of your relationships ever been sexual relationship? Are your sexual activities enjoyable?
- Are you interested in boys? Girls? Both?
- Have you ever been forced or pressured into doing something sexual that you did not want to do?
- Have you ever been touched sexually in a way that you did not want?
- Have you ever been raped, on a date or any other time?
- How many sexual partners have you had altogether?
- Have you ever been pregnant or worried that you may be pregnant? (females)
- Have you ever gotten someone pregnant or worried that that might have happened? (males) What does the term "safe sex" mean to you?
- What do you know about contraception?

Suicide and Depression

- Do you feel sad or down more than usual? Do you find yourself crying more than usual? Are you "bored" all the time? Are you having trouble getting to sleep?
- Does it seem that you have lost interest in things that you used to really enjoy? Do you ever feel so down that life is not worth living?
- Do you find yourself spending less and less time with friends? Would you rather just be by yourself most of the time?
- Have you ever thought a lot about hurting yourself or someone else?
- Have you ever had to hurt yourself (e.g., by cutting yourself) to calm down or feel better?
- Have you started using alcohol or drugs to help you relax, calm down, or feel better?

Safety and Abuse

- Have you ever been seriously injured? Do you always wear a seatbelt in the car?
- Have you ever ridden with a driver who was drunk or high? When? How often?
- Do you use safety equipment for sports and/or other physical activities (e.g., helmets for biking or skateboarding)?

- Is there any violence in your home? Does the violence ever get physical?
- Is there a lot of violence at your school? In your neighborhood? Among your friends?
- Have you ever been physically or sexually abused? Have you ever been raped, on a date or at any other time? (If not asked previously)
- Have you ever been in a car or motorcycle accident? (What happened?)
- Have you ever been picked on or bullied? Is that still a problem?
- Have you gotten into physical fights in school or your neighborhood? Are you still getting into fights?
- Have you ever felt that you had to carry a knife, gun, or other weapon to protect yourself? Do you still feel that way?
- *All communication should be with:* Open-ended questions, affirmations, reflective listening and summary statements (OARS).

WRAPPING UP THE SESSION

At the end of the HEEADSSS assessment, the pediatrician should compliment the young person on their strengths and areas in their life where they are doing well. He should:

- Identify areas for intervention and prevention
- Identify and discuss any issues of concern psychosocial health
- Identify the overall level of risk of the young person and specific risk factors in their lives, as well as protective factors and strengths
- Identify areas for intervention and follow-up
- Provide health education about particular health issues or risk behaviors.

The HEEADSSS assessment is not simply an information gathering exercise; listen carefully to the young person's verbal and nonverbal responses. Adolescents may present with minor complaints but exploring beyond the presenting complaint may detect underlying health concerns and risk factors, thereby providing timely intervention and preventive education.

PRINCIPLES OF INTERVENTION

- Allow time to finish, provide a brief summary, give opportunity for questions
- Discuss options and help the adolescent make choices
- *Based on the level of risk:* Decrease risk factors or increase protective factors
- *Possible foci:* Environment and social context, family, individual.

A pediatrician must seek a collaborative approach and facilitate access to psychological and specialist counseling services once a problem has been identified.

CLINICAL PEARL

- Specific risk behaviors usually occur in clusters. Risk assessment, therefore, must be done continuously throughout the whole interview of the adolescent in order to identify associated factors.

SUGGESTED READING

1. Goldenring JM, Rosen DS. Getting into adolescent heads: an essential update. Contemp Pediatr. 2004;21:64-90.
2. Sanci L. Adolescent Health Care Principles. Melbourne, Australia: The Centre for Adolescent Health, The Royal Australian College of General Practitioners; 2001.
3. SERU. Improving Young People's Access to Health Care Through General Practice: A Guide for General Practitioners and Divisions of General Practice. Melbourne, Australia: Access SERU, Department of General Practice and Public Health, University of Melbourne; 1999.

CHAPTER 21

Adolescent Anemia

Vaishali R Deshmukh

INTRODUCTION

Anemia is a major public health problem in India. It has a special significance in adolescents as it affects final height, cognition, and reproductive health; as well as has intergenerational consequences.

Most of the hereditary or congenital anemias present before the age of adolescence (exceptions—congenital dyserythropoietic anemia, milder forms of hemolytic anemia). Since nutritional anemia, and especially iron deficiency anemia, is the most commonly found anemia in adolescents in India as well as all over the world, it will be discussed here in detail.

Anemia is not a specific entity. It is a condition, which results from an underlying pathologic process.

Surprisingly, in a gradually developing anemia, hardly any symptoms are apparent until hemoglobin reaches a level of 8 gm% or lower because, the body adjusts for anemia in the initial stages by various adaptive mechanisms.

The normal life span of red blood cells (RBCs) is 110–120 days. Adult RBCs do not have a nucleus. This makes them a better oxygen vehicle but gives them a definite life span. Adolescents, beyond the age of 12 years, have hematologic ranges similar to those of adults. At puberty, hemoglobin concentration reaches adult level as a result of effect of androgens on erythropoiesis.

PREVALENCE

According to WHO Global Database, the prevalence of anemia is very high in India putting it in Severe Public Health Problem category.

CLINICAL PEARLS

WHO Global Database:
- Prevalence of anemia in South East Asia—57%
- Global prevalence in school age children—25.4% (305 million)
- Overall prevalence in India—74.3%

According to National Family Health Survey-3 (NFHS-3), the prevalence of anemia in Indian adolescent girls is 56–68% and in adolescent boys—30%. The prevalence went down somewhat during NFHS-4 (2015-16); but when data from NFHS-4 and NFHS-5 (2019-21) is compared, there is a slight increase in the prevalence of anemia among boys and girls between 15 and 19 years; from 29.2 to 31.1%, and from 54.1 to 54.1%, respectively.

DEFINITION

Anemia is defined as reduction in the number of RBCs or reduced PCV (hematocrit) or low hemoglobin, all below the lower limit for the age norm.

The functional definition of anemia is "an insufficient RBC mass to adequately deliver oxygen to peripheral tissues" **(Table 1)**.

Severe anemia is defined clinically as a low hemoglobin concentration leading to cardiac decompensation, that is, to the point that the heart cannot maintain adequate circulation of the blood. There is extreme pallor. If the hemoglobin or hematocrit can be determined, cutoffs of hemoglobin below 7.0 g/dL or hematocrit below 20% should be used to define severe anemia.

ETIOLOGY OF ANEMIA (FLOWCHART 1)

Nutritional anemia: By definition, it is the anemia caused by dietary deficiency of one or more nutrients required

TABLE 1: WHO guidelines for severity of anemia.

Age	*No anemia*	*Mild*	*Moderate*	*Severe*
12–14 years	>12 g%	11–11.9 g%	8–10.9 g%	<8 g%
Nonpregnant >15 years girls	>12 g%	11–11.9 g%	8–10.9 g%	<8 g%
Men	>13 g%	11–12.9 g%	8–10.9 g%	<8 g%

(Guidelines for treatment of iron deficiency anemia—MoHFW, Government of India)

Flowchart 1: Approach to anemia.

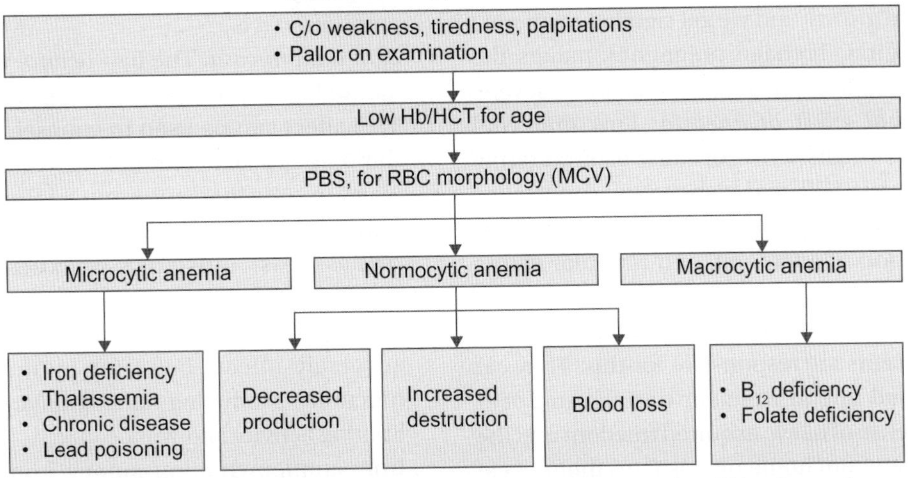

- C/o weakness, tiredness, palpitations
- Pallor on examination

↓

Low Hb/HCT for age

↓

PBS, for RBC morphology (MCV)

↓

Microcytic anemia	Normocytic anemia			Macrocytic anemia
• Iron deficiency • Thalassemia • Chronic disease • Lead poisoning	Decreased production	Increased destruction	Blood loss	• B_{12} deficiency • Folate deficiency

(MCV: mean corpuscular volume; RBC: red blood cell; PBS: peripheral blood smear)

for hemoglobin synthesis. The most common deficiency is that of iron followed by Folate and vitamin B_{12}. This deficiency is usually compounded by intestinal parasites (helminthiasis) and malaria.

Iron deficiency anemia typically shows three phases with increasing severity:

1. *Prelatent phase of iron deficiency:* Reduced serum ferritin, reduced iron stores without reduction in serum iron.
2. *Latent phase:* Iron stores are exhausted but hemoglobin levels are normal. Some symptoms such as fatigue, malaise but no anemia. Increase in total iron-binding capacity (TIBC), reduction in transferrin saturation
3. *Iron deficiency anemia:* Pallor, pica, low hemoglobin, and presence of microcytes

Other causes of anemia in adolescents:
Thalassemia, sickle cell anemia, pernicious anemia, hemorrhagic causes, chronic disease, and bone marrow infiltration

Mechanism of anemia of chronic diseases: In a chronic disease, anemia is caused either due to decreased production or increased destruction of RBCs. The mechanism is as follows:

- Reduced erythropoietin
- Moderate decrease in RBC life span
- Increased RBC destruction by the hyperactive reticuloendothelial system
- Relative failure of bone marrow response
- Defective release of iron from tissues into plasma
- Increased levels of tumor necrosis factor causing suppressed erythroid response

CLINICAL PEARL

Anemia is caused by either reduced or ineffective production of RBCs, blood loss, or increased destruction of RBCs.

SPECIAL FEATURES OF ANEMIA IN ADOLESCENTS

CLINICAL PEARL

The most common anemia in adolescents all over the world is iron deficiency anemia.

Various unique factors contribute to the cause and effect of anemia in adolescence.

Gender difference between normal ranges of hematocrit starts becoming apparent at adolescence. The sudden growth spurt (the third and the last spurt after intrauterine life and gestation) leads to relative deficiency of nutrients and occult deficiencies become apparent. Hormones like testosterone, which affect erythropoiesis, peak during adolescence.

- In adolescent boys, the rapidly increasing muscle mass demands high amount of iron. In addition, the blood volume increases in short span.
- Menstrual losses contribute to iron deficiency in adolescent girls.
- In girls, the beginning of menstruation, i.e., menarche, leads to significant loss of blood on a regular basis. The menstrual flow may be heavier in the initial period

of menarche. Add to this the increased demand for iron due to rapid growth and we get significant anemia in adolescent girls. Teenage pregnancy makes the physiological anemia of pregnancy much more severe.

- *Intergenerational effect of anemia:* Low maternal hemoglobin and weight is a major cause of intrauterine growth restriction (IUGR) and high maternal mortality.
- Changes in thinking patterns and lifestyle lead to food fads, consumption of junk food, and irregular eating habits.

  The changing lifestyle and the peculiar temperament of adolescents are responsible for this. They eat a lot of junk food due to irregular timings and peer pressure. The sense of newly acquired freedom and the need to stay away from home necessitates them to eat outside food.

  - Socioeconomic status of the family, traditional eating habits of the region, the fear of gaining weight, and irregular eating habits are of great importance in development of adolescent anemia.
- Adolescents have poor compliance to treatment.
- "I Don't Care" attitude causes difficulty in convincing them of consequences.
- Occasional or no visits to doctors prevent early detection.

CLINICAL EFFECTS OF ANEMIA

- In a gradually developing anemia, patient may remain asymptomatic until hemoglobin reaches a level of 8 gm% or lower. The symptoms depend upon the magnitude and the rate of reduction in oxygen-carrying capacity of blood and the capacity of the pulmonary and the cardiovascular system to compensate for anemia. The symptomatology also reflects the symptoms of the underlying disease.
- Normally, the body adjusts for anemia in the initial stages by various adaptive mechanisms. The cardiac output increases to increase the oxygen delivery to the tissues. The production of 2,3-DPG in the RBCs increases leading to reduced affinity of hemoglobin to oxygen. This causes shift of oxygen dissociation curve to the left causing release of oxygen to tissues faster. This is also seen at high altitudes. Production of erythropoietin (EPO) increases too, leading to stimulation of bone marrow and increased RBC output.
- A striking feature of iron deficiency anemia is pica. This desire to consume unusual things is very peculiar to iron deficiency anemia, the reason is not clear. Especially seen is pagophagia, i.e., urge to eat unusual amounts of ice.
- *Skin and mucosa:* The hair texture worsens leading to lack of luster, premature graying, and thinning of hair. This effect can be used to counsel the adolescents as this may appeal to them.
- *Neuromuscular symptoms:* Headache, vertigo, tinnitus, faintness, lack of concentration, drowsiness, restlessness, muscular weakness; in pernicious anemia, paresthesias
- *Behavioral and cognitive problems:* Iron deficiency adversely affects behavior by impairing cognitive functions, producing noncognitive disturbances, and limiting activity and work capacity.

Iron supplementation among iron deficient anemic children benefits learning processes as measured by the school achievement test scores.

- Poor physical growth
- High maternal mortality
- Gastrointestinal (GI) symptoms of underlying disorder (duodenal ulcer, Ca, hiatus hernia) especially in adults

INVESTIGATIONS (FLOWCHART 2)

- Hemogram with peripheral blood smear (PBS)—to determine the severity of anemia, affection of other cell lines, RBC morphology, hematocrit level, and presence of parasites such as malaria
- Reticulocyte count—to assess bone marrow response
- Stool for parasites and occult blood
- Hemoglobin electrophoresis
- Serum bilirubin and serum iron studies
- Investigations to rule out underlying diseases

MANAGEMENT (FLOWCHART 3)

Treatment Program (Flowchart 3)

The National Iron+ Initiative guidelines have been developed by the Adolescent Division of the Ministry of Health and Family Welfare (MoHFW), Government of India. The following treatment program has been recommended:

- *Mild anemia:* 60 mg of elemental iron daily for 3 months after which hemoglobin estimation is done.
- *Moderate anemia* is investigated for CBC, PBS, MP, and stool for occult blood and treated in the same way as mild anemia.
- *Severe anemia:* Investigate and treat with 120 mg iron + 400 μg folic acid daily for 3 months

Flowchart 2: Diagnosis of anemia.

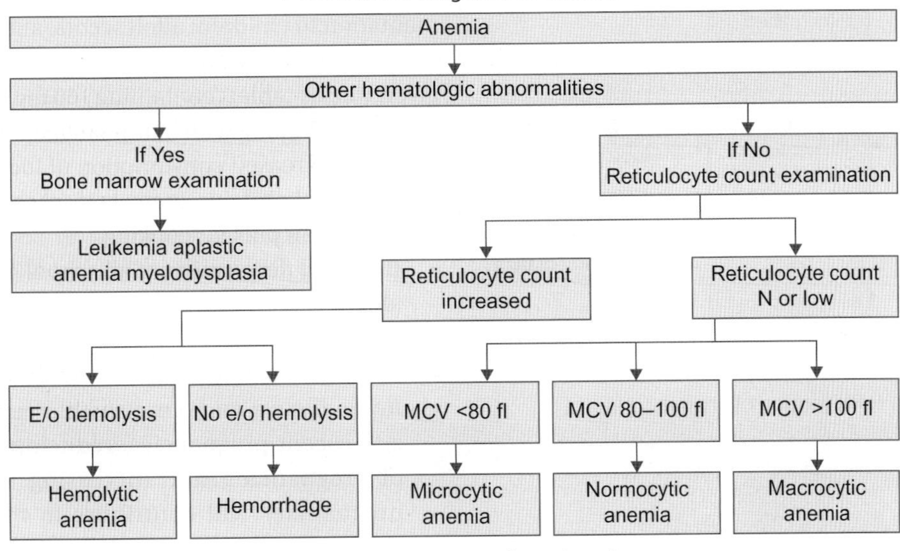

(MCV: mean corpuscular volume)

Flowchart 3: Treatment.

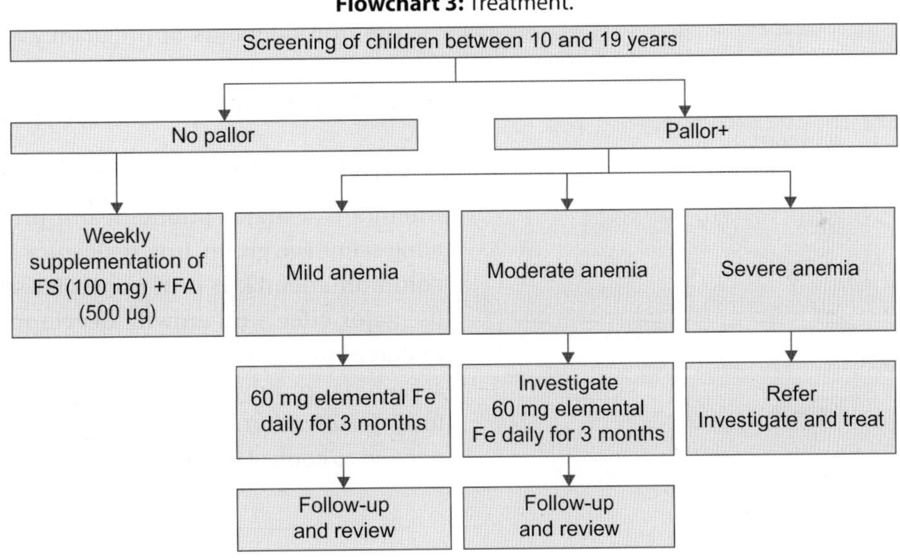

Indications for Blood Transfusion

- All children with Hb ≤4 g/dL
- Children with Hb 4–6 g/dL with complications such as, dehydration, shock, impaired consciousness, heart failure, deep and labored breathing, very high parasitemia (>10% of RBC)
- If packed cells are available, give 10 mL/kg over 3–4 hours preferably. If not, give whole blood 20 mL/kg over 3–4 hours with close monitoring and diuretics.

Prevention (Figs. 1 and 2)

Due to its prevalence across all age groups all over the world, prevention plays a major role in the management of iron deficiency anemia.

- Increased awareness about the magnitude of anemia and its far-reaching consequences among the masses will go a long way to reduce the incidence of it.
- School and college based awareness programs to reduce consumption of junk food and to encourage healthy dietary habits.

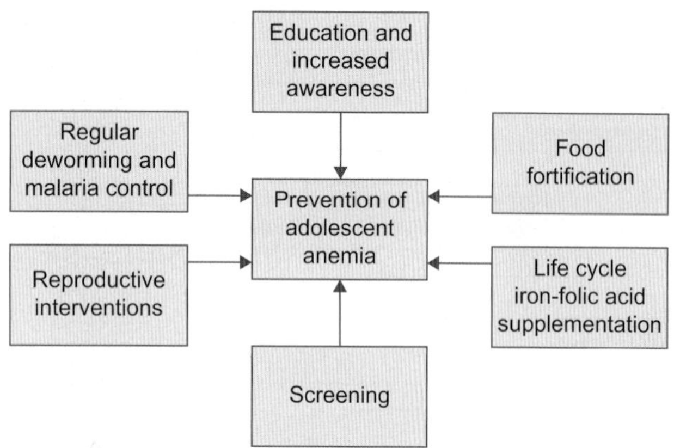

Fig. 1: Prevention of anemia.

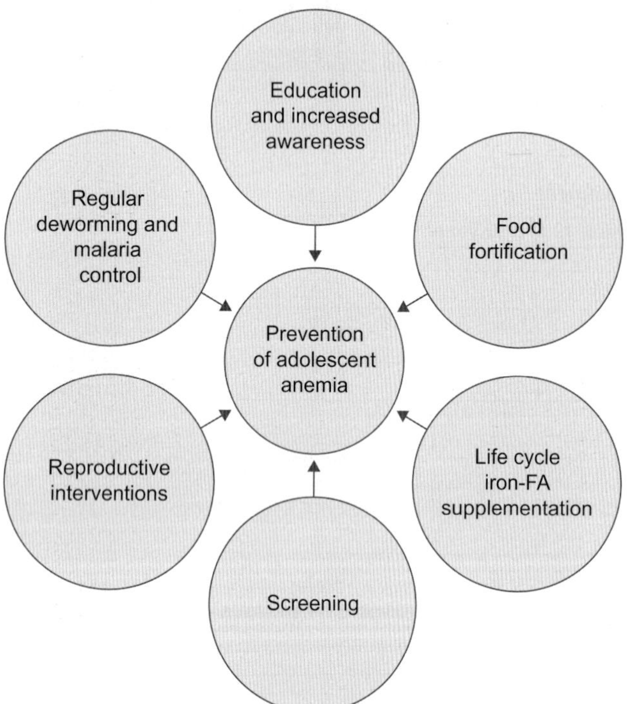

Fig. 2: Prevention of adolescent anemia.

- *Food-based interventions:* Fortification of commonly consumed food such as salt, milk, or atta with iron.
- Screening for anemia in adolescents and other high-risk groups to tap cases of anemia in presymptomatic stage.
- Regular supplementation of iron-folic acid tablets to adolescents and pregnant women.

National iron plus initiative: This is a proposed life cycle iron-folic acid supplementation program by Ministry of Health and Family Welfare, where age specific recommendations are made for prophylactic FSFA supplementation to children, adolescents, and pregnant women.

All adolescent boys as well as girls (10–19 years) are given weekly tablets containing 100 mg elemental iron and 500 µg of FA along with biannual deworming.

- *Diet:* Increased consumption of food rich in iron such as animal proteins, green leafy vegetables, and jaggery. Using iron pots for cooking.
- Biannual deworming of all school going children with albendazole
- Malaria control
- Treatment of underlying condition
- *Reproductive and obstetric interventions:* Preventing adolescent pregnancies, reducing the total number of pregnancies, and increasing the time between pregnancies will contribute to the control of iron deficiency anemia in women. Pregnancy creates a large demand for iron, which is needed to develop the fetus and placenta and to expand a woman's blood volume. Additional iron is lost with blood lost at delivery. When the iron demands of pregnancy are combined with the iron demands of adolescent growth, girls enter adulthood at great risk of iron deficiency.

CONCLUSION

Anemia is a major public health problem in India. In adolescent age group, iron deficiency anemia is the most common anemia. It is of particular significance due to its major effects on growth, development, productivity, maternal mortality, and intergenerational effects. Regular screening, prophylaxis, early detection and treatment, food fortification, and public awareness programs are needed to control iron deficiency anemia.

KEY POINTS

- Iron deficiency anemia is the most common type of anemia in adolescents all over the world.
- Due to the unique stage of growth, adolescent anemia has a significant impact on growth, cognition, reproduction, and general productivity.
- Prevention is the best method of managing iron deficiency anemia.

SUGGESTED READING

1. Adolescent Division, Ministry of Health and Family Welfare, Government of India. (2013). Guidelines for control of iron deficiency anemia. [online] Available from https://

www.nhm.gov.in/images/pdf/programmes/child-health/guidelines/Control-of-Iron-Deficiency-Anaemia.pdf. [Last accessed September, 2024]

2. Bellad A, Kapil R, Gupta A. National Guidelines for Prevention and Control of Iron Deficiency Anemia in India. Indian Journal of Community Health. 2018;30:89-94.
3. Bhave SY, Menon PSN. Bhave's Textbook of Adolescent Medicine. New Delhi: Peepee Publishers; 2016.
4. Chellan R, Paul L. (2010). Prevalence of iron deficiency anemia in India: Results from a large nationwide survey. [online] Available from https://www.cabidigitallibrary.org/doi/pdf/10.5555/20143025694. [Last accessed September, 2024]
5. Daniel WA Jr. Hematocrit: maturity relationship in adolescence. Pediatrics. 1973;52(3):388-94.
6. Greer JP, Foerster J, Rodgers GM, Paraskevas F, Glader B, Arber DA, et al. Wintrobe's Clinical Hematology, 12th edition. Philadelphia: Lippincott Williams & Wilkins; 2009. pp. 779-807.
7. https://main.mohfw.gov.in/sites/default/files/NFHS-5_Phase-II_0.pdf
8. Işık Balcı Y, Karabulut A, Gürses D, Ethem Çövüt I. Prevalence and risk factors of anemia among adolescents in Denizli, Turkey. Iran J Pediatr. 2012;22(1):77-81.
9. Kliegman RM. Nelson's Textbook of Pediatrics. Amsterdam: Elsevier; 2020.
10. Lozoff B. Behavioral alterations in iron deficiency. A review article. Adv Pediatr. 1988;35:331-59.
11. Soemantri AG, Pollitt E, Kim I. Iron deficiency anemia and educational achievement. Am J Clin Nutr. 1985;42(6):1221-8.
12. Stoltzfus RJ, Dreyfuss ML. (1998). Guidelines for the Use of Iron Supplements to Prevent and Treat Iron Deficiency Anemia. International Nutritional Anemia Consultative Group (INACG). [online] Available from https://foodsystems.org/wp-content/uploads/2021/02/INACG_Guidelines_for_the_Use_Of_Iron_Supplements_to_Prevent_and_Treat_Iron_Deficiency_Anemia.pdf. [Last accessed September, 2024]
13. World Health Organization. (2008). Worldwide prevalence of anemia 1993-2005. [online] Available from https://www.who.int/publications/i/item/9789241596657. [Last accessed September, 2024]

Academics and Career Choices in Adolescents: An Approach in the Pediatric Office Setting

Ritu Gupta, Abheet Gupta

INTRODUCTION

Adolescents are a growing area in pediatric practice in both hospital and community settings. They make up for around 25% of the practice of most pediatricians. Adolescence is a phase of transitioning from childhood to adulthood and involves major physical, mental, emotional, and psychological changes. In addition to addressing the physical and mental health issues of the adolescents, pediatricians are also expected to guide and counsel them regarding academics and career. Parents who have been visiting the same pediatrician for all health-related concerns of their child since they were born, have an expectation that the same doctor will address their anxiety related to their adolescent's academic performance and career choices. For many adolescents, their pediatrician is their role model and someone whom they look up to. The role of a pediatrician thus becomes even more important with an added responsibility. Pediatricians who are trained to communicate effectively with adolescents can play an important role in guiding the adolescents in the right direction and refer them to academic and career counselors for further clarity and action. Need of adolescent health experts who can provide anticipatory guidance to the adolescents as well as their parents has increased more than ever.

CAREER CHOICES IN ADOLESCENTS

Importance of Anticipatory Guidance

An adolescent's career choices are influenced by various factors such as life context or purpose, personal aptitude, and educational attainment. The cultural and social context of family and community are found to be instrumental in adolescents' career choices. Moreover, adolescents' career choices are significantly influenced by their parents. Parental expectations, aspirations, and guidance play a pivotal role in shaping career paths of adolescents and a strong emotional bond with parents fosters positive career shaping of youth.

In 21st century India, career options for our young people are plenty. Some of the most popular fields are still the conventional ones such as engineering, medicine, computer science, teaching, journalism, hospitality, law, chartered accountancy, and architecture. Additionally, many new fields have emerged such as data science, artificial intelligence, cybersecurity, social media influencers, and renewable energy that offer promising career opportunities. It is important for the parents and society to understand that the best career choice for a student depends upon their interest, aptitude, skills, and passion. It is important to do research of different fields and industries to find the best fit for one's career goal.

Parents often try to impose their aspirations on their adolescents and expect them to choose what they think is good for them as a career rather than having an open communication with their ward to find out what they want. Pediatricians can play a pivotal role in guiding the parents to actively listen to their adolescents with empathy and compassion. They need to first understand them fully and then guide them appropriately using their own wisdom. Authoritative parenting style where the parents are deeply connected with their children and there is open two way communication amongst them, various career options can be discussed, and the appropriate choice can be made without any pressure or force. When the adolescents feel trusted and encouraged to explore, they are more likely to choose a career that aligns with their true potential and leads to long-term fulfilment. It will be a win-win situation for both the parents and the adolescent. In this way, innumerable suicides and other self-harm behaviors, which we see and read about, so often in the media, could be prevented.

Once the adolescent has made up their mind as to what they want to do, encouraging them to shadow a professional in that field for a few days could be helpful to get more clarity and be sure about their choice. In case, the adolescent is not clear—aptitude test, career counseling, talking to professionals in different fields, and attending workshops and career fairs may help.

An approach to be used by a pediatrician in their office practice, to guide and appropriately refer the adolescents in relation to their academics and career choices is represented in **Flowchart 1**.

Flowchart 1: Academics and career choices.

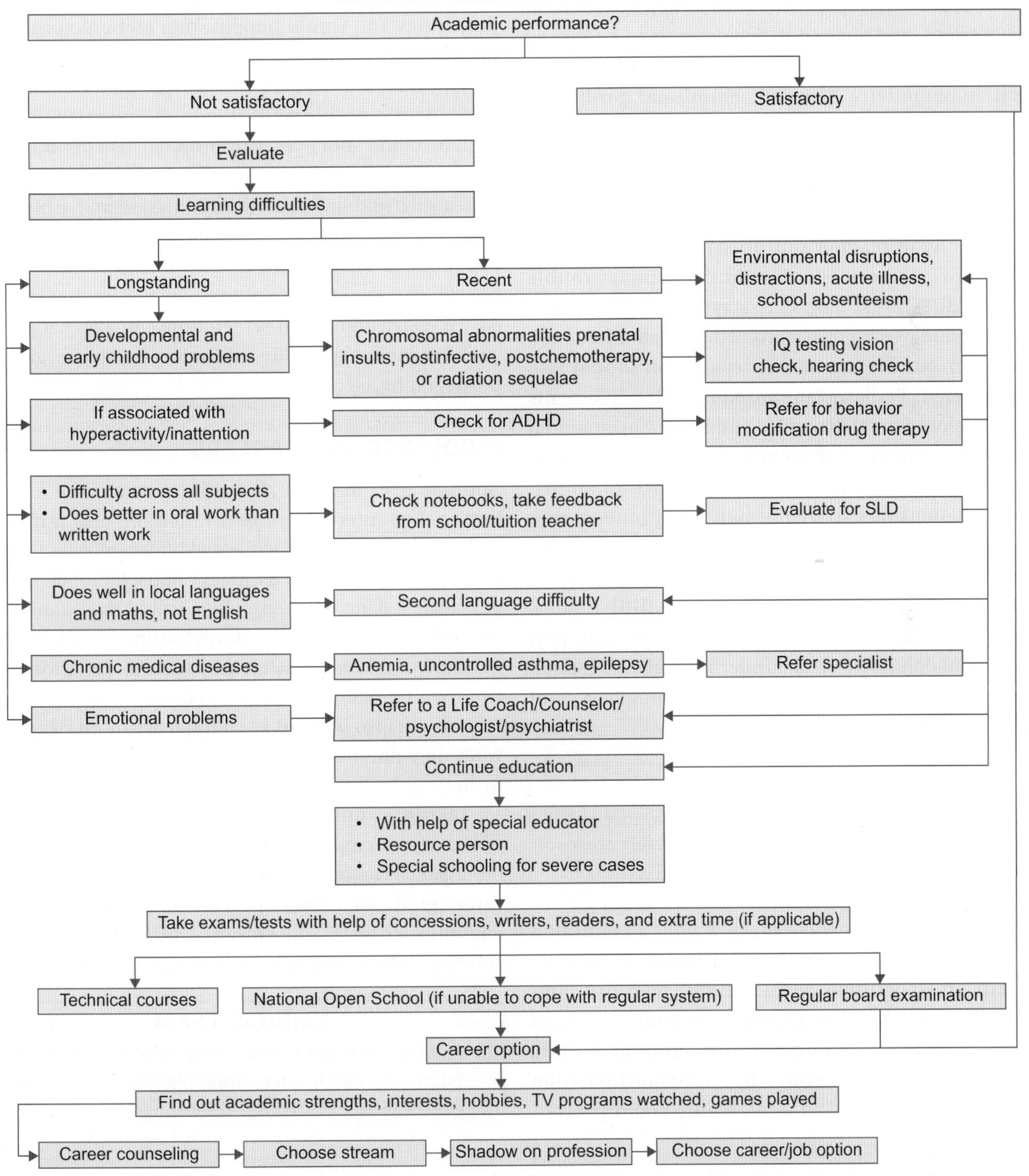

(ADHD: attention-deficit hyperactivity disorder; IQ: intelligence quotient; SLD: specific learning disability; TV: television)

ACADEMIC PERFORMANCE IN ADOLESCENTS

A greater challenge arises when an adolescent presents with academic underachievement. As a pediatrician, one needs to evaluate developmental milestones, study skills, check performance reports, and understand parental expectations. Medical problems such as hypothyroidism, micronutrient, and vitamin deficiencies must be looked for. Checking for specific learning disability, attention deficit hyperactivity disorder, emotional problems, physical problems (defective vision, defective hearing, and absent seizures), poor sociocultural home environment, psychiatric disorders, substance abuse, etc. becomes imperative. Specific learning disabilities usually present with difficulty in reading and/or writing, problem with Math, poor memory, poor attention span, trouble following directions, problems staying organized, etc. Emotional and psychological problems which affect one's self-esteem, confidence, and concentration should also be considered. Pediatricians working with adolescents should explore family dynamics and assess for potential signs of disruption or dysfunction within the family. A weak parent-child bond and the absence of strong, healthy relationship can significantly contribute to poor academic performance. Subnormal intelligence could be due to perinatal infections such as TORCH [toxoplasmosis, others (syphilis, varicella zoster, parvovirus B19), rubella, cytomegalovirus, and herpes] infections, prematurity, meningoencephalitis, or an underlying chromosomal disorder such as Klinefelter syndrome, Fragile X, and Turner's syndrome.

> **CLINICAL PEARL**
>
> - Anemia in adolescent girls and iodine deficiency in hilly areas are often missed and are easily correctable causes of poor school performance.

Micronutrients such as omega-3 poly unsaturated fatty acids, iron, iodine, zinc, and B vitamins contribute to brain and cognitive development, memory, and learning abilities. Nutrient-rich diet positively influences cognitive function, concentration and academic performance. Hence, ensuring a balanced nutritious diet among small children and adolescents could prevent poor scholastic performance. Physical problems such as visual disability (uncorrected refractive errors, squint, or more serious conditions such as chorioretinitis and retinal detachment) and hearing disability (congenital or acquired) need a thorough evaluation. Children with Down syndrome, mild cerebral palsy, and hemiplegic syndromes may also have writing difficulties and would benefit from technological alternatives and communication tools like computers or tablets. Substance abuse should be ruled out as cause of academic problems if there are any tell-tale signs such as blood shot eyes, inappropriate use of sunglasses, wearing long sleeved clothes even in hot weather, increased irritability and mood swings, secretive behavior, avoiding hugging, social disconnect and isolation, unexplained weight gain or loss, unexplained need for pocket money, stealing money, or parental suspicion. An excessive amount of screen time can affect academic performance, especially addiction to online gaming, pornography, etc.

COLLEGE AND CAREERS

Aptitude tests may not always be accurate and enough. Personality, interest and motivation are also important and must be considered while making a career choice. One can also take support of a Career Counselor for clarity and guidance. Asking the teens where would they want to see themselves five or ten years down the line could help them get clarity and decide what they want to do. A road map can then be planned and worked backwards. Exclusion criteria can also be used as children are more clear about what they don't want to do rather than what they want to do.

Taking support of other professionals, experienced seniors and family members, educationists, and professional career counselors could be of great help. Most career guidance centers provide information regarding eligibility criteria and entrance procedure to various colleges and courses, in both India and abroad.

> **CLINICAL PEARL**
>
> - Children with borderline mental retardation should be put in skill-based programs/apprenticeships as early as possible, i.e., after middle school.

KEY POINTS

- Stay alert not to miss learning difficulties, which should be evaluated and managed promptly, to prevent the child getting into a cycle of low self-esteem, worthlessness, dropping out of school, and failure.
- Guide parents of children with specific learning difficulties to seek remediation with a special educator. If detected late, accommodations with concessions and the National Open School are the options.
- The plethora of career choices is confusing. Guide parents to work with their adolescents to access career information from various sources like career guidance centers.
- Guide parents to support their teens in discovering their unique strengths and passions rather than imposing their own expectations.
- Be a catalyst in enabling adolescents reach their full potential. Your role could make a huge difference to an adolescent in being independent, confident, successful and happy or being isolated, depressed, and unproductive.

SUGGESTED READING

1. American Psychiatric Association. Diagnostic Criteria for ADHD DSM-4: Diagnostic and Statistical Manual of Mental Disorders, 5th edition. Arlington, VA, USA: American Psychiatric Association; 2013.
2. Elkind D. All Grown Up and No Place To Go: Teenagers in Crisis. MA, USA: Addison-Wesley; 1998.
3. Emerick LJ. Academic underachievement among the gifted: Students' perception of factors that reverse the pattern. Gifted Child Quarterly. 1992;36(3):140-6.
4. Karande S, Kulkarni M. Poor school performance. Indian J Pediatr. 2005;72(11):961-7.
5. Klegman RM, Stanton BM, St. Geme J, Schor NF. Neurodevelopment function and dysfunction in the school age child. In: Klegman RM, Stanton BM, St. Geme J, Schor NF (Eds). Nelson Textbook of Pediatrics, 20th edition. Philadelphia: Elsevier; 2016. pp. 192-99.
6. Shapiro BK, Gallico RP. Learning disabilities. Pediatr Clin North Am. 1993;40(3):491-505.

WEBSITES FOR PARENTS

- www.careerchoices.com
- www.talkitover.in
- www.onestepup.in
- www.careerage.com
- https://goodmenproject.com/featured-content/how-to-help-your-child-choose-a-career-path/
- https://www.parentcircle.com/helping-children-to-choose-a-right-career-path/article
- https://www.liveabout.com/helping-your-children-make-career-choices-525407

Polycystic Ovarian Syndrome and Menstrual Problems in Adolescents

Roli M Srivastava

INTRODUCTION

Polycystic ovary syndrome (PCOS) is one of the most prevalent endocrinopathies affecting adolescent girls, yet it remains underdiagnosed and often misunderstood in this age group. The manifestations of PCOS in adolescence frequently overlap with normal pubertal changes, presenting a diagnostic challenge for clinicians. Early recognition and intervention are critical to mitigate the long-term consequences of this disorder, including metabolic syndrome, cosmetic, infertility, and psychosocial distress.

This chapter seeks to provide a comprehensive, algorithmic approach to the evaluation and management of PCOS in adolescents. By integrating the latest evidence-based guidelines with practical clinical strategies, it equips healthcare providers to navigate the complexities of this condition. The chapter emphasizes a multidisciplinary approach, addressing the physical, emotional, and social dimensions of care.

In this rapidly evolving field, recent advancements in diagnostic criteria, hormonal therapies, and lifestyle interventions are reshaping the way we understand and treat PCOS. This edition includes updates on these developments, offering readers a contemporary perspective on managing PCOS during adolescence.

The goal of this chapter is not only to inform but also to empower clinicians to make timely and informed decisions, ultimately improving the quality of life for adolescents with PCOS.

POLYCYSTIC OVARIAN SYNDROME

The condition "polycystic ovarian syndrome (PCOS)" was first described in 1935 by Dr Stein and Dr Leventhal; hence its original name Stein-Leventhal syndrome is characterized by an imbalance of hormones in women which can affect menstrual periods and ovulation. Women are often very embarrassed by some of the symptoms associated with this condition, such as excessive hair growth, acne, obesity, and the development of small cysts on the ovaries. Because of these distressing symptoms, women may also experience feelings of depression and anxiety. It is one of the most common female endocrine disorders affecting approximately 5–10% of women of reproductive age and is one of the leading causes of infertility. It is a very common problem amongst young women and teenage girls, sometimes even affecting girls as young as 11 years of age. If not treated early, serious health complications, such as diabetes and cardiovascular disease, can develop and so, the management of the PCOS patient often will vary over time as the patient enters different stages of life with different goals. In contrast, because of the long-term health implications of insulin resistance (IR), the importance of lifestyle modification toward weight management and maintaining adequate physical activity should be the one constant in the management of these patients.

DIAGNOSIS IS BY CLINICAL EXAMINATION, ULTRASOUND, AND LABORATORY

Polycystic ovarian syndrome is most simply clinically defined as the presence of:

- Hyperandrogenism (clinically and/or biochemically)
- Chronic anovulation in the absence of specific adrenal and/or pituitary disease.

Hyperandrogenism

Hyperandrogenism may present clinically as hirsutism, acne, and male-pattern alopecia.

- *Hirsutism:* The growth of coarse hair on a woman in a male pattern (upper lip, chin, chest, upper abdomen, back, etc.)
- *Acne:* Pubertal acne in general is twice as prevalent in adolescent males versus females and males are more likely to have severe disease. Thus, an adolescent

female with moderate-to-severe acne should be investigated for PCOS.

- *Virilization:* Clitoromegaly, deepening voice, increased musculature, or rapidly progressive hirsutism, or alopecia, however, is not a feature of PCOS, but instead of more severe hyperandrogenism.

Chronic Anovulation

It may result in:

- Oligomenorrhea
- Amenorrhea
- Dysfunctional uterine bleeding
- Infertility

However, around 20% of patients with PCOS may have normal menstrual cycles. Often, menstrual abnormalities are long-standing, even since menarche although primary amenorrhea very rare **(Box 1)**.

POLYCYSTIC OVARIAN SYNDROME DIAGNOSTIC CRITERIA

Polycystic ovarian syndrome includes a wide spectrum of clinical symptoms and signs. Three different diagnostic classifications had been proposed to define this disease till November 2015. The first one was published in 1990, and is known as the "National Institute of Health criteria". Later, in 2003, an expert panel met in Rotterdam and added to the previous criteria the presence of polycystic ovarian morphology detected by transvaginal ultrasonography **(Fig. 1)**. Then, the Androgen Excess Society, published in 2006, gave the new diagnostic criteria being applied till late and finally latest in November 2015, the American Association of Clinical Endocrinologists, American College of Endocrinology, and Androgen Excess Society released new guidelines in the evaluation and treatment of PCOS **(Table 1)**.

As PCOS is an umbrella of various signs and symptoms, certain diseases with nearly same presenting features, especially irregular cycles and androgenic features, have to be ruled out to reach the diagnosis **(Flowchart 1)**.

BOX 1: Clinical features of polycystic ovarian syndrome.

- Oligomenorrhea/amenorrhea
- Acne
- Obesity
- Hirsutism
- Acanthosis nigricans
- Male-pattern alopecia

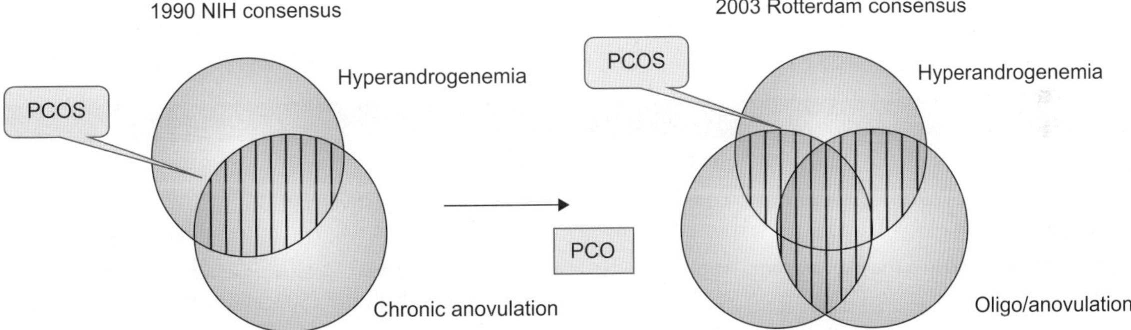

Fig. 1: 1990 National Institute of Health consensus versus 2003 Rotterdam consensus.
(NIH: National Institute of Health; PCOS: polycystic ovarian syndrome; PCO: polycystic ovaries on ultrasound)

TABLE 1: Polycystic ovarian syndrome diagnostic criteria.

NH 1990	***Rotterdam 2003***	***AE-PCOS Society 2006***	***AACE/ACE and AES Society 2015***
• Chronic anovulation • Clinical and/or biochemical signs of hyperandrogenism (with exclusion of other etiologies, e.g., congenital adrenal hyperplasia) (both criteria needed)	• Oligo- and/or anovulation • Clinical and/or biochemical signs of hyperandrogenism • Polycystic ovaries (two of three criteria needed)	• Clinical and/or biochemical signs of hyperandrogenism • Ovarian dysfunction (oligo-anovulation and/or polycystic ovarian morphology) (both criteria needed)	• Chronic anovulation • Hyperandrogenism (clinical/biologic) • Polycystic ovaries (one of the above three criteria)

(AACE: American Association of Clinical Endocrinologists; ACE: American College of Endocrinology; AES: Androgen Excess and PCOS Society; NIH: National Institute of Health)

DIAGNOSIS AND DIFFERENTIAL DIAGNOSIS (TABLE 2)

Not all women with PCOS have polycystic ovaries, nor do all women with ovarian cysts have PCOS; although a pelvic ultrasound is a major diagnostic tool, it is not the only one. The diagnosis is straightforward using the Rotterdam criteria, even when the syndrome is associated with a wide range of symptoms. The number of follicles and ovary volume are both important in the ultrasound evaluation.

RADIOGRAPHIC FEATURES

Ovaries may show sonographic features of polycystic ovaries **(Figs. 2A and B)**, bilateral enlarged ovaries with multiple small follicles: 50%.

- Increased ovarian size (>10 cc)
- 12 or more follicles measuring 2–9 mm
- Follicles of similar size

Flowchart 1: Laboratory investigations.

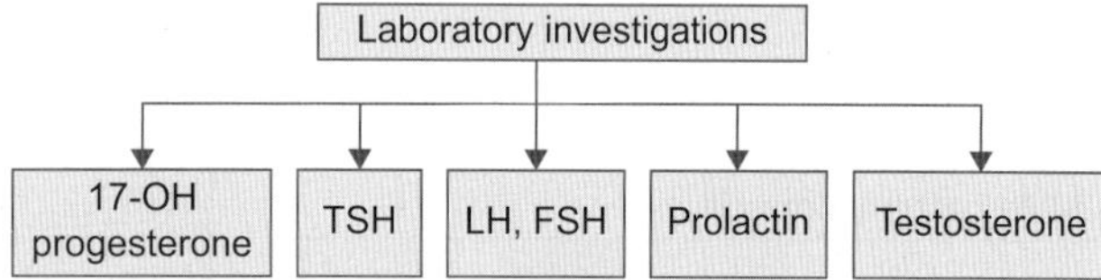

(FSH: follicle-stimulating hormone; LH: luteinizing hormone; 17-OH progesterone: 17-hydroxyprogesterone; TSH, thyroid-stimulating hormone)

- Peripheral location of follicles gives a string of pearl appearance.
- Hyperechoic central stroma

PATHOPHYSIOLOGY OF POLYCYSTIC OVARIAN SYNDROME

Polycystic ovaries develop, when the ovaries are stimulated to produce androgens, either through excess of luteinizing hormone (LH) or through hyperinsulinemia in women whose ovaries are sensitive to this stimulus. Multiple ovarian cysts are seen in ultrasound. These "cysts" are actually immature follicles whose development has arrested at an early-antral stage due to the disturbed ovarian function. PCOS is characterized by a complex set of symptoms, and research to date suggests that IR could be a leading cause. PCOS may also have a genetic predisposition. A majority of patients with PCOS have IR and/or are obese. Their elevated insulin levels contribute to the abnormalities seen in the hypothalamic-pituitary-ovarian axis that lead to PCOS. Adipose tissue possesses aromatase that converts androstenedione to estrone and testosterone to estradiol. The excess of adipose tissue in obese patients creates the paradox of having both excess androgens (which are responsible for hirsutism and virilization) and estrogens [which inhibits follicle-stimulating hormone (FSH) via negative feedback]. Also, hyperinsulinemia increases gonadotropin-releasing hormone (GnRH) pulse frequency,

TABLE 2: Diagnosis and differential diagnosis.

Differential diagnosis	*Test*	*Comments*
Hypothalamic amenorrhea: Weight loss, exercise, anxiety, and chronic illness	Low FSH	LH: FSH >2 is suggestive of PCOS
Pituitary adenoma: Galactorrhea may be present	High prolactin	*Mild-transient hyperprolactinemia (check for hypothyroidism):* Prolactin is generally only 50% above the upper limit of normal
Hypothyroidism: Cold dry skin and constipation	High TSH	
Late-onset congenital adrenal hyperplasia: Rare, mimics PCOS in all regards. The classic forms present in newborn girls as ambiguous genitalia	High 17-OH progesterone	A morning, fasting, level of < 200 ng/dL in the follicular phase excludes late-onset 21-hydroxylase deficiency. Oral contraceptives and glucocorticoids can affect values
Premature ovarian failure	High FSH	
Cushing's syndrome hypertension, purple abdominal striae, prominent dorsal cervical fat pads, and a rounded, plethoric face	High cortisol	Mild elevations can be seen in PCOS values ≥ two times the upper limit of normal (Cushing's syndrome). Oral contraceptive pills should be discontinued before dynamic testing
Adrenal tumor: Extensive signs of virilization	Very high TT	TT values may be normal in PCOS. Oral contraceptive pills lower TT, 3 months off OCPs best to get true value. Most testosterone values in PCOS will be ≤150 ng/dL, i.e., mild elevation, testosterone values of ≥200 ng/dL suggest ovarian or adrenal tumor

(FSH: follicle-stimulating hormone; LH: luteinizing hormone; OCPs: oral contraceptive pills; 17-OH progesterone: 17-hydroxyprogesterone; PCOS: polycystic ovarian syndrome; TSH: thyroid-stimulating hormone; TT: total testosterone)

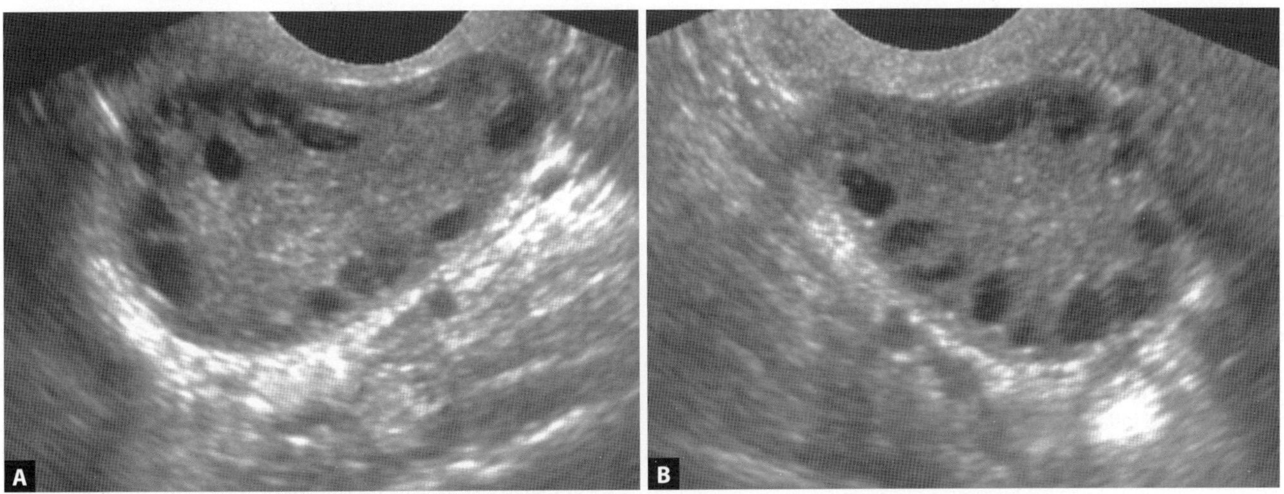

Figs. 2A and B: Characteristic string of pearls sign seen: (A) Left ovary and (B) Right ovary.

Flowchart 2: Pathophysiology of polycystic ovarian syndrome.

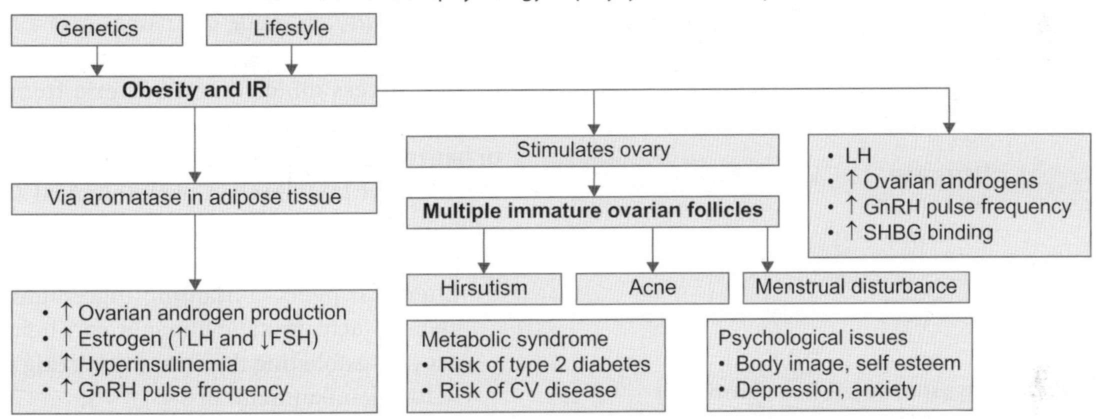

(CV: cardiovascular; FSH: follicle-stimulating hormone; GnRH: gonadotropin-releasing hormone; IR: insulin resistance; LH: luteinizing hormone; SHBG: sex hormone-binding globulin)

LH over FSH dominance, increased ovarian androgen production, decreased follicular maturation, and decreased sex hormone-binding globulin (SHBG) binding; all these steps lead to the development of PCOS. IR is a common finding among patients of normal weight as well as those overweight patients **(Flowchart 2)**.

CLINICAL PEARL

- Polycystic ovarian syndrome should be considered and appropriate assessment should be undertaken before commencement of the oral contraceptive pills in adolescents with irregular periods, i.e., irregular cycles (≥35 days or <21 days), 2 years following menarche. Other causes of irregular cycles, such as thyroid dysfunction or hyperprolactinemia, need to be considered and excluded prior to the diagnosis of PCOS.

POLYCYSTIC OVARIAN SYNDROME

Health consequences of PCOS are given in **Box 2** and **Table 3**.

MANAGEMENT OF POLYCYSTIC OVARIAN SYNDROME

The overall aims of treatment are to:

- Correct the high androgen levels and adverse metabolic effects
- Restore menstrual regularity
- Manage the cosmetic symptoms and signs
- Restore fertility if desired
- *Long-term health:* Chronic disease prevention
- Diabetes prevention

BOX 2: Polycystic ovarian syndrome: Health consequences.

- *Reproductive:*
  - Infertility
  - Increased risk of miscarriage
  - Increased risk of gestational diabetes/preeclampsia
  - Increased risk of endometrial cancer
- *Psychosocial:*
  - Depression and anxiety
  - Cosmetic concerns (hyperandrogenic symptoms)
  - Increased risk of type 2 diabetes
- *Cardiometabolic:*
  - Diabetes hypertension
  - Dyslipidemia
  - Increased inflammation
  - Increased cardiovascular disease risk
  - Nonalcoholic steatohepatitis
  - Sleep apnea

TABLE 3: The spectrum of features of polycystic ovarian syndrome and associated menstrual problems.

Clinical	*Endocrinal*	*Probable complications*
Obesity	Increased insulin	Dyslipidemia
Menstrual disturbance	Decreased sex hormone-binding globulin	LDL increased
Oligomenorrhea	–	HDL increased
Amenorrhea	–	Triglycerides increased
Regular cycle	–	–
Hyperandrogenism	Testosterone increased	Diabetes mellitus
Infertility	LH increased	CV disease and hypertension
Asymptomatic	Prolactin increased	Endometrial carcinoma

(CV: cardiovascular; HDL: high-density lipoprotein; LH: luteinizing hormone; LDL: low-density lipoprotein)

- Cardiovascular disease risk reduction
- Cancer prevention

The medical management of PCOS can be broken into:

- Chronic management
- Acute management **(Flowcharts 3 and 4)**

ADVANCEMENTS IN COSMETIC MANAGEMENT OF PCOS

Polycystic ovary syndrome affects many aspects of a woman's health, including her skin. Cosmetic issues can be very distressful and its management is an important part of the treatment. Below are some cosmetic management strategies for skin issues in PCOS, which includes acne, acanthosis, hirsutism, and hair fall.

Flowchart 3: Medical management of PCOS.

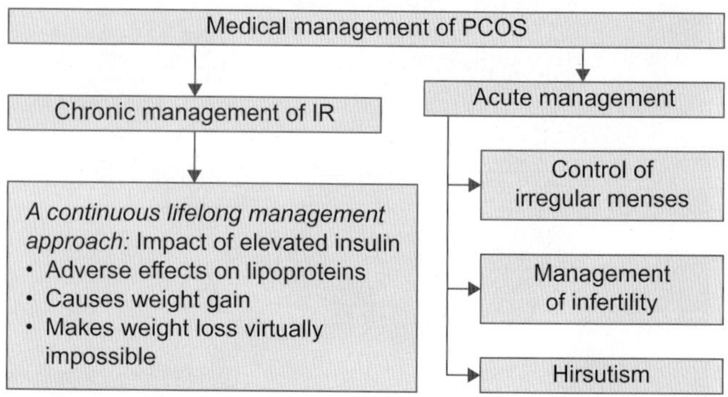

(IR: insulin resistance; PCOS: polycystic ovarian syndrome)

- *Skincare routine:* Gentle cleansing—use a mild, non-comedogenic cleanser morning and evening daily to remove excess oil, dirt, and bacteria from the skin. Using products with ingredients such as salicylic acid or benzoyl peroxide can help with acne.
- *Professional treatments:* Cosmetological treatments such as chemical peels, microdermabrasion, IPL, or chemical peels:
  - Chemical peels containing ingredients such as glycolic acid or salicylic acid can help improve acne by exfoliating the skin, unclogging pores, and reducing inflammation.
  - *Microdermabrasion:* This exfoliating treatment removes dead skin cells and helps improve the appearance of acne scars and skin texture.
- *Laser therapy:* Various laser and light-based treatments, such as laser resurfacing or intense pulsed light (IPL) therapy, can target acne-causing bacteria, reduce oil production, and improve overall skin tone and texture. Microneedling radiofrequency (MNRF) or microneedling alone helps in acne scar reduction and improves overall skin texture. Treatment should be customized as treatment and results vary from individual to individual.
- *Hair removal:* Excessive hair growth (hirsutism) is a common symptom of PCOS. Various hair removal methods such as shaving, waxing, threading, depilatory creams, or laser hair removal can help manage this symptom. Laser hair removal, in particular, can provide long-term reduction in hair growth. Triple wavelength Diode lasers are best in giving results.

Flowchart 4: Acute management: Control of irregular menses.

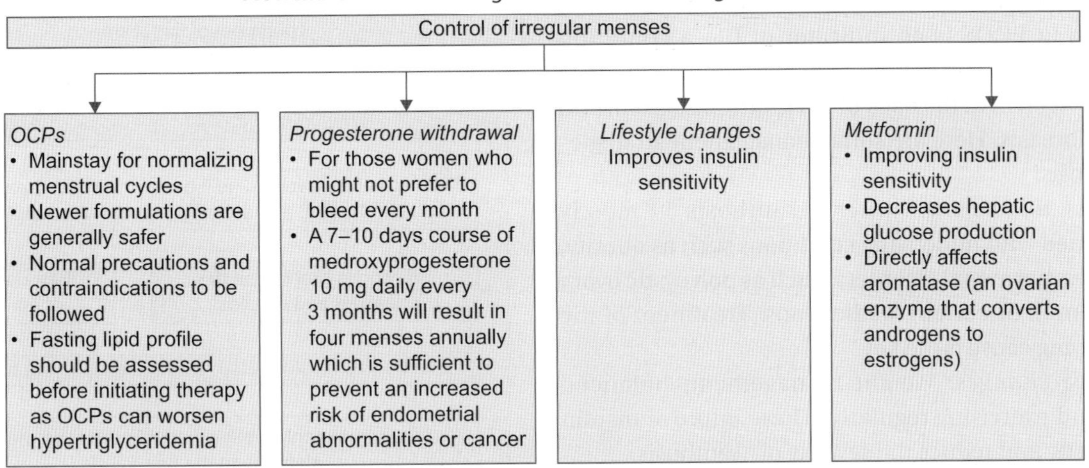

(OCPs: oral contraceptive pills)

- *Makeup techniques:* Using concealers for acne or excess facial hair improves confidence and self-esteem. Color correctors and makeup products which are acne-prone skin friendly can be beneficial.
- *Hormonal therapy:* Oral contraceptives pills (OCPs) are generally used for menstrual cycle regulation and reduce androgen levels in women with PCOS. These medications can also help improve acne and hirsutism over time. Antiandrogen medications, e.g., spironolactone, may be used with OCPs for more severe cases of acne.
- *Topical treatments:* Benzoyl peroxide, salicylic acid, retinoids (e.g., tretinoin and adapalene), or azelaic acid can help reduce acne and new breakouts. These medications act by unclogging pores, reducing inflammation, and increasing skin cell turnover.
    - *Moisturizing:* Using a lightweight, noncomedogenic moisturizer helps in skin hydration without exacerbating acne.
    - *Sun protection:* A broad-spectrum sunscreen with SPF 50 is to be applied daily on skin to prevent sun damage and postinflammatory hyperpigmentation (PIH).
- *Healthy lifestyle:*
    - *Balanced diet:* Adopting a balanced diet rich in fruits, vegetables, whole grains, lean proteins, and healthy fats can help regulate insulin levels and reduce inflammation, which may improve acne symptoms.
    - *Limit sugary and processed foods:* High-glycemic index foods and sugary snacks can exacerbate acne by increasing insulin levels and promoting inflammation. Limiting consumption of these foods may help improve acne in some individuals.
    - *Regular exercise:* Engaging in regular physical activity can help regulate hormone levels, reduce stress, and improve overall skin health.
    - *Stress management:* Stress can worsen acne symptoms by triggering hormonal fluctuations. Incorporate stress-reduction techniques such as mindfulness, meditation, yoga, or deep breathing exercises into your daily routine.
- PCOS is a lifestyle disorder, a healthy lifestyle, with regular exercise and a balanced diet, helps in managing most of the symptoms of PCOS including skin health.
- *Stress management:* Stress increases hormonal imbalance and all the symptoms of PCOS including skin issues. Exercise, mindfulness, yoga, or meditation daily helps reduce Stress and is beneficial for both physical, mental, and emotional wellness.
- *Avoiding certain products and habits:*
    - Avoid using harsh skincare products which may irritate the skin and worsen acne.
    - Avoid picking or squeezing acne lesions, as this can lead to scarring and further inflammation.
    - Avoid makeup and skincare products which are comedogenic, they should be noncomedogenic or oil-free to prevent pore clogging.
    - Avoid three whites—(1) Sugar, (2) salt, and (3) refined flour to regulate insulin levels, which in turn improve acne and hirsutism.

ACANTHOSIS

Acanthosis in PCOS is an indicator of IR—a condition characterized by thickened and darkened skin. It is commonly seen in at the back of neck, armpits, groin, and under the breasts. Here are some management strategies for acanthosis:

- *Address underlying causes:* Acanthosis is mostly associated with underlying conditions such as obesity, diabetes, hormonal disorders (such as polycystic ovary syndrome), or certain medications. Treatment of the underlying cause is the key.
- *Lifestyle changes:* Weight management, balanced diet, and exercising regularly. These improve insulin sensitivity and reduce the severity of acanthosis.
- *Topical treatments:* Topical treatments such as retinoids, alpha hydroxy acids, or salicylic acid improve the appearance of acanthosis by promoting cell turnover and reducing hyperpigmentation.
- *Medications:* In some, medications such as oral retinoids, metformin (for improving insulin sensitivity), or spironolactone (for hormonal disorders) may help.
- *Sun protection:* Sun exposure can worsen the appearance of acanthosis. Patients should use sunscreen regularly and wear protective clothing.
- *Treat complications:* Acanthosis can sometimes lead to skin infections or itching. These should not be ignored and promptly addressed.
- *Regular monitoring:* Patients with acanthosis should be monitored regularly by to assess the effectiveness of treatment and prevent any complications.
- *Patient education:* It provide patients with information about acanthosis, including its causes, management strategies, and the importance of adherence to treatment and lifestyle modifications.
- *Dermatological consultation:* In severe cases or if initial treatments are ineffective, referral to a dermatologist may be necessary for further evaluation and management.
- *Psychological support:* Acanthosis has significant negative impact on a patient's self-esteem and quality of life. Offering psychological support and counseling can help patients cope with the emotional aspects of the condition.

HIRSUTISM

The decision to treat should be based on the patient's perception of the excess terminal hair growth. It can be managed in two ways **(Flowchart 5)**:

Flowchart 5: Management of hirsutism.

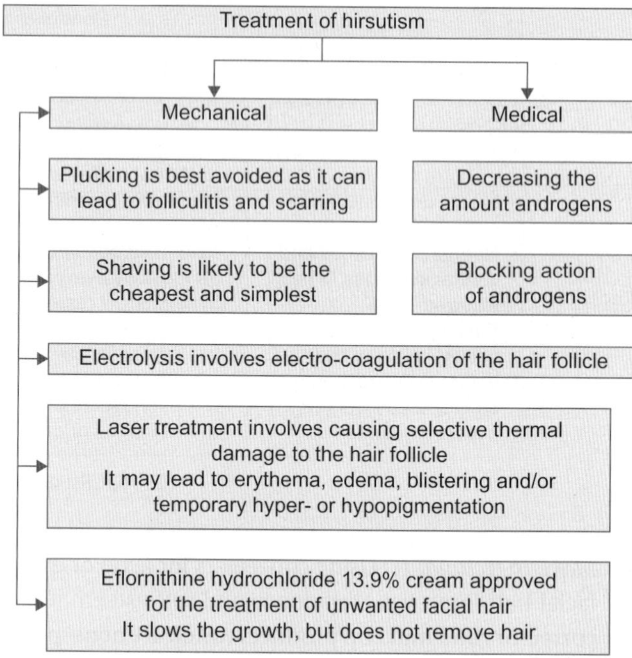

1. *Cosmetic:* Shaving, waxing, electrolysis, and laser hair reduction (LHR)
2. *Medical* management of hirsutism:
   - Decreasing the amount
   - Blocking action of androgens

Mechanical

- Hair removal creams
- Plucking which is best avoided as it can lead to folliculitis and scarring.
- Shaving is likely to be the cheapest and simplest.
- Electrolysis involves electrocoagulation of the hair follicle.
- LHR

Recent diode laser hair reduction popularly called as LHR, is a cosmetic procedure used to reduce unwanted hair growth. It acts by targeting the melanin in the hair follicles, heating them up, and damaging them to inhibit future hair growth. Here is a breakdown of the basis of LHR:

- *Types of lasers:* Different types of lasers are there these days for hair reduction, including alexandrite, diode, Nd:YAG, and ruby lasers. Each type of laser emits light at a specific wavelength, which determines its effectiveness for targeting different skin and hair types.

- *Multiple sessions:* LHR typically requires multiple sessions spaced several weeks apart, because hair grows in cycles, and the laser is most effective when hair is in the active growth phase (anagen phase). Multiple sessions ensure that all hair follicles are targeted during their active growth phases, leading to more effective and long-lasting results

Testosterone Production (Flowchart 3)

- *Oral contraceptive pills:* Gonadotropin production (as testosterone is predominantly ovarian in nature and is caused by both LH and by effect of hyperinsulinemia at the ovary and SHBG)
- Metformin
- Lifestyle modification/weight loss

Medical Management of Hirsutism (Flowchart 6)

Testosterone Action

- *Antiandrogens (spironolactone):*
  - Aldosterone antagonist
  - Antihypertensive agent also has a 67% relative affinity for the testosterone receptors (SHBG by insulin sensitivity):
    - *Spironolactone:* 50 mg twice a day 6–12 months
    - Increase to 100 mg twice a day if required
    - *Side effects:* Menstrual irregularity, nausea

Flowchart 6: Medical management of hirsutism.

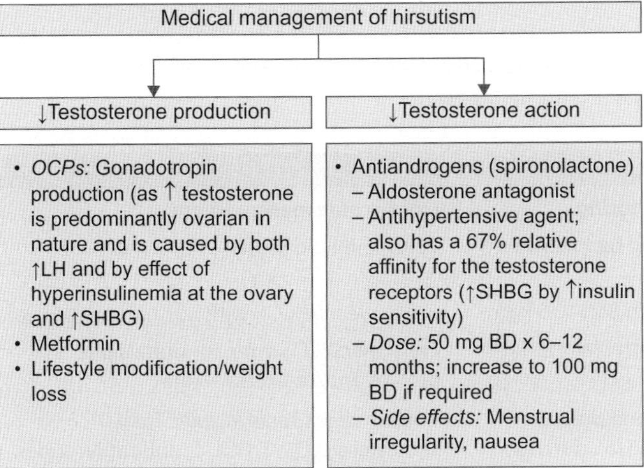

(LH: luteinizing hormone; OCP: oral contraceptive pills; SHBG: sex hormone-binding globulin)

Management of Infertility

It is rarely required in adolescents. It is very difficult to cover its intricacies; therefore, just a brief word on clomiphene, metformin, and lifestyle modifications is being taken up. PCOS accounts for 75% of anovulatory infertility. Additionally, when pregnancies do occur, the first-trimester miscarriage rate is as high as 30–50% **(Table 4)**.

DIABETES RISK AND LONG-TERM MANAGEMENT OF INSULIN RESISTANCE IN POLYCYSTIC OVARIAN SYNDROME (TABLE 5)

Most PCOS patients are inherently IR with the obesity seen in many, with a substantial proportion of patients have abnormalities on the oral glucose tolerance test.

Lifestyle modification:

- 20 minutes of brisk walking
- Daily metformin is found to be useful for significant improvement in insulin sensitivity; causes reduction in the development of type 2 diabetes mellitus.

TABLE 4: Management of infertility.

Clomiphene	*Lifestyle modification/ weight loss*	*Metformin*
• Obese women do not respond to low doses at the rate of 50 mg dose • The degree of obesity correlates with the dose of clomiphene needed to induce ovulation • The higher doses may cause side effects and can increase the rate of multiple gestations, given in combination with metformin	• Lifestyle modification needs to be stressed • 3–6 months trial of aggressive lifestyle modification may be a prudent first step before considering an insulin sensitizer	• Start at 500 mg twice a day and increased to thrice a day if ovulation did not occur by 6 weeks, and add clomiphene 6 weeks later • Use improves the outcome of other infertility therapies • Improves fertilization and pregnancy rates • In the setting of infertility, metformin therapy should likely be continued for as long as fertility efforts are ongoing, even if it "fails" initially • Reduces risk of early pregnancy loss; no birth defects occurred

Cardiovascular Risk Factors and Disease in Polycystic Ovarian Syndrome

- Prevalence of diagnosed hypertension or higher ambulatory blood pressure in PCOS
- The pattern of dyslipidemia in PCOS is in keeping with IR, increased triglycerides, and low high-density lipoprotein cholesterol.

TABLE 5: Indicators and diagnostic tests for insulin resistance: Key signs and optimal testing methods.

Signs of insulin resistance	*Best test for insulin resistance*
• Upper-body obesity • Acanthosis nigricans • However, only 35–50% of polycystic ovarian syndrome patients are obese	• Best test for insulin resistance is 2-hour oral glucose tolerance test • *Interpretation:* – Impaired glucose tolerance: 140–199 mg/dL – Diabetic: ≥200 mg/dL

Assessment of Cardiometabolic Risk (Figs. 3A and B and Table 6)

- *Screen all PCOS for following:* Obesity, lack of physical activity, cigarette smoking, dyslipidemia, hypertension, and impaired glucose tolerance test
- All women with PCOS should be assessed for excess weight at every visit. Age appropriate and gender appropriate body mass index should be considered.

LIFESTYLE MANAGEMENT FOR WOMEN WITH POLYCYSTIC OVARY SYNDROME

Lifestyle management (single or combined approaches of diet, exercise. and/or behavioral interventions) for weight loss, prevention of weight gain, or for general health benefits should be recommended in women with PCOS **(Box 3)**.

Although first-line monotherapy in adolescent age group includes metformin and/or combination therapy with oral contraceptive agents and antiandrogen agents.

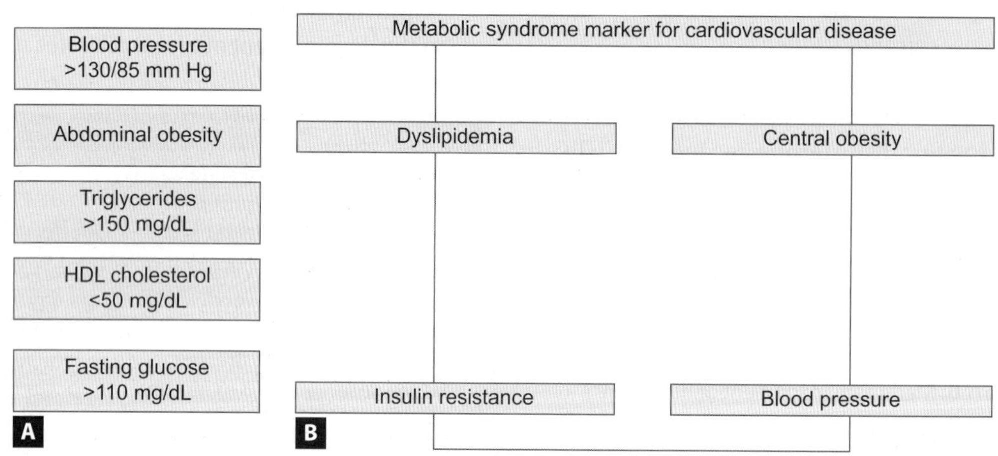

Figs. 3A and B: (A) Metabolic syndrome; (B) Metabolic syndrome marker for cardiovascular disease.

TABLE 6: Assessment of cardiometabolic risk.

Diabetes status	*Blood pressure monitoring*	*Lipid profile measurement*
Prediabetes and/or type 2 diabetes should be assessed	Blood pressure should be measured	Complete lipid profile
Oral GTT should be performed	*Annually:* In PCOS with BMI 18.5 kg/m^2	*Every 2 years:* PCOS with normal lipid profile
Every second year in all women with PCOS	*Every visit:* In PCOS with BMI ≥25 kg/m^2	*Every year:* PCOS with abnormal lipid profiles and/or excess weight
Annually: In those with additional risk factors for type 2 diabetes, e.g., features of IR	The ideal daytime blood pressure should not exceed 135/85 mm Hg	*A lipid profile should include:* Total cholesterol, LDL-C, HDL-C, and triglycerides

(BMI: body mass index; GTT: glucose tolerance test; HDL-C, high-density lipoprotein cholesterol; IR: insulin resistance; LDL-C: low density lipoprotein cholesterol; PCOS: polycystic ovarian syndrome)

BOX 3: Lifestyle management.

- Face-to-face, tailored dietary advice, including education, behavioral change techniques and ongoing emotional support should be provided to women with PCOS and a BMI ≥25 kg/m^2 (overweight/obese)
- Exercise recommendations
- 150 min/week or 20 min/day
- Of this, 90 min/week should be aerobic activity at moderate-to-high intensity (60–90% of maximum heart rate)

(BMI: body mass index; PCOS: polycystic ovarian syndrome)

It is hoped that early and proper diagnosis, will allow more women to be managed properly for their presenting symptoms (hirsutism, irregular menses, etc.), but also to be educated and managed for the continuing health risk of IR throughout their lives.

KEY POINTS

- Polycystic ovarian syndrome is the most common endocrine disorder among young women affecting approximately 5–10%.
- One of the leading causes of infertility
- There is not a single diagnostic test for PCOS
- Associated with a range of metabolic abnormalities which can lead to long-term health problems.
- Lifestyle changes play an important role in management of the syndrome.
- Management should be individually tailored for each patient depending on the type of symptoms and clinical features found.
- Prevent weight gain and address weight loss if needed as body mass index > 30 limits fertility.
- About 5–10% weight loss will greatly assist in symptom control.
- Women with PCOS have increased risk of endometrial cancer with prolonged amenorrhea; aim for >4 periods/year unless on contraception.

SUGGESTED READING

1. Artini PG, Di Berardino OM, Simi G, Papini F, Ruggiero M, Monteleone P, et al. Best methods for identification and treatment of PCOS. Minerva Ginecol. 2010;62(1):33-48.
2. Atiomo WU, Pearson S, Shaw S, Prentice A, Dubbins P. Ultrasound criteria in the diagnosis of polycystic ovary syndrome (PCOS). Ultrasound Med Biol. 2000;26(6):977-80.
3. Broekmans FJ, Knauff EA, Valkenburg O, Laven JS, Eijkemans MJ, Fauser BC. PCOS according to the Rotterdam consensus criteria: change in prevalence among WHO-II anovulation and association with metabolic factors. BJOG. 2006;113(10):1210-7.
4. Dunaif A, Thomas A. Current concepts in the polycystic ovary syndrome. Annu Rev Med. 2001;52:401-19.
5. Farah L, Lazenby AJ, Boots LR, Azziz R. Prevalence of polycystic ovary syndrome in women seeking treatment from community electrologists. Alabama Professional Electrology Association Study Group. J Reprod Med. 1999; 44(10):870-4.
6. Gambineri A, Pelusi C, Vicennati V, Pagotto U, Pasquali R. Obesity and the polycystic ovary syndrome. Int J Obes Relat Metab Disord. 2002;26(7):883-96.
7. http://e-hmr.org/ViewImage.php?Type=F&aid=264837&id=F2&afn=130_ HMR_32_4_197&fn=hmr-32-197-g^{00}2_0130HMR
8. http://www.jarrettfertility.com/PCOS%20patient%20handout.pdf
9. http://www.managingpcos.org.au/pcos-evidence-based-guidelines/algorithms
10. http://www.managingpcos.org.au/pcos-evidence-based-guidelines/algorithms
11. Master-Hunter T, Heiman DL. (2006). Amenorrhea: Evaluation and Treatment. [online] Available from http://www.aafp.org/afp/2006/0415/p1374.html [Last accessed September, 2024].
12. Rebar R, Judd HL, Yen SS, Rakoff J, Vandenberg G, Naftolin F. Characterization of the inappropriate gonadotropin secretion in polycystic ovary syndrome. J Clin Invest. 1976;57(5):1320-9.
13. Sheehan MT. Polycystic ovarian syndrome: diagnosis and management. Clin Med Res. 2004;2(1):13-27.
14. Stein IF, Leventhal ML. Amenorrhea associated with bilateral polycystic ovaries. Am J Obstet Gynecol. 1935;29:181-91.
15. Teede HJ, Misso ML, Deeks AA, Moran LJ, Stuckey BG, Wong JL, et al. Assessment and management of polycystic ovary syndrome: summary of an evidence-based guideline. Med J Aust. 2011;195(6):S65-112.
16. Weissleder R, Wittenberg J, Harisinghani MG, Chen JW, Primer of Diagnostic Imaging, 5th edition. St. Louis, MO: Mosby; 2011.

Approach to a Case of Sexual Abuse in Children/Adolescent

Sushma P Desai

WHAT IS CHILD/ADOLESCENT SEXUAL ABUSE

Child sexual abuse (CSA) is described by the World Health Organization (WHO) as "the participation of a child in sexual activity that he or she does not fully comprehend, is unable to give informed consent to, or for which the child is not developmentally prepared and cannot give consent, or that violates the laws or social taboos of society." It involves the exposure of a child to sexual contact, activity, or behavior and may include an invitation to sexual touching, intercourse, or other forms of exploitation such as juvenile prostitution or pornography".

> **CLINICAL PEARL**
>
> Under the law, CSA is an umbrella term describing criminal and civil offenses in which adult engages in sexual activity with a minor or exploits a minor for the purpose of sexual gratification. It can never be considered normal or socially acceptable behavior.

The WHO defines an adolescent as being between 10 and 19 years.

SEXUAL ABUSE BEHAVIOR DEFINITION

- An adult exposing his/her genitals to or persuading a child or adolescent to do the same
- An adult touching a child or adolescent's genitals or making a child or adolescent touch the adult's genitalia
- An adult involving a child or adolescent in pornography, either by exposing a child or adolescent to create pornographic material
- An adult having oral, vaginal, and anal intercourse with a child or adolescent
- Any verbal or other sexual suggestion made to a child or adolescent by an adult
- An adult persuading a child or adolescent to engage in sexual activity

If an older adolescent manifests such a behavior to a child it will also constitute CSA.

> **CLINICAL PEARL**
>
> The United Nations Children's Fund (UNICEF): "Child marriage represents the most prevalent form of sexual abuse and exploitation of girls".

AGE OF CONSENSUAL SEX

According to the Protection of Children from Sexual Offences (POCSO) Act, the current age of consensual sex in India is 18 years. The age of simple majority is 18 years and the legal age of consent for marriage is 21 years in boys and 18 years in girls.

PEDOPHILE

An adult or older adolescent who experiences a primary or exclusive sexual attraction to prepubescent children is termed as pedophile. Pedophilia is a psychiatric disorder.

INCEST (INTRAFAMILIAL CHILD ABUSE/ CHILD INCESTUOUS ABUSE)

Traditionally "incest" is defined as sexual relations between people classed as being too closely related to marry each other.

> **CLINICAL PEARL**
>
> Incest between a child/adolescent and a related adult has been identified as the most widespread form of CSA with a huge capacity for damage to a child. It leads to serious types of long-term psychological trauma, especially in case of parental incest.

The most often reported form of incest is father-daughter and stepfather-daughter incest, mother/stepmother-daughter form contributes to a small portion of the remaining incest. Sibling incest may also be as common as or more common than other types of incest. The prevalence of parental incest is difficult to assess due to secrecy and privacy. Statistics show that about 30% of all perpetrators are related to the sexual victim, 60% are family acquaintances, and 10% are strangers.

COMMERCIAL SEXUAL EXPLOITATION OF CHILDREN

Commercial sexual exploitation of children is defined as "sexual abuse by an adult accompanied by remuneration in cash or in kind to the child or to the third person(s). Commercial sexual exploitation of children usually takes the form of child prostitution or child pornography and is often facilitated by child sex tourism (also internet child pornography)." It is particularly a problem in developing countries of Asia.

Types of Child Sexual Abuse

Child sexual abuse includes a variety of sexual offenses, including:

- *Sexual assault:* An adult uses a minor for the purpose of sexual gratification, e.g., rape (including sodomy) and sexual penetration with an object.
- *Sexual exploitation:* Offenses in which an adult victimizes a minor for advancement, sexual gratification, or profit, e.g., prostituting a child and creating or trafficking in child pornography.
- *Sexual grooming:* It defines the social conduct of a potential child sex offender who seeks to make a minor more accepting of their advances, e.g., in an online chat room.

VULNERABLE SITUATIONS (RISK FACTORS)

- *Children and adolescents of single parents:* Due to lack of adequate supervision
- *Children and adolescents with low self-esteem:* Due to failure in academic life. If parents persistently keep comparing them with the achievers; this results in low self-esteem and rebellion they may involve in sexual activity considering it as an achievement.
- *Attraction to city life:* Children and adolescents get induced by middlemen and easy access to money/comforts of life.
- *Lack of education:* Children and adolescents due to lack of education lack of being well-informed may get induced into sexual activities by strangers easily. Children and adolescents' education on sex and sexual parts will help them take care of their private parts and sexual life.
- *Poverty:* High risk of getting sexually abused because of poor socioeconomic conditions.
- *Parental factors:* Loss of job and substance abuse such as alcoholism and drug addiction
- *Mentally and physically:* Challenged/retarded children and adolescents
- Unloved, uncared children, and adolescent
- Violence in the community

PROFILE OF THE ADULT SEX OFFENDER

- Children and adolescents living in parents' homes are more likely to be abused by adults from within the family or known friend circle. In 80% of the cases, the perpetrator is either related or known to the victim.
- Children on streets or in observation homes are more likely to be abused by strangers.
- The offender has a special ability to identify vulnerable children, to use that vulnerability to sexually abuse the child.
- They systematically desensitize children to touch.
- They use adult authority to isolate the victim from others and enforce their victim's silence including threats, force, bribery, and acts of cruelty.

TYPES OF OFFENDERS

There are two groups:

- *Situational:* Does not prefer children, but offend under certain circumstances. They can be:
    - *Regressed:* Typically has a relationship with the adults, but a stressor causes them to seek children as a substitute
    - *Morally indiscriminate:* All-round sexual deviant, who may commit other sexual offenses unrelated to children
    - *Naïve/inadequate:* Often mentally disabled in some way, finds children less threatening
- *Preferential:* Has true sexual interest in children

STATISTICS OF CHILD SEXUAL ABUSE IN INDIA

Child sexual abuse in India is a prevalent and devastating issue, with a shocking 28.9% of children experiencing some form of sexual crime. In India, home to 19% of the world's children, it is estimated every second child is exposed to sexual abuse and violence. The Indian National Crimes Records Bureau (NCRB) 2020 reports a child is sexually abused every 15 minute and 53% of children report abuse by a parent, relative, or school teacher. Out of the total child respondents, 20.90% were subjected to severe forms of sexual abuse. Out of these, 57.30% were boys and 42.70% were girls. Andhra Pradesh, Assam, Bihar, and Delhi reported the highest percentage of sexual abuse.

CLINICAL PEARLS

- About 40% of girls and 25% of boys are sexually abused before they reach 16 years of age.
- 42% of Indian girls are sexually abused before 19 years of age: UNICEF.
- One-tenth of children are being sexually abused at any given point of time.

EFFECTS

Psychological Effects

CLINICAL PEARL

- About 51–79% of sexually abused children exhibit psychological symptoms.

The CSA can lead to both long- and short-term harm, including psychopathology in later life. The common effects are anxiety, depression, eating disorders, poor self-esteem, somatization, sleep disturbances, dissociative disorder, and post-traumatic stress disorder. Children may manifest regressive disorders such as thumb sucking and bed wetting.

CLINICAL PEARL

- The strongest indicator of sexual abuse is inappropriate sexual knowledge and interest.

The victim may withdraw from school and normal social activities and exhibit learning and behavioral problems, cruelty to animals, attention deficit hyperactivity disorder, conduct disorder, and oppositional defiant disorder.

Adolescent victims show risky sexual behavior. Self-inflicted harm and teenage pregnancy are some of the important effects. Increased rates of crime in sexually abused teens are observed.

Physical Effects

- *Injury:* Depending on age, the size of the child, and the degree of force used. Internal laceration, bleeding, damage to internal organs, and even death
- *Infection:* Sexually transmitted infections, human immunodeficiency virus/acquired immunodeficiency syndrome
- *Neurological damage:* Traumatic stress, including stress caused by sexual abuse, causes notable changes in brain functioning and development. Increased likelihood of "ictal temporal lobe epilepsy-like symptoms". Short-term memory impairment and lowering of the score of math scholastic aptitude test.

DIAGNOSIS/DISCLOSURE

- Victims are often unable to speak due to different reasons such as threat, fear, shame, and guilt.
- Therefore, indirect nonverbal clues, behavioral disturbances, psychosomatic, psychiatric, and seldom physical symptoms are often the only way to recognize sexual abuse.
- There is no specific symptom/syndrome.
- The most important element of the diagnosis is the disclosure, which depends on our ability to speak with children.
- Children need support and stress-reducing resources after disclosure of sexual abuse. Negative social reactions to the disclosure have been found to be harmful to the survivor's well-being.

CLINICAL PEARL

- Children who received supportive responses after disclosure have less traumatic symptoms and are abused for a shorter period of time.

- The American Academy of Child and Adolescent Psychiatry provides guidelines for what to say to the victim and what to do following the disclosure.

EXAMINATION OF A CASE OF SEXUAL ABUSE

History

- Look for risk factors of victimization/vulnerability for sexual abuse in adolescents such as:
  - Female sex
  - Going alone in lonely places at odd times
  - Going to a friend's house for exchanging notes
  - Parties (especially night parties)
  - Dating
  - Crowded places (e.g., buses, trains, fair, etc.)
  - "Immoral" neighborhood

- Families with a member having personality disorder (sex maniac)
- Single parent/broken homes
- Both parents working and the child alone at home
- Children in foster care, i.e., parents or elders are out and some relative/friend is staying at home
- Drinking/watching pornography/movies with friends
- Heartbreaks, failure, and other situations needing emotional support
- History of past abuse

How to identify victims of child/adolescent sexual abuse/flag signs:
- Fear of being bathed
- Having a great deal of knowledge about sex at a very young age or sexual behavior that seems beyond his or her age
- Feeling depressed
- Anxiety and low self-esteem
- Sudden avoidance of visiting a particular place or a particular person, decreased desire of interaction with peers
- Poor interest in academics
- Fondling with one's genitalia too often
- Drug or alcohol abuse.

Physical Examination

- *Points to remember:*
  - Ensure patient privacy
  - Prepare the child by explaining the examination and showing equipment; this has been shown to diminish fears and anxiety
  - Ask whom he/she would like in the room for support during the examination
- *The examination should include:*
  - Mental maturity—by asking questions such as age and time
  - Physical maturity—with the help of growth parameters
  - Nutrition status
  - Look—vacant/starry/slating/fearful
  - Mental status—confused/clear/apprehensive
  - Clothing—any evidence struggle/trace evidence like hair and stains of forensic importance
  - Oral hygiene and personal hygiene
  - Physical indicator of sexual assault and injuries
- *Indicators of child sexual abuse:*
  - *Sure indicators:*
    - Venereal diseases
    - Pregnancy
    - Presence of semen
    - Gonococcal infection of pharynx, urethra, rectum, and vagina
  - *Probable indicators:*
    - Genital herpes
    - Trichomonas
    - Recurrent urinary tract infection
    - Horizontal hymen opening in relation to age
  - *Near indicators:*
    - Abdominal pains
    - Leaking vagina or anus
    - Difficult walking
    - Sudden withdrawal from normal activities
    - Sudden change in appetite
    - Unusual sexual knowledge
    - Mood variation without any obvious reasons
    - Depression or depersonalization
    - Irritation unprovoked or easily induced
    - Suicide attempts or threats
    - Lack of attachment to parents
    - Torn clothing and/or stained with blood or semen
- *Detail examination of the genitalia:*
  - Genital injuries in adolescents:
    - Scratches over the thigh, genitalia, or body
    - Bruising of the vulva
    - Swelling in the genital area
    - Minor tears in the hymen
    - Minor lacerations
    - Bleeding
    - Laceration of large size in case of age incompatibility
- Sexual abuse signs in sodomy **(Table 1)**

TABLE 1: Sexual abuse signs in sodomy.

Chronic	*Recent*
Proctitis	Tear
Hypotonic sphincters	Bleeding
Anal fistula	Bruising
Anal and perianal skin changes	Semen
Condylomata, warts, and chancre	Gonorrhea

Age Determination

It has a great medicolegal importance as the justice and punishment to the abuser is directly related to the age of the victim. The age determination of an adolescent can be done from a comprehensive examination of the following four aspects:

- General physical features
- *Secondary sexual character:* Tanner's staging
- *Appearance of teeth:* Orthopantomogram is helpful
- Ossification of bones.

Collection of Forensic Samples

The following samples are required to be collected in sexual abuse cases:

- Blood (blood grouping and testing drug intoxication)
- Urine (to test for suspected pregnancy and drug testing)
- Seminal stain (blood grouping)
- Nail scraping (from under the nails, to look for epithelium of the assailant)
- Hair (to look for seminal stain and foreign hair)
- *Vaginal swabs (vulva, low vaginal, and high vaginal):* It is stressed here that it should be made a routine
- Microscopic examination of vaginal slides (motile and immotile sperm)

TREATMENT

The initial approach depends upon following factors:

- Age at the time of presentation
- Circumstances of presentation for treatment
- Comorbid conditions.

The goal of management is:

- To treat current issues
- To prevent future abuse/untoward incidences

There are three modalities of therapy:

1. Family therapy
2. Group therapy
3. Individual therapy.

Treatment of young children requires strong parental involvement and can benefit from family therapy. Adolescents tend to be more independent, they respond well to individual or group therapy. The modalities also shift during the course of therapy, e.g., group therapy is rarely used in initial stages as the subject matter is very personal and/or embarrassing.

PHARMACOLOGICAL MANAGEMENT

Prophylaxis of Sexually Transmitted Diseases

Incidence of sexually transmitted diseases from sexual assault without prophylaxis is:

- *Condyloma:* 1 in 4
- *Chlamydia:* 1 in 10
- *Gonorrhea:* 1 in 30
- *Human immunodeficiency virus:* 1 in 1,000
- *Syphilis:* 1 in 1,000
- *Hepatitis B/herpes simplex virus:* Uncertain

Gonorrhea and Chlamydia

- *Nonpregnant victims:*
  - Doxycycline 300 mg orally, stat, followed by 100 mg twice a day for 3 days (patient >8 years old)
- *Alternative:*
  - Floxacin 400 mg twice a day for 7 days (patient >16 years old)
  - Azithromycin 2 g orally, single dose
- *Pregnancy and adolescent victims:* Erythromycin 1.5 g orally stat, followed by 500 mg four times a day.

Syphilis

Benzathine penicillin 2.4 million units (adults), in children not usually given because of a low incidence of risk of syphilis, instead a follow-up rapid plasma reagent test is done at 6–12 weeks. If seroconversion has occurred therapy is given at that time.

Human Papillomavirus

Not known prophylactic regimen. The human papillomavirus vaccine is recommended for all adolescent girls and the quadrivalent vaccine is for adolescent boys above the age of 9 years.

Human Immunodeficiency Virus

The risk of transmission is very low, risk-benefit ratio should be weighed before giving the drugs.

- Triple-drug therapy including zidovudine, lamivudine (3TC), and famotidine.

Herpes Simplex Virus

Acyclovir 40 mg/kg.

Trichomonas

Metronidazole 2 g orally (single dose).

Pregnancy Prophylaxis

The incidence of pregnancy in rape/sexual assault is 1 per 100.

- Levonorgestrel 0.75 mg two tablets stat or ethinylestradiol 0.05 mg two tablet stat, followed by two tablets after 12 hours

FOLLOW-UP AND REHABILITATION

- Follow-up care must be given to assess the late complications, especially the psychosocial problems.
- Parental support is very important for the rehabilitation. Adolescents can be taken care of at home environment in a better way.
- If parents cannot support their adolescent children, especially in rural areas, supportive social and legal networks should be developed for them to prevent suicidal attempts or fall into the flesh trade.

PREVENTION

- Adults (parents, families, community, and teachers) must help children through nonthreatening and age-appropriate means to participate in their own protection.
- Personal safety curriculum is designed to:
    - Protect children/adolescents from abuse, specifically sexual abuse
    - Empower children/adolescents to take part in their own protection by giving them age-appropriate information, skills, and self-esteem
    - Teach children/adolescents that their body belongs only to them and nobody has the right to touch them in a way they do not like or understand, give them knowledge of sexual organs and function
    - Children not to keep secret
    - To be bold to make friends—but when it comes to sex learn to say no
    - Teach children/adolescents that only the offender is to blame for any inappropriate sexual touch
    - Teach assertiveness skills, helping children to stand up for their own right without violating the right of others
    - Build the support system of each child including the family, school, community, and friends.

HOW TO HELP THE SURVIVOR?

When a survivor tells us that she/he has been sexually abused, she/he is entrusting you with a part of life that is painful, frightening, and vulnerable.

The following guidelines can help us honor that trust and assist in their healing:

- Believe the survivor
- Be clear that abuse is never a child's or young adolescent's fault
- Do not sympathize with the abuser
- Express your compassion
- Validate the survivor's feelings and join with the survivor in validating the damage
- Encourage the survivor to get support
- Seek an expert's help if the survivor is suicidal
- Respect the time and space taken to heal
- Resist seeing the survivor as a victim

SEXUAL ABUSE AND EXISTING LEGAL SYSTEM

- It is necessary to give recognition to child abuse as an offence against innocence and, therefore, the law against child rape needs to be more stringent.
- Since sexual abuse of minors has its own characteristics, it needs to be addressed separately from the offence of sexual assault on an adult person.
- Ironically, existing rape/sexual abuse laws make no distinction between rape of a minor and that of an adult.

CLINICAL PEARL

- The "Protection of Children Against Sexual Offense Bill 2011" was passed in the Indian Parliament on May 22, 2012 which came into force from November 14, 2012.

International Law

Child sexual abuse is outlawed nearly everywhere in the world, generally with severe criminal penalties including in some jurisdictions, life imprisonment, or capital punishment. An adult's sexual intercourse with a child below the age of legal consent is defined as statutory rape, based on the principle that a child is not capable of consent and that any apparent consent by a child is not considered to be legal consent. The United Nations Conventions on the Rights of the Child (CRC) is an international treaty that legally obliges states to protect children's rights in November 2008, 193 countries are bound by the CRC, including every member of United Nations except the United States and Somalia **(Flowchart 1)**.

Flowchart 1: An algorithmic approach to a case of child/adolescent sexual abuse.

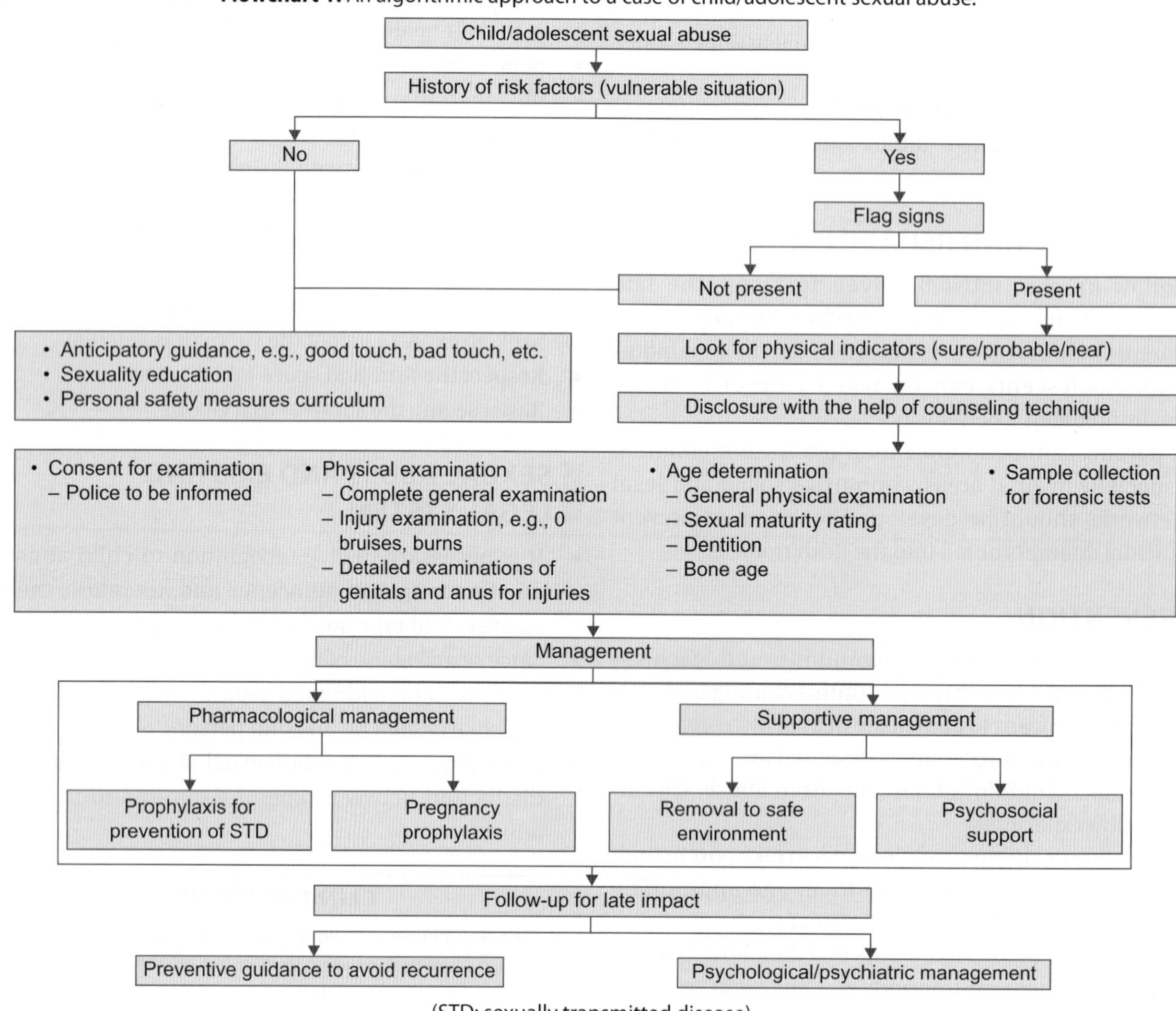

(STD: sexually transmitted disease)

KEY POINTS

- Sexual abuse is rampant and universal as children and adolescents are vulnerable and most often not in a position to voice their protest against the heinous offense against their body/their complains are not taken seriously and many times silenced.
- About 40% of girls and 25% of boys suffer from sexual abuse before they reach 16 years of age. Majority of them are not surfaced.
- Contrary to the common belief, majority of the offenders are known to the victim.
- CSA is one of the most fundamental violations of children's human rights which lead to tremendous psychological trauma having many long-term and short-term effects on their overall development adversely affecting them throughout their life.
- As the survivors are often not able to reveal, high index of suspicion based on nonverbal clues, psychosomatic symptoms, and seldom physical signs are helpful to come to the diagnosis.
- Important aspects of management are helping the survivor in disclosure with the help of counseling and strong psychosocial support.
- Pharmacological therapy is aimed at prevention of pregnancy and prophylaxis against sexually transmitted infection.
- There is a great need to find ways to prevent child/adolescent sexual abuse and to ensure the safety from victimization of any form.
- Self-defense training for every girl has an important role in the prevention of victimization. Schools have the potential to teach protective behaviors effectively, including teaching the parents.
- There is a need for incorporation of CSA in the Indian Penal Code, including incest, sexual abuse of boys, and nonpenetrative sexual abuse.

SUGGESTED READING

1. Aggarwal A. (2000). Age Estimation in the Living: Some Medicolegal Considerations. [online] Available from anilaggrawal.com/ij/vol_001_no_002/ug001.html. [Last accessed September, 2024].
2. American Academy of Child and Adolescent Psychiatry. (2023). Responding to Child Sexual Abuse. [online] Available from: https://www.aacap.org/AACAP/Families_and_Youth/Facts_for_Families/FFF-Guide/Responding_To-Child-Sexual-Abuse-028.aspx#:~:text=Children%20who%20have%20been%20sexually,the%20trauma%20of%20the%20abuse. [Last Accessed September, 2014].
3. American Academy of Pediatrics and Adolescent Psychiatry. Factsheet on Child Sexual abuse.
4. American Psychological Association. (2011). Understanding Child Sexual Abuse: Education, Prevention, and Recovery. [online] Available from https://www.apa.org/pi/about/newsletter/2011/12/sexual-abuse.aspx. [Last accessed September, 2024].
5. Amnesty International. United Nations Convention on the Rights of the Child: Frequently Asked Questions. USA: Amnesty International; 2008.
6. Choudhry V, Dayal R, Pillai D, Kalokhe AS, Beier K, Patel V. Child sexual abuse in India: A systematic review. PLoS One. 2018;13:e0205086.
7. Estes RJ. The sexual exploitation of children: A Working Guide to the Empirical Literature. [online] Available from https://www.researchgate.net/publication/237780283_THE_SEXUAL_EXPLOITATION_OF_CHILDREN_A_Working_Guide_to_the_Empirical_Literature. [Last accessed September, 2024].
8. Gangrade KD, Sooryamoorthy R. Renjini D. Child rape: Facets of a heinous crime. Soc Change. 1995;25:161-76.
9. Hornor G. Child sexual abuse: consequences and implications. J Pediatr Health Care. 2009;24(6):385-64.
10. India Code. (2023). The Protection of Children from Sexual Offences Act. 2012. [online] Available from https://www.indiacode.nic.in/bitstream/123456789/2079/1/AA2012-32.pdf. [Last accessed September, 2024].
11. MedlinePlus. (2008). Child Sexual Abuse. [online] Available from https://medlineplus.gov/childsexualabuse.html. [Last accessed September, 2024].
12. Ministry of Women and Child Development. Manual for Medical Officer dealing with medicolegal cases of victims of trafficking for commercial sexual exploitation and child sexual abuse. New Delhi: Ministry of Women and Child Development; 2005.
13. Ministry of Women and Child Development. Study on Child Abuse: India 2007. New Delhi: Ministry of Women and Child Development; 2007.
14. Parthasarathy A, Nair MK, Menon PS, Bhave SY. Bhave's Textbook of Adolescent Medicine, 1st edition. New Delhi: Jaypee Brothers Medical Publishers; 2006.
15. Pereda N, Guilera G, Forns M, Gómez-Benito J. Prevalence of child sexual abuse in community and student samples: a meta-analysis. Clin Psychol Rev. 2009;29(4): 328-38.
16. Putnam FW. Ten-year research update review: Child sexual abuse. J Am Acad Child Adolesc Psychiatry. 2003;42: 269-78.
17. Teicher MH. Scars that won't heal: the neurobiology of child abuse. Sci Am. 2002;286(3):68-75.
18. Tulir: Center for Treatment of Child Sexual Abuse, Chennai, India.
19. Tyagi S, Karande S. Child sexual abuse in India: A wake-up call. J Postgrad Med. 2021;67(3):125-9.
20. UNICEF. Child Marriage. [online] Available from https://www.unicef.org/protection/child-marriage. [Last accessed September, 2024].
21. Widom CS. Posttraumatic stress disorder in abused and neglected children grown up. Am J Psychiatry. 1999;156(8): 1223-9.
22. Wihbey J. (2011). Global prevalence of child sexual abuse. [online] Available from: https://journalistsresource.org/criminal-justice/global-prevalence-child-sexual-abuse/. [Last accessed September, 2024].
23. World Health Organization (WHO). (2000). Guidelines for Medico-legal Care for Victims of Sexual Violence. [online] Available from https://iris.who.int/bitstream/handle/10665/42788/924154628X.pdf. [Last Accessed September, 2024].
24. World Health Organization. (2012). Understanding and addressing violence against women: Overview. [online] Available from https://www.who.int/publications/i/item/WHO-RHR-12.35. [Last accessed September, 2024].
25. World Health Organization. Report of the Consultation on Child Abuse and Neglect Prevention. Geneva, Switzerland: World Health Organization; 1999.

Adolescent Depression/Suicidal Tendency and Its Management

Paula Goel

INTRODUCTION

Every year about 2 million adolescents (1 in every 12) suffer with an episode of depression; 1 in 5 adolescents experiences depression before they reach adulthood. Depression affects 3.5% of children at any given time, impeding healthy psychosocial development. Diminished self-worth, academic struggles, and difficulties in social relations with family and peers exert a heavy toll on youth who are often unable to communicate the nature of their experience. It is a common and serious problem. It increases the risk for suicide, the third leading cause of death in this age group.

Often, it leads to more poor academic achievement, greater absenteeism, strained relationships with family and friends, interference with extracurricular activities, and substance abuse. Clinical depression during adolescence represents the strongest risk factor for teenager suicide and is linked to significant psychosocial impairment in adulthood.

Periodic screening of children presenting—for any reason—to primary care physicians can improve clinical recognition of these disorders and result in improved rates of treatment.

The importance of detecting and treating depression in adolescents is being increasingly recognized.

Prevalence is related to age, gender, and social class (about 1% between 10 years and 14 years of age and 25% among late teens).

PREDISPOSING FACTORS

- Biological factors
- Endocrinal factors
- Social factors
- Structural factors in brain
- *Environmental factors:* Socioeconomic status, level of family conflict, abuse or neglect, and parental separation or divorce
- Family history of depression

CLINICAL FEATURES

(DSM-V Criteria to be used)

Presence of following symptoms for >2 weeks (Diagnostic and Statistical Manual of Mental Disorders Fourth Edition Text Revision):

- *Depressed mood:* Feels sad, empty, bored, appears tearful, and irritable mood
- Markedly decreased interest or pleasure in almost all activities most of the day, nearly every day
- Significant weight loss or weight gain with increase or decrease in appetite nearly every day
- Poor sleep, insomnia, or hypersomnia nearly every day
- *Psychomotor agitation or retardation almost daily:* Restlessness, pacing, tapping of fingers, abruptly starting and stopping tasks, and meaninglessly moving objects around. Fatigue or loss of energy
- Feelings of worthlessness or excessive or inappropriate guilt nearly daily
- Diminished ability to think or concentrate on academics/indecisiveness almost daily
- Recurrent thoughts of death or suicidal ideation
- Clinically significant distress or impairment in social, occupational, or other important areas of functioning
- Symptoms persist for >2 months or are characterized by morbid preoccupation with feelings of worthlessness, suicidal ideation, psychotic symptoms, marked functional impairment.

Clinical features can also be classified as:

- *Affective:* Depressed mood and feelings of worthlessness or guilt

- *Behavioral symptoms:* Social withdrawal and agitation. Feelings of restlessness, grouchiness, aggression, and sulkiness
- Cognitive symptoms or problems in thinking including difficulty in concentration or making decisions, school difficulties
- *Somatic symptoms:* Insomnia or hypersomnia
- *Prepubertal children:* Somatic symptoms
- *Adolescents:* Affective and behavioral symptoms
- Highly intelligent, academically strong children compensate for mood disorders with increased attention to academics
- *Comorbidities:* Conduct disorder, defiant disorder, panic disorder, attention deficit hyperkinetic disorder, anxiety disorders, and disruptive disorders.

The US Preventive Services Task Force now recommends screening adolescents (12–18 years) for major depressive disorder when systems are in place to assure accurate diagnosis, psychotherapy (cognitive-behavioral or interpersonal) and follow-up.

The American Academy of Pediatrics also strengthened their recommendations for mental health screening and counseling in the latest Bright Futures Guidelines.

The Guidelines for Adolescent Depression in Primary Care (GLAD-PC) were published in 2007 and have been updated in 2010. Guidelines for Adolescent Depression in Primary Care provides a roadmap for enhancing care. This time tool presents important elements from the 2010 GLAD-PC for the identification, assessment, and treatment of adolescent depression in the office setting.

- Systems must be in place to allow effective triage (safety/placement) for:
  - Identification of high-risk cases
  - Screening
  - Assessment and intervention
  - A predetermined "go-to" list of providers and facilities to refer for care when indicated
- The good news:
  - Screening is simple, effective, and well received by patients, parents, and providers.
  - A two-question screening can identify the need for more in depth screening.
  - Adolescents prefer to have their depression addressed in primary care.
  - Most adolescents see their primary doctor at least annually; an estimated 45% of suicide victims reportedly saw their primary doctor in the month prior to the suicide.
  - Most depressed adolescents can be treated in primary care.
  - There are effective treatments and guidelines for using them in primary care.
- *The bad news:*
  - Only about 1 of 3 adolescents with depression is identified (American College of Preventive Medicine, 2011)
  - Fewer than half of primary care clinicians inquire about depression with adolescents; fewer yet use a standardized instrument to assess depression
  - Fewer than half of adolescents who are diagnosed are treated appropriately.
  - Severe cases should be treated by mental health specialists, but there is a severe shortage of child psychiatrists—few of these severe cases are seen by specialists.
  - Reimbursement policies are often a disincentive to treating depression in primary care.
  - Little coordination typically occurs between primary care and mental health specialties.
- *The challenge:*
  - The burden of adolescent depression prevention and management falls squarely on primary care.
  - Most pediatricians and family practitioners believe it is their responsibility to identify depression, but relatively few believe it is their responsibility to treat it.
  - Most do not feel equipped to manage adolescent depression, and their office systems are not set up to handle it.
  - Adolescent depression is different than adult depression due to developmental issues, responses to treatment, issues in psychotherapy, risks of medications, and family dynamics.
- *Steps to integrate care:*
  - *Assess the practice:* Adolescent patient load, prevalence of mental health issues
  - Determine the role you want to play and services to provide for adolescent depression.
  - *Build a network of local resources:* Therapists, peer counseling, group programs, etc.
  - *Determine relation with mental health resources:* Consultation, colocation, and collaboration
  - *Provide training where needed:* Screening/assessing, record keeping, confidentiality (state law), staff roles, insurance coverage including preapprovals or preauthorizations for referrals;

counseling/psychotherapy training for designated staff
  - Assure systems are in place to allow effective triage (safety/placement) that includes a "go-to" list of providers and facilities to send patients as needed
  - Follow guideline recommendations
- *Guide to the office visit:* Mental health or emotional issues as chief complaint, or positive screen on Patient Health Questionnaire-2
- *Staff:* Preparation for visit

IDENTIFY RISK STATUS

- *Assistant:* Perform chart review to ensure—
  - Forms/assessments to be completed by patient in chart
  - Score instrument in chart for clinician

ASSESS FOR DEPRESSION

- Review symptom assessment and scoring.
- Interview with patient and family/caregiver to identify contributing factors.
- Collect collateral information and family history to help distinguish adjustment disorders and family relationship issues.
- Assess for safety/suicide risk and appropriate level of care.
- Refer to crisis or emergency services if necessary.

DIAGNOSE AND RATE SEVERITY

Provide diagnosis; rate severity: Mild, moderate, or severe (based on number of symptoms present).

EDUCATE

- Depression is an illness, not a weakness; very common, no one's fault, usually involves genetic and environmental factors.
- Functional impairment in various domains can be manifestations of the illness.
- Depression can be a recurrent illness—recovery may take a while.
- Key to overcoming depression is staying with the treatment plan long term.
- Stress in the parent-child relationship, if present, may be part of the problem.
- Ask adolescent about future goals—if none, be wary of suicidal ideation.

INITIAL MANAGEMENT

- Discuss limits of confidentiality
- Emphasize monitoring symptoms, especially changes reflecting increasing suicidal ideation.

Primary Care

- Offer referral for peer/family support, community resources, etc.
- Facilitate parental and patient self-management; provide written materials and websites for more information.

CONSIDER CONSULTATION

With mental health specialist: Recommended for severe or complicated depressions, or for interventions not within scope of the pediatric practice—

- Decide to treat in practice or refer to trusted network of mental health providers
- If referred, designate case coordination responsibilities; follow-up plan
- Maintain contact with mental health specialist as long as such treatment continues.

TREATMENT PLAN

If treating in practice:

- *Include family:* Set specific goals for key areas of functioning—home, peer relationships, school, and work.

Mild depression:

- Active support and monitoring for 6–8 weeks, contact every 1–2 weeks

Moderate or severe:

- Initiate shared decision discussion about therapy:
  - Psychotherapy and/or antidepressants
  - Review benefits and risks of each option including the black box warning regarding selective serotonin reuptake inhibitors (SSRIs) and suicide risk
- *Discuss preferences and plan for chosen treatment:*
  - Emphasize importance of finding a therapist one feels comfortable with for psychotherapy
- *Discuss common medication side effects:*
  - Emphasizing temporary nature and importance of not stopping medication without calling first
  - Discuss more serious adverse effects, especially suicidal ideation; emphasize careful monitoring due to increased risk earlier in treatment

- Develop safety plan for acute crisis, deterioration of symptoms
- Consider ongoing mental health consultation
- Evaluate response at 6–8 weeks (American College of Preventive Medicine, 2011).

FOLLOW-UP MANAGEMENT (AT 6–8 WEEKS VISIT)

Mild depression:

- *If persistent:* Institute treatment as moderate cases or refer to mental health
- *If improved:* Continue monitoring monthly for 6 months, regular follow-up for 2 years after resolution of symptoms

Moderate or severe:

- If not improved:
    - Reassess the diagnosis
    - Consider adding a medication, increasing the dosage, or changing medications if already on maximum dosage
    - Add psychotherapy if not already using, or intensifying current therapy
    - Consider referral to mental health
    - Provide further education, review safety plan, continue ongoing monitoring
    - Evaluate response again at 6–8 weeks
- If partially improved:
    - Consider adding a medication or increasing the dosage
    - Add psychotherapy if not already using, or intensifying current therapy
    - Consider referral to mental health
    - Provide further education, review safety plan, continue ongoing monitoring
    - Evaluate response again at 6–8 weeks
- *If improved:*
    - Continue prescribed medication for 1 year after symptom resolution
    - Continue monthly monitoring for 6 months
    - Provide regular follow-up for 2 years after resolution of symptoms

FINAL THOUGHTS

Adolescent depression challenges everyone—from the affected young person to the parents and providers, and the entire healthcare system. The fragmented care and lack of support for primary care undermines early identification and timely treatment.

- *Routine screening and diagnosis:*
    - Periodically screen children and youth for early signs of depression and/or anxiety. Record these results in the patient's problem list.
    - Ask questions of the child (or parent where applicable) when there are red flags including unexplained somatic complaints, unexplained behavioral changes, teenage pregnancy, school absences, and family members with depression, anxiety, alcohol, or other substance abuse.
- *Suggested questions:*
    - Do you find yourself sad, irritable, or worried a lot?
    - Is the child withdrawing from or avoiding their usual activities?
    - Family involvement is invaluable for assisting with and monitoring treatments as well as providing assurance and emotional support for the child or youth. Assure the family that the questions and fact finding are not to assign blame but to better understand the situation.
    - Choose an appropriate diagnostic questionnaire available for download on the internet. If the screen indicates a possible problem then either begin or schedule time to begin a detailed inquiry about anxiety or depressive symptoms, evaluate severity, and the potential for self-harm.
    - Consider that there may be more than one psychiatric disorder when screening because anxiety and depressive disorders are highly comorbid in children and adolescents. All youth with mood or anxiety disorders should be screened for alcohol or drug use.
    - *Note red flags for risk of bipolar depression:* Family history, psychotic depression, mania with SSRIs, hypersexuality, risk-taking behavior, and prepubertal depression. Consider referral if bipolar disorder is suspected. Manage the patient while waiting for referral and provide follow-up.
- *Diagnosis:*
    - Take a medical history and do a physical examination with attention to conditions that may mimic anxiety or depressive disorders. Consider indications for diagnostic tests such as thyroid-stimulating hormone. Consider the family situation and social stressors.

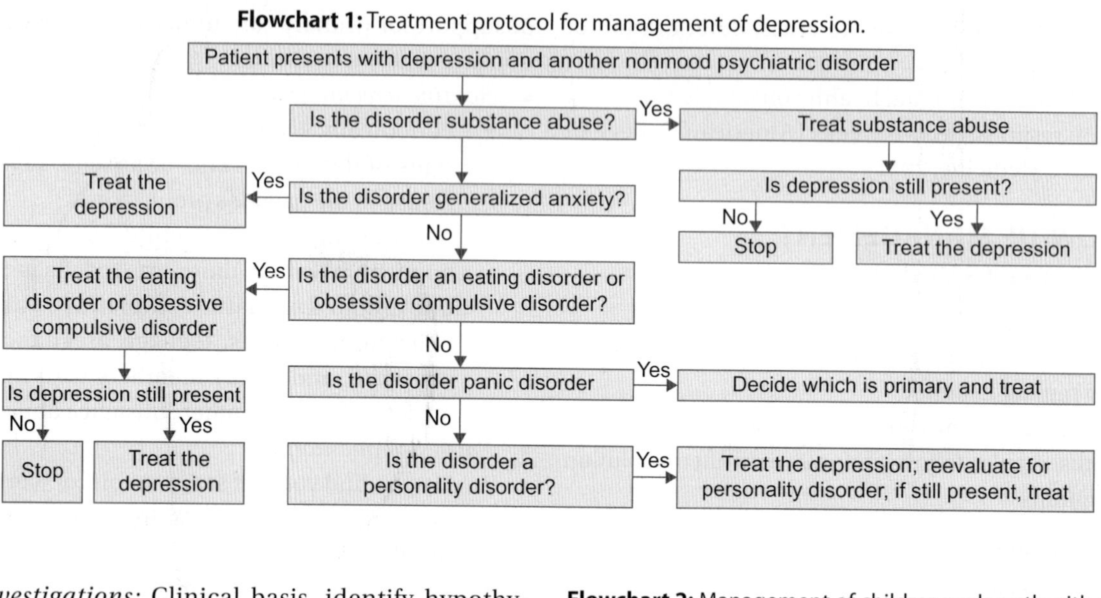

Flowchart 1: Treatment protocol for management of depression.

- *Investigations:* Clinical basis, identify hypothyroidism and anemia
- *Attempt nonpharmacological management strategies first:*
  - Nonpharmacological approaches are essential first-line treatments for both anxiety and depression. If physician counseling, parental involvement, and use of books do not affect a significant improvement, it is appropriate to refer to a specialist or to the child and youth mental health team for treatment **(Flowcharts 1 to 4)**.

INDICATIONS FOR PHARMACOTHERAPY

Indications for pharmacotherapy include persistent depression and/or a comorbid anxiety disorder which have not responded to psychosocial interventions.

Depression: Psychotherapy can be effective for treating depression, particularly in adolescents. If unavailable, medications may be indicated:

- The drug most often used is fluoxetine.
- If bipolar vulnerability, start with a shorter-acting selective serotonin reuptake inhibitor (SSRI) (e.g., sertraline)
- If comorbid anxiety, fluvoxamine or sertraline is possible alternative.

Spontaneous remission in community diagnosed adolescent depression is 50% within 2 months. However, those not remitting in this time period have a high risk of chronicity. Refer to a specialist.

Flowchart 2: Management of children and youth with anxiety or depression.

All levels of severity

↓

Basic interventions—initial step and at any time when needed (Specify text referred to—Attempt nonpharmacological management strategies first)
- Sleep, eating, exercise routines
- Consistency in parenting
- Refer to the list of self-help and community resources including the Ministry of Children and Family Development
- Refer to Guides for Parents
- Emergency safety plan
  Reminder to avoid drugs and alcohol

↓

Moderate severity or persistence of symptoms

↓

After providing basic intervention, follow step 1 then go to step 2 (if necessary)
Step 1: Psychotherapeutic interventions
- CBT for anxiety disorders
  - Practice facing fears (resources)
  - CBT or IPT for depression

Step 2: Medications
- Consider indications for medications particularly if not functioning (not attending school, marked vegetative symptoms)

→ **Specialist referral**
- Diagnostic clarification
- High suicide risk
- Severe OCD and panic
- Persistent school avoidance
- Possible bipolarity

↓

Severe, persistent symptoms despite above interventions

↓

Medications–if severe symptoms persist above interventions (→ Specialist referral)
- Depression–fluoxetine
- OCD–fluoxetine, fluvoxamine, or sertraline
- Mixed anxiety–fluoxetine or fluvoxamine, sertraline

(CBT: cognitive behavioral therapy; IPT: interpersonal psychotherapy; OCD: obsessive compulsive disorder)

Flowchart 3: Pharmacotherapy of major depressive disorder.

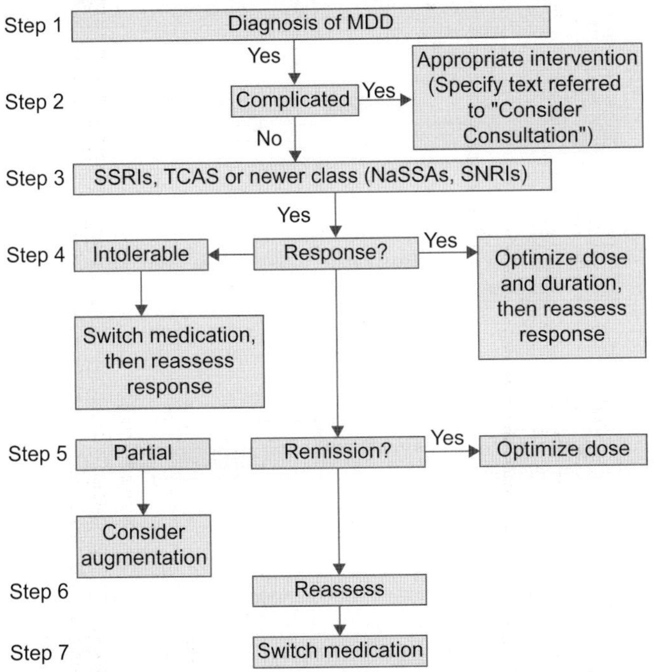

(MDD: major depressive disorder; SSRIs: selective serotonin reuptake inhibitors; TCAs: tricyclic antidepressants; NaSSAs: noradrenergic and specific serotonergic antidepressants; SNRIs: serotonin–norepinephrine reuptake inhibitors)

Medication Dosing and Follow-up for Anxiety and Depression

General Dosing Suggestions

Start with one-fourth or half of the adult dose and wait at least 1 week to increase dosages. For adolescents, the maximum dose can be similar to adults, while the dose is less than the adult dose for children.

- *Anxiety:* Children who are anxious are sensitive to physical sensations. Provide support, reassurance, and monitor frequently. Generalized anxiety disorder may respond at lower doses (e.g., 25–50 mg sertraline), obsessive compulsive disorder (OCD) (100–200 mg sertraline), generally start low and increase slowly. Dosing example: 10 mg daily fluoxetine for an adolescent. For an anxious 6-year-old, start with 5 mg daily and use increments of 5 mg every 2 weeks if needed
- *Depression:* The response often requires full doses for youth and the response to medication is slower. Example, start the first week with 10 mg daily of fluoxetine and increase to 20 mg daily as soon as tolerated. Increase again up 30 mg daily if not improved after 6 weeks to a maximum of 40 mg daily. If not responding after 10–12 weeks, refer to specialist.

Adverse effects: In children, SSRIs and other new antidepressants produce a higher rate of behavioral and emotional adverse effects (such as agitation, disinhibition, irritability, and occasionally thoughts of self-harm). The largest drug-placebo difference in the number of cases of suicidal ideation and behavior is greatest for the under-24 age group. For all ages, the risk is highest during the first few months of drug therapy, therefore, monitor patients closely during this time.

- *Monitoring:* Request assistance of the family and/or teenager, to monitor both symptoms and functions
- *Continuation:* For both anxiety and depression, the usual length of treatment is 6–12 months before a trial of tapering.
- *Discontinuation:* Anxious patients are very sensitive to physical sensations during discontinuation. So, taper off particularly slowly over 1–2 months by approximately 5 mg per reduction.

Antidepressants Commonly Used in Treatment of Major Depressive Disorders (Table 1)

- *Selective serotonin reuptake inhibitors (sertraline, paroxetine, etc.):* These medications are somewhat less toxic in overdosage. As compared to adults, adolescents are a bit more likely to become agitated or to develop a mania while they are taking an SSRI. These medications can decrease libido in both adolescents and adult. Fluoxetine, sertraline, citalopram, and escitalopram are commonly used as an initial medication. Fluoxetine now has Food and Drug Administration (FDA) approval for the treatment of depression in children and adolescents. The other SSRI medications do not as of yet have FDA approval for depression in children. These last two have fewer interactions with other medications.
- *Bupropion (Wellbutrin):* This medication can be helpful for depression and attention deficit hyperactivity disorder but is less effective for comorbid anxiety. It does not seem to cause weight gain.
- *Tricyclics (imipramine, desipramine, and nortriptyline):* These medications are still used if the SSRIs and bupropion do not work. As the tricyclics are more likely to cause rhythm changes in children, baseline

Flowchart 4: Major depression (nonpsychotic).

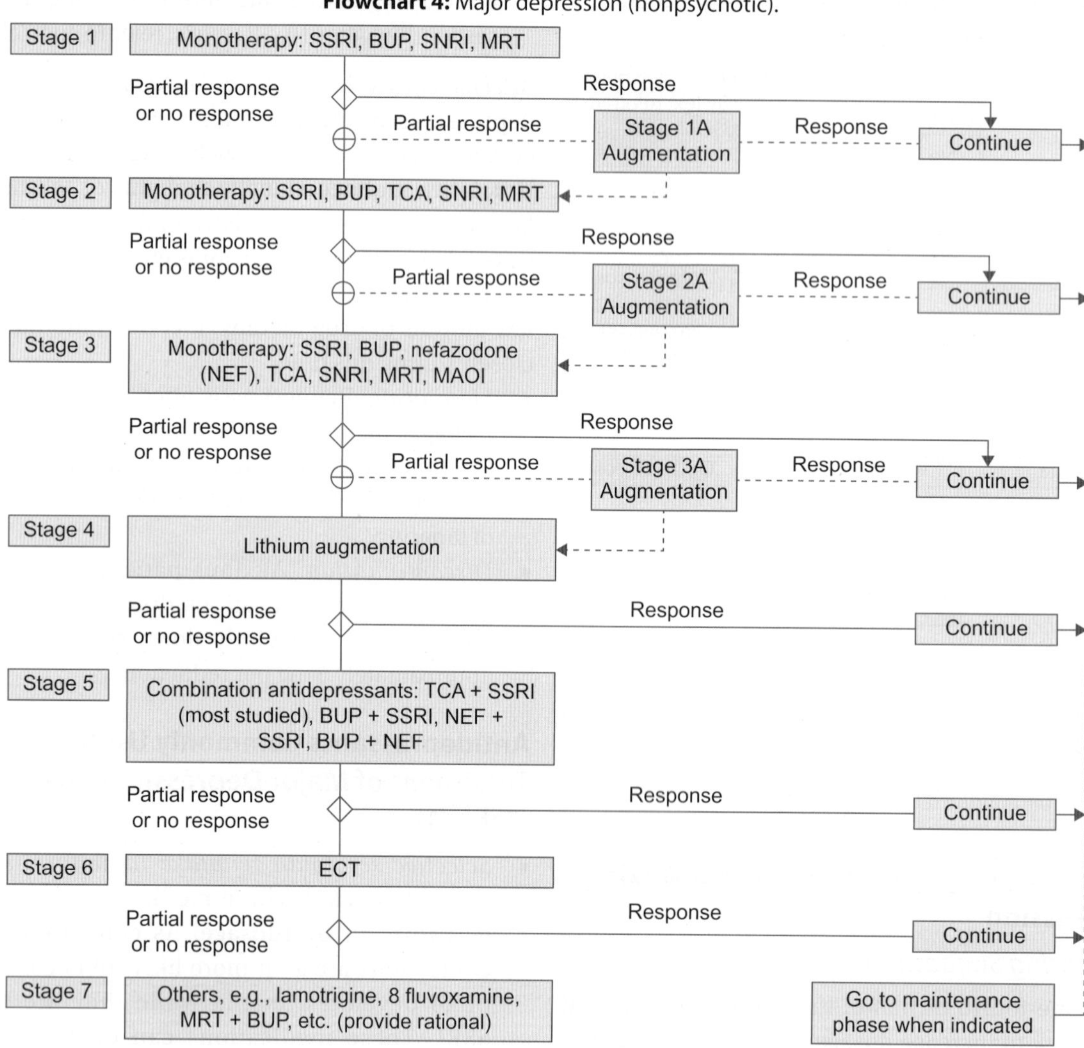

(SSRI: selective serotonin reuptake inhibitor; BUP: bupropion; SNRIs: serotonin–norepinephrine reuptake inhibitors; MRT: mirtazapine; TCAs: tricyclic antidepressants; NEF: nefazodone; MAOI: monoamine oxidase inhibitor; ECT: electroconvulsive therapy)

and periodic electrocardiograms (ECGs) should be considered. Side effects may include dry mouth, dry eyes (problem if contact wearer), dizziness, and ECG, pulse, and rhythm changes. Clomipramine (Anafranil) is quite effective in individuals with OCD.

Prevalence of anxiety disorders in children aged 5–17 is 6.4%. The debilitating nature of these disorders is routinely underestimated and the need for help may not be realized until serious impairment in social and academic functioning has occurred. Untreated anxiety disorders in children and adolescents are associated with higher rates of comorbid depression and substance abuse **(Flowchart 5)**.

TABLE 1: Antidepressants commonly used in treatment of major depressive disorders.

Class	*Drugs*
Selective serotonin reuptake inhibitors	Citalopram, escitalopram, fluoxetine, fluvoxamine, paroxetine, sertraline, vilazodone
Serotonin–norepinephrine reuptake inhibitors	Desvenlafaxine, duloxetine, venlafaxine
Monoamine oxidase inhibitors	Isocarboxazid, phenelzine, selegiline, tranylcypromine
Tricyclic antidepressants	Amitriptyline, desipramine, doxepin, imipramine, nortriptyline
Miscellaneous	Bupropion and mirtazapine

Flowchart 5: Major depressive disorder.

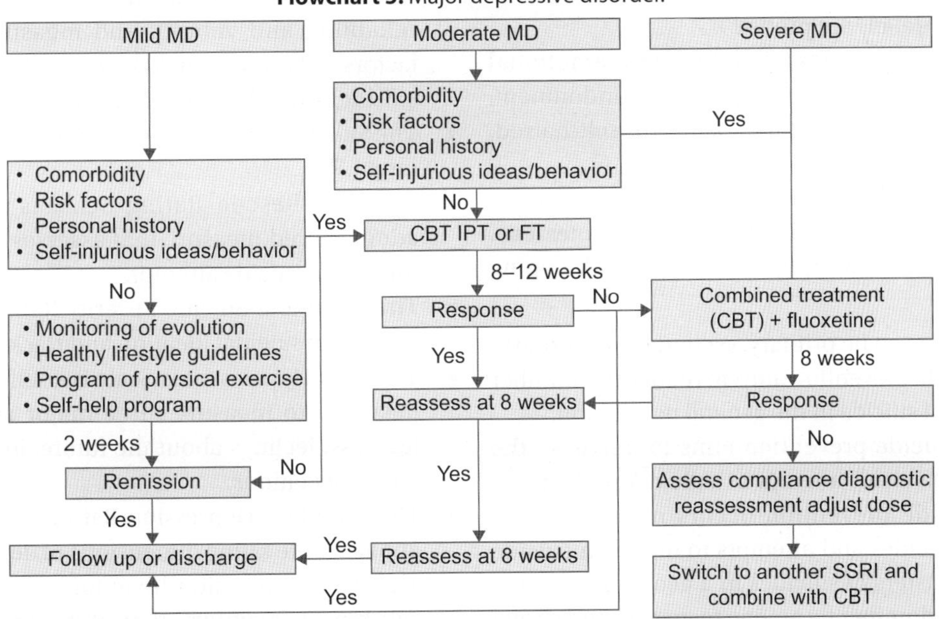

(CBT: cognitive behavior therapy; IPT: interpersonal therapy; FT: family therapy; SSRI: selective serotonin reuptake inhibitor)

SUICIDE

Death due to suicide is more common in boys than girls. Most acts of suicide are preceded by an expression of death wish either to friends or to a trustworthy adult in the previous 24 hours. May be made impulsively without much forethought or can be premeditated. Emotional development is at its peak during middle adolescence, the control of emotions is still incomplete due to evolving and immature prefrontal lobes.

Predisposing Factors

- Adolescents with poor coping skills and problem solving skills. Low levels of serotonin and its major metabolite 5-hydroxyindoleacetic acid (5-HIAA)
- Chaotic childhood with problems during child rearing, domestic violence, abusive adults
- High achiever adolescent may resort to suicide when humiliated for perceived failure. Adolescents with other coexisting mental illnesses may resort to suicide as they are vulnerable to stressors much more than normal population.

Approach to an Adolescent with Suicide Behavior

Adolescents should be posed directly about the existence of suicide ideation. They may not have confided in parents, hence parental history may not be reliable. Questions should be developmentally appropriate as it helps in devising management strategies in form of cognitive behavior therapy and interpersonal therapy. All suicide ideation should be taken seriously and evaluated thoroughly and repeatedly.

What, when, where, how, and why aspects of suicidal behavior should be explored and evaluated.

What:

- Was the action
- Was the thoughts about life after death
- The adolescent expect to happen on completion of suicide
- Any alternative plans thought to accomplish the objective

How:

- Was the plot to suicide conceived
- How were the steps planned
- Any previous attempts?

When and where:

- Was the suicidal action planned
- Where was the place chosen
- Where was the place where the suicidal note if any was planned to be placed. Significant life events are chosen for suicide.

Why:

- Psychological details are probed
- Feelings of worthlessness, helplessness, emotional pain, humiliation, emptiness, rejection, abandonment, fear of death, fear of mental breakdown, self-hatred, and guilt

Adolescents with multiple attempts usually take care to execute the next in a manner which is difficult to intervene. Single attempters usually equip themselves with coping skills with time.

Suicide prevention can be primary, secondary, or tertiary:

- Primary suicide prevention aims to reduce the number of new cases of suicide in the general population.
- Secondary suicide prevention aims to decrease the likelihood of a suicide attempt in high-risk patients.
- Tertiary suicide prevention occurs in response to completed suicides and attempts to diminish suicide contagion (clusters of suicides in a geographical area that occur predominantly among teenagers and young adults) and copycat suicides.

Risk Factors for Suicide

- Biological risk factors for suicide include:
  - Low cerebrospinal fluid 5-HIAA levels
  - Hypothalamic–pituitary–adrenal axis dysregulation
  - Low blood cholesterol levels
  - Medical or neurological illnesses (such as multiple sclerosis, stroke, Huntington disease, and epilepsy)
  - Cigarette smoking
- Psychological risk factors include:
  - Acceptability of suicide
  - A childhood history of physical or sexual abuse
  - Discouraged help-seeking behavior
  - Aggressive/impulsive traits
  - Pessimism
  - Hopelessness
  - Low self-esteem
  - Poor access to psychiatric treatment
  - Relationship problems
  - Financial troubles
  - A family or personal history of suicide
  - Major depression
  - Substance use

Rating Scales for Suicide Behavior and Related Mental Health Conditions

The most widely used scales for rating suicidal behaviors include:

- The Scale for Suicidal Ideation has good reported reliability and validity and measures three major factors—(1) active suicidal desire, (2) specific plans for suicide, and (3) passive suicidal desire.
- The Suicide Intent Scale measures the degree of suicide intent.
- The Risk-Rescue Rating Scale is an interviewer-administered measure that assesses the lethality and intent of a suicide attempt.
- The Columbia-Suicide Severity Rating Scale assesses severity of suicidal ideation and tracks suicidal events.
- The Beck Hopelessness Scale is a self-report inventory designed to measure three major aspects of hopelessness: feelings about the future, loss of motivation, and expectations.
- The Hamilton Depression Rating Scale is a clinician-applied scale rating dimensions of depression.
- The Beck Depression Inventory is a multiple-choice self-report inventory that measures the severity of depression.

Search for Biological Markers for Suicide

Many researchers have been trying to find biological markers related to suicidal behavior that could improve secondary suicide prevention. Several biological features related to failures in neurotransmitter and neuroendocrine systems, such as the serotonergic, noradrenergic, dopaminergic, and hypothalamic–pituitary–adrenocortical (HPA) systems, have been proposed, e.g., considerable evidence accrued using various research approaches suggests a potentially causal association between suicidal behavior and the serotonin neurotransmission system.

To date, the most promising biological predictors of suicidal behavior are low cerebrospinal fluid 5-HIAA (the main serotonin metabolite) and HPA axis dysregulation as indicated by dexamethasone nonsuppression.

What are the Most Effective Secondary Suicide Prevention Strategies?

In a recent systematic review of suicide prevention strategies, Mann et al. found evidence of effectiveness in five secondary suicide prevention methods:

1. Pharmacological interventions
2. Psychological interventions
3. Follow-up care
4. Reduced access to lethal means
5. Responsible media reporting of suicide **(Flowcharts 6 and 7)**.

Flowchart 6: Treatment of bipolar I depression.

Stage 1 — *Treat bipolar I depression for 8 weeks with:*
- Quetiapine >600 mg daily or
- Lithium 0.8 mEq/L daily (or another mood stabilizer) along with lamotrigine 50–200 mg daily. If there is no treatment response, move on to stage 2

↓

Stage 2 — *For treatment-resistant bipolar I depression, use:*
- A combination of olanzapine 6–12 mg plus fluoxetine 25–50 mg (OFC) daily or
- Increase dose to >600 mg of quetiapine along with lamotrigine 50–200 mg daily. If there is no treatment response, move on to stage 3

↓

Stage 3 — *Treat refractory bipolar I depression with:*
- Adjust OFC dose or switch to
- Lithium 0.8 mEq/L daily plus an SSRI 20–40 mg and bupropion 150–300 mg daily or
- Increase dose to >600 mg of quetiapine and 20–40 mg of an SSRI and 150–300 mg of bupropion daily or
- Use novel therapies as adjuncts, such as modafinil or pramipexole. If there is no treatment response, move on to stage 4

↓

Stage 4 — *Treat intractable bipolar I depression with:*
- Electroconvulsive therapy. If there is still no response, the patient may have involution bipolar I disorder

Flowchart 7: Treatment of bipolar II depression.

Stage 1 — *Treat bipolar II depression for 8 weeks with:*
- Lithium 0.8 mEq/L daily (or another mood stabilizer) along with lamotrigine 50–200 mg daily
- Quetiapine 300–600 mg daily or
- If there is no treatment response, move on to stage 2

↓

Stage 2 — *For treatment-resistant bipolar II depression, use:*
- Lithium 0.8 mEq/L daily along with an SSRI 20–40 mg and bupropion 150–300 mg daily or
- Quetiapine 300–600 mg daily along with an SSRI 20–40 mg and bupropion 150–300 mg daily. If there is no treatment response, move on to stage 3

↓

Stage 3 — *Treat refractory bipolar II depression with:*
- Quetiapine 300–600 mg daily and a monoamine oxidase inhibitor (MAOI) such as tranylcypromine 20–100 mg daily or
- Lithium 0.8 mEq/L daily and an MAOI such as tranylcypromine 20–100 mg daily
- Novel therapies as adjuncts, such as modafinil or pramipexole. If there is no treatment response, move on to stage 4

↓

Stage 4 — *Treat intractable bipolar II depression with:*
- Electroconvulsive therapy. If there is still no response, the patient may have involution bipolar II disorder

(SSRI: selective serotonin reuptake inhibitor)

CLINICAL PEARLS

- Counselors and clinicians should actively use specialize tools such as patient health questionnaire.
- An algorithm of nonpharmacological intervention makes it easier to manage depression.
- Pharmacological management, when necessary, should follow correct doses as per body weight and side effects have to be monitored.
- Treatment of adolescent depression/suicidal tendency is a long-term process with regular monitoring and follow-up as small social and psychological trigger factors can produce sudden relapse.

APPENDIX

RECENT INTERVENTIONS (FLOWCHART 8)

Digital Mental Health Interventions

There has been an increasing focus on utilizing technology for mental health interventions. Mobile Apps, online platforms, and telehealth services have become more prevalent, providing adolescents with accessible tools for monitoring and managing their mental health. These interventions leverage the widespread use of smartphones, tablets, and computers to increase access to mental health resources and services. Some of the digital mental health interventions **(Flowchart 9)** include following.

Mobile Applications (Apps)

- *Mood tracking Apps:* These Apps allow users to monitor and track their mood, emotions, and behaviors over time.

Flowchart 8: Recent interventions.

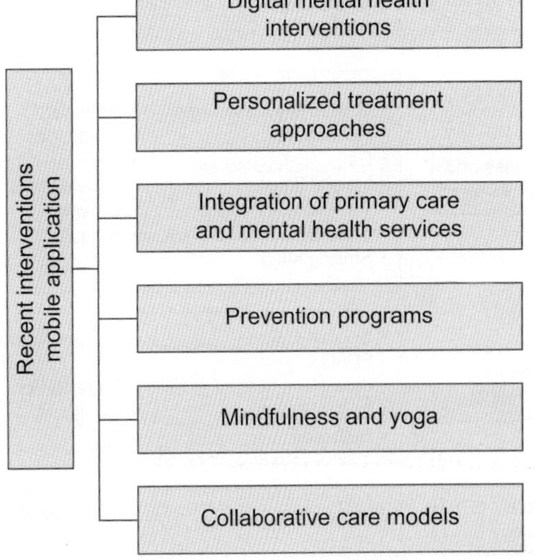

Flowchart 9: Digital mental health interventions.

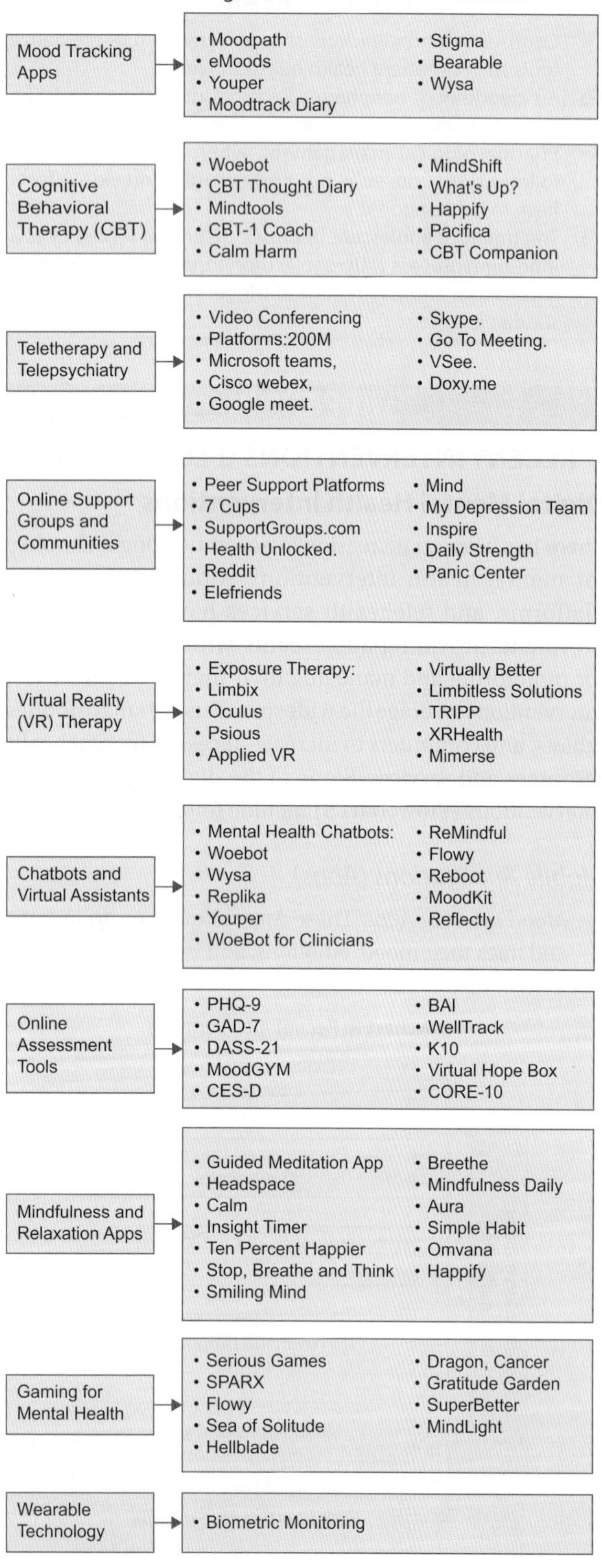

Users can identify patterns and share this information with healthcare providers.

- Moodpath (includes daily mental health assessments and provides feedback based on users' responses)
- eMoods is specifically designed for individuals managing mood disorders, bipolar disorder—track their mood, sleep, medications, and other factors relevant to their mental health.
- Youper combines mood tracking with AI-powered conversations. It uses chatbot technology to engage users in conversations that aim to understand and improve their emotional well-being.
- Moodtrack Diary offers a simple way to track moods, sleep, and medications. Users can create reports to share with their healthcare providers.
- Stigma is a mental health journaling App that allows users to track their mood, thoughts, and experiences. Providing insights into patterns and trends
- Bearable goes beyond mood tracking and includes features for tracking symptoms, habits, and factors that may influence mental health. It aims to help users identify patterns and triggers.
- Wysa is an AI-driven mental health chatbot that offers mood tracking as well as therapeutic conversations. It provides support for managing stress, anxiety, and other mental health concerns.

▪ *Cognitive behavioral therapy (CBT) Apps:* Some Apps offer modules based on CBT principles, providing interactive exercises and tools to help individuals manage their thoughts and behaviors.

- Woebot is an AI-powered chatbot designed to engage users in conversations based on CBT principles. It offers mood tracking, psychoeducation, and interactive exercises to promote emotional well-being.
- CBT Thought Diary helps users identify and challenge negative thought patterns by guiding them through CBT exercises. It includes tools for recording and analyzing thoughts.
- MoodTools is a comprehensive App that incorporates CBT principles for managing depression. It includes features such as a thought diary, activities scheduling, and relaxation exercises.
- CBT-i Coach is specifically designed to address insomnia and sleep difficulties using CBT for

insomnia techniques. It includes tools for tracking sleep patterns and implementing CBT strategies.
- Calm Harm focuses on helping individuals manage self-harm urges through distraction and emotional regulation techniques. It incorporates aspects of CBT.
- MindShift is designed to help users manage anxiety by providing CBT-based tools and coping strategies. It includes relaxation exercises, cognitive restructuring, and mindfulness practices.
- What's Up? is a mental health App that incorporates CBT and acceptance and commitment therapy (ACT) principles. It includes features like a diary, coping strategies, and a grounding technique called the "Get Grounded" page.
- Happify aims to improve emotional well-being through various activities and games based on positive psychology and CBT principles. It includes exercises for stress reduction and building resilience.
- Pacifica offers tools based on CBT and mindfulness to address stress, anxiety, and depression. It includes mood tracking, relaxation exercises, and audio lessons.
- CBT Companion provides users with CBT exercises and tools for managing anxiety and depression. It includes features for tracking mood, setting goals, and challenging negative thoughts.

- *Teletherapy and telepsychiatry:*
  Video conferencing platforms: Mental health professionals can conduct therapy sessions remotely through secure video conferencing platforms, increasing accessibility for individuals who may face barriers to in-person treatment, like *Zoom, Microsoft teams, Cisco Webex, Google Meet, Skype, Go To Meeting, VSee, and Doxy.me (telehealth platform).*
- *Online support groups and communities:*
  - *Peer support platforms:* Online communities and forums provide a space for individuals experiencing similar challenges to share their experiences, offer support, and exchange coping strategies.
  - 7 Cups is an online emotional support platform that connects individuals with trained listeners and volunteers. It offers anonymous chat support for various mental health concerns.
  - SupportGroups.com provides a platform for people to join and create online support groups for a wide range of issues, including mental health, addiction, and chronic illnesses.
  - HealthUnlocked is a social network for health, providing a space for individuals to join communities related to specific health conditions or concerns. Members can share experiences and support one another.
  - Reddit is a large online community with numerous subreddits dedicated to mental health and peer support. Examples include reddit/depression, reddit/anxiety, and others where users can share their experiences and seek advice.
  - Elefriends, developed by the mental health charity
  - Mind is an online community where individuals can connect with others who have experienced mental health challenges. It provides a supportive space for sharing thoughts and experiences.
  - MyDepressionTeam is a social network for individuals living with depression. Members can connect with others, share their experiences, and provide support to those going through similar struggles.
  - Inspire is a platform that hosts various support communities, including those focused on mental health, chronic conditions, and wellness. Members can connect with others for support and information.
  - DailyStrength offers support groups and communities for a wide range of health-related topics, including mental health, addiction, and relationships.
  - Panic Center, previously known as No Panic, is a UK-based platform that provides support and information for individuals dealing with anxiety, panic attacks, and related conditions.
- *Virtual reality (VR) therapy:*
  - *Exposure therapy:* VR can be used for exposure therapy, particularly in the treatment of phobias and post-traumatic stress disorder (PTSD), allowing individuals to confront and manage anxiety-inducing situations in a controlled virtual environment.
  - Limbix offers VR therapy for exposure therapy to treat anxiety disorders, including phobias and post-traumatic stress disorder (PTSD). It provides customizable virtual environments for therapeutic interventions.

- Oculus, owned by Facebook (now Meta), has explored the use of VR for mental health applications. Various VR experiences and applications on the Oculus platform aim to provide relaxation, stress reduction, and mindfulness experiences.
- Psious offers a VR platform for mental health professionals to conduct exposure therapy and relaxation sessions. It provides a range of virtual environments to address anxiety, phobias, and stress.
- AppliedVR focuses on developing VR solutions for pain management and psychological well-being. Their VR programs aim to reduce stress, anxiety, and improve overall mental health.
- Virtually Better develops VR environments for exposure therapy, including scenarios for anxiety disorders, specific phobias, and social anxiety. These environments are used by mental health professionals.
- Limbitless Solutions, known for their work in creating bionic limbs, has developed Relax VR, a virtual reality experience designed to promote relaxation and mindfulness.
- TRIPP is a VR meditation app that uses immersive experiences to promote relaxation and stress reduction. It combines mindfulness principles with virtual environments to create a calming experience.
- XRHealth offers VRHealth, a platform that includes various VR applications for mental health, such as VR therapy for anxiety, stress, and cognitive training exercises.
- Mimerse develops VR applications for exposure therapy, addressing conditions such as social anxiety and phobias. Their platform includes immersive experiences designed to gradually expose individuals to anxiety-provoking situations.

▪ *Chatbots and virtual assistants:*
  - *Mental health chatbots:* AI-driven chatbots provide users with a conversational interface to discuss their feelings and concerns. Some are designed to offer emotional support, psychoeducation, and resources.
  - *Woebot:* Woebot is an AI-powered chatbot that engages users in conversations based on cognitive behavioral therapy (CBT) principles. It offers mood tracking, psychoeducation, and interactive exercises.
  - Wysa is a mental health chatbot that uses evidence-based techniques, including CBT and dialectical behavior therapy (DBT), to provide support for managing stress, anxiety, and mood.
  - Replika is an AI chatbot designed to engage users in conversations and act as a personal AI friend.
  - Youper combines AI with emotional intelligence to engage users in conversations about their emotions and thoughts. It incorporates elements of CBT and acceptance and commitment therapy (ACT).
  - WoeBot for Clinicians is a version of Woebot designed for mental health professionals. It provides additional tools and features to support therapists in their work.
  - ReMindful is a mental health chatbot designed to assist users with stress management and mindfulness. It provides guided mindfulness exercises and stress reduction techniques.
  - Flowy is a chatbot that focuses on mental well-being and emotional intelligence. It engages users in conversations to help them reflect on their emotions and build resilience.
  - Reboot is a chatbot that uses principles from positive psychology and mindfulness to support users in managing stress, building resilience, and fostering well-being.
  - MoodKit is an App that includes a mood tracking feature and a thought journal. While not a chatbot in the traditional sense, it provides tools and exercises based on CBT principles.
  - Reflectly is a journaling App that uses AI to analyze users' entries and provide insights into their emotional well-being. It encourages users to reflect on their thoughts and emotions.

▪ *Online assessment tools:*
  Screening and assessment platforms: Online tools offer self-assessment questionnaires to help individuals evaluate their mental health status. These assessments can guide individuals to seek appropriate professional help.
  - *PHQ-9 (Patient Health Questionnaire-9):* It is a widely used self-report questionnaire for assessing the severity of depression. It includes nine questions about symptoms over the past 2 weeks.
  - *GAD-7 (Generalized Anxiety Disorder 7):* It is a self-report questionnaire used to assess the severity of generalized anxiety disorder. It consists of seven questions about anxiety symptoms.

- *DASS-21 (Depression, Anxiety, and Stress Scale-21):* It is a self-report scale that assesses symptoms of depression, anxiety, and stress. It includes 21 items, with seven items per subscale.
- MoodGYM is an online cognitive behavioral therapy (CBT) program that includes an assessment component. It helps individuals identify and manage symptoms of depression and anxiety.
- *CES-D (Center for Epidemiologic Studies Depression Scale):* It is a self-report scale designed to measure depressive symptoms in the general population. It includes 20 items.
- *BAI (Beck Anxiety Inventory):* It is a self-report inventory that assesses the severity of anxiety symptoms. It includes 21 common symptoms of anxiety.
- WellTrack is an online platform that includes assessments for depression, anxiety, and stress. It also provides tools for self-help and mental health tracking.
- *K10 (Kessler Psychological Distress Scale):* It is a self-report measure of psychological distress. It includes 10 items assessing symptoms of anxiety and depression over the past 4 weeks.
- *Virtual Hope Box:* This is an App designed to help individuals with coping skills and mental health assessment tools. It includes a variety of features for relaxation and mood tracking.
- *CORE-10 (Clinical Outcomes in Routine Evaluation-10):* It is a brief self-report measure that assesses psychological distress and well-being. It includes 10 items covering areas such as well-being, functioning, and risk.

- *Mindfulness and relaxation Apps:*
  - *Guided meditation Apps:* These Apps provide audio-guided meditation sessions, breathing exercises, and relaxation techniques to help individuals manage stress and anxiety.
  - Headspace offers guided meditations, mindfulness exercises, and sleep aids. It is suitable for beginners and includes themed meditation sessions for various aspects of life.
  - Calm provides guided meditations, sleep stories, breathing exercises, and relaxing music. It aims to reduce stress and improve sleep quality.
  - Insight Timer is a meditation App that offers a vast library of guided meditations, music tracks, and talks by meditation teachers. It is suitable for various meditation practices and experience levels.
  - Ten Percent Happier offers guided meditations and mindfulness content. It also includes interviews with meditation teachers and experts, providing insights into the benefits of mindfulness.
  - Stop, Breathe and Think guides users through short mindfulness activities based on their current emotions. It includes meditation exercises and mindful breathing techniques.
  - Smiling Mind is an App designed to teach mindfulness meditation to users of all ages. It includes programs for different age groups and offers mindfulness exercises for stress reduction.
  - Breethe provides guided meditations, calming music, and sleep aids. It aims to help users manage stress, improve focus, and promote relaxation.
  - Mindfulness Daily offers short mindfulness exercises for daily practice. It includes reminders to encourage users to incorporate mindfulness into their routines.
  - Aura focuses on personalized mindfulness with short meditation exercises. Users can choose their mood, and the App provides a tailored meditation session.
  - Simple Habit offers guided meditations for various situations, including stress reduction, sleep, and work-related mindfulness. It is designed for busy lifestyles with short sessions.
  - Omvana provides a variety of meditation tracks, music, and ambient sounds for relaxation and mindfulness. Users can customize their meditation experience.
  - Happify combines mindfulness techniques with positive psychology to promote happiness and well-being. It includes activities and games designed to boost mood.
- *Gaming for mental health:*
  - *Serious games:* Some video games are designed with mental health benefits in mind, incorporating elements of therapy, stress reduction, and cognitive training.
  - SPARX is an interactive game designed to help young people manage symptoms of depression. It combines traditional gaming elements with cognitive behavioral therapy (CBT) techniques.
  - Flowy is a game designed to promote relaxation and mindfulness. It focuses on providing a calming

and visually soothing experience to reduce stress.
    - Sea of Solitude is an adventure game that explores themes of loneliness and mental health. The narrative-driven gameplay aims to foster understanding and empathy.
    - *Hellblade:* Senua's Sacrifice is an action-adventure game that addresses mental health themes, particularly psychosis. It offers a unique and immersive experience to raise awareness and reduce stigma.
    - That Dragon, Cancer is an emotionally impactful game that explores the challenges faced by a family dealing with a child's cancer diagnosis. It provides a reflective and narrative-driven experience.
    - Gratitude Garden is a game that encourages players to focus on positive aspects of their lives and practice gratitude. It is designed to promote well-being and a positive mindset.
    - SuperBetter is a game designed to help individuals build resilience and overcome challenges. It incorporates elements of gamification to motivate users to achieve personal goals.
    - MindLight is a game developed to help children manage anxiety. It uses biofeedback technology to adapt the game world based on the player's stress levels.
- *Wearable technology:*
    - *Biometric monitoring:* Wearables, such as smartwatches, can track physiological indicators like heart rate and sleep patterns, providing data that may be useful for understanding an individual's mental well-being.

Digital mental health interventions offer several advantages, including increased accessibility, anonymity, cost-effectiveness, and the ability to reach individuals who might not otherwise seek traditional forms of mental health support. However, it is important to consider issues of privacy, data security, and the potential limitations of these interventions, as they may not be suitable for all individuals or conditions. Additionally, ongoing research is crucial to assess their efficacy and impact on long-term mental health outcomes.

Personalized Treatment Approaches

Advances in research have highlighted the importance of personalized treatment plans for adolescents. Tailoring interventions to individual needs, considering factors such as family dynamics, cultural background, and personal preferences, can enhance the effectiveness of treatment.

Integration of Primary Care and Mental Health Services

Recognizing the need for a comprehensive approach, there has been an emphasis on integrating mental health services into primary care settings to allow for early identification and intervention in cases of adolescent depression and suicidal tendencies.

Prevention Programs

Preventive interventions target at-risk populations before the onset of severe mental health issues and focus on building resilience, coping skills, and providing education on mental health.

Mindfulness and Yoga

Mindfulness and yoga have gained attention for their potential benefits in managing stress, anxiety, and depression in adolescents. Research has explored the integration of these practices into traditional therapeutic approaches.

Collaborative Care Models

Collaborative care involves a team-based approach, including mental health professionals, primary care providers, and families working together to address the complex needs of adolescents with mental health concerns. This approach aims to improve communication and coordination of care.

KEY POINTS

- Adolescent depression is a common and serious problem increasing the risk of suicide.
- Early detection and treatment is key to effective management.
- Behavioral changes at home among peers and at school should be noticed and acted upon.
- Both nonpharmacological and pharmacological methods have to be used in stepwise integrated approach involving family members and school staff.
- Suicidal ideation needs to be identified early by psychological profiling and the necessary corrective actions have to be initiated.
- Recent advances point toward multidisciplinary approach to adolescent depression and suicidal ideation.

SUGGESTED READING

1. Andersen UA, Andersen M, Rosholm JU, Gram LF. Contacts to the health care system prior to suicide: A comprehensive analysis using registers for general and psychiatric hospital admissions, contacts to general practitioners and practicing specialists and drug prescriptions. Acta Psychiatr Scand. 2000;102(2):126-34.
2. Beck AT, Kovacs M, Weissman A. Assessment of suicidal intention: the scale for suicide ideation. J Consult Clin Psychol. 1979;47(2):343-52.
3. Harith S, Backhaus I, Mohbin N, Ngo HT, Khoo S. Effectiveness of digital mental health interventions for university students: an umbrella review. PeerJ. 2022;10: e13111.
4. Jacobs DG, Baldessarini RJ, Conwell Y, Fawcett JA, Horton L, Meltzer H, et al. Practice Guideline for the Assessment and Treatment of Patients with Suicidal Behaviors. Washington, DC: American Psychiatric Association; 2003.
5. Johansson L, Lindqvist P, Eriksson A. Teenage suicide cluster formation and contagion: implications for primary care. BMC Fam Pract. 2006;7:32.
6. Lattie EG, Adkins EC, Winquist N, Stiles-Shields C, Wafford QE, Graham AK. Digital Mental Health Interventions for Depression, Anxiety, and Enhancement of Psychological Well-Being Among College Students: Systematic Review. J Med Internet Res. 2019;21(7):e12869.
7. Lönnqvist JK, Henriksson MM, Isometsä ET, Marttunen MJ, Heikkinen ME, Aro HM, et al. Mental disorders and suicide prevention. Psychiatry Clin Neurosci. 1995;49(Suppl 1): S111-6.
8. Mann JJ, Apter A, Bertolote J, Beautrais A, Currier D, Haas A, et al. Suicide prevention strategies: a systematic review. JAMA. 2005;294(16):2064-74.
9. Murphy GE. The prediction of suicide: why is it so difficult? Am J Psychother. 1984;38(3):341-9.
10. Oquendo MA, Galfalvy H, Russo S, Ellis SP, Grunebaum MF, Burke A, et al. Prospective study of clinical predictors of suicidal acts after a major depressive episode in patients with major depressive disorder or bipolar disorder. Am J Psychiatry. 2004;161(8):1433-41.
11. Pignone MP, Gaynes BN, Rushton JL, Burchell CM, Orleans CT, Mulrow CD, et al. Screening for depression in adults: a summary of the evidence for the US Preventive Services Task Force. Ann Intern Med. 2002;136(10): 765-76.
12. Posner K, Oquendo MA, Gould M, Stanley B, Davies M. Columbia Classification Algorithm of Suicide Assessment (C-CASA): classification of suicidal events in the FDA's pediatric suicidal risk analysis of antidepressants. Am J Psychiatry. 2007;164(7):1035-43.
13. Sher L, Oquendo MA, Mann JJ. Risk of suicide in mood disorders. Clin Neurosci Res. 2001;1:337-44.
14. Sher L. Preventing suicide. QJM. 2004;9(10):677-80.
15. Van Heeringen K. The neurobiology of suicide and suicidality. Can J Psychiatry. 2003;48(5):292-300.
16. World Health Organization. (2003). World Health Report 2003: Shaping the Future. [online] Available from https://iris.who.int/bitstream/handle/10665/42789/9241562439.pdf?sequence=1&isAllowed=y. [Last accessed October, 2024].

Teen Aggression: Steps in Management

Ritu Gupta, Abheet Gupta

INTRODUCTION

Teenage or adolescence is an important developmental phase in the life of all human beings. It is during this phase of life that a person develops an identity, discovers new emotions, explores new perspectives, and form habits. Many times, unexpressed emotions or suppressed feelings along with poor coping skills can lead to aggression in teenagers which could negatively impact them and their lives.

In psychology, aggression is defined as a wide range of actions and behaviors that can result in mental, emotional, or physical harm to a person, others, or objects. Aggression is centered on purposely (even if subconsciously) hurting another person either emotionally or physically. Aggression can be caused by a variety of reasons, but it is often a result of biological, environmental, or psychological factors.

Aggression often happens as a natural human response to fear, stress or a feeling of losing control. One may also respond aggressively if one feels mistreated, frustrated, or unheard. If someone has never learned how to manage their emotions in an effective way, they are more likely to portray aggressive behaviors. Aggression often results in self-harm behaviors, poor or broken relationships and poor mental health. It is therefore critical to find the root causes of aggression in adolescents and find ways to help teenagers acquire attributes and abilities that will be important for enjoying the adolescent years and assuming adult roles (Kumar et al., 2023).

Aggression is a disruptive behavior. Temper tantrums, physical aggression such as hitting, defiance of authority, and stealing are aggressive behaviors which can be very distressing for the primary care providers and school personnel. The focus of this chapter is to study the definitions, risk factors, related psychiatric disorders, intervention and outcomes of aggressive behaviors in teenagers.

DEFINITIONS

- *Impulsive aggressive behavior:* The type of aggressive behavior which is a reaction to a trigger. It is a reactive aggressive behavior which happens without thinking or planning.
- *Proactive or instrumental aggressive behavior:* The type of aggressive behavior which is premeditated and is done with intention or purpose.

  Both are often shown through either physical aggression (slapping, hitting, or punching) or through harsh emotional outbursts.
- *Oppositional defiant disorder (ODD):* According to the Diagnostic and Statistical Manual of Mental Disorders, Fourth Edition (DSM-IV), children with ODD experience ongoing symptoms of "negativistic, defiant, disobedient, and hostile behavior toward authority figures".
- *Conduct disorder (CD):* This occurs when a child with ODD becomes angrier along with increased behavioral outbursts. According to the DSM-IV, CD is defined as "a repetitive and persistent pattern of behavior in which the basic rights of others or major age-appropriate social rules are violated".
- *Antisocial personality disorder (ASPD):* It is defined by DSM-IV as "a pervasive pattern of disregard for, and violation of, the rights of others that begins in childhood or early adolescence and continues into adulthood". Symptoms include poor school performance, truancy, poor self-esteem, low frustration tolerance, persistent lying or stealing, frequent fighting, and an apparent lack of remorse or empathy. Young adults who have ASPD may have had a history of childhood CD.

Diagnostic features of aggressive behavior in children and adolescents are given in **Table 1**.

TABLE 1: Diagnostic features of aggressive behavior in children and adolescents.

	Oppositional defiant disorder (ODD)	*Conduct disorder (CD)*	*Antisocial personality disorder (ASPD)*
Onset	Usually before age 8 years, no later than early adolescence	• Child onset before age 10 years • Adolescent onset after age 10 years but rarely after age 16 years	Adulthood
Symptoms	Trouble with authority, breaks school rules, always seems angry, argumentative, easily annoyed, and noncompliant	Significant aggression toward others, animal cruelty, destruction of property, theft, setting fires, serious violation of rules, law breaking, substance abuse, and poor school performance	Disregard for others, criminal offenses, substance abuse, and poor school performance
Duration of symptoms for diagnosis	For at least 6 months	3+ incidents within the last 12 months with at least one in the past 6 months	Pervasive pattern since age 15 years

CAUSES OF AGGRESSION

- *Biological causes:* It includes genetics, medical and psychiatric diseases, neurotransmitters, hormones, substances of abuse, and medications.
- *Psychological causes:* It includes numerous DSM-V diagnosis.
- *Environmental causes:* It includes child abuse, poverty, crime, early neglect, antisocial behavior in childhood, exposure to substance abuse and weapons, noise, temperature, overcrowding, violent video games, etc.

RISK FACTORS

Aggression as described by Merriam-Webster dictionary is a "hostile, injurious or destructive behavior or outlook". Aggression is merely a symptom, something which indicates the existence of something else. It is just the tip of the iceberg, what is seen on the surface, and it is of utmost importance to see what is underneath to find the root cause of aggression. It is crucial to study the risk factors which may lead to aggression in teenagers as an attempt to better understand and control them and it could be one of the most efficient ways to limit aggression in teens, in general. With a rapid growth in technology and in other areas of life in the past few decades, it is impossible to cover all things which could lead to aggression in teens. Based on past research, the following are the most common risk factors.

Neglect

Research says that neglect in the first two postnatal years has been found to be the biggest precursor of aggression in teens compared to neglect or physical abuse in any later stages of childhood.

Psychological Maltreatment

Psychological maltreatment could be a result of dysfunctional families with damaging interactions between parents and children or from observing intimate partner violence. Damaging interactions can include belittling, rejecting, and denying emotional attachment which can all destroy a child's sense of self and personal safety.

Parental Discipline/Authoritarian Parenting

A family history of harsh, hostile, and aggressive parental behavior can increase the risk of aggression in teens. Parents' use of physical discipline or punitive treatment creates a model of aggressive behavior for the child. In other words, a child learns what they see or experience.

Media

It is commonly known that exposure to violence in the media can contribute to aggressive behaviors in youth. Various studies have also shown that violence depicted in media has a direct impact on aggression in teens.

Lead Exposure

Lead neurotoxicity can lead to decrease in intelligence quotient (IQ), increase in aggressive symptoms and decrease in balance and hearing. Even low levels of exposure to lead can lead to aggressive behaviors as reported by teachers.

ASSESSMENT

Aggression is not always a sign of abnormal behavior. Aggressive behavior can be a symptom of a normal developmental stage such as rebellion in adolescence. Accurate assessment of a child who exhibits aggressive or disruptive behavior requires determination of the frequency, intensity, and chronicity of the behavior within the developmental stage's context. A thorough evaluation of a child's aggressive behavior is essential to diagnose and intervene appropriately and effectively. Such an evaluation requires knowledge of normal child development; an understanding of the child's and parents' temperaments; and acquisition of information regarding the characteristics, prevalence, and impact of disruptive behaviors. The evaluation should include multiple sources of information, including parent interview, teacher interview, child interview, and the use of standardized rating scales.

Parent Interview

Parent interviews are important sources of the child's developmental history and status. Understanding of a child's developmental level of functioning compared with his or her chronological age helps to determine appropriate behavioral expectations that, in turn, aids in deciding whether a child's aggressive behavior is out of the norm for his or her development. Specific information such as the start of aggressive behavior or presence of psychosocial stressors can be useful pieces of information.

Teacher Interview

Information collected from a teacher interview is like the information collected from a parent interview. It is important to obtain information from both sources to form a comprehensive picture of the child as a child shows different aspects of themselves to different people.

Child Interview

Older children and adolescents may be asked directly about their perceptions of the issue as well as about family and social functioning. Children showing significant aggressive behaviors may be particularly difficult to interview. Often, they are reluctant to talk about their behavior and may be hostile. However, their reports of internalizing symptoms, such as anxiety and depression, are more reliable and likely to be more valid than parent and teacher reports of these symptoms. HEEADSSS assessment, which is a tool to help, understand and assess the physical, emotional and social well-being of adolescents, needs to be done **(Fig. 1)**.

Standardized Rating Scales

Older children, the child's parents, and the teacher should be asked to complete standardized rating scales in addition to providing information during the interviews. Rating scales allow for a comparison of the child's behavior with that of other children the same age. "Broad" rating scales often are administered first that assess for symptoms associated with a variety of disorders, such as depression, anxiety, aggression, withdrawal, inattention, hyperactivity, and delinquent behavior. The Youth Self Report, Child Behavior Checklist (Parent Report Form) and Teacher's Report Form, the Behavior Assessment System for Children, and Conners' Parent and Teacher Rating Scales–Revised are used commonly in primary care settings.

H *Home:* Who lives at home? What are the relationships like? Divorce?

E *Education:* Going to school? Stress of exam/grades? Friends? Bullying?

E *Eating:* Stress from eating habits, weight or body shape change?

A *Activities:* Any hobbies? Meet with friends? Time spent on internet/TV?

D *Drugs: Do you, friends or family use tabacco, alcohol or drugs?*

S *Sexuality: Previous or current relationship? Sexual orientation*

S *Suicide:* Sad? Stressed? Previous or current thoughts? Medication? DSH?

S *Safety: Aware of any risk-taking? Violence at home or school?*

Fig. 1: HEEADSSS assessment chart.

Next Steps

Next steps in the assessment process include figuring out if the behavior is significant and in need of treatment. Factors that necessitate treatment include symptoms that have been troublesome for some time, that are evident in more than one situation, that are relatively severe, and that are likely to impede the child's functioning. Mild behaviors can be treated by providing basic guidance and support. However, serious behaviors may require the doctor to advise the family to seek help of a mental health professional. Furthermore, the pediatrician should help the parents better understand the issue by informing them about the causes of aggression in teens and how it could be a result of improper parenting.

INTERVENTION

Numerous evidence-based interventions are available for tackling disruptive behavior in teens. Past studies show that parent management training and cognitive behavioral therapy (CBT) are the most efficient interventions in

Flowchart 1: Steps in management of teen aggression.

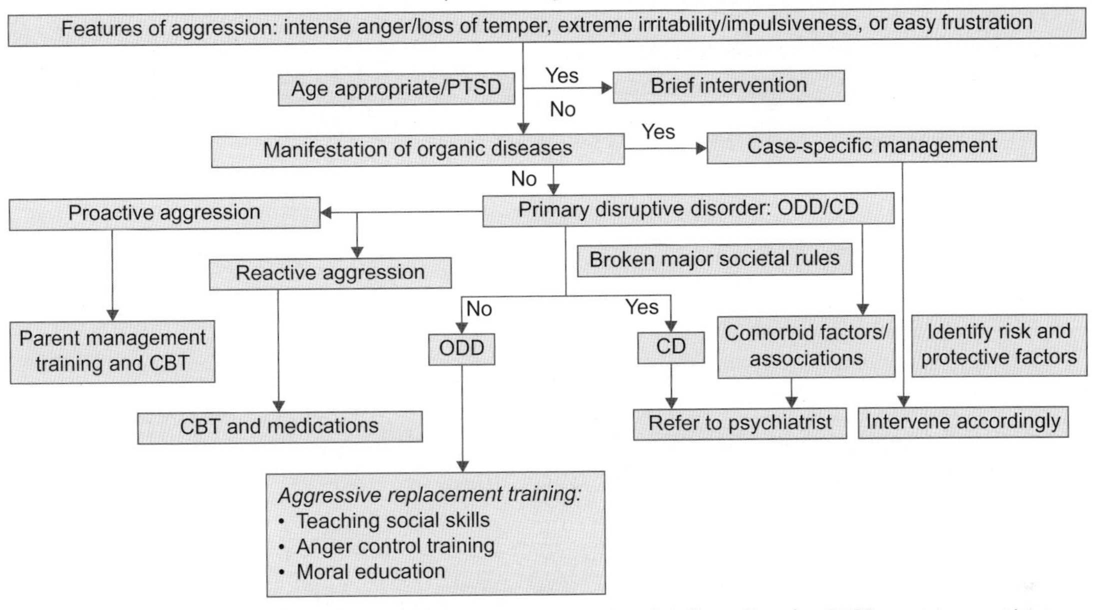

(CBT: cognitive behavioral therapy; CD: conduct disorder; ODD: oppositional defiant disorder; PTSD: post-traumatic stress disorder)

addressing aggression in teens. Furthermore, it is advised to use interventions for both parents and children as both parties can be the cause of the child's disruptive behaviors.

Parent Management Training

It teaches useful techniques and strategies to parents which help them in handling their teens to alter or improve their behavior. The training can be designed for parents from different backgrounds and cultures. It trains the parents to use techniques such as positive reinforcement and differential attention. It is important for parents to first improve their own behavior toward the child as, often, the child learns what they see and positive changes in the parents' behavior play a major role in altering the teen's behavior.

Cognitive Problem-solving Skills Training

Aggressive behavior is not simply a reaction to environmental events. Rather, it is the interpretation, perception, and processing of the event that results in the aggressive response. Thus, cognitive processes, such as perceptions and attributions, often play a large role in the genesis of aggressive behavior. Children showing disruptive behavior focus more on aggressive stimuli, overattribute hostile intent, are deficient in social problem-solving skills, and often lack behavioral self-awareness. Training programs that focus on cognitive problem-solving skills address these issues by teaching children a step-by-step approach to solving interpersonal problems by revealing the cognitive processes that underlie social behavior.

MEDICATION

When behavioral interventions are insufficient or aggressive behavior is severe, the clinician may consider the use of psychotropic drugs as an adjunct to behavioral therapy. Selection of medication should begin with insight into the biologic conditions that predispose the individual to aggression. In addition to the child's history, family history can be very helpful in determining the causes of a child's disordered behavior. Steps in management of teen aggression are depicted in **Flowchart 1**.

SUGGESTED READING

1. American Psychiatric Association. Diagnostic and Statistical Manual of Mental Disorders Fourth Edition Text Revision (DSM-IV-TR). Washington, DC, USA: American Psychiatric Association; 2000. pp. 645-50.
2. Kumar P, Patel SK, Debbarma S, Saggurti N. Determinants of School dropouts among adolescents: Evidence from a longitudinal study in India. 2023;18(3):e0282468.
3. Zahrt DM, Melzer-Lange MD. Aggressive behavior in children and adolescents. Pediatr Rev. 2011;32(8):325-32.

Immunization

Section Editors: *Amar Jeet Chitkara, Jaydeep Choudhury*

CHAPTER 27

Immunization in Childhood

Monjori Mitra

INTRODUCTION

National immunization program (NIP) in India covers about 12 antigens and is on full throttle under The "Indradhanush program" with encouraging results. The Indian Academy of Pediatrics (IAP) on the other hand has all NIP vaccines in their timetable align with new vaccines available in the private sector to provide the most optimal individual immunization. IAP timetable also emphasizes vaccination from neonatal to adolescent age including antenatal immunization in tandem with the global practices. There has been a constant surveillance of the various vaccine-preventable diseases and the data helps IAP to formulate policy decisions for both individual protection and suggestions to the Government stake holders for inclusion in the NIP.

The schedule recommended is based on the best seroprotective outcome of the vaccines which are being continuously studied in various environmental settings. The vaccination providers should try to influence the community or the individual to follow the same to get the best protective efficacy for individual and community.

Optimal response to a vaccine depends on multiple factors, including the type of vaccine, age of the recipient, and immune status of the recipient. Recommendations for the age at which vaccines are administered are influenced by age-specific risks for disease, age-specific risks for complications, age-specific responses to vaccination, and potential interference with the immune response by passively transferred maternal antibodies. Vaccines are recommended for members of the youngest age group at risk for experiencing the disease for which efficacy and safety have been demonstrated.

Certain products, including inactivated vaccines, toxoids, recombinant subunit vaccines, polysaccharide conjugate vaccines, and live vaccines, require two doses or more to elicit an adequate antibody response. Tetanus and diphtheria toxoids require booster doses to maintain protective antibody concentrations. Unconjugated polysaccharide vaccines do not induce T-cell memory, and additional doses (although they elicit the same or a lower antibody concentration) might increase the level of protection. Conjugation with a protein carrier improves the effectiveness of polysaccharide vaccines by inducing T-lymphocyte-dependent immunologic function. Many vaccines that stimulate both cell-mediated immunity and neutralizing antibodies (e.g., live-attenuated virus vaccines) usually can induce prolonged immunity, even if antibody titers decline over time. Subsequent exposure to such viruses usually results in a rapid anamnestic antibody response without viremia.

Approximately, 90–95% of recipients of a single dose of certain live vaccines administered by injection at the recommended age (i.e., measles, rubella, and yellow fever vaccines) develop protective antibodies, generally within 14 days of the dose. For varicella and mumps vaccines, 80–85% of vaccines are protected after a single dose. However, because a limited proportion (5–15%) of measles, mumps, and rubella (MMR) or varicella vaccines fails to respond to first dose, a second dose is recommended to provide another opportunity to develop immunity. Of those who do not respond to the first dose of MMR or varicella vaccine, 97–99% responds to a second dose.

COMBINATION VACCINES AND DRUG CONTROLLER GENERAL OF INDIA LICENSURE

Only combination vaccines licensed by Drug Controller General of India (DCGI) should be used. Vaccination providers should not combine separate vaccines into the same syringe to administer together unless mixing is indicated for the patient's age and is explicitly specified on the DCGI-approved product label inserts. Only two combination vaccines [diphtheria, tetanus, pertussis, polio, and *Haemophilus influenzae* type b (DTaP-IPV/Hib) vaccine] contain separate antigen components for which DCGI approves mixing by the user. The safety, immunogenicity, and effectiveness of unlicensed combinations are unknown and should not be used.

INTERCHANGEABILITY OF FORMULATIONS

Regulatory body generally licenses a combination vaccine based on studies demonstrating that the product's immunogenicity (or efficacy) and safety are comparable or equivalent to monovalent or combination products licensed previously. The combination vaccine may be used interchangeably with monovalent formulations and other combination products with similar component antigens produced by the same manufacturer to continue the vaccination series. For example, DTaP, DTaP/Hib, and future DTaP vaccines that contain similar acellular pertussis antigens from the same manufacturer may be used interchangeably, if licensed and indicated for the patient's age.

Ideally, the doses of vaccine in a series should be from the same manufacturer; however, if this is not possible or if the manufacturer of doses given previously is unknown, providers should administer the vaccines that are available.

VACCINATION ALGORITHM

Bacillus Calmette–Guérin Vaccine

- This should be given at birth before discharge from the hospital or at first contact.
- If missed in the neonatal period the vaccine should be administered at the earliest.
- Catch-up may be given up to 5 years.

Hepatitis B Vaccine

- Minimum age of administration is at birth. Administer monovalent hepatitis B vaccine to all newborns before hospital discharge. Hepatitis B vaccine may also be given in any of the following schedules:
  - At birth, 1, and 6 months (birth weight ≥2,000 g—one dose within 24 hours of birth if medically stable and birth weight <2,000 g—one dose at chronological age 1 month or hospital discharge, whichever is earlier)
  - At birth, 6, and 14 weeks
  - At 6, 10, and 14 weeks
  - At birth, 6, 10, and 14 weeks, etc.
- Monovalent hepatitis B vaccine should be used for doses administered before age of 6 weeks.
- Administration of a total of four doses of hepatitis B vaccine is permissible when a combination vaccine containing hepatitis B is administered after the birth dose.
- Infants who did not receive a birth dose should receive three doses of a hepatitis B containing vaccine starting as soon as feasible.
- The ideal minimum interval between first and second dose is 4 weeks, and between second and third dose is 8 weeks.
- Ideally, the final (third or fourth) dose in the hepatitis B vaccine series should be administered not earlier than the age of 24 weeks and at least 16 weeks after the first dose.
- Routine booster vaccinations are not needed in healthy children who have responded well and have had levels of 10 mIU/mL postvaccination or even if the levels fall below protective levels, as they are protected for life against hepatitis B due to immune memory.

Catch-up Vaccination

- Administer the three-dose series to those not previously vaccinated.
- In catch-up vaccination, use 0, 1, and 6 months schedule.

Poliovirus Vaccines: Oral Polio Vaccine/Inactivated Polio Vaccine

- *Birth dose:* Oral polio vaccine (OPV) before discharge from hospital
  - *Inactivated polio vaccine (IPV):* 6, 10, and 14 weeks. OPV in place of IPV. If IPV is unaffordable or unavailable
- *OPV:* At 6 months with hepatitis B and at 9 months with measles
  - Additional doses of OPV on all national immunization days and subnational immunization days
- *Booster dose:* 18 months with first booster
  - *IPV:* Two instead of three doses can also be used if primary series started at 8 weeks
  - *IPV catch-up schedule:* Two doses at 2 months apart followed by a booster after 6 months

Catch-up Vaccination

- *IPV catch-up schedule*: Two doses at 2 months apart followed by a booster after 6 months of previous dose.

Diphtheria, Tetanus Toxoids, and Pertussis Vaccine

Routine Vaccination

- *Minimum age*: 6 weeks
- Five-dose series (primary series three doses at age 2, 4, and 6 months. Followed by a booster dose at ages 15–18 months and 4–6 years).
- The first booster (fourth dose) may be administered as early as age 12 months, provided at least 6 months have elapsed since the third dose.
- Diphtheria, tetanus, and acellular pertussis (DTaP) vaccine/combinations should preferably be avoided for the primary series.
- Diphtheria, tetanus, and acellular pertussis may be preferred to diphtheria, tetanus, and whole-cell pertussis (DTwP) in children with history of severe adverse effects after previous dose/s of DTwP or children with neurologic disorders.
- First and second boosters may also be of DTwP. However, considering a higher reactogenicity, DTaP can be considered for the boosters.
- If any "acellular pertussis" containing vaccine is used, it must at least have three or more components in the product.
- No need of repeating/giving additional doses of whole-cell pertussis vaccine to a child who has earlier completed their primary schedule with acellular pertussis vaccine-containing products.

Catch-up Vaccination

- *Catch-up schedule*: The second childhood booster is not required if the last dose has been given beyond the age of 4 years
- *Catch-up below 7 years*: DTwP/DTaP at 0, 1, and 6 months
- *Catch-up above 7 years*: Tdap, Td, and Td at 0, 1, and 6 months, respectively. DTwP is not recommended due to increased reactogenicity.

Haemophilus influenzae Type B Conjugate Vaccine

- *Minimum age:* 6 weeks as combination with DTwP/DTaP.
- Primary series includes Hib conjugate vaccine at ages 6, 10, and 14 weeks with a booster at age 12 through 18 months.

Catch-up Vaccination

- *In 6–12 months*: Two doses, 1 month apart and one booster at 16–18 months.
- *In 12–15 months*: One primary and one booster at 16–18 months
- *Above 15 months*: Single dose

If the first dose was administered at age 7 through 11 months, administer the second dose at least 4 weeks later and a final dose at age 12–18 months at least 8 weeks after the second dose.

Patients with comorbidities: According to the Centers for Disease Control and Prevention (CDC) guidelines.

- *For those aged 12–59 months receiving chemotherapy/radiation therapy and are unvaccinated/one dose before age 12 months:* Two doses, 8 weeks apart recommended.
- *If two or more doses are administered before 12 months:* One dose at least 8 weeks after pervious dose is recommended.
- *Hematopoietic stem cell transplant (HSCT):* Three-dose series starting 6–12 months at 4 weeks apart post successful transplant.

Pneumococcal Vaccines

Routine Vaccination

- *Minimum age:* 6 weeks
- Both PCV10 and PCV13 are licensed for children from 6 weeks to 5 years of age (although the exact labeling details may differ by country). Additionally, PCV13 is licensed for the prevention of pneumococcal diseases in adults >50 years of age
- *Primary schedule (for both PCV10 and PCV13):* Three primary doses at 6, 10, and 14 weeks with a booster at age 12–15 months.

Catch-up Vaccination

- Administer one dose of PCV13 or PCV10 to all healthy children aged 24–59 months who are not completely vaccinated for their age
- For PCV13, catch-up in 6–12 months—two doses 4 weeks apart and one booster; 12–23 months—two doses 8 weeks apart; 24 months and above—single dose
- For PCV10, catch-up in 6–12 months—two doses 4 weeks apart and one booster; 12 months to 5 years—two doses 8 weeks apart

- Vaccination of persons with high-risk conditions:
  - Pneumococcal vaccines and pneumococcal polysaccharide vaccine (PPSV) both are used in certain high-risk group of children.
  - For children aged 24–71 months with certain underlying medical conditions, administer one dose of PCV13 if three doses of PCV were received previously, or administer two doses of PCV13 at least 8 weeks apart if fewer than three doses of PCV were received previously.
  - A single dose of PCV13 may be administered to previously unvaccinated children aged 6–18 years who have anatomic or functional asplenia (including sickle cell disease), human immunodeficiency virus (HIV) infection or an immunocompromising condition, cochlear implant, or cerebrospinal fluid leak.
  - Administer PPSV23 at least 8 weeks after the last dose of PCV to children aged 2 years or older with certain underlying medical conditions.
  - The Subject Expert Committee (SEC) of Central Drugs Standard Control Organization (CDSCO) has recommended grant of permission to manufacture 14-valent Investigational vaccine on August 29, 2022. It had proven non inferiority to PCV13 in Phase-3 trials and also is safe and tolerable in comparison to Prevenar 13 vaccine.

Pneumococcal Polysaccharide Vaccine (PPSV23)

- *Minimum age:* 2 years
- Not recommended for routine use in healthy individuals. Recommended only for the vaccination of persons with certain high-risk conditions.
- Administer PPSV at least 8 weeks after the last dose of PCV to children aged 2 years or older with certain underlying medical conditions such as anatomic or functional asplenia (including sickle cell disease), HIV infection, cochlear implant, or cerebrospinal fluid leak.
- An additional dose of PPSV should be administered after 5 years to children with anatomic/functional asplenia or an immunocompromising condition.
- PPSV should never be used alone for prevention of pneumococcal diseases among high-risk individuals.
- Children with following medical conditions for which PPSV23 and PCV13 are indicated in the age group 24–71 months:
  - Immunocompetent children with chronic heart disease (particularly cyanotic congenital heart disease and cardiac failure); chronic lung disease (including asthma if treated with high dose oral corticosteroid therapy); diabetes mellitus; cerebrospinal fluid leaks; or cochlear implant
  - Children with anatomic or functional asplenia (including sickle cell disease and other hemoglobinopathies, congenital or acquired asplenia, or splenic dysfunction)
  - Children with immunocompromising conditions: HIV infection, chronic renal failure and nephrotic syndrome, diseases associated with treatment with immunosuppressive drugs or radiation therapy, including malignant neoplasms, leukemias, lymphomas, and Hodgkin disease; or solid organ transplantation, congenital immunodeficiency.

Rotavirus Vaccines

- Four live oral vaccines licensed and marketed in India: Human Monovalent Live vaccine (RV1), Human Bovine Pentavalent Live vaccine (RV5), Indian Neonatal Rotavirus Live Vaccine (116E), and Bovine Rotavirus Pentavalent Vaccine (BRV-PV)
- *Minimum age:* 6 weeks for both *Rotavirus* (RV)-1 (Rotarix) and RV-5 (RotaTeq)
- Only two doses of RV1 are recommended at present and three doses for RV5
- Three-dose schedule 6-10-14 weeks while two-dose schedule by mouth 6–10 weeks given 4 weeks apart
- The maximum age for the first dose in the series is 14 weeks, 6 days; and 8 months, 0 days for the final dose in the series
- Vaccination should not be initiated for infants aged 15 weeks, 0 days, or older and should not cross 32 weeks.

Catch-up Vaccination

- The maximum age for the first dose in the series is 14 weeks, 6 days.
- Vaccination should not be initiated for infants aged 15 weeks, 0 days or older.
- The maximum age for the final dose in the series is 8 months, 0 days.

Measles, Mumps, and Rubella Vaccine

Routine Vaccination

- *Minimum age:* 9 months or 270 completed days.
- Administer the first dose of MMR vaccine at age 9–12 months, and the second dose at age 15–18 months and the third dose is given at 4–5 years.
- The second dose must follow in second year of life. However, it can be given at any time 4–8 weeks after the first dose.
- No need to give standalone measles vaccine.

Catch-up Vaccination

- Ensure that all school aged children and adolescents have had two doses of MMR vaccine; the minimum interval between the two doses is 4 weeks.
- One dose if previously vaccinated with one dose.
- Standalone measles/measles containing vaccine can be administered to infants aged 6–8 months during outbreaks. However, this dose should not be counted.

Varicella Vaccine

- *Minimum age:* 12 months
- Two-dose series given at age 12–15 months and 4–6 years.
- The risk of breakthrough varicella is lower if given 15 months onward.
- The second dose may be administered before the age of 4 years, provided at least 3 months have elapsed since the first dose.
- For children aged 1–12 years, the recommended minimum interval between doses is 3 months. However, if the second dose was administered at least 4 weeks after the first dose, it can be accepted as valid.
- Children >13 years should receive two doses, 4–8 weeks apart.

Catch-up Vaccination

- Ensure that all persons aged 7–18 years without "evidence of immunity" have two doses of the vaccine.
- For children aged 12 months to 12 years, the recommended minimum interval between doses is 3 months. However, if the second dose was administered at least 4 weeks after the first dose, it can be accepted as valid.
- For persons aged 13 years and older, the minimum interval between doses is 4 weeks.
- For persons without evidence of immunity, administer two doses if not previously vaccinated or the second dose if only one dose has been administered.
- Evidence of immunity to varicella includes any of the following:
    - Documentation of age appropriate vaccination with a varicella vaccine
    - Laboratory evidence of immunity or laboratory confirmation of disease
    - Diagnosis or verification of a history of varicella disease by a healthcare provider
    - Diagnosis or verification of a history of herpes zoster by a healthcare provider
- *Postexposure prophylaxis (PEP):* Vaccine is 90% effective in preventing or modifying the disease if given within 3 days of exposure and 70% effective in preventing if given within 5 days and in both the situation, modification occurs 100%.

Hepatitis A Vaccine

Routine Vaccination

- *Minimum age:* 12 months
- *Killed hepatitis A vaccine:* Start the two-dose hepatitis A vaccine series for children aged 12–23 months; separate the two doses by 6–18 months.
- *Live-attenuated H2-strain hepatitis A vaccine:* Single dose starting at 12 months and through 23 months of age.

Catch-up Vaccination

- Either of the two vaccines can be used in "catch-up" schedule beyond 2 years of age
- Administer two doses for killed vaccine at least 6 months apart to unvaccinated persons
- Only single dose of live-attenuated H2-strain vaccine
- For catch-up vaccination, prevaccination screening for hepatitis A antibody is recommended in children older than 10 years as at this age the estimated sero-positive rates exceed 50%.

Typhoid Vaccine

Routine Vaccination

- Both Vi-PS conjugate and Vi-PS (polysaccharide) vaccines are available
- *Minimum ages:*
    - *Vi-PS (conjugate):* 6 months (preferred)
    - *Vi-PS (polysaccharide) vaccines:* 2 years

- *Vaccination schedule:*
  - *Typhoid conjugate vaccines (Vi-PS):* Single dose at 9–12 through 23 months and a booster during second year of life
  - *Vi-PS (polysaccharide) vaccines:* Single dose at 2 years; revaccination every 3 years
  - An interval of at least 4 weeks with the MMR vaccine should be maintained while administering Vi-PS conjugate vaccine
  - Primary dose of conjugate vaccine should follow a booster at 2 years of age.
  - Either Vi-PS (conjugate) or Vi-polysaccharide (Vi-PS) can be employed as booster
  - Typhoid revaccination every 3 years, if Vi-polysaccharide vaccine is used.
  - No evidence of hyporesponsiveness on repeated revaccination of Vi-polysaccharide vaccine so far.
  - Need of revaccination following a booster of Vi-PS conjugate vaccine is not yet determined.

Catch-up Vaccination

Recommended throughout the adolescent period, i.e., 18 years.

Human Papilloma Virus Vaccine

Routine Vaccination

- *Minimum age:* 9 years
- Human papilloma virus (HPV)-4 (Gardasil) and HPV2 vaccines (Cervarix) are licensed and available.
- Only two doses of either of the two HPV vaccines (HPV4 and HPV2) for adolescent/preadolescent girls aged 9–14 years.
- For girls 15 years and older, and immunocompromised individuals three doses are recommended.
- For two-dose schedule, the minimum interval between doses should be 6 months.
- Either HPV4 (0, 2, and 6 months) or HPV2 (0, 1, and 6 months) is recommended in a three-dose series for females aged 15 years and older.
- HPV4 can also be given in a three-dose series for males aged 11 or 12 years, but not yet licensed for use in males in India
- The vaccine series can be started beginning at age 9 years.
- For three-dose schedule, administer the second dose 1–2 months after the first dose and the third dose 6 months after the first dose (at least 24 weeks after the first dose).

Catch-up Vaccination

- Administer the vaccine series to females (either HPV2 or HPV4) at age 13–45 years if not previously vaccinated.
- Use recommended routine dosing intervals (see above) for vaccine series catch-up.

Influenza Vaccine

- *Minimum age:* 6 months for trivalent inactivated influenza vaccine
- Recommended only for the vaccination of persons with certain high-risk conditions
  - *First time vaccination:* 6 months to below 9 years—two doses 1 month apart; 9 years and above—annual revaccination with single dose
  - *Dosage [trivalent influenza vaccine (TIV)]:* Aged 6–35 months 0.25 mL; 3 years and above 0.5 mL
  - *For children aged 6 months through 8 years:* Administer two doses (separated by at least 4 weeks) to children who are receiving influenza vaccine for the first time
  - All the currently available TIVs in the country contain the swine flu or A (H1N1) antigen; no need to vaccinate separately
- *For children aged 6 months to below 9 years:* For the 2012 season, administer two doses (separated by at least 4 weeks) to those who did not receive at least one dose of the 2010–11 vaccine. Those who received at least one dose of the 2012–13 vaccine require one dose for the 2013–14 season.
- *Best time to vaccinate:* As soon as the new vaccine is released and available in the market and just before the onset of rainy season.

Meningococcal Vaccine

- Meningococcal conjugated and polysaccharide vaccines are available of which when indicated conjugated vaccine is preferred.
- *Minimum age:* 2 years for both the vaccines
  - Recommended only for certain high-risk group of children, during outbreaks, and international travelers, including students going for study abroad and travelers to Hajj and sub-Saharan Africa.
  - Conjugate vaccines are preferred over polysaccharide vaccines due to their potential for herd protection and their increased immunogenicity, particularly in children <2 years of age.

- As of today, quadrivalent conjugate and polysaccharide vaccines are recommended only for children 2 years and above. Monovalent group A conjugate vaccine, PsA–TT can be used in children above 1 year of age. Revaccination only once after 3 years in those at continued high risk for polysaccharide vaccine, conjugate vaccine as of now no booster required.

Cholera Vaccine

- *Minimum age:* 1 year; killed whole cell *Vibrio cholera vaccine (Shanchol)*
- Not recommended for routine use in healthy individuals; recommended only for the vaccination of persons residing in highly endemic areas and traveling to areas where risk of transmission is very high.
- Two doses 2 weeks apart for >1 year.
- For continues risk of exposure, a booster may be administered after 3 years.

Japanese Encephalitis Vaccine

Routine Vaccination

- Recommended only for individuals living in endemic areas
- The vaccine should be offered to the children residing in rural areas only and those planning to visit endemic areas (depending upon the duration of stay)
- Three types of new generation Japanese encephalitis (JE) vaccines are licensed in India; one, live-attenuated, cell culture derived SA 14-14-2, and two inactivated JE vaccines, namely Vero cell culture-derived SA 14-14-2 JE vaccine (JEEV®) and Vero cell culture-derived, 821564XY, JE vaccine (JENVAC®)
- Live-attenuated, cell culture derived SA 14-14-2 (available in National Immunization schedule of Government of India):
  - *Minimum age:* 8 months
  - Two-dose schedule, first dose at 9 months along with measles vaccine and second at 16–18 months along with DTP booster
  - Not available in private market for office use
- Inactivated cell culture derived SA 14-14-2 (JEEV®):
  - *Minimum age:* 1 year (United States Food and Drug Administration: 2 months)
  - *Primary immunization schedule:* Two doses of 0.25 mL each administered intramuscularly on days 0 and 28 for children aged ≥1 year to ≤3 years
  - Two doses of 0.5 mL for children aged >3 years and adults aged 18 years and above at an interval of 4 weeks.
  - Need of boosters still undetermined
- Inactivated Vero cell culture-derived Kolar strain, 821564XY, JE vaccine (JENVAC®):
  - Minimum age: 1 year
  - *Primary immunization schedule:* Two doses of 0.5 mL each administered intramuscularly at 4 weeks interval
  - Need of boosters still undetermined

Catch-up Vaccination

All susceptible children up to 15 years should be administered during disease outbreak/ahead of anticipated outbreak in campaigns.

Rabies Vaccine

- Practically all children need vaccination against rabies.
- Following two situations included in high-risk category of children for rabies vaccination and should be offered preexposure prophylaxis:
  - Children having pets in home
  - Children perceived with higher threat of being bitten by dogs such as hostellers, risk of stray dog menace while going outdoor
- Only modern tissue culture vaccines and intramuscular routes are recommended for both postexposure and preexposure prophylaxis in office practice.
- PEP is recommended following a significant contact with dogs, cats, cows, buffaloes, sheep, goats, pigs, donkeys, horses, camels, foxes, jackals, monkeys, mongoose, squirrel, bears, and others. Domestic rodent (rat) bites do not require PEP in India.
- *PEP:*
  - Modern tissue culture vaccines are recommended for all category II and III bites
  - *Dose:* 1.0 mL intramuscular in anterolateral thigh or deltoid (never in gluteal region) for human diploid cell vaccine, purified chick embryo cell vaccine, purified duck embryo vaccine; 0.5 mL for purified Vero cell vaccine. Intradermal (ID) administration is not recommended in individual practice.
  - *Schedule:* 0, 3, 7, 14, and 28 with day "0" being the day of commencement of vaccination. A sixth dose on day 90 is optional and may be offered to patients with severe debility or those who are immunosuppressed.

- Rabies immunoglobulin (RIG) along with rabies vaccines are recommended in all category III bites.
- Equine RIG (dose 40 U/kg) can be used if human RIG is not available.

- *Preexposure prophylaxis:*
    - Two doses are given intramuscularly in deltoid/anterolateral thigh on days 0, 7 or 2-site ID on day 0 and 7, and 28 (day 21 may be used if time is limited but day 28 preferred).
    - For reexposure at any point of time after completed (and documented) preexposure prophylaxis or PEP, two doses are given on days 0 and 3.
    - RIG is not required during reexposure therapy.

INDIAN ACADEMY OF PEDIATRICS RECOMMENDED VACCINES FOR HIGH-RISK CHILDREN (VACCINES UNDER SPECIAL CIRCUMSTANCES)

Indian Academy of Pediatrics recommended vaccines for high-risk children (vaccines under special circumstances) are as follows:

- Influenza vaccine
- Meningococcal vaccine
- JE vaccine
- Cholera vaccine
- Rabies vaccine
- Yellow fever vaccine
- PPSV23

High-risk category of children:

- Congenital or acquired immunodeficiency (including HIV infection)
- Chronic cardiac, pulmonary (including asthma if treated with prolonged high dose oral corticosteroids), hematologic, renal (including nephrotic syndrome), liver disease, and diabetes mellitus
- Children on long-term steroids, salicylates, immunosuppressive, or radiation therapy
- Diabetes mellitus, cerebrospinal fluid leak, cochlear implant, and malignancies
- Children with functional/anatomic asplenia/hyposplenia
- During disease outbreaks
- Laboratory personnel and healthcare workers
- Travelers

CLINICAL PEARLS

- Constant surveillance is maintained of the various vaccine preventable diseases.
- Vaccine schedule is formulated as per the epidemiology of the disease, need of that particular vaccine, and feasibility.
- Optimal response to a vaccine depends on multiple factors, including the type of vaccine, age of the recipient, and immune status of the recipient.

KEY POINTS

- Certain vaccines are given free of cost to all children in India under NIP.
- IAP has formulated immunization schedule for guiding the members about the available vaccines.
- All the children should be immunized as per the guidelines at specified time and age.

SUGGESTED READING

1. IAP Immunization Timetable 2014-Figure with range and Footnotes. Available from: https://acvip.org/professional/columns/pdf/IAP%20Immunization%20Timetable%202014-Figure%20with%20range%20&%20Footnotes.docx.
2. Plotkin SA, Orenstein WA, Offit PA. Vaccine, 5th edition. Philadelphia: WB Saunders; 2008.
3. Rao MIS, Shivananda S. Immunization in India: past, present, and future. In: Rao MIS, Kasi SG (Eds). Purple book IAP Guidebook On Immunization 2022. New Delhi: Jaypee Brothers Medical Publishers (P) Ltd.; 2023.
4. Yewale V, Choudhury P, Thacker N. IAP Guide Book on Immunization. IAP Committee on Immunization 2009-2011. Mumbai: Indian Academy of Pediatrics; 2011.

Missed Immunization

Ritabrata Kundu, Pratiksha Khatua

INTRODUCTION

Catch-up vaccination is a process of giving missed or delayed vaccinations to individuals who are behind on their immunization schedule to ensure protection against vaccine-preventable diseases. A health care provider evaluates which vaccines are missed and creates an individualized schedule to administer them without unnecessary doses being repeated.

BACILLUS CALMETTE–GUÉRIN VACCINE

If missed at birth, it should be given at the earliest, catch-up can be done till 5 years of age.

HEPATITIS B VACCINE

Hepatitis B vaccine as a 0-1-6 schedule should be given to all children/adolescent who have not been previously vaccinated with hepatitis B/vaccination status not known/administration was inappropriate. Prevaccination screening with anti-hepatitis B surface antigen (HBsAg) antibody is costly and is not recommended routinely.

Catch-up vaccination is important for contacts of HBsAg positive patients. Prevaccination screening should be done in these contacts.

All infants irrespective of birth weight or gestational age born to HbsAg positive mothers should receive a hepatitis B immunoglobulin (HBIG) 0.5 mL on one thigh and a first dose hepatitis B vaccine within 12 hours of birth followed by three doses of hepatitis B containing vaccine at 6-10-14 weeks. Post vaccine testing for HBsAg and anti-HBs should be done at 9–12 months of age.

DIPHTHERIA, TETANUS TOXOIDS, AND PERTUSSIS VACCINE

The recommended schedule is three primary doses at 6, 10, and 14 weeks and two boosters at 15–18 months and 4–5 years.

The second childhood booster is not required if the last dose has been given beyond 4 years of age.

Catch-up <7 years: DTwP/DTaP at 0, 1, and 6 months. The Indian Academy of Pediatrics (IAP)/Advisory Committee on Vaccines and Immunization Practices (ACVIP) does not recommend using Tdap before the age of 7 years.

Catch-up above 7 years: Tdap, Td, and Td at 0, 1, and 6 months. If last dose of Tdap has been administered >9 years the routine adolescent booster (given 10 years through 12 years) is not necessary.

Persons aged 11 years through 18 years who have not received Tdap vaccine should receive a dose followed by tetanus and diphtheria toxoids (Td) booster doses every 10 years.

HAEMOPHILUS INFLUENZAE TYPE B CONJUGATE VACCINE

- Catch-up recommended till 5 years of age.
- *6–12 months:* Two primary doses 4 weeks apart and one booster
- *12–15 months:* One primary dose and one booster dose
- *Above 15 months:* Single dose

PNEUMOCOCCAL CONJUGATE VACCINE

- *6 weeks to 6 months:* Three doses 4 weeks apart plus one booster dose at 12–15 months.
- *7–11 months:* Two doses and one booster dose at second year.
- *12–23 months:* Only two doses "8 weeks apart". No booster required.
- *24–59 months:* One dose of pneumococcal conjugate-13 (PCV13) or two doses of PCV10, 8 weeks apart.
- *24–59 months:* 1 dose of PCV 13 or 2 doses of PCV 10 8 weeks apart. 10v PCV SII (Serum Institute of India) cannot be used after 2 years.

ROTAVIRUS VACCINE

- It can be given from 6 weeks. Maximum age for the first dose in the series is 14 weeks 6 days.
- Vaccination should not be initiated for infants aged 15 weeks 0 days or older.
- The maximum age for the final dose in the series is 8 months 0 days.
- Except RV1 (Rotarix) which has a two-dose schedule, the others are administered in a three-dose schedule (RotaTeq and Rotavac).

MEASLES, MUMPS, AND RUBELLA VACCINE

Catch-up can be done up to 5 years. All school aged children and adolescents should get at least two doses of measles, mumps, and rubella (MMR) vaccine; minimum interval being 4 weeks. One dose is given if previously vaccinated with one dose. During MMR campaign, the vaccine can be administered irrespective of the administration of previous doses.

VARICELLA VACCINE

For catch-up vaccination, children below 13 years should receive two doses 3 months apart and those aged 13 years or more, should receive two doses 4–8 weeks apart.

HEPATITIS A VACCINE

For catch-up vaccination, two doses of the inactivated vaccine (intramuscular) given at 0 month and at 6–18 months or a single dose of the live vaccine can be given (subcutaneous).

For those above 10 years of age, prevaccination screening for hepatitis A antibody is recommended.

TYPHOID VACCINE

Catch-up vaccination, one dose is recommended throughout the adolescent period till 18 years using the conjugate vaccine.

HUMAN PAPILLOMAVIRUS VACCINE VACCINE

CERVAVAC 4-valent human papillomavirus (HPV) vaccine—can be given to males and females 9 years through 26 years. From 9 to 14 years 2 dose schedule (0, 6 months). From 15 to 26 years 3 dose schedule (0, 2, 6 months)

Gardasil 4-valent HPV vaccine—can be given to both males and females 9 years through 26 years as a 3 dose schedule 0, 2, 6 months.

Gardasil 9-valent HPV vaccine—can be given to males from 9 to 14 years and females 9 years through 26 years in a 3 dose schedule (0, 2, 6 months).

JAPANESE ENCEPHALITIS VACCINE

All susceptible children up to 15 years should be administered two doses of either of the two inactivated vaccines at 1 month interval.

KEY POINTS

- Catch-up vaccination aims to provide optimal protection against vaccine-preventable diseases by completing the recommended vaccination schedule.
- Catch-up vaccination not only protects the individual against diseases, but also prevents disease outbreak and therefore acts as a vital tool in global health security.

SUGGESTED READING

1. Hepatitis B vaccines. WHO Position Paper. Weekly Epidemiological Paper Record, No 27.2017.
2. Lokeshwar MR, Singhal T. Immunization against varicella. Immunization in Clinical Practice, 2nd edition. New Delhi: JaypeeBrothers Medical Publishers;2017.
3. Marais BJ, Gie RP, Schaaf HS, Hesseling AC, Obihara CC, Nelson LJ, et al. The clinical epidemiology of childhood pulmonary tuberculosis: a critical review of literature from the pre-chemotherapy era. Int J Tuberc Lung Dis. 2004;8(3):278-85.
4. Panda BK, Mishra S, Awofeso N. Socio-demographic correlates of first dose of measles (MCV1) vaccination coverage in India. BMC Public Health. 2020;20(1):1221.
5. Rotavirus vaccine. WHO Position Paper-July 2021. Weekly epidemiological record. 2021;96:301-19.
6. Sharma H, Yadav S, Lalwani S, Kapre S, Jadhav S, Parekh S, et al. Antibody persistence of two pentavalent DTwP-HB-Hib vaccines to the age of 15-18 months, and response to the booster dose of quadrivalent DTwP-Hib vaccine. Vaccine. 2013;31(3):444-7.
7. WHO. Human Papillomavirus Vaccines: WHO position paper. Wkly Epidemiol Rec. 2017;92(9):241-68.
8. WHO Publication. Pneumococcal vaccines WHO position paper. Vaccine. 2012;14(87):129-44.
9. World Health Organisation. Typhoid vaccines: WHO position paper March 2018. Wkly Epidemiol Rec. 2018; 93:153-72.
10. World Health Organization. Diphtheria vaccine: WHO position paper, August 2017 - Recommendations. Vaccine. 2018;36(2):199-201.
11. Zheng H, Chen Y, Wang F, Gong X, Wu Z, Miao N, et al. Comparing live attenuated and inactivated hepatitis A vaccines: an immunogenicity study after one single dose. Vaccine. 2011;29:9098-103.

CHAPTER 29

Animal Bites

Jaydeep Choudhury

INTRODUCTION

Rabies is a fatal encephalitis. It is a zoonotic disease and transmission to humans occurs by bite of an infected animal. In India, the transmitting animal is dog in more than 95% cases. Though rabies is fatal, once symptoms of the disease develop, it is almost 100% preventable if prophylactic measures are instituted soon after the exposure.

PROBLEMS OF RABIES INFECTION IN CHILDREN

In India and other developing countries, 50–60% of all rabies deaths occur in children (<15 years of age). There are several reasons as to why children are more susceptible:

- Children play in the streets and are more prone for dog bites. Because of their playful nature, they also tend to tease dogs and in consequence, dogs attack them
- Because of their short stature, bites on heads, neck, and upper parts of the body are more common and bites tend to be severe. This results in greater risk for infection with relatively shorter incubation period. Because of their short stature, even bites on lower parts of the body may result in shorter incubation period
- Many times, because of the fear of painful injections that may be given, they even tend to hide the fact that they were bitten
- As children have soft skin, even minor scratches and trivial bites may result in category III exposures.

POSTEXPOSURE PROPHYLAXIS

In rabies endemic country like India, every animal bite is potentially suspected as a rabid animal bite; the treatment should be started immediately. Rabies has long incubation period. Prophylactic postexposure treatment should be started at the earliest to ensure that the individual will be immunized before the rabies virus reaches the nervous system. The classification of animal bite for postexposure prophylaxis (PEP) has been based on these World Health Organization recommendations **(Table 1)**.

Vaccination status of the biting animal: History of rabies vaccination in an animal is not always a guarantee that the biting animal is not rabid. Animal vaccine failures may occur because of improper administration or poor quality of the vaccine, poor health status of the animal, and the fact that one vaccine dose does not always provide long-lasting protection against infection in dogs.

Observation of biting animal: The treatment should always be started immediately after animal bite. The treatment may be modified if animal involved (dog or cat) remains healthy throughout an observation period of 10 days by converting PEP to preexposure vaccination by skipping the vaccine dose on day 14 and administering it on day

TABLE 1: Type of contact, exposure, and recommended post-exposure prophylaxis.

Category	*Type of contact*	*Type of exposure*	*Recommended postexposure prophylaxis*
I	• Touching or feeding of animals • Licks on intact skin	None	None, if reliable case history is available
II	• Nibbling of uncovered skin • Minor scratches or abrasions without bleeding	Minor	Wound management + antirabies vaccine
III	• Single or multiple transdermal bites or scratches, licks on broken skin • Contamination of mucous membrane with saliva (i.e., licks)	Severe	Wound management + rabies immuno-globulin + antirabies vaccine

28 while using Essen schedule. The observation period is valid for dogs and cats only. The natural history of rabies in mammals other than dogs or cats is not fully understood and therefore the 10-day observation period is not applicable.

Approach to Postexposure Prophylaxis

The PEP consists of three parameters and should be done simultaneously as per the category of the bites:

1. Management of animal bite wound(s)
2. *Passive immunization:* Rabies immunoglobulins (RIGs)
3. *Active immunization:* Antirabies vaccines (ARVs).

Management of Animal Bite Wound

Wound toilet: Since the rabies virus enters the human body through a bite or scratch, it is imperative to remove as much saliva as possible. Since the rabies virus can persist and even multiply at the site of bite for a long time, wound toilet must be performed even if the patient reports late **(Table 2)**.

Prompt and gentle thorough washing with soap or detergent and flushing the wound with running water for 10 minutes can do this.

The application of irritants is unnecessary and damaging. In case irritants have been applied on the wound, enough gentle washing with soap or detergent to remove the extraneous material, especially oil, should be done followed by flushing with copious amount of water for 10 minutes immediately.

Application of antiseptic: After thorough washing and drying the wound, any one of the available chemical agents should be applied, viz.: povidone iodine (solution), alcohol, chloroxylenol, chlorhexidine gluconate, and cetrimide solution in appropriate recommended dilution.

TABLE 2: Do's and don'ts of wound management.

Step of wound management	*Purpose*
Do's	
Physical wash under running tap water for at least 10 minutes	Mechanical removal of virus from the wound
Chemical washing the wound with soap and water, dry, and apply disinfectant	Inactivation of the virus
Biological infiltration of immunoglobulins in the depth and around the wound in category III exposures	Neutralization of the virus
Don'ts	
• Touch the wound with bare hand • Apply irritants like soil, chilies, oil, herbs, chalk, betel leaves, etc.	

Local infiltration of RIGs: In category III bites, RIG should be infiltrated in the depth and around the wound to inactivate the locally present virus as described below.

Suturing of wound: It should be avoided as far as possible. If surgical intervention is unavoidable, minimum loose sutures should be applied after adequate local treatment along with proper infiltration of RIGs.

Tetanus toxoid injection (anti-tetanus prophylaxis): This should be given to those children who had not received a booster dose. A properly immunized child can only take one dose of tetanus toxoid if there is a lapse of a period of 5 years from the last dose of tetanus toxoid.

To prevent sepsis in the wound, a suitable course of an antibiotic may be recommended.

Rabies Immunoglobulin

The RIG provides passive immunity to tide over the initial phase of the infection.

Two types of RIGs are available:

1. *Equine rabies immunoglobulin (ERIG):* It is of heterologous origin raised by hyperimmunization of horses. The currently manufactured ERIGs are highly purified and enzyme refined, with these preparations, the occurrence of adverse reaction has been significantly reduced.
2. *Human rabies immunoglobulins (HRIGs):* As it is homologous, HRIG is free from the side effects encountered in a serum of heterologous origin, and because of their longer half-life, are given in half the dose of equine antirabies serum.

Dose of rabies immunoglobulins:

- The dose of ERIG is 40 IU/kg body weight of patient and is given after testing for sensitivity, up to a maximum of 3,000 IU. The ERIG produced in India contains 300 IU/mL.
- The dose of the HRIG is 20 IU/kg body weight (maximum 1,500 IU). HRIG does not require any prior sensitivity testing. HRIG preparation is available in concentration of 150 IU/mL.

Administration of immunoglobulins: As much of the calculated dose of RIG as is anatomically feasible should be infiltrated into and around the wounds. Remaining, if any, after all wounds have been infiltrated, should be administered by deep intramuscular (IM) injection at an injection site distant from the vaccine injection site. The total recommended dose of immunoglobulin must not be exceeded as it may suppress the antibody production by the vaccine.

If immunoglobulin was not administered when vaccination was begun, it can be administered up to the seventh day after the administration of the first dose of vaccine.

In circumstances where no immunoglobulins are available, greater emphasis should be given to proper wound toileting followed by Essen schedule of cell-culture vaccine (CCV) with double dose on day 0 at two different sites intramuscularly (0 day: 2 doses on left and right deltoid, following the single dose on each day, i.e., day 3, 7, 14, and 28). It is emphasized that doubling the first dose of CCV is not a replacement to RIG. A full course of vaccine should follow thorough wound cleansing and passive immunization.

Antirabies Vaccines

Active immunization is achieved by administration of safe and potent CCVs or purified duck embryo vaccines (PDEV). The dosage schedule of cell culture rabies vaccine (CCV/CCRV) is same irrespective of the body weight or age of the children.

- *Storage and transportation:* It is recommended that these vaccines should be kept and transported at a temperature range of 2–8°C. Freezing does not damage the lyophilized vaccine but there are chances of breakage of ampoule containing the diluent. Liquid vaccines should never be frozen
- *Reconstitution and storage:* The lyophilized vaccine should be reconstituted with the diluent provided with the vaccine immediately prior to use. In case of unforeseen delay it should be used within 6–8 hours of reconstitution.

Intramuscular regimen: The currently available vaccines and regimens in India for IM administration are described below.

- *Antirabies vaccines:*
  - Cell-culture vaccines:
    - *Human diploid cell vaccine:* Produced locally in private sector
    - *Purified chick embryo cell vaccine:* Produced locally in private sector
    - *Purified vero-cell rabies vaccine:* Imported and produced locally in public and private sectors
  - Purified duck embryo vaccine:
    - Produced locally in private sector.

Note: All CCRVs and purified duck embryo vaccine used for PEP should have potency (antigen content) greater than 2.5 IU/dose.

- Regimen:
  - *Essen schedule (5-dose IM regimen):* The course for PEP should consist of IM administration of 5 injections on day 0, 3, 7, 14, and 28. Day 0 indicates date of first injection.
  - *Site of inoculation:* The anterolateral thigh region is ideal for the inoculation of these vaccines in infants and younger children, whereas the older children can take in deltoid regions. Gluteal region is not recommended because the fat present in this region retards the absorption of antigen and hence impairs the generation of optimal immune response.

Intradermal (ID) regimens: It consists of administration of a fraction of IM dose of CCVs on multiple sites in the layers of dermis of skin. The use of ID route leads to considerable savings in terms of total amount of vaccine needed for full pre- or postexposure vaccination, thereby reducing the cost of active immunization. In ID route, small amount (0.1 mL) of rabies vaccines/antigen is deposited in the layers of the skin at two or more sites:

- Intradermal vaccine regimen:
  - *Updated Thai Red Cross Schedule (2-2-2-0-2):* This involves injection of 0.1 mL of reconstituted vaccine per ID site and on two such ID sites per visit (one on each deltoid area, an inch above the insertion of deltoid muscle) on day 0, 3, 7, and 28. The day 0 is the day of first-dose administration of intradermal rabies vaccines (IDVR) (ID inoculation of ARV) and may not be the day of rabies exposure/animal bite
  - Antirabies treatment centers which meet the following criteria may use ID administration:
    - Have adequately trained staff to give IDRV
    - Can maintain cold chain for vaccine storage
    - Ensure adequate supply of suitable syringes and needles for ID administration
    - Are adequately well versed in management of open vial and safe storage practices.

Postexposure Therapy for Previously Vaccinated Children

Children who have previously received full PEP or preexposure vaccination (either by IM or ID routes) with a potent CCV should now be given only two booster doses: IM (0.5 mL/1 mL)/ID (0.1 mL at 1 site) on day 0 and 3 irrespective of the duration of previous vaccination. Proper wound toilet should be done. Treatment with RIG is not necessary.

Preexposure Vaccination of Children

As rabies is a 100% fatal disease and children constitute a special risk for getting the infection, it may be advisable to vaccinate children after they attain the age of 3 years and start playing in the streets and may come in contact with street or pet dogs.

Schedule of Preexposure Vaccination

- *Intramuscular:* 3 doses of any CCVs (1 mL or 0.5 mL depending on the brand) administered on the anterolateral thigh on day 0, 7, and 28.

Flowchart 1: Algorithm for management of children exposed to animal bites.

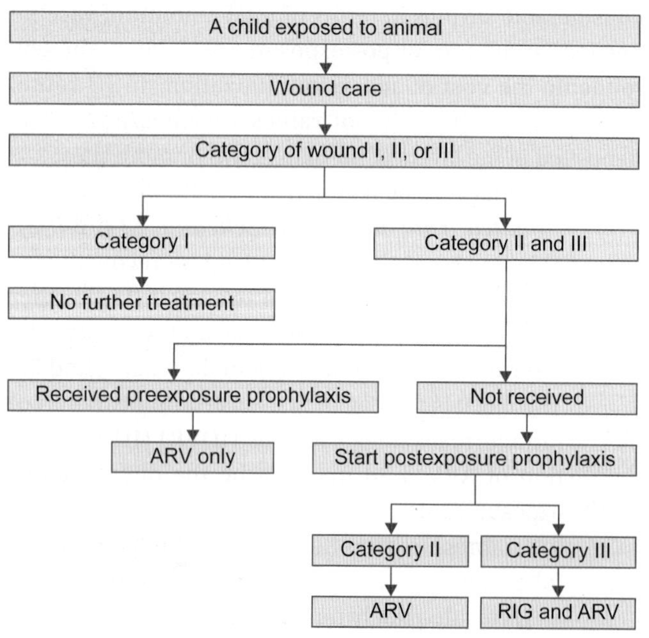

(ARV: antirabies vaccines; PEP: postexposure prophylaxis; RIG: rabies immunoglobulins)

- *Intradermal:* The dose is same for all vaccine brands and 0.1 mL is administered ID over the deltoid on day 0, 7, and 28.

The management of children exposed to animal bites is shown in **Flowchart 1**.

CLINICAL PEARLS

- The transmitting animal of rabies is dog in more than 95% cases.
- Rabies is fatal once symptoms of the disease develop, but it is almost 100% preventable if prophylactic measures are instituted soon after the exposure.
- Intradermal rabies vaccination is given in state run rabies clinics, where many people come for rabies vaccine daily.
- Rabies immunoglobulins is not needed for person who have received full course of rabies vaccine.

KEY POINTS

- In rabies endemic country like India, every animal bite is potentially suspected as a rabid animal bite the treatment should be started immediately.
- Children have soft skin, therefore, even minor scratches and trivial bites may result in category III exposures.
- Prompt and gentle thorough washing with soap or detergent and flushing the wound with running water for 10 minutes.
- Children above 3 years of age may be routinely given preexposure prophylaxis of antirabies vaccines.

SUGGESTED READING

1. Sudarshan MK. (2003). Assessing burden of rabies in India: WHO sponsored National Multi-centric Rabies Survey. [online] Available from: rabies.org.in/rabies-journal/rabies-06/SpecialArticle1.htm. [Accessed November, 2015].
2. Sudarshan MK. Rabies. In: Parthasarathy A, Kundu R, Agrawal R, et al. (Eds). Textbook of Pediatric Infectious Diseases, 1st edition. New Delhi, India: Jaypee Brothers Medical Publishers; 2013.
3. World Health Organization. WHO Expert Consultation on Rabies: First Report. Technical Report Series 931. Geneva, Switzerland: World Health Organization; 2005.
4. World Health Organization. WHO Recommendations on Rabies Post-exposure Treatment and the Correct Technique of Intra-dermal Immunization against Rabies. Geneva, Switzerland: World Health Organization; 1997.

Adverse Event Following Immunization

Amar Jeet Chitkara

INTRODUCTION

Childhood morbidity and mortality has witnessed tremendous decrease following widespread immunization in the last 30–40 years across the globe. Many new vaccines are being developed and introduced in both the public and private sectors. Though the vaccines are of documented safety and efficacy, yet infrequently have adverse events. These adverse events can be a strong deterrent to the acceptability of vaccines; hence it is imperative to have a comprehensive surveillance system to address these concerns, especially with the introduction of many new vaccines/products and that too in a country with 27 million births per year and an extensive expanded program of immunization with constraints of medical care access. The adverse event following immunization (AEFI) is defined as "a medical incident that takes place after immunization, causes concern, and is believed to be caused by the immunization".

WHY REPORT ADVERSE EVENT FOLLOWING IMMUNIZATION?

Vaccines are always administered to healthy infants and children to provide protection against dreadful diseases, hence any alteration in health with a temporal association with the vaccine be it fever, erythema, local pain and swelling, or a major event leading to disability, hospitalization, or death, erodes the confidence of the caregivers in the program and any nonacceptance can have serious outcomes as regards morbidity and mortality by vaccine preventable deaths (VPDs). Ironically, with widespread vaccination, the disease burden decreases and even mild AEFI become noticeable.

NATIONAL ADVERSE EVENT FOLLOWING IMMUNIZATION PROGRAM

Though started along with Universal Immunization Program in 1985, the real thrust started only in 2005 in collaboration with the World Health Organization (WHO)/ National Polio Surveillance Project, India. Operational guidelines were developed and disseminated widely across the country in the public sector by organizing multiple workshops. The program was further strengthened in 2010 with the highest AEFI reports during the year. The initiative by the Indian Academy of Pediatrics (IAP) to collaborate with the national program has been a welcome step. The detailed operational guidelines and standard operating procedures are available in the public domain as well as print. The cases are then taken up for causality assessment as per the standard WHO protocol **(Flowchart 1)**.

Flowchart 1: World Health Organization: Causality assessment of serious adverse event following immunizations.

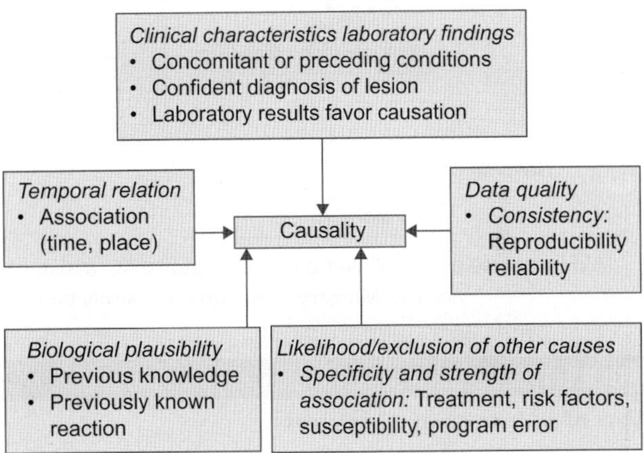

WHAT TO REPORT

Serious AEFI, such as death, disability, and hospitalization, need to be reported immediately while minor AEFI, such as fever and local reactions are reported through monthly reports in the public health. The reporting hierarchy and the timelines are given in **Flowchart 2**. From the programmatic purpose, the AEFIs are classified into five broad categories of AEFI: (1) Programmatic error, (2) vaccine reaction, (3) injection reactions, (4) coincidental, and (5) unknown **(Table 1)**.

Flowchart 2: Reporting framework and timelines.

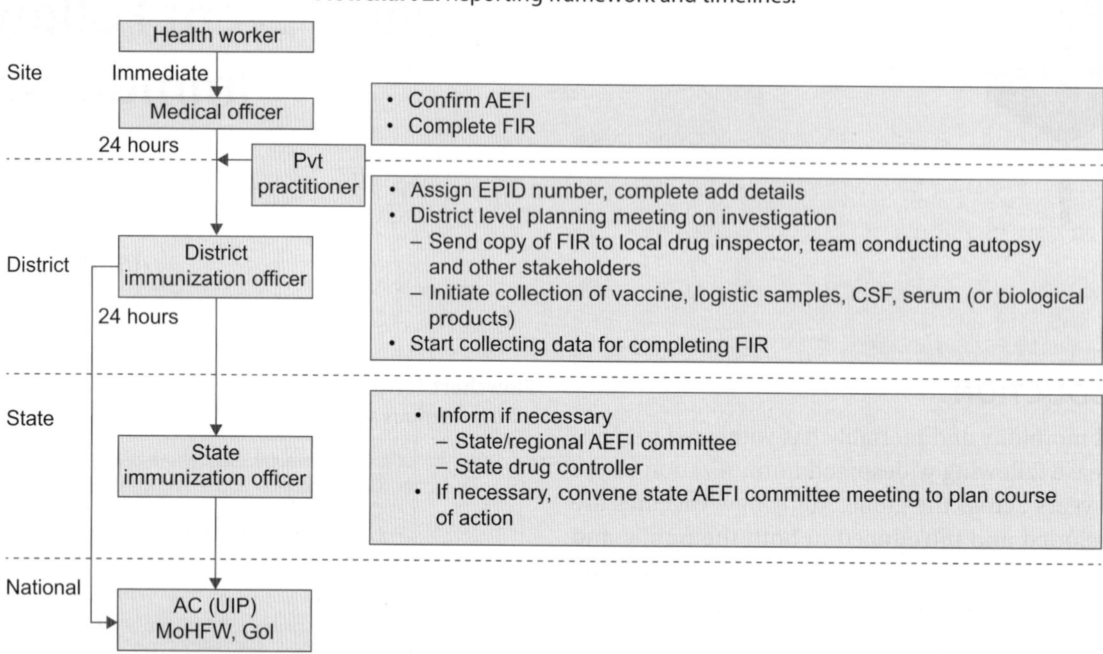

(AEFI: adverse event following immunizations; AC: assistant commissioner; CSF: cerebrospinal fluid; GoI: Government of India; MoHFW: Ministry of Health and Family Welfare; Pvt: private; UIP: Universal Immunization Program)

TABLE 1: Types of adverse event following immunizations.

Types of adverse event	***Examples***
Vaccine reaction	High grade fever following diphtheria, pertussis, and tetanus toxoids vaccination and anaphylaxis
Program error	Bacterial abscess due to unsterile injection/wrong diluent
Coincidental	Pneumonia after oral polio vaccine
Injection reaction	Fainting spell after immunization
Unknown	–

REPORTING FROM PRIVATE SECTOR

It has been estimated that about 9% of the national population gets vaccinated at private facilities and there exists a considerable heterogeneity varying from 10 to 30%, especially being high in urban and metros across the country. The AEFI reporting from private sector has been exceptionally low because of a fear of reporting and harassment following the event. It should also be noted that since all new vaccines evolve from the private sector, the AEFI from this sector has a very high potential for assessing the safety of these vaccines. Since 2011, IAP has taken an initiative to collaborate with national AEFI program to encourage reporting. The infectious disease surveillance, a web and SMS-based surveillance of VPDs has a built in portal of reporting AEFI that follows the standard operating procedures. The information automatically reaches the concerned district immunization officer (DIO), state immunization officer, and Ministry of Health and Family Welfare (MoHFW) for appropriate action. Also, the fear and anxiety of IAP members in reporting has been allayed to a great extent by official communication and talks with MoHFW in this regard. The doctors can also report to their DIOs, medical officer, of nearest primary health center directly. The event is then investigated by DIO and the local AEFI committee; however, the reporting physician is expected to cooperate. The keyword remains creating awareness about utility of AEFI reporting and allaying fears associated with reporting. An increased collaboration with the various AEFI committees and nominating the practicing physicians to these committees can further augment national AEFI program. Another good initiative in the recent years has been the vaccine manufacturer's phase 4/postmarketing surveillance as per the Government of India (GoI)/Central Drugs Standard Control Organisation (CDSCO)/Drugs Controller General of India (DCGI) regulations to map and collect data on AEFI for the recently licensed vaccine through their respective portal.

CLINICAL PEARL

- Report AEFI and feel safe.

KEY POINTS

- Vaccine adverse events are uncommon/rare and can be minor or major.
- Reporting AEFI is an essential component of immunization programs in public/private sectors to ensure public trust and compliance in immunization programs.
- Major AEFI like hospitalization, diasability or death are to be notified to appropriate authorities, to assess the causality.

THE WAY FORWARD

- Collaboration with all professional bodies who vaccinate their patient's across all ages to report AEFI.
- Create awareness among medical fraternity about the strengths of AEFI reporting to evaluate safety aspects of vaccines used and available currently. This can be achieved by a concerted effort through the continuing medical educations, conferences, and print publications of various professional organizations.
- National, state, and district AEFI committees to have representatives from private sector to instill confidence amongst reporting physicians.
- Creating user friendly reporting network, especially an E-network like IDSURV.org and promoting public private partnership toward achieving this.
- Inculcate confidence among practicing doctors in reporting AEFI by strong assurance from the MoHFW and state health departments regarding no harassment following these reports.

SUGGESTED READING

1. Black RE, Counsens S, Johnson HL, Lawn JE, Rudan I, Bassani DG, et al. Global, regional, and national causes of child mortality in 2008: a systematic analysis. Lancet. 2010;375(9730):1969-87.
2. Centers for Disease Control and Prevention (CDC). Global routine vaccine coverage, 2010. MMWR Morb Mortal Wkly Rep. 2011;60(44):1520-2.
3. Chen RT, Rastogi SC, Mullen JR, Hayes SW, Cochi SL, Donlon JA, et al. The vaccine adverse event reporting system (VAERS). Vaccine. 1994;12(6):542-50.
4. Ministry of Health and Family Welfare (MoHFW). Adverse Events Following Immunization: Surveillance and Response Operational Guidelines. New Delhi: Ministry of Health and Family Welfare; 2006.
5. Ministry of Health and Family Welfare (MoHFW). Adverse Events Following Immunization: Surveillance and Response Operational Guidelines. New Delhi: Ministry of Health and Family Welfare; 2010.
6. Ministry of Health and Family Welfare (MoHFW). Adverse Events Following Immunization: Surveillance and Response Standard Operating Procedures. New Delhi: Ministry of Health and Family Welfare; 2010.
7. Ministry of Health and Family Welfare (MoHFW). Multi Year Strategic Plan (MYP) for UIP of India 2005-10. New Delhi: Ministry of Health and Family Welfare; 2010.
8. World Health Organization (WHO), United Nations Children's Fund (UNICEF), World Bank. State of World Vaccines and Immunization, 3rd edition. Geneva, Switzerland: World Health Organization; 2009.
9. World Health Organization. Aide Memoir on AEFI investigation. Geneva, Switzerland: World Health Organization; 2005.
10. World Health Organization. Surveillance of Adverse Events following Immunization: Field Guide for Managers of Immunization Programs. Geneva, Switzerland: World Health Organization; 1997.

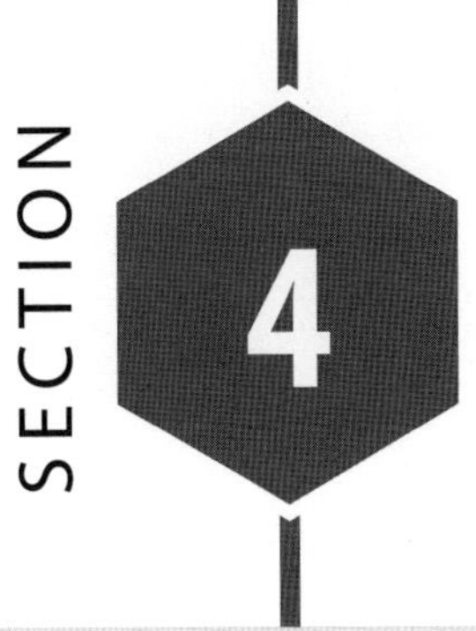

Office Emergencies

Section Editors: *Ajit Gajendragadkar, Rajesh R Chokhani*

Approach to Respiratory Distress in Children

Narendra R Nanivadekar

INTRODUCTION

Respiratory distress is one of the most common complaints presenting to the pediatric emergency department. As many conditions causing respiratory distress have the potential to lead to respiratory failure, it requires a rapid and systematic assessment to facilitate diagnosis and quick efficient management. As the respiratory causes are the most common to cause cardiopulmonary failure in pediatric age. A systematic approach can help us to recognize respiratory distress sufficiently early, before it progresses to respiratory failure, and initiate appropriate supportive and specific management which can improve the outcome.

APPROACH

This section discusses the diagnostic approach to respiratory distress. Management of respiratory distress is dealt with in another section subsequently.

Initial Impression

The first step is a quick audiovisual assessment done within seconds of establishing contact with the child. The aim is to identify the need for cardiopulmonary resuscitation (CPR) and prioritize interventions before proceeding further with a detailed systematic assessment **(Table 1)**.

TABLE 1: Initial impression.

Consciousness	Level of consciousness (e.g., unresponsive, irritable, and alert)
Breathing	Increased work of breathing, absent/ decreased respiratory effort, or abnormal sounds heard without auscultation
Color	Abnormal skin color such as cyanosis, mottling, and pallor

This is followed by a detailed evaluation which consists of primary and secondary assessments and diagnostic tests. This helps us to identify the type and severity of the problem.

Primary Assessment

Primary assessment is a hands-on evaluation of airway, breathing, circulation, disability, and exposure, which includes vital signs and pulse oximetry.

Airway

Airway patency can be checked by looking for the movement of the chest and abdomen and listening for the air movement and breath sounds **(Table 2)**.

A child with a foreign body airway obstruction may require an advanced airway technique such as laryngoscopy or bronchoscopy. Increased inspiratory effort with retractions, abnormal inspiratory sounds (snoring or high-pitched stridor) suggest that the child has an upper airway obstruction (UAO). Episodes where no airway or breath sounds are present despite respiratory effort may suggest complete airway obstruction.

TABLE 2: Assessment of the airway.

Observation	*Inference (airway status)*	*Implication*
Normal chest movement and silent breathing	Clear	Open and unobstructed
Stridor, gurgling, and snoring +/− suprasternal retractions	Partially obstructed/ maintainable	Maintained by simple measures such as position and suction
No chest movement or breath sounds	Complete obstruction/not maintainable	Needs advanced measures such as intubation

Breathing

Evaluation of breathing is helpful to diagnose most causes of respiratory distress. The components are:

- Respiratory rate
- Effort
- Chest expansion and air movement
- Lung and airway sounds
- O_2 saturation by pulse oximetry

Respiratory rate: Respiratory rate should be evaluated before the hands-on evaluation as anxiety and agitation will make it difficult to assess.

Children with respiratory distress are typically tachypneic. Though the normal respiratory rate varies with age, for practical purposes, at any age respiratory rate > 60 indicates abnormality. Though nonspecific, it is the first sign of respiratory distress. Quiet tachypnea (with normal respiratory effort) may be due to nonpulmonary causes such as fever, anemia, pain, sepsis, congestive cardiac failure, or mild metabolic acidosis. Bradypnea may be due to either neuromuscular weakness primarily or after persistent tachypnea leading to fatigue secondarily. Either way it is an ominous sign. Occasionally, it may be due to central causes. Any respiratory rate below 10 per minute requires further evaluation.

CLINICAL PEARLS

- Bradycardia when associated with other signs of decreased perfusion, most commonly indicates hypoxia, and is an ominous sign demanding urgent action.

Respiratory effort: Usually, a child with respiratory distress will have increased effort. Increased effort will be seen as nasal flaring, use of other accessory muscles, retractions, head bobbing, or see-saw respirations. Additionally, we may encounter prolonged inspiration or expiration, open-mouth breathing, or gasping. Grunting indicates that the child has severe respiratory distress.

Nasal flaring will be seen commonly in infants and younger children. Subcostal, substernal, or intercostal retractions indicate mild distress whereas supraclavicular, suprasternal, or sternal retractions suggest severe distress. The type of retractions may also vary with the site of disease—predominant suprasternal retractions are seen in UAO, intercostal retractions in parenchymal lung disease, and subcostal retractions in lower airway obstruction (LAO) **(Table 3)**.

Head bobbing is a sign of respiratory failure and warrants an early intervention. Similarly see-saw respiration is characteristic of neuromuscular weakness in infants and children and indicates that the patient is getting fatigued fast and needs urgent intervention.

TABLE 3: Abnormal sounds and their explanation.

Stridor	An inspiratory, coarse, and high-pitched sound	Upper airway obstruction (extrathoracic)
Grunting	Expiratory short and low-pitched sound	Smaller airway collapse, alveolar collapse, or both
Wheezing	Musical sound heard chiefly during expiration	Lower airway obstruction, chiefly smaller airways (intrathoracic)
Crackles	Sharp, crackling sounds	Wet in a lung tissue disease such as pneumonia or pulmonary edema or dry as in atelectasis or interstitial lung disease
Gurgling	Coarser sounds	Secretions, vomitus, or blood

Chest wall expansion: Decreased or asymmetric chest wall expansion can be due to inadequate effort, airway obstruction, atelectasis, pneumothorax, hemothorax, pleural effusion, mucus plug, or foreign, body aspiration. By and large the diseased side would be moving less.

Air movement: While normal inspiratory sounds will be soft quiet noises with observed inspiratory effort, expiration may be short and quiet, at times inaudible. The presence of abnormal sounds along with respiratory distress often gives clues to the diagnosis.

Pulse oximeter can be considered as another vital sign which may indicate hypoxia long before cyanosis or bradycardia is evident. Preferably it should be done continuously during stabilization of the patient.

Circulation

Circulation assessment consists of evaluation of heart rate and rhythm, pulses (both central and peripheral), capillary refill time, skin color and temperature, and blood pressure. This needs to be done to complete the overall evaluation of the patient and to categorize whether the child also has a circulatory disorder which may be secondary to respiratory insufficiency or may be coexisting.

Disability

The aim is to assess the neurological perfusion/function, either by the alert, voice, pain, unresponsive (AVPU scale), or the Glasgow Coma Scale.

Exposure

This will give an idea about the presence of bruises, petechiae, and the body temperature of the child.

Secondary Assessment

This is to be done after primary assessment is completed and appropriate interventions have been instituted to stabilize the child. It comprises of a focused history and focused physical examination. The focused history can be best remembered by the mnemonic *SAMPLE*: *S*igns and symptoms, *A*llergies, *M*edications, *P*ast medical history, *L*ast meal, and *E*vents. This can be followed with a focused physical examination. This should include careful assessment of the primary area of concern of the illness or injury.

DIAGNOSTIC TESTS

These are performed to confirm the diagnosis or to determine the severity of illness. They are chiefly laboratory evaluation such as complete blood count, arterial blood gas, biochemistry, and radiology such as X-ray and computed tomography scan.

At any point of time, if a life-threatening situation is encountered, one must initiate CPR **(Table 4)**.

In view of the potential life-threatening situation, a detailed history taking may be done only after the child is stabilized **(Table 5)**.

GENERAL APPROACH TO A CHILD IN RESPIRATORY DISTRESS

Children, who present with breathlessness to the emergency department, are likely to be suffering from respiratory, cardiac, or metabolic conditions. History is extremely useful in deciding the probable etiology of breathlessness. A careful evaluation of what the chief complaints are, as well as the onset, duration, and progress of the same, provides valuable clues. Specific findings on physical examination can further suggest the probable diagnosis.

The most common causes of breathlessness are "respiratory". If one identifies the problem to be primarily respiratory, after the assessment one should be able to decide the physiological type of the problem and the severity of the respiratory problem in the patient, which may help us in initiating a specific treatment.

Based on the severity, respiratory problems can be classified into respiratory distress and respiratory failure **(Table 6)**.

Respiratory Distress

Respiratory distress is a clinical state characterized by abnormal respiratory rate or effort. It is commonly characterized by tachypnea and increased respiratory

TABLE 4: Signs of life-threatening illness in a child with respiratory distress.

Airway	Complete or severe airway obstruction
Breathing	Apnea/bradypnea, markedly increased work of breathing
Circulation	Absence of detectable pulse, poor perfusion, hypotension, and bradycardia
Disability	Unresponsiveness
Exposure	Significant hypothermia or bleeding, petechiae, or purpura consistent with septic shock

TABLE 5: Additional diagnostic evaluation that may help in respiratory distress.

History	Time frame	Acute, recurrent, or chronic nature of progression
	Associated symptoms	Cough, fever, rash, and chest pain
	Preceding events	Choking, foreign body inhalation, trauma, exposure to chemical, or environmental irritants
	Family history	Exposure to infections, tuberculosis, and atopy
Diagnostic workup	Direct laryngoscopy	If upper airway obstruction is detected/suspected
	X-rays	Chest, lateral neck, and decubitus
	Arterial blood gas	Hypoxia (PaO_2 < 60 mm Hg), hypercarbia ($PaCO_2$ > 40 mm Hg), and SaO_2 monitoring
		Acidosis (pH < 7.3) and alkalosis (pH > 7.5)
	Sepsis workup	Blood counts and culture studies

(PaO_2: partial pressure of arterial oxygen; $PaCO_2$: partial pressure of carbon dioxide; SaO_2: saturated oxygen of arterial blood)

TABLE 6: Categorization by type and severity.

	Type	*Severity*
Respiratory distress	• Upper airway obstruction • Lower airway obstruction • Lung tissue disease • Disordered control of breathing	• Respiratory distress • Respiratory failure

effort (increased work of breathing). Thus, it is a physiological state in which the child is trying to maintain adequate gas exchange despite a respiratory pathology, by increasing the rate and effort. However, in the absence of effective intervention, a point may be reached at which adequate gas exchange can no longer be maintained despite the increased rate and effort. When this happens, the child is said to have progressed into the state of respiratory failure.

During this progression, at times, the respiratory rate and effort may fall secondary to respiratory fatigue; thus, at times, severe respiratory distress is clinically evident in the form of hypoventilation and is an indication of respiratory failure.

Respiratory Failure

Respiratory failure is defined as inadequate oxygenation, ventilation, or both. Since respiratory distress and respiratory failure represent a continuum, respiratory failure can be identified clinically by recognizing definite clinical signs of hypoxemia or hypercarbia, in addition to the signs of respiratory distress **(Table 7)**.

Though neurological illnesses can lead to "breathlessness", they are unlikely to present with breathlessness as the only/chief complaint. Whether the neurological illness is acute (head injury, encephalitis, or meningitis) or subacute/chronic (Guillain-Barré syndrome or spinal muscular atrophy), there will usually be a prominent history of the initiating/primary events which will suggest the possible cause of hypo/hyperventilation. It is important to note that alteration of sensorium in a child with hypo/hyperventilation does not necessarily mean a primary neurological illness; it could be the end result of any progressive cardiorespiratory pathology as well. Similarly, though see-saw respiration is classically seen in neuromuscular weakness, it could be seen as a preterminal event in any severe respiratory pathology. Therefore, as mentioned above, history is crucial.

If the clinical signs suggest that the type of respiratory problem is "lung tissue disease", the more common causes are pneumonia, acute respiratory distress syndrome (ARDS), and cardiac causes. The detection of cardiac failure, shock, or cyanosis may suggest a cardiac cause of breathlessness **(Table 8)**. Approach to a child with breathing difficulty is represented in **Flowchart 1**.

TABLE 7: Clinical signs of respiratory distress and failure.

Respiratory distress	*Respiratory failure*
• Tachypnea • Tachycardia • Increased respiratory effort • Abnormal airway sounds • Pale cool skin • Changes in mental status	• (Early) Marked tachypnea/ tachycardia • (Late) Bradypnea, apnea/ bradycardia • Increased/decreased/no respiratory effort • Cyanosis agitation, incessant crying, fighting the oxygen mask or combativeness, and diaphoresis • Stupor/coma

TABLE 8: Diagnostic clues to the cause of breathlessness.

"Type" of problem	*Specific features*	*Common causes and their additional clues*
Upper airway obstruction	Stridor, a change in voice, e.g., hoarseness, the presence of a barking cough, drooling, and suprasternal retractions	• Supraglottic—epiglottitis, retropharyngeal abscess • Glottic—acute laryngotracheobronchitis • Infraglottic—bacterial tracheitis
Lower airway obstruction	Wheezing, a particularly increased expiratory effort, subcostal retractions	• Asthma—acute onset, episodic/intermittent breathlessness; fever +/–, and prominent cough Bronchiolitis—infant, prodrome, seasonality, and fever +/–
Lung tissue disease	Grunting, crackles, and diminished breath sounds	• Pneumonia—high fever and chest pain +/– • Pulmonary edema and ARDS (both usually secondary to other causes)
Disordered control of breathing	History of primary illness, significant alteration of sensorium, variable respiratory rate (tachypnea alternating with bradypnea), and poor respiratory effort (shallow breathing, seesaw breathing)	Neurological illnesses

(ARDS: acute respiratory distress syndrome)

Flowchart 1: General algorithmic approach to respiratory distress in children.

Identify breathlessness
↓
Complete assessment
- Initial assessment
- Primary assessment
- Secondary assessment
- Diagnostic tests

↓ Support A, B, C as required
↓
Classify severity
- Respiratory distress
- Respiratory failure

↓
Decide possible cause
↓
- Upper airway obstruction, e.g., croup, retropharyngeal abscess, foreign body
- Lower airway obstruction, e.g., bronchiolitis, asthma foreign body bronchus
- • Parenchymal disease • Pneumonia • ARDS • ILD
- • Disordered control of breathing • GB syndrome • Status epilepticus

For diagnosis of each condition please refer to Table no. 8

- Specific investigations
- Specific management

(ARDS: acute respiratory distress syndrome; GBS: Guillain-Barré syndrome; ILD: interstitial lung disease)

Flowchart 2: Approach to upper airway obstruction.

Feature suggestive of upper airway obstruction
↓
Signs of severe airway obstruction
- Yes → Emergency call for an anesthesiologist and otolaryngologist to assist with securing the airway
- No → Fever
  - No → • Foreign body • Angioedema • Caustic ingestion • Trauma
  - Yes → High-grade fever, toxic appearance
    - Yes → Severe dysphagia with odynophagia with drooling
      - Yes → Neck pain/Stiffness
        - Yes → Retropharyngeal abscess
        - No → Epiglottitis
      - No → • Barking cough • Tracheal tenderness
        - Yes → Bacterial tracheitis
        - No → • Trismus • U/L tonsillar enlargement → Peritonsillar abscess
    - No → Barking cough with hoarseness
      - Yes → Croup
      - No → B/L tonsillar enlargement
        - Yes → Infectious mononucleosis
        - No → Membrane → Diphtheria

CLINICAL PEARLS

- In general, management of respiratory distress does not require an immediate chest radiograph; most conditions are apparent clinically and waiting for radiography to initiate treatment can waste precious time.

KEY POINTS

- *Initial assessment:* Appearance, work of breathing, and circulation
- Manage/restore airway, breathing, and circulation.
- Provide high-flow oxygen.
- Immediate management of specific clinical condition
- Detailed clinical assessment to localize illness to respiratory system (UAO, LAO, and parenchymal illness), cardiovascular system, or neurological illness **(Flowchart 2)**
- If UAO is severe, airway management precedes diagnostic tests.
- X-ray chest is not mandatory in the initial stage in majority of the cases.
- Specific investigations and treatment should be based on the likely cause identified on clinical evaluation.
- Start CPR at any point a life-threatening event is encountered.

SUGGESTED READING

1. Approach to upper airway obstruction—Adapted from https://www.uptodate.com/contents/acute-respiratory-distress-in-children-emergency-evaluation-and-initial-stabilization
2. Fleming S, Thompson M, Stevens R, Heneghan C, Plüddemann A, Maconochie I, et al. Normal ranges of heart rate and respiratory rate in children from birth to 18 years of age: a systematic review of observational studies. Lancet. 2011;377(9770):1011-8.
3. Hazinski MF, Gonzals L, O'Neill L (Eds). BLS for Healthcare Providers. Dallas, TX: American Heart Association; 2006.
4. https://iapindia.org/pdf/Ch-058-stg-acute-epiglottitis.pdf
5. Mathew JL, Singhi SC. Approach to a child with breathing difficulty. Indian J Pediatr. 2011;78:118-26.
6. Mathew JL. Examination of respiratory system. In: Gupta P (Ed). Clinical Methods in Paediatrics. New Delhi: CBS; 2009. pp. 183-218.
7. Meyburg J, Bernhard M, Hoffmann GF, Motsch J. Principles of emergency medical care. Dtsch Arztebl Int. 2009;106:739-47.
8. PALS Providers Manual. Dallals, TX: American Heart Association; 2011.
9. Rajesh VT, Singhi S, Kataria S. Tachypnoea is a good predictor of hypoxia in acutely ill infants under 2 months. Arch Dis Child. 2000;82:46-9.
10. Schuh S, Lalani A, Allen U, Manson D, Babyn P, Stephens D, et al. Evaluation of the utility of radiography in acute bronchiolitis. J Paediatr. 2007:150;429-33.
11. Singhi S, Mathew JL. Acute respiratory distress. In: Singh M (Ed). Medical Emergencies in Children, 4th edition. New Delhi: Sagar Publications; 2007. pp. 352-72.

CHAPTER 32

Recognition of a Child in Shock

Rohit Vohra, Nameet Jerath

INTRODUCTION

Shock is a state of circulatory dysfunction that results in insufficient oxygen delivery and other substrate to meet metabolic demands of the tissues. Inadequate oxygen delivery leads to a shift to anaerobic metabolism, leading to an increase in lactate production and metabolic acidosis. If this state continues to persist, it can lead to multiple organ dysfunction and even death.

PHASES OF SHOCK

If shock is not identified and treated, it typically goes through three stages **(Table 1)**:

1. *Compensated:* The body uses various compensatory mechanisms to preserve homeostasis. In younger children, cardiac output (CO) is maintained by increase in heart rate, resulting in tachycardia; this is due to an increase in systemic vascular resistance (SVR) and CO through sympathetic nervous system activation. By boosting oxygen extraction at the tissue level and preserving blood flow to essential organs (such as the heart, brain, and kidneys), oxygen supply is maximized. Carbon dioxide (CO_2) generation rises with increased oxygen use, which frequently causes an increase in the respiratory rate required to eliminate CO_2. It might be challenging to distinguish the early phases of any kind of shock from the patient's baseline condition. Perhaps the only symptom is tachycardia.
2. *Uncompensated:* Cardiovascular impairment results in insufficient microvascular perfusion despite the body's compensatory measures. An imbalance between oxygen intake (VO_2) and supply (DO_2) characterizes this condition. A decline in oxygen supply compared to oxygen consumption is reflected in declining mixed venous oxygen saturation (SvO_2). Organ system malfunction and metabolic acidosis from lactic acid generation result from the degradation of cellular metabolism and function. Cardiovascular compromise results in the body's inability to sustain blood pressure as this phase progresses. Hypotension in youngsters can indicate a 25–40% reduction in the volume of blood in circulation, making it a concerning symptom.
3. *Irreversible:* Terminal or irreversible shock results from damage to key organs of such magnitude that death occurs. This occurs even if therapy returns cardiovascular parameters to normal.

TABLE 1: Classification of shock.

Type of shock	*Primary derangement*	*Common causes*
Hypovolemic	Decreased circulating blood volume due to internal or external losses	• Hemorrhage • *Fluid losses:* Gastrointestinal, renal • Capillary leak
Distributive	Vasodilation, venous pooling, decreased preload maldistribution of regional blood flow	• Anaphylaxis • Neurogenic • Drug toxicity • Sepsis
Cardiogenic	Decreased myocardial contractility and cardiac pump failure	• Congenital heart disease • Ischemic heart disease • Kawasaki disease • Trauma • Congestive heart failure • Infections; cardiomyopathies • Drug toxicity
Obstructive	Mechanical obstruction to ventricular outflow	• Massive pulmonary embolus • Cardiac tamponade • Tension pneumothorax

RECOGNITION OF SHOCK AND ORGAN FAILURE

Due to the potential for delayed recognition, which can result in organ failure and death, early detection of shock states is essential to treatment and outcome. A complete medical history and examination are necessary. It is essential to perform repeat examinations often, paying close attention to every organ system. The first symptoms of shock could be mild. Shock frequently results in organ failure; thus, any anomalies need to be treated urgently.

RAPID ASSESSMENT

For any child experiencing acute illness, the pediatric assessment triangle (PAT) is a fast assessment that looks at the child's appearance, respiration, and circulation to determine which conditions need immediate attention. The following PAT features are unique for children in shock:

- *Appearance:* Diminished muscular tone, lowered mental state, feeble scream, diminished responsiveness, and aimless or empty gaze. A child's inability to react to discomfort or recognize or acknowledge their parents is a concerning indicator that calls for a quick assessment of the child's oxygenation, ventilation, and perfusion. In the early (compensated) stages of shock, mental status may be normal while the body works to maintain cerebral perfusion until a later stage.
- *Breathing:* There may be stridor or wheezing in anaphylactic shock, tachypnea without respiratory discomfort (effortless tachypnea), and difficulty maintaining airway due to low mental status. Breathing will be more difficult for patients suffering from tension pneumothorax, septic shock with pneumonia, and cardiogenic shock.
- *Circulation:* It is frequently possible to quickly detect poor perfusion before taking a blood pressure reading. Pallor, acrocyanosis, cold extremities, and a mottled look could be present.

  A thorough physical examination that includes vital signs, pulse oximetry, and an electrocardiogram (ECG) should be carried out.
- *Heart rate:* Tachycardia is "the sign" of shock and may be the only sign present in compensated shock. Although tachycardia is not very specific for shock as it is also caused by wide variety of stimuli such as fever, pain, hypoxia, and agitation.

TABLE 2: Hypotension is defined by systolic blood pressure and age.

Age	*Blood pressure*
Term neonates	<60 mm Hg
Infants (1–12 months)	<70 mm Hg
Children (1–10 years of age)	<70 mm Hg + (Child's age in years × 2) mm Hg
Children >10 years	<90 mm Hg

- *Respiratory rate:* Children with shock are usually tachypneic (silent tachypnea). Increased work of breathing (pneumonia, effusions, and pulmonary edema), differential breath sound intensity (tension pneumothorax, pleural effusions, hemothorax, and empyema) present in respiratory conditions as a cause for shock. Apnea, jerky breathing, irregular respiration, and gasping efforts suggest respiratory failure and imminent cardiorespiratory arrest.
- *Quality of central and peripheral pulses:* Pulse volume reflects pulse pressure [systolic blood pressure (SBP)-diastolic blood pressure (DBP)] and CO. Decreased intensity of distal pulses in comparison to central pulses suggests peripheral vasoconstriction and compensated shock (early sign of decreased CO and peripheral perfusion).
- *Skin findings and capillary refill:* Skin findings are the reliable signs of systemic perfusion because it is a visible indicator of SVR and the degree of shunting. Capillary refill time (CFT) greater than 2 seconds suggest vasoconstriction.
- *Blood pressure:* Shock can be defined without reference to blood pressure. Children experiencing shock may have low or normal blood pressure. Hypotension is the result of the body's attempts to sustain SBP and perfusion failing or running out of steam. In most shock types, it is a late finding that may indicate the impending onset of cardiac arrest. However, in septic shock, it may develop early due to mediator-induced vasodilation **(Table 2)**.
- *Mental status:* An altered level of consciousness indicates the need for immediate evaluation of the child's oxygenation, ventilation, and perfusion status.
- *Urine output:* Reduced urine output is the most reliable sign of internal organ perfusion **(Table 3)**.

TABLE 3: Changes in preload, afterload, and cardiac contractility in individual types of shock.

Clinical type of shock	*Preload*	*Cardiac contractility*	*Afterload*	*Capillary refill time*	*Mixed venous oxygen saturation*
Hypovolemic	Low	Normal	Increased	Increased	Low
Cardiogenic	Increased	Low	Increased	Increased	Low
Distributive	Low/normal	Increased	Low	Flash	High
Obstructive	Increased	Low	Increased	Increased	Low

Flowchart 1: Differential diagnosis for shock in a child presenting with signs of impaired perfusion.

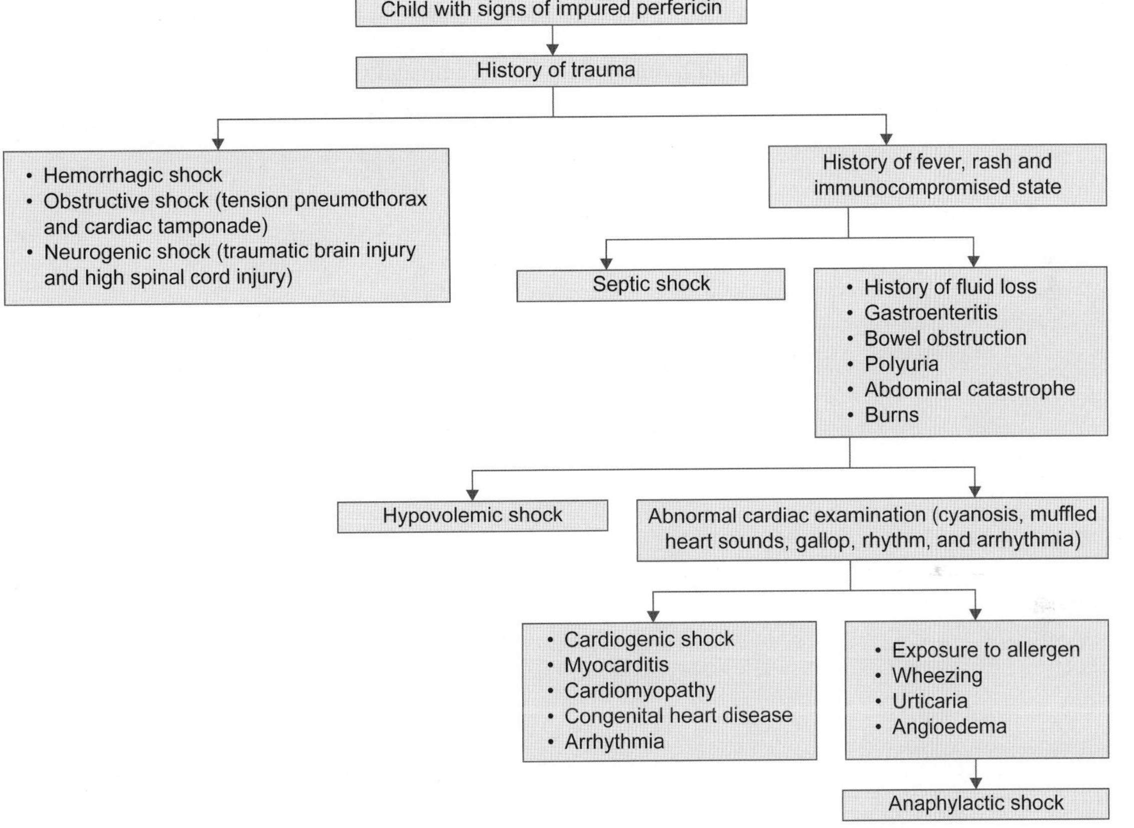

ANCILLARY INVESTIGATIONS (BEDSIDE AND LABORATORY)

Rapid bedside and other selected investigations may be beneficial for identifying the etiology, effective treatment, and monitoring response to treatment **(Flowchart 1)**. These should be simultaneously obtained with rapid assessment and treatment based upon the most likely etiology as follows:

- Rapid blood glucose
- Serum electrolytes
- Complete hemogram
- Hematocrit
- Blood gas measurements
- Ionized calcium
- Blood lactate
- Urine analysis.
- *Bedside echocardiography and ultrasound:* Non-invasive, quick, safe, accurate, and providing visual evaluation of cardiac function, preload status, SVR, CO, lung water, shunt fractions, pulmonary pressures, intra-abdominal findings, pericardial effusion, and improved therapeutic response monitoring, among many other benefits.

KEY POINTS

- Shock is a state of circulatory dysfunction that results in insufficient oxygen delivery and other substrate to meet metabolic demands of the tissues.
- If shock persists, it can lead to multiple organ dysfunction and even death.
- Untreated shock typically goes through three stages: compensated, uncompensated and irreversible.
- Hypotension or low blood pressure is a late feature and is not essential for diagnosis of shock.
- Delayed recognition of shock can result in organ failure and death, early detection of shock states is essential to treatment and outcome.

SUGGESTED READING

1. American Heart Association. (2021). Pediatric advanced life support (PALS) provider manual (6th ed.). American Heart Association.
2. Oczkowski S, Alshamsi F, Belley-Cote E, Centofanti JE, Hylander Møller M, Nunnaly ME, et al. Surviving Sepsis Campaign Guidelines 2021: highlights for the practicing clinician. Pol Arch Intern Med. 2022;132(7-8):16290.

CHAPTER 33

Croup

Kaustubh Mohite

INTRODUCTION

Croup is a one of the most common pediatric respiratory conditions causing inspiratory stridor, cough, and hoarseness. A barking cough is the hallmark of croup. These symptoms result from inflammation in the larynx and subglottic airway. Although croup usually is a mild and self-limited illness, significant upper airway obstruction and respiratory distress can occur.

TERMINOLOGY

The terminology "Croup" has been used to describe a range of upper respiratory conditions in children. For all practical purposes, croup has been used for "viral laryngotracheitis".

Viral Croup

Viral croup refers to the typical croup syndrome that occurs commonly in children 6 months–3 years of age. It is commonly associated with viral respiratory prodromal symptoms such as fever, rhinorrhea, and fatiguability. It is usually a self-limited illness and the symptoms subside by 3–5 days.

Spasmodic Croup

Commonly seen in <3 years old, the child typically gets symptomatic during nighttime. The onset and cessation of symptoms are abrupt, and the duration of symptoms is short, often with symptoms subsiding by the time of presentation for medical attention. Often associated with allergic manifestations as well as a family history of allergies, there may be a familial predisposition to spasmodic croup. Fever is typically absent, but mild upper respiratory tract symptoms may be present. A striking feature of spasmodic croup is its recurrent nature, hence the alternate descriptive term "recurrent croup". Because there is some clinical overlap with atopic diseases, it is sometimes referred to as "allergic croup".

Early in the clinical course, spasmodic croup may be difficult to distinguish from viral croup. One can differentiate spasmodic croup from viral croup as the child is relatively better in between the attacks.

ETIOLOGY

- *Viral (most common)*:
  - Parainfluenza virus (type 1, 2, and 3)
  - Respiratory syncytial virus (RSV)
  - Adenovirus
  - Influenza virus
  - Other [rhinovirus, enterovirus, severe acute respiratory syndrome (SARS) coronavirus 2, and herpes simplex virus (HSV)]
- *Bacterial*: *Staphylococcus aureus*, *Streptococcus pyogenes*, and *Streptococcus pneumoniae*
- Atypical organisms (*Mycoplasma*)

PATHOGENESIS

Viral Croup

Narrowing of the subglottic airway is the anatomic hallmark of croup. In addition to this "fixed" obstruction, dynamic obstruction of the extrathoracic trachea below the cartilaginous ring may occur when the child struggles, cries, or becomes agitated. The dynamic obstruction is attributed to the combination of high negative pressure in the distal extrathoracic trachea and the floppiness of the tracheal wall in children.

Laryngoscopic evaluation typically shows redness and swelling in the area just below the vocal folds **(Figs. 1A and B)**.

Other-associated characteristic findings include mucosal edema and swelling, fibrinous exudates and, occasionally, pseudomembranes over tracheal surfaces and contribute to airway narrowing.

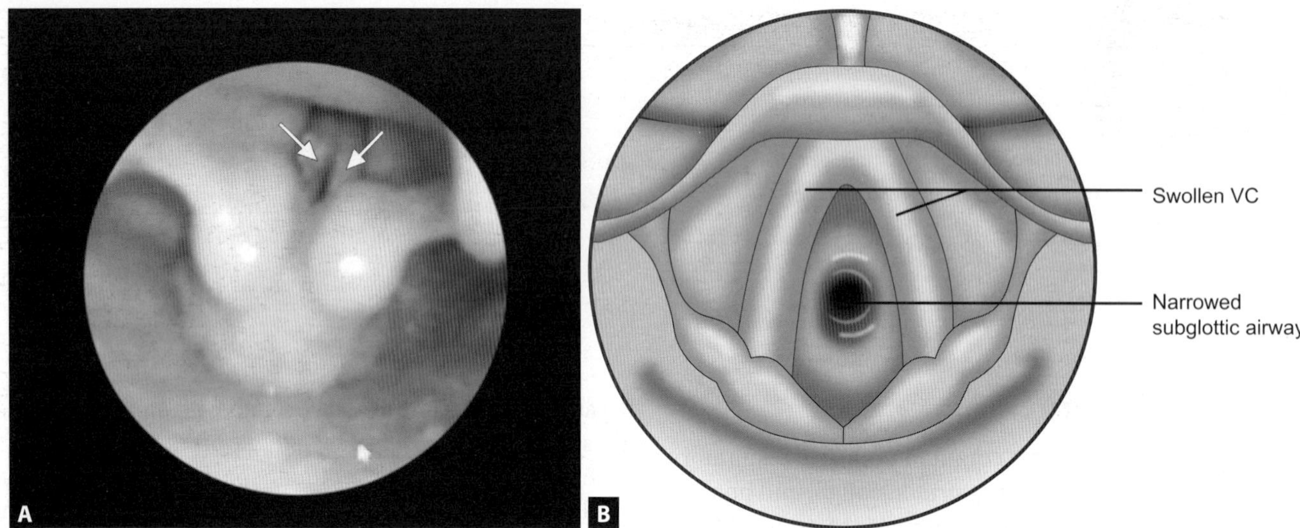

Figs. 1A and B: The vocal cords (VC) are swollen with marked subglottic swelling (arrow), narrowing the opening of subglottic airway. *[For color version (Fig. A), see Plate 1]*

Spasmodic or Recurrent Croup

Spasmodic croup is characterized by noninflammatory edema, suggesting that there is no direct viral involvement but is known to have an association with gastroesophageal reflux disease.

CLINICAL PRESENTATION

The most common age of presentation of croup is between 3 and 6 years of age. The illness begins with typical viral upper respiratory symptoms (rhinorrhea, cough, and congestion) and progresses to signs of airway inflammation and obstruction (barking cough, stridor, and respiratory distress).

Presenting Signs and Symptoms

Upper airway complains such as nasal discharge, congestion, and coryza are the initial complains which further progress to fever, hoarseness, barking cough, and stridor. This noisy breathing is associated with tachypnea with a prolonged inspiratory phase.

Based on the presenting signs and symptoms, croup can be categorized into mild, moderate, severe, and impending respiratory failure as per the Westley croup severity scoring **(Tables 1 and 2)**.

Biphasic stridor (stridor heard on both inspiration and expiration) at rest is a sign of significant airway obstruction. Agitation, which generally is accompanied by increased inspiratory effort, exacerbates the subglottic narrowing by creating negative pressure in the airway. This can lead to further respiratory distress and agitation.

TABLE 1: Clinical features of croup and assigned score as per severity.

Clinical features	*Assigned score*
Level of consciousness	
• Normal	0
• Disoriented	5
Cyanosis	
• None	0
• With agitation	4
• At rest	5
Stridor	
• None	0
• With agitation	1
• At rest	2
Air entry	
• Normal	0
• Decreased	1
• Markedly decreased	2
Retractions	
• None	0
• Mild	1
• Moderate	2
• Severe	3
Total	

INVESTIGATIONS

Croup is a clinical diagnosis, and investigations do not play a major role. However, the following investigations may assist in confirming your diagnosis.

TABLE 2: Westley croup severity scoring.

Total score	*Severity*	*Description*
≤2	Mild	Occasional barky cough, no stridor at rest, mild, or no retractions
3–7	Moderate	Frequent barky cough, stridor at rest, and mild-to-moderate retractions
8–11	Severe	Frequent barky cough, stridor at rest, marked retractions, and significant distress
≥12	Impending respiratory failure	Depressed level of consciousness, stridor at rest, severe retractions, poor air entry, cyanosis, or pallor

Radiograph

In children with croup, steeple sign is observed which is due to subglottic narrowing as observed on a posterior-anterior chest radiograph. The lateral view may demonstrate overdistention of the hypopharynx during inspiration and subglottic haziness **(Figs. 2 and 3)**.

Blood Tests

There are no specific blood investigations for croup. The white blood cell count can be low, normal, or elevated, however, white blood cell counts >10,000 cells/μL are common. As the children with croup have significant tachypnea, there may be associated dehydration which could result in low serum bicarbonate levels and elevated blood urea nitrogen levels.

Microbiology

A polymerase chain reaction (PCR)-based rapid diagnostic test of the nasopharyngeal secretions can isolate the etiological agent of croup in affected children.

DIFFERENTIAL DIAGNOSIS

Conditions which present with stridor at presentation are to be considered during diagnosing croup. These conditions include:

- Acute epiglottitis
- Bacterial tracheitis
- Peritonsillar, parapharyngeal, or retropharyngeal abscesses:
    - Foreign body
    - Allergic reaction or acute angioneurotic edema

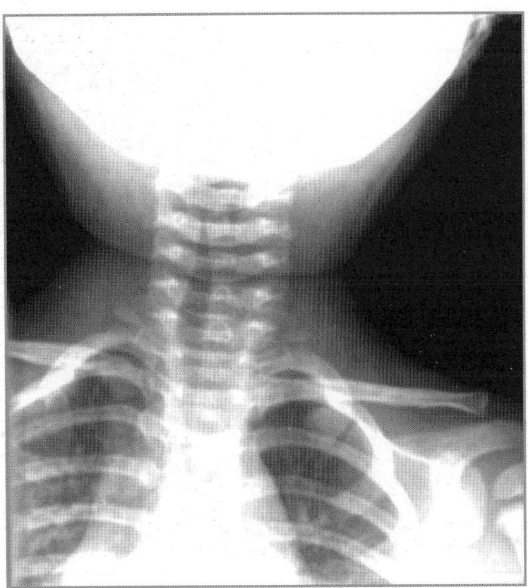

Fig. 2: Anteroposterior (AP) radiograph of the neck in a child with croup, demonstrating the characteristic tapering of the upper trachea "steeple sign".

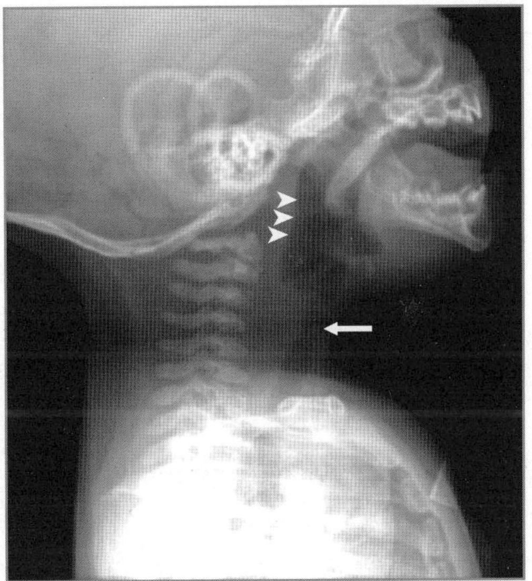

Fig. 3: Lateral neck radiograph showing subglottic narrowing (arrow) and distended hypopharynx (arrowheads) consistent with acute laryngotracheitis.

MANAGEMENT

Management of croup depends on the severity of the condition as mentioned above as per Westley's croup severity scoring **(Flowchart 1)**.

Mild Croup

Children with Westley croup score of <2 are categorized as mild croup and their treatment is mainly

Flowchart 1: Management of croup.

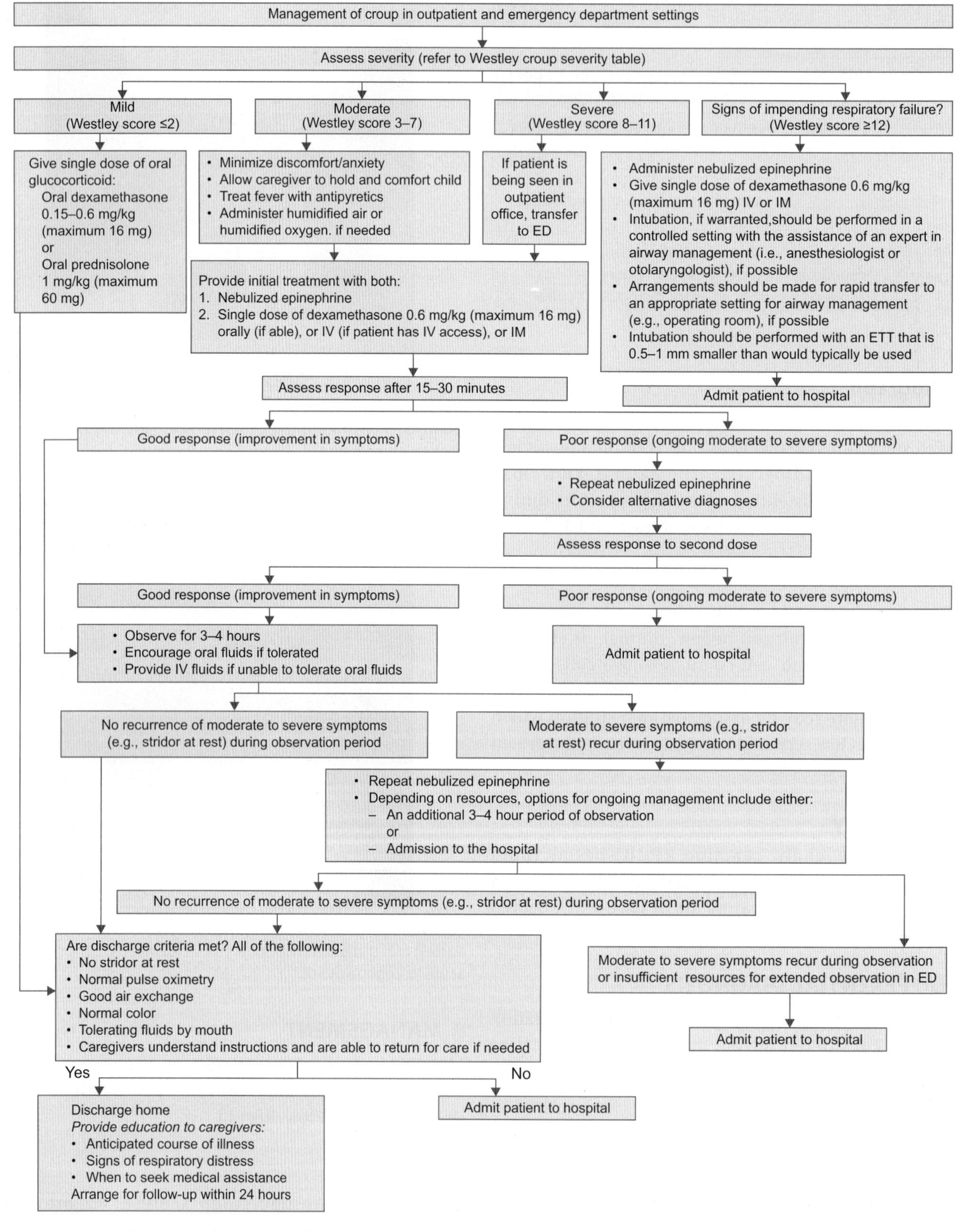

symptomatic management. This involves proper fever control by antipyretics and adequate hydration.

Home Treatment

- Mild croup could be well managed symptomatically at home.
- Supportive care includes antipyretics, encouragement of fluid intake, and exposure to mist or cold outdoor air.
- Instructions should be provided to the caregivers regarding when to seek medical attention, including watching for:
  - Stridor at rest
  - Difficulty breathing
  - Pallor or cyanosis
  - Severe coughing spells
  - Drooling or difficulty swallowing
  - Fatigue
  - Worsening course
  - Persistent or high fever
  - Prolonged symptoms (longer than 7 days)
  - Suprasternal retractions

Outpatient Treatment

A single dose of oral dexamethasone (0.15–0.6 mg/kg) or oral prednisolone (1 mg/kg) has been shown to drastically improve clinical condition of a child with mild croup.

Moderate to Severe Croup

Depending on the severity of the complains, croup could be categorized into moderate (Westley score: 3–7) or severe croup (Westley score > 8).

Initial Treatment

Initial treatment of moderate-to-severe croup includes the following:

- *Dexamethasone:*
  - Dexamethasone has proven to be effective in the treatment of both moderate and severe croup.
  - It is administered at a dose of 0.6 mg/kg, maximum of 16 mg.
  - The least invasive route of administration should be chosen [oral/intravenous/intramuscular (IV/IM)].
- *Nebulized epinephrine:*
  - *L-epinephrine:* 0.5 mL/kg per dose (maximum of 5 mL) of a 1 mg/mL (1:1,000) preservative-free solution
  - *Racemic epinephrine:* 0.05 mL/kg per dose (maximum of 0.5 mL) of a 2.25% solution diluted to 3 mL total volume with normal saline.
  - The drug is administered by nebulizer for over 15 minutes.
  - It has an onset of effect within 10 minutes.

Response to Treatment

The above given medications usually show positive response in a duration of 3–4 hours of initial treatment. The child might show one of the following responses.

- *Improvement:* Children with moderate croup show good response to nebulize epinephrine and glucocorticoids.
- *Recurrent or persistent symptoms:*
  - For children with ongoing severe symptoms, nebulized epinephrine can be repeated every 15–20 minutes, if necessary.
  - It is advisable to admit these children in the hospital wards or pediatric intensive care unit (PICU) based on the clinical assessment of the child.

Indications for Hospital Admission

Indications for inpatient admission include:

- Severe croup with poor air entry, altered consciousness, or impending respiratory failure
- Moderate/severe croup symptoms that recur or persist after initial treatment.
- Toxic appearance
- Requiring supplemental oxygen
- Severe dehydration
- Age < 6 months
- Multiple hospital visits in 24 hours
- Ability of the parents/caregivers to comprehend the instructions regarding recognition of features that indicate the need to return for care.

Admission to the PICU is warranted if any of the following are present:

- Respiratory failure requiring endotracheal intubation
- Persistent severe symptoms requiring frequent nebulized epinephrine dosing
- Underlying conditions placing the child at high risk for progressive respiratory failure (e.g., neuromuscular disease or bronchopulmonary dysplasia)

Inpatient Management

- *Supportive care*:
  - *Fluids*:
    - Children with respiratory distress have decreased oral intake.

- Fever and tachypnoea may increase fluid requirements.
- *Fever control*: Increased core temperature can worsen tachypnea and respiratory distress in children with croup.

- *Respiratory care*:
  - *Nebulized epinephrine*:
    - Multiple doses of nebulized epinephrine may be warranted for children with moderate-to-severe distress.
    - Nebulized epinephrine can be repeated every 15–20 minutes.
  - *Supplemental oxygen*: Oxygen saturation of >92% should be targeted.
  - *Mist*: Mist therapy may provide a sense of comfort and reassurance to both the child and parents.
  - High-flow nasal cannula (HFNC) and noninvasive ventilation (NIV):
    - HFNC works by washing out nasopharyngeal dead space, reducing upper airway resistance, and providing positive distending pressure
    - Primary aim is avoiding the need for intubation and mechanical ventilation.
  - Heliox:
    - Heliox is a mixture of helium and oxygen (70:30).
    - By reducing turbulent airflow, it is postulated to decrease the work of breathing in children with severe croup.
    - A limitation of heliox use is the low fractional concentration of inspired oxygen (FiO_2) in the gas mixture, which may not be adequate for children with hypoxia.
  - Intubation:
    - In children with progressive respiratory failure, the need for intubation should be anticipated.
    - As there is subglottic edema which compromises the airway lumen, endotracheal intubation can be challenging.
    - An endotracheal tube that is 0.5–1 mm smaller than would typically be used should be placed.
- *Atypical course*:
  - Child with croup usually recovers in 36–48 hours.
  - If the child does not respond to the given line of management, there may be an underlying airway abnormality or may be developing a complication of croup.
  - Pulmonary edema, pneumothorax, lymphadenitis, and otitis media are the known complications reported in croup.
- *Discharge criteria*: The child can be planned to be discharged from the hospital once the following criteria are achieved:
  - No stridor at rest
  - Normal pulse oximetry in room air
  - Good air exchange
  - Normal color
  - Normal level of consciousness
  - Demonstrated ability to tolerate fluids by mouth

KEY POINTS

- Croup is commonly a viral respiratory disease affecting the upper airway.
- It is mostly a clinical diagnosis, and investigations do not play a major role.
- It usually is restricted to mild complaints but could progress to moderate–severe disease rarely.
- With proper management, symptoms are controlled within 2–3 days.

SUGGESTED READING

1. Alberta Clinical Practice Guideline Working Group. (2008). Guideline for the diagnosis and management of croup. [online] Available from www.topalbertadoctors.org/download/252/croup_guideline.pdf [Last accessed September, 2024).
2. Alberta Clinical Practice Guideline Working Group. (2015). Guidelines for the diagnosis and management of croup. [online] Available from www.topalbertadoctors.org/download/252/croup_guideline.pdf [Last accessed September, 2015].
3. Cherry JD. Croup (laryngitis, laryngotracheitis, spasmodic croup, laryngotracheobronchitis, bacterial tracheitis, and laryngotracheobronchopneumonitis) and epiglottitis (supraglottitis). In: Cherry JD, Harrison GJ, Kaplan SL, Steinbach WJ, Hotez PJ (Eds). Feigin and Cherry's Textbook of Pediatric Infectious Diseases, 7th edition. Philadelphia: Elsevier Saunders; 2014. pp. 241.
4. Clarke M, Allaire J. An evidence-based approach to the evaluation and treatment of croup in children. Pediatr Emerg Med Pract. 2012;9(9):1.
5. Cooper T, Kuruvilla G, Persad R, El-Hakim H. Atypical croup: association with airway lesions, atopy, and esophagitis. Otolaryngol Head Neck Surg. 2012;147(2):209-14.
6. Coughran A, Balakrishnan K, Ma Y, Vaezeafshar R, Capdarest-Arest N, Hamdi O, et al. The relationship between croup and gastroesophageal reflux: a systematic review and meta-analysis. Laryngoscope. 2021;131(1):209.
7. Elder AE, Rao A. Management and outcomes of patients presenting to the emergency department with croup: Can we identify which patients can safely be discharged from

the emergency department? J Paediatr Child Health. 2019;55(11):1323.

8. Fernandes RM, Oleszczuk M, Woods CR, Rowe BH, Cates CJ, Hartling L. The Cochrane Library and safety of systemic corticosteroids for acute respiratory conditions in children: An overview of reviews. Evid Based Child Health. 2014;9(3):733-47.
9. Gates A, Johnson DW, Klassen TP. Glucocorticoids for Croup in Children. JAMA Pediatr. 2019;173(6):595.
10. Gelbart B, Parsons S, Sarpal A, Ninova P, Butt W. Intensive care management of children intubated for croup: a retrospective analysis. Anaesth Intensive Care. 2016;44(2): 245.
11. Hampton T, Ghazal Asswad R, Bhat J, Stevens K, Whitehall E, Milinis K, et al. Recurrent croup is a good indicator of underlying paediatric airway issues: A 10-year retrospective cohort study of airway endoscopy. Ear Nose Throat J. 2023:1455613231170087.
12. Lee JK, Song SH, Ahn B, Yun KW, Choi EH. Etiology and epidemiology of croup before and throughout the COVID-19 pandemic, 2018-2022, South Korea. Children (Basel). 2022;9(10):1542.
13. McCulloh RJ, Andrea S, Reinert S, Chapin K. Potential utility of multiplex amplification respiratory viral panel testing in the management of acute respiratory infection in children: A retrospective analysis. J Pediatric Infect Dis Soc. 2014;3(2):146.
14. Murata Y, Tomari K, Matsuoka T. Children with croup and SARS-CoV-2 infection during the large outbreak of omicron. Pediatr Infect Dis J. 2022;41(5):e249.
15. Petrocheilou A, Tanou K, Kalampouka E, Malakasioti G, Giannios C, Kaditis AG. Viral croup: Diagnosis and a treatment algorithm. Pediatr Pulmonol. 2014;49(5): 421-9.
16. Rankin I, Wang SM, Waters A, Clement WA, Kubba H. The management of recurrent croup in children. J Laryngol Otol. 2013;127(5):494-500.
17. Rosychuk RJ, Klassen TP, Metes D, Voaklander DC, Senthilselvan A, Rowe BH. Croup presentations to emergency departments in Alberta, Canada: a large population-based study. Pediatr Pulmonol. 2010;45(1): 83.
18. Thompson M, Vodicka TA, Blair PS, Buckley DI, Heneghan C, Hay AD, TARGET Programme Team. Duration of symptoms of respiratory tract infections in children: systematic review. BMJ. 2013;347:f7027.
19. Venn AMR, Schmidt JM, Mullan PC. Pediatric croup with COVID-19. Am J Emerg Med. 2021;43:287.e1.

Approach to a Child with Acute Febrile Encephalopathy

Surpreet BS Nagi

INTRODUCTION

A child presenting with fever and altered sensorium is a common pediatric emergency. Acute febrile encephalopathy (AFE) is a clinical term used to describe an altered mental state that either accompanies or follows a short febrile illness and is characterized by a diffuse and nonspecific brain insult manifested by a combination of coma, seizures, and/or decerebration.

Encephalopathy is a diffuse disease affecting the brain that alters its structure or function and may be caused due to diverse etiology like infective, metabolic, toxic, ischemic, nutritional causes or trauma. In febrile illnesses, encephalopathy may result from pathogenic mechanisms affecting the nervous system directly or systemic complications like hypoglycemia, hypovolemia, hyperpyrexia, hypoxia, anemia, hepatic or renal failure, toxins, vasculitis, and bleeding.

Central nervous system (CNS) infections are the most common cause of AFE in children. Various causes such as viral encephalitis, cerebral malaria, bacterial meningitis, Reye's syndrome, and inflammatory encephalopathies including acute disseminated encephalomyelitis (ADEM), etc. have been implicated in the etiology; and the proportionate contribution of each varies according to the geographical area. In tropical countries like India, cerebral malaria, Japanese encephalitis (JE), herpes simplex encephalitis (HSE), and bacterial meningitis are the common causes of AFE, while tuberculous meningitis (TBM) usually presents with a subacute or chronic history. Even after a detailed diagnostic workup, one may not be able to arrive at a definitive diagnosis in many cases. Nevertheless, a detailed examination and workup is warranted, because many conditions like cerebral malaria and HSE are treatable.

SOME DEFINITIONS

Encephalopathy

Encephalopathy describes a clinical syndrome of altered mental status, manifesting as reduced consciousness or altered behavior, without any inflammation of the brain.

Acute Febrile Encephalopathy

Acute febrile encephalopathy is a clinical diagnosis and is described as a syndrome of altered sensorium associated with fever of less than 1 week duration, and altered consciousness of more than 12-hours duration, with or without seizures in a previously normal child.

Encephalitis

Encephalitis means inflammation of the brain. It is strictly a pathological diagnosis; but surrogate clinical/imaging markers may provide evidence of inflammation.

Acute Encephalitis Syndrome

Clinically, a case of acute encephalitis syndrome (AES) is defined as a person of any age, at any time of year with the acute onset of fever and a change in mental status (including symptoms such as confusion, disorientation, coma, or inability to talk) and/or new onset of seizures (excluding simple febrile seizures). Other early clinical findings may include an increase in irritability, somnolence, or abnormal behavior greater than that seen with usual febrile illness.

PATHOPHYSIOLOGY

The pathophysiology of AFE usually is multifactorial and varies according to the etiology. Encephalopathy generally results from cytotoxic injury or disruption of neurotransmission. However, the final pathway is common, which is interruption of the polysynaptic pathways and altered excitatory-inhibitory amino acid balance, leading to cerebral edema. All forms of acute toxic metabolic encephalopathy interfere with the function of the ascending reticular activating system and/or its projections to the cerebral cortex, thus leading to impairment of arousal and/or awareness, and/or seizures. Despite a wide array of pathophysiologic mechanisms, the clinical manifestations tend to be very similar because of the common final mechanism.

ETIOLOGY

The etiology of AFE varies from infectious etiologies to noninfectious metabolic disorders **(Table 1)**. The following are some of the common causes of AFE:

- Infections:
  - *Meningoencephalitis:* Due to viruses like herpes simplex virus (HSV) 1 and 2, human herpes virus 6, Epstein-Barr virus (EBV), varicella zoster virus, cytomegalovirus, adenovirus, influenza, enterovirus, poliovirus, measles, mumps, rubella, rabies, dengue virus, chikungunya, arboviruses (JE, West Nile virus), and retrovirus [human immunodeficiency virus (HIV)]
  - Bacterial infections like pyogenic meningitis, and other organisms like *Mycobacterium tuberculosis, Mycoplasma pneumoniae, Listeria, Borrelia burgdorferi* (Lyme disease), *Leptospira, Brucella,* and *Salmonella typhi*
  - Rickettsial infections, fungal infections due to cryptococcosis, histoplasmosis, coccidioidomycosis, and candidiasis
  - Cerebral malaria due to *Plasmodium*, and infection with other parasites like *Toxoplasma gondii* and *Schistosoma*
  - Brain abscess, subdural, or epidural empyema
  - Sepsis with disseminated intravascular coagulation or thrombotic thrombocytopenic purpura
- Noninfective causes:
  - *Overproduction of heat:* Neuroleptic malignant syndrome, malignant hyperthermia, nonconvulsive status epilepticus (NCSE), and thyrotoxic encephalopathy
  - *Impaired heat dissipation:* Heat stroke, anticholinergic toxicity
  - *Structural lesions:* Hypothalamic lesion, brainstem lesions, and intraventricular and subarachnoid hemorrhage
- Miscellaneous:
  - Plant toxins like *Cassia occidentalis*
  - Reye's syndrome
  - Infectious or postinfectious ADEM.

TABLE 1: Etiology of acute febrile encephalopathy.

Diagnosis	*Number of cases (%)*
Suspected viral etiology	57 (37.3)
Pyogenic meningitis	51 (33.8)
Tubercular meningitis	12 (7.9)
Cerebral malaria	8 (5.2)
Dyselectrolytemia	6 (4)
Hepatic encephalopathy	3 (2)
DKA	3 (2)
ADEM	2 (1.3)
Septicemia	2 (1.3)
Reye's syndrome	3 (2)
Shigellosis	1 (0.67)
Enteric fever	1 (0.67)
Prolonged coma after seizure	1 (0.67)
IC bleed due to aplastic anemia	1 (0.67)
Total	151 (100)

(ADEM: acute disseminated encephalomyelitis; DKA: diabetic ketoacidosis; IC: intracranial)

EVALUATION

Patients presenting with an AFE can be broadly divided into three categories **(Table 2)**.

A detailed history and physical examination is essential to categorize the patient into one of these groups. At the outset, it is important to differentiate infective from

TABLE 2: Categories of patients presenting with an acute febrile encephalopathy.

Category	*Common causes*
Primary CNS infections	Meningitis, encephalitis (HSV, JE), TBM, and brain abscess
Systemic infections	Shigella, typhoid, malaria, dengue, and rickettsial infections
Noninfectious causes	ADEM, Reye's syndrome, and mitochondrial and other IEMs, drugs and toxins, SOLs

(ADEM: acute disseminated encephalomyelitis; CNS: central nervous system; HSV: herpes simplex virus; IEMs: inborn errors of metabolism; JE: Japanese encephalitis; SOLs: space occupying lesions; TBM: tuberculous meningitis)

non-infective causes, because infection mandates prompt antimicrobial therapy. There are no distinguishing clinical or radiological features to differentiate the various causes of viral encephalitis. The clinical and the radiological findings in encephalitis should be interpreted in the geographical and other epidemiological background.

APPROACH TO ACUTE FEBRILE ENCEPHALOPATHY (FLOWCHART 1)

Step 1: Initiate Resuscitation and Assess Neurological Status

As in any emergency, one needs to quickly evaluate the airway, breathing, and circulation (ABC's). It is during this assessment that alteration of sensorium is first recognized (or confirmed). Initial neurological examination includes only a survey of vital signs, including respiratory patterns, Glasgow Coma Scale (GCS) score, pupillary response, and extraocular muscle examination. The common goal in the treatment of a patient with encephalopathy is to prevent secondary injury by maintaining oxygen delivery and supply of nutrients to the brain. Thus, the ABC's of basic life support supersede all other interventions.

If the initial assessment suggests that the child is unstable, then the management priorities should be directed to ensuring adequacy of airway, breathing, and circulatory function, irrespective of the etiology. Depending on the degree of instability, this initial management may actually precede the assessment of the degree of impairment of consciousness; though usually, both are carried out nearly simultaneously.

The depth of coma can be assessed by the GCS or the AVPU scale (Wherein A-Alert, V-Response to Voice, P-Response to Pain and U-Unresponsive). A modified GCS should be used for infants and young children. In case of any confusion about the assessment, it is preferable to err on the side of recording a lower score initially, since it is easier to withdraw treatment in a child who is improving, rather than to resuscitate a child who is deteriorating.

Assessment of the airway and need for intubation is of paramount importance as the children with impaired consciousness are at a high risk for aspiration **(Box 1)**. These children have loss of tone of the oropharyngeal muscles causing the tongue to fall back and obstruct the airway, and pooling of secretions (leading to aspiration). Measures should be taken to secure the airway. If the child shows signs of airway obstruction, repositioning of the head with the chin lift maneuver may alleviate the obstruction. If cervical spine injury is suspected, a jaw thrust maneuver is preferable and the neck immobilized while securing the airway. An oral airway may be inserted if required and secretions cleared using a large-bore-suction cannula.

Once the airway patency has been established, the adequacy of breathing should be evaluated. Auscultation of the lung fields should assess for air entry, symmetry of breath sounds, and presence of adventitious breath sounds such as crackles or wheezes. Pulse oximetry can be used to evaluate oxygenation. Oxygen should be administered to all seriously-ill children via non-rebreathing face mask. Adequacy of ventilation should be assessed by examination and arterial blood gases. If the airway is patent but the child's respiratory effort is deemed inadequate, positive pressure ventilation should be initiated. The airway interventions should be instituted as nontraumatically as possible, as they may cause spikes in intracranial pressure (ICP). Rapid-sequence intubation is preferred. Moderate hyperventilation (target $PaCO_2$ 30–35 mm Hg) to produce arterial constriction and lower ICP should only be initiated for patients with signs of increased ICP. Extreme hyperventilation has been associated with brain ischemia; the risks of aggressive hyperventilation ($PaCO_2$ <30 mm Hg) are only justified in patients with transtentorial herniation.

Attempt should be made to maintain the cerebral perfusion pressure (CPP), which is the major factor that affects cerebral blood flow and hence, adequate oxygenation. Cerebral perfusion pressure depends on the mean arterial pressure (MAP) and the ICP (CPP = MAP – ICP). Cerebral perfusion pressure can reduce as a result of reduced MAP or raised ICP or a combination of these two. Therefore, adequate MAP should be maintained. If the ICP rises, the blood pressure (BP) rises as a compensatory phenomenon in order to try and maintain the cerebral perfusion. However, there is a limit to such compensation, beyond which the cerebral perfusion may suffer. Cerebral ischemia is the single-most important determinant that decides the outcome of such patients.

Once the airway and breathing have been addressed, circulation must be evaluated. This involves assessment of the cardiac output. Symptoms of shock include tachycardia, cool extremities, delayed capillary refill time, mottled or pale skin, and effortless tachypnea. Hypotension is a late finding in shock. Vascular access is necessary for volume resuscitation in patients with impaired circulation. While establishing an intravenous access, samples should be drawn for various investigations. If there is evidence of circulatory failure, fluid bolus (20 mL/kg of normal saline;

Flowchart 1: Approach to a child with acute febrile encephalopathy.

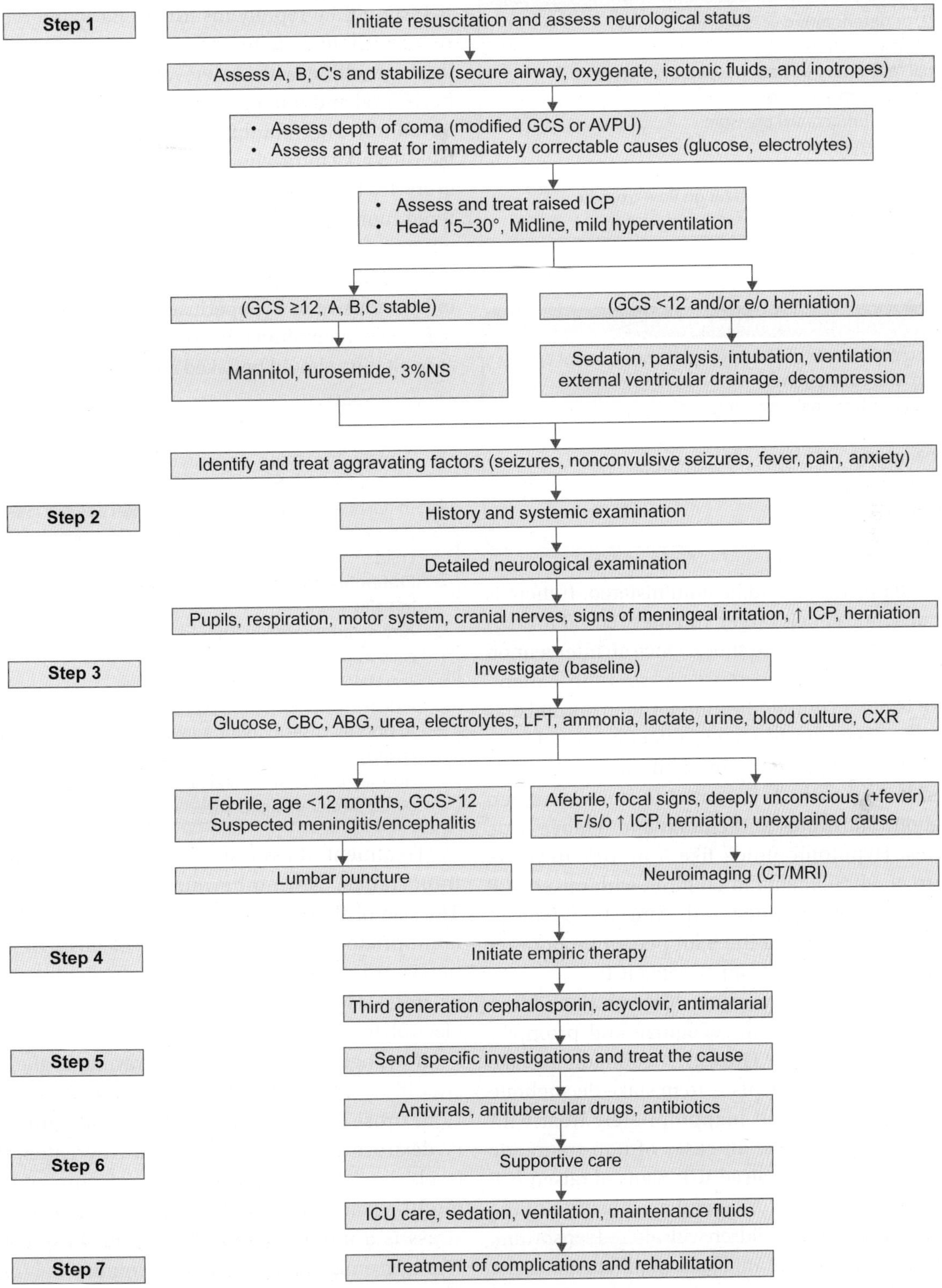

Step 1

Initiate resuscitation and assess neurological status

↓

Assess A, B, C's and stabilize (secure airway, oxygenate, isotonic fluids, and inotropes)

↓

- Assess depth of coma (modified GCS or AVPU)
- Assess and treat for immediately correctable causes (glucose, electrolytes)

↓

- Assess and treat raised ICP
- Head 15–30°, Midline, mild hyperventilation

↓

- (GCS ≥12, A, B,C stable) → Mannitol, furosemide, 3%NS
- (GCS <12 and/or e/o herniation) → Sedation, paralysis, intubation, ventilation external ventricular drainage, decompression

↓

Identify and treat aggravating factors (seizures, nonconvulsive seizures, fever, pain, anxiety)

↓

Step 2

History and systemic examination

↓

Detailed neurological examination

↓

Pupils, respiration, motor system, cranial nerves, signs of meningeal irritation, ↑ ICP, herniation

↓

Step 3

Investigate (baseline)

↓

Glucose, CBC, ABG, urea, electrolytes, LFT, ammonia, lactate, urine, blood culture, CXR

↓

- Febrile, age <12 months, GCS>12 Suspected meningitis/encephalitis → Lumbar puncture
- Afebrile, focal signs, deeply unconscious (+fever) F/s/o ↑ ICP, herniation, unexplained cause → Neuroimaging (CT/MRI)

↓

Step 4

Initiate empiric therapy

↓

Third generation cephalosporin, acyclovir, antimalarial

↓

Step 5

Send specific investigations and treat the cause

↓

Antivirals, antitubercular drugs, antibiotics

↓

Step 6

Supportive care

↓

ICU care, sedation, ventilation, maintenance fluids

↓

Step 7

Treatment of complications and rehabilitation

(ABC's: airway, breathing, and circulation; ABG: arterial blood gas; AVPU: alert, voice, pain, and unresponsive scale; CBC: complete blood count; CT: computed tomography; CXR: X-ray chest; GCS: Glasgow Coma Scale; ICP: intracranial pressure; ICU: intensive care unit; LFT: liver function test; MRI: magnetic resonance imaging; NS: normal saline)

BOX 1: Recommendations for intubation.

- GCS <12, or deteriorating GCS scores
- Impaired airway reflexes
- Abnormal respiratory pattern (respiratory depression)
- Neurogenic hyperventilation
- Signs of raised intracranial pressure
- Evidence of herniation
- Asymmetric or dilated pupils
- Oxygen saturation <92% despite high flow oxygen
- Fluid refractory shock

(GCS: Glasgow Coma Scale)

BOX 2: Signs of raised intracranial pressure.

- Worsening Glasgow Coma Scale despite correction of airway, breathing, and circulation
- Persistence of abnormal posturing
- Abnormal breathing patterns
- Abnormal pupillary response
- Doll's eye reflex
- Cushing's triad (late sign)
- Papilledema

maximum 60 mL/kg) should be administered. If there is evidence of septic shock, larger volumes (60–80 mL/kg) may be needed to correct the shock. Once an intervention is performed, the clinician must reassess the patient. Raised ICP is not a contraindication for fluid administration for the correction of shock. Effective circulation through intravenous isotonic fluid administration and inotropes, if necessary, is essential to deliver oxygen and metabolic substrates to the brain and remove toxic metabolites. Hypotonic fluids like 5 or 10% dextrose can lead to cerebral edema in children with raised ICP and should not be administered. Aim should be to maintain the BP at around the 95th percentile in order to maintain CPP in the face of an elevated ICP.

Raised ICP is a common cause of death in children with AFE. It is important to recognize and promptly manage signs of raised ICP **(Box 2)**. A common mistake in the emergency departments is to mistake decerebrate posturing for seizures, and inappropriately treat with antiepileptic drugs. Almost all cases of non-traumatic coma have an element of raised ICP. Signs of raised ICP should be picked up early. A careful examination of the fundus is mandatory in all children with altered sensorium. Acute elevation of ICP will not cause papilledema in the acute stages. Hence, its absence must not be taken as a reassuring sign. Neither, will a computed tomography (CT) pick up raised ICP in the acute stage.

If there are features of raised ICP, measures to decrease ICP should be rapidly instituted. Early interventions to reduce ICP include treating fever, maintaining the head in the midline with an elevation of 15–30° above the horizontal and moderate hyperventilation (target $PaCO_2$ 30–35 mm Hg). Mannitol should be given in a dose of 0.25–0.5 g/kg intravenously over 15 minutes, and repeated every 4–6 hourly; only if required. It should not be administered round the clock and is unlikely to be effective after 48–72 hours. Furosemide is often used in conjunction with mannitol. Hypertonic saline (3%) may be preferred in hypotensive or hypoperfused patients for reducing the ICP while maintaining the MAP and CPP. A neurosurgical consultation should be asked for.

CLINICAL PEARLS

- Airway, breathing and circulation of basic life support supersede all other interventions.
- Initial management may actually precede the assessment of the degree of impairment of consciousness in an unstable child.
- Preferable to record a lower Glasgow Coma Scale score initially.
- Airway interventions should be instituted as nontraumatically as possible.
- Maintain cerebral perfusion pressure.
- Reassess after every intervention.
- Almost all cases of nontraumatic coma have an element of raised intracranial pressure.
- Normal fundus or normal neuroimaging does not rule out a raised intracranial pressure.

Treatment of associated conditions is of paramount importance. Normothermia should be maintained. The use of therapeutic hypothermia (32–34°C) may be appropriate for children with out-of-hospital arrest and persistent coma or those with ventricular fibrillation or pulseless ventricular tachycardia. Acid-base and electrolyte abnormalities should be corrected.

If hypoglycemia is present, intravenous glucose bolus should be administered. In a neonate, 2 mL/kg of 10% IV dextrose bolus; and in an older child 5 mL/kg of 10% IV dextrose bolus should be given. Thereafter, the sugar levels should be monitored and the glucose infusion rates modified accordingly. Hyperglycemia resulting from stress is a more common finding in these conditions. Hypoglycemia damages the brain immediately and needs urgent correction. Hyperglycemia, on the other hand, is associated with a higher morbidity and mortality if not treated; and hence tight glycemic control should be the aim.

If the child is having seizures, or there is history of a seizure preceding the encephalopathy, anticonvulsants (intravenous benzodiazepine followed by phenytoin loading 20 mg/kg or fosphenytoin) should be administered. The standard protocol for the management of status epilepticus may be followed in case of refractory seizures. Subtle seizures (NCSE) should be identified and treated appropriately, as unrecognized seizure activity increases the ICP and could precipitate herniation. Non convulsive status epilepticus manifests, as an abnormal and fluctuating impairment of consciousness, diminished responsiveness; and may be picked up on an electroencephalogram (EEG), and often showing a delayed response (4–5 days in some patients) to anticonvulsant medications.

Agitation may increase ICP, interfere with respiratory support, and increase the risk of injury. Efforts should be taken to provide pain relief and sedation during painful procedures. Significant sedation, however, may obscure the neurologic examination, may contribute to hypotension and hypoventilation, and should be administered only when the benefits of relieving agitation outweigh the need for close neurologic monitoring by examination.

KEY POINTS

Initial steps in resuscitation:
- Assess airway, breathing and circulation and stabilize.
- Assess level of consciousness (modified Glasgow Coma Scale or Alert, Voice, Pain Unresponsive Scale).
- Secure airway, oxygenation, and ventilation, rapid sequence intubation preferred, maintain cerebral perfusion pressure.
- Secure vascular access, isotonic fluids, inotropes.
- Assess and treat for immediately correctable causes (glucose, electrolytes, acid-base abnormalities).
- Assess and treat raised intracranial pressure: Head 15–30°, midline, mild hyperventilation, mannitol, furosemide, 3% normal saline.
- In case of signs of herniation—sedation, paralysis, intubation, ventilation.
- Identify and treat aggravating factors—seizures, nonconvulsive status epilepticus, fever, pain, anxiety.
- Continuous monitoring of heart rate, respiratory rate, blood pressure, temperature, oxygen saturations, electrocardiogram, Glasgow Coma Scale.

Step 2: Take History and Perform Focused Examination

History (Table 3)

The patient's history may hold the most important and sometimes the only clue to a correct diagnosis. A careful history should be taken with special emphasis on the onset and duration of encephalopathy and the type and degree of fever. The child, who has been apparently well prior to the onset of encephalopathy and has an acute onset of illness, may have suffered from poisonings, drug overdose, metabolic disorders or child abuse, as the probable causes. Central nervous system infections, on the other hand, would present with complaints evolving over a few days associated with a history of fever or recent illness. Disorders in which encephalopathy may be preceded by a febrile illness include ADEM, Reye's syndrome, mitochondrial and other inborn errors of metabolism.

The associated symptoms may indicate the focus of infection. Symptoms such as headache, nausea and vomiting, irritability, seizures, focal deficits, rash, and joint pain should be enquired into in depth.

TABLE 3: Important clues in the history of acute febrile encephalopathy.

History	*Probable etiology*
Geographic area or residence of the child	Endemic for JE, malaria
Recent travel	Malaria, dengue, typhus, arbovirus
Similar illness in the family or locality	Epidemic of AES, HSV, JE
Prodromal symptoms like a URI, flu-like illness or diarrhea	H1N1, enterovirus, polio
Congenital heart disease, chronic ear infections, sinusitis, orbital cellulitis, or dental infection	Brain abscess
Dog bite	Rabies
Insect or mosquito bite	Rickettsial infection, malaria, dengue, JE
Contamination with dirty water	Leptospirosis
Contact with tuberculosis	TBM
Recent immunizations	ADEM
Treatment history prior to the presentation	Partially-treated bacterial meningitis
Exposure to drugs or toxins at home	Poisoning, nonaccidental trauma
Past history of similar episodes	IEM

(ADEM: acute disseminated encephalomyelitis; AES: acute encephalitis syndrome; HSV: herpes simplex virus; IEM: inborn error of metabolism; JE: Japanese encephalitis; TBM: tuberculous meningitis; URI: upper respiratory infection)

Other concurrent systemic illnesses, e.g., jaundice (hepatic failure), pneumonia (hypoxic encephalopathy), diarrhea (dyselectrolytemia), and dysentery (shigella encephalopathy) need to be elicited in the history. Nonaccidental trauma should always be considered in a lethargic infant.

Other history which may offer some aid in the diagnosis:

- History of trauma, recent illness, or surgery (splenectomy, neurosurgery)
- Family history of seizure disorders or previous child deaths
- Comorbid conditions like congenital heart disease, diabetes, chronic liver, or renal diseases
- Premorbid developmental or neurological status of the child
- Immunosuppressive states (HIV), chemotherapy, and prolonged steroids.

Examination

*General examination **(Table 4)**:* The general examination may provide helpful etiological clues. Vital signs are often overlooked but are valuable in assessing ill children. The degree of fever, the presence of tachycardia out-of-proportion to the fever, and the presence of tachypnea and hypotension, when present, are ominous signs.

The presence of fever suggests an infective process (sepsis, pneumonia, meningitis, encephalitis, or brain abscess); but may also indicate heat stroke or abnormality of hypothalamic temperature regulatory mechanisms. Tachycardia may be a result of fever, hypovolemic or septic shock, heart failure, or arrhythmias. Bradycardia may result from raised ICP or a result of myocardial injury (myocarditis, hypoxia, sepsis, or toxins). Tachypnea with respiratory distress indicates lung pathology (pneumonia, pneumothorax, empyema, or asthma). Quiet tachypnea is indicative of acidosis which may be present in diabetic ketoacidosis (DKA), uremia, or some poisonings. Hypotension may be seen in sepsis, cardiac dysfunction, toxic ingestion, or adrenal insufficiency, and may lead to poor cerebral perfusion, resulting in diffuse or watershed hypoxic-ischemic injury. Hypertension may be the cause of altered sensorium in hypertensive encephalopathy or may be a compensatory mechanism to maintain cerebral perfusion in children with increased ICP or stroke.

A thorough systemic examination should be performed to look for a source of sepsis. Systemic examination must be performed to look for hepatosplenomegaly (infections or liver disease), pulmonary involvement such as pneumonia, pleural effusions, and empyema, skin and bone lesions and cardiac involvement such as myocarditis or a pre-existing congenital or rheumatic heart disease (which may predispose to endocarditis and subsequently intracranial abscess).

TABLE 4: Important clues in general examination in acute febrile encephalopathy.

Clinical finding	*Probable etiology*
Pallor	Cerebral malaria, typhoid, intracranial bleed
Icterus	Leptospirosis, cerebral malaria
Generalized lymph-adenopathy	EBV, leptospirosis, HIV
Skin rashes	Meningococcemia, arboviruses, varicella, rickettsia, dengue, measles, enterovirus
Petechiae	Meningococcemia, dengue, viral hemorrhagic fevers
Erythema nodosum	Tuberculosis, histoplasmosis
Parotid swelling and orchitis	Mumps
Mucous membrane lesions and shallow ulcers	Herpes simplex virus
Abnormal odor of breath	Diabetic ketoacidosis, hepatic coma
Myalgia, arthralgia	Leptospirosis, dengue
Hypotension, shock	Dengue, leptospirosis, cerebral malaria
Organomegaly	EBV, dengue, leptospirosis, HIV

(EBV: Epstein-Barr virus; HIV: human immunodeficiency virus)

Detailed neurological examination: The neurological examination is targeted to document the level and localization of brain dysfunction. It may also provide information about the potential causes. This includes assessment of the level of consciousness, patterns of respiration, and signs of meningeal irritation, fundus and pupillary examination, signs of cranial nerve involvement, presence of focal deficits, signs of raised ICP, brainstem signs and autonomic signs.

The level of consciousness must be recorded in the form of an objective scale, such as the GCS or the AVPU score. While the GCS allows efficient, standardized communication of a child's state, a more detailed description of the child's clinical findings is often more useful for relaying detailed information and detecting changes over time.

TABLE 5: Types of abnormal respiratory patterns.

Pattern	*Lesion*	*Presentation*	*Conditions*
Cheyne-Stokes respiration	Deep hemispheric or diencephalic dysfunction	Hyperpnea alternates with apnea	Strokes, traumatic brain injuries, brain tumors, carbon dioxide poisoning, metabolic encephalopathy, high altitude sickness, normal side effect of IV morphine administration
Central neurogenic hyperventilation	Midbrain dysfunction	Sustained, deep, regular, and rapid respiration	Strokes, traumatic brain injuries. Increasing irregularity of this respiratory pattern generally is a sign that the patient will enter into coma
Apneustic	Damage to the pons or upper medulla	Inspiratory pauses, lasting 2–3 seconds, alternating with end-expiratory pauses	Strokes, trauma, pontine infarction, anoxic encephalopathy, and ketamine (temporary)
Ataxic	Damage to the medulla oblongata	Completely irregular breathing pattern with irregular pauses and unpredictable periods of apnea	Trauma, stroke, opioid use This respiratory pattern indicates a very poor prognosis

Respiratory pattern abnormalities signify either a metabolic derangement or a neurological insult **(Table 5)**.

Pupils: Pupillary size, shape, symmetry, and response to light provide valuable clues to brainstem and third nerve dysfunction. The presence or absence of the pupillary reaction to light is one of the most important differentiating features to distinguish between structural and metabolic disorders as metabolic disturbances affect the pupillary pathways late. Usually in metabolic disorders leading to altered level of consciousness, pupils remain reactive in the initial stages. But in structural disorders with increased ICP, signs of herniation syndrome will appear. Topical administration of mydriatics must be avoided, but if done, should be documented to avoid confusion in interpretation. Abnormalities of eye position and movement may provide some clues. Conjugate lateral deviation of the eyes is a sign either of an ipsilateral hemisphere lesion, a contralateral hemisphere seizure focus, or damage involving the contralateral pontine horizontal gaze center (parapontine reticular formation). Lateral gaze palsy may signal central herniation with compression of bilateral sixth nerves. Tonic upward gaze has been associated with bilateral hemispheric damage.

The presence of oculocephalic (doll's eye), oculovestibular, corneal, cough, and gag reflexes must be looked for to check for brainstem function. Brainstem dysfunction is an important feature in some causes of viral encephalitis such as enterovirus 71, mumps, and rabies and in all causes when the ICP has risen progressively.

Fundus examination must be performed to look for papilledema and retinal hemorrhages. Retinal hemorrhages are an important clue for cerebral malaria in endemic setting, being present in nearly a quarter of the patients.

CLINICAL PEARL

- Unilateral pupillary dilatation in the comatose patient should be considered as evidence of oculomotor nerve compression from ipsilateral uncal herniation, unless proved otherwise.

Motor examination ***(Table 6)****:* Assessment of muscle strength, tone, and tendon reflexes should be done for normality and symmetry. The trunk, limb position, spontaneous movements, and response to stimulation must be observed to look for any focal deficits (suggestive of postictal Todd's palsy or structural abnormality), and posturing (decerebrate or decorticate).

Special attention should be given to posturing because it often signals a brainstem herniation syndrome.

- *Decorticate posturing:* Flexion of upper limbs and extension of the lower limbs. It suggests involvement of the cerebral cortex and preservation of brainstem function
- *Decerebrate posturing:* Rigid extension of both arms and legs indicative of cortical and brainstem dysfunction
- *Opisthotonus:* Neck is hyperextended and the teeth are clenched; the arms are adducted and hyperextended; and the legs are extended with feet plantar flexed. It indicates severe brainstem dysfunction
- The flaccid patient with no response to painful stimuli indicates deep brainstem dysfunction
- Monoplegia or hemiplegia, except when in postictal phase, suggests a structural disturbance of the contralateral hemisphere (herniation across falx).

Presence of signs of meningeal irritation (neck rigidity, Kernig's sign, and Brudzinski's sign) must be looked for. Kernig's sign involves flexion of the hip to 90° with subsequent pain on extension of the leg; Brudzinski's sign involves involuntary flexion of the knees and hips after passive flexion of the neck while supine. In younger children, Kernig's and Brudzinski's signs are not consistently present; especially with an open fontanel. Signs of meningeal irritation may be present in meningitis, encephalitis, and subarachnoid hemorrhage. Neck rigidity is present in meningitis, tonsillar herniation, or craniocervical trauma.

The commonly seen focal signs are hemiparesis, ataxia, aphasia, pyramidal signs, and involuntary movements (myoclonus, dystonia, tremors). Cranial neuropathies of the ocular, oculomotor, abducens, facial, and auditory nerve should be looked for.

Signs of increased intracranial tension in children range from headache, vomiting to herniation. It is best to suspect raised ICP and start treating it, on clinical grounds alone. Raised ICP, when untreated, can also lead to herniation of the brain, which causes direct mechanical damage as well as ischemia and hemorrhage secondary to vascular distortion. Brain tissue deforms intracranially and moves from higher to lower pressure when there is asymmetric, unilateral, or generalized increased ICP. This gives rise to the various herniation syndromes. These syndromes, in this order (from higher to lower pressures), signify a progression in severity. Changes from one syndrome to the next, signifies progressive worsening.

The various herniation syndromes can be recognized clinically. The importance lies in recognition and prompt treatment, before the damage becomes irreversible. Treatment of herniation involves removal of the etiologic mass and surgical decompression in the form of external ventricular drainage and hemicraniectomy may be indicated **(Table 7)**.

TABLE 6: Important clues in neurological examination in acute febrile encephalopathy.

CNS signs	*Probable etiology*
Abnormal behavior or psychosis	HSV, NCSE
Meningeal signs	Meningitis, TBM, encephalitis, ADEM
Ataxia	ADEM, varicella, enterovirus
Asymmetric signs and symptoms	TBM, encephalitis, ADEM
Papilledema	SOL, hydrocephalus in TBM
Opisthotonus	JE, autoimmune encephalitis
Cranial nerve palsies	TBM, encephalitis, JE, vasculitis
Bowel and bladder dysfunction	ADEM
Visual loss	Optic neuritis, ADEM, HT encephalopathy
Rapidly changing CNS signs	JE
Acute flaccid paralysis	Enterovirus, poliomyelitis, ADEM
Seizures	JE, cerebral malaria, TBM, meningitis
Dystonia or extra-pyramidal movements	JE, TBM
Myoclonic jerks	Enterovirus

(ADEM: acute disseminated encephalomyelitis; CNS: central nervous system; HSV: herpes simplex virus; HT: hypertensive; JE: Japanese encephalitis; NCSE: nonconvulsive status epilepticus; SOL: space occupying lesion; TBM: tuberculous meningitis)

TABLE 7: Clinical recognition of herniation syndromes.

Type of herniation	*Clinical manifestations*
Uncal	• Unilateral ptosis • Unilateral fixed dilated pupil • Minimal deviation of eyes on oculocephalic/oculovestibular testing hemiparesis
Diencephalic	• Small or midpoint pupils reactive to light • Full deviation of eyes on oculocephalic/oculovestibular testing • Flexor response to pain and/or decorticate posturing • Cheyne-Stokes respiration • Hypertonia and/or hyperreflexia with extensor plantars
Midbrain	• Midpoint pupils, fixed to light
Upper pontine	• Minimal deviation of eyes on oculocephalic/oculovestibular testing • Extensor response to pain and/or decerebrate posturing • Hyperventilation
Lower pontine	• Midpoint pupils, fixed to light • No response on oculocephalic/oculovestibular testing • No response to pain or flexion of legs only • Flaccidity with extensor plantars • Shallow or ataxic respiration
Medullary	• Pupils dilated, fixed to light • Slow, irregular, or gasping respiration • Respiratory arrest with inadequate cardiac output

Step 3: Send Basic Investigations

Basic Investigations

Basic workup like complete blood count with platelet count, peripheral smear, blood culture, blood glucose, liver and renal profile, coagulation parameters, and electrolytes should be obtained in all patients presenting with an AFE. An arterial blood gas, chest X-ray, serum ammonia, and serum lactate should be sent if required.

All patients with febrile encephalopathy should undergo blood cultures. Relative lymphocytosis in the peripheral blood is common in viral encephalitis. Leukopenia and thrombocytopenia are noted in viral hemorrhagic fevers and rickettsial infections. Typhoid fever and cerebral malaria may be associated with severe anemia and thrombocytopenia. Hypoglycemia and electrolyte imbalance are usually associated with CNS infection and they may contribute to altered sensorium. Serum creatinine and blood urea are helpful to assess the renal function and serum bilirubin, transaminases and prothrombin time are indicated if jaundice is present. An X-ray chest may show changes suggestive of tuberculosis, mycoplasma, or legionellosis.

In endemic areas, look for malaria (peripheral smear and rapid detection tests), dengue (serology and NS1 Ag), Leptospira (antibody tests), enteric fever (blood culture), typhus (antibody test), and JE (antibody in serum and CSF) as the probable etiology.

KEY POINTS

Baseline investigations recommended in acute febrile encephalopathy:
- Complete blood count with platelets, peripheral smear
- Blood glucose
- Blood culture, urine examination
- Liver function tests, renal function tests, electrolytes
- Coagulation parameters, chest X-ray
- Arterial blood gas measurement, lactate, ammonia.

Tests which may be done in endemic areas:
- Malaria (peripheral smear and rapid antigen test)
- Dengue (serology and nonstructural protein 1 antigen)
- Leptospira (antibody tests)
- Enteric fever (blood culture)
- Typhus (antibody test)
- Japanese encephalitis (antibody in serum and cerebrospinal fluid).

Lumbar Puncture

Urgent evaluation of CSF is required when there is a suspected infection of the CNS; provided the patient is hemodynamically stable, and has no features of raised ICP. A lumbar puncture is recommended in all patients with suspected CNS infections who are febrile, have a GCS less than 12, and are less than an year old [probably with an open atrial fibrillation (AF)], and those who are clinically stable to undergo the procedure. In patients who are not stable, a neuroimaging study should be obtained prior to the lumbar puncture **(Box 3)**.

BOX 3: Contraindications of lumbar puncture.

Lumbar puncture should be deferred in patients with:
- Abnormal breathing patterns
- Shock
- Bradycardia (HR <60)
- Hypertension (BP >95th percentile)
- GCS <8 or deteriorating GCS
- Convulsive SE or NCSE
- Abnormal doll's eye movement
- Dilated pupils
- Impaired pupillary reaction to light
- Abnormal posture
- Features of raised ICP

(BP: blood pressure; GCS: Glasgow Coma Scale; HR: heart rate; ICP: intracranial pressure; NCSE: non-convulsive status epilepticus; SE: status epilepticus)

Cerebrospinal fluid should be examined for pressure, gross examination for turbidity, cytology, biochemistry, Gram's stain, Ziehl-Neelsen stain for acid fast bacilli, bacterial culture, latex agglutination, polymerase chain reaction (PCR) for HSV 1 and 2, and IgM antibodies for JE and for dengue virus (if suspected), and additional cultures based on clinical suspicion (fungal or tubercular). Concurrent blood sugar must also be measured to look for the CSF to blood sugar ratio.

Usual CSF findings in viral encephalitis include lymphocytic pleocytosis, mild to moderately elevated protein, and normal CSF sugar. Similar findings may occur in tubercular meningitis and partially-treated pyogenic meningitis; however, the CSF sugar is likely to be low in these situations. Neutrophilic predominance is seen in pyogenic meningitis with high protein levels, and a Gram's stain, latex agglutination test or culture may clinch the diagnosis.

Empirical treatment should be started pending the results of lumbar puncture and/or neuroimaging studies. The CSF analysis is an important investigation in children with AES.

Neuroimaging

Decision for imaging should not delay the empiric therapy. CT scan of the brain is of limited value in a patient with

AFE, since it does not definitely indicate either meningeal or parenchymal involvement; however, it may be the only possible option available in an emergency. It is known that CT scan is likely to be normal in many cases of viral encephalitis, especially in the early stages and is more likely to pick up abnormality in the later stages when the pathology is well established. Magnetic resonance imaging is more likely to pick up early lesions in patients with AFE and should be the radiological investigation of choice in such patients as soon as it is available.

Computed tomography (CT): If the child is afebrile and deeply comatose and/or has focal signs, it is preferable to do a CT scan prior to a lumbar puncture. Focal seizures and presence of focal neurological deficits indicate a localized lesion and are expected to be picked up by CT scan. Computed tomography scan may give valuable information such as presence of a bleed, and basal exudates and hydrocephalus in tubercular meningitis. The presence of diffuse edema on CT scan may suggest an underlying parenchymal involvement and focal hypodensities in temporal lobe and basal ganglia or thalamus may point towards a possible diagnosis of viral encephalitis (HSV or JE). Computed tomography may also show brain herniation, effacement of cisterns, and infective collections such as brain abscesses and subdural empyema. Computed tomography should be performed immediately when the examination suggests increased ICP (papilledema, bulging fontanel in infants, or bradycardia with hypertension) or a transtentorial herniation syndrome **(Box 4)**.

Magnetic resonance imaging (MRI): If possible, an MRI should be obtained, as soon as the patient is stable. Magnetic resonance imaging is known to be superior in picking up subtle changes and is likely to be more helpful in establishing a diagnosis by picking up characteristic pattern of gray matter involvement and meningeal enhancement. Magnetic resonance imaging is more sensitive for early evidence of viral encephalitis and may show frontotemporal pathology in HSV infection, thalamic involvement in JE, and midbrain and pons involvement in enterovirus infection. It also picks up infarction, diffuse axonal injury from head injury, petechial hemorrhages, cerebral venous thrombosis and necrotizing lesions in acute necrotizing encephalopathy. Magnetic resonance imaging is also useful for diagnosing alternative etiologies such as ADEM (evident as demyelination on MRI), and antibody associated encephalopathies.

BOX 4: Indications of computed tomography.

- Intracranial bleed
- Basal exudates and hydrocephalus (tuberculous meningitis)
- Herniation syndromes
- Brain abscess
- Subdural empyema

BOX 5: Indications of magnetic resonance imaging.

- Frontotemporal lesions (herpes simplex virus)
- Thalamic involvement (Japanese encephalitis)
- Midbrain and pons (enterovirus)
- Demyelination (acute disseminated encephalomyelitis)
- Infarction, cerebral venous thrombosis

Magnetic resonance imaging may also offer information regarding prognosis in patients with anoxic or traumatic coma.

Magnetic resonance imaging is not needed if the etiology is clear by other investigations, e.g., cerebral malaria, pyogenic meningitis; or if suggestive changes are seen on CT; or in epidemic situations where the likely etiology is already known. In all other patients, MRI provides useful information regarding the etiology and alternative diagnoses. However, the availability, cost, and difficulties in transporting sick and unstable patients for MRI may be limiting factors **(Box 5)**.

CLINICAL PEARLS

- Empirical treatment should be started pending the results of lumbar puncture.
- Decision for imaging should not delay the therapy.
- Magnetic resonance imaging is preferable to computed tomography, if available and affordable.

Step 4: Initiate Empiric Therapy

Empiric antimicrobial treatment is recommended when the diagnosis of bacterial meningitis or herpes encephalitis is strongly suspected, as early treatment improves prognosis of these conditions. Treatment may impair the diagnostic sensitivity of CSF cultures but should not affect other tests (total cell count, Gram's stain, or PCR). The recommended empiric therapy in a case of AFE is a combination of a third-generation cephalosporin, acyclovir and an antimalarial.

A broad-spectrum antibiotic such as ceftriaxone must be given in a dose of 100 mg/kg/day, which can be stopped if no evidence of bacterial meningitis is evident in the subsequent CSF analysis or imaging.

Acyclovir must be started according to age-specific doses, in all cases of suspected viral encephalitis, as HSE is a treatable disease, and can be stopped if the HSV PCR in CSF is negative or the MRI findings are not suggestive of the same. Children beyond the neonatal group should be treated with intravenous acyclovir in a dose of 10 mg/kg every 8 hours given as a 1-hour infusion. A positive MRI scan and EEG have 95% sensitivity in the diagnosis of HSE. However, if the CSF PCR for HSV or MRI have been performed very early after the symptom onset (within 48 hours), these may be falsely negative. Hence, these studies should be repeated before stopping acyclovir if the clinical suspicion of HSE continues to be high.

Empirical antimalarials must be started if there is a suspicion of cerebral malaria. The recommended antimalarial therapy is an artemisinin-based combination therapy consisting of artesunate + sulfadoxine-pyrimethamine or artemether + lumefantrine. Alternatively, quinine may be used with strict monitoring of blood sugar levels and ECG. This should be stopped if the peripheral smear and rapid diagnostic tests are negative.

KEY POINTS

Recommended Empiric therapy for AFE
- Ceftriaxone + Acyclovir + Antimalarial.

Step 5: Send Specific Investigations and Treat the Cause

When the etiology is not clear, other microbiological investigations must be obtained **(Table 8 and 9)**. These samples include urine, throat swab, nasopharyngeal aspirate, serum, and swab from vesicles or rash, if present. In patients having unexplained encephalopathy with fever and rash, testing for rickettsial infections (Weil-Felix test, and rickettsial serology) must be performed. HIV testing should be performed in children with unexplained encephalitis, as rarely, meningoencephalitis may be a presenting feature of primary HIV infection.

Additional studies may be indicated if there are clinical clues suggestive of particular infections. These may include HSV whole blood PCR in suspected cases of disseminated HSV infection and serologic testing for measles, mumps, arboviruses, varicella, EBV, syphilis, and Lyme disease.

TABLE 8: Specific therapy according to the etiology of acute febrile encephalopathy.

Diagnosis	*Specific therapy*
Herpes simplex virus	Acyclovir-DOC, valacyclovir, foscarnet
Varicella zoster	Acyclovir
Human herpes virus 6	Foscarnet, ganciclovir
Cytomegalovirus	Ganciclovir
Enterovirus	Pleconaril
Rickettsia	Doxycycline, erythromycin
Mycoplasma	Azithromycin
Leptospirosis	Penicillin
Tuberculosis	Antitubercular drugs
Pyogenic meningitis	Ceftriaxone + vancomycin
ADEM	Steroids, IVIG

(ADEM: acute disseminated encephalomyelitis; DOC: drug of choice; IVIG: intravenous immunoglobulin)

Identifiable causes like DKA and hypertensive encephalopathy should be treated according to the recommended protocols. The clinician should always be alert to the possibility of child abuse in an infant/toddler with sudden unexplained altered consciousness.

In suspected cases of opioid ingestion, naloxone should be administered; atropine and pralidoxime should be given in suspected organophosphorus poisoning and flumazenil should be given for benzodiazepine overdose. Antivenom is recommended in cases of envenomation.

Other Tests

An EEG must be performed in all children with unexplained altered sensorium to look for suspected NCSE. Periodic epileptiform discharges may occur in NCSE but also in underlying brain injury without seizures. Diffuse theta and delta activity, absence of faster frequencies, and intermittent rhythmic delta activity are characteristic of severe encephalopathies. Periodic lateralized epileptiform discharges suggest herpes encephalitis or infarction. Multifocal or generalized periodic discharges can also be seen with metabolic and infectious etiologies and are characteristic of subacute sclerosing panencephalitis. Triphasic waves indicate a hepatic or uremic encephalopathy. Nonepileptiform features of the EEG, such as slowing or asymmetry, are largely nonspecific findings, but can sometimes provide diagnostic or prognostic information. Continuous EEG

TABLE 9: Diagnostic criteria used for some common etiologies of acute febrile encephalopathy.

Diagnosis	*Criteria*
HSV encephalitis	• Nonspecific prodrome, exanthem ± • Fever with altered sensorium, focal signs +, neck signs + • CSF cytology (predominant lymphocytes), CSF PCR and serology • *EEG:* Periodic lateralized epileptiform discharges • *MRI/CT:* Frontotemporal pathology
Japanese encephalitis	• Disorientation and delirium → somnolence, then progressing to coma • Rapidly changing central nervous system signs, seizures • CSF pleocytosis, PCR, antigen tests • Albuminuria
Pyogenic meningitis	• Fever with altered sensorium, no focal signs, neck signs + • CSF cytology (predominant neutrophils) • *MRI/CT:* Meningeal enhancement
Tubercular meningitis	• *Stage 1:* Nonspecific signs, stage 2—neck signs, signs of ↑ ICP, cranial nerve palsies, focal signs, stage 3—coma, decorticate/decerebrate posturing • CSF compatible with TBM, isolation of AFB, ADA ↑ • *MRI/CT:* Hydrocephalus, basal exudates, tuberculoma
Cerebral malaria	• Fever with altered sensorium ± focal signs, frequent seizures hypoglycemia • Peripheral smear +, rapid antigen test +
ADEM	• Fever much earlier than the onset of encephalopathy • Cranial nerve palsies, visual loss, ataxia, motor and sensory deficits, bladder/bowel dysfunction, and spinal cord demyelination • CSF compatible (↑ proteins, N sugars, N cytology) • *EEG:* Generalized slowing, occipital epileptiform discharges • *MRI:* Diffuse white matter changes
Sepsis associated encephalopathy (SAE)	• Underlying sepsis syndrome • CSF and imaging normal

(ADA: adenosine deaminase activity; AFB: acid-fast bacilli; CSF: cerebrospinal fluid; CT: computed tomography; EEG: electroencephalogram; HSV: herpes simplex virus; ICP: intracranial pressure; MRI: magnetic resonance imaging; PCR: polymerase chain reaction; TBM: tuberculous meningitis)

can be used to assess and titrate the depth of sedation in patients placed under anesthesia for control of status epilepticus or increased ICP. Electrocardiogram may also be helpful in patients with subtle and doubtful seizures, to guide antiepileptic drug management.

In cases of suspected metabolic abnormalities and unexplained or recurrent encephalopathy, blood ammonia, urine and blood samples for amino and organic acid disorders, free fatty acid and carnitine levels should be obtained before starting treatment and stopping feeds. Hyperammonemia may be caused by some inborn errors of metabolism, Reye's syndrome, liver failure, or valproate toxicity. Blood tandem mass spectroscopy, urine gas chromatography-mass spectroscopy can detect common causes of intoxication and drug abuse, and specific drug levels (suspected antiepileptic toxicity) should be obtained if specific ingestions are suspected. In selected cases, a urine toxicology screen, thyroid function tests and thyroid autoantibodies (Hashimoto's encephalopathy), cortisol levels, carboxyhemoglobin levels (carbon monoxide poisoning), autoimmune screen (cerebral vasculitis), and coagulation studies (coagulopathy) are recommended.

Step 6: Supportive Care

After stabilization of the airway, breathing, and circulation, other supportive care measures must be instituted along with the empirical treatment as mentioned above. Timely and appropriate supportive care is of paramount importance to reduce the mortality and morbidity associated with viral encephalitis. Patients with GCS less than 8, having features of raised ICP, status epilepticus, and shock should ideally be managed in an intensive care unit. Full sedation, controlled ventilation, and minimal handling with elevation of the head end of the bed at 30°, should be maintained during transport of the child.

Maintenance Intravenous Fluids

Fluid therapy should be targeted to maintain euvolemia and normoglycemia, and to prevent hyponatremia. Children with acute viral encephalitis should receive fluids at the normal daily requirement. Increased fluids and fluid boluses may be indicated for dehydration and hypotension. Serum sodium should be monitored, and abnormalities of serum sodium should be corrected slowly. Rapid correction of hyponatremia may lead to central pontine myelinolysis.

Other Drugs

Corticosteroids: Steroids are indicated in meningococcemia with shock, enteric encephalopathy, ADEM, Hashimoto's encephalopathy, and autoimmune encephalitis. The role of corticosteroids in the treatment of viral encephalitis is not established. However, corticosteroids may be considered along with acyclovir in patients with marked cerebral edema, brain shift or raised ICP. Dexamethasone is recommended prior to antibiotics in *H. influenzae* B meningitis, as it reduces the incidence of deafness and neurological handicap. However, this benefit is not certain for meningitis due to other organisms like *Pneumococcus*.

If metabolic causes have been identified, e.g., DKA, hepatic encephalopathy, uremia, or hyperammonemia, these should be treated appropriately. Concurrent bacterial infections like pneumonia should be appropriately treated. Haloperidol and phenergan may be used to combat the abnormal or psychotic behavior. Dopamine receptor blocking agents are used to control the choreoathetosis, and muscle relaxants and anticholinergics may help in the management of dystonia.

Step 7: Prevention/Treatment of Complications and Rehabilitation

The clinical course of the child should be monitored closely and documented on a daily basis. Particular attention should be paid to changing level of consciousness, fever, seizures, autonomic nervous system dysfunction, increased ICP, and speech and motor disturbances.

Supportive and rehabilitative efforts are very important after patients recover. Nosocomial infections, aspiration pneumonia, and coagulation disturbances may occur as complications, and should be detected and treated promptly. Motor incoordination, convulsive disorders, total or partial deafness, and behavioral disturbances are commonly seen after viral CNS infections. Visual disturbances due to chorioretinopathy and peripheral amblyopia may also be seen. Myocarditis and pulmonary edema are important complications of enteroviral encephalitis. Subdural effusions develop in 10–30% of patients with meningitis. Other complications include seizures, raised ICP, cranial nerve palsies, stroke, herniation syndromes, and thrombosis of the dural venous sinuses. Pericarditis or arthritis may occur in patients being treated for meningitis, especially that caused by *Neisseria meningitidis*.

Rifampicin chemoprophylaxis is recommended for all close contacts of patients with meningococcal and *H. influenzae* B meningitis. Vaccination for *H. influenzae* B is recommended for all children, and meningococcal and pneumococcal vaccine should be given to the high-risk groups. Vaccination for polio, measles, mumps, rubella and varicella should also be instituted. Control of insect vectors by suitable spraying methods and eradication of insect breeding sites reduces the incidence of arboviral infections and malaria.

Regular posture change must be done to prevent the development of bed sores. The patient should be started on early physiotherapy, to prevent the development of contractures. Neurodevelopmental and audiologic evaluations should be a part of the routine follow-up of children who have recovered from viral meningoencephalitis. Metabolic causes may need long-term dietary treatment. Psychological support needs to be rendered to the patient and family.

PROGNOSIS

The outcome of a child with an AFE depends on the etiology, and the depth and duration of impaired consciousness, the specific cause and the age of the child. Prolonged coma after a hypoxic-ischemic insult carries a poor prognosis. Most children surviving infectious encephalopathies have a comparatively better outcome, often surviving with mild or moderate difficulties only. Outcome has been shown to be worse for patients who were younger, had a lower GCS score on presentation, or had absent brainstem reflexes, poor motor responses, hypothermia, or hypotension. These children should be followed up for early identification of developmental disabilities, learning and behavior problems, as well as other neurological sequelae such as motor, visual, or hearing deficit and seizure disorder. Acute complications like motor deficits and cortical blindness improve with time.

CONCLUSION

Diagnostic approach to a child presenting with an AFE poses a real challenge, especially when the history is not reliable and the clinical findings are not contributory towards a specific etiology. A high index of suspicion should be maintained for a diagnosis in these patients as time is the essence in the management strategy. A systematic approach to the history, thorough physical examination and appropriate investigations aimed at recognition of the etiology could aid in the diagnosis. Early stabilization and institution of nonspecific-supportive measures remain the cornerstone of management, and identification of the cause and its appropriate treatment need to be instituted in order to ensure the survival and also to prevent long-term sequelae, neurological or otherwise.

KEY POINTS

- Acute febrile encephalopathy is an altered mental state manifested by fever, coma, seizures, and/or decerebration.
- Central nervous system infections are the most common cause of acute febrile encephalopathy in children.
- A definitive diagnosis may not be possible even after a detailed diagnostic workup.
- Early recognition, efficient decision making and institution of therapy can be lifesaving.

SUGGESTED READING

1. American Heart Association. 2005 American Heart Association (AHA) guidelines for cardiopulmonary resuscitation (CPR) and emergency cardiovascular care (ECC) of pediatric and neonatal patients: pediatric basic life support. Pediatrics. 2006;117:e989-e1004.
2. Bansal A, Singhi S, Singhi P, Khandelwal N, Ramesh N. Non traumatic coma. Indian J Pediatrics. 2005;72:467-73.
3. Bauer T. Non-convulsive status epilepticus and coma. Epilepsia. 2010;51:177-90.
4. Bhalla A, Suri V, Singh P, Varma S, Khandelwal NK. Imaging in adult patients with acute febrile encephalopathy. Journal of Acute Disease. 2012;1:7-12.
5. Bhalla A, Suri V, Varma S, Sharma N, Mahi S, Singh P, et al. Acute febrile encephalopathy in adults from Northwest India. J Emerg Trauma Shock. 2010;3:220-4.
6. Chandran A, Herbert H, Misurski D, Santosham M. Long-term sequelae of childhood bacterial meningitis. Pediatr Infect Dis J. 2011;30:3-6.
7. Charles G. Prober,LauraLe Dyner: Viral Meningo-encephalitis. In: Kliegman RM, Stanton BM, St. Geme J, Schor N, Behrman RE (Eds). Nelson Textbook of Pediatrics, 19th ed. Saunders Elsevier; 2011. pp. 2095-7.
8. Glaser CA, Honarmand S, Anderson LJ, Schnurr DP, Forghani B, Cossen CK, et al. Beyond viruses: clinical profiles and etiologies associated with encephalitis. Clin Infect Dis. 2006;43:1565-77.
9. Grimwood K, Andersen P, Andersen V, Tan L, Nolan T. Twelve year outcomes following bacterial meningitis: Further evidence for persisting effects. Arch Dis Child. 2000;83:111-6.
10. Hazarika D. Approach to a child with fever and altered sensorium. Indian J Pract Pediatr. 2011;13:193-206.
11. Karmarkar SA, Aneja S, Khare S, Saini A, Seth A, Chauhan BK. A study of acute febrile encephalopathy with special reference to viral etiology. Indian J Pediatr. 2008;75:801-5.
12. Kirkham FJ. Non traumatic coma in children. Arch Dis Child. 2001;85:303-12.
13. Klig JE, O'Malley PJ. Pediatric office emergencies. Curr Opin Pediatr. 2007;19:591-6.
14. Kneen R, Jakka S, Mithyantha R, Riordan A, Solomon T. The management of infants and children treated with acyclovir for suspected viral encephalitis. Arch Dis Child. 2010;95:100-6.
15. Kneen R, Michael BD, Menson E, Mehta B, Easton A, Hemingway C, et al. Management of suspected viral encephalitis in children—Association of British Neurologists and British Pediatric Allergy Immunology and Infection Group National Guidelines. J Infect. 2012;64:449-77.
16. Koelfen W, Freund M, Gückel F, Rohr H, Schultze C. MRI of encephalitis in children: Comparison of CT and MRI in the acute stage with long-term follow-up. Neuroradiology. 1996;38:73-9.
17. Kothari VM, Karnad DR, Bichile LS. Tropical infections in the ICU. J Assoc Physicians India. 2006;54:291-8.
18. Logan SA, MacMahon E. Viral meningitis. BMJ. 2008;336:36-40.
19. Mikati MA. Status epilepticus. In: Kliegman RM, Stanton BM, St. Geme J, Schor N, Behrman RE (Eds). Nelson Textbook of Pediatrics, 19th ed. Saunders Elsevier; 2011. p. 2038.
20. Modi A, Atam V, Jain N, Gutch M, Verma R. The etiological diagnosis and outcome in patients of acute febrile encephalopathy: A prospective observational study at tertiary care center. Neurol India. 2012;60:168-73.
21. Murthy SN, Faden HS, Cohen ME, Bakshi R. Acute disseminated encephalomyelitis in children. Pediatrics. 2002;110:e21.
22. Parke JT. Acute encephalopathies. In: McMillan JA, Feigin RD, DeAngelis C, Jones MD (Eds). Oski's Pediatrics: Principles and Practice, 4th ed. Philadelphia: Lippincott Williams & Wilkins; 2006. p. 2258.
23. Prober CG, Le Dyner L. Acute bacterial meningitis beyond the neonatal period. In: Nelson Textbook of Pediatrics, 19th ed. Saunders Elsevier; 2011:595:2087-2095.
24. Sankhyan N, Vykunta Raju KN, Sharma S, Gulati S. Management of raised intracranial pressure. Indian J Pediatr. 2010;77:1409-16.
25. Saunders M, Gorelick MH. Evaluation of the sick child in the office and clinic. In: Kliegman RM, Stanton BM, St. Geme J, Schor N, Behrman RE (Eds). Nelson Textbook of Pediatrics, 19th ed. Saunders Elsevier; 2011. pp. 275-8.
26. Schor NF. Acute disseminated encephalomyelitis (ADEM). In: Kliegman RM, Stanton BM, St. Geme J, Schor N, Behrman RE (Eds). Nelson Textbook of Pediatrics, 19th ed. Saunders Elsevier; 2011. pp. 2079-80.

27. Sharma S, Kochar GS, Sankhyan N, Gulati S. Approach to the child with coma. Indian J Pediatr. 2010;77:1279-87.
28. Sharma S, Mishra D, Aneja S, Kumar R, Jain A. For the expert group on Encephalitis, Indian Academy of Pediatrics: Consensus Guidelines on Evaluation and Management of Suspected Acute Viral Encephalitis in Children in India. Indian Pediatrics. 2012;49:897-910.
29. Shaw DW, Cohen WA. Viral infections of the CNS in children: imaging features. Am J Roentgenol. 1993;160: 125-33.
30. Singh RR, Chaudhary SK, Bhatta NK, Khanal B, Shah D. Clinical and etiological profile of acute febrile encephalopathy in eastern Nepal. Indian J Pediatr. 2009;76: 1109-11.
31. Stevens RD, Bhardwaj A. Approach to the comatose patient. Crit Care Med. 2006;34:31-41.
32. Taylor DA, Ashwal S. Impairment of consciousness and coma. In: Swaiman KF, Ashwal S, Ferriero DM (Eds). Pediatric Neurology: Principles and Practice, 4th ed. Philadelphia: Elsevier Publications; 2006. p. 1379.
33. Tenembaum S, Chitnis T, Ness J, Hahn JS. Acute disseminated encephalomyelitis. Neurology. 2007;68:S23-S36.
34. Tunkel AR, Hartman BJ, Kaplan SL, Kaufman BA, Roos KL, Scheld WM, et al. Practice guideline for the management of bacterial meningitis. Clin Infect Dis. 2004;39:1267-84.
35. Yeolekar ME, Trivedi TH. Febrile encephalopathy: challenges in management. J Assoc Physicians India. 2006; 54:845-7.

Management of a Child with Respiratory Distress

Sanjay M Bafna, Kochurani Abraham

INTRODUCTION

Respiratory distress (RD) is a manifestation of variety of pulmonary and extrapulmonary conditions. Prompt recognition and early intervention prevent progression of RD to respiratory failure (RF) and cardiorespiratory arrest.

This chapter describes general management approach to RD with main focus on emergency room management. Detailed specific management of conditions causing RD is discussed elsewhere in the book.

DEFINITIONS

Respiratory distress is a clinical state characterized by abnormal respiratory rate or effort. It commonly manifests as tachypnea and increased work of breathing.

A child with neurological illness usually has abnormal pattern of respiration and/or bradypnea.

Respiratory failure is defined as a clinical state of inadequate oxygenation or ventilation or both. It is often the end stage of RD.

PATHOPHYSIOLOGY

Most important function of respiratory system is oxygenation and ventilation. Impaired oxygenation in lungs results in hypoxemia. This may occur due to alveolar hypoventilation, V/Q mismatch or right to left shunt.

Tissue oxygenation depends on oxygenation in lungs, cardiac output, hemoglobin concentration, and tissue perfusion. Impairment of any of these would result in tissue hypoxia.

Inadequate ventilation is seen in airway disease, lung parenchymal disease, and central hypoventilation. This results in hypercarbia.

Conditions causing tissue hypoxia or hypercarbia result in RD as a compensatory mechanism to maintain adequate gas exchange.

When these compensations fail, child develops RF.

INITIAL EVALUATION AND STABILIZATION

The first priority is evaluation and stabilization of airway, breathing, and circulation.

Airway

The airway is assessed to see if it is patent or obstructed. This is done by "look, listen, and feel" for air movement. Abnormal airway sounds and/or poor air entry may indicate obstructed airway.

The airway can be clear, maintainable, or not maintainable.

Clear Airway

Allow the child position of comfort.

Maintainable Airway

This essentially means that the airway may be partially obstructed but is maintainable by simple maneuvers like positioning, suctioning, removal of a visible foreign body from the mouth, or use of airway adjuncts.

- *Head tilt/chin lift:* If the airway is blocked by the falling back of the tongue, it may be opened by this maneuver. The rescuer places one hand on the forehead and applies pressure to tilt the head back gently, to achieve neutral position in an infant and sniffing position in a child. Two to three fingers of the other hand should then be placed under the chin to lift it upwards. The thumb of this hand may be used to part the lips to keep the mouth open.
- *Jaw thrust:* This is used in suspected cervical spine injury as head tilt-chin lift is contraindicated. This is achieved by placing two or three fingers under the angle of the mandible bilaterally, and lifting the jaw upwards.

Not Maintainable Airway

It may need one of the following advanced airway interventions:

- Endotracheal intubation
- Laryngeal mask airway in unconscious patient
- Application of continuous positive airway pressure (CPAP)
- Cricothyrotomy/tracheostomy
- Endoscopic removal of foreign body

Breathing

This can be supported by administration of oxygen or by assisted ventilation. It is important to differentiate RD from RF at initial evaluation. Child with RF has features of hypoxemia and hypercarbia.

> **CLINICAL PEARL**
>
> Respiratory failure is a clinical diagnosis. Arterial blood gas is done for confirmation and monitoring.

In a child with RD, maintenance of airway, administration of oxygen, etiological management, and monitoring may suffice. But in a child with RF, one must take total control of airway and breathing.

Oxygen Delivery

In a child with RD, proper administration of high concentration of oxygen is the mainstay of therapy. Oxygen is given in a nonthreatening manner to a child with RD, avoiding agitation as far as possible, as this increases the work of breathing and makes the flow of air turbulent thereby increasing the resistance to air flow. Taking the mothers help to provide oxygen goes a long way in decreasing the child's agitation. Nasal prongs and a simple face mask do not provide a high concentration of oxygen and are unreliable for use in the emergency room. The devices which can be used are a nonrebreathing mask with a flow rate of 10–12 L/m, an oxygen hood in infants with a flow of 10–15 L/m or a flow inflating bag with a flow rate of three times minute ventilation. Heated humidified high-flow nasal cannula (HHHFNC) and Venturi masks are other devices to deliver high FiO_2.

Assisted Ventilation

Child with severe RD or RF will need advanced airway measures and assisted ventilation. Assisted ventilation can be provided by bag-mask ventilation (BMV), noninvasive ventilation or endotracheal intubation and mechanical ventilation.

In most emergencies, effective BMV usually provides adequate oxygenation and ventilation until definite control of airway can be achieved. BMV can be as effective as ventilation through endotracheal (ET) tube for short periods of time and may be safer when provider is inexperienced in insertion of advanced airway.

Table 1 summarizes the initial management of child with RD.

ASSESSMENT TO DETERMINE THE SEVERITY AND TYPE OF RESPIRATORY PROBLEM (FLOWCHART 1)

Severity

Once oxygenation and ventilation are stabilized, the severity is identified as RD or failure.

TABLE 1: Initial management of respiratory distress/respiratory failure.

Evaluate	*Interventions*
Airway	• Support an open airway or if necessary, open the airway with: – Head tilt-chin lift – Jaw thrust without head tilt if cervical spine injury is suspected. If this maneuver does not open the airway, use the head tilt-chin lift or jaw thrust with gentle head extension • Clear the airway if indicated by suctioning or removal of visualized foreign body • Consider an oropharyngeal airway (OPA) or nasopharyngeal airway (NPA)
Breathing	• Monitor O_2 saturation • Provide humidified O_2. Use a high concentration delivery device like nonrebreathing mask or HFNC for treatment of severe respiratory distress • Administer inhaled medication (e.g., salbutamol, epinephrine) as needed • Assist ventilation with bag mask device and supplementary O_2 if needed • Prepare for endotracheal intubation if indicated
Circulation	• Monitor heart rate, rhythm, and blood pressure • Establish vascular access

(HFNC: high-flow nasal cannula)

Flowchart 1: Step-wise management of a child with respiratory distress.

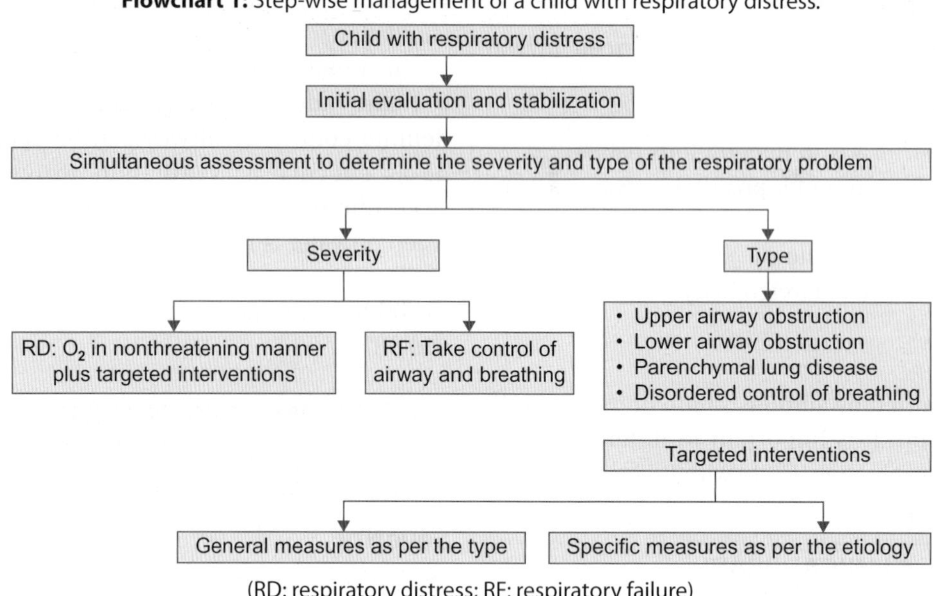

(RD: respiratory distress; RF: respiratory failure)

Type

Respiratory problem is categorized as one of the following:

- Upper airway obstruction (UAO)
- Lower airway obstruction (LAO)
- Lung tissue disease
- Disordered control of breathing

TARGETED INTERVENTIONS

Targeted intervention includes:

- General measures as per the type of respiratory problem
- Specific measures as per the etiology

Following sections describe important emergency room measures in a child with RD. The specific measures depend on the underlying etiology, which are mentioned here briefly. The detailed description is given elsewhere in this book.

UPPER AIRWAY OBSTRUCTION

Acute UAO is an obstruction of large airways outside the thorax.

General Management

The most important priority in UAO is to open and maintain a patent airway. The measures needed to do so are described in **Table 1**.

- When UAO is severe, call for help of a person with expertise in airway management.
- In less severe UAO, children may benefit from insertion of an oropharyngeal airway (OPA) or nasopharyngeal airway (NPA), which may relieve the obstruction caused by the tongue.
- Use OPA only in comatose child.
- A child with intact gag reflex may tolerate an NPA.
- Child with redundant tissues or tissue edema may benefit from application of CPAP.

CLINICAL PEARL

- Failure to aggressively treat a partial upper airway obstruction can lead to complete airway obstruction and cardiac arrest.

Specific Management

Apart from initial interventions mentioned in **Table 1**, additional measures as per etiology focus on relieving the obstruction. **Table 2** summarizes the clinical features of various UAO.

Foreign Body Aspiration

Management depends upon degree of obstruction.

Incomplete Obstruction

(Child is breathing, coughing, and able to make sounds).

- Position of comfort
- Supplemental oxygen
- Rigid bronchoscopy.

TABLE 2: Differential diagnosis of acute upper airway obstruction.

Etiology	*Fever*	*Cough*	*Voice*	*Stridor*	*Dysphagia*	*Others*
Epiglottitis	+++	Ineffective	Hot potato	Soft	+	Drooling of saliva, thumb sign on X-ray
Diphtheria	±	–	Normal to hoarse	In laryngeal involvement	+	Pseudomembrane, toxicity
Retropharyngeal abscess	+++	Ineffective	Muffled	Soft	+	Drooling of saliva, neck stiffness, soft tissue swelling on X-ray
Foreign body	–	Sudden choking	Hoarse	Depends upon level of obstruction	±	–
ALTB	±	Brassy	Hoarse	Harsh	–	Steeple sign on X-ray
Angioedema	–	Dry staccato	Hoarse	Varies	±	Swelling of lip, tongue, mucous membrane
Bacterial tracheitis	+++	Brassy	Hoarse	Harsh	–	Purulent tracheal secretions

(ALTB: acute laryngotracheobronchitis)

CLINICAL PEARL

Do not perform blind finger sweep, it may push the foreign body further into the airway.

Complete Obstruction

(No sound, unable to cough, and unable to breathe adequately). Perform following maneuvers:

- *Less than 1 year:* Five back blows followed by five chest thrusts
- *More than 1 year:* Heimlich maneuver (abdominal thrust)

One of the given outcomes may follow:

- *Relief from obstruction:* Evaluation
- *Incomplete obstruction:* Managed as above
- *Child becomes unresponsive:* Start cardiopulmonary resuscitation (CPR). Before you deliver a breath, look into the mouth. If you a see a foreign body that can be easily removed, remove it.

Angioneurotic Edema

Steps in management of anaphylaxis are summarized in **Box 1**.

CLINICAL PEARL

Hyperacute onset of breathlessness in an alert child should arouse suspicion of foreign body aspiration or anaphylaxis.

Acute Laryngotracheobronchitis

Treatment of child with acute laryngotracheobronchitis depends upon severity as described in **Table 3**.

BOX 1: Management of anaphylaxis.

- Administer adrenaline 1:1,000 IM 0.01 mL/kg, repeated every 10–15 minutes as needed
- Treat bronchospasm with salbutamol metered-dose inhaler or nebulization
- For severe respiratory distress, anticipate further airway swelling and prepare for endotracheal intubation
- To treat hypotension:
  - Place the child in Trendelenburg position as tolerated
  - Administer normal saline bolus 20 mL/kg (repeat as needed)
  - Consider adrenaline drip for hypotension unresponsive to above measures
- Administer diphenhydramine and H2 blocker
- Administer methylprednisolone or equivalent corticosteroid IV

TABLE 3: Management of croup.

Mild	• Careful observation, monitoring • Consider oral dexamethasone
Moderate	• Administer humidified oxygen • Administer nebulized epinephrine • 1:1,000 solution at a dose of 0.5 mL/kg—maximum 5 mL • Administer dexamethasone oral/IM/IV • 0.15–3 mg/kg or budesonide 2 mg nebulization • Observe for at least 2 hours after nebulized epinephrine to ensure continued improvement
Severe	• Administer high concentration of oxygen • Assist ventilation if necessary • Administer dexamethasone IV/IM • Perform endotracheal intubation if indicated • Prepare for surgical airway if needed

CLINICAL PEARL

- In upper airway obstruction with signs of severe obstruction, place an advanced airway early even if SpO_2 is normal, as it drops much later.

LOWER AIRWAY OBSTRUCTION

General Management

- The most important priority is to maintain adequate oxygenation and ventilation.
- The aim is to maintain SpO_2 above 94%.
- Use appropriate oxygen delivery device with optimum flow rate.
- In severe RD, administer oxygen by nonrebreathing mask to provide 100% oxygen or HFNC.
- If assisted ventilation is required, perform BMV at relatively slow rate.
- Prepare for intubation in severe RD.

CLINICAL PEARL

- Ventilating at slow rate in lower airway obstruction reduces the risk of air trapping and complications of high airway pressure.

Specific Management

Common causes of LAO are asthma and bronchiolitis.

Management of Bronchiolitis

- Management is mainly supportive
- Administer humidified O_2
- IV fluids
- Suction oral and nasal secretions
- *Trial of bronchodilators:* Continue only if favorable response is noted
- Severe cases need intensive care unit (ICU) care. Assess and provide ventilatory support if needed
- *Hypertonic saline, steroids, ribavirin:* Conflicting reports, variable response. None have proven benefit.

Table 4 summarizes acute asthma treatment in emergency room.

LUNG TISSUE DISEASE

Common causes of lung tissue disease are:

- Pneumonia
- Cardiogenic pulmonary edema
- Acute respiratory distress syndrome (ARDS)

TABLE 4: Management of acute asthma.

Asthma severity	*Interventions*
Mild to moderate	• Salbutamol MDI with spacer ± mask or nebulized salbutamol every 20 minutes—total three doses • Administer oral prednisolone
Moderate to severe	• Hospitalize and start oxygen • Continue salbutamol nebulization 1–4 hourly or continuously • Administer steroids PO/IV • Add ipratropium bromide nebulization every 20 minutes for three times followed by 6 hourly • Consider magnesium sulfate • Perform diagnostic tests
Impending respiratory failure	• Consider adding following measures: – Start on terbutaline infusion and/or aminophylline infusion – In case of poor response or red flag signs: - Consider HFNC/BiPAP in alert child - ET intubation and mechanical ventilation

(HFNC: high-flow nasal cannula; MDI: metered-dose inhaler; BiPAP: biphasic positive airway pressure; ET: endotracheal)

GENERAL MANAGEMENT

Initial interventions are listed in **Table 1**.

In children with refractory hypoxemia, consider CPAP, noninvasive ventilation or mechanical ventilation with positive end-expiratory pressure (PEEP).

CLINICAL PEARL

- Saturated oxygen of arterial blood less than 90% on 100% oxygen is an indication for assisted ventilation.

Specific Management

Acute Infectious Pneumonia

- Perform diagnostic tests—e.g., complete blood count (CBC), chest X-ray (CXR), blood culture, etc. as indicated
- Administer antibiotic therapy
- Treat wheezing with bronchodilators
- Consider using HFNC or noninvasive ventilation (CPAP/BiPAP). Severe cases need intubation and mechanical ventilation
- *Supportive measures:* Antipyretics, IV fluids, etc.

Cardiogenic Pulmonary Edema

The most common cause of acute cardiogenic pulmonary edema in children is left ventricular myocardial dysfunction.

- Provide ventilatory support as needed.
- Consider diuretics to reduce left atrial pressure.
- Inotropic infusions and afterload-reducing agents to improve myocardial function
- Obtain expert consultation.
- Provide breathing support as discussed above.

Acute Respiratory Distress Syndrome

Early recognition and treatment of bacteremia, shock, and RF may help prevent progression to ARDS.

- Obtain laboratory studies—CBC, arterial blood gas (ABG), serum electrolytes, blood culture, etc. as indicated
- Provide ventilatory support as needed
- Indications for ventilator support:
  - Worsening clinical and radiological lung disease
  - Hypoxemia refractory to high concentrations of fraction of inspired oxygen

DISORDERED CONTROL OF BREATHING

It results from affection of central control of respiration or neuromuscular weakness.

Important Aspects of Treatment

- Airway management
- Management of raised intracranial pressure (ICP)
- Treatment of the cause.

KEY POINTS

- The first priority in the management of a child with RD is to stabilize airway, breathing, and circulation.
- As this is being done, simultaneously the child is assessed to determine the severity and type of respiratory problem.
- Subsequently, detailed evaluation (including investigations) is required to determine the underlying etiology of RD.
- Treatment of RD consists of general measures depending upon the type of the problem and specific targeted intervention as per the etiology.
- Early recognition and a systematic approach to management are crucial for better outcome.

SUGGESTED READING

1. Agarwal R, Singh V, Yewale V. RTI facts; bugs, drugs and you. IAP Consensus Guidelines on Rational Management of Respiratory Tract Infections in Children. IAP Action Plan. Mumbai: Indian Academy of Pediatrics; 2012.
2. American Academy of Pediatrics, American Heart Association. PALS Provider Manual. Dallas: American Heart Association; 2011.
3. Everald ML. Acute bronchiolitis and croup. Pediatr Clin North Am. 2009;56:119-31.
4. Global Initiative for Asthma. Global Strategy for Asthma Management and Prevention—revised 2012. [online] Available from www.ginasthma.org. [Last accessed September, 2024]
5. Helfaer MA, Nichols DG. Roger's Handbook of Pediatric Intensive Care, 4th edition. Philadelphia: Lippincott Williams & Wilkins; 2010.
6. Subramanyam L. Essentials of Paediatric Pulmonology, 3rd edition. PPFI; 2008.
7. Wilmott RW, Boat TF, Bush A, Chernick V, Deterding RR, Ratjen F. Kendig and Chernick's Disorders of the Respiratory Tract in Children, 8th edition. Philadelphia: Saunders; 2012.

CHAPTER 36

Hypovolemic Shock

Paramanand G Andankar, Aditya P Modak

INTRODUCTION

The clinical syndrome of shock is one of the most dramatic, dynamic and life-threatening problems faced by the physician in the critical care setting. Although untreated shock is universally lethal, mortality may be considerably reduced by rapid, proper recognition, diagnosis, monitoring and treatment.

According to hemodynamic profiles, shock states are classified into functional categories; such as—hypovolemic, cardiogenic, etc.

HYPOVOLEMIC SHOCK

Hypovolemia is the most common cause of shock in infants and children. Acute losses of 10–15% of the circulatory blood volume may be well tolerated in healthy children with intact compensatory mechanisms. However, acute loss of 25% or more of the circulating blood volume frequently results in hypovolemic shock that requires immediate management.

ETIOLOGY

Hypovolemia may arise from fluid and electrolyte loss/plasma loss/whole blood loss **(Table 1)**.

PATHOPHYSIOLOGY

Hypovolemic shock is characterized primarily by fluid loss and decreased preload. To maintain adequate cardiac output and tissue perfusion, the body responds by tachycardia and by increase in stroke volume, smooth muscle tone, and systemic vascular resistance (SVR) mediated via increase in sympathetic activity as initial compensatory response. There also occurs renal sodium and water retention mediated by activation of the renin–angiotensin–aldosterone and atrial natriuretic factor axes, cortisol and catecholamine synthesis, antidiuretic hormone secretion; so as to maintain intravascular volume as much as possible.

However, compensatory mechanisms have limitations, beyond which, if adequate and timely intervention is not done, hypotension inevitably develops, leading to tissue ischemia. Also, the underlying shock + host response can itself lead to vascular endothelial cell injury and loss of endothelial adhesion proteins which lead to significant leakage of intravascular fluid into the interstitial extracellular space. Additionally, if patient has preexisting conditions associated with low plasma oncotic pressure (e.g., nephrotic syndrome, malnutrition, hepatic dysfunction, and acute severe burns), further volume loss occurs,

TABLE 1: Causes of hypovolemia.

Whole blood loss			*Plasma loss*	*Fluid and electrolyte loss*
Absolute loss		***Relative loss***	***Burns***	***Vomiting***
External bleeding	Internal bleeding	Barbiturates, vasodilators	Capillary leak syndromes, e.g., inflammation, sepsis, and anaphylaxis	Diarrhea
	Gastrointestinal (GI)/abdominal bleeding	Positive pressure ventilation	Protein-losing syndromes	Excess diuresis
	Intracranial	Sepsis		Adrenal insufficiency
	Fractures	Spinal cord injury		Diabetes insipidus
	Major vessel injury	Anaphylaxis		Diabetes mellitus

and exacerbation of shock may result from worsening vascular leaks.

CLINICAL FEATURES

The clinical presentation depends partly on the underlying etiology. Sympathetic adrenergic system activation and its related signs are among the first physiologic responses.

Cardiovascular system (CVS): Tachycardia, orthostatic hypotension, and depending on severity, peripheral pulses may be normal, decreased, or absent. Hypotension is a late manifestation since the compensatory mechanisms try to maintain blood pressure (BP) so as to preserve tissue perfusion. Hypotension actually reflects advanced state of uncompensated shock. It must be always emphasized to use age-appropriate BP cuffs.

Shock index = ratio of heart rate over systolic BP. Normal is 0.5–0.7. Persistent elevation of shock index >1.0 indicates impaired left ventricular function and is associated with increased mortality.

Skin and mucosae: Dry mucous membranes, dry axillae, poor skin turgor, depending on the degree normal or cool distal extremities. Signs of obvious blood loss may be there in cases of trauma, high output stomies, etc.

Central nervous system (CNS): Alteration of mental status

Renal: Decreased urine output

If unrecognized and untreated, all forms of shock follow a common progression of clinical signs and pathophysiologic changes that may ultimately lead to irreversible organ injury and death. Hence, timely recognition of signs gives a clue to the type of shock.

DIAGNOSIS

Shock is a clinical diagnosis primarily based on history and physical examination as mentioned earlier.

The World Health Organization Criteria for Shock

Cold extremities with capillary refill >3 s and a weak, fast pulse (all signs must be present).

Point-of-care Ultrasound

Increasingly, point-of-care ultrasound (POCUS) is being incorporated into physical examination—helps for assessment of intravascular volume status, myocardial contractility, and likelihood of a positive hemodynamic response to fluids. It also helps to find possible etiologies and severity of pathologies such as pericardial effusion, pneumothorax, and pulmonary embolism.

Blood Lactate Levels

Lactates are indicators of anaerobic metabolism and hence indirectly of tissue perfusion. Levels ≥2 are considered significant. The test is rapidly done and is a good indicator of extent of anaerobic metabolism, irrespective of type of shock.

Oxygen Consumption, Oxygen Delivery and Oxygen Extraction and Central Venous Oxygen Saturation

Hallmark of uncompensated shock is an imbalance between oxygen delivery (DO_2) and oxygen consumption (VO_2). Oxygen delivery normally exceeds oxygen consumption with usual oxygen extraction ratio of approximately 25%. Normal central venous oxygen saturation (SvO_2) is approximately 75%; measured from a catheter at the junction of the superior vena cava and right atrium. SvO_2 values <70% reflect an increased oxygen extraction indicating a decrease in oxygen delivery relative to consumption. This increase in oxygen extraction helps to maintain adequate oxygen delivery at cellular level. However, in very late stages of shock, once cellular death occurs, cells develop reduction in oxygen extraction-leading to hyperlactatemia although SvO_2 remains high.

TREATMENT

Without timely medical intervention, child in shock will inevitably follow a common pathway to multi-organ dysfunction syndrome (MODS) and death. Thus, early recognition and resuscitation are critical to limit morbidity and mortality associated with shock.

Airway and Oxygen

Once shock is recognized, actions should immediately begin to restore oxygen and other nutrient delivery to tissues. It begins with securing a patent airway and providing supplemental oxygen. Children should be given 100% oxygen to begin with so as to maximize oxygen content of blood. In decompensated shock, intubation and mechanical ventilation helps by taking over the work of breathing thereby reducing respiratory muscle demand. Mechanical ventilation also helps to better tackle hypoxemia developing from fluid overload/capillary leak at lungs.

Role of noninvasive ventilation (NIV): In patients who are gradually responding to fluid therapy however starting to develop fluid overload, NIV can be tried with keeping low threshold for intubation.

Vascular Access

Vascular access should be taken within 5 minutes; however, in severe shock, due to collapsed veins, one may not get rapid vascular access. In such case, intraosseous (IO) access should be taken, until more definitive access is established. Central venous access should be considered for patients with unstable peripheral access, persistence of shock despite 40–60 mL/kg fluid bolus therapy (fluid-refractory shock) or need for vasoactive/concentrated dextrose/electrolyte administration. It also helps to measure central SvO_2. It is recommended to have an arterial catheter for accurate measurement of BP as well as for effective and timely titration of vasoactive medications. This also helps for easy sampling for blood tests. It is important to note that placing such catheters may not be possible in certain settings; in such cases resuscitation should be continued with peripheral intravenous (IV)/IO access.

Volume Resuscitation

The primary cause of hypovolemic shock is inadequate preload. Hence, measures should begin with attempts to optimize preload. To begin with, fluid bolus therapy can be started with 10–20 mL/kg of fluid administered as rapidly as possible (within 5–10 minutes, pull and push technique). Patients may require up to 60 mL/kg of fluid in first hour itself. However, the exact volume of bolus to be administered should be decided after response to every bolus—improvement in HR, BP, pulse volume, extremity temperature, urine output, and POCUS examination. Excessive fluids may not be tolerated in cases of associated myocardial dysfunction, where vasoactive medications are the first choice. Hence, clinical assessment should be done before repeating fluid boluses. Fluid responsiveness is not synonymous with fluid requirement.

Choice of Fluid

It depends on the nature of the loss. Hemorrhagic shock should be treated with transfusions of blood components, including emergency transfusion of uncrossmatched blood. Massive transfusion in pediatrics is defined as transfusion of 40 mL/kg of blood product within 24-hour time. Most trauma centers follow transfusions of balanced ratios of plasma, platelets, and packed red blood cells (PRBCs) in hemorrhagic shock. Depending on the source, surgical intervention may be indicated to control the source of bleeding. If the etiology involves ongoing fluid losses from chest tubes, biliary drains, bowel, capillary leak, or other bodily fluids, then resuscitation should be with isotonic or balanced crystalloid solutions. The preferable choice of fluid remains a matter of debate. Isotonic solutions [such as normal saline (NS)] are easily available, cost effective but there are associated concerns of hyperchloremia and metabolic acidosis. Balanced crystalloids [such as Ringer lactate (RL)] have shown improved outcomes in studies; however, convincing pediatric evidence is lacking. Colloids are considered in conditions with low oncotic pressures and ongoing capillary leak; especially when there is a poor response to crystalloids. However, they are also known to cause coagulopathy and nephrotoxicity.

Fluid Refractory Shock

Physicians may come across cases with persistent shock despite adequate fluid therapy. In such cases, additional factors contributing to shock must be actively recognized and addressed, e.g., pneumothorax, myocardial dysfunction, cardiac tamponade, and adrenal insufficiency.

Vasoactive Medications

Pure hypovolemic shock usually responds to fluid therapy, especially in early stages and when therapy is started promptly. However, certain patients may require support of vasoactive medications. This is especially true if a child requires fluid therapy beyond 40 mL/kg. The choice of medication depends on the patient's pathophysiology. This is decided by considering factors such as cardiac contractility and SVR. Adrenaline helps increasing contractility and SVR, noradrenaline predominantly improves SVR, dobutamine increases contractility and has peripheral vasodilatory properties. Choice of vasoactive medication may require to be changed as per the change in pathophysiology of the patient.

Flowchart 1: Approach to hypovolemic shock.

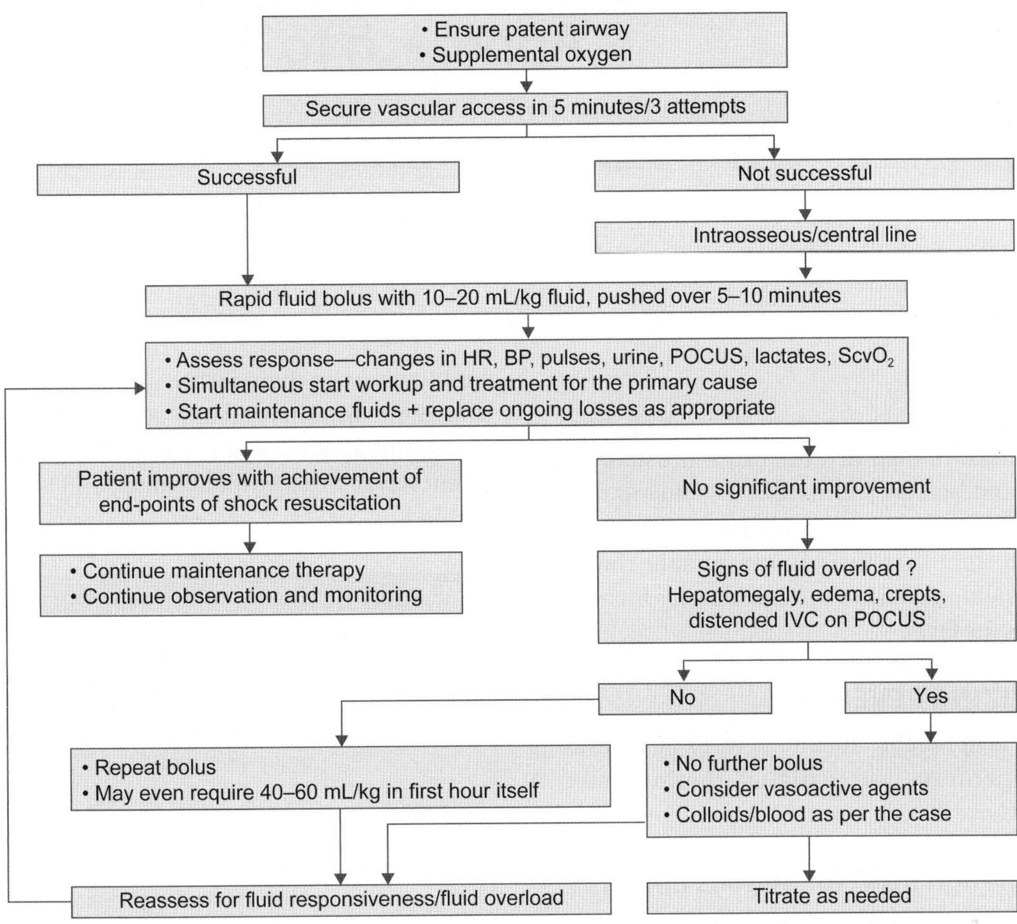

(BP: blood pressure; HR: heart rate; IVC: inferior vena cava; POCUS: point-of-care ultrasound; $ScvO_2$: central venous oxygen saturation)

Treatment of the Primary Cause

Simultaneous work-up and treatment should start depending on the cause of shock, such as surgical treatment for bleeders in case of trauma, specific antidotes in cases of toxins, antibiotics for sepsis.

THERAPEUTIC TARGETS/ENDPOINTS OF SHOCK RESUSCITATION

There is no single parameter to define end point of resuscitation; a combination of multiple parameters should be considered.

- Normalization of HR and BP for age
- Capillary refill <2 seconds
- Normal pulses with warm extremities
- Normal mental status for age
- Urine output >1 mL/kg/h
- Lactates <2
- Central SvO_2 >65%

KEY POINTS

- Need of fluids is obvious, but one must administer supplemental oxygen to optimize arterial oxygen content.
- Crystalloids are effective for fluid resuscitation.
- Always assess response to intervention done and tailor therapy accordingly.
- Simultaneously evaluate and treat the primary cause of hypovolemic shock.
- Timely identification and intervention is the key **(Flowchart 1)**.

SUGGESTED READING

1. Kliegman RM, St Geme JW III. Nelson Textbook of Pediatrics, 22nd edn. Amsterdam: Elsevier Health Sciences; 2024.
2. World Health Organization. Paediatric Emergency Triage, Assessment and Treatment: Care of Critically Ill Children (updated guideline). Geneva: World Health Organization; 2016.
3. Zimmerman JJ, Rotta AT. Fuhrman and Zimmerman's Pediatric Critical Care, 6th edn. Amsterdam: Elsevier; 2021.

Approach to Fever in Children

Rhishikesh P Thakre

INTRODUCTION

Fever is one of the most common distressing signs of childhood illness. In majority, the cause is usually viral, self-limited, and benign, but in few, it is due to serious underlying illness. The clinician's responsibility is to establish a correct diagnosis in reasonable time and initiate treatment, if indicated. This chapter focuses on approach to acute fever.

RECOGNIZING FEVER

The first step is to reliably document fever by measuring axillary temperature using digital thermometer. A temperature above 38°C or 100.4°F is considered as fever.

Identifying "High Risk" for Serious Illness

One should be alert to and identify immediately any life-threatening features, including compromise of the airway, breathing, or circulation, and decreased level of consciousness **(Box 1)**. This identifies seriously ill children in need for urgent referral or treatment.

ASSESSMENT OF FEVER

The main goal of evaluation of febrile children is to distinguish those with mild self-limiting illness from those with serious bacterial infection (SBI).

An enquiry should be made about the nature of fever, defining when was the child last well, activity, sleep pattern, whether the child is getting better or worse, history of exposure to sick contacts, use of antipyretics or antibiotics (with their doses) taken or previous diagnostic tests done and their results. All efforts should be made to enquire about the oral intake, fluid losses, urination, recent travel, prior hospitalization, and vaccination status **(Table 1)**.

BOX 1: Assessing "danger signs" in febrile children.

- A—Arousal, alertness, activity
- B—Breathing difficulty
- C—Color and circulation
- D—Decreased intake and urine output

TABLE 1: Key points on history.

Note	*Comment*
Onset	High fever from the very onset usually suggests viral infection, malaria, or localized bacterial infection at the site of entry of organisms (tonsillitis/UTI)
Duration	Persistent fever beyond day 3 without localizing signs calls for laboratory tests
Progress	Gradually improving fever by day 3 or 4 suggests self-limiting viral infection, while bacterial infections peak by day 3 or 4
Interfebrile state	Children suffering from viral infection or malaria appear normal between fever spikes. If the child continues to appear sick even between fever spikes, the cause is likely to be a bacterial infection
Response to antipyretic	Poor response to optimum doses of paracetamol or ibuprofen may suggest severe bacterial infection
Accompanying symptoms	Bacterial infection usually presents with localization to a part of a system (such as tonsillitis or pneumonia) while viral infection usually affects the entire system or multiple systems (such as respiratory and gastrointestinal system)
Contact with similar illness	Family member with similar illness suggests airborne viral infection
Past history of infective focus	Device (shunt, implant), underlying anomaly (CHD, VUR) predispose to early complication and need urgent evaluation

(UTI: urinary tract infection; CHD: congenital heart defect; VUR: vesicoureteral reflux)

TABLE 2: Key points on general examination.

Look for	*Note*
Appearance	Well or sick based on alertness, interaction, tone, cry, activity, and look. Lack of alertness indicates encephalopathy and underlying serious illness
Breathing	Normal or abnormal, apnea, type of breathing—rate and work of breathing. Breathing difficulty with altered sensorium indicates serious illness
Color	Pink color of extremities is assuring. Mottling, cyanosis, and ashen complexion indicate serious illness
Temperature	Degree and severity
Heart rate	Proportionate or disproportionate to temperature
Hydration	Assess the sensorium, skin turgor, eyes, mucous membrane, and urine pattern

TABLE 3: Common causes of fever.

Fever with localization (<3 days)	*Probable diagnosis*
Watery nasal discharge	Viral URI
Purulent nasal discharge, follicles/ exudates on tonsils, petechiae on palate	Bacterial URI
Ear pain/discharge	Acute otitis media
Tachypnea with chest signs	Pneumonia
Watery stools	Viral AGE
Blood-mucus in stools, tenesmus	Bacterial AGE
Urinary complaints	UTI
Splenohepatomegaly	Malaria, typhoid, hepatitis, or infectious mononucleosis

(URI: upper respiratory infection; AGE: acute gastroenteritis; UTI: urinary tract infection)

EXAMINATION

The purpose of examination is directed at locating a source for fever, with specific attention to potential SBI and resultant complications. Ill-appearing children are more likely than well-appearing children to have SBI, and most well-appearing children do not have SBI.

In addition to temperature, one should record the heart rate, respiratory rate, and capillary refill time as part of the routine assessment **(Table 2)**.

ASSESSMENT FOR LOCALIZING SIGNS

Presence of associated symptoms or signs gives clue to underlying focus of infection **(Table 3)**. Examination of the throat and ear is important and often missed. A systematic examination should then be conducted, including the skin and nails, head and neck, and the cardiovascular, respiratory, abdominal, musculoskeletal, and neurological systems. One should be aware that classical signs of meningitis like neck stiffness are classically seen in older children and are often absent in infants with bacterial meningitis. Hence, one has to have a high index of suspicion and look for subtle signs like bulging fontanel, irritability, high pitched cry, or any other indicator of altered sensorium **(Table 4)**.

An attempt must be made to ensure that possibility of SBI has been ruled out on clinical grounds.

At times, noninfective causes do present with short-duration fever and one should have a high index of suspicion for them (e.g., Kawasaki disease and leukemia).

TABLE 4: Pointers to serious bacterial infections in a febrile child.

Fast respiration (>60/min), chest indrawing, grunt	Pneumonia
Neck stiffness, bulging fontanel, decreased level of consciousness, convulsive status epilepticus	Meningitis
Unexplained vomiting, poor feeding, lethargy, irritability, abdominal pain or tenderness, urinary frequency or dysuria	Urinary tract infections
Disproportionate tachycardia, cool extremities, prolonged capillary refill (>3 seconds), core axillary mismatch, altered sensorium, oliguria suggests systemic inflammatory response causing shock	Septicemia
Non-blanching rash, particularly with one or more of the following—an ill-looking child, lesions >2 mm in diameter (purpura, capillary refill time of ≥3 seconds, and neck stiffness)	Meningococcemia
Swelling of a limb or joint, not using an extremity, nonweight bearing	Septic arthritis/ osteomyelitis

INVESTIGATIONS

Many infections can be identified by history and examination alone, but some infections may be occult. The most common SBIs in infants that may not be clinically apparent are bacteremia, urinary tract infection (UTI),

TABLE 5: Interpreting hemogram.

Hemoglobin	*Total leukocyte count*	*Polymorphs*	*Lymphocytes*	*Eosinophils*	*Platelets*	*Disease*
Normal	+++	+++	–	0	Normal	Acute bacterial infection
Normal	+++	+++	–	+	High	Systemic inflammatory disease
Low	+++	+	+++	–	Low	ALL
Normal	++	++	–	0	Normal/low	Acute viral infection*
Normal	Low	–	++	0	Normal/low	Typhoid*
Low	+/–	–	–	+	Low	Malaria
High	+	–	++	–	Low	Capillary leak
Normal	+	–	++	+	Normal	Tuberculosis, chronic infection

Note: *CBC when done early in an acute viral infection can show high count, high polymorphs and eosinopenia. Similarly, poly or lympho predominance in typhoid can change with the stage of the disease. So, CBC should always be interpreted in correlation with the temporal stage of the illness.
(ALL: acute lymphoblastic leukemia; CBC: complete blood count)

and pneumonia. Tempo and complexity of workup are decided by the pace of illness. Investigations must be done on all sick children and in those without localization by 72 hours.

- *Complete hemogram:* A white blood cell (WBC) count of >15,000/mm^3 or <5,000/mm^3, a band-to-neutrophil ratio ≥0.2 is considered abnormal. An abnormality is a relatively poor surrogate marker for bacteremia **(Table 5)**.
- Urinalysis (dipstick, urinalysis, microscopy, Gram's stain, and culture) must be considered in presence of fever without localization, particularly in younger children or when UTI is suspected. A urine dipstick test positive for nitrite or leukocyte esterase or a finding of >10 WBCs/hpf or organisms seen on Gram's stain is considered abnormal.
- Chest X-ray is useful in children with respiratory localization. Chest film should be considered in an infant with an unexplained WBC count of >20,000, or with prolonged fever or cough.
- In children with no definitive diagnosis beyond day 3 or where antibiotic is to be initiated, blood culture must be done. It is the gold standard for the diagnosis of bacterial infection.
- Cerebrospinal fluid (CSF) examination (cytology, Gram's stain, and culture) is mandatory in every suspected case of meningitis and also in all sick infants without localization. CSF fluid with >8 WBC/mm^3 or organisms on Gram's stain is considered abnormal.

BOX 2: Indications for hospitalization.

- Febrile neonate
- Toxic child
- Presence of "danger signs"
- Admission for period of observation
- Pre-existing medical problem (e.g., congenital heart defect, immunodeficiency, malnutrition)
- Parental preference

- Serial values of C-reactive protein (CRP) and/or procalcitonin are more useful than isolated values in ruling out infection.

No combination of clinical assessment and diagnostic testing will successfully identify all patients who have serious infection at the time of initial presentation; therefore, the importance of timely reassessment with good history, systematic confident clinical examination and intelligent use of laboratory tests, a rational approach cannot be overemphasized.

INDICATIONS FOR HOSPITALIZATION

Most infants and children who have fever and are otherwise healthy, who are well appearing with no localization can be managed on an outpatient basis. The degree of illness should be determined through the child's interactions with the environment; observing their alertness, playfulness and feeding pattern with appearance of any new symptoms **(Box 2)**.

Flowchart 1: Algorithm for acute fever.

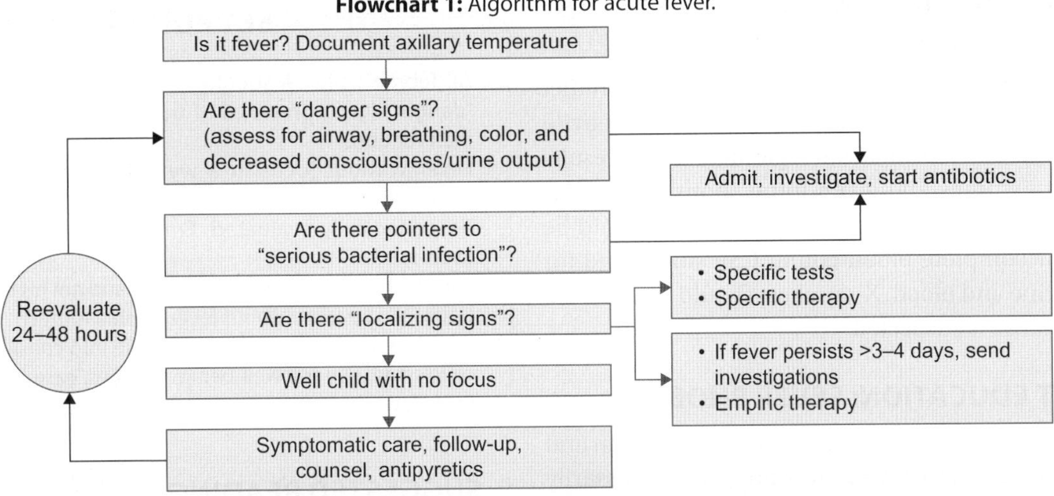

MANAGEMENT OF FEBRILE CHILD (FLOWCHART 1)

Supportive treatment: Supportive treatment of fever is symptomatic. Not all fevers need treatment. Primary goal of treating the febrile child should be to improve the child's overall comfort rather than focus on the normalization of body temperature.

- *Cooling*—involves nursing in cool environment and unbundling the child. Sponging is reserved for patients with hyperthermia (temperature >38.5°C) after 30 minutes of antipyretic dose.
- *Antipyretics:* The use of antipyretics should be individualized and based on the child's well-being, not temperature alone. Antipyretics should be used as "therapy" for fever rather than "control". Treatment for fever with antipyretic is indicated if the child has discomfort, i.e., irritable, drowsy, pain, or excessive crying. Both paracetamol (10–15 mg/kg, 4–6 hourly) and ibuprofen (5–10 mg/kg, 6 hourly) are effective antipyretics **(Table 6)**. *Evidence* comparing ibuprofen and paracetamol shows that ibuprofen has no superior effect or safety profile than paracetamol. Use of mefenamic acid leads to superior antipyretic effect compared to paracetamol but increasing risk of side effects, viz., colitis, renal failure, transaminitis, gastrointestinal bleeding, drug-induced asthma, and drug-induced glaucoma thus compromising safety. The use of antipyretics does not prevent either febrile convulsions or reactions to vaccines.

Hydration should be ensured for all febrile children by increasing oral intake as for every 1°C rise in temperature the fluid requirement increases by 10%.

TABLE 6: Comparison of paracetamol and ibuprofen.

	Paracetamol	*Ibuprofen*
Dose	10–15 mg/kg/dose	5–10 mg/kg/dose
Minimum age	Newborn	6 months
Frequency	4–6 hours	6–8 hours
Duration of action	4–6 hours	6–8 hours
Contraindication	Severe hepatic impairment, allergy to paracetamol	Volume depletion, renal impairment, hepatic impairment, varicella, duct-dependent heart disease, thrombocytopenia, peptic ulcer disease, clotting disorder

Empiric treatment: Empiric treatment is not routinely recommended. It is justified only in toxic children and neonates and that too, only after sending relevant investigations. It is directed toward the probable underlying cause of illness and most probable organism.

Specific treatment: Specific therapy should be directed toward the specific cause identified on evaluation like UTI, pneumonia, etc.

- *Follow-up:* Not all febrile children have a focus identified on first evaluation. All such children should be followed up on outpatient department basis continuing with symptomatic treatment at home. Parents should be made aware about the danger signs and asked to report immediately if there are any concerns or appearance of new symptoms.

SPECIAL CIRCUMSTANCES: FEVER IN NEWBORN (<30 DAYS)

Physical examination has marked limitations to predict accurately a serious infection in neonates. Febrile neonates should be hospitalized regardless of the results of laboratory studies and given intravenous antibiotics till infection is ruled out. All febrile newborns should be screened for complete blood count, CSF study, and for culture of urine and blood. X-ray chest should be done if a respiratory cause is suspected.

PARENT EDUCATION: FEVER PHOBIA

Parents should be made aware that fever is a symptom and not an illness. The severity of fever does not necessarily correlate with seriousness of illness. Child's well-being is more important than the height of the fever. The risk of febrile convulsion is <5% and it is a benign event.

CLINICAL PEARLS

- Clues to the diagnosis are frequently present in the history and physical examination but are not elicited or unappreciated. Therefore, thoroughness and repetition are vitally important.
- Antipyretics should not be combined, or routinely alternated, and be used, if at all, only as long as the child appears distressed.
- Do not use aspirin or nimesulide for control of fever; avoid mefenamic acid.

KEY POINTS

- All febrile children should have periodic assessment for "danger signs"; presence of these should lead to prompt interventions.
- Fever without focus in a well child should be treated symptomatically on OPD basis. Such children should be periodically evaluated. Empiric antibiotics should be avoided.
- The emphasis should be on the child and not his temperature.
- Counseling parents about fever phobia is must.
- Decision-making in fever should take into consideration the child's age, general well-being, facilities, ease and reliability for follow-up.

SUGGESTED READING

1. Barbi E, Marzuillo P, Neri E, Naviglio S, Krauss BS. Fever in Children: Pearls and Pitfalls. Children (Basel). 2017;4(9): 81.
2. Chiappini E, Bortone B, Galli L, de Martino M. Guidelines for the symptomatic management of fever in children: systematic review of the literature and quality appraisal with AGREE II. BMJ Open. 2017;7(7): e015404.
3. Indian Academy of Pediatrics. Rapid approach to common symptoms. Standardization of pediatric office practice. Fever, 13-16. Mumbai: Indian Academy of Pediatrics; 2005.

Approach to Poisoning in Children

Somashekhar M Nimbalkar

INTRODUCTION

Data regarding poison exposure is not well maintained in India, but based on global trends, it can be assumed with fair approximation that poison exposure in children in India would range above 8 million at the least. The US has maintained data since 1972, and deaths due to poison in under five children have dropped to 90% less than that in 1972. In the last decade, publications have doubled, and a move to maintain some registries has been made, but more needs to be done.

ETIOPATHOGENESIS

Common causes of poisoning in India vary geographically and depend on access to various agents. Over the last decade, there has been a significant change in the causes of poisoning in children. Kerosene has been displaced from the top spot in children under five by other causes, such as prescription drugs or liquid mosquito repellants. However, healthcare providers should be familiar with common poisonings in their area as this will vary with urban or rural settings, industrial or farm settings, etc., as access to different chemicals, etc., will vary accordingly. Poor air quality reduces life span and, while not classified as a poison yet, will increasingly contribute to deaths insidiously over the coming decades.

CLINICAL PRESENTATION

Most children present with nonspecific symptoms such as nausea, vomiting, or altered sensorium. However, there are certain toxidromes that, on recognition, can give us a clinical diagnosis **(Tables 1 and 2)**.

TABLE 1: Clinical manifestations of selected toxic ingestions.

Ingestion	***Clinical findings***
Acetaminophen	*Early:* Nausea, vomiting, anorexia; jaundice and liver failure occur later
Antihistamines	Initially CNS depression but stimulation in higher doses (tremors, hyperactivity, hallucinations, seizures)
Aspirin	Tachypnea, respiratory alkalosis, metabolic acidosis, coagulopathies, slurred speech, tinnitus, seizures
β-blockers	Bradycardia, hypotension, coma, convulsions, hypoglycemia, bronchospasm
Calcium channel blockers	Hypotension, bradycardia, junctional arrhythmias, hyperglycemia, metabolic acidosis
Caustics	Coagulation necrosis with acids or liquefaction necrosis with alkali; burning, scarring/strictures, dysphagia, glottic edema
Digoxin	Nausea, vomiting, visual disturbances, lethargy, electrolyte imbalance, hyperkalemia, prolonged AV dissociation, and heart block
Disk batteries	Can cause corrosion if there is contact with mucosal surfaces
Ethanol	• *Early:* Nausea and vomiting, stupor, anorexia; *late:* Coma, hypothermia, hypoglycemia • *Life-threatening:* Cardiorespiratory depression if levels above 400–500 mg/dL
Ethylene glycol	CNS depression, metabolic acidosis, convulsions and coma, renal failure, hypocalcemia, anion gap metabolic acidosis, osmolal gap, oxalaturia

Contd...

Contd...

Ingestion	***Clinical findings***
Hypoglycemic agents	Hypoglycemia, seizures, coma
Iron	Hemorrhagic necrosis of GI mucosa, hypotension, hepatotoxicity, metabolic acidosis, shock, seizure, coma
Isopropyl alcohol	Altered mental status, gastritis, hypotension, osmolal gap elevated, ketonuria without metabolic acidosis or hypoglycemia
Lead	Abdominal pain, constipation, anorexia, listlessness, encephalopathy (peripheral neuropathy), microcytic anemia
Methanol	CNS depression, delayed metabolic acidosis, optic disturbances, anion gap metabolic acidosis, osmolal gap
Tricyclic antidepressants	• Lethargy, disorientation, ataxia, urinary retention, decreased GI motility, seizures, coma • *Cardiovascular alterations:* Sinus tachycardia, widened QRS complex; may progress to hypotension, ventricular dysrhythmias, cardiovascular collapse

(CNS: central nervous system; AV: atrioventricular; GI: gastrointestinal)

TABLE 2: Toxidromes.

	Mental status	***Heart rate***	***BP***	***RR***	***Pupils***	***Laboratory and electrocardiographic findings***
Acetaminophen	• *Early:* nausea, vomiting • *Late:* Confusion, stupor, coma	–	–	–	–	Elevated aspartate transaminase, alanine transaminase, bilirubin after 24-hour
Salicylates	Disorientation, lethargy, convulsions, coma	↑	–	↑	–	Respiratory alkalosis, progressive anion gap metabolic acidosis, hyperglycemia or hypoglycemia, electrolyte imbalances
Anticholinergics	Delirium, psychosis, seizure, coma	↑	↑	–	Large, sluggish	Sinus tachycardia (tricyclic antidepressants increase QRS interval)
Benzodiazepines	Drowsy, lethargy, coma	↓	–	↓	–	–
Calcium channel blockers	Drowsy, confusion	↓	↓	–	–	Heart block, metabolic acidosis, hyperglycemia
Stimulants	Agitation, delirium, psychosis, convulsions	↑	↑	↑	Large, reactive	–
Narcotics	Drowsy, coma	↓	↓	↓	Pinpoint	Respiratory acidosis
Organophosphates	Confusion, coma	↓	↓	↑	Small	–
Sedative/hypnotics	Somnolence, coma	↓	↓	↓	Variable	–

(BP: blood pressure; RR: respiratory rate)

MANAGEMENT OF POISONING

Initial Assessment and Emergency Management—ABCDEF

In a responsive patient, initial management in all patients presenting to the emergency is focused on airway, breathing, and circulation **(Flowchart 1)**.

Airway

Abnormal sounds like stridor, gurgling, or noisy breathing may indicate that the airway is partially obstructed. An altered sensorium indicates that the child's airway is at risk. In such cases, measures to manage the airway should be initiated. These may include positioning, oropharyngeal airways, laryngeal mask airways, or endotracheal intubation.

Flowchart 1: Management of poisoning.

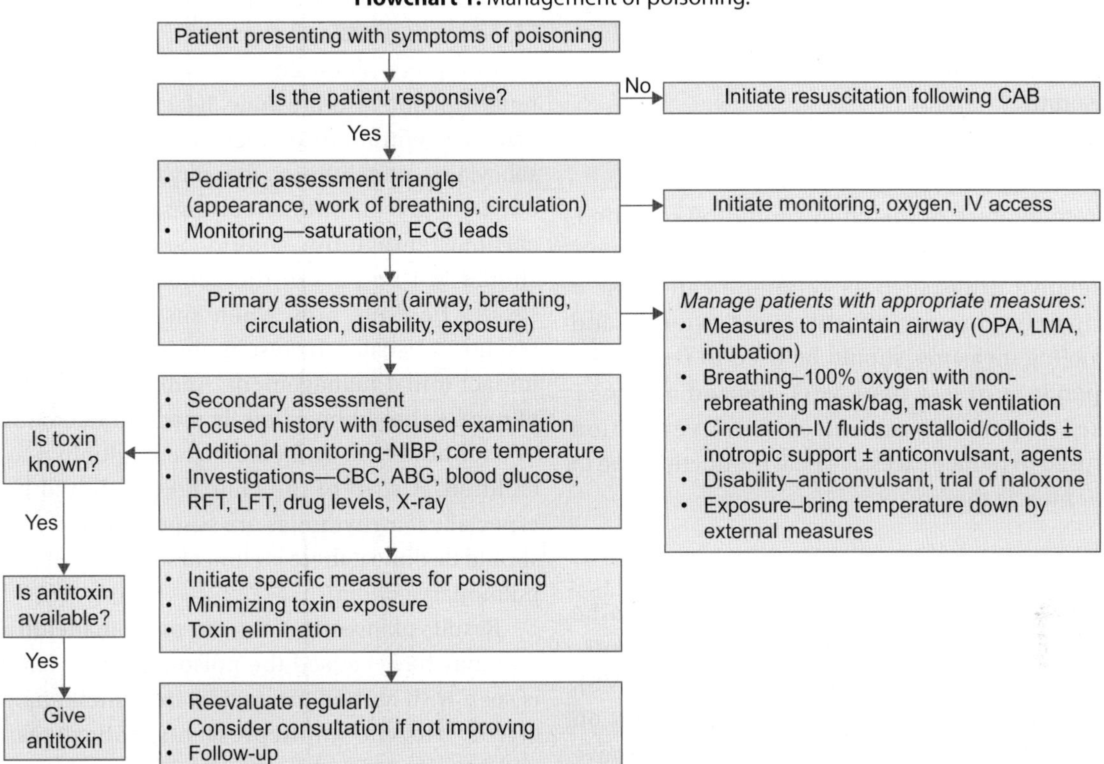

(ECG: electrocardiography; OPA: oropharyngeal airway; LMA: laryngeal mask airway; CBC: complete blood count; NIBP: noninvasive blood pressure; ABG: arterial blood gas; RFT: renal function test; LFT: liver function test; CAB: compressions, airway, breathing)

Caustic agents, angiotensin-converting enzyme inhibitors, and plants containing calcium oxalate crystals can predispose to airway edema and obstruction.

CLINICAL PEARLS

- Abnormal sounds suggest partial airway obstruction.
- If the patient has altered sensorium, the airway should be managed immediately.

Breathing

Respiratory rate, effort of breathing, retractions, breath sounds, chest expansion, and abdominal excursions are noted for the adequacy of breathing and ventilation. Children presenting with respiratory abnormalities or shock should receive high-flow oxygen through a nonrebreathing mask. Children with decreased consciousness and reduced respiratory effort should receive bag-mask ventilation with 100% oxygen. Bag-mask ventilation should be done even with adequate saturation, as children may have high levels of CO_2.

Circulation

The cardiovascular system is assessed by heart rate, pulse volume, capillary refill, blood pressure, coolness of skin, sensorium, and urine output. Crystalloids should be given to manage hypovolemia, followed by inotropes and specific antitoxins, as these can correct hypotension rapidly. In some poisonings, inotropes can worsen hypotension. In a similar fashion, arrhythmias should be managed with specific antidotes, crystalloids, and antiarrhythmics.

Disability

Neurological function is assessed by measuring consciousness, pupillary size, posture, and presence of convulsive movements. The level of consciousness can be measured by using the AVPU scale. Poisoning with opiates, sedatives, antihistamines, and hypoglycemic agents should be considered in children with lower levels of consciousness. Large pupils suggest amphetamines, ecstasy, theophylline, and tricyclic-antidepressant poisoning (all of these cause hypertonia), while small pupils suggest opiates and organophosphorus poisonings. Convulsions can be treated by lorazepam or midazolam. A trial of naloxone should be considered in suspected opiate poisoning.

Exposure

The core temperature of the child should be recorded. Salicylates, anticholinergics, sympathomimetics, cocaine, and dissociative drugs such as ketamine can cause a fever. Antipyretics are not effective, and external and internal cooling measures should be used to reduce the core temperature to less than 39°C. Benzodiazepines, dantrolene, or paralysis and mechanical ventilation should be used to reduce excessive heat production due to agitation or muscle rigidity.

Find

Finding the antidote if it is not known should also be prioritized. The National Poisons Information Centre (NPIC) at All India Institute of Medical Sciences (AIIMS), New Delhi, provides round-the-clock information on the management of poisonings. Poison centers have been established in other cities in India, and having contact details of the one in your region would be important.

Signs and Symptoms

The SAMPLE pneumonic can be used where Signs and Symptoms are sought, Allergies, Medications, Past Medical History, Last meal, and Events leading to current status. This ensures a rapid evaluation. A five W question is also useful. Who: The patient's age, gender, and relationship to others present; **W**hen: The time and date of ingestion; **W**hat: The name and amount of medication(s) or substance(s) of abuse or other coingestants and amount ingested; **W**hy: Whether intentional or accidental and associated details; and **W**here: The route of poisoning. One should be aware that often, history will not be known, unreliable, conflicting, and **W**orse, hidden. The patient may mislead, or be not in a mental state to share correct details or may be hallucinating, etc. Young children may have no idea of what they consume.

Monitoring and Investigations

Monitoring includes pulse oximetry, continuous ECG, noninvasive blood pressure, and core temperature monitoring. Blood investigations should include arterial blood gases and blood glucose.

Complete blood count, urinalysis, and hepatic and renal function tests are done. If facilities exist, then plasma drug concentrations of a few drugs such as paracetamol, salicylates, iron, lithium, theophylline, methanol, digoxin, ethylene glycol, anticonvulsants, methemoglobin, and carboxyhemoglobin should be done. However, they should not be part of the general screen; rather, they should be done only when suspected to confirm the diagnosis. Usually, the results are available later and do not impact initial management. Additionally, interpretation of results should be carefully made in neonates as levels of cholinesterase and carboxyhemoglobin may differ in children. A strip of the child's ECG should be studied, especially if arrhythmias are suspected, and a chest X-ray should be done if there is clinical suspicion of aspiration or pulmonary edema.

Results of investigations can assist in identifying drugs that may have caused the poisoning. Metabolic acidosis is seen with carbon monoxide, iron, methanol, ethylene glycol, tricyclic antidepressants, salicylates, tricyclic antidepressants, and ecstasy. An enlarged anion gap greater than 18 is found in ethanol, iron, methanol, salicylates, and ethylene glycol. Hypokalemia is seen in beta-agonists and theophylline poisoning, while hyperkalemia is seen in digoxin ingestion.

CLINICAL PEARLS

- Interpretation of drug concentrations and enzymes in neonates differs from children.
- Activated charcoal does not absorb iron, metals, lithium, cyanides, petroleum distillates, and alcohol.

Poison Elimination

Minimizing toxin exposure: This step is especially helpful in topical and inhaled toxin exposure cases. External toxin decontamination prevents ongoing toxicity to the child and also protects staff from exposure. The child needs to be disrobed, including removal of jewelry, watches, etc., and the entire body or exposed area washed, preferably in a suitable area in the emergency room. Ocular exposures should be managed by irrigating the eye with copious isotonic saline (such as normal saline or lactated ringers) for at least half an hour or till normal ocular pH is obtained. Prior use of ocular anesthetics such as tetracaine will ensure better irrigation.

Toxin Elimination

The evidence for toxin elimination from the gastrointestinal tract is inconclusive, yet it continues to be used in certain circumstances. It is not required in asymptomatic children with nontoxic ingestions. However, if the ingestion is recent, the child is symptomatic, or there is a possibility of delayed toxicity, then decontamination by various methods is recommended.

Activated Charcoal

Activated charcoal has a surface area of 1,000 m^2/g, is safe, and can be used in the dose of 1 g/kg per dose and is capable of binding a number of poisonous substances without being systematically absorbed. It, however, does not absorb iron, metals, lithium, cyanides, petroleum distillates, and alcohol. The dose is generally 10 times the estimated poison dose, and generally, children are given 25–50 g. Repeated doses can be used in aspirin, barbiturates, and theophylline as they promote drug reabsorption from the circulation into the bowel and thus interrupt enterohepatic cycling. Charcoal is unpalatable, so flavoring may be necessary. This does reduce charcoal's activity. Aspirated charcoal can cause lung damage. Usefulness of activated charcoal beyond 1 hour of ingestion is limited but can be considered if delayed gut absorption is expected.

Emesis

Emesis by administration of ipecac syrup is not recommended for gastrointestinal decontamination.

Gastric Lavage

Lavage is not routinely recommended for decontamination due to variable results, lack of evidence of improved outcomes, and significant adverse effects. Gastric lavage is initiated in children who present within 1 hour. It is contraindicated in poisonings by most hydrocarbons, alkalis, and acids. In children, additional difficulty is encountered as the small size of the lavage tube makes it difficult to remove the toxin. Children often need to be intubated to facilitate the procedure, especially if they have altered sensorium. Most commonly it is effectively used in iron over ingestion and the usual fluid is water or isotonic solution, in aliquots of 10–20 mL/kg. To perform lavage, the child is placed on its left side and a lavage tube is passed into the stomach. Fluid is aspirated and small aliquots of fluid are instilled and reaspirated. This process is continued till the aspirate is clear. After lavage, the tube can be used for instilling specific antidote or activated charcoal.

Whole-bowel Irrigation

This is not routinely indicated but is used in poisoning by sustained-release or enteric-coated drugs, metals such as iron and lithium, and drug packets that have long absorption time or are not bound by charcoal. A large volume (>1 L) polyethylene glycol electrolyte solution is administered at a fast rate, via nasogastric tube. Effectiveness is seen until about 4 hours after ingestion of enteric-coated tablets and sometimes even until about 12–16 hours after administration of some sustained release medications. It causes formation of liquid stools and reduces transit time of intestinal contents.

Cathartics

These are of equivocal efficacy. Saccharide (sorbitol) and saline (magnesium citrate) cathartics have been administered as a single dose.

CLINICAL PEARLS

- Ipecac syrup is not recommended for gastrointestinal decontamination.
- Cathartics are of unknown efficacy.

Other Methods of Elimination

Urinary alkalinization by the administration of sodium bicarbonate effectively increases the elimination of drugs with a low pH such as salicylates and chlorpropamide. Alkalinization increases the ionized fraction of the drug in the tubular lumen, preventing its reabsorption. Hemodialysis is used for salicylates, toxic alcohols, lithium, and theophylline. Charcoal hemoperfusion, plasmapheresis, exchange transfusion, and continuous ultrafiltration techniques may also be used.

Specific Antitoxins

In some poisonings, antidotes that can counter the poison may be available **(Table 3)**.

TABLE 3: Antidotes and management of selected toxic exposures.

Ingestion	*Potential antidote/other management*
Acetaminophen	N-acetylcysteine, activated charcoal within 4 hour
Antihistaminics	Activated charcoal or whole bowel irrigation if extended-release formulations, anticonvulsants, physostigmine
Benzodiazepine	Flumazenil
β-blockers	Glucagon, activated charcoal if early after ingestion, whole bowel irrigation for delayed-release formulations, atropine, IVF, pressors
Calcium channel blockers	Calcium, activated charcoal if early after ingestion, whole bowel irrigation for delayed-release formulations, atropine, IVF, pressors, insulin/glucose
Cholinesterase inhibitors	Atropine, pralidoxime
Digoxin	Digoxin immune fab, activated charcoal, electrolyte management
Iron	Deferoxamine, whole bowel irrigation, hemodynamic support, monitor for possible GI bleed, treat acidosis, hypoglycemia, and hypotension
Isoniazid	Pyridoxine
Opioids	Naloxone
Salicylates	Correct electrolyte imbalance, fluid therapy, urine alkalinizers, hemodialysis
Sulfonylurea	Dextrose, octreotide
Tricyclic antidepressants	Activated charcoal, sodium bicarbonate to reduce cardiotoxicity, pressor support
Cyanide	Ensure airway, breathing, circulation, 100% oxygen inhalation, sodium nitrite/sodium thiosulfate or hydroxocobalamin
Carbon monoxide	100% oxygen inhalation or hyperbaric oxygen
Caustic agents	Ensure airway, breathing, circulation, steroid use in esophageal burns is controversial; hospitalize the patient to monitor for mediastinitis, pneumonitis, and peritonitis
Disk batteries	Removal if in esophagus; if below esophagus, watch for 3 days for passage with stools, if not passed out, consider surgical removal
Ethanol	Respiratory management, correction of hypoglycemia, temperature control, thiamine (in chronic alcoholism)
Ethylene glycol and methanol	Ethanol or 4-methylpyrazole if level >20 mg/dL, sodium bicarbonate, calcium, pyridoxine, thiamine, folate, hemodialysis
Lead	Chelation with edetate calcium disodium, 2,4-dimercaptopropanol, succimer, and anticonvulsants if required
Agents causing methemoglobinemia	Methylene blue

(GI: gastrointestinal)

KEY POINTS

- Providers should be aware of most common poisonings that occur in the area they work.
- Stabilization of the child is of prime importance.
- Awareness of toxidromes will enhance ability to manage complex poisonings.
- Investigations should be tailored to suspected toxins.
- Consultation with a toxicologist is recommended.

SUGGESTED READING

1. Abbruzzi G, Stork CM. Pediatric toxicologic concerns. Emerg Med Clin North Am. 2002;20(1):223-47.
2. Florin TA, Ludwig S. Poisoning. In: Florin T, Ludwig S, Aronson P, Werner H (Eds). Netter's Pediatrics. Philadelphia, PA: Elseiver/Saunders; 2011. pp. 56-61.
3. Jayakrishnan MP, Krishnakumar P, Geeta MG, George B. Changing trends of accidental poisoning in children over the last two decades. Indian J Community Med. 2021;46(2):350-1.

4. Jepsen F, Mary R. Poisoning in children. Curr Paediatr. 2005;15(7):563-8.
5. Kliegman RM, Stanton BF, St Geme JW, Schor NF, Behrman RE. Poisonings. In: Kliegman RM, Stanton BF, St Geme III JW, Schor NF, Behrman RE (Eds). Nelson Textbook of Pediatrics, 19th edition. Philadelphia, PA: Elsevier/Saunders; 2011. pp. 250-70.
6. Penny L, Tony M. Poisoning in children. Continuing Education in Anaesthesia. Crit Care Pain. 2009;9(4):109-13.
7. Pooni PA, Bansal V. Management of Poisonings in Children. J Pediatr Crit Care. 2016;3(2):20-32.
8. Punja M, Hoffman RJ. Approach to poisoning. Critical Care Emergency Medicine. New York: McGraw-Hill Education/Medical; 2011. p. 409.
9. Rezaiyan T. Poisonings. In: Tschudy M, Arcara K (Eds). The Harriet Lane Handbook: A Manual for Pediatric House Officers, 19th edition. Philadelphia, PA: Mosby; 2011. pp. 19-56.
10. Suting E, Bhaskar V, Batra P. Changing epidemiology of poisoning in children: A retrospective study from a tertiary care center in New Delhi, India. Indian J Public Health. 2021;65(4):400-2.
11. The Royal Children's Hospital. (2013). Clinical Practice Guidelines: Paracetamol Poisoning. [online] Available from https://www.rch.org.au/clinicalguide/guideline_index/Paracetamol_Poisoning/. [Last accessed September, 2024]

Burns in Children

Abhaya Gupta

INTRODUCTION

Burns is a health problem concerning countries all over the world. The World Health Organization has estimated that approximately 180,000 deaths occur due to burns. Majority of the patients are from middle- and lower-income countries.

In India, more than a million patients suffer from moderate-to-severe burns. Children and women are more likely to get burned.

Burns are the fifth leading cause of nonfatal childhood injuries. Lack of adult supervision causing accidental burns and child abuse are the major causes of burns in children. The majority of kid burn cases take place in a home setting.

PREVENTION

Burns can lead to both lethal and nonlethal injuries. The mortality figures in developed nations due to burns have decreased significantly. Availability of healthcare services, education, and prevention strategies has contributed to decrease in the number of deaths. Nonfatal burns cause significant morbidity, disability, and economic burden on the country.

Prevention of burns is possible. It requires a multisectoral approach.

Important recommendations for prevention of burns:

- Prior to giving the child a bath, please verify the water's temperature.
- Give bath to children under supervision of an adult.
- Avoid holding an infant while eating, drinking, or preparing hot meals.
- Keep your toddler away from the kitchen as you make meals. If you cannot keep them out, set up a safe area away from the stove for them to play.
- Keep hot foods, drinks, and utensils far away from children.
- Keep matches and lighters out of reach of children.
- Avoid leaving ashtrays with burning cigarettes.
- When holding a youngster, avoid smoking.
- Store all chemicals in a closed cabinet.
- Install safety outlet covers for electrical outlets.
- Educate your kids about the dangers of playing with electrical cables.
- Use only a cold vaporizer, not steam.
- Apply sunscreen with SPF of 30, 30 minutes prior to exposure to sun to prevent sunburns.

FIRST AID

Minor Burns

- Immediately apply running tap water to the burn for 20 minutes. This is effective for up to 3 hours following the burn. Avoid using cold or iced water.
- To relieve a mouth burn, from hot food or drink, place a piece of ice in the mouth for couple of minutes.
- Carefully remove any jewelry or clothes that are not adhered to the burn to avoid causing more skin injury. It is crucial to use cool water just to treat the burn and to keep your child as warm as possible.
- Cover the burnt area loosely with bandage/gauze/cling film/plastic or a dry clean sheet of cloth.
- Avoid rupturing blisters. Blisters aid in infection prevention. Apply an antibiotic ointment and gently wash the affected area with water if a blister does burst.
- Avoid attempting to take off clothing that has been burned.

Major Burns

Please ask for emergency medical services and then begin first aid measures.

- Keep the individual who has been burned safe. Make sure the person you are assisting is not in contact with the burn's source. Before you approach someone, who has been burned by electricity, be sure that the electrical source is turned off.

- Verify the person who was burned is still breathing. If you know how, start rescue breathing if necessary.
- Take off belts, jewelry, and other tight objects.
- The area of burns needs to be covered with sterile gauze or cloth.

Visit the doctor in the following conditions:

- All major burns
- All infantile burns
- All electric and inhalational (smoke) burns
- Minor burns that affect the eyes, mouth, hands, or genitals will require emergency attention
- If the area burns is more than eight centimeters.
- Burns occurring due to chemical injury involving major area
- Burns appear to be deep (dry leathery skin, charred skin appearing white, black, or brown)
- Burns that affect hands, feet, face, groin, buttocks or a major joint, or are circumferential over the limbs
- The need of a tetanus shot depending on the immunization status

CLASSIFICATION OF BURNS

Cutaneous burns are classified depending how deep they are. The depth of the injury helps in decision making for resuscitation, surgical implications, healing time, and prognosis. It is worthwhile to note that children under 5 years of age have thin skin and are more prone to deeper burns.

A method that reflected the requirement for surgical intervention took the place of the previous system of classifying burns as first, second, third, or fourth degree. The terms superficial, superficial partial-thickness, deep partial-thickness, and full-thickness are currently used to describe burn depth **(Fig. 1)**. The most serious burns, which penetrate deeper than the skin into the subcutaneous soft tissue and may affect underlying arteries, nerves, muscle, bone, and joints, are still referred to as fourth degree burns.

The depth of burns can change and can become deeper with time. So, the correct assessment of burns can take several days.

American Burn Association has classified burns into:

- *Superficial:* Burns that are superficial or epidermal only affect the skin's outermost layer. They are painful, dry, red, and blanch when compressed, yet they do not blister. The erythema and pain go away over the course of the following 2–3 days, and by Day 4 or so, the damaged epithelium starts to separate from the freshly repaired epidermis. In most cases, these wounds heal completely in 6 days. Sunburns frequently undergo this phase.

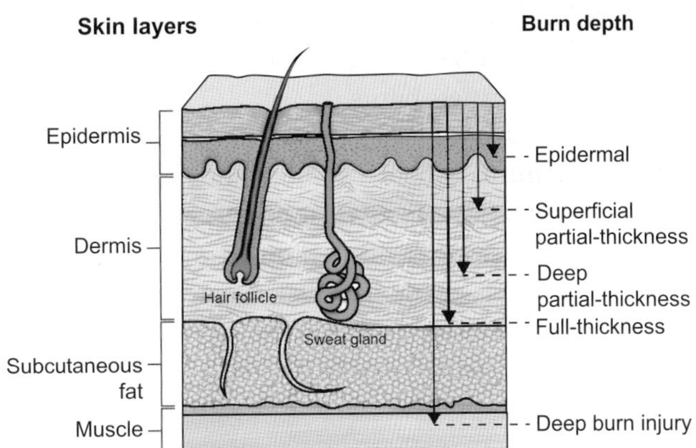

Fig. 1: Classification of burns.

- *Partial-thickness:* Parts of the dermis and the epidermis are affected by partial-thickness burns. They might be classified as deep or superficial.
- *Superficial partial-thickness:* Blisters typically develop between the epidermis and dermis within 24 hours of these burns. When pressure is applied, they blanch, leak, get red, and hurt. After 12–24 hours, burns that at first seem to be just epidermal in depth may be found to be partial-thickness. Although pigment changes may occur, scarring is uncommon with these burns, which typically recover in 7–21 days. The surface may develop a coating of fibrinous exudates and necrotic debris, which could make the burn site more vulnerable to significant bacterial colonization and slowed healing. Usually, these burns heal without causing hypertrophic scarring or functional impairment.
- *Deep partial-thickness:* These burns differ from superficial partial-thickness burns in that they penetrate deeper into the dermis. Hair follicles and glandular tissue are harmed by deep burns. Only pressure causes pain, they are wet or waxy dry, nearly always blister (easily unroofed), and vary in mottled coloration from spotty cheesy white to red. Pressure blanching could be slow. Wounds will heal in 2–9 weeks if infection is avoided and they are left to heal naturally without grafting. Hypertrophic scarring is always the result of these burns. Even with vigorous physical therapy, joint dysfunction is likely if they affect a joint. A deep partial-thickness burn is functionally and aesthetically

equal to a full-thickness burn if it does not cure within 2 weeks. It may be very difficult for it to be differentiated from full-thickness burns.

- *Full-thickness:* All layers of the dermis are destroyed by these burns, which also frequently cause damage to the subcutaneous tissue underneath. The dead and denatured dermis is known as burn eschar. If the eschar is circumferential, it may jeopardize the survival of a limb or torso.

Anesthesia and hypoesthesia are typically used to treat full-thickness burns. The look of skin can range from burnt and black to leathery gray and waxy white. When pressure is applied, the dry, inelastic skin does not blanch. It is simple to extract hairs from hair follicles. Blisters and vesicles do not form.

Pale full-thickness burns may imitate normal skin except that the skin does not blanch with pressure. It could take some time for characteristics that distinguish partial-thickness burns from full-thickness burns to emerge.

Eventually, the eschar breaks from the underlying tissue, exposing a bed of granulation tissue that has not healed. These wounds heal by wound contracture and epithelialization around the wound margins without the need for surgery. Contractures cause extensive scarring; full spontaneous healing is impossible.

Extension to Deep Tissues

Fourth-degree burns are potentially fatal injuries. It may involve not only the subcutaneous tissue but muscles and bones also.

ASSESSMENT OF EXTENT OF BURNS

Since it takes into account the proportion of body surface area (BSA) impacted by growth, the Lund–Browder chart **(Fig. 2)** is the suggested technique for determining the severity of burns in children. The palm approach might work better if the burn is uneven or irregular.

The amount of BSA burned can also be estimated using Barlow's chart **(Table 1)** for various age groups.

Accurate estimation of the percentage of burns is necessary for fluid resuscitation, prognosis, morbidity, and predicting mortality. The area of palm of a child is roughly equal to 1% of surface area. It is especially useful when the burns area is <10%.

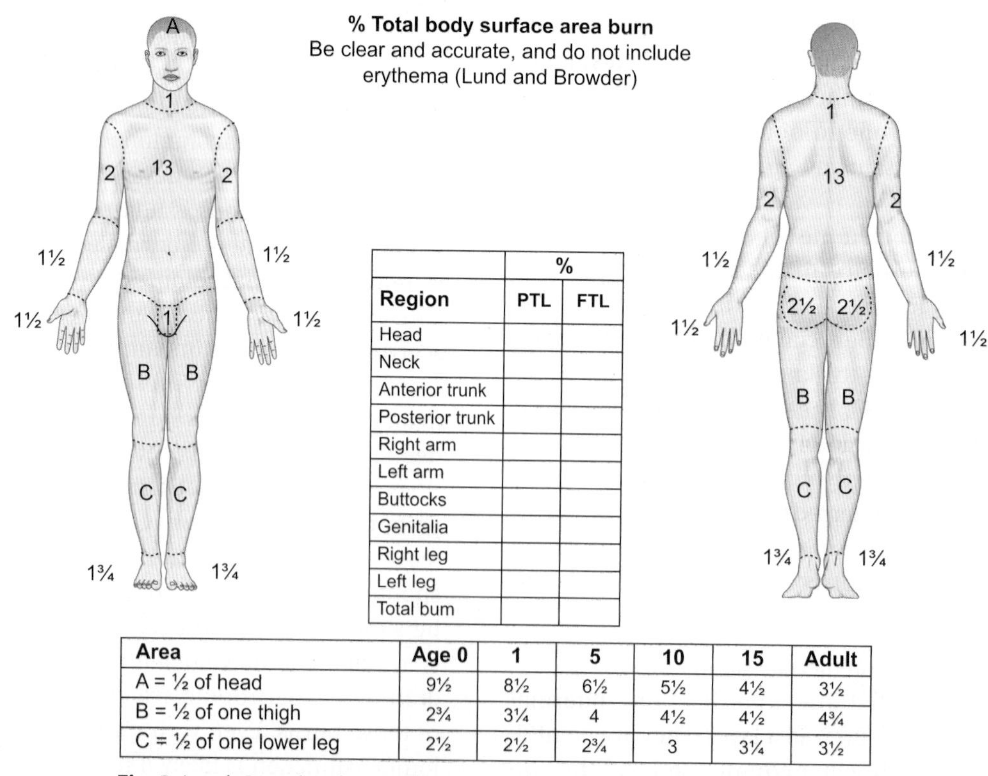

Region	% PTL	% FTL
Head		
Neck		
Anterior trunk		
Posterior trunk		
Right arm		
Left arm		
Buttocks		
Genitalia		
Right leg		
Left leg		
Total bum		

Area	Age 0	1	5	10	15	Adult
A = ½ of head	9½	8½	6½	5½	4½	3½
B = ½ of one thigh	2¾	3¼	4	4½	4½	4¾
C = ½ of one lower leg	2½	2½	2¾	3	3¼	3½

Fig. 2: Lund–Browder chart. (FTL: full-thickness loss; PTL: partial-thickness loss)

TABLE 1: Barlow's chart.

Body part	*0–1 year*	*1–4 years*	*5–9 years*	*10–14 years*	*15–18 years*	*Adult*
Head	19	17	13	11	9	7
Neck	2	2	2	2	2	2
Anterior trunk	13	13	13	13	13	13
Posterior trunk	13	13	13	13	13	13
Right buttock	2.5	2.5	2.5	2.5	2.5	2.5
Left buttock	2.5	2.5	2.5	2.5	2.5	2.5
Genitalia	1	1	1	1	1	1
Right upper arm	4	4	4	4	4	4
Left upper arm	4	4	4	4	4	4
Right lower arm	3	3	3	3	3	3
Left lower arm	3	3	3	3	3	3
Right hand	2.5	2.5	2.5	2.5	2.5	2.5
Left hand	2.5	2.5	2.5	2.5	2.5	2.5
Right thigh	5.5	6.5	8	8.5	9	9.5
Left thigh	5.5	5.5	8	8.5	9	9.5
Right leg	5	5	5.5	6	6.5	7
Left leg	5	5	5.5	6	6.5	7
Right foot	3.5	3.5	3.5	3.5	3.5	3.5
Left foot	3.5	3.5	3.5	3.5	3.5	3.5

MANAGEMENT OF BURNS

Burns should be ideally managed initially in a trauma center. On arrival of a patient, the following history should be noted.

Clinical History

- When did the injury occur (time)?
- How did the injury occur?
- For scald injury ask the liquid's approximate temperature and composition.
- In cases of contact burns, one must know the type of surface and its temperature.
- Friction
- If the patient has suffered burns due to flames or any explosion, then we need to ask the product that was involved and where did it occur, for how long and if there is any suspicion of inhalational injury.
- In cases of electric burns, we need to know the voltage and type of current used.
- We have to ascertain the type of chemical in case of chemical burns
- In case of frost bites, ask for direct exposure to cold.
- History of exposure to sun.
- *History of first aid:*
  - Was the first aid given within 3 hours and for how long?
  - What was used?
  - Ask for history of removal of clothes and ornaments.
  - In cases of chemical burns, were any counter agents used?
- To have a high degree of suspicion of nonburn injury also
- History suggestive of battered child
- Tetanus status

Examination and Initial Management

Avoid becoming sidetracked by the burn injury. As with all injuries, pediatric burn assessments necessitate a primary and secondary survey with the primary goal of identifying and managing immediate life concerns.

Airway

- Signs of an oropharyngeal burn include soot in the mouth, intraoral edema, and erythema; signs of an

airway burn or inhalation damage include stridor, hoarseness, black sputum, respiratory trouble, singed nose hairs, or face puffiness
- Burns involving significant area of the neck.
- If above, think about intubating the patient right away.
- Use high flow oxygen, if there is a possibility of carbon monoxide intoxication or airway burns.
- If there is history of associated trauma, immobilize the cervical spine to protect it.

Breathing

Escharotomy may be necessary for full-thickness and/or circumferential chest burns in order to allow for respiration.

Circulation

- Intravenous (IV) or intraosseous IO access (ideally two points of access)
- IV fluids as needed
- If early shock is apparent, take into account factors other than the burn.
- Assess peripheral circulation and determine whether an escharotomy is necessary for circumferential burns.

Disability

- Consider airway access if patient is unconscious.
- Examine the neurovascular condition of any affected limb.
- Examine the neurovascular condition of any affected limb.
- It is necessary to determine the extent and type of burns following first triage and resuscitation.
- A few clinical indications and symptoms are listed in the **Table 2** to assist the clinician in making decisions about additional care.

Outpatient Treatment

Patients with superficial burns having <10% burnt surface area can be managed on an outpatient basis. Patient will require dressings, pain relief medications, and depending on the immunizations status tetanus vaccine. Topical application of silver sulfadiazine cream on the wound should be applied. Once the blisters have burst, the devitalized skin must be debrided.

Many types of dressing materials can also be applied, e.g., hydrocolloid, collagen, hydrogel, alginate, and medicated gauze.

Inpatient Treatment

Child requiring care in a specialized burns unit:
- Any type of burns involving >10% of BSA
- Child suffering from full-thickness burns
- Particular regions, even if <10%, include the face, ears, eyes, neck, hands, feet, genitalia, perineum, or a major joint.
- Burns that are circumferential in nature
- Any child suffering from chemical burns
- Any burns sustained due to electrical source
- Burns that have coexisting trauma and/or spinal cord injury
- Suspected or sustained inhalation burns
- Children under a year old with burns

In some special situations, depending upon the nature or site of burns things as given in **Table 3** should be considered.

TABLE 2: Clinical signs and symptoms according to depth of burns.

Features	***First-degree burn (superficial)***	***Second-degree, or partial-thickness burn (superficial and deep)***	***Third-degree, or full-thickness burn***
Surface appearance	• Dry, no blisters • Minimal or no edema • Erythematous • Blanches and bleeds	• Moist blebs and blisters • Underlying tissue is mottled, pink and white, and fair capillary refill • Bleeds	• Dry and leathery eschar • Mixed white, waxy, khaki, mahogany, and soot stained • No blanching or bleeding
Pain	Very painful	Very painful	Insensate
Depth of burns	Only epidermis is involved	• Dermis is involved • Some part (domes) of subcutaneous tissue	Down to and may include fat, and deeper tissues also
Healing time	2–5 days with no scarring	• *Superficial:* 5–21 days with no grafting • *Deep partial:* 21–35 days with no infection • *If infected:* Converts to full-thickness burn	• Large areas require grafting • Small areas may heal from the edges after weeks

TABLE 3: Quick guide in burns involving particular type or nature of burns.

Nature/site of burn	*Consideration*
Circumferential deep burn (deep dermal or full-thickness)	Compromise of the nervous system needs to be looked into: • Raise the distal portion of the limb to burn • Track temperature, capillary refill time, and color • Escharotomy might be necessary
Head and neck burns	Nurse head up to reduce swelling and edema
Ocular burns	• Blepharospasm, tears, and conjunctivitis are some of the signs • All facial burns should be assessed using fluorescein. 2% eye drops to check for corneal damage • Treat with extensive irrigation of 0.9% sodium chloride with topical anesthetic in the eye (unaffected eye upward) – Up to 1 hour with acidic contamination or until pain stops – Up to 2 hours with alkaline contamination or until pain stops • Topical chloramphenicol can prevent subsequent infections • Urgent pediatric ophthalmology review
Limb burns	• Raise the limb • Keep an eye on perfusion
Electrical injuries	• Check for wounds at the entrance or exit • Consider spinal precautions • *Dysrhythmia risk:* Think about 24-hour electrocardiogram (ECG) monitoring • Keep an eye out for increased creatine kinase (CK), urine hemoglobin, and hemochromogen levels
Chemical burns	• First aid providers should wear personal protective equipment, such as gloves, a mask, a gown, and eye protection • Take off any contaminated clothing • Brush powdered agent off skin • Cool water should be used to irrigate areas that have come into touch with chemicals • To prevent more injuries from contaminated water, irrigate it in a proper direction

Fluid Management in Burns ≥10% Total Body Surface Area

In order to maximize wound and body perfusion and minimize wound and body edema and their related side effects, the objective is to treat burn shock by replacing fluid losses as efficiently as possible. We should get the requirements based on the burn time rather than the presentation time. Use the modified Parkland formula to get the fluid volume. The preferred fluid is Hartmann's solution; if it is not available, use 0.9% sodium chloride. Use a urinary catheter to maintain strict fluid balance. Keep nil by mouth and think about getting a nasogastric tube because gastric ileus is a possible side effect.

The most used method for determining the initial fluid demand is the modified Parkland formula. The flowing reasoning listed here should serve as a guide. The fluids can be changed based on the patient's needs and urine output, and the patients should be evaluated every 1–2 hours for the first 24 hours. A child should have a urine production of 1 mL per kilogram every hour.

- *24 hours:*
  - 4 milliliters per kilogram of BSA burn of ringer lactate is normally required. Out of which the first half has to be infused in first 8 hours and the remaining in the next 16 hours. All this is calculated from the time of burns.
  - Regular maintenance fluids are also maintained.
- *Second 24 hours:*
  - Ringer lactate is added to 5% dextrose and the quantity being half of first day's requirement.
  - Reduce the amount of sodium in newborns' fluids if their urine sodium levels are increasing.
  - There is currently a debate on the selection of fluids as colloids or crystalloids.
  - Colloids, which should be administered 8–24 hours after the injury, may be recommended for burns that are >85% BSA.

Assessment and Monitoring

Hemogram, urine routine, electrolytes, blood sugar level, renal function test, serum proteins, and other tests (arterial blood gas, prothrombin time, partial thromboplastin time, and cultures, etc.) are performed as needed for the initial investigations.

Electrolytes

If a topical antimicrobial burn treatment containing 0.5% silver nitrate solution is used to treat children who have >20% burns, sodium supplementation may be necessary. To keep sodium levels above 130 mEq/L, 4 g/m^2 BSA/day is administered orally in 4–6 split doses.

Potassium losses are increased in patients in whom 0.5% silver nitrate solution is being used or in patients being treated with aminoglycosides, diuretics, or amphotericin. Keep potassium levels above 3 mEq/L.

Subsequent Fluids and Feeding

Using a nasogastric feeding tube, oral feeding can begin as soon as 48 hours following a burn injury. To maintain a total fluid requirement, IV fluids are reduced in accordance with the oral meals tolerated.

Blood Products: Indications

For hemoglobin levels below 8 g/dL, packed red blood cells are injected. When recurrent grafting is required, patients with hemoglobinopathy, cardiac disease, systemic infection, or expected (or continuing) blood loss with hemoglobin levels below 10 g/dL should be considered for transfusion.

Albumin: To keep the serum albumin level over 2 g/dL, 5% albumin is injected. Beginning on the second day, the following amount is infused throughout the course of 24 hours:

Body surface area (BSA)	30–50%	50–70%	70–100%
Albumin (mL/kg/% BSA)	0.3 mL	0.4 mL	0.5 mL

Children who are bleeding with a disturbed prothrombin time (>1.5 times) or an activated partial thromboplastin time (>1.2 times) and are scheduled for a surgery that could cause more than half of their blood volume to be lost should receive fresh frozen plasma.

Prevention of Infection/Role of Antibiotics

Prophylactic antibiotic use is a contentious topic. Children who have >30% burns should receive treatment in a separate, bacterially controlled facility. Malnutrition, a decrease in host defense, and the metabolic and microbiological effects of a large open wound are the main causes of burn injury mortality. Bloodstream infections, urinary tract infections, pneumonia, and wound infections are examples of specific infection locations. Since fever can be caused by a hypermetabolic reaction, it may not be a sign of infection on its own. Early infection detection requires close monitoring of vital signs and other indicators, as well as serial evaluation of burn wounds. Blood cultures, throat swabs, wound swabs, sputum, urine, and stool are all part of the sepsis screen.

Before beginning empirical treatment, an effort should be made to isolate the organism. It is best to take a broad-spectrum antibiotic that is effective against gram-positive bacteria (staphylococci).

Pain Relief

Reducing early metabolic stress and chronic post-traumatic stress disorders requires adequate analgesics, anxiolytics, and psychological support. Anxiolytics such as lorazepam and opioid analgesics like morphine can work in concert to produce a synergistic effect. The same medications used for the IV route must be utilized to provide sufficient sedation and pain relief for procedures like dressing changes and debridement. Another excellent choice for procedural sedation is ketamine.

Nutritional Support

A hypermetabolic reaction brought on by the burn injury results in the breakdown of fat and protein. Early excision and grafting, regulating humidity and temperature to prevent cold stress, managing pain and anxiety, and allowing for proper sleep cycles can all reduce energy expenditure. Metabolic stress is decreased by high protein intake, i.e., 3–4 g/kg/day, and high calorie support, which includes 1,800 cal/m^2/day plus 2,200 cal/m^2 of burn/day. Zinc, vitamin C, vitamin A, and multivitamins—particularly B group—are also necessary. To satisfy the high calorie requirements, enteral or parenteral alimentation should be initiated as soon as feasible. As soon as possible, enteral feeding should replace parenteral nourishment in order to reduce infection problems.

SURGICAL MANAGEMENT

Early healing is encouraged by wound care and infection avoidance, which also enhances functional and aesthetic results. Mafenide acetate, silver nitrate, or silver sulfadiazine can all be applied topically to burns. These substances have the ability to enter tissues and stop infections. Newer alternatives for treating severe burns include Aquacel-Ag, an absorbent hydrofiber dressing impregnated with silver, and Biobrane, a bilaminate membrane with an inner layer of nylon mesh impregnated with collagen and an outer layer of silicone that promotes neovascularization and epithelialization. In order to eliminate dead tissue and promote early healing in deep second-degree wounds. Accuzyme ointment is used as a topical enzymatic debridement treatment.

Early excision and grafting are recommended for deep second- and third-degree burns. In serious burns, sequential excision and grafting are frequently necessary. Autografts provide rapid excision and wound closure. Allografts, xenografts, and other synthetic skin coverings are alternatives for wound closure that may be helpful in severe burns to minimize loss of fluid, electrolytes, heat, and protein as well as to lessen pain.

Patients may require contracture release and multiple procedures on long-term follow-up.

REHABILITATION

Rehabilitation starts as soon as the acute management is over. A multidisciplinary approach is required. Compression dressings, exercise and stretching to prevent contractures, physiotherapy, and psychotherapy is required. Scar management and help from occupational therapist are required on long-term basis.

SUGGESTED READING

1. Allorto N, Atieh B, Bolgiani A, Chatterjee P, Cioffi W, Dziewulski P, et al. ISBI Practice Guidelines for Burn Care, Part 2. Burns. 2018;44(7):1617-706.
2. Antoon AY, Donovan MK. Burn injuries. In: Kliegman RM, Stanton B, St Geme J, Schor NF, Behrman RE (Eds). Nelson Textbook of Pediatrics, 19th edn. Amsterdam: Elsevier, Saunders; 2011.
3. Bafna VS. Approach to burns in children. In: Shah NK, Vasudev AS (Eds). Algorithms in Pediatrics, 1st edn. New Delhi: Jaypee Brothers Medical Publishers; 2017
4. Broadis E, Chokotho T, Borgstein E. Paediatric burn and scald management in a low resource setting: a reference guide and review. Afr J Emerg Med. 2017;7(Suppl): S27-S31.
5. Mayo Clinic. (2024). Burns: First Aid. [online] Available from https://www.mayoclinic.org/first-aid/first-aid-burns/basics/art-20056649. [Last accessed December, 2024].
6. Nationwide Childrens. (2024). Burn Prevention: Infant and Toddler. [online] Available from https://www.nationwidechildrens.org/family-resources-education/health-wellness-and-safety-resources/helping-hands/burn-prevention-infant-and-toddler. [Last accessed December, 2024].
7. Rode H, Rogers AD. Burns in children. In: Puri P (Ed). Pediatric Surgery. Berlin, Heidelberg: Springer; 2020.
8. The Royal Children's Hospital Melbourne. (2024). Burns—Acute Management. [online] Available from https://www.rch.org.au/clinicalguide/guideline_index/burns/?fbclid=IwAR3y6I9FwR. [Last accessed December, 2024].

Approach to Scorpion Sting Envenomation

Mahesh A Mohite

INTRODUCTION

Scorpion sting envenomation (SSE) is common medical emergency predominantly seen in rural India. It is commonly seen in Konkan region of Maharashtra, northern Karnataka, Andhra Pradesh, Tamil Nadu, and Puducherry. About three decades ago, there was very poor information about its pathophysiology, hence there was no scientific defined protocol for its management and mortality was almost 30% in adults and >50% in children. Dr HS Bawaskar from Mahad, a rural taluka of Maharashtra, did a breakthrough research in understanding the basic pathology based on clinical profile of the disease and first time used Prazosin, an alpha blocker, for SSE treatment successfully. Later on this protocol management brought down the mortality to almost 1%. Recently with further research by Dr Natu from rural Maharashtra and Dr Bawaskar stressed the early use of scorpion antivenom to bring down the mortality to almost zero.

INCIDENCE

The SSE is more common in rural areas, more so in young working males. Scorpions are found in dry farm paddy, house roofs, and soil burrows. The sting happens accidently while working in farms and sting is common on hands and feet. Small children may get stings at home from scorpions dropped from roofs or while playing near house. SSE commonly occurs in early monsoon when rain water enters burrows of scorpion and scorpions come out of the burrows. Stings are common in March to June and October to December.

SCORPION

There are about 1,500 species of scorpion world over of which 50 are poisonous. In India, about 86 species are found of which *Mesobuthus tamulus* and *Palamnaeus dami* are the poisonous ones. *M. tamulus* commonly known as Red scorpion is the poisonous scorpion found in Kokan, Karnataka, and Puducherry. This is predominantly cardiotoxic venom inducing scorpion. Poisonous scorpions are also found in west Asia, south America, and Mexico.

VENOM

The venom contains enzymes and nonenzymatic proteins. The venom of *M. tamulus* causes autonomic storm and leads to predominantly cardiotoxicity. Few American scorpions cause neurotoxicity leading to skeletal muscle paralysis. Few West Indian scorpions cause pancreatitis and severe metabolic derangements.

Flowchart 1: Pathogenesis.

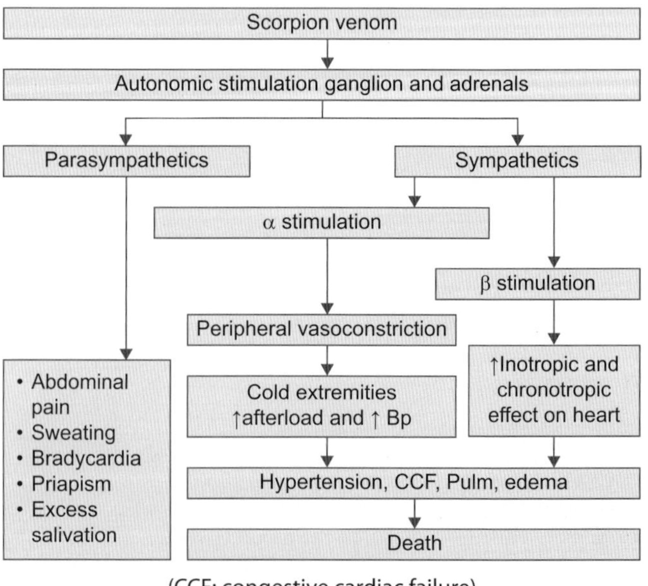

(CCF: congestive cardiac failure)

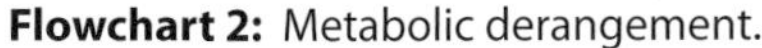

Flowchart 2: Metabolic derangement.

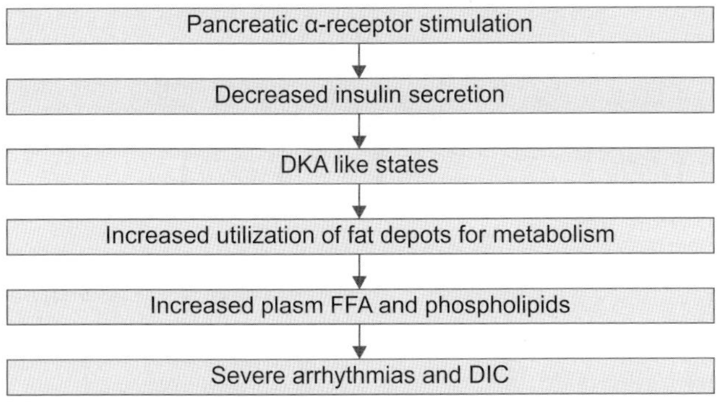

(DIC: disseminated intravascular coagulation; FFA: free fatty acid; DKA: diabetic ketoacidosis)

The Indian Red scorpion causes three major derangements serially or simultaneously:

1. Parasympathetic stimulation
2. Sympathetic storm
3. Metabolic derangements

CLINICAL FEATURES

Clinical features reflect the underlying pathological process. Many times the sting is nonpoisonous and only symptoms are local pain and tingling. The poisonous stings are usually minimally painful or painless and pain may appear after vasodilator treatment is started. In case of poisonous sting initially in parasympathetic phase, there is intense sweating, abdominal pain, vomiting, borborygmi, bradycardia, and priapism, the pathognomonic sign in male victims **(Figs. 1 and 2)**. Usually this stage lasts for first 2–4 hours, but at times, this phase is very short and sympathetic phase may ensue very early. The rapid onset of sympathetic phase may indicate severe envenomation. In sympathetic phase, child will have cold extremity, poor pulses with narrow pulse pressure, hypertension, and tachycardia. This phase usually lasts for 4–6 hours. If not treated appropriately, this phase culminates into cardiac failure and pulmonary edema and death ensues within 12 hours.

DIAGNOSIS

Diagnosis is clinical and there is no laboratory test to confirm the diagnosis. Many times patient is brought with history of sting and scorpion seen at site. The rural population brings killed scorpion for recognition. Sometimes definitive history is not present and the clinical toxidrome of autonomic storm helps to diagnose

Flowchart 3: Clinical presentation.

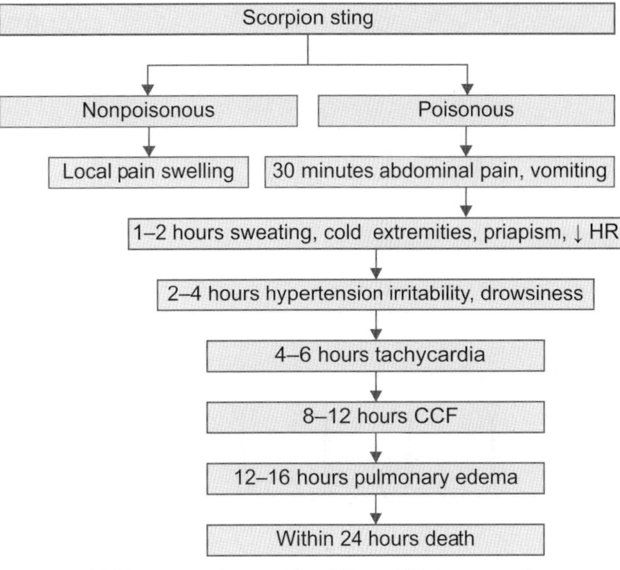

(CCF: congestive cardiac failure; HR: heart rate)

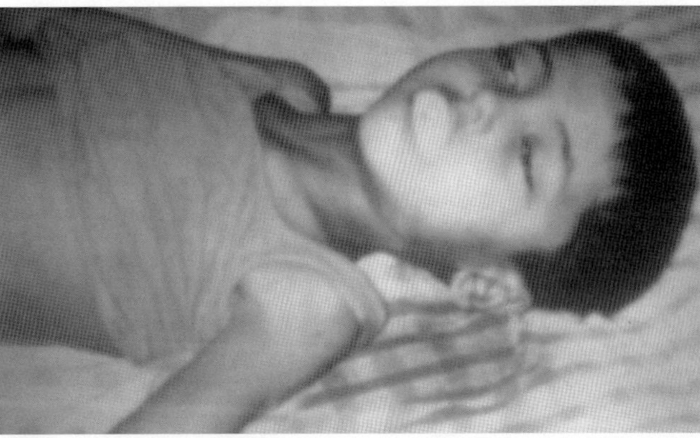

Fig. 1: Pulmonary edema.
(For color version, see Plate 1)

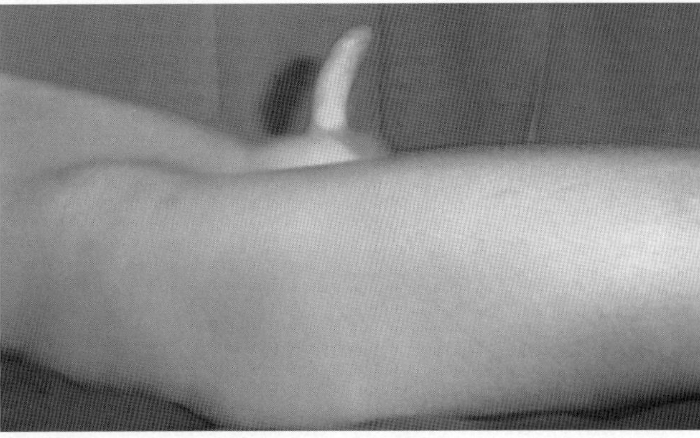

Fig. 2: Priapism.

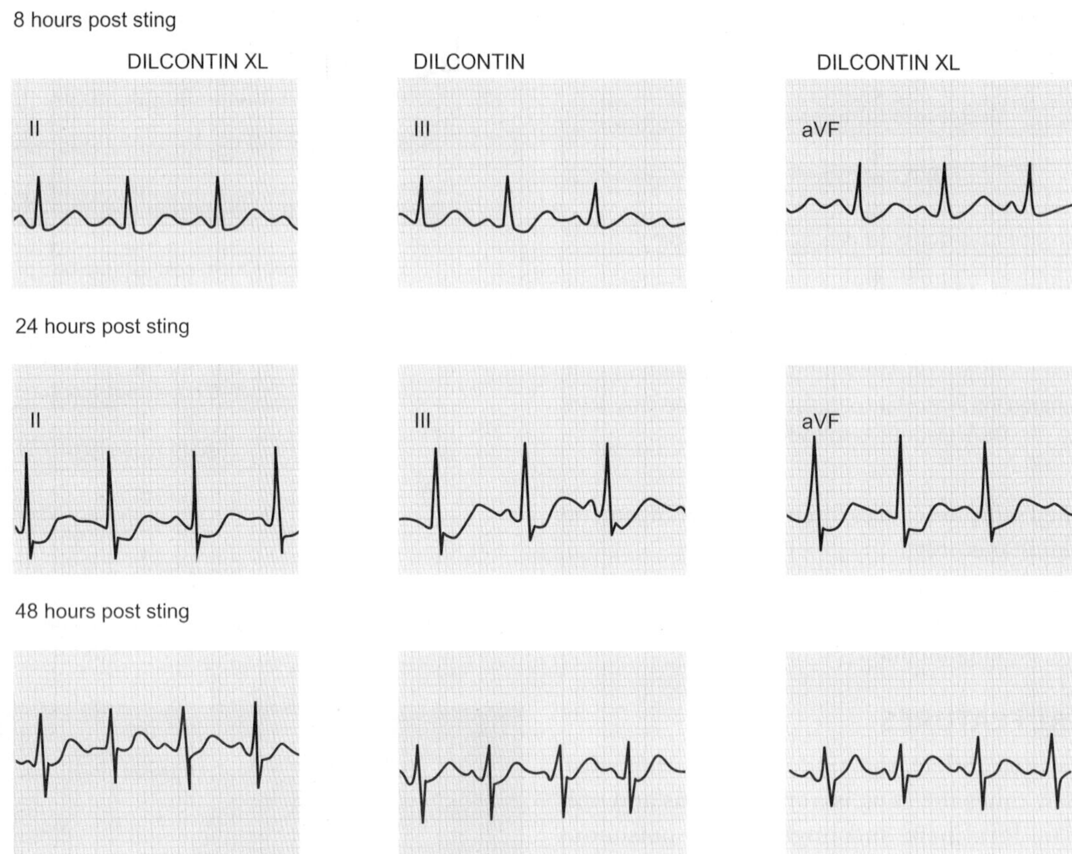

Fig. 3: ECG showing cardiac ischemia.

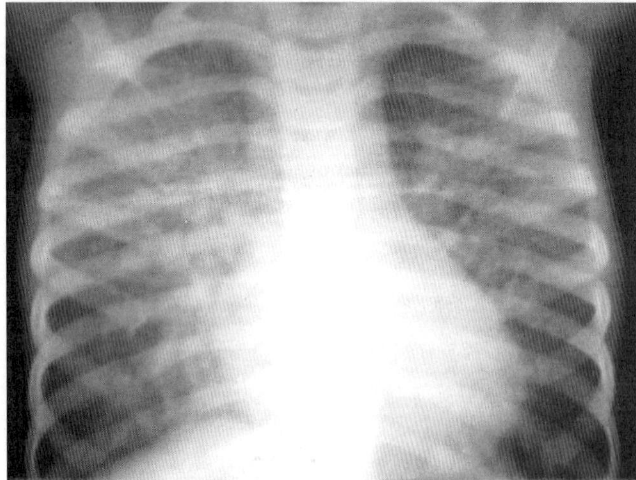

Fig. 4: Pulmonary edema.

the case. In late stage, ECG may show ischemic changes and arrhythmias **(Fig. 3)**. X-ray chest may show signs of pulmonary edema **(Fig. 4)**. Cardiac enzymes may be abnormal, pro-B-type natriuretic peptide (pro-BNP) levels may be raised and can be followed for trends of cardiac function.

TREATMENT

Scorpion sting envenomation is an emergency and treatment depends upon phase of envenomation the patient presents to medical aid. For nonpoisonous sting, usually a pain relief agent, proper hydration and reassurance is sufficient. If any doubt about poisonous venom victim may be observed in the hospital.

In case of poisonous sting, the local treatment has no role. The venom molecule is very small and quickly slips into central circulation, thus there is no role of tourniquet or local suction etc. When patient presents with poisonous envenomation signs, following graph of management can be followed.

Treatment is guided by stage of envenomation:

- *Early parasympathetic stage:* Hydrate well, Prazosin 40 mg/kg stat orally. If patient cannot take orally, give by nasogastric (NG) tube. Monitor patient

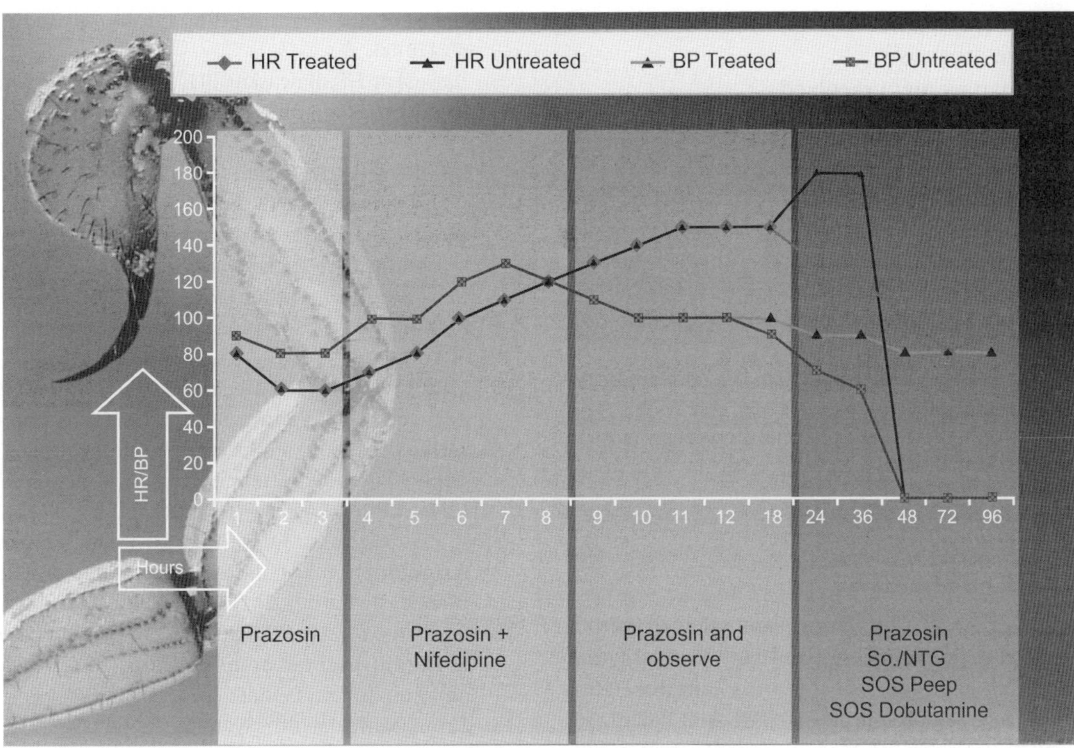

Fig. 5: Pathophysiology-guided management.
(For color version, see Plate 1)

for further progress. Repeat dose of Prazosin after 4–6 hours. Monitor hemodynamics, repeat same dose after next 6 hours. After 24 hours usually no more dose is needed.

- *Patient presents in sympathetic phase:* Prazosin 40 mg/kg stat and subsequent doses as mentioned above. If patient has hypertension congestive cardiac failure (CCF) can be definitely ruled out. In hypertensive patients single dose sublingual Nifedipine can be given at 0.5 mg/kg dose **(Fig. 5)** (maximum 5 mg) and BP is monitored. Repeat dose can be given 4–6 hourly. If there are any signs of CCF, Nifedipine being calcium channel blocker and negative inotropic drug should not be given. Sometimes, it is wise decision to give vasodilators with intense monitoring at this stage to counter the primary pathology directly (the alpha stimulation induced vasoconstriction).
- *If patient comes in cardiac failure:* Prazosin as per protocols with CCF management on ICU protocols is to be done.

Sometimes, patient comes in pulmonary edema with severe vasoconstriction. Here apart from supporting inotropism with adrenaline or dobutamine, small dose of sodium nitroprusside or nitroglycerine can be given under invasive monitoring.

Usually the critical phase lasts for 3–4 days. On recovery, most of the patients have severe bradycardia probably due to adrenaline exhaustion and if patient is hemodynamically stable, no treatment is needed for that. The bradycardia may last for 1 week. In the intensive phase, many metabolic derangements with sugar and electrolytes are observed and they should be managed by ICU protocols.

Recently some trials are showing encouraging results for scorpion antivenom. The antivenom should be derived from local species of poisonous scorpion. It has to be induced in early stages of envenomation. Anti-venom along with prazosin protocol has shown better results.

PROGNOSIS

Following factors determine the prognosis:

- Severity of envenomation
- Post hibernation sting has severe envenomation
- Number of victims in one stage sting. First victim getting maximum dose.

- Stage of presentation—sympathetic stage on presentation, has grave prognosis
- Intensity of management received
- Size of the victim

KEY POINTS

- Scorpion sting envenomation is common rural emergency in India.
- Pathology is autonomic storm...parasympathetic followed by sympathetic.
- Common presentation is cardiocirculatory failure, pulmonary edema and shock.
- Selective alfa blocker Prazosin is pharmacological antidote.
- Antivenom is very effective if used early in course of treatment.

SUGGESTED READING

1. Bawaskar HS, Bawaskar PH. Efficacy and safety of scorpion antivenom plus prazosin compared with prazosin alone for venomous scorpion (mesobuthus tamulus) sting: randomised open label clinical trial. BMJ. 2011;342:c7136.
2. Bawaskar HS, Bawaskar PH. Management of scorpion sting. Heart. 1999;82:253-4.
3. Bawaskar HS, Bawaskar PH. Management of snake bite and scorpion sting. Q Med Rev. 2009;60(4)
4. Bawaskar HS, Bawaskar PH. Management of the cardiovascular manifestations of poisoning by the Indian red scorpion (mesobuthus tamulus). Br Heart J. 1992;68:478-80.
5. Bawaskar HS, Bawaskar PH. Prazosin in the management of cardiovascular manifestations of scorpion sting. Lancet. 1986;1:510-1.
6. Bawaskar HS, Bawaskar PH. Scorpion sting: update. J Assoc Physicians India. 2012;60:46-55.
7. Bawaskar HS. Diagnostic cardiac premonitory signs and symptoms of red scorpion sting. Lancet. 1982;2:552-4.
8. Bawaskar HS. Scorpion sting. TRSTMH. 1984;78(3):414-5.
9. Mahadevan S. Scorpion sting. Indian Pediatr. 2000;27:504-14.
10. Natu VS, Murthy RK, Deodhar KP. Efficacy of species specific anti-scorpion venom serum (ASCVS) against severe, serious scorpion stings (mesobuthus tamulus concanesis pocock)—an experience from rural hospital in western Maharashtra. J Assoc Physicians India. 2006;54:283-7.
11. Prasad R, Misra O, Pandey N, Singh T. Scorpion sting envenomation in children: factors affecting the outcome. Indian J Pediatrics. 2011;5:544-8.
12. Santhanakrishnan BR, Ranganathan G, Ananthasubramanium P. Cardiovascular manifestations of scorpion stings in children. Indian Pediatr. 1977;14:353-6.
13. Tamil Nadu Health Systems Project Health and Family Welfare Department, Chennai. (2008). Handbook on treatment guidelines for snake bite and scorpion sting. [online] Available from https://www.scribd.com/doc/25463309/Hand-Book-on-Treatment-Guidelines-for-Snake-Bite-and-Scorpion-Sting. [Last accessed September, 2024]

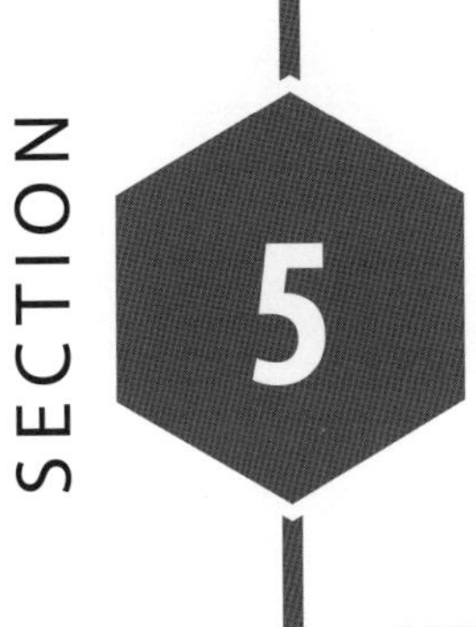

Intensive Care Unit

Section Editor: *Praveen Khilnani*

Recognition and Assessment of Critically Ill Child

Praveen Khilnani

INTRODUCTION

In outpatient practice, pediatric specialist as well as general practitioner comes across common pediatric illnesses frequently. It is important to recognize potentially life-threatening conditions as well as conditions requiring immediate intervention and transfer to a higher-level medical facility.

Besides accidental trauma, poisoning, insect bites, and allergic reactions, common medical problems that bring the child to medical attention are fever, cough, respiratory distress, cyanosis, earache, poor feeding, vomiting, diarrhea, irritability, lethargy, convulsions, and unresponsiveness. Common conditions that require immediate attention are respiratory distress, shock, lethargy, and coma.

Since our main goal as a medical practitioner is to prevent unnecessary mortality and morbidity by prompt and early recognition of potential problems leading to respiratory or cardiorespiratory arrest, it is important to pay attention to the following during history and physical examination done simultaneously.

- Listen carefully to the mother.
- Do not ignore, it will not get better if something is not done.

EVALUATE, IDENTIFY, AND INTERVENE

A carefully performed clinical assessment, including observation, history, and physical examination, will detect serious illness with 90% sensitivity. Each component of the evaluation is effective in identifying serious illness **(Fig. 1 and Flowchart 1)**.

The assessment of a seriously unwell child involves the following:

- Pediatric assessment triangle (initial impression) **(Fig. 2)**

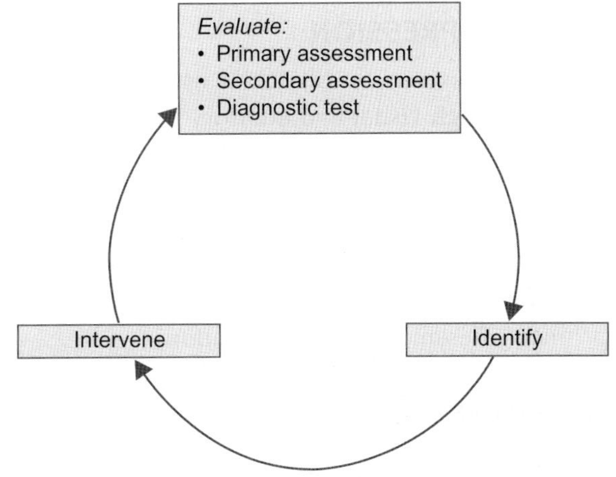

Fig. 1: Action related to pediatric assessment and intervention.

Flowchart 1: Common conditions precipitating cardiac arrest.

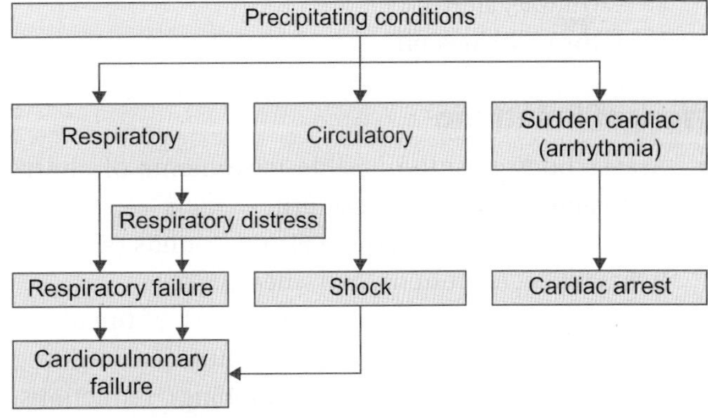

- *Primary assessment:* Airway, breathing, circulation, disability, exposure (ABCDE) assessment
- *Secondary assessment:*
  - Vital signs
  - Focused history
  - Detailed physical examination
- *Diagnostic tests:*
  - Laboratory and radiological

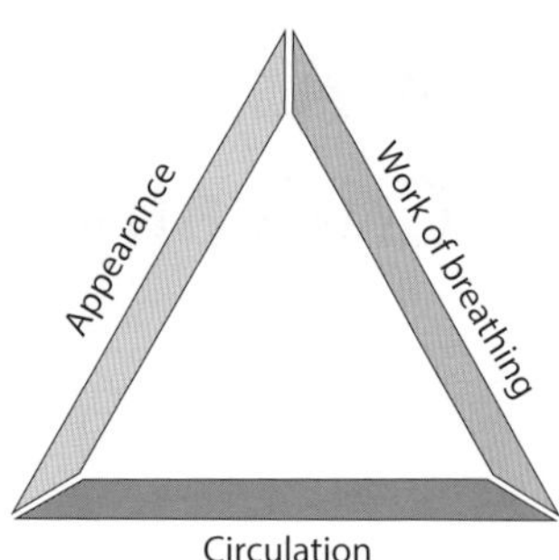

Fig. 2: Pediatric assessment triangle (initial impression).

INITIAL IMPRESSION

It is the rapid assessment of a child with an emergency condition through visual and auditory evaluation of the child's consciousness, work of breathing, and color. It is "from the door" observation to be completed within seconds and no equipment is required. The initial assessment of the child's overall condition is of crucial importance. If the child exhibits abnormal findings, proceed immediately to the primary assessment part of evaluation.

Consciousness

- Reflects the adequacy of ventilation, oxygenation, brain perfusion, body homeostasis, and central nervous system function
- What is the child's state of consciousness: Unresponsive, irritable, alert?
- Does the child look ill?

Work of Breathing

- Assess body position, visible movements of chest/abdomen, and breathing pattern
- Listen for abnormal audible airway sounds (snoring, hoarse speech, grunting, and wheezing)
- Look for visual signs of increased work of breathing such as abnormal position or posture (i.e., sniffing position, tripod position, head bobbing), retractions, nasal flaring, grunting, gasping, and tachypnea
- Reflects the adequacy of airway, oxygenation, and ventilation. Are the airways obstructed? Is the child short of breath?

Coloration of Skin

- Assess skin color
- Look at the skin and mucus membranes for abnormal color (pallor, mottling, and cyanosis)
- Reflects the adequacy of cardiac output and perfusion of vital organs. Is the skin unusually pale, mottled, or cyanotic?

The initial impression will help decide if the child problem is life-threatening or not.

PRIMARY ASSESSMENT

It uses an ABCDE approach. During the evaluation, primary assessment and management occur simultaneously. The primary assessment should be periodically repeated, particularly after major intervention or when a change in the patient's condition is detected (evaluate, identify, and intervene) **(Flowcharts 2 and 3)**.

Airway

The goal is to assess if the airway is patent or if there are signs of obstruction (e.g., stridor, dyspnea, and hoarse voice). If the child is unresponsive and cannot talk, cry, or cough, evaluate for possible airway obstruction. Is the airway noisy (e.g., snoring, stridor, wheeze, grunting, or hoarse speech)? Determine if the airway is patent, and able to be maintained with positioning and suction, or not. If cervical spine injury is suspected, manually stabilize the head and neck in a neutral, inline position (jaw thrust without head tilt maneuver to open the airway).

Look in the mouth for blood, broken teeth, gastric contents, and foreign objects. If solid material is visualized, remove it with a gloved finger covered in gauze under direct vision. If a foreign body is suspected but not visualized, a combination of back blows and chest thrusts is recommended in infants. In an older child back blows in a forward leaning position is recommended. Abdominal thrusts in children are not recommended as their effectiveness and safety have not been established.

Insert an airway adjunct (e.g., oropharyngeal or nasopharyngeal airway, or laryngeal mask airway) as needed to maintain a patent airway. If airway patency cannot be maintained, perform tracheal intubation. Rapid sequence intubation should be considered in all patients, except those in cardiac arrest, to provide optimum conditions and to minimize the potential for aspiration. Cricothyrotomy or emergency tracheostomy can be done as a last resort to maintain airway patency. Not many pediatricians would be familiar with performing these procedures, therefore, in anticipation a consult should be obtained from an airway expert such as anesthesia or an ear, nose, throat consultant.

Flowchart 2: Approach to sick child.

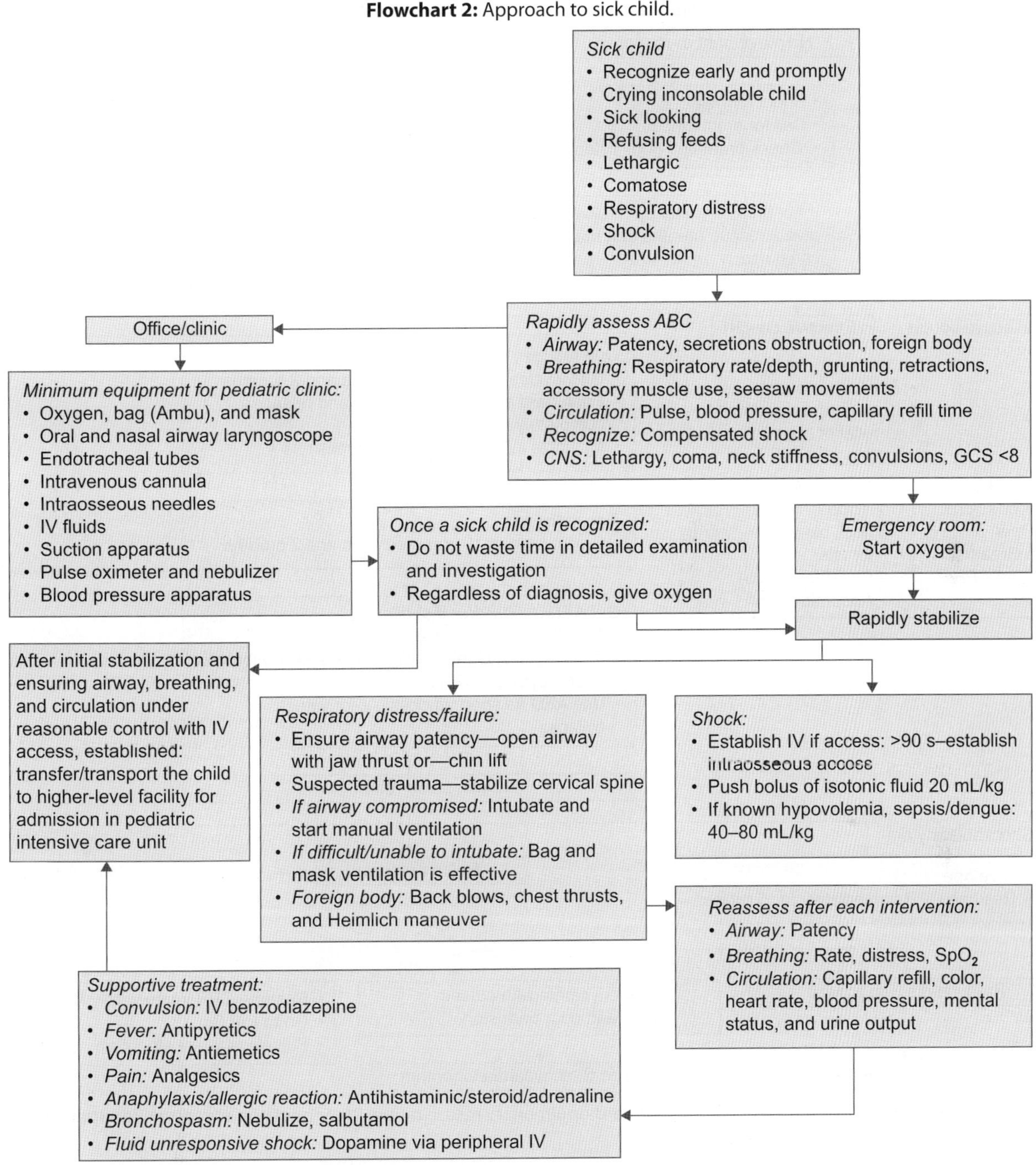

(CNS: central nervous system; GCS: Glasgow coma scale; ET: endotracheal; CPR: cardiopulmonary resuscitation; PICU: pediatric intensive care unit; IV: intravenous)

Breathing

The goal in assessing breathing is to determine whether there is adequate gas exchange.

- Will the child lie flat? Is he in the tripod or "sniffing" position?
- Are accessory muscles being used (head bobbing in infants)? Or is there minimal movement of the chest wall?
- Is there sternal, supraclavicular, substernal, or intercostal recession present?

Flowchart 3: Approach to collapsed child.

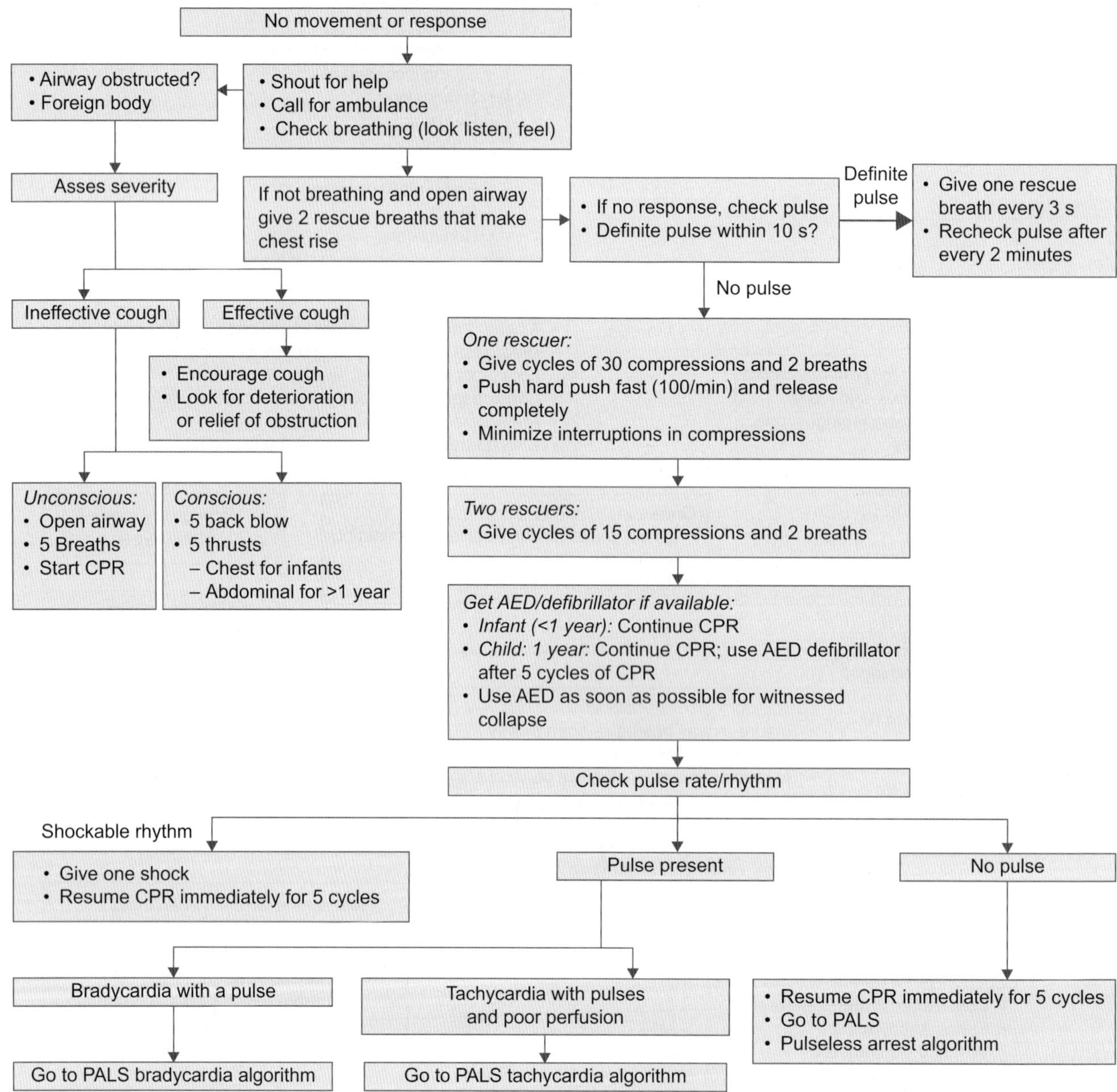

(AED: automated external defibrillator; CPR: cardiopulmonary resuscitation; PALS: pediatric advanced life support)

- Is nasal flaring present?
- Is the respiratory rate fast, slow, or normal?
- Is cyanosis present?
- Is air movement audible on auscultation?
- What is the oxygen saturation (SpO_2)?

Place your cheek near the child's face and mouth and feel/listen for air movement and look at the chest/abdomen for respiratory movement. The child with breathing difficulty often has a respiratory rate outside the normal limits for their age. Normal respiratory rate values according to age are listed in **Table 1**. Initially, the child becomes tachypneic, and as fatigue begins and hypoxia worsens, the child may progress to respiratory failure and bradypnea. On auscultation with a stethoscope over the mid axillary line, try to hear abnormal lung sounds (e.g., wheeze, crackles, and snoring). Palpate the chest for tenderness, instability, and crepitations. **Table 2** shows types and severity of retractions indicating breathing difficulty.

TABLE 1: Normal respiratory rates*.

Age	*Respiratory rates (breaths per minute)*
Infant (<1 year)	30–60
1–3 years	24–40
4–5 years	22–34
6–12 years	18–30
Adolescent (13–18) years	12–16

*>60/min in all ages is abnormal.

TABLE 2: Severity of retractions.

Breathing difficulty	*Location of retraction*	*Description*
Mild-to-moderate	Subcostal	• Abdominal • Retractions below • Rib cage
	Substernal	• Abdominal • Retractions below • The sternum
	Intercostal	• Retractions • Between the ribs
Severe (may include retractions of mild-to-moderate breathings difficulty)	Supraclavicular	Retractions in the neck above the clavicle
	Suprasternal	• Retractions just • Above the sternum
	Sternal	• Inward retraction of sternum towards the anterior spine

Intervention

All children with breathing difficulties should receive high-flow oxygen through a face mask oxygen as soon as the airway has been assessed and demonstrated to be adequate. Pulse oximetry is an excellent tool to use in assessing a child's breathing. A pulse oximetry reading above 94% indicates that oxygenation is probably adequate. A reading below 90% in a child with 100% mask oxygen could be an indication for assisted ventilation.

If the child is breathing adequately but is unresponsive, place the patient in recovery position (lateral recumbent) after assessing ABCD with no other abnormal findings. If breathing is absent or the child is hypoventilating (slow respiratory rate or weak effort), respiration should be supported with oxygen via bag-valve-mask device and an airway adjunct needs to be inserted (e.g., laryngeal mask airway and endotracheal tube).

TABLE 3: Normal heart rates (per minute) by age.

Age	*Awake rates*	*Mean*	*Sleeping rate*
New born to 3 months	85–205	140	80–160
3 months to 2 years	100–190	130	75–160
2 years to 10 years	60–140	80	60–90
>10 years	60–100	75	50–90

Circulation

The goals are to assess adequate cardiovascular function and tissue perfusion, ensure effective circulating volume, and in trauma, control of bleeding. Look for following points:

- Is skin color normal, or is it pale or mottled?
- Is there an increased respiratory rate without increased work of breathing?
- Is it cool peripherally but warm centrally?
- Is the pulse rate fast, slow, or normal?
- Is the pulse volume weak or strong?
- Is the capillary refill time (CRT) normal or prolonged?

It is important to determine the heart rate, pulse quality, skin temperature, CRT, and blood pressure. Normal heart rate varies with age (as noted in **Table 3**); tachycardia can be an early sign of hypoxia or low perfusion, but it can also reflect less serious conditions (e.g., fever, anxiety, and pain). Bradycardia (rate <60/min in children or <100/min in newborns) indicates serious illness and poor myocardial perfusion.

Pulse quality reflects the adequacy of peripheral perfusion. A weak central pulse may indicate decompensated shock, and a peripheral pulse that is difficult to find, weak, or irregular suggests poor peripheral perfusion and may be a sign of shock. Check the femoral pulse in infants and young children, or the carotid pulse in an older child or adolescent. If no pulse is felt, and there are no, or minimal signs of life, commenced cardiopulmonary resuscitation.

Next, evaluate the CRT, skin color, and temperature. Normal CRT is less than 2 seconds. The CRT should be done centrally (e.g., on the chest) to minimize the impact of environmental factors. Blood pressure determination and interpretation can be difficult. Normal blood pressure values in children vary according to age and are difficult to remember. **Table 4** can be very useful in clinical practice. A low blood pressure indicates decompensated shock.

TABLE 4: Normal blood pressure in children by age.

	Systolic blood pressure (mm Hg)		*Diastolic blood pressure (mm Hg)*	
Age	***Female***	***Male***	***Female***	***Male***
Neonates (1st day)	60–74	60–74	31–45	31–44
Neonates (4th day)	76–83	68–84	37–53	35–53
Infant (1 month)	73–91	74–94	36–56	37–55
Infant (3 months)	78–100	81–103	44–63	45–65
Infant (6 months)	82–102	87–105	46–66	48–68
Infant (1 year)	68–104	67–103	22–60	20–58
Child (2 years)	71–105	70–106	27–65	25–63
Child (7 years)	79–113	79–115	39–77	38–78
Adolescent (5 years)	93–127	95–131	47–85	45–85

TABLE 5: Definition of hypotension by age.

Age	*Systolic blood pressure (mm Hg)*
Term neonates (0–28 days)	<60
Infants (1–2 months)	<70
Children (1–10 years)	70 + (age × 2)
Children (>10 years)	<90

An easy formula for determining the lower limit of acceptable blood pressure is: Minimal systolic blood pressure = 70 + (2 × age in years) **(Table 5)**.

Hypertension with hemorrhage: >2–25% acute blood loss.

Blood pressure trends are useful in determining the child's condition and response to treatment.

Disability (Mental Status)

Assess the patient by looking at appearance as part of initial impression and at level of consciousness with the AVPU (Alert, response to Verbal stimuli, response to Pain, Unresponsive) scale **(Table 6)**. The pediatric Glasgow coma scale (GCS) is a second option **(Table 7)**.

Evaluate the brainstem by checking the responses in each pupil to a direct beam of light. A normal pupil will constrict after a light stimulus. Evaluate the motor activity by looking for symmetrical movement of the extremities, seizures, posturing, or flaccidity.

- What is the child's AVPU score?
- Is the child mobile? Or is there limited movement with poor muscle tone?

TABLE 6: AVPU.

A	Alert	• The child is awake, active and appropriately responsive to parents and external stimuli • Appropriate response is assessed in terms of the anticipated response based on the child's age and the setting on situation.
V	Voice	The child responds only when the patient or you call the childs name or speak loudly
P	Painful	The child responds only a painful stimulus, such as pinching the nail bed
U	Unresponsive	The child does not respond to any stimulus

- If the child is crying or speaking, is this strong or weak?
- If crying, can the child be consoled?
- Does the child fix their gaze on the caretaker, or does he/she have a glazed appearance?
- Is the child's behavior normal for their developmental age?
- Is the child having convulsions, is he stiff or floppy?

With knowledge of the child's appearance from the initial appearance and AVPU scale, if the disability assessment demonstrates altered level of consciousness, begin with general life support/monitoring with oxygen, cardiac monitoring, and pulse oximetry. Intubation should be considered if GCS is <8.

Exposure

Proper exposure of the child is necessary for completing the initial physical assessment. The initial impression using pediatric assessment triangle requires removal of part of the child's clothing to allow careful observation. Be careful to avoid rapid heat loss, especially in infants and children in a cold environment.

- Is there fever?
- Is there a nonblanching rash present?

SECONDARY ASSESSMENT

The secondary assessment focuses on advanced life support interventions and management. It is important to perform an additional assessment with a focused history and physical examination in stable patients. Generally, the initial assessment is aimed at detecting immediate

TABLE 7: Glasgow coma scale for adults and modified Glasgow coma scale for infants and children.

Response	*Adults*	*Child*	*Infants*	*Coded value*
Eye opening	Spontaneous	Spontaneous	Spontaneous	4
	To speech	To speech	To speech	3
	To pain	To pain	To pain	2
	None	None	None	1
Best value	Oriented	Oriented	Coos and babies	5
	Confused	Confused	Irritable, cries	4
	Inappropriate words	Inappropriate words	Cries in response to pain	3
	Incomprehensible sound	Incomprehensible words or nonspecific sounds	Moans in response to pain	2
	None	None	None	1
Best motor response†	Obeys	Obeys commands	Moves spontaneously and purposely	6
	Localizes	Localizes painful stimulus	Withdraws in response to pain	5
	Withdraws	Withdraws in response to pain	Withdraws in response to pain	4
	Abnormal flexion	Flexion in response to pain	Decorticate posturing (abnormal flexion)	3
	Extensor response	Extension to response to pain	Decerebrate posturing (abnormal extension with medial rotation in response to pain)	2
	None	None	None	
Total score				*3–15*

†If the patient is intubated, unconscious or preverbal, the most important part of this scale in motor response. Providers should carefully evaluate this component.

life-threatening problems that can compromise basic life functions, as in the primary survey.

The secondary survey is intended to detect less immediate threats to life and has several specific objectives:

- Obtaining a complete history including mechanism of injury or circumstances of the illness. The SAMPLE mnemonic can be helpful:
  - Signs and symptoms
  - Allergies
  - Medications
  - Past medical history
  - Last oral intake
  - Events leading to the injury or illness
- Performing a detailed physical examination

LABORATORY AND RADIOLOGICAL DIAGNOSTIC TESTING

- Establishing a clinical diagnosis: Obtain a quick random blood sugar
- Performing laboratory investigations and imaging

Ongoing Assessment

Always reassess the patient; the purpose is to assess the effectiveness of the emergency interventions provided and identify any missed injuries or conditions. This should be performed in every patient after the detailed physical examination and after ensuring completion of critical interventions.

Categorization by Severity

Respiratory Distress

- Tachypnea
- Tachycardia
- Increased respiratory effort
- Abnormal airway sounds
- Pale cool skin
- Changes in mental status

Respiratory Failure

- *Early*: Marked tachypnea/tachycardia
- *Late*: Bradypnea, apnea/bradycardia

- Increased/decreased/no respiratory effort
- Cyanosis
- Stupor/coma

Shock

Compensated:
- Tachycardia
- Cool pale diaphoretic skin
- Delayed CRT (>2 s)
- Weak peripheral pulses
- Narrow pulse pressure
- Oliguria

Hypotensive:
- All features of compensated shock and blood pressure below the 5th percentile
- Change in mental status.

Initial Stabilization

Things required at all practice locations (hospital or private practice clinic):
- Oxygen source and mask
- Bag valve mask device (Ambu bag)
- Laryngeal mask airway
- Intubating equipment
- Intraosseous needle
- Intravenous cannula, IV fluids
- Suction
- Pulse oximeter
- Nebulizer

Common Initial Interventions

Once the critically ill child is recognized, do not waste time in detailed investigations and diagnosis.

Do the following regardless of diagnosis:
- Start oxygen
- If respiratory distress:
  - Ensure airway open by head tilt, chin lift, jaw thrust
  - If not maintainable, intubate
  - If cannot intubate, ventilate with bag and mask.
  - If cannot intubate or ventilate, then use laryngeal mask airway and call the best expert in airway management.

Foreign Body Obstruction

If known foreign body obstruction:
- Then back blows, chest thrust, and Heimlich maneuver
- Nebulize as required (adrenaline or β2 stimulant). Monitor oxygen saturation if pulse oximeter is available.

Shock

Establish intravenous/intraosseous access.
- Do not waste more than 90 seconds trying for intravenous access or wasting time with attempting to place a central line.
- Intraosseous access can be used in all age groups.
- Push fluid bolus 20 mL/kg up to 60–80 mL/kg of isotonic fluid (normal saline/Ringer's lactate).

After each intervention, reassess airway breathing and circulation (capillary refill, color, heart rate, pulse, blood pressure, mental status, urine output).

OTHER SUPPORTIVE THERAPY

- First dose of antibiotic
- *Anticonvulsants:* If convulsions, use diazepam IV/rectal, lorazepam, or midazolam IV (caution: respiratory depression/arrest)
  - Phenytoin/phenobarbitone intravenously
- Fever control
- Analgesics, if severe pain: nonsteroidal anti-inflammatory agents/narcotics as necessary
- *Antiemetics:* If vomiting
- *Antiallergics:* If allergic reaction/anaphylaxis
- Subcutaneous adrenaline, antihistaminics, and steroids

TRANSPORT

After initial stabilization and ensuring airway, breathing, and circulation under reasonable control with established IV access, transfer/transport to a higher-level facility needs to be arranged.

CLINICAL PEARLS

- Cardiac arrest can be prevented in most children if respiratory distress is assessed and treated.
- Early rapid cardiopulmonary assessment saves life.
- Fluid therapy and antibiotic dose alone can do 80% of the job in a septic child.

KEY POINTS

- Solve immediate problem
- Do not waste time in establishing precise diagnosis
- Recognize critical illness
- Stabilize
- Arrange transfer to a pediatric intensive care unit
- Ensure continued stabilization measures until care is handed over

SUGGESTED READING

1. de Caen AR, Berg MD, Chameides L, Gooden CK, Hickey RW, Scott HF, et al. Part 12: Pediatric Advanced Life Support: 2015 American Heart Association Guidelines Update for Cardiopulmonary Resuscitation and Emergency Cardiovascular Care. Circulation. 2015;132:S526-42.
2. Kleinman ME, de Caen AR, Chameides L, Atkins DL, Berg RA, Berg MD, et al. Pediatric basic and advanced life support: 2010 International Consensus on Cardiopulmonary Resuscitation and Emergency Cardiovascular Care Science with Treatment Recommendations. Pediatrics. 2010;126:e1261-318.

CHAPTER 42

Septic Shock

Vikram Gagneja, Praveen Khilnani

INTRODUCTION

Severe sepsis or septic shock remains a major cause of morbidity and mortality among children, mainly due to acute hemodynamic compromise and associated multiple organ dysfunctions. Emphasis has been on early recognition and early goal-directed therapy of severe sepsis and septic shock by means of aggressive fluid resuscitation (somewhat guarded in malnourished children), use of catecholamines, early antibiotics, and other adjuvant drugs, widely considered of pivotal importance to improve the short- and long-term outcome of these patients. Severe sepsis (septic shock) is defined as sepsis plus sepsis-induced organ dysfunction or tissue hypoperfusion **(Boxes 1 and 2)** as per Surviving Sepsis Campaign 2012. Sepsis-induced hypotension is defined as blood pressure less than two standard deviation below normal for age with no other causes of hypotension. Normal ranges for pediatric age group are given in **Table 1**.

BOX 1: Diagnostic criteria for sepsis.

Infection (documented or suspected), and some of the following:
- *General variables:*
  - Fever (>38.5°C)
  - Hypothermia (core temperature <35°C)
  - Heart rate more than two standard deviation (SD) above the normal value for age
  - Tachypnea
  - Altered mental status
  - Significant edema or positive fluid balance (>20 mL/kg over 24 h)
  - Hyperglycemia (plasma glucose >140 mg/dL or 7.7 mmol/L) in the absence of diabetes
- *Inflammatory variables:*
  - Leukocytosis (WBC count >12,000 μL^{-1})
  - Leukopenia (WBC count <4,000 μL^{-1})
  - Normal WBC count with greater than 10% immature forms
  - Plasma C-reactive protein more than two SD above the normal value
  - Plasma procalcitonin more than two SD above the normal value
- *Hemodynamic variables:*
  - Arterial hypotension less than two SD below normal for age
  - Organ dysfunction variables
  - Arterial hypoxemia (PaO_2/FiO_2 <300)
  - Acute oliguria (urine output <0.5 mL/kg/h for at least 2 h despite adequate fluid resuscitation)
  - Creatinine increase >0.5 mg/dL or 44.2 μmol/L
  - Coagulation abnormalities (international normalized ratio >1.5 or activated partial thromboplastin time >60 s)
  - Ileus (absent bowel sounds)
  - Thrombocytopenia (platelet count <100,000 μL^{-1})
  - Hyperbilirubinemia (plasma total bilirubin >4 mg/dL or 70 μmol/L)
- *Tissue perfusion variables:*
  - Hyperlactatemia (>1 mmol/L)
  - Decreased capillary refill or mottling (normal filling in early warm shock)

MANAGEMENT

Airway, Breathing, and Circulation

Patient should be given 100% oxygen by facemask if airway is maintainable or high flow nasal cannula/nasopharyngeal continuous positive airway pressure (CPAP) if there is increase work of breathing to maintain their functional residual capacity. The decision to intubate and ventilate is based on clinical assessment of increased work of breathing, hypoventilation, or impaired mental status. Waiting for confirmatory laboratory tests is discouraged. However, during intubation and mechanical ventilation, increased intrathoracic pressure and drugs used for sedation can reduce venous return and lead to worsening shock if the patient is not adequately volume-loaded. Mechanical ventilation should be done using lung protective strategies (tidal volume 4–6 mL/kg of ideal body weight, plateau pressure ≤30). Appropriate sedation and analgesia should be provided to a patient on mechanical ventilation.

Getting intravenous access may be difficult early in the course of shock especially in small children, rapid use of intraosseous access should be utilized which can be used to give any type of medication. Time should not be wasted in attaining central line. Rapid fluid boluses of 20 mL/kg (isotonic crystalloid or colloids) can be administered by push or rapid infusion device (pressure bag) while observing for signs of fluid overload (i.e., the development of increased work of breathing, rales, gallop rhythm or hepatomegaly). In the absence of these clinical findings, repeated fluid boluses can be administered. Children commonly require 40–60 mL/kg in the first hour (some children may require 180–200 mL/kg). Each fluid bolus should be followed by quick assessment of clinical parameters like improvement in heart rate as per age **(Table 1)**, capillary refill time (CRT) (normal CRT <2 s), normal pulses with no differential between peripheral and central pulses, normal blood pressure for age, sensorium, and urine output. Thereafter, central venous oxygen saturation ($ScvO_2$) greater than or equal to 70% and cardiac index between 3.3 and 6.0 L/min/m^2 should be targeted, if facilities for such monitoring are available. Fluid responsiveness techniques can be applied wherein fluid administration is continued as long as there is hemodynamic improvement either based on dynamic (e.g., change in pulse pressure, stroke volume variation) or static (e.g., arterial pressure, heart rate) variables. Noninvasive measures, such as echocardiography, may be utilized to assess for adequacy of fluid resuscitation by assessing inferior vena cava collapse.

BOX 2: Severe sepsis

Any of the is following thought to be due to infection:
- Sepsis-induced hypotension
- Lactate above upper limits laboratory normal
- Urine output <0.5 mL/kg/h for more than 2 h despite adequate fluid resuscitation
- Acute lung injury with PaO_2/FiO_2 <250 in the absence of pneumonia as infection source
- Acute lung injury with PaO_2/FiO_2 <200 in the presence of pneumonia as infection source
- Creatinine >2.0 mg/dL (176.8 µmol/L)
- Bilirubin >2 mg/dL (34.2 µmol/L)
- Platelet count <100,000 µL
- Coagulopathy (international normalized ratio >1.5)

TABLE 1: Heart rates and systolic blood pressure and perfusion pressure (MAP-CVP) for age.

Age group	*Heart rate (bpm) (Range 5th–95th percentile)*	*Systolic blood pressure (mm Hg), 5th percentile (Perfusion pressure = MAP-CVP)*
Up to one month	140 (120–180)	<60 (55)
2 months to 1 year	130 (80–180)	<70 (60)
1–5 years	80 (60–140)	<70 + [2× age in years] (65)
6–10 years	80 (60–130)	<70 + [2× age in years] (65)
>10 years	75 (90–100)	<90 (65)

Fifth percentile is the minimum acceptable. MAP (mean arterial pressure) = diastolic pressure + 1/3 pulse pressure (mm Hg)

Fluid Refractory Shock

If despite of 60 mL/kg of fluid, therapeutics endpoints like CRT less than 2 seconds, threshold heart rates, normal pulses with no differential between the quality of the peripheral and central pulses, warm extremities, urine output more than 1 mL/kg/h, normal mental status, and blood pressure more than fifth centile for age are not met, shock is defined as fluid refractory and child should be shifted to pediatric intensive care unit (PICU) for further monitoring. Vasoactive drugs can be started through peripheral or intraosseous line till the central line is established. Shock is further defined into warm or cold shock, catecholamine resistant, and refractory shock as shown in **Table 2**. Further management of septic shock in PICU is guided as per **Flowchart 1**.

TABLE 2: Hemodynamic definitions of shock as per American College of Critical Care Medicine.

Cold or worm shock	Decreased perfusion manifested by altered decreased mental statue, capillary refill >2 s (cold shock) or flash capillary refill (warm shock), diminished (cold shock) or bounding (warm shock) peripheral pulses, mottled cool extremities (cold shock), or decreased urine output <1 mL/kg/h
Fluid-refractory/ dopamine-resistant shock	Shock persists despite ≥60 mL/kg fluid resuscitation (when appropriate) and dopamine infusion to 10 mg/kg/min
Catecholamine-resistant shock	Shock persists use of the direct-acting catecholamines; epinephrine or norepinephrine
Refractory shock	Shock persists despite goal-directed use of inotropic agents, vasopressors, vasodilators, and maintenance of metabolic (glucose and calcium) and hormonal (thyroid, hydrocortisone, insulin) homeostasis

Flowchart 1: Algorithm for time sensitive, goal-directed stepwise management of hemodynamic support in infants and children. Proceed to next step if shock persists. 1) First hour goals—Restore and maintain heart rate thresholds, capillary refill ≤2 seconds, and normal blood pressure in the first hour/emergency department. Support oxygenation and ventilation as appropriate. 2) Subsequent intensive care unit goals—If shock is not reversed, intervene to restore and maintain normal perfusion pressure (mean arterial pressure-central venous pressure) for age, central venous oxygen saturation >70%, and CI >3.3, <6.0 L/min/m^2 in pediatric intensive care unit.

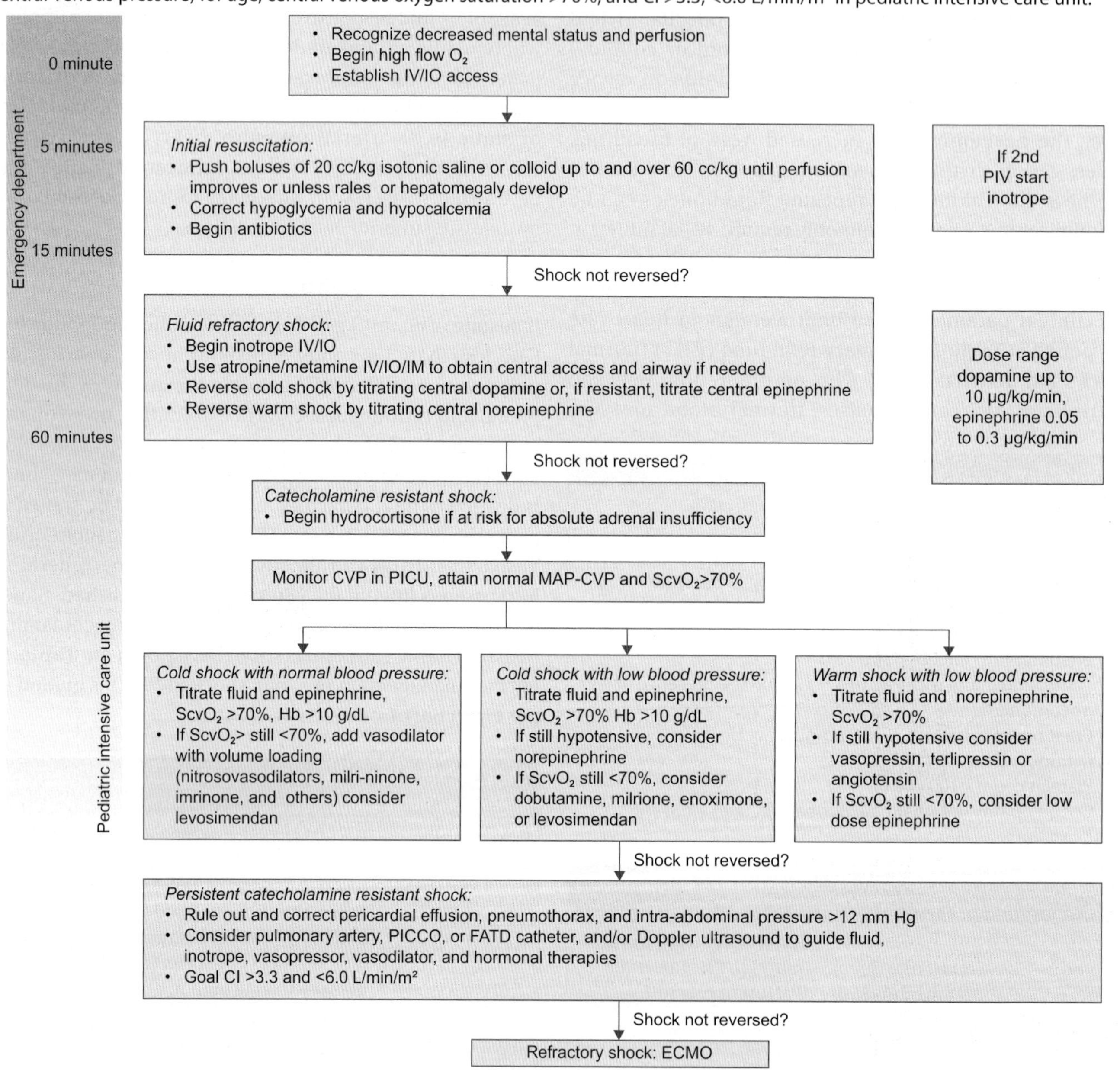

(CI: cardiac index; CVP: central venous pressure; FATD: femoral arterial thermodilution; Hb: hemoglobin; IM: intramuscular; IO: interosseous; IV: intravenous; MAP: mean arterial pressure; PICCO: pulse contour cardiac output; PIV: peripheral intravenous)

Antibiotics and Source Control

Broad-spectrum antibiotics should be administered early preferably within first hour of therapy after taking appropriate cultures but should not delay therapy, as each passing hour increase chances of mortality. Antimicrobials can be given intramuscularly or orally (if tolerated) until intravenous line access is available. Antibiotics should be chosen based on suspected community acquired or hospital-acquired infection, local resistance pattern of organism, site of infection, and whether immune-compromised or immune-competent and past history of chronic illness. The choice of empiric drugs should also take into consideration the ongoing epidemic and endemic (e.g., H1N1, methicillin-resistant *Staphylococcus aureus*, chloroquine-resistant malaria, and penicillin-resistant pneumococci). Clindamycin, to decrease toxin production and intravenous immunoglobulin in refractory toxic shock syndrome may be considered. Any site of localized pus collection or any other source of infection should be taken care of once child is stable enough for procedure. Antibiotics may de-escalated later according to culture sensitivity report.

Steroid Therapy

If a child is at risk of suspected or proven absolute adrenal insufficiency (random cortisol level <18 μg/dL) or adrenal pituitary axis failure (e.g., purpura fulminans, congenital adrenal hyperplasia, prior recent steroid exposure, hypothalamic/pituitary abnormality) and remains in shock despite epinephrine or norepinephrine infusion, then hydrocortisone can be administered. Hydrocortisone may be administered as an intermittent or continuous infusion (preferable in view of decrease incidence of hyperglycemia and hyponatremia) at a dosage of 50 $mg/m^2/24$ h titrated to reversal of shock and tapered once vasopressor support is not required.

Glycemic Control

Hypoglycemia should be prevented by providing appropriate glucose delivery rate to the child. Associations have been reported between hyperglycemia and an increased risk of death and longer length of hospital stay. Two consecutives values of more than or equal to 180 mg/dL should be managed with insulin infusion in addition to glucose to avoid hypoglycemic episodes.

Blood Products and Plasma Therapies

Packed cell transfusion may be given to maintain hemoglobin of 10 gm/dL if child is hemodynamically unstable ($ScvO_2$ <70% during resuscitation) and target of 7–9 g/dL is reasonable after stabilization and recovery from shock and hypoxemia. Fresh-frozen plasma may be used as infusion not as bolus, if international normalized ratio is prolonged and bleeding tendency is present. In patients with severe sepsis, platelets be administered prophylactically when counts are less than or equal to $10{,}000/mm^3$ ($10 \times 10^9/L$) in the absence of apparent bleeding, as well when counts are less than or equal to $20{,}000/mm^3$ ($20 \times 10^9/L$) if the patient has a significant risk of bleeding. Higher platelet counts ($\geq 50{,}000/mm^3$ [$50 \times 10^9/L$]) are advised for active bleeding, surgery or invasive procedures.

Nutrition

Providing early enteral nutrition to maintain gut integrity and to prevent gut translocation of bacteria should be the goal once hemodynamic stability is achieved. Partial or complete total parenteral nutrition can be given, where enteral feeding cannot be established.

Protein C and Activated Protein Concentrate

No benefit of recombinant human activated protein C in patients with septic shock.

Deep Vein Thrombosis and Stress Ulcer Prophylaxis

There is no role of deep vein thrombosis and stress ulcer prophylaxis in prepubertal children with severe sepsis. However, stress ulcer prophylaxis is commonly used in children who are mechanically ventilated and high risk for bleeding with H2-blockers or proton pump inhibitors, although its effect is not known.

Diuretics and Renal Replacement Therapy

Fluid overload in severe sepsis has been associated with increased risk of mortality, so effort to reverse fluid overload with diuretics when shock has resolved and if unsuccessful, then continuous venovenous hemofiltration or intermittent dialysis to prevent greater than 10% of total body weight fluid overload has met with improved survival in severe sepsis.

Extracorporeal Membrane Oxygenation

Extracorporeal membrane oxygenation may be used to support children and neonates with septic shock or sepsis-associated respiratory failure. The survival of septic patients supported with ECMO is 73% for newborns and 39% for older children, and is highest in those receiving venovenous ECMO. Forty-one percent of children with a diagnosis of sepsis requiring ECMO for respiratory failure survive to hospital discharge. Venoarterial ECMO is also useful in children with refractory septic shock, with one center reporting 74% survival to hospital discharge using central cannulation via sternotomy. ECMO has been used successfully in critically ill H1N1 pediatric patients with refractory respiratory failure.

CONCLUSION

Optimum treatment of severe sepsis or septic shock is a dynamic and evolving process. Early diagnosis, allowing rapid therapeutic intervention, is essential in improving the outcome of these patients. Current treatment includes early fluid resuscitation, early appropriate antibiotics, tailored use of inotropes and vasopressors, lung protective strategy for acute respiratory distress syndrome, and use of adjuvant treatments such as low-dose hydrocortisone **(Table 3)**. Early recognition of organ failure and supportive therapy especially renal replacement therapy to prevent further injury helps in reversal of organ dysfunction.

TABLE 3: Summary of pediatric recommendations of surviving sepsis guidelines 2012.

A. Initial resuscitation	• For respiratory distress and hypoxemia, start with face mask oxygen, or if needed and available, high flow nasal cannula oxygen or nasopharyngeal continuous positive airway pressure. For improved circulation, peripheral intravenous access or intraosseous access can be used for fluid resuscitation and inotrope infusion when a central line is not available. If mechanical ventilation is required then cardiovascular instability during intubation is less likely after appropriate cardiovascular resuscitation • Initial therapeutic endpoints of resuscitation of septic shock: capillary refill of ≤2 s, normal blood pressure for age, normal pulses with no differential between peripheral and central pulses, warm extremities, urine output >1 mL/kg/h, and normal mental status. Central venous oxygen saturation ≥70% and cardiac index between 3.3 and 6.0 L/min/m^2 should be targeted thereafter • Follow American College of Critical Care Medicine-Pediatric Life Support guidelines for the management of septic shock • Evaluate for and reverse pneumothorax, pericardial tamponade, or endocrine emergencies in patients with refractory shock
B. Antibiotics and source control	• Empiric antibiotics be administered within 1 hour of the identification of severe sepsis. Blood cultures should be obtained before administering antibiotics when possible but this should not delay administration of antibiotics. The empiric drug choice should be changed as epidemic and endemic ecologies dictate (e.g., H1N1, MRSA, chloroquine resistant malaria, penicillin-resistant pneumococci, recent ICU stay, and neutropenia) • Clindamycin and antitoxin therapies for toxic shock syndromes with refractory hypotension • Early and aggressive source control (grade 1D) • *Clostridium difficile* colitis should be treated with enteral antibiotics if tolerated. Oral vancomycin is preferred for severe disease
C. Fluid resuscitation	In the industrialized world with access to inotropes and mechanical ventilation, initial resuscitation of hypovolemic shock begins with infusion of isotonic crystalloids or albumin with boluses of up to 20 mL/kg crystalloids (or albumin equivalent) over 5–10 minutes, titrated to reversing hypotension, increasing urine output, and attaining normal capillary refill, peripheral pulses, and level of consciousness without inducing hepatomegaly or rales. If hepatomegaly or rales exists then inotropic support should be implemented, not fluid resuscitation. In nonhypotensive children with severe hemolytic anemia (severe malaria or sickle cell crises) blood transfusion is considered superior to crystalloid or albumin bolusing
D. Inotropes/ vasopressors/ vasodilators	• Begin peripheral inotropic support until central venous access can be attained in children who are not responsive to fluid resuscitation • Patients with low cardiac output and elevated systemic vascular resistance states with normal blood pressure be given vasodilator therapies in addition to inotropes
E. Extracorporeal membrane oxygenation (ECMO)	Consider ECMO for refractory pediatric septic shock and respiratory failure
F. Corticosteroids	Timely hydrocortisone therapy in children with fluid refractory, catecholamine resistant shock, and suspected or proven absolute (classic) adrenal insufficiency
G. Protein C and activated protein concentrate	No recommendation as no longer available

Contd...

Contd...

H. Blood products and plasma therapies	• Similar hemoglobin targets in children as in adults. During resuscitation of low superior vena cava oxygen saturation shock (<70%), hemoglobin levels of 10 g/dL are targeted. After stabilization and recovery from shock and hypoxemia, a lower target >7.0 g/dL can be considered reasonable • Platelet transfusion targets as described in text • Use plasma therapies in children to correct sepsis-induced thrombotic purpura disorders, including progressive disseminated intravascular coagulation, secondary thrombotic microangiopathy, and thrombotic thrombocytopenic purpura
I. Mechanical ventilation	Lung-protective strategies during mechanical ventilation
J. Sedation/analgesia/ drug toxicities	• We recommend use of sedation with a sedation goal in critically ill mechanically ventilated patients with sepsis • Monitor drug toxicity labs because drug metabolism is reduced during severe sepsis, putting children at greater risk of adverse drug-related events
K. Glycemic control	Control hyperglycemia using a similar target as in adults ≤180 mg/dL. Glucose infusion should accompany insulin therapy in newborns and children because some hyperglycemic children make no insulin whereas others are insulin resistant
L. Diuretics and renal replacement therapy	Use diuretics to reverse fluid overload when shock has resolved, and if unsuccessful then continuous venovenous hemofiltration or intermittent dialysis to prevent >10% total body weight fluid overload
M. Deep vein thrombosis prophylaxis	No recommendation on the use of deep vein thrombosis prophylaxis in prepubertal children with severe sepsis
N. Stress ulcer prophylaxis	No recommendation on the use of stress ulcer prophylaxis in prepubertal children with severe sepsis
O. Nutrition	Enteral nutrition given to children who can be fed enterally, and parenteral feeding in those who cannot

CLINICAL PEARLS

- Septic patients may have warm shock or cold shock with or without respiratory distress.
- Source control (debridement, drainage) should be considered in all septic patients.
- Isotonic solution such as normal saline or Ringers lactate for all initial fluid therapy.
- First dose of antibiotics to be stored in outpatient department and emergency areas.
- If persistent hypotension despite fluids and inotropes, one should look for mechanical causes, such as tamponade due to raised intra-abdominal pressure, pleural or pericardial effusion, or tension pneumothorax.

KEY POINTS

- Early fluid resuscitation, early appropriate antibiotics, tailored use of inotropes and vasopressors, use of hydrocortisone in catecholamine resistant shock, known adrenal insufficiency (chronic steroid therapy, example nephrotic syndrome, autoimmune disorders).
- Lung protective strategy for acute respiratory distress syndrome should be used.
- Early recognition of fluid overload, organ failure, and supportive therapy, especially renal replacement therapy to minimize fluid overload and further injury helps should be considered in all patients with every sepsis once hemodynamic stability has been achieved.
- Inborn errors of metabolism can mimic sepsis, therefore, anion gap and urine metabolic screen should be considered especially in infants.

SUGGESTED READING

1. Amado VM, Vilela GP, Queiroz A Jr, Amaral AC. Effect of a quality improvement intervention to decrease delays in antibiotic delivery in pediatric febrile neutropenia: A pilot study. J Crit Care. 2011;26:103.e9-12.
2. Aneja RK, Carcillo JA. Differences between adult and pediatric septic shock. Minerva Anestesiol. 2011;77: 986-92.
3. Arikan AA, Zappitelli M, Goldstein SL, Naipaul A, Jefferson LS, Loftis LL. Fluid overload is associated with impaired oxygenation and morbidity in critically ill children. Pediatr Crit Care Med. 2012;13(3):253-8.
4. Branco RG, Garcia PC, Piva JP, Casartelli CH, Seibel V, Tasker RC. Glucose level and risk of mortality in pediatric septic shock. Pediatr Crit Care Med. 2005;6(4): 470-2.
5. Brierley J, Carcillo JA, Choong K, Cornell T, Decaen A, Deymann A, et al. Clinical practice parameters for hemodynamic support of pediatric and neonatal septic shock:

2007 update from the American College of Critical Care Medicine. Crit Care Med. 2009;37:666-88.
6. Dellinger R, Levy M, Rhodes A, Annane D, Gerlach H, Opal SM, et al. Surviving sepsis campaign: international guidelines for management of severe sepsis and septic shock: 2012. Crit Care Med. 2013;41(2):580-637.
7. Foland JA, Fortenberry JD, Warshaw BL, Pettignano R, Merritt RK, Heard ML, et al. Fluid overload before continuous hemofiltration and survival in critically ill children: A retrospective analysis. Crit Care Med. 2004;32:1771-6.
8. Goldstein B, Giroir B, Randolph A; International Consensus Conference on Pediatric Sepsis, International pediatric sepsis consensus conference: Definitions for sepsis and organ dysfunction in pediatrics. Pediatr Crit Care Med. 2005;6:2-8.
9. Khilnani P, Singhi S, Lodha R, Santhanam I, Sachdev A, Chugh K, et al. Pediatric sepsis guidelines: summary for resource-limited countries. Indian J Crit Care Med. 2010; 14(1):41-52.
10. Khilnani P. The pediatric BUS has arrived: Is bedside ultrasound in the pediatric intensive care unit a feasible option? Pediatr Crit Care Med. 2011;12(6)681-3.
11. Pizarro CF, Troster EJ, Damiani D, Carcillo JA. Absolute and relative adrenal insufficiency in children with septic shock. Crit Care Med. 2005;33:855-9.
12. Randolph AG. Management of acute lung injury and acute respiratory distress syndrome in children. Crit Care Med. 2009;37:2448-54.
13. Skinner SC, Iocono JA, Ballard HO, Turner MD, Ward AN, Davenport DL, et al. Improved survival in venovenous vs venoarterial extracorporeal membrane oxygenation for pediatric noncardiac sepsis patients: a study of the Extracorporeal Life Support Organization registry. J Pediatr Surg. 2012;47:63-7.

Status Epilepticus

Soonu Udani

INTRODUCTION

Status epilepticus (SE) is a brain damaging emergency that needs prompt and targeted therapy in a protocolized manner if good outcome is to be expected. Several algorithms may be available, and units must make one most suitable for their setting.

DEFINITIONS AND TIMELINES

Refer **Tables 1 to 3** and **Boxes 1 to 4**.

CLASSIFICATION OF STATUS EPILEPTICUS BASED ON ETIOLOGY

- *Symptomatic:* Acute/remote/progressive:
  - *Acute symptomatic SE (acute symptom of a medical or neurologic disease):*
    - Central nervous system infections (meningitis and encephalitis)
    - Acute hypoxic–ischemic insult (cardiopulmonary resuscitation, drowning, and hypotension)
    - Metabolic disease (hypoglycemia, inborn error of metabolism)
    - Electrolyte imbalances (hyponatremia)
    - Traumatic brain injury
    - Drugs, intoxication, and poisoning
    - Cerebrovascular event (infarcts, bleeds)
  - Remote symptomatic epilepsy/seizures—caused by an insult early in life:
    - Perinatal hypoxic–ischemic injury
    - Trauma
    - Infection
    - Congenital brain malformation
  - *Progressive brain tumors:*
    - Progressive myoclonic epilepsy
    - Syndromic epilepsies
    - Inherited disorders

TABLE 1: Definitions and correlation with timeline.

Epilepsy	*Definition*	*Correlation with timeline*
SE (also called impending SE)	Any seizure lasting longer than 5 minutes, without a return to normal consciousness, or recurrent seizures without a return to normal consciousness between seizures	Stabilization phase 0–5 minutes
Established SE	Seizure(s) that continue(s) following first-line medications (benzodiazepines)	Initial treatment phase 5–30 minutes
RSE	Seizures that do not resolve following benzodiazepines plus one or two anticonvulsants	Second therapy phase 30–60 minutes
SRSE	Drug-resistant status that persists or recurs despite continuous intravenous	Third therapy phase >60 minutes (ill defined)

(RSE: refractory status epilepticus; SE: status epilepticus; SRSE: super-refractory status epilepticus)

- *Unknown or cryptogenic*—no known or identifiable cause

MANAGEMENT OF STATUS EPILEPTICUS

Magnetic resonance imaging and etiology seeking tests (as in encephalopathy) should be performed even with the patient on ventilation.

CLINICAL PEARLS

- Prolonged status injures the brain.
- Accelerated protocol saves 20–30 minutes.
- Treat within the facility's capabilities and transfer early.

TABLE 2: Suggested protocol for management of SE and RSE based on stage and proposed timeline.

Stage	*Management*
Impending SE, 0–5 minutes *AES stabilization stage*	• *No IV access/casualty:* Consider buccal midazolam or rectal diazepam • *Benzodiazepines:* – Lorazepam, 0.1 mg/kg IV (maximum, 5 mg) over 1 minute – Allow 5 minutes to determine whether seizure terminates • *Supportive measures:* All supportive care as needed—metabolic and hemodynamic • *Monitoring:* Begin EEG monitoring
Established SE, 5–10 minutes *AES initial therapy stage*	• *Antiepileptics:* – Repeat benzodiazepine administration – Administer fosphenytoin PE 30 mg/kg IV at 2–3 mg/kg/min (maximum 150 mg/min) – If a patient's age is <2 years, consider pyridoxine 100 mg IV push • *Testing:* – Bedside glucose, CBC, cultures, electrolytes, Ca, Mg, P, and LFT – Toxicology screen if indicated (serum and urine; preserve till further clarity) – AED levels, PT, and PTT • *Urgent neuroimaging:* If treatable cause is suspected. MRI is preferred • *Supportive measures:* – Support airway, respiration, and hemodynamics as needed – Consult neurology service
Initial refractory SE *AES secondary therapy stage*	• *Anticonvulsants:* – If seizure continues 10 minutes after fosphenytoin infusion, repeat 10 mg/kg dose of fosphenytoin – Wait 10 minutes – Administer levetiracetam 60 mg/kg IV at 5 mg/kg/min (maximum, 3 g) – If contraindication to levetiracetam and no specific concern regarding liver/metabolic/mitochondrial disease, then administer valproate 40 mg/kg at 5 mg/kg/min (in 8–10 minutes) • *Consider "accelerated protocol":* Midazolam infusion—directly
Established RSE	• *Anticonvulsants:* If seizure continues 5 minutes after levetiracetam or valproate, administer phenobarbital 20–30 mg/kg IV at 2 mg/kg/min (maximum rate 60 mg/min) • *Admit to PICU and go to "accelerated protocol":* Midazolam infusion—directly • *Supportive measures:* Prepare to secure airway, mechanically ventilate, and obtain central venous access and continuous hemodynamic monitoring through arterial line • *Monitoring:* After clinical seizure terminates, will likely need EEG monitoring to assess for subclinical seizures
Coma induction AES third therapy stage SRSE	• *Coma induction:* – If seizure continues 10 minutes after completion of phenobarbital infusion, then initiate coma with midazolam 0.2 mg/kg bolus (maximum, 10 mg) over 2 minutes, and then initiate infusion at 0.1 mg/kg/hour – If clinical seizures persist 5 minutes after initial midazolam bolus, then administer additional midazolam bolus of 0.2 mg/kg bolus – Continue infusion – Repeat and escalate midazolam • *Supportive measures:* – Intubate, and secure ABP and CVP lines – Prepare inotrope on standby • *Start: Thiopental* – Dose 4–5 mg/kg load and 1–2 mg/kg/h – Increase only on advice of consultants and under EEG for burst suppression according to neurology service • *Consider high-dose phenobarbital therapy and immunotherapy*

Contd...

Contd...

Stage	*Management*
Coma phase	• *Continue pharmacologic coma* for 24 hours after last seizure, with EEG goal of burst suppression • Continue EEG monitoring with at least 8-hourly reviews • Continue initial medications (phenytoin goal level, 20–30 µg/mL; phenobarbital goal level, 40–50 µg/mL) • (Daily) phenobarbital and free phenytoin levels • Continue levetiracetam at 40–80 mg/kg IV, divided every 6 hours (maximum, 3 g) • *Consider high-dose phenobarbitone therapy instead of thiopental* • Ketogenic diet if not already on
Weaning phase If no electrical/clinical seizures for >48 hours	• Reduce midazolam by 0.05 mg/kg/hour every 3 hour, with frequent EEG review • If no clinical or electrographic seizures, then wean until off • Continue EEG for at least 24 hours after end of infusion, to evaluate for recurrent electrographic seizures **(Figs. 1A and B)**
Repeat coma phase	• If clinical or subclinical seizures occur, reinstitute coma with midazolam for 24 hour • Similarly for thiopental • *NB:* Midazolam does not cause burst suppression, the endpoint is loss of seizure activity
Repeat weaning phase	• Reduce midazolam by 0.06 mg/kg/hour every 6 hours • If seizures persist, then manage as guided by neurology consultation for advanced therapies

(ABP: arterial blood pressure; AED: antiepileptic drug; AES: American Epilepsy Society; Ca: calcium; CBC: complete blood count; CVP: central venous pressure; EEG: electroencephalogram; LFT: liver function tests; Mg: magnesium; MRI: magnetic resonance imaging; P: phosphorus; PICU: pediatric intensive care unit; PT: prothrombin time; PTT: partial thromboplastin time; RSE: refractory status epilepticus; SE: status epilepticus; SRSE: super-refractory status epilepticus)

TABLE 3: Drugs used in the management of SE and refractory status epilepticus.

Drugs	*Loading dose*	*Maintenance dose*	*Side effects*
Midazolam	0.2 mg/kg	0.2–1 mg/kg/hour	• Hypotension • Respiratory depression • Tolerance
Propofol	2 mg/kg	1–5 mg/kg/hour	• Hypotension • Respiratory depression • Propofol infusion syndrome (PRIS)—acute refractory bradycardia leading to asystole evidenced by rhabdomyolysis, shock, and metabolic acidosis • Increased risk with ketogenic diet • Monitor lactate, triglycerides (>400 mg/dL), CPK, and potassium • Avoid in Infants
Thiopental	2–4 mg/kg	1–5 mg/kg/hour	• Hypotension • Respiratory depression • Tolerance
High-dose phenobarbital	30 mg/kg	Repeat 10–20 mg/kg/day over 4–5 days. Do not worry about levels	• Hypotension • Respiratory depression • Avoid in NCSE and epilepsia partialis continua
Ketamine	2–3 mg/kg bolus of ketamine every 5 min x	10–60 µg/kg/min for several days	Can be used as second line after MDZ. Increased secretions. High/low BP
Ketogenic diet	ASAP	Advance to 4:1 fast	Blood sugar, acidosis, infection. Will be less effective with steroid use

(CPK: creatinine phosphokinase; NCSE: nonconvulsive status epilepticus)

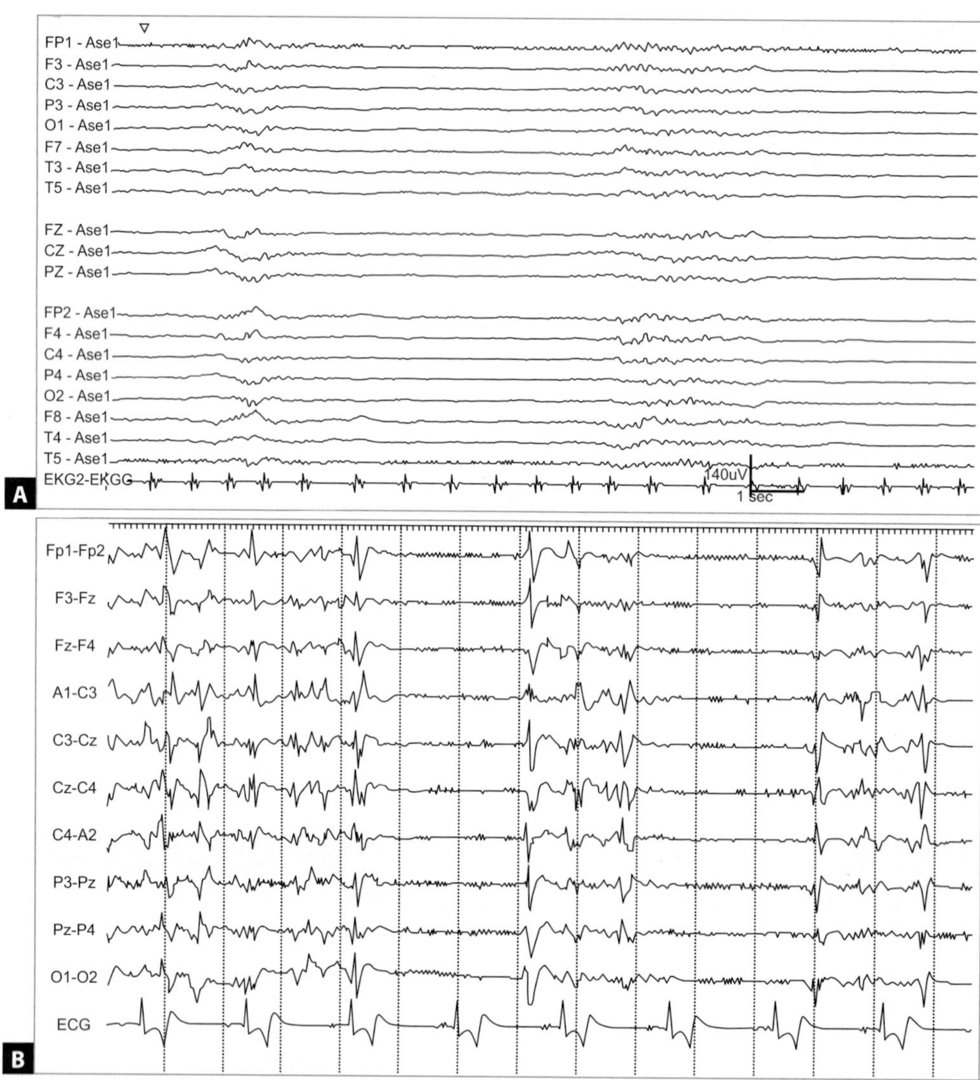

Figs. 1A and B: Continuous EEG monitoring. (A) Oversuppressed with very low amplitude; (B) Adequately suppressed with short suppression.

BOX 1: Initial management.

- Brief physical examination is done to assess respiratory and circulatory status
- Establish an adequate airway immediately if there is respiratory compromise
- Place an intravenous (IV) catheter for sampling of blood and administration of medications
- Supportive therapy (e.g., oxygen, mechanical ventilation) instituted as needed
- Initiate ongoing monitoring of vital signs
- Rapid neurologic examination
- Preliminary classification of the type of status epilepticus (SE)
- History obtained from a witness may help to determine the cause and semiology of the seizures

BOX 2: Laboratory studies.

- Random blood glucose by fingerprick
- Serum electrolytes, calcium, and magnesium levels
- Arterial blood gases
- Complete blood counts
- Urine and blood toxicology (if suspected)
- Serum drug levels (*Subtherapeutic levels are found in almost one-third of children presenting in SE and dosing can be rationalized once the levels are known*) in those already on treatment
- *Other investigations:* Imaging, metabolic screen, etc., as per clinical profile for suspected metabolic, genetic, or structural disorders

BOX 3: Management for positive CSF antibodies in the autoimmune panel or cryptogenic refractory status: Immunotherapy.

1. Consider methylprednisolone (30 mg/kg daily, max 1 g, for 3–5 days); IV immunoglobulin (IVIG, 2 g/kg divided over 2–3 days)
2. If no response, try plasmapheresis, rituximab, or cyclophosphamide
3. Send serum, and CSF, if available, for cytokine assays (specifically IL-1B, IL-6, and neopterin)
4. Consider IL-1 RA anakinra (subcutaneous injection 2–8 mg/kg). Consider other antiepileptic drugs (AEDs) including cannabidiol (CBD oil)
5. This may take up to 4 weeks and after that consider other immunomodulation such as tocilizumab (subcutaneous or intravenous injection 8–12 mg/kg) or canakinumab (subcutaneous injection 2–3 mg/kg)
6. *Day 7–21:* Avoid prolonged burst suppression coma with barbiturates, ketamine, lidocaine, or propofol infusion. Extended trial of anakinra (3–4 weeks) may be necessary before response is seen. Continue immunomodulatory therapy if positive response noted

Note: Anakinra, canakinumab, and cannabidiol are not easily available but can be imported under special license.
Adjunctive therapy like cannabinoids and electroconvulsive therapy is not standardized and cannot be part of a protocol.
(CSF: cerebrospinal fluid; IVIG: intravenous immunoglobulin; RA: rheumatoid arthritis)

BOX 4: PICU care.

- 1:1 nursing care with multimodal monitoring
- Mechanical ventilation
- Inotropes
- Continuous EEG monitoring
- Temperature
- Arterial line for BP monitoring and maintenance
- Central line as many drugs cannot be given for long periods peripherally
- Indwelling urinary catheter for good output monitoring
- Attention to downstream markers of tissue perfusion—lactate, bicarbonate, mixed venous oxygen saturation, etc.
- Dietician for ketogenic diet
- Neurologist to guide therapy

(BP: blood pressure; EEG: electroencephalogram; PICU: pediatric intensive care unit)

KEY POINTS

- Status epilepticus is a common pediatric as well as critical care emergency.
- Attention to the timeline is essential as early cessation of seizure activity is vital.
- Good supportive care goes hand-in-hand with prompt seizure termination.
- Immunotherapy needs to be considered.
- Attention to oxygenation and blood pressure will prevent further brain damage.
- Optimization of doses before adding new drugs should be attempted.
- Every unit must make its own implementable protocol within available guidelines.
- A multidisciplinary approach is needed in refractory status epilepticus (RSE) with high level monitoring.
- There should be no hesitation to transfer if optimal care cannot be delivered.

SUGGESTED READING

1. Alkhachroum A, Der-Nigoghossian CA, Mathews E, Massad N, Letchinger R, Doyle K, et al. Ketamine to treat super-refractory status epilepticus. Neurology. 2020; 95(16):e2286-94.
2. Glausser T, Shinnar S, Gloss D, Alldredge B, Arya R, Bainbridge J, et al. Evidence-based guideline: treatment of convulsive status epilepticus in children and adults: Report of the Guideline Committee of the American Epilepsy Society. Epilepsy Curr. 2016;16(1):48-61.
3. Trinka E, Cock H, Hesdorffer D, Rossetti AO, Scheffer IE, Shinnar S, et al. A definition and classification of status epilepticus—Report of the ILAE Task Force on Classification of Status Epilepticus. Epilepsia. 2015;56(10):1515-23.

Cardiogenic Shock

Nameet Jerath, Praveen Khilnani

INTRODUCTION

Children with congenital heart disease, cardiomyopathy, various arrhythmias, viral myocarditis, postcardiac surgery or severe sepsis can have severe myocardial dysfunction and cardiogenic shock. It is a commonly encountered problem in pediatric age group and early diagnosis and initiation of treatment can prevent mortality and severe morbidity. This chapter covers algorithmic approach to a child with cardiogenic shock with systematic differential diagnosis and broad management of various etiologies leading to cardiogenic shock.

DEFINITION

Shock is a state of imbalance between the metabolic supply and demands of the body. Cardiogenic shock is the subset when the cardiac function is responsible for the failure of cardiovascular system to meet the metabolic demands of the body.

Shock on presentation has similar signs and symptoms, like tachycardia, tachypnea, poor perfusion, and decreased urine output with or without drop in blood pressure (hypotension), and it may be impossible to identify shock to be cardiogenic on presentation.

The initial management of any child who presents with shock, irrespective of the etiology, remains the same. The aim is quick identification of shock status and an early appropriate response to improve outcomes.

Cardiac function can be depressed in patients with any type of shock, even of noncardiac origin. Myocardial dysfunction could be responsible for worsening of shock state as in massive sepsis. We shall restrict ourselves to only the cardiac causes of cardiogenic shock in this chapter **(Flowchart 1)**.

PATHOPHYSIOLOGY

It pays to remember the determinants of substrate delivery to the tissues **(Flowchart 2)**. Cardiac output is dependent on heart rate (HR) and stroke volume, and the stroke volume itself is dependent on preload, contractility, and afterload of the heart.

The oxygen content of blood is dependent on the hemoglobin concentration and its oxygen saturation (SpO_2).

Preload, contractility, afterload, hemoglobin, SpO_2, and to some extent, HR can be optimized with drugs or other interventions and help tilting the metabolic balance back to normal.

As the shock progresses, body's compensatory mechanisms, like increase in systemic vascular resistance (SVR) and HR start to kick in. These compensatory responses can be detrimental and can worsen the cardiogenic shock by increasing afterload and worsening cardiac output. As the critical point is reached, patient can switch from a "warm" state of adequate perfusion to a "cold" state. Patients now show signs of poor cardiac output and are tachycardic, hypotensive, diaphoretic, oliguric, acidotic, and poorly perfused. Extremities are cool and mental status is altered. Hepatomegaly, jugular venous distension, rales, and peripheral edema may be observed.

Diastolic Dysfunction

Diastolic dysfunction is poorly understood and often overlooked. It can be associated with normal systolic ventricular function. Impaired myocardial relaxation during diastole increases left ventricular end diastolic pressure (LVEDP). This is transmitted to the lung and results in pulmonary edema and dyspnea. Elevated LVEDP reduces the perfusion pressure in the coronaries which further hampers cardiac perfusion and function.

Recognition of Cardiogenic Shock

There are often subtle clues to suggest that the shock could be cardiogenic and it is important to identify such patients, as their management plan would differ from the routine management of shock.

Flowchart 1: Cardiogenic shock management according to cause.

High index of suspicion:
- History
- Clinical features
- Newborn in shock
- Radiological features

Initial management:
- *Cautious fluid bolus:* 5–10 mL/kg
- Check rhythm
- Rule out arrhythmias (SVT, atrial fibrillation, ARVD)
- *Normalize*: Glucose, calcium, magnesium
- Arrange for m/m at appropriate place with adequate facilities

Shock persistent →

Consider early ventilation:
- Ventilate to normal pH and CO_2 SpO_2 >95%

Close hemodynamic monitoring:
- Rhythm, HR, BP, SpO_2, RR
- Consider early central venous and invasive arterial lines

Newborn:
- Consider duct dependent lesions
- Start PGE1 infusion @ 0.05–0.1 µg/kg/min, until proven otherwise

- Start dopamine @ 10 µg/kg/min
- Investigations if not done including CXR, Echo

Optimize cardiac function:
- *Preload optimization:* Cautious fluid boluses, CVP-guided
- *Contractility enhancement:* Dopamine, dobutamine, adrenaline
- *Afterload reduction:* Milrinone, dobutamine, ventilation

- Titrate vasoactive drugs based on physiological state (cold/warm shock)
- Avoid pure vasopressors alone (noradrenaline, vasopressin)
- Target therapy based on CVO_2, CVP, BP

Refractory cardiogenic shock:
- *Consider:* Ventricular assist devices or ECMO

(ARVD: arrhythmogenic right ventricular dysplasia; BP: blood pressure; CO_2: carbon dioxide; CVO_2: central venous oxygen saturation; CVP: central venous pressure; CXR: chest X-ray; Echo: echocardiography; ECMO: extracorporeal membrane oxygenation; HR: heart rate; PGE1: prostaglandin E1; RR: respiratory rate; SpO_2: saturation of peripheral oxygen; SVT: supraventricular tachycardia)

Flowchart 2: Pathophysiology of cardiogenic shock.

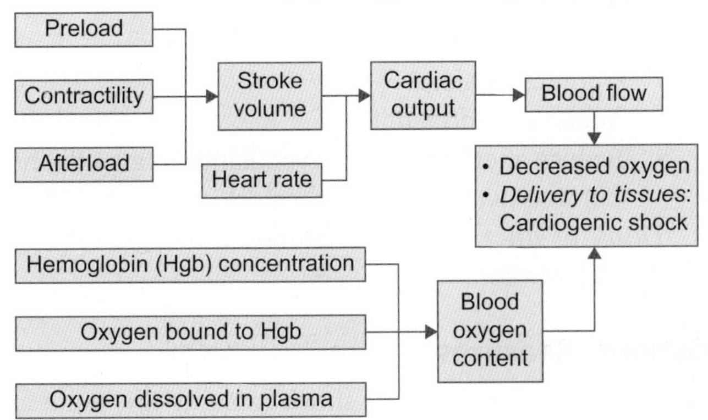

Though there are often overlap of symptoms with other noncardiogenic conditions, the following symptoms should alert one to the possibility of cardiogenic origin of shock:

- Insignificant fevers compared to the distress, illness
- Excessive sweating
- Excessive irritability
- Breathlessness while feeding
- History of fast breathing at all times
- Dramatic, sudden onset of illness
- Any shock state in an infant
- Central cyanosis.

Often clues towards cardiogenic shock can be found on careful monitoring and trend of vitals and response to interventions during resuscitation. The response to a fluid bolus should be improvement of the HR and improvement in blood pressure as the venous return [and central venous pressure (CVP)] improves. Contrary to expectation, if the HR starts rising and/or the blood pressure drops in response to a fluid bolus, one should be alerted and cautiously review the scenario. Excessive and too fast fluid bolus in a child with cardiogenic shock could worsen the hemodynamic state. Such children may still be hypovolemic and require fluid boluses but these should be slower and in smaller aliquots. The importance of assessment and reassessment after each intervention cannot be overemphasized.

Causes of Cardiogenic Shock

- *Arrhythmias:* Supraventricular tachycardia (SVT), arrhythmogenic right ventricular dysplasia
- *Myocarditis/cardiomyopathy:* Hypoxia, infectious, metabolic, toxic, neuromuscular disorders
- Congenital heart diseases
- Postoperative low cardiac output state (LCOS)
- Trauma.

Neonatal period undergoes significant transitions in pulmonary and systemic circulations immediately to a few weeks after birth. Congenital heart diseases with duct dependent circulations can present dramatically with collapse. Any newborn who presents in shock should be suspected to have a duct dependent circulation.

Congenital heart diseases are a significant group of patients who can present in shock. A chest X-ray can help group them into either well, overly or poorly perfused lung fields. Lesions with generous pulmonary blood flows (like large ventricular septal defect) present with tachypnea and respiratory distress and need measures to restrict the pulmonary blood flow.

Investigations

After initial stabilization, laboratory investigations that may be ordered include complete blood count, arterial blood gas, electrolytes including ionized calcium, renal and liver functions, serum lactate, and cardiac enzymes if indicated.

Once a central venous line is in place, measurement of central venous oxygen saturation (CVO_2) is a good marker of cardiac output. Central venous oxygen saturation measured from superior vena cava reflects the adequacy of oxygen delivery, and therefore, cardiac output (Fick's Principle).

Chest Radiography

The chest radiograph should be evaluated for the size of heart and pulmonary vasculature, both of which provide essential information regarding the possible causes of shock.

Electrocardiography

An electrocardiogram can be diagnostic in certain conditions like anomalous origin of left coronary artery from pulmonary artery. The rhythm on the monitor should be carefully assessed. Long-standing SVT, ventricular tachycardia, atrial fibrillation, or atrioventricular block could be the reason of shock.

Echocardiography

This is the most effective way of a comprehensive assessment of cardiac structure and function. It also helps in the calculation of cardiac output and systemic vascular resistance index. A quick, limited assessment should be in the armamentarium of each critical care specialist.

More specialized tests, like cardiac catheterization or magnetic resonance imaging, are sometimes needed for detailed assessment and management of certain conditions.

Management

Principles of management:

- Minimize myocardial oxygen demands
  - Intubation and mechanical ventilation
  - Reduce agitation, anxiety with judicious sedation
  - Blood transfusion
- Improve myocardial function
  - Optimize preload
  - Augment contractility
  - Reduce afterload (think of ventilation as a modality)
  - Correct rhythm disturbances
- *Think of duct dependent states:* Prostaglandin E1 (PGE1) infusion.

General Measures

The initial management of shock remains the same as outlined in the guidelines elsewhere, as many times it is impossible to discern the cause of shock on presentation.

The history, clinical features, and response to resuscitation efforts often have enough clues to primary cardiac involvement. Once cardiogenic shock has been identified, the management should be tailored to the suspected condition.

Fluid boluses should be carefully given in small aliquots of 5–10 mL/kg. Most children will have concomitant dehydration too because of poor oral intake, respiratory losses, and sometimes associated diarrhea and vomiting, and will benefit from fluid boluses. At any stage, if the desired hemodynamic response is not seen, no more fluid boluses should be administered.

Maintain normal sugar levels, temperature, and a calm state by judicious use of sedation to reduce the metabolic demands of the body. The electrolytes including magnesium and calcium should be normalized.

Ventilation should be thought of early in patients with cardiogenic shock. It has the advantages of reducing metabolic demands of the body by reducing the work of breathing, allowing sedation and muscle relaxation, and by reducing afterload. Ventilated patients should be targeted to normal pH and CO_2 with adequate oxygenation.

Monitoring is a vital part of management of cardiogenic shock. Most such children will require invasive arterial pressure monitoring and central venous lines for CVP and for infusion of vasoactive drugs.

CARDIOGENIC SHOCK IN A NEWBORN

The newborn period presents a specific subgroup as this is a period of transition from fetal to extrauterine circulation. Many duct dependent lesions can present with dramatic shock with the closure of the patent ductus arteriosus. All circulatory shocks in newborns should be treated as duct dependent lesion unless proven otherwise and efforts should be targeted to keep the duct patent by PGE1 infusion (0.05–0.1 mg/kg/min).

Preload

Preload assessment and titrating fluid management can be very challenging. The idea is to optimize preload to help the cardiac output by shifting up on the Frank-Starling curve. Judicious small volume fluid boluses are recommended, sometimes as small as 5 mL/kg with subsequent fluid being guided by hemodynamic response. Crystalloids remain the fluid of choice.

In a fluid overloaded child with stable blood pressure, diuretics may be judiciously used later on in the course of the management.

Myocardial Contractility, Inotropic Agents

The choice of vaso-cardioactive drugs will depend on the clinical state and no one prescription fits all.

Dopamine and adrenaline are good inotropic agents and increase the contractile force of the heart pump and increase the SVR. They thus increase the cardiac output and the blood pressure. Both also increase the metabolic demands of the heart.

Dobutamine and milrinone are inodilators that improve the pump function and also cause dilation of systemic vessels [reduced SVR and hence blood pressure (BP)]. The combined effects of improved contractility and reduction in afterload improves cardiac output albeit with some drop in BP. Milrinone and to smaller extent dobutamine has excellent lusitropic effect, which allows for relaxation of heart, improving the diastolic dysfunction.

Noradrenaline and vasopressin are primarily vasoconstrictors and their use alone in a failing heart is not appropriate. They both increase blood pressure but with increased workload (afterload) for the heart. They can help improve coronary perfusion.

Vasoactive Drugs

The clinical effects and recommended doses of few vasoactive drugs are given in **Table 1**.

Diastolic Blood Pressure

The left heart gets its perfusion through coronary arteries during diastole across a pressure gradient (diastolic blood pressure–LVEDP). Maintenance of adequate diastolic blood pressure is, therefore, necessary to maintain the coronary perfusion to fuel the heart.

TABLE 1: Vasoactive drugs.

Drug	*Dose*	*Clinical effect*
Dopamine	5–20 mg/kg/min	↑ contractility, vasoconstricts, ↑ heart rate
Dobutamine	5–20 mg/kg/min	↑ contractility, vasodilates
Adrenaline	0.01–1 mg/kg/min	↑ contractility, vasoconstricts, ↑ heart rate
Noradrenaline	0.01–1 mg/kg/min	Vasoconstricts+++, ↑ contractility, heart rate
Milrinone	0.25–0.75 mg/kg/min	↑ contractility, lusitropic
Vasopressin	0.0001–0.008 U/kg/min	Vasoconstricts +++

Afterload Reduction

Positive end expiratory pressure in a child with adequate venous filling has the effects of reducing afterload making it easier for the heart to pump. This, amongst others, is an important reason to consider early ventilation of such children.

Inodilators (dobutamine, milrinone, amrinone) or pure vasodilators (nitroprusside, nitroglycerine) will reduce afterload and may be used to augment cardiac output. They should be avoided as monotherapy in acute early phase of shock due to the risk of uncontrolled hypotension. They are sometimes used together with an inotrope.

SPECIFIC THERAPY

Intravenous immunoglobulin is often used in patients with myocarditis to modulate the immune response. There is not enough literature support for this practice though.

Postoperative LCOS is the state of low cardiac output after cardiac surgeries because of many factors including tissue edema, cytokine release, cardiac stun, etc. This needs careful monitoring and management on the lines described above. Most carefully managed hearts will start showing improvement in about 48 hours.

Surgical Correction

Some congenital heart diseases may need urgent surgical correction. Cardiac lesions with torrential pulmonary blood flow benefit from pulmonary artery banding procedures.

Extracorporeal Cardiac Support

Cardiogenic shock refractory to the above mentioned therapies can be supported on extracorporeal support systems, like ventricular assist devices (e.g., Berlin Heart, Thoratec) or extracorporeal membrane oxygenation. These are used as temporary measures while awaiting spontaneous recovery or as a bridge to transplant.

CARDIAC TRANSPLANT

Heart transplant is the last option for refractory and terminal heart failure. Organ supply remains the biggest hurdle in our country for this option to be exercised.

CLINICAL PEARLS

- Cardiogenic shock in children can present as respiratory distress.
- Newborns cardiogenic shock due to congenital heart disease present when ductus closes, as a corollary prostaglandin drip to keep ductus open may be life-saving.
- Metabolic/endocrine problems, such as hypoglycemia, hypocalcemia, and hypothyroidism, can present as cardiogenic shock.
- Septic shock is an important cause of cardiogenic shock.

KEY POINTS

- Tachycardia and worsening of blood pressure in response to a fluid bolus in any child with shock should alert to a likely cardiogenic cause.
- Central venous oxygenation is a good surrogate for cardiac output assessment.
- Fluid bolus of 5–10 mL/kg should be cautiously used in children suspected to have cardiogenic shock.
- Echocardiography is invaluable in diagnosis of cardiac lesions/conditions.
- All newborns with shock should be suspected to have a duct-dependent lesion.
- Early ventilation should be considered in cardiogenic shock.

SUGGESTED READING

1. Arikan AA, Citak A. Pediatric shock. Signa Vitae. 2008; 3(1):13-23.
2. Lincoln S Smith, Lynn J Hernan. Shock states. In: Fuhrman BP, Zimmerman JJ (Eds). Pediatric Critical Care. 4th ed. Philadelphia: Elsevier Saunders; 2011. p. 364.
3. Reynolds HR, Hochman JS. Cardiogenic shock: current concepts and improving outcomes. Circulation. 2008; 117(5):686-97.
4. Rossano JW, Price JF, Nelson DP. Treatment of heart failure in infants and children: Medical management. In: Nichols DG (Ed). Rogers' Textbook of Pediatric Intensive Care. Lippincott Williams and Wilkins; 2008. p. 1093.
5. Smith KA, Bigham MT. Cardiogenic shock. The Open Pediatric Medicine Journal. 2013;7(Suppl 1: M5): 19-27.
6. Woods WA, McCulloch MA. Cardiovascular emergencies in the pediatric patient. Emerg Med Clin North Am. 2005; 23(4):1233-49.

Head Injury in Infants and Children

Bhaskar Saikia, Praveen Khilnani

INTRODUCTION

Traumatic brain injury in children is prevalent universally with potentially poor outcomes. Domestic accidents, motor vehicle accidents, recreational injuries, and sports mishaps are the common causes; however, child abuse must be kept in mind in children, especially in toddlers. The reported mortality in developed countries in hospital setting is 9–35%.

The incidence in developing countries is poorly documented, however, mortality is higher in developing countries.

Primary brain injury is the direct result of the physical trauma. It may result in uncomplicated concussion with quick recovery and no residual deficit or in serious hemorrhage, contusion or hematomas. While these are all visible on a computed tomography (CT) scan, diffuse axonal injury can be a severe condition where the initial CT scan may look deceptively benign. Secondary brain injury may occur after the primary event due to potentially preventable causes like hypoxia, hypoperfusion, hypercarbia, and hematoma.

MANAGEMENT

Management of head injury and control of intracranial pressure (ICP) **(Flowchart 1)** or maintenance of cerebral perfusion pressure (CPP) is to be started right from the site of accident to include prevention of hypotension by active control of bleeding and fluid therapy. Immediate stabilization of the airway, breathing, and circulation (ABC) with cervical spine immobilization should be done followed by detailed evaluation of the following:

- Mode of injury
- Time of injury
- Neurological condition of the child
- Seizures may occur immediately or soon after the injury.

Loss of consciousness of more than 5 minutes warrants imaging and evaluation. Recovery from early loss of consciousness with a secondary lapse may be indicative of extradural hematoma.

Vomiting after even trivial head injury is not uncommon in children, but observation for this is usually advisable.

Neurological deficit may be transient after an impact such as a short seizure. If the child presents with coma, deficit cannot be assessed, a previous observation by parents or doctor is noted and needs to be followed closely.

The AVPU (Alert, Responds to Verbal commands, Responds to pain, Unresponsive) scale can provide valuable information.

Glasgow Coma Scale

The Glasgow Coma Scale (GCS) is used to assess the depth of coma after head injury in adults and children above 5 years of age. In those below 5 years, modified GCS should be used **(Table 1)**.

Classification of head injury using GCS:

- *13–15:* Mild
- *9–12:* Moderate
- *3–8:* Severe.

Clinical criteria for discharge from emergency room after 2 hours of observation:

- No loss of consciousness
- No vomiting
- No amnesia
- Normal mental status
- No focal neurological deficit
- No neurological deterioration
- No post-traumatic seizure including impact seizure
- No otorrhea or rhinorrhea or bleeding
- No shock or other organ involvement that would preclude discharge

Flowchart 1: Pediatric head trauma.

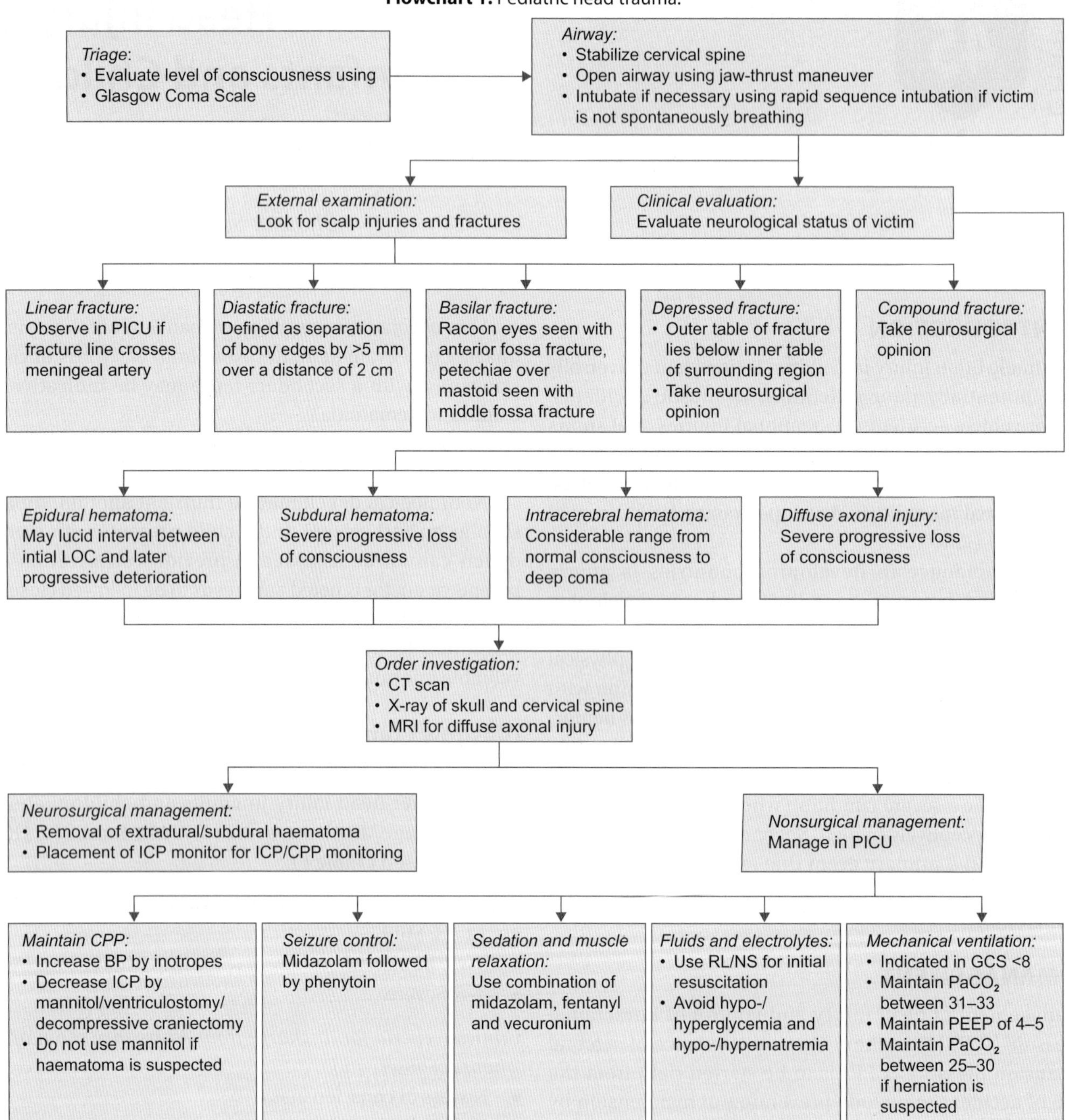

(BP: blood pressure; CPP: cerebral perfusion pressure; CT: computed tomography; GCS: Glasgow Coma Scale; ICP: intracranial pressure; LOC: loss of consciousness; MRI: magnetic resonance imaging; $PaCO_2$: partial pressure of carbon dioxide; PEEP: positive end-expiratory pressure; PICU: pediatric intensive care unit; RL/NS: Ringer's lactate/normal saline)

- No anticoagulant, anti-inflammatory drug, or bleeding diathesis
- No suspicion of child abuse, no matter how trivial the injury
- Radiological criteria for minor head injury
- No intracranial abnormality related to the head injury on CT scan.

TABLE 1: Modified Glasgow Coma Scale in pediatrics.

Eye opening		***Score***
Spontaneous		4
To verbal stimuli		3
To pain		2
None		1
Nonverbal children	***Best verbal response***	
Verbal response		***Score***
Smiles, oriented to sounds, follows objects, interacts	Oriented and converses	5
Consolable when crying and interacts inappropriately	Disoriented and converses	4
Inconsistently consolable and moans; makes vocal sounds	Inappropriate words	3
Inconsolable irritable and restless; cries	Incomprehensible sounds	2
None	None	1
Motor response		***Score***
Obeys commands		6
Localizes pain		5
Flexion withdrawal		4
Abnormal flexion (decorticate rigidity)		3
Extension (decerebrate rigidity)		2
None		1

Skull fractures are acceptable except:

- Those that cross the middle meningeal artery
- Those that cross the dural sinuses
- Those that are depressed more than the thickness of the adjacent skull.

In children fulfilling the above criteria for minor head injury, delayed deterioration is extremely uncommon and can be safely discharged. All other patient should be admitted.

Care Upon Admission

Tracheal intubation is indicated for children with GCS ≤8. Children with multi-trauma, inhalation injury, airway/facial injury, and shock with inaccessible head injury should be intubated, especially if at risk for increased ICP from pain and agitation. The cervical spine must be protected.

Pain, fever, and retention of urine should be treated immediately. Constrictive cervical collar or large-bore internal jugular catheter should be avoided. Supine position with the head end elevated to 30° is preferred for adequate venous drainage. All unnecessary touch, rough handling, moving, and noise should be controlled or kept to minimum. Severe hyperglycemia greater than 180 mg/dL and hypoglycemia should be avoided.

Orotracheal intubation is preferred as it is quicker, requiring less manipulation of the neck, avoids aggravating any anterior basilar skull fracture, or introducing infection into the anterior cranial vault.

All patients should be presumed to be full stomach. The jaw thrust maneuver is used during bag mask ventilation and head tilt and chin lift maneuver should be avoided. Common medications used during intubation include thiopentone and lidocaine. It should be emphasized that even comatose patients must have good sedation and muscle relaxant during intubation to avoid sudden rise in ICP.

Hypotension is common and blood loss should never be attributed to the head injury alone.

A diligent search should be made for the source of bleeding.

Scalp and head trauma can cause hypotension only in children below 2 years of age. Rapid and aggressive treatment is needed to prevent secondary damage from hypoxic-ischemic injury. A low blood pressure at the time of presentation is associated with poor prognosis. Hypotension of neurogenic origin is rare and indicates severe brainstem or cervical spine injury. Hypertension as part of Cushing's triad—hypertension, bradycardia, and hypoventilation—are more common. This indicates raised ICP. Hypertension may mask hypovolemia, therefore, blood pressure measurement alone should not be accepted as a sign of normovolemia. Normal saline is the best choice for initial resuscitation.

Radiological Investigations

There is no real role for skull X-ray in head injury as far as prognostication or severity of injury is concerned. Normal ultrasound cranium in an infant may give false sense of security as it will miss details. Computed tomography scan is very helpful and threshold should be low for ordering a CT in patients with:

- Any focal deficit
- Any history of loss of consciousness >5 minutes
- GCS persistent <13
- Unable to examine the patient because of sedation, paralysis, or intubation for other reasons
- Pupillary inequality
- Cerebrospinal fluid (CSF) leak

- Depressed skull fracture
- Vomiting more than three times.

It is not necessary to repeat a scan after 24–48 hours if there is no clinical deterioration or change in the GCS.

A quick cross table lateral X-ray can help to visualize at least the top three vertebrae. Cervical spine should also be scanned during the CT head to avoid repeated radiation exposure.

Other associated injuries should be ruled out and should be treated simultaneously if required. The following conditions warrant early surgical intervention:

- Acute extra-axial hematomas of 1 cm or more in thickness
- Subdural or epidural hematomas of more than 5 mm in thickness with midline shift
- Hematomas more than 5 mm with midline shift in patients with moderate brain injury with effacement of the basal cisterns
- Depressed skull fractures.

Cerebrospinal fluid rhinorrhea and otorrhea need conservative approach avoiding packing of ears and nose. Almost all cases resolve spontaneously over 7–10 days. Cerebrospinal fluid leaks less likely to heal are:

- Developing after days or weeks
- Postsurgical repair or accidental trauma
- Massive leaks immediately after surgery
- Gunshot injury
- With normal CSF pressure.

Antibiotic prophylaxis remains controversial.

Intracranial Pressure

Intracranial vault is a closed compartment—although with some potential for expansion in the infant, follows the Monro-Kellie doctrine hypothesis. Intracranial pressure should be monitored in facilities are available. Brief increases in ICP for less than 5 minutes are not associated with significant damage. Sustained increases of >20 mm Hg that do not return to base line in 5 minutes probably require attention. Most of the evidences in adults and children set the acceptable high ICP level at 20 mm Hg. In a study by Esparza, an ICP more than 40 mm Hg was associated with a 100% mortality and those between 20–40 mm Hg had a 28% mortality, and with 0–20 mm Hg had 7% mortality or disability. The current recommendation is to keep the ICP less than 20 mm Hg.

Cerebral Perfusion Pressure

This is the critical determinant of cerebral blood flow (CBF) and brain perfusion. It is defined as the difference between mean arterial pressure and the ICP. Studies showing outcomes at various CPP levels confirm that a higher CPP level usually above 60 mm Hg is associated with worse outcome. However, there does not seem to be difference of outcome in 40–60 mm Hg. Guidelines for the acute medical management of severe traumatic brain injury in infants, children, and adolescents (2012) recommended CPP of 40 mm Hg as the threshold for infants and younger children and 50 mm Hg for older children.

Monitoring Devices

Intraventricular catheter, intraparenchymal pressure transducer, and subdural bolt can be used as invasive devices and transcranial Doppler can be used as noninvasive device. Advanced monitoring like jugular venous oxygenation and brain tissue oxygenation are technologies measuring the adequacy of oxygen delivery to the brain directly. Regional oxygenation can be noninvasively measured with near infrared spectroscopy if available.

Steroids have no benefit in head injury as the edema is cytotoxic in nature.

Hypocapnia reduces the CBF by vasoconstriction and hence reduces ICP. However, it will also reduce CBF to the point of reducing CPP and cause ischemia. Hyperventilation for a brief period of <10 minutes may be employed in the setting of a sudden rise in ICP or impending herniation preferably under ICP and CPP monitoring. The goal of therapy is to maintain eucapnia with $PaCO_2$ of 32–35 mm Hg.

Mannitol 0.25–1 g/kg is still the most commonly used agent by reducing the blood viscosity reduces the cerebral vasoconstriction, improves the cerebral blood flow, and prevents stasis. This action is immediate and last about 75 minutes. It takes 15 minutes to 6 hours for osmotic reduction of brain water in an intact blood-brain barrier. It may also get deposited in injured brain cells after prolonged use for less than 48 hours, resulting in rebound edema.

Three to seven percent saline has been successfully used in the treatment of traumatic brain injury. The hyperosmolar state induced is more sustained and the reduction in ICP tends to be more sustained with fewer peaks requiring intermittent measures. The exact dosage is still unclear and bolus doses from 6.5 mL–10 mL/kg have been advocated followed by an infusion of 0.1–2.5 mL/kg/h. Serum sodium levels up to 160 mmol/L have been reported with no side effects. Serum osmolarity rather than sodium level should be monitored for effect, with a target osmolarity of 340–360 mOsm/kg. Gradual tapering of about 10% every 6 hours is required if continuous infusion is used for more than 48–72 hours.

Barbiturates are used for reducing the metabolic activity of the brain, thereby its oxygen consumption. Short-acting barbiturates like thiopentone in a loading dose of 4 mg/kg followed by 2–4 mg/kg/h as an infusion is most commonly used. Significant side effect includes hypotension in 54% requiring fluids and vasopressors, anergy, pneumonia, sepsis, and hyponatremia.

Moderate hypothermia with a core temperature of 32–34°C may be useful but did not improve outcome in children.

A seizure does worsen ICP and the severe head injury patient has a high incidence of early symptomatic seizure; prophylactic medication like fosphenytoin, valproate or levetiracetam should be administered. Seizures may occur even in minor trauma. Immediate seizure may occur on impact or within the first 24 hours. Most seizures appear within the first 3 hours, are short-lived, generalized, and without any CT scan abnormality. They do not predict future epilepsy, require no treatment, and bear a good prognosis. If the seizure is complex, prolonged, or localized, further observation and treatment is warranted.

Decompressive craniectomy may be required for severe head injury and medically refractory intracranial hypertension in conditions like:

- Diffuse cerebral swelling on cranial CT imaging
- Sustain ICP more than 40 mm Hg before surgery
- Glasgow Coma Scale 3 at some point of subsequent to injury
- Secondary clinical deterioration
- Evolving cerebral herniation syndrome.

Delayed lethargy and behavioral changes may be seen after head injury in a child with normal CT scan and normal neurological examination known as post-concussive syndrome.

CLINICAL PEARLS

- Vomiting, migraine, and cortical blindness can occur with concussion with complete recovery in most cases of closed head injury.
- Jaw thrust should be used for cervical spine protection.
- Bleeding or clear fluid (cerebrospinal fluid) from ear or nose indicates fracture base of skull.
- Persistent hypotension in multitrauma patient may not be due to head injury; look for other causes such as long bone fracture, and abdominal bleeding due to visceral injury.

KEY POINTS

- All patients with head injuries with loss of consciousness should be admitted for observation.
- Computed tomography head is the investigation of choice in patients with loss of consciousness or neurological symptoms following head injury.
- Glasgow Coma Scale less than 8 is an indication for intubation.
- Hypotension must be treated by control of bleeding and fluid therapy.

SUGGESTED READING

1. Adelson PD, Bratton S, Carney NA, Chesnut RM, du Coudray HE, Goldstein B, et al. Guidelines for the acute medical management of severe traumatic brain injury in infants, children and adolescents. Pediatr Crit Care Med. 2003;4(Suppl. 3):S72-5.
2. Coles JP, Minhas PS, Fryer TD, Smielewski P, Aigbirihio F, Donovan T, et al. Effect of hyperventilation on cerebral blood flow in traumatic head injury: clinical relevance and monitoring correlates. Crit Care Med. 2002;30(9):1950-9.
3. Hutchinson JS, Ward RE, Lacroix J, Hebert PC, Barnes MA, Bohn DJ, et al. Hypothermia therapy after traumatic brain injury in children. N Engl J Med. 2008;358(23):2447-56.
4. Ichai C, Armando G, Orban JC, Berthier F, Rami L, Samat-Long C, et al. Sodium lactate versus mannitol in the treatment of intracranial hypertensive episodes in severe traumatic brain-injured patients. Intensive Care Med. 2009;35(3):471-9.
5. Jagannathan J, Okonkwo DO, Dumont AS, Ahmed H, Bahari A, Prevedello DM, et al. Outcome following decompressive craniectomy in children with severe traumatic brain injury: a 10-year single-center experience with long-term follow up. J Neurosurg. 2007;106(Suppl. 4):268-75.
6. Kochanek PK, Carney N, Adelson PD, Ashwal S, Bell MJ, Bratton S, et al. Guidelines for the acute medical management of severe traumatic brain injury in infants, children and adolescents—Second edition. Pediatr Crit Care Med. 2012;13(Suppl. 1):S1-82.
7. McHugh GS, Engel DC, Butcher I, Steyerberg EW, Lu J, Mushkudiani N, et al. Prognostic value of secondary insults in traumatic brain injury: results from the IMPACT study. J Neurotrauma. 2007;24(2):287-93.
8. Muizelaar JP, Marmarou A, Ward JD, Kontos HA, Choi SC, Becker DP, et al. Adverse effect of prolonged hyperventilation in patients with severe head injury: a randomized control trial. J Neurosurg. 1991;75(5):731-9.
9. Muizelaar JP, Wei EP, Kontos HA, Becker DP. Mannitol causes compensatory cerebral vasoconstriction and vasodilation in response to blood viscosity changes. J Neurosurg. 1983;59(5):822-8.
10. Wakai A, Roberts I, Schierhout G. Mannitol for acute traumatic brain injury. Cochrane Database Syst Rev. 2007;24(1):CD001049.

Trauma in Children

Soonu Udani

INTRODUCTION

Polytrauma is defined as trauma to more than one area of the body and the term is usually reserved for moderate-to-severe injury requiring multiple interventions, e.g., head ± orthopedics ± abdominal ± plastic surgery and includes burns.

The length should be used for the rapid determination of weight for appropriate drug doses and equipment size.

BE PREPARED!!!

UNIQUE ANATOMY OF PEDIATRIC PATIENTS

- Cranium is larger relatively → more space between brain and bone, hence bridging veins have less support.
- Thinner musculature and padding, thus less protection to organs
- Ribs are more flexible, hence less dissipation of energy and lung contusion can occur.
- Solid organs are comparatively larger than adults, so, less protected by the rib cage.
- Kidney more mobile, hence more commonly injured.
- Larger surface area relative to volume predisposes children to thermal evaporative loss. Result is hypothermia and dehydration.

PRIMARY SURVEY (FLOWCHART 1)

Goals of primary survey are:

- Identify immediate/potential threats to life and initiate treatment.
- Identify the disposition of the patient (e.g., operating room, intensive care unit, and trauma facility).
- Continuous reassessment is essential.

Stabilize and transfer/triage only after the following:

- A—airway
- B—breathing
- C—circulation
- D—disability
- E—exposure

Airway

- Priority → choking will kill faster than anything else.
- Assess for obstruction due to position, injury, blood, teeth, vomitus, and foreign object **(Boxes 1 and 2)**.
  - Level of consciousness
  - Maxillofacial injury
  - Stridor or cyanosis

Hemodynamics → initial fluids: normal saline (NS). Packed cell transfusions if hypotension persists after 2–3 boluses. Attempt to control hemorrhage by bandages.

Breathing Assessment

- Rate
- *Chest wall movement:* Paradoxical breathing; flail segment
- Oxygen status
- Percussion note
- Tracheal deviation
- Crepitus
- Open wounds

Management will be specific to the findings:

- Warm humidified oxygen
- Gastric decompression
- Appropriate mechanical ventilation → avoid barotrauma and volutrauma
- Chest tube(s) if indicated.

Circulation/Hemodynamics

- Blood volume = 70–90 mL/kg
- Systolic blood pressure (SBP) = 70 + 2 (age in years); In years old, will be 70 + 10 = 80 mm Hg
- Diastolic blood pressure = 2/3 SBP

Flowchart 1: Primary survey meant to discover life-threatening conditions and stabilize patient.

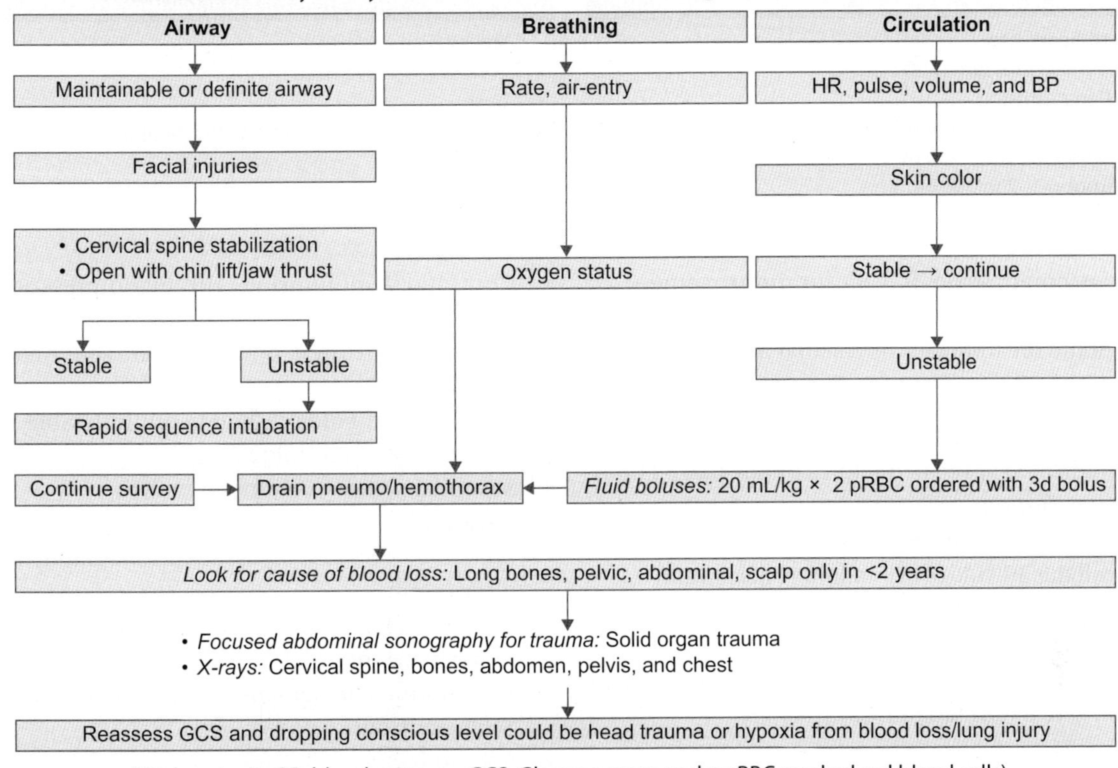

(HR: heart rate; BP: blood pressure; GCS: Glasgow coma scale; pRBC: packed red blood cells)

BOX 1: Structure of the pediatric airway.

- Passive flexion due to large occiput → airway obstruction
- Relatively larger tongue → airway obstruction
- Mass of adenoidal tissues → nasopharyngeal (NP) airways difficult to pass
- U-shaped, floppy epiglottis → may necessitate use of a straight blade
- Anterior and cephalad larynx → visualization more difficult
- Airway narrowest at the cricoid ring → uncuffed tubes up to 6 mm or ~ 8 years
- Narrow tracheal diameter and distance between the rings
- Needle cricothyroidotomy over surgical for a difficult airway
- Short tracheal length (4 cm NB; 8 cm toddler) → RMS intubation and dislodgment
- More narrow large airways → greater airway resistance (R = 1/r4)

BOX 2: Indications for a definitive airway.

- Lack of a patent/protected airway
- Impending loss of the airway
- Comatose patient Glasgow coma scale <9
- Inability to oxygenate
- Inability to ventilate
- Full/impending cardiac arrest
- Head injury

Pediatric vasculature readily constricts and increases systemic vascular resistance to maintain perfusion.

Tachycardia and poor skin perfusion may be the only keys to hypovolemia.

Hypotension in a child = decompensated shock and estimated blood loss ≥45% and may be abruptly followed by bradycardia.

Circulation with Hemorrhage Control

- Heart rate (HR)
- Systolic blood pressure and pulse pressure
- Peripheral pulses
- Skin condition/perfusion/capillary refill
- Sensorium
- Potentially "deadly" bleeding checks.

After initial resuscitation done → reassess, check for the following **(Box 3)**:

- Cervical spine must be stabilized
- Chest has to be reassessed
- Fractures long bones and pelvis
- Abdominal injuries
- Bleeding from the ear and nose

BOX 3: Repeatedly check for optimal response to resuscitation.
- Slowing of heart rate
- Increased pulse pressure (>20 mm Hg)
- Normal skin perfusion
- Improvement in level of consciousness
- Systolic blood pressure >80 mm Hg (age based)
- Urine output = 1–2 mL/kg/hour

BOX 4: Check these areas for potential threats to other organs.
- Maxillofacial and head
- Cervical spine and neck
- Chest
- Abdomen, perineum, rectum, and vagina
- Neurological

- Glasgow coma scale (GCS) for improvement or deterioration

No child should die from lack of vascular access.

Intraosseous access: Anything can be given for this site.
- *Maximal flow rate:* 25 mL/min
- Contraindicated at site of fractures or devitalized limb
- *Fluid resuscitation:*
  - 20 mL/kg warmed NS = first-line therapy
  - Recall the 3:1 rule of crystalloid resuscitation
- Consider packed red blood cells (pRBCs) if:
  - Obvious exsanguination injury
  - Initiating third bolus (10 mL/kg of type specific or O-negative warmed pRBCs)

Disability Assessment

- Alert/verbal/painful/unresponsive (AVPU)/modified GCS
- Pupil size and reactivity
- Extremity movement and tone
- Posturing
- Reflexes

Management: Address findings in keeping with increased intracranial pressure and/or spinal cord injury without radiological abnormality.

Exposure with Environmental Control

- Logroll to examine back
- Look under hair, collar, and splints
- Survey repeatedly

SECONDARY SURVEY

This commences once the injured child is stabilized.

Goals to identify any new/potential threats to life organ and limb are discussed in **Box 4**.
- Identify injuries that may impact the child later (e.g., minor fractures, dislocations, and lacerations).
- Obtain a more complete history.
- Continuous monitoring (HR, blood pressure, T, and $SaO_2 \pm etCO_2$)
- Achieved through a well-organized head-to-toe examination
- Placement of Foley catheter with inflatable retaining device only when child >5 kg
- Secondary survey continued
- Review labs
- *Radiology:* Focused assessment sonography in trauma ultrasound:
  - Chest, pelvis, and lateral C-spine if not done with primary survey
  - Additional images on the basis of threat to life/limb
- Tetanus toxoid
- Antibiotics
- Analgesia (systemic and local)
- Continuous reassessment; tracking of vitals and urine output

Head Trauma

- Leading cause of death
- Results in significant morbidity
- Hypotension and hypoxia from concurrent injury adversely affect the outcome from intracerebral injury.

Spinal Cord Injury without Radiological Abnormality

- If spinal cord injury is suspected on the basis of mechanism or clinical examination, do not be dissuaded by normal X-rays.
- A normal X-ray and initial examination are not enough
- Be aware of local pain and torticollis.

Management:
- Avoid secondary and iatrogenic injury.
- Corticosteroids are currently not recommended.

Chest and Abdomen

Pliable chest wall so lung contusions may occur without obvious external injury.

Clinical examination improved with gastric and bladder decompression. Clinical findings may underestimate problems. Therefore, diagnostic adjuncts:

- *Computed tomography:* Less sensitive for bowel, spleen, early pancreas, and liver
- *Ultrasound:* Good for hepatic and splenic injury.

Visceral injuries specific to the pediatric population:

- Pancreatic injury
- Small bowel perforation (ligament of Treitz)
- Mesenteric and small bowel avulsion
- Duodenal hematoma
- Spleen, liver, and kidney disruption
- Bladder injury

Missed abdominal trauma is the leading cause of preventable morbidity and mortality.

Clinical findings associated with intra-abdominal injury:

- Initial hematocrit (Hct) <30%
- Abdominal tenderness
- Femur fracture
- Aspartate transaminase (AST) >200 U/L and/or alanine transaminase (ALT) >125 U/L
- Urine with >5 RBCs/hpf

INDICATIONS FOR SURGERY

- Hemodynamic instability despite maximal resuscitative measures ± a positive diagnostic study
- Falling Hct
- Transfusion of >50% of total blood volume
- Radiographic evidence of pneumoperitoneum, intraperitoneal bladder rupture, grade V renovascular injury
- Peritonitis or the development to peritoneal signs
- Evisceration of intraperitoneal contents
- Evidence of fecal or bowel contamination on diagnostic peritoneal lavage.

Nonoperative approach mandates pediatric intensive care unit accessibility.

CLINICAL PEARLS

- Cervical spine should be always taken care of in a child with polytrauma.
- Patients with persistent shock despite initial resuscitation may have neurogenic shock, cardiac contusion, or cardiac tamponade.
- Multidisciplinary approach with one team leader.

KEY POINTS

- Trauma is leading cause of morbidity and mortality in developed world.
- Blunt trauma is most common mechanism of injury in children.
- ABCDE sequence of initial assessment should be followed in every child with multiple trauma.
- Continuous monitoring following initial resuscitation is mandatory to detect further deterioration.
- *Fatal:* Pediatric Trauma score <0, transport to nearest facility.

SUGGESTED READING

1. ATLS Subcommittee; American College of Surgeons' Committee on Trauma; The International ATLS Working Group. Advanced Trauma Life Support (ATLS®); The 9th edn. J Trauma Acute Care Surg. 2013;74(5):1363-6.
2. Nichols DG. Roger's Textbook of Pediatric Intensive Care, 4th edn. Philadelphia: Lippincott Williams & Wilkins; 2008.

Poisoning in Children

Pradeep K Sharma, Praveen Khilnani

INTRODUCTION

Various Indian studies report kerosene (30–50%), drugs (11%), pesticides (11%), snakebites (10–20%), corrosives, and household cleaning products as the common substance causing poisonings. Certain household items often ingested by children are proven to be nontoxic and harmless **(Box 1)**. However, ingestion of excessive amount of these substances may lead to toxicity.

EVALUATION OF CHILDREN WITH SUSPECTED TOXIN INGESTION

The acute management generally begins in the emergency department with triage and the determination of appropriate decontamination and treatment regimens. Immediate attention to the patient's airway, breathing, and circulation (ABC) should be done and following the establishment of lifesaving supportive care, a detailed evaluation can be performed **(Flowchart 1)**.

HISTORY

A comprehensive history may be obtained from witnesses, family members, and friends. Nature of substance ingested, its amount, time of ingestion, circumstances preceding, smells or unusual items, occupation of those in home, and queries regarding the presence of a suicide note is pivotal to management. Obtaining an accurate history in adolescent is especially challenging due to the potential use of multiple substances, possible drug abuse, prolonged time between ingestion and presentation, and attempts at concealing information. Additional information includes the maximum amount of toxin available and the minimum amount per kilogram that produces symptoms. Quantity of liquid toxins swallowed can be estimated as 5–10 mL in a young child and 10–15 mL in an adolescent. Product containers or medication labels are helpful to identify specific toxic contents. A number of medications have been determined to be potentially lethal to a child who weighs 10 kg and ingests just one tablet, capsule, or teaspoonful **(Table 1)**.

BOX 1: Nontoxic substances.

- Silica gel
- Ball pen inks
- Candle
- Modeling clay
- Crayons
- Lipstick
- Shampoo
- Chalk
- Pencil lead
- Shaving cream and lotions
- Soaps and detergents
- Bath oils
- Thermometer mercury
- Saccharin
- Water colors
- Petroleum jelly
- Toothpaste

PHYSICAL EXAMINATION

A comprehensive physical examination is crucial in determining the involved agents and allows for specific initial treatment. The signs and symptoms that suggest specific classes of poisoning are generally grouped into syndromes and referred to as toxidromes **(Table 2)**. A vitals recording also helps in determining the particular toxidrome **(Table 3)**.

SYSTEMIC EXAMINATION

Frequent neurologic examination is especially important, as many toxins can depress the consciousness. Symmetrical pupillary changes are typical of toxic exposures, with asymmetry most commonly evidencing a structural or focal neurologic abnormality. Detailed general physical and systemic examinations help in pointing to a specific toxin as shown in **Table 4**.

LABORATORY EVALUATION

The laboratory generally confirms a diagnosis and also based upon quantitative drug or toxin levels helps in deciding about therapy. The drug or toxin levels are available for acetaminophen, ethanol, methanol, ethylene

Flowchart 1: Approach to a child with poisoning.

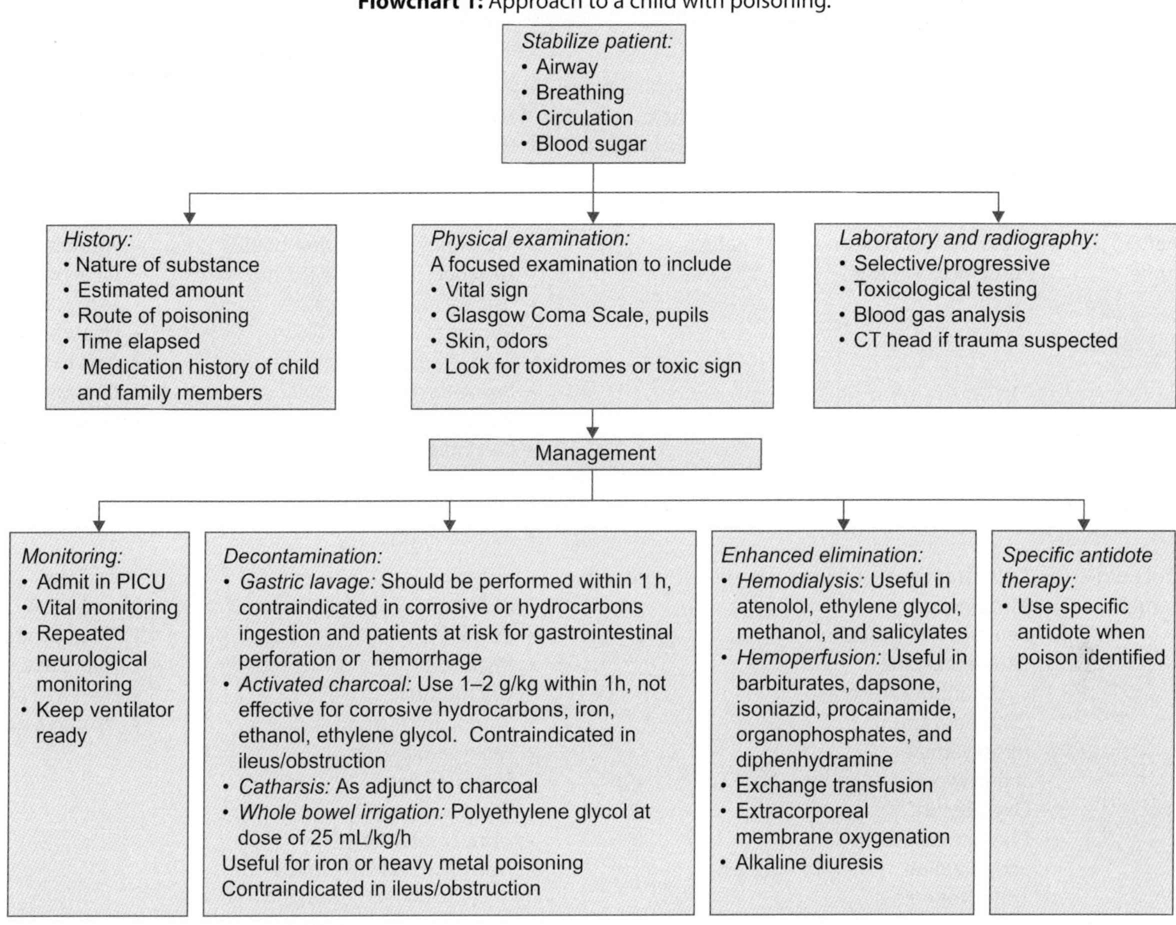

TABLE 1: Toxicity levels of selected medication and medication classes.

Agents	*Minimum lethal dose*	*Potential maximum available*	*Dose potentially fatal units in a 10 kg child*
Antimalarial			
• Chloroquine	20 mg/kg	500 mg	1
• Hydroxychloroquine	20 mg/kg	200 mg	1
Camphor	100 mg/kg	200 mg/mL	5 mL
Imidazolines			
• Clonidine	0.01 mg/kg	0.3 mg, 7.5 mg/patch	1
• Tetrahydrozoline	2.5–5 mL	0.1%	2.5–5 mL
Methyl salicylates	150–200 mg/kg	1400 mg/mL	1.1–1.4 mL
Sulfonylureas			
• Glipizide	0.1 mg/kg	5 mg	1
• Glyburide	0.1 mg/kg	10 mg	1

glycol, lithium, salicylates, iron, lead, mercury, arsenic, phenobarbital, carbon monoxide, methemoglobin, and theophylline. A negative toxicology screen by no means excludes the possibility of toxic exposure.

Arterial blood gas analysis evaluates acid-base status and anion gap metabolic acidosis. Agents with elevated anion gap can be summarized by the mnemonic MUDPILES as given below.

TABLE 2: Toxidromes and agents.

Toxidrome	*Agents*	*Clinical manifestations*	
Sympathomimetic toxidrome*	Albuterol; amphetamines; caffeine; catecholamines; cocaine; ephedrine; ketamine; lysergic acid diethylamide; methamphetamine; phencyclidine; phenylephrine; phenylpropanolamine; pseudoephedrine; terbutaline; theophylline	• Agitation; seizures; mydriasis; tachycardia • Hypertension • Diaphoresis	• Pallor • Cool skin • Fever
Cholinergic toxidrome	• Organophosphate and carbamates • Pesticides, nicotine	• Muscarinic effects (dumbbells) • Diarrhea • Urinary incontinence • Miosis • Bradycardia • Bronchorrhea • Emesis • Lacrimation • Salivation • Nicotinic effects • Fasciculations	• Weakness • Paralysis • Tachycardia • Hypertension • Agitation • Central effects • Lethargy • Coma • Agitation • Seizures
Anticholinergic toxidrome*	• Antihistamines—diphenhydramine, hydroxyzine • Atropine • Benztropine mesylate • Carbamazepine • Cyclic antidepressants • Cyclobenzaprine • Hyoscyamine • Jimsonweed • Oxybutynin • Phenothiazines • Scopolamine • Trihexyphenidyl	• Agitation • Delirium • Coma • Mydriasis • Dry mouth • Warm, dry, flushed skin • Tachycardia • Hypertension • Fever • Urinary retention • Decreased bowel sounds	Associated expressions • "Mad as a hatter" • "Blind as a bat" • "Red as a beet" • "Hot as a hare"
Opioid toxidrome	Morphine, methadone, dextromethorphan, fentanyl, pentazocine, heroin, codeine	Central nervous system depression, respiratory depression, coma, miosis, hypothermia, bradycardia, constipation	

*Both have almost similar clinical features except diaphoresis, cool skin, and hyperactive bowel sounds in sympathomimetic toxidrome and warm, dry skin and diminished bowel sounds in anticholinergic toxidrome.

TABLE 3: Common clinical findings in toxidrome.

Physical findings	*Sympathomimetic*	*Anticholinergic*	*Cholinergic*	*Opioid*	*Sedative-hypnotic*
Pulse rate	Increased	Increased	Decreased	Decreased	Decreased
Respiratory rate	Increased	No change	No change	Normal/decreased	Normal/decreased
Body temperature	Increased	Increased	No change	Normal/decreased	Normal/decreased
Blood pressure	Increased	No change/increased	No change	Normal/decreased	Normal/decreased
Mental state	Agitated	Agitation/delirium	Depressed	Depressed	Depressed
Pupils	Mydriasis	Mydriasis	Miosis	Miosis	Normal
Mucous membranes	Wet	Dry	Wet	Normal	Normal
Skin	Diaphoretic	Dry	Diaphoretic	Normal	Normal

MUDPILES: Methanol, uremia, diabetic ketoacidosis, paraldehyde and phenformin, isoniazid and iron, lactic acidosis, ethanol and ethylene glycol, salicylates.

Electrocardiogram is invaluable in detecting dysrhythmias and conduction abnormalities. Increased serum osmolality is seen with methanol, ethanol, ethylene glycol,

TABLE 4: Clinical manifestations of poisoning.

Clinical manifestations	***Suspected toxins***
Skin	
Cyanosis unresponsive to oxygen	Nitrates, nitrites, phenacetin, benzocaine
Red flush	Carbon monoxide, cyanide, boric acid, anticholinergics
Sweating	Amphetamines, LSD, organophosphates, cocaine, barbiturates
Dry	Anticholinergics
Bullae	Barbiturates, carbon monoxide
Jaundice	Acetaminophen, mushrooms, carbon
Purpura	Aspirin, warfarin, snakebite
Temperature	
Hypothermia	Sedative hypnotics, ethanol, carbon monoxide, phenothiazines, TCAs, clonidine
Hyperthermia	Anticholinergics, salicylates, phenothiazines, TCAs, cocaine, amphetamines, theophylline
Blood pressure	
Hypertension	Sympathomimetics (especially phenylpropanolamine in over-the-counter cold remedies), organophosphates, amphetamines, PCP
Hypotension	Narcotics, sedative hypnotics, TCAs, phenothiazines, clonidine, β-blockers, calcium channel blockers
Pulse rate	
Bradycardia	Digitalis, sedative hypnotics, β-blockers, ethchlorvynol, calcium channel blockers
Tachycardia	Anticholinergics, sympathomimetics, amphetamines, alcohol, aspirin, theophylline, cocaine, TCAs
Arrhythmia	Anticholinergics, TCAs, organophosphates, phenothiazines, digoxin, β-blockers, carbon monoxide, cyanide, theophylline
Mucous membranes	
Dry	Anticholinergics
Salivation	Organophosphates, carbamates
Oral lesions	Corrosives, paraquat, lacrimation
Lacrimation	Caustics, organophosphates, irritant gases
Respiration	
Depressed	Alcohol, narcotics, barbiturates, sedative/hypnotics

Contd...

Contd...

Clinical manifestations	***Suspected toxins***
Tachypnea	Salicylates, amphetamines, carbon monoxide
Kussmaul	Methanol, ethylene glycol, salicylates
Pneumonia	Hydrocarbons
Pulmonary edema	Aspiration, salicylates, narcotics, sympathomimetics
Central nervous system	
Seizures	TCAs, cocaine, phenothiazines, amphetamines, camphor, lead, salicylates, isoniazid, organophosphates, antihistamines, propoxyphene, strychnine
Miosis	Narcotics (except demerol and lomotil), phenothiazines, organophosphates, diazepam, barbiturates, mushrooms (muscarine types)
Mydriasis	Anticholinergics, sympathomimetics, cocaine, TCAs, methanol, glutethimide, LSD
Blindness, optic atrophy	Methanol
Fasciculation	Organophosphates
Nystagmus	Diphenylhydantoin, barbiturates, carbamazepine, PCP, carbon monoxide, glutethimide, ethanol
Hypertonia	Anticholinergics, strychnine, phenothiazines
Myoclonus, rigidity	Anticholinergics, phenothiazines, haloperidol
Delirium, psychosis	Anticholinergics, sympathomimetics, alcohol, phenothiazines, PCP, LSD, marijuana, cocaine, heroin, methaqualone, heavy metals
Coma	Alcohols, anticholinergics, sedative hypnotics, narcotics, carbon monoxide, tricyclic antidepressants, salicylates, organophosphates, barbiturates
Weakness, paralysis	Organophosphates, carbamates, heavy metals
Gastrointestinal symptoms	
Vomiting, diarrhea, pain	Iron, phosphorus, heavy metals, lithium, mushrooms, fluoride, organophosphates, arsenic
Constipation	Lead, narcotics, botulism
Hematemesis	Aminophylline, corrosives, iron, lead, salicylates

(LSD: lysergic acid diethylamide; PCP: phencyclidine; TCA: tricyclic antidepressant)

acetone, and isopropanol. Complete blood cell count with platelets and leukocyte differential, prothrombin time, partial thromboplastin time, liver function tests, and electroencephalogram may prove useful. Urine color may be helpful in the identification of a number of toxins. It is important to obtain urine pregnancy tests on patient of childbearing age.

RADIOLOGIC IMAGING

Radiographic evaluation is useful for certain foreign bodies, radiopaque drugs, metals, and chemicals. Serial chest/abdominal X-rays identify the movement of the disc batteries through the gastrointestinal (GI) tract. Radiopaque compounds may be grouped by the mnemonic "COINS": chloral hydrate and cocaine packets, opiate packets, iron and heavy metals (lead, arsenic and mercury), neuroleptics, and sustained-release or enteric coated tablets.

MANAGEMENT

The approach includes:

- Emergency stabilization
- Decontamination
- Enhanced elimination
- Antidote and poison specific therapy.

Emergency Stabilization

This begins with checking the ABC and stabilization. Because the patient's status can change rapidly, it is essential to reassess the patient often and monitor the need for ventilator support. Blood glucose should be obtained from patient with ingestion of oral hypoglycemic agents, alcohol, and with altered sensorium. Symptoms of hypoglycemia may be rapidly reversed with intravenous dextrose. Intravenous thiamine (10 mg for infants, 10–25 mg for children) should be given before dextrose administration to prevent Wernicke encephalopathy. Although altered mental status in a child may be presumed to be from poisoning, traumatic head injury should also be considered. Any child with coma, altered sensorium, seizures, agitation, impaired vital parameter—tachycardia/bradycardia, arrhythmia, hypotension/hypertension, respiratory distress or depression, and organ failure should be managed in pediatric intensive care unit.

Decontamination

Decontamination may be individualized, depending upon the type and amount of substance ingested, potential toxicity, time elapsed since ingestion, and the symptoms exhibited.

Gastric Lavage

A mainstay of gastric decontamination, involves insertion of a large-bore orogastric tube into the stomach, followed by repeated administration and aspiration of 10–15 mL/kg saline until aspirates is clear. This can be particularly traumatizing to a young child. Contraindications include compromised upper airway protection, ingestion of corrosive substances or hydrocarbons, and patients at risk for GI perforation or hemorrhage. Possible complications are aspiration, respiratory compromise, mechanical injury/perforation, and electrolyte imbalances. The American Academy of Clinical Toxicology (AACT) and European Association of Poison Centers and Clinical Toxicologists discourage its routine use unless performed within 1 hour of the ingestion.

Syrup of Ipecac

In 2003, the American Academy of Pediatrics released a policy statement advising that syrup of ipecac should no longer be used.

Activated Charcoal

It works by adsorbing the toxin and preventing enterohepatic and enteroenteric recirculation. A charcoal/drug ratio of 10:1 is recommended (1–2 g/kg). Activated charcoal (AC) is helpful in carbamazepine, dapsone, phenobarbital, quinine, theophylline, salicylates, phenytoin, or valproic acid ingestion. AC is unpalatable, messy, and poorly accepted by young children often causing vomiting. AC does not bind well with xenobiotics that are highly ionized (e.g., metals, electrolytes, acids, and alkali). In addition, AC is contraindicated in patients who have ingested corrosives or hydrocarbons, in those with bowel obstruction or perforation, and in patients with a depressed level of consciousness.

The AACT discourages the routine use except within 1 hour of ingestion. The first dose is often given with a cathartic agent, such as sorbitol, to improve taste and transit through the intestinal tract. Multiple doses should not include sorbitol because of possible electrolyte and fluid abnormalities.

Whole-bowel Irrigation

Whole-bowel irrigation (WBI) involves administration of large volumes of polyethylene glycol solution orally to decontaminate the GI tract. The pediatric dose is 25 mL/kg/h, up to 500 mL/h in young children and up to 1 L/h in adolescents. It may be useful when a drug or toxicant does not have an antidote or treatment and the substance ingested is an enteric pill, sustained release preparation, or agents poorly adsorbed by AC. Examples are lithium, iron, and lead. Adverse effects of WBI include vomiting, abdominal cramps, bloating, and rarely, aspiration pneumonitis.

Surgical Decontamination

Surgical intervention is usually indicated for mechanical bowel obstruction or bowel ischemia due to heroin or cocaine drug packets and also for massive iron ingestion with failure to evacuate the GI tract.

Enhanced Elimination

Active elimination techniques should be considered only in ingestion of a potentially lethal dose of toxin, progressive clinical deterioration refractory to aggressive supportive care, and blood concentrations that indicate serious intoxication and impaired organ function. Hemodialysis (HD) is useful for drugs with small volume of distribution, poor plasma protein binding, low molecular weight, and weak lipid solubility, e.g., atenolol, ethylene glycol, methanol, and salicylates. Hemoperfusion, using a charcoal filter in a HD machine, can remove toxins with high molecular weight, e.g., barbiturates, carbamazepine, chloral hydrate, dapsone, isoniazid, procainamide, organophosphates, and diphenhydramine.

Exchange transfusion is an alternative procedure for a small group of children who are not eligible for HD. Beneficial effects are seen with salicylate, theophylline, phenobarbital, chloramphenicol, lithium, aniline, chloral hydrate, salicylate, quinine, and methemoglobinemia. Extracorporeal membrane oxygenation has been used for hydrocarbon-induced lung injury, bupropion, amiodarone, calcium channel blocker overdose, and a severe ibuprofen poisoning.

Diuresis

Drug elimination may be facilitated by ensuring adequate renal flow 2–5 mL/kg/h. Elimination of drugs with pKa values of 3.0–7.2 may be enhanced by alkalinizing the urine, e.g., salicylate, phenobarbital, chlorpropamide, and the chlorophenoxy herbicides. Complications are fluid overload, with cerebral edema, pulmonary edema, and hyponatremia.

Toxin-specific Treatments

If physical examination or laboratory findings suggest a specific toxidrome, then consider toxin specific treatments, such as an antidote **(Table 5)**. Antidotes are usually given after the patient is stable, preferably within a few hours of ingestion and may require multiple doses because of short durations of action.

TABLE 5: Selected antidotes.

Antidote	***Toxin***
Atropine	Organophosphate, carbamate poisoning, bradydysrhythmias
Calcium (chloride or gluconate)	Calcium channel blocker overdose, hydrofluoric acid ingestion/exposure
Cyanide antidote package, Amyl nitrite, Sodium nitrite, Sodium thiosulfate	Cyanide, acetonitrile (artificial nail remover), amygdalin (peach, apricot pits), nitroprusside (thiosulfate only)
Deferoxamine	Iron
Digoxin-specific antibody	Digoxin, digitoxin, natural cardiac glycosides (e.g., oleander, red squill, *Bufo* toad venom)
Flumazenil	Benzodiazepines
Fomepizole	Toxic alcohols (ethylene glycol, methanol)
Glucagon	Calcium channel blocker, β-blocker toxicity
Glucose (dextrose)	Sulfonylureas, insulin, hypoglycemia (multiple toxins)
Hydroxocobalamin (vitamin B_{12})	Cyanide, acetonitrile, amygdalin, nitroprusside
Insulin (high dose)	Calcium channel blocker, β-blocker toxicity
Methylene blue	Methemoglobinemia
N-acetylcysteine	Acetaminophen, pennyroyal oil, carbon tetrachloride
Naloxone	Opioid toxicity
Octreotide	Sulfonylurea toxicity
Physostigmine	Antimuscarinic delirium (as a diagnostic tool only)
Pralidoxime	Organophosphate poisoning (insecticides, nerve agents)
Protamine sulfate	Heparins
Pyridoxine	Isoniazid, *Gyromitra* mushrooms
Thiamine	Deficiency states (e.g., alcoholism, anorexia nervosa)
Sodium bicarbonate	Sodium channel blocking cardiotoxins, salicylates

CONCLUSION

Poison prevention remains a challenge and a necessity to prevent the most vulnerable population from becoming exposed to potentially lethal drugs and toxins.

The evaluation of a child presumed to have been exposed to a toxic substance should include a precise history of the exposure, a physical examination, and knowledge of current ingestions and recreational practices. Poison centers and medical toxicologists should be consulted to assist with the diagnosis and management of medicinal/drug overdoses.

CLINICAL PEARLS

- Common toxidromes can identify many poisonous substances **(Tables 2 and 3)**.
- Causes of high anion gap—MUDPILES: methanol, uremia, diabetic ketoacidosis, paraldehyde and phenformin, isoniazid and iron, lactic acidosis, ethanol and ethylene glycol, salicylates.

KEY POINTS

- Precise history is very important in all cases of poisonings.
- Management of most poisonings is supportive.
- Induction of vomiting (syrup ipecac) is no longer recommended due to risk of aspiration in comatose patients and all patients with suspected hydrocarbon ingestion.
- Poison control centers are helpful in guiding therapy and observation period.
- All unknown poisonings or unknown causes of coma are medicolegal cases.

SUGGESTED READING

1. American Academy of Pediatrics Committee on Injury, Violence, and Poison Prevention. Policy statement: poison treatment in the home. American Academy of Pediatrics Committee on Injury, Violence, and Poison Prevention. Pediatrics. 2003;112(5):1182-5.
2. Bronstein AC, Spyker DA, Cantilena LR, Rumack BH, Dart RC. 2011 Annual report of the American Association of Poison Control Centers' National Poison Data System (NPDS): 29th Annual Report. Clin Toxicol (Phila). 2012; 50(10):911-1164.
3. Gupta SK, Peshin SS, Srivastava A, Kaleekal T. A study of childhood poisoning at National Poisons Information Centre, All India Institute of Medical Sciences, New Delhi. J Occup Health. 2003;45(3):191-6.
4. McGregor T, Parkar M, Rao S. Evaluation and management of common childhood poisonings. Am Fam Physician. 2009;79(5):397-403.
5. National Poisons Information Centre (NPIC), All India Institute of Medical sciences. [online] available from http://www.aiims.edu/aiims/departments/pharmacology/NPIC/home.htm [Accessed December, 2015].
6. Nichols DG, Ackerman AD, Argent AC, et al. (Eds). Rogers' Textbook of Pediatric Intensive Care, 4th edition. Philadelphia: Lipincott Williams and Wilkins; 2008.
7. Rathore S, Verma AK, Pandey A, Kumar S. Pediatric poisoning trend in Lucknow District, India. J Forensic Res. 2013;4:179.

CHAPTER 48

Snake Bite in Children

Mahesh A Mohite

INTRODUCTION

Snake bite is a common rural emergency, causing approximately 45,000 deaths annually. There are not many advances in the last few decades in management.

There are about 3,500 species of snake worldwide of which 200 are poisonous. In India about 216 species of snakes are seen of which 52 species are poisonous (Fauna of British India 1943—Dr Malcom Smith).

Almost 60% bites are nonpoisonous or dry bites (nonvenomous bite by poisonous snake). Toxicity of same snake varies in different bites according to age of snake, size of victim, intactness of fangs, site of bite, etc. **(Table 1)**. There are three major groups of poisonous snakes **(Fig. 1 and Table 2)**:

1. *Elapids:* Neurotoxic: Cobra and Krait
2. *Vipers:* Hemorrhagic and vasculotoxic
3. *Sea snakes:* Neurotoxic, myolytic

In rural areas the killed snake is often brought with the victim. Recognizing whether it is poisonous or nonpoisonous and if poisonous, what type of poison, helps in providing early specific treatment to the victim which improves survival.

One can also look at the number of fang marks: 2–4 suggest poisonous bite as against multiple fang marks in nonpoisonous bites.

TABLE 1: Gross identifying characteristics.

	Poisonous	*Nonpoisonous*
Head	Triangular, scale pattern	Blunt
Tail	Pointed	Blunt
Scales	Specific pattern	No pattern
Belly scales	Multiple scales	Single transverse scale
Pupils	Specific pattern	Circular

Clinical Features of Bites

Local features appear within 10–30 minutes of bite. They are severe in viper bites. Sea snake bites have minimal local swelling and pain. Nonpoisonous bites also cause local symptoms but usually they are not progressive.

Systemic manifestations usually start within 15 minutes–1 hour but may appear as late as 12 hours in elapids, and up to 48 hours in vipers. Hence, a confirmed elapid bite should be observed for at least 24 hours and a viper bite for at least 72 hours. Clinical features in a nutshell are:

- *Krait:* Usually night bites, may start as abdominal pain, early morning presentation with respiratory failure, ptosis. No other systems affected, no local signs, fang marks not seen usually.
- *Cobra:* Thick fang marks seen, local hemorrhage with edema, may have local lymph node swelling and pain, progressive cellulitis. Main feature is progressive neuro-paralysis in 2–8 hours leading to respiratory failure and death. May develop systemic coagulopathy. Few victims may develop myocardial injury and failure.
- *Russel's viper:* Local toxin leading to progressive cellulitis, hemorrhage, and lymphadenopathy. Later it progresses to systemic coagulopathy and hemorrhage. It may develop superimposed bacterial infections.
- *Saw scaled viper:* Presentation is almost similar to Russel's viper.
- *Sea snake bites:* They present with severe body aches and progressive weakness due to myolysis. They may progress to renal injury due to myoglobinuria.

Victim presents with severe fear and anxiety due to prejudiced information.

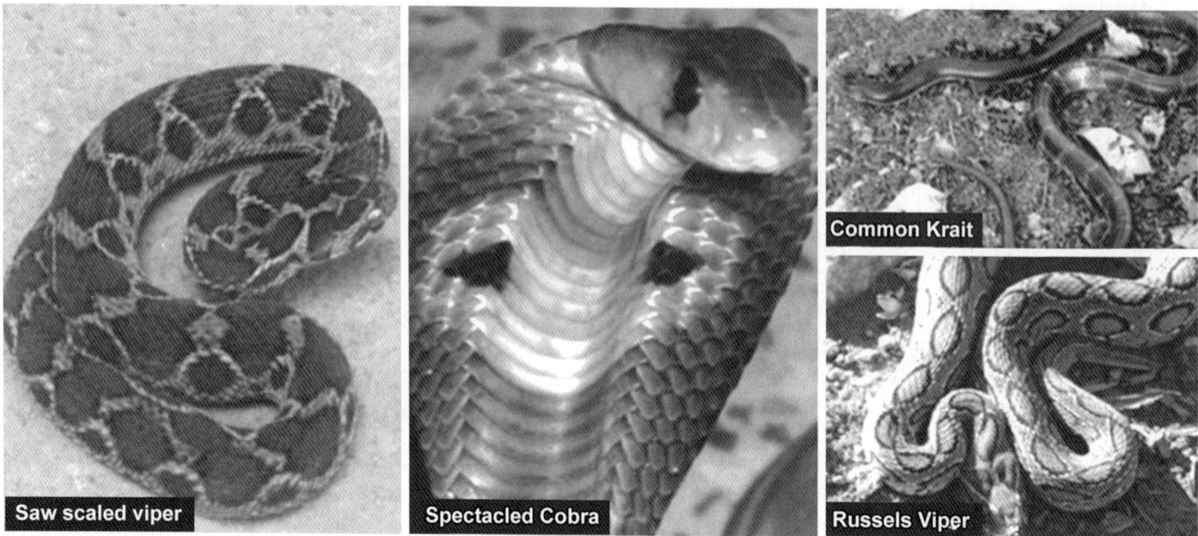

Fig. 1: Three major groups of poisonous snakes.

TABLE 2: Even elapids and vipers have specific identification marks.

	Cobra	*Krait*	*Saw scaled V*	*Russel's V*
Head	Narrow	Narrow blunt	Triangular	Triangular
Tail	Pointed	Pointed	Pointed	Pointed
Scales	3rd labial scale touch eye	Black, banded or nonbanded	Saw like scales	Diamond bands on back
Length	4–6 feet	5–8 feet	2–3 feet	6–8 feet bulky
Fangs	Short thick	Hypodermic needle like	Large soft	Large soft

DIAGNOSIS

It is based upon:

- Information given by attendants.
- Inspection of the killed snake.
- Clinical presentation and progress as provided in the following text.
- Few specific tests.

Clinician working in rural area should have high level of suspicion for snake bites.

Lab tests done in snake bites are:

- *20 minutes whole blood clotting test:* It is a bedside test. Collect 3–5 mL blood in a test tube. After 20 minutes turn it upside down. If no clot has been formed, it suggests hemorrhagic toxin of viper. It can be repeated after 6 hours of antivenom injection to monitor the coagulopathy and guide further doses of antivenom.
- Other standard lab tests appropriate for critical care management need to be performed during management.

TREATMENT (FIG. 2)

- If victim is sick on initial and primary assessment, basic airway, breathing, and circulation support needs to be given to stabilize to optimum level.
- If patient is stable on presentation, counseling to allay the anxiety is very important to avoid psychological complications.
- *Immobilization:* It is very important to immobilize the bitten part to delay spread of venom proximally.
- Tight tourniquet should be avoided to avoid vascular compromise especially on the background of progressive cellulitis.
- *Position of the limb:* Till the antivenom is not given, bitten limb should be kept below the level of the heart. After antivenom is given, if there is severe local tissue damage (viper bite), limb should be at the level of the heart.
- All wounds should be cleaned with soap and water.

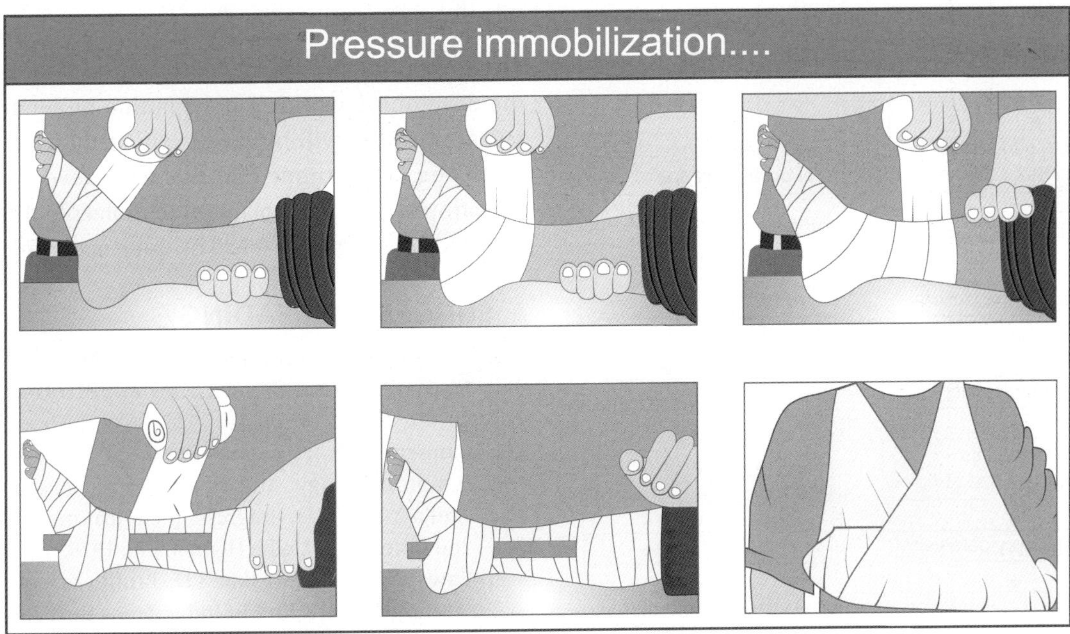

Fig. 2: Pressure immobilization of the bitten limb.

- *Don'ts:* Avoid cuts, suction, tight bandage, etc., which is harmful.
- *Specific treatment is antisnake venom (ASV):* In India only polyvalent ASV is available effective against common four snake bites, i.e., Cobra, Krait, Russel's Viper, and Saw scaled viper.
- A poisonous snake injects various amounts of venom irrespective of size of the victim, and each mL of antivenom neutralizes a specific amount of the venom (depending on the type of snake). So antivenom dose is to be calculated according to amount of venom injected which can only be indirectly assessed clinically by the severity of envenomation; it is not per kg weight of the child.
- Doses can be repeated after 6–8 hours depending upon clinical improvement. In Elapids usually ASV is given in smaller periodic doses for 48 hours. In Viper bites ASV repeated doses may be needed for 7 days **(Table 3)**.
- ASV being animal protein can evoke serious allergic reactions including anaphylaxis. Provision to counter such reactions should be kept ready.
- In neurotoxic snake bite if antivenom is not showing improvement cholinesterase inhibitor neostigmine can be used. This works only in postsynaptic pathologies. Neostigmine is to be given in doses of 50 μg/kg IV first dose and every 30 minutes for 5 doses followed by 25 μg/kg every 2 hourly till neurorecovery. Every fourth dose of neostigmine should be preceded by atropine (20 μg/kg) to counter the muscarinic effect.
- Early induction of treatment leads to neurorecovery within 48 hours. Hemorrhage and cellulitis may take longer times.
- If victim is brought late, is neuro paralyzed and has not received ASV, neurorecovery may take 2–3 weeks.

TABLE 3: Antivenom: Recommended doses (each vial 10 mL).

Severity	*Clinical features*	*Dose*
Mild	Only local signs with or without lymphadenitis	5–10 vials
Moderate	Mild systemic signs, bleeding tendency, hypotension	10–20 vials
Severe	Severe local signs, DIC, shock, paralysis	20–30 vials

(DIC: Disseminated intravascular coagulation)

Supportive therapy:

For critical patient appropriate intensive care unit (ICU) support may be needed:

- Mechanical ventilation
- Blood component therapy
- Renal replacement therapy
- Surgical debridement
- Limb compartment syndrome release therapy

Flowchart 1: History of snake bite or suspected snake bite.

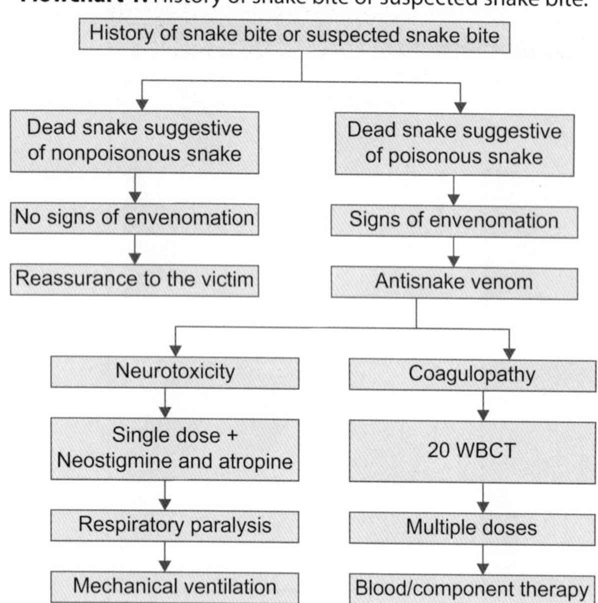

(WBCT: whole blood clotting test)

Algorithm of management after counseling, immobilization, and ASV therapy is given in **Flowchart 1**.

TO SUMMARIZE

- If possible identify whether poisonous or non-poisonous bite.
- Immobilize the limb.
- If medial facility far away, put tourniquet.
- Give antivenin primary dose as soon as possible.
- Shift to a center with all back up facility after giving antivenin immediately.

ADVANCES

The cost of antivenin is exorbitant and prohibitive in the developing world. A polypeptide molecule is under research which will bind the venom molecule before it binds the target tissue and this will prevent the further catastrophe. Being a polypeptide molecule that is manufactured commercially it will be quite economical.

SUGGESTED READING

1. Alirol E, Sharma SK, Bawaskar HS, Kuch U, Chappuis F. Snake bite in South Asia: a review. PLoS Negl Trop Dis. 2010;4:e603.
2. Bannerjee RN. Poisonous snakes in India, their venoms, symptomatology, and treatment of envenomation. In: Ahuja MMS (Ed). Progress in clinical medicine in India, 2nd series. New Delhi: Heinemann; 1978. pp. 136-76.
3. Bawaskar HS, Bawaskar PH. Profile of envenoming in Western Maharashtra in India. Trans Royal Soc Trop Med Hyg. 2002;96:79-84.
4. Bhat RN. Viperine snake bite poisoning in Jammu. J Indian Medical Association. 1974;63:383-92.
5. Dayal S, Lall SB. In: Lall SB (Ed). Management of common Indian snake and insect bites. New Delhi: Noble Vision. 1997. pp. 17-23.
6. Simpson ID, Tanwar PD, Andrade C, Kochar DK, Norris RL. The Ebbinghaus retention curve: training does not increase the ability to apply pressure immobilisation in simulated snake bite—implications for snake bite first aid in the developing world. Trans R Soc Trop Med Hyg. 2008;102(5):451-9.
7. Warrel DA, venom, toxins, and plant poisons. In: Weatneral DS (Ed). Oxford textbook of medicine. NY: Oxford University Press; 1996. pp. 1124-39.

Initial Approach to a Comatose Child

Soonu Udani

INTRODUCTION

Whatever the initiating event that results in altered sensorium, it is the "secondary injury" (which results from hypoxia and hypoperfusion), that has huge impact on the eventual outcome. The approach to a child with altered sensorium, therefore, focuses on the efforts to prevent or limit this secondary injury, while trying to offer specific treatment.

Rapidly evaluate the appearance, breathing, and circulation. Confirm the altered sensorium and proceed with further assessment only if the child is stable. If the child is unstable, "the initial management priorities are to stabilize and support the airway, breathing, and circulation, irrespective of the etiology".

- Detailed, focused physical examination—fundamental
- Earliest signs of evolving injuries—repetitive observations
- Serve as screening tool for further testing

Awake nonintubated child: Specific reliable accurate

Not so reliable in sedated/comatose patients. Therefore numerical scales like the Glasgow coma scale (GCS) give reference points for changing caregivers **(Box 1)**.

Noninvasive and clinical bedside monitoring: Easy to interpret.

- *Non-neurological:*
  - Vital signs:
    - Temperature
    - Heart rate
    - Blood pressure (BP)
    - Pattern of respiration
  - *General examination:*
    - Pallor and icterus
    - Rash
    - Signs of trauma
- *Neurological—repeat frequently:*
  - *Glasgow coma scale three points ↓ in GCS:* Indicates clinical change warrants further investigation escalation of treatment
    - Pupils especially for asymmetry
    - Fundus
    - Cranial nerve examination
    - *Motor examination:* Tone, power, reflexes, and primitive reflexes
  - *Posturing:*
    - Sensory changes
    - Meningeal signs

BOX 1: Indications for intubation (use full analgesia, sedation, and muscle relaxant).

- Glasgow coma scale ≤12 or AVPU [A (alert) V (responds to voice) P (responds to pain) U (unresponsive)]
- Features of herniation
- Abnormal respiration
- Asymmetric or dilated pupils
- Inability to handle secretions (absent gag, gurgling sounds)

Every patient of altered sensorium/coma should be treated as having increased intracranial pressure (ICP) until proved otherwise: An unstable airway leads to hypoxia → cerebral vasodilation → increase in cerebral blood flow → increase in ICP.

Open with "jaw thrust" or "chin lift" method if the spine is deemed unaffected.

IMMEDIATE TREATMENT

- *Treatment for raised ICP:* Mannitol 1.25–2 mL/kg. Do not write continuing orders for mannitol.
- Hypertonic saline 1–2 mL/kg and 1–2 mL/kg/hour to 155 mEq/L Na and to osmolarity of 300–330 mOsm/L
- Controlled ventilation to partial pressure of oxygen (PaO_2) >65 mm Hg and CO_2 35–40 mm Hg
- Supportive nursing management
- Specific treatment, if cause is known.

- More broad-based treatment covering meningitis, herpes, malaria, and other treatable infections, if cause is not known or till results are available.
- If noninfectious/unknown/postinfectious—immune therapy [steroids/intravenous immunoglobulin (IVIG)]
- Early imaging with magnetic resonance imaging (MRI) valuable

Focus on:

- *Oxygenation:* PaO_2 <60 mm Hg (>95% SpO_2)
- *Ventilation:* Partial pressure of carbon dioxide ($PaCO_2$) → mid-30s overzealous hyperventilation → CO_2 too low → danger of hypoperfusion, and drop in cerebral perfusion
- Cerebral perfusion pressure = Mean arterial pressure (MAP) - ICP
- Target MAPs to 70 mm Hg minimum considering a target CPP of 50 mm Hg
- Isotonic fluids, inotropes maintain BP = 95th centile. In head injury, avoid glucose infusion in the first 24 hours.
- When monitoring of ICP/MAP unavailable, avoid hypo-osmolar/hyperosmolar fluids—no role of fluid restriction.
- High BP at presentation → effect/cause—reduce slowly after ICP ruled out.
- Glycemic control <180 mg/dL.

BEWARE HYPOGLYCEMIA

Worsening Glasgow Coma Scale Despite Correction of Airway, Breathing, and Circulation (Box 2)

Chasing the cause: The list is exhaustive; "obvious causes" can be remembered by the "mnemonic COMA **(Table 1 and Flowchart 1)**":

- *C:* Convulsions (status epilepticus)
- *O:* O_2 depriving events—resuscitation following episodes such as drowning, electrocution, and foreign body

BOX 2: Signs of raised intracranial pressure in coma.

- Abnormal posturing
- Abnormal breathing pattern
- Abnormal oculocephalic (Doll's eye) or oculovestibular reflex
- Abnormal pupillary response
- Cushing's triad

TABLE 1: Quick guide to causes of coma.

Febrile	*Afebrile*
Bacterial meningitis	*Well child:* Poisoning
Tuberculous meningitis	Metabolic
Herpes meningoencephalitis	Child abuse
Malaria	*Sick child:* Tumor
Dengue	Hypertension
Immune mediated (ADEM)	Diabetic ketoacidosis
Onset in hours—drugs, poisoning	–
Onset in days—CNS infections	–
Onset in weeks—tumor, DKA, and HTN	–

(ADEM: acute disseminated encephalomyelitis; CNS: central nervous system; DKA: diabetic ketoacidosis; HTN: hypertension)

Flowchart 1: Simplified approach to coma.

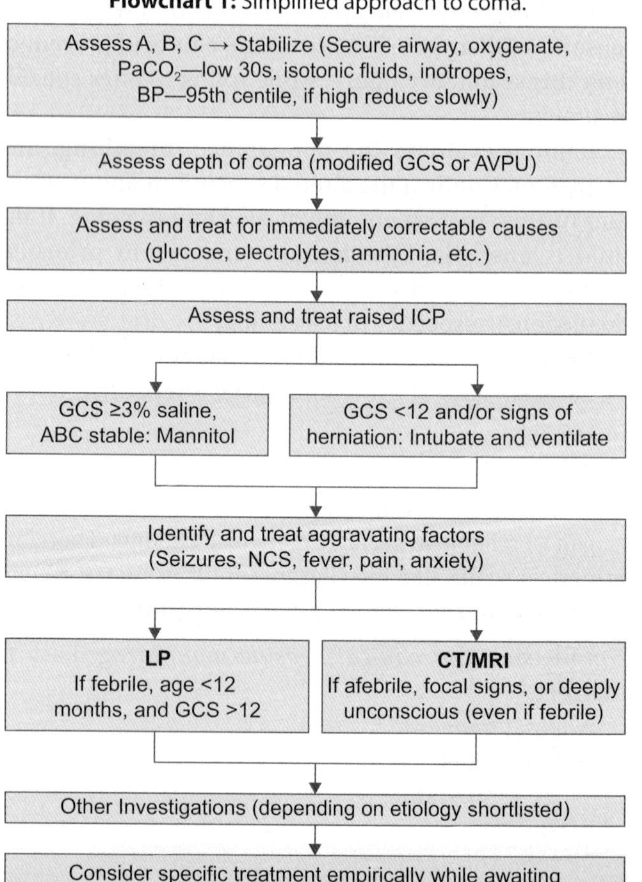

(AVPU: alert, voice, pain, unresponsive; BP: blood pressure; CT: computed tomography; GCS: Glasgow coma scale; ICP: intracranial pressure; LP: lumbar puncture; MRI: magnetic resonance imaging; NCS: nonconvulsive seizures; $PaCO_2$: partial pressure carbon dioxide)

- *M:* Major illnesses, e.g., diabetes, hypertension (secondary), viral hepatitis, etc.
- *A:* Accidents (trauma)

INVESTIGATIONS

- Complete blood count, peripheral smear for malarial parasites (MP), cultures, blood sugar, blood urea nitrogen, electrolytes, liver function test, ammonia, lactate, and arterial blood gas—keep extra samples for further tests.
- Prioritize as per working diagnosis
- *Imaging:* If signs of raised ICP, no lumbar puncture—MRI preferable. If not, computed tomography to check edema and impending herniation.

Second tier:

- Blood and cerebrospinal fluid (CSF) autoimmune panel
- CSF polymerase chain reaction (PCR) panel for infectious etiology—save samples for further tests if needed.
- Electroencephalogram (EEG)—continuous if possible for nonconvulsive status

Order prompt: Helps to remember all aspects of care:

- 30° head up unless a shock is present.
- Hourly pupil and GCS check and recording
- Eye care with lubricant and closure to prevent exposure keratitis
- Sedation and analgesia orders
- Suctioning with premedication with intravenous (IV) and/or endotracheal (ET) lignocaine
- Prevention and prompt treatment of fever
- Feeding orders, H_2 blockers
- Watching for development of autonomic dysfunction—sweating, tachy-/bradycardia, and anisocoria
- Swings in BP and temperature—in concurrent spinal injury, watch for seizures. Check for posturing, eye deviation
- Deep venous thrombosis (DVT) prevention in older, heavier children
- Bed sore and other pain check as pain will raise ICP.
- Bladder and bowel attention—internal stimulus
- Cluster care to avoid multiple handling
- Severe traumatic brain injury (TBI) so seizure prophylaxis for 7 days for acute symptomatic seizures. Continue if seizures have occurred.

CLINICAL PEARLS

- Every patient of altered sensorium/coma should be treated as having increased ICP until proved otherwise.
- Raised ICP should be presumed until proven otherwise.
- Overzealous hyperventilation → CO_2 too low → danger of hypoperfusion and drop in cerebral perfusion.
- Hypertonic saline replaces mannitol as the osmolar agent of choice.
- No role of fluid restriction.

KEY POINTS

- Neuroprotective strategies should be employed from the time of first contact.
- Supportive care is as important as specific treatment.
- Repeated assessment is important.
- Prevention and rapid treatment of aggravating causes.
- Institute early rapid empirical treatment of probable causes.
- Eye on good outcome, not only on survival.

SUGGESTED READING

1. Kirkham FJ. Non-traumatic coma in children. Arch Dis Child. 2001;85(4):303-12.
2. Udani S. Advances in neurocritical care. Indian J Pediatr. 2015;82(3):272-6.
3. Udani S. The comatose child. In: Udani S, Chugh K, Ugra D, Khilnani P (Eds). IAP Specialty Series Textbook on Pediatric Intensive Care, 2nd edition. New Delhi: Jaypee Brothers Medical Publishers; 2013. pp. 341-451.

Infectious Diseases

Section Editors: *Shyam Kukreja, Tanu Singhal*

Fever without Focus in Infants Less than 3 Months of Age

S Balasubramanian

INTRODUCTION

The differential diagnosis involving fever in neonates and young infants 29–60 days of age includes both infectious and noninfectious causes. Although self-limited viral infections are the most common cause of fever, the incidence of serious bacterial infections (SBIs) may be higher in this population compared to older children; neonates have been shown to be at particularly high risk. SBIs include bacteremia (e.g., sepsis), cellulitis, osteomyelitis, septic arthritis, meningitis, pneumonia, and urinary tract infection (UTI).

Among these, UTI is the most common type of SBI. Among bacterial pathogens causing SBI in infants less than 90 days of age, gram-negative bacteria such as *E. coli* and *Klebsiella* are most frequently identified. Other common pathogens are *Streptococcus pneumoniae, Haemophilus influenzae, Neisseria meningitidis, S. aureus* and less commonly Group B streptococcus and *Listeria monocytogenes*. Neonatal herpes simplex virus (HSV) is an important consideration in infants 0–28 days of age. Neonates with cutaneous vesicles, seizures, and/or elevated transaminases present a high index of suspicion for HSV infection; however, it is rare for a neonate with HSV to present with fever of uncertain source (FUS).

Because the clinical examination alone is unable to reliably predict serious illness in infants less than 60 days of age with FUS and culture results are not immediately available, clinicians must often approach management of patients with fever by relying on a combination of history, physical examination findings, and diagnostic screening tests.

DEFINITION

The term fever without focus or fever without localizing Signs or FUS is defined as an acute febrile illness in which the etiology of the fever is not apparent after a thorough history and physical examination. A rectal temperature higher than 38°C (100.4°F) has been defined as fever in literature.

EPIDEMIOLOGY

Risk of SBI varies with age. Risk is greatest during the immediate neonatal period and through the first month (and is heightened in the infant born prematurely). Even among neonates, only 7% of those who have fever without focus have an SBI.

LABORATORY DIAGNOSIS

Various diagnostic tests to quantify the risk of bacteremia and its complications have been assessed including the white blood cells count and differential, microscopic examination of buffy coat of blood, erythrocyte sedimentation rate, C-reactive protein, procalcitonin serum levels, morphologic changes in peripheral blood neutrophils, and quantitative cultures of blood. In addition, clinical scales have been developed to help identify the febrile child with a serious illness.

The outcome of primary concern is not occult bacteremia but meningitis. An ideal diagnostic test would specifically identify febrile children at risk of a serious complication, because many focal infections after bacteremia (e.g., most cases of either pneumonia or cellulitis) can be treated when they become apparent and are not usually associated with serious sequelae. Unfortunately, there is no such test. Lowering the risk of serious complications by preventing infections through use of conjugate vaccines has proven to be the most effective strategy.

MANAGEMENT

There is general agreement that febrile children who are "very young" (variably considered to be younger than 3, 2,

Flowchart 1: Management algorithm.

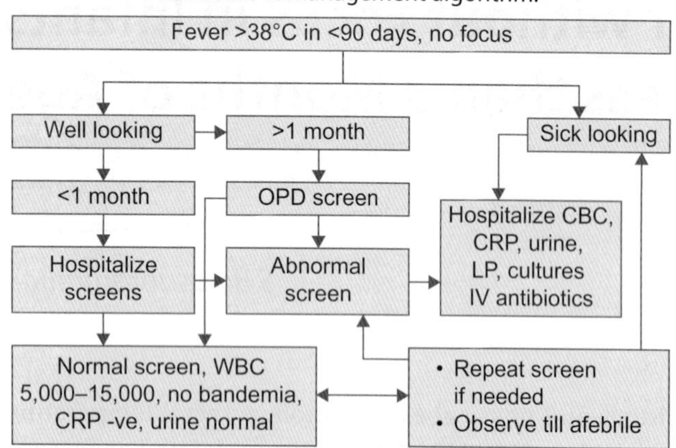

(CBC: complete blood count; CRP: c-reactive protein; IV: intravenous; LP: lumbar puncture; OPD: outpatient department; WBC: white blood cell)

or 1 month of age) should be managed differently from the way in which older children are managed **(Flowchart 1)**. Some clinicians adhere to a protocol of treating all young infants with fever and no apparent focus of infection with broad-spectrum antimicrobial agents administered intravenously in the hospital until the results of cultures of the blood, urine and cerebrospinal fluid (CSF) are known. Although sometimes perceived as the "safe" approach, such management incurs considerable financial cost and risk of iatrogenic complications and of diagnostic misadventures associated with hospitalization.

These risks include errors in the type and dosage of drugs, complications of venous cannulation (such as phlebitis and sloughing of the skin), and nosocomial infections. many experts believe that febrile infants from 2 to 3 months of age with no apparent focus of infection who appear well and/or who have a laboratory-documented viral infection can be managed without either additional laboratory tests or hospitalization, provided that careful follow-up is ensured.

If an antimicrobial agent is to be administered, cultures of the blood, urine and CSF should be obtained first. Rapid tests for specific viral pathogens, which now are widely available, may aid decisions about managing patients and may reduce the need for and/or the duration of hospitalization.

Febrile infants at low risk of SBI for whom adequate home observation and follow-up cannot be ensured should be hospitalized and can be observed without antimicrobial treatment. Doing so (if the child appears well) is reasonable and avoids the adverse side effects of antimicrobial agents and intravenous cannulation, shortens the duration of hospitalization, and saves money without placing the child at significant risk of complications.

Most febrile infants with no apparent focus of infection who are younger than 1 month should be hospitalized and treated with antimicrobial therapy. The choice of antibiotic would depend on local epidemiological data and antibiotic susceptibility patterns in the area of practice. A third generation cephalosporin with an aminoglycoside would be generally sufficient for initial empiric therapy in most infants with community acquired infection.

PITFALLS AND PEARLS IN ASSESSMENT AND DIAGNOSIS

- Parental report of fever via palpation is unreliable as a sole method of determining fever.
- Practice guidelines recommend that if a neonate has had a fever recorded at home by a reliable parent, the patient should be treated as a febrile neonate.
- If excessive clothing and blankets encasing the infant are suspected of falsely elevating the body temperature, then the excessive coverings should be removed and the temperature retaken in 15–30 minutes. If body temperature is normal after the covers are removed, then the infant is considered afebrile.
- A response to antipyretic medication does not change the likelihood of an infant having an SBI.
- Clinical assessment include a thorough history and physical examination (include questions about recent symptoms, vaccinations, exposure to sick contacts, and the child's birth history in the patient history).
- The large majority of children with fever without localizing signs in the 1–3 months age group likely have a viral syndrome.
- Ill-appearing (toxic) febrile infants less than or equal to 3 months of age require prompt hospitalization and immediate parenteral antimicrobial therapy after cultures of blood, urine, and CSF are obtained. It is recommended that the following laboratory studies be performed in neonates with FUS, complete blood count, differential, blood culture urinalysis and urine culture. cerebrospinal fluid studies:
  i. *Tube 1:* Protein and glucose
  ii. *Tube 2:* Culture, sensitivity, Gram stain
  iii. *Tube 3:* Cell count and differential
  iv. *Tube 4:* Hold for additional studies. Stool culture if diarrhea is present.

- Well-appearing infants 1–3 months of age can be managed safely using low-risk laboratory and clinical criteria if reliable parents are involved and close follow-up is assured.
- Among SBIs, pyelonephritis is the most common and may be seen in well-appearing infants who have fever without a focus or in those who appear ill. Urinalysis may be negative in infants less than 2 months of age with pyelonephritis.
- Analysis of CSF for HSV using polymerase chain reaction (PCR) may be considered in neonates with CSF pleocytosis and a negative Gram stain.
- Delaying or omitting a lumbar puncture for CSF analyses may be considered in young infants 29–60 days of age with FUS who meet all applicable low-risk clinical and laboratory criteria **(Box 1)**.
- If antimicrobial therapy will be initiated in infants who meet low-risk criteria, CSF specimens need to be collected prior to treatment.
- A chest X-ray may be performed in neonates and young infants 29–60 days of age who manifest one or more of the following clinical findings: tachypnea more than 60 breaths/min, crackles in the chest, retractions, nasal flaring, cyanosis or oxygen saturation less than 95%.
- In patients who are not responding to antimicrobial therapy, the clinician should consider additional evaluation and treatment options, including: alternative antimicrobial therapy for resistant organisms (in neonates only) CSF HSV PCR (if not completed previously) and empiric treatment with acyclovir.

BOX 1: Low-risk criteria for infants with fever 1–3 months of age.

Low-risk clinical criteria:
- Well-appearing
- Previously healthy
- No focal source of infection

Low-risk laboratory criteria:
- Urinalysis
  - ≤10 WBC/hpf
  - No bacteria on Gram's stain
- Complete blood count
  - WBC 5,000 to 15,000/mm^3
  - ≤1,500 band cells/mm^3
- Chest radiograph (if obtained)
  - No evidence of discrete infiltrate
- Stool smear (when diarrhea is present)
  - Negative for blood
  - ≤5 WBC/hpf

(WBC: white blood cell)

KEY POINTS

- Although controversy remains as how to best manage acutely febrile infants and children, there are several areas of near consensus.
- Infants aged less than or equal to 60 days continue to have the highest rates of serious bacterial infections (SBIs) and pose a challenge to practitioners attempting to determine how extensive an evaluation to perform in a non-toxic appearing child.
- Urinary tract infections (UTIs) are the most common SBIs in all age groups.
- Assessment for UTI should be part of any evaluation for all but the lowest-risk patients (i.e., circumcised boys).
- New technologies can more rapidly diagnose common viral and bacterial infections and recommendations to simplify the management of these febrile infants and children are needed.

SUGGESTED READING

1. Huppler AR, Eickhoff JC, Wald ER. Performance of low-risk criteria in the evaluation of young infants with fever: review of the literature. Pediatrics. 2010;125(2):228-33.
2. Jhaveri R, Byington CL, Klein JO, Shapiro ED. Management of the non-toxic-appearing acutely febrile child: a 21st century approach. The Journal of Pediatrics, 2011; 159(2):181-5.
3. Kramer, Michael S, Steven G. Rothrock, Andy Jagoda. "The young febrile child: evidence-based diagnostic and therapeutic strategies" An Evidence-Based Approach to Infectious Disease; 2015.
4. Olaciregui I, Hernández U, Muñoz JA, Emparanza JI, Landa JJ. Markers that predict serious bacterial infection in infants under 3 months of age presenting with fever of unknown origin. Arch Dis Child. 2009;94(7):501-5.

CHAPTER 51

Acute Viral Encephalitis

Jaydeep Choudhury

INTRODUCTION

Acute viral encephalitis is an important cause of mortality and morbidity in children. Most of the times acute viral encephalitis is a clinical diagnosis and laboratory confirmation is not possible due to lack of availability of diagnostic testing for most of the agents. A period of up to 14 days is considered to define "acute". Acute encephalitis syndrome (AES) including Japanese B encephalitis (JE) is a group of clinically similar neurologic manifestation caused by several different viruses, bacteria, fungus, parasites, spirochetes, chemical/toxins, etc. There is seasonal and geographical variation in the causative organism. It may be sporadic like herpes simplex encephalitis (HSE) or epidemic such as JE. The outbreak of JE usually coincides with the monsoon and post-monsoon period when the density of mosquitoes increases while encephalitis due to other viruses especially enteroviruses occurs throughout the year as it is water borne disease. For surveillance purposes, all the acute encephalitis cases to be reported under the heading of acute encephalitis.

The case fatality rate of AES is very high and those who survive may suffer with various neurological sequelae. Children are at risk of highest attack rates because of lack of cumulative immunity due to natural infection. Encephalitis, usually caused by a virus, cannot be treated with antibiotics. A good clinical management is important to reduce the risk of disability or death from the disease.

Clinically, a case of AES is defined as a person of any age, at any time of year with the acute onset of fever and a change in mental status (including symptoms such as confusion, disorientation, come, or inability to talk) and/or new onset of seizures (excluding simple febrile seizures). Other early clinical findings may include an increase in irritability, somnolence or abnormal behavior greater than that seen with usual febrile illness.

It is important to note that in an epidemic situation fever with altered sensorium persisting for more than 2 hours with a focal seizure or paralysis of any part of body is encephalitis. Presence of rash on body excludes Japanese encephalitis. AES with symmetrical signs and fever is likely to be cerebral malaria.

A suspected case that meets the clinical case definition for AES may be classified in one of the following four ways as shown in **Flowchart 1**.

- *Laboratory-confirmed JE:* A suspected case that has been laboratory-confirmed as JE
- *Probable JE:* A suspected case that occurs in close geographic and temporal relationship to laboratory-confirmed case of JE, in the context of an outbreak
- *Acute encephalitis syndrome (due to agent other than JE):* A suspected case in which diagnostic testing is performed and an etiological agent other than JE virus is identified
- *Acute encephalitis syndrome (due to unknown agent):* A suspected case in which no diagnostic testing is performed or in which testing was performed but no etiological agent was identified or in which the test results were indeterminate.

CLINICAL MANIFESTATIONS

A case of viral encephalitis including JE presents with a prodrome of fever, headache, nausea, diarrhea, vomiting, and myalgia lasting for 1–5 days. It is followed by irritability, altered behavior, convulsions, and coma. The progression of disease is rapid. Features of raised intracranial tension are commonly present in acute stage of illness. The patient may develop difficulty of speech and other neurological deficits like ocular palsies, hemiplegia, quadriplegia and may have extrapyramidal signs in the form of dystonia, choreoathetosis, and coarse tremors.

All the cases of AES should be reported as they have similar clinical manifestations. Their case management usually follows a common protocol along with situation specific treatment.

Flowchart 1: Causes of acute encephalitis syndrome.

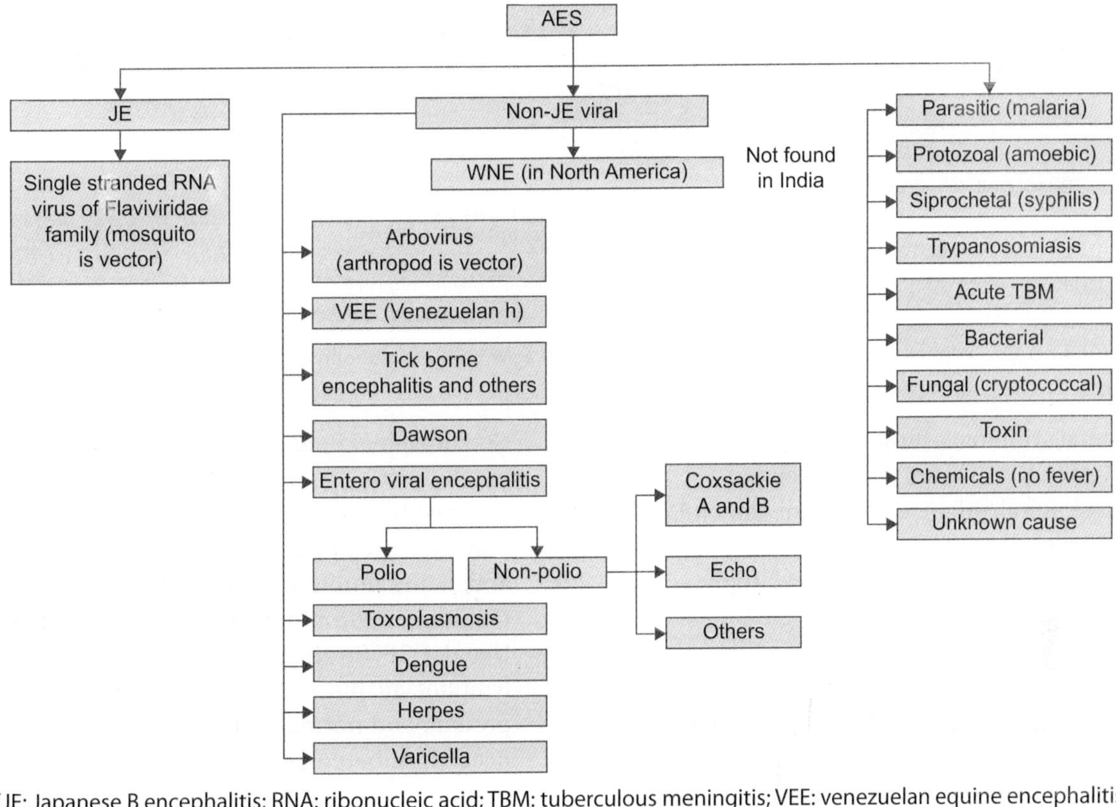

(JE: Japanese B encephalitis; RNA: ribonucleic acid; TBM: tuberculous meningitis; VEE: venezuelan equine encephalitis; WNE: West Nile encephalitis)

MANAGEMENT

Acute encephalitis syndrome is a medical emergency and it requires immediate consideration of vital functions including life support, identification of cause and institution of specific therapy if available. Management of AES including Japanese encephalitis is essentially symptomatic. To reduce severe morbidity and mortality, it is important to identify early warning signs and refer patients to health facility.

The step-wise management of AES is as follows.

Step I: Rapid Assessment and Stabilization

- *Establish and maintain airway:* The child has to be intubated if Glasgow Coma Scale (GCS) less than 8, there is impaired airway reflexes, abnormal respiratory pattern, signs of raised intracranial pressure (ICP), oxygen saturation less than 92% despite high flow oxygen and fluid refractory shock
- Ventilation, adequate oxygenation
- *Circulation:* Intravenous (IV) access has to be established, samples to be collected for investigation (complete blood count, blood sugar, liver function test, renal function test, electrolytes, blood gas, lactate, peripheral smear and rapid diagnostic test for malarial parasite, serology for viruses). Fluid bolus to be given if in circulatory failure (20 mL/kg 0.9% NaCl), inotropes if required
- Signs of cerebral herniation or raised ICP should be identified
- *Temperature:* Fever and hypothermia should be treated
- *Ongoing seizures:* Benzodiazepine, followed by phenytoin loading if required.

Step II: Clinical Evaluation—History and Examination

The following are the important aspects in history and examination. The approach to a suspected case of AES is shown in **Flowchart 2**.

- Fever, headache, vomiting, seizures, abnormal posturing
- Altered behavior, cognition, personality changes, altered consciousness

Flowchart 2: Approach to a child with acute encephalitis syndrome.

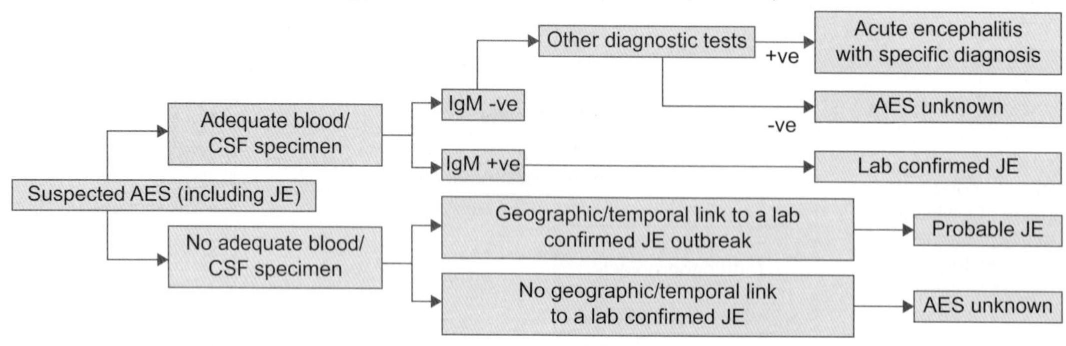

(AES: acute encephalitis syndrome; CSF: cerebrospinal fluid; IgM: immunoglobulin M; JE: Japanese B encephalitis)

- Prodromal symptoms, flu-like illness, diarrhea
- Rash, vesicles, past history of chicken pox
- *Residence:* Rural/urban, endemic for cerebral malaria, any epidemic of AES in neighborhood
- History of animal contact, insect bite, dog bite
- Drug or toxin exposure
- Recent history of travel
- History of trauma
- Personal or family history of seizure disorder
- Recent immunizations
- *History of recurrent episodes of encephalopathy:* These are characteristic of some inborn errors of metabolism (urea cycle defects, organic acidemias, and fatty acid oxidation defects). It may also be present in migraine, epilepsy and substance abuse
- Other concurrent systemic illness, e.g., jaundice (hepatic failure), pneumonia (hypoxic encephalopathy), diarrhea (dyselectrolytemia), dysentery (shigella encephalopathy)
- *Past medical illness:* Diabetes, congenital heart disease, chronic kidney or liver disease
- Family history of previous infant/child deaths
- Pre-morbid developmental/neurological status of the child
- *Risk factors for immunodeficiency:* HIV risk factors, cancer treatment and steroid/immunosuppressant treatment.

Step III: Investigation/Samples to be Collected

- *Cerebrospinal fluid (CSF):* In hemodynamically stable patients without any features of raised intracranial pressure, lumbar puncture should be performed. Cerebrospinal fluid should be examined for cytology, biochemistry, Gram stain, Ziehl–Neelsen stain for acid fast bacilli, bacterial culture, latex agglutination, polymerase chain reaction for herpes simplex virus 1 and 2, and immunoglobulin M antibodies for JE and for dengue virus depending on clinical suspicion. Usual CSF findings in viral encephalitis include lymphocytic pleocytosis, mild to moderately elevated protein, and normal CSF sugar. Similar findings may occur in tubercular meningitis and partially treated pyogenic meningitis; however, the CSF sugar is likely to be low in these situations
- *Blood/serum, urine:* Complete blood count including platelet count, blood glucose, serum electrolytes, liver and kidney function tests, blood culture, arterial blood gas and lactate. Peripheral smear for malarial parasite and rapid diagnostic test for malaria should be obtained. Chest X-ray should also be obtained
- *Neuroimaging:* Magnetic resonance imaging (MRI) or computed tomography scan may give valuable information such as presence of bleed, cerebral edema, temporal lobe hypodensities in HSE, thalamic abnormalities in JE, and basal exudates and hydrocephalus in tubercular meningitis. Computed tomography may also show brain herniation, effacement of cisterns, infective collections such as brain abscesses and subdural empyema. Neuroimaging is not needed if the etiology is clear by other investigations, e.g., cerebral malaria, pyogenic meningitis. Suggestive MRI findings are present in some conditions of viral encephalitis such as HSE, JE, and enterovirus encephalitis
- Throat swab, nasopharyngeal swab.

Step IV: Empirical Treatment

Empirical treatment must be started, pending the results of investigations.

- *Ceftriaxone:* A broad spectrum antibiotic, such as ceftriaxone must be given, which can be stopped if there is no evidence of bacterial meningitis
- Acyclovir (should be started in all suspected sporadic viral encephalitis). Dose of acyclovir 3 months to 12 years is 500 mg/m^2 8 hourly. In children above 12 years 10 mg/kg 8 hourly. Duration of treatment in confirmed cases should be 14–21 days intravenous treatment and minimum 21 days for those aged 3 months to 12 years
- Artemether combination therapy: in cerebral malaria.

Step V: Supportive Care and Treatment

- Euglycemia should be maintained, fever should be controlled and hydration maintained
- Raised ICP to be treated with mild head-end elevation by 15–30°. Mannitol 20% IV 5 mL/kg over 30 minutes as first dose then 2.5 mL/kg at 6 hourly intervals up to 48 hours. Injection furosemide IV 1 mg/kg up to 40 mg can be given
- *Seizures:* Anticonvulsant to be given if history of seizures or if GCS less than 8, or child has features of raised ICP
- *Steroids:* Pulse steroids (methylprednisolone or dexamethasone) to be given in children with suspected acute disseminated encephalomyelitis.

Step VI: Prevention/Treatment of Complications and Rehabilitation

- Physiotherapy, posture change, prevention of bed sores, and exposure keratitis
- Complications like aspiration pneumonia, nosocomial infections, and coagulation defects to be treated accordingly
- *Nutrition:* Early feeding should be initiated
- Psychological support to patient and family.

PREVENTION OF ACUTE ENCEPHALITIS SYNDROME

Prevention and/or control of AES require a multipronged strategy. It consists of:

- Surveillance for cases of AES
- Vector control
- Reduction in man-vector contact
- Vaccination.

KEY POINTS

- Acute encephalitis syndrome (AES) may be due to different viruses including Japanese B encephalitis, bacteria, fungus, parasites, spirochetes, chemical/toxins, etc.
- Clinically acute onset of fever (period of up to 14 days is considered acute) and a change in mental status and/or new onset of seizure.
- Case fatality is high and survivors often have neurologic sequelae.
- Acute encephalitis syndrome is a medical emergency, requires immediate consideration of vital functions, identification of cause, and institution of specific therapy, if available.
- All AES cases should be reported.

SUGGESTED READING

1. Guidelines: Clinical Management of Acute Encephalitis Syndrome including Japanese Encephalitis. Government of India. Directorate of National Vector Borne Disease Control Programme. Directorate General of Health Services, Ministry of Health & Family Welfare, 2009.
2. Japanese Encephalitis Clinical Care Guidelines. PATH, November, 2006. [online] Available from: www.path.org/vaccineresources/filesJE_clinical_care_guidelines_PATH.pdf. [Accessed November, 2013].
3. John TJ. Outbreak of killer brain disease in children: mystery or missed diagnosis? Indian Pediatr. 2003;40:863-9.
4. Kneen R, Michael BD, Menson E, Mehta B, Easton A, Hemingway C, et al. Management of suspected viral encephalitis in children—Association of British Neurologists and British Pediatric Allergy Immunology and Infection Group National Guidelines. J Infect. 2012;64:449-77.
5. Kumar R, Tripathi P, Singh S, Bannerji G. Clinical features in children hospitalized during the 2005 epidemic of Japanese encephalitis in Uttar Pradesh, India. Clin Infect Dis. 2006;43:123-31.
6. Ministry of Health and Family Welfare, Government of India. Facility-based IMNCI (F-IMNCI) Participants Manual. Government of India, New Delhi, 2009. [online] Available from: www.unicef.org/india/FBC_Participants_Manual.pdf. [Accessed November, 2013].
7. Sharma S, Mishra D, Aneja S, Kumar R, Jain A, Vashishtha VM. Consensus Guidelines on Evaluation and management of Suspected Acute Viral Encephalitis in Children in India. Indian Pediatr. 2012;49:897-910.
8. World Health Oraganization. Acute Encephalitis Syndrome. Japanese encephalitis surveillance standards. January 2006. From WHO-recommended standards for surveillance of selected vaccine-preventable diseases. WHO/V&B/03.01. [online] Available from: http://www.who.int/vaccines-documents/DocsPDF06/843.pdf. [Accessed November, 2013].

CHAPTER 52

Acute Osteomyelitis

Baldev S Prajapati, Rajal B Prajapati

INTRODUCTION

Acute osteomyelitis in children is an important condition because of its potential to cause permanent disability. It is common in infants and toddlers than in older children. Early recognition of acute osteomyelitis in young patients before extensive infection develops and prompt institution of appropriate medical and surgical therapy minimize permanent damage. Acute osteomyelitis in neonates and infants is commonly associated with septic arthritis due to peculiar vascularity of the physis and epiphysis. The risk is greatest if the physis (the growth plate of bone) is damaged. Once the growth plate forms, it acts as a barrier and in toddlers and children the infection is usually confined to the metaphysis.

PATHOGENESIS

The unique anatomy and circulation of the ends of long bones result in the predilection for localization of blood borne bacteria. In the metaphysis, nutrient arteries branch into non-anastomosing capillaries under the physis, which make a sharp loop before entering venous sinusoids draining into the marrow **(Fig. 1)**. Blood flow in this area is sluggish and provides an ideal environment for bacteria seeding. Once a bacterial focus is established, phagocytes migrate to the site and produce inflammatory exudates (metaphyseal abscess). The generation of proteolytic enzymes, toxic oxygen radicals, and cytokines result in decreased oxygen tension, decreased pH, osteolysis, and tissue destruction. As the inflammatory exudate progresses, pressure increases spread through the porous metaphyseal space via the Haversian system and Volkmann canals into the subperiosteal space. Purulence beneath the periosteum may lift the periosteal membrane of the bony surface, further impairing blood supply to the cortex and metaphysis.

In the newborns and young infants, transphyseal blood vessels connect the metaphysis and epiphysis **(Fig. 2)**.

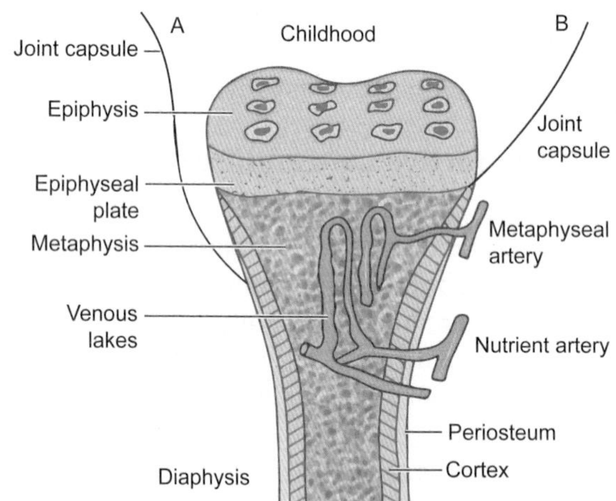

Fig. 1: Anatomy and circulation of the ends of long bones—the hair-pin bend (sharp loop) of the blood vessels resulting in sluggish blood flow and stasis of bacteria.

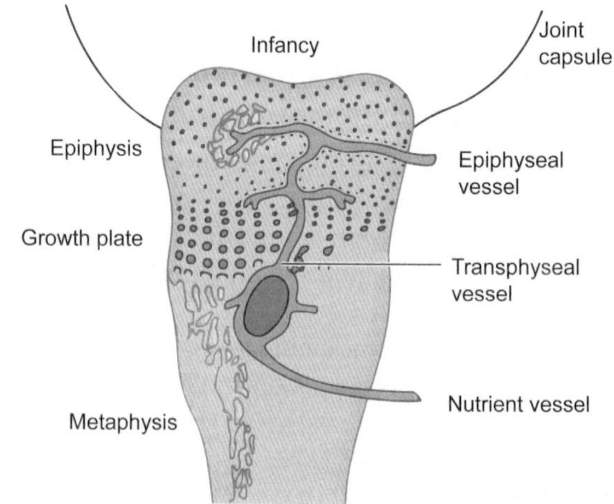

Fig. 2: In the new born and young infant, transphyseal blood vessels connect the metaphysic and epiphysis resulting in osteomyelitis with septic arthritis.

So it is common for pus from the metaphysis to enter the joint space. This extension through the physis (growth plate) has the potential to result in abnormal growth and bone or joint deformity. During the later part of infancy, the physis forms, obliterating the transphyseal blood vessels. Joint involvement once the physis forms may occur in joint where the metaphysis is intraarticular (hip, ankle, shoulder, and elbow) and subperiosteal pus ruptures into the joint space.

In the later childhood, the periosteum becomes more adherent, favoring pus to decompress through the periosteum. Once the growth plate closes in the late adolescence, hematogenous osteomyelitis more often begins in diaphysis and can spread to the entire intramedullary canal. With trivial trauma, the hematoma which forms in the metaphysis acts as a perfect soil for bacteria to seed.

ETIOLOGY

Bacteria are the most common pathogens in acute osteomyelitis. *Staphylococcus aureus* is the most common infecting organism in all age groups, including new borns. *Escherichia coli*, *Klebsiella*, and Group B streptococci are also prominent pathogens in neonates. Group A streptococci constitutes less than 10% of all cases. After the age of 6 years, most cases of acute osteomyelitis are caused by *S. aureus*, *streptococcus* or *Pseudomonas aeruginosa*. *Salmonella* species and *S. aureus* are the two most common causes of osteomyelitis in children with sickle cell anemia. *Pneumococcus* may also cause osteomyelitis in children with sickle cell anemia.

Infection with atypical mycobacteria, *S. aureus* or *Pseudomonas* can occur after penetrating injuries. Fungal infection usually occurs as part of multisystem disseminated disease. Candida osteomyelitis sometimes complicates fungemia in neonates with indwelling vascular catheters.

Overcrowded neonatal nursery, poor aseptic precautions while insertion of indwelling catheters and other procedures and their poor maintenance are common factors responsible for hematogenous spread acute osteomyelitis in neonates and young infants. It is very common scenario at our set up that a neonate presents with acute osteomyelitis after few days of discharge from nursery. Nosocomial infections are also very common in this group.

Community acquired Methicillin-resistant *Staphylococcus aureus* (MRSA) is also emerging as a potent cause of acute osteomyelitis in children in many parts of the world, including India.

Acute osteomyelitis following skin infection like pyoderma or pneumonia is also known in our patients **(Table 1)**.

CLINICAL MANIFESTATIONS

The signs and symptoms of acute osteomyelitis are highly dependent on the age of the patient **(Box 1)**.

- Abrupt onset of high grade fever. Fever is present in only 50% of neonates
- Signs of toxemia and irritability, like generalized manifestations, are more common in neonates
- Pain with movement of the affected extremity. Pseudoparalysis (restriction of movement) is very common in neonates and young infants due to pain
- Limp or refusal to walk in older children with involvement of lower extremities
- Affected limb held in position of flexion of adjacent joints
- Local edema, erythema and tenderness
- Focal tenderness over a long bone
- Local swelling and redness indicate infection has spread out of the metaphysis into the subperiosteal space.

TABLE 1: Shows organisms causing acute osteomyelitis and their association with different conditions.

Common clinical association	*Microorganism*
Frequent microorganism in any type of osteomyelitis	*Staphylococcus aureus* (MSSA or MRSA)
Sickle cell disease	*Salmonella* species, *S. aureus* and *S. pneumoniae*
Foreign body associated infections (catheters)	CONS (coagulase negative staphylococcus)
Nosocomial infections	Enterobacteriaceae, *Pseudomonas, Candida*
HIV	Bartonella
Immunocompromised	*Aspergillus* species, *Candida albicans, Mycobacteria* species

(HIV: human immunodeficiency virus; MRSA: methicillin resistant *staphylococcus aureus*; MSSA: methicillin sensitive *staphylococcus aureus*)

BOX 1: Common clinical manifestations.

- Abrupt onset of high grade fever. Fever only in 50% of neonates
- Signs of toxemia, irritability more common in neonates
- Pain with movement of affected extremity
- Restriction of movement—pseudoparalysis
- Limp or refusal to walk
- Limb held in flexion of adjacent joints
- Local edema, erythema, tenderness, cellulitis

It represents secondary soft tissue inflammatory response (cellulitis)

- Long bones are commonly involved in acute osteomyelitis. Femur (27%), tibia (22%), and humerus (12%) are common bones involved in osteomyelitis. The femur and tibia together constitute almost half of the cases. Flat bones are less commonly affected
- Single site of bone or joint involvement is common. The exception is osteomyelitis in neonates, in whom two or more bones are affected in almost half of the cases
- Subacute symptoms and focal findings in metaphyseal area over tibia may be due to a Brodie abscess.

LABORATORY INVESTIGATIONS (BOX 2)

- No specific laboratory tests for osteomyelitis
- Complete blood count (CBC), erythrocyte sedimentation rate (ESR), and C-reactive protein (CRP) are sensitive for bone infections but are non-specific and cannot distinguish between skeletal infections and other inflammatory conditions. Leukocytosis with increased polymorphs is very common. Acute phase reactants, like ESR, and CRP are significantly raised
- Blood culture should be routine in all cases of suspected osteomyelitis. It may be positive in 50% of cases with hematogenous osteomyelitis
- Aspiration for Gram stain and culture is the definitive diagnostic technique.

RADIO IMAGING STUDIES (BOX 3)

Radio imaging studies play a crucial role in evaluation of osteomyelitis. Conventional radiographs, ultrasonography, computed tomography, magnetic resonance imaging and radionuclide studies may all contribute to establishing the diagnosis. Plain radiographs are often used for initial evaluation to exclude other causes such as trauma and foreign bodies. Magnetic resonance imaging has emerged as a very sensitive and specific test and is widely used for diagnosis. The sequence of radionuclide studies or MRI is often determined by age, site and clinical presentation.

Plain Radiographs

- Overlying soft tissue edema after 3–5 days infection may be suggesting osteomyelitis
- Lytic bone changes are evident on radiographs after 7–14 days of onset of infection in tubular long bones. Flat and irregular bones can take longer time. Lytic bone changes are not visible on radiographs until 30–50% of bony matrix is destroyed.

BOX 2: Laboratory investigations.

- No specific laboratory tests
- Leukocytosis with raised polymorphs
- Significantly raised erythrocyte sedimentation rate and C-reactive protein
- Blood culture
- Aspiration for Gram stain and culture

BOX 3: Radio imaging studies.

- Plain radiograph shows lytic bone changes after 7–14 days of onset of infection. It is very late. Do not wait for radiographical changes for diagnosis
- Ultrasonography (USG)—simple and inexpensive. Very sensitive. USG guided aspiration has found positive in 70–80% of cases
- Magnetic resonance imaging is best radiographic imaging, effective in early detection and surgical localization, sensitivity 90–100%

Ultrasonography

- Simple and inexpensive
- Very sensitive, can diagnose subtle signs like subperiosteal edema soft tissue swelling within 2–3 days of infection
- USG guided aspiration can be attempted to determine presence of infection. Aspiration has found positive results in 70–80% of cases.

Computed Tomography Scan

- CT can demonstrate osseous and soft tissue abnormalities and is ideal for detecting gas in soft tissues
- Can depict abnormal calcification, ossification and intra-cortical abnormalities
- Most useful in the evaluation of spinal vertebral lesions, pelvis, sternum, etc.

Magnetic Resonance Imaging

- Best radiographic imaging technique for identification of abscess and differentiation between bone and soft tissue infection
- Effective in early detection and surgical localization of osteomyelitis
- Sensitivity ranges from 90 to 100%.

Radionuclide Bone Scanning

- Useful when osteomyelitis is suspected but difficult to ascertain clinically
- Can detect osteomyelitis within 24–48 hours after onset of symptoms
- Three phase imaging with 99 m Tc has 85–100% sensitivity and 75–95% specificity in hematogenous osteomyelitis
- Sensitivity in neonates is much lower due to poor bone mineralization.

Radio nuclide bone scanning is useful when osteomyelitis is suspected but difficult to ascertain clinically, can detect in 24–48 hours, less sensitive in neonates.

DIFFERENT DIAGNOSIS

- Trauma
- Leukemia
- Sickle cell disease
- Hemophilia
- Collagen disorders
- Neuroblastoma

TREATMENT

The treatment of osteomyelitis comprised of:

- Antibiotic therapy
- Surgical therapy
- Physiotherapy.

Antibiotic Therapy (Box 4)

The primary treatment for osteomyelitis is parenteral antibiotics that penetrate bone and joint cavities and most effective to the likely organisms.

- *Neonates:*
  - Cefotaxime 200 mg/kg/day divided in three doses Intravenous (IV) + Injection cloxacillin 150–200 mg/kg/day divided in four doses IV
  - If MRSA is considered as likely organism → injection vancomycin is substituted for cloxacillin
  - If neonate is a preterm baby or has a central vascular catheter → Possibility of nosocomial bacteria like pseudomonas or coagulase negative staphylococcus or fungi should be considered
- *In older infants and children:*
  - Common organisms are *S. aureus* and *streptococcus* → injection cefazolin 100–150 mg/kg/day divided in three doses or injection cloxacillin 150–200 mg/kg/day in divided four doses
  - If MRSA is suspected → vancomycin is substituted for cloxacillin
  - Injection cefotaxime 200 mg/kg/day in three divided doses or inj. ceftrixone 100 mg/kg/day in two divided doses may be used to cover *Haemophilus influenzae* type B (Hib) and other organisms
- Patients of sickle cell disease with osteomyelitis, *Salmonella* and *S. aureus* should be covered → inj. cefotaxime 200 mg/kg/day divided in three doses IV or inj. ceftraixone 100 mg/kg/day divided in two doses IV → inj. clindamycin 40 mg/kg/day divided in four doses IV is useful alternative for sensitive to beta lactam drugs. In addition to good anti-staphylococcus activity, clindamycin has broad activity against anaerobes and is useful for the treatment of infection secondary to penetrating injuries or compound fractures
- Injection vancomycin and injection clindamycin are alternatives for MRSA
- Immunocompromised patients with osteomyelitis:
  - Injection vancomycin + inj. ceftzidime or inj. piperacillin - tazobactam + inj. amikacin
- Changes of antibiotics should be considered, once pathogens are identified

BOX 4: Antibiotic therapy.

Neonates
- Inj. cefotaxime 200 mg/kg/day divided in three doses IV + inj. cloxacillin 150–200 mg/kg/day divided in four doses IV
- If MRSA suspected → inj. vancomycin is substituted for inj. cloxacillin
- If preterm or central vascular catheter → consider antibiotics to cover CONS, pseudomonas and fungi

Older infants and children
- Injection cefazolin 100–150 mg/kg/day divided in three doses IV or inj. cloxacillin 150–200 mg/kg/day in four divided doses IV
- If MRSA suspected → vancomycin is substituted by cloxacillin
- Injection cefotaxime or inj. ceftriaxone for Hib and other organisms

Sickle cell
- Injection cefotaxime or inj. ceftriaxone or inj. clindamycin
- Immunocompromised children:
- Injection vancomycin + inj. ceftizidime or Inj. piperacillin – tazobactam + Inj. amikacin
- Intravenous antibiotics 2–3 weeks → oral antibiotics. Total duration 4–6 weeks

(CONS: coagulase negative staphylococcus; Hib: haemophilus influenzae type B; Inj.: injection; MRSA: methicillin-resistant *staphylococcus aureus*)

- *Sequential antibiotics therapy:*
  - Intravenous antibiotics duration varies from 10 days to 3 weeks. Appropriate antibiotic respond includes clinical and laboratory improvement. A decreasing CRP and white blood cell count with absence of local signs and symptoms should initiate to oral antibiotics.
- *Duration of antibiotic therapy:*
  - For *S. aureus* or gram-negative bacillary infections, the minimal duration of antibiotics is 28 days, but 6 weeks therapy is desirable.
  - For Group A *streptococcus* and *S. pneumoniae* or Hib, the minimal duration is 14 days.

Surgical Therapy

Indications for surgical therapy should be defined **(Box 5)**.

- *Interventions:*
  - Drainage of subperiosteal abscess
  - Decompression of intra-medullary cavity

BOX 5: Indications for surgical therapy.

- Soft tissue or periosteal abscess
- Sinus tract formation
- Presence of necrotic or non-viable bone
- Prolonged fever, swelling, pain and erythema
- Possibility of foreign body
- Involvement of joint

Flowchart 1: Management of acute osteomyelitis.

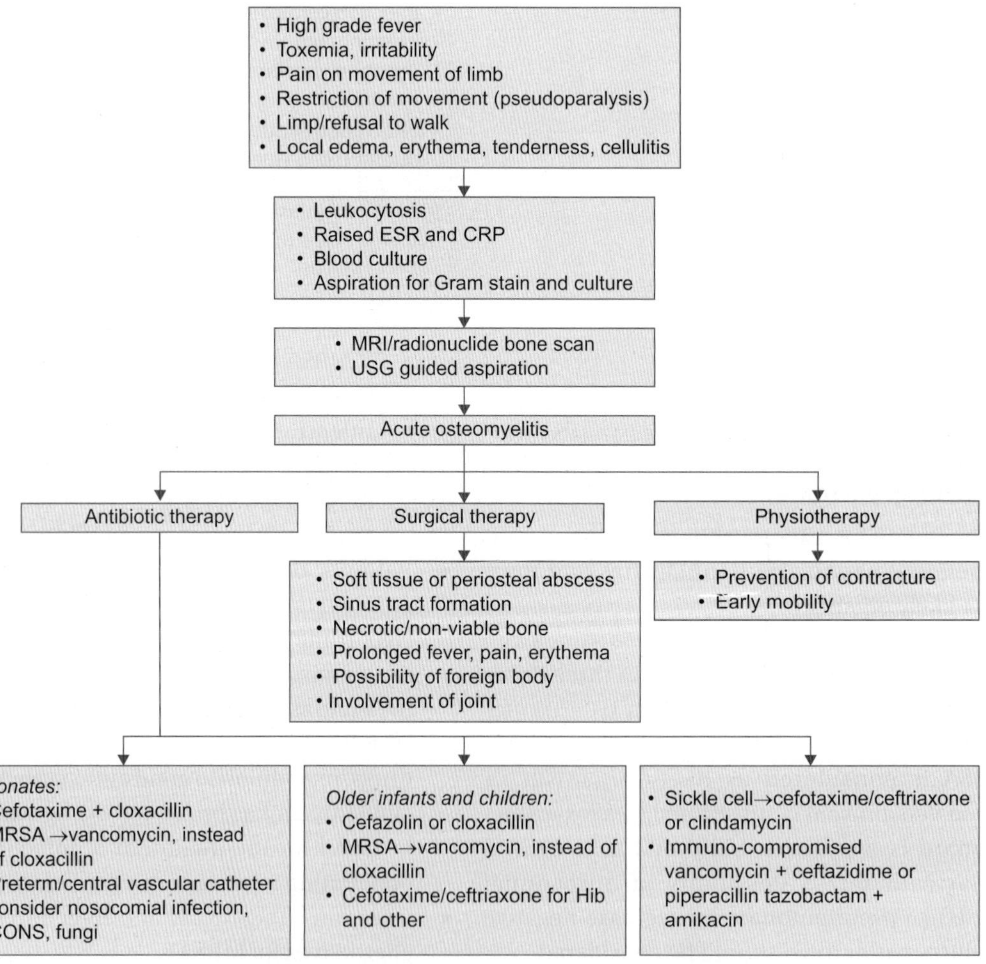

(CONS: coagulase negative staphylococcus; CRP: c-reactive protein; ESR: erythrocyte sedimentation rate; IV: intravenous; MRI: magnetic resonance imaging; MRSA: methicillin-resistant *staphylococcus aureus*; USG: ultrasonography)

- Complete removal of all necrotic tissues
- Splint application to prevent muscle spasm and pathological fractures.

Physiotherapy for Prevention of Contractures and Early Mobility

Prognosis

- When the pus is drained and appropriate antibiotic therapy is given, improvement in signs and symptoms is rapid
- Failure to improve or worsening by 72 hours, requires review of the appropriateness of antibiotic therapy, need for surgical intervention or correctness or diagnosis
- Acute phase reactants (ESR and CRP) may be helpful for monitoring the response to therapy. Long-term follow-up is necessary for sequelae like contractures and bone length
- Meticulous following to **Flowchart 1** is quite rewarding in most cases.

Complications

- Septicemia
- Chronic osteomyelitis
- Septic arthritis
- Pathological fracture
- Growth plate disturbances.

CONCLUSION

Acute osteomyelitis in children is an important condition because of its potential to cause permanent disability. Long bones are commonly involved in acute osteomyelitis in children. The unique anatomy and circulation of the ends of long bones (hair-pin bend of blood vessels) result in sluggish circulation and localization of blood borne bacteria. Acute osteomyelitis in neonates and infants is commonly associated with septic arthritis due to peculiar vascularity of physis and epiphysis. Bacteria are the most common pathogens in acute osteomyelitis in children. *Staphylococcus aureus* is the most common infecting organism in all age groups, including newborns. Sickle cell anemia, penetrating injuries, nosocomial infections, certain skin infections, and immunocompromised like conditions are known to have association with very specific organisms responsible for acute osteomyelitis.

The clinical manifestations of acute osteomyelitis in children are highly dependent on the age of the patient. Fever, signs of toxemia, and irritability are more common in neonates. Pain, pseudoparalysis, limp, refusal to walk, local edema, erythema, tenderness, and cellulitis are other manifestations. There are no specific laboratory tests for osteomyelitis. Leukocytosis with polymorphonuclear reactions, significantly raised ESR and CRP are very common. Blood culture should be routine in all cases of suspected osteomyelitis. Aspiration for Gram stain and culture is the definite diagnostic technique.

Radio imaging studies play a crucial role in evaluation of osteomyelitis. Plain radiograph shows lytic bone changes after 7–14 days of onset infection. Do not wait for plain radiographical changes for diagnosis of acute osteomyelitis, it is very late. Soft tissue edema may be evident after 5 days of infection. Ultrasonography is simple, inexpensive and very sensitive for subtle signs like subperiosteal edema and soft tissue swelling. Ultrasonography guided aspiration is rewarding, positive in 70–80% of cases. Magnetic resonance imaging is considered as best radio imaging technique for effective early detection and surgical localization of osteomyelitis. Sensitivity ranges from 90 to 100% Radionuclide bone scanning is useful when osteomyelitis is suspected but difficult to ascertain clinically. It is less sensitive in neonates.

The treatment of acute osteomyelitis is comprised of proper antibiotics in optimum doses by specific route of administration, for defined duration, usually 4–6 weeks, surgical intervention if required and physiotherapy. Early diagnosis and prompt, efficient management favor good prognosis.

CLINICAL PEARLS

- Acute osteomyelitis is an important condition because of its potential to cause permanent disability.
- Long bones are commonly involved in acute osteomyelitis in children. In neonates and infants, it is commonly associated with septic arthritis due to peculiar vascularity of physis and epiphysis.
- Bacteria are the most common pathogens in acute osteomyelitis in children. *Staphylococcus aureus* is the most common organism. Association of different organisms with very specific condition is known.
- Fever, toxemia, and irritability are common clinical manifestations in neonates. Pain, pseudoparalysis, limp, refusal to walk, local edema, erythema, tenderness, and cellulitis are other manifestations.

- Leukocytosis with raised polymorphonuclear cells and raised erythrocyte sedimentation rate and C-reactive protein are very common. Blood culture should be routinely done in all cases.
- Radioimaging studies play a crucial role in evaluation of osteomyelitis. Plain radiograph shows lytic bone changes after 7–14 days of onset of infection. Do not wait for radiological changes for diagnosis, it is very late. Ultrasonography is simple, inexpensive, and very sensitive for subtle signs. Ultrasonography guided aspiration is rewarding, positive in 70–80% of cases. Magnetic resonance imaging is considered as the best radioimaging technique. Radionuclide bone scanning is useful when osteomyelitis is suspected but difficult to ascertain.
- The treatment of acute osteomyelitis is comprised of appropriate antibiotics in optimum doses by specific route of administration, for 4–6 weeks duration, surgical intervention if required, and physiotherapy.
- Early diagnosis along with prompt and efficient management favor the good prognosis.

KEY POINTS

- Acute osteomyelitis in children is an important condition because of its potential to cause permanent disability.
- Long bones are commonly involved in acute osteomyelitis in children.
- *Staphylococcus aureus* is the most common infecting organism in all age groups, including newborns.
- Fever, signs of toxemia, and irritability are more common in neonates. Pain, pseudoparalysis, limp, refusal to walk, local edema, erythema, tenderness, and cellulitis are other manifestations.
- Blood culture should be routine in all cases of suspected osteomyelitis. Aspiration for Gram stain and culture is the definite diagnostic technique.
- Plain radiograph shows lytic bone changes after 7–14 days of onset infection. Magnetic resonance imaging is considered as the best radio imaging technique.
- The drug of choice for treating osteomyelitis is cefazolin/cloxacillin for 4–6 weeks. Intravenous antibiotics can be switched to oral once acute signs of inflammation have subsided.

SUGGESTED READING

1. Bhaskar A. Acute osteomyelitis in children. In: Shah MA, Vekariya PM, Chowdhary J (Eds). Challenges in the Management of Pediatric Bone & Joint Infections. pp. 81-3.
2. Gutierrez KM. Osteomyelitis In: Long SS, Pickering LK, Prober C. (Eds). Principles & Practice of Pediatric Infectios Diseases, 3rd edition. 2008. pp. 474-82.
3. Kaplan S. Osteomyelitis. In: Kliegman RM, Stanton BF, Geme III JWS, et al. (Ed.). Nelson Textbook of Pediatrics. 19th ed. India. Elsevier Saunders. 2012. pp. 2394-98.
4. Mitra M. Skeletal infections. In: Ghosh TK, Yewale V, Parathasarathy A, Shah NK (Eds). IAP Speciality Series on Pediatric Infectious Diseases (Under IAP Action Plan, 2006), 1st edition. 2006. pp. 111-22.

Algorithmic Approach to Short Duration Fever without Focus in Older Infants and Children

Suhas V Prabhu

INTRODUCTION

Fever in an older infant and child (>3 months of age) is one of the most common cases presenting to the pediatrician (up to half of outpatient visits). The causes may vary from something as innocuous as a nonspecific viral infection needing only symptomatic treatment to more dangerous ones such as dengue, malaria, or bacteremic infections requiring correct diagnosis and prompt intervention.

CAUSES

Bacteremia will be seen in between 3 and 5% of children with fever without focus in this age group, especially if the fever is >39°C. While bacteremia due to organisms such as *Streptococcus pneumoniae, Staphylococcus,* and *Haemophilus influenzae* is more common in children younger than 2 years, in older children, typhoid and paratyphoid fevers account for the majority of bacterial causes. Parasitic infestations like malaria also account for a large percentage of fevers in this age group in certain parts of the country in certain seasons.

APPROACH

The clinician's approaches to these patients need to be one of a cautious balance between over investigation and/or unnecessary usage of antibiotics versus the other extreme of missing the child with serious infection who will suffer because of delayed diagnosis and intervention. While the majority of cases will need only symptomatic treatment and observation for the first 2 or 3 days, the clinician needs to be alert to pick up those who are more likely to have serious illnesses bacterial or otherwise that need to be investigated promptly.

The first step therefore is to assess for toxicity (degree of severity of illness). Signs of severe infection/sepsis or danger signs requiring immediate workup and possible hospitalization can be easily remembered by the mnemonic ABCD:

- *A*ctivity and *A*lertness (reduction of or *A*ltered sensorium)
- *B*reathing (difficult or fast)
- *C*olor (cyanosis, pallor, decreased capillary fill time) and *C*ry (weak or high pitched)
- *D*ehydration (poor intake and oliguria)

Additional factors may exist that need to be considered such as an immune-compromised patient (human immunodeficiency virus, asplenia, etc.), child with an indwelling foreign body (port, shunt, prosthesis, etc.), condition predisposing to subacute bacterial endocarditis (bicuspid aortic valve, small ventricular septal defect, etc.), compromised due to chronic cardiovascular disease or severe protein energy malnutrition, latent cortisol deficiency congenital adrenal hyperplasia, and so on. This subset of patients should be investigated and treated more aggressively than the general population.

The second step is to ensure that it is truly a fever without focus. Make an extra effort to look for a focus although in the history or on cursory examination there is no apparent one. In particular, look for otitis media, joint involvement, local skin infections, rash, urinary symptoms, etc., if found appropriate investigation and treatment should be done.

If no focus is found after a thorough history and physical examination, and the child is not toxic, there are no risk factors, and the temperature is <39°C, it is safe to observe the child with antipyretics alone and reassess after 48–72 hours. Parents must be informed about danger signs (ABCD listed earlier) that should prompt them to return for medical reevaluation earlier. However, if the child is already suffering with fever for the past 2–3 days and there is no focus found on the day of presentation, then the child should be investigated straightaway.

Even this early in the fever episode, in the context of an ongoing viral epidemic, or even on grounds of high clinical suspicion, an attempt can be made to diagnose a viral infection. This would be by molecular testing for specific viral antigens or nucleic acid. Some examples of this are the rapid strip test for severe acute respiratory syndrome coronavirus 2 (SARS-CoV-2) ribonucleic acid (RNA) on a throat swab, NS1 antigen of dengue virus in a blood sample, etc. While there is no specific antiviral treatment to be offered even on diagnosis of these conditions, a definite etiological diagnosis will enable the child to be observed for progress of the illness and possible complications. It will also allay the pediatrician's anxiety of a possible missed bacterial infection and ensure antimicrobial stewardship by offering firm ground to withhold antibiotics. Newer modalities of array testing for multiple deoxyribonucleic acid (DNA)/RNA are available and some of these commercial kits include bacterial and malarial pathogen testing too. But they are too expensive for widespread use and should be used selectively. Also, proper interpretation is required if multiple pathogens test positive, in order to correctly identify the actual pathogen in that particular patient.

Once a decision is made to look for a bacterial infection, the initial investigations should consist of the following: Complete blood count (CBC), an acute phase reactant marker like C-reactive protein (CRP), urinalysis and, where feasible, blood and urine cultures. Tests for malaria (smear for malarial parasite and/or rapid malarial antigen test) or dengue (NS1 antigen ± dengue immunoglobulin G and immunoglobulin M) should be added if the epidemiology warrants.

However, additionally, if the child is severely toxic or dehydrated or has signs of early sepsis, hospitalization is mandatory for observation, stabilization, and prompt empirical administration of antibiotics. Ceftriaxone at 100 mg/kg/day is usually an appropriate initial choice. On the other hand, in situations where availability or affordability is a problem and the child is not too sick, the initial step may be only a CBC with (where appropriate) smear for malarial parasite and a routine urinalysis. If the white cell count is >15,000/mm^3 or bandemia or toxic granulation is present, a blood culture would be advisable. Similarly, if the urinalysis shows pyuria, urine culture should be asked for before the first dose of antibiotic is administered. If there is leukopenia [white blood cell (WBC) count below 4,000] then possibilities of enteric fever, malaria, dengue, and viral infection should be considered and appropriate investigations asked for. If the WBC count is normal and low with absolute eosinopenia and there is a very high CRP enteric fever should be considered and blood cultures sent before starting antibiotics **(Flowchart 1)**.

The CBC needs to be evaluated in detail rather than only looking for leukocytosis. **Table 1** indicates possible clues to the diagnosis from the humble CBC.

The CRP (if done) can help to distinguish bacterial from viral fevers even on the second or third day of illness. But a mildly elevated CRP can be seen in some viral infections like adenovirus or viral infections with secondary bacterial complications. However, a very high CRP (>40 mg/L)

Flowchart 1: Approach to short duration fever without focus in older infants and children.

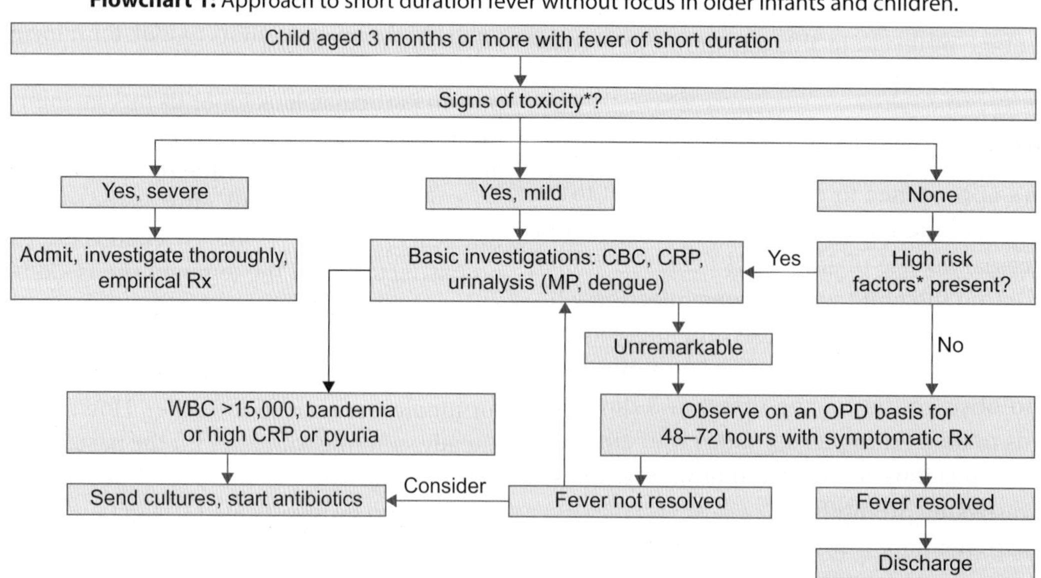

*See text for details.

(CBC: complete blood count; CRP: C-reactive protein; WBC: white blood cell)

TABLE 1: Clues to the diagnosis from the humble complete blood count.

Parameter	*Enteric fever*	*Malaria*	*Dengue fever*	*Other viral fevers*
Hemoglobin/hematocrit	Normal	Low	Normal/high	Normal
Total white blood cell	Normal/Low	Normal/Low	Low/very low	Normal/Low
Differential white blood cell	Polys predominant, Eosinopenia	Monocytosis	Lymphocytosis	Lymphocytosis, activated lymphocytes
Platelets	Normal/Low	Low	Low	Normal/Low

is more likely to be due to a bacterial infection and a clue to further investigation or empirical antibiotic therapy.

KEY POINTS

- Examine thoroughly to rule out an occult focus.
- In all sick children or in those with no focus even after 2–3 days of fever, perform investigations including CBC, smear for malarial parasite, CRP, and urine routine.
- Molecular tests for viruses and other pathogens are available and can be done on clinical suspicion. Multiple (array) testing should be restrictively used and correctly interpreted.
- Other investigations that may be asked for depending on findings on initial investigations or clinical setting include urine and blood cultures and dengue serology.
- Careful interpretation of the CBC is important, often repeat testing is required.
- Mildly elevated CRP can be seen in viral infections.
- Widal test is of no value in the first 7 days. Blood culture is the most reliable method to diagnose enteric fever.

In certain circumstances, the first CBC may be unremarkable but repeat CBCs might yield the diagnosis, e.g., in dengue, serial CBC shows decline in the WBC and platelet count and rising hematocrit. The Widal test is of no utility in evaluation of fever of <7 days duration.

SUGGESTED READING

1. Baker MD. Evaluation and management of infants with fever. Pediatr Clinics North Am. 1999;46:1061-72.
2. Lorin MI. Fever: Pathogenesis and treatment. In: Feigin RD, Cherry J (Eds). Textbook of Pediatric Infectious Diseases, 4th edition. Philadelphia, WB Saunders; 1998. pp. 89-94.
3. Manabe YC, Betz J, Jackson O, Asoala V, Bazan I, Blair PW, et al. Clinical Evaluation of the BioFire Global Fever Panel for the identification of malaria, leptospirosis, chikungunya and dengue from whole blood a prospective, multicentre cross-sectional diagnostic accuracy study. Lancet Infect Dis. 2022;22(9):1356-64.

Fever with Rash

Ritabrata Kundu, Aniruddha Ghosh

INTRODUCTION

Skin is the mirror of many internal ailments which may manifest as rashes. At the outset one should determine the types of rashes which are as follows.

Macules are flat lesions of altered color in the skin. Papules are raised flat topped lesions with diameter of <5 mm, whereas nodules are >5 mm in diameter with raised rounded configuration. Vesicles are fluid filled lesions <5 mm in diameter and are known as bullae when they are >5 mm in diameter. Pustules are raised pus filled lesions. Purpuras are bleeding into the skin which are nonblanchable. When they are <5 mm in diameter they are known as petechiae and if they are >5 mm in diameter they are known as ecchymoses.

A good history in all cases must include site of onset of rash, rate, and direction of its spread. Inquire about medications taken in recent months, history of travel, exposure to insects and animals, immune status, and immunization history. It should also include history of any cardiac abnormality including prosthesis, exposure to ill individual, and sexually transmitted diseases.

Next one should determine the type of rash, i.e., its morphology, distribution, and arrangement of the lesions. At times, the morphology might change with passage of time for instance in dengue the initial diffuse flushing may give away to maculopapular rash. Also the spread of lesions should be taken into account as maculopapular rash of dengue which starts in the trunk spreads centrifugally to extremities and face.

CLASSIFICATION OF RASH WITH FEVER

It is broadly classified as follows:

- Centrally distributed maculopapular rash
- Peripheral rash
- Confluent desquamative rash
- Vesiculobullous rash
- Urticarial rash
- Nodular rash
- Purpuric rash
- Rashes with ulcer

Centrally Distributed Maculopapular Rash

They are most common type of rash which is mainly truncal. Most common viral infections seen in children belong to this group are discussed in **Table 1**.

Peripheral Rash (Table 2)

These rashes start at the periphery (acral) and then spread centripetally.

Confluent Desquamative Rash (Table 3)

They start with diffuse erythema often followed by desquamation.

Vesiculobullous Rash (Table 4)

They are mostly due to virus or bacterial infections.

Urticarial Rash (Table 5)

Classic urticaria (hives) is not associated with fever. They do not last at a particular location for >24 hours, does not have purpuric or pigmented component and itch rather than burn.

Purpuric Rash (Table 6)

Nonpalpable purpura is flat lesion due to bleeding in the skin. If <3 mm in diameter then it is known as petechiae whereas >3 mm in diameter then called ecchymoses. Palpable purpura is due to inflammation of the vessel wall (vasculitis) with subsequent hemorrhage causes raised lesions.

TABLE 1: Centrally distributed maculopapular rash.

Diseases	*Common recognizing features*
Measles	Respiratory prodrome; Koplik's spot in buccal mucosa which gradually wanes after onset of rash, maculopapular rash starting from hairline and behind the ears, spread down the trunk, and limbs. Rash fades in the order in which it appeared with brownish discoloration and desquamation
Rubella	Prodrome of fever and malaise, followed by posterior auricular, cervical and suboccipital lymphadenopathy, fever, and rash. Rash, maculopapular begins on face and spreads downward
Erythema infectiosum	Common in children between 3 and 12 years; bright (fifth disease) red "slapped cheek" appearance following a minor febrile prodrome
Exanthema subitum	Common in children below 3 years; diffuse (roseola) truncal maculopapular rash sparing face following resolution of fever
Infectious	• Common in older children and adolescents. Fever, mononucleosis sore throat, and lymphadenopathy are most common • Morbilliform or papular rash develops usually on trunk and arms
Drug rash	• Usually maculopapular common in trunk and symmetrical • Intensely pruritic, absence of respiratory catarrh and enanthems helps to distinguish from a viral eruption
Dengue	• Initially diffuse red flushing with pruritus followed by maculopapular rash on trunk which spreads centrifugally to extremities and face • Petechiae may be seen in some cases on extremities
Systemic lupus erythematosus	• Photosensitive butterfly rash on check and nose • Discoid, urticarial, or bullous lesion may also be seen
Juvenile rheumatoid arthritis	Evanescent erythematous papules on trunk appearing at the height of fever
Multisystem inflammatory syndrome in children (MIS-C)	Children, adolescents, and young adults after suffering from coronavirus disease 2019 (COVID-19) develop fever along with maculopapular rash and/or nonpurulent conjunctivitis, gastrointestinal symptoms, cardiovascular symptoms, etc., after developing an autoimmune response

TABLE 2: Peripheral rash.

Diseases	*Common recognizing features*
Erythema multiforme (infection and drugs)	• Target lesions symmetrical on palms, soles, knee, and elbow • The center of the lesion dusky violet color or petechiae • In erythema multiforme major, there is usually involvement of ocular, nasal oral, or genital mucous membrane
Hand-foot and mouth disease (coxsackievirus and enterovirus)	• Tender maculopapular lesion on hand, fingers, feet, buttocks and groin • Vesicular lesions are also seen • Involvement of buccal mucosa, pharynx, gingiva, and palate
Secondary syphilis	• Maculopapular rash frequently involving palms and soles • They are dark colored, nonpruritic, and discrete • Constitutional symptoms other than fever include malaise, sore throat, weight loss, and headache • There is also involvement of mucous membrane
Bacterial endocarditis	• Erythematous or hemorrhagic macules on palms and soles are painless (Janeway lesions) • Petechiae on skin and mucosa; tender red nodules on finger and toe pads (Osler's node) • Associated heart murmur

TABLE 3: Confluent desquamative rash.

Disease	*Common recognizing features*
Scarlet fever	• Blanchable erythema over face and upper trunk to start • Minute papules which give the skin a sandpaper feel • Associated feature include strawberry tongue • Subsidence of rash is followed by desquamation
Streptococcal toxic shock syndrome	• Generalized erythematous macular rash which desquamate • May develop other features which usually include hypotension, renal impairment, respiratory distress syndrome, coagulopathy, or soft tissue infection
Staphylococcal scalded skin syndrome	• Seen in infants and children below 5 years • Scarlatiniform erythema develops followed by sterile flaccid blisters • Nikolsky sign is positive with skin peeling off leaving moist and glistening denuded areas • Patient may appear well despite marked skin tenderness
Staphylococcal toxic shock syndrome	• Acute onset with high fever, erythematous macular rash which desquamates later and associated with hypotension • Multisystem involvement with thrombocytopenia, renal failure, liver, and central nervous system abnormality are seen
Kawasaki disease rashes	• Maculopapular, scarlatiniform, or erythema multiforme with accentuation in the groin area • Associated feature includes fissuring of the lips, conjunctivitis, strawberry tongue, edema of hands and feet with periungual desquamation of finger and toes • Illness predominantly in young children with majority under 5 years
Stevens–Johnson syndrome (SJS) and toxic epidermal necrolysis (TEN)	• SJS start as erythematous macule which develops central necrosis to form vesicles, bullae, and skin denudation • Extend of involvement is <10% of body surface area • Skin lesions are accompanied by two or more mucous membrane involvement like conjunctivitis, oral ulceration, or anogenital inflammation • TEN has involvement >30% of body surface area with more systemic symptoms like pulmonary or gastrointestinal involvement • In SJS/TEN, involvement is between 10 and 30%

TABLE 4: Vesiculobullous rash.

Disease	*Common recognizing feature*
Varicella	• Macules appears on trunk and face that rapidly spreads to other areas of the body • Lesions have an erythematous base which quickly evolves to vesicles, pustules and then crust formation • Lesions appear in crops with different stages of development • In healthy children it is usually associated with mild fever and malaise
Herpes simplex virus (HSV) infection	• Cutaneous lesions usually involve face, lips, gingiva, tongue, and palate • Erythema followed by grouped vesicles, which progress to pustules and crust formation • There is regional lymphadenopathy but systemic symptoms are usually absent
Herpes zoster	• Clustered vesicular lesions confined to one or two dermatomes • Pain, hyperesthesia, and fever are mild as compared to adults • Lesions completely resolve within 1 or 2 weeks

TABLE 5: Urticarial rash.

Disease	*Common recognizing feature*
Urticarial vasculitis	• Raised erythematous lesions with flat top • They are indurated, painful and sometimes lesions are purpuric • May have burning sensation and individual lesion lasts up to 5 days

TABLE 6: Purpuric rash.

Disease	*Common recognizing feature*
Acute meningococcemia	• Initial maculopapular lesion involving trunk and lower extremities • Lesions quickly evolving to petechiae and purpura may spread to involve upper extremities and face • Large ecchymoses with hemorrhagic bullae (purpura fulminans) indicate disseminated intravascular coagulation (DIC) • Associated features of meningitis and shock may be evident
Dengue hemorrhagic fever	• After a relatively benign first stage with fever, malaise, and headache patient suddenly collapses with cold extremities and irritability • Petechiae and purpura may be seen in extremities and face followed by ecchymoses
Rickettsial infections	• Indian spotted fever is associated with an initial maculopapular and then petechial/purpuric rash with peripheral distribution and involvement of palms and soles • In scrub typhus a necrotic rash is seen at the bite site and a centrally distributed rash

Nodular Rash

The most common nodular rash with fever is erythema nodosum. They are violaceous, tender, and large subcutaneous nodules seen particularly on lower legs above the shin bone. It may be due to drugs (penicillin and sulfonamide) infection (streptococcal, mycobacterial, and fungal) or idiopathic. Common associated feature include arthralgias.

KEY POINTS

- Fever with rash is a common and vexing problem.
- It may signify a serious disorder such as meningococcemia or dengue hemorrhagic fever or may be associated with a minor drug allergy.
- The most important factor that helps to determine the etiology of an exanthematous febrile illness is the nature of rash.
- All efforts should be made to diagnose the serious entities first and institute immediate treatment.
- For stable children, a specific diagnosis may not be always be possible. In this situation, symptomatic therapy, close observation, explanation of danger signs to parents, and staying away from school until the rash resolves are recommended.

SUGGESTED READING

1. Cherry JD. Cutaneous manifestations of systemic infections. In: Feigen RD, Cherry JD (Eds). Textbook of Pediatric Infectious Diseases, 4th edition. Philadelphia: WB Saunders; 1998. pp. 713-37.

Approach to Managing New-onset Fever in the Intensive Care Unit

Tanu Singhal

INTRODUCTION

New-onset fever is defined as fever occurring after 48 hours of admission to the intensive care unit (ICU) in a patient who was previously afebrile. It is generally considered as a sign of a hospital acquired/healthcare associated, or nosocomial infection. However, an infection may occur without fever and not all fever is due to infection. In certain circumstances, a new-onset fever may also be a continuum or a complication of a previously acquired infection. Approach to diagnosis and management of this clinical entity is discussed in this chapter **(Flowchart 1)**.

GENERAL PRINCIPLES IN DIAGNOSIS

Distinguishing Infectious from Noninfectious Causes of Fever

It must be remembered that fever can often be the result of noninfectious causes including postoperative atelectasis, drug fever, thrombophlebitis, transfusions, deep venous thrombosis, central fever, etc. Similarly, leukocytosis may not always be due to an infection; noninfectious causes include stress, bleeding, atelectasis, and steroids.

Flowchart 1: Algorithmic approach to new-onset fever in intensive care unit.

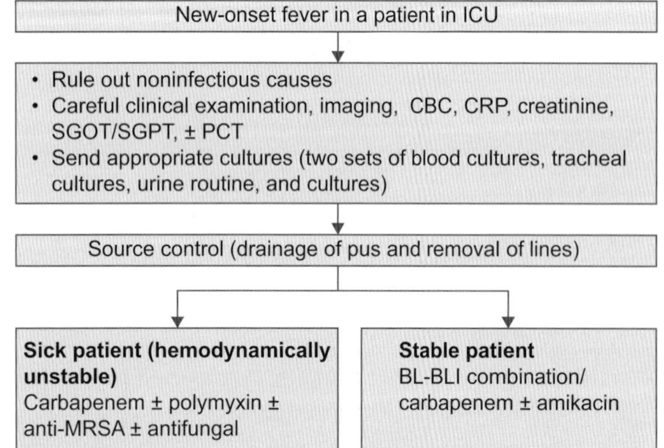

(BL-BLI: beta-lactam/beta-lactamase inhibitor; CBC: complete blood count; CRP: C-reactive protein; MRSA: methicillin-resistant *Staphylococcus aureus*; PCT: procalcitonin)

Determining the Site of Infection

Once, major noninfectious causes are excluded a thorough clinical assessment should be made for determining the site of infection. Common sites if infections in the ICU are bloodstream infections, especially in patients who have central lines, sinusitis/tracheobronchitis/pneumonia in patients on invasive ventilation, urinary tract infections in those who have indwelling catheters, surgical site infections in postsurgical patients, and sometimes enteric infections. *Clostridium difficile*-associated infection (CDAI) is less common in children as compared to adults. Central nervous system (CNS) infections and intra-abdominal sepsis should be also considered in children with predisposing procedures/interventions at these sites. Occult sites of infection include sinusitis, osteomyelitis, and septic arthritis. Eliciting symptoms referable to a particular system is often difficult in very sick children but should be done. A head to toe assessment should be done with careful inspection of the central line, exit site of central venous, respiratory system, nature of tracheal secretions, abdomen, bones, joints, examination of neck stiffness and surgical sites, and the skin. It is important to disrobe and examine the entire skin as these might show areas of cellulitis and pustules which indicate bacteremia/fungemia.

Distinguishing Infection from Colonization in the Nosocomial Setting

An important issue in managing nosocomial infections is to differentiate infection from colonization. In several ICUs, surveillance cultures are sent from nonsterile sites such as endotracheal tubes, central line ports, urinary catheters, and drains external ventricular drains (EVDs). These will always grow microbes as these sites are inevitably colonized. It is important that these colonizations are not treated with antibiotics as treating colonization will not prevent infection and only contributes to selection of resistant organisms. Unless an infection is suspected, no surveillance cultures should be sent. More difficult is to differentiate infection from colonization, in the setting when fever is associated with positive cultures from nonsterile sites. Here, careful interpretation is needed to ascertain whether the positive culture is colonization or true infection.

INVESTIGATIVE APPROACH

The initial investigations include a complete blood count and peripheral smear evaluation with acute phase reactants such as C-reactive protein (CRP)/procalcitonin. Signs of sepsis include neutrophilia/neutropenia, thrombocytopenia, shift to left/bandemia, and toxic granules in the neutrophils. Rise in acute phase reactants such as CRP and procalcitonin may indicate an infection. However, both of these may also increase due to noninfectious causes like previous surgery.

At least two sets of blood cultures each including one aerobic and one anaerobic culture should be sent. If there is a central catheter then one culture should be sent from the catheter lumen and the other from peripheral venipuncture. The total blood cultured should be 1% of the circulating blood volume. Confirmation of the diagnosis of a catheter-related bloodstream infections (CRBSIs) involves isolation of the identical organism with the same antibiogram from simultaneous cultures; one obtained through peripheral venipuncture and the other either catheter lumen blood culture or culture of the catheter tip. A positive lumen culture alone has poor positive predictive value for CRBSI as it may just indicate colonization; but high negative predictive value (90%).

In those with suspected urinary tract infection, a routine urine analysis and culture should be sent. Results of these investigations should be interpreted carefully as some degree of pyuria and significant bacteriuria (colony count of $>10^5$/mL) may be seen in any catheterized patient with no urinary tract infection.

For suspected hospital-acquired pneumonia, cultures of the respiratory secretions should be sent. Several methods such as quantitative endotracheal aspirates, bronchoalveolar lavage, and protected specimen brush have been recommended for diagnosis of pneumonia. Generally speaking, quantitative cultures of endotracheal secretions are easily done and of almost comparable yield as those of the bronchoscopic methods. Hence, in suspected ventilator-associated pneumonia (combination of fever/leukocytosis/purulent secretions/new infiltrates) quantitative endotracheal cultures should be sent and empirical antibiotic therapy initiated.

Cultures should also be sent from other suspected sites of infection such as surgical sites, cerebrospinal fluid (CSF), and abscesses. Care should be taken to send deep samples; skin swabs and cultures from drains may just indicate colonization. Since targeted therapy in sick improves outcomes, use of matrix-assisted laser desorption ionization-time of flight (MALDI-ToF) and molecular methods such as BCID panel/Xpert Carba for quicker identification of pathogens and resistance is recommended, if available. Molecular identification of pathogens directly from blood is not sufficiently validated and is not recommended at this time.

Imaging also assists in diagnosing site of infections. Basic imaging includes chest X-ray and ultrasonography abdomen. Presence of a new infiltrate on chest imaging is also not specific enough for a pneumonia as it may be due to atelectasis, progression of underlying lung disease, or due to thoracic surgery. In some patients, computerized scans of the thorax and abdomen may be needed to detect site of infection.

TREATMENT

The most important component of treatment of a nosocomial infection is appropriate antimicrobial therapy administered as soon as possible once sepsis is considered. At the same time, source control such as removal of an infected central line and drainage of pus and supportive therapy are also crucial.

Factors Determining Choice of Empiric Antimicrobial Therapy

Various factors determine the empiric choice of antibiotics and include:

- *Local epidemiologic data:* Knowledge of common microbial pathogens and their resistance profile in a particular ICU helps in making empirical choice of antibiotics till cultures are available. The most common etiologic agents for nosocomial infections in India are gram-negative pathogens including *Klebsiella*,

Escherichia coli, Pseudomonas, Acinetobacter, and *Enterobacter*. These are followed by gram-positive including *Staphylococcus aureus, S. epidermidis*, and enterococci. There is an increase in infections due to *Candida*. The most common species are *C. tropicalis, C. albicans, C. parapsilosis, C. krusei*, and *C. glabrata. C. auris* is an emerging super bug in ICUs and is characterized by its hardiness, transmissibility, and drug resistance. Most of the nosocomial pathogens are multidrug resistant. Most significant is drug resistance in gram-negative pathogens with 80% of nosocomial gram-negative isolates being resistant to third-generation cephalosporins by virtue of production of extended-spectrum beta-lactamases (ESBL) and beta-lactam/beta-lactamase inhibitor (BL-BLI) combinations by production of AmpC. The fall out of ESBL and AmpC-mediated resistance has been excessive use of carbapenems in ICU settings. Consequently, a significant proportion of gram-negative isolates (up to 50%) are now resistant to even carbapenems. Carbapenem-resistant gram-negative isolates have limited treatment options and associated with 50% mortality. *S. aureus* isolates are often methicillin resistant and the coagulase negative *S. aureus* are always methicillin resistant. Vancomycin resistance in enterococci is becoming increasingly common. Also seen is increasing fluconazole resistance in *Candida*.

- *Previous antibiotic usage:* This again helps in predicting the likely resistance profile of the microbe till culture results are available. Additionally, it helps in guessing what pathogens have not been appropriately covered till now.
- *Severity of infection:* For a patient who is critically sick or in septic shock, empiric therapy with a carbapenem with/without polymyxin may be needed till cultures are available as there is no leeway for making an error in choice of antibiotic nor is their time to upgrade. On the other hand, if there is doubt about the presence of infection or there is mild infection a BL-BLI combination may suffice.
- *Associated comorbidities:* These are important considerations. For instance if there is associated renal compromise, nephrotoxic drugs such as aminoglycosides, vancomycin, and colistin should be avoided or used with caution.
- *Site of the infection:* In the presence of a CNS infection a drug with good CSF penetration must be used.

Initial Empirical Antimicrobial Regimes

Since most nosocomial infections in Indian ICUs are due to resistant gram-negative pathogens, the initial empirical regime should comprise of an adequate gram-negative cover such as BL-BLI combinations or carbapenems. In units with high rates of carbapenem resistance, upfront use of aminoglycosides/polymyxins is also recommended in sick patients. An anti-methicillin-resistant *S. aureus* (MRSA) cover should be added to the regime if there is a high incidence of MRSA in that unit, if there are gram-positive cocci in the Gram stain of secretions or if there are other features suggesting a gram-positive infection. If risk factors for fungal infections are present such as prolonged ICU stay, prolonged antibiotic use, gut surgery, renal failure, use of corticosteroids, use of total parenteral nutrition, immunocompromised status, extreme prematurity, and isolation of candida from multiple nonsterile sites then an antifungal should be added either upfront or of there is failure to respond in 48 hours. The choice of antifungal depends on previous azole exposure, the local patterns in the unit, and the severity of infection and associated comorbidities and includes fluconazole/amphotericin B or echinocandin.

Dosing of Antibiotics

Adequate attention is needed toward administration of appropriate doses. Loading doses are indicated for drugs such as colistin, polymyxin B, vancomycin, and tigecycline. Higher doses may be needed for serious infections. Time-dependent antibiotics such as beta-lactams should be dosed frequently to maintain serum levels continuously above the minimum inhibitory concentration. Recent data supports administration of beta-lactams like piperacillin tazobactam/meropenem by prolonged infusion over 3–4 hours instead of the usual 30 minutes. On the other hand, concentration-dependent antibiotics, such as aminoglycosides, may be effectively dosed once a day.

Source Control

This is paramount and includes drainage of pus and removal of lines. If the patient is sick image-guided drainage of abscesses/collections can be done.

TABLE 1: Preferred targeted therapy based on organism.

Organism	*Preferred treatment*
ESBL GNB	BL-BLI or in sick patients carbapenems
CR *E. coli*	Fosfomycin + minocycline/amikacin
CR *Klebsiella*	Ceftazidime avibactam ± aztreonam
CR *Pseudomonas*	Polymyxin B/colistin
CR *Acinetobacter*	Polymyxin B/colistin ± sulbactam ± minocycline
Elizabethkingia/Stenotrophomonas	Cotrimoxazole ± minocycline
MSSA	Cloxacillin/cefazolin
MRSA	Vancomycin/teicoplanin/daptomycin/linezolid
Enterococcus faecalis	Ampicillin ± gentamicin/ceftriaxone
Enterococcus faecium	Vancomycin/teicoplanin
Vancomycin-resistant enterococcus	Daptomycin ± ceftaroline/ampicillin/linezolid
Azole-sensitive *Candida*	Fluconazole
Azole-resistant *Candida*	Amphotericin B/echinocandin

(CR: carbapenem resistant; ESBL: extended-spectrum beta-lactamase; GNB: gram-negative bacilli; MRSA: methicillin-resistant *Staphylococcus aureus;* MSSA: methicillin-sensitive *Staphylococcus aureus*)

Modification of Initial Empiric Therapy (Optimization/De-escalation/Escalation)

The antimicrobial therapy should be reviewed at 48–72 hours depending on the clinical situation and culture reports. If an alternate noninfectious cause has been identified antibiotics should be stopped. If representative cultures are positive then decisions of optimization/de-escalation/escalation are easy and antibiotics should be modified to the preferred drug **(Table 1)**. If the cultures are negative and the patient is improving the same antibiotics can be continued; however if given empirically, anti-MRSA antibiotics can be stopped. De-escalation is an important strategy to reduce cost of therapy/adverse effects/preserve future antibiotic options and reduce antimicrobial resistance. If cultures are negative and the patient is deteriorating then escalation to the next level may be warranted. However, other causes of non-response including noninfectious causes/inadequate source control should also be considered.

Duration of Therapy

New data supports the use of short-term antibiotic therapy (usually 7 days) for most nosocomial infections (exception *S. aureus*, fungal infections, and necrotizing pneumonias). This helps in reducing costs, reducing the antibiotic pressure in the unit and chances of selection of resistant pathogens.

CONCLUSION

A new-onset fever in the ICU is usually due to a serious drug resistant infection and is a medical emergency. A systematic approach should be followed to identify the site of infection and causative organism. Empiric antibiotics should be correctly chosen and suitably modified once the culture results are back. Due attention should be paid to source control and efforts should be made to limit duration of therapy. Finally, it is paramount to implement comprehensive infection control strategies so that such an event can be prevented.

CLINICAL PEARLS

- A robust infection control program is crucial in preventing healthcare-associated infections.
- Knowledge of local microbial flora and susceptibility helps in designing empirical regimes.
- Appropriate antimicrobial therapy is essential for improving outcomes and reducing the burden of antimicrobial resistance.

KEY POINTS

- New-onset fever in ICUs is usually due to infection.
- A careful examination is needed to identify the source of fever.
- Relevant cultures should always be sent prior to starting antimicrobial therapy.
- The empirical antimicrobial therapy should be guided by local susceptibility patterns, severity of illness, and prior antibiotic use. It should be broad enough, especially in sick patients.
- Results of investigations including cultures from nonsterile sites should be carefully interpreted.
- Efforts should be made to de-escalate antimicrobials at the earliest.
- Infection control strategies are paramount.

SUGGESTED READINGS

1. Garner JS, Jarvis WR, Emori TG, Horan TC, Hughes JM. CDC definitions for nosocomial infections. Am J Infect Control. 1988;16:128-40.
2. Indian Council of Medical Research. (2021). Antimicrobial Resistance Research and Surveillance Network: Annual Report January 2021 to December 2021. [online] Available from https://main.icmr.nic.in/sites/default/files/upload_documents/AMR_Annual_Report_2021.pdf. [Last accessed September, 2024].
3. Lodha R, Natchu UC, Nanda M, Kabra SK. Nosocomial infections in pediatric intensive care units. Indian J Pediatr. 2001;68:1063-70.
4. Sick-Samuels AC, Booth LD, Milstone AM, Schumacher C, Bergmann J, Stockwell DC. A Novel Comprehensive Algorithm for Evaluation of PICU Patients With New Fever or Instability. Pediatr Crit Care Med. 2023;24(8):670-80.
5. Tamma PD, Aitken SL, Bonomo RA, Mathers AJ, van Duin D, Clancy CJ. Infectious Diseases Society of America 2022 guidance on the treatment of extended-spectrum beta-lactamase producing enterobacterales (ESBL-E), carbapenem-resistant enterobacterales (CRE), and Pseudomonas aeruginosa with difficult-to-treat resistance (DTR-P. aeruginosa). Clin Infect Dis. 2022;75:187-212.

CHAPTER 56

Infant Born to Human Immunodeficiency Virus Infected Mother

Ira Shah, Noella Maria Delia Pereira

INTRODUCTION

Human immunodeficiency virus (HIV) in children is predominantly acquired vertically through mother-to-child transmission (MTCT). Without intervention, the transmission rate of HIV from mother to child has varied from 20 to 45%. However, this risk can be decreased to <2% with effective prevention strategies implemented in both mother and baby through the elimination of vertical transmission of HIV introduced by World Health Organization (WHO) and National AIDS Control Organization (NACO). The current MTCT rate of HIV in India is 24.25%. Vertical transmission of HIV can occur at three stages—(1) *in utero* through placental transmission, (2) intrapartum through contact with the infected birth canal secretions, and (3) postpartum through breastfeeding. Without intervention, nearly 15–30% of babies are infected during pregnancy and labor with an additional risk of 15–20% associated with breastfeeding and an estimated 15–30% of vertically infected infants die in the first year of life.

CLINICAL PEARLS

- Mother-to-child transmission of infant born to HIV infected mother occurs in 20–45% children without intervention.
- Without intervention, nearly 15–30% of babies are infected during pregnancy and labor with an additional risk of 15–20% associated with breastfeeding.

PREVENTION MODALITIES

Human immunodeficiency virus transmission from mother to child is mainly prevented by antiretroviral therapy (ART) to the mother and antiretroviral drug (ARV) prophylaxis to the baby along with exclusive breastfeeding replacement feeding when feasible. Although normal vaginal delivery is considered in most cases, an elective cesarian section is considered in special circumstances such as obstructed labor and fetal distress in India. ART acts by decreasing the viral load in the mother and ARV prophylaxis helps to decrease the vertical transmission of HIV to the newborn baby. Routine cesarean section with an aim to reduce intrapartum transmission of HIV is no longer recommended.

The aim of effective elimination of vertical transmission of HIV from mother to child is to ensure mother's safety and health as well as reduce the transmission of HIV to the infant. The PROMISE trial conducted in sub-Saharan Africa and India as well as the HIVNET 012 study conducted in Uganda showed that maternal ART along with infant ARV prophylaxis reduced the MTCT rate significantly. In 2015, WHO recommended starting ART in all HIV-infected adults, children, and pregnant women irrespective of their clinical stage or CD4 count.

CLINICAL PEARLS

Prevention modalities include three ART to mother during pregnancy and while feeding:

1. Antiretroviral prophylaxis to baby postdelivery
2. Choice of feeding
3. Mode of delivery

ELECTIVE CESAREAN SECTION

Elective cesarean section (ECS) was found to decrease transplacental hemorrhage during labor, reduce the length of exposure of baby to vaginocervical secretions, as well as decrease the chances of ascending infection of HIV transmission. Earlier studies had found that among HIV-1 infected women not taking ARV during pregnancy, ECS was efficacious for prevention of MTCT of HIV-1, and decreased transmission as compared to other modes of delivery.

However, ECS is no longer recommended routinely as a mode of delivery in HIV-positive mothers and is only indicated if there an obstetric indication for the same. Normal vaginal delivery is considered in most cases with minimal use of instrumentation and safe delivery practices. When ART is given to the mother and ARV prophylaxis given to the child exclusive breastfeeding can be given to the infant. There is no added advantage to ECS as a mode of delivery in the era of ART being given to all mothers irrespective of their CD4 count and clinical staging and ARV prophylaxis given to the infant.

ANTIRETROVIRAL PROPHYLAXIS

Many trials have demonstrated a sharp decrease in the *in utero* and intrapartum transmission rates with an increasing length of duration of ART during pregnancy and the increased potency of drug combinations used during pregnancy and at delivery. In all countries of the world, highly active ART (triple-drug therapy) is used as prophylaxis in pregnant women.

CHOICE OF FEEDING

Human immunodeficiency virus can be transmitted through breastmilk as cell free and cell-associated virus. Even if intrauterine and intrapartum transmission are significantly reduced, postnatal transmission through breastfeeding still remains an additional risk for transmission of HIV varying from cell associated 15–20%. A high viral load in the breastmilk can increase the transmission and this risk is further increased with, maternal nipple lesions, mastitis, oral thrush, and prolonged breastfeeding. It has also been seen that transmission can occur with undetectable viral loads further questioning the role of viral reservoirs present in breastmilk.

Replacement feeding reduces the risk of transmission of HIV through breastmilk. However in low and middle income countries, replacement feeding may not be affordable and requires the available of safe and portable water. It has been seen that replacement feeding can increase the risk of diarrheal diseases and malnutrition thus increasing mortality and morbidity. Hence replacement feeding should only be advised when it is acceptable, feasible, affordable, sustainable, and safe.

Exclusive breastfeeding for up to 6 months, however, is associated with a threefold to fourfold decreased risk of transmission of HIV with ART given to the mother and ARV prophylaxis is given to the infant, mixed feeding on the other hand can pose a risk for postnatal transmission, and should therefore be avoided. However with ART given to the mother and ARV prophylaxis administered to the infant, this risk remains low. Various recent clinical trials have now shown that the risk of HIV transmission with breastfeeding is reduced to 2% when ART is administered to the mother during pregnancy and postpartum. This approach has provided hope for mothers with HIV infection who can now safely breastfeed their babies. Breastfeeding not only improves the chances of infants remaining free from HIV but will also keep them healthy as it provides optimal nutrition and protects against other fatal childhood diseases such as pneumonia and diarrhea.

WORLD HEALTH ORGANIZATION 2015 GUIDELINES

The new WHO 2015 guidelines as well as NACO guidelines 2021 have suggested a once daily three-drug fixed dose combination of tenofovir and lamivudine (or emtricitabine), and dolutegravir (DTG) as first-line ART in HIV-infected pregnant and breastfeeding women which should be continued lifelong. Infants of these mothers should receive 6 weeks of infant prophylaxis with daily nevirapine if low risk and (and dual prophylaxis with nevirapine and twice daily zidovudine if the infant belongs to the high-risk category). Infant prophylaxis should begin at birth or when HIV exposure is recognized postpartum **(Table 1 and Flowchart 1)**.

In all pregnant, plasma viral load should be done between 32 and 36 weeks of pregnancy (regardless of the duration of the ART), to assess the risk of HIV transmission to the infant. Mothers with a high viral of >1,000 copies/mL have a high risk of HIV transmission to their infants and those with a viral load of <1,000 copies/mL have a low risk of HIV transmission. Both WHO and NACO recommend a single-drug ARV prophylaxis to infants with a low risk and dual prophylaxis to infants with a high risk of transmission as follows.

When single prophylaxis is to be given, in the event that zidovudine is not available, syrup lopinavir/ritonavir should be used after 14 days of birth. When dual prophylaxis is to be given and zidovudine syrup is not available, syrup nevirapine should be used for the first 14 days after birth following which syrup lopinavir/ritonavir can be added thereafter. An alternative to dual prophylaxis may be a fixed dose combination of zidovudine + lamivudine+ nevirapine in pediatric formulation.

TABLE 1: HIV risk assessment of infants born to HIV infected mothers and infant ARV prophylaxis options as per NACO guidelines 2021.

High-risk status	*Option for ARV prophylaxis*
Low-risk infants: Infants born to mothers with suppressed plasma viral loads (<1,000 copies/mL) assessed any time after 32 weeks of pregnancy up to delivery	• Syrup Nevirapine • Syrup zidovudine (in situations where nevirapine will not be effective): – Infant born to a mother with confirmed HIV-2 or HIV-1 and HIV-2 combined infections – Infant born to a mother who had received single dose of nevirapine during earlier pregnancy or delivery – Infant born to a mother who is on PI-based ART regime due to treatment failure *Duration:* From birth till 6 weeks of age
High-risk infants: • Infants born to HIV-positive mother not on ART • Maternal viral load not done after 32 weeks of pregnancy • Maternal plasma viral load not suppressed after 32 weeks of pregnancy • Mother newly identified HIV positive within 6 weeks of delivery	*Options for dual prophylaxis:* • Syrup nevirapine + syrup zidovudine • *Duration:* – In case of exclusive replacement feeding, from birth till 6 weeks of age – In case of exclusive breastfeeding, from birth till 12 weeks of age

(ART: antiretroviral therapy; ARV: antiretroviral drug; HIV: human immunodeficiency virus; NACO: National AIDS Control Organization)

Flowchart 1: Algorithm risk assessment at the time of delivery to help identify infants at high risk and low risk (taken from WHO guidelines 2021).

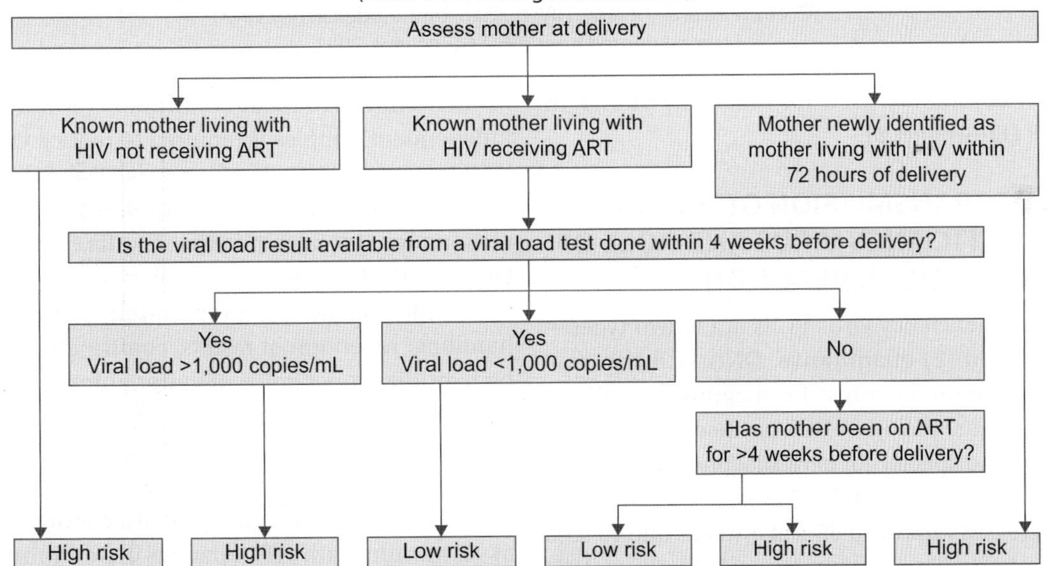

(ART: antiretroviral therapy; HIV: human immunodeficiency virus; WHO: World Health Organization)

DIAGNOSIS OF HUMAN IMMUNODEFICIENCY VIRUS IN INFANTS BORN TO HUMAN IMMUNODEFICIENCY VIRUS INFECTED MOTHERS

Infants born to HIV-infected mothers carry HIV antibodies transmitted from the mother until 12–15 months of age. Some of these antibodies are also transmitted through breast milk from mother to child. Hence serological testing in children is reliable only after 18 months of age. Infants <18 months of age are tested for HIV using nucleic acid testing. Nucleic acid testing can include HIV RNA or HIV deoxyribonucleic acid (DNA) polymerase chain reaction (PCR) as well as HIV RNA qualitative and quantitative assay.

Flowchart 2: Simplified infant diagnosis algorithm.

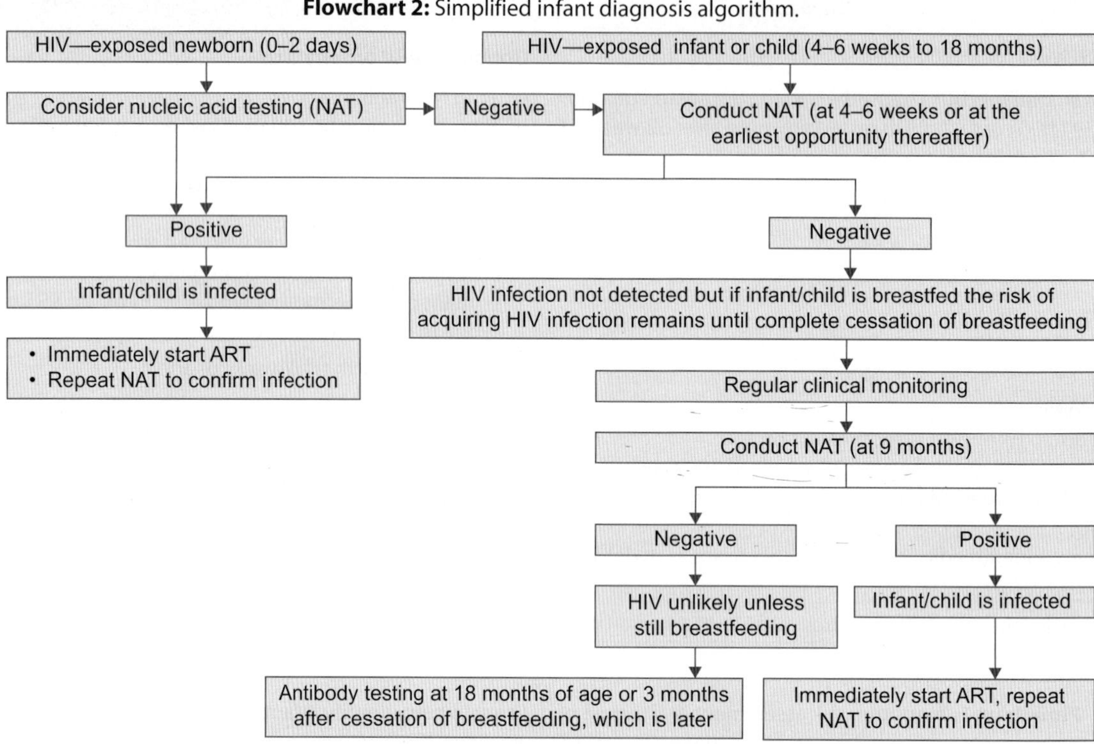

(ART: antiretroviral therapy; HIV: human immunodeficiency virus)
Source: Adapted from WHO Guidelines, 2021.

Thus, the test commonly used for diagnosis of HIV in infants is PCR **(Flowchart 2)**.

TIMING OF TRANSMISSION OF HUMAN IMMUNODEFICIENCY VIRUS AND ROLE OF POLYMERASE CHAIN REACTION

Human immunodeficiency virus PCRs are of two types—(1) qualitative and (2) quantitative. DNA PCR has now become the recommended test for diagnosis of HIV in HIV-exposed infants. HIV DNA PCR has been found to be highly sensitive and specific for early diagnosis of pediatric HIV infection. Sensitivity of HIV PCR is less at birth and sensitivity increases rapidly to 95% at 4 weeks and to 99% at 6 months of age. Thus, in nonbreastfed infants, HIV PCR can be done at 4–6 weeks after birth. In breastfeeding populations, HIV testing should be done after 3 months after cessation of breastfeeding. HIV DNA PCR testing requires a dried blood sample on a filter paper or a sample whole blood sent to the laboratory.

False positive and false negative results with HIV DNA PCR are known to occur. The authors have reported a very high incidence of false positive HIV DNA PCR (80%) especially in younger infants born to HIV-infected mothers in their study. A repeat confirmatory DNA PCR test on independent samples is required to reduce the test errors. WHO recommends a confirmatory DNA PCR test prior to the initiation of ART in HIV-exposed infants. One of the reasons for the false positive results is contamination. Optimal PCR conditions, inclusion of control samples, strict rules on sample preparation, pre- and post-PCR handling, repetition of results, confirmation of specificity by hybridization, choice of material from which HIV-1 is amplified, and the primers used for amplification will all predict the reliability of HIV DNA PCR. Thus, diagnosis of HIV should never be based on one result but should always be confirmed by a repeat test. Serological diagnosis at 18 months with HIV enzyme-linked immunosorbent assay would also be useful.

DIAGNOSIS OF HUMAN IMMUNODEFICIENCY VIRUS IN CHILDREN ABOVE 18 MONTHS OF AGE

Enzyme-linked immunosorbent assay is the time-tested reliable method for detection of anti-HIV antibodies with a sensitivity of >99.5% and specificity of 99% **(Flowchart 3)**.

Flowchart 3: Testing HIV-exposed children >18 months of age.

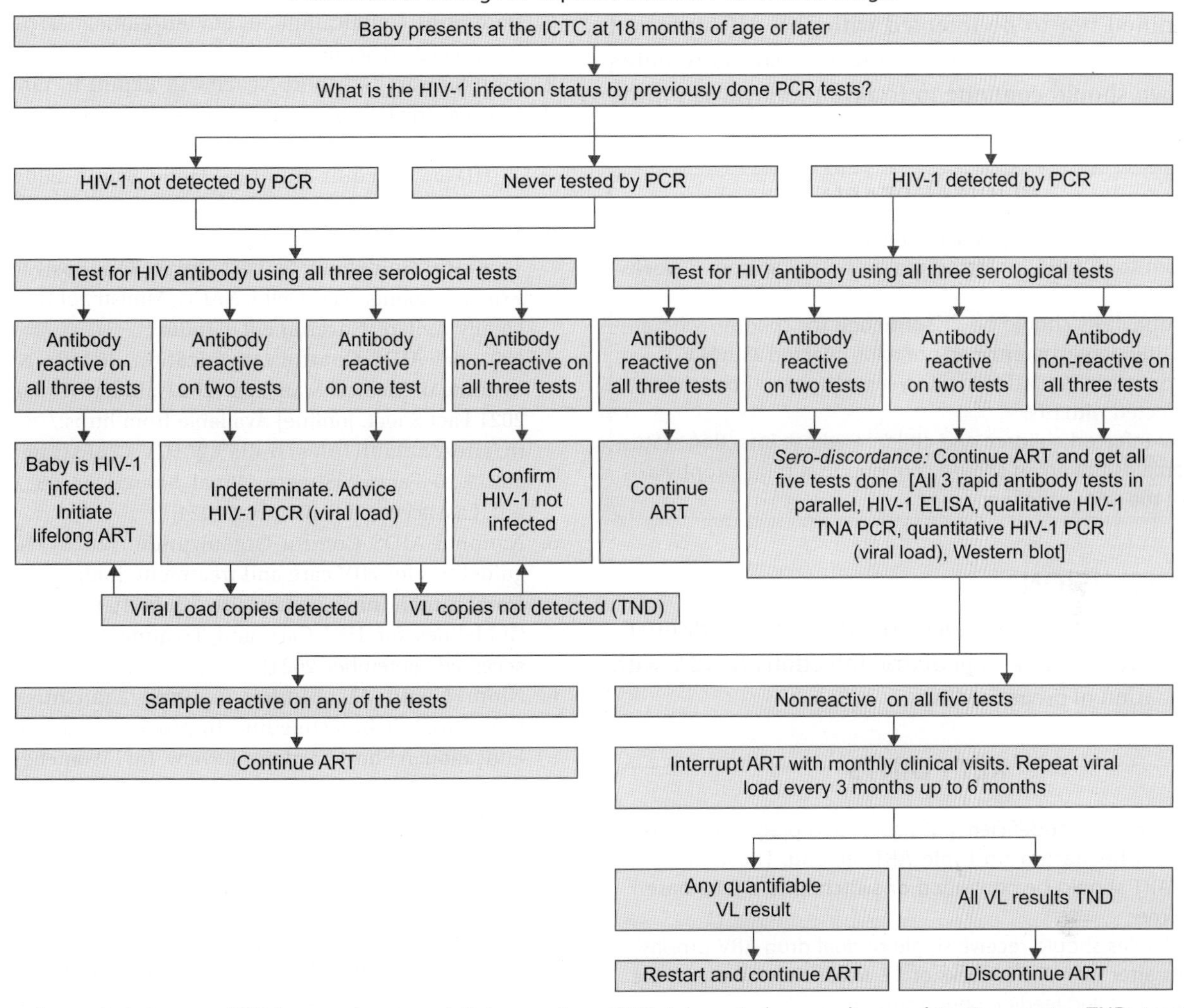

(ART: antiretroviral therapy; HIV: human immunodeficiency virus; ICTC: integrated counseling and testing center; TND: target not detected)

Source: Adapted from the EID Algorithm -Laboratory Technical Guidelines on Early Infant Diagnosis for HIV Exposed Infants. NACO. 2023.

CLINICAL PEARLS

- Diagnosis in children <18 months—HIV–total nucleic acid (RNA and DNA) or DNA PCR
- Diagnosis in children above 18 months—HIV enzyme-linked immunosorbent assay

COTRIMOXAZOLE PROPHYLAXIS

Cotrimoxazole prophylaxis is safe, inexpensive, and highly effective in reducing morbidity and mortality among HIV-infected infants and children, as well as in adolescents and adults. Ideally, all infants exposed to HIV should be started on cotrimoxazole prophylaxis at 6 weeks of age, as recommended by the WHO and NACO. This period is particularly critical for HIV-infected infants. Providing cotrimoxazole prophylaxis protects against serious, often fatal, opportunistic infections (OIs). It has also been recognized that cotrimoxazole prophylaxis provides benefits beyond the prevention of pneumocystis pneumonia including malaria and severe bacterial infections. The prophylaxis is given to all HIV-exposed infants till 18 months of age if not infected and till 5 years of age if found to be infected provided they are clinically stable, with evidence of immune recovery and HIV infected virally suppressed on ART at that time.

Children born to HIV-infected mothers should be administered prophylaxis with trimethoprim sulfamethoxazole beginning at age 4–6 weeks. Prophylaxis should be discontinued for children who are subsequently determined not to be infected with HIV. HIV-infected children and children whose infection status remains unknown should continue to receive prophylaxis for the first year of life.

CLINICAL PEARLS

- Cotrimoxazole prophylaxis should be given to all children born to HIV (HIV) infected mothers starting from 6 weeks of age.
- Prophylaxis should be discontinued for children who are subsequently determined not to be infected with HIV.
- Prophylaxis is continued till 5 years of age for those children infected with HIV.
- HIV-infected children and children whose infection status remains unknown should continue to receive prophylaxis for the first year of life.

CONCLUSION

While interventions to prevent MTCT of HIV can dramatically reduce the risk of pediatric infections to <2% with continuation of breastfeeding.

KEY POINTS

- Human immunodeficiency virus-infected pregnant women should be started on triple ART lifelong. Those already on ART should be continued or switched to a DTG-based regime.
- All babies should receive single or dual drug ARV prophylaxis after birth for 6 weeks or 12 weeks depending on the risk status and feeding option chosen.
- Exclusive breastfeeding is recommended for all HIV-exposed newborns.
- Early diagnosis consists of HIV DNA PCR in infants <18 months and serological testing for those 18 months of age.

SUGGESTED READING

1. Department of Health and Human Services. (2023). Recommendations for the Use of Antiretroviral Drugs During Pregnancy and Interventions to Reduce Perinatal HIV Transmission in the United States. [online] Available from https://clinicalinfo.hiv.gov/en/guidelines/perinatal [Last accessed September, 2024].
2. John-Stewart G, Mbori-Ngacha D, Ekpini R, Janoff EN, Nkengasong J, Read JS, et al; Ghent IAS Working Group on HIV in Women Children. Breast-feeding and Transmission of HIV-1. J Acquir Immune Defic Syndr. 2004;35(2): 196-202.
3. National AIDS Control Organization (2023). Laboratory Technical Guidelines on Early Infant Diagnosis for HIV-Exposed Infants. New Delhi: NACO, Ministry of Health and Family Welfare, Government of India.
4. National AIDS Control Organization, ICMR—National Institute of Medical Statistics. (2022). India HIV Estimates 2021 Fact Sheet. [online] Available from https://naco.gov.in/sites/default/files/India%20HIV%20Estimates%202021%20_Fact%20Sheets__Final_Shared_24_08_2022_0.pdf [Last accessed September, 2024].
5. National AIDS Control Organization. (2021). National guidelines for HIV care and treatment. [online] Available from https://naco.gov.in/sites/default/files/National_Guidelines_for_HIV_Care_and_Treatment_2021.pdf [Last accessed September, 2024].
6. Njom Nlend AE. Mother-to-Child Transmission of HIV Through Breastfeeding Improving Awareness and Education: A Short Narrative Review. Int J Womens Health. 2022;14:697-703.
7. Volmink J, Marais B. HIV: mother-to-child transmission. BMJ Clin Evid. 2008;2008:0909.
8. WHO. (2015). Guideline on when to start antiretroviral therapy and on pre-exposure prophylaxis for HIV. [online] Available from https://www.who.int/publications/i/item/9789241509565 [Last accessed November, 2024].
9. WHO. (2021). Consolidated guidelines on HIV prevention, testing, treatment, service delivery and monitoring; Recommendations for a public health approach. [online] Available from https://www.who.int/publications/i/item/9789240031593 [Last accessed September, 2024].
10. World Health Organization. (2010). Antiretroviral drugs for treating pregnant women and preventing HIV infection in infants: recommendations for a public health approach. [online] Available from https://www.who.int/publications/i/item/9789241599818 [Last accessed September, 2024].

Fever of Unknown Origin

Raju C Shah, Tanu Singhal

INTRODUCTION

Fever of unknown origin (FUO) or pyrexia of unknown origin (PUO) is still a diagnostic challenge for many pediatricians especially practicing in remote placed or resource limited settings. Following simple protocol and going stepwise will help the pediatrician in reaching the diagnosis.

DEFINITION

The definition of FUO is fever >101°F lasting for 3 weeks or more for which no cause is apparent after 1 week of outpatient investigation. A practical definition of FUO is simply fever >101°F measured on several occasions over a 7-day period.

CAUSES

The principal causes of FUO are listed in **Box 1**. Infections account for most of the cases of FUO in children (60–70%). Most common among infectious causes are enteric fever, malaria, pulmonary or extrapulmonary tuberculosis, and urinary tract infections (UTIs). Malignancies, especially leukemia and autoimmune diseases chiefly juvenile rheumatoid arthritis (JRA), account for the remaining cases. Relatively rare causes include drug fever, temperature dysregulation, diabetes insipidus, sarcoidosis, ectodermal dysplasia, sensory autonomic neuropathies, etc. Even with extensive investigations the cause of FUO remains undiagnosed in 10–20% of the cases.

BOX 1: Causes of fever of unknown origin.

Infectious causes: Enteric fever, malaria, urinary tract infections, tuberculosis, chronic hepatitis, human immunodeficiency virus (HIV), hidden abscesses (liver and pelvic), mastoiditis, sinusitis, osteomyelitis, meningitis, infectious mononucleosis, infective endocarditis, brucellosis, cytomegalovirus (CMV), toxoplasmosis, and kala-azar

Autoimmune causes: Systemic onset juvenile rheumatoid arthritis, Kawasaki disease, systemic lupus erythematosus, inflammatory bowel disease, and polyarteritis nodosa

Malignant causes: Leukemia, lymphoma, Langerhans cell histiocytosis, and Kikuchi's disease

APPROACH TO FEVER OF UNKNOWN ORIGIN

The first step is to identify sick patients who need stabilization and urgent referral to a tertiary care center. Subsequently, all attempts should be made to reach an etiologic diagnosis. A detailed history is of paramount importance. History should include:

- Whether and how fever was documented (it is not uncommon to find children with history of prolonged fever not to have fever documented by a thermometer)
- Duration and pattern of fever (distinguish from recurrent fever)
- Symptoms referable to all organ systems and weight loss
- History of recurrent infections and oral thrush [human immunodeficiency virus (HIV) infection]
- History of joint pain, rash, and photosensitivity (autoimmune disease)
- History of contact with tuberculosis and animals (brucellosis)
- Travel to endemic zones (kala-azar)
- Drug history particularly anticholinergics (drug fever)

History is followed by a complete physical examination. Documentation of fever is necessary, followed by assessment of general activity, nutritional status, and vitals. A head-to-toe examination, after removing all clothes, is vital. The physical examination should be repeated on daily basis as new findings may emerge that provide a clue to the etiology. One must keep Kawasaki disease (though a relatively uncommon illness) in mind as here diagnosis before the 10th day of fever is crucial to prevent coronary complications.

INVESTIGATIONS AND MANAGEMENT

Preliminary investigations, which should be repeated in all patients with FUO (even if done earlier) include complete blood count (CBC), peripheral smear (PS), malarial parasite, erythrocyte sedimentation rate (ESR), blood cultures, Widal test, chest X-ray, tuberculin test, urinalysis and culture, hepatic transaminases, and abdominal ultrasound. The CBC and PS will help in the differential diagnosis. If the counts are low or normal, enteric fever, malaria, and viral infections are a possibility. A high white blood cell (WBC) count with neutrophilia indicates a bacterial infection/pus collection, possible Kawasaki's disease, systemic onset JRA, or even tuberculosis. A high WBC count with lymphocytosis suggests a mononucleosis syndrome or a hematologic malignancy. Absolute eosinopenia is indicative of an acute bacterial/viral infection particularly enteric fever. A low platelet count points toward malaria, enteric fever, or a malignancy whereas a very high platelet count is present in Kawasaki's disease or systemic onset JRA. The usefulness of an ESR as an investigative modality in prolonged fever is often debated. It is not a sensitive or specific investigation. Studies show that one-third of pulmonary tuberculosis had a normal ESR. Exceptionally, a very high ESR is indicative of an autoimmune process such as Kawasaki disease or JRA. The C-reactive protein (CRP) parallels ESR and may not help to differentiate a viral from bacterial etiology. However, a very high CRP points to a bacterial infection or autoimmune disease. Evaluation for malarial parasite is a must. Repeated thick smears are gold standard for diagnosis and may be sent irrespective of the fever spike. However, in a setting where reliable microscopy is not available, the malarial antigen tests may be used; the parasite lactate dehydrogenase tests score over the histidine-rich protein 2-based tests. The blood culture is a crucial investigation in this setting as enteric fever is the most common differential. Though, it should be sent prior to starting antibiotics, the yield is fair for *Salmonella* even if the patient is on antibiotics. If infective endocarditis is suspected then three blood cultures at 30 minutes interval should be sent and if brucellosis is being considered as a differential then the laboratory should be informed so that the cultures are incubated for longer and not discarded within 5 days. Widal may be sent as it is the 7th day of fever, but the results should be carefully interpreted. It may be considered positive if both TO and TH/TA titers are 1:120/1:160 or more. Either TO/TH being positive or titers of 1:40/80 should be considered as false positive. Similarly, a negative Widal does not rule out enteric, especially if the patient has been on antibiotics. Typhidot-M or Tubex tests do not offer any advantage over the Widal and are not routinely recommended. Liver enzymes both aspartate aminotransferase (SGOT) and alanine aminotransferase (SGPT) should be assayed as these are often elevated in malaria, enteric, infectious mononucleosis, and brucellosis; SGOT being higher than SGPT. UTI is a diagnostic possibility and hence urine routine is mandatory. Features of UTI include presence of one or more of the following: >10 pus cells/hpf of centrifuged urine, positive leukocyte esterase, positive nitrite tests, and presence of bacteria on the Gram stain. If the urine routine is suggestive of a UTI then urine culture should be sent before starting antibiotics. This is to confirm the diagnosis and also to know the antibiotic susceptibility of the isolate. A chest X-ray should also be done to pick up pneumonia or features of pulmonary tuberculosis. An ultrasonography abdomen with pelvis is recommended as an initial investigation as it helps in detecting a liver abscess, gallbladder wall thickening and sludge (often seen in enteric fever), pyelonephritis, and retroperitoneal adenopathy. Nonspecific mesenteric lymphadenopathy is a common finding and usually merits no consideration. The author does not recommend doing a tuberculin test at this point if there is no clinical or radiologic suspicion of tuberculosis and unless more common causes such as enteric are ruled out. This is because a positive tuberculin test at this juncture may be indicative of latent tuberculosis infection and may not be causally associated with the fever.

If a diagnosis is established on the basis of the earlier mentioned approach, appropriate treatment should be instituted. If no diagnosis is made, clinical reassessment and further investigations are merited. While second-line investigations are being planned and executed, treatment with intravenous ceftriaxone may be considered as enteric fever is an important cause of FUO in our country, especially in those cases with negative clinical/preliminary investigations **(Flowchart 1)**.

Second-line investigations include HIV enzyme-linked immunosorbent assay, contrast-enhanced computed tomography of chest and abdomen, bone marrow histology and cultures, 2D echocardiogram, complement level, antinuclear and rheumatoid factors, and tissue biopsies, if indicated. Other serologic tests that may be done

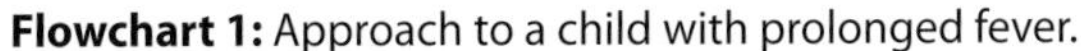

Flowchart 1: Approach to a child with prolonged fever.

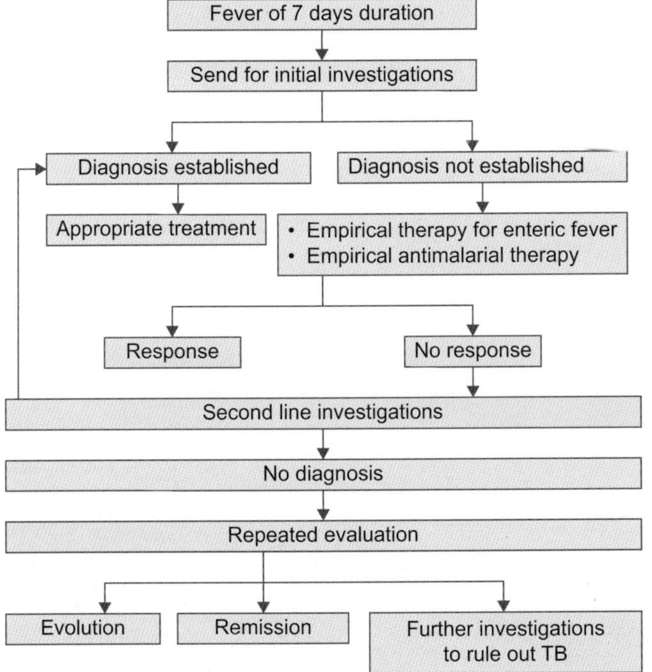

include *Brucella* serology, hepatitis B surface antigen, Paul Bunnell/Monospot test/immunoglobulin M viral capsid antigen (VCA) for infectious mononucleosis. Tests which are of no clinical value include serology and polymerase chain reaction in blood for *Mycobacterium tuberculosis* or other organisms.

CLINICAL PEARLS

- Infections particularly tuberculosis is the most common cause for FUO in India.
- A high index of suspicion should be kept for diagnosis of Kawasaki disease.
- Empirical therapy should be avoided as far as possible.
- The diagnosis often evolves with time and patience is the key.

KEY POINTS

- A practical definition of FUO is fever for which a cause cannot be established despite 1 week of investigations.
- A detailed history and physical examination is most crucial. This should include travel history, contact with tuberculosis and animals.
- The primary objective is to identify sick children and prompt referral to an appropriate center.
- Kawasaki disease should always be considered as a possibility in young children.
- Investigative approach should be stepwise starting with basic investigations and proceeding to more complex ones.
- Tuberculosis serology has no place in the diagnosis of FUO.
- With patience and application of methods, it should be possible to make a diagnosis of the etiology of FUO in most cases.
- In a small number of cases, it may not be possible to arrive at the etiologic diagnosis. In such cases, periodic reassessments should be done as the disease may finally surface (e.g., lymphoma and systemic-onset juvenile rheumatoid arthritis). Some cases of FUO may self-resolve over time.
- Empirical use of steroids should be avoided.

SUGGESTED READING

1. Campbell J. Fever of unknown origin in a previously healthy child. Semin Pediatr Infect Dis. 2002;13:64-6.
2. Edwards K. Fever: From FUO to PFAPA to recurrent or persistent. San Francisco, California: Program and abstracts from the American Academy of Pediatrics National Conference and Exhibition; 2004.
3. Miller L, Sisson B, Tucker L, Schaller J. Prolonged fevers of unknown origin in children: patterns of presentation and outcome. J Pediatr. 1996;12:419-23.
4. Miller ML, Szer I, Yogev R, Bernstein B. Fever of unknown origin. Pediatr Clin North Am. 1995;42:999-1015.
5. Steele R. Fever of unknown origin. A time for patience with your patients. Clin Pediatr. 2000;39:719-20.

Hematology/Oncology

Section Editors: *Nitin K Shah, Sangeeta Mudaliar*

CHAPTER 58

A Mass in the Abdomen: The Way to Diagnosis

Gauri Kapoor

INTRODUCTION

The identification of an abdominal mass in a neonate or child is a cause for concern because of the possibility of malignant disease. In addition, even benign conditions can be serious and warrant prompt evaluation and treatment. Hence, the pediatrician needs to be wary of these masses and give them urgent attention.

Although abdominal masses could be any one of the following:

- Fluid
- Fat
- Flatus
- Solid mass

For the purpose of this chapter, we will focus on solid abdominal masses.

PRESENTATION

Evaluation of an abdominal mass includes a thorough history and examination to detect important clinical findings, potential clues to the diagnosis, and issues that may need to be addressed promptly. A short, acute history is likely to be suggestive of an aggressive, rapidly growing mass, and warrants prompt review, whereas the presence of symptoms for many months is more consistent with a benign process.

At presentation children with abdominal masses may be asymptomatic (coincidental finding) or symptomatic (e.g., abdominal pain or distension and presence of hematuria) as shown in **Box 1**. The asymptomatic cases may be incidentally picked up on a routine prenatal ultrasound or detected by a family member or alert pediatrician during an immunization visit. The general presentation varies depending on the underlying pathology of the abdominal mass. Patients can present with difficulty with urination or defecation if the mass physically obstructs the gastrointestinal (GI) or genitourinary (GU) tract. Patients presenting with constitutional symptoms such as fever and weight loss with an abdominal mass are more likely to be suffering from a malignant condition. Neuroblastoma and Wilms' tumor are two conditions pediatricians must be vigilant about as they are the two malignant tumors in children where abdominal mass is commonly the initial presentation.

BOX 1: Presentation of abdominal mass.

Asymptomatic:
- Incidentally detected
- Prenatal ultrasound
- Immunization visit—alert pediatrician

Symptomatic:
- Abdominal distension (right upper quadrant and epigastric mass)
- Respiratory distress
- Weight loss, fever, and anorexia
- Easy fatigability and paleness
- Congestive heart failure, hydramnios, and fetal hydrops
- Bowel obstruction and urinary retention

Although it is imperative that a child be referred quickly to the appropriate specialist (e.g., pediatric oncologist, pediatric surgeon, nephrologist, gastroenterologist, and gynecologist), evaluation by the pediatrician is of great value in deciding on initial management and in making the most appropriate referral. The evaluation of a child with an abdominal mass involves a number of possibilities and depends to some extent on the age and sex of the patient, the location of the mass, and the presence or absence of other potentially related signs and symptoms, as well as features of the physical examination. Determination of the organ or tissue of origin of the mass can narrow down the diagnostic possibilities considerably. Thus, a completion of a careful history and physical examination, baseline laboratory studies, and limited diagnostic imaging studies can provide sufficient information to determine the diagnosis or to choose the appropriate subspecialist and counsel the family.

Clues to diagnosis based on:

- Age and sex
- Location of the mass
- Organ of origin
- Signs and symptoms
- Examination findings
- Investigative workup (limited)

Some of the common conditions that might produce an abdominal mass in a child are listed in **Table 1** and are categorized by the organ of origin. Abdominal masses in the neonatal age group are often benign as shown in **Table 2**, and will be further discussed in the section on age. Not all of these possibilities need be considered in every patient; many can be eliminated on the basis of the age

TABLE 1: Differential diagnosis based on organ of origin in the non-neonatal age group.

Organ	*Malignant disease*	*Nonmalignant disease*
Adrenal	• Adrenal carcinoma • Neuroblastoma • Pheochromocytoma	• Adrenal adenoma • Adrenal hemorrhage
Gallbladder	Leiomyosarcoma	• Choledochal cyst • Gallbladder obstruction • Hydrops (e.g., leptospirosis)
Gastrointestinal tract	• Leiomyosarcoma • Non-Hodgkin lymphoma	• Appendiceal abscess • Intestinal duplication • Fecal impaction • Meckel's diverticulum
Kidney	• Lymphomatous nephromegaly • Renal cell carcinoma • Peripheral neuroectodermal tumor (PNET) of kidney • Wilms' tumor	• Hydronephrosis • Multicystic kidney • Polycystic kidney • Mesoblastic nephroma • Renal vein thrombosis • Hamartoma
Liver	• Hepatoblastoma • Hepatocellular carcinoma • Embryonal sarcoma • Liver metastases • Hemangioendothelioma • Hemangiomas • Mesenchymoma	• Focal nodular hyperplasia • Hepatitis • Liver abscess • Storage disease
Lower genitourinary tract	• Ovarian germ cell tumor • Rhabdomyosarcoma of bladder • Rhabdomyosarcoma of prostate • Rhabdomyosarcoma and Ewing sarcoma of pelvis	• Bladder obstruction • Ovarian cyst • Hydrocolpos
Spleen	• Acute or chronic leukemia • Histiocytosis • Hodgkin lymphoma • Non-Hodgkin lymphoma	• Congestive splenomegaly • Histiocytosis • Mononucleosis • Portal hypertension • Storage disease
Miscellaneous	• Hodgkin lymphoma • Non-Hodgkin lymphoma • Pelvic neuroblastoma • Retroperitoneal neuroblastoma • Retroperitoneal rhabdomyosarcoma • Retroperitoneal germ cell tumor	• Teratoma • Abdominal hernia • Pyloric stenosis • Omental or mesenteric cyst

TABLE 2: Common abdominal masses in the newborn.

Masses	*Frequency*
Retroperitoneal masses: Polycystic kidneys, hydronephrosis, dysplastic kidneys, neoplasms, and other	65%
Gastrointestinal masses: Things that cause obstruction, hepatic masses, and other	25%
Genitosacral masses: Teratomas, congenital genital anomalies, ovarian cysts, and other	10%

and sex of the patient, the location and type of mass, and features of the history or physical examination.

The differential for an abdominal mass can be extensive and quite daunting, as it incorporates many systems including the GI, GU, and endocrine system. An organized approach to abdominal masses includes thinking about possible etiologies based on the location of the mass with regards to the underlining abdominal anatomy as well as discerning likely pathologies based on the age of the patient and associated symptoms or signs.

CLINICAL PEARL

- Solid abdominal masses are rare in neonates and account for <2% of childhood tumors.

TABLE 3: History: special points.

History	*Clue*
Age of the child	Neonates (rarely malignant) and children (more likely to be malignant)
How long has it been there	Months to years (benign)
How fast is it growing	Faster growing (malignant)
Pressure symptoms	Constipation and urine retention
Constitutional symptoms	Fever, weight loss, pallor, and bruising (infection vs. marrow infiltrative)
Watery diarrhea	Neuroblastoma secreting vasoactive intestinal peptide
Hematuria	Renal pathology (Wilms' tumor)
Opsomyoclonus	Neuroblastoma
Periorbital ecchymosis and ptosis	Neuroblastoma (raccoon eye)
Acute abdomen	Intussusception (benign or ileocecal lymphoma)
Cushing's syndrome	Adrenal adenoma and adrenocortical carcinoma
Genetic syndrome or inherited predisposition	Familial adenomatous polyposis, Gardner's, Beckwith–Wiedemann (Wilms', hepatoblastoma, and adrenocortical carcinoma), aniridia (Wilms'), and hemihypertrophy (Wilms')

HISTORY

When approaching an abdominal mass, a proper history with a focused physical examination is necessary to direct you to the proper diagnostic tests to order, or the right specialist to refer too (i.e., pediatric oncologist, surgeon, gastroenterologist, nephrologists, or gynecologist).

Age

The age of the patient is very important when approaching abdominal masses in the pediatric population and should be the first question asked. Malignant tumors are uncommon in the newborn period. These conditions are often related to the kidney. Posterior urethral valves are manifested during the newborn period by a very large urinary bladder. Hydronephrosis secondary to distal obstruction may result in a unilateral or bilateral flank mass. A multicystic kidney also may be found at this time. Other considerations include developmental abnormalities, such as duplications or cysts of abdominal organs. Among the malignant conditions, neuroblastoma and extragonadal germ cell tumors are most common, followed by hepatoblastoma and Wilms' tumor. Moreover, of the malignant conditions, children younger than 2 years are more likely to suffer from neuroblastoma and hepatoblastoma, whereas older children more frequently have Wilms' tumor, hepatocellular carcinoma, GU tract tumors, and germ line tumors.

Other important points to be noted in history are detailed in **Table 3**.

CLINICAL PEARLS

- Abdominal masses in older children are usually malignant and need prompt evaluation.

EXAMINATION

The importance of a thorough physical examination with vitals (including temperature and blood pressure) cannot be overemphasized. **Table 4** highlights the salient features to look for in a child with abdominal mass. One must be

TABLE 4: Points to be considered during examination.

System	*Clinical features*
General appearance	Well, ill, cachexic, anxious, and in pain
Weight and height	Plot on growth chart
Vitals	Include blood pressure and temperature
Skin	Jaundice, café-au-lait, nevi, freckles, skin nodules, petechiae, and purpura
Head, neck, eyes, and nose throat	Pallor, aniridia, periorbital ecchymosis, ptosis, and lymphadenopathy
Abdomen	Details of mass, quadrant, consistency, tenderness, mobility, bruit, veins over it, possible organ of origin, and bowel sounds
Cardiovascular	Murmurs
Respiratory	Wheeze and superior vena cava syndrome
Genitalia	Normal/abnormal
Others	Stigmata of congenital syndrome (e.g., hemihypertrophy)

patient as physical examination in young children can be a difficult proposition. **Table 5** lists some of the important clinical findings to look for during examination.

INVESTIGATIONS

All children with abdominal masses should have a complete blood count and peripheral smear examination as it may throw up important clues to diagnosis. Further investigations would include baseline chemistries and specific tumor markers on the basis of the clinical differential diagnoses **(Table 5)**.

IMAGING

An abdominal mass in children is often first assessed by a plain abdominal radiograph to rule out GI obstruction. Next, an ultrasound study is helpful and can be done without sedation. It is noninvasive, easily available and fairly inexpensive, and is sometimes the first investigation done for an abdominal mass. It can usually identify the organ of origin of the mass, such as the kidney, adrenal gland, or liver, and helps differentiate solid from cystic masses. Further information is provided in **Table 6**.

An algorithmic approach to evaluation of a child with abdominal mass is depicted in **Flowchart 1**.

TABLE 5: Laboratory investigations.

Test	*Indication/clues*
Complete blood count with differential	Anemia, neutropenia, or thrombocytopenia can indicate bone marrow infiltration
Coagulation profile (pre-biopsy)	PT, PTTK, and INR
Bone marrow biopsy and/or aspiration	Indicated if one or more bone marrow cell lines are compromised
Chemistry panel electrolytes uric acid and lactate dehydrogenase	• Electrolyte abnormality indicates pathology with the kidney or tumor lysis syndrome • Elevated uric acid or lactate dehydrogenase suggest a high grade malignancy
Urinalysis	Hematuria or proteinuria suggest renal involvement
Urinary homovanillic acid and vanillylmandelic acid	Elevated levels indicate neuroblastoma or pheochromocytoma
Tumor markers: Serum B human chorionic gonadotropin and α-fetoprotein	Elevated levels may occur in teratomas, liver tumors, and germ cell tumors

(INR: international normalized ratio; PT: prothrombin time; PTTK: partial thromboplastin time with kaolin)

TABLE 6: Imaging studies.

Test	*Indication/clue*
Plain abdominal X-ray	• First imaging study to be ordered • Helps determine the location and density of the abdominal mass • Multiple air fluid levels or absence of air in the rectum—indicate obstruction • Calcification may indicate a neuroblastoma, teratomas, kidney stones, or biliary stones
Ultrasound	• Inexpensive and safe modality • Useful for discerning between solid versus cystic mass
Computed tomography scan	• Used to attain more specific anatomic information about the abdominal mass • CT scan can be used to determine organ of origin, characteristics of the mass, and invasion of malignant lesion into adjacent structures
Magnetic resonance imaging	• Used for greater anatomic details • Especially for imaging of brain and spine in patients presenting with neurologic deficits

Flowchart 1: Algorithmic approach to diagnosis of an abdominal mass in a child.

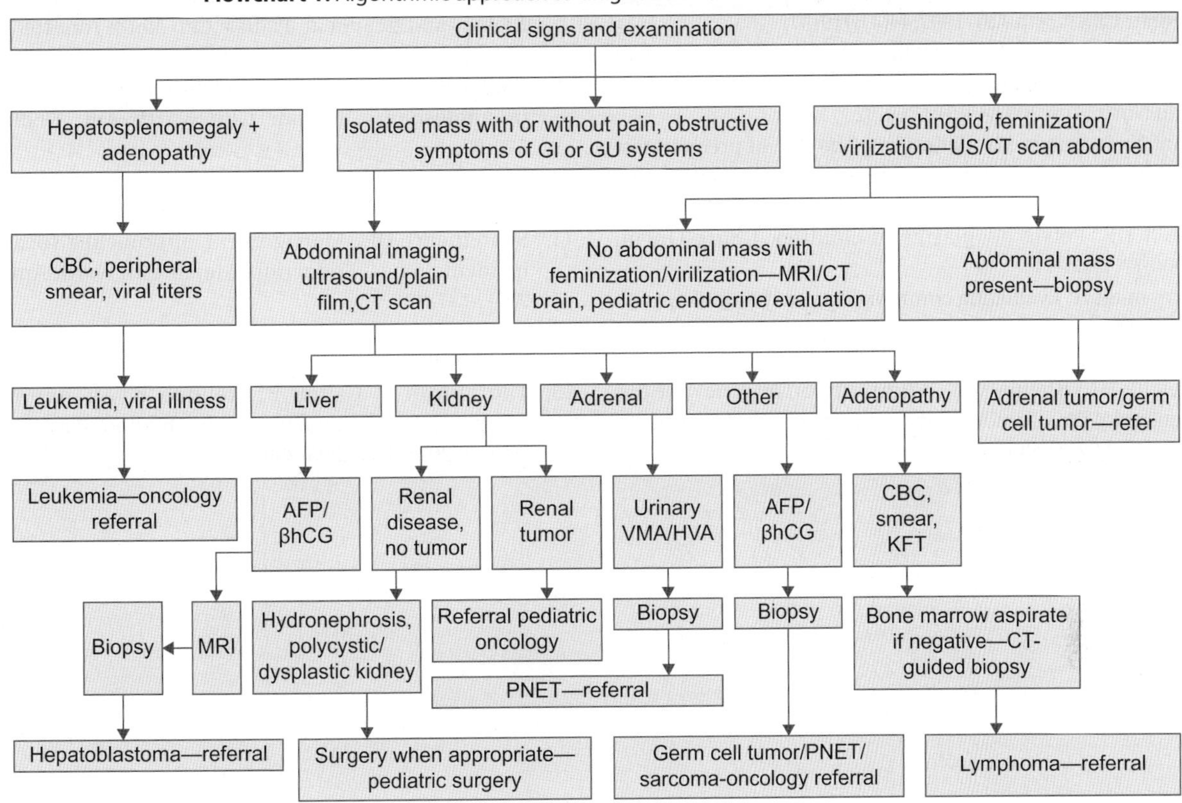

(AFP: alpha-fetoprotein; βhCG: β-human chorionic gonadotropin; CBC: complete blood count; CT: computed tomography; GI: gastrointestinal; GU: genitourinary; HVA: homovanillic acid; KFT: kidney function test; PNET: primitive neuroectodermal tumor; US: ultrasound; VMA: vanillylmandelic acid)

Once a malignancy is suspected it is recommended that the child be referred to a pediatric oncology unit, since early diagnosis of pediatric cancers are associated with very good cure rates. Delayed diagnosis not only reduces the chances of cure but is also associated with higher complication rate. Parents should, therefore, be appropriately counseled at this time and the pediatrician has a very important role to play in bridging the gap between the family and the oncology center.

COMMUNICATION WITH THE FAMILY

Communicating with families about the possible diagnosis is very important. However, it is important to gently explain to the parent(s)/guardian(s), using nonmedical terminology, that a diagnosis of a benign/cancer is suspected or needs to be ruled out, prior to transfer/referral to the tertiary oncology center. Reassurance and guidance are needed. Age-appropriate information also needs to be given to the child as well.

KEY POINTS

- Abdominal masses in children are a cause for concern because of the possibility of malignant disease and need prompt evaluation.
- Most abdominal masses in neonates are benign unless they are solid.
- Age of the patient, along with history and examination findings provide important clues to the possible organ of origin and underlying pathology.
- Neuroblastoma and Wilms' tumor are the two most common malignant conditions that present as abdominal masses in young children.
- The pediatrician plays an important role in early diagnosis, prompt evaluation, and appropriate referral.
- Most childhood cancers have good cure rates if diagnosed in time and treated properly.

SUGGESTED READING

1. Broecker B. Non-Wilms' renal tumors in children. Urol Clin North Am. 2000;27(3):463-9.

2. Castleberry RP. Biology and treatment of neuroblastoma. Pediatr Clin North Am. 1997;44(4):919-37.
3. Golden CB, Feusner JH. Malignant abdominal masses in children: quick guide to evaluation and diagnosis. Pediatr Clin North Am. 2002;49(6):1369-92.
4. Graf N, Tournade MF, deKraker J. The role of preoperative chemotherapy in the management of Wilms tumor: The SIOP Studies. Urol Clin North Am. 2000;27(3):443-54.
5. Groff DB. Pelvic neoplasms in children. J Surg Oncol. 2000;77(1):65-71.
6. Grossman H. Evaluating common intra-abdominal masses in children—a systematic roentgenographic approach. CA Cancer J Clin. 1976;26(4):219-35.
7. Neville HL, Ritchey ML. Wilms' tumor, overview of the National Wilms Tumor Study Group results. Urol Clin North Am. 2000;27(3):435-42.
8. Pappo AS, Shapiro DN, Crist WM. Rhabdomyosarcoma. Biology and treatment. Pediatr Clin North Am. 1997;44(4): 953-72.
9. Pfeifer SM, Gosman GG. Evaluation of adnexal masses in adolescents. Pediatr Clin North Am. 1999;46(3): 573-92.
10. Rahhal RM, Eddine AC, Bishop WP. A Child with an Abdominal Mass. Pediatr Rounds. 2006;42:37-42.
11. Schteingart DE. Management approaches to adrenal incidentalomas. Endocrinol Metab Clin North Am. 2000; 29(1):127-39.
12. Stringer MD. Liver tumors. Semin Pediatr Surg. 2000; 9(4):196-208.
13. Thorbinson C, Calton E, Brennan B. An approach to oncological abdominal masses in children, Paediatr Child Health. 2021;31(7):295-299.

Approach to a Child with Persistent Anemia

Tushar Idhate

INTRODUCTION

Anemia is the most common hematologic abnormality identified in infants and children. Anemia is associated with increased morbidity and mortality in children, particularly children of preschool age. The statistics from the National Family Health Survey (NFHS-5; 2019–21) have raised a red flag highlighting the rising prevalence of anemia across all ages. The highest spike in anemia was reported among children (6–59 months) with a rise to 67.1% (NFHS-5) from 58.6% (NFHS-4, 2015–16) followed by girls aged 15–19 years. The Comprehensive National Nutrition Survey (CNNS) conducted in 2016-2018 revealed that 41% of preschoolers (1–4 years), 24% school-age children (5–9 years), and 28% of adolescents (10–19 years) in India have anemia.

DEFINITION OF ANEMIA

Anemia is defined quantitatively as a decreased number of circulating erythrocytes or functionally as a condition where numbers of erythrocytes, carriers of oxygen, are insufficient to meet metabolic demands. In practice, anemia is defined by hemoglobin (Hb), hematocrit, or red blood cell count levels lower than the normal age- and sex-adjusted ranges.

Table 1 gives the normal values (normal mean, lower limit) of various hematological parameters at different age groups.

The initial diagnostic approach to the anemic patient should include detailed history, physical examination, and screening laboratory tests followed by specific laboratory tests as indicated to confirm the diagnosis.

HISTORY IN THE DIAGNOSIS OF ANEMIA

Age

Anemia manifesting in the neonatal period is generally as a result of blood loss, including fetomaternal hemorrhage, fetofetal hemorrhage and occult hemorrhage, or due to hemolysis as a result of isoimmunization, uncommonly glucose-6-phosphate dehydrogenase (G6PD) deficiency, spherocytosis, or due to congenital infections.

Nutritional anemia is uncommon below the age of 6 months (especially in term breastfed infants), except in preterm infants. Most common cause of anemia in the age group of 6 months to 3 years is nutritional anemia.

TABLE 1: Normal blood values at different age groups.

Age	*Hb g/dL*	*RBC million/mm^3*	*Hct %*	*MCV femtoliters (fL)*	*MCH (pg)*	*MCHC (%)*	*Reticulocyte (%)*
1 day	18.0	5.14	61	119	36.0	31.6	3.2
4 weeks	14.2	4.0	43	106	35.5	33.5	0.6
1 year	11.6	4.6	35	77	25.0	33.0	0.9
10–12 years	13.0	4.8	39	80	27.0	33.0	1.0
Adult men	16.0	5.4	47	87	29.0	34.0	1.0
Adult women	14.0	4.8	42	87	29.0	34.0	1.0

(Hb: hemoglobin; Hct: hematocrit; MCH: mean corpuscular hemoglobin; MCHC: mean corpuscular hemoglobin concentration; MCV: mean corpuscular volume; RBC: red blood cell)

Faulty complementary feeding, intake of junk foods, and worm infestation remain major causes of iron deficiency anemia (IDA) in this age group. Adolescent age group children also have nutritional anemia including megaloblastic anemia due to dietary deficiencies.

Hemoglobinopathies such as thalassemia major commonly present during 6–18 months of age and rarely before that age.

Gender

Nutritional anemia incidence is equal in both genders during childhood.

Family History

Certain inherited anemias are transmitted as X-linked recessive and hence are commonly seen in male children such as G6PD deficiency. Hence, similar history of anemia should be enquired in other male siblings, maternal male cousins, maternal uncles, and maternal grandfather. Hereditary spherocytosis is an autosomal dominant disorder, whereas hemoglobinopathies like thalassemia, sickle cell anemia, etc. are inherited as autosomal recessive conditions. It is important to enquire about family history of anemia, jaundice, gallstones, splenectomy, etc. in the other members of the family. A history of consanguineous marriage is also helpful in recessive conditions. Hence, a detail pedigree chart including the family members, who have expired, should be obtained.

Birth History

Review of birth history should include labor, delivery, and neonatal course, including the history of anemia, jaundice, phototherapy, or blood transfusion.

Dietary History

Nutritional anemias are associated with poor dietary intake of iron, B_{12}, and folic acid in the diet. Inadequate iron containing complementary foods and/or predominantly milk-based diet beyond 4–6 months of age contribute significantly to occurrence of IDA. Megaloblastic anemia due to folate deficiency may be seen in children fed predominantly goat's milk and B_{12} deficiency seen in pure vegetarians.

Other Relevant History

History of trauma, infections, surgery, travel, and exposure to drugs, chemicals, toxins, or oxidants should be sought, as should sources of blood loss such as epistaxis, gastrointestinal (GI) bleeding, or in young women, dysmenorrhea.

EXAMINATION FINDINGS AS A CLUE TO THE DIAGNOSIS OF ANEMIA

General Examination Findings

Presence of platynychia and/or koilonychias is pathognomonic of IDA. Hyperpigmentation of knuckles is common with megaloblastic anemia. Glossitis is seen in vitamin B_{12}, folate, and iron deficiency; angular stomatitis and bald tongue are seen in iron deficiency. Blue sclera is often a feature of IDA. Presence of hemolytic facies is seen in congenital hemolytic anemias such as thalassemia major, sickle cell anemia. Fanconi's anemia may have microphthalmia and microcornea, besides microcephaly, triangular facies.

Thumb anomalies suggest constitutional hypoplastic anemias (Diamond–Blackfan anemia, Fanconi's anemia). Lymphadenopathy would prompt one to consider various malignant disorders, such as leukemias, lymphomas, metastatic malignancies such as neuroblastoma, infections such as tuberculosis, infectious mononucleosis, human immunodeficiency virus, cytomegalovirus (CMV), etc.

Systemic Examination

Hepatosplenomegaly

Presence of hepatosplenomegaly almost always rules out hypoplastic anemia except the infiltrative causes of marrow suppression. It suggests hemolytic anemias, the infiltrative causes such as leukemias, osteopetrosis, myelofibrosis, myelodysplasia.

LABORATORY APPROACH TO ANEMIA

The investigations in children with anemia should be done in a phased manner as expensive confirmatory tests may be useless and unnecessary in concluding the cause of anemia, unless done judiciously. Therefore, it is imperative to follow a stepwise testing to get a better yield without spending the patient's money unnecessarily.

Investigations should be done as follows:

- Screening tests
- Definitive diagnostic tests

Screening Tests

Screening tests include:

- Complete blood count including hematocrit and blood indices

- Reticulocyte count
- Examination of the peripheral smear

Complete Blood Counts

- *Hemoglobin:* The severity of anemia can be gauged with the value of hemoglobin.
- *Red cell indices:* These include mean corpuscular volume (MCV), mean corpuscular hemoglobin (MCH), mean corpuscular hemoglobin concentration (MCHC), and red cell distribution width (RDW). This helps in typing the anemia.

Based on MCV, MCH, and MCHC, anemias can be classified into three categories to give a morphologic classification. Besides, the RDW further elucidates the cause of anemia. Along with the findings of the peripheral smear findings, most anemias can be categorized completely with a few specific confirmatory tests.

- Microcytic, hypochromic anemia—MCV <80 μ^3, MCH <27 pg, and MCHC <32%
- Macrocytic anemia—MCV >95 μ^3
- Normocytic, normochromic anemia—MCV 80–95 μ^3, MCH 27–32 pg, and MCHC 32–36%.

Red cell distribution width: It is the measure of the degree of anisocytosis. This is calculated from the histogram of MCV and expressed as a coefficient of variation. The normal values are 11.5–14.5%. Along with MCV, it can help categorize anemias further. The relationship of MCV and RDW is given in **Table 2**.

Reticulocyte Count

Reticulocyte count is considered to be a window to the bone marrow. As reticulocytes are the immediate precursors of mature red blood cells (RBCs), their presence in the peripheral blood reflects the marrow activity in response to anemia. Reticulocyte count is expected to be high in children with anemia if they have a responsive marrow. Therefore, one needs to consider whether the reticulocytes have increased proportionate to the degree of anemia. This is done by calculating the corrected reticulocyte count as:

$$\frac{\text{Reticulocyte count} \times \text{Observed Hct}}{\text{Desired Hct}}$$

Example: If the reticulocyte count of a child is 6% and the hematocrit (Hct) is 15%, the corrected reticulocyte count would be as follows: 6 × 15/45 = 2%, which is not as high as it seems.

TABLE 2: Relationship of mean corpuscular volume and red cell distribution width.

RDW	*Low MCV*	*Normal MCV*	*High MCV*
Normal	Thalassemia trait	Normal lead poisoning	Aplastic anemia
High	• Iron deficiency • HbH disease • HbS/thalassemia trait	• Early IDA • Liver disease • Mixed nutritional deficiency	• Newborns • Vitamin B_{12}/ folate deficiency

(IDA: iron deficiency anemia; MCV: mean corpuscular volume; RDW: red cell distribution width)

Polychromasia and basophilic stippling on peripheral smear are indirect evidences of reticulocytosis.

Points to note:

- Reticulocyte count is a window to the bone marrow and if normal to increased suggests the pathology does not exist in the marrow.
- Red blood cell indices along with red cell distribution width and reticulocyte count can help diagnose many of the causes of anemia.

Peripheral Smear Examination

This is the single most important, cost-effective test for anemia. It not only suggests the type of anemia but also gives the clue to the underlying cause and disease.

The peripheral smear may provide insights into the diagnosis such as spherocytes in hereditary spherocytosis or autoimmune hemolytic anemia, elliptocytes in hereditary elliptocytosis, fragmented cells, schistocytes, and helmet cells in microangiopathic hemolytic anemia, target cells in hemoglobinopathies, liver disease, and postsplenectomy, and inclusions of various types seen in malaria.

Confirmatory Tests

These would be based on the screening test results. As per the algorithms given below and the suspected diagnosis, these confirmatory tests should be performed or ordered.

Coombs test, G6PD estimation, osmotic fragility and flow cytometry, bone marrow aspiration and biopsy, high-performance liquid chromatography, serum iron studies, Sr vitamin B_{12} and folate levels are required to reach to specific diagnosis. Besides these, certain corroborative tests such as serum bilirubin, lactate dehydrogenase (LDH), haptoglobins, etc. also assist in diagnosing the cause of anemia.

Flowchart 1: Microcytic and hypochromic anemia.

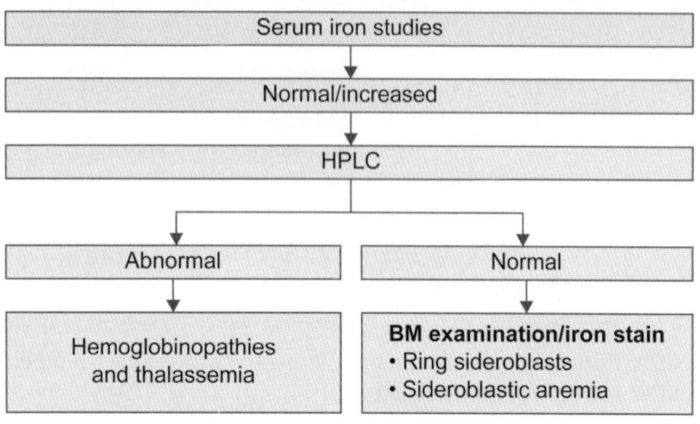

(BM: bone marrow; HPLC: high-performance liquid chromatography)

Flowchart 2: Macrocytic anemia.

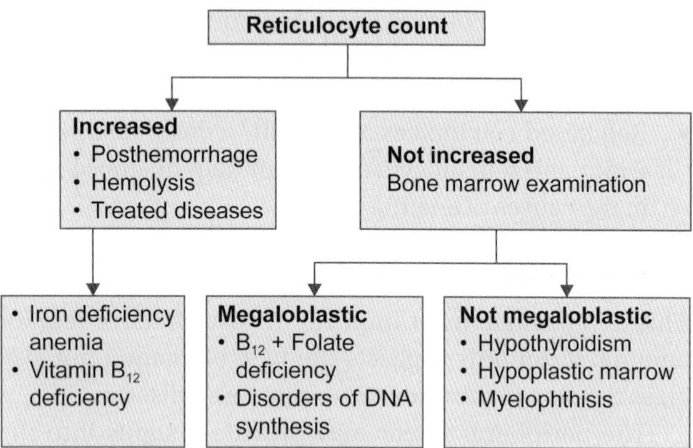

Flowchart 3: Normocytic and normochromic.

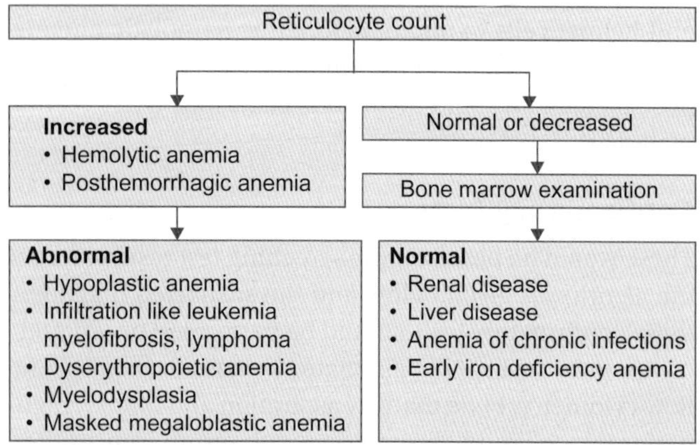

Occasionally, workup for alfa-thalassemia, unstable hemoglobins, rare hemoglobin variants, cytogenetics, and other RBC enzyme levels may be required.

In today's era, genetic studies including NGS have vital importance in establishing final diagnosis in many of anemias.

ALGORITHMS TO DIAGNOSE ANEMIA BASED ON VARIOUS INVESTIGATIONS

Methods to diagnose anemia based on various investigation are represented in **Flowcharts 1 to 3**.

CONCLUSION

With detailed history taking and relevant clinical examination, basic screening tests, and minimum specific tests, it is possible to diagnose the type of anemia and institute appropriate treatment. This approach would definitely help in minimizing the need for useless and expensive tests in children with anemia.

KEY POINTS

- Hemoglobin range varies as per age, so age is very important parameter in children to decide whether Hb is normal or low.
- Presence of lymphadenopathy and hepatosplenomegaly should prompt exclusion of malignancies especially in presence of affection of other cell lines, i.e., white cells and platelets.
- Reticulocyte count is increased in hemolysis, hemorrhage, or after starting therapy for nutritional deficiencies. However, it is low or normal in nutritional anemias and it is below 1% in bone marrow suppression.
- Detailed history and good clinical examination is essential to the diagnosis of anemia.
- Screening tests give you direction. A proper evaluation of the complete blood count especially red cell indices along with red cell distribution width, peripheral smear, and reticulocyte count would help in directing type of anemia in almost all patients.
- Confirmatory tests are essential to establish final diagnosis. A stepwise approach helps in limiting the investigations required to reach a diagnosis.

SUGGESTED READING

1. Bessman JD, Feinstein DI. Quantitative anisocytosis as a discriminant between iron deficiency and thalassemia minor. Blood. 1979;53:288-93.
2. Bessman JD, Gilmer PR, Gardner FH. Improved classification of anemia by MCV and RDW. Am J Clin Pathol. 1983; 80:322-6.
3. Beuttler E. The red cell indices in the diagnosis of iron deficiency anemia. Ann Intern Med. 1959;50:313-22.

4. Buch AC, Karve PP, Panicker NK, Singru SA, Gupta SC. Role of red cell distribution width in classifying microcytic hypochromic anemia. J Indian Med Assoc. 2011;109:297-9.
5. de Benoist B, McLean E, Egli I, Cogswell M. (2008). Worldwide prevalence of anaemia 1993–2005: WHO global database on anaemia. [online] Available from https://iris.who.int/bitstream/handle/10665/43894/9789241596657_eng.pdf?sequence=1. [Last accessed October, 2024]
6. DeMaeyer EH, Adiels-Tegman M. The prevalence of anemia in the world. World Health Stat Q. 1985;38:302-16.
7. Hermiston ML, Mentzer WC. A practical approach to the evaluation of anemic child. Pediatr Clin North Am. 2002;49:877-91.
8. Irwin JJ, Kirchner JT. Anemia in children. Am Fam Physician. 2001;64:1379-86.
9. Janus J, Moerschel SK. Evaluation of anemia in children. Am Fam Physician. 2010;81:1462-71.
10. Lee GR. Iron deficiency and iron deficiency anemia. In: Lee GR, Bithel TC, Foester J, Athens JW, Lukens JN (Eds). Wintrobe's Clinical Hematology, 9th edition. Philadelphia: Lea & Febiger; 1993. pp. 808-39.
11. Lokeshwar MR, Manglani M. Antenatal supplementation-effect on iron status of infants. Indian Pediatr. 1990;27:677-80.
12. Manglani M, Lokeshwar MR, Vani VG, Bhatia N, Mhaskar V. 'NESTROFT'-an effective screening test for beta-thalassemia trait. Indian Pediatr. 1997;34:702-7.
13. Mehta BC. Approach to a patient with anemia. Indian J Med Sci. 2004;58:26-9.
14. Orkin SH, Fisher DE, Look AT, Lux SE, Ginsburg D, Nathan DG. Nathan and Oski's Hematology of Infancy and Childhood, 7th edition. Philadelphia: Saunders, an imprint of Elsevier Inc.; 2009.
15. Vasanta G, Pawashi AR, Susie H, Sujatha T, Raman L. Iron nutritional status of adolescent girls from rural area and urban slum. Indian Pediatr. 1994;31:127-32.

Algorithmic Approach to Thrombocytopenia in Children

Purva Kanvinde, Purvaja Kubde

INTRODUCTION

The normal platelet count for children ranges from approximately 150,000 to 450,000/μL. Thrombocytopenia is defined as platelet count of <150,000/cumm. However, clinically significant thrombocytopenia is defined as any count $<100 \times 10^9$/L; furthermore, it is considered severe if the platelet count is below 30×10^9/L, moderate if it is between 30×10^9/L and 50×10^9/L, and mild (and usually asymptomatic) if above 50×10^9/L.

The risk of bleeding does not increase until the platelet count falls well below 100,000/μL, and significant spontaneous bleeding is not likely to occur until the platelet count falls below 20,000/μL. The lifespan of platelet ranges from 7 to 10 days, after which they are removed from the circulation by cells of the monocyte-macrophage system.

CAUSES OF THROMBOCYTOPENIA

Causes of thrombocytopenia are given in **Table 1**.

TABLE 1: Causes of thrombocytopenia.

Destructive thrombocytopenias	***Decreased platelet production***
Immune-mediated: • Immune thrombocytopenia (ITP) • Drug-induced thrombocytopenia • Systemic autoimmune disorders and immune dysregulation syndromes (secondary ITP) • Systemic lupus erythematosus (SLE) • Autoimmune lymphoproliferative • Syndrome (ALPS) and ALPS like • Antiphospholipid antibody syndrome • Common variable immunodeficiency • DiGeorge (22q11.2 deletion) syndrome • Post-transfusion purpura • Malignancy-associated ITP • Neonatal immune thrombocytopenia (including alloimmune and autoimmune)	*Infection:* Epstein–Barr virus, cytomegalovirus, bacterial sepsis, parvovirus, varicella, rickettsia, and dengue virus *Nutritional deficiencies:* Folate, B_{12}, and iron
Platelet activation and consumption: • Microangiopathic disorders • Hemolytic-uremic syndrome • Thrombotic thrombocytopenic purpura • Disseminated intravascular coagulation • Major surgery or trauma • Kasabach–Merritt syndrome	*Acquired disorders:* • Aplastic anemia • Myelodysplastic syndromes • Medications (e.g., chemotherapy) • Radiation • Infiltrative bone marrow diseases • Leukemias • Lymphomas • Metastatic cancers • Infectious granulomas • Storage diseases

Contd...

Contd...

Destructive thrombocytopenias	*Decreased platelet production*
Mechanical destruction: Extracorporeal therapies (e.g., cardiopulmonary bypass)	*Genetic causes of impaired thrombopoiesis:* • Wiskott–Aldrich syndrome/X-linked thrombocytopenia • Inherited bone marrow failure syndromes • Secondary to transcription factor defects • May–Hegglin anomaly
Sequestration and trapping: • Hypersplenism • Platelet-type von Willebrand disease	

CLINICAL FEATURES

The clinical features of thrombocytopenia are due to the defect in primary hemostasis. It is clinically suspected when there is history of easy bruising or bleeding. Petechiae, purpura, epistaxis, gum bleeding, gastrointestinal (GI) bleeds, hematuria, and menorrhagia are some of the important presenting features. Intracranial bleeding, though rare, is one of the dreaded complications of low platelet counts.

Patients with thrombocytopenia are more likely to have bleeding after minor cuts and less likely to have deep bleeding into tissues, muscles, and joints. In patients with thrombocytopenia, posttraumatic or postoperative surgical bleeding usually responds to local measures.

CLINICAL APPROACH TO THE PATIENT WITH THROMBOCYTOPENIA

Detailed History

A detailed history should be documented regarding age of onset, present as well as past history of type and site of bleeding, presence of symptoms suggestive of underlying etiology of thrombocytopenia, and a focused family history regarding thrombocytopenia and bleeding to rule out underlying inherited causes of thrombocytopenia.

- *Age at presentation:* Early age of presentation points toward an inherited cause of thrombocytopenia.
- *Sex of the child:* Male sex would be important in cases of thrombocytopenia which is inherited in an X-linked pattern such as Wiskott–Aldrich syndrome.
- A detailed history documenting the *number of episodes, type and site of bleeding, and intervention required to control the bleeding episode.*
- A *focused history* should be documented to look for the *underlying etiology of thrombocytopenia* which includes:
  - A history of recurrent respiratory tract infections or diarrhea would provide a clue to an underlying primary immune deficiency.
  - History of receiving vaccination or an episode of viral illness 4–6 weeks prior to an episode of thrombocytopenia would be typically seen in cases with immune thrombocytopenia (ITP).
  - History of bloody diarrhea followed by oliguria is typically seen in cases of hemolytic uremic syndrome (HUS).
  - History of hearing loss and renal disorder would indicate underlying hereditary macrothrombocytopenia disorders.
  - A history of rash and joint pain would be seen in children with autoimmune disorders such as systemic lupus erythematosus (SLE).
  - History of bone pains, increasing pallor, abdominal distension and constitutional symptoms like fever, and weight loss would be suggestive of hematolymphoid malignancy.
  - History suggestive of malaria and dengue
  - History of medications such as heparin, aspirin, and anticonvulsants should be taken to rule out drug induced thrombocytopenia.
  - History/risk for human immunodeficiency virus (HIV)
  - Detailed dietary history including consumption of nonvegetarian food should be taken to rule out causes of nutritional deficiencies.
- A detailed *family history* of thrombocytopenia, bleeding disorder, history of symptoms suggestive of primary immunodeficiency disease, inherited marrow failure syndrome, and platelets disorders should be taken.

Physical Examination

The extent of the bleeding should be evaluated and documented in detail. Sites of bleeding in each episode should be noted, especially mucosal areas such as oral cavity, gums, and dependent parts of the body.

Physical examination that may provide clues to the underlying cause of thrombocytopenia includes:

- *Head, neck, eyes, and ears:*
  - Microcephaly, bird like facies, and micrognathia would be seen with inherited marrow failure syndromes such as Fanconi anemia.
  - Sensorineural hearing loss and cataracts are commonly seen with hereditary macrothrombocytopenia syndromes such as May–Hegglin anomaly.
- *Skin and oral cavity manifestations:*
  - Cafe au lait spots, hypo-, or hyperpigmentation is seen with Fanconi anemia.
  - Chronic eczema is a common manifestation of Wiskott–Aldrich syndrome.
  - Nail dystrophy and oral leukoplakia can be seen with dyskeratosis congenita (DKC).
  - Butterfly rash and oral ulcers provide a clue to diagnosis of SLE.
  - Presence of vascular malformations point toward a Kasabach–Merritt syndrome.
- *Orthopedic abnormalities:*
  - Absent radius with functional thumbs, radioulnar synostosis, and mainly upper limb deformities are seen with disorders such as thrombocytopenia absent radius (TAR) and amegakaryocytic thrombocytopenia with radioulnar synostosis (ATRUS).
  - Absent or hypoplastic, supernumerary or bifid thumb, hypoplastic thenar eminences, absent or hypoplastic radi, clinodactyly, and lower limb anomalies are commonly seen with Fanconi anemia.
  - Arthralgia and arthritis is suggestive of collagen vascular diseases.
- *Constitutional symptoms:*
  - Short stature is seen with inherited marrow failure syndromes.
  - Fever could be a presentation of infections as well as malignancy.
  - Features of renal failure such as edema and hypertension may be noted in HUS.
  - Presence of pallor may be seen with Evans syndrome, HUS, and malignancies.
  - Bony tenderness points toward malignancy.
- *Systemic examination:*
  - Lymphadenopathy or hepatosplenomegaly may suggest malignancy, HIV, and infectious mononucleosis.
  - Abnormal neurological examination should alert one to the possibility of an intracranial bleed or thrombotic thrombocytopenic purpura (TTP).
- *Others:* Well child with absence of splenomegaly, stigmata of inherited marrow failure will suggest ITP.

DIAGNOSTIC EVALUATION

The initial step in the evaluation of suspected thrombocytopenia in children is verification of a low platelet count. A platelet count that is inconsistent with the clinical presentation of the patient (such as a platelet count <20,000/μL in a patient with no petechiae or other abnormalities) should be confirmed before extensive evaluation.

Spurious thrombocytopenia can be caused by improper collection, delayed processing, or inadequate anticoagulation of the blood sample, resulting in platelet clumps that are counted as leukocytes by automated cell counters. In addition, agglutination of platelets by ethylenediaminetetraacetic acid (EDTA)-dependent antibodies, which are normally present in 0.1% of adults, may cause a falsely low platelet count. The presence of pseudothrombocytopenia can also be confirmed by collecting a blood sample in a non-EDTA anticoagulant tube such as sodium citrate or on a peripheral smear made by direct finger prick.

Laboratory Evaluation

The laboratory evaluation of thrombocytopenia begins with a complete blood count (CBC), which includes the platelet count and mean platelet volume (MPV), and evaluation of the peripheral blood smear.

- *Complete blood count:* In addition to measuring the platelet count, the CBC assesses for other cytopenias (anemia and leukopenia) and it estimates the newer parameters such as MPV and immature platelet fraction (IPF).
  - *Other cytopenias:*
    - Presence of macrocytic anemia could point toward an inherited marrow failure syndrome, Evans syndrome, and microangiopathic anemia.
    - Presence of leukopenia could point toward a viral infection, inherited marrow failure syndrome.
    - Presence of leukopenia or leukocytosis with presence of blasts would be suggestive of malignancy.
  - *MPV:*
    - Normal MPV value is 7–10 fL

    - High MPV is seen in ITP, Bernard–Soulier syndrome and hereditary macrothrombocytopenia syndromes.
    - Low MPV is seen in Wiskott–Aldrich syndrome and X-linked thrombocytopenia.
  - *Immature platelet function (IPF):*
    - IPF is normal to low in patients with bone marrow failure syndrome and high in patients with immune destruction like ITP.
- *Peripheral blood smear examination* **(Figs. 1 to 5)** should include:
  - Estimated platelet count: To confirm presence and severity of thrombocytopenia
  - Characterization of platelet size and morphology: Large platelets will be seen with ITP, Bernard–Soulier syndromes and other hereditary macrothrombocytopenias. Small platelets will be seen in Wiskott–Aldrich syndrome.
  - Presence of platelet clumping
  - Associated white and/or red blood cell abnormalities: Presence of circulating blasts points toward diagnosis of hematolymphoid malignancies.

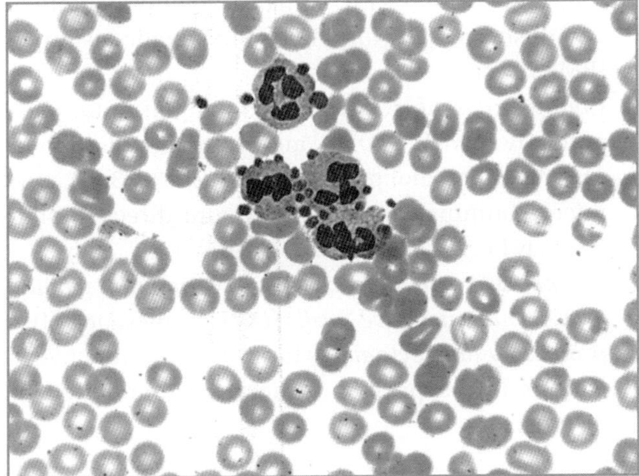

Fig. 1: Pseudothrombocytopenia due to platelet satellitism. *(For color version, see Plate 2)*

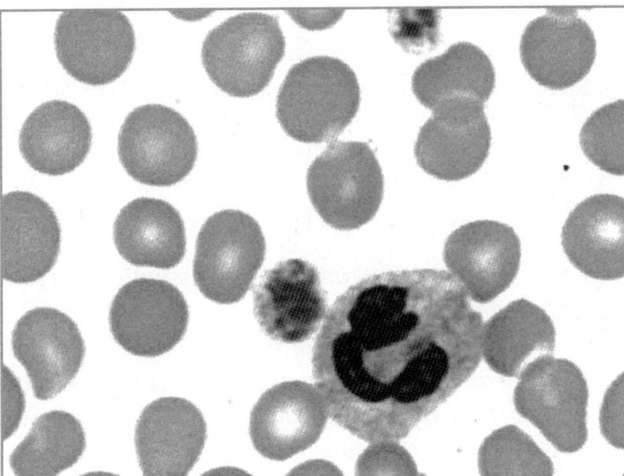

Fig. 3: May–Hegglin anomaly: Neutrophil contains multiple prominent, light blue, and round Dohle bodies, which are intracytoplasmic inclusions that consist of RNA and giant platelets. *(For color version, see Plate 2)*

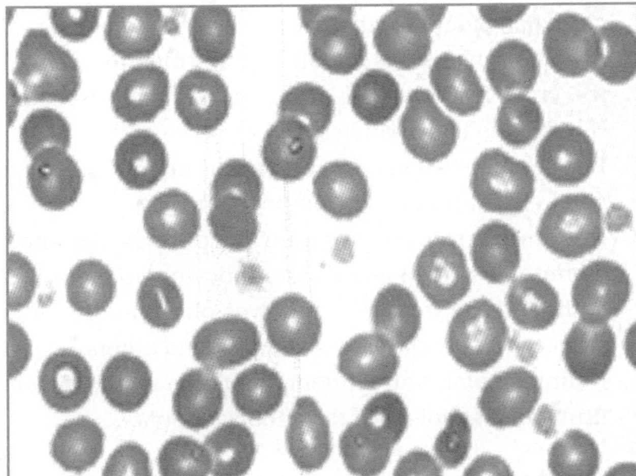

Fig. 2: Gray platelet syndrome: Large platelets which look colorless (due to absence of alpha granules), giving it a grey appearance on peripheral smear. *(For color version, see Plate 2)*

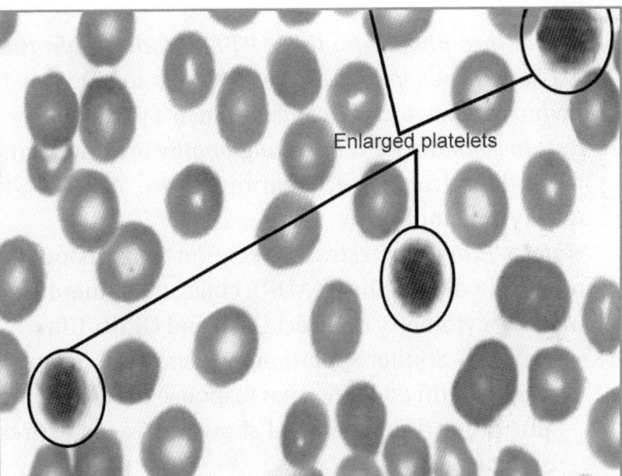

Fig. 4: Bernard–Soulier syndrome: Large platelets on peripheral smear. *(For color version, see Plate 2)*

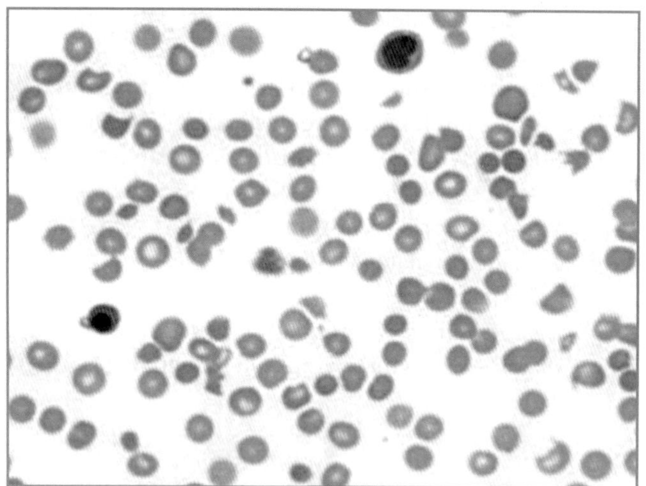

Fig. 5: Microangiopathic hemolytic anemia (HUS/TTP): Schistocytes, spherocytes, polychromasia, and thrombocytopenia on peripheral smear. (HUS: hemolytic uremic syndrome; TTP: thrombotic thrombocytopenic purpura) *(For color version, see Plate 2)*

- *Bone marrow aspirate and biopsy* is essential in certain conditions like:
  - *Symptoms and signs of inherited marrow failure syndromes:* To look for marrow cellularity and megakaryocytes. Megakaryocytes will be absent in cases with congenital amegakaryocytic thrombocytopenia (CAMT).
  - *Suspicion of hematolymphoid malignancies:* To confirm the diagnosis of leukemia by flow cytometry.

Other Tests

- *Partial thromboplastin time (PTT), prothrombin time (PT), D-dimer, and fibrinogen levels* are useful to diagnosis intravascular coagulation in a patient.
- *Tests to evaluate for a microangiopathy* include serum lactic dehydrogenase, creatinine, and ADAMTS13 activity and antibody.
- *Platelet functions tests:* Aggregation with ristocetin, adenosine diphosphate (ADP), collagen, epinephrine, and flow cytometry to detect GPIb and GPIIb-IIIa.
  - Bernard–Soulier syndrome will show no response to ristocetin and a normal response to ADP, epinephrine, and collagen and show decreased expression of GPIb.
- *Type 2B von Willebrand disease (vWD) and platelet-type vWD* typically show decrease in von Willebrand factor (vWF) protein (VWF:Ag), vWF: RCo and increased response to low-dose ristocetin-induced platelet aggregation (LD-RIPA)
- Patients with giant platelets and/or family history of thrombocytopenia should undergo testing for inherited platelet disorders, including MYH9-related disorder and Bernard–Soulier syndrome.
- Many of the *inherited thrombocytopenias* can be identified by genetic testing either with a targeted panel or single-gene testing if a particular diagnosis is suspected.
- *Inherited bone marrow failure syndromes (IBMFS)* can be diagnosed by mitomycin-induced chromosomal breakage studies (for Fanconi anemia), telomere length shortening (for DKC), and genetic testing for IBMFS panel.
- *Collagen vascular diseases:* Looking at antinuclear antibody (ANA), DsDNA, antiphospholipid antibody (APLA), anticardiolipin antibody (ACLA), C3, C4, urine microalbuminuria/proteinuria, and direct Coombs test may help to clinch the diagnosis.
- *Lymphocyte subset analysis (LSSA), immunoglobulin levels, double negative T cells (DNT), expression of WAS protein by flow cytometry* form the first-line investigations for suspected primary immunodeficiency disorders.

TREATMENT

Treatment involves management of the underlying cause:
- Mild bleeding may be controlled with local pressure and antifibrinolytics.
- Serial monitoring of platelet count may be required in cases of incidentally discovered thrombocytopenia.
- Platelet transfusions are often performed to tide over the crisis in cases with inherited platelet disorders, IBMFS, and malignancies.
- Platelet transfusions are contraindicated in HUS, TTP, and heparin-induced thrombocytopenia.
- Immune thrombocytopenic purpura is the most common cause of acute thrombocytopenia in a well child and the treatment involves observation, intravenous immunoglobulins, steroids, and others.
- Definitive plan of treatment should be made on confirmation of etiology of thrombocytopenia.

ALGORITHM

Algorithm for approach to thrombocytopenia is given in **Flowchart 1**.

Flowchart 1: Approach to thrombocytopenia.

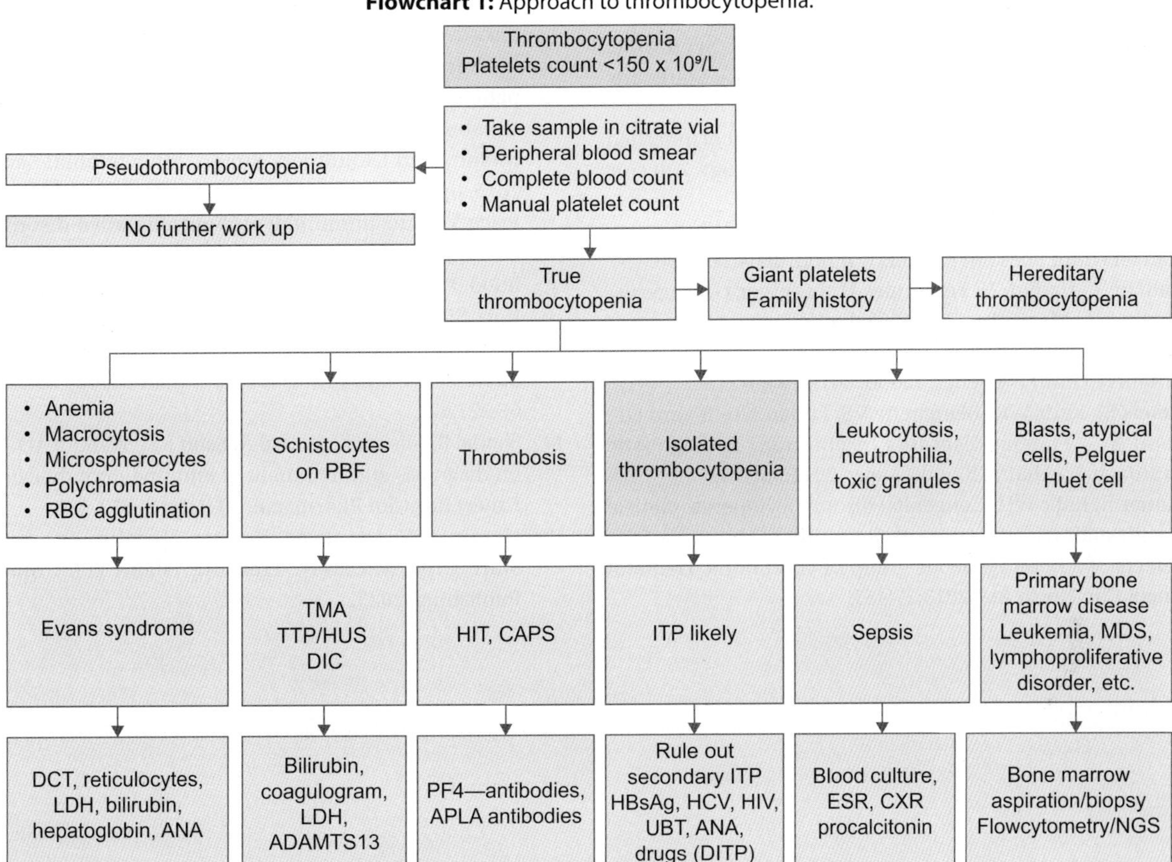

(ANA: antinuclear antibody; APLA: antiphospholipid antibody; CXR: chest X-ray; DCT; distal convoluted tubule; DIC: disseminated intravascular coagulation; HBsAG: hepatitis B surface antigen; HCV: hepatitis C virus; HIV: human immunodeficiency virus; HUS: hemolytic uremic syndrome; ITP: immune thrombocytopenia; LDH: Lactate dehydrogenase; MDS: myelodysplastic syndrome; NGS: next-generation sequencing; PBF: peripheral blood film; TMA: thrombotic microangiopathy; TTP: thrombotic thrombocytopenic purpura)

KEY POINTS

- Thrombocytopenia is defined as platelet count below 150,000/µL. Spontaneous bleeding does not occur until the platelet count is <20,000/µL.
- Most common cause of thrombocytopenia in children is immune thrombocytopenia.
- Autoimmune thrombocytopenia in younger children can be a manifestation of primary immune deficiency.
- Underlying autoimmune disease should be ruled out as a cause of immune thrombocytopenia in adolescents and young adult patients.
- Detailed family history can give clue to early diagnosis.
- Symptomatic patients generally presents with muco-cutaneous bleeding such as petechiae, purpura, ecchymoses and epistaxis. Intracranial bleeding is rare and it is often preceded by history of head trauma.
- Initial diagnostic evaluation includes complete blood count (CBC), peripheral blood smear. Bone marrow examination is not routinely required for the initial evaluation in most cases of isolated thrombocytopenia. It is indicated if there is evidence of other cell lines involvement or if child has systemic symptoms or abnormal physical finding such as lymphadenopathy, hepatosplenomegaly.
- Avoid unnecessary platelet transfusions unless bleeding is severe and treat the underlying cause.
- Platelet transfusions are contraindicated in HUS, TTP, and heparin-induced thrombocytopenia.
- Persistent thrombocytopenia or refractory cases may require long-term monitoring and specialist input.

SUGGESTED READING

1. Almomani MH, Mangla A. Bernard-Soulier Syndrome. In: StatPearls [Internet]. Treasure Island (FL): StatPearls Publishing; 2023.
2. Alter BP. Diagnosis, genetics, and management of inherited bone marrow failure syndromes. Hematology Am Soc Hematol Educ Program. 2007:29-39.
3. Drachman JG. Inherited thrombocytopenia: When a low platelet count does not mean ITP. Blood. 2004;103:390.
4. Hadjadj J, Aladjidi N, Fernandes H, Leverger G, Magérus-Chatinet A, Mazerolles F, et al. Pediatric Evans syndrome is associated with a high frequency of potentially damaging variants in immune genes. Blood. 2019;134:9-21.
5. Israels SJ, Kahr WH, Blanchette VS, Luban NL, Rivard GE, Rand ML. Platelet disorders in children: A diagnostic approach. Paediatric Blood Cancer. 2011;56:975.
6. Kumar R, Kahr WH. Congenital thrombocytopenia: clinical manifestations, laboratory abnormalities, and molecular defects of a heterogeneous group of conditions. Hematol Oncol Clin North Am. 2013;27:465.
7. Lambert MP. Updates in diagnosis of the inherited platelet disorders. Curr Opin Hematol. 2020;27:333.
8. Lusher JM. Clinical and laboratory approach to the patient with bleeding. In: Nathan DG, Orkin SH, Look AT, Ginsburg D (Eds). Nathan and Oski's Hematology of Infancy and Childhood, 8th ed, Philadelphia: Saunders; 2015. pp. 1515.
9. Price V. Auto-immune lymphoproliferative disorder and other secondary immune thrombocytopenias in childhood. Pediatr Blood Cancer. 2013;60 Suppl 1:S12.
10. Rotz SJ, Ware RE, Kumar A. Diagnosis and management of chronic and refractory immune cytopenias in children, adolescents, and young adults. Pediatr Blood Cancer. 2018; 65:e27260.
11. Sandal R, Mishra K, Jandial A, Sahu KK, Siddiqui AD. Update on diagnosis and treatment of immune thrombocytopenia. Expert Rev Clin Pharmacol. 2021;14(5):553-568.
12. Untanu RV, Vajpayee N. May-Hegglin Anomaly. In: StatPearls [Internet]. Treasure Island (FL): StatPearls Publishing; 2023.

CHAPTER 61

Algorithmic Laboratory Approach to a Child with Anemia

Sneha Shinde, Ritika Khurana

INTRODUCTION

Anemia is a condition in which the total circulating red cell mass is reduced below normal limits resulting in decreased oxygen carrying capacity that is insufficient to meet the body's physiologic needs. Anemia is a sign of a disease rather than being a diagnosis, hence efforts should be made to reach the cause of anemia. It is a common problem in India, and the National Family Health Survey III data showed the prevalence of anemia among children <5 years of age to be around 70% with nearly 73 million children below the age of 3 (79%) suffering from varying degrees of anemia.

Anemia is measured by reduction in the volume of packed red cells as measured by the hematocrit and reduction in the hemoglobin concentration below the normal for the age and gender of the individual. These values correlate with the red cell mass, except when there is change in the plasma volume caused by fluid retention or dehydration.

DIAGNOSIS OF ANEMIA

Basic investigations are done to document the presence of anemia and classify it according to morphology and function. Thereafter, based on the differential diagnosis and clinical features, specific diagnostic tests are indicated that help establish the etiology and pathophysiology of anemia. **Table 1** presents age based cut-offs of hemoglobin and hematocrit for diagnosis of anemia in children. The initial laboratory studies should include a complete blood count with red cell indices, reticulocyte count, and study of a well-prepared peripheral blood smear.

TABLE 1: Hemoglobin and hematocrit cut-offs for a diagnosis of anemia in children.

Age (years)/gender	*Hemoglobin (g/dL)*	*Hematocrit (%)*
Both sexes		
1–1.9	11.0	33
2–4.9	11.2	34
5–7.9	11.4	34.5
8–11.9	11.6	35
Females		
12–14.9	11.8	35.5
Males		
12–14.9	12.3	37

BOX 1: Red blood cell indices and their normal values.

- MCV = Hematocrit (%)/RBC count ($\times 10^{12}$/L) × 10
- Normal value: 70–84 fL at 1 year. Mean 80 fL by 5 years
- MCH = Hemoglobin (g/dL)/RBC count ($\times 10^{12}$/L) × 10
- *Normal value:* 26–34 pg. Changes parallel to MCV in infancy and childhood
- MCHC = Hemoglobin (g/dL)/hematocrit (%) × 100
- *Normal value:* 32–36 g/dL
- Increased MCHC seen in hereditary spherocytosis, dehydrated cells in sickle cell anemia, hereditary xerocytosis, and spuriously in immune hemolytic anemias

(MCH: mean corpuscular hemoglobin; MCV: mean corpuscular volume; MCHC: mean corpuscular hemoglobin concentration; RBC: red blood cell)

CLASSIFICATION OF ANEMIA

The common mechanisms of anemia are decreased production, decreased lifespan of red cells, blood loss, and splenic pooling. Detailed history and diligent general and systemic examination are prudent to delineate underlying cause of anemia before ordering investigations. However, if the cause is not readily apparent from clinical features, evaluation based on morphology and function is a well-established approach. Morphological classification of anemia is based on the red blood cell (RBC) indices **(Box 1)** that reflect the RBC volume [mean corpuscular volume (MCV)] and hemoglobin content [mean corpuscular hemoglobin concentration (MCHC)] and divided into microcytic hypochromic, normocytic, normochromic, and macrocytic anemia. As children (other than neonates) have smaller erythrocytes than adults the determination of MCV and subsequent classification of anemia must be determined by age-related ranges. Morphological classification is useful as the differential diagnoses of microcytic hypochromic anemia and macrocytic anemia are limited.

The functional classification is based on the number of reticulocytes produced as a response to anemia. Reticulocyte count can be corrected depending on the degree of anemia and the extent of stress/shift reticulocytosis to derive the reticulocyte production index (RPI), an index of bone marrow proliferation and its response to the degree of anemia. In hyperproliferative anemias seen in blood loss and hemolytic anemias, the RPI is >2. In untreated thalassemia major, however, the reticulocyte count may be low. In hypoproliferative anemias and maturation defects seen in deficiency anemias, anemia of chronic disease, endocrine deficiencies, sideroblastic anemias, aplastic anemia, and myelodysplasia, the RPI is <2. The morphological classification combined with the functional classifications and the differential diagnoses thereof are applicable to the majority of anemias. Unusual patterns may occur while the anemia is not fully developed, when there is a combination of causes, the patient is under treatment or in an unusual cause of anemia **(Flowchart 1)**.

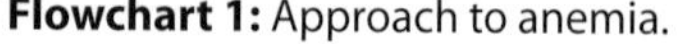

Flowchart 1: Approach to anemia.

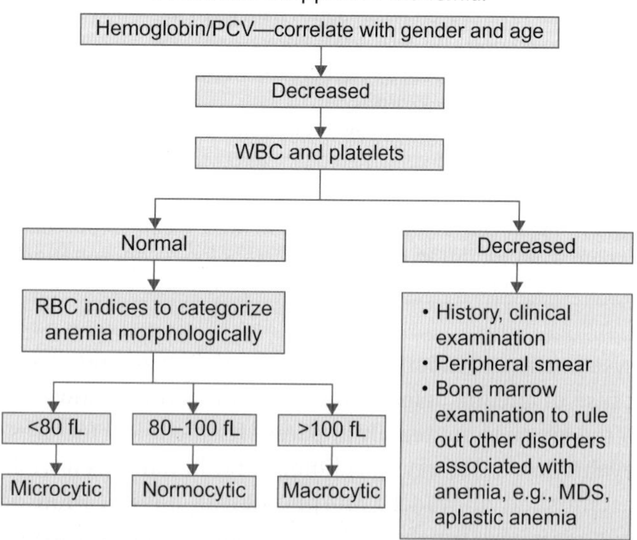

(MDS: myelodysplastic syndrome; PCV: packed cell volume; RBC: red blood cell)

USE OF AUTOMATED BLOOD COUNTING INSTRUMENTS IN ANEMIA

Automated counters are widely available and have improved accuracy, precision, and reliability compared to manual methods. Most modern automated blood-counting instruments give the complete blood count which includes hemoglobin, hematocrit, RBC indices, white blood cell (WBC), and platelet counts which are useful in the initial morphological diagnosis of anemia. Red cell distribution width (RDW) is a measure of anisocytosis and normally between 11.5 and 14.5%. A value of >14.5% indicates a heterogeneous RBC population. Study of the volume histograms gives a guide to the RBC morphology as well as distribution, which can be correlated with the peripheral smear. Absolute reticulocyte count reflects the increased production of reticulocytes as a response of the erythropoietic elements of the bone marrow to anemia or treatment and is more useful than the manually counted reticulocyte percentage. In some automated counters, the immature reticulocyte fraction (IRF), which reflects the early reticulocyte fraction and the reticulocyte hemoglobin, which reflects the iron supply in the bone marrow, are also available **(Box 2)**.

Certain indices either numerical or computational can be calculated from data derived from automated counters, e.g., Mentzer index, which is useful in the differentiation of thalassemia minor from iron deficiency anemia (IDA) can be calculated **(Box 3)**.

BOX 2: Data that are useful in anemia from automated blood-counting instruments.

- Complete blood counts hemoglobin, PCV, MCV, MCH, MCHC, RDW, WBC, and platelet counts
- *Volume histograms*: Help to diagnose dimorphic patterns which can be present in combined nutritional anemias, sideroblastic anemia, MDS, post-transfusion, and during treatment.
- Automated counters give data on the leukocytes and platelets which can be correlated with the RBC parameters.
- Absolute reticulocyte count and immature reticulocyte fraction is an indication of the proliferation of the bone marrow and response to treatment

(MCH: mean corpuscular hemoglobin; MCV: mean corpuscular volume; MCHC: mean corpuscular hemoglobin concentration; MDS: myelodysplastic syndrome; PCV: packed cell volume; RBC: red blood cell; RDW: red cell distribution width; WBC: white blood cell)

EXAMINATION OF THE PERIPHERAL SMEAR (FIG. 1)

Examination of RBC morphology on a blood smear is important in diagnosing the type of anemia, assessing anisocytosis, and correlating it with the RDW. Meticulous smear examination supplemented with detailed history can help delineate cause of anemia as nutritional deficiency, hemolysis, hemoglobinopathies, membrane defects, etc. Erythrocyte inclusions when present are at times useful in determining the cause of anemia such as Howell–Jolly bodies seen in some hemolytic anemias and pappenheimer bodies in sideroblastic anemia. Evaluating the morphology of the WBCs may be useful in diagnosing certain anemias such as megaloblastic anemia and other hematological diseases where anemia is secondary to another cause, e.g., leukemia. Examination of a peripheral smear is also invaluable in the diagnosis of malaria, a common cause of anemia. Data from automated counters may be correlated with peripheral smear findings.

BOX 3: Calculated indices which may be useful.

- *Mentzer's index = MCV/RBC count*
- <13 suggests thalassemia trait
- >13 suggests iron deficiency
- It is a sensitive but less specific test; therefore, confirmatory tests must be carried out
- *Reticulocyte production index =*

$$\frac{\text{Patient hematocrit (\%)}}{\text{Normal hematocrit (\%)}} \times \frac{\text{Reticulotyte (\%)}}{\text{Maturation days}}$$

- *Maturation days* depend on the hematocrit and are calculated as follows:
  - Hematocrit 0.25–0.35, maturation days: 1.5
  - Hematocrit 0.15–0.25, maturation days: 2
  - Hematocrit <0.15, maturation days: 2.5
- <2 indicates hypoproliferative anemia
- >2 indicates hyperproliferative anemia

(MCV: mean corpuscular volume; RBC: red blood cell)

APPROACH TO MICROCYTIC HYPOCHROMIC ANEMIA

Microcytic RBCs are usually associated with decreased MCHC and are, therefore, microcytic hypochromic. **Table 2** summarizes differential diagnoses of hypochromic microcytic anemia. Iron deficiency is the most common cause of microcytic hypochromic anemia but microcytic hypochromic anemia can also occur in thalassemia minor (both α and β), in the late stages of anemia of chronic disease, sideroblastic anemia, hemoglobin C and hemoglobin E, and other rare causes. Beta-thalassemia major and intermedia and hemoglobin H disease also cause microcytic hypochromic RBCs; however, their clinical features and peripheral smear findings are usually significant enough for them not

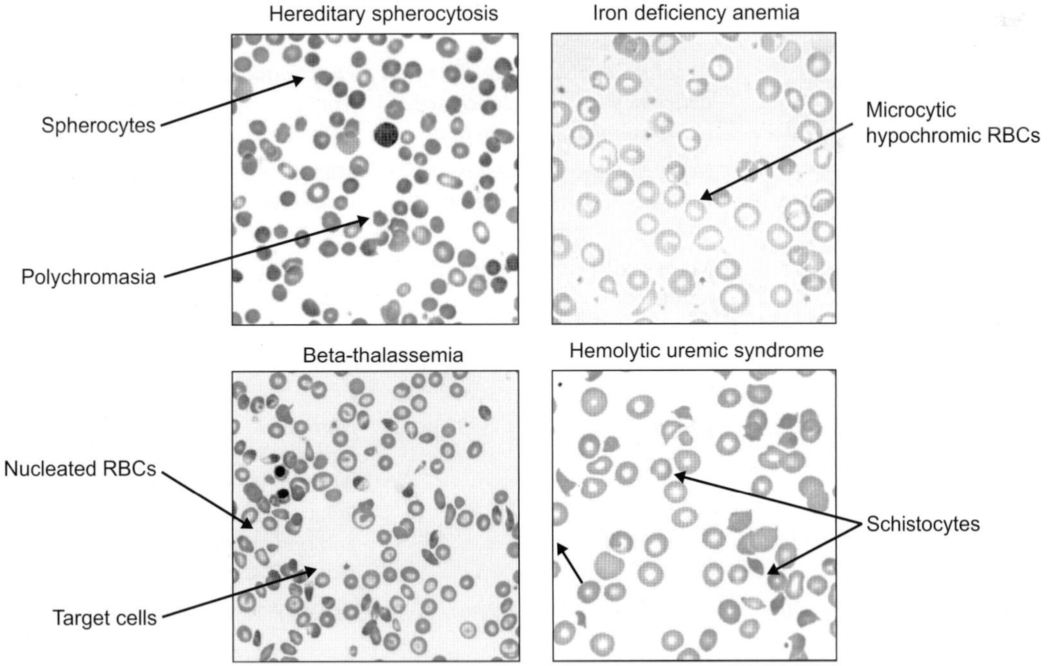

Fig. 1: Peripheral smear examination in common disorders with anemia. *(For color version, see Plate 3)*

to be included in the differential diagnosis of iron deficiency anemia. In iron deficiency anemia, the RBCs are microcytic hypochromic with moderate anisopoikilocytosis. The platelet count is usually on the upper level of normal and reticulocyte response is usually identified 3 days after institution of iron therapy. Iron studies will show decreased serum iron and ferritin and increased total iron binding capacity. Serum transferrin receptor assay (sTFR) is useful in detecting and differentiating IDA from anemia of chronic disease; it is raised in patients with IDA in comparison to anemia of chronic disease, where levels are almost identical to normal individuals. **Table 3** outlines the spectrum of iron deficiency and associated laboratory parameters.

In both α- and β-thalassemia trait, the peripheral smear will show microcytic hypochromic RBCs with minimal anisocytosis which is reflected as a decreased RDW. The RBCs are increased in number and both these

TABLE 2: Differential diagnosis of iron deficiency anemia.

	Iron deficiency	*Beta-thalassemia minor*	*Anemia of chronic disease*	*Sideroblastic anemia*
Serum ferritin	Low*	Normal/high	Normal/high	High
Serum iron	Low	Normal/high	Normal/low	Normal/high
Total iron binding capacity	High	Normal/low	Normal	Normal/low
RDW/anisocytosis	High	Normal	Normal	High/dimorphic population
Special tests for confirmation	Serum transferrin receptor assay—increased	HbA2 estimation >4%	Serum transferrin receptor assay— normal	Ringed sideroblasts in bone marrow

*Serum concentrations of ferritin are lower in children than in adults and ferritin <12 µg/L is considered appropriate for detecting iron deficiency.
(HbA2: hemoglobin A2; RDW: red cell distribution width)

TABLE 3: Spectrum of iron deficiency anemia.

	Iron repletion	*Low iron stores*	*Absolute iron deficiency (non-anemic)*	*Absolute iron deficiency (anemia)*	*Functional iron deficiency*	*Functional iron deficiency with absolute iron deficiency*	*Iron-refractory iron deficiency anemia due to TMPRSS6 variants*
Hemoglobin	Normal	Normal	Normal or low-normal	Reduced (anemic)	Mild-to-moderate anemia	Mild-to-moderate anemia	Reduced (anemic)
Mean cell volume and mean cell hemoglobin concentration	Normal	Normal	Normal or reduced	Reduced	Normal or mild reduction	Reduced	Reduced
Ferritin	>30–60 µg/L	15–30 µg/L	<15–30 µg/L	<15–30 µg/L	Normal or increased depending on inflammation and body iron stores	<70–100 µg/L depending on degree of inflammation	Typically 20–50 µg/L
Transferrin saturation	>20%	Usually >20%	<20%	<15%	Usually <20%	<20%	<20%, usually <5%

Contd...

Contd...

	Iron repletion	*Low iron stores*	*Absolute iron deficiency (non-anemic)*	*Absolute iron deficiency (anemia)*	*Functional iron deficiency*	*Functional iron deficiency with absolute iron deficiency*	*Iron-refractory iron deficiency anemia due to TMPRSS6 variants*
Reticulocyte hemoglobin content	Normal	Normal	Low	Low	Low	Low	Low
Soluble transferrin receptor	Normal	Normal	Increased	Increased	Normal	Normal or increased	Increased
Hepcidin	Normal	Low-normal	Low	Very low	Increased relative to transferrin saturation	Normal or reduced	High relative to transferrin saturation
Bone marrow stainable iron	Normal	Detectable or absent	Absent	Absent	Detectable	Absent	Absent or trace

are reflected in the Mentzer's index. While investigating for β-thalassemia trait, estimation of hemoglobin A2 is important as an increase (usually a value of between 4 and 7%) is considered diagnostic of β-thalassemia trait. If, after evaluation of the common causes, a diagnosis has not been reached, unusual causes such as lead toxicity may be considered **(Flowchart 2)**.

APPROACH TO MACROCYTIC ANEMIA

Macrocytic anemias are defined by a MCV more than two standard deviations above the normal mean for age and sex. Macrocytic anemias may be megaloblastic or nonmegaloblastic.

In megaloblastic anemia, examination of the peripheral smear will show macro-ovalocytes and hypersegmented neutrophils (defined as five neutrophils with more than five lobes or one with six lobes) and there may be decrease in the RBC, WBC, and platelet counts. Increase in serum lactate dehydrogenase, unconjugated bilirubin, and decreased haptoglobin indicate ineffective erythropoiesis and hemolysis. The bone marrow in megaloblastic anemia shows nuclear—cytoplasmic asynchrony and giant metamyelocytes, however, bone marrow examination may not be essential for the diagnosis of megaloblastic anemia. Megaloblastic anemia may be due to folic acid, vitamin B_{12} deficiency which may be due to decreased absorption, inadequate nutrition, defects in metabolism, or increased requirements. Other causes include defects in purine and pyrimidine synthesis either inherited or acquired as in myelodysplastic syndrome (MDS), drug induced or associated with human immunodeficiency virus infection.

In nonmegaloblastic anemia, the MCV is usually mild and between 100 and 110 fL and the WBC and platelets are usually normal. Causes of nonmegaloblastic macrocytic anemia include hypothyroidism, liver disease, and rare conditions such as pure red cell aplasia and aplastic anemia. The smear shows round macrocytes and may show features of the underlying cause such as target cells and stomatocytes in liver disease. Correlation with clinical and laboratory tests for the causative disease must be done to confirm the cause **(Flowchart 3)**.

Hemolytic anemias and blood loss may also have raised MCV due to reticulocytosis which can be excluded by reticulocyte count and peripheral smear examination **(Flowchart 4)**.

NORMOCYTIC NORMOCHROMIC ANEMIA

Normocytic normochromic anemia can be caused by a hematological disorder or an underlying systemic condition. Depending on the RPI, they can be categorized into anemia with hyperproliferative or hypoproliferative marrow. Normocytic anemia with hyperplastic marrow (>2 RPI) present from birth is usually due to some nonthalassemic hemoglobinopathies, RBC enzyme, or membrane defects. In addition to peripheral smear examination and tests

Flowchart 2: Approach to microcytic hypochromic anemia.

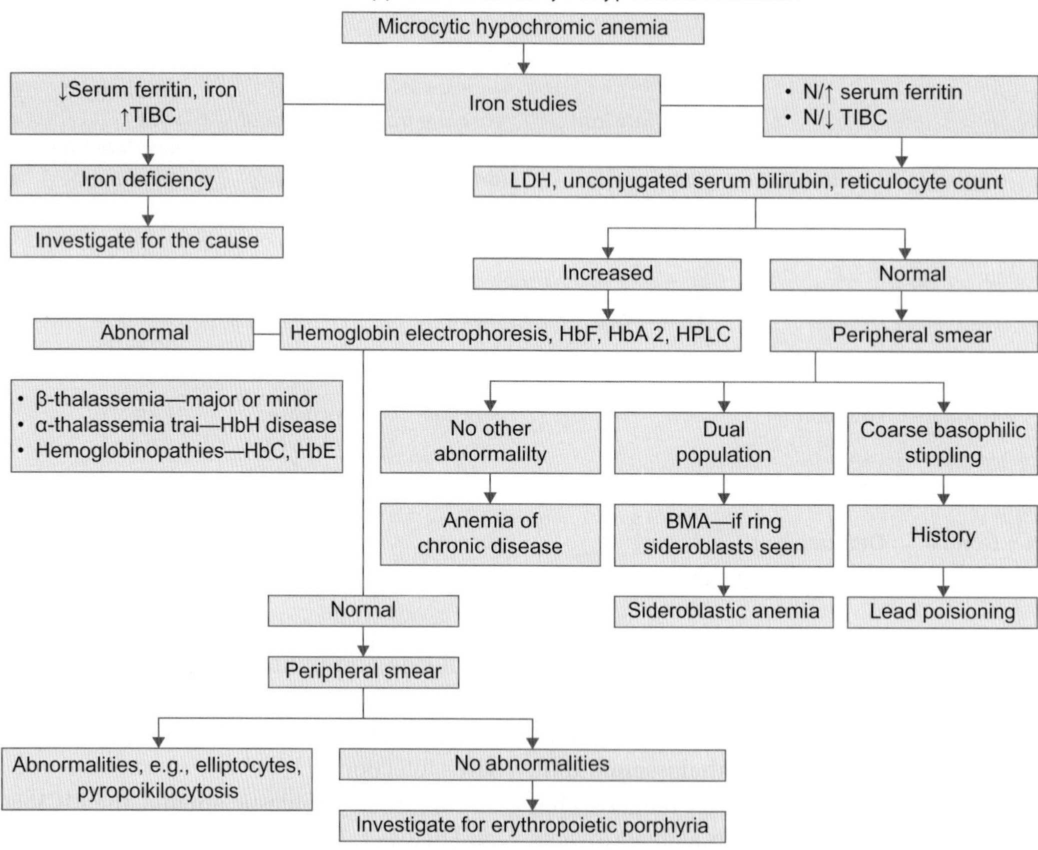

(BMA: bone marrow aspiration; LDH: lactate dehydrogenase; TIBC: total iron binding capacity)

for increased turnover of cells, further tests such as hemoglobin electrophoresis can characterize the disease. Rare causes of hemolysis including paroxysmal nocturnal hemoglobinuria and Wilson disease must be confirmed by specific tests. Normocytic anemia with hypoplastic marrow (<2 RPI) can be seen early in the course of iron deficiency, renal disease, liver disease, endocrine disorders, chronic inflammatory disease, and anemia secondary to medications. In these conditions, specific tests following clinical evaluation will confirm the diagnosis. Primary hematological conditions may also present with normochromic anemia and these include MDS, aplastic anemia, pure red cell aplasia, and leukemia. Evaluation of the bone marrow will be useful in confirming these diagnoses **(Flowchart 5)**.

ANEMIA IN THE NEWBORN

Anemia in the newborn differs from those in children in that the level of hemoglobin is higher (16–22 g/dL at birth), the MCV is higher (average 107 fL at birth) and the reticulocyte count is higher (3–7%) in the newborn compared to children. The etiologies that are uncommon in older children that need to be considered in a newborn include congenital disorders, metabolic disorders, intrauterine infections, ABO/Rh-incompatibility, and internal hemorrhage. **Table 4** outlines the different causes of anemia in children based on age.

NEWER RED BLOOD CELL INDICES AND RETICULOCYTE PARAMETERS

Red Blood Cell Indices

Red blood cell indices are available in automated hematology analyzers.

- *% Hypochromic red cells:*
  - % of red cells with a hemoglobin content of <17 pg
  - Reflects iron status in the last 2–3 months and assessment of iron availability for erythropoiesis
- *% Hyperchromic red cells:*
  - % of red cells with a hemoglobin content of >49 pg.
  - Increased in hereditary/immune-mediated spherocytosis. Used as an effective screening tool

Flowchart 3: Approach to macrocytic anemia.

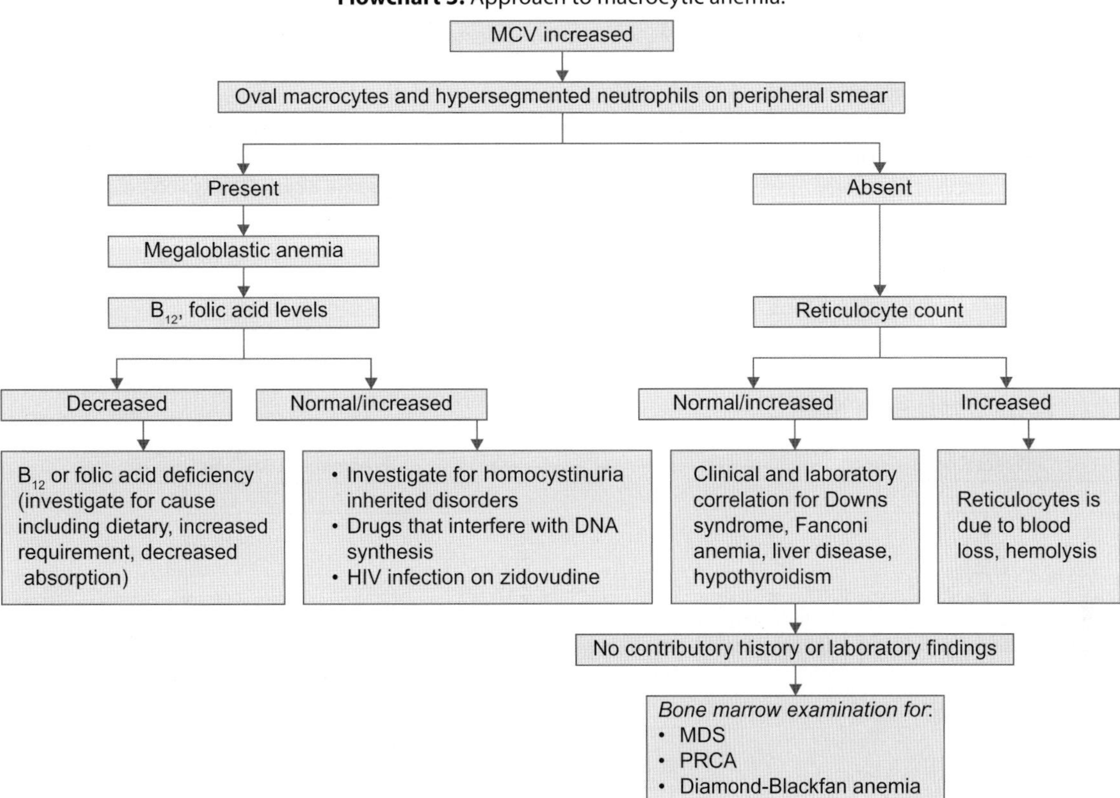

Note: Autoagglutination can cause spurious increase in MCV in automated counters. This can be ruled out by examination of the peripheral smear and direct Coombs test.

(DNA: deoxyribonucleic acid; MCV: mean corpuscular volume; HIV: human immunodeficiency virus; MDS: myelodysplastic syndrome; PRCA: pure red cell aplasia)

Flowchart 4: Approach to normocytic anemias.

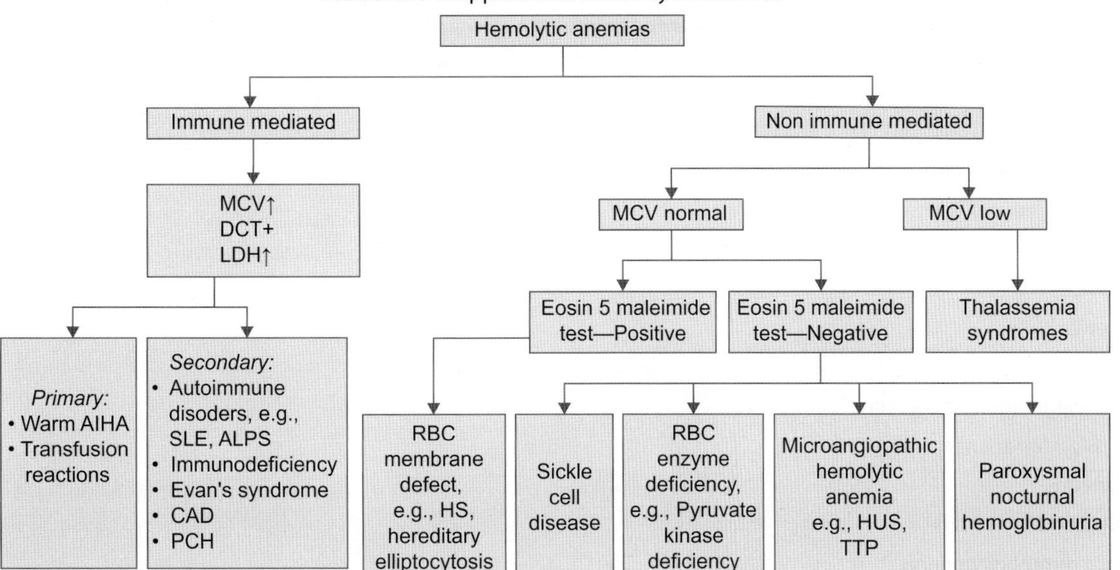

(AIHA: autoimmune hemolytic anemia; CAD: cold agglutinin disease; HS: hereditary spherocytosis; HUS: hemolytic uremic syndrome; LDH: lactate dehydrogenase; MCV: mean corpuscular volume; PCH: paroxysmal cold hemoglobinuria; PNH: paroxysmal nocturnal hemoglobinuria; SLE: systemic lupus erythematosus)

Flowchart 5: Approach to hemolytic anemia.

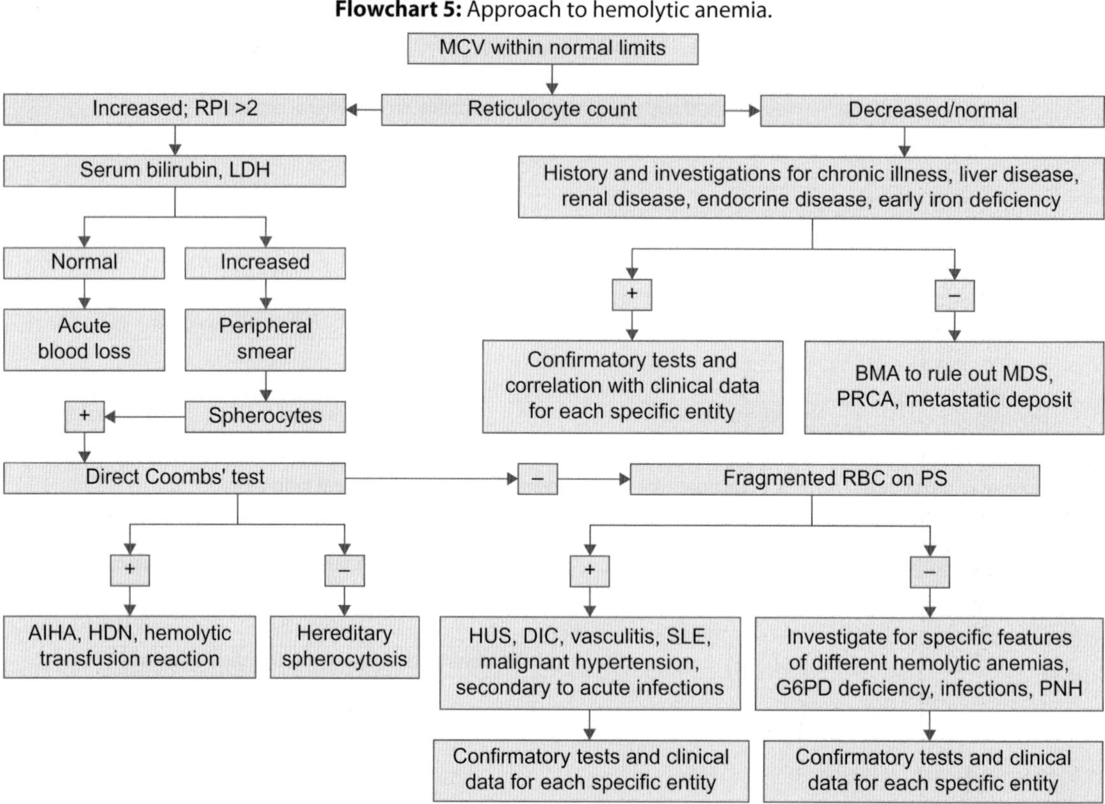

AIHA: autoimmune hemolytic anemia; BMA: bone marrow aspiration; DIC: disseminated intravascular coagulation; HDN: hemolytic disease of the newborn; HUS: hemolytic uremic syndrome; LDH: lactate dehydrogenase; MCV: mean corpuscular volume; MDS: myelodysplastic syndrome; PRCA: pure red cell aplasia; PNH: paroxysmal nocturnal hemoglobinuria; SLE: systemic lupus erythematosus)

TABLE 4: Agewise causes of anemia (The darker, the more common in that age group).

	Anemia in infants and children						
Age disorder	***Newborn (0–30 days)***	***Infant (0–1 year)***	***Toddler (2–3 years)***	***Preschool (4–5 years)***	***Child (6–9 years)***	***Preteen (10–12 years)***	***Teenager (13–18 years)***
Membrane defects							
Abnormalities of metabolism							
Unstable hemoglobin							
Sideroblastic anemia							
α-Thalassemia							
β-Thalassemia							
Sickle cell disease							
Congenital diaphragmatic anemia							
Diamond-Blackfan anemia							
Fanconi anemia							
Hemolytic uremic syndrome							
Thrombotic thrombocytopenic purpura							

Contd...

Contd...

	Anemia in infants and children						
Age disorder	***Newborn (0–30 days)***	***Infant (0–1 year)***	***Toddler (2–3 years)***	***Preschool (4–5 years)***	***Child (6–9 years)***	***Preteen (10–12 years)***	***Teenager (13–18 years)***
Disseminated intravascular coagulation							
Hemorrhage							
Chronic inflammation							
Malignancies							
Neonatal alloimmune hemolytic disease							
Primary autoimmune hemolytic anemia							
Secondary autoimmune hemolytic anemia							
Aplastic anemia							
Iron deficiency							
B_{12} deficiency							
Folate deficiency							

Source: Gallagher PG. Anemia in the pediatric patient. Blood. 2022;140(6):571-93.

- *% Microcytic red cells:*
  - % of red cells with MC <60 fL
  - Differential diagnosis of microcytic anemias
- *% Macrocytic red cells:* % of red cells with MCV >120 fL

RETICULOCYTE INDICES

The reticulocyte count is important in classification of anemia based on pathophysiology as well as to look for the erythropoietic/marrow response to treatment. However, it may miss the early erythropoietic activity in certain cases.

Immature Reticulocyte Fraction (IRF)

It is a new parameter available on automated hematology analyzers. It is an early and sensitive index of erythropoiesis and constitutes the RNA rich, more immature fraction of reticulocyte which can serve as an indicator of effective erythropoiesis. Increase in IRF precedes the increase in total reticulocyte count by several days. **Table 5** illustrates the application of IRF in identifying the cause of anemia.

TABLE 5: Reticulocyte count versus immature reticulocyte fraction.

Condition	***Reticulocyte count***	***IRF***
Aplastic/hypoplastic anemia	Low	Low
Early bone marrow regeneration	Low	High
Chronic disease	Low	High
Iron deficiency/vitamin B_{12} deficiency	Low	High
Myelodysplasia	Low/normal	High
Acute infections	Low/normal	High
Engraftment post-BMT (early)	Low/normal	High

(BMT: bone marrow transplantation; IRF: immature reticulocyte fraction)

Uses:
- It can serve as a marker for hematological recovery postchemotherapy.
- Indicator for engraftment following bone marrow transplant and precedes neutrophil recovery, immature platelet fraction (IPF) and retic count.
- Evaluating response to erythropoietin therapy in patients with chronic renal failure
- Evaluating response to therapy in nutritional anemias. In intravenous (IV) iron therapy, it can be found to be increased as early as Day 1.

Reticulocyte Hemoglobin Equivalent

It is a marker to assess iron incorporation into erythrocyte hemoglobin. It is used to distinguish between iron deficiency and IDA as reticulocyte hemoglobin equivalent (RHE) will be significantly reduced in IDA as compared to iron depleted state without anemia.

Uses:

- Diagnosis of iron deficiency in adults and children
- Measure of bone marrow response to iron therapy within a short period of time (5–7 days)

RETICULOCYTE HEMOGLOBIN CONTENT

- Hemoglobin content of reticulocytes
- Product of cellular volume × cellular Hb content. Expressed in pg/cell
- Reliable and early indicator of bone marrow iron stores and can detect functional iron deficiency. It can be used to monitor early treatment response.

Mean Reticulocyte Volume

- Decreased in iron-deficient erythropoiesis and increased in macrocytic anemia
- Normalizes rapidly with treatment and can be used to evaluate therapy response.
- Hematocrit of reticulocytes = Mean reticulocyte volume × Number of reticulocytes

ROLE OF GENETIC TESTING IN ANEMIA

Genetic mutation analysis has revolutionized the diagnostic and therapeutic approaches in certain inherited and atypical diseases. In the current era, genetic testing involves next-generation sequencing (NGS) which includes phenotype-based predefined panel of target genes or whole exome sequencing in more rare and complex cases. It has an important role to play in certain situations such as:

- *RBC membrane defects:* Presence of deficiency in 5' eosin maleimide is a screening test to detect RBC membrane defects but cannot differentiate between hereditary spherocytosis, hereditary stomatocytosis, hereditary elliptocytosis, hereditary pyropoikilocytosis, and south Asian ovalocytosis and can also be deranged in congenital dyserythropoietic anemia; treatment of each of these may differ.
- *Alpha-thalassemia:* It cannot be diagnosed on the basis of conventional high-performance liquid chromatography (HPLC) and alpha-gene mutation analysis is required.
- *Congenital anemias* such as congenital dyserythropoietic anemias and inherited bone marrow failures such as Diamond–Blackfan anemia (DBA).
- *Iron metabolism defects:* NGS can be used to diagnose inherited disorders of iron metabolism such as hemochromatosis, iron refractory IDA (IRIDA), atransferrinemia, and sideroblastic anemias.
- *Rare disorders* such as Ghosal hematodiaphyseal syndrome characterized by increased bone density and steroid responsive anemia and osteopetrosis (marble bone disease).

CLINICAL PEARLS

- The final diagnosis in anemia must be done after correlating the laboratory test results with patient history, symptoms, and physical examination.
- Results of laboratory tests should be interpreted with an understanding of the limitations of the test and the variations with respect to age, gender, sample collection, etc.
- All laboratory investigations should be interpreted in relation to the reference range established in that individual laboratory using blood samples from the local population.

KEY POINTS

- The morphological classification of anemia is based on red cell indices and correlated with the RBC morphology on peripheral smear examination.
- The differential diagnosis of microcytic hypochromic anemia and macrocytic anemias is limited.
- Based on the morphology and clinical features, further investigations can be done to help establish the etiology and pathophysiology of anemia; after which appropriate treatment can be given.

SUGGESTED READING

1. Bain BJ, Bates I, Laffan MA, Lewis SM. Dacie and Lewis Practical Haematology, 11th edition. Churchill Livingstone: Elsevier; 2012.
2. Brugnara C, Platt OS. The Neonatal Erythrocyte and its Disorders. In: Orkin SH, Nathan DG, Ginsburg D, Look AT, Fisher DE, Lux SE (Eds). Nathan and Oski's Hematology of Infancy and Childhood, 7th edition. Philadelphia: Saunders Elsevier; 2009.
3. Brugnara C. Reticulocyte cellular indices: a new approach in the diagnosis of anemias and monitoring of erythropoietic function. Crit Rev Clin Lab Sci. 2000;37(2):93-130.
4. Buttarello M. Laboratory diagnosis of anemia: are the old and new red cell parameters useful in classification and

treatment, how? Int J Lab Hematol. 2016;38 (Suppl 1): 123-32.
5. Camaschella C, Poggiali E. Inherited disorders of iron metabolism. Curr Opin Pediatr. 2011;23(1):14-20.
6. Centers for Disease Control (CDC). CDC criteria for anemia in children and childbearing aged women. MMWR Morb Mortal Wkly Rep. 199;38(22):400-4.
7. Dallman PR, Simes MA. Percentile curves for hemoglobin and red cell volume in infancy and childhood. J Pediatr. 1979;94(1):26-31.
8. Khoury MJ, Rhodes M. How to approach chronic anemia? Hematology Am Soc Hematol Educ Program. 2012;2012: 183-90.
9. Kotecha PV. Nutritional anemia in children with focus on Asia and India. Indian J Community Med. 2011;36(1):8-16.
10. McKenzie SB, Williams JL. Clinical laboratory hematology, 3rd edition. New Jersey: Pearson Education Inc.; 2015.
11. Osta V, Caldirola MS, Fernandez M, Marcone MI, Tissera G, Pennesi S, et al. Utility of new mature erythrocyte and reticulocyte indices in screening for iron-deficiency anemia in a pediatric population. Int Jnl Lab Hem. 2013; 35:400-5.
12. Russo R, Marra R, Rosato BE, Iolascon A, Andolfo I. Genetics and Genomics Approaches for Diagnosis and Research Into Hereditary Anemias. Front Physiol. 2020;11:613559.
13. Tkachuk DC, Hirschmann JV. Wintrobe's Atlas of Clinical Hematology. Philadelphia: Lippincott Williams and Wilkins; 2007.
14. Voulgaridou A, Kalfa TA. Autoimmune hemolytic anemia in the pediatric setting. J Clin Med. 2021;10(2):216.

CHAPTER 62

Recurrent Unusual Infections in a Child: The Way Forward

Tulika Seth

INTRODUCTION

Children are immunologically immature more prone to many infections compared to adults. More than six infections per year are suspicious of an immunodeficiency status, though some studies report 4–8 may be normal. So when is it warranted to do special and extra investigations in a child? Repeated infections with the same bacterial organism, serious infections of the lower respiratory tract, repeated diarrhea, recurrent urinary tract infection, and repeated pyogenic infections all warrant a detailed history and evaluation. Unusual organisms causing an infection should also get special attention. Before we discuss recurrent unusual infections, it is important to understand what are recurrent infections and unusual organisms.

RECURRENT OR REPEATED INFECTIONS: COMMON CAUSES

The child referred for repeated or recurrent infection needs a detailed history. Often a common mistake is to assume cases of repeated infections, when in fact it is a case of inadequate, improper, or incomplete treatment of a previous infection. Compliance, dosage of antibiotics, and all culture reports should be checked. Home environment, smoker at home, going to a crèche, etc. can predispose to recurrent infections in an otherwise normal child. The vaccination history and documentation of vaccines is important. Malnutrition is the most common cause of decreased immunity, hence nutritional parameters should be checked. Any anatomic malformation, gastroesophageal reflux, congenital masses, and foreign body aspiration may also be a cause of repeated infections. Atopic dermatitis may lead to skin infections due to scratching the pruritic rash. Other systemic disease, e.g., sickle cell, nephritic syndrome, etc., needs to be evaluated, if previous illness, then medications should be checked as the child may be on steroids or other immune-suppressants. Check if on complementary medicines, as they have been found to sometimes also contain steroids. Occasionally, the recurrent infection can lead to the diagnosis of an unsuspected condition like cystic fibrosis or a previously missed congenital heart disease, etc. Most common infections in children are viral, of short duration, and do not compromise growth. Children with inherited conditions like Down syndrome, DiGeorge syndrome, etc. are also more susceptible to infections. Family history of other family members prone to infections (siblings and parents) and history of human immunodeficiency virus (HIV) need to be taken. If none of the above, then a primary immunodeficiency disorder may be the cause of the condition.

In neutropenic patients, there are frequent bacterial and fungal infections. Though they present with fever, the classic signs of infection are often less marked due to neutropenia, hence a high index of suspicion is needed.

UNUSUAL INFECTIONS: CAUSES

An unusual infection may be either an uncommon setting, or a rare organism. These are warning flags to investigate a child for immunodeficiency disorders or undiagnosed systemic disease like malignancy. Certain signature infections can help pinpoint the type of immune defect **(Box 1)**.

- If presented with an unusual organism, rule out contamination and obtain a detailed history of travel, exposure to pets, medication leading to immune-suppression, and previous courses of broad-spectrum antibiotics.
- If a usual setting, rule out underlying undiagnosed disease such as malignancy, metabolic or systemic disease, HIV, malnutrition, or undisclosed use of steroids or other immune-suppressive medicines.

As seen by the above discussion, all children with recurrent infections do not have a primary immune

BOX 1: Clinical features of primary immunodeficiency disorders.

Adaptive immunity:

- *B-cell defects:*
  - Recurrent bacterial sinopulmonary infections, with polysaccharide encapsulated organisms (*Streptococcus pneumoniae, Haemophilus influenzae* type b) or bronchiectasis
  - Chronic or recurrent gastroenteritis (Giardia/enteroviruses)
  - Chronic enteroviral meningoencephalitis
  - Failure to thrive and/or autoimmune disease
- *T-cell defects:*
  - Lymphopenia as a neonate or infant
  - Repeated severe, or unusual viral infections (varicella-zoster, CMV, HSV)
  - Chronic candidiasis
  - Chronic diarrhea
  - Opportunistic infections like *Pneumocystis pneumonia*
  - Severe seborrheic rashes (skin rash, desquamating skin, abnormal liver function tests, and cytopenias)
  - *Associated features*: Failure to thrive

Innate immunity:

- *Phagocytic defects:*
  - Delayed separation of the umbilical cord
  - Lymphadenitis or soft tissue abscesses
  - Repeated infections due to catalase-positive bacteria and/or fungi
  - Recurrent gastrointestinal or genitourinary tract obstruction
  - Poor wound healing, oral ulcers
- *Complement defects:*
  - Angioedema of face, GI tract, etc.
  - Autoimmune disease
  - Pyogenic bacterial infections (e.g., *Neisseria meningitidis*), Herpes simplex meningoencephalitis in infancy
  - Papilloma virus infections of skin, including extensive warts
  - Autosomal dominant inheritance

(CMV: cytomegalovirus; HSV: herpes simplex virus; GI: gastrointestinal)

deficiency disorder. It is important to rule out secondary immunodeficiency as these can be treated easily **(Box 2)** leaving the primary immunodeficiency child who needs a more detailed investigation.

WARNING SIGNS OF IMMUNODEFICIENCY (BOX 2)

Presence of oral candidiasis, tissue or organ abscesses, and opportunistic infections all warrant investigation. A complication from a live vaccine, in the child or elder siblings and family history of siblings with history of early death or similar presentation are important.

BOX 2: The Jeffrey Modell Foundations' 10 warning signs of primary immunodeficiency.

Warning signs observed in children:

1. ≥4 new ear infections within 1 year
2. ≥2 serious sinus infections within 1 year
3. ≥2 months on antibiotics without benefit
4. ≥2 pneumonias within last 1 year
5. Failure of an infant to gain weight or grow normally
6. Recurrent, deep skin or organ abscesses
7. Persistent thrush in mouth or fungal infection on skin
8. Need for IV antibiotics to clear infections
9. ≥2 deep-seated infections including septicemia
10. A family history of primary immunodeficiency disorder

Source: From Jeffrey Modell Foundation (JMF). [online] Available from http://www.info4pi.org/library/educational-materials/10-warning-signs. [Last accessed September, 2024]

The immunodeficiency may be secondary or primary. Secondary immunodeficiencies are due to contributing malnutrition, chronic disease, prematurity, cancer, HIV, etc. The type and pattern of recurring infections depend on which components of the immune system are affected **(Box 1)**. History **(Table 1)** and examination **(Box 3)** give clues and signature infections help highlight disorders **(Table 2)**. Initial steps with workup of the child are represented in **Flowchart 1**.

GENERAL EXAMINATION

Physical examination in children with recurrent infections provides information as to their general health and may suggest the presence of allergy, chronic disease, or immunodeficiency. A dysmorphic appearance may signify an underlying genetic syndrome. Dark circles under the eyes, a transverse nasal crease, and congested nasal turbinates suggest presence of allergy. Mouth ulcers, gingivitis, and mucosal candidiasis may be due to an immunodeficiency state. Diminished or absent tonsils and cervical lymphadenopathy with a history of recurrent respiratory infections suggest an antibody deficiency diagnosis. The presence of nasal polyps suggests cystic fibrosis, and confirmatory testing should be performed.

KEY FEATURES OF UNUSUAL RECURRENT INFECTIONS

Not all children with recurrent infections have a primary immunodeficiency disorder. A simplified checklist for immunodeficiency to be suspected if there are:

- Six or more new infections within 1 year
- Two or more sinus infections or pneumonias in 1 year

- Two or more episodes of sepsis or meningitis
- Two or more months of oral antibiotics without resolution of problem

A more detailed comprehensive guideline is given in **Box 2**. Probing history clues are summarized in **Table 1**.

Boxes 1 and 3 provide clinical clues and examination evidence that needs to be sought. With a detailed history and examination, a high index of suspicion necessitates investigation. This can be done in an algorithmic way to arrive at a diagnosis promptly.

TABLE 1: Historical details useful in differentiating between cases of suspected primary and secondary immunodeficiency.

Primary immunodeficiency	***Secondary immunodeficiency***
History details:	
• Poor feeding history or history of food allergies (common in high IgE conditions like DOCK8, IPEX, etc.) • Delayed detachment of the umbilical cord should be noted since persistent attachment beyond 30 days is suggestive of a leukocyte adhesion defect	*Birth history:* Pregnancy history should be explored for maternal illness (e.g., HIV, CMV), birth history should include length of gestation, birth weight, and neonatal problems such as jaundice, respiratory distress, or need for intensive care. Transfusions in the neonatal period should be recorded
Growth:	
• Weight, height, and head circumference should be plotted and followed over time. • Children with chronic disease or immunodeficiency often have poor weight gain or even weight loss. • Children with chronic lung, heart, or gastrointestinal disease are often small because of anorexia, high energy expenditure, or malabsorption caused by infection or bacterial overgrowth	
Development:	
• Children with ataxia–telangiectasia and DiGeorge syndrome can have delayed developmental milestones • Progressive neurologic dysfunction is seen in Chédiak–Higashi syndrome	• Children with HIV, and TORCH may have delays in milestones • Children with other chronic disease may also lag in development
Immunization history:	
See for adverse effects from a vaccine, particularly live virus. The immunization record is valuable to see vaccine titers to evaluate antibody function	The immunization record is valuable to see vaccine titers to evaluate antibody function
Medications:	
• If immunoglobulin has been given • The route, dose, frequency, and adverse effects should be noted	• Current and past medications should be recorded, including duration, effectiveness, and adverse reactions • Use of any immunosuppressive medications, such as glucocorticoids, should be noted
Other illnesses:	
• Other immune problems such as allergies, anaphylaxis, arthritis, or autoimmunity may give a clue to diagnosis • Autoimmune disorders are seen with many primary immunodeficiency conditions • Ask about surgery and hospitalizations (abscess, poor wound healing, pneumonia, etc.)	• Severity of prior chickenpox, roseola, and other febrile illnesses should be noted • Ask about surgery and hospitalizations (abscess, poor wound healing, pneumonia, etc.) (common for both primary and secondary)
Family history:	
• Consanguinity, sibling death due to recurrent infections, unexplained deaths, family members with similar infections, or autoimmune disease • Autosomal recessive pattern in ataxia–telangiectasia • X-linked transmission (e.g., agammaglobulinemia, chronic granulomatous disease)	• HIV, TB • Parental health or other family members ill • Parents' occupation

Contd...

Contd...

Primary immunodeficiency	***Secondary immunodeficiency***
Infection history:	
The infection history should include the age of onset, duration, frequency, sites, organisms, treatment, and response to therapy	
Age of onset:	
Birth to 6 months: • Several immunodeficiencies: congenital neutropenia, severe combined immunodeficiencies, and complete DiGeorge syndrome • Persistent diarrhea, chronic cough, or failure to thrive suggests cystic fibrosis or a primary immunodeficiency • Inherited antibody deficiencies present at 7–9 months, as the maternal IgG decreases. Infants with TLR3 transduction may present with herpes simplex encephalitis	*Birth to 6 months:* • Infections shortly after birth may be due to prolonged rupture of membranes, congenital infection, or aspiration • Premature infants are at high risk for sepsis
2–6 years: • Less serious antibody deficiencies (e.g., immunoglobulin A deficiency and selective antibody deficiency) present at this age. • Two or more episodes of bacterial meningitis or sepsis suggest a complement or other innate immune defect	*2–6 years:* • Secondary immunodeficiencies resulting from underlying malignancy, nephrotic syndrome, or gastrointestinal problems, malabsorption often start at this age • Daycare or school will result in frequent respiratory and gastrointestinal infections, these are normal

(HIV: human immunodeficiency virus; CMV: cytomegalovirus; TORCH: toxoplasmosis, other, rubella, cytomegalovirus, and herpes infections; TB: tuberculosis)

BOX 3: Examination findings to look for in a child with recurrent infections.

Skin:
- See breach of skin barriers due to prematurity, atopy, chronic eczema, burns, wounds, fistula, and sinuses. Several immunodeficiency syndromes are also associated with eczema, including Wiskott–Aldrich, hyperimmunoglobulin E, Omenn syndrome, and severe combined immunodeficiency disease (SCID)
- Cutaneous granulomas, impetigo, or nonhealing ulcers suggest the diagnosis of an antibody or phagocytic disorder. Pyogenic abscesses are common in chronic granulomatous disease, or leukocyte adhesion defects
- Oculocutaneous albinism is seen in Chédiak–Higashi disease
- *Rashes*: Seborrheic dermatitis and alopecia can be seen in some forms of SCID, or may be found in other conditions like Langerhans cell histiocytosis. Lupus-like rash in the children with early complement component defects. A dermatomyositis-like rash is found in X-linked agammaglobulinemia (XLA)
- Extensive warts or molluscum contagiosum occurs in T cell disorders, innate immune defects, or a rare entity called warts, hypogammaglobulinemia, infections, and myelokathexis syndrome

Lymphadenopathy, hepatosplenomegaly:
- Immunodeficiency disorders can be characterized by paucity or even overabundance of lymphoid tissue (e.g., tonsils, lymph nodes, adenoids, spleen). The absence of lymph tissue suggests XLA or SCID
- Lymphadenopathy and hepatosplenomegaly can be seen in B-cell disorders (e.g., common variable immune deficiency, IgA deficiency) and also in children with human immunodeficiency virus infection
- Suppurative adenitis is common in chronic granulomatous disease

LABORATORY EVALUATION

Laboratory evaluation of children with recurrent infection should be directed by history and physical examination findings **(Boxes 2 and 3, and Flowchart 2)**, before evaluating for primary immunodeficiency diseases exclude secondary immunodeficiency, which are more common.

General screening tests should include the following to exclude systemic disease: complete blood count with differential electrolytes, glucose, renal and liver function tests, urinalysis, autoimmune workup, and HIV testing. The evaluation for primary immunodeficiency should focus on the component of the immune system that is most likely to be involved based upon the screening tests.

TABLE 2: Signature infections in certain immunodeficiencies.

Type of infection/organism	*Immune defect*
Recurrent sinopulmonary infections, pneumococcus, *Haemophilus influenza* type b	B-cell abnormalities
Enteroviral meningoencephalitis	X-linked agammaglobulinemia
Severe oral candidiasis	Abnormal T-cell immunity
Staphylococcus aureus, coagulase-negative staphylococci, *Serratia marcescens, Aspergillus*	Chronic granulomatous disease
Neisseria species (*Neisseria meningitidis, Neisseria gonorrhoeae*)	Deficiencies of the late components of complement (C5–C9)
Infection with vaccine strains following live vaccines, e.g., oral polio, measles, varicella, or BCG	Primary immunodeficiency
Some infections can occur in both primary and secondary immunodeficiency states:	
Recurrent pneumococcal disease	Primary immunodeficiency such as agammaglobulinemia or complement defect or secondary immunodeficiency, due to sickle cell disease, asplenia, HIV/AIDS, or nephritic syndrome, also results in recurrent pneumococcal disease
Pneumocystis jirovecii (carinii) pneumonia	Severe combined immunodeficiency, primary or secondary T-cell immunodeficiencies—HIV or immunosuppressive therapy
Pseudomonas infection	Neutropenia, skin burns, trauma, Cystic fibrosis

(BCG: bacillus Calmette–Guérin; HIV: human immunodeficiency virus; AIDS: acquired immunodeficiency syndrome)

General Screening Tests

- The total absolute lymphocyte count is a useful test (lymphopenia is defined as a count of <1,500 cells/μL in patients over 5 years and <2,500 cells/μL in younger children). The presence of anemia, thrombocytopenia, or an abnormal differential count warrants further investigation.

Flowchart 1: Initial evaluation with workup of a child with unusual recurrent infections.

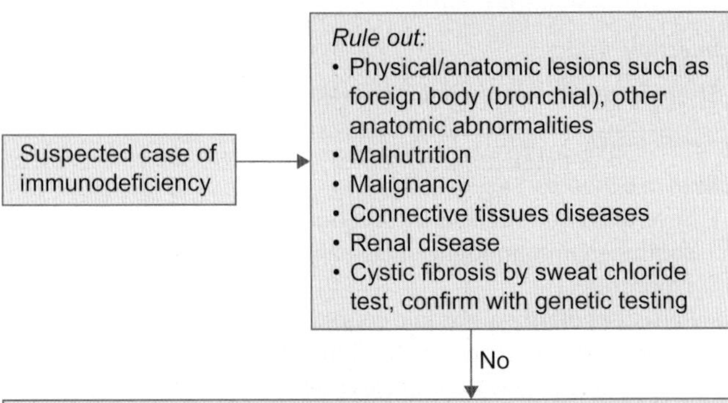

- Neutropenia and absolute neutrophil count should be checked:

$$\text{ANC} = \frac{\text{WBC (cells/}\mu\text{L)} \times \text{percent (PMNs + bands)}}{100}$$

  Other important blood cells to be evaluated are eosinophils; if increased, suggest an allergic state. Platelet size and number should be seen as they are useful—small platelets seen in Wiskott-Aldrich syndrome, etc. However, thrombocytosis is less specific and only points to chronic inflammation.
- *Chest X-ray, computed tomography scan:* This will assist in documenting serious infections like pneumonia, thymus size, presence of mass in chest predisposing to infection, bronchiectasis, etc. This may suggest a diagnosis of previously unsuspected etiology.
- *Immunoglobulin levels:* Immunoglobulin G (IgG), IgM, IgA, and IgE must be compared with age-matched controls for children. An antibody deficiency is suggested by an IgG <200 mg/dL and a total Ig (IgG plus IgM plus IgA) <400 mg/dL, or by the complete absence of IgM or IgA (after infancy). A small increase of IgE (>100 IU/mL) can occur due to allergy, eczema, or with phagocytic dysfunction. In hyper-IgE syndrome, the level of IgE is generally >2,000 IU/mL.
- *Antibody titers, complement screening test:* Functional assessment of the antibody system can be done by checking antibody titers to vaccines that the child has been documented to have received. Titers to tetanus,

Flowchart 2: Investigations guided by symptoms in a patient with recurrent infection.

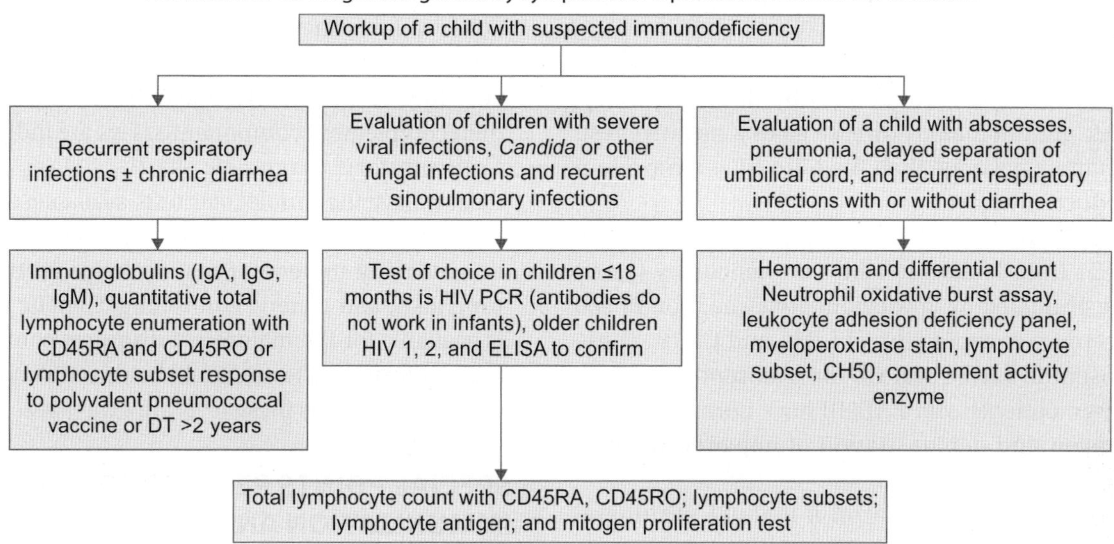

(ELISA: enzyme-linked immunosorbent assay; HIV: human immunodeficiency virus; PCR: polymerase chain reaction)

diphtheria, and *Haemophilus influenzae* type b are available for reference. Response to polysaccharide antigens can be determined by measurement of pneumococcal titers (12–14 serotypes) in children over the age of 2 years.

- Complement activity needs to be evaluated in patients with recurrent sepsis due to Neisserial infections as meningococcal vaccination and prophylaxis with ciprofloxacin can be offered. A screening test is a total hemolytic complement determination (CH50). A normal CH50 level excludes nearly all hereditary complement deficiencies. More detailed evaluation can be done by an immunologist.

Confirmatory and Diagnostic Tests

Specific testing is indicated when screening tests are abnormal or if there is a convincing history or family history suggestive of an immunodeficiency. The patients with confirmed immunodeficiencies should be referred to a special center for diagnostic tests and management by an immunologist or hematologist. Hematopoietic stem cell transplant, gene therapy, and other modalities are providing cure to many affected patients. Hence, diagnosis is essential. Genetic testing has made the diagnosis and confirmation of these conditions more accessible. This is important for genetic counseling of families of affected patients.

- *Lymphocyte subset analysis:* By flow cytometry for CD3 (total T cells), CD4 (T helper), CD8 (T cytotoxic), CD19 (B cells), and CD16/56 (natural killer cells), compared with age-matched controls (B or T cell defect)
- An absolute CD4 count of <500 cells/μL in a child over 5 or <1,000 cells/μL in younger children (suggests a cellular immunodeficiency)
- An absolute B-cell (CD19) count of <100 cells/μL can be seen in children with agammaglobulinemia.
- Low levels of any lymphocyte subset should be repeated and if still decreased, followed by functional analysis of the respective subset.
- Immunoglobulin G subset levels can be tested if the patient has low total IgG levels and poor antibody response to vaccinations. A complete absence of IgG1, IgG2, or IgG3 suggests immune dysregulation, and may indicate the early onset of common variable immunodeficiency. However, a low level of only one or more IgG subclasses does not make a diagnosis if an antibody deficiency, for such a diagnosis functional antibody studies are needed.
- Delayed cutaneous hypersensitivity is a good functional in vivo test of T cells; however, it is limited in utility as it can be performed only in older children.
- Lymphoproliferative assays are in vitro assays used to evaluate the cellular immune system. This examines proliferative response of lymphocytes to mitogens (phytohemagglutinin, pokeweed), stimulatory

monoclonal antibodies (anti-CD3), etc. Defects in this assay suggest a T cell defect.

- Phagocytic oxidative response is evaluated by a fluorescent dye (dihydrorhodamine) by flow cytometry. Chronic granulomatous disease gives a negative test. This is more accurate than the nitro-blue tetrazolium dye reduction assays.
- *Leukocyte adhesion defect testing:* Cases presumed to suffer from leukocyte adhesion deficiency (LAD) can be evaluated by flow cytometry evaluation of cell surface marker expression of CD11 and CD18. These are absent in LAD-I and CD15a is absent in LAD-II. However, patients with LAD-III have normal integrin expression and demonstration of impaired integrin activation is needed.
- Confirm the neutropenia on a manual peripheral smear stained with Wright–Giemsa stain and perform a bone marrow test. For cyclic neutropenia, there will be recurrent infections and a regular oscillation in the neutrophil count at approximately 21-day intervals. Other causes of neutropenia are given in **Table 3**.
- *Complement component:* If the screening test shows very low or absent CH50 activity on repeat testing then complement component assays are indicated.
- *Confirmatory diagnostic studies:* Many immune defects have their molecular tests available; these tests are usually performed in specialized labs. A definite diagnosis by molecular testing helps in treatment, prognosis, and genetic counseling. Genetic diagnosis is available for the majority of disorders commercially and confirmatory tests should be done in conjunction with a specialist as these tests are expensive.

TABLE 3: Causes of isolated neutropenia.

Acquired neutropenia disorders	***Congenital neutropenia conditions***
Postinfectious: Mechanisms are sequestration, aggregation, or destruction of neutrophils by the circulating antibodies	Kostmann's syndrome
Drug induced: Immune-mediated destruction, drug-induced antibodies or by direct toxic effects on bone marrow granulocyte precursors	Shwachman–Diamond syndrome
Primary immune disorders: Antineutrophil antibodies inpatients of systemic lupus erythematosus, rheumatoid arthritis	Chédiak–Higashi syndrome
Isoimmune neonatal neutropenia: Due to transplacental passage of immunoglobulin G antibodies against specific paternal neutrophil antigens in the infant	Cyclic neutropenia
Chronic autoimmune neutropenia occurs in infants and children and is a benign entity	*Rule out other diseases:* Fanconi anemia, reticular agenesis, myelodysplastic syndrome (may precede pancytopenia), glycogen storage disease type 1

SPECIAL POINTS RELATED TO IMMUNIZATION AND PROPHYLAXIS OF CHILDREN WITH IMMUNODEFICIENCY DISORDERS

Immunizations: Children with immunodeficiencies also require to be vaccinated against common childhood illnesses. Those with severe B-cell defects such as agammaglobulinemia and severe common variable deficiency have poor response to vaccines and the IVIG they receive also interferes with the antibody production. But routine vaccines can be given to these children except for live oral polio, live attenuated influenza, BCG. If milder deficiency disorders, e.g., selective IgG subclass or IgA deficiency then all vaccines are safe and recommended. In primary T-cell deficiency disorders and phagocytic disorders, avoid all live vaccines, also avoid in malignancy patients or those on immunosuppressive medicines till the immunosuppression treatment is reduced. Patients with complement deficiency should be given vaccines against encapsulated organisms—pneumococcal and meningococcal.

Antimicrobial prophylaxis: Since infections cause morbidity, prophylaxis has been tried for many PID. Evidence of benefits is available for some conditions **(Table 4)**. Neutropenic diets have not been shown to impact survival or infection. Good hygiene and cooked food is recommended.

CLINICAL PEARLS

- Opportunistic infections can be due to neutrophil defects, T cell deficiency, or human immunodeficiency virus.
- Recurrent sinopulmonary infections may be due to antibody defects.

TABLE 4: Evidence supporting antibiotic, antifungal, immunoglobulin prophylaxis in some patients with primary immunodeficiencies.

	Disease	*Antibiotic prophylaxis (bacteria/PJP)*	*Level of evidence*	*Antifungal prophylaxis*	*Level of evidence*	*IVIG*	*Level of evidence*
1	CGD	Daily cotrimoxazole prophylaxis	AIII	Itraconazole	AI	Not recommended	
2	Severe congenital neutropenia	Cotrimoxazole	AIII	Itraconazole only if persistent severe neutropenia despite G-CSF	BIII	Not recommended	
3	Complement deficiency	Penicillin intra-muscularly (2.4 million units every 2–3 weeks)	AIII	NR		Not recommended	
4	Asplenia	Penicillin VK	AIII	NR		Not recommended	
	Agammaglobulinemia	Cotrimoxazole or azithromycin	BIII	NR		400 mg/kg every 3 weeks	AII
5	CVID	None recommended		None recommended		None recommended	
6	Hyper-IgM	Cotrimoxazole	No data	NR		Conflicting data	
7	SCID	Cotrimoxazole	AII	±		Recommended 400 mg/kg every 3 weeks Till definitive therapy	AII
8	STAT3	Cotrimoxazole Cloxacillin (for *Staphylococcus aureus*)	AII AIII	Itraconazole	AIII	NR	

Note: Level of evidence from RCT is level highly supportive (AIII).
(CGD: chronic granulomatous disease; CVID: common variable immunodeficiency; SCID: severe combined immunodeficiency disease)
Source: Modified from DR Syndman, Aguilar C, Malphettes M, Donadieu J, Chandesris O, Coignard-Biehler H, et al. Prevention of infections during primary immunodeficiency. Clin Infect Dis. 2014;59:1462-70.

KEY POINTS

- A single episode of unusual infection (rare organism or unusual severity of infection of common organism) should be taken seriously and investigated.
- History of sibling death, family history of PID, recurrent or unusual infections features should raise suspicion for a PID and appropriate testing should be ordered. Early diagnosis and treatment is lifesaving.

SUGGESTED READING

1. Buckley RH. Diagnostic and clinical care guidelines for primary immunodeficiency diseases: Immune Deficiency Foundation 2006. [online] Available from www.primaryimmune.org. [Last accessed September, 2024]
2. Butte MJ, Stiehm ER. (2022). Approach to the child with recurrent infections. [online] Available from https://www.uptodate.com/contents/approach-to-the-child-with-recurrent-infections. [Last accessed September, 2024]
3. Grüber C, Keil T, Kulig M, Roll S, Wahn U, Wahn V, et al. History of respiratory infections in the first 12 yr among children from a birth cohort. Pediatr Allergy Immunol. 2008;19(6):505-12.
4. Jeffrey Modell Foundation (JMF). [online] Available from http://www.info4pi.org/library/educational-materials/10-warning-signs. [Last accessed September, 2024]
5. Skoda-Smith S, Barrett DJ. When earaches and sore throats become more than a pain in the neck. Contemp Pediatr. 2000;17:156.
6. Snydman DR, Aguilar C, Malphettes M, Donadieu J, Chandesris O, Coignard-Biehler H, et al. Prevention of Infections During Primary Immunodeficiency. Clin Infect Dis 2014;59(10):1462-70.
7. Stiehm ER, Ochs HD, Winkelstein JA. Immunodeficiency disorders: general considerations. In: Stiehm ER, Ochs HD, Winkelstein JA (Eds). Immunologic disorders in infants and children, 5th edition. Philadelphia: Saunders/Elsevier; 2004. p. 289.
8. Stiehm ER. (2015). Approach to the child with recurrent infections. [online] Available from http://www.uptodate.com/contents/approach-to-the-child-with-recurrent-infections. [Last accessed September, 2024]

Approach to Persistent Fever with Hepatosplenomegaly in a Child

Anupam Sachdeva, Srijib Mukherjee, Manas Kalra, Divij Sachdeva

INTRODUCTION

Infants and children with fever can sometimes present with hepatosplenomegaly. There can be a multitude of causes of hepatosplenomegaly which include infections, hematological, oncological, connective tissue disorders, storage disorders, and cardiac. Fever can be a common associated complaint in most of these disorders. It is pertinent to take a thorough history, a good clinical examination and appropriate laboratory investigations to further narrow down the diagnosis and to initiate early therapy. This chapter will discuss in detail the approach to a child with hepatosplenomegaly and fever.

HEPATOMEGALY

It is not uncommon to have a clinically palpable liver, especially in practically "healthy" infants and young children and it can range from 1 to 2 cm below the costal margin. Furthermore, the liver being in close proximity to the diaphragm and thoracic organs, diseases affecting them can cause the liver to be palpable falsely giving the impression of hepatomegaly. Hence, liver examination is incomplete without percussing the chest and looking for liver dullness. The upper border of the dull note to the point where the liver is palpable is a true indicator of hepatomegaly. The liver span varies according to the age of the child and is usually around 4.5–5 cm in neonates, 5–6 cm for infants, 5–6.5 cm for children aged 1–5 years, 6–7 cm between 5 and 10 years, and in older children it can range between 8 and 10 cm. As mentioned earlier, there can be multiple causes of hepatomegaly, but they can be grouped to the following pathophysiological mechanisms:

- Inflammatory
- Infectious
- Storage disorders
- Infiltrative
- Congestive
- Obstructive

Infections causing hepatomegaly can range from viruses and bacteria in an immunocompetent individual to fungi and parasites in immunocompromised children. In addition, toxins, radiation therapy, and autoimmune disorders cause inflammatory changes in the liver which in turn leads to Kupffer cell hyperplasia resulting in hepatomegaly. Malignant disorders such as leukemia, lymphoma, neuroblastoma, and histoplasmosis can all lead to infiltrative hepatomegaly. Chronic transfusion-dependent anemia can lead to extramedullary hematopoiesis resulting in hepatomegaly.

> **CLINICAL PEARL**
>
> ♦ Liver can normally be palpable in young children. Enlarged liver span signifies hepatomegaly.

SPLENOMEGALY

The clinical manifestation of splenomegaly is seen manifested once the spleen enlarges two to three times in size. It can be classified as mild (1–3 cm), moderate (4–7 cm), and massive (>7 cm) based on the degree of enlargement below the left costal margin. An enlarging spleen first grows upward; hence, it is important to percuss the intercostal spaces to look for splenic dullness. A spleen of 1–2 cm in infants is a normal finding and can be found in up to 10–15% of them.

> **CLINICAL PEARL**
>
> ♦ A soft, thin spleen can be palpable in 15% of neonates, 10% of normal children, and 5% of adolescents.

Persistent fever with hepatosplenomegaly is depicted in **Flowchart 1**.

Flowchart 1: Approach to persistent fever with hepatosplenomegaly in a child.

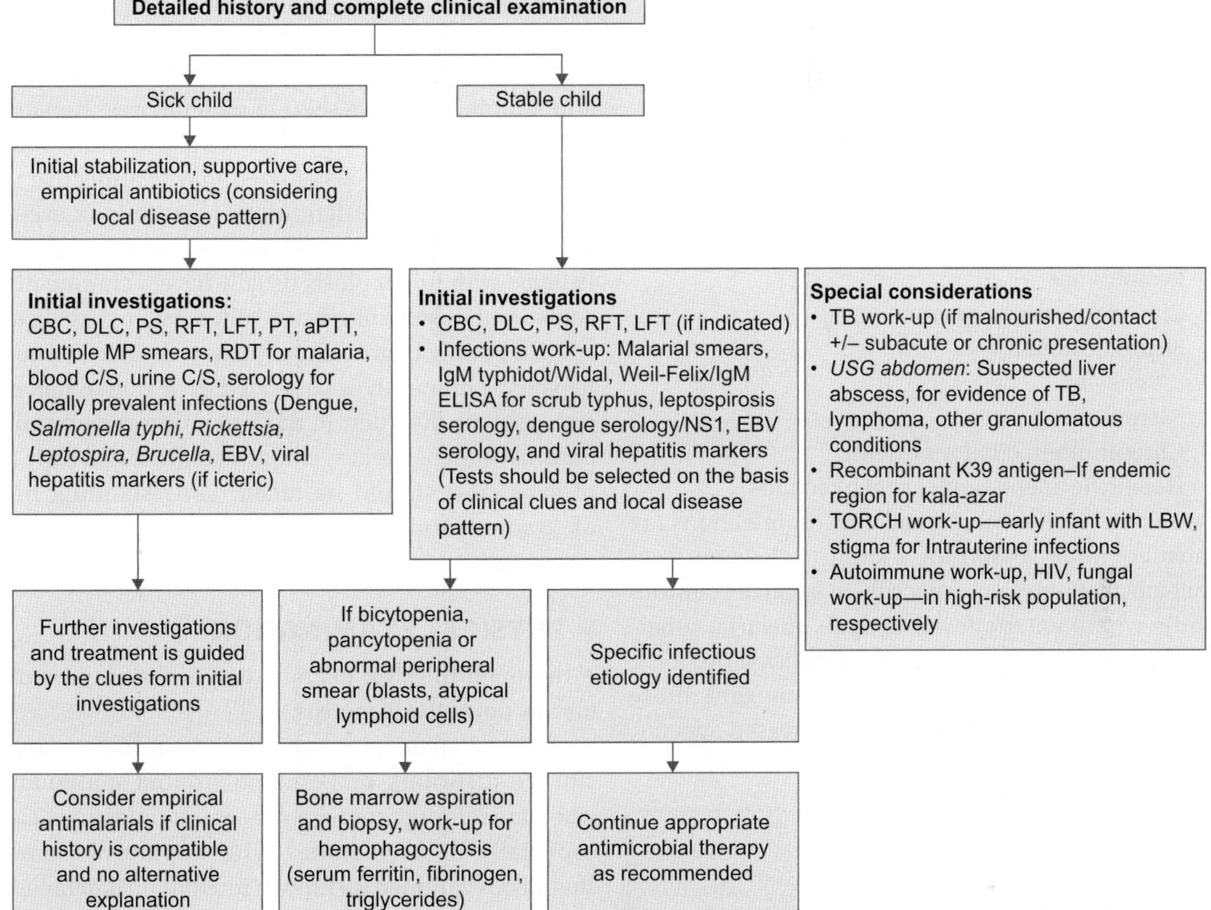

(aPTT: activated partial thromboplastin time; CBC: complete blood count; DLC: differential leukocyte count; EBV: Epstein–Barr virus; ELISA: enzyme-linked immunosorbent assay; HIV: human immunodeficiency virus; LBW: low birth weight; LFT: liver function test; PS: peripheral smear; PT: prothrombin time; RDT: rapid diagnostic test; RFT: renal function test; TB: tuberculosis; TORCH: toxoplasmosis, other agents, rubella, cytomegalovirus, and herpes simplex virus; USG: ultrasonography)

- *Infections:*
  - *Viral:*
    - Hepatitis A and E infection
    - Dengue infection
    - Epstein–Barr virus (EBV) infection
    - Toxoplasmosis, rubella, cytomegalovirus, and herpes simplex virus (TORCH) infection
    - Human immunodeficiency virus (HIV)
  - *Bacterial:*
    - Typhoid fever
    - Tuberculosis
    - Rickettsia
    - Pyogenic liver abscess
    - Brucellosis
    - Borreliosis
    - Infective endocarditis
    - Bacterial sepsis
    - Leptospirosis
  - *Parasitic:*
    - Malaria
    - Kala-azar
    - Toxoplasmosis
    - Toxocariasis
  - *Fungal:*
    - Histoplasmosis
    - Systemic candidiasis (in immunosuppressed)

- *Connective tissue disorders:*
  - Systemic lupus erythematosus
  - Systemic onset juvenile idiopathic arthritis
- *Hemophagocytic syndromes:*
  - Postinfectious
  - Familial
  - Connective tissue disorder related
- *Malignancies:*
  - Acute leukemia
  - Lymphomas
  - Chronic myeloid leukemia
  - Neuroblastoma
- *Miscellaneous:*
  - Sarcoidosis
  - Chronic granulomatous disease
  - Hemolytic anemia with acute infections

Among the earlier-mentioned causes, infections are the most common reason for a child to develop fever with hepatosplenomegaly, especially in tropical countries like India where enteric fever, dengue, malaria, tuberculosis, and viral hepatitis account for significant numbers. In addition to fever with hepatosplenomegaly, these children also have associated jaundice, decreased appetite, and abdominal distension.

> **CLINICAL PEARL**
>
> In tropical regions, infections remain the common cause of fever with hepatosplenomegaly.

HISTORY

The most important initial step toward evaluation of such a child is by taking a thorough and complete history. Different disorders present at different ages. Acute leukemia is common in the age group of 2–10 years. In children younger than 1 year of age, perinatally acquired infections such as TORCH, HIV, hepatitis B, and enteroviruses should be excluded. Whereas in older children, history pertaining to toxin exposure, travel, and drug intake may yield further clues to the etiology. There can be geographic alteration in the incidence of some infectious diseases, such as kala-azar is more common in Bihar and eastern Uttar Pradesh and rickettsia infections are common in hilly regions (Himachal Pradesh and Uttarakhand).

In a child with failure to thrive, repeated infections should be evaluated for a possible HIV infection and an inborn error of immunity. EBV infection is heralded by a prodrome of upper respiratory illness. Other viral illnesses are associated with myalgia or arthralgia. Patients with acute leukemia have a classical history of bony pains and tenderness. Acute onset of anorexia, vomiting, fever, and abdomen pain is seen in patients with hepatitis A. Brucellosis is commonly transmitted to individuals by the intake of raw unpasteurized milk. Connective tissue disorders and autoinflammatory conditions are associated with systemic and multisystem involvement. Patients with tuberculosis usually have a chronic disease course with history of contact with a patient having tuberculosis. Family history should always be taken when the hepatosplenomegaly is suspected to be due to hereditary or hemolytic disorder; in the latter, history pertaining to transfusion dependency, chronic jaundice, and early onset of gallstones should be taken. Long-standing history of gradual abdominal distension indicates storage disorders.

PHYSICAL EXAMINATION

A thorough physical examination is the cornerstone to narrow down the diagnosis.

A firm hepatosplenomegaly is seen in patients with storage disorders or hematolymphoid malignancies, whereas, soft organomegaly is seen in infectious causes, especially EBV. Neonates with hepatosplenomegaly should be examined for growth retardation, microcephaly, and any purpuric spots on the body, a fundus examination should also be done to look for chorioretinitis to rule out TORCH infections. The skin should also be examined for any possible rashes. Most of the viral infections are associated with an exanthem. In patients with hepatosplenomegaly along with fever and rash, diagnosis of dengue fever and dengue-like illness should be considered. Other infections associated with an exanthem are infectious mononucleosis, herpes simplex, typhoid fever, leptospirosis, rickettsial infections, and borreliosis. Among the noninfective causes, connective tissue disorders such as systemic lupus erythematosus and systemic-onset juvenile idiopathic arthritis should be ruled out. Other skin findings in such patients include petechia and ecchymosis which are commonly seen in patients with dengue fever, hematological malignancies, disseminated intravascular coagulation (DIC), and sepsis (attributed to the low platelet count). Lymphadenopathy can be a common associated finding in febrile patients with hepatosplenomegaly. Lymphomas should also be considered in the differential if the lymphadenopathy is generalized and associated with other "B" symptoms or a rapid course.

Other clinical findings include pallor, jaundice, edema, and evidence of third spacing, evidence of malnutrition, and involvement of other organ systems.

> **CLINICAL PEARL**
>
> Detailed history, complete physical examination, and having knowledge about infections prevalent in the locality and their mode of presentations help in guiding initial investigations.

INVESTIGATIONS

Investigations act as an adjunct to the clinical findings and they should be specific and tailored to what disorder is being suspected. A host of investigations leads to diagnostic dilemma and can be misleading. Hence, narrowing the investigatory workup not only leads to better diagnosis but helps in reducing undue expenditure.

Initial Investigations

Initial laboratory work-up in most patients:

- A complete blood count with differential and a peripheral smear examination gives us vital information about affliction of any hematological cell lines and helps in quantifying cytopenias. Information pertaining to etiology can be relayed by a good peripheral smear examination. Presence of abnormal cells like blasts can be seen in patients with leukemia, transformed or activated lymphocytes are seen in viral infections like EBV, evidence of hemolysis in the form of spherocytes, schistocytes, bite cells and reticulocytosis and infections like malaria can also be picked up by a peripheral smear. In patients with suspected malaria, repeating multiple smears during the febrile episodes might increase the yield of finding the parasite. Most patients with malaria will have parasites that show up of thick smear within 48 hours of the symptom onset.
- Liver functions tests and renal function tests should be done in patients with a liver disorder or for patients who are sick with multisystem involvement.
- *Infectious screening:* Common infections that are predominant in the particular region should be screened for. A blood and urine culture is a must before starting a patient on antibiotics. Serological investigations are important diagnostic tests for infections such as enteric fever, brucellosis, rickettsial fever, leptospiral infections, dengue fever, viral hepatitis, HIV, and EBV infections. It is important to note that a full "host" of infectious screen should not be done for all patients and investigations should be warranted based on clinical cues and epidemiological patterns. Rapid diagnostic kits are available for diagnosis of malaria, enabling bedside results without a difficult training period to interpret along with good sensitivity and specificity.

Imaging of Abdomen

A child having tender hepatomegaly and is unwell can be rapidly diagnosed by the help of an ultrasound examination as having a pyogenic liver abscess. In addition, an ultrasound examination helps in diagnostic testing by image-guided biopsies for ruling out malignant, storage, and infective causes. Taps from the liver or other infective foci can be sent for microbiological testing. CT scanning with or without contrast should be done in patients where CT helps delineate the pathology better. Careful attention to who really requires CT imaging should be done to avoid radiation exposure.

Other Investigations

- Serology for congenital infections like TORCH in a neonate with low birth weight and stigmata of the earlier mentioned infections
- Tubercular work-up for malnourished children with a chronic presentation and contact with a tuberculosis case should be done. Work-up includes a chest X-ray, Mantoux, sputum, and gastric lavage for acid-fast bacilli and nucleic acid testing should be sent.
- HIV testing
- Kala-azar infections can be rapidly diagnosed by antigen RK39 testing, especially when the individual comes from an endemic area. The sensitivity and specificity of the test is around 100%.
- Antinuclear antibody and extended nuclear antigen profile should be done in children having associated characteristic rashes, joint pains, polyserositis, and alopecia.
- Children undergoing immunosuppressive therapy including chemotherapy and other myelosuppressive

agents need testing for opportunistic organisms. Fungal workup includes cultures from urine and blood and serological markers.

- In patients with associated pancytopenia/bicytopenia or the peripheral smear showing abnormal cells a bone marrow aspiration and biopsy can be done to rule out malignancy or hemophagocytosis. In addition, cultures can be sent from the bone marrow to rule out occult infections. Kala-azar can also be picked by the help of a bone marrow showing the characteristic Leishman-Donovan (LD) bodies. Storage disorders like Gaucher disease can also show characteristic Gaucher cells which can be picked up by a bone marrow evaluation sent.
- Image-guided biopsies from liver and the lymph nodes, fine-needle aspiration from abscesses can be helpful for diagnosis of patients with infective, malignant, and infiltrative disorders.
- Rheumatological causes are usually a diagnosis of exclusion after ruling out common causes.

TREATMENT

Treatment of the underlying etiology remains the mainstay of therapy. However, in a sick child presenting to emergency with fever and hepatosplenomegaly, initial stabilization, supportive care followed by intravenous (IV) antibiotics against the common infections prevailing in the community such as enteric fever and rickettsial infections should be initiated after sending the initial etiological work-up. Measures have to be taken to demonstrate malaria parasite before starting empirical antimalarial therapy. However, if clinical presentation indicates severe malaria and there is no alternative explanation these patients should be treated accordingly. Investigations should be continued simultaneously till a definitive diagnosis is made and specific therapy must be initiated.

KEY POINTS

- Hepatosplenomegaly is a common clinical finding seen in infants and children presenting with fever.
- Fever with hepatosplenomegaly can be caused by infectious (viral, bacterial, parasitic, and fungal), connective tissue disorders, malignancies, hemophagocytic syndromes, and other rare conditions.
- In tropical regions, infections remain the most common cause of fever with hepatosplenomegaly.
- Detailed history, complete physical examination, and having knowledge about infections prevalent in the locality and their presentations help in guiding initial investigations.
- Complete blood count with a good peripheral smear examination and work-up for common infectious etiologies give a clue to diagnosis in a majority of cases.
- Treatment of the underlying etiology remains the mainstay of therapy. However, in a sick child, initial empirical therapy is justified pending investigation reports.

SUGGESTED READING

1. Anusha G, Somaiah G, Siddique AM, Srikanth B, Suresh Babu M, Vamsidhar NS. Study of etiological and clinical profile of hepatosplenomegaly in children between 1 month and 15 years of age. Sch J App Med Sci. 2014;2(2A):554-7.
2. Kliegman RM, Stanton BF, Geme JW, Schor NF, Behrman R. Nelson Textbook of Pediatrics, 19th edn. Amsterdam: Elsevier; 2011.
3. Lakshmanaswamy A. Clinical Paediatrics. History Taking and Case Discussion, 3rd edn. Philadelphia: Wolters Kluwer Health; 2012.
4. National Institute of Malaria Research. Guidelines for Diagnosis and Treatment of Malaria in India, 2nd edn. New Delhi: National Institute of Malaria Research; 2011.
5. Paul V, Bagga A. Ghai Essential Paediatrics, 8th edn. New Delhi: CBS Publishers; 2013.
6. Sarkar R, Mishra K, Garg VK. Fever with rash in a child in India. Indian J Dermatol Venereol Leprol. 2012;78(3): 251-62.
7. Wolf AD, Lavine JE. Hepatomegaly in neonates and children. Pediatr Rev. 2000;21(9):303-10.

Approach to a Bleeding Child

Nitin K Shah

INTRODUCTION

Bleeding in a child is a common presentation of benign disorders like idiopathic thrombocytopenic purpura (ITP). However, doubt always remains is it a more sinister disease like hemophilia or malignancy? Systematic approach will lead to correct diagnosis with minimum tests and lead to effective therapy.

INTERPRETATION OF ALGORITHM (FLOWCHART 1)

Hemostasis is a delicate balance between fluidity of blood so that it can circulate freely within blood vessels and coagulation so that any breach in continuity of blood vessels can be sealed efficiently and immediately so as not to exsanguinate the body. This delicate balance is

Flowchart 1: Approach to a bleeding child.

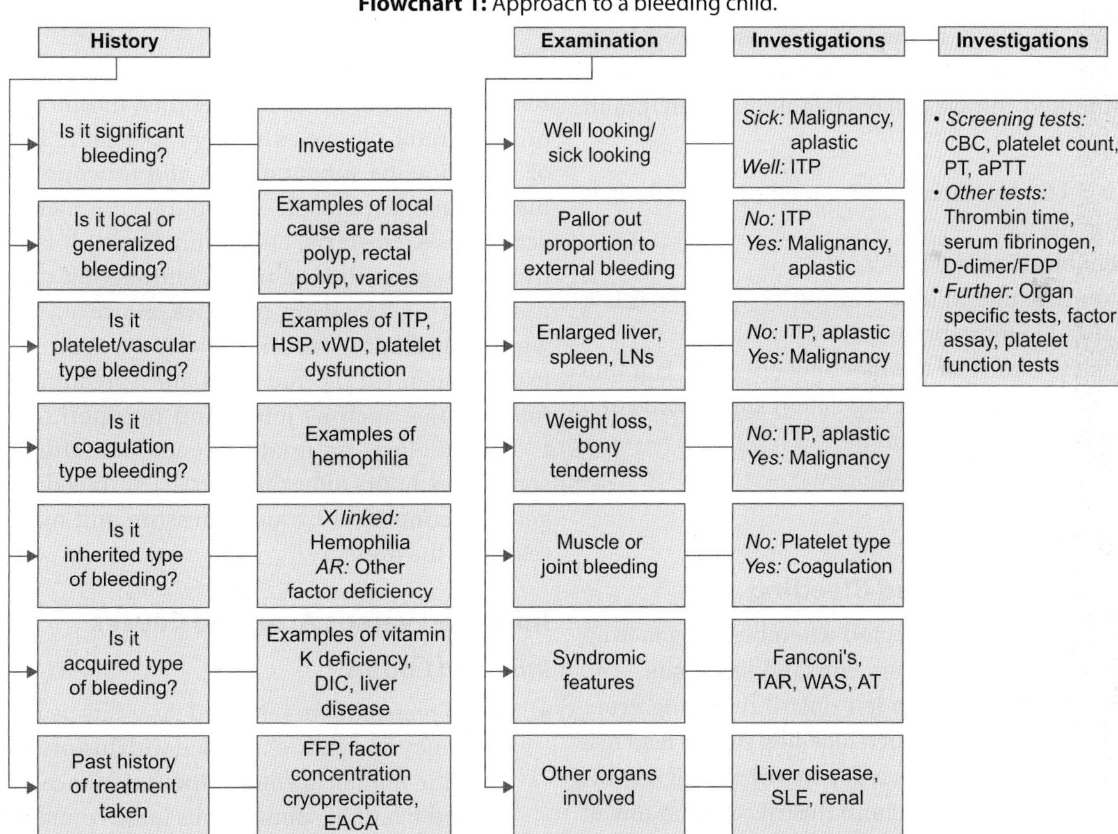

(AR: autosomal recessive; aPTT: activated partial thromboplastin time; CBC: complete blood count; DIC: disseminated intravascular coagulation; EACA: epsilon aminocaproic acid; FDP: fibrinogen/fibrin degradation product; FFP: fresh frozen plasma; HSP: Henoch–Schönlein purpura; ITP: idiopathic thrombocytopenic purpura; LN: lymph node; PT: prothrombin time; SLE: systemic lupus erythematosus; TAR: thrombocytopenia and absent radius; WAS: Wiskott-Aldrich syndrome; vWD: von Willebrand disease)

maintained mainly by three factors, namely, vascular and extravascular tissues, platelets, and plasma factors. Any disturbance in these three factors will lead to either bleeding or excessive clotting (thromboembolism).

Successful management of an acute bleeding episode in a child mainly depends on the ability to make a rapid diagnosis and prompt implementation of therapeutic measures. Proper detailed history and thorough clinical examination often suggest the presence and type of bleeding disorder. However, accurate diagnosis which is required for specific therapy depends on laboratory tests. A careful history also provides critical information in selecting subsequent tests thus avoiding a battery of investigations. Further workup becomes necessary when there is:

- *A recent bout of bleeding:* Spontaneous or after injury or surgery—usually prolonged and disproportionate to extent of injury
- Family history of bleeding episodes
- Preparation for surgery or invasive procedures
- Systemic diseases known to be associated with bleeding disorders, e.g., liver disorder, renal disorder, disseminated intravascular coagulation (DIC), and sepsis

Whenever a child presents with bleeding episode it is necessary to decide:

- Whether bleeding is significant?
- Whether it is due to local causes, or whether it is a generalized hemostatic defect?
- What is the nature of the bleeding episode? Is it due to vascular, platelet, or a coagulation abnormality or a combination of two or more?
- Is it congenital or acquired?

CLINICAL HISTORY

Local versus Generalized Bleeding

Local cause should be suspected when bleeding is from a single site and recurs often from the same site, e.g., epistaxis with bleeding from left nostril recurring every time from the same nostril. Such bleeding should lead to a suspicion of local causes such as a polyp or a foreign body. However, if bleeding is from both nostrils or from any of the nostrils and patient gives history of hematuria or a past history of excessive bleeding after tooth extraction, then it is more likely to be due to a systemic defect. Common local causes of bleeding are shown in **Table 1**.

TABLE 1: Common local causes of bleeding based on site of bleeding.

Site of bleeding	*Local cause of bleeding*
Epistaxis	Deviated septum, hypertrophic turbinate, and ectatic vessel
Oral	Poor dental hygiene
Upper gastrointestinal	Swallowed blood in newborn, varices, and hemangioma
Lower gastrointestinal	Rectal polyp, Meckel's diverticulum, anal fissure
Hematuria	Cystitis, bladder stone, and renal tumor
Umbilicus	Slipped ligature and granuloma

In generalized bleeding disorders, bleeding is spontaneous or greater than expected for extent of injury or the site of bleeding and bleeding is from multiple sites such as skin and mucous membrane, bleeding into interstitial tissue, muscles, and joints.

Platelet/Vascular Type versus Coagulation Type of Bleeding

Bleeding following vascular disorder, thrombocytopenia, or functional platelet disorders is usually in the form of spontaneous subcutaneous and mucous membrane bleeds such as petechiae, purpura, superficial, and few ecchymosis, epistaxis, and menorrhagia. It is often controlled by pressure and once controlled; it usually does not recur on releasing pressure. However, in patients with coagulation factor deficiency, hematomas are usually deep (in the muscles) and spreading, bleeding into cavities such as joints and retroperitoneal space is known. Post-traumatic bleeds are often delayed, sometimes hours after the injury. This bleeding may not get well controlled by local pressure and may recur on releasing the pressure.

Inherited versus Acquired Causes

Inherited Causes

- *Age of presentation:* Inherited disorders usually present in infancy and early childhood with history of bleeding from the umbilical cord, without evidence of sepsis or slipped ligature; spontaneous large cephalhematoma during early neonatal period, bleeding during the eruption or fall of deciduous tooth, etc.; exception being mild hemophilia though inherited cause of bleeding presenting late in life say following a surgery.

Whereas acquired bleeding disorders present at any age, usually later in life, like ITP presenting at 3–5 years of age, exception being hemorrhagic disorder of newborn due to vitamin K deficiency though being acquired cause of bleeding presenting in first week of life.

- *Family history:* Proper family history of bleeding disorders of at least two to three generations on each side of parents (including those who might have died) and noting the pedigree chart helps in realizing the mode of transmission of the disorder such as sex-linked recessive, autosomal recessive, or autosomal dominant
    - *X-linked recessive inheritance:* Females are carrier and males are affected. Only male siblings, males on maternal side including maternal male cousins, maternal uncles, and maternal grandfather are affected. This is typically seen in hemophilia A and B or Wiskott–Aldrich syndrome.
    - *Autosomal recessive inheritance:* Both parents of affected person are heterozygotes and often there is a history of consanguinity. Siblings of either sex and both maternal as well as paternal cousins of either sex are affected (horizontal transmission). This pattern is typical of disorders of factor II, V, VII, X, XI, XII, and XIII deficiency.
    - *Autosomal dominant inheritance:* There is vertical transmission as the proband is affected, one of the parents is affected and grandparents may be affected with variable penetrance and variable severity within families. This is seen typically in von Willebrand disease, some types of qualitative platelet defects, dysfibrinogenemia, and hereditary hemorrhagic telangiectasia. Some of the cases may be spontaneous mutation with negative family history.
    - Although a positive family history is of great value in the diagnosis of bleeding disorders, a negative family history does not rule out the possibility of inherited bleeding disorders. Family history might be negative, if the coagulation defect is mild or there is a spontaneous mutation, as is seen in 20% of patients with hemophilia A.
- *Site of bleeding:* Superficial bleeding is more common in platelet type of bleeding and most common platelet disorder is ITP which is acquired cause of bleeding whereas deep bleeding especially muscle hematoma or joint hematoma are typically seen in coagulation factor deficiency like hemophilia which are inherited causes of bleeding.

Acquired Causes

Conversely, patients with acquired disorders usually present later in life and have a negative family history. They may be associated with underlying systemic disorders such as kidney diseases, liver disorders, and infections. Previous history of operations such as circumcision, dental extraction, tonsillectomy, or major operation practically rules out the possibility of a moderate to severe inherited bleeding disorder. Absence of bleeding from previous trauma, however, does exclude an inherited bleeding disorder. Patients of mild hemophilia with factor level around 10–25% may bleed only after severe trauma. Subject with normal hemostasis may also have bleeding from nonhematological causes as seen in females with menorrhagia or of molar tooth extraction. History of ingestion of drugs like aspirin in the recent past should lead to the suspicion of a transient drug-related hemostatic defect. Similarly, history of oral contraceptives or pregnancy may temporarily increase factor VIII and von Willebrand factor levels and thus increasing the hemostatic competency in women with von Willebrand disease.

Associated Underlying Disorders

Certain characteristic hemostatic defects are associated with specific clinical conditions, e.g., liver diseases with factor II, VII, IX, and X deficiency and fibrinolysis due to decreased clearance of activators and hypercoagulable state because of antithrombin III and protein C deficiency. Malabsorption states may be associated with vitamin K deficiency. Acute promyelocytic leukemia is known to be associated with DIC due to increased cellular procoagulant activities. Myeloproliferative disorder may have platelet defects, thrombocytopenia, and thrombocythemia. Amyloidosis may be associated with factor X deficiency and capillary fragility. Systemic lupus erythematosus (SLE) and antiphospholipid antibody (APLA) syndromes may be associated with thrombocytopenia, acquired hemophilia or acquired von Willebrand disease or on the other hand with hypercoagulable states.

CLINICAL PEARLS

Questions to be asked while history taking in a bleeding child:

- It the bleeding significant?
- Is the bleeding due to local cause or systemic cause?
- Is the bleeding platelets/vascular type or coagulation type?
- Is the bleeding due to congenital or acquired cause?

EXAMINATION

Well versus Sick Child

Well child with no fever, pain, organomegaly, bleeding, bone pains, or weight loss would suggest ITP, whereas sick child would suggest other causes like bone marrow failure or infiltrates.

Pallor and Organomegaly

Sick child with presence of pallor out of proportion of external bleeding would suggest bone marrow suppression such as in malignancies and aplastic anemia. Presence of organomegaly such as hepatomegaly, splenomegaly, and significant lymphadenopathy, weight loss, and bony tenderness would suggest malignancies whereas absence of organomegaly and bony tenderness would suggest aplastic anemia.

Site of Bleeding

Presence of superficial bleeds such as petechiae, purpura, and few superficial ecchymosis suggest ITP, vascular cause, or platelet dysfunction. Deep bleeding such as muscle hematoma, exsanguinating hematomas, retroperitoneal bleeds, and joint bleeds are pathognomonic of coagulation disorders like hemophilia.

Associated Syndromes

There are some specific systemic disorders which have bleeding as a significant problem and have pathognomonic tell-tale signs as shown in **Table 2**. This includes presence of:

- Skeletal deformities, mental retardation, hypogonadism, short stature, hyperpigmentation, and renal anomalies in Fanconi anemia
- Absent radius in thrombocytopenia with absent radius (TAR) syndrome
- Ataxia, mucosal telangiectasia, and mental subnormality in ataxia telangiectasia
- Partial albinism in Heřmanský–Pudlák syndrome
- Syndactyly or lobster hand in factor V deficiency
- Keloids in children with afibrinogenemia and factor XIII deficiency
- Cigarette paper scar, hyperextensible joints, cutis elastic in Ehlers–Danlos syndrome
- Hematochezia, thrombocytopenia, recurrent infection, otitis media, and eczema in a male child with Wiskott–Aldrich syndrome
- Giant hemangioma associated with evidence of clinical and subclinical DIC and thrombocytopenia in Kasabach–Merritt syndrome.

TABLE 2: Syndromes associated with specific bleeding disorders.

Associated condition	*Interpretation*
Oral or nasal telangiectasia and ataxia	Hereditary telangiectasia
Partial albinism	Heřmanský–Pudlák syndrome
Syndactyly	Factor V deficiency
Skeletal malformation and short stature	Fanconi anemia
Absent radius	Thrombocytopenia-absent radius syndrome
Injury marks, rib fractures, and subdural hemorrhage	Battered baby syndrome
Linear purpura at accessible sites	Fictitious purpura
Keloids	Afibrinogenemia
Cigarette paper scar and hypermobile joints	Ehlers–Danlos syndrome
Thrombocytopenia, eczema, and ear discharge	Wiskott–Aldrich syndrome
Giant hemangioma	Kasabach–Merritt syndrome

CLINICAL PEARLS

Questions to be asked while examining a bleeding child:
- Is he a well or a sick child?
- Is there organomegaly?
- Are there other systemic disorder signs?
- Are there physical anomalies, especially skeletal deformities?

INVESTIGATIONS

No single test is suitable for the laboratory evaluation or the overall process of hemostasis and blood coagulation. Laboratory tests can be conveniently divided into screening tests and special tests. Screening tests are applied only after evaluating the nature and clinical circumstances of bleeding and prior to surgery, so as to know the presence and nature of bleeding disorder so that special tests can be done to confirm the diagnosis thus avoiding a battery of unnecessary tests.

Screening Tests

Screening tests include:

- Complete blood count (CBC) and peripheral smear (PS) examination
- Platelet count
- Prothrombin time (PT) and activated partial thromboplastin time (aPTT)
- Thrombin time (TT)
- Bleeding time (BT), clotting time (CT), and clot retraction (rarely)

Interpretation of the screening tests is always done together and never in isolation as shown in the **Table 3**.

Complete blood count and PS examination: CBC tells the involvement of red blood cell series [hemoglobin (Hb) and red cell indices], white blood cell series (total leukocytes and absolute neutrophil count), and platelet series. PS examination will confirm all the three cell series involvement and give clue to the probable diagnosis like leukemia. For platelets, PS is more reliable than machine reports. Presence of 10–15 platelets per high power field and presence of platelet clumps will suggest normal platelet counts. Large platelets are seen in regenerative thrombocytopenia as seen in ITP, normal size platelets are seen as in aregenerative cause of thrombocytopenia like aplastic anemia, giant platelets are seen as in Bernard–Soulier syndrome, microplatelets are seen as in Wiskott-Aldrich syndrome, and presence of normal platelets but not in clumps will indicate absence of aggregation, suggesting platelet functional disorder. Immature platelet fraction (IPF) is useful to differentiate between regenerative thrombocytopenia like ITP where IPF is high versus aregenerative thrombocytopenia like aplastic anemia or leukemia where IPF is low. IPF also helps in predicting marrow recovery like in dengue where rising IPF forecasts rise in platelet count in coming days.

Platelet count: It is a simple first step in evaluating the cellular aspect of hemostasis. However, manual count is not reliable and not reproducible and hence platelet count should be done on particle cell counter or using phase contrast microscope. In platelet type of bleeding, if platelet count is normal or marginally low, vascular or platelet functional disorders should be kept in mind.

Prothrombin time, aPTT, and TT: aPTT is an excellent screening test for determining abnormality of intrinsic clotting pathway and common pathways and is sensitive to activities of approximately 20% or less of factor VIII

TABLE 3: Interpretation of screening tests for bleeding.

Clinical bleeding	*aPTT*	*PT*	*TCT*	*Bleeding time*	*Platelet count*	*Possible defects*
Absent	Abnormal	Normal	Normal	Normal	Normal	High-molecular-weight kininogen, prekallikrein, factor XII, and lupus inhibitor
Present	Abnormal	Normal	Normal	Normal	Normal	Factor XI, IX, VIII deficiency
Present	Abnormal	Abnormal	Normal	Normal	Normal	Factor V, X, II, coumarin, vitamin K deficiency, and mild hepatic disease
Present	Normal	Abnormal	Normal	Normal	Normal	Factor VII deficiency
Present	Abnormal	Normal	Normal	Abnormal	Normal	von Willebrand disease
Present	Abnormal	Abnormal	Abnormal	Abnormal	Normal	Afibrinogenemia
Present	Normal	Normal	Normal	Abnormal	Abnormal	Thrombocytopenia
Present	Normal	Normal	Normal	Abnormal	Normal	Qualitative platelet disorder (aspirin, thrombasthenia, and Bernard–Soulier syndrome)
Present	Normal	Normal	Normal	Normal	Normal	Factor XIII deficiency
Present	Abnormal	Abnormal	Abnormal	Abnormal	Abnormal	Disseminated intravascular coagulation and severe liver disease
Variable	Normal	Normal	Abnormal	Normal	Normal	Dysfibrinogenemia, myeloma, and fibrinogen/fibrin degradation products
Present	Abnormal	Normal	Abnormal	Normal	Normal	Heparin

(aPTT: activated partial thromboplastin time; PT: prothrombin time; TCT: thrombin clotting time)

and IX or XI. aPTT is prolonged during deficiency or abnormalities of extrinsic pathway clotting factors such as high molecular weight, kininogen, prekallikrein, factor XII, XI, IX, VIII; or of common pathway clotting factors like X, V, II, and fibrinogen; or by inhibitors of blood coagulation such as lupus inhibitors, heparin, and fibrin/fibrinogen degradation product. aPTT of test >10 seconds over control is considered abnormal.

Prothrombin time measures extrinsic clotting system and the common pathway. It is measured as International Normalized Ratio (INR) and is considered abnormal when INR is >1.2, however, if INR is not available it is considered abnormal when test PT is >3 seconds over control. PT is prolonged with deficiencies of intrinsic pathway clotting factor like VII; or common pathway factors like X, V, II, and fibrinogen and inhibitors of these factors.

Thrombin time measures thrombin-induced conversion of fibrinogen to fibrin and is abnormal in patients with hypofibrinogenemia whether acquired or congenital or dysfibrinogenemia and in presence of inhibitors such as heparin, myeloma proteins, and fibrin degradation products which block either thrombin cleavage of fibrinopeptide or fibrin monomer polymerization.

A prolongation of PT with normal partial thromboplastin time (PTT) that is corrected by adding normal pooled plasma indicates factor VII deficiency that occurs with congenital deficiency, early during oral anticoagulant therapy, vitamin K deficiency, or liver diseases. This is further confirmed by factor VII assay.

A prolonged aPTT with normal PT which is corrected by adding normal pooled plasma will suggest deficiency of factor VII, IX, XI, or XII, however, factor XII deficiency does not manifest clinically with bleeding and in fact presents with thromboembolism hence leaving deficiency of factor VIII, IX or XI as the cause. This can be confirmed further by doing factor VIII, factor IX, and factor XI assay in that order based on their incidence.

Prolongation of both PT and aPTT would suggest common pathway factor deficiency like factor X, V, II, or fibrinogen; or multiple factor deficiency of intrinsic as well as extrinsic pathways as seen in chronic liver disease or vitamin K deficiency.

Prolonged TT would suggest fibrinogen deficiency or dysfunction. Prolonged TT with normal serum fibrinogen would suggest dysfibrinogenemia, and with low or absent fibrinogen levels would suggest hypo- or afibrinogenemia.

Prolonged aPTT should be screened for presence of inhibitor doing correction study where 1 mL of test plasma is mixed with 1 mL of pooled normal plasma and aPTT is repeated at zero and 4 hours. If aPTT corrects by >50%, it suggests factor deficiency. If aPTT does not correct and even worsens after 4 hours of incubation, it suggests of presence of inhibitor which is then confirmed by doing inhibitor assay. In such cases, one must also rule out autoimmune disorders such as APLA syndrome and SLE by doing appropriate tests.

Others

Bleeding Time

This test evaluates primary hemostatic stage and is ideally done with the help of template. The normal BT is 4–7 minutes and prolongation of BT usually occurs at platelet count less than 50,000/mm^3. At counts below 10,000/mm^3, BT is usually prolonged and is often 15 minutes or longer and hence BT in severe thrombocytopenia is not required and can be hazardous as it can lead to scarring.

Qualitative platelet disorders have prolonged BT with nearly normal platelet count as seen in Glanzmann's thrombasthenia, Bernard–Soulier syndrome, storage pool disorder, Wiskott–Aldrich syndrome, and with various drugs like aspirin and nonsteroidal anti-inflammatory agents like ibuprofen, etc. Even in von Willebrand disease, BT is usually prolonged as von Willebrand factor is involved in binding of platelets to matrix protein or to other cells. One can do platelet aggregation study to prove platelet functional disorders as shown in **Table 4**. This can be confirmed by doing platelet surface receptor studies for gpIIB/IIIA or gpIX which are now widely available **(Flowchart 2)**.

Clot Retraction

Retraction and exudation of the serum after 1 hour is observed in the clotting tube. Normally, 50% exudation at the end of 1 hour of the original blood volume is taken as normal retraction. However, with the advent of platelet aggregation study and platelet receptor study, this test has become obsolete.

Factor XIII Assay

Factor XIII deficiency presents with delayed umbilical cord falling, intracranial bleeds, or delayed bleeding from wounds with poor healing. Screening tests for bleeding are normal in such cases; one can do 5 molar urea solubility test to prove factor XIII deficiency.

TABLE 4: Platelet aggregation study (for platelet dysfunction).

Disorder	*ADP*		*Collagen*	*Adrenalin*	*Ristocetin*	*Arachidonic acid*
	Primary	*Secondary*				
Thrombasthenia	ABN	ABN	ABN	ABN	N	ABN
Bernard–Soulier syndrome	N	N	N	N	ABN	N
von Willebrand disease	N	N	N	N	ABN	N
Cyclooxygenase deficiency and thromboxane synthetase deficiency	N	—	ABN	ABN	N	ABN
Storage pool disorder	N	ABN decreased	ABN	ABN	N	N or decreased
Aspirin defect	N	ABN decreased	ABN	ABN	N	ABN

(ABN: impaired aggregation; N: normal aggregation)

Flowchart 2: Correction studies when activated partial thromboplastin time is prolonged.

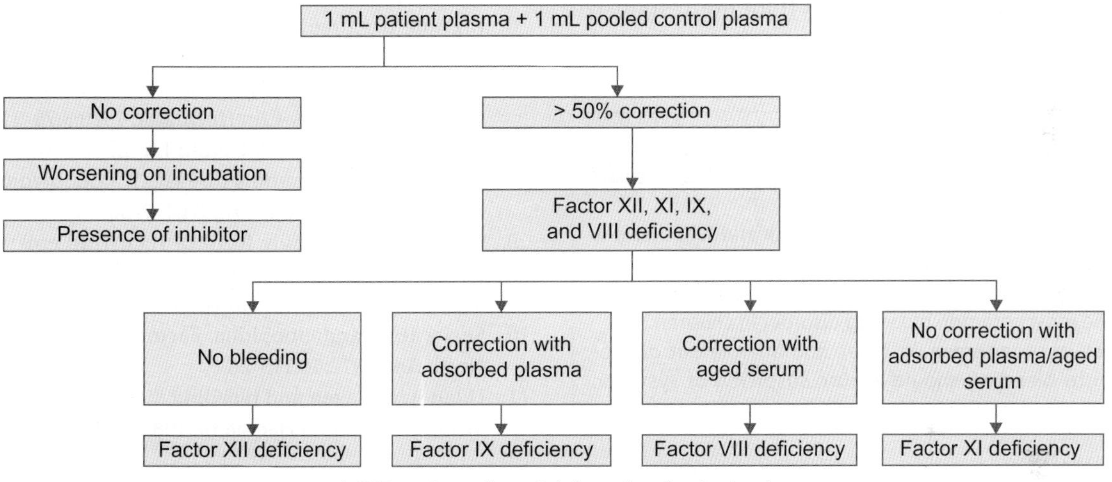

(aPTT: activated partial thromboplastin time)

CLINICAL PEARLS

Never do BT and CT as screening tests.
Always do following tests:
- CBC with platelets counts and a PS for platelet morphology
- PT
- aPTT
- TT with serum fibrinogen

Bleeding Disorders with Normal Screening Tests

Bleeding disorders not associated with any abnormalities in screening tests are:
- Vascular causes such as Henoch-Schönlein purpura, hereditary telangiectasia (Pender-Osler-Weber syndrome), scurvy, Ehlers-Danlos syndrome, senile purpura, and simple purpura (seen in 10% of women)
- Factor XIII deficiency (unless one does factor XIII assay)
- Fibrinolytic pathway defects like a-2 antiplasmin deficiency
- Amyloidosis (may or may not be associated with factor X deficiency)
- Mild clotting factor deficiency
- Nonaccidental hemorrhage like in child abuse
- Fictitious or self-inflicted purpura

MANAGEMENT OF BLEEDING CHILD

Management of a bleeding child will include general supportive care and specific supportive care and treatment of primary disease (the list is vast and beyond the scope of this chapter).

General Supportive Care

This will include volume expansion using crystalloids and colloids, inotropes for falling blood pressure, oxygen to improve tissue oxygenation, and treatment of primary disease if any.

Specific Supportive Care

It includes packed red blood cells to maintain hemoglobin in physiological range, platelets to arrest bleeding in a case of thrombocytopenia (mainly in cases due to decreased production), DIC [along with fresh frozen plasma (FFP)] and platelet dysfunction; FFP in cases with coagulopathy; specific factor replacement in a case of known clotting factor deficiency; use of cryoprecipitate to increase fibrinogen levels; use of factor eight inhibitor bypassing activity or activated prothrombin complex concentrates in hemophilia with inhibitor; plasma exchange in a case of any inhibitors; and activated factor VII for nonresponsive bleeding due to any cause.

KEY POINTS

- Ascertain whether bleeding is significant, platelet/vascular/coagulation type
- Ascertain whether the child is well or sick and whether it is inherited or acquired in origin
- Always to complete screening tests and not BT/CT
- ITP is the most common bleeding disorder in children.
- Presence of organomegaly, fever, and anemia out of proportion to bleeding should arouse suspicion of systemic disease.

SUGGESTED READING

1. Bachmann HF. Diagnostic approach to mild bleeding disorders. Semin Hematol. 1980;17:292-305.
2. Bithell TC. Bleeding disorders caused by vascular abnormalities. In: Lee GR (Ed). Wintrobe's Clinical Hematology, 9th edition. Philadelphia: Lea & Febiger; 1993. pp. 1374-89.
3. Bowie EJ, Owen CA. Significance of abnormal preoperative hemostatic test. Pros Hemost Thromb. 1980;5:179-209.
4. Fisher S, Rikover M, Noor S. Factor XIII deficiency with severe hemorrhagic diathesis. Blood. 1966;28:34.
5. Gilbert C, White II, Marder VJ, Colman RW. Approach to bleeding patient. In: Colman RW, Hirsh J, Marder VJ, Salzman EW (Eds). Hemostasis and Thrombosis. Philadelphia: JB Lippincott & Co.; 1987. pp. 1048-960.
6. Ingram GI. Investigation of a long-standing bleeding tendency. Br Med Bull. 1977;33:261-4.
7. Lowe GD, Forbes CD. Laboratory diagnosis of congenital coagulation defects. Clin Haematol. 1979;8:79-94.
8. Miller CH, Graham JB, Goldin LR, Elston RC. Genetics of classic von Willebrand's disease. I. Phenotypic variation within families. Blood. 1979;54:117-36.
9. Osler W. On a family form of recurring epistaxis, associated with multiple telangiectases of skin and mucous membranes. Bull John Hopkins Hosp. 1901;7:333-7.
10. Seeler RA. Parahemophilia. Factor V deficiency. Med Clin North Am. 1972;56:119-25.
11. Uden A. Collagen and bleeding diathesis in Ehlers–Danlos syndrome. Scand J Haematol. 1982;28:425-30.

Clinicopathological Approach to Coagulation Disorder

Sangeeta Mudaliar, Bharat Agarwal

INTRODUCTION

Bleeding in a child can be a diagnostic challenge because of the wide range of possible causes. Evaluation of a child presenting with bleeding should include a comprehensive medical and bleeding history, a complete family history, a detailed physical examination and selected laboratory tests. Investigations and laboratory tests should be requested based on history and clinical findings.

This chapter will be focused on interpretation and significance of laboratory tests for arriving at a diagnosis in various bleeding disorders. Bleeding disorders can be inherited or acquired, and include coagulation factor deficiencies, platelet deficiencies, and/or dysfunctions and von Willebrand disease (vWD).

Flowchart 1 represents the differential diagnosis of various clinical conditions which may present with purpura or bleeding. The various disease conditions have been grouped as nice (benign course) or nasty (malignant or life-threatening or prolonged course).

Flowchart 1: Clinical differential diagnosis of purpura/bleeding in a child.

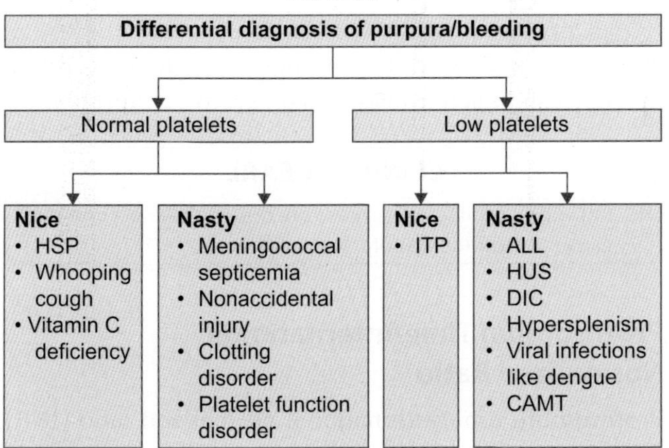

(ALL: acute lymphocytic leukemia; CAMT: congenital amegakaryocytic thrombocytopenia; DIC: disseminated intravascular coagulation; HSP: Henoch–Schönlein purpura; HUS: hemolytic uremic syndrome; ITP: immune thrombocytopenia)

Flowchart 2 gives an approach to causes of mucosal and superficial skin bleeding while **Flowchart 3** gives an approach to conditions which present with large ecchymosis and/or joint bleeding.

Flowchart 4 explains a comprehensive approach to a child presenting with bleeding and/or abnormal coagulation screening test.

SCREENING TESTS

Initial tests to screen for bleeding disorders should include a complete blood count (CBC) with platelet counts, blood film, prothrombin time (PT), and activated partial thromboplastin time (aPTT).

Sample Collection

Improperly collected sample is the most common cause of falsely elevated clotting time. Also, samples collected from indwelling catheters give spuriously abnormal values due to contamination with heparin or intravenous fluids.

Samples should be collected in tubes containing citrate (3.2 or 3.8%) as anticoagulant. The ratio of citrate to whole blood should be 1:9. This needs to be adjusted if patient has high hematocrit. For infants and children, small 3 mL tubes (2.7 mL blood to 0.3 mL citrate) should be used.

Samples should be tested within 2 hours of collection if at room temperature or within 4 hours if kept cold.

Complete Blood Count

Complete blood count [blood collected into ethylenediaminetetraacetic acid (EDTA)] is performed to exclude thrombocytopenia. CBC also provides information about additional cytopenias and other white blood cell (WBC) and red blood cell (RBC) abnormalities. Peripheral blood film provides additional information regarding platelet number,

Flowchart 2: Workup of a patient with a defect in primary hemostatic mechanism.

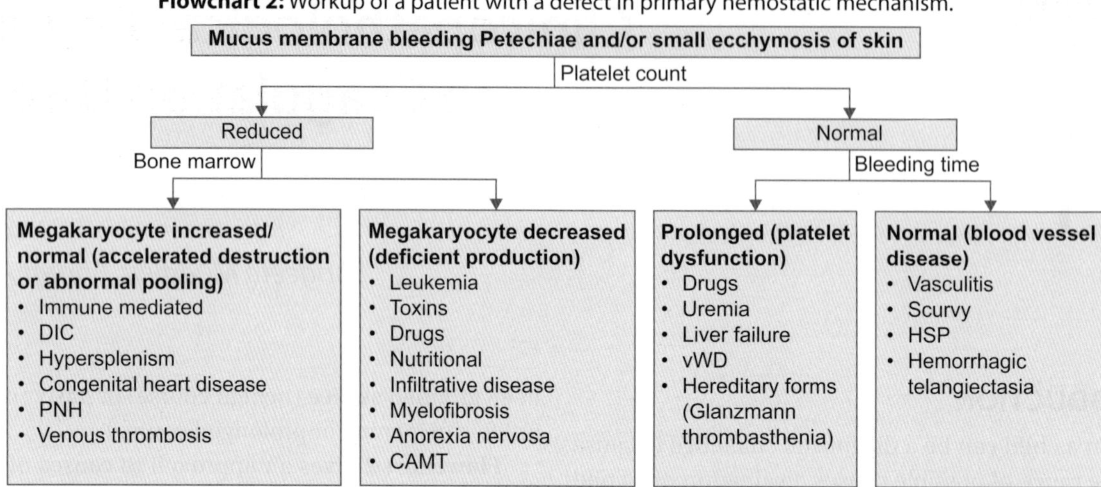

(DIC: disseminated intravascular coagulation; CAMT: congenital amegakaryocytic thrombocytopenia; HSP: Henoch–Schönlein purpura; PNH: paroxysmal nocturnal hemoglobinuria; vWD: von Willebrand disease)

Flowchart 3: Approach to defects in plasma phase laboratory.

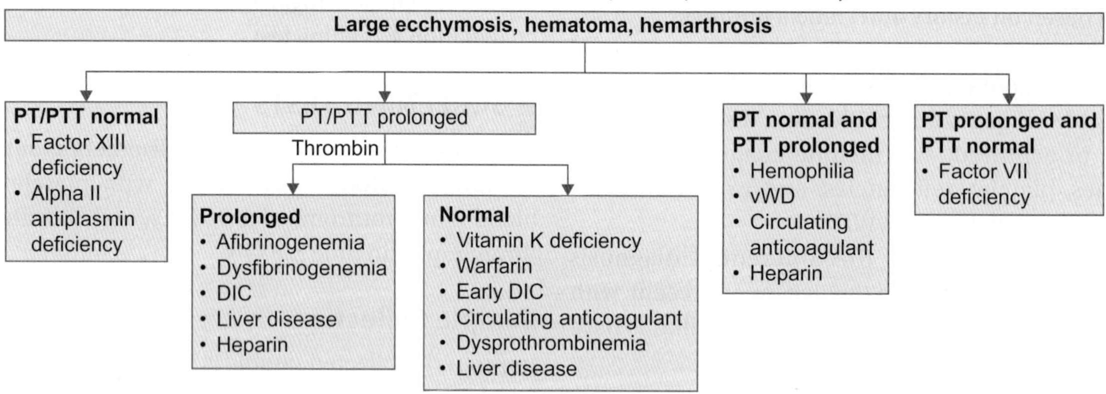

(DIC: disseminated intravascular coagulation; PT: prothrombin time; PTT: partial thromboplastin time; vWD: von Willebrand disease)

size, clumping, and granularity (the platelet count can be estimated by the number of platelets per × 100 field multiplied by 20×10^9/L).

Pseudothrombocytopenia resulting from clumping of platelets collected in EDTA anticoagulant can be identified by examination of the blood film, and confirmed by recollecting a specimen in citrate anticoagulant in which clumping will not occur. If true thrombocytopenia is diagnosed, the next step is to differentiate between new-onset acquired thrombocytopenia, chronic acquired thrombocytopenia, and congenital thrombocytopenia.

Evaluation of WBC morphology allows identification of malignant blasts, granulocyte inclusions such as Döhle-like bodies, or other WBC abnormalities. Evaluation of RBC morphology is important to exclude a microangiopathic process as evidenced by presence of fragmented RBCs, microcytosis, macrocytosis, and other RBC abnormalities.

CLINICAL PEARL

- Improperly collected samples are one of the most common causes of spurious laboratory results.

Prothrombin Time/International Normalized Ratio

Prothrombin time/international normalized ratio (INR) (blood collected into citrate) measures the extrinsic and common pathway in the coagulation cascade (tissue factor, FVII, FX, FV, FII, and fibrinogen). Results should be compared with age-specific laboratory reference intervals,

Flowchart 4: Evaluation of a child with bleeding or abnormal coagulation screening tests.

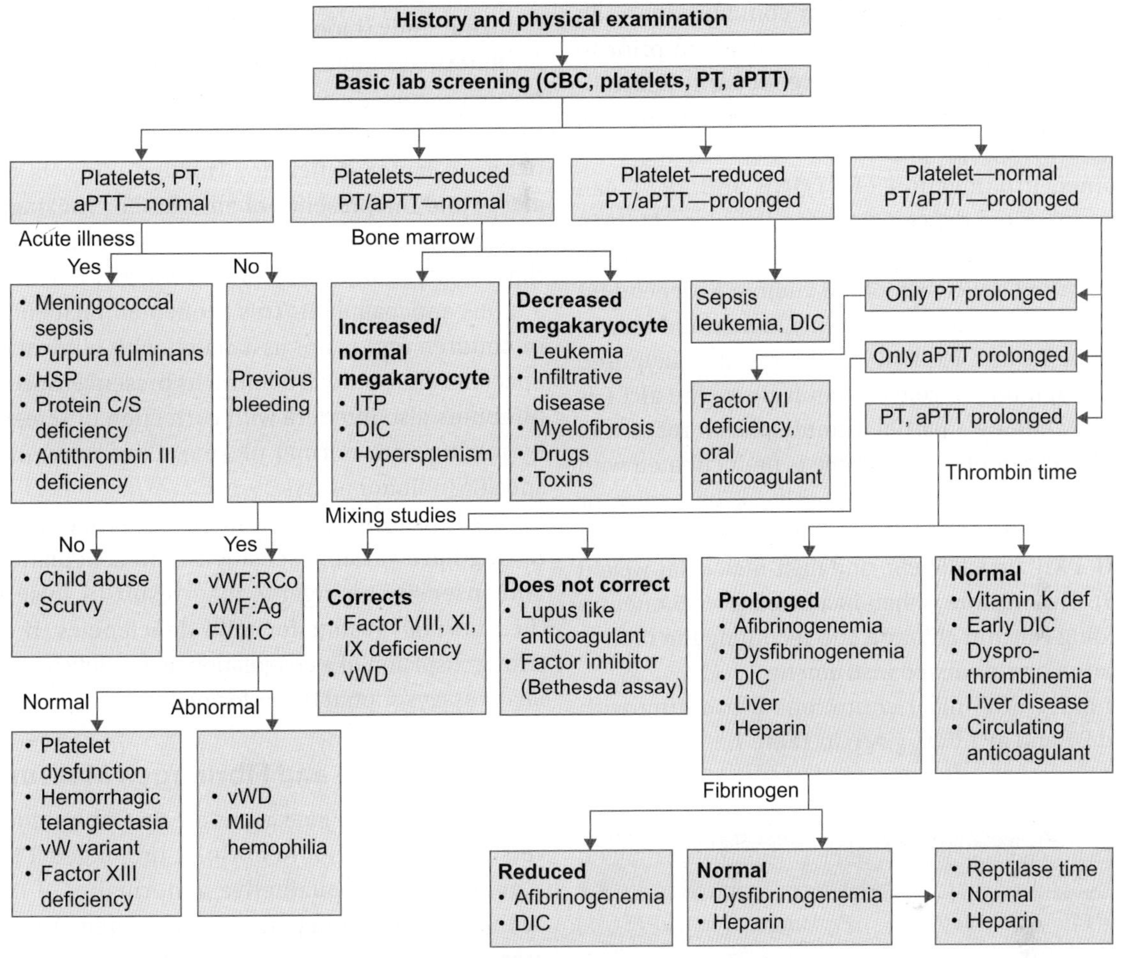

(aPTT: activated partial thromboplastin time; CBC: complete blood count; DIC: disseminated intravascular coagulation; ITP: immune thrombocytopenia; PT: prothrombin time; vWD: von Willebrand disease; vWF: von Willebrand factor; vWF:RCo: vWF:ristocetin; vWF:Ag: vWF:antigen)

and are reported in seconds and/or as a percentage of a normal control sample. The INR is the ratio of a patient's PT to a normal control sample, raised to the power of the ISI value for the analytical system used: INR = (observed PT/control PT) ISI, where ISI = international sensitivity index (sensitivity of thromboplastin).

A prolonged PT/high INR (with normal aPTT) suggests FVII deficiency, or use of vitamin K analogs such as warfarin. The PT is performed by adding a thromboplastin reagent that contains calcium chloride to the citrated plasma sample of patient. The time required for clot formation is recorded using an automated instrument.

Activated Partial Thromboplastin Time

Activated partial thromboplastin time measures the intrinsic and common pathways of coagulation (FXII, FXI, FIX, FVIII, FX, FV, FII, and fibrinogen). The aPTT is less sensitive than the PT to deficiencies of the common pathway factors. Results should be compared with age-specific laboratory reference intervals, and results are reported in seconds.

An abnormally prolonged aPTT (with normal PT/INR) suggests FVIII, FIX, FXI, or FXII deficiency. An aPTT within the reference range does not reliably exclude mild FVIII, FIX, or FXI deficiency. Therefore, factor assays should be performed if specific deficiencies are suspected.

Factor XII deficiency causes a prolonged aPTT, but is not associated with clinical bleeding. A prolonged aPTT can occur in severe vWD, as a result of the associated FVIII deficiency.

The aPTT is also prolonged in the presence of inhibitors including heparin. Heparin contamination occurs most often in specimens drawn from arterial or central venous catheters. To avoid heparin contamination, an adequate volume of blood should be removed prior to sampling. Where that is not possible, heparin neutralization can be performed, usually by the addition of heparinase to the sample plasma.

Combined prolongation of PT/INR and aPTT can result from inherited deficiencies of individual factors in the common pathway: FX, FV, FII, and fibrinogen, or from the rare inherited deficiency of the vitamin K-dependent coagulation factors. More commonly, combined abnormalities of aPTT and PT/INR are the result of acquired deficiencies of multiple coagulation factors. The aPTT is performed by adding a partial thromboplastin reagent to citrated plasma sample. The sample is preincubated with a surface activating reagent (such as celite, kaolin, silica, or ellagic acid) to introduce controlled activation of contact factor (FXI, FXII, prekallikrein, and high-molecular weight kininogen). This mixture is then incubated for 2–5 minutes before adding calcium chloride and recording the time to clot formation by automated instrument.

A summary of clinical conditions presenting with prolonged PT and aPTT are given in **Table 1**.

TABLE 1: Causes of prolonged prothrombin time and activated partial thromboplastin time.

Prolonged PT	*Prolonged aPTT*	*Prolonged PT and aPTT*
Inherited		
Factor VII deficiency	vWF, factor VIII, IX, XI, or XII deficiency	Prothrombin, fibrinogen, factor V, X, or combined factor deficiency
Acquired		
Vitamin K deficiency	Heparin use	Liver disease
Liver disease	Inhibitor of vWF, factors VIII, IX, XI, or XII	DIC
Warfarin use	Antiphospholipid antibodies	Supratherapeutic heparin or warfarin
Factor VII inhibitor	—	• Combined heparin or warfarin use • Inhibitor of prothrombin, fibrinogen, factor V or X • Direct thrombin inhibitor

(aPTT: activated partial thromboplastin time; DIC: disseminated intravascular coagulation; PT: prolonged prothrombin time; vWF: von Willebrand factor)

Mixing Study

A mixing study (blood collected into citrate) is done when an abnormal PT and/or an aPTT is identified. The patient's plasma is mixed with normal plasma in a 1:1 ratio, and the screening tests are repeated. This test differentiates between factor deficiency (mixing corrects the PT or aPTT) and the presence of an inhibitor (mixing does not correct the PT or aPTT). The most common inhibitor that results in noncorrection of the aPTT with mixing is a lupus anticoagulant. This is often an incidental finding in children and is not associated with clinical bleeding. Specialized assays will confirm its presence. Specific factor inhibitors also interfere with correction of screening tests by mixing with normal plasma. Confirmation requires specific inhibitor assays.

Prothrombin time and aPTT reagents used for testing have variable sensitivities to coagulation factors and insensitive reagents may result in false negative (i.e., normal) results for mild deficiencies. If there is a strong suspicion of a coagulation factor deficiency, specific factor assays should be performed.

Thrombin Time and Fibrinogen Measurement

Thrombin time (TT) measures the thrombin-induced conversion of fibrinogen to fibrin. A prolonged TT suggests a quantitative or qualitative abnormality of fibrinogen or the presence of heparin in the sample. A quantitative measurement of fibrinogen should also be performed.

Prothrombin time, aPTT, and TT do not screen for factor XIII deficiency.

Thrombin time is the time to clot formation after the addition of thrombin to citrated blood. The TT is prolonged by heparin, direct thrombin inhibitors, fibrin degradation products, paraproteins, and fibrinogen deficiency (qualitative and quantitative). Protamine is added to neutralize the heparin so that the TT can be interpreted without heparin interference. This assay has been used to establish the presence of adequate fibrinogen but is not being used as widely now.

Reptilase Time

Reptilase time measures time to clot formation after the addition of reptilase, a thrombin-like snake enzyme, to citrated blood. Unlike the TT, it is not affected by heparin. It can be useful to determine whether heparin is the cause of the prolonged TT.

Urea Clot Lysis Test

Urea clot lysis test (blood collected into citrate) measures the solubility of the clot with the addition of urea. The urea clot solubility test relies on the ability of urea to dissolve unstable clots, which are formed in the absence of factor XIII. Normal clots are not dissolved by urea or monochloroacetic acid, unlike clots in patients with factor XIII deficiency.

An abnormal test suggests severe FXIII deficiency or hypofibrinogenemia. Clot solubility is increased only at very low levels of FXIII levels (<3%) and, therefore, does not detect mild/moderate deficiencies. A quantitative assay of FXIII should be used to confirm the result of this screening test.

Fibrinogen

Fibrinogen's normal levels range from 200 to 400 mg/dL. It is an acute phase reactant and higher levels are seen with acute illness and stress. Fibrinogen levels can be measured immunologically or by a chemical method. The level of function of fibrinogen or fibrinogen activity can also be measured using von Clauss kinetic assay.

Fibrinogen Degradation Products or D-dimer

Fibrin degradation products are fragments resulting from the action of plasmin on fibrin or fibrinogen and reflect high fibrinolysis states [such as disseminated intravascular coagulation (DIC)], when their levels are elevated.

D-dimers are formed when cross-linked fibrin is degraded. They can be measured specifically by enzyme-linked immunosorbent assay. Their level is usually higher in DIC and in thrombotic conditions, such as deep venous thrombosis and pulmonary embolism. Their elevation in the absence of symptoms does not imply the presence of these disorders.

Fibrinolysis Inhibitors

Abnormalities of fibrinolysis inhibitors (blood collected into citrate), such as α2-antiplasmin (α2-AP) and plasminogen activator inhibitor 1 (PAI-1), can cause rare bleeding disorders because of increased fibrinolysis.

Genetic Testing

The genetic mutations associated with inherited hemostatic disorders are gradually being revealed. If available, mutational analysis aids in accurate diagnosis and helps in genetic counseling and prenatal diagnosis.

Specific Coagulation Factors

A specific factor assay measures the clotting time of a mixture of diluted test plasma and a specific factor deficient substrate plasma that supplies all the factors except the one being measured.

Euglobulin Clot Lysis Test

It is a screening test for excessive fibrinolysis. It is shortened in conditions characterized by increased fibrinolysis like systemic fibrinolysis, PAI-1 deficiency, and α2-AP deficiency.

Bleeding Time (Using a Device Appropriate for Size of Child)

A lancet device is used to make a standardized cut on the volar surface of the forearm, and the time it takes for bleeding to stop is measured. The bleeding time assesses the function of platelets and their interaction with the vascular wall. The bleeding time test was widely used as a screening test for primary hemostasis disorders, but is less often used now because of difficulties in standardization.

Platelet Function Analyzer

Platelet function analyzer, PFA-100 (blood collected into citrate) is an instrument in which primary and platelet-related hemostasis is simulated. A small sample of anticoagulated whole blood (0.8 mL) is aspirated via a narrow diameter capillary through a microscopic aperture cut into a membrane coated with the platelet agonists collagen and epinephrine or collagen and adenosine 5'-diphosphate. The high shear rate generated under standardized flow conditions and presence of chemical stimuli result in platelet adhesion, activation, and aggregation at the aperture, building a stable platelet plug. The time required to obtain full occlusion of the aperture is reported as the closure time. The closure time is prolonged by low levels of von Willebrand factor (vWF), thrombocytopenia, decreased hematocrit, and by some platelet function abnormalities (e.g., severe disorders such as Bernard–Soulier syndrome and Glanzmann thrombasthenia).

Due to issues of both sensitivity and specificity, use of the PFA-100 as a routine screening test is still debated. However, the small blood volume needed for this test compared with the much larger volume required for platelet function testing by aggregometry (10 mL or more) is an advantage, especially for screening very young children for vWD or severe platelet function disorders.

Testing for Defects in Primary Hemostasis von Willebrand Factor Antigen and Activity

These tests help in making diagnosis of vWD by measuring the level of von Willebrand antigen and ristocetin cofactor activity.

Platelet Function Testing

The most common method of assessing platelet function is light transmission aggregometry, in which the increase in light transmission through a rapidly stirred sample of citrated platelet-rich plasma is recorded as platelets aggregate. As a fresh blood sample is needed for aggregation testing, the patient may have to be referred to a center with a specialized laboratory. Specialized testing includes measurement of granule secretion, dense granule enumeration by whole mount electron microscopy, flow cytometric assessment of surface receptors, and evaluation of platelet ultrastructure by transmission electron microscopy.

Screening platelet function for detecting vWD has a low negative predictive value and may require repeat testing. One also may measure von Willebrand factor antigen (vWF:Ag) by immunoassay and vWF activity by measuring the ability of patient's vWF to agglutinate normal platelets in the presence of ristocetin (vWF:RCo) or by its ability to bind collagen (vWF:CB). Factor VIII:C activity is a functional assay for factor VIII that is measured by mixing normal plasma with factor VIII-deficient plasma. Levels of vWF:Ag and vWF:RCo may be elevated during pregnancy, oral contraceptive use, and liver disease. They may decrease with hypothyroidism and type O blood.

Platelet Aggregometry

The rapidity and extent of platelet agglutination are graphically recorded after adding a variety of agonists [ristocetin, epinephrine, collagen, adenosine diphosphate (ADP), and arachidonic acid].

Platelet aggregation studies remain the most sensitive method for detecting and distinguishing platelet function defects. In these tests, platelet aggregation is tested by measuring changes in optical density as platelets respond to various agents such as ADP, epinephrine, collagen, arachidonic acid, and ristocetin. Different disorders will show different patterns. For example, platelets of patients with Glanzmann thrombasthenia (dysfunctional or deficient glycoprotein IIb/IIIa complex in platelets) only aggregate with ristocetin, whereas platelets of patients with Bernard–Soulier syndrome (absent or decreased glycoprotein Ib complex on platelets) have no aggregation with ristocetin, reduced aggregation with collagen, and normal aggregation with ADP, arachidonic acid, and epinephrine.

Thromboelastography

Thromboelastography provides the whole dynamic process of hemostasis from clot formation to its dissolution and also provides information about platelet function.

KEY POINTS

- Improperly collected sample is the most common cause of abnormal coagulation results.
- Initial tests to screen for bleeding disorders include—complete blood count (CBC) with platelet counts, blood film, prothrombin time (PT), and activated partial thromboplastin time (aPTT).
- Further investigations can be planned based on the screening test reports.

SUGGESTED READING

1. Leung LK. Antithrombotic therapy: problems and issues. Hematology. 2006;457-62.
2. Rajpurkar M, Lushar JM. Clinical and laboratory approach to the patient with bleeding. In: Orkin SH, Nathan DG, Ginsburg D, Look AT, Fisher DE, Lux S (Eds). Nathan and Oski's Hematology of Infancy and Childhood, 7th ed. Philadelphia: Saunders Elsevier; 2009.
3. Revel-Vilk S, Rand ML, Israels SJ. An approach to the bleeding child. In: Blanchette VS, Breakey VR, Revel-Vilk S (Eds). SickKids Handbook of Pediatric Thrombosis and Hemostasis. Basel: Karger Publishers; 2013. pp. 14-22.
4. Stasi R. How to approach thrombocytopenia. Hematology Am Soc Hematol Educ Program. 2012;2012:191-7.

Algorithmic Approach to Eosinophilia in Children

ATK Rau, Sangeetha Shenoy

INTRODUCTION

Eosinophilia is probably the second most common hematologic abnormality in children in the tropics after anemia. The normal eosinophil count ranges from 0.04×10^9 to 0.4×10^9/L and the percentage in relation to the total leukocyte count ranges from 1 to 6%. Eosinophilia is defined as eosinophil count $>0.4 \times 10^9$/L. The count has a diurnal variation, with the lowest value in the morning and the highest being at night. For standardization, the morning value at 8 AM is taken as the baseline eosinophil count. The count also varies with age **(Table 1)**, exercise, and environmental stimuli (allergen exposure).

Eosinophilia can further be classified as mild ($<1.5 \times 10^9$/L), moderate ($1.5–5 \times 10^9$/L), and severe ($>5 \times 10^9$/L). The peripheral eosinophil count does not correlate with the level of organ damage. The counts may be normal in conditions where there is significant recruitment of eosinophils into organs as in eosinophilic pneumonia. On the other hand, a high eosinophil count may not have associated organ damage. But an eosinophil count of $>1.5 \times 10^9$/L is considered the level above which organ damage is more likely to occur. Eosinophilia can also be masked because of pyogenic inflammation which can lower the eosinophil counts, as well as by exogenous administration of medications like corticosteroids, estrogen, and epinephrine.

The development and terminal differentiation of eosinophils are controlled by several cytokines like interleukin-3 (IL-3), granulocyte-macrophage colony-stimulating factor, and IL-5, of which the IL-5 is the one which is primarily responsible for the production. Hence, diseases like extrinsic asthma and helminthiasis which stimulate the T-helper 2 mediated immune response have associated eosinophilia.

After transendothelial migration, eosinophils can invade target organs, secreting their products into surrounding tissues causing local inflammation and tissue remodeling.

TABLE 1: Eosinophil counts based on age.

Age	*Eosinophil count* $\times 10^9$/L
Birth	0.1–1.0
Day 3	0.1–2.0
1 month	0.2–1.0
2 months to 12 years	0.1–1.0

Marked changes in the microenvironment subsequently leading to chronic organ damage may be caused by the eosinophil-derived substances. This may lead to fibrosis and/or thrombosis in some of the patients. Certain organs like heart, lung, skin, spleen, gastrointestinal tract (GIT), and central nervous system are the ones predominantly affected.

ETIOLOGY

Causes of eosinophilia can be divided into primary, secondary, and idiopathic.

- *Primary:*
  - *Clonal:* There can be neoplastic proliferation as part of an underlying myeloid malignancy. There is histologic, cytogenetic, or molecular evidence of underlying myeloid malignancy.
- *Secondary/reactive:* This is the most common cause of eosinophilia:
  - Infectious diseases like helminthiasis and fungal infections
  - Drugs including herbal remedies
  - Allergic disorders like asthma, atopic dermatitis/eczema, seasonal allergic disorders like hay fever, and rhinitis syndromes. Allergic vasculitis, allergic angiitis, and Churg–Strauss disease
  - Respiratory diseases like eosinophilic pneumonias [including allergic bronchopulmonary eosinophilia (ABPA), Loeffler's syndrome, and sarcoidosis]

- Gastrointestinal diseases like eosinophilic esophagitis, chronic pancreatitis, celiac disease, and inflammatory bowel disease
- Rheumatologic disease like systemic lupus erythematosus, rheumatoid arthritis, and dermatomyositis
- Neoplastic diseases like solid tumors, lymphomas and acute lymphocytic leukemia, and mastocytosis
- Immunologic disorders
- Endocrine

- *Idiopathic eosinophilia:* This is considered once primary and secondary causes are ruled out.

Infections: Worldwide, helminthiasis is the most common cause of eosinophilia. It can be associated with tissue nematodes, cestodes, and trematodes. All parasitic infections, including hookworm, roundworm, tapeworm, filariasis, *Trichinella*, *Strongyloides*, and visceral larva migrans, have moderate to marked eosinophilia. Parasites elicit eosinophilia when they or their products come in contact with immune effector cells in tissues which happen during migration. Hence, it is seen in infestation with worms that migrate through extraintestinal organs. Parasites that are wholly intramural like adult tapeworm or contained in a cystic structure like hydatid cyst do not cause eosinophilia unless the cyst wall ruptures and its contents leak.

Other infections like scabies, fungal diseases like disseminated coccidioidomycosis, and aspergillosis [when presenting as allergic bronchopulmonary aspergillosis (ABPA)] can also be associated with marked eosinophilia. Tropical pulmonary eosinophilia is the result of immunologic hyper-responsiveness to the filarial parasite.

Allergic diseases: In Western countries, allergic diseases are the leading cause of eosinophilia. Asthma generally is not associated with moderate or severe eosinophilia. If there is moderate to severe eosinophilia in asthma, possibility of Churg–Strauss disease or ABPA has to be considered.

Drug-related eosinophilia: It is a common cause of persistent eosinophilia in parts of the world where helminthiasis is uncommon. It can be asymptomatic or associated with some symptoms as follows:

- *Asymptomatic:* Quinine, penicillin, cephalosporins, and quinolones
- *Associated pulmonary infiltrates:* Nonsteroidal anti-inflammatory drugs, sulfa drugs, and nitrofurantoin
- *Hepatitis:* Tetracyclines and antipsychotics
- *DRESS (Drug Reaction with Eosinophilia and Systemic Symptoms) syndrome:* Sulfasalazine, hydantoin, carbamazepine, and D-penicillamine

Neoplastic diseases: Lymphoid malignancy (Hodgkin's lymphoma), B- or T-cell leukemia or lymphoma, Langerhans cell histiocytosis, solid tumors, and mastocytosis are associated with eosinophilia. It could be a paraneoplastic feature of solid tumors like adenocarcinoma of lung, cervix, and gastrointestinal tract (GIT) because of ectopic production of IL-5 and other cytokines by malignant cells.

Immunologic disorders like Omenn syndrome, hyper-IgE syndrome, graft-versus host disease

Endocrine: Eosinophilia is seen in conditions with hypoadrenalism because of loss of endogenous glucocorticosteroids as in Addison's disease, adrenal hemorrhage, hypopituitarism.

Hypereosinophilic syndrome: It is characterized by persistent eosinophilia $>1.5 \times 10^9/L$ for >6 months, evidence of end organ damage but no explanation after investigations. It has two variants—myeloproliferative variant hypereosinophilic syndrome (M-HES) and lymphocytic variant hypereosinophilic syndrome (L-HES). Myeloproliferative-HES is associated with other features of myeloproliferative diseases like increased serum vitamin B_{12} levels, hepatosplenomegaly, anemia, thrombocytopenia, and increased bone marrow cellularity. Lymphocytic-HES is associated with cutaneous manifestations, increased serum IgE levels and hypergammaglobulinemia. There is overproduction of IL-5 by deregulated T cells leading to polyclonal eosinophil expansion.

Clonal eosinophilia: There are two subcategories in World Health Organization classification of hematologic malignancies: chronic eosinophilic leukemia, not otherwise specified and myeloid/lymphoid neoplasms with eosinophilia and mutations involving platelet-derived growth factor receptor, and or fibroblast growth factor receptor. It might also be seen in other myeloid malignancies like myelodysplastic syndromes and systemic mastocytosis.

Rare syndromes with eosinophilia:

- Gleich's syndrome
- Churg–Strauss syndrome
- Eosinophilia–myalgia syndrome
- Omenn syndrome
- Hyper-IgE syndrome

Pulmonary infiltrates with eosinophilia syndrome:

- Loeffler's syndrome
- Allergic angiitis and granulomatosis

- Hypersensitivity vasculitis
- *Allergic bronchopulmonary aspergillosis:* Asthma, positive skin test to *Aspergillus* and *Aspergillus* precipitating antibodies
- In addition, drug reaction, HES, and parasitic infections may be associated with pulmonary symptoms.

APPROACH TO A PATIENT WITH EOSINOPHILIA (FLOWCHART 1)

Firstly, an attempt should be made to rule out any underlying treatable cause like parasitic infections or drug reaction. Secondly, any evidence of target organ damage should be looked for.

History:

- Travel history, particularly to tropical countries
- Occupational history
- Drug history
- Family history
- Allergy history
- Cardiorespiratory and gastrointestinal symptoms
- *Constitutional symptoms:* Fever, night sweats, weight loss, and pruritus

Physical examination of skin, liver, spleen, lungs, and soft tissues.

Laboratory investigations ***(Table 2):*** Patients with mild-to-moderate eosinophilia who are otherwise asymptomatic need not be subjected to further testing. However, those with persistent eosinophilia (at least 1.5×10^9/L) should be investigated for underlying etiology.

Flowchart 1: Evaluation of a child with eosinophilia.

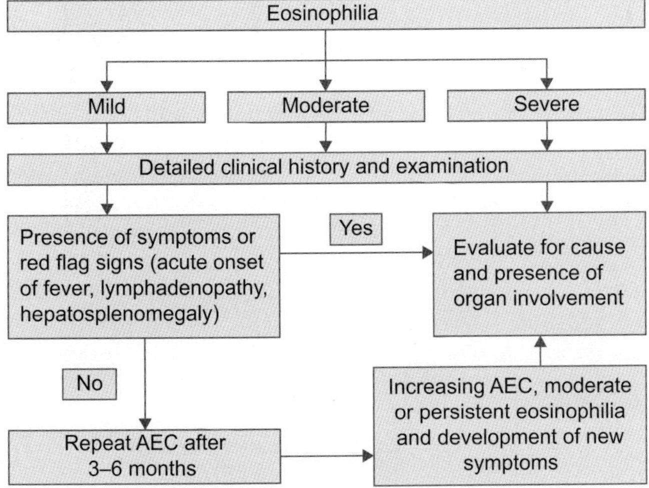

(AEC: absolute eosinophil count)

- *Investigations in all patients with eosinophilia:*
  - Complete blood count with peripheral smear
  - Liver function test (LFT) and renal function test (RFT)
  - Erythrocyte sedimentation rate (ESR) and C-reactive protein (CRP)
  - Bone profile
  - Lactate dehydrogenase (LDH)
  - Serum vitamin B12
- *Investigations to rule out secondary causes in patients with persistent eosinophilia or those with systemic symptoms or those with suspected organ damage:*
  - *Infectious cause:* Stool for ova and cysts and parasites, serological tests for parasitic infections
  - *Allergic cause:* Serum IgE and skin prick tests
  - *Gastrointestinal cause:* Upper GI endoscopy, serum amylase, anti-tissue transglutaminase for celiac disease
  - *Rheumatologic cause:* Antinuclear activity (ANA), anti-dsDNA
  - *Respiratory cause:* Imaging, bronchoscopy with bronchoalveolar lavage
- *Investigations in severe eosinophilia with no obvious underlying cause:*
  - Blood tryptase levels
  - Bone marrow morphology
  - Cytogenetic analysis

TABLE 2: Laboratory investigations in a case of eosinophilia.

Laboratory parameter	***Significance***
Peripheral smear	Parasites, circulating blasts, dysplastic cells, monocytosis
ESR/CRP	Inflammatory or reactive pathology
Vitamin B_{12} levels	Elevated in myeloid disorder
Bone marrow	To exclude hematological and nonhematological malignancies
Cytogenetic analysis	
Molecular studies	F1L1P1-PDGFRA using FISH or RT-PCR
Serum tryptase	Systemic mastocytosis and other vasculitides
ANCA	Churg–Strauss disease

(CRP: C-reactive protein; ESR: erythrocyte sedimentation rate; PDGFRA: platelet-derived growth factor receptor-alpha; FISH: fluorescence in situ hybridization; RT-PCR: reverse transcriptase polymerase chain reaction; ANCA: antineutrophil cytoplasmic antibodies)

- *Molecular studies:* F1L1P1-PDGFRA using fluorescence *in situ* hybridization (FISH) or nested reverse transcription polymerase chain reaction (RT-PCR)

- *Investigations to look for evidence of target organ damage:*
  - Chest X-ray, echocardiography, and troponin levels
  - Pulmonary function tests
  - Gastrointestinal endoscopy
  - Skin biopsy
  - X-ray paranasal sinuses
  - Neuroimaging

CLINICAL PEARLS

- Untreated eosinophilia can lead to chronic organ damage due to fibrosis and/or thrombosis and hence should be treated.
- Presence of moderate to severe eosinophilia in a child with asthma points toward the possibility of Churg–Strauss disease or allergic bronchopulmonary aspergillosis.
- Eosinophilia can also be associated with neoplastic diseases like lymphomas, B- or T-cell leukemia, Langerhans cell histiocytosis, solid tumors, and mastocytosis which need to be excluded in persistent cases.
- Evaluation should include cause of the eosinophilia as well as assessment for eosinophil associated end organ damage.
- Presence of acute onset of fever, adenopathy, organomegaly, and evidence of organ dysfunction are red flag signs which require immediate referral and evaluation irrespective of severity of eosinophilia.

KEY POINTS

- The most common cause for eosinophilia worldwide is helminthiasis whereas allergic diseases are the leading causative factor in western countries.
- An eosinophil count of $>0.4 \times 10^9$/L is considered as eosinophilia and is further classified into mild ($<1.5 \times 10^9$/L), moderate ($1.5–5 \times 10^9$/L), and severe ($>5 \times 10^9$/L) eosinophilia. A count of $>1.5 \times 10^9$/L is generally associated with organ damage.
- Hypereosinophilic syndrome (HES) is defined by persistent eosinophilia $>1.5 \times 10^9$/L for >6 months, evidence of end organ damage but no explanation after investigations. The two variants of HES are myeloproliferative variant HES (M-HES) and lymphocytic variant HES (L-HES).

SUGGESTED READING

1. Butt NM, Lambert J, Ali S, Beer PA, Cross NC, Duncombe A, et al. Guideline for the investigation and management of eosinophilia. Br J Haematol. 2017;176:553-72.
2. Costagliola G, Marco SD, Comberiati P, D'Elios S, Petashvili N, Di Cicco ME, et al. Practical approach to children presenting with eosinophila and hypereosinophilia. Curr Pediatr Rev. 2020;16(2):81-8.
3. Opper CE, Simeonsson KL, Hillenbrand K. Eosinophilia. Pediatr Rev. 2022;43(8):476-8.
4. Schwartz JT, Fulkerson PC. An Approach to the Evaluation of Persistent Hypereosinophilia in Pediatric Patients. Front Immunol. 2018;9:1944.

Pulmonology

Section Editors: *Ankit Parakh, Varinder Singh*

CHAPTER 67

Approach to a Child with Respiratory Distress

Soumya Tiwari, Parmarth Chandane

INTRODUCTION

Respiratory distress is the most common presentation in children visiting a hospital emergency. It initially, may manifest only as fast breathing (rate more than the normal upper limit for that age group; see **Table 1**), and signs of increased work of breathing in the form of nasal flaring and/or lower chest indrawing, and/or head nodding can follow. It may also be associated with stridor or wheeze suggestive of upper and lower airway obstruction, respectively. There is a need of urgent assessment of airway patency and breathing, when a child with respiratory distress is first evaluated. Stabilization of vital parameters may require proper positioning, oronasal suctioning, and intubation if the airway patency cannot be maintained and use of oxygen by hood/nasal prongs. Supportive therapy in the form of maintaining temperature or correction of hyperthermia/hypothermia; intravenous fluid boluses; correction of hypoglycemia; nebulization with bronchodilator; intercostal tube drainage of any air or fluid collection in the pleural cavity, etc. Such initial treatment coupled with a thorough history, physical examination, and relevant investigations, is followed by establishing a provisional diagnosis and instituting appropriate empirical treatment in the emergency ward itself. Uncommonly, a serious terminally sick child may show bradypnea (decreased heart rate) instead of tachypnea.

TABLE 1: The cut offs for respiratory rate marking significant lower chest disease (World Health Organization).

Age group	*Respiratory rate cut-off*
Young infant (<2 months)	>60/min
Infant (2 months–1 year)	>50/min
Children (1–5 years)	>40/min
School children (>5 years)	>30/min

DEFINITION

Any unusual pattern of breathing, causing a subjective feeling of discomfort, in a previously well child is termed as respiratory distress. It includes abnormally fast or slow breathing, shallow or labored efforts, or noisy breathing.

ETIOLOGY OF RESPIRATORY DISTRESS

Respiratory distress may not always result from a lung disease. Rapid breathing may be physiological, e.g., exercise induced, or pathological due to pulmonary or nonpulmonary causes. The respiratory rate cut offs given in **Table 1** are seen in pathological conditions and these could be seen in many different clinical situations as detailed in **Box 1**.

CLINICAL FEATURES

A child with respiratory distress may have tachypnea with increased work of breathing (suggested by use of accessory muscles), cyanosis, and lethargy or altered sensorium. Alteration in sensorium (in the form of irritability, agitation, lethargy, or coma) indicates brain hypoxia and is one of the earliest indicators of impending respiratory failure. While fast breathing is commonly associated with respiratory diseases, it may also occur with fever, crying, or metabolic acidosis. However, normal or decreased respiratory rate may be more ominous if it is associated with severe retractions (paradoxical breathing), cyanosis, grunting, or altered sensorium. Central cyanosis is a late sign but may not be detected in presence of severe pallor (low hemoglobin) and dark skin color.

Stridor is a harsh inspiratory sound that indicates upper airway obstruction. Grunt is a loud noise produced by a forceful expiration against a partially closed glottis. Grunt is a sign of alveolar or interstitial lung involvement. Wheeze (a musical sound) are suggestive of lower airway obstruction.

BOX 1: Causes of respiratory distress in children.

Upper respiratory tract involvement:
- Croup, acute epiglottitis, and Ludwig's angina
- Retropharyngeal abscess
- Foreign body aspiration
- Diphtheria
- Laryngospasm

Lower respiratory tract involvement:
- Pneumonia
- Bronchiolitis
- Asthma
- Pleural effusion or empyema and hemothorax
- Pneumothorax
- Atelectasis
- Hypersensitivity pneumonitis

Nonpulmonary causes:
- Congestive heart failure due to heart disease or severe anemia
- CNS infections, cerebral edema, tumor (raised ICT, compression of the brainstem), spinal cord injury, and Guillain–Barré syndrome
- *Metabolic acidosis:*
  - Renal failure
  - Renal tubular acidosis
  - Lactic acidosis
  - Poisonings
  - Diabetic ketoacidosis
  - Psychogenic hyperventilation, anxiety, and panic attacks

(CNS: central nervous system; ICT: intracranial tension)

A complete history including the onset, duration, progression of dyspnea, the aggravating and relieving factors as well as the associated symptoms, such as fever, cough, sore throat, chest pain, choking episodes, and accidental ingestion of poisons can help in short listing the likely cause **(Table 2)**.

CLINICAL PEARLS

Symptoms of impending respiratory failure:
- Cyanosis
- Silent chest
- Poor respiratory efforts
- Fatigue/exhaustion
- Agitation or reduced level of consciousness

Preterminal signs:
- Bradycardia, desaturation, and altered sensorium

INVESTIGATIONS

Laboratory investigations help to confirm the diagnosis but the immediate management of a patient should not be delayed pending the reports of the investigations. Use of noninvasive devices, such as pulse oximeter and end-tidal carbon dioxide detector lessen the need for repeated invasive tests for monitoring of the child. **Table 3** shows the relevant investigations to ascertain the cause of respiratory distress in a child.

TABLE 2: Clinical feature based diagnostic clues.

Clinical features	***Diagnosis***
Fever, cough, and rapid breathing	Lower respiratory tract infections, such as pneumonia, bronchiolitis and virus and associated wheeze
Exercise-induced dyspnea	Asthma, congestive heart failure, and severe anemia
Nocturnal cough, orthopnea, and dyspnea	Congestive heart failure
Fever, sore throat, and stridor	Acute epiglottitis
Severe chest pain with rapid, shallow breathing, and decreased air entry	Pneumonia, pneumothorax, and pulmonary embolism
Persistent wheezing, recurrent vomiting, and failure to thrive	Gastroesophageal reflux disease
Acute respiratory distress after sudden choking, hyperinflated chest	Foreign body inhalation
Fever with altered sensorium, headache, vomiting, convulsions, and fast breathing	Encephalitis involving brain stem
Chest-wall retractions, paraplegia	Acute flaccid paralysis
Acute respiratory distress with vomiting, altered sensorium	Poisoning
Fast breathing usually without other signs of respiratory distress, may be associated with oliguria or anuria	Acute kidney injury/chronic kidney disease with metabolic acidosis
Fast breathing, altered sensorium, polyuria, and dehydration	Diabetic ketoacidosis

TABLE 3: Laboratory investigations.

Investigation	*Suggested diagnosis*
Complete blood count with peripheral smear	Leukocytosis/leukopenia, toxic granules, shift to left, anemia/polycythemia, eosinophilia-pneumonia, sepsis, and TPE
CRP and ESR	Raised-pneumonia, bronchiolitis
Blood culture	Sepsis with pneumonia
Kidney function tests	Acute/chronic kidney disease
Arterial blood gas	Hypoxemia, hypercarbia, acidosis (metabolic/respiratory)—pneumothorax, and AKI
Chest X-ray and X-ray soft tissue neck	Pneumonia, pneumothorax, effusion, foreign body, acute epiglottitis, and CHF
Bronchoscopy	Foreign body
Echocardiography	Cardiac disease
24-hour pH monitoring	GERD
Pleural tap	Pleural effusion (bacterial and tubercular)

(AKI: acute kidney injury; CHF: congestive heart failure; CRP: C-reactive protein; ESR: erythrocyte sedimentation rate; GERD: gastroesophageal reflux disease; TPE: therapeutic plasma exchange)

Flowchart 1: Management of a child with respiratory distress.

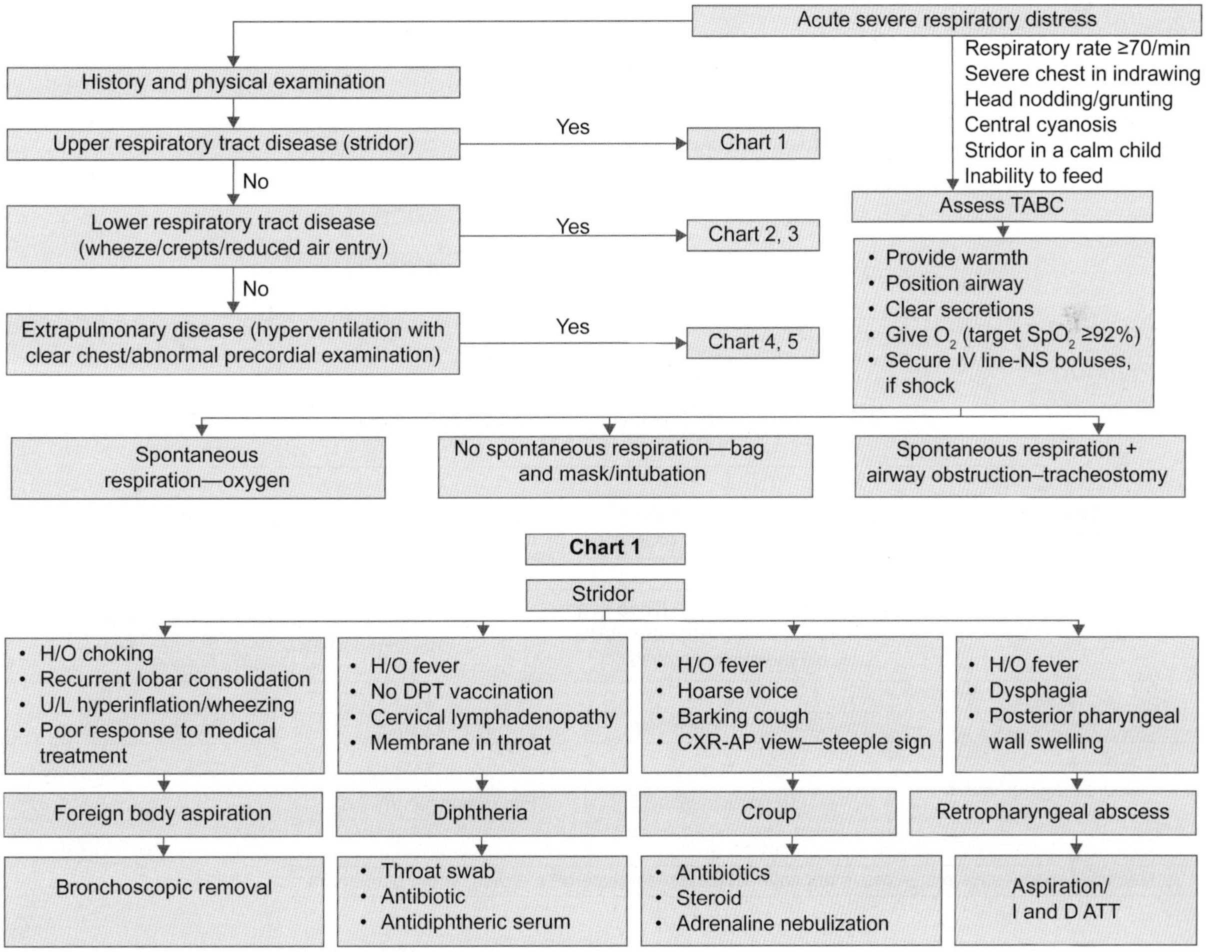

Acute severe respiratory distress

Respiratory rate ≥70/min
Severe chest in indrawing
Head nodding/grunting
Central cyanosis
Stridor in a calm child
Inability to feed

History and physical examination

Upper respiratory tract disease (stridor) → Yes → Chart 1

No

Lower respiratory tract disease (wheeze/crepts/reduced air entry) → Yes → Chart 2, 3

No

Extrapulmonary disease (hyperventilation with clear chest/abnormal precordial examination) → Yes → Chart 4, 5

Assess TABC

- Provide warmth
- Position airway
- Clear secretions
- Give O_2 (target SpO_2 ≥92%)
- Secure IV line-NS boluses, if shock

Spontaneous respiration—oxygen

No spontaneous respiration—bag and mask/intubation

Spontaneous respiration + airway obstruction–tracheostomy

Chart 1

Stridor

- H/O choking
- Recurrent lobar consolidation
- U/L hyperinflation/wheezing
- Poor response to medical treatment

Foreign body aspiration

Bronchoscopic removal

- H/O fever
- No DPT vaccination
- Cervical lymphadenopathy
- Membrane in throat

Diphtheria

- Throat swab
- Antibiotic
- Antidiphtheric serum

- H/O fever
- Hoarse voice
- Barking cough
- CXR-AP view—steeple sign

Croup

- Antibiotics
- Steroid
- Adrenaline nebulization

- H/O fever
- Dysphagia
- Posterior pharyngeal wall swelling

Retropharyngeal abscess

Aspiration/
I and D ATT

Contd...

Contd...

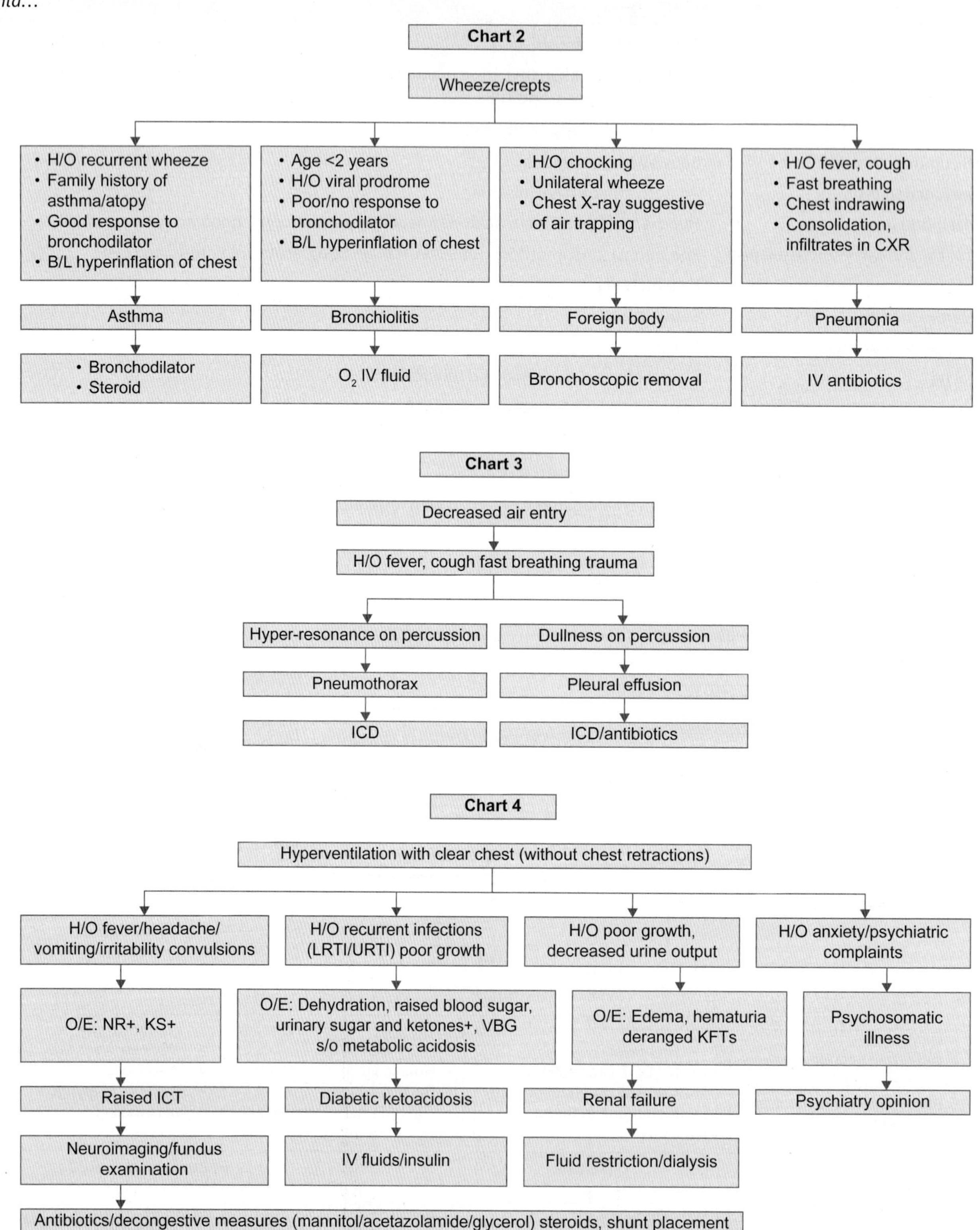
Chart 2
Wheeze/crepts
• H/O recurrent wheeze
• Family history of asthma/atopy
• Good response to bronchodilator
• B/L hyperinflation of chest
Asthma
• Bronchodilator
• Steroid
• Age <2 years
• H/O viral prodrome
• Poor/no response to bronchodilator
• B/L hyperinflation of chest
Bronchiolitis
O_2 IV fluid
• H/O chocking
• Unilateral wheeze
• Chest X-ray suggestive of air trapping
Foreign body
Bronchoscopic removal
• H/O fever, cough
• Fast breathing
• Chest indrawing
• Consolidation, infiltrates in CXR
Pneumonia
IV antibiotics
Chart 3
Decreased air entry
H/O fever, cough fast breathing trauma
Hyper-resonance on percussion
Pneumothorax
ICD
Dullness on percussion
Pleural effusion
ICD/antibiotics
Chart 4
Hyperventilation with clear chest (without chest retractions)
H/O fever/headache/ vomiting/irritability convulsions
O/E: NR+, KS+
Raised ICT
Neuroimaging/fundus examination
Antibiotics/decongestive measures (mannitol/acetazolamide/glycerol) steroids, shunt placement
H/O recurrent infections (LRTI/URTI) poor growth
O/E: Dehydration, raised blood sugar, urinary sugar and ketones+, VBG s/o metabolic acidosis
Diabetic ketoacidosis
IV fluids/insulin
H/O poor growth, decreased urine output
O/E: Edema, hematuria deranged KFTs
Renal failure
Fluid restriction/dialysis
H/O anxiety/psychiatric complaints
Psychosomatic illness
Psychiatry opinion

Contd...

Contd...

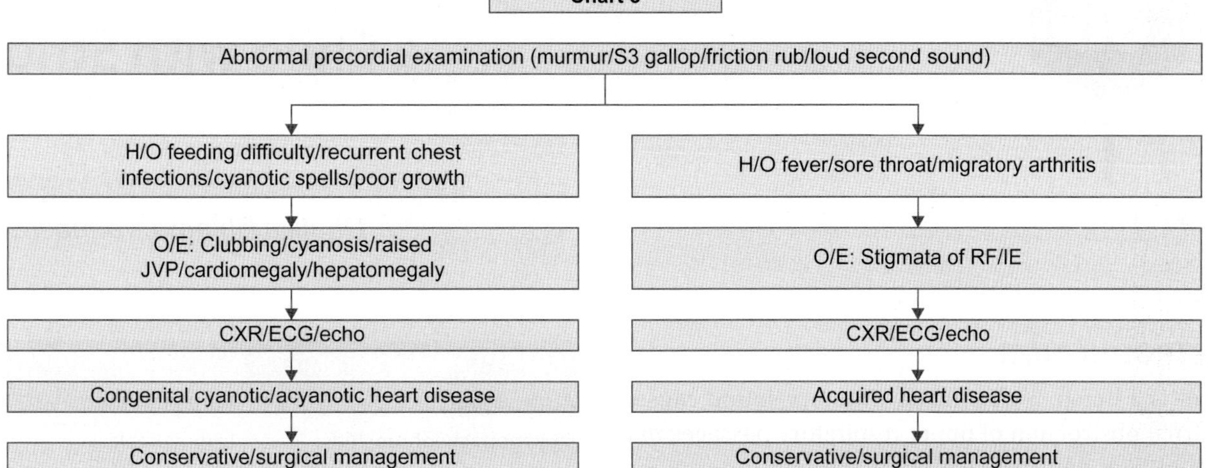

(AP: anteroposterior; ATT: antitubercular treatment; B/L: bilateral; CXR: chest X-ray; DPT: diphtheria-pertussis-tetanus; ECG: electrocardiogram; echo: echocardiogram; ICD: implantable cardioverter-defibrillator; ICT: intracranial tension; I&D: incision and drainage; IE: infective endocarditis; IV: intravenous; JVP: jugular venous pressure; KFT: kidney function test; LRTI: lower respiratory tract infection; NS: normal saline; RF: rheumatic fever; TABC: temperament assessment battery for children; URTI: upper respiratory tract infection; VBG: venous blood gas; U/L: unilateral)

TREATMENT

The management of a child with respiratory distress includes supportive treatment in the form of stabilization of vital parameters, i.e., airway, breathing, and circulation followed by definitive treatment by instituting appropriate respiratory support, antibiotics, chest tube drainage, decongestive measures, etc. The algorithmic approach to management of such a child is shown in **Flowchart 1**.

CONCLUSION

It is essential to promptly triage children with impending respiratory failure and quickly institute supportive management, simultaneously searching for the etiology and planning a definitive treatment. The above mentioned approach will improve the outcome of children, especially the under-five ones, in whom respiratory infections lead to the highest number of mortalities.

KEY POINTS

- Respiratory distress may not always be due to respiratory diseases, nonpulmonary causes should be carefully evaluated.
- Stabilization of vital signs is the first step in the management of a child with respiratory distress.
- Signs of impending respiratory failure should prompt immediate respiratory support.
- Clinical features guide further investigations and definitive treatment.

SUGGESTED READING

1. Fallot A. Respiratory distress. Pediatr Ann. 2005;34(11):885-91.
2. Kilham H, Gillis J, Benjamin B. Severe upper airway obstruction. Pediatr Clin North Am. 1987;34(1):1-14.
3. Mathew JL, Singhi SC. Approach to a child with breathing difficulty. Indian J Pediatr. 2011;78(9):1118-26.
4. Singh V, Tiwari S. Respiratory problems. In: Gupta P (Ed). Textbook of Pediatrics. India: CBS publishers; 2013. pp. 335-68.

Assessing and Managing a Child with Stridor

Dhulika Dhingra, Varinder Singh

INTRODUCTION

Stridor is a harsh, high-pitched vibratory sound caused by partial obstruction of upper respiratory passages that result in turbulent passage of air through the airways. It can be often heard without stethoscope. Stridor is usually heard during inspiration or may be biphasic but rarely it may appear expiratory when the child breathes through semi-approximated vocal cords causing resistance to exhalation and biphasic stridor may result due to severe obstruction of subglottic, glottic, or the extrathoracic airway.

Loudness of the sound is poor marker of the degree of obstruction, while its presence even when the patient is quiet or biphasic stridor is associated with significant compromise. Stridor must be differentiated from stertor, which is produced by an obstruction in the nose or nasopharynx and is a characteristic low-pitched sound.

Stridor is the sound caused by abnormal obstruction to air passage in upper airways during breathing. The cause of stridor can usually be located in extrathoracic airway (larynx) or may be intrathoracic (commonly congenital disorders involving tracheal narrowing). Stridor may be acute (caused by inflammation/infection or foreign body inhalation) or chronic. It may be congenital or acquired. Stridor is a sign and not a diagnosis and the cause for which must be ascertained. This chapter aims to educate the pediatrician faced with an infant or child with stridor to determine the severity or respiratory compromise and the need for immediate intervention. A comprehensive history and clinical examination can indicate if a significant lesion is suspected and can help to plan further investigations and management strategies of the underlying lesion for subsequent management of the child and follow-up.

PATHOPHYSIOLOGY

Gases produce pressure equally in all directions; however, when a gas moves in a linear direction, it produces pressure in the forward vector and decreases the lateral pressure. When air passes through a narrowed flexible airway in a child, the lateral pressure that holds the airway open can drop precipitously (venturi principle) and cause the tube to collapse. A similar process obstructs airflow and produces stridor in cases with upper-airway obstruction.

The most common causes of stridor are summarized in **Table 1**.

TABLE 1: Causes of stridor.

Acute stridor	*Chronic stridor*
Laryngotracheobronchitis	Laryngomalacia
Epiglottitis	Congenital or acquired subglottic stenosis
Diphtheria	Laryngeal webs
Bacterial tracheitis	Congenital laryngeal cysts
Retropharyngeal abscess	Tracheal stenosis or complete tracheal rings
Allergic reactions	Tracheomalacia
Vocal cord palsy	Subglottic hemangioma
Acquired subglottic stenosis (following prolonged intubation)	Posterior laryngeal cleft

HISTORY AND CLINICAL EXAMINATION

A good history and clinical examination are the key to localization of the cause of stridor. A child presenting with stridor should be inquired about the onset of stridor (onset in first few weeks of life usually indicate a congenital cause), postural variation, feeding difficulties, any change in voice quality, pattern of fever if any, history of foreign body inhalation in form of sudden choking, any neurological symptoms, history of trauma to head and neck (neurogenic stridor), immunization history, and history of similar illness in the neighborhood (diphtheria). It is, however, emphasized that parents may not have noticed the choking episode hence, a high index of suspicion is warranted if stridor has appeared all of a sudden without any other attendant symptoms, such as fever and coryza. Character of stridor may also be an important clue. A constant stridor indicates a fixed lesion pathology while intermittent symptoms may be indicative of conditions such as laryngomalacia **(Table 1)**.

Detailed clinical examinations may also help in identifying the cause. Onset of stridor, presence/absence of fever, voice change, and ability of patient to handle secretions will aid in determining the site. Stridor present since birth most often indicates a congenital pathology such as laryngeal webs or bilateral vocal cord paralysis, whereas a more gradual onset over days/weeks points toward laryngomalacia **(Table 2)**. Positional change in severity of stridor may also indicate laryngomalacia. A child with choanal atresia may have increased distress as he closes his mouth and with crying his distress may be relieved. Voice quality should also be observed during the examination; however, it must be remembered that a normal voice quality does not rule out laryngeal or pharyngeal pathology though presence of changes in voice quality does. **Table 3** summarizes important voice changes associated with different pathologies.

TABLE 2: Causes of stridor on the basis of age of onset of stridor.

Age	*Common causes*
Neonates	Congenital anomalies like laryngomalacia, tracheomalacia, and subglottic stenosis
Infants and toddlers	• Croup—most common • Epiglottitis—less common • Foreign body inhalation
School-aged children	• Vocal cord dysfunction • Peritonsillar abscess
All ages	Anaphylaxis and bacterial tracheitis

TABLE 3: Voice changes with localization of site of stridor.

Change in voice	*Localization of lesion*	*Differential diagnosis*
Hoarseness of voice	Vocal cords	• Laryngeal webs • Abductor palsy • Croup • Retropharyngeal abscess • Diphtheria
Muffled voice	Supraglottic involvement	• Tonsillitis • Parapharyngeal abscess • Peritonsillar abscess
Weak voice	Subglottic obstruction	Subglottic stenosis (congenital or acquired)

Clinical examination must also include a detailed neurological examination and inspection of the spine to rule out neurogenic stridor. Neck should be examined for any lymph node masses or for any evidence of trauma. Note should also be made of craniofacial anomalies including macroglossia, retrognathia, and maxillary hypoplasia. Throat examination may reveal the presence of a membrane, tonsillar enlargement, or presence of exudates. Throat examination should not be attempted for a child who is drooling, has high-grade fever, and is agitated. Skin examination may also give important clues. Presence of urticarial rashes may point to allergic etiology while presence of skin hemangiomas may be associated with similar lesions in the airway.

Apart from ascertaining the diagnosis, clinical examination should also aim at assessing the severity of respiratory distress. Retractions/use of accessory muscles are better clinical signs than degree of stridor when assessing degree of respiratory distress. Cyanosis is a late finding and is a sign of impending respiratory failure.

CLINICAL PEARL

- Onset of stridor, presence/absence of fever, voice change, and ability of patient to handle secretions will aid in determining the diagnosis.

INVESTIGATIONS

Establishing a patent airway is of utmost importance. No laboratory investigation or imaging should take precedence over establishing airway. If the child has an acute stridor in the absence of severe respiratory distress, one may go for a chest X-ray or soft-tissue lateral neck imaging depending upon the history. A clinician capable of establishing airways should accompany such a patient to the X-ray department.

If the patient has chronic stridor, has no or minimal respiratory distress, he/she may be taken up for flexible laryngoscopy or bronchoscopy to look for underlying abnormalities. The procedure may also rule out secondary airway lesions.

CLINICAL PEARL

- Establishing a patent airway must take precedence over imaging and bronchoscopy in evaluating patients with stridor.

Chest X-ray of soft tissue of neck in a child with history of epiglottis may reveal a swollen epiglottis (thumbprint sign), while in a child with laryngotracheobronchitis, it shows subglottic narrowing (Steeple sign).

MANAGEMENT

As stridor is not a diagnosis by itself, the management of stridor shall be determined by the underlying pathology, hence we discuss these as per the etiology of stridor.

Laryngotracheobronchitis/Croup

Croup is a heterogeneous group of acute and infectious processes in children (between 6 months and 6 years of age) that manifest most commonly with characteristic inspiratory stridor, barking cough, hoarse voice, and varying degrees of respiratory distress. Parainfluenza viruses type 1 (50%), 2, and 3; respiratory syncytial virus, influenza A and B, and rhino virus account for the majority of cases. The illness usually starts with a common cold, such as illness with symptoms of rhinorrhea, cough, sore throat, and fever with symptoms being worse in evening and night especially in the mild cases. Features of upper airway obstruction, i.e., inspiratory stridor, hoarseness, and barking cough develop over next 2–3 days.

Treatment is dependent upon the severity of croup and includes humidified oxygen, oral or parenteral steroids, and inhaled adrenaline.

- *Humidified air:* It has been widely advocated in the past without any scientific validation, but it still can be used as home remedy in children with mild croup.
- *Oxygen therapy:* Oxygen is the most important treatment for a child with a moderate or severe croup who has considerable upper-airway obstruction or SpO_2 <92%.
- *Oral or inhaled steroids:* Steroids can improve the symptoms of croup within 6–8 hours after starting the treatment. They also result in shorter duration of hospital stay, lesser need of endotracheal intubation, and decreased need for adrenaline nebulization. Oral corticosteroids are preferred as they are inexpensive, easy to administer, readily available, as effective, and produce measurable improvements within hours. The recommended dose of dexamethasone is 0.15–0.3 mg/kg body weight (oral or IM) and prednisolone (suspension or tablets) is 1 mg/kg body weight. Nebulized budesonide (2 mg) has been shown to be equally efficacious. This can be repeated 12 hourly for up to 48 hours. The choice of route is based upon the cost and the child's condition.
- *Nebulized adrenaline:* It is indicated in children with moderate-to-severe croup with stridor at rest and marked intercostal or subcostal indrawing. One needs to administer 1:1,000 dilution solution of nebulized adrenaline 0.5 mL/kg of body weight (maximum of 5 mL). It has a rapid onset of action on bronchial and tracheal epithelial vascular permeability, thereby decreasing airway edema, which, in turn, increases the airway radius and improves airflow, with improvement in croup severity score within 30 minutes. However, it has a temporary action on the airway obstruction and only gives time for the underlying basic pathology to resolve and may delay or decrease the need for intubation/tracheostomy. If the severity recurs, the dose can be repeated after 2–4 hours.
- *Antimicrobials:* These have no role in the treatment of viral croup, even to prevent secondary bacterial infection.
- *Airway management:* In a small subset of patients, a severely obstructed airway leading to signs of impending respiratory failure will need either endotracheal intubation or tracheostomy. Intubation with a size smaller than the most appropriate size based on the age of the child is preferred as there is significant edema of the airway. Tracheostomy can often be avoided if an experienced pediatrician/anesthetist is available for rapid-sequence intubation **(Flowchart 1)**.
- *Discharge:* Child can be sent home when there is no stridor at rest. Parents need to be educated for monitoring worsening of symptoms.

Epiglottitis

Epiglottitis is a medical emergency occurring most commonly in children aged 2–7 years, due to fulminant inflammation of the supraglottic structures—epiglottis, arytenoids, aryepiglottic folds, and uvula, due to infection by *Haemophilus influenzae* type B. With the introduction of Hib vaccination in the National immunization Schedule, other organisms are now being implicated including groups A, B, C, and G β-hemolytic *Streptococcus, H. parainfluenzae, Staphylococcus aureus, Moraxella catarrhalis*, and *Streptococcus pneumoniae*. It is not often reported from India. Clinically, the child appears toxic. The disease is characterized by an abrupt onset of high-grade fever, sore throat, stridor, dysphagia, respiratory distress, and drooling of saliva. Children tend to sit in a

Flowchart 1: An approach to management of a child with laryngotracheobronchitis (LTB).

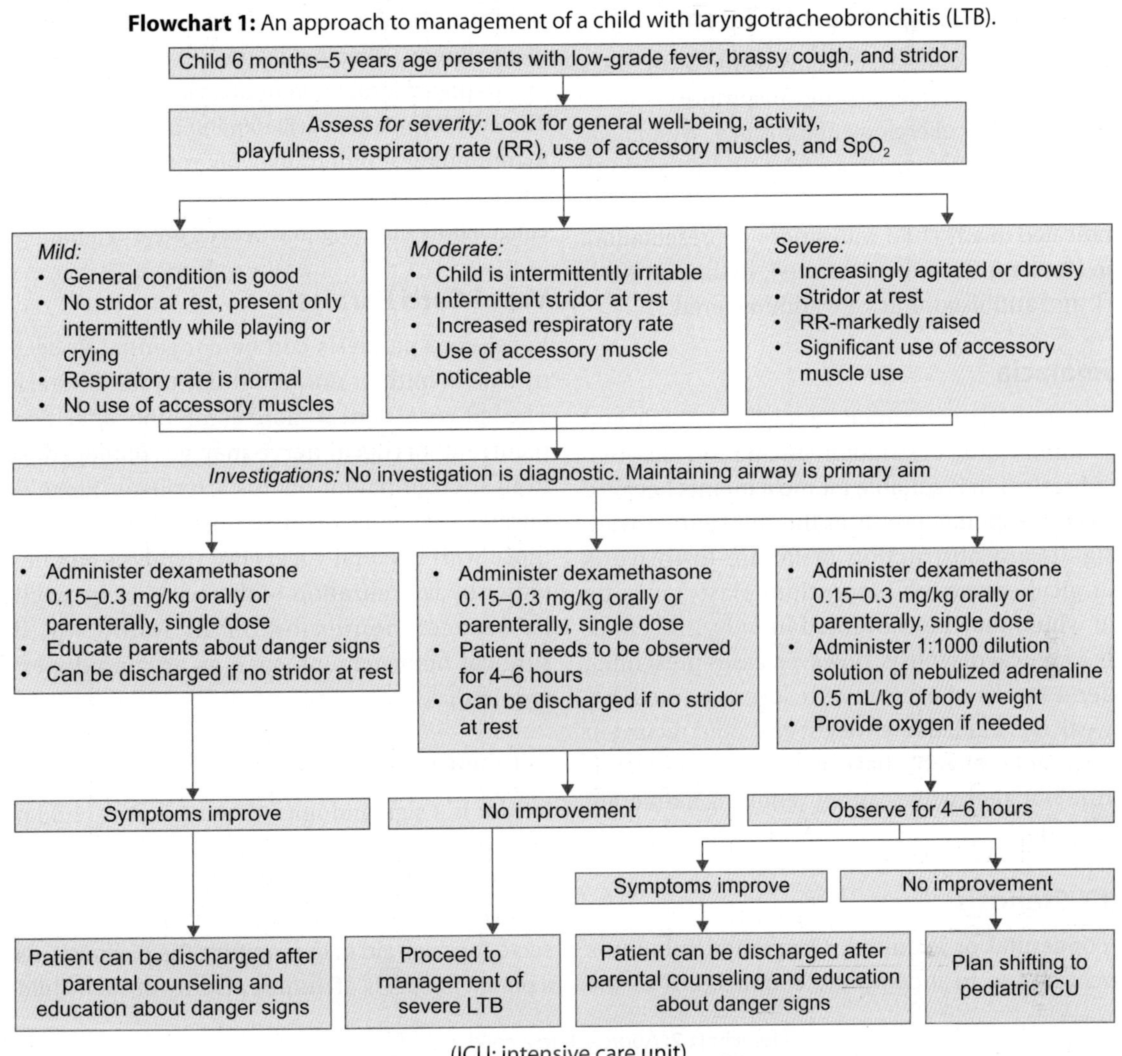

(ICU: intensive care unit)

tripod fashion. Establishing an airway by nasotracheal intubation or less often, by tracheostomy is indicated. In general, children with acute epiglottitis are intubated for 2–3 days, because the response to antibiotics is usually rapid.

Diphtheria

Diphtheria is commonly seen in partially or completely unimmunized children. Throat examination reveals a thick pharyngeal membrane spreading to the adjacent larynx. This results in airway obstruction. It is important not to agitate the child as this may precipitate aspiration or airway obstruction. Child may be administered oxygen. Emergency intubation is to be avoided and early tracheostomy to establish a patent airway should be done. Diphtheria antitoxin [80,000–120,000 IU, intravenous (IV)] should be administered and child should be treated with crystalline penicillin (40,000 U/kg/dose 6 hourly for 14 days).

Retropharyngeal Abscess

Retropharyngeal abscess is a complication of bacterial pharyngitis observed in children younger than 6 years. The child presents with abrupt onset of high fever, difficulty in swallowing, refusal to feed, sore throat, hyperextension of the neck, stridor, and respiratory distress. Most often they are polymicrobial; usual pathogens include group A Streptococci, oropharyngeal anaerobic bacteria, and *Staphylococcus aureus*. Treatment options include IV antibiotics, such as coamoxyclavulanic acid with or without surgical drainage. Endotracheal intubation is indicated in any child with stridor at presentation.

Allergic Reactions/Angioneurotic Edema

Allergic reaction (i.e., anaphylaxis) occurs within 30 minutes of adverse exposure. Hoarseness and inspiratory stridor maybe accompanied by allergic symptoms (e.g., dysphagia, nasal congestion, itching eyes, sneezing, and wheezing). Oxygen should be administered and endotracheal intubation is indicated in any child with stridor at presentation. Adrenaline (0.01 mL/kg subcutaneous), hydrocortisone (10 mg/kg), and antihistaminics are administered.

Laryngomalacia

It is the most common congenital laryngeal anomaly and the most common cause of stridor in infants and children. Expectant observation is suitable for most infants because symptoms resolve spontaneously as the child and airways grow. If significant obstruction or failure-to-thrive is present, surgical correction (supraglottoplasty) may be considered which may be warranted in only 10% cases. It is usually a clinical diagnosis, however, cases presenting early (under 4 weeks of age) or with severe retractions, cyanosis, weak cry, inadequate weight gain, and recurrent aspirations should preferably have an early airway examination to rule-out alternative causes, requiring a different treatment approach.

Subglottic Stenosis

It can be congenital or acquired. Congenital subglottic stenosis occurs due to incomplete canalization of the subglottis and cricoid rings leading to narrowing of the subglottic lumen. Acquired stenosis is most commonly caused by prolonged intubation or due to a neglected foreign body. The symptomatology will depend on the degree of stenosis. Symptomatic children may be tracheotomized. Definitive surgical management includes endoscopic methods, laser coagulation, or laryngotracheal reconstruction.

Vocal Cord Paralysis

Vocal cord paralysis can be congenital or secondary to trauma at birth or during cardiac or intrathoracic surgery. The left vocal cord is more commonly affected as the left recurrent laryngeal nerve may get damaged, secondary to ligation of patent ductus arteriosus. Since vocal cord paralysis usually resolves in 6–18 months in infants, those with bilateral vocal cord paralysis can be managed either by lateralization of the cords or by tracheostomy. In case of nonresolution in follow-up, definitive surgical management, such as arytenoidopexy may be required.

CONCLUSION

Stridor is a sign and not a diagnosis. Any child presenting with stridor should be evaluated to determine the cause **(Flowchart 2)**. The onset of stridor, presence/absence of fever, voice change, and ability of patient to handle secretions will aid in determining the diagnosis. Establishing a patent airway is of utmost priority in such children.

Flowchart 2: Approach to a child with stridor.

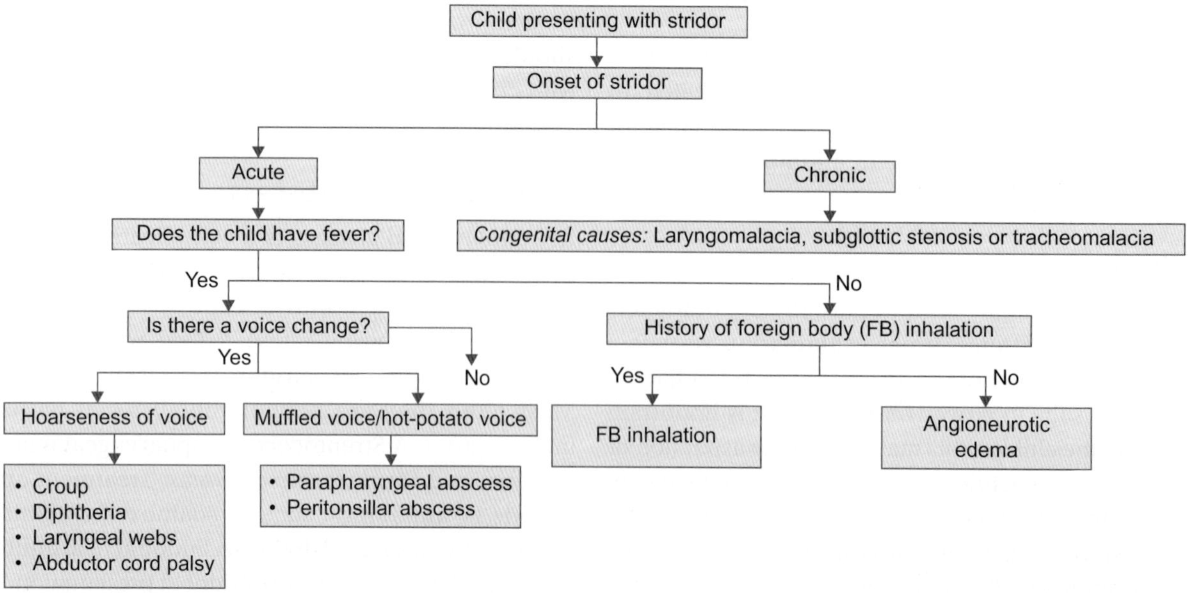

Child presenting with stridor
Onset of stridor
Acute
Chronic
Does the child have fever?
Congenital causes: Laryngomalacia, subglottic stenosis or tracheomalacia
Yes
No
Is there a voice change?
History of foreign body (FB) inhalation
Yes
No
Yes
No
Hoarseness of voice
Muffled voice/hot-potato voice
FB inhalation
Angioneurotic edema
- Croup
- Diphtheria
- Laryngeal webs
- Abductor cord palsy

- Parapharyngeal abscess
- Peritonsillar abscess

KEY POINTS

- Stridor is a harsh, high-pitched vibratory sound caused by partial obstruction of respiratory passages that result in turbulent passage of air through the airways.
- Stridor is a sign and not diagnosis. Hence, every effort should be made to identify the cause of this sign.
- Maintenance of airway should take precedence over making a diagnosis.
- A detailed history and clinical examination will help in determining the cause at the earliest.
- Neurogenic stridor is an important entity which is often ignored. Hence, a detailed neurological examination should not be ignored while examining a patient with stridor.

SUGGESTED READING

1. Bluher AE, Darrow DH. Stridor in the Newborn. Pediatr Clin North Am. 2019;66:475-88.
2. Boudewyns A, Claes J, Vande Heyning P. Clinical practice: an approach to stridor in infants and children. Eur J Pediatr. 2010;169:135-41.
3. D'Agostino J. Pediatric airway nightmares. Emerg Med Clin North Am. 2010;28:119-26.
4. Leung AK, Cho H. Diagnosis of stridor in children. Am Fam Physician. 1999;60:2289-96.
5. Rudman DT, Elmaraghy CA, Shiels WE, Wiet GJ. The role of airway fluoroscopy in the evaluation of stridor in children. Arch Otolaryngol Head Neck Surg. 2003;129(3):305-9.
6. Skirko J. Childhood Respiratory Conditions: Stridor. FP Essent. 2022;513:25-31.
7. Sly PD, Collins RA. Physiological basis of respiratory signs and symptoms. Paediatr Respir Rev. 2006;7:84-8.
8. Tibballs J, Watson T. Symptoms and signs differentiating croup and epiglottitis. J Paediatr Child Health. 2011;47:77-82.

CHAPTER 69

Recurrent Wheezing in Infants and Preschool Children

Ankit Parakh, Varinder Singh

INTRODUCTION

Recurrent wheezing in children less than five years of age is a common childhood respiratory problem and possibly the most common indication for referral to pediatric respiratory physicians. Asthma in school-age child is due to cellular airway inflammation and inhaled corticosteroids (ICS) are pivotal to management in school-age children with asthma. However, much less is known about pathophysiology of pre-school wheeze and its management has been extrapolated from studies on older children. The present chapter deals with the phenotypes, causes, investigations, and management under-five childhood wheezing with a focus on practical aspects.

PHENOTYPES OF PRESCHOOL WHEEZE

The conventional teaching was to classify children into wheeze associated lower respiratory tract infection and early onset asthma. This distinction was based on whether there were afebrile episodes, personal/family history of atopy and response to bronchodilators. Although this distinction could be useful in clinical practice; a significant overlap between phenotypes made it less useful. These terms, however, are still commonly used in clinical practice.

The largest epidemiological data comes from the work of Fernado Martinez and colleagues from the Tucson children's cohort with a follow up into adulthood. Children were classified as transient early wheezers, late onset wheezers and persistent wheezers. Although this has been extremely important in understanding of childhood wheezing, the classification system is retrospectively based on the follow-up of the child. What a clinician needs and the parents want is to know whether the index case shall develop asthma early in disease. They need a prognostication as soon as possible and not a retrospective epidemiological tool. An Asthma Predictive Index (API) has been suggested based on the association between certain risk factors with certain types of early child wheezing. The API has a moderate positive predictive value and a very high negative predictive value. Hence, an early childhood wheezer with a negative API has very low chance of developing asthma later in life.

European Respiratory Society task force recommended classifying these children in a more pragmatic clinically relevant syndrome based on their temporal pattern, named as episodic viral wheeze (EVW) and multiple-trigger wheeze (MTW) **(Table 1)**. The task force agreed not to use term asthma to describe preschool wheezing illness since

TABLE 1: New classification of phenotypes of wheezing by the European Respiratory Society.

	Episodic viral wheeze	*Multiple-trigger wheeze*
Definition	Wheezing during discrete time periods, often in association with clinical evidence of a viral cold	Wheezing that shows discrete exacerbations but also symptoms between episodes
Triggers	Viral infections	Viral infections, tobacco smoke, allergen exposure, mist-exposure, crying, exercise
Possible underlying factors	Pre-existent impaired lung function, tobacco smoke exposure, prematurity, atopy	Eosinophilic inflammation?
Continues treatment with ICS	Little or no benefit	Significant fewer days with symptoms
Treatment with montelukast	Moderate benefit	Moderate reduction in exacerbations
Long-term outcome	Declines over time (<6 years), can continue as episodic viral wheeze into school age, can change in multiple-trigger wheeze	Can continue as asthma into adulthood

(ICS: inhaled corticosteroid)

there was insufficient evidence showing that pathophysiology of preschool wheezing is similar to childhood asthma. Inflammation has been poorly studied in preschool children and might be absent in very young children who wheeze. However, easy as it seems, yet these divisions do not remain as distinct compartmental entities and there is a shift of phenotypes in many cases. The temporal pattern of wheeze during preschool years (EVW or MTW) is a relatively poor predictor of long-term outcome (transient versus persistent wheeze). Frequency and severity of wheezing episodes are stronger predictors of long-term outcome and should be taken into consideration when deciding treatment. As a result of which GINA guidelines 2015 suggests a probability-based approach to assess which under-five children with viral induced wheezing are more likely to have asthma and hence are more likely to respond to controller therapy.

Causes

The forgoing discussion of the under-five wheezers is not for an atypical wheezer. Unlike a typical wheezer, the atypical wheezer is always marking an underlying disorder. A detailed description of various form of atypical wheezing is out of scope of the present chapter but the common differential diagnosis, clinical pointers, and investigations are summarized in **Table 2**.

CLINICAL PEARLS

- Preschool wheeze is a very common disorder and usually does not need to be investigated.
- Clinicians should try and clinically differentiate these typical wheezers from children having atypical wheezing.
- Red flag signs need to be identified.
- Children with atypical wheezing would need a pediatric pulmonology referral and will have to be investigated further.
- Further investigation can be decided on a case-to-case basis and might need (one or multiple) sweat chloride, studies for gastroesophageal reflux disease, flexible bronchoscopy, immune studies and computed tomography chest.

HISTORY AND EXAMINATION

A detailed history should be obtained including the age of onset of the first episode, frequency of episodes, severity of episodes [requiring out-patient department, and emergency visits, admissions, and intensive care unit (ICU) admissions], association with viral upper respiratory infection (URI), and nature of drugs used including response should be sought. Seasonal variation and severity

TABLE 2: Causes of atypical wheezing in preschool children.

Differential diagnosis	*Clinical pointers*	*Investigations*
Infections		
Protracted bacterial bronchitis (PBB)	Wet cough for >4 weeks, no wheezing, complete response to co-amoxiclav for 14 days	Clinical features usually suffice, cough swabs or BAL might be considered
Chronic suppurative lung disease	Recurrent episodes for wet cough, wet cough lasting for >6 months, clubbing	Usually clinical diagnosis, HRCT chest normal
Bronchiectasis	Recurrent episodes for wet cough with or without wheezing, wet cough lasting for >6 months	HRCT changes of bronchial wall thickening and dilatation
Tuberculosis	Prolonged fever, weight loss, anorexia, contact with TB case	Mantoux, gastric aspirates, chest X-ay
Chronic rhino-sinusitis	Chronic cough with upper airway signs (postnasal drip, chronic pharyngeal congestion) with no wheezing	Sinus X-ray, CT useful but required only in resistant cases for surgical intervention
Adenoid hypertrophy	Chronic mouth breathing, adenoid facies	X-ray lateral soft-tissue neck
Bronchiolitis obliterans	Usually post infectious are viral bronchiolitis, persistent wheezing lasting for >60 days	Pulmonary functions tests suggestive of non-reversible severe obstruction, HRCT pattern of mosaic perfusion, lung biopsy in atypical cases
Congenital problems		
Tracheobronchomalacia	Onset of symptoms since birth, usually symptoms persists during interval periods, monophonic wheezing	Flexible bronchoscopy: dynamic airway compression
Cystic fibrosis	Features of CSLD/bronchiectasis, malabsorption, failure to thrive	Sweat chloride, mutation analysis

Contd...

Contd...

Differential diagnosis	*Clinical pointers*	*Investigations*
Bronchopulmonary dysplasia	Preterm birth, HMD, oxygen requirement during neonatal period, ventilation	Chest X-rays, CT chest
Primary ciliary dyskinesia	Features of CSLD/bronchiectasis, rhinitis since birth, chronic otitis, situs inversus	Ciliary motility and ultrastructural studies
H type tracheoesophageal fistula	Cough with feeding since birth, recurrent pneumonias	Flexible bronchoscopy, contrast study
Vascular airway compression	Onset of symptoms since birth, usually symptoms persist during interval periods, monophonic wheezing, feeding difficulties	Flexible bronchoscopy: non dynamic airway pulsatile compression
Non-vascular airway compression (lymph node, cardiomegaly, tumors, cyst)	Congenital cardiac disease, other suggestion of TB, lymphoma, monophonic wheezing, feeding difficulties	Flexible bronchoscopy, Chest X-rays, CT chest
Mechanical problems		
Gastroesophageal reflux disease (GERD)	Early onset symptoms (<6 months), severe wheezing episodes, gastroesophageal symptoms, features of aspiration on chest X-ray	24 hours pH study, GER scan
Foreign body aspirations	Choking while feeding, monophonic wheezing, lateralizing signs	Flexible bronchoscopy

(BAL: bronchoalveolar lavage; CSLD: chronic suppurative lung disease; CT: computed tomography; GER: gastroesophageal reflux; HMD: hyaline membrane disease; HRCT: high resolution computed tomography; TB: tuberculosis)

trend should also be seen. It would be extremely important to elicit details regarding symptoms during interval period (any cough, wheezing, etc.), symptoms with activity, and any aeroallergen sensitization. History of feeding difficulty, choking, and regurgitation of feeds should be asked. History for allergic rhinitis and conjunctivitis should be elicited. A detailed family history including grand parents would also be useful. All details of the previous medicines taken should be recorded.

Examination should focus particularly on the growth velocity of the baby, since children who have failure to thrive could have an underlying serious illness, like cystic fibrosis (CF). Presence of clubbing indicates an underlying suppurative lung disease and should be carefully seen.

Adenoid facies, Dennie-Morgan Folds, transverse nasal creases, nasal examination (nasal mucosa, turbinate, deviated nasal septum) are also important features on physical examination. Respiratory examination should focus on shape of chest (any increased anteroposterior diameter), symmetry, and type of wheeze (monophonic or polyphonic). Presence of monophonic wheeze would indicate a lesion/compression of the intrathoracic airway and if persistent, should be investigated further, e.g., endoscopic evaluation. The examination should also cover the cardiovascular, abdominal, and nervous systems.

INVESTIGATIONS: HOW AND HOW FAR?

Most children with recurring wheezing (EVW or MTW) do not require any investigations. A detailed history and complete physical examination usually is sufficient. As a rule, wheeze should be documented as clinical mimickers, like recurrent or back to back URI (nursery school syndrome) and protracted bacterial bronchitis do not have a wheeze but have ruttles. Children who are asymptomatic during intervals and have a normal examination (normal respiratory rate, no noisy breathing, no wheeze) are unlikely to have any atypical cause of wheeze.

The role of investigations to differentiate the phenotype of preschool wheeze and predict whether this child might go on to develop asthma or remit is still a matter of research. Preschool pulmonary function testing techniques (impulse oscillometry/interrupter technique), fractional exhaled nitric oxide and biomarkers on exhaled breath condensate have been used. Since there is no final conclusion on any of these modalities their routine use in clinical practice needs to wait.

Gastroesophageal reflux disease (GERD) has been evaluated as a cause of wheezing in children but still many questions remain unanswered. Gastroesophageal reflux disease is physiological and whether the "D: the disease" can be attributed to reflux or is just a co-traveler, needs to be defined for each case. Children with severe episodes,

BOX 1: Red flag signs.

- Failure to thrive
- Clubbing
- Presence of persistent wet cough
- Persistent wheezing >4 weeks
- Stridor/noisy breathing
- Age of onset <6 months
- Severe wheeze episodes

especially less than 6 months are more likely to have GERD as the sole or one of the reasons of persistent or recurrent wheezing.

Investigations are required only in children suspected to have atypical causes of wheezing. The red flag signs in **Box 1** should prompt referral for a detailed evaluation. Focused investigations would be required and might include GER scan/24 h pH study, flexible bronchoscopy, sweat chloride test, and computed tomography chest.

TREATMENT

Acute Episode

Inhaled short-acting β2-agonists remain the cornerstone of therapy although nebulized and oral route are also acceptable although inferior options. Inhaled or nebulized ipratropium may be added in severe wheezy episodes. Systemic steroids short course (either patient initiated or doctor initiated) have not shown to reduce the symptom scores, hospital admission rate or duration of hospital stay. It might be considered for a very severe episode as a counsel of despair but its routine use is not recommended. Routine use of nebulized steroids has shown to be ineffective and is not recommended.

Recent studies have evaluated the role of pre-emptive therapy, i.e., treatment started at the beginning of a URI to prevent a wheezy episode. Both inhaled fluticasone and oral montelukast have been shown to have an only modest effect on reduction in number of wheezing episodes and the number needed to treat is high. Hence, their routine use is not justified and might be reserved for children with severe EVW episodes.

Regular Prophylaxis

The key issues while considering long-term treatments are:

- Can we identify a child who is more prone to be an asthmatic in the future?
- Can we modify the natural history of the disease with any intervention?
- Can we modify lung function levels in adult life?

Three landmark trials (Peak, Ifwin, and PAC) over the last 10 years have shown that ICS only improves symptoms with no long-term benefit in the form of modification of the natural course of disease or alteration in lung function. Interested readers could refer to these very important studies mentioned under Suggested Reading.

What does all this Mean in and what are the Implications for Clinical Practice?

Preschool children with recurrent wheeze, selected based on the API do respond to ICSs as a group although the effect size is less as compared to older children with asthma. There are no studies on non-atopic MTW, but recent data showed that the pathology of non-atopic and atopic MTW can be similar. Recent meta-analysis suggests no difference in response between atopic versus nonatopic, although this awaits further studies.

The *NHLBI-EPR 3 Guidelines* has recommended using prophylaxis in the following subset of children with recurrent wheezing less than 5 years of age:

- Greater than 4 episodes of wheezing in past 1 year lasted more than 1 day and affected sleep and who have risk factors for developing persistent asthma: positive API
- Consistently require symptomatic treatment more than 2 days per week for a period of more than 4 weeks
- Second asthma exacerbation requiring systemic corticosteroids within 6 months.

Although, these guidelines are also based on expert opinion but appears to be useful.

There is no clear consensus on the type of ICS, dose at which ICS to be started, maximum dose and when to label therapy as ineffective. Also there are no studies on the addition of leukotriene receptor antagonist (LTRA) to ICS. Since long-acting β-agonist are Food and Drug Administration (FDA) approved for more than 6 years of age due to concerns on safety, there are no studies on the use of LABA in preschool children with wheezing in addition to ICS.

Given the significant shift between the phenotypes, ICS/LTRA may be considered on a trial basis in preschool child with recurrent wheeze (MTW or EVW with severe and recurrent episodes), but should be discontinued if there is no clear clinical benefit. Children treated with a low-dose ICS have an average of 5% fewer days with symptoms (or 18 days per year) than children receiving placebo. Hence, it is arguable whether this increase in symptom-free days is clinically significant. The increase cost of therapy, negative impact on height and other unrecognizable adverse effects should also be considered. Hence, the use of preventer regimen should be reserved for only those with very troublesome symptoms and needing repeated

Flowchart 1: Approach to management of wheezing in preschool children.

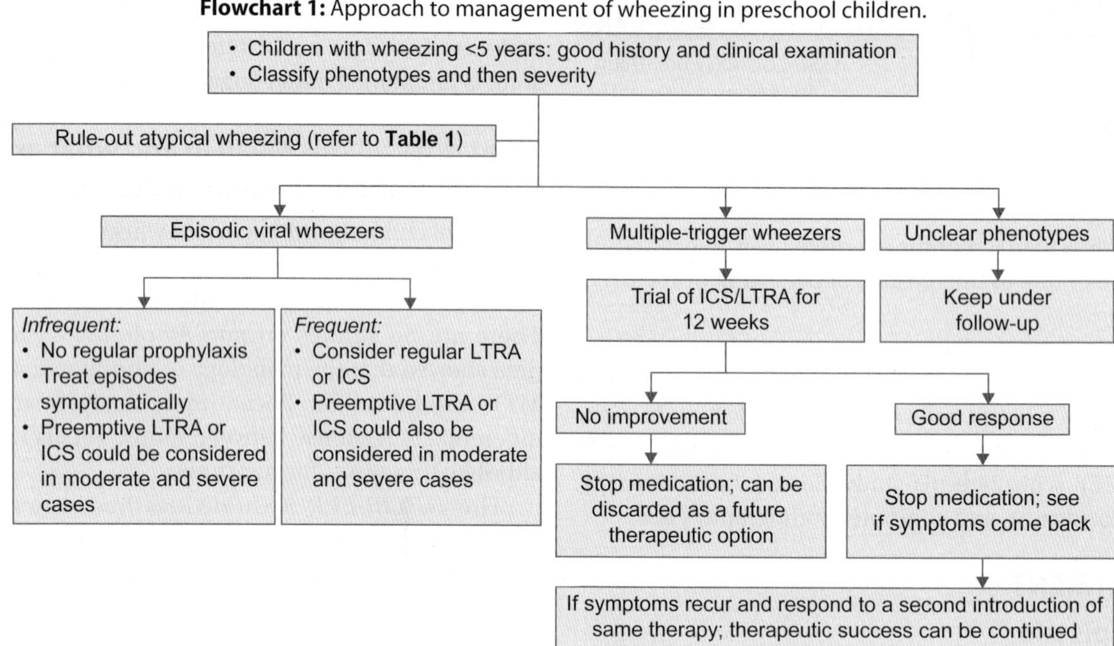

(ICS: inhaled corticosteroids; LTRA: leukotriene receptor antagonist)

oral steroids. The management algorithm is discussed in **Flowchart 1**.

KEY POINTS

- Most children wheeze only when they have upper respiratory infection, are usually nonatopic, and outgrow symptoms by 6 years of age.
- A good history and physical examination would suffice in most cases. Invasive investigations would be only required for atypical cases.
- Most children would require only symptomatic therapy.
- Some with very frequent or severe symptoms require some prophylaxis: either pre-emptive or regular.
- Inhaled corticosteroids (ICS) do control symptoms but do not seem to alter the natural history of wheezing (benefit not as much as children with school asthma).
- Efficacy of ICS with episodic viral wheeze remains controversial, while with multiple-trigger wheeze (MTW) appears to be at least somewhat effective. However, the effect size in preschool children with MTW is smaller than the effect size in school-aged children with asthma.
- Treatment of children with recurrent wheezing in <5 years still remains practice imperfect.

SUGGESTED READING

1. Bacharier LB, Guilbert TW. Diagnosis and management of early asthma in preschool-aged children. J Allergy Clin Immunol. 2012;130(2):287-96.
2. Brand PL, Baraldi E, Bisgaard H, Boner AL, Castro-Rodriguez JA, Custovic A, et al. Definition, assessment and treatment of wheezing disorders in preschool children: an evidence-based approach. Eur Respir J. 2008;32(4):1096-110.
3. Brand PL, Caudri D, Eber E, Gaillard EA, Garcia-Marcos L, Hedlin G, et al. Classification and pharmacological treatment of preschool wheezing: changes since 2008. Eur Respir J. 2014;43(4):1172-7.
4. Castro-Rodriguez JA, Pedersen S. The role of inhaled corticosteroids in management of asthma in infants and preschoolers. Curr Opin Pulm Med. 2013;19(1):54-9.
5. Castro-Rodriguez JA, Rodrigo GJ. Efficacy of inhaled corticosteroids in infants and preschoolers with recurrent wheezing and asthma: a systematic review with meta-analysis. Pediatrics. 2009;123(3):e519-25.
6. Global Initiative for Asthma. (2015). Global Strategy for Asthma Management and Prevention. [online] Available from: www.ginasthma.org [Accessed December 2015].
7. Guilbert TW, Morgan WJ, Zeiger RS, Mauger DT, Boehmer SJ, Szefler SJ, et al. Long-term inhaled corticosteroids in preschool children at high risk for asthma. N Engl J Med. 2006;354(19):1985-97.
8. Rosenfeld M, Allen J, Arets BH, Aurora P, Beydon N, Calogero C, et al. An official American Thoracic Society workshop report: optimal lung function tests for monitoring cystic fibrosis, bronchopulmonary dysplasia, and recurrent wheezing in children less than 6 years of age. Ann Am Thorac Soc. 2013;10(2):S1-S11.

CHAPTER 70

Managing Acute Severe Asthma

Ankit Parakh, Shalu Gupta, Varinder Singh

INTRODUCTION

Acute severe asthma or acute exacerbations are acute episodes of progressive deteriorating shortness of breath, cough, wheezing, chest tightness, or a combination of these symptoms. These acute episodes of asthma are an important cause of morbidity, school absenteeism, and frequent hospital admissions in children. The severity of these episodes varies from mild to severe and each episode has the potential to progress to respiratory failure. The term "critical asthma syndrome" is now used to describe any child who is at high risk of fatal asthma and includes acute severe asthma, refractory asthma, status asthmaticus, and near fatal asthma. Status asthmaticus refers to an acute asthma exacerbation in which bronchial obstruction is severe and continues to worsen or not improve despite the institution of adequate standard therapy, leading to respiratory fatigue and finally to respiratory failure.

A stepwise approach is required for the early recognition, coordinated evaluation, and prompt treatment by an experienced healthcare provider team.

EPIDEMIOLOGY

In USA more than 3.5 million children have greater than or equal to 1 exacerbation/year, resulting in approximate 1.75 million total emergency department (ED) visits, including 0.64 million for children aged 0–17 years. Children younger than 4 years old age have the highest rate of hospitalizations. Children aged 5–17 years missed 10.5 million school days owing to asthma, and activity limitations were reported in 5.5% as well.

In the Indian subcontinent as per the phase 3 ISAAC study, in children aged 13–14 and 6–7 years, the prevalence of asthma increased per year by +0.02 and +0.06%, respectively. Although there is little change in the overall prevalence of the current wheeze, the percentage of children reported to have had asthma increased significantly, possibly reflecting a greater awareness of this condition and/or changes in diagnostic practice. No country wide or large series data exist regarding burden of disease due to acute exacerbations.

CLINICAL FEATURES

A rapid initial assessment is a must to determine degree of airway obstruction and hypoxia. Immediately identify severe or life-threatening attack in children and institute immediate measures to treat it **(Box 1)**.

A detailed and rapid clinical assessment is done on the basis of history, physical examination, and relevant investigations. A clinical history should include episodes/duration of respiratory distress, fever, cough, noisy breathing, abnormal respiratory sounds, episodes of lethargy and cyanosis, records of past treatment and current treatment, any previous hospitalization or intensive care unit admission, use of steroids, and exposure to any allergen or trigger which could have triggered this attack. A child with asthma will present with bouts of cough, wheezing, dyspnea, and increases work of breathing. Because early recognition is important for improving outcomes, various risk factors are defined for early identification of fatal asthma **(Box 2)**.

Detailed clinical examination should include level of consciousness and degree of agitation, respiratory rate, heart rate, temperature, peripheral pulses, blood pressure, pulsus paradoxus, use of accessory muscles including chest retractions and nasal flaring, chest auscultation (wheeze), and oxygen saturation. Categorization of the acute attack can be done into mild, moderate, or severe **(Table 1)**.

BOX 1: Identification of life-threatening attack.

- Silent chest with increasing respiratory effort
- Agitation with decreased level of consciousness
- Central cyanosis
- Inability to speak
- Diaphoresis
- Inability to lie down
- Hypotension
- Bradycardia

Chest radiography is not routinely indicated in a child with previous history of asthma. Indications for chest radiography may include clinical suspicion for pneumothorax, atelectasis, foreign body aspiration, after endotracheal intubation or failure to respond to standard therapy.

Arterial blood gas measurement provides objective assessment of gas exchange. Early in the course of asthma, hypoxemia and hypocapnia are found due to ventilation/perfusion mismatch and hyperventilation. With the progression of airflow obstruction, $PaCO_2$ measurement returns to normal values, though in a tachypneic and hyperventilating child, a normal $PaCO_2$ value should be interpreted as a sign of early muscle fatigue. With further progression of the disease mixed respiratory and metabolic acidosis occurs. Lactic acidosis indicates a combination of excess production from respiratory muscles, tissue hypoxia (due to hypoxemia and decreased cardiac output), and dehydration (due to decreased intake and increased insensible losses). The decision to intubate a child with severe acute asthma should be based on the child's clinical status and not simply the arterial blood gas values.

BOX 2: Risk factors for potentially fatal asthma in children.

- Previous near fatal asthma
- Previous admission to a PICU for asthma
- Admission for asthma in the last year
- Excessive use of or overdependence on β2 agonists
- Current use or recent use of oral corticosteroids
- Repeated attendances at emergency unit for asthma treatment, especially if in the last year
- "Brittle" asthma (sudden onset of acute severe asthma attacks)
- Poor adherence to medication
- Psychosocial and/or family problems

(PICU: pediatric intensive care unit)
Source: Adapted from Global Initiative for Asthma, British Thoracic Society/Scottish Intercollegiate Guidelines Network

CLINICAL PEARLS

- Clinical signs correlate poorly with the severity of airways obstruction. Some children may have very severe airways obstruction without appearing to be obviously distressed
- In a tachypneic and hyperventilating child, a normal $PaCO_2$ value should be interpreted as a sign of early muscle fatigue
- The decision to intubate a child with severe acute asthma should be based on the child's clinical status and not simply the arterial blood gas values.

TABLE 1: Acute asthma severity assessment.

Examination	*Mild*	*Moderate*	*Severe*
Breathing frequency (awake)	Increased	Increased	>30/min
Wheezing	None or mild end expiratory	Throughout expiration	Both inspiratory and expiratory
Work of breathing and use of auxiliary muscles	Normal or minimal retractions	Intercostals retractions	Suprasternal retractions, present
Expiration	Normal or minimally prolonged	Moderately prolonged	Severely prolonged
Pulsus paradoxus	Absent	Can be present	Often present
Pulse pressure fluctuation	<10 mm Hg	10–25 mm Hg	20–40 mm Hg
Air entry	Normal	Decreased at bases	Wide-spread decrease
Breathlessness	With activity or walking	While at rest *For infants:* Soft or shorter cry, difficulty feeding, prefers sitting	While at rest *For infants:* Stops feeding, sits upright
Talks	Sentences	Phrases	words
Alertness	Alert/can be agitated	May be agitated	agitated
Investigations			
Pulse oximetry (room air)	>95%	91–95%	<91%
$PaCO_2$ (KPa)	<5.6	<5.6	≥5.6
PaO_2 (KPa)	Normal	>8	<8, possible cyanosis
PEF (% of predicted for height)	≥70%	40–69%	<40%

(PEF: peak expiratory flow)

TREATMENT

There is good evidence supporting recommendations for the initial treatment of acute asthma. Most children would respond to these measures although a small proportion of children would need further therapy. There is less evidence to guide the use of second-line therapies to treat the small number of severe cases poorly responsive to first-line measures.

The details regarding assessment, first-line treatment, second-line treatment, algorithm, further evaluation and drug doses should be present in all emergency and pediatric intensive care unit as a ready to use tool. A suggested algorithm is shown in **Flowchart 1** and drugs with doses, delivery methods, and adverse effects are summarized in **Table 2**. After each step in the algorithm the child should be reclassified. Children moving down

Flowchart 1: Algorithm for management of acute severe asthma.

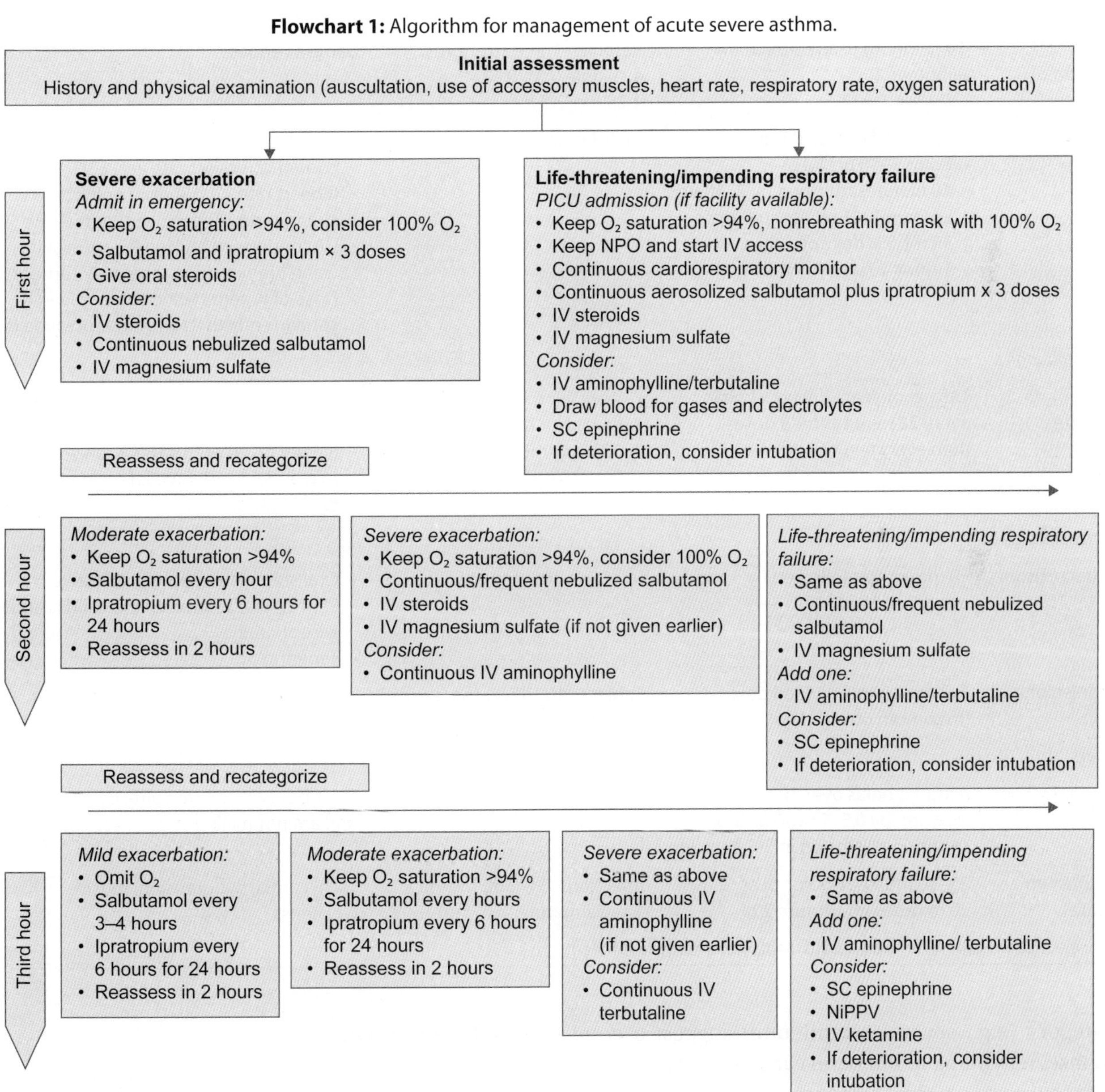

(IV: intravenous; IV: intravenous; NiPPV: nasal intermittent positive pressure inhibitors; NPO: nil per os; PICU: pediatric intensive care unit; SC: subcutaneous)

TABLE 2: Doses of common drug used in acute severe asthma.

	Dose	***Available formulations***	***Adverse effects and comments***
Short-acting β-agonists			
Salbutamol	• *Nebulized:* 0.15 mg/kg (minimum dose 2.5 mg) every 20 minutes for 3 doses then 0.15–0.3 mg/kg up to 10 mg every 1–4 hours as needed, or 0.5 mg/kg/hour by continuous nebulization • *MDI:* 2–4 puffs (up to 10 puffs) at the same intervals as above	• *Respules:* 2.5 mg/2.5 mL • *Respirator solution:* 5 mg/mL • *MDI:* 100 µg/puff	Tachycardia, palpitations, headache, hypokalemia, hyperglycemia
Levo salbutamol	0.075 mg/kg usage similar to salbutamol	*Respules:* Three strengths available 0.31/0.63/1.25 mg/2.5 mL	Same as above
Terbutaline	• 0.01 mg/kg subcutaneous • Bolus 5–10 µg/kg over 10 minutes followed by 2–10 µg/kg/hour IV (1 mL terbutaline + 50 mL 5% dextrose, thus, 1 mL = 10 µg terbutaline)	Inj 0.5 mg/mL	• IV terbutaline drip necessitates continuous heart rate and ECG • If heart rate, i.e.,180/min or if ECG changes develop, halve the drip rate • Discontinue nebulized β2 agonist if using high infusion rates of IV terbutaline • Dose of IV terbutaline to be halved if concurrently used with theophylline drip
Anticholinergics			
Ipratropium bromide	125 µg <1 year; 250 µg >1 year every 20 minutes for 3 doses, then every 6–8 hours	• *Respules:* 0.5 mg/2 mL • *Respirator solution:* 0.25 mg/mL; • *MDI:* 20 µg/puff	• Dryness of mouth increased wheezing in some • Slower onset of than β2 agonists but may provide additive effect in severe exacerbations
Corticosteroids			
Hydrocortisone	10 mg/kg stat followed by 5 mg/kg every 6 hourly IV	Injection 100 mg/vial	• Oral steroids are equally effective • Shift to oral as soon as the child is able to accept orally • Tapering not required for short courses
Prednisolone	1–2 mg/kg in 2 divided doses (maximum 60 mg/day)	Tablet 5, 10, 20, 30 mg, syrup 5 mg/mL and 15 mg/mL	
Others			
Aminophylline	6 mg/kg bolus over 30 minutes followed by 0.5–1 mg/kg/hour continuous infusion in 5% dextrose	Injection 250 mg/10 mL	Omit bolus in children already on oral aminophylline
Magnesium sulfate	25–50 mg/kg IV bolus over 20 minutes (maximum 2 g)	Injection 50% (500 mg/mL), 1 mL ampoule	Tachycardia, hypotension, muscle weakness

(ECG: electrocardiogram; IV: intravenous; MDI: metered-dose inhaler)

a category (e.g., severe to moderate) suggest a good response; remaining in the same category (e.g., severe to severe) suggests a partial response; and children moving up a category (e.g., severe to life threatening) suggest a poor response.

First-line Treatment

Oxygen

All children with severe and life-threatening asthma or SpO_2 less than 92%, should receive supplemental oxygen via a face mask or nasal cannula at sufficient flow rates to achieve normal saturations. Partial rebreathing and non-rebreathing masks are useful in providing high concentration of fraction of inspired oxygen in children not maintaining on simple/venturi face mask.

Short-acting β-2 Agonists

Short-acting β-2 agonists (salbutamol, levosalbutamol, terbutaline) are the bronchodilators of choice for acute exacerbations of asthma across all severity. Children with severe or life-threatening asthma should receive frequent doses of nebulized bronchodilators (2.5–5 mg salbutamol) driven by oxygen, repeated every 20–30 minutes; although metered-dose inhaler with spacers can be used (10–12 puffs of salbutamol 100 μg repeated every 2–4 minutes titrated according to clinical response). Continuous nebulized β-2 agonists are of no greater benefit than the use of frequent intermittent doses in the same total hourly dosage.

Anticholinergics

Children with severe exacerbation or moderate exacerbation with poor response to the initial dose of β-2 agonists, are usually nebulized with combination with nebulized ipratropium bromide. There is good evidence for the safety and efficacy of frequent doses of ipratropium bromide (every 20–30 minutes) used in addition to β-2 agonists for the first two hours of a severe asthma attack. Benefits are more apparent in the most severe patients.

Corticosteroids

Systemic corticosteroids are pivotal in the management of acute severe asthma and reduce the need for hospital admission and prevent a relapse in symptoms after initial presentation. Benefits can be apparent within 3–4 hours. Both oral as well as intravenous (IV) steroids have similar efficacy. Intravenous hydrocortisone (4 mg/kg repeated 4-hourly) should be reserved for severely affected children who are unable to retain oral medication.

Second-line Treatment

Children with continuing severe asthma, despite frequent nebulized β-2 agonists and ipratropium bromide plus oral steroids, and those with life-threatening features, need transfer to a high dependency unit or PICU to receive second-line IV therapies. There are three options to consider: (1) Magnesium sulfate, (2) aminophylline and (3) continuous IV salbutamol/terbutaline.

Intravenous or Nebulized Magnesium Sulfate

Magnesium sulfate is a physiological calcium antagonist that acts by inhibiting the contraction, mediated by the bronchial smooth muscle. In addition, it interferes with the para-sympathetic stimulation and prevents acetylcholine release to the axon terminal; therefore promoting a bronchodilating effect. It has been usually recommended as an add-on therapy after the first hour of treatment with salbutamol and steroids (GINA 2015, Evidence level A). One large open-labeled trail from Argentina has shown that magnesium sulfate when used in the first hour itself can reduce significantly, the percentage of children who required mechanical ventilation support. There is now evidence to support use of nebulized isotonic magnesium sulfate.

Intravenous Aminophylline

There is no evidence that aminophylline is of benefit for mild-to-moderate asthma and side effects are common and troublesome. One well-conducted study has shown evidence of benefit in severe acute asthma unresponsive to multiple doses of β-2 agonists and steroids, although the loading dose used was double that currently recommended in UK and one-third of patients were withdrawn from active medication because of vomiting. Two studies have compared IV β-2 agonists with IV theophylline/aminophylline. One demonstrated equivalence. The other resulted in a shorter period of inpatient treatment among the children receiving an aminophylline bolus followed by infusion but in the salbutamol arm of the study an infusion was not given after the bolus dose.

Intravenous Terbutaline

A continuous IV infusion of terbutaline could be used in children not responding to the above mentioned drugs. This should be given in a high dependency unit or PICU with continuous electrocardiogram (ECG) monitoring and twice daily electrolyte monitoring. Nebulized bronchodilators should be continued while the patient is receiving IV bronchodilators. Once the patient is improving the IV infusion should be reduced before reducing the frequency of nebulized bronchodilators. Currently, the availability of this drug is poor across our country.

Other Modalities

Children not responding to the above measures should be considered for noninvasive ventilation, IV ketamine, and if required, intubation and mechanical ventilation.

The use of a helium-oxygen gas mixture is another potentially attractive therapy for the treatment of status asthmaticus in children. The use of helium-oxygen–driven aerosolized therapy increases drug delivery by improving gas exchange to the distal airways.

KEY POINTS

- Acute asthma management involves prompt recognition of severity and treatment using short-acting β-agonists, anticholinergics, and systemic corticosteroids.
- Children with severe exacerbations should receive high-dose short-acting β-agonists mixed with ipratropium bromide as well as systemic steroids.
- Children with less-severe exacerbations might benefit from systemic steroids.
- Patients not improving after multiple high-dose systemic steroids should receive adjunctive therapy, such as intravenous magnesium.
- Prepare a written asthma action plan. Ensure proper follow-up after discharge with an aim to implement a long-term management plan.

SUGGESTED READING

1. Camargo CA Jr, Rachelefsky G, Schatz M. Managing asthma exacerbations in the emergency department: summary of the National Asthma Education And Prevention Program Expert Panel Report 3 guidelines for the management of asthma exacerbations. Proc Am Thorac Soc. 2009; 6(4):357-66.
2. Carroll CA, Sala KA. Pediatric status asthmaticus. Crit Care Clin. 2013;29(2):153-66.
3. Kling S, Zar HJ, Levin ME, Green RJ, Jeena PM, Risenga SM, et al. Guideline for the management of acute asthma in children: 2013 update. S Afr Med J. 2013;103(3 Pt 3): 199-207.
4. Koninckx M, Buysee C, dee Hoog M. Management of status asthmaticus in children. Paediatr Respir Rev. 2013; 14(2):78-85.
5. Nelson KA, Zorc JJ. Asthma update. Pediatr Clin North Am. 2013;60(5):1035-48.
6. Nievas IF, Anand KJ. Severe acute asthma exacerbation in children: a stepwise approach for escalating therapy in a pediatric intensive care unit. J Pediatr Pharmacol Ther. 2013;18(2):88-104.

CHAPTER 71

Management of Bronchiolitis

Savneet Kaur, Preeti Singh, Varinder Singh

INTRODUCTION

Bronchiolitis accounts for significant number of hospital admissions worldwide especially in the age group of <2 years. The American Academy of Pediatrics Clinical Practice Guideline defines bronchiolitis as "a constellation of clinical symptoms and signs including a viral upper respiratory prodrome followed by increased respiratory effort and wheezing in children less than two years of age".

EPIDEMIOLOGY

Bronchiolitis is primarily a disease of infancy, with the first (and the most severe) episode occurring between 2 and 6 months of age. Respiratory syncytial virus (RSV) is the most common etiological agent and accounts for 50–80% of cases worldwide as well as in India. Other viruses responsible include rhinovirus, adenovirus, coronavirus, enterovirus, parainfluenza virus type 3, influenza, and human metapneumovirus (HMPV). Molecular diagnostic techniques have also revealed that young children with bronchiolitis have mixed viral infections (10–30%), most common being with RSV and either HMPV or rhinovirus. There has been no evidence for role of bacteria in the etiology of bronchiolitis. Data on synergistic viral-bacterial infections also are unconvincing. Bronchiolitis shows a seasonal pattern with highest rates occurring during winter season in most locations. However, a change in epidemiology of RSV was seen due to the COVID-19 pandemic. The public health measures taken to prevent the COVID-19 infection like social distancing, hand washing, using masks, lock down, etc. have led to significant decrease in number of cases of bronchiolitis worldwide. In addition, when these measures were lifted, resurgence of RSV was seen especially during the atypical time of the year.

PATHOGENESIS

Bronchiolitis is characterized by acute inflammation of the bronchiolar epithelium, with peribronchial infiltration of white blood cells, mostly mononuclear cells, edema of the submucosa and adventitia, necrosis of small airway epithelial cells, increased mucus production, and bronchospasm. Plugs of sloughed, necrotic epithelium and fibrin in the airways cause partial or total obstruction to airflow. A "ball-valve" mechanism results in air trapping distal to the obstructed areas, with subsequent absorption, atelectasis, and a ventilation perfusion mismatch leading to hypoxemia. The degree of obstruction may vary as these areas are cleared, resulting in rapidly changing clinical signs. Certain underlying conditions, such as prematurity, chronic lung disease, cardiac disease, immunodeficiency, and neuromuscular disorders, can predispose a child to a more turbulent course while certain clinical clues suggest a more likely severe course **(Table 1)**.

CLINICAL PEARL

- Bronchiolitis is primarily a disease of infancy with RSV being responsible for >50% of cases. Host, anatomical, immunological, and environmental factors along with nature of the viral pathogen play an important role in severity of clinical syndrome.

CLINICAL FEATURES AND COURSE

Bronchiolitis typically starts with fever and rhinorrhea. After 1–3 days, a prominent staccato-like cough and wheeze develop. The clinical presentation of bronchiolitis can be quite variable, both over time and between patients. It can range from mild respiratory distress with cough, coryza, to a more severe illness with increased respiratory distress with increased work of breathing, and respiratory failure. Excessive nasal secretions can cause upper airway obstruction, with both inspiratory and expiratory sound

TABLE 1: Factors associated with an increased risk and severity of bronchiolitis.

Personal risk factors	***Environmental risk factors***	***Clinical factors***
• Male gender • Prematurity <34 weeks • Age <6 months • Absence of breastfeeding • Chronic pulmonary disease • Hemodynamically significant congenital heart disease • Immunodeficiency • Family or personal history of atopy • Congenitally small airways • RSV-specific IgE responses	• Having school age or younger siblings • Passive smoke • Household crowding • Child-care attendance	• Toxic or ill appearance • Oxygen saturation <95% on room air • Respiratory rate ≥70 breaths per minute • Moderate/severe chest retractions • Atelectasis on chest radiograph

(IgE: immunoglobulin E; RSV: respiratory syncytial virus)

TABLE 2: Severity of bronchiolitis.

	Mild	***Moderate***	***Severe***
Respiratory rate	Normal or slightly increased	Increased	Markedly increased
Respiratory effort	Mild chest retractions	Moderate chest retractions, tracheal tug, nasal flaring	Marked chest retraction, nasal flaring, grunting
Oxygen saturation	No supplemental oxygen required, O_2 saturation >95% on room air	O_2 saturation 90–95%	O_2 saturation <90% on room air
Feeding	Normal to slightly decreased	50–75% of normal feeds	Unable to feed, <50% of feeds
Apnea	Absent	Occasional, brief episodes	Frequent and prolonged episodes

on auscultation. Other manifestations of upper respiratory tract infection (URTI), like mild conjunctivitis, otitis media, and pharyngitis, may be present. Concurrent presence of similar respiratory symptoms in other family members is common. On examination, child has tachypnea, varying degree of hypoxemia due to ventilation perfusion mismatch and increased work of breathing manifested as nasal flaring, intercostal retractions, subcostal retractions, and use of other accessory muscles of respiration. On auscultation, diffuse bilateral wheeze and crackles are often present. In mild cases, a prolonged expiratory phase of respiration may be seen. The liver and spleen may be palpable due to hyperinflation of the lungs secondary to air trapping. The severity of bronchiolitis can be classified into mild, moderate, and severe depending on respiratory distress and oxygen saturation on room air **(Table 2)**.

The mean duration of illness with bronchiolitis is 15 days, and the majority of these infections resolve spontaneously within 3–4 weeks. The mortality rate is <1%, being attributable to apnea or respiratory failure. While RSV bronchiolitis actually leads to long-term changes in the lungs in a proportion of patients, in others, RSV infection simply may serve as a marker for a genetic or physiologic/anatomic predisposition to wheezing.

DIAGNOSIS

The diagnosis of bronchiolitis is essentially clinical and does not require any diagnostic testing. The use of complete blood counts has not proved to be useful in either diagnosing bronchiolitis or guiding its therapy. A blood gas (capillary, venous, or arterial) can aid with assessment of gas exchange in a child with moderate to severe respiratory distress. If a child has poor oral intake, one can assess electrolyte abnormalities and extent of dehydration by measuring the plasma blood urea nitrogen, creatine, and electrolytes. The typical findings on chest radiograph are hyperinflation with peribronchial infiltrates. Areas of atelectasis are not uncommon. Indian Academy of Pediatrics as well as American Academy of Pediatrics does not recommend the routine use of chest radiography for diagnosis and management of bronchiolitis. Chest imaging may be useful when the hospitalized child does not improve at the expected rate, or, if the severity of disease requires further evaluation, or, if another diagnosis is suspected. Laboratory testing of nasopharyngeal aspirates for identification of viruses can aid with syndromic surveillance, but has limited utility and does not aid individual case management.

The differential diagnosis is broad and usually there are multiple clinical clues to differentiate between them **(Box 1)**.

CLINICAL PEARL

- The diagnosis of bronchiolitis is essentially clinical, particularly in a previously healthy infant with first episode of wheezing.

MANAGEMENT

The treatment of bronchiolitis is often debated and no consistently effective therapy has shown to alter the course of the disease or its major outcomes. It is critical to remember that most infants with mild bronchiolitis improve and resolve spontaneously and hence can be successfully treated at home. Children with moderate-to-severe bronchiolitis and well-known risk factors for developing severe bronchiolitis must be considered for hospital admission. The cornerstone of therapy for bronchiolitis is supportive care. Supportive treatment is either for hypoxemia necessitating supplemental oxygen or the inability to take adequate fluids by mouth. Monitoring the child with bronchiolitis for disease progression and complications is a vital part of supportive care. **Table 3** details the current evidence for the management of acute bronchiolitis. **Flowchart 1** provides the steps of management of a child with acute bronchiolitis while the following text details the management further.

BOX 1: Differential diagnoses for acute bronchiolitis.

- Virus-induced wheeze of infancy
- Viral and bacterial pneumonias
- Other pulmonary infections (e.g., *Mycoplasma*, *Chlamydia*, tuberculosis)
- Gastroesophageal reflux disease
- Congestive heart failure
- Structural abnormalities, like congenital vascular ring, laryngotracheomalacia, mediastinal mass, bronchogenic cyst, etc.
- Tracheoesophageal fistula
- Foreign body aspiration
- Cystic fibrosis

TABLE 3: Evidence-based recommendations for treatment of bronchiolitis.

Intervention	*Recommendation*
• Supportive care: Fluid and hydration management • Nasal decongestion using saline drops and gentle nasal suction • Use of supplemental oxygen if SpO_2 <90% RA: • Nasal prongs • Noninvasive respiratory support: CPAP, high flow nasal canula, BiPAP • Mechanical ventilation	Strong recommendation
Nebulized bronchodilators (epinephrine/beta-2 agonists)	Consider trial under strict monitoring but use of either drug continued only if benefit is demonstrated
Nebulized hypertonic saline	Can be used effectively
Corticosteroids—no role	Not recommended for routine use
Antibiotics	Specific indications in case of coexisting bacterial infection suspected in very sick or toxic looking baby
Antiviral: Ribavirin	Not recommended for routine use
• Surfactant • Heliox	Possibly effective for most severe cases and areas of future research
• Leukotriene receptor antagonists/montelukast • Oral bronchodilators • Chest physiotherapy • Inhaled furosemide/inhaled interferon α-2a/inhaled recombinant human DNase	Possibly ineffective, hence not recommended

(BiPAP: bi-level positive airway pressure; CPAP: continuous positive airway pressure; DNase: deoxyribonuclease)

Flowchart 1: Algorithmic approach and management of a child with bronchiolitis.

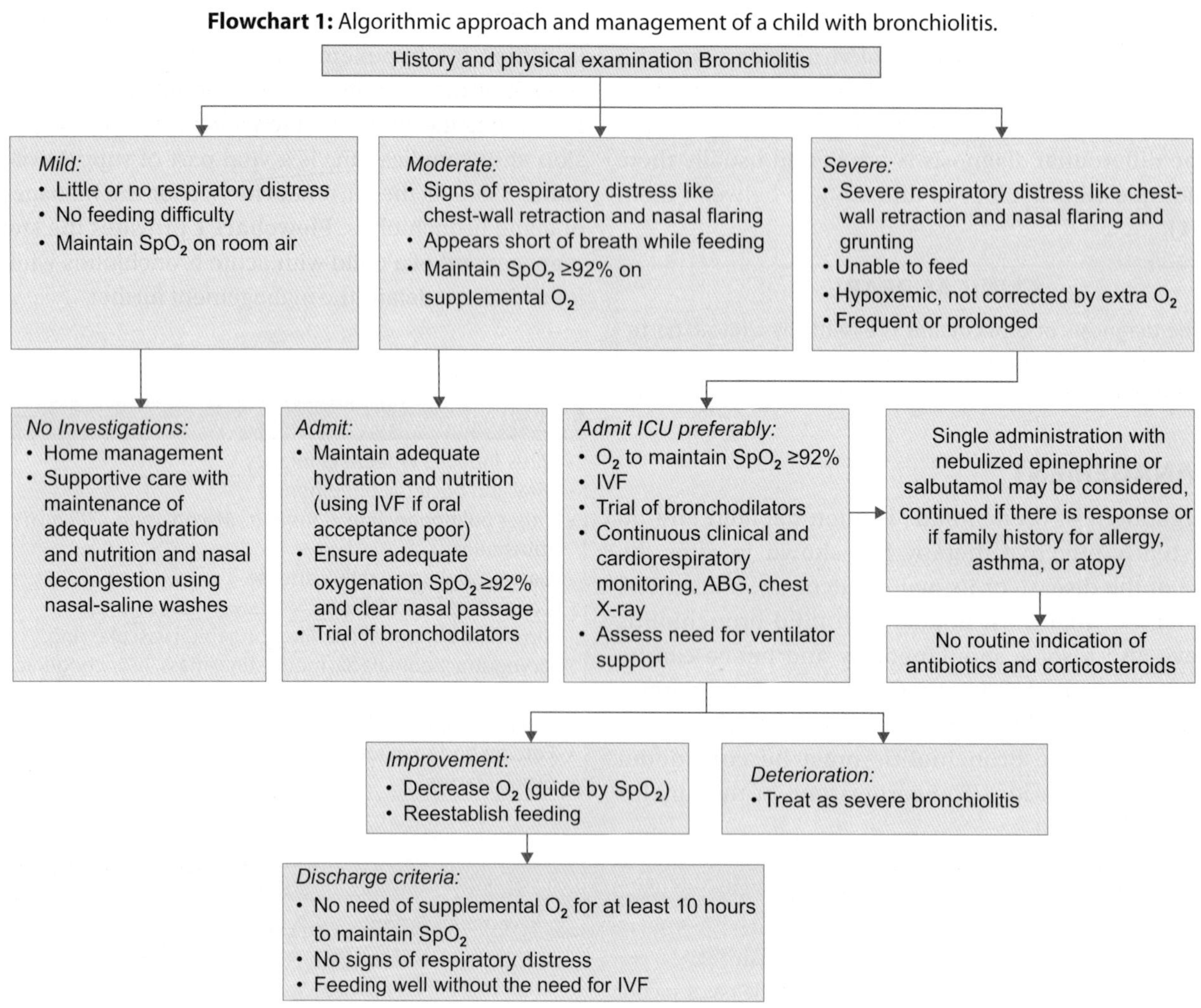

(ABG: arterial blood gas; ICU: intensive care unit; IVF: in vitro fluid; SpO_2: oxygen saturation)

Supportive Care

Fluid and Hydration Management

Children with bronchiolitis often have potential problem of dehydration because of decreased intake and increased needs (due to fever and tachypnea), so body hydration should be properly maintained. Care should be taken not to overhydrate these babies because edema is an important part of the pathology of bronchiolitis (excessive antidiuretic hormone production), which can lead to pulmonary congestion. Breastfeeding should be encouraged as soon as the distress starts setting, as it provides hydration and confers immunological protection. Nasogastric feedings may be considered for a child who has decreased oral intake, with mild-to-moderate respiratory distress. In infants with difficulty in feeding, persistent vomiting, or with moderate-to-severe respiratory distress, intravenous fluids should be considered to maintain hydration as oral feeds are withheld. Usual maintenance fluids are needed.

Nasal Decongestion

Children with bronchiolitis suffer from nasal blockade due to thick copious nasal secretions. Cleaning of nostrils by instilling saline drops and gentle nasal suction may help to relieve nasal block and facilitate feeding.

Oxygen Supplementation

The keystone of therapy for bronchiolitis is maintaining oxygenation by administration of oxygen in moderate-to-severe cases. Humidified oxygen should be administered using nasal prongs, face mask, or head box and the patient's respiratory status is monitored along with pulse oximetry.

In an irritable child, one may have to accept the least threatening but most acceptable manner of oxygen therapy (like nasal blow by) which the baby tolerates. The American Academy of Pediatrics (AAP) recommends supplemental oxygen if the hemoglobin oxygen saturation is persistently below 90%. Their suggested point of discontinuation of oxygen therapy is when the child's oxygen saturation can be maintained at or above 90% with room air and the child is feeding well, with minimal respiratory distress. Premature or low birth weight infants, as well as those with chronic lung disease or congenital heart disease, have lower tolerance for hypoxemia and a higher likelihood of severe disease, so one needs to be careful while discontinuing oxygen.

Noninvasive Respiratory Support: Continuous Positive Airway Pressure, High-flow Nasal Cannula, and BiPAP

Assisted ventilation is indicated in infants with moderate-to-severe bronchiolitis with progressive clinical deterioration, i.e., increasing respiratory distress, apnea, and poor peripheral perfusion. In severe bronchiolitis, early intervention in form of continuous positive airway pressure (CPAP), bi-level positive airway pressure (BiPAP), or high-flow nasal cannula (HFNC) can be used. Use of CPAP has not produced any conclusive evidence in decreasing the need for intubation and the current evidence is inconclusive regarding routine use of CPAP in children with acute bronchiolitis. However, HFNC is an emerging modality and clinical trials for its effectiveness in bronchiolitis are encouraging. The use of chest physiotherapy is discouraged in children with bronchiolitis as it does not reduce supplemental oxygen requirement, or length of hospital stay, rather it may increase the distress and irritability of ill infants.

High flow nasal cannula: The use of humidified heated HFNC in the treatment of patients with bronchiolitis not responding to conventional oxygen therapy by nasal prongs is increasing. It decreases the work of breathing in a child of bronchiolitis with severe respiratory distress. It provides positive airway pressure which helps maintain functional residual capacity, decreases nasopharyngeal edema and secretions and decreases physiologic dead space. Hence, using HFNC in a child with severe bronchiolitis decreases the need for mechanical ventilation. However, no correlation is seen with usage of HFNC and duration of hospital stay of the patients with bronchiolitis. Therefore, it should only be considered in children not responding to conventional oxygen therapy by nasal prongs and should not be used as first-line modality for treatment of bronchiolitis. Randomized controlled trials have shown decreased need of intubation with use of noninvasive respiratory support.

Mechanical Ventilation

Patients with severe respiratory distress usually respond to supportive measures and noninvasive respiratory support. But around 2–10% of all bronchiolitis patients do not respond well to these measures and develop hypoxemia, hypercarbia, and respiratory failure requiring need for invasive mechanical ventilation. According to a retrospective cohort study, there are multiple risk factors associated with higher risk for need of invasive mechanical ventilation which includes younger age group, history of prematurity, pre-existing chronic disease, and multimicrobial infections. Studies show that early intubation has a better prognosis with lesser hospital stay. Overall, mechanical ventilation is safe and associated with good outcome in patients of acute bronchiolitis.

CLINICAL PEARL

- The cornerstone of therapy for bronchiolitis is supportive care with maintenance of adequate hydration and nutrition, ensuring adequate oxygenation, and nasal decongestion using nasal saline drops and gentle nasal suction.

Bronchodilators

Bronchodilators are one of the most commonly used therapy for bronchiolitis. The evidence to support the routine use of bronchodilators in the management of bronchiolitis is not very strong, and the practice remains controversial.

Epinephrine

Epinephrine stimulates alpha-adrenergic, beta-adrenergic, and beta-2-adrenergic receptors, resulting in bronchodilatation. Nebulized epinephrine (0.1–0.5 mL/kg of 1:1,000 diluted in 3 mL saline) is found to be more efficacious than short-acting beta-2 agonists.

Short-acting Beta-2 Agonists: Salbutamol

Salbutamol is a short-acting beta-2 agonist, causing bronchodilatation.

The Cochrane review does not show any benefit of short-acting beta-2 agonists for the management of bronchiolitis. Another meta-analysis demonstrated superiority of epinephrine compared to placebo for short-term outcomes for outpatients. If the decision is made to use an inhaled bronchodilator, it should be based on personal or family history of atopy or asthma; if present, salbutamol inhalation may be given, otherwise a trial of epinephrine inhalation may be given. Further doses of either medication may be continued only on documentation of improvement.

Mucolytics: Nebulization with Hypertonic Saline

Mucous plugging plays a significant role in the small airway obstruction of bronchiolitis and interventions like nebulization with hypertonic saline decrease epithelial edema and elasticity and viscosity of mucus which could improve clinical outcomes. Hypertonic saline inhalation may be considered as potential treatment for bronchiolitis. Recent randomized controlled trial reported that high volume normal saline was as effective as 3% saline in children with mild bronchiolitis.

Corticosteroids

The use of systemic corticosteroid in bronchiolitis remains without merit. Meta-analyses show that corticosteroids are not effective in treatment of bronchiolitis. However, it has been used in patients of bronchiolitis with risk factors for asthma, but in a recent study it is seen that using corticosteroids does not improve the outcome in patients with bronchiolitis who are later hospitalized with asthma. Hence, currently, there is no definitive evidence to support the use of inhaled corticosteroids for acute or long-term benefit in bronchiolitis.

Antibiotics

As bronchiolitis is a viral disease, antibiotics are not useful or necessary. Use of antibiotics should be considered only when a change in course of illness suggests the possibility of secondary bacterial infection. A recent review did not find sufficient evidence to support the routine use of antibiotics for bronchiolitis, but concluded that research may be justified to identify a subgroup of patients who may benefit from antibiotics. It was also stressed that the future research should focus on determining the reasons that clinicians use antibiotics so readily for bronchiolitis, so that the antibiotic usage in bronchiolitis is reduced and also the clinician anxiety about not using antibiotics is reduced.

Antiviral

Ribavirin is the only antiviral agent licensed for use with RSV bronchiolitis. Routine use of ribavirin is not recommended for children with bronchiolitis. It may be considered in high-risk infants (immunocompromised and/or hemodynamically significant cardiopulmonary disease) and in infants requiring mechanical ventilation.

Others

Currently some evidence suggests that surfactant therapy may have potential use in acute severe bronchiolitis requiring mechanical ventilation in decreasing duration of mechanical ventilation and intensive care unit stay. There is a need for larger trials with adequate power and to establish beneficial role of administration of surfactant in infants with severe bronchiolitis. Currently, there is insufficient evidence to recommend leukotriene modifier and heliox use for bronchiolitis.

LONG-TERM IMPACT

It has been seen that infants who need hospitalization due to severe bronchiolitis have high risk (up to 30%) to subsequently develop childhood asthma. However, risk of developing childhood asthma in future also varies with different phenotypes of bronchiolitis patients. The risk is particularly higher in bronchiolitis patients with previous breathing problems and eczema and patients infected with rhinovirus than RSV.

PREVENTION

There is no effective therapy that can improve outcome, if administered early in course of bronchiolitis. Hand decontamination is the most important step in preventing nosocomial spread of RSV. Clinicians should educate health personnel and family members on hand sanitation.

Monoclonal Antibodies

Passive immunoprophylaxis can be given using polyclonal or monoclonal antibodies to high-risk infants **(Table 4)** before RSV season, which has been documented to markedly reduce the rate of hospitalization and reduction in the severity of illness. Palivizumab [humanized mouse immunoglobulin G1 (IgG1) recombinant monoclonal antibody (mAb)] has been used for passive immunoprophylaxis

TABLE 4: Recommendations for respiratory syncytial virus immunoprophylaxis with mAbs.

High-risk group	*Details*
Prematurity	• Infants born at 28 weeks of gestation or earlier who are younger than 12 months of age at the start of the RSV season • Infants born at 29–32 weeks of gestation who are younger than 6 months of age at the start of the RSV season • Infants born between 32 and 35 weeks of gestation, who have 2 or more of the following risk factors (child care attendance, school-aged siblings, exposure to environmental air pollutants, congenital abnormalities of the airways, or severe neuromuscular disease) and are younger than 6 months of age at the start of the RSV season
Chronic lung disease (CLD)	Required medical therapy for CLD within 6 months before onset of RSV season
Congenital heart disease	• Cyanotic heart disease • Taking medications for congestive heart failure

(mAb: monoclonal antibody; RSV: respiratory syncytial virus)

in high-risk infants. A systematic review conducted on patients with advanced disease has shown marked reduction in rate of hospitalization, however, no benefit on survival rates is seen. It is administered intramuscularly at a dose of 15 mg/kg monthly (every 30 days) during the RSV season with maximum of 5 doses being required for prophylaxis during one season. Motavizumab is a second-generation mAb derived from palivizumab, which has more potent RSV neutralizing activity. A randomized trial did not show any reduced severity of illness in patients who received motavizumab.

Newer long-acting mAbs like recently introduced Nirsevimab need to be administered as a single intramuscular dose and provide protection for 5–6 months, sufficient to cover entire RSV season. In recent studies, it has been seen that mAbs decrease RSV-related lower respiratory tract infection (LRTI) by 70% and RSV-related hospitalization by 78% in healthy preterm infants. These new long-acting mAbs are effective in protecting young infants entering their first RSV season. However, considering the high cost, routine use of mAb in preventing patients against acute bronchiolitis is not recommended.

Immunization

Another effective strategy used is passive immunization against RSV infection by maternal vaccination and active immunization of older infants. Recently, RSV vaccine (Abrysvo) has been approved in august 2023 for active immunization of pregnant females of 32–36 weeks' gestation to prevent severe LRTI caused by RSV in infants from birth till 6 months of age.

KEY POINTS

- Bronchiolitis is a disease of infancy with essentially clinical diagnosis.
- The cornerstone of therapy for bronchiolitis is supportive care with maintenance of adequate hydration and nutrition, ensuring adequate oxygenation, and nasal decongestion.
- Bronchodilators should not be routinely used in the management of bronchiolitis. A carefully monitored trial of either α- or β-adrenergic inhalation is an option.
- Hand decontamination is the most important step in preventing nosocomial spread of RSV.
- Breastfeeding is recommended to decrease a child's risk of having LRTI.

SUGGESTED READING

1. Alansari K, Toaimah FH, Almatar DH, El Tatawy LA, Davidson BL, Qusad MIM. Monoclonal Antibody Treatment of RSV Bronchiolitis in Young Infants: A Randomized trial. Pediatrics. 2019;143(3):e20182308.
2. American Academy of Pediatrics Subcommittee on Diagnosis and Management of Bronchiolitis. Diagnosis and management of bronchiolitis. Pediatrics. 2006;118(4):1774-93.
3. Anil AB, Anil M, Saglam AB, Cetin N, Bal A, Aksu N. High volume normal saline alone is as effective as nebulized salbutamol-normal saline, epinephrine-normal saline, and 3% saline in mild bronchiolitis. Pediatr Pulmonol. 2010;45(1):41-7.
4. Beem M, Wright FH, Fasan DM, Egerer R, Oehme M. Observations on the etiology of acute bronchiolitis in infants. J Pediatr. 1962;61:864-9.
5. Bharaj P, Sullender WM, Kabra SK, Mani K, Cherian J, Tyagi V, et al. Respiratory viral infections detected by multiplex PCR among pediatric patients with lower

respiratory tract infections seen at an urban hospital in Delhi from 2005 to 2007. Virol J. 2009;6:89.
6. Bisgaard H, Flores-Nunez A, Goh A, Azimi P, Halkas A, Malice MP, et al. Study of montelukast for the treatment of respiratory symptoms of post-respiratory syncytial virus bronchiolitis in children. Am J Respir Crit Care Med. 2008;178(8):854-60.
7. Davison C, Ventre KM, Luchetti M, Randolph AG. Efficacy of interventions for bronchiolitis in critically ill infants: a systematic review and meta-analysis. Pediatr Crit Care Med. 2004;5(5):482-9.
8. Donlan M, Fontela PS, Puligandla PS. Use of continuous positive airway pressure (CPAP) in acute viral bronchiolitis: a systematic review. Pediatr Pulmonol. 2011;46(8):736-46.
9. Farley R, Spurling GK, Eriksson L, Del Mar CB. Antibiotics for bronchiolitis in children under two years of age. Cochrane Database Syst Rev. 2014;(10):CD005189.
10. Fernandes RM, Bialy LM, Vandermeer B, Tjosvold L, Plint AC, Patel H, et al. Glucocorticoids for acute viral bronchiolitis in infants and young children. Cochrane Database Syst Rev. 2010;(10):CD004878.
11. Gadomski AM, Scribani MB. Bronchodilators for bronchiolitis. Cochrane Database Syst Rev. 2014;(6):CD001266.
12. Gupta S, Shamsundar R, Shet A, Chawan R, Srinivasa H. Prevalence of respiratory syncytial virus infection among hospitalized children presenting with acute lower respiratory tract infections. Indian J Pediatr. 2011;78(12):1495-7.
13. Hammitt LL, Dagan R, Yuan Y, Baca Cots M, Bosheva M, Madhi SA, et al. Nirsevimab for Prevention of RSV in Healthy Late-Preterm and Term infants. N Engl J Med. 2022;386(9):837-46.
14. Hartling L, Bialy LM, Vandermeer B, Tjosvold L, Johnson DW, Plint AC, et al. Epinephrine for bronchiolitis. Cochrane Database Syst Rev. 2011;(6):CD003123.
15. Jat KR, Chawla D. Surfactant therapy for bronchiolitis in critically ill infants. Cochrane Database Syst Rev. 2012;(9):CD009194.
16. Jat KR, Mathew JL. Continuous positive airway pressure (CPAP) for acute bronchiolitis in children. Cochrane Database Syst Rev. 2015;(1):CD010473.
17. Kampmann B, Madhi SA, Munjal I, MATISSE Study Group. Bivalent Perfusion F Vaccine in Pregnancy to Present RSV Illness in Infants. N Engl J Med. 2023;388(16):1451-64.
18. Kwon JW. High-flow nasal cannula oxygen therapy in children: a clinical review. Clin Exp Pediatr. 2020;63(1):3-7.
19. Liet JM, Ducruet T, Gupta V, Cambonie G. Heliox inhalation therapy for bronchiolitis in infants. Cochrane Database Syst Rev. 2010;(4):CD006915.
20. Loda FA, Clyde WA Jr, Glezen WP, Senior RJ, Sheaffer CI, Denny FW Jr. Studies on the role of viruses, bacteria, and M. pneumoniae as causes of lower respiratory tract infections in children. J Pediatr. 1968;72(2):161-76.
21. Maitreyi RS, Broor S, Kabra SK, Ghosh M, Seth P, Dar L, et al. Rapid detection of respiratory viruses by centrifugation enhanced cultures from children with acute lower respiratory tract infections. J Clin Virol. 2000;16(1):41-7.
22. Mansbach JM, Clark S, Christopher NC, LoVecchio F, Kunz S, Acholonu U, et al. Prospective multicenter study of bronchiolitis: predicting safe discharges from the emergency department. Pediatrics. 2008;121(4):680-8.
23. McConnochie KM, Roghmann KJ. Parental smoking, presence of older siblings, and family history of asthma increase risk of bronchiolitis. Am J Dis Child. 1986;140(8):806-12.
24. Meissner HC. Selected populations at increased risk from respiratory syncytial virus infection. Pediatr Infect Dis J. 2003;22(2 Suppl):S40-4.
25. Mejías A, Ramilo O. Review of palivizumab in the prophylaxis of respiratory syncytial virus (RSV) in high-risk infants. Biologics. 2008;2(3):433-9.
26. Paranhos-Baccalà G, Komurian-Pradel F, Richard N, Vernet G, Lina B, Floret D. Mixed respiratory virus infections. J Clin Virol. 2008;43(4):407-10.
27. Pickering, Baker CJ, McMillanassociate JA. Red Book: 2006 Report of the Committee on Infectious Diseases, 27th edition. Elk Grove, Illinois: American Academy of Pediatrics; 2006.
28. Plint AC, Johnson DW, Patel H, Wiebe N, Correll R, Brant R, et al. Epinephrine and dexamethasone in children with bronchiolitis. N Engl J Med. 2009;360(20):2079-89.
29. Shaw KN, Bell LM, Sherman NH. Outpatient assessment of infants with bronchiolitis. Am J Dis Child. 1991;145(2):151-5.
30. Smyth RL, Openshaw PJ. Bronchiolitis. Lancet. 2006;368(9532):312-22.
31. Steven LS, Alexandre TR, Richard S, Katherine NS, Benjamin G. Corticosteroid therapy during acute bronchiolitis in patients who later develop asthma. Hosp Pediatr. 2017;7(7):403-9.
32. van Steensel-Moll HA, Hazelzet JA, van der Voort E, Neijens HJ, Hackeng WH. Excessive secretion of antidiuretic hormone in infections with respiratory syncytial virus. Arch Dis Child. 1990;65(11):1237-9.
33. Verma N, Lodha R, Kabra SK. Recent advances in management of bronchiolitis. Indian Pediatr. 2013;50(10):939-49.
34. Voets S, van Berlaer G, Hachimi-Idrissi S. Clinical predictors of the severity of bronchiolitis. Eur J Emerg Med. 2006;13(3):134-8.
35. Wang EE, Law BJ, Stephens D. Pediatric Investigators Collaborative Network on Infections in Canada (PICNIC) prospective study of risk factors and outcomes in patients hospitalized with respiratory syncytial viral lower respiratory tract infection. J Pediatr. 1995;126(2):212-9.
36. Wright AL, Taussig LM, Ray CG, Harrison HR, Holberg CJ. The Tucson Children's Respiratory Study. II. Lower respiratory tract illness in the first year of life. Am J Epidemiol. 1989;129(6):1232-46.
37. Zhang L, Mendoza-Sassi RA, Wainwright C, Klassen TP. Nebulized hypertonic saline solution for acute bronchiolitis in infants. Cochrane Database Syst Rev. 2013;(7):CD006458.

Management of Bronchiectasis

Kana R Jat

INTRODUCTION

Bronchiectasis is a disease of conducting airways characterized clinically by chronic moist or productive cough, airway hyperreactivity, recurrent respiratory infections, and failure to thrive and radiologically by dilated airways. Chronic suppurative lung disease (CSLD) is a broad category with sign and symptoms similar to bronchiectasis with or without radiological evidence of dilated airways. There is lack of consensus whether bronchiectasis and CSLD represent a spectrum of common disease or are different entities. Empyema and lung abscess are considered different from both bronchiectasis and CSLD.

CLINICAL PEARL

- Never ignore a child with chronic wet cough.

The prevalence of bronchiectasis had decreasing trend in developed countries, but it is still an important chronic respiratory disease in developing countries including India. In early 90s, bronchiectasis was present in approximate 1% children at pediatric respiratory centers in developed countries.

CAUSES OF BRONCHIECTASIS

Bronchiectasis is secondary to many diseases or conditions that injure the conducting airways with recurrent respiratory infections **(Table 1)**. Bronchiectasis may be grouped in two major categories: (1) Associated with cystic fibrosis (CF) and (2) non-CF bronchiectasis. The both group may differ in age of onset, airway colonization, disease severity and distribution, extrapulmonary manifestations, treatment strategies, and overall prognosis. Bronchiectasis is mainly secondary to CF in industrialized countries, whereas in developing countries, postinfectious bronchiectasis forms a major chunk. In a study from Korea, the underlying etiology was identified in 85.8% (79/92) patients that included bronchiolitis obliterans (32.6%), childhood respiratory infection (20.6%), interstitial lung disease (17.3%), immunodeficiency (8.6%), primary ciliary dyskinesia (PCD) (4.3%), and CF (2%). In a study from India of 80 cases of non-CF bronchiectasis, postinfective (23.8%)

TABLE 1: Causes of bronchiectasis*.

Postinfectious: After severe LRTI—tuberculosis, pertussis, measles, and severe viral pneumonia	*Airway obstruction (intraluminal or external compression):* Foreign body, granulation tissue, lymph node, tumor, vascular ring	Yellow nail lymphedema syndrome
Primary ciliary dyskinesia	Bronchiolitis obliterans (postviral, post-transplant)	Marfan syndrome
Immune deficiencies: Both primary and secondary	Cystic fibrosis	Usher syndrome
Congenital airway malformation: Tracheomalacia, bronchomalacia, etc.	*Recurrent aspiration:* Tracheoesophageal fistula, gastroesophageal reflux	Alpha-1 trypsin deficiency
Allergic bronchopulmonary aspergillosis	Neuromuscular weakness	Eosinophilic lung disease
Interstitial lung disease	Asthma	Idiopathic

Note: *Not in order of incidence or prevalence.
(LRTI: lower respiratory tract infection)

was most common cause followed by suspected PCD (15%) and allergic bronchopulmonary aspergillosis (ABPA) (7.5%) and in about one-third, the etiology was identified.

PATHOPHYSIOLOGY OF BRONCHIECTASIS

Bronchiectasis is characterized by tortuous and dilated airways filled with infected secretions with airway obstruction. There is neutrophilic inflammation, peribronchial fibrosis, and accompanying pulmonary and bronchial vascular changes. Pathologically, bronchiectasis may be classified as cylindrical (or tubular), varicose (or fusiform), and cystic (or saccular). Cystic bronchiectasis mostly reflects advanced irreversible disease.

CLINICAL FEATURES

Chronic wet sounding cough with or without sputum expectoration is hallmark of bronchiectasis. Other clinical features include failure to thrive, hemoptysis, exertional dyspnea, wheezing, recurrent respiratory infections, clubbing, and/or chest hyperinflation. Auscultation of chest may reveal coarse crackles and/or rhonchi or it may be normal. Cyanosis and pulmonary hypertension are late ominous signs of bronchiectasis.

CLINICAL PEARL

- Detailed history and clinical examination is a never ending weapon for a physician: Get alerted if you find clubbing and coarse crackles in a child with respiratory symptoms.

Bronchiectasis may be generalized or localized to one or more lobes. In localized form, left lower lobe is most commonly affected followed by right upper lobe. Airway hyperreactivity is not uncommon in children with bronchiectasis ranging from 26 to 74%. Presence of cough and wheezing may not always suggest asthma, rather it may be due to airway obstruction and increased secretion in bronchiectasis. Gastroesophageal reflux disease (GERD) may coexist with bronchiectasis and should be looked for and treated when clinically indicated. Complications of bronchiectasis may include pulmonary hypertension with/without cor pulmonale, hypertrophic osteoarthropathy, systemic amyloidosis, scoliosis, and social problems.

DIAGNOSIS

Once bronchiectasis is suspected clinically, child should be evaluated to confirm the diagnosis, to find extend and severity of disease, and to identify underlying cause.

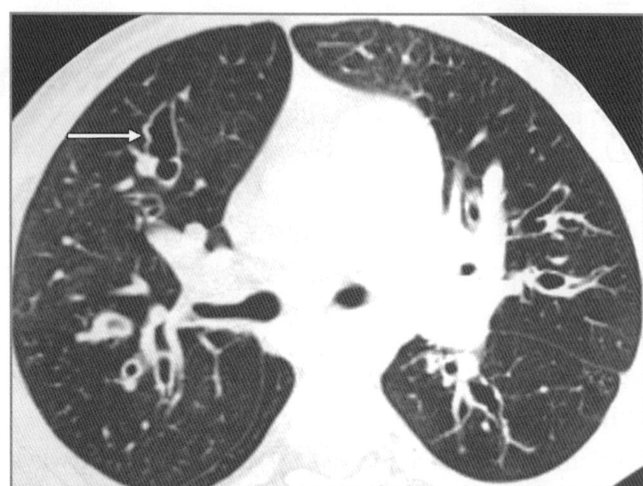

Fig. 1: Bronchiectasis in a child with allergic bronchopulmonary aspergillosis (arrow: dilated central bronchus).

Bronchiectasis may be suspected on chest X-ray but high-resolution computed tomography (HRCT) scan of the chest is investigation of choice to diagnose and to define extend of bronchiectasis. Chest X-ray may reveal peribronchial thickening, bronchial crowding, atelectasis, and persistent infiltrates in early stages; and cystic spaces, air-fluid levels, dilated thick-walled bronchi, and mucus plugging in advanced stage.

Diagnostic criteria for bronchiectasis are based on HRCT chest findings. A dilated bronchus having size greater than nearby artery is considered diagnostic of bronchiectasis in HRCT chest **(Fig. 1)**. This appears as signet rings or tramlines depending on precise orientation of bronchi to the plane of section.

CLINICAL PEARL

- High-resolution computed tomography (HRCT) chest is useful to confirm and to define extent of bronchiectasis, but do not delay treatment if facility for HRCT is not available. If treated at very early stage, much of the disease can be reversed.

Other HRCT chest findings in bronchiectasis may include mucus plugs, bronchial wall thickening, lack of normal airway tapering toward lung periphery, visualization of the peripheral bronchi within 1 cm of the costal pleural surface, air-fluid levels in dilated bronchi, a linear array or cluster of cysts, mosaic perfusion, string of pearls (ectatic bronchi with beaded appearance), and air trapping.

After diagnosing bronchiectasis, try to identify underlying etiology by performing sweat test, immunological workup, sputum analysis, workup for tuberculosis and other infections, bronchoscopy, tests for PCD, gastroesophageal reflux (GER), or ABPA. The all these tests are not required in each child; the test should be tailored by clues from history and examination. There are many scoring systems to assess severity of bronchiectasis based on chest X-ray and HRCT chest findings, but later ones are preferred (Bhalla HRCT score, Reiff scoring system, etc.). Pulmonary function tests (PFTs) may also be performed to assess the severity of bronchiectasis, but there is lack of good correlation between PFTs and HRCT scores. A parent cough-specific quality of life questionnaire is available to assess quality of life in children with bronchiectasis.

Isolation rate for microorganism from sputum or bronchoalveolar lavage (BAL) in children varies between 53 and 67%. Common pathogens isolated in children with non-CF bronchiectasis include *Streptococcus pneumoniae*, *Staphylococcus aureus*, and *Haemophilus influenzae* non-type b, *Pseudomonas aeruginosa*, and *Moraxella catarrhalis*. Exacerbation in bronchiectasis may be suggested by increased sputum production, purulent sputum, increase in cough severity, and/or cough changing from dry to weight.

TREATMENT

Therapy for bronchiectasis may be needed for acute exacerbations, chronic therapy for persistent bronchiectasis, and treatment of underlying disease. The chronic therapy is different for CF- and non-CF-related bronchiectasis. Early diagnosis and aggressive treatment of bronchiectasis and underlying etiology has paramount importance in reducing morbidity and mortality associated with bronchiectasis.

> **CLINICAL PEARL**
>
> - If you diagnose bronchiectasis, do not look for higher center; it may reasonably be managed at any center.

Management of bronchiectasis requires a team approach comprising pediatrician, nurse, physiotherapist, social worker, nutritionist, etc. The general management for bronchiectasis is discussed here. The therapeutic options for bronchiectasis include: (1) Rational use of antibiotics (for maintenance and exacerbation), (2) airway hydration and mucoactive drugs, (3) effective chest physiotherapy (airway clearance methods), (4) use for anti-inflammatory, (5) bronchodilators, (6) good nutritional support, (7) treatment of comorbid conditions and complications, (8) surgical intervention if required, (9) education and social support, and (10) prevention.

Rational Use of Antibiotics

Long-term antibiotics may be used as aerosol or orally for bronchiectasis. Data regarding efficacy of antibiotics for chronic maintenance in children with non-CF bronchiectasis are limited. Till further evidence is available, chronic maintenance antibiotics should be used for a group of selected children only, e.g., with frequent exacerbations, children having severe lung disease with documented pseudomonas endobronchial infection (inhaled tobramycin may be useful) and CF. Long-term use of oral macrolide therapy is found to be beneficial for both CF and non-CF children with bronchiectasis; mainly because of its anti-inflammatory and antisecretagogue properties, rather than due to antimicrobial properties. Acute exacerbations must be treated with antibiotics based on isolated pathogen and local antibiotic sensitivity pattern.

Airway Hydration and Mucoactive Drugs

Mucus clearance is impaired more in children with CF and PCD as compared to idiopathic bronchiectasis. Use of inhaled hypertonic saline (6–7%) is associated with decreased exacerbation and improved lung function in CF bronchiectasis, but data is limited for non-CF bronchiectasis. Risk of bronchospasm following hydrating agents can be minimized with pre-treatment with inhaled salbutamol. To further enhance mucus clearance, mucolytic agents may be used. Recombinant human deoxyribonuclease (rhDNase) is efficacious in CF, but is contraindicated in non-CF-related bronchiectasis as it had worsening of symptoms in non-CF bronchiectasis. Alternative to rhDNase is N-acetylcysteine, but there is lack of evidence for its efficacy. Role of anticholinergics and bromhexine is not established either.

Chest Physiotherapy (Airway Clearance Methods)

Airway clearance techniques (ACTs) with spontaneous or directed cough help in improving mucus clearance. A recent Cochrane review revealed that ACTs appear to be safe and beneficial for both adults and children with stable bronchiectasis. The role of these techniques in people with an acute exacerbation of bronchiectasis is unknown. There are many ACTs, but data is lacking to suggest superiority of one over other and choices may be individualized. Regular physical activity is also encouraged for children with bronchiectasis.

Anti-inflammatory Agents

There is lack of evidence for or against use of inhaled nonsteroidal anti-inflammatory agents in the management of bronchiectasis in adults or children; one small trial of inhaled indomethacin in adults reported a reduction in sputum production and improved dyspnea. Use of high-dose ibuprofen for 4 years in children with CF showed a reduction in the rate of lung function decline and improved weight gain but no change in the frequency of pulmonary exacerbations. There are no randomized controlled trials regarding efficacy of oral nonsteroidal anti-inflammatory drugs (NSAIDs) in patients with non-CF bronchiectasis. Inhaled corticosteroids (ICS) failed to benefit in adults with stable bronchiectasis; therefore, routine use is not recommended. There is lack of trials of ICS for children and for acute exacerbation of bronchiectasis. ICS may be beneficial if there is associated reactive airway disease. Long-term oral steroids in CF bronchiectasis improved lung function, but with significant adverse effects; therefore, not recommended to treat CF-related bronchiectasis. There is lack of trials for use of oral steroids in acute and stable non-CF bronchiectasis both in children and adults except for ABPA, where steroids are indicated whether bronchiectasis is present or absent. Thus, steroid therapy in children with bronchiectasis is related to etiology and its use should be individualized.

Bronchodilators

There is insufficient evidence for or against use of short- or long-acting β-2 agonists, adrenergics, and leukotriene receptor antagonists for management of bronchiectasis and their use should be individualized. Increased cough or wheezing in children with bronchiectasis should be treated as exacerbation at first instance.

The sequence of therapy in bronchiectasis should be bronchodilator, hypertonic saline, ACT, and ICS and inhaled antibiotics if child getting.

SURGICAL TREATMENT

There are no randomized trials comparing medical versus surgical treatment. Usual indication of surgery is failure of medical therapy in localized disease. Other indications for surgery may include severe persistent hemoptysis uncontrolled by bronchial artery embolization, severe chronic symptoms, and growth failure in localized disease. Surgery should not be considered for generalized disease,

Flowchart 1: Approach to a child with suspected bronchiectasis.

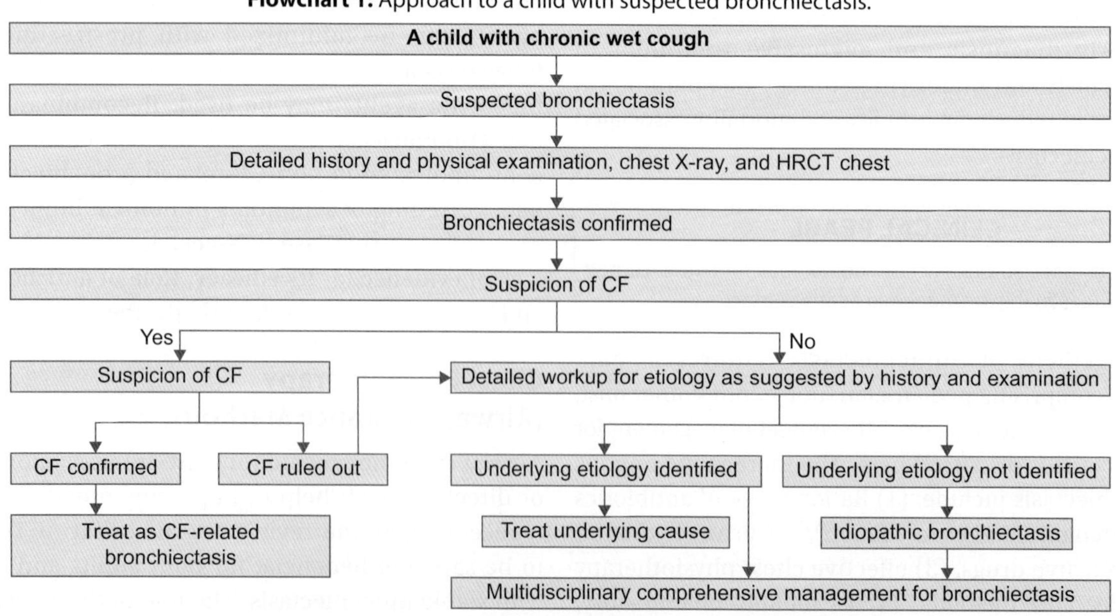

(HRCT: high-resolution computed tomography; CF: cystic fibrosis)

children below 6 years of age, and in bronchiectasis with mild to moderate symptoms. At present, perioperative morbidity and mortality is minimum after lobectomy or pneumonectomy. Outcome after lung transplantation in children with non-CF bronchiectasis is not available.

PREVENTION

Children with bronchiectasis should receive routine vaccination as per national schedule. Limited evidence suggests that routine 23-valent pneumococcal vaccination in children with bronchiectasis may be useful, though robust trials are needed. Role of new 13-valent pneumococcal vaccine requires further trials for young children. Although, there is neither evidence for, nor against, routine influenza vaccination for children and adults with bronchiectasis, it may be used if affordability is not the problem. Children with bronchiectasis should have no/minimal environmental tobacco-smoke exposure as it increases susceptibility to respiratory infections.

An approach to a child with suspected bronchiectasis is shown in **Flowchart 1**.

Prognosis of bronchiectasis depends on underlying etiology; extent and severity of disease at diagnosis, frequency of exacerbations; baseline lung function; rate of decline in FEV1, bacterial density and neutrophils in sputum; and nature of treatment. Delayed diagnosis, presence of reactive airway disease, bilateral lung involvement, and saccular bronchiectasis are some of poor prognostic factors. Bronchiectasis may be reversible in certain situations, e.g., after removal of chronic foreign body. Although lack of mortality data for pediatric bronchiectasis, nearly one-fourth children had respiratory failure in an about 7 years follow-up. With availability of better and inhaled antibiotics, ACTs, and good nutrition support, the prognosis of bronchiectasis has improved with time.

CONCLUSION

Bronchiectasis is chronic disease of conducting airways with a variety of underlying conditions. Data is lacking for effective treatment in children with non-CF bronchiectasis. Early diagnosis and aggressive multidisciplinary therapy with good nutritional and social support has improved prognosis of bronchiectasis in children. More robust clinical trials for various treatment options are required especially for children with non-CF bronchiectasis. In developing countries, control of infectious diseases is needed to curb the load of postinfectious bronchiectasis.

KEY POINTS

High index of suspicious is required to diagnose bronchiectasis at early stage in children:

- Multidisciplinary comprehensive management is key for both CF- and non-CF-related bronchiectasis.
- Pathogen-directed inhaled antibiotics, inhaled hypertonic saline, and oral macrolides are important component of therapeutic regimen for children with CF-related bronchiectasis.
- Data is lacking for use of inhaled antibiotics, airway hydrating treatments, mucolytic agents, inhaled anti-inflammatory agents, and bronchodilators in children with non-CF-related bronchiectasis.

SUGGESTED READING

1. Anuradha KWDA, Gunathilaka PKG, Wickramasinghe VP. Effectiveness of hypertonic saline nebulization in airway clearance in children with non-cystic fibrosis bronchiectasis: A randomized control trial. Pediatr Pulmonol. 2021;56(2):509-15.
2. Chang AB, Bush A, Grimwood K. Bronchiectasis in children: diagnosis and treatment. Lancet. 2018;392(10150):866-79.
3. Eralp EE, Gokdemir Y, Atag E, Ikizoglu NB, Ergenekon P, Yegit CY, et al. Changing clinical characteristics of non-cystic fibrosis bronchiectasis in children. BMC Pulm Med. 2020;20(1):172.
4. Hnin K, Nguyen C, Carson KV, Evans DJ, Greenstone M, Smith BJ. Prolonged antibiotics for non-cystic fibrosis bronchiectasis in children and adults. Cochrane Database Syst Rev. 2015;2015(8):CD001392.
5. Kim HY, Kwon JW, Seo J, Song YH, Kim BJ, Yu J, et al. Bronchiectasis in children: 10-year experience at a single institution. Allergy Asthma Immunol Res. 2011;3(1):39-45.
6. Kumar A, Lodha R, Kumar P, Kabra SK. Non-cystic fibrosis bronchiectasis in children: clinical profile, etiology and outcome. Indian Pediatr. 2015;52(1):35-7.
7. Lee AL, Burge A, Holland AE. Airway clearance techniques for bronchiectasis. Cochrane Database Syst Rev. 2013;(5): CD008351.
8. Lee E, Sol IS, Kim JD, Yang HJ, Min TK, Jang GC, et al. Long-term macrolide treatment for non-cystic fibrosis bronchiectasis in children: a meta-analysis. Sci Rep. 2021;11(1):24287.
9. Newcombe PA, Sheffield JK, Chang AB. Parent cough-specific quality of life: development and validation of a short form. J Allergy Clin Immunol. 2013;131(4):1069-74.
10. O'Grady KF, Cripps AW, Grimwood K. Paediatric and adult bronchiectasis: Vaccination in prevention and management. Respirology. 2019;24(2):107-14.
11. Poeta M, Maglione M, Borrelli M, Santamaria F. Non-cystic fibrosis bronchiectasis in children and adolescents: Neglected and emerging issues. Pediatr Neonatol. 2020;61(3):255-62.
12. Reiff DB, Wells AU, Carr DH, Cole PJ, Hansell DM. CT findings in bronchiectasis: limited value in distinguishing between idiopathic and specific types. AJR Am J Roentgenol. 1995;165(2):261-7.

SECTION 9

Cardiology

Section Editor: *Vikas Kohli*

Management of Heart Failure in Infants and Children: An Algorithmic Approach

M Zulfikar Ahamed

INTRODUCTION

Heart failure (HF) in infancy and childhood is "a clinical syndrome which reflects the inability of the heart to pump blood to meet the metabolic requirements of the body, including those needs incurred by growth; or able to do so at a higher filling pressure". It is a complex syndrome that can result from any structural or functional disorder that can impair the ability of ventricle(s) to fill with or eject blood.

While adult HF is often due to coronary artery disease (CAD), hypertension, valvar heart diseases and cardiomyopathies, infants and children have HF primarily due to congenital heart disease (CHD), valvar heart diseases, and cardiomyopathies. Overall, 75% of HF in pediatric population is due to CHD and the rest due to acquired heart diseases. 80% of HF occurs in infants (below 1 year). While in market economies, cardiomyopathies, CHD, and postoperative CHD cause HF in that order, in India the leading causes of pediatric HF are CHD, rheumatic fever/rheumatic heart disease (RF/RHD) and cardiomyopathies.

Pathophysiologically HF can be divided into three types:

1. *Type I:* HF due to abnormal loading conditions. It can be due to preload abnormality or afterload problem. This is the most common variety of congestive heart failure (CHF) in infants.
    - *Preload: Ventricular septal defect (VSD), patent ductus arteriosus (PDA), mitral regurgitation (MR)*
    - *Afterload: AS, coarctation of aorta*
2. *Type II:* HF due to abnormality of contractility (inotropy)
    - *Dilated cardiomyopathy (DCM)*
3. *Type III:* HF due to abnormality of diastolic function (Lusitropy)
    - *Hypertrophic cardiomyopathy (HCM)*

In addition, heart rate abnormalities (very slow or fast rate) can also cause HF—complete heart block (CHB) and supraventricular tachycardia (SVT)

Type I HF:

- *L → R shunt:* VSD, PDA, aortopulmonary window (APW), atrioventricular septal defect (AVSD)
- *Admixture CHD:* Total anomalous pulmonary venous connection (TAPVC), single ventricle, double outlet right ventricle (DORV), truncus arteriosus
- *Valvar regurgitation:* MR and aortic regurgitation (AR)
- *Left ventricular outflow tract (LVOT) obstruction:* AS and coarctation of aorta (CoA)
- Rheumatic fever and carditis

Type II HF:

- Dilated cardiomyopathy (DCM)
- Myocarditis
- Postoperative CHD
- Tachycardia-associated cardiomyopathy syndrome (TACS)
- Chronic RHD with LV dysfunction

Heart failure can be caused mostly by *structural* lesions. Occasionally *functional* heart diseases can also cause HF. They could be either remediable or nonremediable **(Flowchart 1)**.

Flowchart 1: Heart failure: Causes.

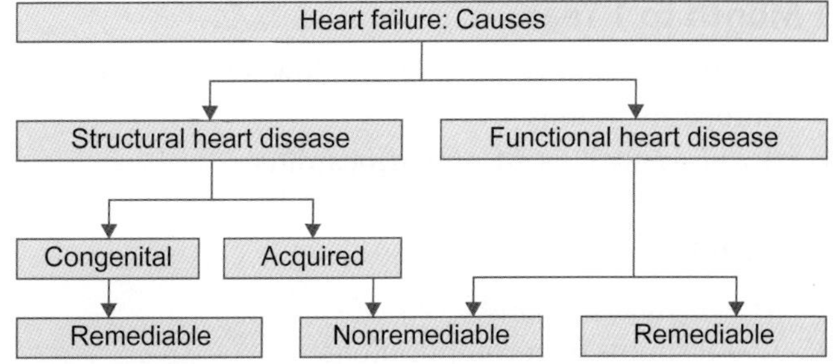

Most congenital structural heart diseases are remediable either surgically or by intervention. Many acquired heart diseases are also amenable to correction, e.g., MS and MR. Some are not—DCM and HCM. Tachycardia-associated cardiomyopathy is a remediable functional heart disease, by conversion to sinus rhythm.

CAUSES

Causes of HF in infancy and childhood have a chronological order. This phenomenon is quite useful, looking for and identifying a cause for HF in childhood.

Fetal Causes

- *CHD:* Ebstein anomaly, systemic AV fistula
- *Others:* Intrauterine myocarditis
- *Arrhythmia:* Complete heart block, SVT

Day One Causes (0–24 Hours)

- Ebstein anomaly, systemic AV fistula, absent pulmonary valve syndrome, severe MR, and myocarditis
- CHB and SVT

First Week Causes (1–7 Days)

- *Critical left heart obstruction:* AS, hypoplastic left heart syndrome (HLHS), coarctation of aorta and interrupted aortic arch
- Obstructed TAPVC
- Extension of *day one causes*

7–28 Days

- *Large L → R shunts:* VSD, PDA, and AVSD
- *Admixture lesions:* TAPVC, DORV, single ventricle, and truncus arteriosus
- *Less critical CHD:* Coarctation and AS
- *Rare defects:* Pompe, anomalous left coronary artery from the pulmonary artery (ALCAPA), and endocardial fibroelastosis (EFE)

1 Month to 1 Year

- *Left to right shunts:* PDA, AP window, VSD, and AVSD
- Admixture lesions
- *Acquired:* SVT, DCM, and myocarditis

1–6 Years

- Viral myocarditis and DCM
- L → R shunts with complications:
    - Infective endocarditis
    - Kawasaki disease

6–12 Years

- Rheumatic fever/RHD
- Infective endocarditis
- CHD—postoperative/complications
    - Viral myocarditis/DCM

MANIFESTATIONS OF HEART FAILURE

These are also *age* and *etiology* dependent. It may present as:

- *Shock:* In newborn—conditions presenting are duct-dependent left-sided critical lesions, sepsis, hypoxemic ischemic problems and arrhythmia.
- *Acute/subacute HF:* It occurs in post-tricuspid L → R shunts, obstructive lesions, admixture lesions, and cardiomyopathies.
- *Chronic HF:* It occurs due to cardiomyopathies, valvar heart disease, and moderate L → R shunts.

RECOGNITION OF HEART FAILURE IN INFANTS

Clinical recognition of HF in infancy is different from that of an older child. The classical quartet of findings are *tachycardia, tachypnea, tender hepatomegaly, and cardiomegaly.* Others are S_3 gallop, prolonged capillary refill time, and bibasal crepitation. Elevated jugular venous pressure (JVP), pedal edema, and hypotension are less common manifestations **(Fig. 1)**.

Functional assessment in an infant or child with HF will be based on the NYHA (older child) or Ross (infants) classification.

Modified Ross Classification

- *Class 1:* No symptom, no feeding difficulty, and normal growth
- *Class 2:* Tachypnea on feed, sweating on feed, and normal growth

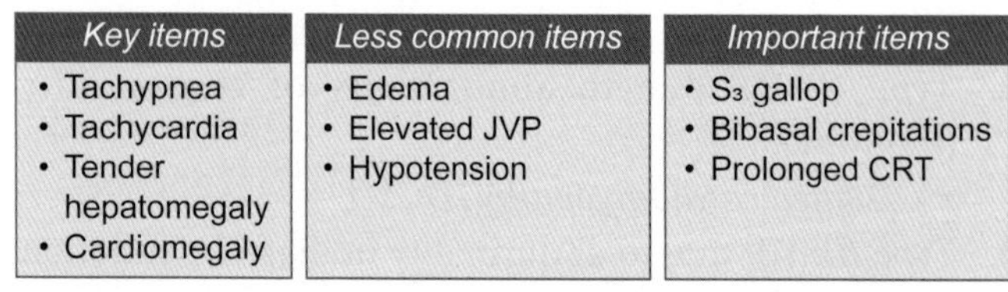

Fig. 1: Recognition of HF in infants. (HF: heart failure; CRT: capillary refill time; JVP: jugular venous pressure)

- *Class 3:* Significant tachypnea/sweating on feed, retractions at rest, and growth failure
- *Class 4:* All the above on rest also

EVALUATION

Evaluation of HF includes recognition and characterization of CHF and investigations **(Flowchart 2)**. The investigations can be either definitive or nondefinitive.

One has to decide whether HF is *acute or chronic*. Acute CHF could be either primary or decompensated. Both chronic and acute CHF can be either responsive or nonresponsive (refractory) **(Flowchart 3)**.

- *Chest X-ray* still is useful in preliminary evaluation of HF at any age. It looks at heart size, lung blood flow, presence of pulmonary arterial hypertension (PAH), and the "typical" look (e.g., figure of 8 in TAPVC). It can also sort out primary or additional lung issues.
  Practically all causes of HF in infancy will cause cardiomegaly (CTR ≥ 50% in a child, >55% in infants, and ≥60% in neonates). The exceptions could be obstructed TAPVC or cor triatriatum.
- *Electrocardiography:* A 14-lead ECG with or without a rhythm strip (lead II) is quite useful. It is a must in all forms of HF. ECG can be a pointer to a specific CHD (e.g., biventricular hypertrophy in large VSD) or characteristic of a CHD (e.g., LAD and RVH in AVSD). It can diagnose tachyarrhythmia as the cause of HF (e.g., SVT leading to "DCM" like picture) and can pick up drug toxicity (e.g., digitalis toxicity).
- *Echocardiography:* This is the most useful tool in evaluating HF in infants and children. It can virtually diagnose all structural heart lesions, both congenital and acquired. It can pick up diastolic abnormalities and hemodynamic problems such as PAH.

Flowchart 2: Evaluation of heart failure.

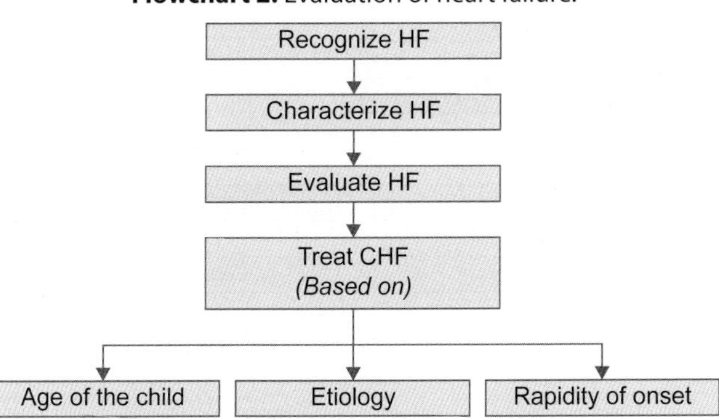

(CHF: congestive heart failure; HF: heart failure)

Flowchart 3: Acute and chronic heart failure.

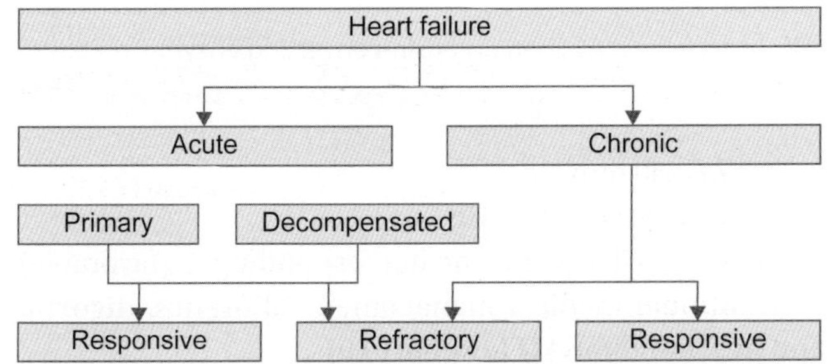

Echo:

- *Structural CHD:* Coarctation and VSD
- *Ventricular function:* DCM and myocarditis
- *PAH:* PPHN and IPAH
- *Mechanical heart disease:* Acute MR and acute AR

Others: B-type natriuretic peptide (BNP) is useful in assessing HF in infants, especially recent onset (acute). It will help in differentiating between cardiac and respiratory causes of distress. The normal value is <30 picograms/mL. An abnormal value (≥100 picograms) will indicate cardiac cause of respiratory distress with high sensitivity and specificity.

Troponins, either Trop T or Trop I, can be useful in conditions like myocarditis.

Radionuclide studies, CMR and CT, are occasionally useful in evaluating cause of CHF, especially in adult CHD—postoperative catheterization could be utilized in evaluating cause of HF and also endomyocardial biopsy **(Flowchart 4)**.

TREATMENT

Treatment of HF involves three facets:

1. Treating the cause
2. Treating the precipitating cause
3. Treating the congestive state

"Mostly causes of HF in infancy are mechanical problems which need mechanical solutions—either surgical or interventional."

Monitoring is an important factor in treating HF. We can monitor.

- Heart rate, respiratory rate, BP, capillary refill time
- Cardiomegaly, S_3, murmur, lungs
- Urine output, pulse oximetry/ABG, renal function

Drug therapy in HF in infants and children is a temporary measure which could be a short-term on long-term bridge. It is also an initial life saver. In addition,

Flowchart 4: Investigations of heart failure.

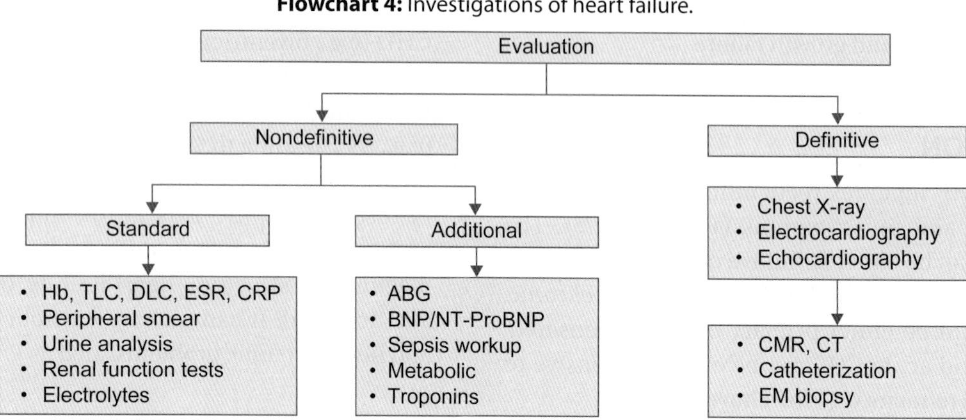

(ABG: arterial blood gas; BNP: B-type natriuretic peptide; CMR: cardiac magnetic resonance; CRP: C-reactive protein; CT: computed tomography; DLC: differential leukocyte count; ESR: erythrocyte sedimentation rate; proBNP: pro brain natriuretic peptide; EM: endomyocardial; TLC: total leukocyte count)

some drugs may eventually "correct" the abnormality, e.g., prostaglandin E1 (PGE1) or adenosine.

Management of Chronic Heart Failure/Subacute Heart Failure

It is the most common situation. It can be treated in the wards or in OPD. Initial general measures include rest, Fowler position, oxygen when indicated, correction of electrolytes and Hb abnormalities, and volume depletion.

Drug therapy primarily uses four drugs—*diuretics, digoxin, angiotensin-converting enzyme (ACE) inhibitors, and β-blockers* **(Flowcharts 5 to 7)**.

Acute Heart Failure

Acute HF can be either primary or decompensated **(Flowchart 8)**.

Management of acute HF will include admission into pediatric intensive care unit (PICU). General measures include temperature control, oxygen supply, alkali therapy, sepsis management, and metabolic correction.

Specific measures will be by using IV inotrope, IV diuretic, and IV vasodilators. Targeted therapy will be using PGEI, sildenafil, adenosine, or ibuprofen, according to indications. Additional measures will be IV access, multiorgan protection, and mechanical ventilation **(Flowchart 9)**.

Hypotension (SBP):

- *Newborn:* <60 mm Hg
- *Infant:* >70 mm Hg
- *Child:* <80 mm Hg
- *Adolescent:* <90 mm Hg

Refractory HF is the one not responding to (favorably) conventional medical management (diuretics, digoxin, and ACE inhibitors) **(Flowchart 10)**.

Flowchart 5: Heart failure scenario I.

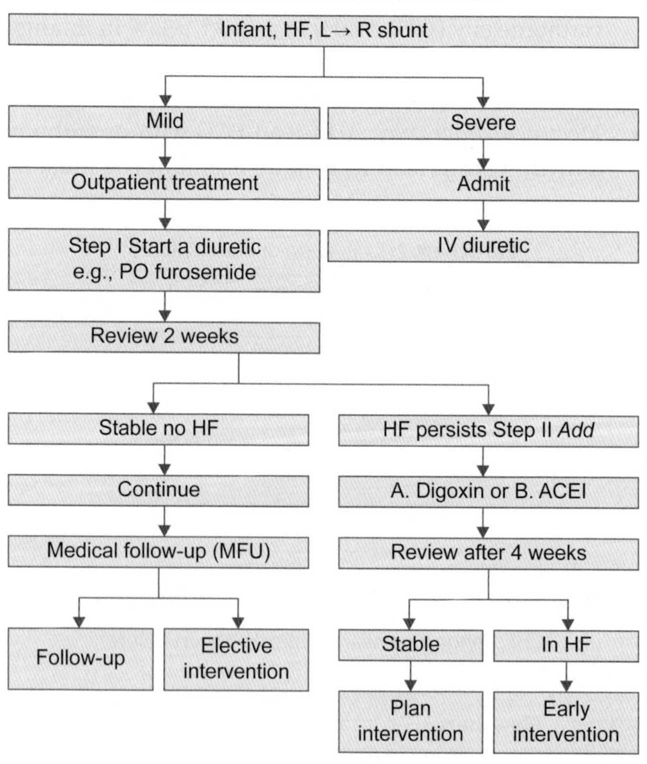

(HF: heart failure; ACEI: angiotensin-converting enzyme inhibitor)

Flowchart 6: Scenario III.

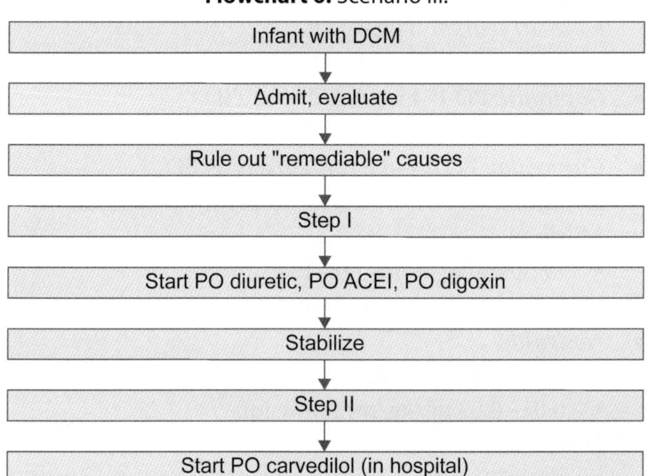

(ACEI: angiotensin-converting enzyme inhibitor; DCM: dilated cardiomyopathy)

Flowchart 7: Acute heart failure.

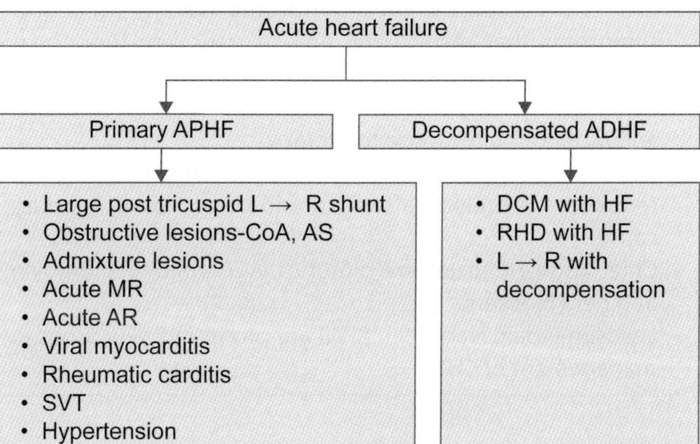

(ADHF: acute decompensated heart failure; APHF: acute primary HF; AR: aortic regurgitation; CoA: coarctation of aorta; DCM: dilated cardiomyopathy; HF: heart failure; MR: mitral regurgitation; RHD: rheumatic heart disease; SVT: supraventricular tachycardia)

Heart failure: Specific situations—

- *Newborn, HF, PPHN:* IV milrinone, IV sildenafil
- *Newborn, HF, CHB:* IV dobutamine
- *Newborn, HF, sepsis:* IV dobutamine
- *Newborn, HF, preterm PDA:* Indomethacin/ibuprofen
- *Postoperative CHD: HF, PAH:* IV milrinone, sildenafil, NO
- *Hypertensive HF:* IV NTP, IV diuretic
- *IE, acute MR:* IV NTP, IV antibiotics
- *DCM on β-blockers, HF:* IV milrinone
- *Viral myocarditis HF:* IVIG
- *Postoperative ventricular dysfunction:* ACEI

Flowchart 8: Management of acute heart failure.

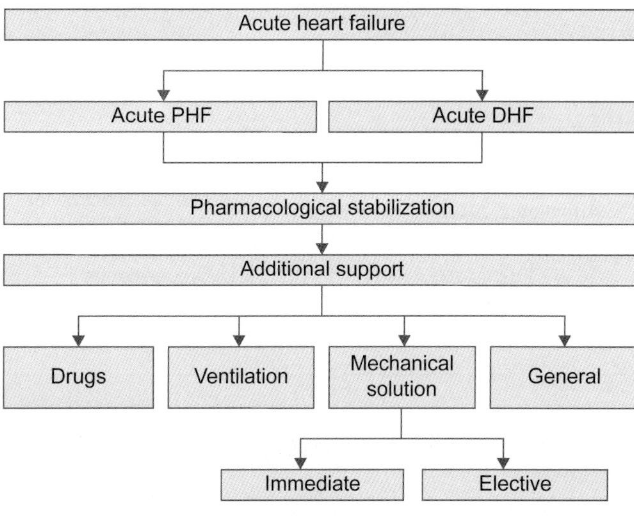

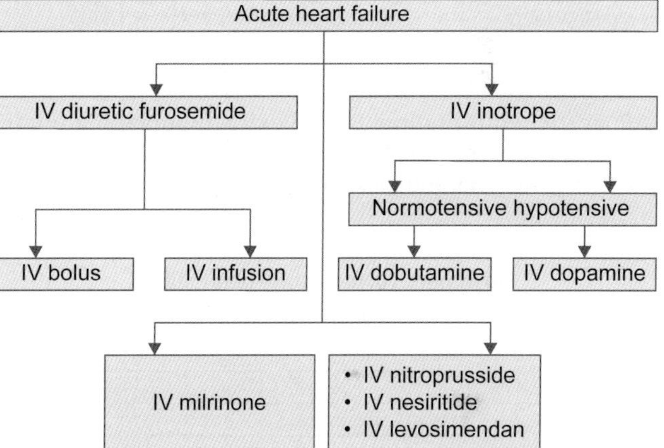

(PHF: primary heart failure; DHF: decompensated heart failure; IV: intravenous)

Two new kids in the block treating HF in children are:

1. *Ivabradine:* Situation—Child with DCM in HF. Persistent tachycardia in spite of β-blocker
   2.5–5 mg daily
2. *ARNI (ARB/neprilysin inhibitor):* Sequentially block both RAAS system and neuropeptide cleaving system
   Situation: DCM on full medication, as an alternative to ACEI
   Pediatric doses have been established.

Drugs and Doses

- *Furosemide:*
  - PO 1 mg/kg OD/BD/TID
  - IV 1 mg/kg OD/BD/TID
  - *Infusion:* 0.1–1.0 mg/kg/hour

Flowchart 9: Refractory heart failure.

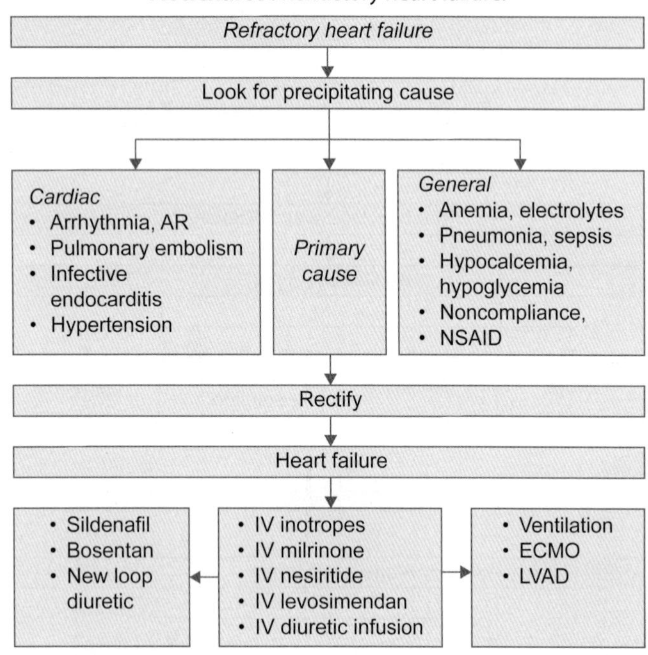

(AR: aortic regurgitation; ECMO: extracorporeal membrane oxygenation; HF: heart failure; LVAD: left ventricular assist device; NSAID: nonsteroidal anti-inflammatory drug)

Flowchart 10: Refractory heart failure.

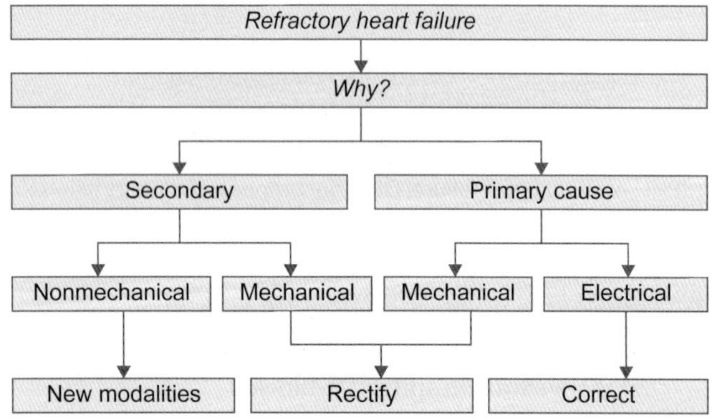

- *Torsemide:*
  - PO 0.25–0.5 mg/kg
  - IV 2.5–5 mg OD
- *Bumetanide:* PO 0.45–0.1 mg/kg BD
- *Digoxin (maintenance) PO: (Per oral)*
  - Preterm newborn: 5 µg/kg OD
  - *Term newborn:* 7.5 µg/kg OD
  - *Infant:* 10 µg/kg BD
  - *2–10 years:* 7.5 µg/kg OD
  - *≥10 years:* ½–1 tablet OD
- *Captopril:* PO 1–4 mg/kg/day as TID
- *Enalapril:* PO 0.1–0.3 mg/kg/day as OD/BD
- *Carvedilol:* PO 0.1–0.5 mg/kg/day as BD
- *Dobutamine:* IV 2–20 µg/kg/hour for 72–96 hours
- *Milrinone:*
  - IV 50 µg/kg/bolus (10–15)
  - 0.375–0.75 µg/kg/min infusion
- *Nesiritide:*
  - IV 1–2 µg/kg/bolus
  - 0.01– 0.03 µg/kg/min infusion
- *Levosimendan:*
  - IV 6–12 µg/kg/bolus
  - 0.05–0.60 µg/kg/min infusion
- *Dopamine:* IV 2–20 µg/kg/hour for 72–96 hours

KEY POINTS

- CHF is a complex clinical syndrome having signs and symptoms that result from any structural or functional impairment of ventricular filling or ejection of blood.
- Echocardiography is crucial in quantification of problems and monitoring response to therapy.
- Mainstay of treatment is improving cardiac contractility, reduction of preload/afterload and correction of primary cause.
- Chief anti-CHF drugs are diuretics, ACE inhibitors, digoxin and beta blockers.
- Levosimendan, Ivabradin, ARNI are promising new drugs in management of CHF.

SUGGESTED READING

1. Burch M. Heart failure in the young. Heart. 2002;88(2): 198-202.
2. Chaturvedi V, Saxena A. Heart failure in children: clinical aspect and management. Indian J Pediatr. 2009;76(2): 195-205.
3. Kantor PF, Lougheed J, Dancea A, McGillion M, Barbosa N, Chan C, et al. Presentation, diagnosis, and medical management of heart failure in children: Canadian Cardiovascular Society Guidelines. Can J Cardiol. 2013;29(12):1535-52.
4. Kay JD, Colan SD, Graham TP Jr. Congestive heart failure in pediatric patients. Am Heart J. 2001;142(5):923-8.
5. Opie LH, Gersh BJ. Drugs for The Heart, 7th edition. Philadelphia: Saunders; 2009.

6. Ross RD. Medical management of chronic heart failure in children. Am J Cardiovasc Drugs. 2001;1(1):37-44.
7. Shaddy RE, Penny DJ. Chronic Cardiac Failure: Physiology and Treatment in Pediatric. In: Anderson RH, Baker EJ, Penny DJ, Redington AN, Rigby ML, Wernovsky G (Eds). Cardiology, 3rd edition. London: Churchill Livingstone (Elsevier); 2010.
8. Shaddy RE, Tani LY. Chronic Heart failure on children. In: Allen HD, Driscoll DJ, Shaddy RE, Felters TF (Eds). Moss and Adams' Heart Disease in Infants, Children and Adolescents, 8th edition. Philadelphia: Lippincott Williams Wilkins; 2013.
9. Working Group on Management of Congenital Heart Diseases in India; Saxena A, Juneja R, Ramakrishnan S. Drug therapy of cardiac diseases in children. Indian Pediatr. 2009;46(4):310-38.
10. World Health Organization. 17th Expert Committee on the Selection and Use of Essential Medicines. Geneva: WHO; 2009.

Approach to Pediatric Chest Pain

Vikas Kohli, Priya Tomar

INTRODUCTION

Chest pain is not an uncommon complaint in children visiting a healthcare provider. Chest pain is chronic in one-fourth to one-third of children, 40% miss some school, 70% have activities restricted. Cardiac origin of chest pain is not the most common cause, but it is definitely one of the most serious causes. Rarely, it can be an indicator of a serious cardiac condition. Chest pain should be thoroughly assessed in presence of pain with exertion. This algorithm gives you a plan how to approach such a patient.

The evaluation should be focused on ruling out cardiac and other serious causes of chest pain. The following risk factors could point toward serious underlying causes **(Box 1 and Table 1)**.

Family history of sudden cardiac death, cardiomyopathy, or congenital heart disease (CHD) especially bicuspid aortic valve is very relevant ***(Table 2)***.

BOX 1: Causes of chest pain.

Chest wall: Commonly seen—
- *Trauma to chest:* New strenuous physical activity, peaks in 48 hours, reproducible by actions
- *Costochondritis:* Pain localized to costal cartilage, elicited by tenderness at costochondral junction. There is no joint inflammation, involves two to four joints, unilateral, and exacerbated by deep breathing.
- *Precordial catch:* Brief, sharp, sudden onset often at rest. Lasts for few seconds and exacerbated by deep breath.
- *Muscular pain:* School bag, weightlifting, and new sport
- *Breast tenderness:* During thelarche or infection/inflammation causing mastitis
- *Herpes zoster of chest wall:* Unilateral dermatome distribution, pain usually precedes skin changes
- *Slipping rib syndrome:* The medial fibrous attachments of the 8th, 9th, 10th ribs are inadequate or ruptured. Unusual cause of chest pain.

Gastric: Very common—
- *Esophagitis:* Temporal association with food intake
- Gastritis
- *Esophageal dysmotility:* Spasm or achalasia
- Strictures, foreign body, caustic ingestions
- Referred pain from abdominal trauma—Kehr's sign positive

Respiratory: Not uncommon—
- *Infections:* Pneumonia and bronchitis
- *Asthma:* Chronic history present. Exercise-induced or undertreated patient. Cough, dyspnea, and chest pain
- *Pleuritis/effusion:* Pleuritic, positional
- Pneumothorax—following pneumonia/trauma or Marfan syndrome. This should be suspected in case of unexplained tachypnea, dyspnea, or decreased breath sound.

Cardiac: Rare—
- Arrhythmias
- Coronary artery disease (anomalous coronary arteries), acute Kawasaki disease (coronary arteritis), premature atherosclerosis (e.g., dyslipidemia), congenital coronary artery aneurysm, coronary artery vasospasm (toxic ingestion as cocaine/marijuana)
- *Mitral valve prolapse:* Overdiagnosed but when present may be associated with arrhythmias also

Contd…

Contd…

- *LVOT obstruction:* Hypertrophic cardiomyopathy, aortic valvular stenosis, coarctation of aorta
- *Aortic disease:* Marfan, Turner, and Noonan syndromes
- Ruptured sinus of Valsalva aneurysm
- Myocarditis, pericarditis—infection/autoimmune
- Infective endocarditis
- Pulmonary hypertension, pulmonary valve stenosis

Hematologic:

- Sickle cell crisis
- *Chest wall or mediastinal tumors:* Fatigue, weight loss, and growing mass

Psychiatric:

- *Bulimia nervosa:* Seen in children > 12 years, eating disorder
- *Anxiety/conversion disorder:* Stressful event, other somatic complaints, insomnia
- Hyperventilation

(LVOT: left ventricular outflow tract)

TABLE 1: Diagnostic clues in history.

Pain often localized and sharp, and exacerbated by deep breath/palpation	Chest wall pain
Pain accentuated with inspiration or cough, although pain is less likely to be well-localized	Pleural (sharp and superficial)/ pulmonary pain (deep and diffuse pain)
• Midsternal or precordial pain that worsens after eating or when lying down • History of drooling or reluctance to swallow	• Esophageal pain • Esophageal foreign body
Temporal association with fever	Myocarditis, pericarditis, or pleural effusion/pneumonia
• Pressure/crushing or squeezing pain, radiation to back, jaw, left arm, or left shoulder • Association with exertion or exertional syncope	• Typical cardiac pain • Cardiac origin
Pain relieved by sitting up and leaning forward	Pericarditis
Vague, poorly localized, varying in location, and associated with other somatic complaints	Psychogenic
History of systemic inflammatory disease, malignancy, hypercoagulable state myopathy or coagulable state, myopathy or prolonged immobilization	Pulmonary embolism

TABLE 2: Risk factors for serious or life-threatening conditions.

Cardiac	*Respiratory*	*Pulmonary embolus*	*Gastric*
• First episode severe chest pain • Pain radiating to arm or back • Associated dizziness or syncope • Sudden cardiac death or arrhythmia • Kawasaki disease • Connective tissue disease	• Fever • Cough • Lethargy • Pleuritic chest pain • Chronic respiratory disease	• Immobility • Recent surgery • Hypercoagulability • Central venous catheter • Pleuritic pain • Hemoptysis	• Chest pain after vomiting • Recurrent vomiting • Odynophagia/dysphagia • Other atopic history • Epigastric pain or discomfort • Ingested foreign body • Suspected button battery ingestion

TABLE 3: Examination of child with chest pain.

General examination	• Skin and extremities for evidence of trauma, chronic disease, or dysmorphology • Xanthomas on the hands, elbows, knees, and buttocks—characteristic of familial dyslipidemia • Markers for Marfan syndrome or other connective tissue disorders
Chest wall and respiratory examination	• Signs of trauma, pectus carinatum/excavatum, costosternal swelling • Tenderness of chest wall, costochondral junction, or costosternal junction • Subcutaneous emphysema in neck area due to pneumomediastinum • *Auscultation:* Reduced breath sounds, crepts, wheeze may suggest pneumonia or asthma
CVS	• Presence of an irregular rhythm, murmur, rub, gallop, or muffled heart sounds • 4 limb BP essential if coarctation of aorta is suspected • Tachycardia, gallop rhythm, displaced point of maximal impulse, or a murmur of mitral regurgitation in myocarditis • Rub of pericarditis is best appreciated when the patient is leaning forward
Gastric	Epigastric tenderness found in gastric cause of pain

(CVS: cardiovascular system)

INVESTIGATIONS (TABLE 3)

- Chest X-ray to rule out bony issues or pleural/pericardial collections
- Echocardiography to rule out CHD, pericardial disease, or specifically aortic stenosis
- ECG to rule out ST elevation seen in pericarditis or in ischemia. Also to rule out arrhythmias

Gastrointestinal (GI) referral in case of gastrointestinal cause for chest pain should be made.

CONCLUSION

The differential diagnosis of chest pain is exhaustive. The clinician should keep in mind the broad differential diagnosis and order further investigations when the history and physical examination are not conclusive.

KEY POINTS

- Pediatric chest pain is most often of benign etiology.
- Commonest causes of chest pain are musculoskeletal, gastric or respiratory; rarely cardiac disorders.
- Goal of evaluation is to rule out serious causes and manage pain appropriately.
- Diagnostic tests may include ECG, chest X-ray, echocardiography commonly.
- Management depends on etiology, reassurance is important.

SUGGESTED READING

1. Barbut G, Needleman JP. Pediatric Chest Pain. Pediatr Rev. 2020;41(9):469-80.
2. Huang SW, Liu YK. Pediatric Chest Pain: A Review of Diagnostic Tools in the Pediatric Emergency Department. Diagnostics. 2024;14(5):526.
3. O'Meara D. Chest Pain in Children. JAMA Pediatr. 2023; 177(10):1112.
4. Pissarra R, Pereira M, Amorim R, Neto BP, Lourenço L, Santos LA. Chest pain in a pediatric emergency department: clinical assessment and management reality in a third-level Portuguese hospital. Porto Biomed J. 2022;7(3): e150.

Systemic Hypertension in Children: An Algorithmic Approach

Vikas Kohli, Priya Tomar

INTRODUCTION

Hypertension is defined as average systolic blood pressure (SBP) and/or diastolic blood pressure (DBP) that is ≥95th percentile for gender, age, and height in children or >130/80 mm Hg in adolescents; measured on ≥3 occasions.

CAUSES (TABLE 1)

- *Primary hypertension:* More common in children >6 years or those with obesity
- *Secondary hypertension:* More common <6 years age

TABLE 1: Causes of hypertension in children.

Primary causes			
• Genetic/familial • Low birth weight • Sedentary lifestyle • Obesity • Dietary habits (increased salt intake) • Smoking			
Secondary causes			
Renal: • Parenchymal lesions • Glomerulonephritis • Pyelonephritis • Reflux nephropathy • Hydronephrosis • Renal dysplasia • Polycystic kidney disease • Chronic renal failure • Renal tumor • Postrenal trauma • Systemic lupus erythematosus	*Renovascular:* • Renal artery stenosis • Fibromuscular dysplasia • Renal vein thrombosis • Umbilical artery catheter-related thrombosis • Takayasu's arteritis • Moyamoya disease	*Cardiac:* • Coarctation of the aorta *Central nervous system:* • Intracranial mass • Hemorrhage • Quadriplegia	*Endocrine:* • Hyperthyroidism • Hyperparathyroidism • Congenital adrenal hyperplasia • Cushing syndrome • Pheochromocytoma • Catecholamine excess • Neuroblastoma • Iatrogenic steroid
Transient hypertension causes			
Renal: • Post-streptococcal glomerulonephritis • Acute tubular necrosis • Postrenal transplant • Post-blood transfusion • Pyelonephritis	*Central nervous system:* • Increased intracranial pressure • Guillain–Barré syndrome • Burn • Familial dysautonomia • Stevens–Johnson syndrome • Porphyria • Poliomyelitis		*Drugs:* • Cocaine • Oral contraceptive pills • Amphetamine • Cyclosporine • Tacrolimus • Vitamin D toxicity

CLINICAL FEATURES

The children are mostly asymptomatic. Nonspecific symptoms are irritability, excessive sweating, feeding issues in small baby, and failure to thrive. Specific symptoms are:

- Features of cardiac failure
- Headache
- Vomiting
- Altered sensorium
- Convulsion
- Facial hemiparesis
- Clinical symptoms may be on the basis of system involved.

APPROACH TO PATIENT WITH HYPERTENSION

Blood Pressure Measurement

Blood pressure (BP) should be measured annually in children and adolescents ≥3 years of age and at each visit in children with risk factors.

In children <3 years, BP should be measured in presence of following risk factors:

- History of prematurity <32 week's gestation or small for gestational age, very low birth weight, other neonatal complications requiring intensive care, and umbilical artery line
- Congenital heart disease (repaired or unrepaired)
- Recurrent urinary tract infections, hematuria, or proteinuria
- Known renal disease or urologic malformations
- Family history of congenital renal disease
- Solid organ transplant
- Malignancy or bone marrow transplant
- Neurofibromatosis, tuberous sclerosis, and sickle cell disease
- Evidence of elevated intracranial pressure

Method

Neonate: In hospitalized neonate, arterial monitoring is done preferably or oscillometric method [noninvasive blood pressure (NIBP)]

Children: Cuff bladder length should encircle 80–100% of the arm circumference; width should be 40%.

- Take good history including perinatal events, systemic illness
- Anthropometry, BMI calculation
- Classify into stages as shown in **Table 2**
- Detailed physical examination **(Table 3)**
- Relevant investigations **(Table 4)**
- *Lifestyle modifications:* Decrease sedentary lifestyle for all ages. This is the main line of management for elevated BP and stage 1 hypertension.
- Age-appropriate salt intake. Reduce junk food. Follow DASH diet (dietary approaches to stop hypertension)
- Antihypertensive drugs **(Table 5)** as indicated

Indications for Antihypertensive Drug Therapy in Children

- Symptomatic hypertension
- Secondary hypertension
- Hypertensive target organ damage
- Diabetes
- Persistent hypertension despite nonpharmacologic measures

HYPERTENSIVE CRISIS

- *Hypertensive urgency:* Severe elevation in BP in absence of end organ damage
- *Hypertensive emergency:* When signs of end organ damage are present like acute left ventricular (LV) failure, acute encephalopathy or kidney failure, papilledema or elevated LFTs along with severely elevated BP.

TABLE 2: Classification of hypertension in children.

BP categories	*Children aged 1–12 years (percentile based)*	*Adolescents ≥13 years (mm Hg based)*
Normotensive	<90th centile	<120/80 mm Hg
Elevated BP (prehypertension in older classification)	≥90th percentile to <95th centile or 120/80 mm Hg to <95th centile (whichever is lower)	120/<80 to 129/<80 mm Hg
Stage 1	≥90th percentile to <95th centile + 12 mm Hg or 130/80 to 139/89 mm Hg (whichever is lower)	130/80 to 139/89 mm Hg
Stage 2	≥95th percentile + 12 mm Hg, or ≥140/90 mm Hg (whichever is lower)	≥140/90 mm Hg

Source: Adapted from AAP guidelines, 2017.

TABLE 3: Physical findings giving due to etiology of hypertension.

• Moon facies • Elfin facies • Webbing of neck	• Cushing syndrome • Williams syndrome • Turner syndrome
Pallor, edema, and growth retardation	Chronic renal failure
Webbing of neck, low hairline, widely spaced nipple	Turner syndrome
Moon facies, buffalo hump, hirsutism, truncal obesity	Cushing syndrome
Thin built	Hyperthyroidism, renal disease, pheochromocytoma
Presence of virilization	Congenital adrenal hyperplasia
Ophthalmic findings—proptosis	Hyperthyroidism
Café-au-lait spots, tubers, rashes, striae	Neurofibroma
Goiter	Thyroid
Asymmetric limb pulses, bruits	Arteritis
Weak lower limb pulses	Coarctation of aorta
Acute congestive heart failure	Acute nephritis
Adenotonsillar hypertrophy	Suggestive of sleep apnea

TABLE 4: Investigations for hypertensive child/adolescent.

First line	***Second line***	***Document target organ damage***
• Complete blood count • Blood urea nitrogen • Creatinine • Electrolytes • Urine—routine examination, culture and sensitivity • Ultrasound—kidneys, ureters, bladder	• Antineutrophil antibodies • C3, C4, antineutrophil cytoplasmic antibody • DMSA scan • Doppler scan • Urinary—VMA, catecholamine, spot urine test	• 12-lead electrocardiogram • Echocardiography evaluation • Ophthalmic evaluation • Urinary microalbuminuria
Special tests for endocrine function	***Confirmatory test***	
• Hormonal profile • Serum cortisol • Catecholamine • Renin activity • Aldosterone estimation	• Renal biopsy • MCUG • Renal arteriography • CT scan	

(DMSA: dimercaptosuccinic acid; VMA: vanillylmandelic acid; MCUG: micturating cystourethrogram)

TABLE 5: Classes of antihypertensive drugs.

Class	***Drug***	***Initial dose***	***Dose per 24 hours***
Calcium channel blockers	Amlodipine	• 0.1–0.2 mg/kg • Maximum 5 mg OD	0.6 mg/kg/day
	Nicardipine LP	0.25–0.5 mg/kg/dose BD	1–3 mg/kg/day
	Felodipine	5 mg OD	10 mg
ACE inhibitors	Enalapril	• *Newborns:* 0.05 mg/kg/dose • *Infants:* 0.05 mg/kg/dose • *Older children:* 0.08 mg/kg/dose	0.8 mg/kg/day
	Lisinopril	0.08 mg/kg	0.6 mg/kg/day

Contd...

Contd...

Class	Drug	Initial dose	Dose per 24 hours
ARBs	Losartan	0.7 mg/kg/dose	1.4 mg/kg/day
	Irbesartan	2 mg/kg/dose	• 6–12 years <35 kg • 75–150 mg/day ≥13 years • >35 kg: 150–300 mg/day OD
	Valsartan	3 mg/mL drug with liquid formulation	• *1–6 years:* 1 mg/kg/day and <4 mg/kg/day • *6–18 years:* <35 mg
Beta-blockers	Acebutolol	1.5–3 mg/kg/day	5–15 mg/kg/day OD/BD
	Propranolol	1 mg/kg/day	4 mg/kg/day
	Atenolol	0.1–1 mg/kg/day	2 mg/kg/day
Alpha- and beta-blocker	Labetalol	1–3 mg/kg/day	10–15 mg/kg/day
Alpha-blockers	Prazosin	• 0.05–0.1 mg/kg/day • Maximum 0.5 mg × 2 per day	0.5 mg/kg/day
	Clonidine	5 μg/kg/day	30 μg/kg/day
Diuretics	Hydrochlorothiazide	0.5–1 mg/kg/day	3 mg/kg/day
	Furosemide	0.5–2 mg/kg/day	6 mg/kg/day
	Spironolactone	1 mg/kg/day	3.3 mg/kg/day

(ACE: angiotensin-converting enzyme; ARB: angiotensin receptor blocker)

TABLE 6: Management strategy.

Category	Frequency of blood pressure measurement	Therapeutic lifestyle changes	Pharmacologic therapy
Normal	Recheck at next schedule physical examination	Encourage healthy diet, sleep, and physical activity	No
Elevated BP	Recheck in 6 months	Weight management, physical activity, diet management. ABPM should be ordered if available	None unless compelling indications such as chronic kidney disease, diabetes mellitus, heart failure, or left ventricular hypertrophy
Stage 1 hypertension	Recheck in 1–2 week or early if symptomatic; if persistently elevated on two occasions, evaluate or refer to source of care within 1 month	Weight management, physical activity, diet management. ABPM; if available	Initiate treatment based on indications or if compelling indications
Stage 2 hypertension	Evaluate or refer to source of care within 1 week or immediately if the patient is symptomatic	Weight management, physical activity, diet management	Initiate therapy

(ABPM: ambulatory blood pressure monitoring)

Treatment for Hypertensive Urgency and Hypertensive Emergency

Aim of treatment ***(Table 6)****:*

- Urgent reduction of blood pressure
- Reduction by 25% over the next 1 hour
- Gradual reduction to 95th percentile over the next 24 hours
- Below 90th percentile or <130/80 mm Hg achieved by 48–72 hours.

Drugs of choice:

- Intravenous labetalol—bolus 1 mg/kg/dose, infusion 2 mg/kg/h, maximum 30 μg/kg/min
- Sodium nitroprusside—0.3–8 μg/kg/min
- Nifedipine—1–2 mg/kg/hour
- Rapid acting diuretics
- Seizure control with intravenous diazepam—0.2 mg/kg

KEY POINTS

- Incidence of pediatric hypertension is increasing among children and adolescents.
- Children >3 years age visiting pediatrician should have annual BP checked.
- Primary hypertension is becoming more common owing to obesity and lifestyle changes.
- ACEi, ARBs, long-acting calcium channel blocker and thiazide diuretics are well-tolerated in children.

SUGGESTED READING

1. Flynn JT, Kaelber DC, Baker-Smith CM, Blowey D, Carroll AE, Daniels SR, et al. Subcommittee on Screening and Management of High Blood Pressure in Children. Clinical Practice Guideline for Screening and Management of High Blood Pressure in Children and Adolescents. Pediatrics. 2017;140(3):e20171904.
2. Lurbe E, Agabiti-Rosei E, Cruickshank JK, Dominiczak A, Erdine S, Hirth A, et. al. 2016 European Society of Hypertension guidelines for the management of high blood pressure in children and adolescents. J Hypertens. 2016;34(10):1887-920.
3. Göknar N, Çalışkan S. New guidelines for the diagnosis, evaluation, and treatment of pediatric hypertension. Turk Pediatri Ars. 2020;55(1):11-22.
4. Raina R, Mahajan Z, Sharma A, Chakraborty R, Mahajan S, Sethi SK, et al. Hypertensive crisis in pediatric patients: an overview. Front Pediatr. 2020;8: 588911.

Follow-up of a Postoperative Child: Pediatrician's Perspective

Vikas Kohli

INTRODUCTION

Children after cardiac intervention procedures and cardiac surgery are under care of their pediatricians. Common concerns are discussed here.

GENERAL CARE

- *General hygiene and isolation:* Parents are always counseled regarding respiratory hygiene. The emphasis on hand washing and separation from other family member especially small children ensures the avoidance of chest infection or skin infection.
- *Fever and cough:* Any fever of >100°F always needs evaluation. If cause of fever is obvious, such as dehydration, upper respiratory tract infection (URTI), and gastroenteritis then can be treated accordingly or else further investigation in form of white blood cell (WBC) count, C-reactive protein (CRP), chest X-ray, or urine examination may be required for localizing the focus of infection. Mild cough with clear expectoration is not uncommon after heart surgery. But persistent or cough with fever, crepitation's, increased rate, and/or work of breathing needs attention.
- *Feeding:* Feeding and eating advice are no different from routine care. Adequate intake has to be maintained especially in the care of a small baby.

WOUND CARE

- *Dressing:* The children discharged after 5–7 days of surgery, need dressing change once in 2–3 days.
- *Discharge:* Any redness, swelling, discharge, or opening of the wound is signs that need reporting to cardiac unit.
- *Sutures:* The skin sutures used to close sternotomy and thoracotomy wound are dissolvable and do not need removal. The sutures used to close the drain sites need removal at first follow-up visit.
- *Scar:* The nature of skin scar after surgery depends on individual propensity of scaring. The scar can be a thin white line or to large with keloid. Some children have lot of itching and warmth over scar tissue; they can be advised calamine lotion or coconut oil along with cotton clothing to decrease friction and avoidance of direct sun exposure.

PAIN RELIEF

Most of the children at the time of discharge are on round the clock or as per need base pain medications. In case of the child having more pain or excessive crying, non-steroidal anti-inflammatory drug (NSAID) combination can be used. Parents of infants and toddlers are always counseled regarding holding the baby. For the first 2 weeks after surgery, they should avoid picking the baby from under the arms, so that rib cage issues do not aggravate the pain.

INITIAL FOLLOW-UP

Most of the children are called for follow-up couple of days after discharge and then 5–7 days later. At this visit, child is assessed for cardiac status, any deterioration in respiratory issues, medication adjustment, weight gain and any signs of infection, adequacy of oral intake, and the status of wound. Stitches are removed, if any present, analgesics are discontinued and cardiac medicines are adjusted as needed.

FOLLOW-UP

- *Corrective surgeries:* If no significant issues are noted during the initial follow-up, the further follow-up are planned after 3–6 months depending on institutional policy. After that usually annual follow-up is required; subsequent to adolescence the follow-up is usually decreased to 2 yearly and then to 5 yearly.

- *Palliative surgeries:* These include children who have undergone Blalock–Taussig (BT) shunts or single ventricle palliation. These children require close follow-up along with oxygen saturation monitoring.

MEDICATIONS

- *Antibiotics:* Not infrequently, children are discharged on antibiotics for non-bloodstream infection.
- *Diuretics and vasodilators:* After cardiac surgeries children are frequently discharged on diuretics which are usually stopped by 4–6 weeks. Angiotensin-converting enzyme (ACE) inhibitor, ARB and beta-blockers are given to some children for remodeling of ventricles usually which are stopped by 3–6 months.
- *Aspirin and INR drugs:* The patients of BT shunt and those with the suture lines exposed to systemic circulation are sent home on aspirin. Whereas aspirin is stopped after 3–6 months in later case, it is continued throughout the duration of BT shunt or Glenn shunt. Patients with artificial conduit and prosthetic valve remain on anticoagulants (warfarin or nicoumalone) for lifetime. The INR should be monitored and adjusted by the cardiac unit only, although bleeding complication may need immediate attention.

VACCINATIONS

Variation in Vaccination after Heart Surgery

Factors that should be considered before immunization before surgery:

- *In general, vaccination can be started 6 weeks post-surgery.*
- Most open heart surgeries [ventricular septal defect (VSD) closure and tetralogy of Fallot (ToF)] will require high-dose methylprednisolone to be given at the time of anesthesia prior to cardiopulmonary bypass. This attenuates the live vaccine responses for 6 weeks.
- DPT or DPaT can cause fever within days of administration.
- Rash and fever can cause by vaccine such as measles or measles, mumps, and rubella (MMR) as late as 2 weeks and by varicella vaccine as late as 4 weeks.
- Blood product administration can interfere with the antibody response to live-attenuated vaccine like measles, rubella and varicella, so should not be given within 6 weeks of cardiac surgery, else repeat dose will be required later.
- Oral polio vaccine (OPV) should be avoided in hospital inpatients.

CLINICAL PEARLS

Vaccination plan before surgery:
- No vaccine in the week preceding surgery.
- No measles, rubella, or varicella vaccine in 6 weeks prior to surgery as the immune response may be decreased (due to high-dose steroids given during surgery).

Factors that should be considered related to immunization before surgery:

- According to CDC "general recommendations on immunization", blood products can interfere with antibody response to measles, rubella, and varicella vaccine for 3–6 months so these vaccinations should be delayed at least by 3 months. Vaccines Ty21a typhoid, yellow fever, live-attenuated influenza vaccine (LAIV), zoster, and rotavirus vaccines may be administered at any time before, concurrent with, or after administration of any blood or immune product.
- The chance of a vaccine associated fever complicating postoperative management.

CLINICAL PEARLS

Vaccination plan after surgery:
- No vaccine for first 4–6 weeks.
- No measles, rubella, or varicella for 3 months.

- *Additional vaccine:* Children with corrected or uncorrected congenital heart diseases (CHDs) are higher risk for lower respiratory tract infection (LRTI), should be considered for pneumococcal and influenza vaccine at appropriate time. Influenza vaccine is a must for all patients on aspirin.

DENTAL PROCEDURE

- No dental cleanings or scheduled surgeries for 3 months after heart surgery
- Between 3 and 6 months after surgery, antibiotics should be taken before any dental procedures.

ACTIVITY

Infants

- Baby can sleep on back and sides from beginning and also prone after skin healing (2–3 weeks).
- Bath can be given without a soiling wound during the first week, and all over after with soft soap.

Children

- Should not be send to daycare or school for first 2–3 weeks.
- Swimming can be allowed (if no other contraindication) to private pool after 4 weeks and to the public pool and sea after 6 weeks.
- Games, or bike riding can be allowed after 6 weeks, although contact sports should be avoided for up to 3–6 months in most cases and forever when on anticoagulants.
- Lifting weight, backpack, or items >10 pound should be avoided for 6 weeks.

Young Adults

Similar to children except can be given more leverage on weight up to 10 kg.

AIR TRAVEL

Air travel is usually safe after 2–3 weeks except few contraindications such as severe pulmonary arterial hypertension, saturations <80%, and significant ventricle dysfunction. Children with pacemakers and ICD have different security check guidelines, which need to be followed.

INFECTIVE ENDOCARDITIS PROPHYLAXIS

- For palliative shunts and conduits
- Completely repaired congenital heart defect with prosthetic material or device, whether placed by surgery or by catheter intervention, during the first 6 months after the procedure.
- Repaired CHD with residual defects at the site or adjacent to the site of a prosthetic patch or prosthetic device (which inhibit endothelialization).

NEXT CHILD

- *Counseling of genetic studies:* Counseling for 22q-screening in families with children with heart disease, e.g., ToF, truncus, and interrupted aortic arch.
- *Fetal echo:* It should be done in all the subsequent pregnancies after a child with heart disease is born. There is a three times increased risk of heart disease in next child.

KEY POINTS

- No vaccine for first 4–6 weeks. No measles, rubella, or varicella for 3 months.
- No dental cleanings or scheduled surgeries for 3 months after heart surgery.
- Between 3 and 6 months after surgery, antibiotics should be taken before any dental procedures.
- Should not be sent to daycare or school for the first 2–3 weeks.

SUGGESTED READING

1. Gupta AK, Singh VK, Varma A. Approach to postoperative fever in pediatric cardiac patients. Ann Pediatr Cardiol. 2012;5(1):61-8.
2. Harvey KA, Kovalesky A. Post-operative pain and comfort in children after heart surgery: a comparison of nurses and families pre-operative expectations. J Pediatr Nurs. 2018;43:9-15.

SECTION 10

Gastroenterology

Section Editors: *Aathira Ravindranath, Anupam Sibal*

Chronic Diarrhea in Children Less than 3 Years of Age

Moinak S Sarma, Surender K Yachha

INTRODUCTION

This topic will address only the relatively common causes of chronic diarrhea in children <3 years of age that are of practical importance to the physician and also the emerging entities that are often missed. Management of persistent diarrhea is beyond the scope of this chapter.

Chronic diarrheas may arise from intestinal diseases (small or large bowel), pancreatic, hepatobiliary, or systemic causes. Their differentiation is elaborated in the next chapter "Chronic Diarrhea in Children More than 3 Years of Age".

Gastrointestinal (GI) and systemic causes of chronic diarrhea in children across all ages are shown in **Figures 1 and 2** and **Box 1**.

DEFINITIONS

Before embarking upon the details of this topic, a few clarifications regarding the terminologies used in diarrhea need to be understood.

While describing diarrhea of a fairly large duration, the terms "chronic", "persistent", "protracted", and "intractable" are loosely interchanged in literature and creates confusion in the minds of the pediatricians.

Chronic Diarrhea

Chronic diarrhea is defined as an insidious onset diarrhea of >2 weeks duration in children rarely leading to dehydration with a wide range of underlying structural

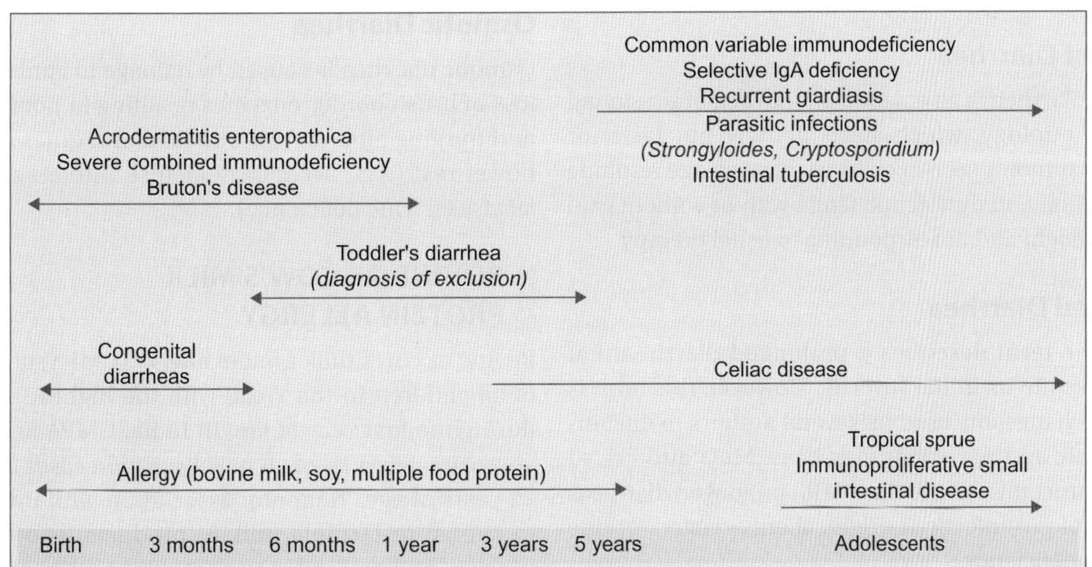

Fig. 1: Timeline showing onset of the age-specific presentations of the major causes of chronic diarrhea. (IgA: immunoglobulin A)

Across All Age Groups

- *HIV:* Opportunistic infections and enteropathy
- Intestinal lymphangiectasia
- Inflammatory bowel disease (including very early onset)
- Eosinophilic gastroenteritis and colitis
- *Pancreatic insufficiency:* Cystic fibrosis; Schwachmann-Diamond synd
- Short bowel syndrome
- *Anatomical causes:* Malrotation of gut, duodenocolic fistulae
- Autoimmune enteropathy
- Small intestinal bacterial overgrowth syndrome (diagnosis of exclusion)

Birth 3 months 6 months 1 year 3 years 5 years Adolescents

Fig. 2: Causes of chronic diarrhea that may present at any age. (HIV: human immunodeficiency virus)

BOX 1: Systemic causes of chronic diarrhea that may present at any age.

Systemic causes across all ages:
- Nephrotic syndrome
- *Drugs:* Laxatives, antacids, and antineoplastic
- Endocrinal causes, e.g., Addison's disease and hypoparathyroidism
- Neuroblastoma and ganglioneuroblastoma
- Constrictive pericarditis and restrictive cardiomyopathy (causing secondary lymphangiectasia)

or chronic inflammatory causes (acquired or congenital) causing malabsorptive or maldigestive states.

Persistent Diarrhea

Persistent diarrhea is an episode of diarrhea of presumed infectious etiology, which starts acutely but lasts for >14 days commonly seen in children <2 years age resulting in dehydration and dyselectrolytemia with or without gain or loss in weight and not responding to usual therapy.

Protracted Diarrhea

Usually, the term describes a prolonged diarrhea that resolves despite its initial severity. However, this term is often interchangeably used by several authors to encompass chronic and persistent diarrheas. Most authors, at present, restrict this term to those with prolonged diarrheas in infancy of postinfectious origin, allergy-related, or due to immunodeficiency.

Intractable Diarrhea

Prolonged diarrhea of >2 weeks occurring in infants <3 months of age. The term is used to describe a specific group of severe diarrheas of congenital nature that persist despite bowel rest and often require total parenteral nutrition for survival. This is a distinct entity and has been briefly discussed here.

Secretory Diarrhea

Secretory diarrhea refers to a diarrhea with profound losses of water and electrolytes in stools that persists despite bowel rest. It occurs due to sodium pump failures at the enterocyte as a result of toxins, drugs, bile acid, inflammatory cytokines or various mediators (e.g., bile acid diarrhea and neuroblastoma).

Osmotic Diarrhea

Osmotic diarrhea is caused by damage to epithelium and loss of brush border enzymes resulting in poor tolerance and purging after an osmotic load and quiescence with bowel rest (e.g., secondary lactose intolerance due to lactase enzyme deficiency).

BOVINE OR COW'S MILK PROTEIN ALLERGY

Bovine or cow's milk protein allergy (CMPA) affects 2–5% of all children in the West, with the highest prevalence during the first year of life. In India, CMPA accounts for approximately 13% of all malabsorption cases in children <2 years of age. Temporal association with introduction to animal or formula milk (± products) is often noted. Wheeze, eczema, and atopy (20–30%) with similar history in family members (10%) may be associated. Nearly 50% children outgrow the allergy by 1 year and approximately 90% by 5 years of age. It is the most common food allergy in small children who are top fed.

There are two kinds of reactions to cow's milk:

1. *Immediate [immunoglobulin E (IgE) mediated]:* It occurs within minutes of milk intake and is characterized by anaphylaxis-like features such as vomiting, pallor, shock-like state, urticaria, and swelling of lips seen in 10–20% cases.
2. *Delayed (T-cell, non-IgE mediated):* It has an indolent course and presents mainly with GI symptoms. This is more common in India and seen in 80–90% of cases.

Symptoms

The most common presentation is diarrhea with blood and mucus. Depending upon the site and extent of involvement, the child may have small bowel, large bowel, or mixed type diarrhea. Diarrhea and colitis is seen in 80% cases. They may have iron deficiency anemia and failure to thrive rarely as a clinical manifestation (especially those presenting as predominant small bowel diarrhea).

Diagnosis

Gold standard for diagnosis is double blind placebo controlled food challenge, but it is cumbersome to execute. A simpler yet conclusive way in India is to document the disease by the following methods:

- *Flexible proctosigmoidoscopy:* Aphthous ulcers (80% cases)
- *Rectal biopsy:* More than six eosinophils per high power field + eosinophilic cryptitis (97% cases)
- Symptom resolution after withdrawal of animal milk or milk products (including formula feeds).

The new European Society of Pediatric Gastroenterology, Hepatology, and Nutrition, 2012 guidelines recommend the following:

- *Non-IgE mediated CMPA:* A response to a trial of elimination diet for 2–4 weeks, followed by relapse of symptoms in next 2 weeks of oral challenge with cow's milk protein diagnoses the condition without any biopsy. Thereafter a therapeutic elimination diet is given
- *IgE-mediated disease:* CMP-specific IgE and skin-prick tests. However these tests are not reliable in India due to lack of standardized laboratories.

These recommendations reserve rectal biopsy and histopathology in scenarios of diagnostic dilemma, complicated disease, and nonresponse to elimination diet.

Treatment

All animal milk/milk products have to be eliminated from the diet. Breast milk should be continued. Calcium supplementation is mandatory as milk that has been withdrawn is a rich source of calcium. Explaining the natural history of the disease to parents, counseling, vigilance, and compliance are the cornerstones.

Child Less than 4 Months of Age

An exclusive extensively hydrolyzed formulation (EHF) is prescribed at this age group. In case of nonresponse to EHF (10%), severe symptoms, or anaphylaxis (IgE mediated), an elemental (amino acid formula) is used. Soy formulations in infants <6 months of age are not recommended in the West (the European Society of Pediatric Gastroenterology, Hepatology, and Nutrition and the American Academy of Pediatrics). Concomitant soy allergy is seen in 10–15% due to allergens (conglycinin and glycinin). Other problems with soy are high amounts of phytoestrogens that may interfere with neuroendocrine functions, high phytates that limit zinc, iodine, and iron absorption, and, manufacturing related aluminum contamination. If EHF or elemental formulae are not available or affordable, then the physician may be compelled to prescribe a noncasein-based soy formulation. Breastfeeding always should be continued. In very rare circumstances, where transmission of antigen is suspected through breast milk, mother's milk ingestion can be discontinued with supplementation of calcium.

Child More than 4 Months of Age

Formula feeds, animal milk, and milk products are stopped. Children >4 months of age are at an appropriate age for weaning and hence, dietary supplementation with cereals and pulses (region specific) is started. Rice gruel which is relatively hypoallergenic may be tried. If the child is >6 months of age, then, soy formulae can be permitted. **Flowchart 1** outlines the management of CMPA.

SECONDARY LACTOSE INTOLERANCE

This condition is commonly seen as a cause of persistent diarrhea (secondary to viral gastroenteritis). However, it may be associated with underlying chronic diarrhea (celiac disease, Crohn's disease, and giardiasis) due to villous atrophy and secondary deficiency of brush border enzymes (including lactase). It manifests as explosive

Flowchart 1: Approach and management of food protein allergy.

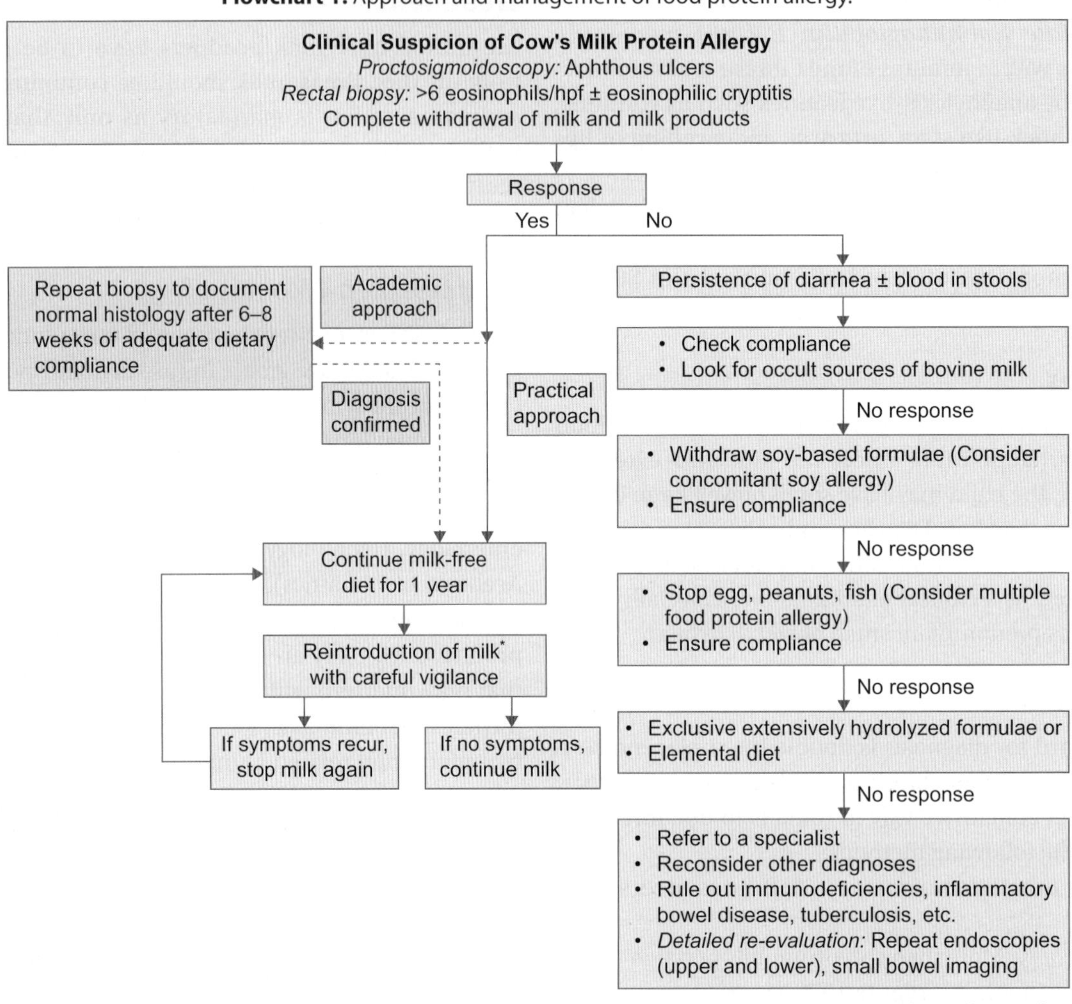

#In an academic setting, biopsy is repeated twice after initial milk withdrawal. First assessment is at 6–8 weeks as shown above to confirm normalization of histology. Second assessment is at 48 hours of reintroduction of milk to decide whether it is safe to continue milk or not by: (1) clinical symptoms and (2) histologic changes. Milk-free diet is continued if symptoms or histological changes reappear. If histology is normal and symptoms do not reappear, then, child can be continued on milk. However, in practical setting, both the repeat biopsies are not feasible due to the cumbersome process.

**Reintroduction of milk:* Child is given 10 mL/kg cow's milk (0.3 g/kg milk protein) initially and watched for 1 hour. If there are no adverse events, then, 20 mL/kg cow's milk is given again watched for another 1 hour. If there are no symptoms, such as diarrhea, vomiting, etc., then, normal milk feeding is continued.

(gaseous and noisy) stools and perianal excoriation that resolves on lactose-free diet. Persistent diarrhea causes damage to enterocyte and causes deficiency of the lactase enzyme located at the top of brush border epithelium. Hence, lactose is not broken down to glucose and galactose. Unabsorbed dietary lactose delivered to colon is converted to hydrogen and lactic acid by colonic bacteria. Lactic acid results in decreased stool pH, hydrogen gives explosive stool, and unabsorbed lactose gives positive reducing substances if tested. Lactose increased the osmolality (osmotic diarrhea). Fungal infection of the perineum in fungal diarrhea may mimic secondary lactose intolerance. In fungal infections, there are curdy white, satellite lesions and extension into the genitalia and groin flexures.

Confirmation is not required if stools are explosive and perianal area is excoriated. In doubtful cases, the diagnosis is confirmed by stool pH <6.0 and reducing substances >0.5%. Withdrawal of lactose containing milk for 3 weeks is the mainstay of treatment. Perianal area is managed by nursing on soft cloth, avoiding diapers, maintaining proper hygiene, and applying local emollients (coconut oil and liquid paraffin zinc oxide).

IMMUNODEFICIENCY STATES

Common presenting features and brief management of immunodeficiency has been discussed in detail in the next chapter. Additionally, there are few more immunodeficiency states with GI manifestations that are seen in younger children.

X-linked Agammaglobulinemia

- Onset after 6 months of age
- Chronic rotavirus infection
- Absent tonsils
- Panhypogammaglobulinemia + B-cells <1%. Normal T-cells.

Severe Combined Immunodeficiency

- Onset in first few months
- Cytomegalovirus colitis and mucocutaneous candidiasis
- Absent tonsils
- Leukopenia, hypogammaglobulinemia, absent T-cells ± B-cells

In both the groups, most children die by 1–2 years of age, if untreated. Treatment is specific; antimicrobials and intravenous immunoglobulin 400–600 mg/kg to tide over the crisis. Allogenic bone marrow transplantation is curative.

VERY EARLY ONSET INFLAMMATORY BOWEL DISEASE

Very early onset inflammatory bowel disease (VEO-IBD) is defined as IBD starting <2 years age. This comprises of <5% of all pediatric IBD and requires detailed immunological workup for immunodeficiencies of monogenic inheritance. Some of the notable genetic defects associated with the infantile onset IBD are interleukin-10 (IL-10), IL-10 receptor A, IL-10 receptor B, ADAM-17, XIAP, TTC7A (apoptotic enterocolitis), immune dysregulation, polyendocrinopathy, enteropathy, X-linked (IPEX) syndrome, atypical severe combined immunodeficiency (Omenn syndrome), Wiskott–Aldrich syndrome, agammaglobulinemia, hyper IgM syndrome, common variable immunodeficiency (CVID), and chronic granulomatous disease. These diseases are primary immunodeficiencies which manifest as recurrent infections and IBD. Setting to suspect monogenic IBD is shown in **Table 1**. The very early onset, infantile, and neonatal IBD have marked poor prognosis. They have severe course, fistulizing disease, resistance to biological therapy and often require colectomy or colonic diversion. Allogeneic hematopoietic stem cell transplants (HSCTs) have shown to produce 80% remission in those who do not respond to standard therapy. Due to the significant risk associated with HSCT, including graft-versus-host disease and severe infections, it is important to determine the genetic basis for each patient's VEO-IBD before selecting HSCT as a treatment approach.

TABLE 1: Settings to suspect monogenic IBD (one or more features).

Feature	*Comment*
Very early onset of symptoms	Most commonly <2 years age
Family history	• Consanguinity, sib death, and affected sib or multiple family members • Known immunodeficiency state in family
Atypical endoscopy or histology	Apoptotic enterocolitis, unusual and coalescent pattern of ulcers
Resistance to conventional therapies	Failure of response to steroids, immunomodulators, and biological therapy
Ectodermal defects	Skin lesions (epidermolysis bullosa and eczema), nail dystrophy, and hair abnormalities (wooly hair and trichorrhexis nodosa)
Early onset perianal disease	Deep-fistula (mucocutaneous and rectogenitourinary) and abscess
Reticuloendothelial abnormalities	Lymph node abscesses, splenomegaly, and cyclical neutropenia
Recurrent infections or unexplained fever	Deep seated infections, atypical infections (intestinal or nonintestinal), and multisystemic life-threatening infections
Hemophagocytic lymphohistiocytosis	Induced by Epstein–Barr virus or cytomegalovirus
Associated autoimmunity	Arthritis, serositis, thyroiditis, and type 1 diabetes
Early onset tumors	Non-Hodgkin's lymphoma and hamartomas

NONSPECIFIC OR TODDLER'S DIARRHEA

This is a diagnosis of exclusion and contributes to 16% of all chronic diarrheas in preschool children. It is seen usually in thriving children of 6–20 months of age and spontaneously resolves by 3 years of age in majority. The diarrhea worsens with high osmolar feeds, e.g., juices, nectar fruits (grapes, melons, etc.). Occasionally, undigested food particles are seen in stool. No nocturnal symptoms or red flags are associated. The family history of irritable bowel syndrome may be present. Normal anthropometry and absence of anemia differentiate this condition from common conditions such as celiac disease and CMPA. Treatment consists of reassurance, high fat, and high fiber diet with reduced intake of juices. Antimotility agents should not be prescribed.

Celiac disease and intestinal lymphangiectasia are discussed in detail in next chapter.

Box 2 shows brief clinical pointers and management of other pertinent causes of chronic diarrheas in children <3 years of age.

INTRACTABLE DIARRHEA OF INFANCY

These are very rare causes of chronic diarrhea that are of congenital nature, severe in their course, often dependent on parenteral nutrition and most requiring small bowel transplant.

Setting to Suspect Intractable Diarrhea of Infancy

- Dehydrating diarrhea in an infant beginning in neonatal period or <3 months of age and
- Prolongation of diarrhea beyond 2 weeks despite extensive hospital therapy with one or more of the following:
  - At least three negative stool cultures for bacterial pathogen
  - Family history of consanguinity, sibling death, or polyhydramnios
  - Associated dysmorphism or systemic features
  - Common conditions such as food protein allergy, intestinal lymphangiectasia, and antibiotic-associated diarrhea ruled out
  - No response to empirical elemental diet

Common causes of intractable diarrhea of infancy (IDI) with their salient features are shown in **Table 2**. Brief approach to IDI is shown in **Flowchart 2**.

Except congenital alactasia which has favorable prognosis with absolute restriction of lactose in diet, the rest of the disorders have no definitive treatment; often require lifelong parenteral nutrition or small bowel transplant. IDI patients have very high mortality.

BOX 2: Salient features and management of common causes of chronic diarrhea in children <3 years of age.

- *Short gut syndrome:*
  - History of intestinal resection for small bowel obstruction or necrotizing enterocolitis in infancy
  - *Functional definition:* Massive small bowel resection >75% or dependence on parenteral nutrition for >6 weeks
  - Symptoms occur when >150 cm small bowel + no colon
  - <70 cm small bowel + intact colon (older children/adults)
  - Long-term total parenteral nutrition requirement
  - *Treatment:* Small bowel lengthening surgeries or small bowel transplant
  - Loperamide can be selectively used to slow the small bowel transit time
- *Anatomical defects:*
  - *Duodenocolic fistula or small bowel fistulas:*
    - May be idiopathic or secondary to inflammatory conditions, e.g., IBD and TB
    - Passage of undigested food particles soon after intake
    - Fistulous tract delineated by barium studies
    - Duodenocolic fistulous openings seen on UGIE ± colonoscopy
  - *Malrotation:* Bacterial overgrowth and secondary lymphangiectasia
- *Acrodermatitis enteropathica:*
  - May be primary (symptoms after weaning) or secondary to persistent diarrhea
  - Eczematous exfoliative rash in perioral, and perianal areas and extremities
  - Associated alopecia and sinopulmonary infections
  - Oral supplementation of 2–3 mg/kg or 50–150 mg zinc sulfate or gluconate daily

Contd...

Contd...

- *Shwachman–Diamond syndrome:*
  - Exocrine pancreatic insufficiency (steatorrhea) beginning in infancy
  - Cyclical neutropenia with risk of recurrent bacterial infections ± thrombocytopenia
  - Dental and skeletal abnormalities including short stature
  - Transient hepatomegaly ± transaminitis till 5 years of age
  - *Diagnosis:* Abnormal pancreatic function tests, cyclical neutropenia, hypoplastic pancreas on computed tomography, and genetic testing for abnormal Shwachman–Bodian–Diamond syndrome gene
  - *Treatment:* Enzyme supplements, granulocyte colony-stimulating factor, and regular skeletal monitoring
- *Hirschsprung enterocolitis:*
  - Explosive diarrhea or colitis in a background history of constipation from birth or after pull through surgery for Hirschsprung disease
  - History of delayed passage of meconium. Distension, tenderness, fever, and shock
  - *Erect X-ray abdomen:* Intestinal cut-off sign
  - In the setting of enterocolitis, barium enema is also contraindicated for the risk of perforation
  - *Treatment:* Intravenous antibiotics, rectal irrigation (saline washes). Colonic decompression (diversion colostomy) in severe cases

- *Hirschsprung enterocolitis:*
  - Explosive diarrhea or colitis in a background history of constipation from birth or after pull through surgery for Hirschsprung disease
  - History of delayed passage of meconium. Distension, tenderness, fever, and shock
  - *Erect X-ray abdomen:* Intestinal cut-off sign
  - In the setting of enterocolitis, barium enema is also contraindicated for the risk of perforation
  - *Treatment:* Intravenous antibiotics, rectal irrigation (saline washes). Colonic decompression (diversion colostomy) in severe cases

- *Wolman disease:*
  - Stormy neonatal course in first 2 weeks of life, rapid deterioration, and death within 6 months
  - Associated with hepatosplenomegaly, liver failure, and intractable ascites
  - Consanguinity and sibling death
  - Bilateral adrenal calcification on abdominal imaging and foamy histiocytes on bone marrow studies
  - *Enzymatic studies:* Deficient lysosomal acid lipase in white blood cells and fibroblasts
  - Corticosteroids for adrenal insufficiency
  - Bone marrow transplant may not be useful in all cases
- *Abetalipoproteinemia:*
  - Diarrhea begins within the first year of life, worsens with a high fat diet, and some improvement is noted when a patient learns dietary aversion
  - Neurologic symptoms (ataxia, areflexia, loss of vibration, and position) appear after first decade
  - Retinitis pigmentosa seen in adulthood
  - Absence of chylomicron, low density lipoprotein and very low-density lipoprotein in plasma (fasting lipid profile)
  - Hemolytic anemia and acanthocytosis in peripheral smear
  - *UGIE (fat loading):* White duodenal mucosa
  - *Small bowel histology:* Lipid droplet filled enterocytes at villus tips
  - *Treatment:* Restricted fat intake with supplementation of all fat-soluble vitamins. High-dose vitamin E (1,000–2,000 mg/day)

(IBD: inflammatory bowel disease; TB: tuberculosis; UGIE: upper gastrointestinal endoscopy)

TABLE 2: Common causes of intractable diarrhea of infancy and their characteristic features.

Condition	***Characteristic features***
Congenital sodium diarrhea	• Elevated levels of fecal Na^+ and HCO_3^- • Antenatal polyhydramnios
Congenital chloride diarrhea	• Elevated levels of fecal Cl^- (>90 mmol/L) • Antenatal polyhydramnios
Microvillous inclusion disease	Absent microvilli with inclusions in enterocytes
Tufting enteropathy	• Epithelium of villi arranged in "tufts" • Associated with choanal, esophageal, or anal atresia

Contd...

Contd...

Condition	*Characteristic features*
• Autoimmune enteropathy • Part of immune dysregulation, polyendocrinopathy, enteropathy, X-linked (IPEX) syndrome	• Eczema, type I diabetes mellitus, and polyendocrinopathy • High serum immunoglobulin E and anti-enterocyte antibody positive
Syndromic diarrhea	Facial dysmorphism, trichorrhexis nodosa (woolly hair), immunodeficiency, and cirrhosis of liver
Congenital alactasia (primary lactase deficiency)	• Improvement on lactose-free diet • Deficient lactase activity in a duodenal or jejunal biopsy when the other disaccharidases are normal
Glucose-galactose malabsorption	• Elimination of glucose and galactose (and lactose) from the diet results in the complete resolution of diarrhea • Diagnosis of exclusion

Flowchart 2: Approach to intractable diarrhea of infancy.

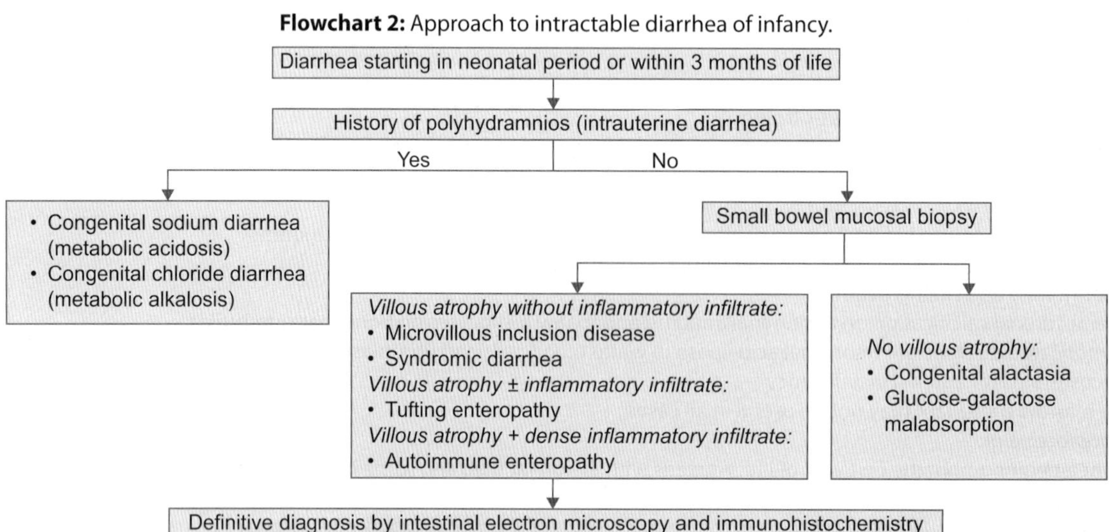

CLINICAL PEARLS

- *Relatively thriving child with colitis:* Think of bovine (cow's) milk protein allergy.
- *Severe colitis with failure to thrive not responding to milk-free, soy-free, hydrolyzed, or elemental diet:* Think of infantile IBD.
- *Small bowel diarrhea + perianal erythema + explosive stool:* Think of secondary lactose intolerance.
- *Severe intractable diarrhea beginning just after neonatal period:* Think of congenital diarrheas.
- *Diarrhea + fever:* Think of urinary tract infections and sepsis.
- *Chronic diarrhea with recurrent systemic infections:* Think of immunodeficiency states.

Note: Diarrhea in an underlying surgical setting are short gut syndrome, Hirschsprung enterocolitis, duodenocolic fistula, and bacterial overgrowth syndrome (due to malrotation and blind-loop syndrome)

KEY POINTS

- CMPA is the most common cause of colitis in children <3 years of age.
- Algorithm approach of management of CMPA is to be followed.
- Secondary lactose intolerance, celiac disease, and intestinal lymphangiectasia are common causes of small bowel diarrhea in children <3 years of age.
- Urinary tract infections and sepsis are important systemic causes.

SUGGESTED READING

1. Avery GB, Villacivencio O, Lilly JR, Randolph JG. Intractable diarrhea in early infancy. Pediatrics. 1968;41:712-22.

2. Bhatia J, Greer F. American Academy of Pediatrics Committee on Nutrition. Use of soy protein based formulas in infant feeding. Pediatrics. 2008;121(5):1062-8.
3. ESPGHAN Committee on Nutrition, Agostoni C, Axelsson I, Goulet O, Koletzko B, Michaelsen KF, et al. Soy protein infant formulae and follow-on formulae: a commentary by the ESPGHAN Committee on Nutrition. J Pediatr Gastroenterol Nutr. 2006;42(4):352-61.
4. Goldman AS, Anderson DW, Sellers WA, Saperstein S, Kniker WT, Halpern SR. Oral challenge with milk and isolated milk proteins in allergic children. Pediatrics. 1963; 32:425-43.
5. Goulet O, Philips AD. Congenital enteropathy involving intestinal mucosa development. In: Walker AW, Goulet O, Kleiman RE, Sherman PM, Shneider BL, Sanderson RI (Eds). Pediatric Gastrointestinal Diseases, 4th edn. Hamilton, Ontario: BC Decker; 2004. pp. 922-31.
6. Guarino A, Spangnuolo MI, Russo S, Albano F, Guandalini S, Capano G, et al. Etiology and risk factors of severe and protracted diarrhea. J Pediatr Gastroenterol Nutr. 1995;20: 173-8.
7. Høst A, Halken S, Jacobsen SP, Christensen AE, Herskind AM, Plesner K. Clinical course of cow's milk protein allergy/ intolerance and atopic diseases in childhood. Ped Allergy Immunol. 2002:13 (Suppl 15):23-8.
8. Høst A. Frequency of cow's milk allergy in childhood. Ann Allergy Asthma Immunol. 2002;89(6 Suppl 1):33-7.
9. Kneepkens CM, Hoekstra JH. Chronic nonspecific diarrhea of childhood: pathophysiology and management. Pediatr Clin North Am. 1996;43:375-90.
10. Kotlarz D, Beier R, Murugan D, Diestelhorst J, Jensen O, Boztug K, et al. Loss of interleukin-10 signaling and infantile inflammatory bowel disease: implications for diagnosis and therapy. Gastroenterology. 2012;143:347-55.
11. Matthai J, Sathiasekharan M, Poddar U, Sibal A, Srivastava A, Waikar Y, et al; Indian Society of Pediatric Gastroenterology, Hepatology and Nutrition; Pediatric Gastroenterology Chapter of Indian Academy of Pediatrics. Guidelines on Diagnosis and Management of Cow's Milk Protein Allergy. Indian Pediatr. 2020;57(8):723-9.
12. Matthai J, Yachha SK. Pediatric Gastroenterology Chapter, Indian Academy of Pediatrics. Chronic and Persistent Diarrhea in Infants and Young Children: Status Statement. Ind Pediatr. 2011;48:37-42.
13. Poddar U, Agarwal J, Yachha SK, Srivastava A. Toddler's diarrhea: is it an under recognized entity in developing countries? J Trop Pediatr. 2013;59:470-5.
14. Poddar U, Yachha SK, Krishnani N, Srivastava A. Cow's milk protein allergy (CMPA): an entity for recognition in children in developing countries. J Gastroenterol Hepatol. 2010;25:178-82.
15. Uhlig HH, Schwerd T, Koletzko S, Shah N, Kammermeier J, Elkadri A, et al; COLORS in IBD Study Group and NEOPICS. The diagnostic approach to monogenic very early onset inflammatory bowel disease. Gastroenterology. 2014; 147(5):990-1007.e3.
16. Wales PW, Christison-Lagay ER. Short bowel syndrome: epidemiology and etiology. Semin Pediatr Surg. 2010;19: 3-9.
17. Yachha SK, Misra S, Malik A, Nagi B, Mehta S. Spectrum of malabsorption syndrome in North Indian children. Indian J Gastroenterol. 1993;12:120-5.

Chronic Diarrhea in Children More than 3 Years of Age

Surender K Yachha, Moinak S Sarma

INTRODUCTION

Chronic diarrhea is defined as an insidious onset diarrhea of >2–3 weeks duration in children. Causes of chronic diarrhea in older children (>3 years) and adolescents are distinctly different from those in younger age.

APPROACH TO CHRONIC DIARRHEA

Approach to chronic diarrhea should be considered with the following points in mind:

- *Small or large bowel type of diarrhea:* Features in history and examination that help in differentiating small from large bowel diarrhea shown in **Table 1**. To summarize, large volume diarrhea without blood and mucus suggests "small bowel type" and small volume stools with blood and mucus suggests "large bowel type" of diarrhea.
- *Gastrointestinal (GI) versus systemic causes:* Commonly, diarrhea is of intestinal origin and sometimes due to pancreatic etiology, and rarely, hepatobiliary causes. Cholestasis due to biliary obstruction or intrahepatic cause can cause diarrhea due to fat malabsorption as a result of deficiency of bile. Diarrhea may be caused due to liver diseases having genetic or metabolic defects mostly prevalent among young children. Pruritus, fat soluble vitamins (A, D, E, and K), and calcium malabsorption are commonly associated with hepatobiliary diseases. Maldigestion due to deficiency of pancreatic enzymes results in clinical steatorrhea in cystic fibrosis, Shwachman-Diamond syndrome (cyclical neutropenia and skeletal dysplasia), or chronic pancreatitis. Diarrhea may also be a systemic manifestation of other conditions such as nephrotic syndrome, sepsis, or collagen vascular disorders. **Box 1** enumerates the common and uncommon causes of diarrhea in children > 3 years of age.

TABLE 1: Differentiating small versus large bowel diarrhea.

Features	*Small bowel diarrhea*	*Large bowel diarrhea**
Stool volume	Large	Small
Blood in stool	No	Usually present
Rectal symptoms (urgency, tenesmus)	No	Yes
Carbohydrate malabsorption	Yes, explosive	No
Protein malabsorption	Yes	No
Pain (if any)	Periumbilical, no reduction after passage of stool	Hypogastric, reduced after passage of stool
Color of stool	Pale	Normal
Smell of stool	Unusually offensive	Normal
Nutrient deficiency (iron, calcium, and multivitamins)	Frequent	Can occur due to blood loss

*Large bowel diarrhea in exceptional cases may not necessarily have blood in stools or rectal symptoms.

WHAT SHOULD YOU LOOK FOR IN HISTORY?

- Details of duration of symptoms, nature, frequency and consistency of stools, and presence of blood/mucus/clinical steatorrhea (stool floating in water, greasy oily droplets)
- Age of onset, dietary details, i.e., introduction of wheat/wheat products and their relationship with onset of diarrhea. Relationship with milk intake and quantity
- Family history of atopy (food allergy, asthma, or allergic rhinitis), celiac disease, inflammatory bowel disease (IBD), or cystic fibrosis

BOX 1: Causes according to age of onset (in order of priority).

- *Common causes:*
  - Celiac disease
  - *Parasites:* Giardiasis and others
  - Lymphangiectasia
  - Gastrointestinal tuberculosis
  - Inflammatory bowel disease (Crohn's disease; ulcerative colitis* unclassified IBD)
  - Immunodeficiency syndromes
  - Pancreatic insufficiency
  - Bacterial overgrowth syndrome (diagnosis of exclusion) in a nonsurgical setting
- *Uncommon causes:*
  - Tropical sprue
  - Immune proliferative small intestinal disease (IPSID)
  - Anatomical causes (malrotation of gut)
  - Intestinal fistulae (duodenocolic the most common)
  - Late-lactose intolerance (very rare)
  - Autoimmune enteropathy
  - *Systemic causes:*
    - Nephrotic syndrome[#]
    - Constrictive pericarditis[$]
  - *Endocrine causes:*
    - Hyperthyroidism
    - Addison's disease

*Ulcerative colitis presents as bloody diarrhea. Crohn's disease may present either as colitis or small bowel diarrhea or both.
[#]Diarrhea in nephrotic syndrome is presumed to be due to bowel wall edema (hypoalbuminemia).
[$]Secondary lymphangiectasia due to chronic back pressure is the cause of diarrhea in constrictive pericarditis, can also occur due to other causes.

- History of abdominal surgery, systemic disease, features of intestinal obstruction, pedal edema, anasarca, recurrent infections at multiple sites, previous blood transfusion, and coexisting medical problems which predispose the child to diarrhea such as congenital immunodeficiency, diabetes mellitus, hyperthyroidism, and cystic fibrosis.

WHAT SHOULD YOU LOOK FOR IN PHYSICAL EXAMINATION?

- Growth parameters
- Volume status and rarely, presence of dehydration
- Signs of vitamin and mineral deficiencies anemia, tetany, (conjunctival xerosis, Bitot's spots, angular stomatitis, glossitis, cheilitis, rickets, and phrynoderma)
- *Edema:* Symmetric and pitting (hypoalbuminemia) or asymmetric and nonpitting (lymphedema)
- Fever and other signs of toxicity
- Extra-GI manifestations in eye, skin, joints, and oral cavity (particularly aphthous ulcers) in IBD
- Inspection of perianal area for fissures, anal tags, and fistulae in IBD
- Oral thrush and scars of recurrent skin infections in immunodeficiency
- *Abdominal examination:* Abdominal distention, localized or generalized tenderness, masses, hepatosplenomegaly, and ascites.

The common etiologies are elaborated below. **Flowchart 1** shows an approach to chronic diarrhea >3 years of age (major etiologies).

CELIAC DISEASE

It is an enteropathy caused by permanent sensitivity to gluten in genetically susceptible subjects. It is the most common cause of chronic diarrhea in children over 2 years of age in North India. **Boxes 2 and 3** summarize the diagnosis and management of the same.

INTESTINAL LYMPHANGIECTASIA

It is characterized by ectasia of the bowel lymphatic system, which on rupture causes leakage of lymph in the bowel. **Box 4** summarizes the diagnosis and management of the same.

IMMUNODEFICIENCY

Both congenital and acquired immunodeficiency can cause chronic diarrhea. It should be suspected if there is history of recurrent infections at multiple sites (chest/GI/skin) and wasting. The common immunodeficiency conditions in children >3 years of age presenting with diarrhea are human immunodeficiency virus (HIV) infection, selective immunoglobulin A deficiency, common variable immunodeficiency, and chronic granulomatous disease. **Boxes 5 and 6** summarize the diagnosis and management of the same. Diarrhea is either due to opportunistic enteric infections or due to bacterial overgrowth.

INFLAMMATORY BOWEL DISEASE

Inflammatory bowel disease is a chronic inflammatory disease of the GI tract and is of two main types—(1) Crohn's disease (CD) and (2) ulcerative colitis (UC). In approximately 10% cases, the findings are nonspecific and subjects cannot be classified into one of the above two groups. These cases are labeled as IBD unclassified.

Flowchart 1: Approach to management of chronic diarrhea in children >3 years of age: Major etiologies.

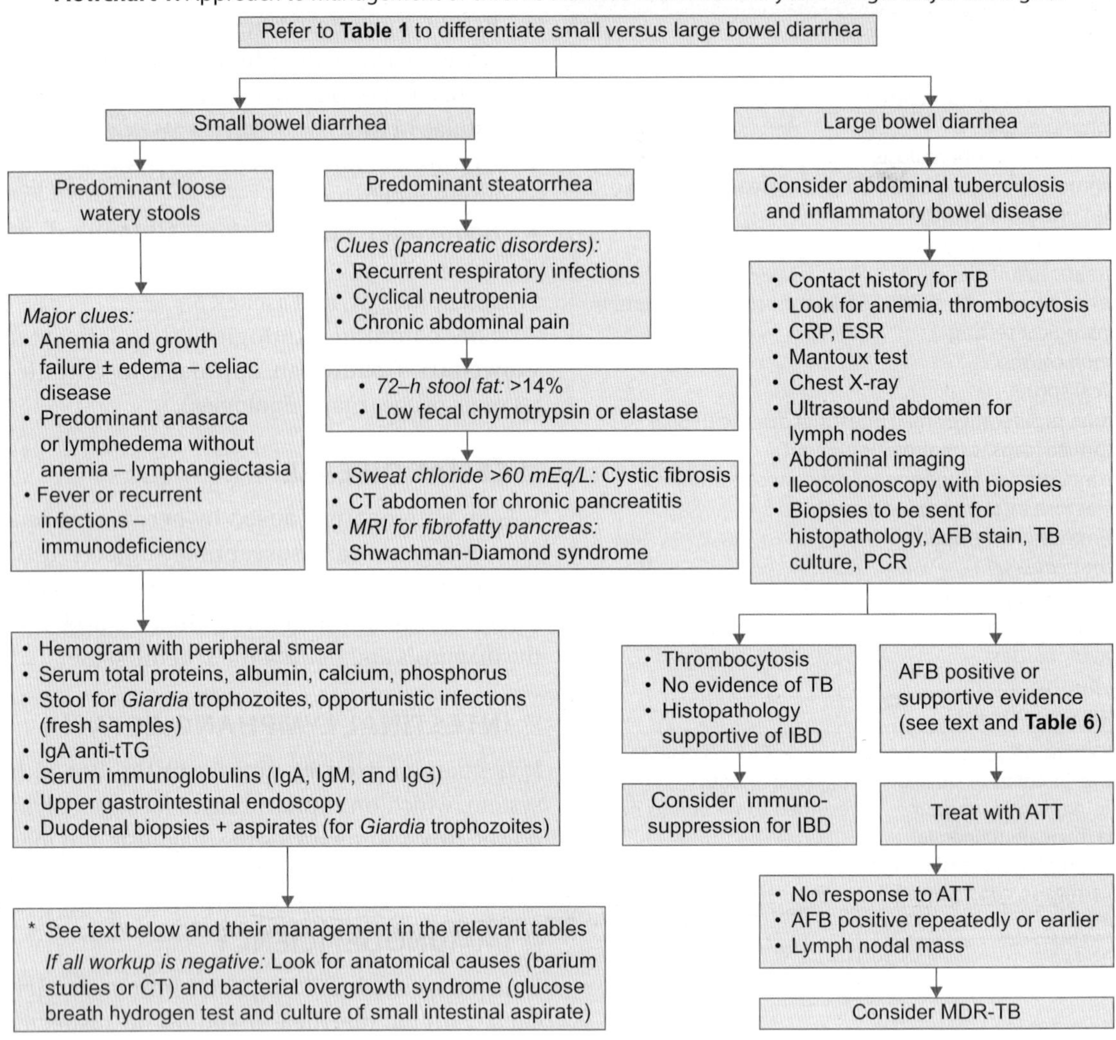

*Note:**
- *Selective IgA deficiency:* Recurrent giardiasis
- IgA anti-tTG positive + villous atrophy + other biopsy changes **(Box 2)**: Celiac disease
- IgA anti-tTG negative + low IgA level + villous atrophy + other biopsy changes **(Box 2)**: Celiac disease
- Dilated lacteals on duodenal biopsies: intestinal lymphangiectasia (**Box 4** for other supportive features)
- Low IgA, IgM, and IgG ± villous atrophy ± paucity of plasma cells on duodenal biopsies: Immunodeficiency workup as shown in **Box 5**.

(AFB: acid-fast bacilli; ATT: antitubercular therapy; CT: computed tomography; CRP: C-reactive protein; ESR: erythrocyte sedimentation rate; IBD: inflammatory bowel disease; IgA: immunoglobulin A; IgG: immunoglobulin G; IgM: immunoglobulin M; MRI: magnetic resonance imaging; MDR-TB: multidrug resistance tuberculosis; PCR: polymerase chain reaction; TB: tuberculosis; tTG: tissue transglutaminase).

Nearly 25% of all IBD patients present in the pediatric age group. Worldwide, the incidence of IBD is increasing in children with increase in recent reports of both UC and CD from India. The average age of presentation in children is nearly 10–11 years. Genetics is a very important risk factor for IBD and up to 30% patients may have an affected family member with IBD. **Box 7** summarizes the disease distribution of UC and CD.

CLINICAL FEATURES

Children with CD present with abdominal pain, diarrhea (with or without blood), and constitutional symptoms

BOX 2: Classical clinical features and workup of celiac disease.

- *Presentation:*
  - Onset after weaning when gluten is introduced
  - Small bowel diarrhea, failure to thrive, short stature, and gaseous abdominal distension
  - Anemia, rickets, and multivitamin deficiencies
- *Workup:*
  - *Positive serology:* IgA anti-tTG (screening), and IgA anti-EMA
  - *Upper gastrointestinal endoscopy:* Scalloping ± reduced number of duodenal folds, mosaic pattern, and cobblestoning of duodenal mucosa (not specific)
  - Endoscopic duodenal biopsy (Marsh 2–3):*
    - Partial to total villous atrophy
    - Hyperplastic crypts
    - Increased intraepithelial lymphocytes (>25/100 enterocytes)
    - Lymphoplasmacytic infiltrates
- *Workup:* Supportive
  - HLA-DQ2 or 8 positive (not done routinely). Only in exceptional cases where diagnosis is doubtful
  - *Serum IgA levels:*
    - Suspect if serology is negative and clinical suspicion is high
    - Levels <5 mg/dL suggests IgA deficiency
  - *Serum IgG anti-DGP:*
    - Children < 2 years of age if tTG or EMA is negative
    - Concomitant IgA deficiency

*Between 4 and 6 biopsies should be obtained (at least 4 from second part of duodenum and one from first part). Biopsies should be directly immersed in formalin solution for best orientation under microscope.
(DGP: deamidated gliadin peptide; EMA: endomysial antibody; HLA: human leukocyte antigen; IgA: immunoglobulin A; tTG: tissue transglutaminase antibody)

BOX 3: Diagnosis and treatment of celiac disease.

Diagnosis of celiac disease based on the modified ESPGHAN 1990 criteria:
- Clinical picture consistent with celiac disease
- Changes in intestinal biopsy as described above (+ serology*)
- Unequivocal response to GFD within 12 weeks of initiation of GFD

New ESPGHAN 2020 guidelines for diagnosis:
- Small bowel biopsy may be omitted when anti-tTG ≥ 10 times upper limit and anti-EMA positive
- Small bowel biopsy should be done if either (1) discrepant serology, (2) anti-tTG <10 time supper limit of normal or (3) negative anti-EMA antibody. Anti-tTG and anti-EMA should be done in separate blood samples
- False negative serology can occur in (1) low or short duration of gluten intake, (2) on immunosuppressive medication, and (3) extraintestinal manifestations such as gluten ataxia and dermatitis herpetiformis
- False negative IgA Anti-tTG or IgA Anti-EMA can occur if (1) selective IgA deficiency, (2) panhypogammaglobulinemia, or (3) children <3 years. In selective IgA deficiency, alternative test is IgG anti-tTG or anti-EMA. In children <3 years, alternative test is IgA or IgG DGP
- False negative histology or Marsh 0-1 histology can occur if poor quality of biopsy (small bits of tissue), poor orientation of biopsy, sampling from noninvolved areas or inexperienced pathologist. In such cases, a repeat biopsy is recommended
- If serology is strongly positive yet histology is negative, the label as potential celiac disease. Need to be regularly screened or keenly watched for development of symptoms
- However, due to certain limitations in India (cost, unreliability of laboratory reports, and overlap with other chronic diarrheal diseases), the above guideline is difficult to implement currently. Hence, small bowel biopsy is still recommended for diagnosis irrespective of antibody titers. Hence nonendoscopy-biopsy pathway in India is not recommended (personal view)

Contd...

Contd...

Treatment:
- Gluten-free diet (GFD) (wheat and barley) should never be started without a positive histology
- Lifelong GFD, vigilance, and counseling. Region-specific dietary chart
- Hematinics, folic acid, and multivitamin supplementation for 3 months
- Response to GFD should be assessed at 8–12 weeks to label the patient having celiac disease as per diagnostic criteria

New ESPGHAN 2022 guidelines for follow-up:
- *At follow-up:* Compliance with repeated reinforcement of GFD, symptomatic, anthropometric, and laboratory (hemoglobin, albumin, and transaminases) normalization to be assessed
- One-third of potential celiacs can progress to symptomatic celiacs in 10 years
- *IgA TTG:* Surrogate marker for mucosal healing. Normalize in 18–24 months
- If persistently high, look for noncompliance and test from same manufacturer as baseline
- Small bowel biopsy healing is not routinely recommended. Only in doubt
- *Routine bone density screening:* Not recommended
- *Stool/urinary gluten immunogenic peptides (GIP):* Further data required
- *Catchup growth:* First assessment at 6 months
- Failure to gain height by 1 year of GFD requires workup
- Lactose reduced diet only in those with lactose intolerance on GFD

New ESPGHAN 2022 guidelines for gluten challenge:
- To be done only in those patients who are already on GFD but diagnosis is in doubt
- Should not be done <7 years (affects dentition) and >12 years (affects puberty)
- HLA testing is mandatory before gluten challenge
- Intestinal biopsy is mandatory before gluten challenge
- Give 10–15 g gluten/day for 12 months
- Serology test at first month and thereafter every 3 months
- If positive serology or symptomatic at any time, then biopsy
- If normal serology and asymptomatic, then continue gluten. Follow up annually

*In India, positive serology (IgA-tTG) should be demonstrated as there are other conditions that may result in villous atrophy mimicking celiac disease.

(ESPGHAN: European Society for Pediatric Gastroenterology, Hepatology, and Nutrition; EMA: endomysial antibody; GFD: gluten-free diet; HLA: human leukocyte antigen; IgA: immunoglobulin A; tTG: tissue transglutaminase)

BOX 4: Features and management of intestinal lymphangiectasia.

Presentation:
- Small bowel diarrhea with anasarca ± lymphedema of peripheries
- Abdominal or thoracic chylous effusions may be associated.
- Usually, absence of anemia and rickets (in contrast to celiac disease)
- Hypocalcemic tetany

Diagnosis:
- Panhypoproteinemia, low immunoglobulins, hypocalcemia, and lymphopenia
- *Upper gastrointestinal endoscopy:* White patches in duodenum (snow-flake appearance), better appreciated after overnight fat (butter) loading 2 g/kg
- *Small bowel biopsy:* Dilated lacteals in the villi

Treatment:
- *Diet:* Low fat, high medium chain triglyceride with high protein (2–4 g/kg)
- Medium chain triglycerides should be 85% of total fat intake
- Calcium supplementation
- Intravenous albumin (1 g/kg) during acute exacerbations
- In refractory cases, subcutaneous octreotide 15–20 µg daily twice or 10–20 µg depot preparation once in 4 weeks
- Resection if localized segment of small bowel is involved by identifying the segment by 99Tc albumin scintigraphy

BOX 5: Clinical features of common immunodeficiency states (above 3 years of age).

Common features:
- Positive family history, affected sib, or sib death
- Associated systemic infections (sinopulmonary, skin, urinary, meningeal, etc.)
- Small bowel, large bowel, or mixed diarrhea depending on the opportunistic pathogen
- *Recurrent GI infections:* Cryptosporidia, *Isospora*, *Giardia*, *Cytomegalovirus*, and fungal

Human immunodeficiency virus infection:
- Hepatosplenomegaly, lymphadenopathy, thrombocytopenia, and hypergammaglobulinemia
- Enzyme-linked immunosorbent assay and Western blot tests positive
- Opportunistic infections depending upon the level of CD4 count

Selective IgA deficiency:
- Recurrent giardiasis
- Serum IgA <5 mg/dL

Common variable immunodeficiency:
- Age of onset variable usually after 2 years of age
- Low serum IgG ± low IgA or M with variable B-cell numbers

Chronic granulomatous disease:
- Multifocal abscess (skin and liver), colitis
- Blood nitro-blue tetrazolium reduction test positive

(IgA: immunoglobulin A; IgG: immunoglobulin G)

BOX 6: Common infections and management of immunodeficiency states.

- *Common infections include:*
  - Viral: *Cytomegalovirus*, herpes simplex, and adenovirus
  - Bacterial: *Salmonella*, *Shigella*, *Mycobacterium avium complex* (MAC), *Campylobacter jejuni*, and *Clostridium difficile*
  - *Fungal:* Candidiasis, histoplasmosis, and cryptococcosis
  - *Protozoa:* Microsporidium, *Isospora belli*, *Cryptosporidium*, *Entamoeba histolytica*, *Giardia lamblia*, *Cyclospora*, and *Blastocystis hominis*
  - Parasites: *Strongyloides*
- *Diagnosis:*
  - Serum immunoglobulin, B-cell, and T-cell assays
  - Colonic biopsies, duodenal fluid examination, and multiple stool samples for opportunistic infections (special stains, polymerase chain reaction, and fungus)
- *Treatment:*
  - Specific antimicrobials for the isolated organisms
  - *Acquired immunodeficiency syndrome:* Highly active antiretroviral therapy (HAART)
  - *Common variable immunodeficiency:* Intravenous immunoglobulin therapy 400–600 mg/kg every 3–4 weeks to maintain serum immunoglobulin G levels >500–700 mg/dL

BOX 7: Disease distribution.

- *Ulcerative colitis:*
  - *Distal colitis (proctitis/proctosigmoiditis):* 5–20%
  - *Left side colitis (up to splenic flexure):* 10–40%
  - *Pancolitis:* 50–90%
- *Crohn's disease:*
  - *Ileocolonic disease:* 50–70%
  - *Isolated colonic involvement:* 10–20%
  - *Small bowel:* 10–15%
  - *Associated:*
    - *Upper gastrointestinal involvement:* 30–40%
    - *Perianal disease:* 20–25%

Note: Crohn's disease is also classified as predominantly inflammatory, fistulizing, or stricturing disease based on the clinical features.

(fever, anorexia, and growth failure). In contrast, children with UC present with only recurrent or prolonged episodes of bloody diarrhea, commonly without constitutional symptoms. **Table 2** summarizes the clinical, histologic, and endoscopic differences between UC and CD.

Extraintestinal manifestations are seen in 25–30% of children with IBD. They can precede, follow, or occur concurrently with the intestinal disease and may be related or unrelated to the activity of the intestinal disease. Arthralgia/arthritis is the most common manifestation seen in 15–17% of cases. Uveitis, erythema nodosum, and sclerosing cholangitis are the other manifestations.

DIAGNOSIS

The initial evaluation of a child with suspected IBD includes a detailed clinical, family, and treatment history. Also, a complete examination with growth charting, perianal and rectal examination for fistulae, tags, and fissures to be done. Laboratory tests may reveal anemia and thrombocytosis (67%), low albumin, high erythrocyte sedimentation rate (ESR) and C-reactive protein in 40–60% cases. Hence, IBD must be suspected in any child presenting with constitutional symptoms, chronic large bowel diarrhea (± blood), and thrombocytosis. **Table 3** summarizes the diagnostic modalities available for IBD.

TREATMENT

The goal of treatment is to control inflammation, mucosal healing, improve growth, and ensure a good quality of life with the least toxic therapeutic regimen. Ensuring proper nutrition with caloric supplementation (~120% of recommended dietary allowances) is a necessity for children with IBD. Calcium and vitamin D supplementation should be given as these children are at an increased risk

TABLE 2: Differentiation between Crohn's disease and ulcerative colitis.

Parameters	*Crohn's disease*	*Ulcerative colitis*
Distribution	Entire GI tract	Colon only
	Transmural inflammation	Mucosal disease
	Discontinuous (skip) lesions	Continuous involvement
Bloody diarrhea	Less common	Common
Abdominal pain	Common	Less common
Growth failure	Common	Less common
Perianal disease (abscess/fistulae)	Present	Absent
Histopathology	Noncaseating granuloma (any part of GI tract)	Widespread crypt architectural distortion
	Transmural involvement	Diffuse inflammatory infiltrate
	Focal discontinuous crypt architectural distortion	Basal plasmacytosis
	Focal discontinuous chronic inflammation	Goblet cell depletion
	Focally enhancing gastritis (stomach)	Crypt abscess
	Pyloric gland metaplasia (terminal ileum)	Paneth cell metaplasia
Endoscopy	Deep irregular serpiginous or aphthous ulcers	Diffuse superficial ulceration
	Normal intervening mucosa (skip lesion)	Granularity, loss of vascular pattern, friability
	Ileal involvement, rectal sparing (60%)	Rectal involvement and ileal sparing (unless back-wash ileitis)

TABLE 3: Diagnostic modalities available for inflammatory bowel disease.

Diagnostic modality	*Importance*
• Colonoscopy with ileal intubation • Multiple biopsies from disease sites	Most important to differentiate ulcerative colitis vs. Crohn's disease
Upper gastrointestinal endoscopy with biopsies	To look for granulomas (40%)
Small bowel imaging	For small bowel strictures fistula
Barium enteroclysis, CT, or magnetic resonance enteroclysis	Extramural complications may be seen in CT/MRI
MRI pelvis	Fistula, pelvic and genitourinary abscess
Capsule endoscopy	Ideal to evaluate small bowel involvement after excluding intestinal stricture that may result in retention of capsule. Disadvantage—biopsies cannot be taken
Enteroscopy	Limitation of not able to pass bigger diameter enteroscopes in younger children

(CT: computed tomography; MRI: magnetic resonance imaging)

of osteoporosis. As IBD is a chronic disease with remissions and exacerbations, proper counseling of both, patient and family, at diagnosis is essential. The main drugs used for IBD are listed in the **Tables 4 and 5**. Additionally, for perianal fistulizing CD, antibiotics (ciprofloxacin 20 mg/kg, metronidazole 10–20 mg/kg, azithromycin 10 mg/kg, or rifaximin 10–30 mg/kg) for 4–6 weeks have shown good short-term response.

Surgery is indicated in UC patients with severe acute colitis refractory to medical disease. Uncontrolled hemorrhage, perforation, toxic megacolon, abscesses, and obstruction are the other indications for surgery. Nearly 40% pediatric patients with UC require total colectomy within 5–10 years of diagnosis. Risk of adenocarcinoma colon is 8% after 20 years of disease in pediatric UC.

TABLE 4: Drugs used in inflammatory bowel disease (first-line therapy).

Drug	*Dosage and route*	*Indication*	*Main side effects*
• Sulfasalazine or • 5-aminosalicylic acid or mesalamine (active moiety of sulfasalazine)	• 40–60 mg/kg/day oral • 50–100 mg/kg/day oral • Enema	• Anti-inflammatory (local action) in mild ulcerative colitis and maintenance • Enema in mild-to-moderate left-sided colonic disease	• Folate deficiency • Pancreatitis • Steven–Johnson syndrome • Hepatotoxicity • Oligospermia (with sulfasalazine)
Prednisolone	1–2 mg/kg oral	Induction therapy (first line) in all types of inflammatory bowel disease	• Cushingoid facies • Hypertension • Glaucoma • Cataract • Fractures • Hyperglycemia • Growth impairment
Thiopurines:			
• Azathioprine • 6-Mercaptopurine (active moiety of azathioprine)	• 2–3 mg/kg/day oral • 1–2 mg/kg/day oral	• Frequent relapses* • Steroid dependence# • Steroid resistance† • Maintenance in moderate-to-severe disease	• Myelosuppression • Hepatotoxicity • Pancreatitis

**Frequent relapses:* 2–3 relapses per year.
#Steroid dependency: Initial remission but recurrence while tapering or inability to stop steroids in 14–16 weeks of initiation.
†Steroid resistance: Nonresponse to optimal doses of oral steroids within 7–14 days of initiation and good compliance.

TABLE 5: Drugs used in inflammatory bowel disease (second-line therapy).

Drug	*Dosage and route*	*Indications*	*Main side effects*
Methotrexate	15 mg/m^2 IM weekly	• Steroid sparing • Refractory disease and/or intolerant to thiopurines	• Hepatotoxicity • Myelosuppression • Folate deficiency
Cyclosporine	2–4 mg/kg/day IV infusion followed by 5–8 mg/kg/day oral	Rescue therapy for maximum 4 weeks in severe refractory ulcerative colitis	• Nephrotoxicity • Hypertrichosis • Gum hyperplasia • Hypertension • Paresthesia
Tacrolimus	0.1 mg/kg oral		
Biological agents (infliximab and adalimumab)	5 mg/kg IV at 0, 2, 6 weeks and thereafter need based	• Fistulizing CD • Severe disease not responding to immunomodulators	• Autoimmunity • Demyelination • Psychiatric problems • Flare infections (especially tuberculosis) • Hepatosplenic T-cell lymphoma (in combination with azathioprine)
Thalidomide	1.5–2.5 mg/kg oral	Refractory CD and intolerant to biological agents (very selective group)	• Irreversible peripheral neuropathy • Agitation • Hallucination

(CD: Crohn's disease; IM: intramuscular; IV: intravenous)

ABDOMINAL TUBERCULOSIS

High index of suspicion for abdominal tuberculosis is to be considered in any child with:

- Constitutional symptoms (prolonged fever, anorexia, and weight loss) + any of the features in **Table 6**
- Contact with open case of tuberculosis (adult)
- Mantoux test positivity (≥5 mm in HIV and ≥10 mm in non-HIV patients irrespective of age at 48–72 hours of tuberculin injection)
- *Contributory laboratory features:* High ESR, lymphocytosis.

Diagnosis

- *Definitive:* Demonstration of acid-fast bacilli (fine needle aspiration cytology from lymph nodes, ascitic fluid, and endoscopic biopsies) on Ziehl-Neelsen (ZN) staining or culture (BACTEC or Lowenstein-Jensen media). If adequate tissue is sampled and processed, a definitive diagnosis is achievable in up to 64% of pediatric cases.
- *Supportive:* Tubercular granuloma with caseation in the biopsies (endoscopic/peritoneal/liver)
- In the absence of above features, a probable diagnosis of abdominal tuberculosis is made when suggestive clinical features and response to antitubercular therapy (ATT) without relapse after completion of therapy is observed
- Due to emergence of multidrug resistance tuberculosis (MDR-TB) and delay in obtaining culture sensitivity, World Health Organization recommends "Line Probe Assay" from all acid fast bacilli positive tissue samples (ZN stain or culture). Line probe assay provides drug sensitivity within 6 hours and differentiates *Mycobacterium tuberculosis* from nontubercular mycobacteria.

Treatment

Antitubercular drugs are the mainstay of treatment of abdominal tuberculosis as per the current pediatric guidelines in India. Surgery is indicated if there is bowel perforation, obstruction, or massive hemorrhage.

TABLE 6: Presentation and specific workup in abdominal tuberculosis.

Involvement	*Features*	*Tissue sampling and specific workup (laboratory and abdominal imaging)*
Peritoneum	• *Dry:* Adhesive intestinal obstruction lump (cocoon abdomen) • *Wet:* Exudative ± loculated ascites • "Doughy" feel of abdomen	• *Peritoneoscopy/laparoscopy:* Peritoneal tubercules • *Ascitic fluid:* Lymphocytosis with high adenosine deaminase
Lymph nodes	Lump (lymph nodal mass)	Fine needle aspiration from necrotic, enlarged (>10 mm) and/or calcified, conglomerate lymph nodes
Gastrointestinal tract (luminal)	• *Ulcerative:* Abdominal pain, GI bleed, and anemia • *Hypertrophic:* Intestinal obstruction • *Ulcerohypertrophic:* Combination of above 18–64% present as chronic diarrhea or colitis	• Features on colonoscopy* • Colonic and ileal biopsies by endoscopy# • Laparotomy and surgical biopsy of small bowel
Hepatic	• Systemic symptoms with hepatomegaly • Nonresolving liver abscess	• Raised serum alkaline phosphatase • Multiple hypodense ± calcified foci in liver
Combination	Nodal ± peritoneal ± GI	Tissue sampling and workup as above
Disseminated	Abdominal + other organs (lungs, peripheral LN, and bone marrow)	

*Ab.TB is a close differential of Crohn's disease. Some major endoscopic features (though not discriminatory) may favor Ab.TB:
- Segmental involvement (as compared to skip areas in CD)
- Deep circular transverse ulcers (as compared to deep linear serpiginous ulcers in CD)
- Short colonic strictures (as compared to multiple long strictures in CD).

#Due to significant overlap between the two diseases, all biopsy specimens should be simultaneously sent for histopathology, ZN staining, TB culture and TB-PCR (polymerase chain reaction). Culture positivity may be seen despite initial ZN stain negativity. Tissue TB-PCR (nested or real time) has high specificity (98%) but lower sensitivity (68–75%).

(GI: gastrointestinal LN: lymph node)

It is important to differentiate intestinal tuberculosis from CD as they mimic each other in clinical presentation but have different treatment. One should also suspect MDR-TB in patients with a definite diagnosis of abdominal tuberculosis but a poor response to standard ATT. MDR-TB presents mostly as refractory lymph nodal masses in the abdomen with close differential diagnosis of non-Hodgkin's lymphoma.

CLINICAL PEARLS

Small bowel diarrhea:

- Small bowel diarrhea + anemia and rickets: Think of celiac disease
- Small bowel diarrhea + predominant edema without anemia: Think of intestinal lymphangiectasia
- Small bowel diarrhea + recurrent infections: Think of immunodeficiency
- Abdominal tuberculosis rarely presents as small bowel diarrhea
- In celiac disease, do not start gluten-free diet without confirmation of diagnosis (serology + histopathology).

Large bowel diarrhea:

- Large bowel diarrhea in an older child: Think of IBD and tuberculosis.
- Workup for both should be sent together as they may mimic each other.
- Necrotic or calcified lymph node in chest or abdomen and exudative ascites is specific for tuberculosis.
- Attempt to obtain tissue diagnosis in abdominal tuberculosis before starting ATT.

KEY POINTS

- Differentiating small from large bowel diarrhea, malabsorption from maldigestion clinically provides a clue to diagnosis.
- Common causes of chronic small bowel diarrhea in children above 3 years of age are celiac disease (in North India), giardiasis, intestinal lymphangiectasia, and immunodeficiency.
- Celiac disease and lymphangiectasia require life-time therapy whereas giardiasis and opportunistic infections in immunodeficiency states require antimicrobials. Immunodeficiency needs to be treated as per cause.
- Common causes of small bowel diarrhea in children above 3 years of age are abdominal tuberculosis and IBD.
- Antitubercular therapy is the mainstay of therapy in abdominal tuberculosis. MDR-TB should be considered if there is nonresponse and acid-fast bacilli are positive in tissue. Usually, abdominal MDR-TB presents as large abdominal lymph nodal masses.
- Immunosuppression is the mainstay of treatment in IBD. Only a small proportion requires surgeries in select situations.

SUGGESTED READING

1. Al Sinani S, Rawahi YA, Abdoon H. Octreotide in Hennekam syndrome-associated intestinal lymphangiectasia. World J Gastroenterol. 2012;18:6333-7.
2. Baldassano RN, Piccoli DA. Inflammatory bowel disease in pediatric and adolescent patients. Gastroenterol Clin North Am. 1999;28:445-58.
3. Husby S, Koletzko S, Korponay-Szabó I, Kurppa K, Mearin ML, Ribes-Koninckx C, et al. European Society Paediatric Gastroenterology, Hepatology and Nutrition Guidelines for Diagnosing Coeliac Disease 2020. J Pediatr Gastroenterol Nutr. 2020;70(1):141-56.
4. Husby S. For ESPGHAN Working Group on Coeliac Disease. European Society for Pediatric Gastroenterology, Hepatology, and Nutrition guidelines for the diagnosis of coeliac disease. J Pediatr Gastroenterol Nutr. 2012;54:136-60.
5. Kumar A, Gupta D, Nagaraja SB, Singh V, Sethi GR, Prasad J, et al. Updated National Guidelines for Pediatric Tuberculosis in India, 2012. Indian Pediatr. 2013;50:301-6.
6. Lee HS, Park KU, Park JO, Chang HE, Song J, Choe G, et al. Rapid, sensitive, and specific detection of M. tuberculosis complex by real-time PCR on paraffin- embedded human tissues. J Mol Diagn. 2011;13:390-4.
7. Magro F, Langner C, Driessen A, Ensari A, Geboes K, Mantzaris GJ, et al. European Consensus on the histopathology of inflammatory bowel disease. J Crohns Colitis. 2013; 7:827-51.
8. Malik R, Srivastava A, Yachha SK, Poddar U, Lal R. Childhood abdominal tuberculosis: Disease patterns, diagnosis, and drug resistance. Indian J Gastroenterol. 2015;34(6): 418-25
9. Mearin ML, Agardh D, Antunes H, Al-Toma A, Auricchio R, Castillejo G, et al.; ESPGHAN Special Interest Group on Celiac Disease. ESPGHAN Position Paper on Management and Follow-up of Children and Adolescents With Celiac Disease. J Pediatr Gastroenterol Nutr. 2022;75(3):369-86.
10. Ruemmele FM, Veres G, Kolho KL, Griffiths A, Levine A, Escher JC, et al. Consensus guidelines of ECCO/ESPGHAN on the medical management of pediatric Crohn's disease. J Crohns Colitis. 2014;8(10):1179-207.
11. Sabery N, Bass D. Use of serologic markers as a screening tool in inflammatory bowel disease compared with elevated erythrocyte sedimentation rate and anemia. Pediatrics. 2007;119:e193-9.
12. Sandhu BK, Fell JM, Beattie RM, Mitton SG, Wilson DC, Jenkins H; on Behalf of the IBD Working Group of the British Society of Paediatric Gastroenterology, Hepatology, and Nutrition. Guidelines for the Management of Inflammatory Bowel Disease in Children in the United Kingdom. J Pediatr Gastroenterol Nutr. 2010;50:S1-13.
13. Sari S, Baris Z, Dalgic B. Primary intestinal lymphangiectasia in children: Is octreotide an effective and safe option in the treatment? J Pediatr Gastroenterol Nutr. 2010; 51:454-7.

14. Sauer CG, Kugathasan S. Pediatric inflammatory bowel disease: Highlighting pediatric differences in IBD. Med Clin North Am. 2010;94:35-52.
15. Sawczenko A, Sandhu BK. Presenting features of inflammatory bowel disease in Great Britain and Ireland. Arch Dis Child. 2003;88:995-1000.
16. Thapa BR, Yachha SK, Mehta S. Abdominal tuberculosis. Indian Pediatr. 1991;28:1093-100.
17. Turner D, Levine A, Escher JC, Griffiths AM, Russell RK, Dignass A, et al. Management of pediatric ulcerative colitis: joint ECCO and ESPGHAN evidence-based consensus guidelines. J Pediatr Gastroenterol Nutr. 2012;55:340-61.
18. Van Limbergen J, Russell RK, Drummond HE, Aldhous MC, Round NK, Nimmo ER, et al. Definition of phenotypic characteristics of childhood-onset inflammatory bowel disease. Gastroenterology. 2008;135:1114-22.
19. Walker Smith JA. For working group of European Society of Pediatric Gastroenterology and Nutrition. Revised criteria for diagnosis of celiac disease. Report of Working group of ESPGHAN. Arch Dis Child. 1990;65: 909-11.
20. Yachha SK, Poddar U. Celiac disease in India. Indian J Gastroenterol. 2007; 26:230-7.

CHAPTER 79

Approach to Upper Gastrointestinal Bleed in Children

Anshu Srivastava, Vignesh V

INTRODUCTION

Upper gastrointestinal bleeding (UGIB) is a commonly encountered problem in children that usually manifests as hematemesis or melena. The incidence in pediatric intensive care unit (ICU) is reported to vary from 6 to 25% and approximately 5% of upper gastrointestinal (UGI) endoscopies in children are done for UGIB. The overall mortality is ~2% with higher mortality in children with secondary UGIB, i.e., those with other comorbid conditions than children with primary UGIB (no comorbidity, 2.6% vs. 0.37%).

Medical attention is sought early in majority of the cases with UGIB due to its alarming nature and this helps in prompt diagnosis and management. Children tolerate UGIB better than adults due to absence of systemic comorbidities but are at greater risk of developing shock due to their smaller blood volumes.

Etiology of UGIB depends on the age of the patient, setting (ward, ICU, and home) and geographical location. In India, esophageal varices secondary to extrahepatic portal venous obstruction (EHPVO) is the most common cause while in the West, it is the ulcer disease often secondary to nonsteroidal anti-inflammatory drugs (NSAIDs) intake. Stress ulcers are an important cause and should be suspected in any child with significant stress such as septic shock, organ failure, burns, and trauma. UGIB is an important cause of unexplained anemia, especially iron deficiency anemia, in children.

The important causes of UGIB in children are given in **Table 1** and clues in history and physical examination toward the likely cause are shown in **Table 2**.

TABLE 1: Causes of upper gastrointestinal bleeding.

Neonate	*Infant-small child*	*Older child and adolescent*
Swallowed maternal blood	Esophagitis	Esophagitis—reflux, infections, and pill
• Vitamin K deficiency • Coagulopathy	Gastritis and gastroduodenal ulcer/erosion	Mallory–Weiss tear
Sepsis	Foreign body ingestion and caustic ingestion	Caustic ingestion
Stress gastritis or gastroduodenal ulcer	Sepsis/coagulopathy/stress erosions	Foreign body ingestion
Esophagitis	Cow's milk protein allergy	Portal hypertension—esophageal/gastric varices; congestive gastropathy; and gastric antral vascular ectasia
Vascular malformation	Hemorrhagic disease of newborn	Gastritis, peptic ulcer (duodenal/gastric), Dieulafoy lesion, Cameron lesion, hemobilia, and hemosuccus pancreaticus
Less common—nasogastric tube-related trauma	• Vascular malformation • Esophageal varices	Arteriovenous malformation and coagulation disorders

Contd...

Contd...

Neonate	*Infant-small child*	*Older child and adolescent*
Gastrointestinal duplication	Upper gut duplication	Henoch–Schönlein purpura, Crohn's disease, and stress/sepsis/coagulopathy-related erosions
	Uncommon: Trauma (nasogastric tube), gastric cardia prolapse, and heterotopic pancreatic tissue	Tumors—leiomyoma and lymphoma Polys and gastric mucosal prolapse
	Munchausen's syndrome by proxy	*Rare:* Gastrointestinal duplication, radiation gastritis, and Munchausen's syndrome by proxy

TABLE 2: Clues in history and examination toward etiology of upper gastrointestinal bleeding.

Likely diagnosis	*Clinical signs/symptoms*
Variceal bleeding	Painless significant bleed, similar episode in the past, splenomegaly, jaundice, ascites, and other stigmata of chronic liver disease
Esophagitis	Presence of heart burn/regurgitation/dysphagia/odynophagia, placement of Ryle's tube, corrosive intake, and drug intake (e.g., doxycycline)
Mallory–Weiss tear	Repeated retching and vomiting followed by hematemesis
Gastritis/erosions/ulcer	• History of drug ingestion like aspirin/nonsteroidal anti-inflammatory drugs/steroids • Epigastric pain • Intensive care unit patient on mechanical ventilation • Family history of peptic ulcer disease
Vascular malformation	Painless bleed and presence of hemangiomas at other sites
Cow's milk protein allergy	Introduction of animal milk, presence of diarrhea/eczema, and family history of atopy
Munchausen's syndrome by proxy	Complaints disproportionate to examination findings, absence of anemia, and negative stool occult blood during active bleeding
Hemobilia	Setting of hepatobiliary intervention, associated jaundice, and pain abdomen
Hemosuccus pancreaticus	Setting of acute/chronic pancreatitis

DEFINITIONS

Upper Gastrointestinal Bleeding

This denotes bleeding from a site in the gastrointestinal (GI) tract above the ligament of Treitz (esophagus to duodenojejunal flexure).

The common terms used to describe UGIB are as follows:

- *Hematemesis* is presence of bright red or altered coffee-ground blood in vomiting. Majority of UGIB presents as hematemesis (~73% children) while ~21% present with melena and 6% with coffee-ground colored vomiting.
- *Melena* is passage of black, tarry, and sticky stools with an offensive smell and suggests a UGI or small bowel site of bleeding.
- *Hematochezia* is passage of bright red blood in stools and is usually seen with bleeding in colon but very brisk UGIB with fast gut transit may also present with hematochezia.
- *Hemobilia* refers to bleeding from the biliary tree and *hemosuccus pancreaticus* to bleeding from the pancreas. In both these conditions, blood enters the duodenum from the common bile duct or pancreatic duct through the ampulla of Vater.

Obscure Gastrointestinal Bleeding

Obscure gastrointestinal bleeding (OGIB) is defined as bleeding from GI tract that persists or recurs without any obvious etiology after a diagnostic esophagogastro-duodenoscopy, colonoscopy, and small bowel evaluation with video capsule endoscopy and/or enteroscopy and radiographic testing. It accounts for ~5% of all GI bleeds and is classified into two types:

1. *Occult OGIB:* Presents as stool occult blood positivity and iron deficiency anemia
2. *Overt OGIB:* Presents as visible blood in stool and/or vomitus

APPROACH

A detailed history, followed by physical examination, is helpful in determining the most probable cause of UGIB. Management includes simultaneous stabilization of the child and determination of etiology of UGIB, followed by definitive therapy **(Flowchart 1)**.

- *The first question is if the hematemesis and/or melena is due to blood or not, especially in an otherwise healthy child.*
  - The food items looking like blood in vomitus are shown in **Box 1**.
  - An Apt-Downey test is used to differentiate the swallowed maternal blood from hematemesis in a neonate.
  - **Box 2** shows ingested items which may present as melena. The differentiation is made by performing a guaiac [detects "heme" component of hemoglobin (Hb)] or fecal immunochemical testing (detects "globin" component of Hb) in stool.
- *The next step is to differentiate UGIB from epistaxis, oropharyngeal bleeding, and hemoptysis:*
  - History of chronic cough and passage of bright red blood associated with sputum indicates toward hemoptysis.
  - Nose and oropharynx should be examined to rule out other sites of bleed.
  - It is important not to confuse onset of menarche with melena.

Flowchart 1: Approach to a patient with acute upper gastrointestinal bleeding.

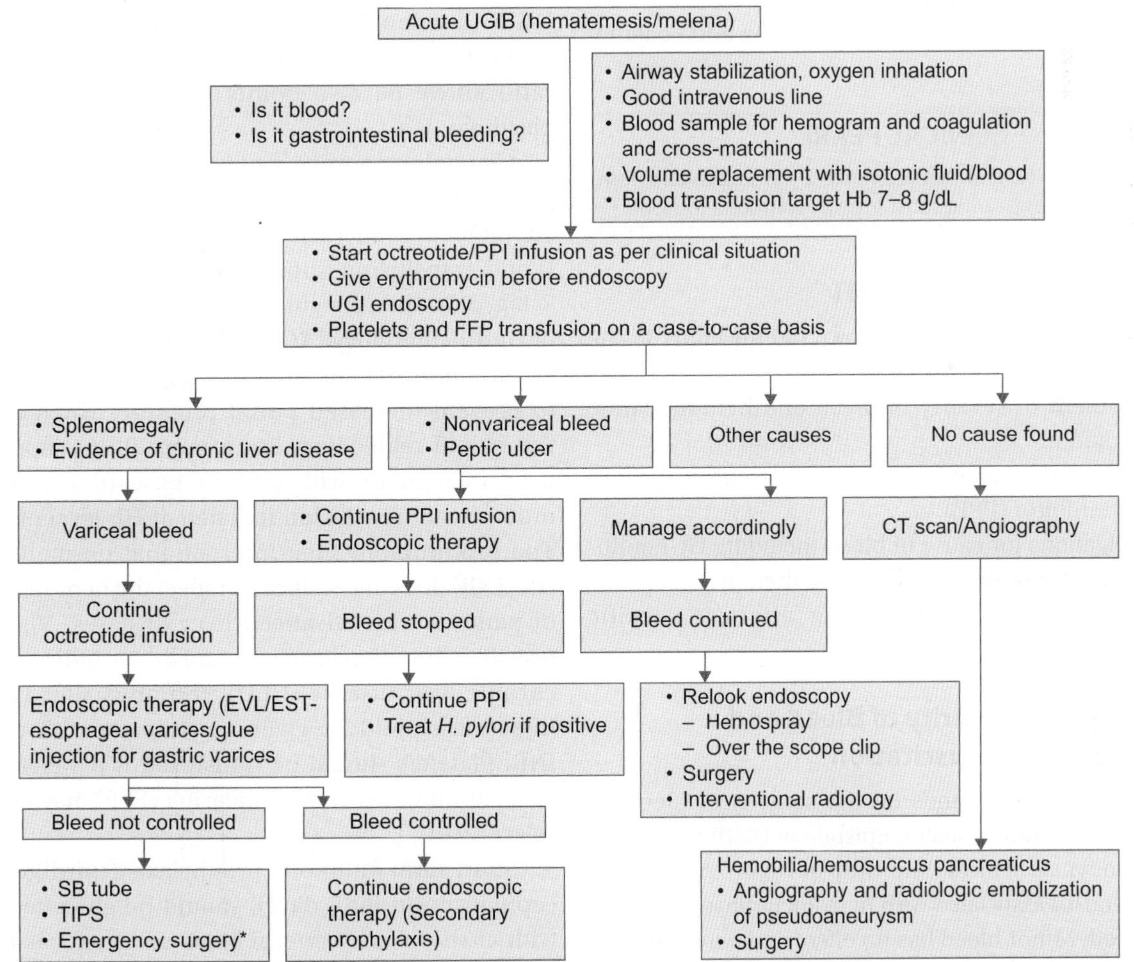

*As per the discussion in the text.

(EST: endoscopic sclerotherapy; EVL: endoscopic variceal ligation; FFP: fresh frozen plasma; Hb: hemoglobin; PPI: proton pump inhibitor; SB: Sengstaken–Blakemore; TIPS: transjugular intrahepatic portosystemic shunt; UGIB: upper gastrointestinal bleeding)

BOX 1: Causes of red colored vomitus (other than upper gastrointestinal bleeding).

- Food items such as tomatoes, strawberries, beetroot, and cranberries or those containing red food coloring agents (jelly, candies, and juices)
- Ingestion of maternal blood (in neonates)
- Drugs (rifampicin)

BOX 2: Causes of melena like stools (other than upper gastrointestinal bleeding).

- *Food items:* Ingestion of spinach, licorice, grape juice, and blueberries
- *Drugs:* Bismuth/iron preparations
- Ingestion of maternal blood (in neonates)

History of bleeding from multiple sites points toward systemic causes such as thrombocytopenia and coagulopathy.

CLINICAL PEARL

- Tests for occult blood are required to distinguish blood from other similar appearing substances in vomitus and stool.

STEPWISE MANAGEMENT

The management approach is shown in **Flowchart 1**. The main steps include:

- Assessment of severity of bleed and hemodynamic resuscitation
- Initiation of vasoactive therapy [octreotide/proton pump inhibitor (PPI)]
- Investigations for cause of bleed including UGI endoscopy and appropriate endoscopic therapy
- Supportive therapy including etiology specific treatment

Assessment of Severity of Bleed and Hemodynamic Resuscitation

The management depends on the severity of bleeding which can be minor or major. Episode of UGIB associated with hemodynamic instability, drop of Hb of >2 g/dL or to <8 g/dL, and/or associated with hematochezia is labeled as major bleed. Minor bleed has no effect on heart rate (HR) and blood pressure, moderate bleed is associated with postural hypotension and tachycardia whereas massive bleed is associated with shock (defined in children as tachycardia with signs of decreased organ or peripheral perfusion).

Assessment of severity of bleed and hemodynamic status is done by monitoring of HR, blood pressure, postural change in blood pressure (decrease in systolic blood pressure of ≥10 mm Hg) and HR (increase by 20 beats/min), pulse volume, capillary refill time, oxygen saturation (pulse oximetry), and urine output. Central venous oxygen saturation and venous blood lactate levels are good indicators of adequacy of tissue perfusion.

Presence of blood on nasogastric (NG) tube aspiration confirms a UGI source of bleeding. NG tube is also useful in monitoring the bleeding in children with variceal bleeding as well as removing blood which may predispose to development of hepatic encephalopathy in children with chronic liver disease and variceal bleeding. However, absence of blood on NG aspiration does not rule out a UGIB (duodenal source or intermittent bleeding from stomach/esophagus). A serum urea nitrogen to creatinine ratio above 30 also points toward a UGI source of bleeding.

General supportive measures include establishing a good venous access, intake output monitoring, oxygen supplementation (if required), and charting of vitals. Blood transfusion should be given to achieve Hb of 7–8 g/dL as per the guidelines of the American College of Gastroenterology (ACG) and the European Society for Gastrointestinal Endoscopy (ESGE). Avoid overtransfusion to prevent increased portal pressure which increases the risk of rebleeding. But a more liberal approach is used in patients with underlying cardiovascular disorders, with transfusion initiated at Hb level of >8 g/dL. The prothrombin time/international normalized ratio (PT/INR) does not accurately reflect the hemostatic status of patients with advanced liver diseases. Viscoelastic tests like thromboelastogram are better indicators of the chronic liver disease (CLD). Intramuscular vitamin K injection should be given in children with deranged INR. Platelets should be transfused if platelet count is <20,000/mm^3. Fresh frozen plasma (FFP) may be used in select cases.

Short-term antibiotic prophylaxis (third-generation cephalosporin for 7 days), should be given to children with cirrhosis and variceal bleed as it reduces bacterial infection, variceal rebleeding and mortality. Lactulose (oral/enema) may be considered to decrease ammonia absorption, in children with CLD and UGIB.

CLINICAL PEARLS

- Children with UGIB should be admitted in the high dependency or ICU.
- Resuscitation and stabilization first, followed by early endoscopy within 12–24 hours of presentation. More urgent endoscopy is advised in children requiring continuous circulatory support.
- Injectable erythromycin should be given prior to (30–120 minutes) endoscopy for better visualization.

Initiation of Vasoactive Therapy (Octreotide/Proton Pump Inhibitor)

Medical treatment should be started at the earliest prior to endoscopy with either vasoactive drugs like octreotide, in patients with variceal bleeding or, high dose PPI infusion in suspected ulcer bleeding. PPI infusion has been shown to decrease incidence of endoscopic stigmata in children with peptic ulcer related bleeding and thus reducing need for endoscopic therapy. However, it is not associated with reduced mortality, rebleeding, or need for surgery. It is especially useful as a cost-effective therapy in patients with a probable nonvariceal cause of UGIB and possibility of delay in endoscopy.

Sucralfate should be avoided as it may obstruct the view during endoscopy (but may be given after endoscopy). Prokinetics like erythromycin (3 mg/kg/dose, given 30–120 minutes before endoscopy) may help in stomach emptying and thus endoscopic visualization as well as reduce the need for relook endoscopy.

Predictor for Endoscopy

In adults, there are validated scoring systems that can predict the necessity of endoscopic hemostatic intervention and risk stratification for rebleed and mortality. Recently Sheffield scoring was assessed to predict children who are at high risk and need endotherapy. It is based on presence of clinical factors such as melena, large volume hematemesis, HR > 20 beats/min from the mean HR for age, prolonged capillary refill, Hb drop of >2 g/dL, need for a fluid bolus, or red blood cell (RBC) transfusion. The total score is 24 and a cutoff of 8 had sensitivity of 88.57%, specificity of 91.18%, positive predictive value (PPV) of 91.18%, and negative predictive value (NPV) of 88.57% to predict the need for endotherapy in children with acute GI bleed.

Investigations for Cause of Bleed Including Upper Gastrointestinal Endoscopy

Investigations are aimed at establishing the site, severity, and cause of bleeding. Hematocrit (Hct) should be monitored frequently to assess severity of blood loss as the Hb falls only after a few hours, after hemodilution. A complete hemogram including platelet count, coagulation profile [PT/activated partial thromboplastin time (aPTT)], liver function tests, urea, creatinine, electrolytes, and cross matching should be done in all patients at admission.

The UGI endoscopy is the investigation of choice both for diagnosing the cause and providing therapy. It should preferably be done under general anesthesia or conscious sedation with airway protection to avoid aspiration and only after the patient is hemodynamically stable. Intubation is preferred in patients with active hematemesis and those with altered sensorium and the patient can be considered for extubation as soon as possible/once the sensorium improves. The yield of UGI endoscopy is best if it is done within 24 hours of onset of UGIB. A complete examination of esophagus, stomach, and duodenum with retroflexion to inspect the fundus and gastroesophageal junction is essential **(Figs. 1 to 3)**. Biopsy should always be taken in patients with gastric/duodenal ulcers, esophagitis, and gastritis. These help in diagnosing *Helicobacter pylori* infection and other entities

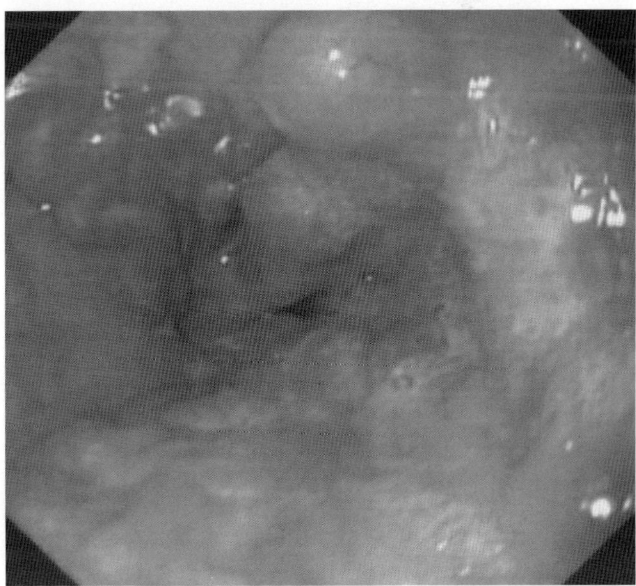

Fig. 1: Upper gastrointestinal endoscopy showing large esophageal varices. *(For color version, see Plate 3)*

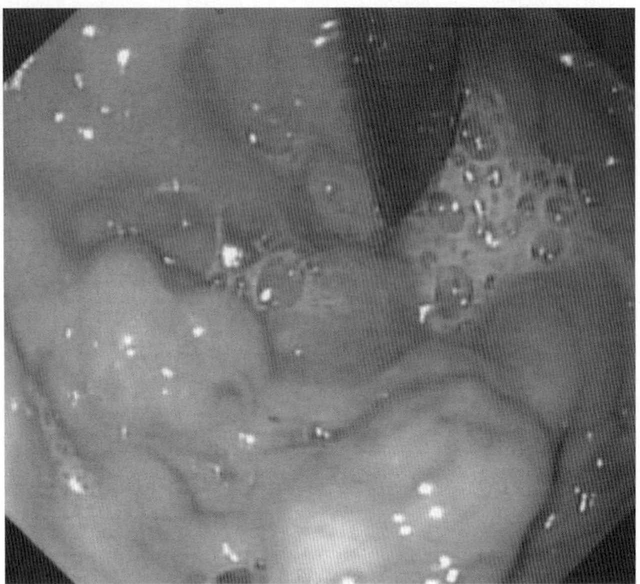

Fig. 2: Upper gastrointestinal endoscopy showing gastric varices with red color signs on retroversion. *(For color version, see Plate 3)*

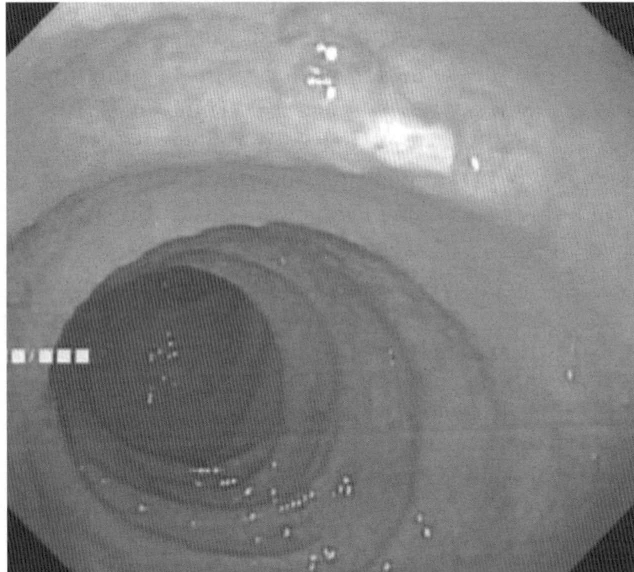

Fig. 3: Upper gastrointestinal endoscopy showing duodenal ulcer without signs of active bleeding. *(For color version, see Plate 4)*

such as infections (cytomegalovirus and herpes) and Crohn's disease.

The important checklist for endoscopy before scoping a sick child with UGIB includes:

- Control of airway
- Availability of blood and blood products
- Check the irrigation method and suction of the scope
- Ensure availability of band ligator, sclerosant, adrenaline (1:10,000), glue and needle for sclerotherapy, bipolar cautery and/or argon plasma coagulation, hemoclips, and hemospray
- Backup endoscope in case of malfunction
- Backup of interventional radiology and/or surgeon if endoscopic hemostasis fails

The other investigations which help in reaching a diagnosis include:

- *Ultrasonography with Doppler:* This provides information about portal vein, hepatic veins, inferior vena cava, presence of collaterals, etc., and helps in diagnosis of portal hypertension (EHPVO and chronic liver disease).
- *Contrast-enhanced computed tomography scan:* This is useful in evaluation of patients with mass lesions, suspected hemobilia, or hemosuccus pancreaticus. Selective angiography of celiac trunk/superior mesenteric artery is required in patients where a vascular lesion like pseudoaneurysm is suspected. Therapy with coil/gel embolization can be done at the time of angiography.
- *Nuclear scintigraphy* (technetium-99m labeled pertechnetate scan) is helpful in children suspected to have duplication cyst of proximal GI tract.
- *Enteroscopy (single/double balloon)/capsule endoscopy:* It is required in some cases for evaluation of lesions in distal duodenum (third and fourth part) if the etiology cannot be determined on standard UGI endoscopy.

CLINICAL PEARLS

- Hct should be monitored to assess severity of bleeding as Hb falls later, after hemodilution.
- The yield of UGI endoscopy in patients with UGI endoscopy is maximum if done within 24 hours of onset of bleed.
- Intermittently bleeding lesions (e.g., hemobilia and Dieulafoy's lesion) may be missed if endoscopy is done after the bleed has stopped.

Management of Upper Gastrointestinal Bleed

The choice of treatment depends upon the patient's condition, available facilities, and expertise of the personnel. Specific treatment can be broadly divided into management of variceal and nonvariceal bleed.

Variceal Bleeding

In a child with portal hypertension, esophageal varices are the most common cause of UGIB **(Fig. 1)**. Gastric varices (GV), congestive gastropathy, and gastric antral vascular ectasia can also present with hematemesis.

Somatostatin and octreotide: These drugs decrease the splanchnic and azygous blood flow and reduce portal venous inflow, thus reducing the portal pressure. Somatostatin and octreotide both are equally effective. Limited studies in children have shown control of bleeding in 64–71% children. Overall, this therapy is well tolerated with mild side effects such as hyperglycemia, abdominal discomfort, nausea, and diarrhea which often resolve spontaneously. Infusion should be given for at least 24–48 hours after the bleeding has stopped to prevent recurrence and infusion should not be stopped abruptly. The doses are shown in **Table 3**. Vasopressin and terlipressin are also useful in management of variceal bleed but data are largely limited to adults.

CLINICAL PEARLS

- In patients with UGI endoscopy, transfusion should be given for a target Hb of 7–8 g/dL.
- Intravenous (IV) antibiotic for 7 days should be given to all patients with chronic liver disease and variceal bleeding.

Endoscopic Therapy for Variceal Bleed

Esophageal varices: Endoscopic variceal ligation (EVL) and endoscopic sclerotherapy (EST) are the two main methods. The varices are inspected and their location, size, and extent are documented. In EST, 2–3 mL of sclerosant (1% ethoxysclerol) is injected into each variceal column. EVL is done with a device called multiple band ligator. The variceal column is sucked into a cylinder attached at the tip of the endoscope and the band is deployed by pulling the trip wire around the varix. Both EST and EVL have a 90–100% efficacy in controlling acute bleeding. The major complications include esophageal ulceration, stricture esophagus, and rarely perforation. EVL is preferred over EST due to lesser side effects and quicker eradication with a smaller number of sessions. However, EVL cannot be done in children <2 years due to technical reasons and in them EST is the only option.

Gastric varices: Endoscopic injection of tissue adhesive glue, i.e., N-butyl-2-cyanoacrylate or isobutyl-2-cyanoacrylate is done for GV **(Fig. 2)**. These agents harden within 20 seconds of contact with blood, and lead to a more rapid control of active bleeding. Only a small volume (0.5–1 mL) of glue is injected at a time and multiple injections can be done in a single session. Appropriate care must be taken to avoid damage to the endoscope during glue injection. Another technique is endoscopic ultrasound (EUS)-guided coiling or coiling combined with cyanoacrylate glue injection for large fundal varices as it reduces the risk of systemic embolization.

Endoscopic therapy either with argon plasma coagulation or band ligation can be used for bleeding due to portal hypertensive gastropathy (PHG) and/or gastric antral vascular ectasia.

TABLE 3: Drugs used to control upper gastrointestinal bleeding.

Drugs for acid suppression	
Ranitidine	• PO 2–4 mg/kg/day q 8–12 h, maximum 10 mg/kg/d (300 mg) • IV 2–4 mg/kg/day q 8–12 h
Proton pump inhibitors	• Omeprazole 0.7–3.3 mg/kg/day single or two divided doses • Lansoprazole 15 mg/day if weight <30 kg; 30 mg if weight >30 kg • Esomeprazole 10 mg/day if weight <20 kg; 20–40 mg if weight >20 kg • Proton pump inhibitors infusion for ulcer bleed—intravenous pantoprazole 2 mg/kg (maximum 80 mg) loading followed by 0.2 mg/kg/h infusion (maximum 8 mg/h)
Drugs for variceal bleeding	
Vasopressin	Start at 0.002–0.005 U/kg/min, increase to a maximum dose of 0.01/U/kg/min
Octreotide	1 µg/kg bolus and then 1 µg/kg/h infusion, maximum 5 µg/kg/h
Somatostatin*	250 µg bolus and then 250 µg/h infusion in adults
Terlipressin*	2 mg (20 µg/kg maximum) every 4 hours IV till a bleed free period of 24–48 hours

*Limited experience in children.
(IV: intravenous; PO: per oral)

Tamponade of varices: This is required only when the endoscopic and pharmacologic measures have failed. Sengstaken-Blakemore tube (SBT) is a triple lumen tube with connection to an esophageal balloon, a gastric balloon and one distal end which helps in aspiration of the stomach contents. The SBT has efficacy of ~75% in controlling acute variceal bleeding (AVB). Both pediatric and adult size SBTs are available. The tube is passed through the nose and allowed to reach the stomach. Thereafter, the gastric balloon is inflated with 75–150 mL of air depending on the size of the patient (stomach) and the tube is gently pulled outward so that it sits snugly against the fundus and gastroesophageal junction. A plain X-ray of the abdomen is done to check the proper placement of gastric balloon in the stomach. If the bleeding continues after inflation of gastric balloon, then the esophageal balloon is inflated. Esophageal necrosis and perforation, pulmonary aspiration, and rebleeding on deflation of balloon are important complications. The esophageal balloon should be deflated after 12–24 hours, and in case of continued bleeding it can be reinflated. However, it should be remembered that SBT is a temporary treatment and efforts should be done to arrange for endoscopic therapy at the earliest.

Transjugular intrahepatic portosystemic shunt: Transjugular intrahepatic portosystemic shunt (TIPS) effectively reduces portal pressure by creation of a communication between the hepatic vein and portal vein and is indicated in children who have failed medical and endoscopic therapy. TIPS can be done in cirrhotic patients with a patent splenoportal axis. It involves insertion of a multipurpose catheter through the jugular vein and superior vena cava. The catheter is thereafter passed via hepatic vein into a branch of portal vein through the hepatic parenchyma. The passage is dilated by a balloon and an expansile metallic mesh prosthesis is placed to maintain the communication directly between the portal vein and hepatic vein. Experience in children is limited. In a recent meta-analysis with 284 children, TIPS was technically successful in 93.3% of patients, with a major adverse event rate of 3.2% and hepatic encephalopathy rate of 2.9%. Stent dysfunction with need of reintervention is a drawback of TIPS.

In refractory esophageal variceal bleeding, self-expanding metallic stents have been tried in adults but the data in children is lacking. In patients with gastroesophageal type 2 and type 1 isolated GV, and ectopic varices, balloon-occluded retrograde transvenous obliteration (BRTO) or coil-assisted retrograde transvenous obliteration is an alternative to TIPS. The data in children is limited.

Surgical management: Emergency surgery is required when all the other therapeutic measures have failed or when bleeding is from ectopic varices inaccessible to endoscopic procedures. Surgery can be done either in the form of portacaval shunt (selective or nonselective) or devascularization with esophageal staple transection. This is especially useful for children with noncirrhotic portal hypertension such as EHPVO, idiopathic portal hypertension, and congenital hepatic fibrosis.

Acute variceal bleeding is a serious and life-threatening complication of patients with portal hypertension. Standard of care mandates early administration of vasoactive drugs followed by endoscopic therapy preferably within 12 hours of bleed. Balloon tamponade followed by TIPS or surgery may be done in patients who fail endoscopic and drug therapy.

All patients surviving an episode of AVB should undergo further secondary prophylaxis with EST/EVL to prevent rebleeding.

Nonvariceal Bleeding

The etiology of nonvariceal UGIB is diverse and management largely depends on the cause. Most common cause is peptic ulcer disease (PUD). The Forrest classification (to identify features associated with increased risk of continuous bleeding) is useful in deciding the management protocol. EUS and through the scope Doppler may help identify the lesions for endoscopic therapy and are more objective than visual assessment of the presence of stigmata.

Medical Therapy

Proton pump inhibitors promote clot stability and facilitate hemostasis by raising the intragastric pH. PPI infusion should be initiated in any patient suspected to have nonvariceal bleeding (NVB) from the UGI. Drugs like NSAID should be stopped in patients with UGIB.

Specific therapy: Antifungal (fluconazole) in esophageal candidiasis and specific antiviral therapy (acyclovir/ganciclovir) in esophagitis due to herpes/cytomegalovirus infection is essential. Immunosuppressants and antitubercular drugs is given for UGI Crohn's and tuberculosis, respectively.

Helicobacter pylori infection should be looked for and treated in all patients with bleeding peptic ulcers. The high false-negative rate for *H. pylori* testing in the setting of acute UGIB should be remembered. Triple therapy [PPI plus two of the three antibiotics (amoxicillin, clarithromycin, and metronidazole)] for 14 days is the treatment of choice [the European Society for Paediatric Gastroenterology Hepatology and Nutrition (ESPGHAN)].

Dietary changes: Stoppage of milk and milk products is required for infants with UGIB due to cow's milk protein allergy.

Endoscopic Therapy for Nonvariceal Bleed

Endoscopic treatment is effective in patients with NVB and includes multiple options such as injection (adrenaline or hypertonic saline), electrocoagulation, heater probes, hemoclips [through the scope or over-the-scope clip (OTSC)] and hemospray.

Peptic ulcer bleeding: Endoscopic hemostasis using thermal or mechanical therapies alone or in combination with injection should be done in all patients with high-risk ulcers [Forrest Ia (active spurting bleeding), Ib (active oozing bleeding), IIa (nonbleeding visible vessel)]. PPI infusion is given for 72 hours and thereafter twice daily PPI is given for 2 weeks after index endoscopy as it decreases rebleeding, need for surgery and mortality. If there is adherent clot (Forrest IIb), there is no recommendation for or against endoscopic therapy, but needs high dose PPI therapy. Cases with flat pigmented spot and clean based ulcer require only standard PPI therapy.

Over-the-scope clips are used for patients who develop recurrent bleeding due to ulcers after previous successful endoscopic hemostasis. Patients who have hemodynamic instability, active bleeding at endoscopy, ulcer size >2 cm, ulcer located in high lesser gastric curvature or posterior duodenum, Hb < 10 g/dL, and need for transfusion are at a higher risk of having rebleeding after endoscopic hemostasis. The therapeutic options for patients with post endotherapy rebleeding include repeat endoscopic hemostasis, radiologic transcatheter arterial embolization of the bleeding vessel and surgery. Choice of therapy is to be decided on case-to-case basis and expertise in surgical and interventional techniques.

Some of the other causes of NVB and their management are discussed here.

Mallory-Weiss tear (MWT): Antiemetics and PPI infusion is given. Patients with active bleeding may be treated with local adrenaline (1:10,000 dilution) injection along with thermal coagulation or endoscopic clips.

Visceral artery aneurysm: True visceral artery aneurysm is defined as focal arterial dilatation >1.5 times the diameter of the original vessel and involving all three layers of the arterial wall, whereas pseudoaneurysm is due to a tear in the vessel wall with extravasated blood contained by only one or two layers of the arterial wall. It may be secondary to trauma, abscess, pancreatitis, cholecystitis, and/or iatrogenic injury (surgical, endoscopic, and interventional radiological procedures). Endovascular treatment (coil embolization) is the first-line treatment modality. Surgical intervention is reserved in case of anatomically unfeasible or failed endovascular coiling.

Dieulafoy's lesion: It is a vascular abnormality consisting of a dilated submucosal caliber-persistent artery which protrudes through a small 2–5 mm mucosal defect and erodes into the GI lumen, in the absence of ulcers, erosions, or aneurysms. Mucosal disruption due to the mechanical pressure perpetrated by the underlying submucosal ectatic artery. The most common site is proximal lesser curvature of gastroesophageal junction. Treatment includes combination endoscopic therapy with epinephrine injection followed by mechanical therapy with band ligation or endoclip placement.

Cameron lesions: Cameron lesions are linear gastric erosions or ulcerations located on the crest of mucosal folds in cases with large hiatal hernia near the diaphragmatic pinch. It occurs due to mechanical trauma and ischemia, secondary to repetitive movement of the hernia sac against the diaphragm during respiratory movements. Endoscopic hemostasis is indicated in case of active bleeding, visible vessel, or adherent clot. In refractory Cameron lesion, laparoscopic or open fundoplication should be considered.

Hemosuccus pancreaticus: The classical Sandblom's triad consists of abdominal pain radiating to the back (due to increase in intraductal pressure due to blood clot), intermittent UGIB (melena/hematemesis), and hyperamylasemia. It is seen in patients with a history of acute or chronic pancreatitis and less frequently pancreatic neoplasms. The most common cause is ruptured pseudoaneurysm formed secondary to leakage of proteolytic enzymes with destruction of the arterial wall. Mortality rate is high, reaching up to ~90% in untreated cases. Endovascular treatment is preferred with surgery being reserved for patients with unsuccessful embolization.

Hemobilia: Hemobilia is defined as bleeding into the intra- or extrahepatic biliary system and into the duodenum *via* the major duodenal papilla. The classic clinical presentation is Quincke's triad, consisting of right upper quadrant pain, jaundice, and UGIB. Bleeding can be intermittent and difficult to visualize endoscopically, even with side-viewing endoscope. EUS/ultrasound abdomen can detect aneurysm or pseudoaneurysm in the hepatic vasculature, blood within the gallbladder and common bile duct, and biliary radicle dilation. In the presence of vascular lesions and refractory bleed, transcatheter arterial embolization is treatment of choice. In the absence of these, management includes endoscopic retrograde cholangiography and biliary stenting which can provide tamponade and maintain patency of the duct.

Other rare causes include aortoenteric fistula, especially in children with button battery ingestion due to aortoesophageal fistula. This can be fatal and can occur weeks after button battery removal.

CLINICAL PEARLS

- IV octreotide and PPIs infusion should be given to all patients with UGIB due to varices and peptic ulcer, respectively.
- Endotherapy (EVL/endoscopic sclerotherapy for esophageal varices and glue injection for GV) is the main stay for management of variceal bleeding.

PREVENTION

- Stress ulcers, erosions of the stomach, and duodenum are well-known complications of critical illness in children admitted to the pediatric ICU **(Fig. 3)**. Nearly 10% of pediatric intensive care unit (PICU) subjects have UGIB but it is clinically significant only in <2% cases. Children with coagulopathy, respiratory failure, and high pediatric risk of mortality score >10 are at an increased risk of bleeding. Although literature is limited, pooled data from two randomized controlled trials shows that prophylactic acid neutralizing treatment was significantly more effective in preventing UGIB compared with no treatment [two studies = 300 participants; relative risk, 0.41; 95% confidence interval (CI) 0.19–0.91].
- Secondary prophylaxis for variceal bleeding by EST/EVL as discussed earlier.
- *H. pylori* eradication therapy to prevent recurrence of peptic ulcer. Eradication should be ensured by repeat testing.

CONCLUSION

Acute UGIB is a potentially serious problem in children and presents with hematemesis or melena. As the causes of UGIB vary with age, it is important to evaluate children for the age specific etiologies. Esophagitis, gastritis, PUD, and varices are the most common causes of UGIB in children. The approach to diagnosis is largely dictated by the child's condition. Prompt hemodynamic stabilization is of utmost importance and physical examination and blood investigations are done simultaneously. UGI endoscopy is the most useful diagnostic and therapeutic tool for children presenting with UGIB. Medications such as octreotide and PPI are useful in variceal and ulcer bleed respectively with radiological intervention and surgery being reserved for cases with continued bleed and failure of endoscopic therapy.

KEY POINTS

- UGIB is a common emergency in children and presents as hematemesis or melena.
- Hemodynamic stabilization, identifying the cause and providing specific treatment is the aim.
- Octreotide/PPI infusion to be started at admission depending on clinical suspicion of varices or nonvariceal UGIB, respectively.
- UGI endoscopy should be done after hemodynamic resuscitation.
- Erythromycin should be given 30–120 minutes before endoscopy for better visualization.
- In patients with variceal bleeding (esophageal or gastric):
  - Octreotide infusion should be continued for 2–5 days. Endotherapy (EVL/EST/glue injection) is done.
  - Blood transfusion should be given to target a Hb of 7–8 g/dL. However, ongoing bleed, hemodynamic status, and associated cardiac disease should be kept in mind.
  - Antibiotic should be given in patients with chronic liver disease and variceal bleeding.
  - Secondary prophylaxis for esophageal varices till eradication
- UGIB due to peptic ulcer disease:
  - Endotherapy (adrenaline injection, mechanical, thermal, and hemospray) as per Forrest classification.
  - PPI to be continued after endotherapy. *H. pylori* eradication is essential in patients with ulcer and *H. pylori* infection to prevent recurrence.
- If the source of bleeding is not identified at UGIE, angiography is done.
- Radiologic intervention/surgery is recommended for children with UGIB and failed medical and endoscopic therapy.

SUGGESTED READING

1. Acharyya BC, Mukhopadhyay M, Chakraborty H. Changing trend in the spectrum of upper gastrointestinal bleeding in children-A multicentre experience. Indian J Gastroenterol. 2023;42:562-8.
2. de Franchis R, Bosch J, Garcia-Tsao G, Reiberger T, Ripoll C. Baveno VII—Renewing consensus in portal hypertension. J Hepatol. 2022;76:959-74.
3. Eroglu Y, Emerick KM, Whitingon PF, Alonso EM. Octreotide therapy for control of acute gastrointestinal bleeding in children. J Pediatr Gastroenterol Nutr. 2004;38:41-7.
4. Franciosi JP, Fiorino K, Ruchelli E. Changing indications for upper endoscopy in children during a 20-year period. J Peadiatr Gastroenterol Nutr. 2010;51:443-7.
5. Garcia-Pagán JC, Barrufet M, Cardenas A, Escorsell A. Management of gastric varices. Clin Gastroenterol Hepatol. 2014;12:919-28.
6. Hegade VS, Sood R, Mohammed N, Moreea S. Modern management of acute non-variceal upper gastrointestinal bleeding. Postgrad Med J. 2013;89:591-8.
7. Herrera JL. Management of acute variceal bleeding. Clin Liver Dis. 2014;18:347-57.
8. Hospital JH, Engorn B, Flerlage J. The Harriet Lane Handbook, 6th edition. Missouri, United States: Mosby; 2002.
9. Khamaysi I, Gralnek IM. Acute upper gastrointestinal bleeding (UGIB)—initial evaluation and management. Best Pract Res Clin Gastroenterol. 2013;27:633-8.
10. Kim SJ, Kim KM. Recent trends in the endoscopic management of variceal bleeding in children. Pediatr Gastroenterol Hepatol Nutr. 2013;16:1-9.
11. Laine L, Barkun AN, Saltzman JR, Martel M, Leontiadis GI. ACG Clinical Guideline: Upper Gastrointestinal and Ulcer Bleeding. Am J Gastroenterol. 2021;116:899-917.
12. Martino A, Di Serafino M, Orsini L, Giurazza F, Fiorentino R, Crolla E, et al. Rare causes of acute non-variceal upper gastrointestinal bleeding: A comprehensive review. World J Gastroenterol. 2023;29:4222-35.
13. Molleston JP. Variceal bleeding in children. J Pediatr Gastroenterol Nutr. 2003;37:538-45.
14. Quintero J, Juampérez J, Mercadal-Hally M, King ML, Ortega J, Molino JA, et al. Endoscopic variceal ligation as primary prophylaxis for upper GI bleeding in children. Gastrointest Endosc. 2020;92:269-75.
15. Reveiz L, Guerrero-Lozano R, Camacho A, Yara L, Mosquera PA. Stress ulcer, gastritis, and gastrointestinal bleeding prophylaxis in critically ill pediatric patients: a systematic review. Pediatr Crit Care Med. 2010;11:124-32.
16. Yachha SK, Khanduri A, Sharma BC, Kumar M. Gastrointestinal bleeding in children. J Gastroenterol Hepatol. 1996;11:903-7.

Management of Lower Gastrointestinal Bleed

Malathi Sathiyasekaran

INTRODUCTION

Lower gastrointestinal bleed (LGIB) is a common problem seen in pediatric practice. The etiological spectrum ecompasses several disorders which may vary with age of the child. Endoscopy and Imaging have revolutionized the approach to the management of LGIB. It is essential that the definite etiology is identified for definitive therapy which may include simple diet modifications, antimicrobials, endotherapy, interventional radiology or surgery.

DEFINITION

Lower gastrointestinal bleed (LGIB) indicates bleeding from sites distal to the ligament of Treitz presenting as bleeding per rectum (PR).

The introduction of capsule endoscopy and double balloon enteroscopy in the diagnostic armamentarium of LGIB has given rise to a new term mid gastrointestinal bleeding (MGIB) for a bleed occurring anywhere distal to the ampulla of Vater up to the ileocecal valve. In this chapter, both small bowel bleed (MGIB) and colonic bleed have been included as LGIB.

TYPES OF BLEED

Lower gastrointestinal bleed may be overt or occult. Overt bleeding can be acute massive or chronic intermittent and can present as hematochezia (passage of frank blood PR), melena, or streaks of blood. Occult bleeding is not clinically apparent but becomes manifest by laboratory evidence of iron deficiency or chemical evidence of blood in the stool. Obscure gastrointestinal bleeding refers to a bleed where the bleeding site is not obvious even after evaluation by upper gastrointestinal endoscopy, an ileocolonoscopy, or a contrast radiological study of the small intestine.

INCIDENCE

Lower gastrointestinal bleeding in infants and children is common in clinical practice yet its epidemiology has not been well studied. It constitutes 0.3% of cases reporting to the emergency room.

ETIOLOGY

The common causes of LGIB in children depend on the age of presentation. In this chapter, the neonatal causes of LGIB have not been included. In India, the common causes of LGIB are polyp, colitis, and fissure-in-ano.

The causes of LGIB may be classifies as:

- Gastrointestinal (**Table 1** shows the gastrointestinal causes of LGIB)
- *Hematological:* Bleeding disorders, coagulation defects, disseminated intravascular coagulation (DIC), thrombocytopenia (dengue and idiopathic thrombocytopenic purpura)
- *Vasculitic disorders:* Henoch-Schönlein purpura
- *Connective tissue disorders:* Ehlers–Danlos syndrome and cutis laxa
- *Factitious:* Various coloring agents, jelly, beetroot, and drugs such as phenolphthalein or rifampicin can color the stool

CLINICAL EVALUATION

A focused and detailed history and physical examination are essential in the evaluation of all children with LGIB.

HISTORY

A meticulous history including details such as whether bleed is major or minor, chronic recurrent or acute massive, treatment, and associated symptoms should be taken. Details of the bleed such as duration, number of episodes,

TABLE 1: Gastrointestinal causes of lower gastrointestinal bleed (LGIB).

1 month to 2 years	*2–12 years*	*12–18 years*
Anal fissure	Anal fissure	Anal fissure
Cow's milk protein allergy	Juvenile polyp	Infection colitis
Infectious/allergic colitis	Infectious colitis	Inflammatory bowel disease
Lymphonodular hyperplasia	Inflammatory bowel disease	Solitary rectal ulcer
Meckel's diverticulum	Solitary rectal ulcer	Colonic polyp
Intussusception	Intussusception	Hemorrhoids
Volvulus	Intestinal duplication	Intestinal duplication
Segmental enteritis	Segmental enteritis	Segmental enteritis
Vascular malformations	Vascular malformations	Vascular malformations

Flowchart 1: Simple approach to LGIB based on age and stool frequency.

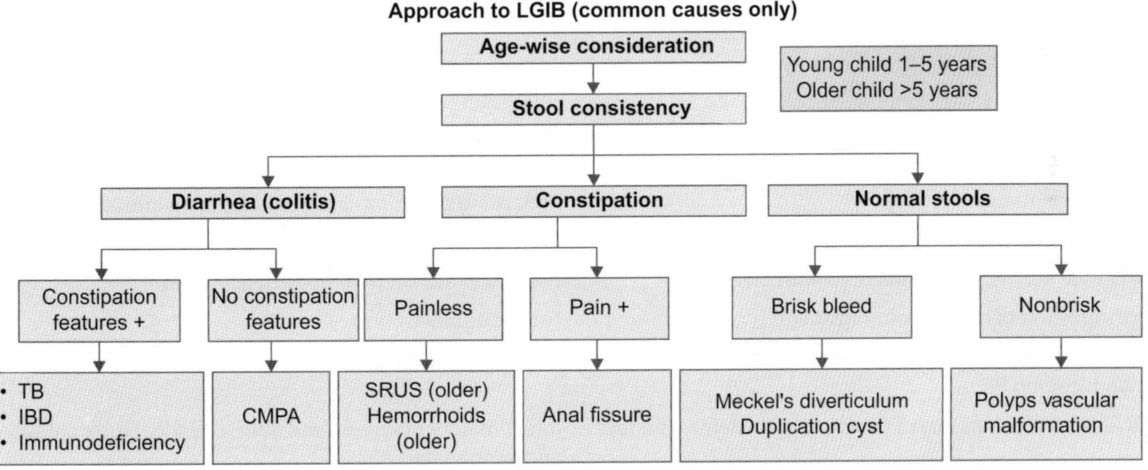

(CMPA: cow's milk protein allergy; IBD: inflammatory bowel disease; LGIB: lower gastrointestinal bleed; SRUS: solitary rectal ulcer syndrome; TB: tuberculosis)

frequency, volume, color, presence of clots, mucus, frank bleed, or mixed with feces, painful or painless should be obtained. The age of the child and frequency of stools **(Flowchart 1)** will also help in establishing the site and probable etiology.

Site of Bleed

About 10% of UGIB may present with bleeding PR. Hematemesis is suggestive of UGIB. Similarly, melena is more often seen in UGIB, whereas hematochezia is usually from small bowel or colon. Specks or streaks of bright red blood indicate bleed from anorectal region.

Etiology

Acute massive bleed may be due to Meckel's diverticulum, intestinal duplication, or arteriovenous malformation. Historically eliciting certain associated symptoms in addition to bleeding PR assists in determining the etiology of LGIB **(Table 2)**.

EXAMINATION

- *General:* All children with acute LGIB whether major or minor require a complete examination including documentation of vital signs.
- *Skin:* Examination of the skin for petechiae, ecchymosis, palpable purpura **(Figs. 2 and 3)** and hemangiomas, buccal pigmentation **(Figs. 4A and B)**, and café au lait spots to exclude familial polyposis syndromes.
- *Abdomen:* Splenomegaly may indicate portal hypertension. Right upper quadrant mass may indicate intussusception. Distended abdomen with dilated bowel loops suggests intestinal obstruction, volvulus, gangrene, or segmental enteritis.

TABLE 2: Diagnostic clues for lower gastrointestinal bleed (LGIB) in history and examination.

Clues in history	*Possible diagnosis*
Crampy abdominal pain and frequent loose stools mixed with mucus and blood	Infectious, inflammatory, or ischemic colitis
Painless bleeding per rectum (PR)	Colonic polyp, Meckel's diverticulum, ulcerated duplication, or vascular malformation
Painful defecation with streaks of blood	Anal fissure
Colicky abdominal pain, vomiting, red currant jelly stool, and mass abdomen	Intussusception
Constipation, mucorrhea, small rectal bleed, with or without digital evacuation, and rectal prolapse	Solitary rectal ulcer syndrome (SRUS)
Recent antibiotic administration followed by passage of blood and mucus in stools	Antibiotic-associated colitis or pseudomembranous colitis
An infant with stools mixed with blood following introduction of bovine milk protein	Cow's milk protein allergy
An infant of normal weight on breast milk with blood in the stool	Benign allergic proctocolitis due to transfer of allergen through breast milk
Passage of large volume and maroon or bright red blood requiring blood transfusions	Meckel's diverticulum, intestinal duplication, or arteriovenous malformation
Mass prolapsing PR with bleeding	Prolapsing polyp, prolapse rectum, or an intussusceptum
A family history of bleeding PR requiring surgical intervention	Polyposis coli
Failure to thrive and recurrent infections with bleeding PR	Primary or acquired immune deficiencies
History of ingestion of beet or coloring agents	Factitious bleed
History of recurrent petechiae, ecchymosis, or epistaxis in addition to bleeding PR	Hematological disorder
Abdominal pain, diarrhea, loss of weight, pedal edema, and fever	Inflammatory bowel disease (IBD), intestinal tuberculosis, and lymphoma
History of abdominal pain, bleeding PR with rash on legs and gluteal region	Henoch–Schönlein purpura
History of fever, rash, features of third spacing, and bleeding PR	Dengue fever
Bluish cutaneous hemangiomas with bleeding PR	Blue rubber bleb nevus syndrome **(Flowchart 1)**
Telangiectasia on fingers and lips with bleeding PR	Hereditary hemorrhagic telangiectasia
Family history of bleeding PR and buccal pigmentation	Peutz–Jeghers syndrome **(Figs. 1A and B)**

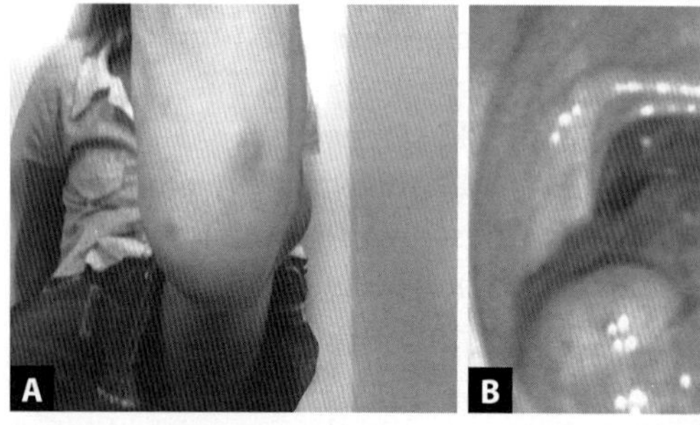

Figs. 1A and B: Bluish black hemangiomas on the sole and hemangiomas on colonoscopy (Blue rubber bleb nevus syndrome). *(For color version, see Plate 4)*

- *Perianal examination:* The presence of skin tags, perianal fistula, or fissure may be markers of inflammatory bowel disease (IBD).

INVESTIGATIONS

Laboratory Studies

Basic investigations such as hemoglobin, total and differential white blood cell count, platelet, bleeding time, clotting time, and prothrombin time, C-reactive protein, and serum albumin are included in the investigative

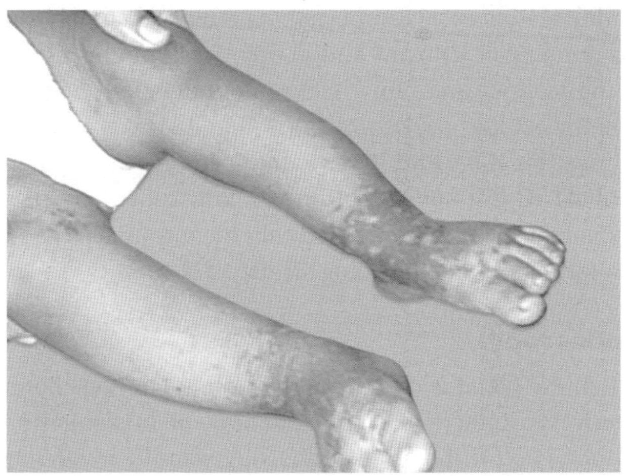

Fig. 2: Infant with dengue and thrombocytopenia with ecchymosis both ankles. *(For color version, see Plate 4)*

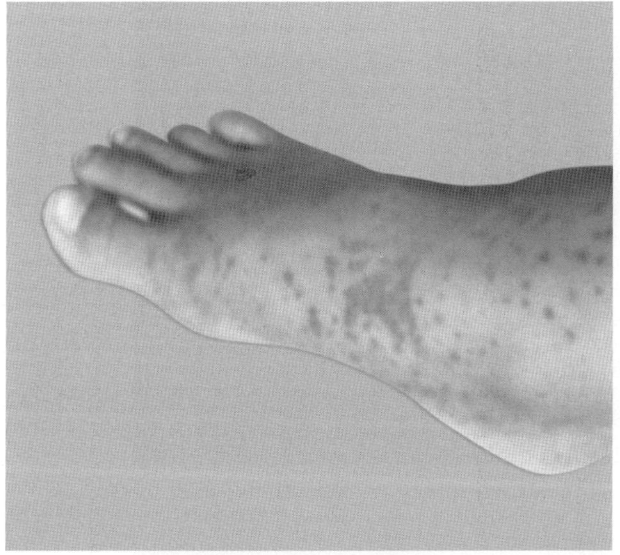

Fig. 3: Palpable Henoch–Schönlein purpura. *(For color version, see Plate 4)*

panel. Refractory iron deficiency anemia is an important manifestation of occult gastrointestinal bleed and should be evaluated diligently. Fecal Calprotectin is a specialised test to detect presence of inflammation and monitior inflammatory bowel disease (IBD). It is usually elevated during active IBD but normal in children with irritable bowel syndrome.

Stool Examination

A simple macroscopic examination of the stool is essential before considering sophisticated investigations.

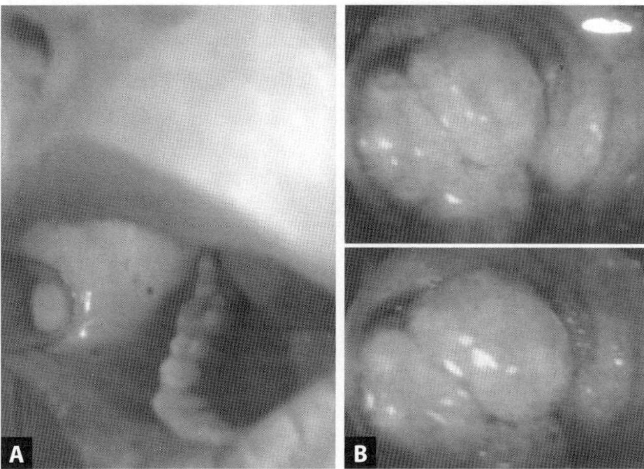

Figs. 4A and B: Oral buccal mucosal pigmentation and colonic polyps (Peutz–Jeghers syndrome). *(For color version, see Plate 4)*

Microscopic Examination

If the stools show more than 10 pus cells/high power field it may indicate an invasive form of colitis. Presence of numerous eosinophils would suggest an allergic colitis or cow's milk protein allergy (CMPA). The presence of trophozoites with hemophagocytosis would be diagnostic of *Entamoeba histolytica* infection. If the clinical setting is suggestive of infectious colitis then stool culture for *Shigella, Salmonella,* and *Campylobacter jejuni* may be helpful. Occult bleeding is identified by testing stool for occult blood.

Radiology

Plain X-ray abdomen is done when there is pain, bilious vomiting, or features of intermittent intestinal obstruction **(Fig. 5)**. Ultrasonography can detect bowel wall thickening pseudokidney appearance or identify characteristic features of intussusception such as target sign **(Figs. 6A and B)**. Air contrast or saline contrast enema helps not only to confirm but also treat ileocolonic intussusception. Computerized tomography or magnetic resonance angiography is generally reserved for evaluation of intestinal duplications **(Figs. 7A and B)**, mass lesions, or complex vascular anomalies. Endosonography helps in the visualization of submucosal lesions and arteriovenous malformations.

Radionuclide Studies

Scintigraphy is useful in the evaluation of children with obscure but active LGIB of at least 0.1 mL/min. In young children with acute massive bleed if Meckel's diverticulum

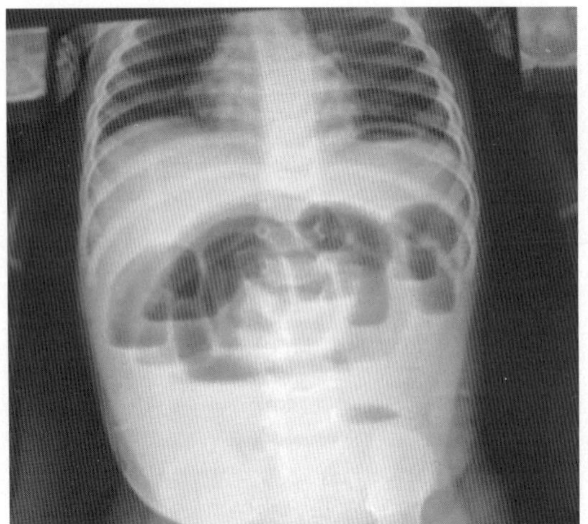

Fig. 5: Plain X-ray abdomen showing features of intestinal obstruction.

or duplication cyst is suspected, radionuclide studies may be done even prior to endoscopy. Radionuclide study using technetium-99m (Tc99m) pertechnetate helps to identify ectopic gastric mucosa within a Meckel's diverticulum **(Figs. 8A and B)** or a duplication cyst **(Figs. 9A and B)** with a sensitivity of 85% and specificity 95%. Technetium-labeled red blood cells identify arteriovenous malformations and bleeding ulcers.

Endoscopy

When the bleed is chronic and intermittent, ileocolonoscopy is preferred as the first line of investigation. Upper gastrointestinal endoscopy should always be done along with ileocolonoscopy since 10% of upper gastrointestinal bleed can present as bleeding PR.

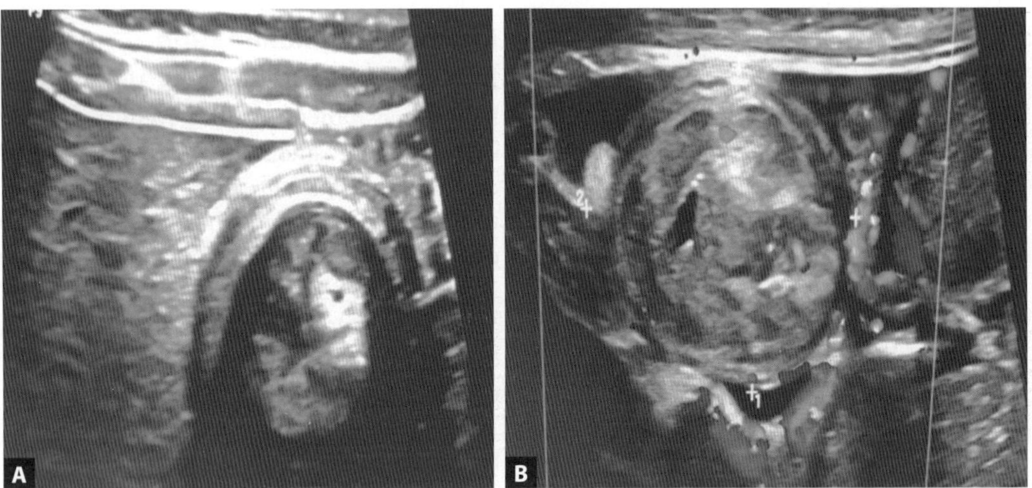

Figs. 6A and B: Ultrasound and Doppler study showing target sign of intussusception. *[For color version (Fig. B), see Plate 4]*

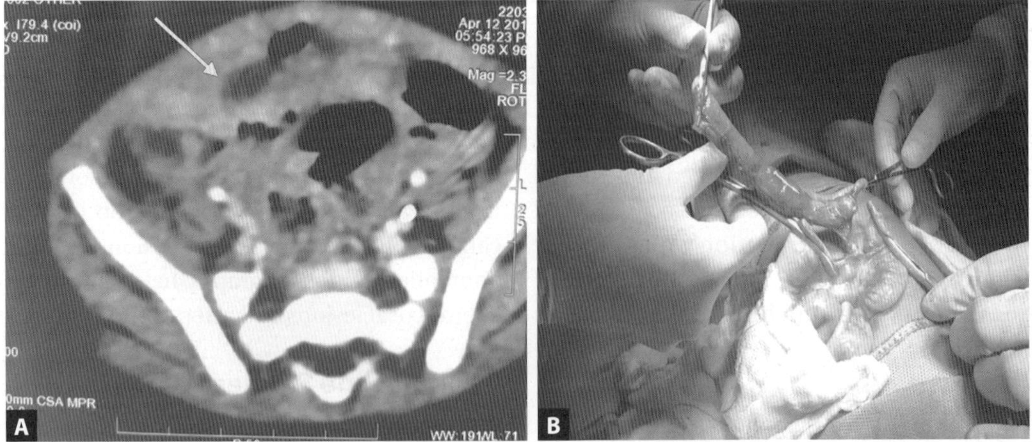

Figs. 7A and B: Contrast-enhanced computed tomography (CECT) abdomen demonstrating the ileal duplication confirmed on surgery. *[For color version (Fig. B), see Plate 5]*

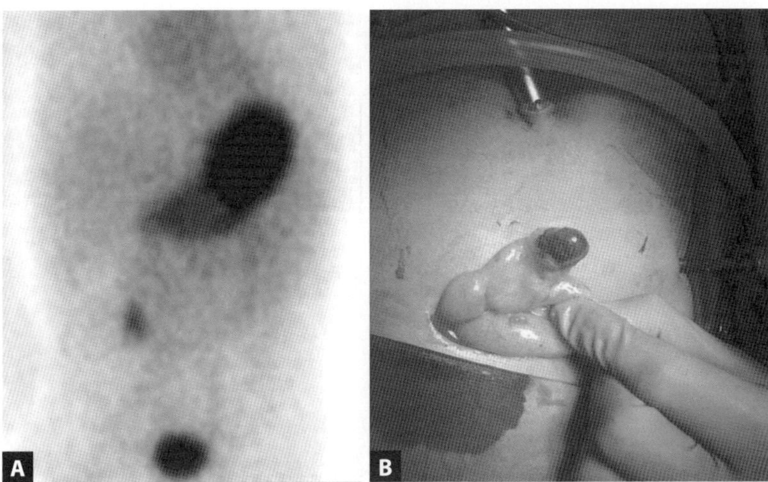

Figs. 8A and B: Radionuclide study technetium-99m pertechnetate scan demonstrating the Meckel's diverticulum confirmed on surgery. *[For color version (Fig. B), see Plate 5]*

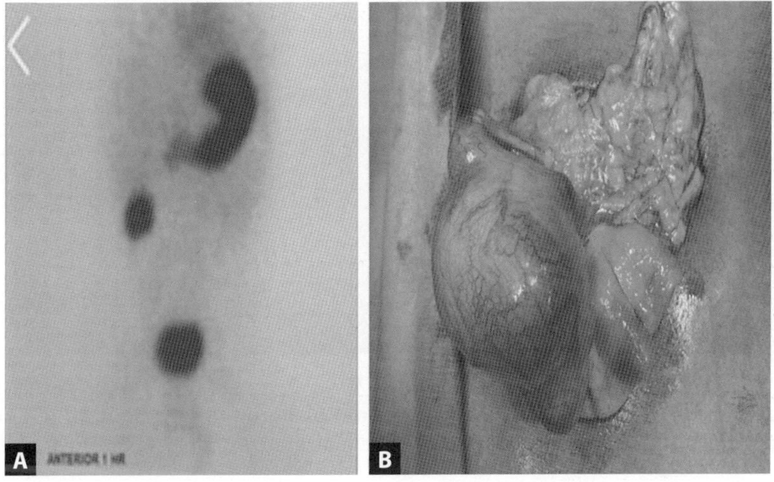

Figs. 9A and B: Radionuclide technetium-99m pertechnetate scan showing uptake of ileal duplication cyst confirmed on surgery. *[For color version (Fig. B), see Plate 5]*

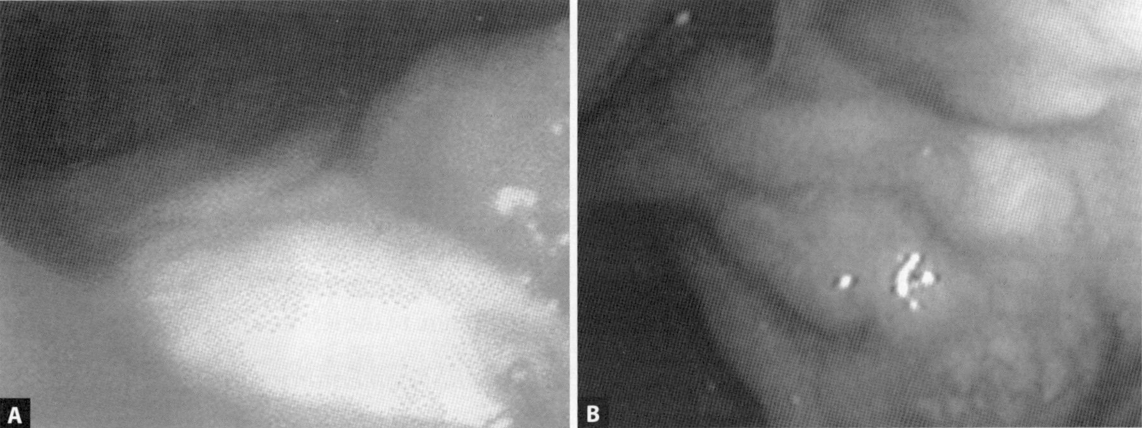

Figs. 10A and B

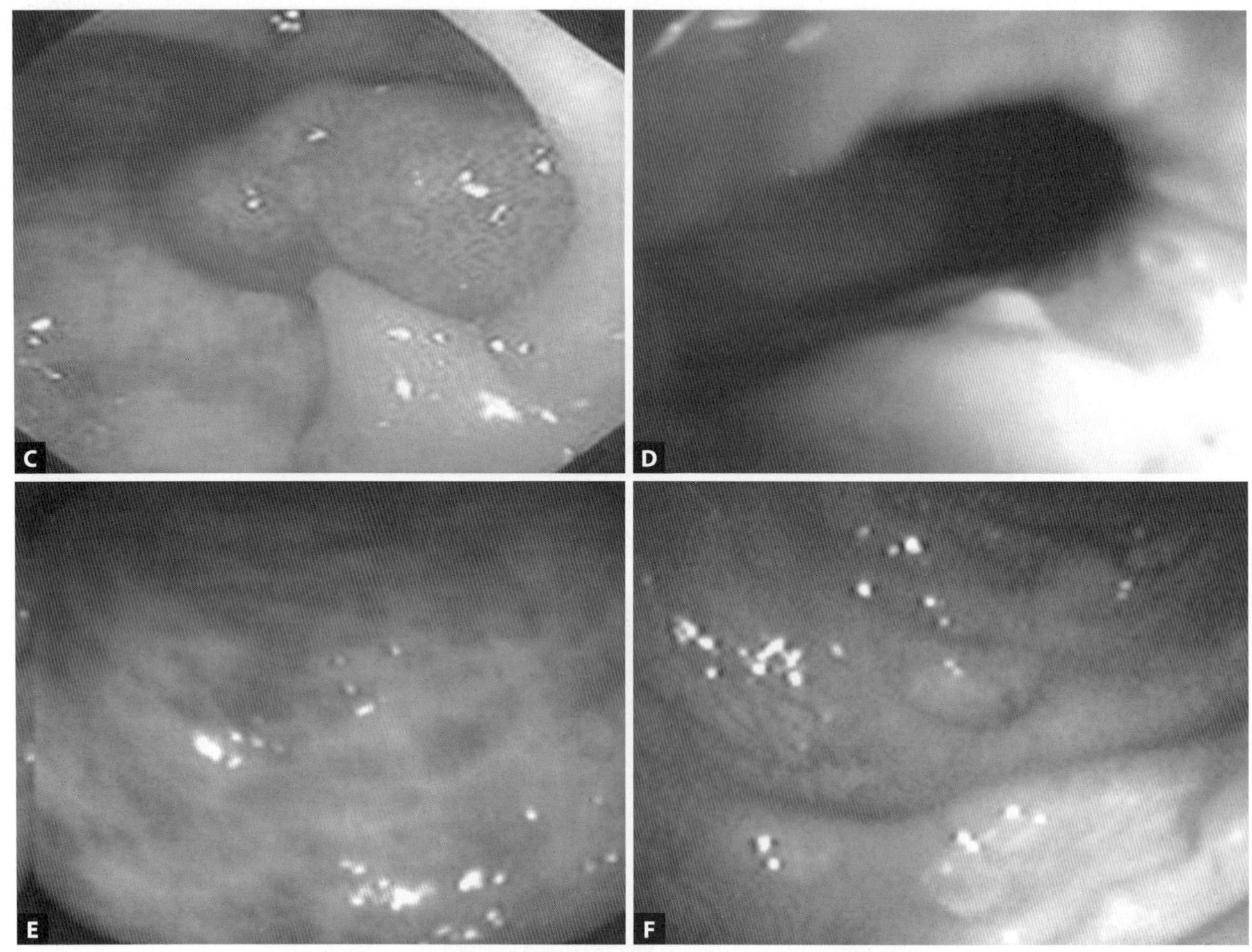

Figs. 10C to F

Figs. 10A to F: Colonoscopy images seen in lower gastrointestinal bleed (LGIB). (A) Solitary rectal ulcer; (B) Rectal varices; (C) Pedunculated cherry red rectal polyp; (D) Fissure-in-ano; (E) Severe ulcerative colitis; (F) Irregular ulcers seen in Crohn's disease. *(For color version, see Plate 6)*

Ileocolonoscopy

An early ileocolonoscopy helps both in diagnosis and therapy of mucosal lesions of the colon presenting as LGIB. The overall yield ranges from 69 to 80%. Bowel preparation is safely achieved in children using a standard oral polyethylene-glycol electrolyte solution. The majority of mucosal lesions, such as allergic colitis, polyps, solitary rectal ulcer, IBD, vascular malformations, rectal varices, and portal colopathy **(Figs. 10A to F)**, can be diagnosed on colonoscopy. Biopsy of the mucosal lesions will help in confirming the etiology.

Additional Procedures

The earlier mentioned investigations will suffice to identify the source of bleeding in the majority of children with LGIB. However, in a small percentage (3–5%), the source will remain obscure necessitating small bowel examination, either with triple vessel arteriography, capsule endoscopy, magnetic resonance enteroclysis, enteroscopy, or intraoperative enteroscopy.

Triple Vessel Arteriography

This is rarely necessary in children with LGIB. It is, however, useful in obscure small bowel bleed if there is active bleeding of at least 0.5 mL/min. The advantage of arteriography is that it helps both in localization and embolization of the lesion.

Double Balloon Enteroscopy

This procedure helps in visualizing the entire small bowel up to the ileocecal valve. It is not regularly used in pediatrics but may be warranted in older children and adolescents with obscure LGIB.

Capsule Endoscopy

Children >5 years of age can swallow the capsule and in younger children, it can be introduced endoscopically. Capsule endoscopy is an excellent modality for identifying obscure gastrointestinal bleed. The detection rate is higher (87–92%) if the procedure is done during active bleed. Impaction of the capsule may occur if there is an underlying stricture.

Intraoperative Enteroscopy

In this procedure, both surgeon and endoscopist work as a team in the evaluation of a child with LGIB. A pediatric colonoscope or enteroscope can be negotiated through an operative enterotomy and the small bowel visualized. It helps in detecting the majority >85% of obscure small bowel bleeding lesions. The surgeon guides the intestine over the scope and examines the outer serosa by palpation and transillumination while the endoscopist examines the inner mucosa.

Diagnostic Laparoscopy/Laparotomy

In children with recurrent gastrointestinal bleed, and if investigations are futile, it may be worthwhile performing a diagnostic laparoscopy to identify lesions such as enteric duplication cyst.

MANAGEMENT

The management of LGIB includes prompt resuscitative measures and treatment of the specific condition by five distinct modalities such as diet modification, medications, endotherapy, radiological intervention, and surgery.

Diet

- *CMPA:* Avoidance of bovine milk protein and milk products till the age of 9 months to 1 year is recommended for all infants diagnosed as having significant CMPA. The child is given hypoallergenic formula either amino acid formula (in severe CMPA or infants <6 months not on breast milk) or extensively hydrolysed formula. Majority will be able to tolerate cow's milk protein by the age of 3–5 years.
- *Fissure-in-ano and solitary rectal ulcer syndrome (SRUS):* Child is encouraged to eat food rich in fiber and to add fruits and vegetables which will benefit children with fissure-in-ano or SRUS.

Medications

- *Bacillary dysentery:* In India, the recommendation is to consider infectious colitis as *Shigella colitis* and treat with oral cefixime 10 mg/kg/day for 7 days if child is ambulant and with intravenous ceftriaxone 100 mg/kg for those hospitalized.
- *Amoebic colitis:* Routine antiamoebic medication should not be prescribed for children with acute colitis. Metronidazole 10 mg/kg/day thrice a day for 5 days is given only if trophozoite with hemophagocytosis suggestive of *Entamoeba histolytica* is identified. It is also prescribed if the child has persistence of symptoms in spite of two antibiotics which are known to be sensitive for *Shigella* have been administered.
- *Ulcer bleeds:* Proton pump inhibitors like omeprazole at a dose of 0.7–1 mg/kg/day or H2 blockers, such as ranitidine at a dose of 4–6 mg/kg/day, can be administered or orally if the bleed is secondary to duodenal ulcer, gastric ulcer, or nonsteroidal anti-inflammatory drugs-induced gastrointestinal injury. In children with active major bleed, proton pump inhibitors score over ranitidine in controlling ulcer bleeds and is recommended at a dose of 1 mg/kg and given slow intravenous followed by infusion.
- *Coagulopathy:* Injection of vitamin K (1 mg/year of age, maximum 10 mg) intravenous/intramuscular is given when the bleed occurs in individuals with portal hypertensive colopathy and hepatocellular dysfunction. Fresh frozen plasma (FFP) may be necessary in children with prolonged international normalized ratio not responding to injection of vitamin K.
- *Thrombocytopenia and coagulopathy:* In children with LGIB secondary to thrombocytopenia as in dengue fever or dengue shock syndrome platelet transfusion, FFP and rarely recombinant factor V may be required.
- *Variceal bleed:* The role of octreotide and somatostatin is well established in acute variceal bleed. When the bleed is nonvariceal, somatostatin and its analog octreotide (1–2 μg/kg bolus followed by 1 μg/kg/h continuous intravenous or 1 μg/kg every 8–12 hours subcutaneously for 24–48 hours) may reduce the risk of continued or recurrent bleeding. These vasoactives act by reducing the splanchnic flow and may help in tiding over the crisis till active intervention is available.
- *IBD:* In IBD, the bleeding stops once the activity of the disease is controlled. IBD is managed according to the severity of disease. 5-aminosalicylic acid 40–50 mg/kg/

day is initiated in children with mild ulcerative colitis (UC) and mild Crohn's disease (CD). Steroids at a dose of 1 mg/kg/day is given for induction of remission and tapered over a period of 12 weeks in moderate UC or CD. Immunomodulators such as azathioprine 6 mercaptopurine are excellent steroid sparing agents and used in the phase of maintenance.
- Anal fissure can be managed with stool softeners and high fiber diet.
- SRUS is managed by encouraging the child to increase fiber in the diet and thus avoiding constipation and straining during defecation. The child is trained to acquire a proper and regular bowel habit. In some situations, several sittings of biofeedback therapy may be required. Various modalities of topical therapy have been tried such as 5-aminosalicylic acid suppository and sucralfate enema. When the bleed is severe and not responding to dietary modifications argon plasma coagulation and surgery may be recommended.

Endotherapy

- If SRUS does not respond to medications, endoscopic argon plasma coagulation can be attempted.
- Colonic polyps are managed by endoscopic polypectomy.

Interventional Radiology

- Intussusception in infants <2 years can be reduced either with air or saline enema.
- When the bleed occurs due to an arteriovascular malformation or a bleeding, aneurysm embolization using coils is an excellent method to arrest the bleed.

Surgery

- Children with familial polyposis coli are advised total colectomy to prevent malignancy.
- Intussusception which has not been reduced by pneumatic reduction should be tackled surgically.
- Meckel's diverticulum, volvulus, and duplication are all managed surgically.

CONCLUSION

Lower gastrointestinal bleed presenting as bleeding PR is a common problem in children and may be due to several causes. The bleed may be very insignificant or sinister. A careful detailed history and clinical examination will help in diagnosis. Since acute massive bleed in young children is usually due to Meckel's diverticulum or duplication cysts, radionuclide scan using Tc99m pertechnetate may be done as a precedent to ileocolonoscopy. The given **Flowchart 2**

Flowchart 2: Simple algorithm approach to child with LGIB presenting as bleeding PR.

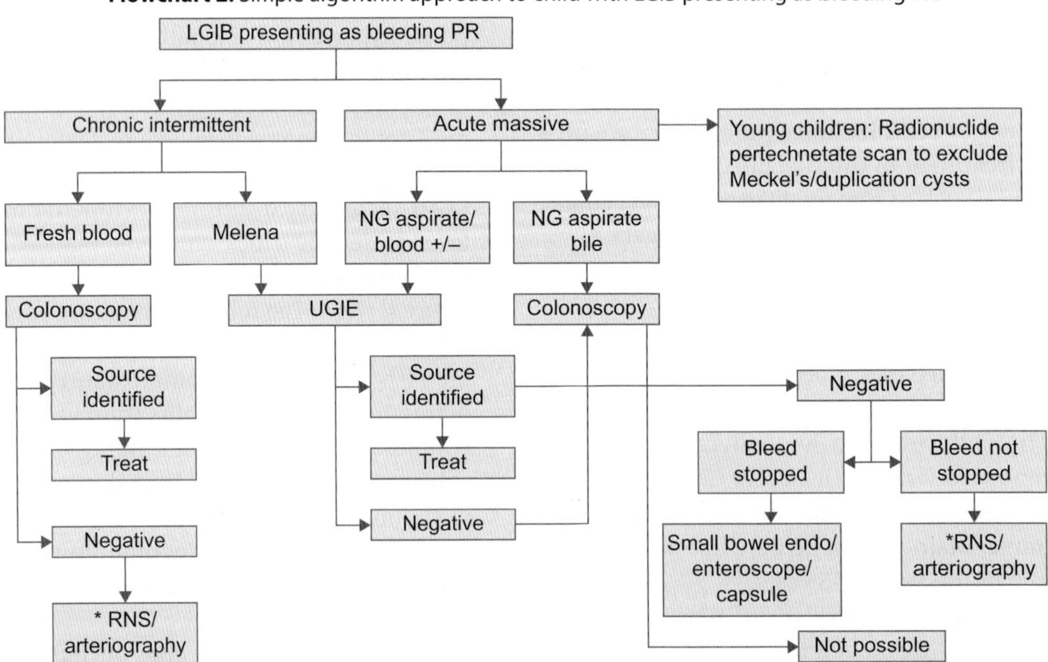

*RNS may be RBC tagged or with pertechnetate
(LGIB: lower gastrointestinal bleed; NG: nasogastric; PR: per rectum; RBC: red blood cell; RNS: radionuclide studies; UGIE: upper gastrointestinal endoscopy)

for LGIB should be modified according to the age of the child, clinical presentation, and feasibility of investigation.

CLINICAL PEARLS

- LGIB may be insignificant or sinister in presentation.
- Detailed history and simple macroscopic examination of stool are the most important tools in evaluation.
- Meckel's scan should be included in the initial diagnostic workup of infants with acute massive bleed.
- Ileocolonoscopy is a safe procedure for both diagnosis and therapy of LGIB.

KEY POINTS

- LGIB may be due to gastrointestinal and nongastrointestinal causes.
- LGIB may be chronic intermittent or acute massive.
- It is essential to evaluate in detail and identify the etiology in all children presenting with LGIB.
- In acute massive nongastrointestinal bleed, radionuclide scan may be done prior to endoscopy.
- Ileocolonoscopy should be included in the protocol.
- Surgery is indicated in some select conditions of LGIB.

SUGGESTED READING

1. Arguelles-Arias F, Caunedo A, Romero J, Sánchez A, Rodríguez-Téllez M, Pellicer FJ, et al. The value of capsule endoscopy in pediatric patients with a suspicion of Crohn's disease. Endoscopy. 2004;36:869-73.
2. Balachandran B, Singhi S. Emergency Management of Lower Gastrointestinal Bleed in Children. Indian J Pediatr. 2013;80(3):219-25.
3. Ell C, May A. Mid-gastrointestinal bleeding: capsule endoscopy and push-and-pull enteroscopy give rise to a new medical term. Endoscopy. 2006;38(1):73-5.
4. Fox VL. Gastrointestinal bleeding in infancy and childhood. Gastroenterol Clin North Am. 2000;29:36-64.
5. Lacroix J, Nadeau D, Laberge S, Gauthier M, Lapierre G, Farrell CA. Frequency of upper gastrointestinal bleeding in a pediatric intensive care unit. Crit Care Med. 1992;20: 35-42.
6. Leung Alexander KC, Wong AL. Lower gastrointestinal bleeding in children. Pediatr Emeg Care. 2002;18: 319-23.
7. Pandey S, Srivastava A, Lal R, Yachha SK, Poddar U. Enteric duplication cysts in children: A target in algorithm for evaluation of lower gastrointestinal bleeding. Indian J Gastroenterol. 2014;33:285-8.
8. Poddar U, Thapa BR, Vaiphei K, Singh K. Colonic polyps: experience of 236 children. Am J Gastroenterol. 1998;93: 619-22.
9. Romano C, Oliva S, Martellossi S, Miele E, Arrigo S. Pediatric gastrointestinal bleeding: Perspectives from the Italian Society of Pediatric Gastroenterology. World J Gastroenterol. 2017;23(8):1328-37.
10. Siafakas C, Fox VL, Nurko S. Use of octreotide for the treatment of severe gastrointestinal bleeding in children. J Pediatr Gastroentrol Nutr. 1998;26:356-9.
11. Strate LL. Lower GI bleeding: epidemiology and diagnosis. Gastroenterol Clin North Am. 2005;34:643-64.
12. Vinton NE. Gastrointestinal bleeding in infancy and childhood. Gastroenterol Clin North Amer. 1994;23:93-122.
13. Yachha SK, Khanduri A, Sharma BC, Kumar M. Gastrointestinal bleeding in children. J Gastroenterol Hepatol. 1996;11:903-7.

CHAPTER 81

Acute Liver Failure

Karunesh Kumar, Jaswinder Kaur, Anupam Sibal

INTRODUCTION

Acute liver failure (ALF) is a rare life-threatening syndrome associated with high mortality mainly due to rapid death or injury to a large proportion of hepatocytes, leaving insufficient functional hepatocytes to sustain life. ALF is a multisystem disorder wherein liver cell function dysfunction and coagulopathy exists with or without the presence of encephalopathy.

DEFINITION AND DIAGNOSIS

Understanding and definition of ALF has evolved in the last few decades, especially in children. Earlier definitions were an extrapolation of adult definitions for which the duration of illness and presence of encephalopathy was an essential part of the definition. However, those definitions failed to capture the complexities associated with pediatric acute liver failure (PALF). Since in most young children and infants, it is difficult to define and classify encephalopathy, the current definition relies more on coagulopathy as an index of liver function **(Box 1 and Table 1)**. Chronic liver diseases such as Wilson disease (WD) and autoimmune hepatitis (AIH) may acutely present with PALF phenotype, these conditions may have different management approaches, prompting to define PALF separately from adults.

BOX 1: PALF study group definition of acute liver failure is as follows (all three components are needed).

1. Acute onset of liver disease without evidence of chronic liver disease
2. Biochemical evidence of severe liver injury
3. *Coagulopathy not corrected by vitamin K:* Prothrombin time (PT) ≥ 15 seconds or INR ≥ 1.5 with evidence of hepatic encephalopathy or PT ≥ 20 seconds or INR > 2 with or without encephalopathy

(INR: international normalized ratio; PALF: pediatric acute liver failure)

TABLE 1: Assessment of encephalopathy in pediatric acute liver failure (PALF).

Grade	*Mental status*
Age <4 years	
Early (Stage 1 and 2)	Inconsolable crying, sleep reversal, and inattention to task
Mid (Stage 3)	Somnolence, stupor, and combativeness
Late (Stage 4)	Comatose, arouses with painful stimuli, or no response
Age >4 years	
Stage 1, prodromal	*Mood swing:* Euphoria/depression; confusion; slowness of mentation and affect; untidiness; slurred speech; and disordered sleep
Stage 2	Accentuation of stage 1; lethargy; moderate confusion; inappropriate behavior; and inability to maintain sphincter control
Stage 3, stupor	Marked confusion; sleepy but arousable; and incoherent speech
Stage 4, coma	May or may not respond to painful stimuli

CLINICAL PEARL

- Encephalopathy is not essential to make a diagnosis of ALF in children.

ETIOLOGY OF ACUTE LIVER FAILURE IN INDIA

The incidence of ALF in the developed world has been stable in the last decade but is increasingly higher in developing countries, possibly due to a higher rate of infectious hepatitis. Acute viral hepatitis is the most common cause of ALF either alone or in combination with other etiologies in developing countries including India.

Metabolic etiologies are increasingly being recognized especially in the younger age group. The other underlying causes of ALF are given in **Box 2**.

DIAGNOSTIC WORKUP

Table 2 summarizes the diagnostic workup necessary to establish the etiology of ALF. It is important to stratify investigations depending on the demographic status of the child. Not all investigations are needed in every child.

BOX 2: Underlying etiology of acute liver failure in children.

- *Infections:* Acute viral hepatitis (A, E, and B), severe dengue, HSV, EBV, adenovirus, *Enterovirus*, and leptospirosis
- *Drugs:* Valproate, isoniazid, and paracetamol
- *Toxins:* Iron and complementary and alternative medicines (CAMs) mushroom
- *Metabolic:* Wilson disease, galactosemia, tyrosinemia type 1, HFI, mitochondrial hepatopathy, and FAOD
- *Vascular:* Budd–Chiari syndrome and veno-occlusive disease
- *Immunological:* Autoimmune liver disease, HLH, and GALD
- Idiopathic

(EBV: Epstein–Barr virus; FAOD: fatty acid oxidation disorder; GALD: gestational alloimmune liver disease; HFI: hereditary fructose intolerance; HLH: hemophagocytic lymphohistiocytosis; HSV: herpes simplex virus)

TRANSPORT AND INITIAL MANAGEMENT

Management of ALF in children is often challenging due to rapid deterioration and multisystemic involvement necessitating intensive care management and a multidisciplinary approach. Children with coagulopathy and worsening encephalopathy should be timely transferred to a tertiary care unit with facilities for liver transplantation. It is important to act early because the risks involved with patient transport may increase or even preclude transfer as encephalopathy progresses. Any child who develops grade III encephalopathy should be intubated to secure the airway, sedated well, and resuscitated for any hemodynamic instability before the transport and transported in a well-equipped ambulance with continuous monitoring of vital parameters.

CLINICAL PEARL

- Sedation should be given to a child only when support for intubation and ventilation is available.

TABLE 2: Diagnostic workup for acute liver failure in children.

General workup	• Total and conjugated bilirubin, AST, ALT, GGTP, alkaline phosphatase, prothrombin time and INR, PTTK, fibrinogen, hemogram, peripheral smear, serum electrolytes, magnesium, serum phosphate, blood urea, creatinine, blood and urine cultures, blood group, serum α-fetoprotein, lactate, lactate dehydrogenase, blood ammonia, ABG, urine for reducing substances, and G6PD levels • Chest X-ray and ultrasound abdomen with liver Doppler
Specific workup	
Infectious	• IgM anti-HAV, IgM anti-HEV, and HBsAg • *Leptospira* and dengue serology • Serology or PCR for CMV, Epstein–Barr virus, HIV 1 and 2, *Enterovirus*, adenovirus, human herpesvirus 6, herpes simplex virus 1/2, and parvovirus
Wilson disease	Serum ceruloplasmin, 24 urinary copper estimation, and KF ring
Metabolic (in younger children)	Pyruvate, serum amino acid profile, urine amino acids/organic acids, urine succinylacetone, carnitine level and acylcarnitine profile, creatine phosphokinase, urine for reducing substance and ketone (urine dipstick examination), GALT assay, and alpha-fetoprotein
Autoimmune	Direct Coombs test, antinuclear antibody (>1:40), liver kidney microsomal antibody, smooth muscle antibody (>1:20), and IgG levels
Hemophagocytic lymphohistiocytosis	Serum triglyceride, cholesterol, ferritin, and bone marrow biopsy
Drug overdose	Acetaminophen level and urine toxicology

(ABG: arterial blood gas; ALT: alanine transaminase; AST: aspartate transaminase; CMV: cytomegalovirus; G6PD: glucose-6-phosphate dehydrogenase deficiency; GALT: galactose-1-phosphate uridyltransferase; GGTP: gamma-glutamyl transpeptidase; HAV: hepatitis A virus; HBsAg: hepatitis B surface antigen; HEV: hepatitis E virus; Ig: immunoglobulin; INR: international normalized ratio; KF: Kayser–Fleischer; PCR: polymerase chain reaction; PTTK: partial thromboplastin time activated with kaolin)

SUPPORTIVE MANAGEMENT

The management of a child with ALF should always be done in the intensive care unit of a center with experience in liver transplantation. Hepatic encephalopathy (HE), hypoglycemia, multiorgan dysfunction, and cardiovascular instability warrant continued care in the pediatric intensive care unit. Frequent neurological, cardiorespiratory assessment, and biochemical parameters monitoring are needed which is best available in an intensive care setting.

Initial management includes maintenance of airway and respiratory support, if required, volume resuscitation and vasopressor support depending upon hemodynamic status, and most importantly measures for raised intracranial pressure (ICP). Intravenous fluids should be initially restricted to 90% of total maintenance with 10% dextrose and half normal saline being the fluid of choice.

Overhydration can precipitate pulmonary and peripheral edema, ascites, and cerebral edema, while underhydration can precipitate hepatorenal syndrome, acute tubular necrosis, worsening encephalopathy, and hypotension. Glucose infusion rates as high as 10–15 mg/min per kg body weight may be required to achieve stable serum glucose levels (between 90 and 120 mg/dL). N-acetyl cysteine (NAC) has been used in the management of ALF secondary to acetaminophen poisoning but its use in nonacetaminophen causes of ALF lacks evidence. NAC can be used in the dose of 100 mg/kg/24 hours. Prophylactic administration of proton pump inhibitors in ALF is found to be useful as it is helpful in the prevention of gastrointestinal hemorrhage. Patients with PALF are likely catabolic and require more calories than basal needs. Enteral feeding is often preferred over total parenteral nutrition (TPN). Protein restriction (1 g/kg protein daily) can be considered if hyperammonemia is present. Additionally, lipids should be utilized unless a disorder of fatty acid oxidation or mitochondrial disease is suspected.

The cardiovascular changes in ALF consist of peripheral vasodilatation (cytokine release), low vascular resistance, and intravascular volume depletion, leading to decreased tissue oxygenation and multiorgan dysfunction. Resuscitation should start with adequate volume replacement with intravenous normal saline and if there is persistent hypotension, vasoconstrictor medications should be started. Norepinephrine is usually the preferred agent as it best enhances peripheral organ perfusion while minimizing tachycardia and preserving splanchnic circulation. Vasopressin and its analogs can be used to potentiate the effect of norepinephrine on patients who do not respond to the combination of volume challenge and norepinephrine.

Acute kidney injury (AKI) often accompanies ALF and may lead to increased morbidity as well as mortality. It is estimated that up to 17.5% of children with ALF may have associated AKI. The etiology is multifactorial and includes intrarenal vasoconstriction, shock, nephrotoxic medicines, sepsis, and tubular necrosis. The management consists of maintaining fluid balance and avoiding nephrotoxic medicines and few may require continuous venovenous hemofiltration or renal replacement therapy to maintain fluid balance.

All medications that can decrease the level of consciousness should be avoided to prevent the worsening of encephalopathy. If sedation is mandatory (e.g., for intubation) a short-acting agent like propofol can be given. Once the patient has been stabilized, further management includes close monitoring and supporting the organ systems, managing complications, age-appropriate diagnostic evaluation, and optimizing treatment to maximize health and survival.

Age-appropriate diagnostic evaluation should be considered to identify the underlying etiology for ALF as few may be amenable to specific therapies. Specific therapy should be administered if the underlying cause of ALF has been determined **(Box 3)**.

MANAGEMENT OF RAISED INTRACRANIAL PRESSURE

Raised ICP occurring because of cerebral edema is one of the leading causes of mortality in ALF. Sustained severe hypertension, bradycardia, pupillary changes, reflexes (brisk–sluggish), muscle tone changes, and decerebrate posturing are clinical indicators of the presence of cerebral edema. Definitive pathogenesis continues to be debated, and various toxins have been implicated, including bile acids, aromatic amino acids, cytokines, and chemokines; however, among all potential causative agents, ammonia assumes an essential role.

Children with lower-grade encephalopathy (I–II) should be managed in a quiet environment, minimally stimulated and general measures such as treating fever, dyselectrolytemia, infection, and seizures must be implemented. However, if encephalopathy progresses to

BOX 3: Specific therapy of common causes of pediatric acute liver failure.

- *Gestational alloimmune liver disease:*
  - High dose of intravenous immunoglobulin in combination with exchange transfusion
  - Liver transplantation if no improvement is seen
- *Herpes simplex:* High dose IV acyclovir 60 mg/kg/day for 21 days
- *Type 1 tyrosinemia:*
  - Nitisinone 1 mg/kg/day per os divided bid
  - Dietary restrictions of phenylalanine and tyrosine
  - Liver transplantation if no improvement is seen
- *Galactosemia:* Lactose-free diet, avoid galactose containing dietary items
- *Hereditary fructose intolerance:* Fructose-free diets, avoid fructose and sorbitol infusions
- *Acetaminophen poisoning:* N-acetyl cysteine
- *Mitochondrial cytopathies:*
  - *Electron acceptors and cofactors:* Coenzyme Q10: 3–5 mg/kg
  - *Antioxidants:* Vitamin E: 25 IU/kg
  - *Carnitine:* 50–100 mg/kg
- *Autoimmune hepatitis:*
  - IV methylprednisolone
  - Liver transplantation
- *Wilson disease (therapy based on the scoring system):*
  - Plasmapheresis
  - D-penicillamine/trientine (20 mg/kg/day) may be administered
  - Liver transplantation
- *Hemophagocytic lymphohistiocytosis:*
  - Corticosteroids
  - Chemotherapy
  - Bone marrow transplantation
- *Budd–Chiari syndrome:* Transjugular intrahepatic porto-systemic shunt (TIPS)

a higher grade, endotracheal intubation must be done. Ammonia is an accepted triggering factor in cerebral edema. Lactulose and antibiotics like rifaximin or neomycin are commonly used as ammonia-lowering agents, but evidence is debatable. Protein restriction in children with HE is no longer recommended. Energy intakes should be increased appropriately to counter the catabolic state. Osmotic agents such as hypertonic saline (HTS) and mannitol play an important role in reducing cerebral edema. HTS (3–30%) reduces ICP by decreasing cerebral water content through its osmotic effect and improves cerebral blood flow by reducing endothelial swelling by dehydration. Prophylactic administration of HTS (3% saline is commonly available in India) to maintain sodium at 145–155 mmol/L in patients with severe encephalopathy is recommended over mannitol. However, once obvious neurological signs develop, a bolus of intravenous mannitol (0.25–1 g/kg, 20% mannitol) over 15 minutes must be given. This can be repeated if serum osmolality is <320 mOsm/L. Mannitol is a hyperosmolar agent and acts by increasing serum osmolality which leads to the movement of water from the swollen astrocytes into serum. Mannitol use has only been recommended for acute increase in ICP and it should not be used prophylactically. There is no data in PALF to support the use of therapeutic hypothermia; active normothermia (36–37°C), with aggressive management of hyperthermia, is recommended. Seizures further increase ICP and reduce cerebral perfusion pressure. Clinical seizures may occur in 15–20% of patients and subclinical seizures may occur even more often. Prophylactic anti-epileptics to prevent subclinical seizures have often been used. Continuous renal replacement therapy (CRRT) plays an important role in lowering ammonia. Electroencephalogram (EEG) may be used as a sensitive tool to screen for declining neurological status or subclinical seizures, especially for patients with grade III or IV encephalopathy. Bedside measurement of optic nerve sheath diameter (ONSD) using ultrasound is a new and safe tool for early detection of raised ICP. Several studies have shown its correlation with the grade of HE. Normal ONSD in children (>4 years) is <4.5 and a value of >5.1 mm in ALF requires urgent attention.

CLINICAL PEARL

- HTS is preferred to 20% mannitol for decreasing raised ICP in children with ALF.

COAGULOPATHY

Patients with ALF develop failure of synthesis of clotting factors, altered platelet number and function, intravascular coagulation, and altered blood vessel wall integrity. Notably, abnormalities in these synthetic markers do not equate with bleeding risk in PALF as both procoagulant proteins (e.g., factors V, VII, and X and fibrinogen) and anticoagulant proteins (e.g., antithrombin, protein C, and protein S) are reduced. The age- and weight-appropriate dose of vitamin K ranging from 1 mg in infants to 10 mg in older adolescents should be administered to all children as vitamin K deficiency may also contribute to coagulopathy. Routine correction of coagulopathy or thrombocytopenia is not recommended. Prophylactic fresh frozen plasma (FFP) is not recommended, as it does not reduce the risk of significant bleeding or transfusion requirements and obscures the trend of international normalized ratio (INR) as a prognostic marker. However, replacement with FFP is recommended in patients with clinically significant bleeding, while performing invasive procedures or in situations where INR > 7. A single dose of vitamin K1 (5–10 mg, slowly not >1 mg/min) is recommended empirically in all patients with ALF. Platelet transfusion is not recommended unless a threshold platelet count of 10,000/mm^3 is reached or there is significant bleeding with a platelet count of <50,000/mm^3. A platelet count of 50–70,000/mm^3 is usually considered adequate when an invasive procedure is to be performed. Cryoprecipitate may be used for low fibrinogen levels (e.g., <100 mg/dL) Recombinant factor VIIa may be used if there is a concern about volume overload with FFP or refractory life-threatening bleeding. Thromboelastography may play an important role in guiding decisions as it incorporates all coagulation phases.

CLINICAL PEARL

- Prophylactic FFP is only recommended when any invasive procedure is attempted.

SEPSIS

Infection remains one of the major causes of death in patients with ALF. The liver performs multiple immune-related functions, and its impairment leads to immune dysfunction and makes individuals susceptible to infections. Invasive procedures, mechanical ventilation, bone marrow suppression, and deranged neutrophil function may contribute as well.

The most isolated organisms are gram-positive cocci (staphylococci and streptococci), enteric gram-negative bacilli, and *Candida albicans*. Prophylactic antibiotics or antifungals have not been shown to improve outcome or survival in patients with ALF and there are no clear guidelines for its use. Close monitoring and surveillance for infection is needed and cultures should be obtained with any evidence of clinical deterioration and antibiotics should be initiated. Evidence of infection may be subtle, such as tachycardia, bleeding (e.g., intestinal and pulmonary), reduced renal output, or mental status changes. Fever may not be present. It is reasonable to consider empiric antibiotic therapy in patients exhibiting systemic inflammatory response syndrome (SIRS) and in those who are in advanced coma grade 3 or 4. Some centers routinely place patients on antibiotic prophylaxis while waiting for liver transplantation. Coverage with a third-generation cephalosporin and an antifungal may be considered.

LIVER ASSIST DEVICES

The high cost of liver transplantation, lifetime immunosuppression, limited availability of donors, and risk of death while awaiting liver transplantation have stimulated the development of extracorporeal therapies or liver assist devices. Liver support devices have been shown to improve biochemical parameters, neurological status, and hemodynamical stability by lowering ammonia and maintaining fluid balance as well as cytokine homeostasis. The most common extracorporeal therapies are CRRT and therapeutic plasma exchange (TPE) or plasmapheresis. Others include extracorporeal membrane oxygenation (ECMO) and molecular absorbent reticulating system (MARS). Plasmapheresis removes cytokines and other drivers of systemic inflammation and curbs the inflammatory cascade and early CRRT may successfully manage both AKI and hyperammonemia. Indications for CRRT include AKI, fluid overload severe hyperammonemia, or hyperlactatemia. Early CRRT can successfully manage both AKI and hyperammonemia. There are no standard guidelines for the duration and number of sessions of CRRT and TPE, respectively. Many studies both in children as well as adults have shown better native liver survival with the deployment of these modalities.

HEPATOCYTE TRANSPLANTATION

Hepatocyte transplantation provides, at least theoretically, synthetic, and detoxifying function and has been performed in patients with ALF as a potential alternative or bridge to liver transplantation. Hepatocytes are derived from unsuitable donated grafts, can be cryopreserved, and are usually infused into the intrahepatic portal vein or peritoneum. Encapsulating these hepatocytes in a bioinert material, which also serves as a scaffold, such as an alginate microbead can prevent clearance by the immune system and allow free passage in the system.

PROGNOSTIC SCORES AND LIVER TRANSPLANTATION

Liver transplantation is the only definite treatment available for ALF. PALF is a rapidly evolving clinical condition with no current satisfactory tools to predict outcomes although improved prognostic models capable of predicting outcomes would greatly benefit the community. Several prognostic scores have been used to identify children who may benefit from early liver transplantation. These include King's College Hospital criteria, pediatric end-stage liver disease (PELD) score, Acute Physiology and Chronic Health Evaluation (APACHE) II, and Clichy criteria. Recently Peds-HAV model, a novel prognostic score in children with hepatitis A induced ALF was introduced. The presence of two out of three criteria (INR > 3.1, jaundice to encephalopathy interval >10 days, or presence of Grade 3–4 HE) predicts mortality with 90% sensitivity and 81.4 % specificity. However, an INR > 4 or factor V concentration of <25% is by far the best available criterion for listing for liver transplantation. Acute fulminant WD has a high mortality necessitating liver transplantation in most cases. A special prognostic score (new Wilson Index) is now available for these children and a score of 11 or more indicates mortality, with 93% sensitivity and 98% specificity. Recently, artificial intelligence-based scoring systems have also been proposed to predict native liver survival or death/requirement for liver transplantation (CHLA-ALF score). Despite all these, significant limitations to the current prognostic models persist and decisions to pursue liver transplantation remain complex, based on the alignment of physician experience, clinical assessment, and suitable organ availability.

Up to 10.3% of all pediatric liver transplantations are now performed in the setting of PALF. Most liver transplants in developing countries are living related, as cadaveric donation is scarce. A welcome development has been the increasing number of fathers willing to come forward as donors. Another positive aspect has been the involvement of the community in arranging funds for those who cannot afford liver transplantation. The availability of generic immunosuppressant drugs and consumables has greatly aided in bringing down costs to about one-fifth to one-tenth of the cost in the West. The paucity of facilities for liver transplantation in several regions of the world has prompted many foreign nationals to come to India for liver transplants. India has now become a major center for liver transplantation for international patients because of the high-quality and low cost value proposition.

OUTCOME

Improved understanding of pathophysiology, intensive care management, and use of liver assist devices have greatly improved native liver survival in the last few decades. Survival has improved from 15% in 1985–1993 to 73% in the current era. The prognosis of ALF in children varies greatly with the underlying etiology, type of presentation, and disease progression. Paracetamol poisoning and viral hepatitis have relatively better prognoses whereas WD as well as AIH presenting as ALF are fatal and do not respond to medical management and warrant liver transplantation. Unknown etiology, high grade (III/IV) of encephalopathy, time to onset of encephalopathy >7 days, higher bilirubin (>17.5 mg/dL), lower alanine transaminase (ALT) (≤2,384 IU/L), uncorrected prothrombin time >55 seconds, and clinical signs of cerebral edema are considered unfavorable prognostic markers. Children with encephalopathy and coagulopathy have a poorer outcome than those with coagulopathy alone.

KEY POINTS

- Infectious hepatitis is the most important cause of ALF in India.
- Raised ICP, infections, and multiorgan failure are the major causes of mortality in children with ALF.
- Early referral and early initiation of high-quality supportive and cause-based treatment at a liver transplant center is vital for survival.
- Extracorporeal therapies including continuous kidney replacement therapy and extracorporeal liver support systems are increasingly being used in PALF.
- Serial evaluation of laboratory coagulation variables (prothrombin time) is central to prognostic evaluation.
- Administration of coagulation factors should be avoided, except when needed to treat bleeding or before invasive procedures.
- Liver transplantation remains the only definite therapy for ALF in children.

SUGGESTED READING

1. Alam S, Khanna R, Sood V, Lal BB, Rawat D. Profile and outcome of first 109 cases of paediatric acute liver failure at a specialized paediatric liver unit in India. Liver Int. 2017;37(10):1508-14.
2. Berardi G, Tuckfield L, DelVecchio MT, Aronoff S. Differential Diagnosis of Acute Liver Failure in Children: A Systematic Review. Pediatr Gastroenterol Hepatol Nutr. 2020;23(6):501-10.
3. Bischoff SC, Bernal W, Dasarathy S, Merli M, Plank LD, Schütz T, et al. ESPEN practical guideline: Clinical nutrition in liver disease. Clin Nutr Edinb Scotl. 2020;39(12):3533-62.

4. Das MC, Srivastava A, Yadav RK, Yachha SK, Poddar U. Optic nerve sheath diameter in children with acute liver failure: A prospective observational pilot study. Liver Int. 2020;40(2):428-36.
5. Jain V, Dhawan A. Prognostic modeling in pediatric acute liver failure. Liver Transpl. 2016;22(10):1418-30.
6. Jørgensen MH, Rasmussen A, Christensen VB, Jensen AB, Fonsmark L, Andreassen BU, et al. Safety of High-Volume Plasmapheresis in Children With Acute Liver Failure. J Pediatr Gastroenterol Nutr. 2021;72(6):815-9.
7. Larsen FS, Schmidt LE, Bernsmeier C, Rasmussen A, Isoniemi H, Patel VC, et al. High-volume plasma exchange in patients with acute liver failure: an open randomised controlled trial. J Hepatol. 2016;64:69-78.
8. Lenz D, Hørby Jørgensen M, Kelly D, Cardinale V, Geerts A, Gonçalves Costa I, et al. Etiology and Outcome of Adult and Pediatric Acute Liver Failure in Europe. J Pediatr Gastroenterol Nutr. 2023;77(1):115-20.
9. Lutfi R, Abulebda K, Nitu ME, Molleston JP, Bozic MA, Subbarao G, et al. Intensive care management of pediatric acute liver failure. J Pediatr Gastroenterol Nutr. 2017; 64:660-70.
10. Malhotra S, Sibal A, Goyal N. Pediatric Liver Transplantation in India: 22 Years and Counting. Indian Pediatr. 2020;57(12):1110-3.
11. Mann JP, Lenz D, Stamataki Z, Kelly D. Common mechanisms in pediatric acute liver failure. Trends Mol Med. 2023;29(3):228-40.
12. Mieli-Vergani G, Vergani D, Baumann U, Czubkowski P, Debray D, Dezsofi A, et al. Diagnosis and Management of Pediatric Autoimmune Liver Disease: ESPGHAN Hepatology Committee Position Statement. J Pediatr Gastroenterol Nutr. 2018;66(2):345-60.
13. Nagral A, Sarma MS, Matthai J, Kukkle PL, Devarbhavi H, Sinha S, et al. Wilson's Disease: Clinical Practice Guidelines of the Indian National Association for Study of the Liver, the Indian Society of Pediatric Gastroenterology, Hepatology and Nutrition, and the Movement Disorders Society of India. J Clin Exp Hepatol. 2019;9(1):74-98.
14. Ng VL, Li R, Loomes KM, Leonis MA, Rudnick DA, Belle SH, et al. Outcomes of Children With and Without Hepatic Encephalopathy From the Pediatric Acute Liver Failure Study Group. J Pediatr Gastroenterol Nutr. 2016;63(3): 357-64.
15. Pediatric Gastroenterology Chapter of Indian Academy of Pediatrics; Bhatia V, Bavdekar A, Yachha SK; Indian Academy of Pediatrics. Management of acute liver failure in infants and children: consensus statement of the pediatric gastroenterology chapter, Indian academy of pediatrics. Indian Pediatr. 2013;50(5):477-82.
16. Poonacha P, Sibal A, Soin AS, Rajashekar MR, Rajakumari DV. India's first successful pediatric liver transplant. Indian Pediatr. 2001;38(3):287-91.
17. Sibal A, Malhotra S, Guru FR, Bhatia V, Kapoor A, Seth S, et al. Experience of 100 solid organ transplants over a five-yr period from the first successful pediatric multi-organ transplant program in India. Pediatr Transplant. 2014;18(7):740-5.
18. Socha P, Janczyk W, Dhawan A, Baumann U, D'Antiga L, Tanner S, et al. Wilson's Disease in Children: A Position Paper by the Hepatology Committee of the European Society for Paediatric Gastroenterology, Hepatology and Nutrition. J Pediatr Gastroenterol Nutr. 2018;66(2):334-44.
19. Squires JE, Alonso ME, Ibrahim SH, Kasper V, Kehar M, Martinez M, et al. North American Society for Pediatric Gastroenterology, Hepatology, and Nutrition Position paper on the diagnosis and management of Pediatric Acute Liver Failure. J Pediatr Gastroenterol Nutr. 2022;74: 138-58.
20. Squires RH, Dhawan A, Alonso E, Narkewicz MR, Shneider BL, Rodriguez-Baez N, et al. Intravenous N-acetylcysteine in pediatric patients with nonacetaminophen acute liver failure: a placebo-controlled clinical trial. Hepatol Baltim Md. 2013;57(4):1542-9.
21. Squires RH, Shneider BL, Bucuvalas J, Alonso E, Sokol RJ, Narkewicz MR, et al. Acute liver failure in children: the first 348 patients in the pediatric acute liver failure study group. J Pediatr. 2006;148(5):652-8.
22. Sundaram SS, Alonso EM, Narkewicz MR, Zhang S, Squires RH; Pediatric Acute Liver Failure Study Group. Characterization and outcomes of young infants with acute liver failure. J Pediatr. 2011;159(5):813-818.e1.
23. Walayat S, Shoaib H, Asghar M, Kim M, Dhillon S. Role of N-acetylcysteine in non-acetaminophen-related acute liver failure: an updated meta-analysis and systematic review. Ann Gastroenterol. 2021;34(2):235-40.
24. Young AM, Guilfoyle MR, Donnelly J, Scoffings D, Fernandes H, Garnett M, et al. Correlating optic nerve sheath diameter with opening intracranial pressure in pediatric traumatic brain injury. Pediatr Res. 2017;81: 443-7.
25. Zellos A, Debray D, Indolfi G, Czubkowski P, Samyn M, Hadzic N, et al. Proceedings of the European Society for Pediatric Gastroenterology, Hepatology and Nutrition Monothematic Conference, 2020: "Acute Liver Failure in Children": Treatment and Directions for Future Research. J Pediatr Gastroenterol Nutr. 2022;74(3):338-47.
26. Zoica BS, Deep A. Extracorporeal renal and liver support in pediatric acute liver failure. Pediatr Nephrol. 2021; 36:1119-28.

CHAPTER 82

Corrosive Injury in Children

Barath Jagadisan, Vibhor Borkar

INTRODUCTION

In pediatric emergency rooms, the ingestion of corrosive substances by children and adolescents is a frequent cause for visits. Children aged between 1 and 6 years, who are mobile, curious, and capable of drinking from bottles, are particularly vulnerable to accidental ingestion. One significant factor contributing to these incidents is the common practice of storing acidic toilet cleaners in containers typically used for beverages or water. In contrast to adults, who may ingest corrosives intentionally for self-harm, such cases are primarily observed in adolescents. According to data from the American Association of Poison Control Centers, children under 6 years old account for 51% of corrosive ingestion cases. Unfortunately, similar data is scarce in developing countries due to under-reporting, which stems from the lack of effective poison control centers and systematic data collection.

TYPES OF CORROSIVES

Corrosives ingested by children can include common household products such as toilet cleaners, bleach, laundry detergents, drain cleaners, and oven cleaners. Additionally, farm and industrial chemicals stored in homes pose significant risks. The occupation of parents also plays a role in the incidence of corrosive injuries; for instance, paraquat, a widely used herbicide in rural households, is corrosive and often stored in nonchild proof containers. Children from families involved in goldsmithing may accidentally ingest aqua regia, a mixture of hydrochloric and nitric acid. Generally, these corrosives can be categorized into two main types: (1) Acids and (2) Alkalis. Notably, acid ingestion is more prevalent in developing countries like India due to the easy availability of these substances.

PATHOGENESIS OF CORROSIVE INJURY

The nature and severity of corrosive injuries depend on several factors—the type of corrosive (acid or alkali), the amount ingested, its concentration, and its physical state (solid or liquid). **Table 1** summarizes the differences between the acid and alkali corrosive injury. Acidic substances typically cause coagulative necrosis of the mucosal tissue, leading to eschar formation on the esophagus's surface. If a smaller amount of acid is consumed, this eschar may limit further penetration into deeper tissues. Conversely, alkalis induces liquefactive necrosis, saponification, and thrombosis of underlying vessels, allowing them to penetrate deeply into tissues and potentially cause transmural injury and perforation. While it is generally observed that self-harm cases involve larger volumes of ingestion compared to accidental cases—resulting in a higher proportion of severe injuries among adolescents—children are still at risk. Alkalis tends to inflict more damage on the esophagus due to their higher viscosity and slower clearance from that area; acids are usually cleared more rapidly into the stomach, leading to predominant gastric injury. However, severe esophageal injuries from acid ingestion are not uncommon. The concentration of a corrosive substance significantly influences the depth of injury and the timeline for clinical deterioration. Solid corrosives tend to remain in contact with the mouth and esophagus longer than liquids, which are quickly cleared into the stomach. The antrum and pylorus are typically the first areas affected by corrosives entering from the esophagus; thus, perforations and strictures are more frequently observed in these regions. In addition to local effects, acids can lead to serious systemic complications such as disseminated intravascular coagulation and organ dysfunction (e.g., renal or hepatic failure). For example, acute lung injury is a common cause of death following paraquat ingestion.

TABLE 1: Difference between injury from alkalis and acids.

Injury	*Acids*	*Alkalis*
Type of necrosis	Coagulative necrosis	Liquefactive necrosis
Formation of eschar/coagulum	Yes	No
Depth of injury	Limited by coagulum formation	Deep, transmural
Risk of perforation	Lower	Higher
Location of injury	Predominantly stomach due to rapid esophageal clearance. However, strong acids would also damage esophagus significantly.	Predominantly esophagus due to viscous nature and slow esophageal clearance

Following corrosive ingestion, the sequence of events is critical for understanding the management of such injuries. Before 4 weeks postingestion, the tensile strength of the affected tissue is significantly reduced. Consequently, late endoscopies—particularly those conducted beyond 96 hours—carry a heightened risk of perforation. For similar reasons, stricture dilation is generally not attempted until at least 3 weeks postinjury. The process of fibrosis can continue even after epithelialization, leading to worsening strictures over time. Delayed follow-up endoscopies often reveal mature, tight strictures where visualization of the lumen for cannulation and dilation becomes increasingly difficult. **Flowchart 1** has summarized the pathogenesis of corrosive injury.

Flowchart 1: Pathogenesis of corrosive ingestion.

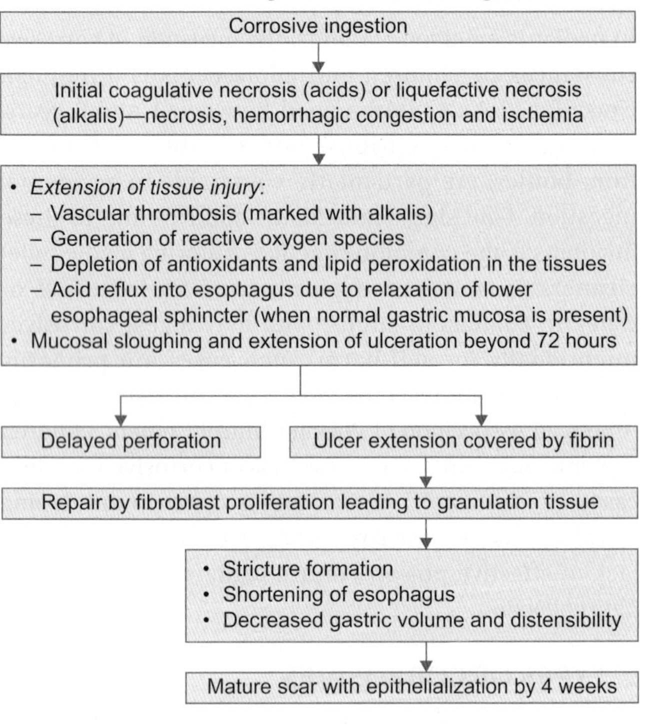

Clinical Manifestations

The clinical manifestations of corrosive injury can be varied and include:

- *Airway injury:* Stridor and dyspnea
- *Feeding refusal:* Reluctance to eat
- *Drooling:* Excessive saliva production
- *Dysphagia:* Difficulty swallowing
- *Odynophagia:* Painful swallowing
- *Retrosternal pain:* Pain behind the sternum
- *Abdominal pain:* Discomfort in the abdomen
- *Vomiting:* Often accompanied by hematemesis; large volumes indicate extensive gastric injury
- *Oral cavity injuries:* Erythema, edema, bleeding, and ulceration
- *Systemic complications:* Acute lung injury, renal and hepatic failure, and disseminated intravascular coagulation
- *Severe outcomes:* Perforation and mediastinitis leading to death

It is essential to note that the clinical presentation in a tertiary care center may not fully represent the spectrum of corrosive injuries. Children with extensive injuries and rapid deterioration may not reach medical facilities in time. Research indicates that symptoms and oral cavity injuries do not consistently correlate with endoscopic findings. In a study involving 378 children with corrosive injuries, 82% of symptomatic children exhibited no esophageal injury, while 12% of asymptomatic children had severe esophageal damage. Although an increase in symptoms may suggest a higher likelihood of significant injury, deep mucosal injuries can occur without overt symptoms. Airway injury indicated by stridor often correlates with esophageal injury; however, no single symptom or combination of symptoms reliably predicts esophageal or gastric damage. Moreover, the absence of oral lesions does not exclude the possibility of esophageal injury; up to 61% of children without oral lesions still exhibit esophageal damage. Conversely, significant oral cavity lesions may occur without any distal injury. These observations underscore the necessity for endoscopic assessment in all children with corrosive injuries, regardless of their symptoms, or oral manifestations. While clinical examination remains vital—especially in identifying respiratory issues that require prompt management—computed tomography (CT) is more relevant for diagnosing perforations than endoscopy alone. Given that perforation can occur at any point within the first 2 weeks postingestion, any clinical deterioration or emergence of new symptoms should be thoroughly evaluated.

INVESTIGATIONS IN THE ACUTE PHASE

Chest and Abdominal Radiographs

Radiographs may reveal mediastinal air, subcutaneous emphysema, or subdiaphragmatic air indicative of esophageal or gastric perforation.

Laboratory Investigations

Laboratory tests should focus on identifying acidosis, electrolyte imbalances, disseminated intravascular coagulation, and multiple organ dysfunctions—particularly in critically ill children prior to surgical intervention.

Early Endoscopic Evaluation

Endoscopy plays a crucial role in assessing mucosal injury extent and estimating its severity concerning potential transmural damage. Historically, endoscopic evaluation timing has varied; however, due to ongoing mucosal necrosis and tissue friability, early endoscopy between 24 and 72 hours is now preferred to reduce perforation risks. Endoscopy within 24 hours may underscore the mucosal damage. Endoscopic assessment should be performed by experienced practitioners under sedation—deep sedation without intubation is ideal unless respiratory issues necessitate intubation. Endoscopy is contraindicated in cases of severe hypopharyngeal injury or perforation. Gentle maneuvering, use of thin scope (ultraslim endoscope 5.5 mm external (diameter) and minimal air insufflation is essential during the procedure. **Table 2** describes endoscopic grades of corrosive mucosal injury. It is advised not to navigate beyond severe circumferential mucosal injuries (grade 3b). The primary purpose of endoscopy is to grade mucosal injury according to established classifications, predict the likelihood of strictures and inserting a nasoenteral tube if possible.

TABLE 2: Endoscopic grading of mucosal injury during endoscopy.

Grade of injury	*Endoscopic findings*
0	Normal appearance
1	Edematous and hyperemic mucosa
2A	Superficial injury—friability, hemorrhagic areas, erosions with whitish exudates and membranes, and superficial ulceration
2B	Grade 2A with deep discrete ulcers or circumferential involvement
3A	Multiple scattered areas of ulceration and necrosis seen as brown/black/gray areas
3B	Extensive areas of necrosis
4	Perforation

Many cases of corrosive ingestion may not result in gastrointestinal damage—especially in accidental ingestion scenarios—allowing for early discharge in identified patients. Injury grading correlates well with morbidity and mortality; children with grades 1 and 2A injuries typically do not develop strictures, while stricture rates in grade 3 injuries can approach 75%. Mortality rates are notably higher in grade 3 injuries, emphasizing the importance of endoscopic grading in determining treatment strategies such as feeding jejunostomy or emergency surgical interventions for extensive grade 3b and grade 4 injuries.

Computed Tomography

Computed tomography offers advantages over endoscopy by providing comprehensive information about the extent of transmural injuries. In cases where clinical assessments suggest a high likelihood of perforation—despite no obvious signs on chest or abdominal radiographs—CT should be prioritized as the initial investigation. CT grading of corrosive injuries has been implemented to predict stricture formation, although it is not routinely used for this purpose alone.

MANAGEMENT (FLOWCHART 2)

Management in the Acute Phase

Effective management of corrosive injuries begins with adherence to fundamental emergency care principles. Patients must be evaluated for respiratory distress, and airway intubation or tracheostomy may be necessary

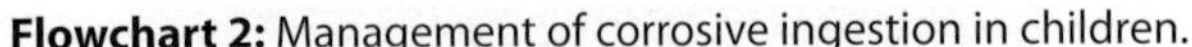

Flowchart 2: Management of corrosive ingestion in children.

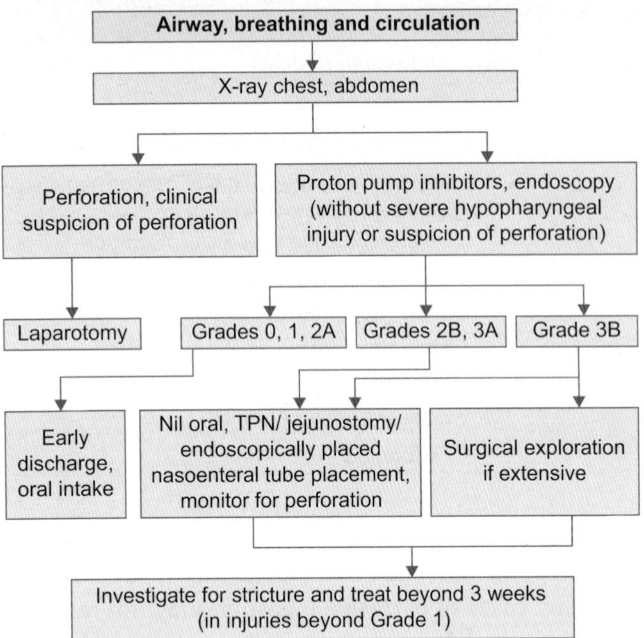

in cases exhibiting airway compromise. Edema in the epiglottic and supraglottic regions can signal impending airway obstruction, even if symptoms are absent at presentation. Additionally, patients with perforations may require ventilation and hemodynamic support. There is no justification for gastric lavage or inducing emesis to eliminate corrosives; such actions can lead to repeated exposure of the proximal mucosa and increase the risk of aspiration and esophageal mucosa damage. Attempts to neutralize corrosives with weak acids or bases are also counterproductive. Administration of milk, activated charcoal or any other agent should be avoided. The blind placement of nasogastric tubes is discouraged due to the risk of perforation. Some medical centers prefer using endoscopically guided nasojejunal tubes for feeding, which may also serve as stents to maintain a narrow lumen for cannulation during stricture dilation. However, this approach is controversial; some argue that it can increase reflux and lead to longer strictures, while other studies indicate that nasojejunal feeding is equivalent to jejunostomy feeding in maintaining nutrition without increasing stricture frequency. In summary, while endoscopic evaluation remains crucial for assessing corrosive injuries, careful consideration must be given to management strategies to minimize complications and optimize patient outcomes.

Based on the data indicating lower esophageal sphincter relaxation and a high frequency of acid reflux into the esophagus, along with preliminary findings showing significant healing of corrosive injuries through proton pump inhibitor (PPI) infusion, it has become standard practice to administer PPIs, at least in bolus doses. However, the use of systemic steroids to prevent strictures is discouraged. Meta-analyses have demonstrated that steroids do not confer this benefit and may increase the risk of infections. Additionally, there is a theoretical risk that steroids could mask signs of inflammation resulting from bowel perforation. Systemic steroids should only be considered in cases involving airway edema. Antibiotic therapy is not routinely indicated for corrosive injuries and is reserved for cases with perforation and invasive procedures. Broad-spectrum antibiotics may be warranted for patients receiving steroids due to airway edema.

Management of Perforation

In instances where there is clear clinical or radiological evidence of perforation, emergency laparotomy is necessary. If there is a high suspicion of perforation despite the absence of radiological confirmation, laparotomy may still be warranted. In clinically stable patients with ambiguous signs regarding perforation, CT scans can provide valuable insights. If both clinical and radiological assessments do not suggest perforation, endoscopic evaluation of mucosal injury should be performed. The decision for early surgical intervention should not rely solely on overt signs of perforation; if acidosis, renal injury, or hemodynamic instability is present, early surgery is critical due to the strong suspicion of perforation. Any clinical suspicion of perforation based on the patient's overall condition and the quantity of corrosive ingested should prompt early surgical exploration.

Endoscopic Assessment and Management

Following endoscopic assessment, the grade of injury will guide subsequent management strategies. Children with normal mucosa can be discharged immediately, while those with grades 1 and 2A injuries may resume oral intake and can be discharged after a brief observation period if their intake remains satisfactory. Conversely, children with grades 2B and 3 injuries must refrain from oral intake. For grades 2B and 3A injuries where oral intake is restricted, nutritional support options include total parenteral nutrition (TPN), jejunostomy feeding, or endoscopically placed nasoenteral tube feeding. In many developing countries, TPN is often avoided due to its high cost and associated infection risks. Research by

Kochhar et al. demonstrated that nasoenteric feeding could maintain comparable nutritional status without increasing stricture rates; the tube also facilitates guidewire passage during future dilatations. In cases where perforation or massive hemorrhage occurs, immediate surgical intervention becomes critical. Esophagectomy and cervical esophagostomy may be required for esophageal perforations, while areas of the stomach exhibiting transmural involvement may necessitate resection. Complete gastrectomy may also be necessary in some cases. A gastrostomy during surgery allows for accurate assessment of the extent of involvement; however, surgical closure of perforations is not indicated. Distal jejunostomy is essential for maintaining nutrition. In extensive grade 3B injuries, laparotomy may be needed to assess for transmural necrosis that could indicate impending perforation. Surgical procedures may involve varying degrees of resection along with jejunostomy for feeding support. The role of laparoscopy in these situations remains controversial due to longer operating times and challenges in thoroughly assessing injury extent.

Management of Strictures

Stricture formation is more frequent with higher grades of mucosal injury, and systemic steroids do not prevent this complication. Esophageal strictures typically present with dysphagia and aspiration pneumonia, while strictures in the antral and pyloric regions manifest as gastric outlet obstruction. Prior to endoscopic evaluation for strictures, obtaining a contrast radiograph is advisable to assess the position, number, length of strictures, and potential presence of diverticula. On radiography using oral contrast, strictures appear as narrowed areas with proximal contrast hold-up; chronic strictures may exhibit varying degrees of proximal dilatation. While barium is generally preferred as a contrast agent, it should be avoided in children with severe dysphagia due to aspiration risks. Stricture dilatation within 3 weeks postinjury is inadvisable due to a heightened risk of perforation; however, delaying dilatation can result in nonvisualization for treatment and malnutrition issues. Long strictures are common after corrosive injuries. Savary–Gilliard (bougie) dilators or balloon dilators can be used depending upon the location, number, length of the stricture, and tortuosity of the lumen. For refractory strictures, local triamcinolone injections or mitomycin applications or esophageal stent placements may be necessary. In instances presenting months after corrosive injury where dilatation proves impossible, surgical correction may become the sole option. Esophageal resection and jejunal or colonic transposition may be required. For gastric strictures, partial resection, gastrojejunostomy may be required.

Long-term Complications

Long-term complications following corrosive injury include dysmotility and an increased risk of dysplasia or malignancy in affected tissues.

Patient Educations

Parents should be educated about children's safety practices when corrosives, toxic substances, and poisonous substances are stored at home. The manufacturing industry should package these substances in children's proof bottles. Hazardous substances should be kept at a height beyond the reach of the children and should be locked properly.

CONCLUSION

The optimal management of corrosive injuries hinges on adherence to life support principles, avoidance of gastric lavage or emesis, timely selection for emergency surgical resection based on endoscopic evaluations, careful attention to nutritional needs, and prompt detection and management of strictures. The widespread availability of corrosives in unregulated markets poses significant risks in many developing countries where these substances are commonly used as household cleaners. Strict regulations regarding the concentration of household caustics and child-resistant packaging for corrosives must be enforced to mitigate these risks effectively.

CLINICAL PEARLS

- Oral manifestations and symptoms do not predict the degree of esophageal and gastric mucosal injury.
- Blind nasogastric tube insertion, lavage, emesis, charcoal, and milk should be avoided after corrosive ingestion.
- Endoscopic NG tube insertion helps in maintaining enteral nutrition, helps in avoiding prolong parental nutrition and hospital admission.
- Steroids are indicated only in cases of airway edema.
- Esophagogastroduodenoscopy between 24 and 48 hours is indicated in all children with corrosive ingestion who do not have perforation or severe hypopharyngeal injury.
- Children with significant mucosal injury required multiple endoscopic stricture dilatation or surgical resection of the damaged gut.

KEY POINTS

- Early recognition of airway compromise and perforation is essential to ensure survival.
- Endoscopic assessment of severity of mucosal injury directs early management and prognosticates the likelihood of strictures.
- Existing data is insufficient to support use of systemic corticosteroids for prevention of strictures.
- Routine barium esophagogram at 3 weeks after corrosive ingestion is necessary for early diagnosis and management of strictures.

SUGGESTED READING

1. Ananthakrishnan N, Parthasarathy G, Kate V. Acute corrosive injuries of the stomach: a single unit experience of thirty years. ISRN Gastroenterol. 2011;2011:914013.
2. Betalli P, Falchetti D, Giuliani S, Pane A, Dall'Oglio L, de Angelis GL, et al. Caustic ingestion in children: is endoscopy always indicated? The results of an Italian multicenter observational study. Gastrointest Endosc. 2008;68:434-9.
3. Chirica M, Resche-Rigon M, Bongrand NM, Zohar S, Halimi B, Gornet JM, et al. Surgery for caustic injuries of the upper gastrointestinal tract. Ann Surg. 2012;256: 994-1001.
4. Doğan Y, Erkan T, Cokuğraş FC, Kutlu T. Caustic gastroesophageal lesions in childhood: an analysis of 473 cases. Clin Pediatr. 2006;45:435-8.
5. Gaudreault P, Parent M, McGuigan MA, Chicoine L, Lovejoy FH Jr. Predictability of esophageal injury from signs and symptoms: a study of caustic ingestion in 378 children. Pediatrics. 1983;71:767-70.
6. Kochhar R, Poornachandra KS, Puri P, Dutta U, Sinha SK, Sethy PK, et al. Comparative evaluation of nasoenteral feeding and jejunostomy feeding in acute corrosive injury: a retrospective analysis. Gastrointest Endosc. 2009;70: 874-80.
7. Kochhar R, Ray JD, Sriram PV, Kumar S, Singh K. Intralesional steroids augment the effects of endoscopic dilation in corrosive esophageal strictures. Gastrointest Endosc. 1999;49:509-13.
8. Lakshmi CP, Vijayahari R, Kate V, Ananthakrishnan N. A hospital based epidemiological study of corrosive alimentary injuries with particular reference to the Indian experience. Natl Med J India. 2013;26(1):31-6.
9. Oliva S, Romano C, Angelis P, Isoldi S, Mantegazza C, Felici E, et al. Foreign Body and caustic ingestion in children: a clinical practice guideline. Dig Liver Dis. 2020; 52(11):1266-81.
10. Uhlen S, Fayoux P, Vachin F, Guimber D, Gottrand F, Turck D, et al. Mitomycin C: an alternative conservative treatment for refractory esophageal stricture in children? Endoscopy. 2006;38:404-7.
11. Watson WA, Litovitz TL, Rodgers GC Jr, Klein-Schwartz W, Reid N, Youniss J, et al. 2004 Annual Report of the American Association of Poison Control Centers Toxic Exposure Surveillance System. Am J Emerg Med. 2005;23: 589-666.
12. Zargar SA, Kochhar R, Mehta S, Mehta SK. The role of fiberoptic endoscopy in the management of corrosive ingestion and modified endoscopic classification of burns. Gastrointest Endosc. 1991;37:165-9.

CHAPTER 83

Chronic Abdominal Pain

Sarah Paul, John Matthai

INTRODUCTION

Chronic (recurrent) abdominal pain is the most common abdominal symptom that a pediatrician confronts in his practice. Modifying the conventional terminology by Apley, the preferred term is chronic abdominal pain (CAP) or functional abdominal pain disorders (FAPDs). Advances in investigative facilities over the years have failed to yield a cause in a majority of children. This has led to the concept that the pain is real and not imaginary, and may be related to stress, environmental, and familial factors.

CLASSIFICATION

Functional gastrointestinal disorders (FGIDs) as a group have now been renamed as disorders of gut brain interaction (DGBI) according to Rome IV criteria laid down in 2016. FAPD in children categorizes pain-related disorders into four main groups with H2a being subdivided **(Table 1)** and has diagnostic criteria for each.

TABLE 1: Rome IV criteria-H2: Functional abdominal pain disorders (FAPD).

H2a	Functional dyspepsia
• H2a1 • H2a2	Postprandial distress syndrome Epigastric pain syndrome
H2b	Irritable bowel syndrome
H2c	Abdominal migraine
H2d	*Functional abdominal pain:* Not otherwise specified

Red Flag Signs

Chronic abdominal pain may not always be functional. The red flag signs that suggest a possible organic basis are given in **Box 1**.

BOX 1: Red flag signs in chronic abdominal pain.

- Clearly localized/radiating pain
- Pain that wakes the child from sleep
- Gastrointestinal blood loss
- Deceleration of linear growth
- Family history of inflammatory bowel disease
- Celiac disease or peptic ulcer
- Perirectal disease
- Dysphagia
- Persistent vomiting
- Nocturnal diarrhea
- Unexplained fever
- Arthralgia and rash
- Delayed puberty
- Weight loss

CLINICAL PEARL

- Do not ignore red flag signs in abdominal pain. Investigate children with any of them.

H2a: Functional Dyspepsia

Diagnostic Criteria

Diagnostic criteria must include one or more of the following (at least four times a month for at least 2 months):

- Postprandial fullness
- Early satiation
- Epigastric pain or burning not associated with defecation
- After appropriate medical evaluation, symptoms cannot be attributed to another medical condition

H2a1: Postprandial distress syndrome: Postprandial fullness or early satiation, which prevents finishing a full meal. May have upper abdominal bloating, nausea, or belching.

H2a2: Bothersome pain or burning localized to the epigastrium (without any generalization or radiation) and not relieved by defecation or passage of flatus. It need not have a retrosternal component and can be induced or relieved by a meal, but may also occur while fasting.

Evaluation

The dyspeptic symptoms may follow a viral infection. An upper gastrointestinal (GI) endoscopy is not mandatory for making a diagnosis, except in the following situations: (1) Patient has dysphagia, (2) symptoms improve with antacids, but relapse on withdrawal of the drug, and (3) *Helicobacter pylori* disease is suspected.

Treatment

Avoidance of drugs (particularly analgesics) and specific foods that aggravate symptoms are important. Antacids and prokinetics may offer symptom relief in some patients, but their routine use is not recommended without an upper GI endoscopy. A search for psychological factors may be made in appropriate settings.

H2b: Irritable Bowel Syndrome

Diagnostic Criteria

Abdominal pain (at least 4 days per month and for at least 2 months) associated with one or more of the following:

- Symptoms are related to defecation
- Change in frequency of stool (four or more stools per day and two or less stools per week)
- Change in appearance of stool
- If associated with constipation, then resolution of constipation does not result in disappearance of pain
- Symptoms cannot be attributed to another medical condition after appropriate medical evaluation

Evaluation

Visceral hypersensitivity related to genetic predisposition and early stressful events are a likely cause. Anxiety, depression, and multiple somatic complaints are often reported not only by the patient, but also by the parents. In the absence of red flag signs, a positive diagnosis of irritable bowel syndrome (IBS) can be made without any investigations. Inflammatory bowel disease has similar clinical features and should be considered in older children.

Treatment

A confident diagnosis, reasonable explanation of pain experience, and reassurance are by themselves therapeutic. Antidepressants have not been proven useful.

CLINICAL PEARL

- Abdominal discomfort associated with a change in frequency or form of the stool and related to defecation suggests IBS if no red flag signs are present.

H2c: Abdominal Migraine

Diagnostic Criteria

Must include all of the following occurring at least twice for at least 6 months:

- Paroxysmal episodes of intense acute periumbilical, midline, or diffuse pain that lasts for 1 hour or more
- Episodes are separated by weeks to months
- The pain interferes with normal activities
- Stereotypical pattern in an individual patient
- The pain is associated with two or more of the following: Anorexia, nausea, vomiting, headache, photophobia, and pallor
- After appropriate medical evaluation, symptoms cannot be attributed to another medical condition

Evaluation

Cyclic vomiting syndrome, migraine headache, and abdominal migraine are believed to be the spectrum of the same disease with overlap. Family history of migraine and motion sickness may be present. In appropriate settings, subacute obstruction of the intestine, urinary and biliary tract, as well as chronic pancreatitis and porphyria should be ruled out. Response to migraine prophylactic drugs is supportive evidence.

Treatment

Avoidance of potential triggers, such as caffeine, prolonged fasting, sleep deprivation, and exposure to flickering lights, may be suggested. In those with recurrent episodes, propranolol, cyproheptadine, and sumatriptan can be tried.

H2d: Functional Abdominal Pain—Not Otherwise Specified

Diagnostic Criteria

Must include all of the following at least four times per month:

- Episodic or continuous abdominal pain unrelated to physiologic events like eating or menses
- Insufficient criteria for other FAPDs
- After appropriate medical evaluation, symptoms cannot be attributed to another medical condition

Evaluation

These children are not troubled by their symptoms and parental anxiety is the main compounding factor. No investigations are necessary in the absence of any red flag signs, provided the parents can be convinced.

Treatment

Parents need to be reassured that there is no organic basis. Placebo drugs should be discouraged. Psychological evaluation is not necessary.

APPROACH TO A CHILD WITH CHRONIC ABDOMINAL PAIN

Children presenting with CAP can broadly be classified into three groups, based on the pattern of pain **(Table 2)**:

1. Isolated paroxysmal periumbilical CAP
2. CAP with dyspepsia
3. CAP with altered bowel habits

CLINICAL PEARL

- Isolated paroxysmal periumbilical pain in children is most commonly functional pain.

TABLE 2: Classification of chronic abdominal pain based on the pattern of pain.

Isolated paroxysmal periumbilical abdominal pain	
Functional 95%	*Organic causes (<5%):* • *Intestinal:* Malrotation, Crohn's disease, and adhesions • *Renal:* Stone colic and PUJ obstruction • *Infection:* Tuberculosis and *Yersinia* • *Others:* Food allergy and dysmenorrhea
CAP with dyspepsia	
Functional 90%	*Organic causes (10%):* • GERD, *Helicobacter pylori*, and *Giardia* • Pancreatitis and biliary disease • Food intolerance and drugs
CAP with altered bowel habits	
Functional 75%	*Organic causes (25%):* • Constipation, IBD, TB, and parasites • Lactose intolerance and food allergy • Gynecological and drugs

(CAP: chronic abdominal pain; GERD: gastroesophageal reflux disease; IBD: inflammatory bowel disease; PUJ: pelviureteric junction; TB: tuberculosis)

MANAGEMENT OF FUNCTIONAL PAIN

The first step in management is making a positive diagnosis. Parental counseling should be well planned with an unequivocal reassurance that there is no organic disease and that the prognosis is good. They need to understand that the pain is real and the child is not feigning, but there is no need for medication. Hospitalization is best avoided, since it is likely to reinforce pain behavior. The treatment aims to normalize lifestyle (school attendance, extracurricular activities, and sleep) by benign negligence or distraction techniques. It is also important to identify and reduce stress/triggers at home, neighborhood, or with peers. Preventing the child from using the pain to avoid unpleasant but essential responsibilities should minimize any form of secondary gain. Diet changes have little role in reducing pain, but a regular balanced diet with adequate fibers must be insisted on. Though some small studies have reported benefits, most do not show any statistically significant difference between amitriptyline and placebo in functional GI diseases in children. Interaction with the teachers may help identify children with special needs (specific learning disability and attention deficit hyperactivity disorders). They can be informed directly or through the parents that they need to be sympathetic to the child while not creating panic. Consultation with a psychiatrist is not recommended unless there are compelling reasons to do so, since it can affect the morale and outlook of the parents and the child.

CLINICAL PEARL

What to tell the parents?

- The pain in functional abdominal pain is real, not imaginary. Do not deny the presence of pain. The reassurance is only that there is no organic basis.

KEY POINTS

- Functional GI disorders are the most common cause of CAP in children.
- Functional dyspepsia, IBS, and functional abdominal pain are the most common causes.
- Look for red flag signs before considering functional disorders.
- Isolated paroxysmal periumbilical pain is most likely functional.
- CAP with dyspepsia or altered bowel habits warrant consideration of upper/lower GI disorders.
- Children with functional pain need reassurance and return to normal lifestyle at the earliest, after an attempt to correct or reduce trigger/stress factors.

SUGGESTED READING

1. Benninga MA, Faure C, Hyman PE, St James Roberts I, Schechter NL, Nurko S. Childhood functional gastrointestinal disorders: neonate/toddler. Gastroenterology. 2016:150;1443-55.e2.
2. Bhaskar R, Ghosh M, Pal S, Gupta SD. Recurrent (chronic) abdominal pain in children. In: Bavdekar A, Matthai J, Sathiyasekaran M, Yachha SK (Eds). Pediatric Gastroenterology, 2nd edition. New Delhi: Jaypee Brothers Medical Publishers (P) Ltd.; 2013. pp. 22-36.
3. Drossman DA. Functional gastrointestinal disorders: history, pathophysiology, clinical features and Rome IV. Gastroenterology. 2016;150:1262-79.
4. Hyams JS, Di Lorenzo C, Saps M, Shulman RJ, Staiano A, van Tilburg M. Functional disorders: children and adolescents. Gastroenterology. 2016:150;1456-68.e2.
5. Schmulson MJ, Drossman DA. What is new in Rome IV. J Neurogastroenterol Motil. 2017;23(2):151-63.

CHAPTER 84

Approach to Vomiting

D Venkata Umesh Reddy, Dimple Jain

INTRODUCTION

Vomiting is a very common complaint in children presenting to outpatients as well as emergency rooms. Its presence alone does not always indicate a serious illness, as it may be seen in benign conditions such as overfeeding, rumination syndrome, functional nausea and vomiting, etc. Vomiting can be a presenting symptom of both gastrointestinal and nongastrointestinal diseases. Gastrointestinal causes range from most commonly acute gastritis or gastroenteritis to more complex ones such as pancreatitis, cholecystitis, inflammatory bowel disease, and intestinal obstruction. Nongastrointestinal causes include raised intracranial pressure, meningitis, renal colic, uremia, inborn errors of metabolism, diabetic ketoacidosis, etc. Tweezing out the underlying cause requires thorough detailed history-taking and examination. The right approach will expedite work up toward specific etiologies thus helping in timely diagnosis and management.

DEFINITIONS

Vomiting is an organized, protective reflex that results in the forceful expulsion of gastric contents through the mouth. It may be preceded by nausea, retching, and autonomic manifestations. It needs to be differentiated from regurgitation, a passive effortless movement of gastric contents into the mouth without abdominal wall contractions.

Rumination involves effortlessly bringing up recently ingested food through an increase in abdominal pressure, chewing, and sometimes re-swallowing. Though definitions make our understanding easier, analyzing the symptoms in a child is a challenge in itself and a clear distinction between the above conditions cannot be made, and often put in the basket of "vomiting."

ETIOLOGY

The etiology of vomiting is diverse and depends on the age, characteristics of vomiting, and the presence or absence of other associated symptoms **(Table 1)**.

APPROACH

History and examination is the key to making the right diagnosis. Acute vomiting usually has an abrupt onset and a duration of <1 week. Infectious causes such as acute gastroenteritis and viral gastritis predominate. Some of the causes of acute vomiting may have a prolonged course such as cholecystitis, pancreatitis, meningitis, raised intracranial pressure, etc., or can complicate and change to recurrent or chronic vomiting, e.g., pseudocyst which is a known complication of acute pancreatitis, hydrocephalus in a child with meningitis. Though the ROME IV criteria define the duration of chronic nausea and vomiting in children as 2 months, a more practical cutoff would be to take 4 weeks so that evaluation is not delayed.

A basic three-step process can be used **(Fig. 1)** for any child presenting with vomiting. Age at presentation, characteristics of vomiting including onset, duration, nature of vomiting whether bilious **(Fig. 2A)**, nonbilious, blood mixed **(Fig. 2B)**, or feculent, projectile or nonprojectile, and associated symptoms and signs such as fever, pain abdomen, headache, jaundice, cough, burning micturition, head trauma, drug or foreign body ingestion, relevant significant past history including any previous surgery, triggers like fasting or postmeal, acidotic breathing, etc., give clues to the diagnosis **(Table 2)**. Although there are some benign causes such as overfeeding, functional vomiting, rumination syndrome, etc., most often it is a result of an organic etiology and the presence of red flags warrants immediate evaluation and management as outcomes are time-bound **(Box 1)**. An algorithm for the approach to a child with vomiting is presented in **Flowchart 1**.

TABLE 1: Etiology (system-wise) of vomiting based on the age at presentation.

Etiology	*Neonate*	*Infant*	*Toddler/older child*	*Adolescent*
Infections (usually a cause of acute vomiting; any infection in general can trigger vomiting response)	• Urinary tract infection (UTI) • Systemic infections including sepsis, meningitis, etc.	• Acute gastroenteritis • UTI • Systemic infections including sepsis, meningitis, etc.	• Acute gastroenteritis • Gastritis • Hepatitis • Parasitic worm infestation • Otitis media • UTI • Systemic infections including sepsis, meningitis, etc.	• Acute gastroenteritis • Gastritis • Hepatitis • UTI • Otitis media • Pharyngitis • Systemic infections
Gastro-intestinal	• GERD • CMPA • Intestinal malrotation • Hypertrophic pyloric stenosis • Intestinal atresia • Esophageal atresia • Feed intolerance (prematurity, sepsis, NEC) • Hirschsprung's disease • Hiatus hernia • Duodenal web • Annular pancreas • Congenital esophageal stenosis • Duplication cyst • Intestinal pseudobstruction • Intestinal-aganglionosis • Congenital microgastria	• GERD • CMPA • Overfeeding • Post-tussive • Hypertrophic pyloric stenosis • Intestinal malrotation • Cholelithiasis • Intussusception • Hirschsprung's disease • Choledochal cyst with cholangitis • Eosinophilic esophagitis • Esophageal stricture • Duodenal web • Annular pancreas All the three diseases can cause vomiting in infancy. They need to be arranged one below another separately: • Very early onset inflammatory bowel disease • Gastroparesis • Duplication cyst • Intestinal pseudobstruction • Postsurgical adhesions	• Gastritis and/or peptic ulcer (Food/drug related) • Post-tussive • Appendicitis • Cholecystitis/ cholelithiasis • Pancreatitis • Foreign body ingestion • Acute corrosive ingestion • Celiac disease • GERD • CMPA • Crohn's disease • Intestinal tuberculosis • Choledochal cyst with cholangitis • Rumination syndrome • Intussusception • Intestinal malrotation • Esophageal stricture Pyloric stricture • Achalasia cardia • Functional vomiting • Gastrointestinal lymphoma • Intestinal malrotation • Duplication cyst • Superior mesenteric artery syndrome • Intestinal pseudobstruction • Postsurgical adhesions	• Gastritis or peptic ulcer (Food/drug/*H. pylori* related) • Appendicitis • Cholecystitis/ cholelithiasis • Pancreatitis • Rumination syndrome • GERD • Crohn's disease • Intestinal tuberculosis • Celiac disease • Achalasia cardia • Acute corrosive ingestion • Eosinophilic esophagitis • Esophageal stricture, Pyloric stricture • Gastroparesis • Functional vomiting • Gastrointestinal lymphoma • Trichobezoar • Superior mesenteric artery syndrome • Intestinal malrotation • Duplication cyst • Intestinal pseudobstruction • Postsurgical adhesions
CNS	• Congenital hydrocephalus • Intracranial bleed • Arnold–Chiari malformation • Pseudotumor cerebri	• Intracranial tumors • Pseudotumor cerebri • Head trauma	• Cyclical vomiting syndrome • Intracranial tumors • CNS tuberculosis Neurocysticercosis • Head trauma	• Cyclical vomiting syndrome • Intracranial tumors • CNS tuberculosis Neurocysticercosis • Bulimia nervosa • Migraine

Contd...

Contd...

Etiology	*Neonate*	*Infant*	*Toddler/older child*	*Adolescent*
Metabolic	• Urea cycle defects • Fatty acid oxidation defects • *Organic acidemia:* In newborn period, it mainly manifests as encephalopathy, seizures; but vomiting has been described. Hence we included it • *Mitochondrial hepatopathy:* In newborn, it mainly presents as liver failure with multi system involvement including neurological symptoms like seizures, vomiting, floppiness etc. • *Gluconeogenic disorders and galactosemia:* They can cause hypoglycemia which may inturn cause vomiting but not a direct/major symptom. Hence these two disorders can be removed from the box • Phenylketonuria Congenital lactic acidosis	• Hereditary fructose intolerance • Urea cycle defects • Fatty acid oxidation defects • Organic acidemias • Mitochondrial hepatopathies	• Hereditary fructose intolerance • Urea cycle defects • Fatty acid oxidation defects • Organic acidemias • Mitochondrial hepatopathies	• Urea cycle defects • Fatty acid oxidation defects • Acute intermittent porphyria
Endocrine	• Congenital adrenal hyperplasia • Neonatal thyrotoxicosis • Hypercalcemia	• Hypercalcemia • Addison's disease	• Diabetic ketoacidosis • Hypercalcemia • Hyperthyroidism • Addison's disease	• Diabetic ketoacidosis • Hypercalcemia • Hyperthyroidism • Addison's disease
Others	• Hydronephrosis • Dyselectrolytemia (of any cause) • VUR • Neonatal abstinence syndrome • Munchausen syndrome by proxy	• Hydronephrosis • Dyselectrolytemia (of any cause) • Uremia • VUR • Drugs (antibiotics, iron, zinc, opioids, etc.) • Renal tubular acidosis • Munchausen syndrome by proxy	• Dyselectrolytemia (of any cause) • Uremia • Hydronephrosis Vestibular disorders • Drugs (chemotherapeutics, antibiotics, iron, zinc, NSAIDs, opioids, etc.)	• Dyselectrolytemia (of any cause) • Uremia • Vestibular disorders • Drug-induced (e.g., chemotherapy, NSAIDs, iron, etc.) • Testicular/ovarian torsion • Cannabinoid hyperemesis syndrome • Glaucoma

(CMPA: Cow milk protein allergy; CNS: Central nervous system; GERD: Gastroesophageal reflux disease; NEC: Necrotizing enterocolitis; NSAIDs: Nonsteroidal anti-inflammatory drugs; UTI: Urinary tract infection; VUR: Vesico ureteric reflux)

Step 1
History (age, characteristics of vomiting, associated symptoms) and examination

Step 2
Localize to a system/s and make a list of possible differential diagnosis

Step 3
Evaluate based on working differentials and manage

Fig. 1: Basic three-step process for a child with vomiting.

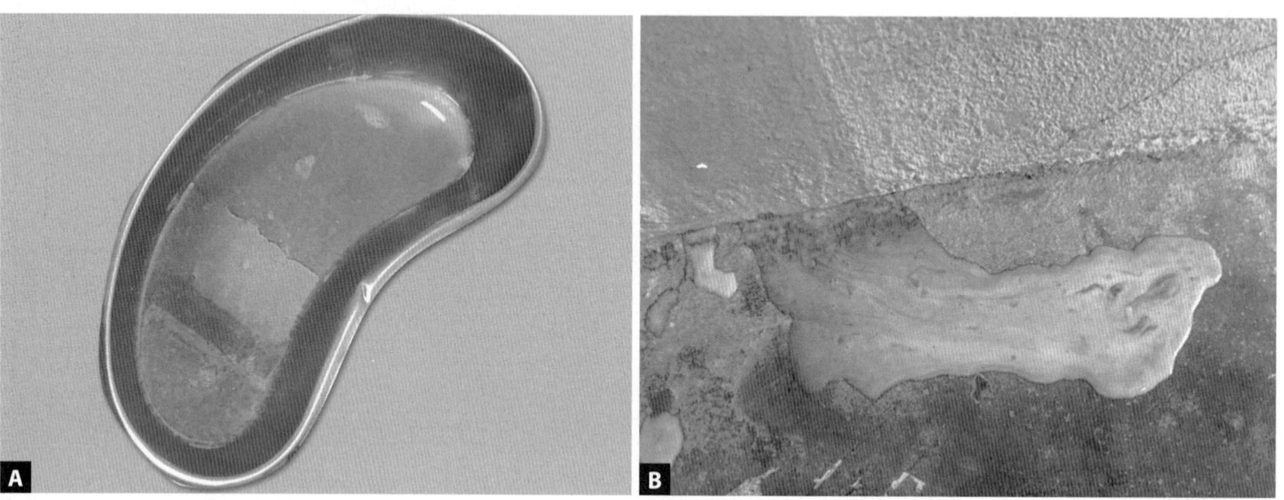

Figs. 2A and B: (A) Image showing bilious (greenish) vomiting in a 3-year-old with malrotatio; (B) Small volume of blood-stained (hematemesis) vomitus in an infant with cow milk protein allergy. *(For color version, see Plate 7)*

TABLE 2: Clues in history and examination toward etiology of vomiting.

Blood in vomitus, epigastric pain, tenderness	Gastritis/Peptic ulcer disease
Blood in vomitus, splenomegaly, no abdominal pain, with or without jaundice, ascites	Portal hypertension
Bilious (greenish) vomiting, abdominal distension, abdominal pain (colicky), increased bowel sounds	Intestinal obstruction (distal to ampulla of Vater)
Bilious vomiting, abdominal distension, decreased bowel sounds	• Ileus (paralytics, sepsis) • Pseudobstruction
Stale food, nonbilious, large volume, may be projectile	Gastric outlet obstruction (Hypertrophic pyloric stenosis, postcorrosive pyloric stricture, pancreatic pseudocyst)
Feculent, generalized abdominal distension, constipation	Colonic obstruction
Undigested food or uncurdled milk, dysphagia	Esophageal stricture, Achalasia cardia
Regurgitation, retrosternal burning, failure to thrive, aspirations, recurrent respiratory infections	Gastroesophageal reflux disease
Vomiting, food bolus impaction, dysphagia, retrosternal pain	• Eosinophilic esophagitis • Esophageal stricture (e.g., peptic)
Postprandial regurgitation, chewing, re-swallowing	Rumination syndrome
Vomiting increases after food intake, epigastric pain	Gastritis, Cholecystitis, Pancreatitis (Pain radiates to back; gets better on stooping forward)
Vomiting followed by watery loose stools (acute history), crampy abdominal pain (diffuse/periumbilical)	Acute gastroenteritis

Contd...

Contd...

Periumbilical pain followed by vomiting, pain may shift to McBurney's site in RIF (with sharp parietal nature),	Acute appendicitis
Vomiting, loose stools associated with blood and mucus, urgency, Tenesmus	Colitis
Abdominal distension, diffuse tenderness, guarding, decreased bowel sounds, minimal abdominal movement	Peritonitis
Burning micturition, vomiting	Urinary tract infection
Prodrome of anorexia, vomiting, pain abdomen, and/or fever followed by jaundice with high colored urine, hepatomegaly	Acute viral hepatitis
Headache, early morning vomiting, focal neurological deficits	Raised intracranial pressure
Fever, headache, vomiting, meningeal signs	Meningitis
Vomiting only during travel, family history of migraine, or motion sickness	Motion sickness
Rash	• Infective (fever, acute onset) • Vasculitis [e.g., Henoch-Schönlein purpura (HSP)] • Drug-induced • Connective tissue disorders • Porphyria
Head trauma	Intracranial bleed with raised intracranial pressure
Indigenous medication use	• Hepatitis • Gastritis
Temporal relation to drugs	• Chemotherapy related • Doxycycline • NSAIDs, etc.
Encephalopathy, vomiting triggered by infections or fasting, acidotic breathing, concern for hypoglycemia	Metabolic disorders
Stereotypical pattern, intense nausea and vomiting (often bilious especially the terminal bouts), interval period normal	Cyclical vomiting syndrome
Infant or toddler with vomiting, chronic diarrhea (watery or blood and mucus), atopy, rash(eczema)	Cow milk protein allergy
Chronic diarrhea, failure to thrive, pallor	Celiac disease
Weight loss, fever, anorexia, vomiting, pain abdomen	• Intestinal tuberculosis • IBD • Malignancies (e.g., lymphoma)
Weight loss, vomiting, fatigue, dehydration, low blood pressure, hyperpigmentation, concern for hypoglycemia	Addison's disease/CAH (ambiguous genitalia in female infants)
Polyuria, failure to thrive, vomiting	• RTA • Diabetes mellitus • Diabetes insipidus
History of abdominal surgery	• Adhesions (usually present as intestinal obstruction) • Recurrence
Binge eating, self-induced vomiting, and purging	• Bulimia nervosa • Psychiatric
Vomiting, visual disturbances, headache, and pallor during episodes; often brief limited or no motor activity, can be diagnosed as migraine	Occipital epilepsy

(RTA: Renal tubular acidosis; IBD: Inflammatory bowel disease; CAH: Congenital adrenal hyperplasia)

BOX 1: Red flags in a child with vomiting warranting urgent evaluation.

- Bilious vomiting (*Note:* Benign conditions like cyclical vomiting syndrome often have bilious vomiting, a terminal bout after multiple vomits can have a bilious nature)
- Blood in vomitus
- Altered sensorium (cause or effect)
- Dehydration
- Concern for symptomatic hypoglycemia or documented hypoglycemia
- Acute severe abdominal pain (acute abdomen) and abdominal tenderness
- Toxic look/sepsis
- Inconsolable cry or irritability
- Abdominal distension, guarding, stillness with avoidance of unnecessary movement
- Bulging fontanelle or features suggestive of raised intracranial pressure

Flowchart 1: Algorithm showing an approach to a child presenting with vomiting.

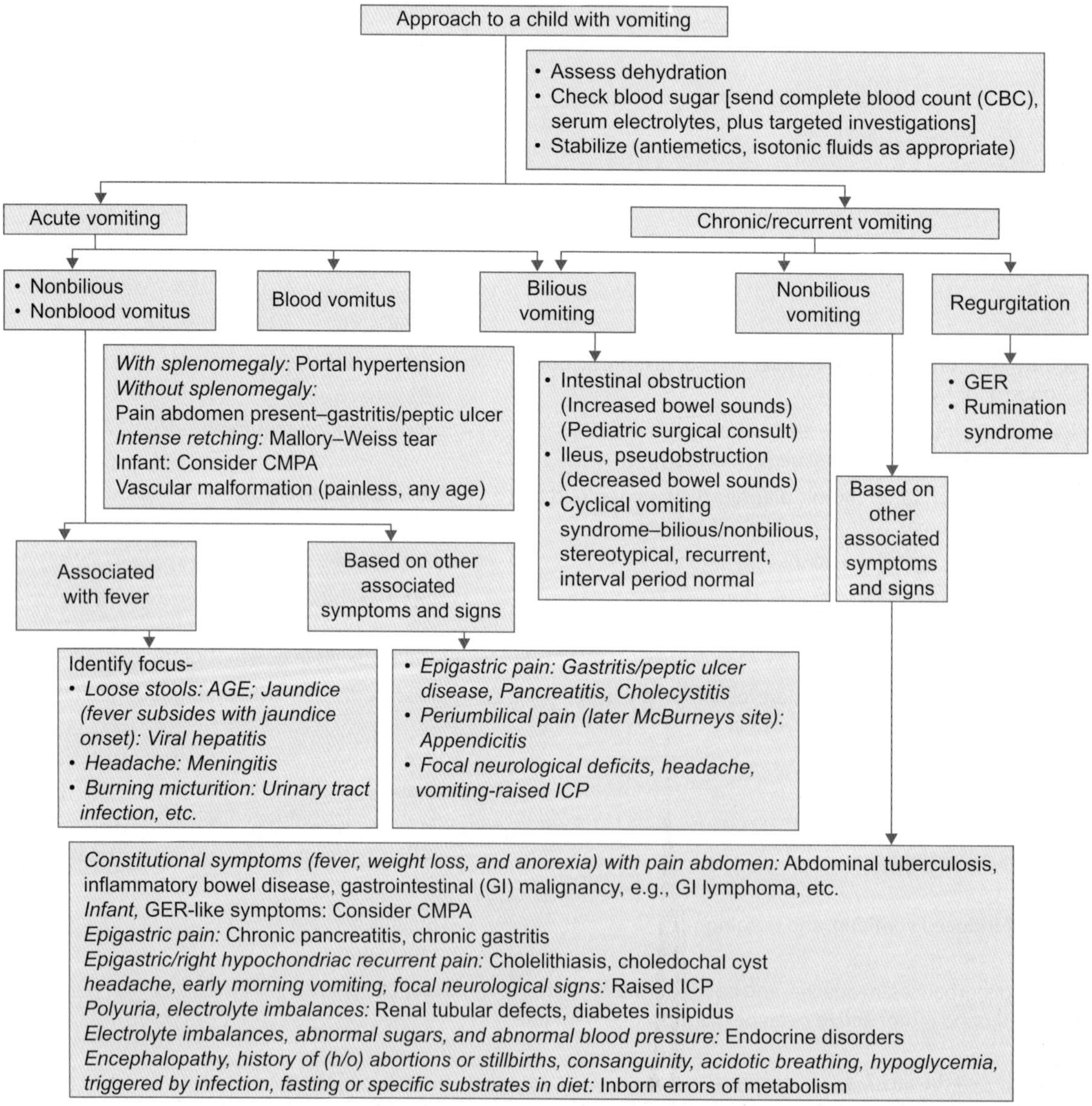

Approach to a child with vomiting

- Assess dehydration
- Check blood sugar [send complete blood count (CBC), serum electrolytes, plus targeted investigations]
- Stabilize (antiemetics, isotonic fluids as appropriate)

Acute vomiting

- Nonbilious
- Nonblood vomitus

→ Associated with fever → Identify focus-
- *Loose stools: AGE; Jaundice (fever subsides with jaundice onset): Viral hepatitis*
- *Headache: Meningitis*
- *Burning micturition: Urinary tract infection, etc.*

→ Based on other associated symptoms and signs →
- *Epigastric pain: Gastritis/peptic ulcer disease, Pancreatitis, Cholecystitis*
- *Periumbilical pain (later McBurneys site): Appendicitis*
- *Focal neurological deficits, headache, vomiting-raised ICP*

Blood vomitus

With splenomegaly: Portal hypertension
Without splenomegaly:
Pain abdomen present–gastritis/peptic ulcer
Intense retching: Mallory–Weiss tear
Infant: Consider CMPA
Vascular malformation (painless, any age)

Bilious vomiting (acute and chronic/recurrent)

- Intestinal obstruction (Increased bowel sounds) (Pediatric surgical consult)
- Ileus, pseudobstruction (decreased bowel sounds)
- Cyclical vomiting syndrome–bilious/nonbilious, stereotypical, recurrent, interval period normal

Chronic/recurrent vomiting

Nonbilious vomiting → Based on other associated symptoms and signs →

Constitutional symptoms (fever, weight loss, and anorexia) with pain abdomen: Abdominal tuberculosis, inflammatory bowel disease, gastrointestinal (GI) malignancy, e.g., GI lymphoma, etc.
Infant, GER-like symptoms: Consider CMPA
Epigastric pain: Chronic pancreatitis, chronic gastritis
Epigastric/right hypochondriac recurrent pain: Cholelithiasis, choledochal cyst
headache, early morning vomiting, focal neurological signs: Raised ICP
Polyuria, electrolyte imbalances: Renal tubular defects, diabetes insipidus
Electrolyte imbalances, abnormal sugars, and abnormal blood pressure: Endocrine disorders
Encephalopathy, history of (h/o) abortions or stillbirths, consanguinity, acidotic breathing, hypoglycemia, triggered by infection, fasting or specific substrates in diet: Inborn errors of metabolism

Regurgitation →
- GER
- Rumination syndrome

INVESTIGATIONS

Owing to the diverse nature of the etiologies, investigations have to be tailored based on the most likely differential diagnosis made clinically. Routine blood investigations in a child with nonbilious vomiting with moderate-to-severe dehydration include complete blood counts, serum electrolytes, liver enzymes, blood sugar, and renal functional tests.

> **CLINICAL PEARLS**
>
> Since vomiting is a very common presentation of many nonspecific illnesses, it is important not to do unnecessary investigations (only do specific for the cause) and directly go to trial of treatment if a clinical diagnosis warrants:
>
> *Examples:*
> - Well child with no dehydration and clear etiology of acute gastritis or acute gastroenteritis.
> - Infections, e.g.,: Urinary tract infection
> - Infant with typical gastroesophageal reflux
> - Suspected cow milk protein allergy-related vomiting
> - Classical rumination syndrome

Specific Investigations

Blood Investigations

Typical blood picture abnormalities can point to specific etiologies such as elevated liver transaminases in hepatitis; elevated serum amylase, and lipase in pancreatitis, hypochloremic hypokalemic metabolic alkalosis in pyloric stenosis/gastric outlet obstruction; hyponatremia with hyperkalemia in congenital adrenal hyperplasia/Addison's disease; metabolic acidosis with a normal anion gap in renal tubular acidosis. When suspecting metabolic diseases, it is important to send a critical sample as changes may be seen only during acute episodes. Metabolic workup includes arterial blood gas with lactate, blood ammonia, serum transaminases, serum electrolytes, random blood sugar, urine ketones, urine nonglucose reducing substances, urine porphyrins, blood tandem mass spectrometry, and urine gas chromatography-mass spectrometry.

Radiological Investigations

X-ray erect abdomen: This should be done in all cases where intestinal obstruction is suspected. In infants, single-bubble and double-bubble signs may be seen in pyloric and duodenal obstruction, respectively. More distal intestinal obstruction results in multiple air-fluid levels **(Fig. 3A)**, which can also be seen in cases of paralytic ileus.

Ultrasound of abdomen: Very useful, does not give radiation, and has diagnostic potential in many cases. In congenital hypertrophic pyloric stenosis, a pyloric thickness of >3 mm (most accurate), pyloric length >15–17 mm, and pyloric diameter >14 mm is significant **(Fig. 3B)**. It can detect intussusception [target sign **(Fig. 3C)**, Doppler can assess vascularity], appendicular inflammation in appendicitis, and bulky pancreas with or without pancreatic collections in pancreatitis. The superior mesenteric artery and superior mesenteric vein relationship can help in the detection of malrotation. Hepatomegaly with gall bladder wall edema in hepatitis, gall bladder wall thickening, and pericholecystic fluid in cholecystitis, gall stones in cholelithiasis, and increased common bile duct diameter in choledochal cyst. Hydronephrosis, hydroureter in obstructive uropathy, and bladder wall thickening with irregularities in cystitis.

Upper gastrointestinal (GI) contrast series: Barium swallow can detect esophageal strictures, timed barium swallow shows hold up of contrast along with bird's beak appearance in achalasia **(Fig. 3D)**. Barium meal follow-through provides small bowel anatomical evaluation and can diagnose malrotation.

Cross-sectional imaging: Computed tomography (CT) abdomen as cross-sectional imaging gives a more detailed evaluation of intestinal as well as extraintestinal structures. Indicated in patients with suspected intestinal tuberculosis, and Crohn's disease where contrast-enhanced CT enterography (using oral negative contrast with mannitol or polyethylene glycol along with intravenous contrast) or magnetic resonance (MR) enterography (in an older child who is cooperative) is necessary. CT triple-phase (angio) enterography is needed in cases with suspicion of SMA syndrome, malignancy, or vasculitis. CT/MRI brain in cases with suspected meningitis or raised intracranial pressure. Magnetic resonance cholangiopancreatography (MRCP) is useful in chronic pancreatitis and biliary abnormalities.

Endoscopy

Upper gastrointestinal endoscopy (UGIE) can give both diagnostic and therapeutic advantages. Conditions that

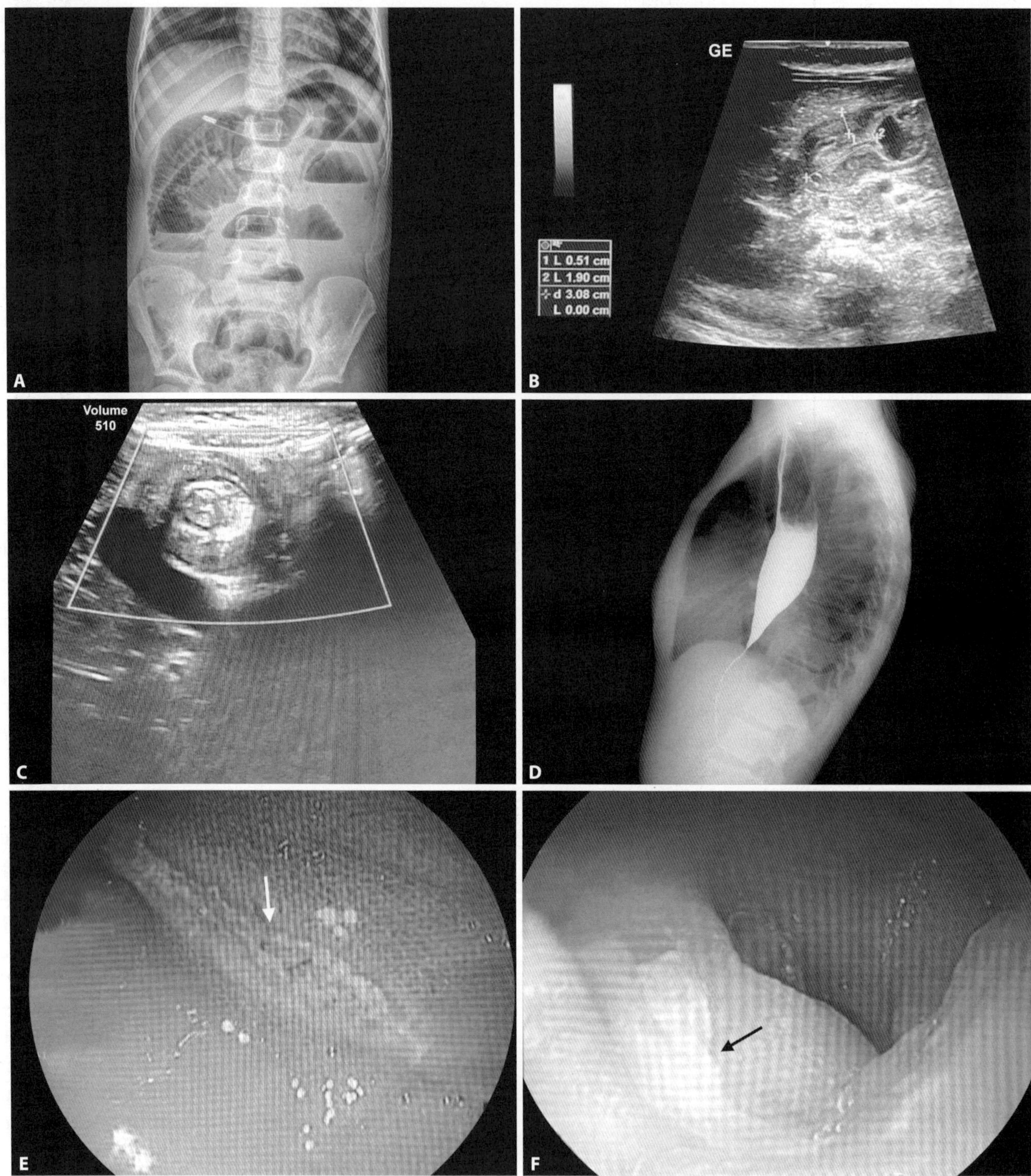

Figs. 3A to F: (A) Multiple air-fluid levels seen in a 9-year-old child with intestinal obstruction; (B) A 3-month-old infant with ultrasound abdomen showing hypertrophic pyloric stenosis (thickness 5.1 mm, length 19 mm); (C) Target sign of intussusception in an 18 month old child; (D) Barium swallow showing hold up of contrast in the esophagus with a characteristic bird's beak/rat tail sign in a child with achalasia cardia; (E) A 10-year-old with a large linear gastric ulcer (white arrow; *Helicobacter pylori* positive); (F) A 6-year-old with peptic duodenal (D1 part) clean based ulcer (black arrow; *H. pylori* negative). *[For color version (Figs. B, C, E and F), see Plate 7]*

can be diagnosed (or add support to management) on UGIE include eosinophilic esophagitis (with biopsy), esophageal stricture (therapeutic as well), achalasia cardia, reflux esophagitis, hiatus hernia, esophageal foreign body, severe acute gastritis, chronic gastritis/peptic ulcer disease **(Figs. 3E and 3F)** not responding to proton pump inhibitors with biopsies taken to rule out *Helicobacter pylori* infection, trichobezoar, Vasculitis, e.g., Henoch-Schönlein purpura (HSP). Colonoscopy (along with UGIE) in suspected inflammatory bowel disease and intestinal tuberculosis.

Manometry

High-resolution esophageal manometry can diagnose and classify achalasia cardia and other causes of esophageal dysmotility. For antroduodenal manometry, there are limited indications as in intestinal pseudo-obstruction, rumination syndrome, and gastroparesis.

Other Appropriate Investigations

The Ph impedance metry monitoring for gastroesophageal reflux. For gastroparesis, gastric emptying scintigraphy can be done apart from manometry. In children with associated headaches and suspected raised intracranial pressure (ICP) fundus examination for papilledema should be done along with neuroimaging. Lumbar puncture for cerebrospinal fluid analysis and pressure studies for suspected meningitis and pseudotumor cerebri, respectively. Breath tests can be performed including a urea breath test (noninvasive, but has low specificity, useful for monitoring before and after treatment, especially in a setting where endoscopy is not feasible) for *H. pylori* infection, glucose hydrogen breath test for small intestinal bacterial overgrowth. Urine pregnancy test in teenage girls with vomiting, amenorrhea. Bulimia nervosa, psychogenic vomiting, rumination syndrome, abdominal migraine, and cyclic vomiting syndrome are generally diagnosed clinically but additional tests often are necessary to rule out organic etiology.

TREATMENT

Initial Treatment

It should be directed primarily at correcting abnormalities such as dehydration, electrolytes and acid-base imbalance, and hypoglycemia. Thereafter, management strategies depend on the underlying cause.

Specific Treatment Strategies

Gastrointestinal causes: In cases presenting with intestinal obstruction keep the child nil orally, nasogastric tube for gastric decompression, intravenous fluids, and antibiotics have to be started, along with surgical consultation. In superior mesenteric artery (SMA) syndrome, most improve with conservative management by hyperalimentation, and nasojejunal feeding, and only the resistant cases require duodenojejunostomy. In CMPA, therapeutic elimination of milk and milk products has to be done for a minimum of 6 months or till 1 year of age whichever is later. In exclusively breastfed babies, the mother should be advised to eliminate milk and milk products in her diet. In formula-fed babies, an extensively hydrolyzed formula (EHF) should be started. In severe CMPA or children not responding to EHF, an aminoacid-based formula should be considered. In infants with GERD, if there is no improvement after correction of feeding techniques and thickening of feeds, then a 2–4-week trial of milk elimination should be done treating as possible CMPA. If there is still no improvement then a 4–8-week trial of proton-pump inhibitors (PPIs) should be given, along with an early introduction of semisolids and a pediatric gastroenterologist consult. In children, if the PPI trial is not successful or if weaning off PPI is difficult then eosinophilic esophagitis (EoE) is a possibility. Six food elimination (animal milk, wheat, nuts, egg, soy, and seafood) can achieve remission in three-fourths of children with EoE. Thereafter, sequential reintroduction will aid in identifying specific triggers. In the subset of children who do not respond to PPI or elimination diet, viscous budesonide or oral fluticasone has good efficacy. For achalasia cardia, pneumatic balloon dilatation, Hellers myotomy, or the recently developed third space endoscopic technique per-oral endoscopic myotomy (POEM) is equally effective. For type 3 achalasia cardia, POEM has shown to be better than the other modalities, however, there may be an increased risk of gastroesophageal reflux. Endoscopic bougie or balloon dilatation is the first-line treatment for managing esophageal or pyloric strictures. Diaphragmatic breathing exercise is the mainstay of treatment in rumination syndrome; other behavioral modifications such as distraction, aversion techniques, and psychological counseling are beneficial. For gastroparesis, management includes dietary modification by giving small frequent feeds with low fat, low fiber, and prokinetics (erythromycin, domperidone, and metoclopramide). In refractory cases,

TABLE 3: Pharmacologic therapy of vomiting in children.

Disorder	*Drug*	*Dosage*
GERD	Dopamine antagonist—Domperidone	0.2–0.3 mg/kg/dose Tid
Chemotherapy-induced vomiting/ postoperative nausea/vomiting	Dopamine antagonist—Domperidone 5Ht3 antagonist—Ondansetron • Phenothiazines • Chlorpromazine In refractory cases • Steroids—Dexamethasone	 0.15–0.3 0.5 mg/kg 0.15 mg/kg
Motion sickness/vestibular disorders	Antihistaminic— • Dimenhydrinate • Diphenhydramine • Promethazine	 1 mg/kg PO Tid 1.25 mg/kg/dose Tid/Qid >2 years—0.25–1 mg/kg can be repeated 8–12 hourly
Adrenal crisis	Cortisol	2 mg/kg IV bolus f/b 0.2–0.4 mg/kg/h IV
Gastroparesis	Dopamine antagonist—Domperidone Motilin agonist—Erythromycin	0.2–0.3 mg/kg/dose Tid 3–5 mg/kg PO Tid/Qid
Intestinal pseudoobstruction	Somatostatin analog— Octreotide Dopamine antagonist—Domperidone Motilin agonist—Erythromycin	 1 ug/kg SC Bid/Tid 0.2–0.3 mg/kg/dose Tid 3–5 mg/kg PO Tid/Qid
Cyclic vomiting syndrome	Abortive therapy Ondansetron *Prophylaxis:* Cyproheptadine <5 years Amitriptyline >5 years (ECG monitoring)	 0.3–0.4 mg/kg/dose 0.1–0.25 mg/kg/day in 2 divided dose 0.5–1 mg/kg/day

(GERD: Gastroesophageal reflux disease)

gastric-per-oral endoscopic myotomy (G-POEM) is the treatment of choice.

Nongastrointestinal causes: For acute attacks of cyclical vomiting syndrome, supportive strategies with dextrose-containing fluids (10%D with 0.45 normal saline with KCL) initially at 1.25–1.5 times the maintenance should be started, along with antiemetics such as ondansetron at higher doses and sedation **(Table 3)**. For prophylaxis, it is important to avoid triggers; and maintain good sleep hygiene, healthy eating habits including regular meals and snacks, and good hydration. Drugs for prophylaxis include [*first-line:* Cyproheptadine in <5 years and amitriptyline in >5 years of age), *second line:* Propranolol] and supplements such as carnitine, co-enzyme Q. For other systemic diseases such as renal tubular acidosis, endocrine disorders, raised intracranial pressure, inborn errors of metabolism, etc., specific treatment along with team management including the concerned pediatric super-specialties is essential.

CONCLUSION

Vomiting in children has a whole array of causes that affect different organ systems. Age at presentation, meticulous history, and examination help in reaching a clinical differential diagnosis which guides further investigations for confirmation. Management involves stabilization, symptomatic control, identifying conditions in which immediate medical or surgical intervention is needed, and specific treatment strategies as appropriate.

KEY POINTS

- Vomiting is a common presenting problem in children seen in our day-to-day practice.
- Identifying clinically when a child requires emergency management is important.
- Bilious, clinically significant blood vomitus, features of raised ICP, and associated red flags warrant an emergency management
- Etiology depends on the age at presentation and associated symptoms and signs
- Vomiting is a result of a whole gamut of causes, and a methodical clinical approach is necessary for the right diagnosis
- Targeting investigations should be based on the clinical differential diagnosis
- Initial stabilization should be directed towards correcting dehydration, electrolytes, acid-base imbalance, hemodynamics, and/or hypoglycemia
- Symptomatic control can be achieved with drugs like antiemetics, e.g., ondansetron, prokinetics, e.g.; domperidone, etc.
- Treatment should be channelized and be specific to the disease (gastrointestinal or nongastrointestinal) once the etiology is made.
- Clinically, when an intestinal obstruction is present keep the child nil orally, nasogastric tube for decompression, intravenous (IV) fluids, stabilize hemodynamics, start antibiotics, and a pediatric surgical consult.
- Consulting pediatric superspecialist/s is helpful as part of team management where appropriate.

SUGGESTED READING

1. Kliegman RM, St. Geme III JW. Chp 332. In: Maqbool A, Liacouras CA. Major symptoms and signs of digestive tract disorders: Nelson Textbook of Pediatrics, 21st edition. Gurugram: Elsevier; 2023.
2. Koletzko S, Niggemann B, Arato A, Dias JA, Heuschkel R, Husby S, et al. Diagnostic approach and management of cow's-milk protein allergy in infants and children: ESPGHAN GI Committee practical guidelines. J Pediatr Gastroenterol Nutr. 2012;55(2):221-9.
3. Mokha J. Vomiting and Nausea: Wylie Textbook of pediatric Gastrointestinal and Liver disease; 6th edition; 2021. pp. 70-87.
4. Ravindranath A. Chronic vomiting in children: Etiology, diagnosis, and management. Indian J Gastroenterol. 2020; 39(2):117-22.
5. Rosen R, Vandenplas Y, Singendonk M, Cabana M, DiLorenzo C, Gottrand F, et al. Pediatric gastroesophageal Reflux Clinical Practice Guidelines: Joint Recommendations of the North American Society for Pediatric Gastroenterology, Hepatology, and Nutrition and the European Society for Pediatric Gastroenterology, Hepatology, and Nutrition. J Pediatr Gastroenterol Nutr. 2018;66(3):516-54.
6. Singhi SC, Bansal A, Shah R, Jayashree M. Management of a child with vomiting. Indian J Pediatr. 2013;80(4):318-32.

Neonatal Cholestasis Syndrome: An Algorithmic Approach

Seema Alam, Bikrant Bihari Lal

INTRODUCTION

Neonatal cholestasis syndrome (NCS) is the term used to describe conjugated hyperbilirubinemia (conjugated bilirubin >20% of total bilirubin if total bilirubin is >5 mg/dL or conjugated bilirubin >1 mg/dL if total bilirubin is <5 mg/dL. Dark urine staining the diapers is a clinical indicator to differentiate it from neonatal unconjugated jaundice. Whenever evaluating a neonate with jaundice, fractionation of bilirubin should be done at least once so as to not miss conjugated hyperbilirubinemia. NCS encompasses a wide etiological spectrum ranging from structural defects like biliary atresia (BA) and choledochal cyst, genetic intrahepatic cholestasis, metabolic liver diseases (MLDs), congenital and postnatal infections, and endocrinal and other less common causes **(Fig. 1)**. During evaluation, the emphasis should be on timely identification of surgically manageable causes such as BA or choledochal cyst, and medically treatable conditions such as hypothyroidism, urinary tract infection, sepsis, galactosemia, and tyrosinemia. BA singularly accounts for 25–60% of cases presenting as NCS. It is always wise to classify NCS as those with or without acholic stools. BA accounts for 80–95% of NCS presenting with persistent or intermittent acholic stools. It is not easy for parents to interpret stool color and occasionally acholic stools may get mixed with urine giving false impression of pigmented stool.

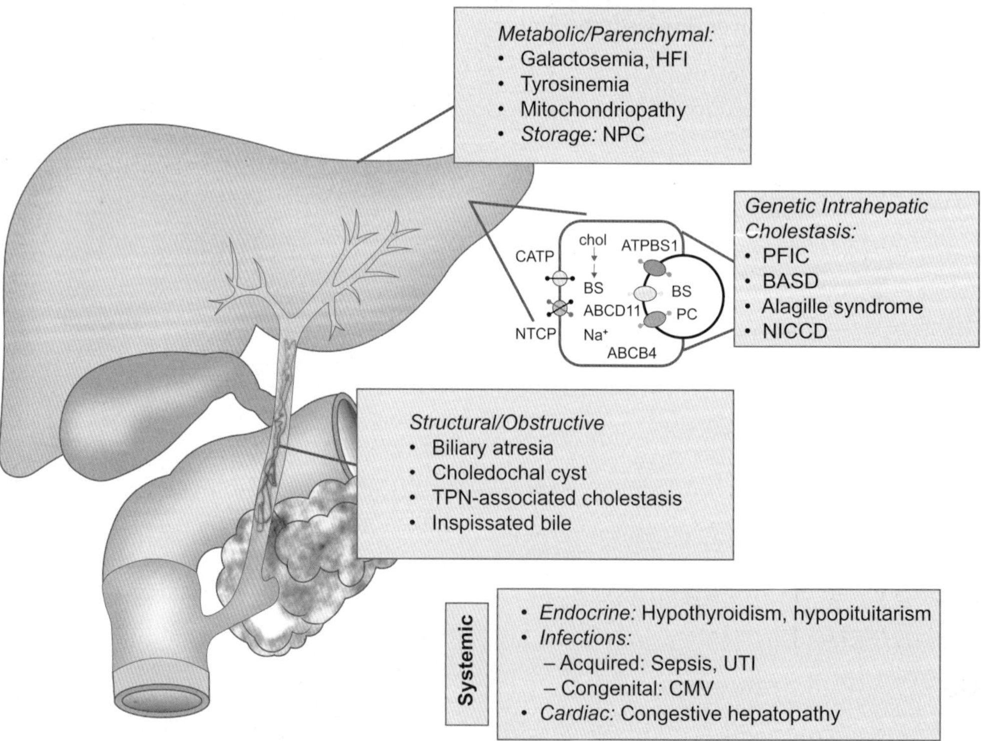

Fig. 1: Common causes of neonatal cholestasis syndrome.

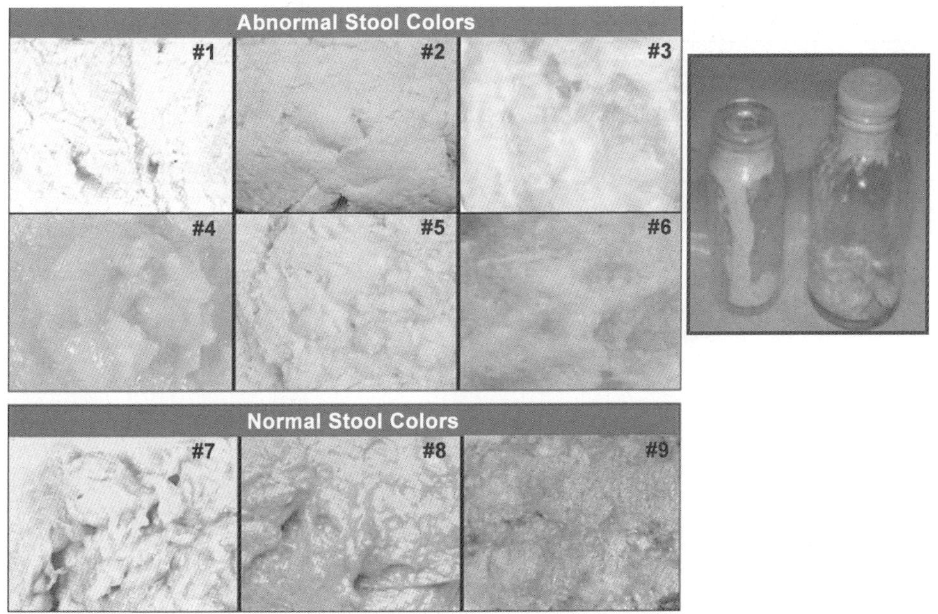

Fig. 2: Stool color chart. *(For color version, see Plate 8)*

Parents should be shown stool color chart **(Fig. 2)** for better elicitation of response and clinicians should themselves check stool color. In case of doubt, a gentle digital per rectal examination may be done to assess stool color. Screening of BA by stool color chart given to parents in Taiwan led to early diagnosis and improved outcome. Other conditions which may have intermittent or persistent acholic stools are Alagille syndrome (AGS), parenteral nutrition (PN)-associated cholestasis or multifactorial causes (MCs) of neonatal sclerosing cholangitis (NCS), NCS, few cases of choledocal cysts, and progressive familial intrahepatic cholestasis (PFIC). **Flowchart 1** shows a basic clinical algorithm which is widely used by pediatric hepatologists to guide the basic work-up. **Flowchart 1** describes more detailed work up of an infant with NCS. Nevertheless, all treatable causes should be evaluated as a part of screening procedure when a child presents with NCS. A focused history and examination may narrow the differentials and expedite diagnosis and therapy. **Table 1** shows the important pointers in history taking and examination of these children with NCS.

NEONATAL CHOLESTASIS SYNDROME WITH ACHOLIC/FLUCTUATING STOOL

Biliary Atresia

Structural defects form a major chunk of the cases with neonatal cholestasis. It is very important to make an early diagnosis in these cases as the outcome is dependent upon the timing of intervention in these cases. The prevalence of BA is approximately 1:5,000 in Taiwan and 1:20,000 in Europe and America. BA is the most common cause of NCS and requires expedited diagnosis followed by Kasai portoenterostomy surgery. Early diagnosis and surgery are the key as success rates are good when Kasai surgery is performed early before advanced fibrosis sets in the liver. Most children diagnosed beyond 90–100 days of life have advanced fibrosis or ascites and are listed for primary liver transplantation (LT) **(Table 2)**. Most of these children fail to ultimately receive LT due to logistic issues, lack of technical expertise, and lack of robust organ donation program in the country. Liver histopathological findings have close to 90% sensitivity and 90% specificity for diagnosis of BA and should be performed as an emergency procedure. High gamma-glutamyl transpeptidase (GGT) cholestasis with pale stools in good weight baby with enlarged firm to hard liver and splenomegaly are the clinical pointers. Characteristic findings on USG abdomen are triangular cord sign, small gallbladder (<19 mm), and common bile duct not visible. The typical liver biopsy findings of BA include bile ductular proliferation, bile plugs and portal expansion, and fibrosis. BA can be classified into three clinical variants. The isolated or perinatal form accounts for 80–90% of BA cases. Syndromic or embryonic form is known as BA splenic malformation (BASM) syndrome, which is more common

Flowchart 1: Approach to a child with neonatal cholestasis syndrome.

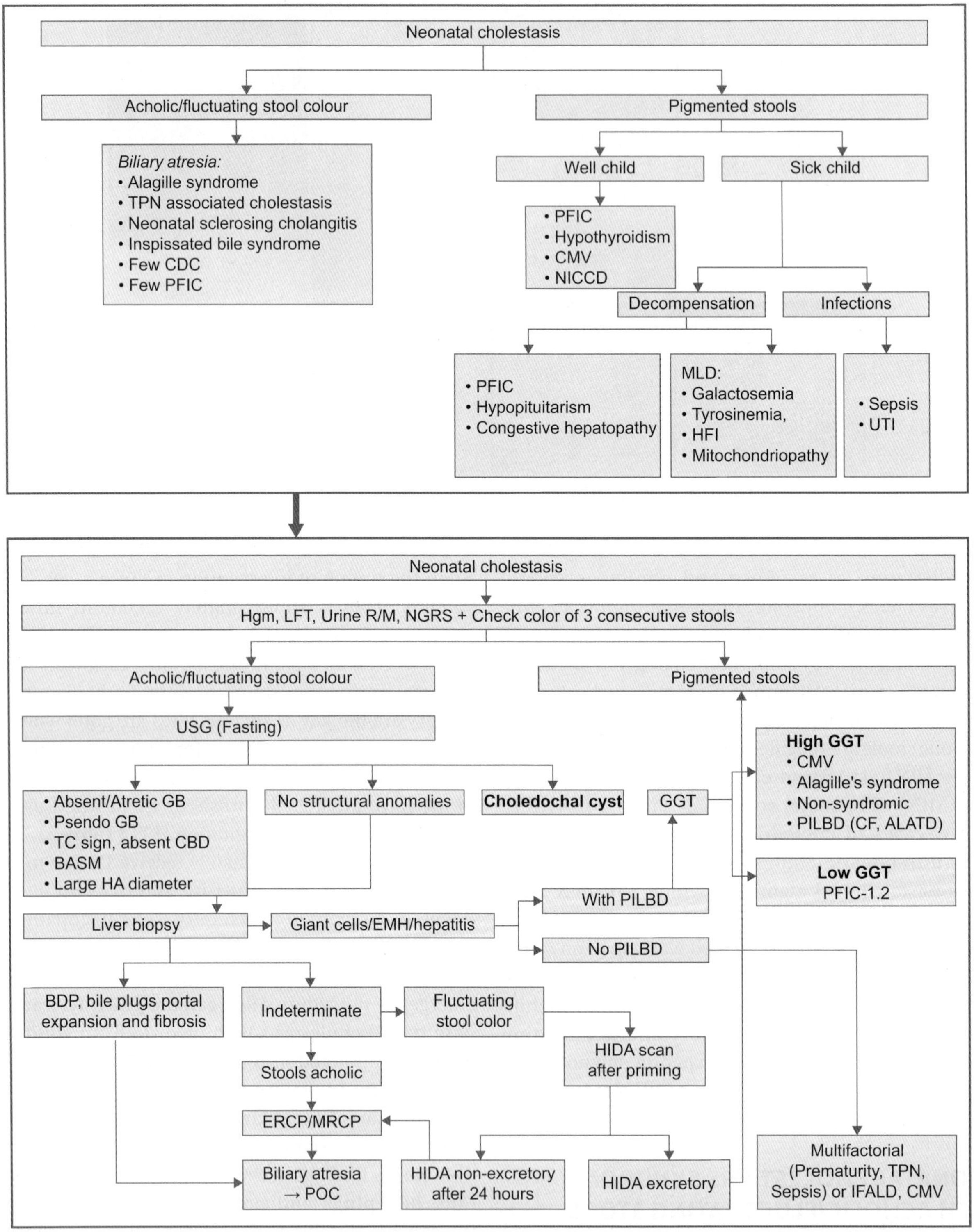

Neonatal cholestasis

Acholic/fluctuating stool colour

Biliary atresia:
- Alagille syndrome
- TPN associated cholestasis
- Neonatal sclerosing cholangitis
- Inspissated bile syndrome
- Few CDC
- Few PFIC

Pigmented stools

Well child
- PFIC
- Hypothyroidism
- CMV
- NICCD

Sick child

Decompensation
- PFIC
- Hypopituitarism
- Congestive hepatopathy

MLD:
- Galactosemia
- Tyrosinemia,
- HFI
- Mitochondriopathy

Infections
- Sepsis
- UTI

Neonatal cholestasis

Hgm, LFT, Urine R/M, NGRS + Check color of 3 consecutive stools

Acholic/fluctuating stool colour

USG (Fasting)

- Absent/Atretic GB
- Psendo GB
- TC sign, absent CBD
- BASM
- Large HA diameter

No structural anomalies

Choledochal cyst

Liver biopsy

Giant cells/EMH/hepatitis

With PILBD

No PILBD

GGT

High GGT
- CMV
- Alagille's syndrome
- Non-syndromic
- PILBD (CF, ALATD)

Low GGT
PFIC-1.2

Pigmented stools

BDP, bile plugs portal expansion and fibrosis

Indeterminate

Fluctuating stool color

HIDA scan after priming

Stools acholic

ERCP/MRCP

Biliary atresia → POC

HIDA non-excretory after 24 hours

HIDA excretory

Multifactorial (Prematurity, TPN, Sepsis) or IFALD, CMV

(BASM: biliary atresia associated splenic malformations; CBD: common bile duct; CMV: cytomegalovirus; CBD: common bile duct; ERCP/MRCP: endoscopic/magnetic retrograde cholangiopancreatography; GB: gallbladder; GGT: gamma-glutamyl peptidase; HA: hepatic artery; HIDA: hepatobiliary iminodiacetic acid; IFALD: intestinal failure associated liver disease; LFT: liver function test; NGRS: nonglucose reducing sugar; PILBD: paucity of bile duct; TC: triangular cord)

TABLE 1: Salient points in history taking and clinical examination in a child with neonatal cholestasis.

Clinical pointers	*Relevance*
History	
Dark urine with diaper staining	Conjugated hyperbilirubinemia
Acholic stools	Possible obstruction to biliary tree/structural biliary disorders
Vitamin K responsive bleeds	Cholestasis
Stormy perinatal course, parenteral nutrition	Suggests total parenteral nutrition (TPN)-associated cholestasis, multifactorial
Pointers toward metabolic liver diseases	• Consanguinity, abortions, previous sib deaths • Failure to thrive, diarrhea, and vomiting • Recurrence during periods of catabolic stress (*fatty acid oxidation defects*) • Seizures, early morning irritability, and lethargy • Developmental delay, hypotonia, cataract (*galactosemia*) • Aversion to sugars (HFI) or proteins (*urea cycle defects*)
Maternal history	ICP in PFIC/AFLP or HELLP in FAOD
Family history	Pedigree analysis/history of gallstones in <35 years of age
Examination	
Facial dysmorphism	Alagille syndrome; Zellweger syndrome; and other trisomies like Down's syndrome
Eye examination	• Cataract in galactosemia, congenital rubella syndrome • Posterior embryotoxon (on slit lamp), optic nerve drusen in Alagille syndrome • Fundus (cherry red spot in Niemann–Pick disease, chorioretinitis in cytomegalovirus, and optic nerve hypoplasia in hypopituitarism) • Coloboma in biliary atresia
Hearing	Affected in congenital rubella infection and ATP8B1and USP53 defects
Visible acholic stools/per rectal	Strong likelihood of biliary atresia
Genitalia	Hypogonadism, midline defects in hypopituitarism
Skin	Pruritus marks, excoriations and shiny nails in intrahepatic cholestasis; ecchymosis in cholestatic bleed
Rickets, renal enlargement	Tyrosinemia, hereditary fructose intolerance, and Caroli syndrome
Firm liver with splenomegaly	Portal hypertension
Palpable lump in right hypochondrium	Choledochal cyst
Splenohepatomegaly	Lipid storage disorders
Apraxia/Gaze palsy	Neimann–Pick disease
	Mitochondropathy
Speech and developmental delay	USP53 and LSR
Optic atrophy, peripheral neuropathy, ataxia, tremor, and intellectual disability	CALFAN (SCYL1 defect)

(AFLP: acute fatty liver of pregnancy; FAOD: fatty acid oxidation disorder; HELLP: hemolysis, elevated liver enzymes and low platelets; ICP: intrahepatic cholestasis of pregnancy; PFIC: progressive familial intrahepatic cholestasis)

in Europe and America (10–15%). BASM is characterized by distinct visceral anomalies, including polysplenia, situs inversus, preduodenal portal vein, and absence of the intrahepatic vena cava. Cardiac anomalies are also present in approximately half of the cases. Cystic BA (CBA) is characterized by the cystic dilatation of the extrahepatic bile ducts and fibrosing obstruction of the duct segments. CBA must be differentiated from choledochal cyst, which can be seen in prenatal ultrasonography but have different clinical courses. Jaundice, and acholic stools may manifest shortly after birth or following a variable period. In a comprehensive review of BA cases, CBA was observed in approximately 8% of patients. Hepatobiliary iminodiacetic acid (HIDA) scan is time consuming, does not give any

TABLE 2: Outcome versus timing (age of the infant) of Kasai portoenterostomy.

Study	*Outcome*	*<30 days*	*30–60 days*		*60–90 days*	*90–120 days*	*>120 days*
USA (1976–1989)	5-year overall survival	63%	44%		40%	29%	29%
CANADA (1985–2002)	4-year transplant free survival	49%	36%			28%	
FRANCE (1986–2002)	5-year transplant free survival	58%	<45 day 41%	>45 day 42%	36%	36%	27%
USA (1997–2000)	2-year transplant free survival	70%	54%		50%	50%	

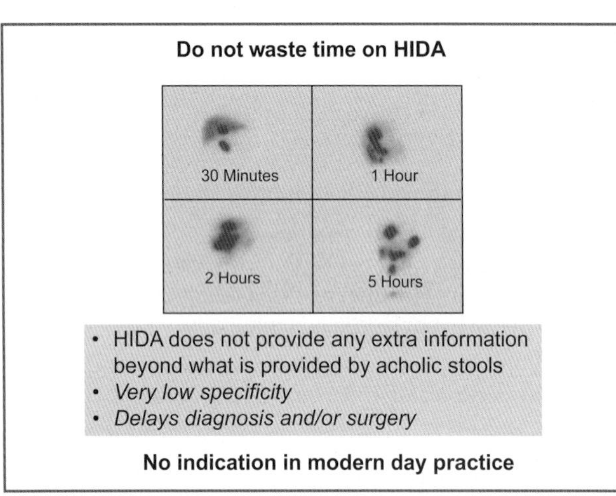

Fig. 3: Why we should not do HIDA for patients where you suspect biliary atresia? (HIDA: hepatobiliary iminodiacetic acid)

additional information, and has very low specificity, yet continues to be used at several centers delaying the diagnosis **(Fig. 3)**. Percutaneous cholecystocholangiogram is a good tool in hands of experienced intervention radiologist in cases with equivocal histopathological findings. When in doubt, intraoperative cholangiogram should be done which is the gold standard for diagnosis and should proceed to Kasai surgery if dye injected through gallbladder does not opacify the distal or the proximal bile ducts. **Figures 4A to C** describe endoscopic retrograde cholangiopancreatography/magnetic resonance cholangiopancreatography (ERCP/MRCP) in cases where liver biopsy if not conclusive of BA but more recently it is percutaneous cholecystocholangiogram **(Figs. 4A to C)** which is done in such a situation at most tertiary centers. In CBA, cholangiography may reveal an abnormal, tenuous connection with the intrahepatic ducts or ductules, which is often described as "cloud-like".

Multifactorial Cause

Multifactorial causes are common conditions seen in neonatal intensive care units (NICU) and can present in up to 20% of neonates receiving PN for >2 weeks with absence of enteral feeds, neonatal sepsis, and prematurity. Longer duration of PN and intestinal failure is independent risk factors for development of cholestasis. Use of fish oil-based lipids rich in omega-3 fatty acids has anti-inflammatory activity and has shown to result in improvement of cholestasis in these infants. Other treatment involves discontinuation of PN, early initiation of enteral feeds, and use of ursodeoxycholic acid (UDCA) apart from treatment of sepsis. These babies have decreasing trend of bilirubin, high GGT cholestasis with fluctuating to pigmented stools with no splenomegaly. If you find decreasing trend of bilirubin then wait and monitor the patient. The cholestasis subsides within weeks to months. This cause of NCS have good prognosis if PN has not caused intestinal failure.

Alagille Syndrome

Alagille syndrome is an autosomal dominant genetic disorder that affects multiple body systems. AGS is primarily caused by JAGGED1 (JAG1) mutation, which is responsible for producing the Jagged protein in the notch signaling pathway. Over 90% of patients have a detectable mutation in JAG1. However, the rest have NOTCH2 mutations. Even with the same genetic mutations, individuals within a family show different AGS characteristics. The traditional diagnosis criteria for AGS involved liver histology showing reduced bile ducts and three of the five major clinical features: Cholestasis, eye abnormalities, distinct facial features (Broad forehead, deep-set eyes, up-slanting palpebral fissure, prominent ears, straight nose with bulbous tip, and pointed chin, and triangular facies),

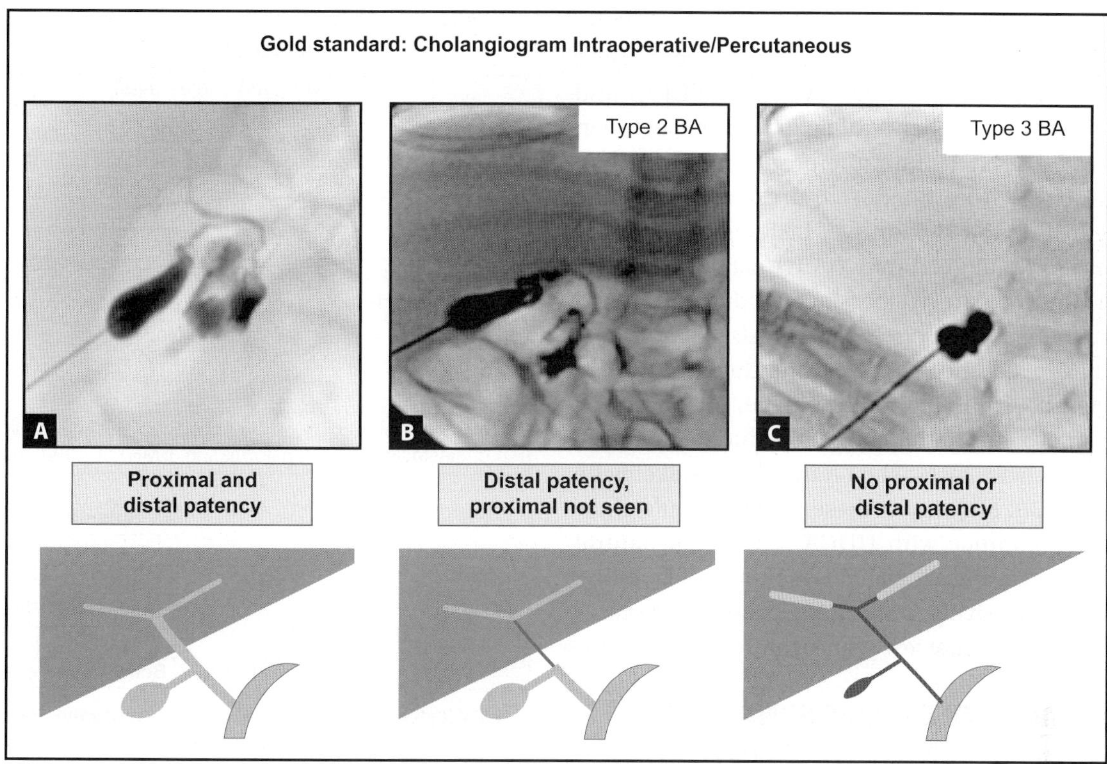

Figs. 4A to C: Role of percutaneous cholangiogram.

cardiac defects, and skeletal abnormalities. Recent findings have expanded the criteria, and liver biopsy is no longer mandatory; cholestasis alone is sufficient for diagnosis. For diagnosing bile duct hypoplasia, a bile duct to hepatic artery ratio of <0.5, is observed in at least 10 portal tracts in a liver biopsy. Moreover, ≥4 major criteria are required for the diagnosis of AGS. In the presence of a familial history of AGS, the presence of JAG1 mutation is diagnostic of AGS even if the above criteria are nonexistent. If either a genetic mutation or familial history is positive, at least one major criterion is needed to make the diagnosis. Xanthoma is a sign of hypercholesterolemia in AGS. Patients with AGS with mild hyperbilirubinemia (TB <5.8 mg/dL) have high levels of low density lipoprotein cholesterol (LDL-C) and high-density lipoprotein cholesterol. Medical intervention for pruritus typically combines choleretics, antihistamines, rifampin, and opiate antagonists such as naltrexone. Recently, apical sodium-dependent bile acid transporters (ASBT) inhibitors have been studied for pruritus treatment in AGS. Maralixibat, an ASBT inhibitor, showed promising results in reducing pruritus in children with AGS. Similarly, odevixibat, another ASBT inhibitor, improved pruritus, and reduced serum bile acids. In severe cases, surgical biliary diversion may be considered. Partial external biliary diversion (PEBD) is a frequently performed procedure in which the gallbladder is externally drained through a jejunal conduit. PEBD can help improve total serum cholesterol, pruritus severity, and xanthoma. Dietary recommendations in AGS include initiating vitamin D supplementation and providing calcium at a dosage of 50–100 mg/kg/day and phosphorus at 25–50 mg/kg/day are essential. Chronic cholestasis leads to osteopenia and fractures, particularly in the long bones. This is worsened by genetic abnormalities in JAG1 and NOTCH2, which are crucial for bone formation and regulation. Uncontrollable pruritus and frequent fractures often signal the need for LT in patients with AGS. Patients should undergo brain magnetic resonance imaging (MRI)/magnetic resonance angiography, abdominal computed tomography (CT), and echocardiography as part of the assessment for LT. Regarding living-related LT, donors with JAG1 or NOTCH2 mutations must be avoided.

Neonatal Sclerosing Cholangitis

Neonatal sclerosing cholangitis are a group of monogenic disorders characterized by abnormal strictures of the intrahepatic and/or extrahepatic biliary tree leading to NCS with acholic stools and high GGT cholestasis. Defects in three genes have been associated with development of NSC which include two genes coding for microtubule-associated proteins [doublecortin domain containing protein 2 (DCDC2), zinc finger YVE19 (ZFVE19)] and 1 associated with maintenance of tight junctions between hepatocytes (claudin 1). Infantile-onset NSCs are often indistinguishable from BA due to presence of acholic stools, high GGT, and similar liver histological findings. Percutaneous cholangiography (PCC) may be useful at times as it can show the dye passing into duodenum and into the intrahepatic biliary tree. PCC can also demonstrate irregular narrowed and strictured bile ducts. However, the dye often does not fill into the smaller ducts such as left, right, and common hepatic ducts due to extensive structuring in severe cases when it may be mistakenly be interpreted as BA. Majority of these patients would show resolution of jaundice with UDCA. The usual natural course of NSC may show a gradual resolution of jaundice, but there is progressive portal hypertension. Severe cases may require LT in the first few years of life.

NEONATAL CHOLESTASIS SYNDROME IN A WELL LOOKING INFANT WITH PIGMENTED STOOL

If the infant has NCS with pigmented stool and is well looking then follow **Flowchart 2** to work-up the patient.

Flowchart 2: Approach to a well-looking infant with pigmented stool.

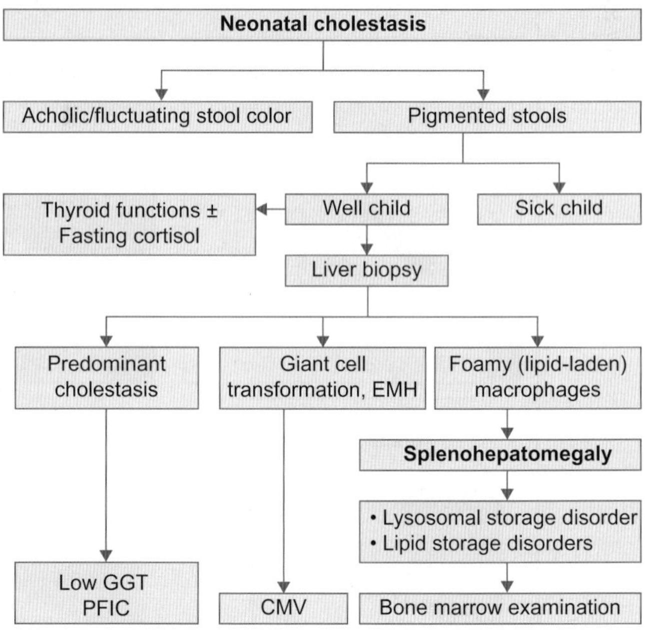

(CMV: cytomegalovirus; GGT: gamma-glutamyl transferase; PFIC: progressive familial intrahepatic cholestasis)

Genetic Intrahepatic Cholestasis

Genetic intrahepatic cholestasis, widely known as PFIC, is a group of disorders characterized by monogenic defects in secretion or transport of either bile salts or other components of bile. Bile acid synthetic defects (BASDs) are a closely related group of disorders involving monogenic defects in synthesis of bile acids leading to accumulation of abnormal, toxic bile in the hepatocytes leading to hepatocyte injury. >10 genes have been identified as sites of mutations leading to the clinical phenotype of PFIC, of which the common ones include: (1) bile salt exporter pump (BSEP), (2) multidrug resistance protein 3 (MDR3), (3) tight junction protein 2 (TJP2), and (4) familial intrahepatic cholestasis-1 (FIC1). Other less common variants of PFIC which can present with NCS include defects in ubiquitin specific peptidase 53 (USP53), farnesoid X receptors (FXR), motor head of myosin 5b (MYO5B), kinesin family member-12 (KIF12), etc. >75% children with defects in FIC1, BSEP, TJP2, and FXR present with NCS within first 3 months of life. On the other hand, children with defects in USP53, MYO5B, and MDR3 may present with transient NCS or may present for the first time in late infancy or beyond. About half of them develop pruritus usually starting around 4–6 months of life. Significant genotype-phenotype correlation has been described in children with BSEP and TJP2 deficiency where those with biallelic protein truncating mutations (PTM) have earlier onset of jaundice, progressive course, and early decompensation. Patients with biallelic missense variants usually have some residual protein activity and are thus responsive to medical therapy with UDCA. PFIC spectrum should be suspected in all children with NCS having cholestatic symptoms and elevated serum bile acids, especially in presence of low GGT cholestasis (all PFIC except MDR3 and KIF12). BASD may be clinically and biochemically indistinguishable from PFIC spectrum disorders but characteristically demonstrate low-to-normal serum bile acids in contrast to highly elevated values seen in PFIC. Liver histology may help in differentiating these from other causes of NCS, especially if immunostaining is available. However, with targeted and whole exome sequencing becoming widely available and affordable, the role of histology is rapidly shrinking. Exome sequencing is necessary for definitive diagnosis and classification as well as for prognostication. UDCA is the only definitive medical therapy which is useful in patients with residual functional protein. The newer ASBT inhibitors have been shown to improve pruritus and decrease bilirubin in patients with PFIC. Surgical biliary diversion may be considered if ASBT inhibitors are not available in the region. Supplementation with fat soluble vitamins is indicated at doses 3–10 times the recommended daily allowance (RDA). Urgent LT is indicated in those not responding to medical therapy and those progressing to end-stage liver disease with decompensation. Of note, patients with FIC1 deficiency may experience chronic diarrhea, graft steatosis, and graft failure after LT which can be ameliorated by total biliary diversion during or after LT or by using ASBT inhibitors post-LT. Patients with severe BSEP deficiency may develop antibodies to the BSEP from donor liver leading to recurrence of BSEP disease post-LT. **Flowchart 3** describes the approach to diagnosis and management of a case of suspected genetic intrahepatic cholestasis.

Congenital Infections

TORCH profile [IgM and IgG antibodies to toxoplasma, rubella, cytomegalovirus (CMV) and herpes] is another widely used test with little relevance to this clinical entity. A diagnosis of CMV hepatitis should only be made in

Flowchart 3: Approach to diagnosis and management of a suspected case of genetic intrahepatic cholestasis.

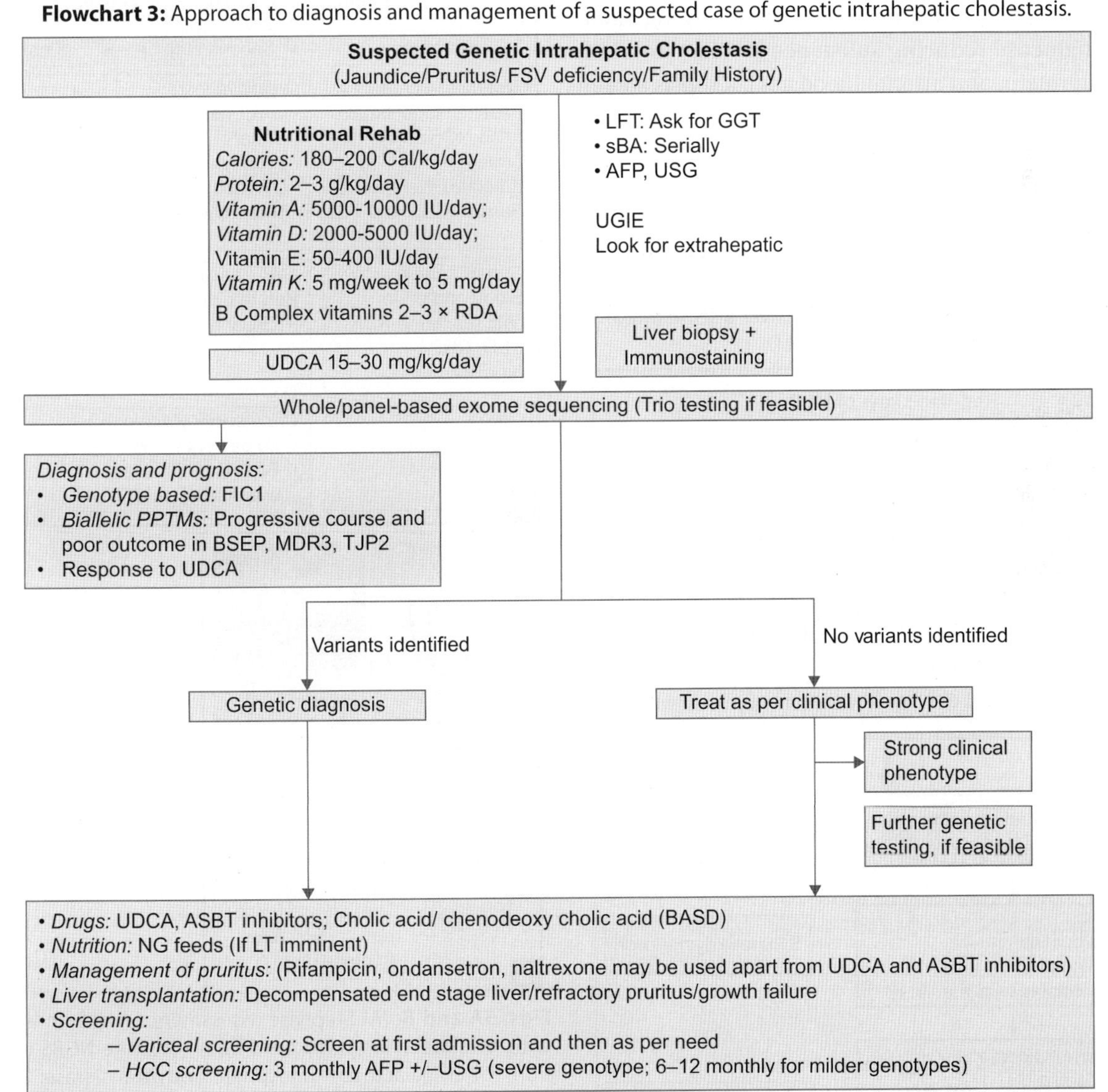

(AFP: alpha-fetoprotein; ASBT: apical sodium-dependent bile acid transporters; BASD: bile acid synthetic defects; BSEP: bile salt exporter pump; FIC1: familial intrahepatic cholestasis 1; FSV: fat soluble vitamin; GGT: gamma-glutamyl peptidase; LFT: liver function test; MDR3: multidrug resistance protein 3; PPTM: predicted protein-truncating mutation; RDA: recommended daily allowance; TJP2: tight junction protein 2; UDCA: ursodeoxycholic acid; UGIE: upper gastrointestinal endoscopy; USG: ultrasonography)

presence of relevant clinical findings and liver histology showing cytopathic changes and inclusions along with a positive CMV DNA by polymerase chain reaction (PCR).

NEONATAL CHOLESTASIS SYNDROME IN A SICK LOOKING INFANT WITH PIGMENTED STOOL

In case of the presence of red flag signs for MLD **(Flowchart 4)**, and if the child is sick with pigmented stools, then suspect MLD. MLDs are more likely if synthetic dysfunction is prominent with family history of sib death and abortions. As depicted in **Figures 5A and B**, in a sick child with NCS, a first-line metabolic screen (fasting blood sugar, nonglucose reducing substance (NGRS) in urine, alpha-fetoprotein, and arterial blood gas), a sepsis screen (urine routine and culture, leukocyte count, C-reactive protein/procalcitonin, and blood cultures), and plasma cortisol should be immediately done and further specific investigations should be guided based on these results. It is essential to do Benedict's test (to detect reducing substance in urine) as well as urine dipstick test (to detect urinary glucose) to confirm nonglucose nature of the reducing substance in urine, most likely urinary galactose or fructose. It is essential to ensure that child is on mother's feeds/other galactose containing feeds when the test is done. If suspecting galactosemia, galatose-1-PO4-uridyl transferase (GALT) assay should be immediately sent and child should be immediately shifted to galactose free diet after testing for urine NGRS awaiting the final GALT assay report. Previous blood transfusions may alter the

Flowchart 4: Red-flag signs of metabolic liver disease (MLD) and when to suspect MLD.

Red-flag signs of MLD

- Consanguinity, abortions, prev sib deaths
- Failure to thrive, diarrhea and vomitings
- Recurrence during periods of catabolic stress (FAOD)
- Seizures, early morning irritability, lethargy
- Developmental delay, hypotonia, cataract (galactosemia)
- Rickets and renal tubulopathy (Tyrosinemia, HFI)
- Synthetic dysfunction disproportionate to jaundice
- Hypoglycemia, lactic acidosis, hyperammonemia
- Aversion to sugars (HFI) or proteins (urea cycle defects)

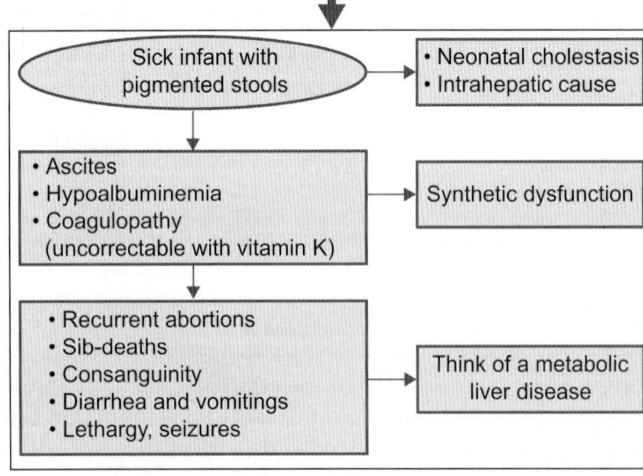

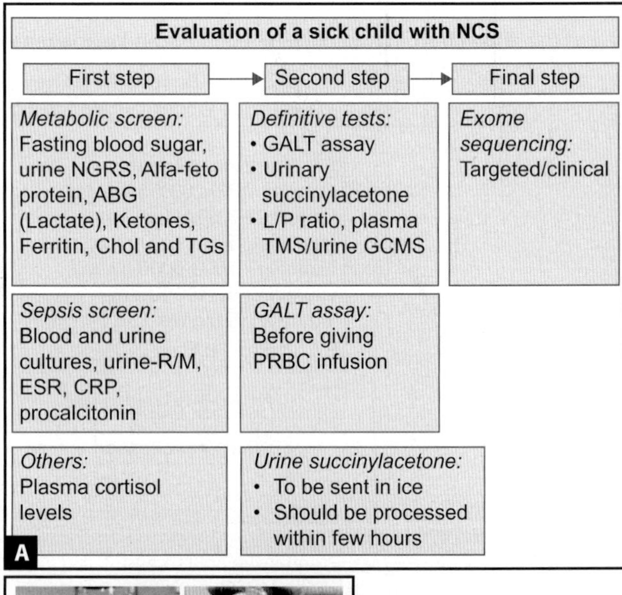

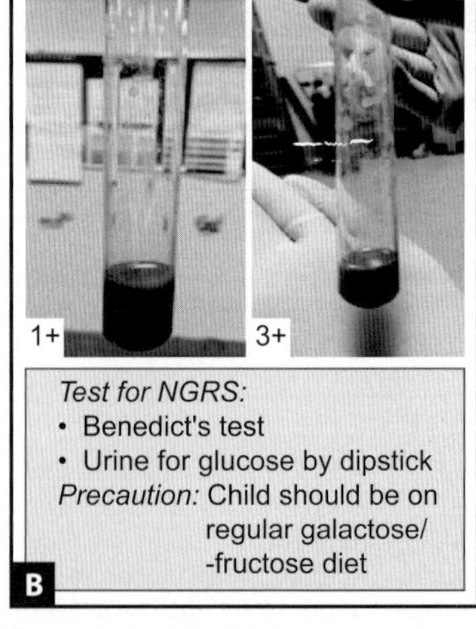

Figs. 5A and B: (A) Stepwise assessment of MLD In a sick child with neonatal cholestasis syndrome; (B) Urine NGRS interpretation. (GALT: galactose-1-phosphate uridyltransferase; GCMS: gas chromatography mass spectrophotometry; L/P: lactose/pyruvate ratio; MLD: metabolic liver disease; NGRS: nonglucose reducing substance; PRBC: packed red blood cell; TMS: tandem mass spectrophotometry)

Flowchart 5: Approach in a sick Infant with neonatal cholestasis syndrome and pigmented stool.

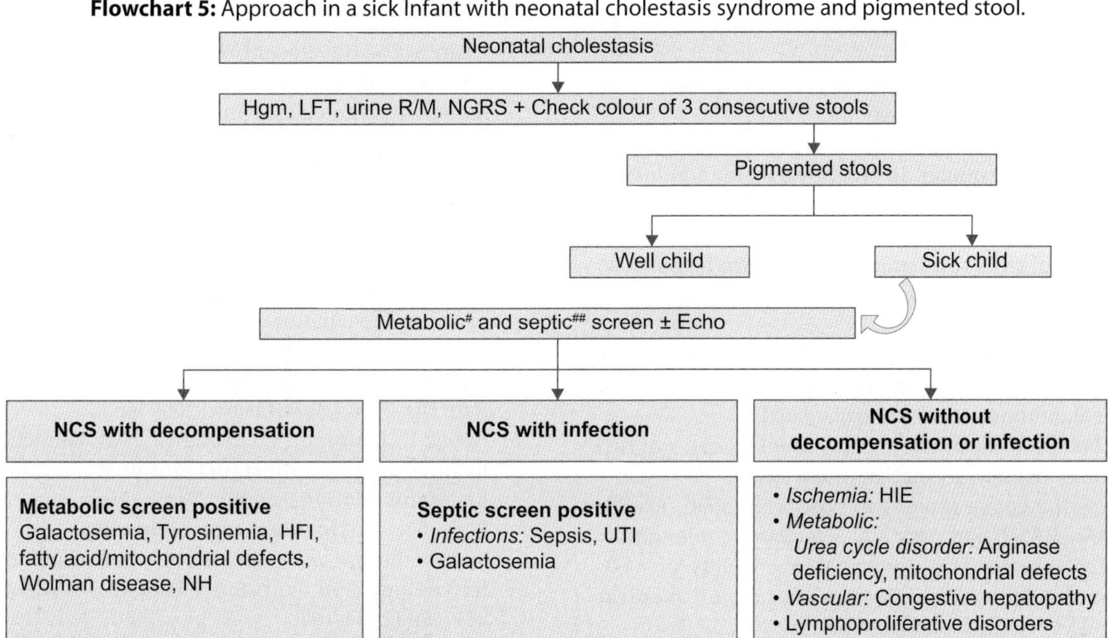

#*First line:* Fasting blood sugar, urine NGRS, NH_3, ABG (+ lactate), ketones, AFP, ferritin, cholesterol, and TGs
Second line: GALT, Urinary succinylacetone, L/P ratio, plasma/urine aminoacidogram, carnitine/acylcarnitine
##*Sepsis screen:* Blood and urine cultures, urine-R/E, ESR, CRP, procalcitonin, chest X-ray
(ABG: arterial blood gas; AFP: alpha-fetoprotein; CRP: C-reactive protein; ESR: erythrocyte sedimentation rate; GALT: galactose-1-phosphate uridylyltransferase; NGRS: nonglucose reducing sugar; TG: triglyceride)

GALT assay report and such children require confirmation by genetic sequencing. International normalized ratio (INR) should always be checked along with other liver biochemical tests as INR changes quickly with changes in liver status and increased INR is suggestive of poor liver synthetic functions. Children with INR >1.5 should receive one or two 10 mg doses of vitamin K for coagulopathy correction. As seen in **Flowchart 5**, sick infants with NCS and pigmented stools should undergo metabolic and sepsis screen to further decide the differential diagnosis. GALT assay (galactosemia) and urinary succinylacetone (tyrosinemia) decide the diagnosis of two important causes in MLD. While Hereditary fructose intolerance will show urine NGRS positive but with GALT normal and will have postprandial hypoglycemia. Both the diagnosis should be confirmed with whole exome sequencing. As can be seen in **Flowchart 5**, NCS with decompensation and without decompensation are listed out. Also NCS with pigmented stool can be an infant with sepsis. Galactosemia and hereditary fructose intolerance can be treated with early exclusion of the incriminating substance from the diet. The drug of choice for tyrosinemia is nitisinone (NTBC). If detected late these cases will need LT.

To summarize, NCS represents conjugated hyperbilirubinemia in newborn and encompasses a wide spectrum of etiologies. Classifying them based on stool color and sick status allows focused and expedited work-up. Emphasis should be on identifying treatable causes and instituting timely treatment. BA needs expedited diagnosis and early Kasai portoenterostomy. A protocol-based systematic approach to the work-up of each case helps in establishing a specific diagnosis in most with minimum but relevant investigations in stepwise approach. This is especially important in a resource limited country such as India. Our protocol has rational use of liver histopathology as a tool for diagnosis and hence accurate characterization of the disease process has been possible in most. The only exception for biopsy in our study being a sick child passing pigmented stools. We have also used cholangiopancreatography whenever biopsy was indeterminate but index of suspicion for BA was high. With the advent and widespread use of genetic diagnosis, a large number of cases previously labeled as neonatal hepatitis are now being diagnosed with genetic intrahepatic cholestasis which includes monogenic disorders leading to PFIC, BASD, AGS, and NSC.

KEY POINTS

- Neonatal cholestasis (NCS) is defined by presence of conjugated hyperbilirubinemia.
- Biliary atresia is the most common surgically correctable cause of NCS and should be urgently excluded in infants with persistent acholic stools. Early Kasai portoenterostomy significantly improves outcomes.
- Assessment of stool color using a standardized stool color chart is a simple, non-invasive tool that facilitates early detection of BA.
- Classifying NCS based on stool color and the infant's clinical condition (well vs. sick) enables a focused, stepwise, and efficient algorithmic approach to diagnosis.
- A metabolic and sepsis screening is useful in cases of NCS with pigmented stools, especially those sick.
- Genetic intrahepatic cholestasis—including PFIC, Alagille syndrome, BASD, and neonatal sclerosing cholangitis—is increasingly diagnosed with the availability of next-generation sequencing and requires tailored medical, nutritional, or surgical interventions.
- Treatable medical causes such as galactosemia, tyrosinemia, hereditary fructose intolerance, congenital hypothyroidism, and infections should be ruled out early in the evaluation.
- A protocol-based, algorithmic approach enhances diagnostic accuracy and ensures timely treatment.

SUGGESTED READING

1. Alam S, Lal BB. Recent updates on progressive familial intrahepatic cholestasis types 1, 2 and 3: Outcome and therapeutic strategies. World J Hepatol. 2022;14(1):98-118.
2. Bezerra JA. The next challenge in pediatric cholestasis: deciphering the pathogenesis of biliary atresia. J Pediatr Gastroenterol Nutr. 2006;43(Suppl 1):S23-S29.
3. Bhatia V, Bavdekar A, Matthai J, Waikar Y, Sibal A. Management of neonatal cholestasis: consensus statement of the Pediatric Gastroenterology Chapter of Indian Academy of Pediatrics. Indian Pediatr. 2014;51(3):203-210.
4. Davit-Spraul A, Gonzales E, Baussan C, Jacquemin E. Progressive familial intrahepatic cholestasis. Orphanet J Rare Dis. 2009;4:1. Published 2009 Jan 8.
5. Fawaz R, Baumann U, Ekong U, et al. Guideline for the Evaluation of Cholestatic Jaundice in Infants: Joint Recommendations of the North American Society for Pediatric Gastroenterology, Hepatology, and Nutrition and the European Society for Pediatric Gastroenterology, Hepatology, and Nutrition. J Pediatr Gastroenterol Nutr. 2017;64(1):154-168.
6. Feldman AG, Mack CL. Biliary Atresia: Clinical Lessons Learned. J Pediatr Gastroenterol Nutr. 2015;61(2):167-175.
7. Harpavat S, Aucott SW, Karpen SJ, et al. Guidance for the Primary Care Provider in Identifying Infants With Biliary Atresia by 2-4 Weeks of Life: Clinical Report. Pediatrics. Published online February 18, 2025.

Neurology

Section Editors: *Shekhar Patil, Vrajesh Udani*

Approach to Global Developmental Delay

Pratibha D Singhi, Naveen Sankhyan

DEFINITION

Global developmental delay (GDD) is an umbrella term used to describe young children with developmental delay. Conventionally, the term developmental delay is reserved for children under 5 years of age. The term mental retardation or more appropriately, "intellectual disability (ID)" is usually applied to older children (>5 years), when intelligent quotient testing is valid and reliable. GDD implies a significant delay in two or more areas of developmental performance—defined as gross fine motor, speech language, cognition, social personal, and activities of daily living. Significant delay is defined as a developmental level two standard deviations or more below the mean on age-appropriate, standardized, and norm-referenced tests. Contrary to popular use, GDD is not a diagnosis by itself and so it should be used only as a basis for reaching a diagnosis. The prevalence of ID is estimated to be around 1–3% of the population.

APPROACH TO DIAGNOSIS

A systematic approach to a child with GDD will help in the proper and optimum evaluation. The essential components of the diagnostic evaluation of a child with GDD or ID include the following:

- *History:* Including prenatal and birth history, family history, and construction of a pedigree of three generations
- *Physical examination (special emphasis on dysmorphism):* Neurologic examination, organomegaly
- *Psychometric evaluation:* To document and objectify the functional level in various domains
- *Laboratory tests:* Radiological evaluation (X-rays and neuroimaging), genetic testing, metabolic tests, etc., as indicated.

CLINICAL ASSESSMENT

History

The clinical assessment of a child with GDD/ID begins with a thorough and directed history **(Box 1)**.

A detailed history is essential to elicit antenatal and perinatal risk factors for GDD/ID. The history should be focused on maternal health during the first trimester of pregnancy including fever, drug intake or toxin exposures, and clues to intrauterine difficulties (oligohydramnios, preeclamptic toxemia, poor growth, antenatal bleeding, reduced fetal movements, etc.). The timing and mode of delivery, birthweight, APGAR scores, head circumference at birth, time to independent feeding, and duration of postnatal hospital stay are important objective markers of newborn health status. One needs to remember that a history of delayed cry, although an important clue is insufficient to conclude perinatal hypoxia, unless there is definite suggestion of neonatal encephalopathy (e.g., excessive lethargy, seizures, and feeding difficulties requiring orogastric/nasogastric feeding). Other insults like hypoglycemia, hyperbilirubinemia, meningitis and other severe infections in the neonatal period can also adversely affect brain.

BOX 1: Questions to be answered after history in a child with global developmental delay/intellectual disability.

- Is it a static or progressive disorder?
- Is there an obvious etiologic cause?
- What is the timing of the possible underlying cause?
- What is the developmental and functional level of the child?
- What are the associated comorbid medical or behavioral conditions (e.g., epilepsy and attention-deficit hyperactivity disorder)?
- In what socioeconomic and sociocultural milieu is the child being raised?

CLINICAL PEARL

- Remember that a history of delayed cry, although an important clue is insufficient to conclude perinatal hypoxia, unless there is definite suggestion of neonatal encephalopathy (e.g., excessive lethargy, seizures, and feeding difficulties requiring orogastric/nasogastric feeding).

Postnatal insults such as neuroinfections are common in the resource-poor countries and account for a large number of children with acquired GDD/ID. A detailed developmental history and past history should be elicited for the presence of seizures, hospitalizations, and other acute or chronic conditions. Peculiar to India is the severe deficiency of vitamin B_{12} that can lead to infantile tremor syndrome, and permanently affect cognitive abilities. A family history of ID can point toward a genetic cause of GDD/ID, for example fragile-X syndrome or other X-linked mental-retardation syndromes. Family history may also point toward an unrecognized metabolic disorder such as phenylketonuria. Feeding history to look at infants of vegetarian mothers who are at risk for vitamin B_{12} deficiency is important in Indian setting.

CLINICAL PEARL

- A three-generation family history should be carefully elicited in all children with developmental delay to unearth possible inherited causes.

To recognize patterns of inheritance, it is essential that a carefully elicited history is used to construct a three-generation pedigree and identify consanguinity.

Examination

A child with GDD/ID evaluation with special focus on dysmorphic features. Special attention is to be paid to the size and shape of head, facies, eyes, stature, skin, hearing, hair, and organomegaly. Any abnormalities in the head shape, sutures, and fontanels should be noted. In children with abnormal head size, head circumferences of both parents should be obtained. The head circumference has to be assessed over a period of time to understand the trajectory of head growth. When a child is noted to have an unusual appearance, a diagnosis is significantly more likely. Neurological examination is important to identify cerebral palsy, muscle tone abnormalities, weakness, paresis, ataxia, and other specific neurological signs. A good physical examination, particularly to look for organomegaly, is also essential. Such abnormalities on neurologic examination assist in determining the need for additional investigations such as electroencephalography, neuroimaging or molecular genetic testing, or referral to other specialists such as psychologists, or geneticists for further assessment.

The history and examination provide essential clues to the diagnosis, which can be later confirmed by additional studies, for example, in patients with Pradder-Willi syndrome, the history and examination may be contributory to the diagnosis and the molecular genetic analysis confirms it. Typical signs of hypothyroidism and infantile vitamin B_{12} deficiency will help pick these treatable conditions.

DEVELOPMENTAL ASSESSMENT

The clinical history should be supplemented with standardized testing of developmental level by a clinical psychologist. Standardized tools include screening tests such as the Denver's Development Screening Test, and the Ages and Stages Questionnaire, and more detailed tests such as the Gesell Development Schedules and the Bailey's Developmental Scales. When there is a concern about developmental delay in a child, a developmental quotient should be calculated for each developmental stream. It is a means to simply express a developmental delay in quantifiable terms. The "developmental quotient" is the ratio of the child's developmental age over the chronological age. Typical development is a developmental quotient >70%, and atypical development is a developmental quotient of <70%. The term GDD delay is used if a child—younger than 5–6 years of age—has a developmental quotient <70% in two or more domains.

INVESTIGATIONS

The choice and the sequence of investigations should be guided by the clinical evaluation, cost of investigations, and availability **(Flowchart 1)**. Some investigations are a part of complete evaluation (e.g., standardized vision, hearing testing, ultrasound, and skeletal X-rays) while other tests offer means to establish the diagnosis (genetic and metabolic testing).

In the absence of a universal thyroid screening in India, thyroid function tests should be done in all children with GDD/ID. Additionally, keeping in mind that large numbers of children in resource-poor countries have acquired causes for GDD/ID, it is prudent to opt for imaging studies as the initial diagnostic testing. Magnetic resonance imaging is the imaging modality of choice, given the higher resolution and better resolution to pick up dysgenesis and white-matter abnormalities.

Flowchart 1: Approach to diagnosis in a child with global developmental delay/intellectual disability.

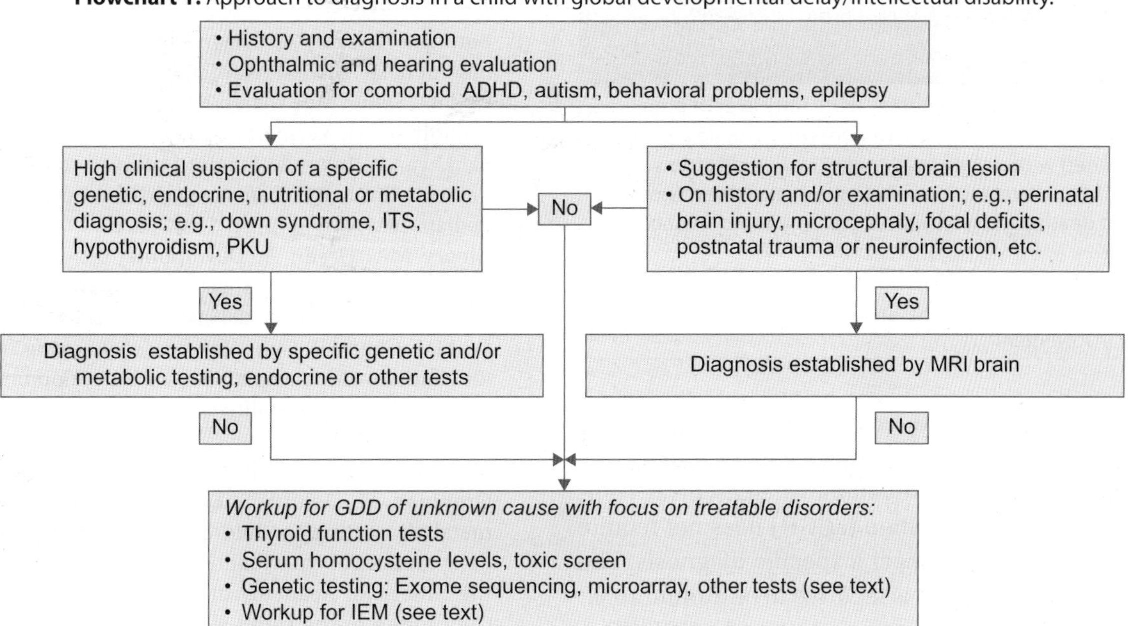

(GDD: global developmental delay; ID: intellectual disability; MRI: magnetic resonance imaging; aCGH: array comparative genomic hybridization; ITS: infantile tremor syndrome, Microarray-aCGH, PKU: phenylketouria)

Genetic Testing

It is preferable to involve experts in clinical genetics whenever possible for the genetic evaluation of GDD/ID.

Exome Sequencing

The exome sequencing platforms have developed immensely in the past decade and have become affordable too. Current data suggests that the overall yield of exome sequencing in GDD/ID is in the range of 35%. In populations with high consanguinity, the yield of this test may be even higher. It can be considered as the test with the highest yield and as the first-line test for GDD/ID. Many Exome sequencing platforms also do analysis for copy number variants and this further increases the yield of this test.

Cytogenetic Studies

Chromosome abnormalities are found in all categories of ID, mild to profound and in both sexes. The reported frequency of chromosomal anomalies detected by high-resolution karyotyping (i.e., 550 bands) in patients evaluated for ID or developmental delays is around 10%. This test is reported to be a valuable test for evaluation of GDD after a negative exome sequencing result.

Testing for *FMR1* Gene

Fragile -X is a disorder that is an important cause of GDD/ID in boys and to a lesser extent in girls. This disorder is not picked up by exome sequencing. A targeted variant analysis by PCR is used to determine the number of triple repeats and confirm the diagnosis. The yield of this test in GDD/ID is 2% in boys and 1% in girls.

Fluorescent in situ Hybridization Testing

About half of all structural chromosome abnormalities include the telomere of the chromosome. Many of these abnormalities may be missed by the standard karyotype. Fluorescent in situ hybridization (FISH) techniques have been applied to examine the subtelomeric regions of each chromosome for abnormalities that are known to cause ID. The yield is higher among familial cases as compared with sporadic cases.

Array Comparative Genomic Hybridization Techniques

It is a better technique to evaluate chromosomal abnormalities.

It identifies deletions and/or duplications of chromosome material with a high degree of sensitivity in a more

BOX 2: Indications for screening for inborn errors of metabolism in children with global developmental delay/intellectual disability.

- *Pregnancy:* A history of maternal acute fatty liver of pregnancy or hemolysis, elevated liver enzymes, and low platelets is associated with several fatty acid oxidation disorders
- *Family history:* Parental consanguinity, unexplained neonatal or infant deaths, and family history of suspected metabolic disorder
- *Others:* Unexplained hypoglycemia, recurrent encephalopathy, protein aversion, multisystem involvement, and possible white matter involvement

efficient manner than FISH techniques. Furthermore, the FISH test is used to confirm a specific clinical diagnosis suspected, after clinical evaluation, whereas, array comparative genomic hybridization (aCGH) does not require an expert clinician to suspect a specific diagnosis. The yield of this test in GDD/ID is reported to be around 15%.

The combined yield of genetic testing in GDD/ID is 50% or more.

Metabolic Testing (Box 2)

Both genetic testing and metabolic testing are expensive; hence their judicious use is warranted. It would be wise to obtain an expert consultation before proceeding with these tests. Importantly interpretation of advanced genetic testing and metabolic testing requires experience and expertise. A proper a-priory consultation with an expert is hence suggested before such testing.

KEY POINTS

- Global developmental delay means a significant delay in two or more areas of developmental performance.
- The term mental retardation or more appropriately, "ID" is usually applied to older children (>5 years). The essential components of the diagnostic evaluation include history (including prenatal and birth history), family history, physical and neurologic examinations, laboratory tests, including metabolic, and genetic testing, and imaging.

SUGGESTED READING

1. Battaglia A, Carey JC. Diagnostic evaluation of developmental delay/mental retardation: an overview. Am J Med Genet C Semin Med Genet. 2003;117C(1):3-14.
2. Chaudhary H, Verma S, Bhatia P, Vaidya PC, Singhi P, Sankhyan N. Infantile Tremor Syndrome or a Neurocutaneous Infantile B12 Deficiency (NIB) Syndrome? Indian J Pediatr. 2020;87(3):179-84.
3. Cleary MA, Green A. Developmental delay: when to suspect and how to investigate for an inborn error of metabolism. Arch Dis Child. 2005;90:1128-32.
4. Ko MH, Chen HJ. Genome-wide sequencing modalities for children with unexplained global developmental delay and intellectual disabilities-a narrative review. Children (Basel). 2023;10(3):501.
5. Michelson DJ, Shevell MI, Sherr EH, Moeschler JB, Gropman AL, Ashwal S. Evidence report: Genetic and metabolic testing on children with global developmental delay: report of the Quality Standards Subcommittee of the American Academy of Neurology and the Practice Committee of the Child Neurology Society. Neurology. 2011;77(17):1629-35.
6. Savatt JM, Myers SM. Genetic Testing in Neurodevelopmental Disorders. Front Pediatr. 2021;9:526779.
7. Schroeder S, Gerry M, Gert G, Velazquez F. Final Project Report: Usage of the term "Intellectual disability:" Language, Image and Public Education, in American Association of Intellectual Disability Resource Network International. Center on Developmental Disabilities; Center for the Study of Family, Neighborhood and Community Policy. Kansas: University of Kansas; 2001. pp. 1-216.
8. Sherr EI, Shevell MI. Global developmental delay and mental retardation/ intellectual disability. In: Swaiman KF, Ashwal S, Ferriero DM, Schor NF (Eds). Pediatric Neurology: Principles and Practice, 5th edition. Philadelphia: Saunders, Elsevier; 2012. pp. 554-74.
9. Srivastava S, Love-Nichols JA, Dies KA, Ledbetter DH, Martin CL, Chung WK, et al; NDD Exome Scoping Review Work Group. Meta-analysis and multidisciplinary consensus statement: exome sequencing is a first-tier clinical diagnostic test for individuals with neurodevelopmental disorders. Genet Med. 2019;21(11):2413-21.
10. Williams J. Global developmental delay—globally helpful? Dev Med Child Neurol. 2010;52:227.

CHAPTER 87

Approach to Psychomotor Regression in Children

Shekhar Patil, Omkar P Hajirnis

INTRODUCTION

Neurodevelopmental regression is often challenging to clinicians in terms of diagnosis and management. The purpose of this chapter is to outline a systematic approach to a child presenting with suspected neurodevelopmental regression. Reaching a specific diagnosis is of pivotal importance for providing appropriate early therapy, prognosis, and genetic counseling. Although the causes of psychomotor retardation are individually rare, the combined estimate can be as high as about 1 in 2,000 live births.

DEFINITION

Neuroregression is defined as loss of previously achieved milestones in a previously healthy child with progressive loss of speech, hearing, vision, locomotion, bulbar function, and cognitive abilities. They are often associated with seizures. It is also extended to a decrease in the normal rate of acquisition of developmental milestones, followed by a developmental plateau.

CLINICAL APPROACH

A history of loss of skills helps distinguish the neurodegenerative from static, nonprogressive conditions. The onset may be insidious but is sometimes acute and may hence cause diagnostic confusion. The regression may thereafter progress at varying speeds or also have an intermittent plateauing of milestones prior to the next period of deterioration, which may be triggered by factors like viral infections. The presentations can be varied from behavioral changes to recurrent seizures mimicking epileptic encephalopathies. It is a dictum that greater the genetic deficiency, earlier and more aggressive is the presentation. Knowing the age at which signs first appear helps enormously in narrowing the diagnosis. The diagnostic process begins with a detailed family history as inheritance patterns are disease specific and a history of consanguinity is especially important in autosomal recessive disorders **(Flowchart 1)**.

> **CLINICAL PEARL**
>
> It is important to differentiate between developmental delay and developmental regression.

The four-step approach described below provides a useful strategy for initial evaluation of patients with neurodegenerative diseases:

1. *Identify the form of inheritance:* Autosomal recessive, autosomal dominant, X-linked, and mitochondrial inheritance
2. *Age at onset of regression:* Based on this, the disorders can be divided into neonatal, infantile, late infantile, and childhood or juvenile onset
3. *Determine from the history the predominant neuro-anatomical system involved:* Gray matter, white matter, basal ganglia, cerebellar, spinal cord, etc.
4. *Review other system involvements:* Involvement of skin, liver, spleen, dysmorphic features, ophthalmic changes, presence of seizures, peripheral neuropathy, etc.

Step 1: Inheritance

A detailed family tree or a pedigree chart helps to define different modes of inheritance. The most common modality of inheritance is autosomal recessive, seen commonly in our circumstances due to high degree of consanguineous marriages. It is important to note that mitochondrial disorders can be inherited by maternally-transmitted modalities or an autosomal pattern of inheritance. This is because mitochondria contain two types of genetic material, namely mitochondrial deoxyribonucleic acid (DNA) which can only be passed on from the mother and nuclear DNA which is passed on from both parents.

Flowchart 1: Approach to psychomotor regression in children.

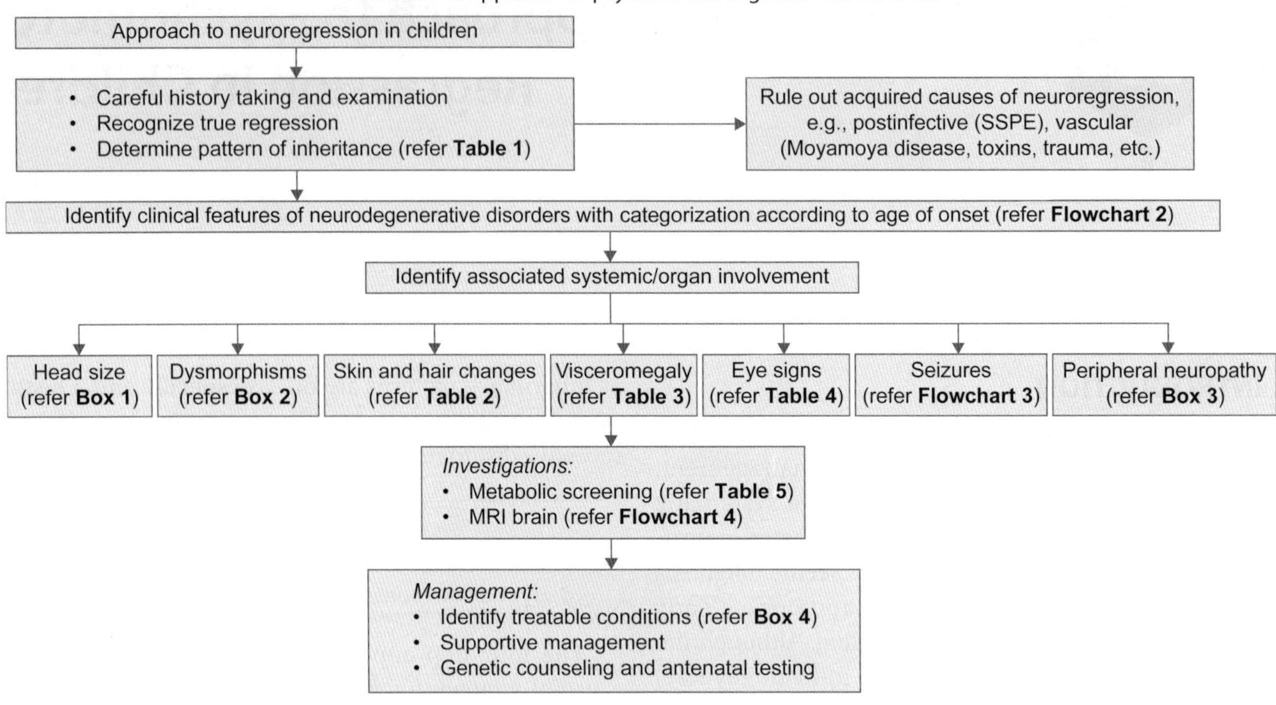

(SSPE: subacute sclerosing panencephalitis)

A few examples of neurodegenerative disorders with their modes of inheritance are listed in the **Table 1**.

Step 2: Age of Onset

The age of onset of neuroregression helps us classify the disorders. It goes without saying that the earlier the onset, the more severe and progressive is the disorder. Those who manifest late in childhood or adolescence usually have milder symptoms and the progress is slower as compared to those who manifest early and progress faster. Age of onset is divided into neonatal (0–1 month), infantile (1–12 months), late infantile (1–5 years), childhood (5–10 years), and adolescent or juvenile onset (5–15 years).

Age-related Presentations

Neonatal onset (0–1 month): Acute encephalopathy presents early in life with recurrent vomiting, poor feeding, lethargy, and dehydration. This suggests a gray matter involvement initially representing a toxic or intoxication encephalopathy. Liver involvement may be evident in few disorders presenting with jaundice, liver failure, and failure to thrive.

Infancy onset (1–12 months): Onset at this age usually presents with loss of interest in surroundings which can be either visual or in nonverbal communication. The inability to roll over, sit, use the hands in play, and vocalize suggests neurologic difficulties at this age.

Late infantile age group onset (1–5 years): The changes noted in this age group are more commonly in the speech and behavior along with motor disabilities. They may exhibit clumsiness, tremors, and gait abnormalities. They can present primarily with seizures.

Juvenile age group onset (5–15 years): In disorders of childhood and adolescence, the onset is more insidious and the progression slower than in disorders appearing earlier. Regression in this age group can present with seizures along with deterioration of school performance, lack of new learning skills, handwriting changes, poor concentration, and memory.

Step 3: Neuroanatomical Localization

The next most important feature to assess from the history and examination is the onset of symptoms and progression to the present state. The first sign or symptom of neuroregression usually but not always gives a clue to the neuroanatomical localization. For example, gait or motor regression at the onset is suggestive of white matter pathologies, whereas seizures, dementia, and cognitive decline is more suggestive of gray-matter pathologies. Those who start with chorea, dystonia, and involuntary movements

TABLE 1: Neurodegenerative disorders and their inheritance patterns.

Inheritance	*Neurodegenerative disorders*
Autosomal recessive	• Disorders involving white matter – Canavan's disease – Krabbe's disease – Metachromatic leukodystrophy • Disorders involving gray matter – Progressive myoclonic epilepsies (Lafora body disease, etc.) – Progressive infantile poliodystrophy – Sialidosis type 1 – Neuronal ceroid lipofuscinosis (variable) • Disorders involving predominantly basal ganglia – Wilson's disease – Pantothenate kinase-associated neurodegeneration • Spinocerebellar degeneration/spinal cord and peripheral nerve conditions – Friedreich's ataxia – Spinal muscular atrophy – Infantile neuroaxonal dystrophy – Refsum's disease
Autosomal dominant	• Juvenile Huntington's disease • Dystonia musculorum deformans • Spinocerebellar ataxia • Familial spastic paraplegia • Charcot-Marie-Tooth disease
X-linked recessive	• Pelizaeus-Merzbacher disease • Adrenoleukodystrophy • Menke's kinky hair syndrome
Mitochondrial	• Alpers–Huttenlocher syndrome • Leigh's syndrome • Kearns-Sayre syndrome • Myoclonic epilepsy with ragged red fibers • Leber's hereditary optic neuropathy • Mitochondrial encephalomyopathy with lactic acidosis and stroke like episodes

suggest that the primary area of involvement is the basal ganglia. Over a period of time, symptoms evolve to involve multiple neuroanatomical sites; e.g., Krabbe's disease starts with increase in tone or loss of motor milestones suggestive of white matter pathology. There may also have some dystonia, indicative of basal ganglia involvement and over time, the child will become loose with absent reflexes suggestive of additional peripheral neuronal involvement.

Hence by careful history taking and detailed general and nervous system examination, it is easier to determine which pathways are involved and the range of diagnostic possibilities is more easily circumscribed **(Flowchart 2)**.

CLINICAL PEARL

- The first sign of neuroregression usually correlates best with neuroanatomical localization.

Step 4: Identifying Associated System/ Organ Involvement

Multiple systems get involved with different degenerative disorders. The physician needs to carefully screen other associated systemic involvements beginning with a detailed head-to-toe general examination. The examination should begin with height, weight, and head-circumference measurements. Many disorders eventually lead to acquired microcephaly due to brain atrophy; others are noted for megalencephaly. Dysmorphisms may be evident at birth or may be noted later as the disorder manifests **(Boxes 1 and 2)**.

A careful observation of the skin and hair and a full assessment of the chest, abdomen, and extremities are part of the examination **(Tables 2 and 3)**.

A detailed ophthalmologic examination with fundoscopy is pivotal and the various disorders associated with eye abnormalities are listed in **Table 4**.

Seizures may be a presenting complaint or may present as the disease progresses. The age of onset and also the seizure type provides useful information to arrive at the diagnosis **(Flowchart 3)**. The peripheral nervous system may be involved in certain neurodegenerative disorders giving rise to diminution or absence of deep-tendon reflexes and sensation **(Box 3)**.

Thus, all the features and clues mentioned above along with a careful history and examination help to arrive at a diagnosis. Each associated system needs to be examined in detail to be able to put all the pieces of the puzzle together.

INVESTIGATIONS

The investigations should cater to the common causes seen in each age group and proceed from common to rarer causes. All disorders that are potentially treatable or have genetic implications should be screened in all cases. For example, thyroid function tests should be done as hypothyroidism can present with no obvious signs in infancy. Although below mentioned is an exhaustive list of investigations, the physician should prioritize from specific clues in the history and physical examination. The basic metabolic screen which includes blood, urine, and sometimes the cerebrospinal fluid examination should

Flowchart 2: Clinical features of neurodegenerative disorders with categorization according to age of onset.

Neurodegenerative disorders

Detailed history and neurological examination

Neuroanatomical classification Signs/symptoms	**White matter** (+/–peripheral neuropathy) • Spasticity • Gait disturbances	**Gray matter** • Dementia • Seizures • Visual impairment • Speech impairment • Behavior/psychiatric disturbances	**Basal ganglia** • Involuntary movements (chorea, athetosis, tremors, etc.) • Dyskinesias • Dystonia • Bradykinesia	**Cerebellum** • Ataxia • Nystagmus • Tremor • Hypotonia
Age of onset	**Leukodystrophies**	**Poliodystrophies**	**Corencephalopathies**	**Spinocerebellopathies**
Infantile 1–2 months	• Krabbe's disease • PMD and PMD-like disorders • Canavan's disease • VWM disease • MLC • Aicardi Goutieres syndrome • CDG • MLD	• Urea cycle defects • MSUD • Aminoacidopathies • Organic acidurias • FAO defects • Galactosemia • MCAD deficiency • Menkes disease • Infantile NCL	• Biotin responsive basal ganglia disease • Lesch Nyhan syndrome • Cockayne's syndrome • Pyruvate dehydrogenase deficiency • Mitochondrial disorders • Fahr's disease	• Pontocerebellar hypoplasias • Pyruvate dehydrogenase deficiency • Cockayne's syndrome • Infantile NCL • CDG
Late infantile 1–5 years	• MLD • Alexander's disease • Mitochondrial disorders • VWM disease • Late infantile NCL • H-ABC	• Lysosomal storage disorders, e.g., Tay Sach's disease Niemann-Pick disease type A, sialidosis • Mitochondrial disorders, e.g., Alper's poliodystrophy	• Lesch Nyhan syndrome • Mitochondrial disorders • Methylmalonic aciduria • Propionic aciduria • PKAN • Wilson's disease • CSF neurotransmitter disorders • H-ABC	• Late infantile NCL • H-ABC • VWM disease • H-ABC • Ataxia telangiectasia *Spinal cord:* • Infantile onset SCA • INAD
Juvenile 5–15 years	• X-linked ALD • MLD • VWM disease • MLC • Alexander's disease • LBSL	• Lysosomal storage disorders • NCL's • Niemann-Pick disease • Gaucher's Type III	• Wilson's disease • PKAN • Huntington's (Westphal variant) • DRPLA Neuroacanthosis • Juvenile Parkinson's disease	• Ataxia telangiectasia • Friedrich's ataxia • Refsum's disease • Spinocerebellar ataxia • Late onset gangliosidosis *Spinal cord and peripheral nerve:* • HMSN • HSP's

(ALD: adrenoleukodystrophy; CDG: congenital defects of glycosylation; DRPLA: dentatorubral-pallidoluysian atrophy; FAO: fatty acid oxidation; H-ABC: hypomyelination with atrophy of the basal ganglia and cerebellum; HMSN: hereditary motor sensory neuropathy; HSP: hereditary spastic paraplegia; INAD: infantile neuroaxonal dystrophy; LBSL: leukoencephalopathy with brainstem and spinal cord involvement and lactate elevation; MCAD: medium chain acyl-coa dehydrogenase; MLC: megalencephalic leukoencephalopathy with subcortical cysts; MLD: metachromatic leukodystrophy; MSUD: maple syrup urine disease; NCL: neuronal ceroid lipofuscinosis; PKAN: pantothenate kinase-associated neurodegeneration; PMD: Pelizaeus-Merzbacher disease; SCA: spinocerebellar ataxia; VWM: vanishing white matter disease)

BOX 1: Neurodegenerative disorders with megalencephaly.

- Alexander disease
- Tay-Sachs disease
- Canavan's disease
- Sandhoff's disease
- Glutaric aciduria type 1

BOX 2: Neurodegenerative disorders with dysmorphic features.

- Zellweger's syndrome
- Inclusion-cell disease
- Smith-Lemli-Opitz syndrome
- 18 q syndrome
- Pyruvate dehydrogenase deficiency
- Mucopolysaccharidoses
- Oligosaccharidoses
- Mucolipidosis
- Prader–Willi syndrome
- Cockayne's syndrome
- GM1 gangliosidosis

TABLE 2: Hair and skin changes in neurodegenerative disorders.

Hair changes	***Skin changes***

• Menkes syndrome (kinky, colorless or steel-colored and easily broken—Pili torti)
• Biotinidase deficiency (alopecia and fine, brittle hair)
• Homocystinuria (thin and fair hair)
• Cockayne's syndrome (fine, thin, and dry hair)
• Mucopolysaccharidosis (alopecia areata and pale-colored hair)
• Argininosuccinic acidurias (sparse brittle hair)
• Ataxia telangiectasia (progeroid changes like premature graying of hair)
• Multiple sulfatase deficiency (hypertrichosis)
	• Phakomatosis
	  – Neurofibromatosis
	  – Tuberous sclerosis
	  – Sturge-Weber syndrome
	• Angelman's syndrome
	• Hypomelanosis of Ito
	• Incontinentia pigmenti
	• Homocystinuria (pale, pink skin, malar rash, livedo reticularis)
	• Ataxia telangiectasia (vitiligo, warts, granulomas)
	• Cockayne's syndrome (photosensitivity)
	• Multiple sulfatase deficiency (ichthyosis)

TABLE 3: Visceromegaly associated with neurodegenerative disorders.

Hepatosplenomegaly
• Lipid storage disorders
  – Gangliosidosis
  – Mucolipidosis
  – Farber disease
• Mucopolysaccharidosis
  – Hurler's syndrome
  – Hunter's syndrome
• Glycogen storage disorders (GSD)
  – GSD type IV
	Hepatomegaly
	• GSD type I
	• GSD type II, VI, IX
	• Wolman's disease
	• Zellweger's syndrome
	• Hunter's syndrome
	• Glycogenosis type II

Splenohepatomegaly • Gaucher's disease • Niemann-Pick disease	*Splenomegaly* • Alpha mannosidosis • Hurler's syndrome and other mucopolysaccharidosis • Tangier disease • Sandhoff's disease

TABLE 4: Eye abnormalities associated with neurodegenerative disorders.

Eye abnormalities	
Cornea • Wilson's disease • Hurler's disease • Maroteaux-Lamy syndrome • Morquio's disease • Mucolipidosis type IV • Mannosidosis • Fucosidosis • Aspartylglucosaminuria	*Pigmentary retinopathy* • Fetal cytomegalovirus infection • Fetal toxoplasmosis • Hallervorden-Spatz disease • Kearns–Sayre syndrome • Neuronal ceroid lipofuscinosis • Zellweger's syndrome • Cockayne's syndrome • Congenital disorder of glycosylation • Abetalipoproteinemia
Conjunctiva • Ataxia telangiectasia	*Cherry-red macula* • GM1 gangliosidosis • Niemann-Pick disease, types A and B • Tay-Sachs disease • Sialidosis type I
Lens • Homocystinuria • Myotonic dystrophy • Galactosemia • Lowe syndrome • Fabry's disease • Cerebrotendinous xanthomatosis	*Optic atrophy* • Adrenoleukodystrophy • Metachromatic leukodystrophy • Globoid cell leukodystrophy • Pelizaeus-Merzbacher disease • Mitochondrial–MELAS, LHON • Canavan disease • Sulfite oxidase deficiency • 3-methylglutaconicaciduria III
Cortical blindness • MELAS syndrome	*Abnormal eye movements* • Opsoclonus myoclonus syndrome (with progressive ophthalmoplegia) • AD spinocerebellar ataxias • Ataxia telangiectasia • Gaucher's disease, types 2 and 3 • Kearns–Sayre syndrome • Niemann-Pick disease type C • Pelizaeus-Merzbacher disease

(AD: autosomal dominant; LHON: Leber's hereditary optic neuropathy; MELAS: mitochondrial encephalomyopathy, lactic acidosis, and stroke-like episodes)

be done initially along with neuroimaging [magnetic resonance imaging (MRI) brain] for suspected metabolic disorders. More advanced tests should be prioritized according to the condition suspected. Now genetic diagnosis is the gold standard of diagnosis and wherever possible should be attempted as it is useful not only for diagnosis but also for future genetic counseling **(Table 5)**.

The workup involves neuroimaging in most cases. Magnetic resonance imaging with or without contrast is preferred over computed tomography. It is useful for visualizing cerebral malformations and for documenting the degree of cerebral atrophy or white matter changes, such as those that occur in various leukodystrophies. Magnetic resonance imaging with contrast is ordered in suspected adrenoleukodystrophy, Alexander's disease, etc. Specific spectroscopy is useful in mitochondrial disorders, Canavan's disease, and creatine deficiency. Increased N-acetylaspartate peak is detected in Canavan's disease,

Flowchart 3: Epilepsies associated with neurodegenerative disorders.

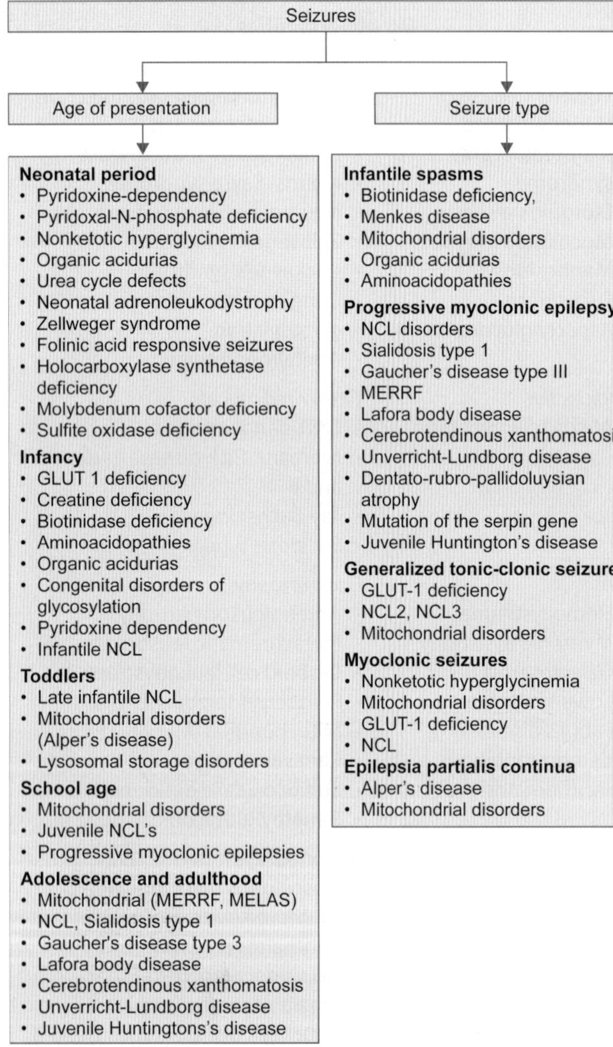

(GLUT: glucose transporters; MELAS: mitochondrial encephalomyopathy lactic acidosis and stroke-like episodes; MERRF: myoclonic epilepsy with ragged red fibers; NCL: neuronal ceroid lipofuscinosis)

and in mitochondrial disorders a high lactate peak may be found. Magnetic resonance imaging with angiography is done in suspected Menke's disease to demonstrate tortuous vessels.

Thus, the MRI is an important ancillary test in approaching neuroregression and helps the clinician to delineate disorders based on the findings on it **(Flowchart 4)**.

CLINICAL PEARL

- Carefully planned investigations are needed rather than ordering a battery of tests.

BOX 3: Peripheral neuropathies associated with neurodegenerative disorders.

Episodic neuropathy
- Acute intermittent porphyrias
- Tyrosinemia type I

Progressive neuropathy
- Metachromatic leukodystrophy
- Refsum's disease
- Mitochondrial neuropathy/myopathy (Leigh's syndrome, neuropathy ataxia and retinitis pigmentosa syndrome, etc.)
- Abetalipoproteinemia
- Pyruvate dehydrogenase deficiency
- Friedreich's ataxia
- Juvenile GM2 gangliosidosis
- Krabbe's disease (late infantile form)
- Adrenomyeloneuropathy
- Cockayne's syndrome
- Methylenetetrahydrofolate reductase deficiency
- Carbohydrate deficient glycoprotein syndrome
- 3-hydroxy dicarboxylic aciduria
- Familial dysautonomia

MANAGEMENT

The specific cause of regression in childhood can be difficult to elucidate and a large number of children remain undiagnosed. It is essential to maintain the child's quality of life and help in supportive care. Careful attention to nutrition helps in maintaining general well-being. Symptomatic treatment of disturbed sleep, behavior and mood disturbances should be done. A small number of disorders have specific treatment and maximum effort should be made to diagnose these conditions. They can be enumerated as in the **Box 4**.

Bone marrow transplantation has been tried in various disorders and has shown promise when it has been done at a stage where irreparable brain damage has not occurred. This includes lysosomal storage disorders, metachromatic leukodystrophy, Gaucher's disease, mucopolysaccharidosis, and adrenoleukodystrophy.

Every effort should be made to prevent the family from having another affected child with the help of antenatal screening.

ANTENATAL TESTING AND COUNSELING

Having an accurate genetic diagnosis helps immensely for genetic counseling and antenatal testing. A clear explanation of the inheritance pattern will clear up misunderstandings in the family about who is "at fault".

TABLE 5: Investigations for suspected metabolic/neurodegenerative disorders.

Test/Study	***Abnormalities of interest***
Urine	
• Collect each fresh sample separately in clean container and store at 4°C (short term) • Freeze at –20°C for long-term storage. Compare samples collected before and after treatment	• Smell (special odor), look (special color) • Acetone • Reducing substances • Ketoacids (DNPH) • pH • Electrolytes • Sulfite oxidase • Uric acid • Aminoacids • Organic acids (quantitative) • 24-h urine copper excretion • MPS screening and electrophoresis
Blood	
• 5 mL plasma (heparinized or plain tube) • 5–10 mL whole blood in EDTA (for molecular DNA studies) • Blood on filter paper (Guthrie's test)	• Complete blood count • Electrolytes (for anion gap, glucose, calcium) • Blood gas (pH, pCO_2, HCO_3^-, pO_2) • Uric acid • Prothrombin time • Liver function tests • Thyroid function tests • Plasma ammonia (on ice) • Lactic acid (on ice; stat processing) • Pyruvic acid (requires specialized deproteinization tube) • Serum ketones • Serum homocysteine • Serum vitamin B_{12} levels • Serum copper and ceruloplasmin • Free fatty acids • Plasma amino acids • Plasma organic acids • Acylcarnitine profile
Advanced workup	• Very long-chain fatty acids • Immunoglobulin levels • Autoantibodies • White cell enzyme studies to look for vacuolation of lymphocytes • Isoelectric focusing of transferrin
Cerebrospinal fluid	
Neurotransmitters are collected in specific tubes and transported in dry ice; collect minimum 2 mL stat (on ice) for chemistries and lactate	• Opening and closing pressures • Cell count, protein, glucose with simultaneous blood glucose (For suspected GLUT1 deficiency—4 h minimum fasting needed) • Lactate • Pyruvate • Neurotransmitters

Contd...

Contd...

Test/Study	***Abnormalities of interest***
Genetic analysis	DNA analysis of specific suspected disorders
Bone marrow examination	For foam cells, sea blue histocytes, etc.
Skin biopsy	• Enzyme analysis in cultured fibroblasts (lysosomal disorders) • Staining for lipids, glycogen, cholesterol, fatty acids • NP-C (cholesterol esterification, filipin staining) • DNA analysis • Electron microscopy for storage inclusions (lysosomal, mitochondrial NCL)
Muscle biopsy	Light and electron microscopy, immunohistochemistry, trichrome for ragged red fibers, lipid storage, etc.
Liver biopsy	Staining for accumulation of lipids, glycogen, cholesterol, fatty acids, immunohistochemistry
EMG/SSEP	• Lower motor neuron disease patterns • Neuropathies • Myopathies
EEG	Associated seizures (clinical and sub-clinical) and their pattern
ERG	In suspected retinitis pigmentosa
BERA	In suspected hearing loss
USG abdomen	Organomegaly, nephrocalcinosis, renal cysts
2D echocardiography	Cardiomyopathy in storage disorders, rhabdomyosarcomas in tuberous sclerosis
X-ray screening	For dysostosis multiplex in MPS, assessment of bone age

(BERA: brainstem evoked response audiometry; DNPH: 2 4-dinitrophenylhydrazine; EEG: electroencephalogram; EMG/SSEP: electromyography/somatosensory evoked potentials; ERG: electroretinography; GLUT: glucose transporter; MPS: mucopolysaccharidosis; NCL: neuronal ceroid lipofuscinosis; NP-C: Niemann-Pick type C disease; NTBC: nitisinone)

Once a genetic diagnosis is made, this should be used to screen other family members. This is especially important for younger, as yet asymptomatic, siblings who might benefit greatly from specific therapies if these are instituted prior to the development of symptoms or in the early symptomatic period.

Flowchart 4: Approach to neuroregression according to major neuroimaging pattern.

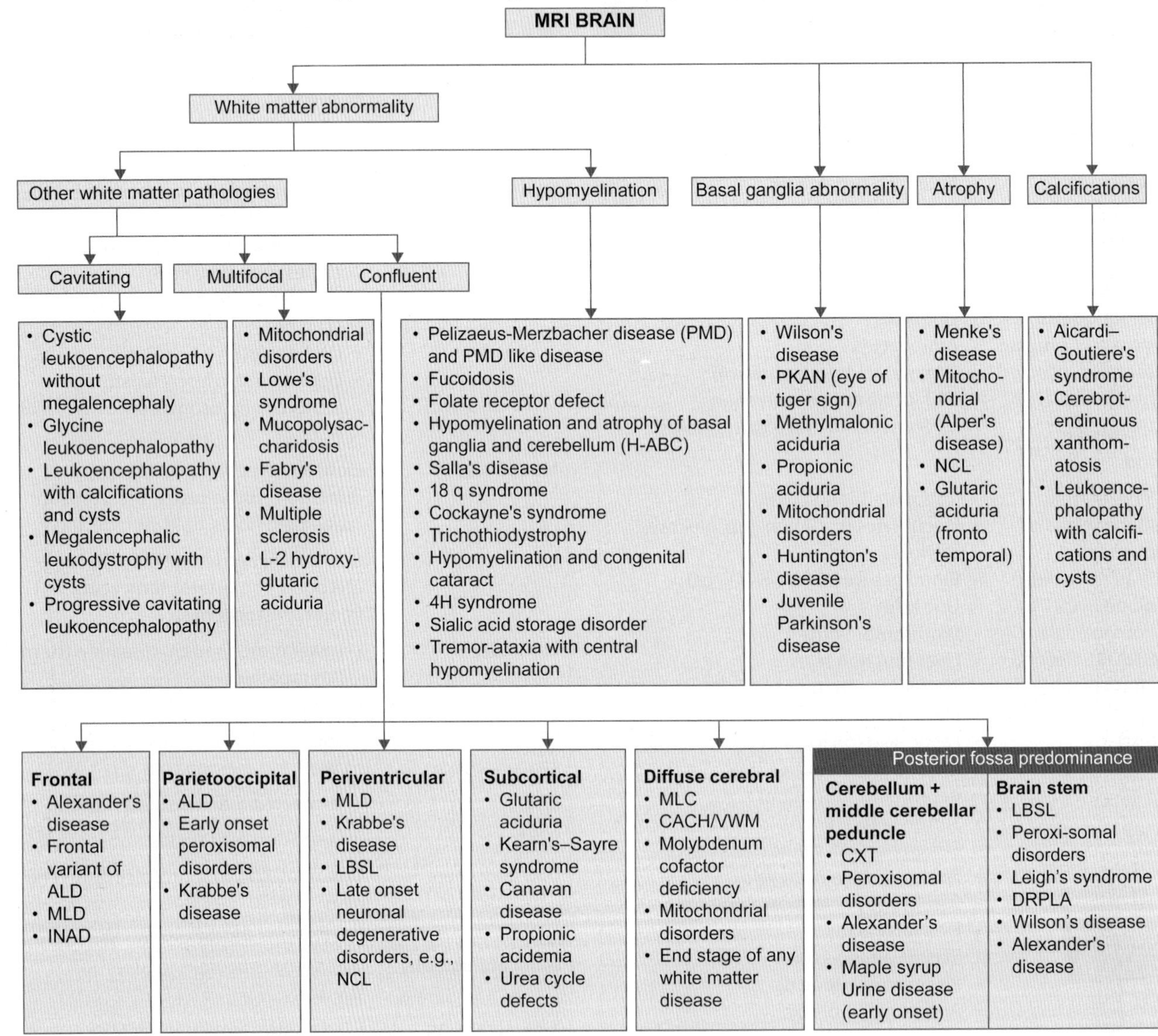

(ALD: adrenoleukodystrophy; CACH/VWM: childhood ataxia with central hypomyelination/vanishing white matter; CXT: cerebrotendinous xanthomatosis; INAD: infantile neuroaxonal dystrophy; LBSL: leukoencephalopathy with brainstem and spinal cord involvement and lactate elevation; MLC: megalencephalic leukoencephalopathy with cysts; MLD: metachromatic leukodystrophy; NCL: neuronal ceroid lipofuscinosis; PKAN: pantothenate kinase-associated neurodegeneration)

BOX 4: Treatable neurodegenerative/metabolic conditions.

- Wilson's disease—D-Penicillamine and other chelating agents
- Aminoacidopathies—specific diets. Nitisinone in tyrosinemia
- Pyridoxine and pyridoxal phosphate dependent seizures—pyridoxine
- Biotinidase deficiency and biotin responsive basal ganglia disease—biotin
- Glucose transporter-1 deficiency—ketogenic diet
- Folinic acid responsive seizures—folinic acid
- Creatine deficiency syndromes—creatine
- Serine biosynthesis disorders—L-serine and glycine
- Neurotransmitter disorders—dopamine in some cases
- Inborn errors of folic acid and cobalamin synthesis—folic acid and vitamin B_{12}
- Homocysteinemia, methylenetetrahydrofolate reductase—B_{12}, folic acid, pyridoxine
- Gaucher's disease, Fabry's disease, mucopolysaccharidosis, Pompe's disease—enzyme replacement

CLINICAL PEARL

- Every effort should be taken to diagnose treatable causes of psychomotor regression.

The following is an algorithmic flowchart to aid the physician in approaching a child with psychomotor regression. However, significant overlaps exist and also disorders with atypical presentations can confuse the physician. A systematic clinical approach with a sound theoretical knowledge helps in reducing the investigative burden on the patient.

KEY POINTS

- Never ignore a parent's concerns. A history of loss of milestones helps distinguish neuroregression from developmental delay.
- A detailed pedigree chart helps to identify different modes of inheritance. The most common modality in neurodegenerative conditions is autosomal recessive type.
- The dictum is earlier the onset, more severe and aggressive is the disorder due to greater genetic deficiency. The regression may progress at varying speeds and some may evolve with time.
- The presenting symptom is usually but not always a pivotal clue to the neuroanatomical localization. Magnetic resonance imaging with or without contrast is preferred over computed tomography as the neuroimaging of choice and is an important ancillary test in approaching neuroregression.
- The disorders that have specific treatment should always be looked out and diagnosed promptly.
- Although most disorders do not have specific treatment, maximum effort should be made to reach a genetic diagnosis for genetic counseling and antenatal testing later. Every effort should be made to prevent the family from having another affected child.

SUGGESTED READING

1. Barkovich AJ. An approach to MRI of metabolic disorders in children. Journal of Neuroradiology. 2007;34:75-88.
2. Cognitive and motor regression. In: Swaiman KF, Ashwal S, Ferriero DM, Schor NF (Eds). Swaiman's Pediatric Neurology: Principles and Practice, 5th edition. Elsevier Saunders; 2012. pp. 575-603.
3. Metabolic and heredodegenerative disorders of central nervous system. In: Aicardi J (Ed). Diseases of the Nervous System in Childhood, 3rd edition. Mac Keith Press; 2009. pp. 243-371.
4. Metabolic disorders and leukodystrophies. In: Sims KB, Peters JM, Musolini PL, Elibol MZ (Eds). Handbook of Pediatric Neurology. Lippincotts Williams and Wilkins; 2014. pp. 155-91 and 206-20.
5. Neurology—degenerative brain disorders. In: Forfar & Arneil's Textbook of Pediatrics, 7th edition. Churchill Livingstone; 2008. pp. 898-903.
6. Psychomotor retardation and regression In: Fenichel's Clinical Pediatric Neurology: A Signs and Symptoms Approach, 6th ed. Elsevier Saunders; 2009. pp. 119-52.
7. Schiffmann R, van der Knaap MS. An MRI-based approach to the diagnosis of white matter disorder. Neurology. 2009; 72(8):750-9.

Approach to a Child with First Seizure

Anju Aggarwal, Shekhar Patil

INTRODUCTION

In 2005, a Task Force of the International League Against Epilepsy (ILAE) formulated conceptual definition of a "seizure" where an epileptic seizure is defined as a transient occurrence of signs and/or symptoms due to abnormal excessive or synchronous neuronal activity in the brain.

Epilepsy was defined as a disorder of the brain characterized by an enduring predisposition to generate epileptic seizures. This definition is usually practically applied as having two unprovoked seizures more than 24-hour apart. A seizure that is provoked by a transient factor acting on an otherwise normal brain to temporarily lower the seizure threshold, does not count toward a diagnosis of epilepsy. However, conceptually, epilepsy also exists after at least one unprovoked seizure, when there is high risk for another, although the actual required risk is debatable.

The term "provoked seizure" is considered being synonymous with a "reactive seizure" or an "acute symptomatic seizure".

NEWER DEFINITIONS

In the need to address circumstances with high risk for future seizures after a first unprovoked seizure, the ILAE commissioned a Task Force in December 2013 to formulate an operational definition of epilepsy for the purposes of clinical diagnosis **(Box 1)**.

STATISTICS

About 2–5% of children experience a seizure one time or the other in their lifetime. This includes both febrile and afebrile seizures. After a single unprovoked seizure, risk for another is 40–52%. With two unprovoked nonfebrile seizures, the chance by 4 years of having another is 73%, with a 95% confidence interval (CI) of 59–87%, subsequently herein portrayed as approximately 60–90%.

BOX 1: Operational (practical) clinical definition of epilepsy.

Epilepsy is a disease of the brain defined by any of the following conditions:

- At least two unprovoked (or reflex) seizures occurring >24 hours apart
- One unprovoked (or reflex) seizure and a probability of further seizures similar to the general recurrence risk (at least 60%) after two unprovoked seizures, occurring over the next 10 years
- Diagnosis of an epilepsy syndrome
- Epilepsy is considered to be resolved for individuals who had an age-dependent epilepsy syndrome but are now past the applicable age or those who have remained seizure-free for the last 10 years, with no seizure medicines for the last 5 years

Risks of Recurrence after First Status Epilepticus

- The recurrence risk after a prolonged event or status epilepticus is the same as that of a brief seizure.
- However, if they do recur, they have a higher chance of getting a repeat status epilepticus.

CLINICAL PEARLS

- If an event is ambiguous, it is better to wait for a recurrence for clarification.
- Misdiagnosis of an "epileptic" seizure may be more stigmatizing than a delayed diagnosis of epilepsy.

High-risk Factors Associated with Recurrence after First Unprovoked Seizure

- Pre-existing static brain abnormalities
- Focal neurological deficits
- Focal seizure semiology (including Todd's paresis)
- Focal/generalized epileptiform activity on electroencephalogram (EEG)
- Tumors or other progressive lesions
- Status epilepticus
- Family history of epilepsy
- Previous febrile seizures.

Factors Known to Provocate Seizures and Epilepsy

Factors known to provocate seizures and epilepsy are given in **Table 1**.

Clinical Evaluation after a First Seizure in a Child

Whenever a child comes with first episode of seizure, what we need to know is:

- Is it a seizure or other events which mimic seizures?
- What is the type of seizure?
- What is the possible etiology?
- What investigations are required?
- Does he or she require therapy?
- Prognosis in terms of recurrence of seizure or remission of epilepsy.

HISTORY

A good clinical history is what is going to help us decide the type of seizure and distinguish it from nonepileptic events. Best is to elicit history from the caretaker or parent who has witnessed the seizure. If not possible, history should be elicited again after the initial control of seizure activity.

Questions that need to be addressed are:

- What was the child doing when he had a seizure?
- What happened in intricate detail?
- Did the eyes turn to one side?
- Did the child become stiff?
- Did the child have clonic movements or jerks or just brief flickering of eyes?
- How long the seizure did last?
- Was the child unconscious after that and for how long?
- Did the child experience any weakness of any limb after the seizure?
- Did the child pass urine and stool during the episode?
- Did the child suffer any injury during the seizure?

TABLE 1: Factors provoking seizures and epilepsy.

Acute symptomatic seizures	*Susceptible to epilepsy*
• Fever • Head injury • Hypoglycemia • Electrolyte disturbance • Brain infections • Stroke • Hemorrhage • Drugs • Minor risk of epilepsy (3–10%)	• Sleep deprived • Severe psychological stress • Extremes of emotion • Fatigue • Infections • Family history • Higher risk of epilepsy (50–70%)

History should include a detailed antenatal history of mother, birth history, and developmental history to find out any associated risk factors or etiology of seizures.

EXAMINATION

In addition to the vitals including a blood pressure reading and general physical examination, one should look for neurocutaneous markers, microcephaly, dysmorphic features, and signs of raised intracranial pressure. Detailed neurological examination is required to detect neurological deficit, altered sensorium and meningeal signs should be looked for.

> **CLINICAL PEARL**
>
> Determination of type of seizure and distinction from non-epileptic events is best done by clinical history (preferably from the person who has witnessed the seizure).

DIFFERENTIAL DIAGNOSIS

The differential diagnosis of seizures can range from a variety of clinical presentations. Understanding the occurrence and nature of minor events is crucial to make an accurate diagnosis. These are principally:

- Loss of awareness
- Generalized convulsive movements
- Drop attacks
- Transient focal motor attacks
- Transient focal sensory attacks
- Facial muscle and eye movements
- Psychic experiences
- Aggressive or vocal outbursts
- Episodic phenomena in sleep
- Prolonged confusional or fugue states.

Some of the common differential diagnoses are described below:

Syncope with Secondary Jerking Movements

People who faint often have small, brief myoclonic twitches of the extremities which can be prominent with prolonged cerebral hypoperfusion.

Nonepileptic Attack Disorder

Nonepileptic attack disorder (NEAD), previously known as pseudoseizures typically gives rise to episodes of two broad types:

1. Attacks involving motor phenomena
2. Attacks of lying motionless.

A child with NEAD will have a seizure-like-episode only during the awake state, may remember the sequence of events well, will not have any injury during seizure, may have family history of seizure and may not have seizure-like-movements of any particular seizure type. They may talk during the seizure like activity, usually will not have cyanosis or incontinence. They usually do not have any postictal changes. Seizure can be precipitated or mimicked on suggestion.

Breath-holding Spells

Children of breath-holding spells will have seizure like activity only during awake period when the child is not attended, usually not followed by neurological deficit; may be associated with anemia, usually seem to occur in children less than 2 years.

Sleep Disorders

At times sleep disorders as night terrors mimic seizures usually seen in children 4–8 years of age. Child wakes up with sweating, tachycardia, tachypnea, fear, and anxiety. They do not remember the event. These are usually self-limiting. Nightmares occur in children 5–12 years, who suddenly get up during rapid eye movement sleep with an unpleasant dream; they have autonomic activity and are able to describe the event.

Primary Cardiac or Respiratory Abnormalities Presenting with Secondary Anoxic Seizures

Episodes of complete heart block may have syncopal features followed by collapse and secondary anoxic seizures. Usually the attacks last for less than 1 minute.

Involuntary Movement Disorders and Other Neurological Conditions

There is no alteration in consciousness. Some of the common examples include paroxysmal kinesigenic choreoathetosis, idiopathic torsion dystonia, etc.

Hyperekplexia

Attacks are characterized by excessive startle, may cause stiffening, and collapse with a sudden jerk of all four limbs. Attacks are provoked by sudden unexpected stimuli, usually auditory. Hyperekplexia needs to be distinguished from seizures induced by startle.

ROLE OF INVESTIGATIONS

Investigations after first unprovoked seizure:

- *Routine labs:* Complete blood counts, serum electrolytes, blood urea nitrogen, serum creatinine, glucose, calcium, and magnesium based on individual clinical circumstances—based on suggestive history, clinical findings or failure to return to baseline alertness
- *Lumbar puncture:* Nonfebrile seizure does not warrant a lumbar puncture
  - In less than 6-month-old or with persistent alteration of alertness and meningeal signs, lumbar puncture should be performed
- Electroencephalogram is recommended as part of the diagnostic evaluation of a child with a first unprovoked seizure, preferably 5–7 days after the seizure
- Neuroimaging
  - *Emergency imaging:*
    - Computed tomography (CT) scan is equally effective as magnetic resonance imaging
    - Child of any age who experiences postictal focal deficit not resolving/not returned to baseline after many hours
    - Suspicion of structural lesion
  - *Nonemergency imaging:*
    - Magnetic resonance imaging is routinely much better for all epilepsies
    - Some indications for CT scan especially in our country where cost is a major issue.

CLINICAL PEARL

A normal electroencephalogram does not rule out and an abnormal electroencephalogram does not prove epilepsy; it is only a supportive investigation.

TREATMENT RECOMMENDATIONS

- Treatment with antiepileptic drugs is not indicated for the prevention of epilepsy after the first unprovoked seizure
- Treatment is considered in circumstances where the benefit of reducing risk of second seizure outweighs the risk of pharmacologic and psychosocial side effects.

CLINICAL PEARL

Treatment decision is made depending on the risk of recurrence of seizure in a particular situation.

Flowchart 1: Management of first unprovoked seizure.

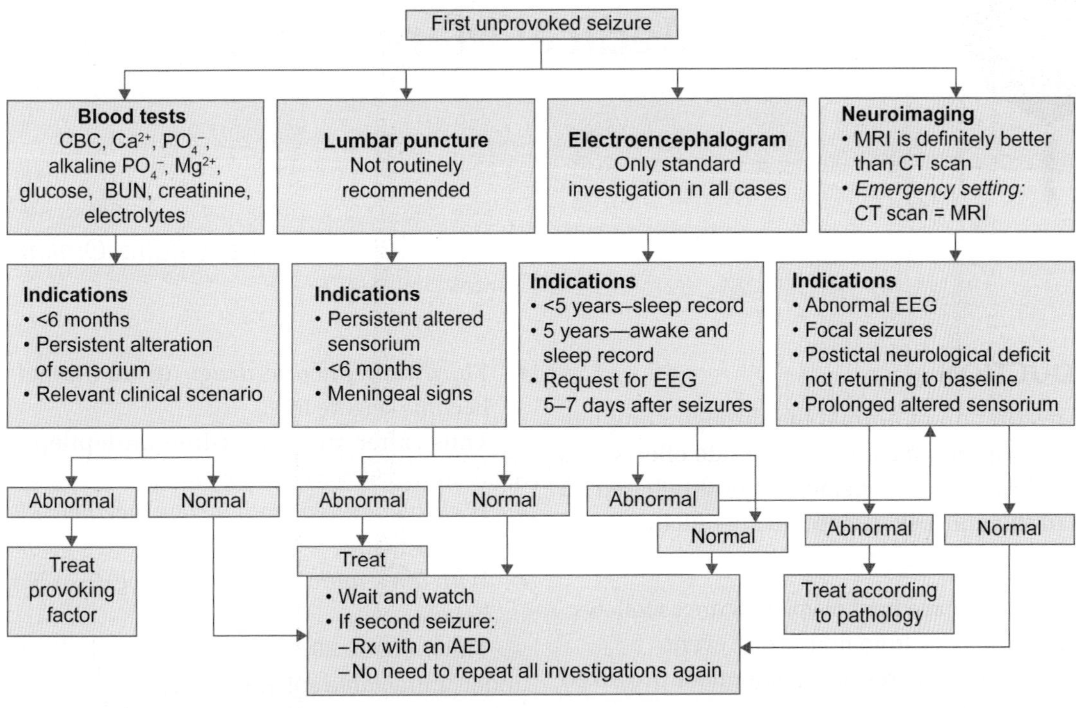

(AED: antiepileptic drugs; PO_4^-: phosphatase; BUN: blood urea nitrogen; CBC: complete blood count; CT: computed tomography; EEG: electroencephalogram; MRI: magnetic resonance imaging)

COUNSELING AND EMERGENCY HOME MANAGEMENT

Education of the child and parents about seizures, epilepsy and, medication plays an important part in reducing the emotional stress on the family. Providing the child and family with written material on epilepsy and antiepileptic medications can be very helpful.

It is important to review appropriate seizure precautions with the family, including proper positioning of a child during a seizure and issues regarding water safety and driving. The parents and other care givers can be taught the emergency management of a seizure when prolonged beyond 3–4 minutes with usage of intranasal or buccal midazolam or rectal diazepam as per the age and weight of the child.

The following is an algorithmic approach **(Flowchart 1)** to management of a first unprovoked seizure in a child.

KEY POINTS

- Simple febrile seizures do not require any investigates as magnetic resonance imaging or electroencephalogram (EEG). Investigations as to the cause of fever should be carried out
- First nonfebrile seizure requires a detailed clinical evaluation, electroencephalogram, and neuroimaging whenever possible
- There is no long-term difference if treated after the first or second seizure
- Antiepileptic drug treatment is not usually started after a first unprovoked seizure, unless the clinical or EEG features suggest a high risk of recurrence
- Patient education is perhaps the most important and often neglected aspect of management of seizures and hence needs to be stressed on when explaining to the care givers.

SUGGESTED READING

1. Arzimanoglou A, Guerrini R, Aicardi J. In: Arzimanoglou A, Guerrini R, Aicardi J (Eds). Aicardi's Epilepsy in Children, 3rd edition. Lippincott Williams & Wilkins; 2004. pp. 11-114.
2. Freeman JH. Practice parameter: evaluating a first nonfebrile seizure in children: Report of the Quality Standards Subcommittee of the American Academy of Neurology, the Child Neurology Society, and the American Epilepsy Society. Neurology. 2001;56:574.
3. Michoulas A, Farrell K, Connolly M. Approach to a child with a first afebrile seizure. BCMJ. 2011;53:274-7.
4. Waite Sehelly R, Chu-shore CJ, Neumeyer AM. Pediatric First Seizure. [online]. Available from: emedicine.medscape.com/article/1179097 [Last accessed December, 2015].

Medical Management of Epilepsy

Veena Kalra, Omkar P Hajirnis

INTRODUCTION

The aim is restoration of normal life through complete seizure control with minimal or no drug side effects. It is imperative to develop a management algorithm based on knowledge of the epilepsy disease, likely outcome, and rational use of antiepileptic drugs.

The basic steps in management of epilepsy are as follows:

- Differentiate a seizure from nonseizure event
- Identify cause of seizures and distinguish provoked seizure
- Diagnose epilepsy and epilepsy syndrome
- Distinguish benign and severe epilepsy syndromes.

CLINICAL PEARLS

- The first step in approaching a child with seizure disorder is to determine whether the event in the patient is truly a seizure or not.
- It is surprising to note that many other paroxysmal events are misdiagnosed as seizures and the consequences of this can be disastrous.

DEFINITIONS

First-line-antiepileptic drug: It is a drug internationally recognized as appropriate treatment for pediatric epilepsy as monotherapy.

Add-on-antiepileptic drug: It is a drug recognized internationally as appropriate for treatment of pediatric epilepsy not as monotherapy but in addition to another already existing antiepileptic drug.

STATISTICS

- *First antiepileptic drug:* Will make 50% of children seizure free
- *Second antiepileptic drug:* An additional 15% will become seizure free
- *Third antiepileptic drug:* An additional 1–3% will become seizure free.

Thus, after three first-line-antiepileptic drugs, a maximum of 66% will be seizure free.

- *With two antiepileptic drugs together:* 3% more will be seizure free
- *With three antiepileptic drugs together:* No additional benefit seen.

Thus, about 30% of patients by definition will fall under "intractable epilepsy".

CLINICAL PEARL

- Children with treatment-resistant epilepsy are defined as "failure of adequate trials of two tolerated, appropriately chosen and used antiepileptic-drug schedules (whether as monotherapies or in combination) to achieve sustained seizure freedom".

MANAGEMENT OF THE FIRST SEIZURE

- The first seizure is not designated epilepsy and management approach is to treat the seizure and identify its cause
- The first generalized seizure may not recur in 50–60% cases. Anticonvulsant therapy, is therefore, not indicated for the first generalized seizure
- Predicts high recurrence risk (80%) in symptomatic seizures and in patients with abnormal electroencephalogram (EEG) versus a 40% risk with a normal EEG.

Anticonvulsant therapy is started after the first episode in the following situations:

- If first seizure is a partial seizure—it merits anticonvulsant therapy as the recurrence risk is high (60–80%) and it may be symptomatic
- Examples of first seizures which merit treatment are myoclonic seizures and absence attacks
- Acute symptomatic seizures, e.g., ring-enhancing lesions, etc.

Indications of Electroencephalogram

Electroencephalogram is recommended as part of the diagnostic evaluation of a child with a first unprovoked seizure, preferably 5–7 days after the seizure.

Table 1 highlights the clinical usefulness of an EEG in epilepsy management.

Neuroimaging

Conventional radiography has no place in epilepsy management. Magnetic resonance imaging scan with epilepsy protocol is the preferred modality. It is far superior to computed tomography scan for epileptogenic lesion identification, focal cortical dysplasias, etc. and thus helps to distinguish symptomatic epilepsies of partial/generalized nature from idiopathic epilepsy. In intractable epilepsy, advanced MRI techniques, volumetric evaluation of hippocampi, etc. are useful. However, a large number of epilepsies do not require neuroimaging, e.g., absence attacks.

TABLE 1: Indications of electroencephalogram.

Usefulness	*Remarks*
Differentiate seizures from nonseizures	Interictal electroencephalogram (EEG) may be normal in epilepsy (30%) and abnormal in normal children (7–10%). Ictal record must show epileptiform activity
Classify seizures and epilepsy type	Interpreter fallacies are common
To identity background rhythm and origin of epileptic focus	*Background rhythm data important:* • Hyperventilation, photic stimulation, and sleep/sleep deprived record essential • Helps to locate epilepsy-related-lesion
Classify epileptic syndromes and to distinguish: • Complex-partial-seizures • Absence seizures • Epileptic syndromes	Ictal recording is necessary
In intractable epilepsy, to localize epileptogenic focus	Helps to take therapy decision, identify nonconvulsive status
Monitoring of status epilepticus and nonconvulsive status	EEGs essential for diagnosis of epilepsy syndromes
Underlying disease state identification	May point to metabolic/genetic basis of epilepsy

Functional scans like positron emission tomography/single-photon emission computed tomography scans are useful in presurgical evaluation of patients in addition to MRI scans.

WHEN TO LOOK BEYOND ANTIEPILEPTICS

- If patient has a clear-cut, well-defined focal cortical dysplasia—surgery is best option
- Identifiable unilateral structural lesions on MRI
- Hemiatrophy due to congenital, perinatal, or acquired causes
- Tumors
- Suspected Rasmussen's encephalitis
- Conditions listed for ketogenic diet.

The above conditions require early referral to specialized centers.

DRUG TREATMENT OF EPILEPSY

How to Start Treatment?

- Start low, go slow
- Reach maximum dose/side effects before you discard the drug
- Dosage to ideally once-a-day or twice-a-day
- Adjust to the child's daily activity
- Add a second (first-line-drug); achieve control; then try and taper off the first antiepileptic drug
- If seizure frequency is decreased but not stopped after the first antiepileptic drug, add a second drug; use rational polytherapy.

The following logistic approach provides a simple clinical approach to drug for the treatment of epilepsy:

How to Choose the First Drug?

Start with the correct "first line" antiepileptic drug. "Correct"—good efficacy (effectiveness) and low on side-effects (tolerability).

Efficacy is the time to "repeat seizure" after starting the drug while tolerability is the time to "withdrawal" due to ineffectiveness or side-effects.

CLINICAL PEARLS

- Effectiveness = Efficacy + Tolerability.
- When two drugs are equally effective, tolerability is the deciding factor.

Table 2 provides a useful guide to choose and start the appropriate first-line antiepileptic drug. However, the

TABLE 2: Choosing the appropriate antiepileptic drug.

Partial seizures		*Generalized seizures*			
First line	***Add on***	***First line***	***Add on***	***Absence***	***Myoclonics***
• Carbamazepine • Oxcarbazepine • Sodium valproate • Topiramate • Lamotrigine • Levetiracetam • Phenytoin • Gabapentin	• Clobazam • Clonazepam • Levetiracetam • Zonisamide • Tiagabine • Pyridoxine	• Valproate • Topiramate • Levetiracetam • Lamotrigine • Phenobarbitone • Vigabatrin (IS) • Gabapentin	• Clobazam • Clonazepam • Levetiracetam • Pyridoxine	• Valproate • Ethosuximide • Lamotrigine	• Valproate • Lamotrigine • Topiramate • Zonisamide • Levetiracetam

TABLE 3: Dosing guidelines for established and new antiepileptic drugs in children.

Established AED	*Starting dose (mg/kg/day)*	*Maintenance dose (mg/kg/day)*	*Dosing interval*
Phenobarbital	3–5	3–5	OD or BD
Phenytoin	5–8	5–8	OD or BD
Carbamazepine	5–10	20–30	BD or TDS
Valproate	10–15	20–60	OD or BD
Clonazepam	0.025	0.025–0.1	BD or TDS
Clobazam	0.25	0.5–1	OD or BD
Ethosuximide	10	15–30	OD or BD
New antiepileptic drugs			
Oxcarbazepine	5–10	10–50	BD or TDS
Lamotrigine • Monotherapy • With valproate	 0.4 0.15	 2–8 1–5	 BD BD
Topiramate	1–3	3–8	BD
Levetiracetam	10	20–60	BD or TDS
Vigabatrin	40	50–150	OD or BD
Zonisamide	2–4	5–6	BD
Gabapentin	10	20–50	TDS

(BD: twice-a-day; OD: once-a-day; TDS: thrice-a-day)

decision regarding specific drug depends upon the age, seizure type, side effects, cost, and lifestyle of the patient.

CLINICAL PEARL

- Whenever in doubt as to seizure type or syndrome, sodium Valproate is the best first choice for first-line therapy.

Table 3 enumerates the dosing guidelines for the various commonly used antiepileptic drugs.

Do I Use an Established Antiepileptic Drug or Try a Newer Antiepileptic Drug?

Evidence-based medicine proves that the efficacy is similar in most first-line antiepileptic drugs, new or old. Thus, it is important to choose your drug by identifying the seizure type and knowing the common side effects of the drug in relation to your patient.

What are the Common Side Effects of Each Drug I should Know?

The usual dose-related side-effects of most antiepileptic drugs include drowsiness, dizziness, nystagmus, cognitive decline, gastrointestinal dysfunction, etc.

Specific side effects

- *Carbamazepine:* Diplopia, dizziness, cognition, or counts
- *Sodium valproate:* Weight gain, hair loss, or liver dysfunction
- *Phenytoin:* Hirsutism, coarse facies, gingival hyperplasia, drowsy, ataxia, cognition, or nausea—toxic range
- *Phenobarbitone:* Drowsiness, cognitive decline, ataxia, withdrawal seizures
- *Lamotrigine:* Rash with danger of Stevens-Johnson syndrome, or hair loss
- *Topiramate:* Weight loss, cognition issues, or incontinence, hypohidrosis leading to pyrexia
- *Vigabatrin:* Visual field cuts
- *Levetiracetam:* Mood swings, or drowsiness
- *Benzodiazepine:* Drowsiness, low tone, or tolerance.

What do I do if there is no Response to First-line Antiepileptic Drug?

- Firstly use all tests available to confirm the seizure type

TABLE 4: Preferred drugs for different epileptic syndromes.

Severe myoclonic epilepsy of infancy (Dravet syndrome)	*Benign rolandic epilepsy with centrotemporal spikes*	*Juvenile myoclonic epilepsy*	*Myoclonic astatic epilepsy*	*Childhood absence epilepsy*
• Clobazam • Valproate • Topiramate • Stiripentol • Levetiracetam • Lamotrigine	• Carbamazepine • Oxcarbazepine • Valproate • Topiramate • Levetiracetam	• Valproate • Lamotrigine • Levetiracetam • Clonazepam	• Clonazepam • Clobazam • Valproate • Lamotrigine • Topiramate • Levetiracetam	• Valproate • Clobazam

TABLE 5: Preferred drugs for different malignant epileptic syndromes.

Lennox-Gastaut syndrome	*Infantile spasms*	*Landau-Kleffner syndrome*	*Rasmussen's syndrome*	*Progressive myoclonic epilepsies (metabolic epilepsies)*
Combination of: • Valproate (VPA) + • Lamotrigine (LMT) + • Topiramate (TPM)) • Zonisamide (ZNS) • Levetiracetam (LVT) • Clobazam (CLBZ) • Clonazepam (CLNZ)	• ACTH • Oral steroids • Vigabatrin • Nitrazepam • Valproate • Topiramate • Clonazepam	• Intravenous immunoglobulin • Steroids • Antiepileptic drugs	• Steroids • Antiepileptic drugs • Surgery	• Zonisamide • Levetiracetam • Valproate

(ACTH: adrenocorticotropic hormone)

TABLE 6: Drugs worsening certain epilepsies.

Drug	*Syndrome*	*Worsening*
Carbamazepine	Absence seizures, juvenile myoclonic epilepsy, progressive myoclonic epilepsies, benign rolandic epilepsy	Absence seizures, myoclonic seizures, or continuous slow wave in sleep
Phenytoin	Absence, progressive myoclonic epilepsies	Absences, cerebellar syndrome
Phenobarbitone	Absence seizures	At high doses, absences
Benzodiazepines	Lennox-Gastaut syndrome	Tonic seizures
Vigabatrin	Absence, myoclonic seizures	Absences, myoclonic seizures
Lamotrigine	Severe myoclonic epilepsy of infancy, juvenile myoclonic epilepsy	At high doses, myoclonic seizures

- Choose a drug with a different mechanism of action to your first-line antiepileptic drug.

The following drug combinations are effective and recommended:

- Valproate + Lamotrigine
- Topiramate + Carbamazepine
- Topiramate + Valproate
- Valproate + Carbamazepine
- Carbamazepine + Phenytoin

Identify an epileptic syndrome and choose a drug known to work on the identified syndrome.

Tables 4 and 5 list the various epileptic syndromes and the preferred drugs for the same.

It is prudent to remember some antiepileptic drugs are known to worsen certain epilepsies. **Table 6** depicts the drugs to avoid in certain epilepsies.

DISCONTINUATION OF ANTIEPILEPTIC THERAPY

Epilepsy therapy need not be life-long in most subjects. In most epilepsies, the antiepileptic drug is withdrawn after 2 years of seizure-free period. However, about 20–29% subjects relapse after antiepileptic drugs withdrawal. Drug withdrawal is over 3–6 months and is one drug at a time in cases of polytherapy. When withdrawing on abnormal EEGs, adolescent epilepsies or remote symptomatic epilepsies adequate counseling is required to parents and patient with regards to chances of relapse.

Flowchart 1 depicts the approach to withdrawing anti-epileptic drugs.

Flowchart 2 depicts the newly diagnosed epilepsy.

DRUG MONITORING

Therapeutic range is the optimum level of a drug in the body which is effective, but not toxic. However, there are wide variations in blood levels are observed at the same dosage in different patients. Also, there is no correlation between efficacy and toxicity of the anti-epileptic drug in the blood for a given patient. There is also a difference between total drug and free drug in the system—total is what is being tested, free is what is effective.

Timing of collection is most important as the trough levels are determined for efficacy and peak levels for toxicity **(Table 7)**.

> **CLINICAL PEARLS**
>
> - Treat the patient, not the drug level.
> - If a value does not make sense—ignore it or repeat it.

PARENTAL COUNSELING

Explain the Disease

- Explain the nature of the disease and alleviate fears of supernatural involvement
- In vast majority of cases (80%), epilepsy would improve with first-line drug therapy
- Most children are normal and their mental development would not be affected by drugs or disease
- Remind about seizure precipitants:
  - Sleep deprivation
  - Exhaustion
  - *Excessive emotion:* Stress/anxiety/anger/tear/excitement
  - Illness/infection
  - Usually a combination of two or more factors
  - *Days to be careful:* Birthday, exam, festivals, holiday, travelling, or illness
- Must explain how to abort an event at home. Draw, write, whatever is easier for the parent to understand
- The use of intranasal midazolam spray or buccal midazolam or rectal diazepam should be explained to the parents and caretakers in detail

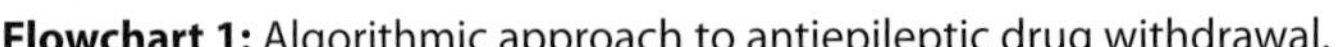

Flowchart 1: Algorithmic approach to antiepileptic drug withdrawal.

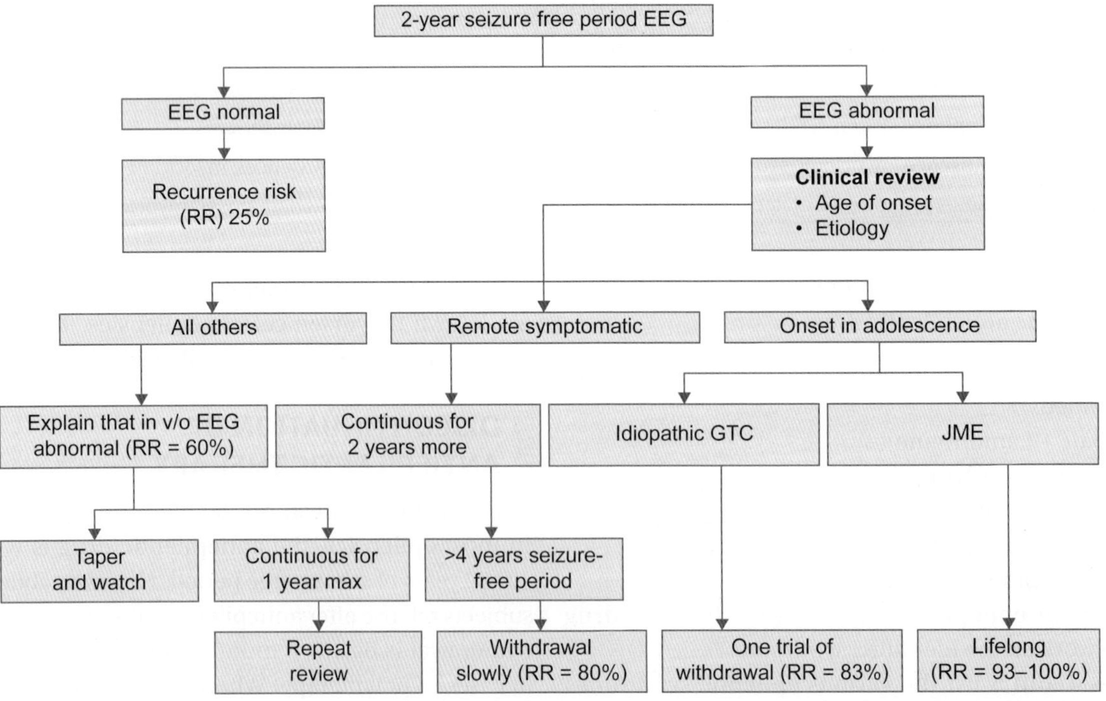

(EEG: electroencephalogram; GTC: generalized tonic-clonic seizure; JME: juvenile myoclonic epilepsy; v/o: view of)

Flowchart 2: Algorithm for a newly diagnosed epilepsy.

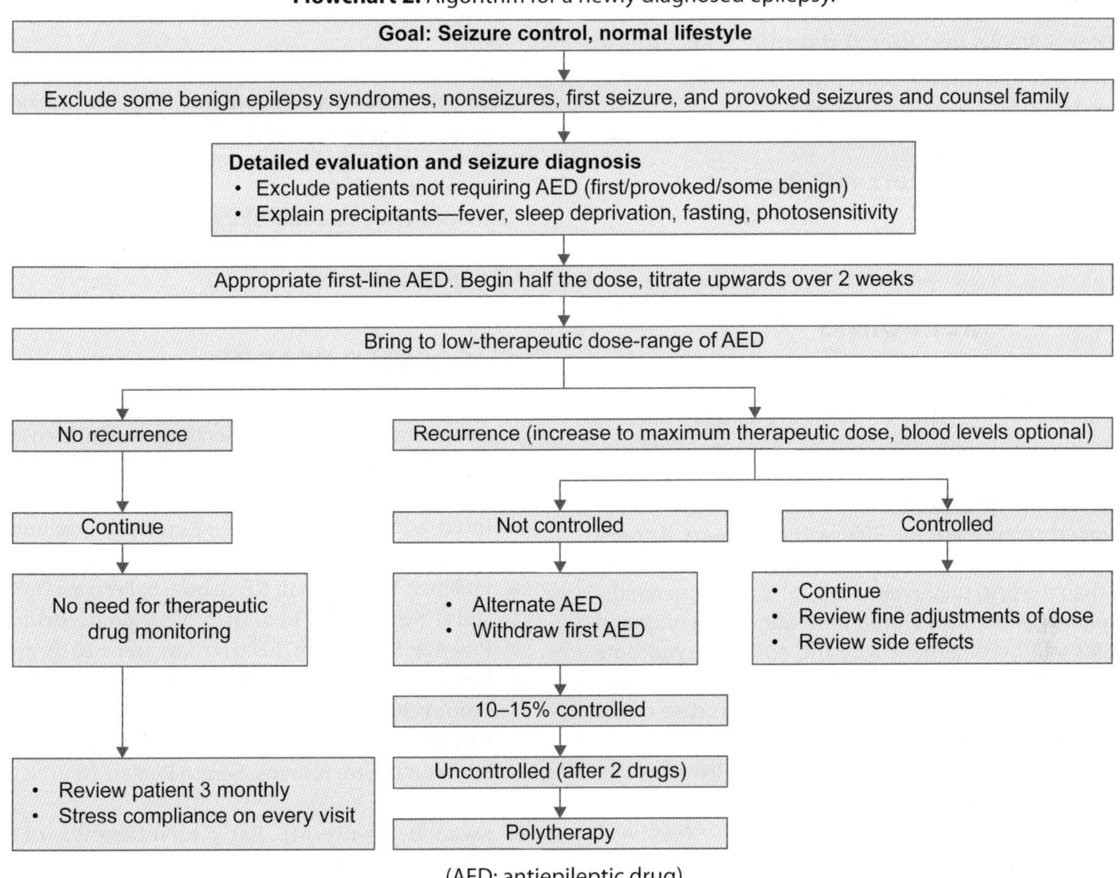

(AED: antiepileptic drug)

TABLE 7: Drugs for which therapeutic drug monitoring is available.

Drug	*Effective plasma concentration (mg/mL)*
Carbamazepine	6–12
Lamotrigine	2–16
Phenobarbital	15–40
Phenytoin	10–20
Valproate	50–120

- Explain the need to keep medication near the patient and not at a different venue so that when he/she seizures, the drug is readily available
- Answer all their queries and alley their anxiety regards academics, medicines, social stigmas, marriage, and children.

Drug Therapy

- *Compliance:* Regular drug treatment is the corner stone of therapy
- *Safety:* The drugs should be kept out-of-reach of children to avoid inadvertent ingestion
- *Empowerment:* Parents should be explained the domiciliary management of acute breakthrough seizures
- *Follow-up:* Appropriate timely drug withdrawal.

Lifestyle

- Maintain a normal healthy lifestyle
- No food restrictions needed
- School teachers should be informed
- Children should carry a card displaying their diagnosis
- Caution is advocated in dangerous activities such as cycling, swimming. and fire particularly during early therapy.

CLINICAL PEARLS

- Domiciliary management of seizures is extremely important and should be taught to every family.
- Facility of intranasal midazolam should be available in all schools.

FOLLOW-UP

Initially after 6 weeks and then 3 monthly if seizures are controlled. Refer to a higher center if:

- Uncontrolled seizures/side effects
- Suspected syndromes
- Suspected inborn errors of metabolism
- Deteriorating cognition
- Fresh neurological deficits.

KEY POINTS

- The first step in approaching a child with suspected epilepsy is to confirm that the reported spells are actually seizures rather than another condition such as syncope, migraines, tics, or behavioral events.
- After a second unprovoked seizure, the chances of a third unprovoked seizure are 80–90% within 2 years if treatment is not initiated. Therefore, treatment after the second (rather than the first) unprovoked seizure is recommended.
- The choice of antiepileptic drug in treating the childhood epilepsies will be determined by the epilepsy syndrome (and hence the specific seizures help to define the syndrome), side effects profile and, to an extent, its ease of use (formulation and dosing regimen).
- Sodium valproate appears to remain the most effective antiepileptic drug in treating most seizure types.
- It is important to be aware of drugs that may exacerbate some seizure types.
- The temptation should be strongly resisted to indulge in polytherapy, as it is always easier to add another drug than to withdraw one.
- There are no convincing data that the simultaneous use of three antiepileptic drugs results in better seizure control than two drugs.
- In order to assess response to treatment, information on baseline seizure frequency and intervals between initial seizures is crucial. Tracking response to seizures is important, either with paper diaries or with online seizure-tracking tools.
- A trial of epilepsy medication discontinuation is usually recommended after 2 seizure-free years. Medications should be discontinued over at least a 6-week period, and if the patient is on polytherapy, only one medication should be weaned at a given time.
- Children with pharmacologically-resistant epilepsy and seizures due to focal abnormalities are potential candidates for epilepsy surgery.

SUGGESTED READING

1. Arhan E, Serdaroglu A, Kurt AN, Aslanyavrusu M. Drug treatment failures and effectivity in children with newly diagnosed epilepsy. Seizure. 2010;19(9): 553Y557.
2. Commission on Classification and Terminology of the International League against Epilepsy. [online] Available from: http://www.ilae.org/[Last accessed December, 2024].
3. Epilepsy. In: Swaiman KF, Ashwal S, Ferriero DM, Schor NF. (Eds) Swaiman's Pediatric Neurology: Principles and Practice, 5th edition. Elsevier Saunders; 2012. pp. 811-35.
4. Jerome Engel Jr. Seizures and Epilepsy, 2nd edition. Oxford; 2012.
5. Kossoff EH. Intractable childhood epilepsy: choosing between the treatments. Semin Pediatr Neurol. 2011;18(3): 145-9.
6. Kwan P, Brodie MJ. Early identification of refractory epilepsy. N Engl J Med. 2000; 342(5):314-9.
7. Pestian J, Matykiewicz P, Holland-Bouley K, Standridge S, Spencer M, Glauser T. Selecting anti-epileptic drugs: a pediatric epileptologist's view. Acta Neurol Scand. 2013; 127(3):208-15.
8. Vendrame M, Loddenkemper T. Approach to seizures, epilepsies, and epilepsy syndromes. Sleep Med Clin. 2012: 7(1):59-73.
9. Wallace S, Farrell K. Epilepsy in Children, 2nd edition. London: Arnold; 2004.

Approach to Drug-resistant Epilepsies

Neelu Desai, Vrajesh Udani

INTRODUCTION

Drug-resistant epilepsy (DRE) or intractable or pharmacoresistant epilepsy is epilepsy which does not successfully respond to antiseizure drug (ASD) therapy. About one-third of children with newly diagnosed epilepsy are likely to subsequently develop DRE which has tremendous implications not only on the child but also on the patient's family members and caregivers. Aggressiveness in the diagnosis and treatment of DRE in children is imperative given the adverse effect of recurrent seizures on early brain development, learning, and memory.

DEFINITION

Conventionally, therapeutic failure of three ASDs defined intractability. Frequency, duration, and severity of seizures are less commonly included in definition of DRE. The International League Against Epilepsy (ILAE) defines DRE as failure of adequate trials of two well tolerated and appropriately chosen and used ASD schedules (monotherapies or in combination) to achieve sustained seizure freedom.

INTERNATIONAL LEAGUE AGAINST EPILEPSY DEFINITION OF DRUG REFRACTORY EPILEPSY

Failure of adequate trials of two well tolerated and appropriately chosen and used ASD schedules (monotherapies or in combination) to achieve sustained seizure freedom.

EPIDEMIOLOGY

Incidence and prevalence of DRE are uncertain due to unstandardized definitions as well as misdiagnoses. Though 20–40% of epilepsy cases present as DRE, the figure for true DRE has been estimated to be significantly less as many are pseudoresistant. Data from various studies on DRE reveal that with the first drug trial, 50% patients would become seizure-free. A second medication trial produced remission in an additional 13%, while with the third drug, only a further 4% would become seizure-free.

> **CLINICAL PEARL**
>
> Appropriately chosen first ASD will control half the cases of new-onset epilepsy while only one-third of these will be drug resistant.

WHAT ARE THE CONSEQUENCES OF DRUG-RESISTANT EPILEPSY?

Recurrent seizures are associated with a range of deleterious consequences including death. Uncontrolled epilepsy in infants and children has deleterious effect on early brain development, learning, and memory. Refractory seizures restrict patients' social activities, academic achievements, and in adults reduce the ability to hold a driving license or keep a job. It is a great economic burden for society through expenditures in healthcare and unemployment.

Patients with epilepsy have a mortality rate significantly higher than that of the general population. Sudden unexpected death in epilepsy (SUDEP) accounts for 8–17% of deaths in people with epilepsy.

COMPLICATIONS OF DRUG-RESISTANT EPILEPSY

- *Mortality*—underlying neurological disorder, status epilepticus, and seizure-related accidents; treatment related deaths and SUDEP
- *Morbidity:* Increased cognitive, behavioral, and psychiatric problems
- *Nonfatal injuries*—head injury, burns, drowning, and fractures

- *Diminished quality of life*—developmental delay, poor academic performance, unemployment, and other lifestyle restrictions
- Social stigma

RISK FACTORS OF DRUG-RESISTANT EPILEPSY

A number of prospective studies have attempted to identify factors that predict the risk of true DRE. Some of these factors are as follows:

- The response to the first-antiepileptic drug trial has been found as the most consistent and vital predictive factor for DRE. As mentioned before, half of patients with new-onset epilepsy respond to the first appropriate ASD prescribed. With a subsequent ASD trial, ~20% are likely to respond. High-seizure frequency prior to treatment is consistently identified risk factor for DRE.
- Etiology of epilepsy and syndrome classification is also a relevant factor deciding prognosis. Self-limiting epilepsy syndromes have a better prognosis than structural etiologies. Certain pediatric epilepsy syndromes that are usually medically intractable include early (neonatal) myoclonic encephalopathy, early infantile epileptic encephalopathy, Lennox–Gastaut syndrome, etc. Some of these are now known as developmental and epileptic encephalopathies (DEE) and underlying genetic defects are now increasingly recognized.
- Other variables such as electroencephalographic findings and the presence or absence of psychiatric comorbidities have been correlated with outcomes in some analyses.
- Some findings such as status epilepticus, a long duration of epilepsy, a family history of epilepsy and febrile convulsions are variable determinants of prognosis. Some studies have also identified an abnormal neurologic examination and/or developmental delay/intellectual disability as risk factors for DRE.
- Some studies, but not all, suggest that age at presentation may be a factor in the development of DRE. Age of onset of seizures < 5 years was found to be associated with the development of drug resistance than seizures with onset between the ages of 5 and 10 years. One series found onset in the neonatal time period associated with DRE.

PREDICTORS OF TRUE DRUG-RESISTANT EPILEPSY

- Lack of efficacy with first appropriate ASD
- High number of seizures prior to treatment
- Underlying etiology—structural/presumed structural
- *Others:* Early age of onset, abnormal development/neurological examination, electroencephalogram (EEG) abnormality, presence of status epilepticus, co-morbidities

DIFFERENTIAL DIAGNOSIS

Pseudodrug-resistant Epilepsy

Very often in practice, medical intractability is not true. This apparent treatment failure could be due to:

- *Wrong diagnosis:* Some paroxysmal events appear like seizures but are not due to abnormal electrical discharges. They could be physiological or psychogenic in nature and do not respond to ASDs. Video EEG is a golden tool to prove or disprove them. In one study almost 20% of patients seen at epilepsy referral centers were nonepileptic attack disorder (NEAD). Some common seizure mimics are mentioned in the **Table 1**.
- *Wrong choice of drug:* Inappropriate drug selection is often responsible for intractability. For example, a narrow-spectrum ASD such as carbamazepine can

TABLE 1: Common seizure mimics in childhood.

Neonates	*Infants*	*Children*	*Adolescents*
• Jitteriness • Benign sleep myoclonus • Hyperekplexia	• Breath holding spells • Colic • Self-gratification • Benign paroxysmal vertigo • Benign paroxysmal torticollis • Sandifer syndrome (GERD) • Shuddering attacks	• Stereotypies • Self-gratification • Sleep disorders • Tics	• Pseudoseizures • Syncope • Migraine • Tics

worsen seizure frequency in generalized epilepsy, e.g., absence or myoclonic jerks. Precision medicine with next-generation sequencing can often aid choice of ASDs. Certain genetic defects respond dramatically with certain ASDs (SCN2a associated epilepsy with sodium channel blockers) while others may worsen with certain ASDs (SCN1a-associated epilepsy with sodium channel blockers).

- *Wrong dosage:* Inappropriate dosages and frequency can also lead to pseudo DRE, e.g., giving short half-life ASDs, e.g., syrup carbamazepine in once or twice daily doses or suboptimal daily dosage.
- *Wrong lifestyle:* Recreational drug or alcohol abuse, sleep deprivation, or noncompliance and self-adjustment of drug doses can also lead to improper seizure control.

MANAGEMENT OF DRUG-RESISTANT EPILEPSY

The treatment of children with DRE is both challenging and rewarding. True DRE needs referral to a *Comprehensive Epilepsy Care Center* for optimal evaluation and management. This comprises of a Pediatric Neurologist/Epileptologist, Electrophysiologist, Epilepsy surgeon, Neuropsychologist, and counsellor.

If initial history, examination and videos suggest DRE, appropriate steps should be taken to resolve them. This would include discontinuing ASDs in NEAD and counseling.

Antiseizure Drugs

Medical management with ASDs remains the first-line treatment in patients with epilepsy. A good number of patients respond to small changes in treatment such as switching to appropriate monotherapy according to seizure/syndrome, increasing dose, frequency, and assuring strict compliance. Rational polytherapy is recommended in nonresponders to monotherapy, e.g., synergistic combinations such as valproate and lamotrigine; ASDs with different mechanisms of action like a sodium channel blocker carbamazepine with a gamma-aminobutyric acid (GABA)-ergic drug like clobazam. Tapering drugs such as carbamazepine or oxcarbazepine in generalized epilepsies are rewarding. Drug levels may sometimes help in adjustment of drug dosages. Cannabidiol has also been found effective in Dravet's syndrome, Lennox-Gastaut syndrome, and tuberous sclerosis with significant seizure reduction in >50% of cases. Other newer drugs such as perampanel and brivaracetam are also found effective in several epilepsies.

Seizure Diary

A seizure diary is a very helpful tool in all patients with DRE to document seizure frequency and intensity with specific interventions, e.g., a new ASD. This improves drug compliance and helps to identify triggers such as menstrual cycle. It often would help to avoid unnecessary polytherapy with ineffective ASDs and identify scenarios where the ASD itself leads to paradoxical increase in seizures.

CLINICAL PEARL

- Seizure diary is an essential tool kept by patient or caregivers of DRE recording frequency and intensity of seizures along with ASDs and precipitants.

As mentioned before, of the 20–40% of individuals with DRE about half will continue their seizures despite three appropriate drugs being tried to their full therapeutic potential. Though new ASDs have undoubtedly reduced drug interactions and adverse effects the number of DRE patients who become seizure free after the first 2–3 drugs is not >5%. These patients should be evaluated for possibility of epilepsy surgery, ketogenic diet (KD), or vagus nerve stimulation (VNS).

CLINICAL PEARL

- The DRE represents a significant portion of all pediatric epilepsies and should be referred early to a comprehensive epilepsy center where all treatment options including epilepsy surgery and the KD are available for optimal management.

Epilepsy Surgery

Surgery has the potential of altering the natural history of epilepsy by improving or eliminating seizures in carefully selected patients. Epilepsy surgery should be considered early in appropriate patients with DRE when seizures are sufficiently frequent or severe as to significantly disrupt the patient's quality of life.

Presurgical evaluation would need video-EEG monitoring and high-resolution magnetic resonance imaging (MRI) of brain in all cases. The sensitivity of MRI can be substantially improved by an epilepsy protocol including

3D acquisition of T2-fluid-attenuated inversion recovery (FLAIR)/T1-spoiled gradient echo (SPGR) sequences to delineate subtle malformations of cortical development such as focal cortical dysplasias (FCD) which often underlie DRE. Functional neuroimaging such as ictal single photon emission computed tomography (SPECT) can help delineate the ictal-onset zone and often complements MRI in the search of the epileptogenic zone (EZ), critical for planning any surgical intervention. Similarly, positron emission tomography (PET) is very useful as a tool to map out glucose metabolism in the interictal state as many EZs are hypometabolic. Postprocessing techniques coregistering MRI and functional images and diffusion tensor imaging enhance the information. Another very important consideration in presurgical evaluation is defining the eloquent cortex for sensorimotor, language, and visual functions. If this overlaps with the EZ, post-operative deficits may be unacceptable.

Neuropsychological evaluations help understand the specific cognitive defects a patient has, e.g., verbal or visual memory deficits in hippocampal sclerosis when planning surgery in older children and teenagers.

Unlike potentially curative *resective surgeries* (discussed above), VNS and deep brain stimulation are *palliative* neuromodulation procedures which can potentially improve seizure control and improve quality of life. Corpus callosotomy is another palliative procedure most useful for drop attacks.

Flowchart 1: Surgical approach in drug refractory epilepsy.

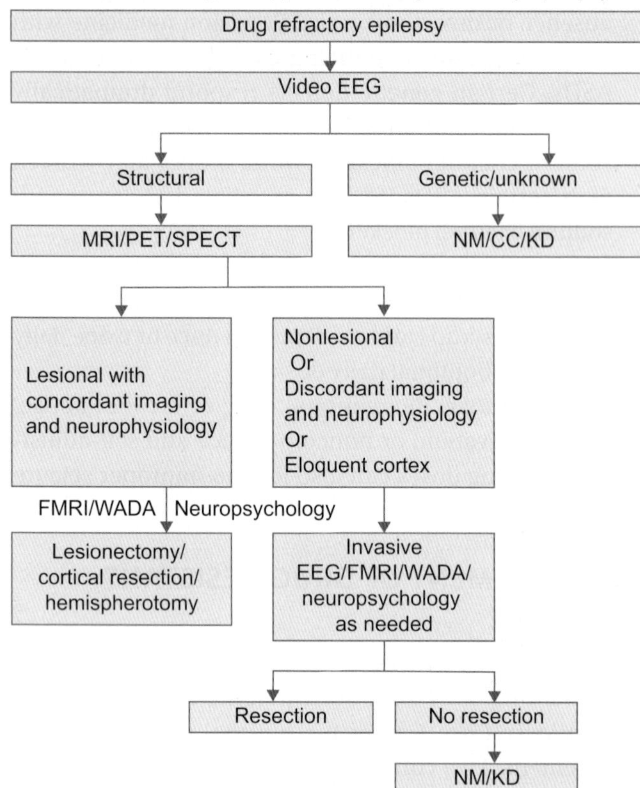

(CC: corpus callosotomy; FMRI: functional magnetic resonance imaging; KD: ketogenic diet; NM: neuromodulation; PET: positron emission tomography; SPECT: single photon emission computed tomography; VNS: vagus nerve stimulation)

Ketogenic Diet

If surgical procedures are not feasible, there are several KDs available which also improve seizure control and quality of life. These KDs include the classic KD, medium-chain triglyceride diet (MCTD), modified Atkins diet (MAD), and the low-glycemic index diet (LGID). These all include significant reduction in carbohydrate content with significant increase in calories derived from lipid and only moderate increases in protein. Recent studies have documented fairly similar improvements in seizure control in all the different diets used. Also there has been significant simplification in diet preparation and in the pragmatic use of this useful fairly affordable therapy **(Flowchart 1)**.

Surgical options in DRE are either resective or palliative epilepsy surgery.

- *Resective epilepsy surgery* has the best-established efficacy for individuals with lesional epilepsy. Patients with concordant abnormalities on MRI, EEG, SPECT, and PET have a rate of seizure remission as high as 90%.
- *Disconnective surgery* is sometimes employed for palliative treatment in children with catastrophic epilepsy syndromes with no resectable lesion **(Table 2)**.

Dietary Therapies

Ketogenic diet (high-fat, low protein) in children with DRE is an effective therapy with more than one-third experiencing a 50% or greater reduction in seizures. Behavioral improvements is often an additional bonus. It is tried for about 3 months and if effective, is continued for 2–3 years. Less restrictive modifications such as the MAD can be used in older children, though with less success.

KETOGENIC DIET

Ketogenic diet is given in **Table 3**.

TABLE 2: Surgical options in drug-resistant epilepsy.

Resective surgery (curative)	***Disconnective surgery (palliative)***
• Children with recognized resectable lesions (FCD, MTS) and failed appropriate AED trial • Improvement of seizure control with developmental, cognitive and behavioral improvement, e.g., lesionectomy; hemispherotomy for hemispheric epilepsies	• Severe uncontrolled epilepsy with no resectable lesion • Prevents falls/injuries, e.g., corpus callosotomy in Lennox–Gastaut syndrome

(AED: antiepileptic drug; FCD: focal cortical dysplasia; MTS: mesial temporal sclerosis)

TABLE 3: Ketogenic diet.

Indication	Any drug-resistant epilepsy, West syndrome, epilepsy associated with tuberous sclerosis complex, Dravet syndrome, Doose syndrome, Lennox-Gastaut syndrome (LGS), and glucose transporter 1 (GLUT-1) deficiency
Response	One-third experiencing 50% or greater reduction in seizures, one-sixth achieve seizure freedom; behavioral improvements
Side effects	Gastrointestinal or metabolic side effects, drowsiness, and increased susceptibility to infections
Duration	3 months trial; if effective continued for 2–3 years

NEUROMODULATION

These include VNS, responsive neurostimulation (RNS), and deep brain stimulation (DBS). VNS has been approved for adjunctive treatment of DRE in adults and children over 12 years of age. Approximately 30-40% of patients achieve a >50% reduction in seizure frequency. Serious adverse events are rare. VNS is efficacious in patients with well-documented DRE, who are not candidates for intracranial surgery, or whose seizures were not benefitted by prior epilepsy surgery. In resectable lesions, resective surgery is preferred over VNS because of the greater potential for complete seizure remission **(Flowchart 2)**. Responsive neurostimulation and deep brain stimulation though approved for adults above 18 years have recently been used in children as well for seizures arising from multiple foci or from eloquent cortex.[11]

Flowchart 2: Approach to drug refractory epilepsy.

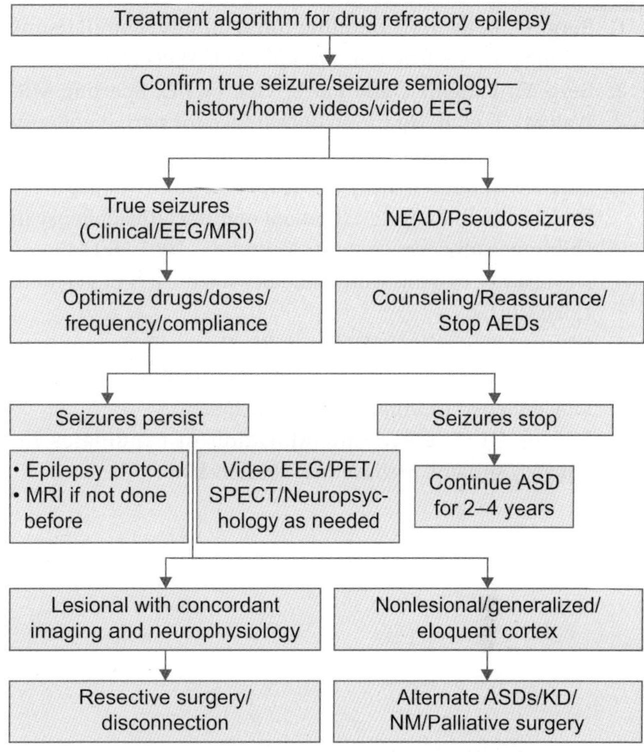

(KD: ketogenic diet; NM: neuromodulation)

KEY POINTS

- 20–40% of patients with epilepsy have incomplete seizure control with ASD therapy alone.
- Most patients with DRE can be identified early in their presentation, after a failure of two appropriate ASD trials.
- As many as 20% of patients with apparent DRE will have a nonepileptic paroxysmal disorder. Video EEG monitoring is the gold standard to confirm.
- Predictors of true DRE: Lack of efficacy of a first appropriate ASD trial, a high number of seizures prior to treatment, and a structural/presumed structural epilepsy syndrome.
- Individuals with DRE have an increased risk of mortality as well as morbidity. Hence aggressive treatment is imperative.
- Patients with true DRE should have a high-resolution MRI study to identify a potential surgical lesion. Other neuroimaging studies (e.g., SPECT and PET) can be helpful for maximum localization.
- For patients in whom epilepsy surgery is not an option or whose seizures persist after surgery, treatment trials with other ASDs appropriate for their epilepsy syndrome/genetic defect or KD or neuromodulation is suggested.

SUGGESTED READING

1. Berg AT, Kelly MM. Defining intractability: comparisons among published definitions. Epilepsia. 2006;47:431.
2. Berg AT, Langfitt J, Shinnar S, Vickrey BG, Sperling MR, Walczak T, et al. How long does it take for partial epilepsy to become intractable? Neurology. 2003;60:186.
3. Berg AT, Shinnar S, Levy SR, Testa FM, Smith-Rapaport S, Beckerman B. Early development of intractable epilepsy in children: a prospective study. Neurology. 2001;56:1445.
4. Devinsky O. Patients with refractory seizures. N Engl J Med. 1999;340:1565.
5. Dlugos DJ, Sammel MD, Strom BL, Farrar JT. Response to first drug trial predicts outcome in childhood temporal lobe epilepsy. Neurology. 2001;57:2259.
6. Dlugos DJ. The early identification of candidates for epilepsy surgery. Arch Neurol. 2001;58:1543.
7. Kwan P, Arzimanoglou A, Berg AT, Brodie MJ, Hauser WA, Mathern G, et al. Definition of drug resistant epilepsy. Consensus proposal by the ad hoc Task Force of the ILAE Commission on Therapeutic Strategies. Epilepsia. 2010; 51(6):1069-77.
8. Kwan P, Brodie M. Issues of Medical Intractability for Surgical Candidacy. In: Wyllie E, Gupta A, Lachhwani D (Eds). The Treatment of Epilepsy and Practice, 4th edition. Philadelphia: Lippincott, Williams & Wilkins; 2006. pp. 983.
9. Kwan P, Brodie MJ. Early identification of refractory epilepsy. N Engl J Med. 2000;342:314.
10. Kwan P, Schachter SC, Brodie MJ. Drug-resistant epilepsy. N Engl J Med. 2011;365:919.
11. Singhal NS, Numis AL, Lee MB, Chang EF, Sullivan JE, Auguste KI, et al. Responsive neurostimulation for treatment of pediatric drug-resistant epilepsy. Epilepsy Behav Case Rep. 2018;10:21-4.

Acute Flaccid Paralysis

V Viswanathan, Ayesha Mariam

INTRODUCTION

Acute flaccid paralysis (AFP) is something that most pediatric neurologists see on a regular basis particularly during certain seasons (mostly during the winter seasons) although they seem to occur most of the year round. These children, who are previously healthy, develop weakness in both legs to start with and then progressing to involve the breathing muscles quickly over a few hours to days. They then develop difficulties in swallowing and invariably end up getting admitted to hospital. In some cases, they may follow mild upper respiratory illnesses or fever. The etiologies are diverse. With the advent of newer diagnostic tests including MRI and serological testing for antibodies a newer set of possible autoimmune demyelination should always be considered.

Acute flaccid paralysis can be defined as acute onset of flaccid weakness, <4 weeks, reaching its maximum severity in days to weeks. The term "flaccid" indicates the absence of spasticity or other signs of disordered central nervous system and a lower motor neuron lesion. The latest recommendations of reporting a case of AFP surveillance are of utmost importance in today's era **(Flowchart 1)**.

CAUSES OF ACUTE FLACCID PARALYSIS

When one looks at various causes of such paralysis in children, there are many and sometimes very difficult for one to identify the clear cause. Some of these are listed below.

Nerve Roots (Radiculopathy)

Guillain-Barré syndrome (GBS) and variants

Peripheral Neuropathy

- GBS and other variants
- Toxic neuropathy—diphtheria, tick bite paralysis
- Metabolic neuropathies (hypokalemia and hypophosphatemia)
- Heavy metal poisoning (lead and arsenic)
- Acute intermittent porphyria
- Traumatic neuritis

Anterior Horn Cell Disease

- Acute poliomyelitis presently eradicated in India
- Vaccine-associated poliomyelitis
- Other neurotropic viruses such as Japanese B, rabies, and nonpolio enteroviruses

Acute Myelopathies

- Transverse myelitis
- Acute-disseminated encephalomyelitis
- Spinal cord ischemia
- Spinal cord injury
- Spinal cord compression (abscess, space occupying lesions, and postoperative hematomas)

SYSTEMIC DISEASE

Critical illness neuropathy/myopathy.

Muscle Disorders

- Polymyositis and dermatomyositis
- Trichinosis
- Periodic paralysis
- Corticosteroids and blocking agents
- Mitochondrial diseases (infantile type)

Disorders of Neuromuscular Transmission

- Immune myasthenia gravis presenting in crisis
- Botulism
- Insecticide (organophosphate poisoning)
- Snake bite.

Flowchart 1: Approach to a case with acute flaccid paralysis.

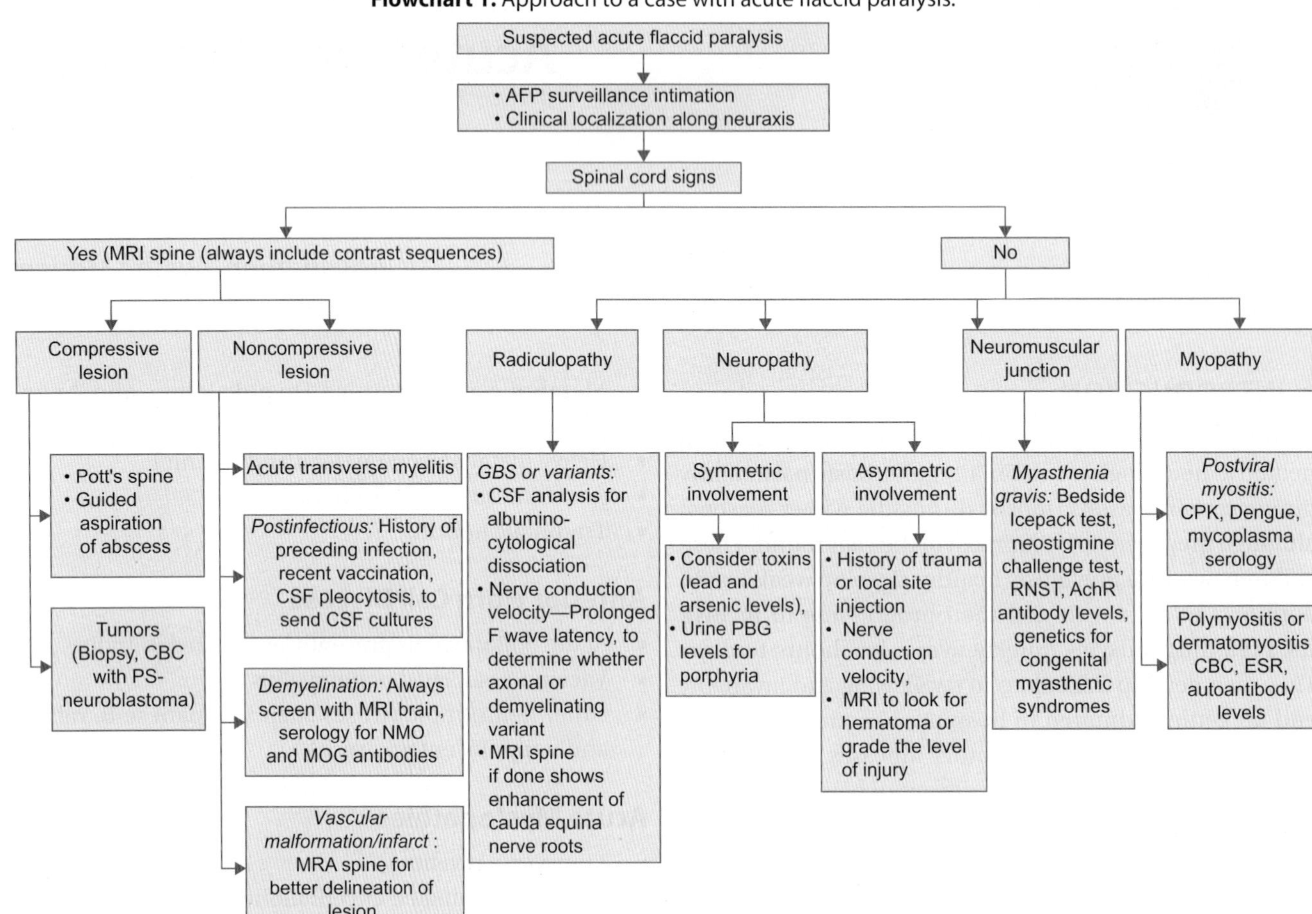

(AFP: acute flaccid paralysis; CBC: complete blood count; CPK: creatine phosphokinase; ESR: erythrocyte sedimentation rate; GBS: Guillain–Barré syndrome; MRA: magnetic resonance angiography; MRI: magnetic resonance imaging; MOG: myelin oligodendrocyte glycoprotein; NMO: neuromyelitis optica; PBG: porphobilinogen)

Others

- Traumatic neuritis
- Conversion reaction

CLUES IN HISTORY AND EXAMINATION

- *Fever at onset:* Polio or enteroviral myelitis, transverse myelitis, myositis, epidural abscess, and Pott's spine (prolonged history) **(Table 1)**
- *Trauma:* Head/neck trivial trauma may lead to spinal compression in patients with cervical vertebral instability (patients with Down's syndrome, congenital cervicovertebral anomalies, or juvenile idiopathic arthritis).
- *Exposure toxins:* Lead, Arsenic, or snake envenomation
- *Dog bite:* Rabies and postrabies-vaccine encephalomyelitis

Preceding Infectious Prodrome/Vaccination

- GBS or transverse myelitis
- *Sore throat and neck swelling:* Diphtheritic polyneuropathy (non/partly immunized)

Precipitating Factors

- *Diarrhea:* Hypokalemia and enteroviral myelitis
- *Exertion or postprandial:* Hypokalemic periodic paralysis
- *Intramuscular injection:* Polio and traumatic sciatic neuritis
- *Sensory loss:* Compressive myelopathy and transverse myelitis
- *Early bowel/bladder involvement:* Compressive myelopathy and transverse myelitis
- *Constipation in <1 year:* Botulism (history of honey exposure).

Prominent Autonomic Signs/Symptoms

- GBS, rabies, and acute myelopathy
- *Ascending weakness:* GBS, rabies, varicella zoster virus, and ascending myelitis
- *Descending weakness:* Diphtheria and botulism

TABLE 1: MRI spine findings in various cases of acute flaccid paralysis.

Pott's spine	Marrow edema, localized destruction of intervertebral disk, vertebral bodies and end plates, and pre-/paravertebral or epidural abscess
MOGAD	• Single or multiple longitudinal extensive lesions, gray matter involvement (H sign) • Conus lesions
NMOSD	Single longitudinal extensive lesion, bright spotty appearance of entire transverse diameter of the cord
GBS	Gadolinium enhanced nerve roots
Poliomyelitis like syndrome	Involvement of ipsilateral anterior horn cells, with T2 hyperintense lesions, do not enhance on gadolinium contrast unless there is radicular involvement

(GBS: Guillain–Barré syndrome; MOGAD: myelin oligodendrocyte glycoprotein antibody-associated disease; NMOSD: Neuromyelitis optica spectrum disorder)

Prominent and Early Ptosis

- Myasthenia gravis, botulism
- *Facial weakness:* GBS, myasthenia gravis and botulism
- *Fluctuating symptoms, fatigability:* Myasthenia gravis
- *Muscle tenderness:* Myositis and inflammatory myopathy (myalgias may be severe in GBS)

Muscle Stretch Reflexes

- *Absent:* GBS, poliomyelitis, diphtheria, spinal shock, and at level of spinal cord damage
- *Preserved:* Myasthenia gravis, periodic paralysis, and botulism
- *Exaggerated:* Below level of spinal lesion/upper motor neuron lesion

Spinal Tenderness, Painful Spine Movement

- Spinal trauma, epidural abscess, or other extradural compression
- *Neck stiffness:* Poliomyelitis, enteroviral myelitis, GBS, and transverse myelitis

Localization Based on Clinical Examination

A detailed clinical examination should be performed to localize the cause along the neuraxis **(Table 2)**.

TABLE 2: Clinical pointers to localize along the neuraxis and possible etiologies.

Localization along the neuraxis	***Clinical clues***	***Possible etiologies***
Anterior horn cell	Rapid progressive Asymmetric LMN weakness, arreflexia, no bladder bowel involvement, no sensory level, and fever at onset	Non polio viruses—enterovirus 71, coxsackie, echovirus, and West Nile virus
Radicles	• LMN weakness and arreflexia • Symmetric ascending weakness with no fever at onset, no sensory level, transient bladder involvement, cranial nerves 7, 9, 10, 11, and 12 involved occasionally	GBS and variants
Spinal cord	Symmetrical weakness, bladder involvement, LMN at the level of lesion and UMN signs below the level of lesion, and plantar extensor after the spinal shock stage	• Transverse myelitis—postinfective, demyelination • Vascular events • Spinal cord injury
Peripheral nerve	Sensory loss, glove and stocking sensory involvement, and loss of ankle reflex	• GBS variants • Metabolic neuropathy • Toxin induced neuropathy • Critical illness neuropathy
Neuromuscular junction	Diurnal variation, fluctuating weakness	Myasthenia gravis
Muscle	Hypotonia, LMN weakness, and reflexes elicitable	Polymyositis, dermatomyositis, and postviral myositis

(GBS: Guillain–Barré syndrome; LMN: lower motor neuron; UMN: upper motor neuron)

Guillain–Barré Syndrome

This is one of the most common causes of AFP in children. Peripheral nerves are the target of an abnormal immune response. In most cases, there is a history of an antecedent viral infection. The most common viral infection that precipitates this is usually respiratory infection, although in some gastrointestinal infections may be the cause. Enteritis caused by specific strains of *Campylobacter jejuni* is more often the cause of the acute axonal form of GBS, rather than the demyelinating variety.

The common subtypes include acute inflammatory demyelinating polyradiculoneuropathy (AIDP), acute motor axonal neuropathy (AMAN), acute motor sensory axonal neuropathy (AMSAN), and Miller Fisher syndrome.

The clinical presentation is usually with progressive motor weakness involving more than one limb—usually the legs. Mild sensory symptoms are usually present characterized by dysesthesia and muscle tenderness in the limbs. The weakness progresses to reach a nadir by about 2–3 weeks. Deep tendon reflexes are absent in all the weak muscles. Bilateral facial weakness occurs in about half of the children. Autonomic dysfunction such as arrhythmia, labile blood pressure, and gastrointestinal dysfunction may be seen. Respiratory involvement is not uncommon in this condition during the initial progressive phase of the illness and so needs close monitoring and appropriate intervention. Miller Fisher syndrome is characterized by ataxia, ophthalmoplegia, and arreflexia.

Recovery usually begins about 2–3 weeks after the progression stops and is usually complete in most children but takes even as much as 2–3 months in some cases. The prognosis is best when recovery begins early and also in children with the demyelinating variety rather than the axonal type.

Diagnosis is best with the help of nerve-conduction studies, which will help to distinguish the axonal variety from the demyelinating type. The earliest changes in AIDP are delayed or absent F and H responses, suggestive of demyelination with prolonged distal latencies and decreased conduction velocities. These changes are present in 50% of children by 2 weeks and in 85% by 3 weeks. Cerebrospinal fluid (CSF) examination during the second week may show mild elevation in CSF protein and a few mononuclear leukocytes (usually <10), albuminocytological dissociation.

Management is primarily supportive with careful monitoring for respiratory function and adequate support including ventilation in some during the initial phase. Intravenous immunoglobulin and plasma exchange hasten the recovery of GBS.

All cases of AFP should be notified in the appropriate form to the corporation health officials, as it is mandatory that we take samples for polioviruses from the stool specimen, soon after the diagnosis and then they will follow-up the cases and do the needful.

ACKNOWLEDGMENTS

We thank Indian Journal of Pediatrics for allowing us to reproduce charts from their publication.

KEY POINTS

- AFP is a neurological emergency, which requires urgent and detailed evaluation for the array of differential diagnoses.
- A detailed and quick clinical localization is important for ordering appropriate and tailored investigations, and planning management to reduce long-term morbidities.
- It is very important from the public health perspective to identify, notify cases for maintaining a strict and vigilant AFP surveillance system.

SUGGESTED READING

1. Banwell B, Bennett JL, Marignier R, Kim HJ, Brilot F, Flanagan EP, et al. Diagnosis of myelin oligodendrocyte glycoprotein antibody-associated disease: International MOGAD Panel proposed criteria. Lancet Neurol. 2023;22(3): 268-82.
2. Kliegman R, Behrman RE, Nelson WE. Nelson textbook of pediatrics, 20th edition. Philadelphia, PA: Elsevier; 2016. pp. 2.
3. Kunju M, Subir A, Eapen M. Acute flaccid paralysis beyond polio- a case based approach. Indian J Prac Pediatr. 2020; 22(1):36.
4. Leonhard SE, Mandarakas MR, Gondim FAA, Bateman K, Ferreira MLB, Cornblath DR, et al. Diagnosis and management of Guillain–Barré syndrome in ten steps. Nat Rev Neurol. 2019;15(11):671-83.
5. Van Doorn PA, Van den Bergh PYK, Hadden RDM, Avau B, Vankrunkelsven P, Attarian S, et al. European Academy of Neurology/Peripheral Nerve Society Guideline on diagnosis and treatment of Guillain–Barré syndrome. J Peripher Nerv Syst. 2023;28(4):535-63.
6. Wakerley BR, Yuki N. Mimics and chameleons in Guillain–Barré and Miller Fisher syndromes. Pract Neurol. 2015; 15(2):90-9.

Approach to Floppy Infant

Sarbani S Raha, Vrajesh Udani

INTRODUCTION

Floppiness or hypotonia is a common symptom and/or sign in infants presenting to a pediatric outpatient department (OPD) for complaints of developmental delay. Hypotonia may be secondary to diseases involving brain, spinal cord, nerves, or muscles. A systematic approach helps us decide appropriate investigations as well as reach the correct diagnosis without unwanted delays.

Weak infants always have hypotonia but hypotonic infants may not always be weak.

DEFINITION

Hypotonia is an impairment of the ability to sustain posture and control movement against gravity. Floppy infants exhibit delayed motor skills and hypotonic motor movement patterns.

Phasic tone is a rapid contraction in response to a high-intensity stretch. Postural tone is the prolonged contraction of antigravity muscles in response to the low-intensity stretch of gravity. The maintenance of normal tone requires intact central and peripheral nervous system.

A detailed history and neurological examination help differentiate between central hypotonia of upper motor neuron origin and motor unit disorders.

Infants who show delay in all aspects of development and have other evidence of brain dysfunctions abnormal eye movements or seizures, dysmorphic features, or exaggerated deep-tendon reflexes probably have a central cause of hypotonia. On the other hand, an alert and active infant who has significant motor weakness and absent deep-tendon reflexes is most likely to have a peripheral cause of hypotonia involving anterior horn cells, nerve, neuromuscular junction, or muscle **(Box 1)**.

BOX 1: Salient points in history-taking.

- Consanguineous marriage
- Reduced fetal movements
- Feeding difficulty in neonatal period
- Family history of sibling death/ similar illness
- Static versus progressive course
- Choking episodes
- Increased respiratory efforts, hospitalization for pneumonia

EXAMINATION OF A HYPOTONIC INFANT

- *Posture:* Lack of/reduced spontaneous movements; full abduction of legs; and arms either extended at the sides of the body or flexed at elbow with hands beside the head **(Fig. 1A)**
- *Skeletal:* Fixed deformities such as clubfoot, arthrogryposis, and pectus excavatum; hyperlaxity of skin and joints
- Dysmorphic features
- *Evidence of hypotonia:*
  - *Horizontal suspension:* The infant is suspended in prone position with the examiner's palm underneath the chest. The hands and legs of a hypotonic infant lie limply forming an inverted "U" posture.
  - *Vertical suspension:* An infant who has hypotonia "slips through" at the shoulders when the examiner grasps him/her under the arms in an upright position.
  - *Traction response:* Head lag or hyperextension is evident when the infant is pulled by the arms from a supine to sitting position **(Fig. 1B)**.
  - *Scarf sign:* In a hypotonic infant, on grasping the infant's hand and pulling it across the chest, the elbow can easily be brought well beyond the midline.

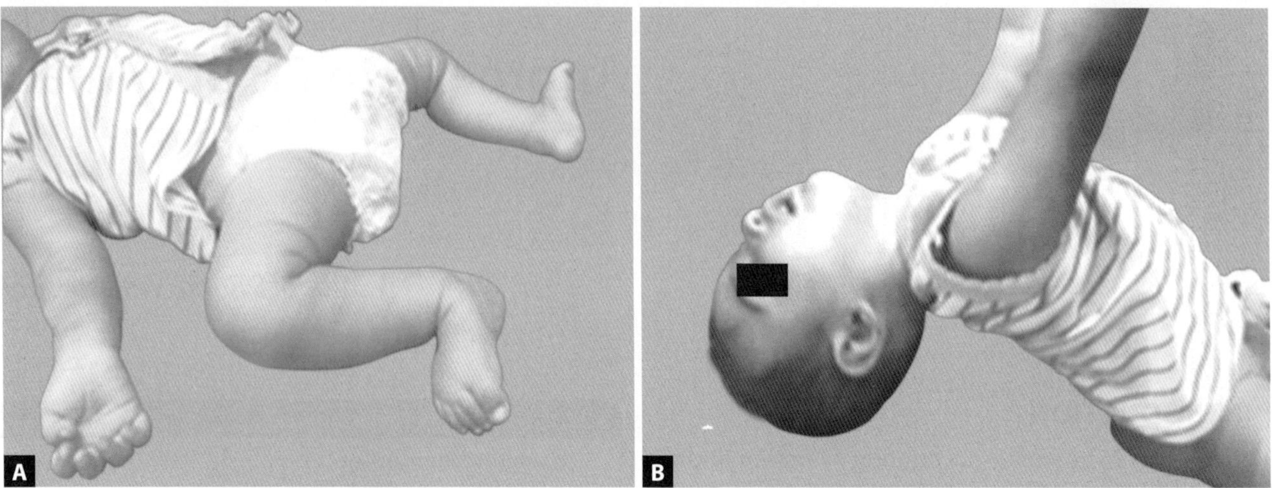

Figs. 1A and B: (A) Posture of a hypotonic infant; (B) Traction response.

Flowchart 1: Suggested approach to a floppy infant and stepwise investigations that would help reach a dagnosis.

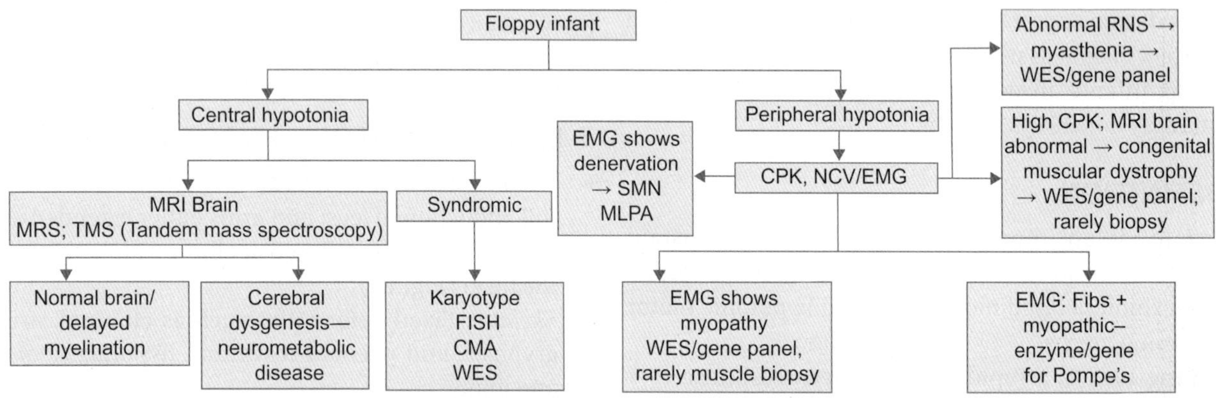

(CPK: creatine phosphokinase; EMG: electromyography; FISH: fluorescence *in situ* hybridization; MRI: magnetic resonance imaging; MRS: magnetic resonance spectroscopy; NCV: nerve conduction velocity; RNS: repetitive nerve stimulation; survival motor neuron)

- *Wheelbarrow:* In prone position when the child is raised holding his legs in the air, whether he/she can support his weight on hands is tested.

- A complete neurological examination should be performed. Of particular importance are the following:
  - Measurement of head circumference
  - *Facies:* Myopathic/hypotonic
  - Hypophonia
  - *Power:* Presence of antigravity movements
  - Tongue fibrillations, polyminimyoclonus
  - Paradoxical respiration
  - Examination of mother for myotonia.

A systematic approach and stepwise investigations will go a long way in diagnosing the underlying disorder in a floppy infant **(Flowchart 1)**.

BOX 2: Points favoring central hypotonia.

- Global developmental delay
- Dysmorphic features
- Increased tone of neck extensor
- Normal or brisk tendon reflexes
- Other organ involvement

CEREBRAL HYPOTONIA

Neonatal and infantile hypotonia is common in most cerebral disorders. But in some of them, hypotonia is one of the most prominent features, making it difficult to differentiate between a central versus peripheral cause **(Box 2)**.

SYNDROMIC HYPOTONIA

An infant with dysmorphism and hypotonia may require chromosomal analysis fluorescence *in situ* hybridization (FISH) studies to diagnose the appropriate syndrome. In selected cases whole exome sequencing may be diagnostic.

Prader-Willi Syndrome

This is caused by deletion of paternally-contributed proximal long arm of chromosome 15 or maternal disomy (both chromosomes 15 received from mother). Hypotonia at birth along with severe feeding problems requiring nasogastric tube feeding is a significant neonatal history in patients of Prader–Willi syndrome (PWS). Delayed milestone is the usual presenting feature. Hyperphagia and obesity develop later in childhood.

Joubert Syndrome

Classic Joubert syndrome is characterized by distinct cerebellar and brainstem malformations, hypotonia, and developmental delays. Often there is presence of oculomotor apraxia and episodic tachypnea. Cognitive disabilities are variable.

Many other syndromes have central hypotonia. Among them, Down syndrome is usually diagnosed early due to presence of typical facies.

NONSYNDROMIC CENTRAL HYPOTONIA

There are patients who have anomalies or abnormalities of central nervous system in absence of any particular syndrome. The neurological examination may reveal global or motor delay in presence of signs suggestive of central hypotonia. These patients may have presence of minor anomalies of the brain broadly classified as cerebral dysgenesis, some of them may have delayed myelination or even normal neuroimaging findings.

Systemic Disease

In a newborn and sometimes in infants, systemic disease can cause hypotonia. Presence of congenital heart disease and in an acute setting, sepsis may be responsible for hypotonia.

Craniocervical Junction Lesions

Obstetric injuries to the cord result in neonatal hypotonia. Later patients may have flexion of arms with flaccid paraplegia. A distended bladder with overflow incontinence is highly suggestive of cord injury in such cases.

CONGENITAL HYPOTONIA WITH FAVORABLE OUTCOME

This is a nonprogressive neurological disorder characterized by generalized flaccidity of muscles and hypermobile joints. Deep-tendon reflexes are normal or mildly exaggerated. An increased incidence of intellectual disability, learning disability, and likewise is evident later in life. A high family incidence is reported. This is a diagnosis of exclusion, and all routine investigations are normal.

CLINICAL PEARL

- Hypotonia without weakness may suggest a syndromic diagnosis (Down's and Prader-Willi).

MOTOR UNIT DISORDERS

There may be many clues in history and neurological examination that suggest a peripheral cause of hypotonia. A maternal account of reduced fetal movements and polyhydramnios; "myopathic" facies; tongue fasciculations or polyminimyoclonus; low-pitched cry; and lack of antigravity movements are all markers of a lower motor neuron cause of a floppy infant **(Box 3)**.

Differential Diagnosis (Table 1)

Spinal Muscular Atrophy

These are progressive group of disorders associated with deletions or mutations in exons 7 and 8 of the telomeric copy of the *survival motor neuron* gene (*SMN1*). The centromeric copy (SMN2) is the disease-modifying gene with milder cases having more copies.

In type 1, onset of weakness is before 6 months of age; most patients do not achieve sitting. In type 2, onset is

BOX 3: Evaluation of motor unit disorders.

- Creatine phosphokinase
- Neostigmine test
- *Electrodiagnosis:* Nerve conduction study, electromyography, and repetitive nerve stimulation
- *Genetic test:* SMN polymerase chain reaction (PCR) (for spinal muscular atrophy); CES or WES (clinical or whole exome sequencing)
- Enzyme analysis—alpha glucosidase (acid maltase)
- Muscle biopsy
- Nerve biopsy

TABLE 1: Differential diagnosis of peripheral hypotonia depending on the component of motor unit involved.

Motor neuron	*Nerve*	*Neuromuscular junction*	*Muscle*
Spinal muscular atrophy	• Congenital hypomyelinating neuropathy • Hereditary motor sensory neuropathy-familial dysautonomia	Congenital and transient myasthenia	• Congenital myotonic dystrophy • Congenital muscular dystrophy • Pompe's disease • Congenital myopathy

between 6–18 months; most patients can sit but never walk. In type 3, onset is after 18 months and such patients may be difficult to diagnose and confused with limb-girdle muscular dystrophy.

In spinal muscular atrophy (SMA), there is presence of proximal more than distal weakness and despite of intrauterine hypotonia, arthrogryposis is not present. Electromyography study reveals fibrillations and fasciculations.

Once the genetic testing confirms SMA, the same should be performed in chorionic villi biopsy sample for prenatal diagnosis in every subsequent pregnancy.

Gene replacement therapy called Zolgensma, and two drugs, called nusinersen (Spinraza) and risdiplam (Evyrsdi) are now available for treating SMA.

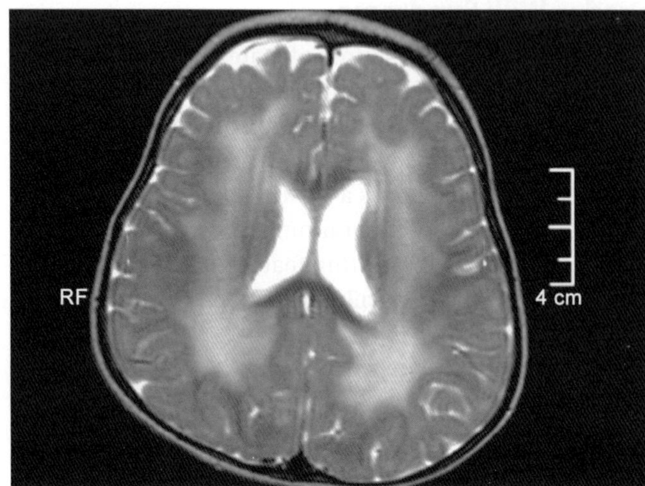

Fig. 2: T2-weighted axial sections of magnetic resonance imaging of brain in a patient with merosin deficient congenital muscular dystrophy demonstrating hyperintensities in periventricular white matter suggesting cerebral demyelination.

Congenital Muscular Dystrophy

This group is classified into syndromic and, nonsyndromic forms. The nonsyndromic form may have merosin-deficient congenital muscular dystrophy (CMD) or merosin-positive CMD. This is now called LAMA2 associated CMD.

Delayed motor milestones, hypotonia, contractures, and high creatine phosphokinase (CPK) values help to diagnose this condition. In merosin deficient CMD MRI brain shows abnormal T2 hyperintensity giving an impression of leukodystrophy **(Fig. 2)**.

Syndromic CMD is characterized by anomalies of cortical migration, ocular abnormalities such as cataract, and muscle disease with high CPK.

Congenital Myotonic Dystrophy

Prominent clinical feature of this autosomal dominant disorder includes facial diplegia; significant neonatal feeding difficulty; and mental retardation. The mother is usually the affected parent when a child has the disease. There is unstable trinucleotide (CTG) expansion with 300–1,000 CTG repeats and hence genetic anticipation is common in myotonic dystrophy type 1. Cardiac dysrhythmias and cataract may also be present.

Pompe's Disease

Hypotonia in Pompe's disease is the result of glycogen storage in brain, spinal cord, and skeletal muscles. The presence of cardiomegaly with abnormal electrocardiogram is highly suggestive of alpha glucosidase deficiency.

After establishing the diagnosis with the help of enzyme analysis, patient should be offered enzyme-replacement therapy which is available at certain centers in India.

Myasthenic Syndromes

Transitory neonatal myasthenia usually presents as hypotonia and feeding difficulty; the cry of such an infant is weak and there is lack of facial expression. Anti-acetylcholine receptor (AChR) antibody is high and such newborns respond to neostigmine.

Familial infantile myasthenia with prominent respiratory and feeding difficulty at birth and congenital myasthenia with predominant ocular findings are genetic myasthenic syndromes with negative anti-AChR antibodies. These patients may have episodic apneas which could be life threatening.

CLINICAL PEARL

- A very high CPK value usually points toward a muscular dystrophy.

NEONATAL HYPOTONIA

Hypotonia is a manifestation of many acute neonatal injuries.

The profile of disorders presenting with neonatal hypotonia to the neonatal intensive care unit was studied in an 11-year retrospective cohort of neonates admitted to the Neonatal Intensive Care Unit at the Montreal Children's Hospital (Montreal, Québec). Of the 50 neonates, who met the inclusion criteria, hypotonia was classified as central in 33 patients (66%) and peripheral in 17 (34%). Hypoxic-ischemic encephalopathy (n = 13), PWS (n = 6), myotonic dystrophy (n = 6), other muscle disorders (n = 6), chromosomal disorders (n = 4), and peripheral nerve disorders (n = 3) were the most common diagnoses. The genetic tests of highest yield were FISH and DNA methylation studies for PWS, CTG repeat testing for myotonic dystrophy, and karyotype analysis (Richer et al. 2001).

KEY POINTS

- Differentiating between central and peripheral hypotonia is the first step.
- Targeted investigations will yield better results.
- Many of the diseases are inherited, hence genetic counseling is important.
- Neonatal hypotonia can be specially challenging to investigate.

SUGGESTED READING

1. Bodensteiner JB. The evaluationof the hypotonic infant. Semin in Pediatr Neurol 2008;15:10-20.
2. Fenichel Gerald. Clinical Pediatric Neurology A signs and symptoms approach(5th edition). Elsevier; Philadelphia:2005.p.149-169.
3. Peredo DE, Hannibal MC. The floppy infant: evaluation of hypotonia. Pedaitr in Review 2009;30(9):66-76.
4. Prasad AN, Prasad C. Genetic evaluation of the floppy infant. Semin Fetal Neonatal Med 2011;16: 99-108.

Approach to Ataxia

Jayakumar Vaikundam

INTRODUCTION

Ataxia is a common symptom manifesting as unsteady gait, frequent falls, and clumsiness in walking or in using the hands due to derangement in posture control, movement, and coordination.

Ataxia can occur as a result of:

- Cerebellar dysfunction
- Posterior column dysfunction
- Vestibular dysfunction

Hence, as a first step one should be able to identify which is the main structure that is affected to result in ataxia. **Table 1** will help in the differentiation.

SENSORY ATAXIA

The most common cause of sensory ataxia in children is vitamin B_{12} deficiency. It is more commonly seen in vegetarians. Apart from the dietary insufficiency and malabsorptive state, lack of intrinsic factor can also lead to vitamin B_{12} deficiency state.

It is clinically characterized by anemia, lethargy, poor cognitive performance, hypotonia, sensory ataxia, and involuntary movements especially in infants. Neurological examination will reveal hyporeflexia, posterior column involvement, and bilateral extensor plantar response due to additional pyramidal tract involvement.

TABLE 1: Differentiating features of different structures involved in the causation of ataxia.

Features	*Posterior column*	*Vestibular*	*Cerebellar*
Headache/vomiting	–	+/–	+/–
Tinnitus/vertigo	–	Often present	+/–
Speech	Normal	Normal	Slurring/Scanning/Staccato
Titubation	–	–	+/–
Nystagmus	–	• Seen in primary position often with rotary component with direction of the fast phase away from the side of lesion • Positional nystagmus is common	• Usually not seen in primary position Gaze evoked (fast component to the direction of gaze) • Rebound nystagmus is also a sign of intrinsic cerebellar lesion • Positional nystagmus is not common
Clumsiness and incoordination of upper limb	–	–	Common
Hypotonia	+/–	–	Often seen in acute lesions
Romberg sign	+	–	–
Gait	Sensory ataxia more prominent on eye closure or in darkness	Tendency to lurch to one side	Wide based, staggering, lurching, and drunken ataxia
Other signs	Other signs of peripheral nerve or cord involvement	Positional vertigo and blocking feeling in the ear	Dysdiadochokinesia, dyssynergia, and dysmetria

One important clinical clue for vitamin B_{12} deficiency state is the presence of hyperpigmentation over the dorsum of interphalangeal joints, knuckles, palmar creases, intertriginous areas, and recent scars. The mechanism for hyperpigmentation is not known and it is reversible disappearing with treatment.

Peripheral smear studies will show macrocytic anemia, hypersegmented polymorphs, bone marrow showing megaloblastic reaction. Serum vitamin B_{12} level is low. Magnetic resonance imaging studies usually show the picture of subacute combined degeneration causing increased signal intensity in T2W images in the posterior columns of cervical and thoracic spinal cord. Treatment may reverse these changes.

CLINICAL PEARL

- Hyperpigmentation over the knuckles, interphalangeal joints in an ataxic child should suggest the possibility of vitamin B_{12} deficiency which is eminently treatable.

VESTIBULAR ATAXIA

Recurrent attacks of vertigo with unsteadiness, nystagmus, and vomiting sometimes can occur in infants and preschool children as a part of benign paroxysmal vertigo. The episode lasts for few minutes and may recur irregularly.

It is often considered as a variant of migraine and nearly one-fourth of them subsequently develop migraine. There is often a family history of migraine.

CEREBELLAR ATAXIA

Cerebellar dysfunction appears to be the most common cause for ataxia and is characterized by the following clinical features which will help to some extent to identify which portion of the cerebellum is the most affected, although there is a considerable overlap.

- *Ataxia:*
  - Vermis lesions produce truncal ataxia and titubation
  - Hemispherical lesions produce limb ataxia with a tendency to lurch to the side of lesion
  - Anterior lobe lesions produce gait ataxia
- *Kinetic tremor and incoordination:* Seen in hemispherical lesions involving dentate nucleus
- *Hypotonia:* Seen mostly in acute lesions than in chronic
- *Nystagmus and eye movement abnormalities:* Seen commonly in flocculonodular lobe and vermis lesions
- *Dysarthria:* Slurring, scanning, and staccato speech are commonly in left cerebellar hemispherical lesions.

CLINICAL PEARLS

- Nystagmus, dysarthria, incoordination suggest cerebellar ataxia.
- Hypotonia is usually seen in acute lesions than in chronic.

Table 2 describes the localizing features of different signs.

CLINICAL PEARLS

- Nystagmus is a sign of flocculonodular lobe lesion.
- Truncal ataxia is a sign of vermis lesion.
- Limb incoordination is a sign of cerebellar hemispherical lesion.
- Gait ataxia is a sign of involvement of anterior lobe of cerebellum.

Clinical Approach to Cerebellar Ataxia

Cerebellar ataxia can be acute, intermittent/episodic or chronic. **Flowchart 1** describes the different causes.

Acute Cerebellar Ataxias

Acute cerebellar ataxias due to infective/parainfective causes:

- Often occur following infections with varicella, mumps, and other viral infections
- Occur either immediately following fever or within 6 weeks, characterized by headache, vomiting, a severe

TABLE 2: Cerebellar ataxia: localizing features.

Site of involvement	*Clinical features*
Midline: • Upper vermis lesion • Lower vermis lesion • Fastigial nuclear lesion	Abnormal stance, truncal ataxia, titubation abnormal head-posture and eye-movement abnormalities • Abasia, gait ataxia are prominent • Nystagmus is prominent • Abasia (difficulty in maintaining the stance)
Intermediate (lesions affecting interposed nuclei)	Rebound response, titubation, dysdiadochokinesia, finger nose, heel-knee shin incoordination, kinetic tremor, proximal limb oscillation of outstretched arms
Lateral hemispherical (lesions affecting dentate nuclei)	Cerebellar dysarthria (especially in left-sided lesions), limb ataxia, hypotonia, kinetic tremor and eye-movement abnormalities

Flowchart 1: Approach to an ataxic child (acute/episodic intermittent cerebellar ataxia).

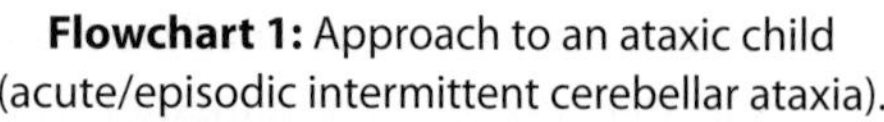

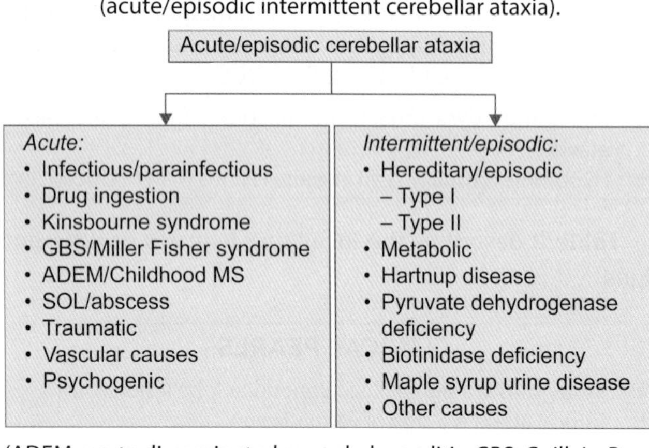

(ADEM: acute disseminated encephalomyelitis; GBS: Guillain-Barré syndrome; MS: multiple sclerosis; SOL: space occupying lesion)

gait disturbance, nystagmus, and behavioral changes with increased cerebrospinal fluid (CSF) cell count in viral cerebellitis and normal cell count in postinfectious ataxia along with mild increase in proteins

- Although there is no specific therapy, most of them respond well to antiviral (acyclovir) drugs, steroids, and intravenous immunoglobulin therapy.

Ataxia due to drugs:

- Overdose of phenytoin, phenobarbitone, carbamazepine, phenothiazines, benzodiazepines, and sometimes anthelmintic drugs like piperazine; antihistamine are well-known to produce acute ataxias
- Some helpful clues are drowsiness, vomiting, or nystagmus which is less prominent on downward gaze and absence of fever
- Electroencephalogram in some of these patients may show diffuse fast activity, indicative of sedative drug overdose
- The treatment depends on the identification of the specific causative drug. In certain life-threatening situations, dialysis and vital support function may be required.

Kinsbourne syndrome (opsoclonus myoclonus syndrome): It is characterized by—

- Acute or subacute onset of peculiar dancing eye movements in different directions and planes (opsoclonus) due to unwanted spontaneous saccades. Opsoclonus may persist during sleep
- Myoclonic jerking of the trunk and limbs which may be stimulus sensitive and may increase with action
- Child is often irritable and ataxic and may require support with hands and may be even afraid of standing or sitting without support
- Nearly about 50% of the children with opsoclonus-myoclonus may have occult neuroblastoma and these symptoms can precede the diagnosis of the tumor
- May need abdominal ultrasonogram; urinary vanillylmandelic acid and homovanillic acid estimation; and in some cases computed tomography chest, abdomen; metaiodobenzylguanidine; or Dotatoc scan may be required
- Injection adrenocorticotropic hormone is useful in some patients.

Guillain-Barré syndrome/Miller Fisher syndrome

- Early stages of Guillain-Barré syndrome (GBS) can present with ataxia and subsequently patient may develop weakness
- A variant of GBS—viz. Miller Fisher syndrome characterized by acute ataxia, ophthalmoplegia, and areflexia can present with acute ataxia
- Ophthalmoplegia in Miller Fisher syndrome starts initially with upward gaze restriction followed by lateral gaze and finally down gaze restriction
- Intravenous immunoglobulin therapy is useful.

Acute disseminated encephalomyelitis:

- Acute disseminated encephalomyelitis is usually a monophasic illness following a viral infection, immunization or vaccination usually after an afebrile period following the initial febrile illness
- Usually characterized by altered mental status, irritability and lethargy, seizures, and focal neurological deficits
- Some children may present with brainstem signs, limb ataxia, nystagmus, and bilateral optic neuritis (in multiple sclerosis the optic neuritis is unilateral)
- In MRI, T2W/FLAIR images will show multiple subcortical lesions (usually at the junction of deep cortical gray and subcortical white matter) with smudging of edges (in contrast the multiple sclerosis lesions will have sharp clear margins)
- Treatment involves mainly intravenous methyl prednisolone and in some cases intravenous immunoglobulin.

Childhood multiple sclerosis:

- Around 4–5% of them can occur in children (mostly around 10–15 years of age)
- Visual disturbances are common apart from brainstem, cerebellar, and long tract disturbances

- In contrast to adult type of multiple sclerosis, seizures and mental status changes are common in children
- Magnetic resonance imaging typically shows hyperintense T2W lesions in cerebellum, brainstem, periventricular, and pericallosal white matter
- Evoked potentials studies and CSF immunoglobulin G index and CSF analysis for oligoclonal bands are useful
- Treatment involves intravenous methyl prednisolone.

Psychogenic: The following clues help in the diagnosis of acute psychogenic ataxia—

- Ataxia occurs immediately on standing
- Bizarre and gross
- Absence of wide based stance
- Tendency to move from one object to another in a room to get a support
- Absence of other neurological signs.

Other causes:

- Space-occupying-lesions—cerebellar abscess
- Traumatic
- Vascular—cerebellar hemorrhage, infarct, or arterial dissection
- Basilar migraine.

CLINICAL PEARLS

- Drug-induced ataxia should always be considered first in acute ataxia.
- Past history of chicken pox should always be asked.
- Guillain-Barré syndrome should be considered when there is ataxia with absent deep tendon reflexes.
- In a febrile ataxic child with history of chronic suppurative otitis media, always rule out cerebellar abscess.
- Past history of similar episode could suggest the possibility of episodic ataxias.

Episodic/Recurrent/Intermittent Ataxias

Recurrent attacks of ataxia can occur either as a form of hereditary episodic ataxia or due to some metabolic disorders.

Hereditary episodic ataxia: Although there are four types of hereditary ataxias Type I and Type II are more common and their differentiating features are outlined in the **Table 3**.

Metabolic disorders producing intermittent ataxia: The usual clues are—lethargy, vomiting and occasional ICT. The following metabolic disorders can present with intermittent ataxia.

- Hartnup disease
- Pyruvate dehydrogenase deficiency
- Biotidinase deficiency
- Maple syrup urine disease
- Certain urea cycle—ornithine transcarbamylase deficiency

Other causes of intermittent ataxia: Children with Down syndrome can present with ataxia, transient weakness of the limbs, especially after sudden flexion of the neck usually after vigorous toweling of the head after head bath due to recurrent atlanto-axial subluxation.

CLINICAL PEARLS

- Pellagra like pigmentation suggest the possibility of Hartnup disease.
- Increased blood pyruvate and lactate suggest pyruvate dehydrogenase deficiency.
- Alopecia, dermatitis, and deafness suggest biotinidase deficiency.
- Acetazolamide is useful for Type I and Type II hereditary episodic ataxias.
- Always rule-out atlanto-axial subluxation in an ataxic Down syndrome child.

TABLE 3: Hereditary episodic ataxias.

Features	*Type I*	*Type II*
Age	5–7 years	School going/adolescents
Precipitating factors	Exercise, fever, sudden movement, carbohydrate meal	–
Duration	Few seconds to minutes	Few minutes to few days
Frequency	Several times per day	1–3 times per month
Attacks	Mainly ataxia	Ataxia, dysarthria, diplopia, vertigo
Useful clinical clue in between the attacks	Myokymia (seen in periorbital, facial, and hand muscles)	Nystagmus
Ion channel involved	Potassium channel gene KCNA1 linked to chromosome 12p13	Calcium channel CACNA1A in Chromosome 19p
Treatment	Acetazolamide, phenytoin	Acetazolamide, flunarizine, 4-aminopyridine

Chronic Ataxias

Chronic ataxia can be nonprogressive or progressive and the various causes are outlined in the **Flowchart 2**.

Chronic nonprogressive cerebellar ataxias: There are two major conditions which can cause nonprogressive cerebellar ataxias, viz.

1. Congenital malformations of the brain
2. Ataxic form of cerebral palsy.

1. *Congenital malformations of the brain:* The following malformations often cause nonprogressive cerebellar ataxia—

- Cerebellar hypoplasia
- Vermian hypoplasia:
  - Joubert's syndrome
  - Dandy-Walker syndrome
  - Chiari malformation
  - Rhombencephalosynapsis
- Congenital cerebellar hypoplasia:
  - Autosomal recessive disorder
  - Characterized by hypotonia, ataxia, nystagmus
  - Magnetic resonance imaging (MRI) of brain will show mainly cerebellar hemispherical atrophy
  - It should be differentiated from other progressive conditions by serial MRI and involvement of brainstem and other neurological findings.
- *Cerebellar vermian hypoplasia:* The vermis of the cerebellum is maximally involved in the following conditions:
  - Joubert's syndrome:
    - Autosomal recessive disorder with partial or total agenesis or hypoplasia of the vermis
    - Characteristic facies, squint, ataxia, oculomotor apraxia, and breathing abnormalities are typical
    - MRI brain will show the following characteristic findings:
      - Molar tooth appearance of the brainstem
      - Bullet-shaped upper-fourth ventricle
      - Horizontal superior cerebellar peduncle
      - Bat-wing appearance of the lower fourth ventricle.
  - Dandy-Walker malformation:
    - Clinically patients present with hydrocephalus and large posterior fossa
    - Vermian hypoplasia (mainly caudal vermis) and cystic dilatation of the fourth ventricle are characteristic imaging findings
  - Chiari malformation:
    - Clinically patients present with vague pain in the neck, suboccipital headache, and ataxia
    - The characteristic clinical clues are presence of down beat nystagmus, oscillopsia
    - May be associated with syrinx, lower cranial nerves palsy and skeletal abnormalities
    - Magnetic resonance imaging of craniovertebral junction will show downward displacement of the cerebellar tonsil which is peg shaped. Coexistent syrinx may be seen
    - Treatment involves surgical decompression.

Flowchart 2

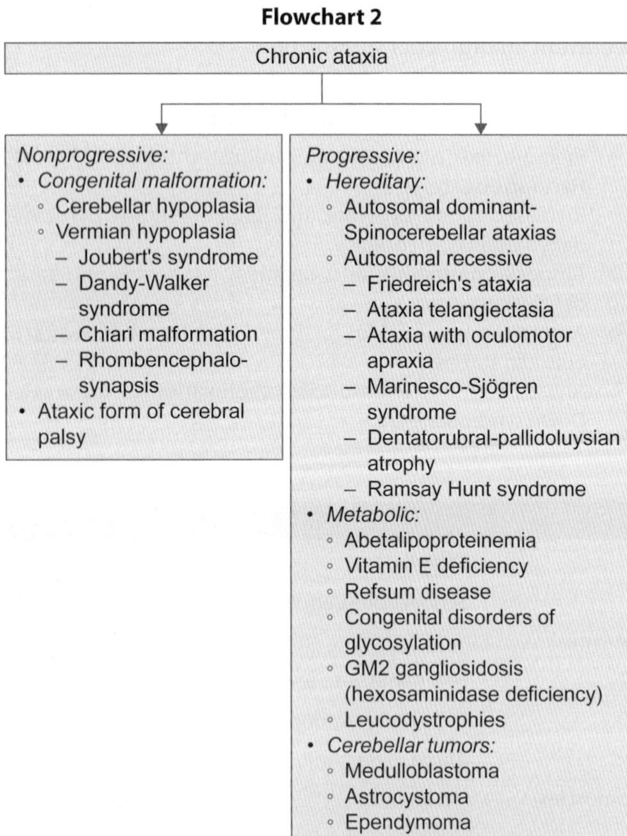

2. *Ataxic form of cerebral palsy:*

- Accounts for 5–10% of all forms of cerebral palsy
- 50% of them are autosomal recessively inherited
- History of birth asphyxia, mild spasticity, brisk reflexes, and ataxia
- Lack of correlation between imaging and clinical findings
- Recent gene mapping to chromosome 9p12-q12 is useful to differentiate this from other conditions.

CLINICAL PEARLS

- Most of the congenital cerebellar malformations cause nonprogressive ataxias.
- Brisk deep tendon reflexes in a child with nonprogressive ataxia suggest the possibility of ataxic form of cerebral palsy.
- Imaging findings do not correlate with clinical picture in ataxic cerebral palsy.

Chronic progressive cerebellar ataxias: Chronic progressive cerebellar ataxias could be due to—

- Hereditary ataxias which could be autosomal dominant or autosomal recessively inherited
- Metabolic disorders
- Cerebellar tumors
- Chronic hydrocephalus.
- Hereditary ataxias:
    - Autosomal dominant variety is mostly seen in adults
    - Autosomal recessive disorders include:
        - Friedreich's ataxia
        - Ataxia telangiectasia
        - Ataxia with oculomotor apraxia
        - Abetalipoproteinemia
        - Vitamin E deficiency
        - Congenital disorder of glycosylation
        - Refsum disease
        - Marinesco-Sjogren syndrome.
    - Autosomal recessive hereditary ataxias:
        - Friedreich's ataxia:
            - Autosomal recessive disorder due to defective expression of "frataxin" encoded by X25 gene at chromosome 9
            - Onset around puberty
            - Pes cavus, loss of deep tendon reflexes; extensor plantar and posterior column sensory loss, apart from cerebellar signs are the cardinal features
            - In 25% of them deep-tendon reflexes may be normal
            - Magnetic resonance imaging brain will show atrophy of cerebellum, cervical cord and abnormal signals in the posterior and lateral columns
            - Nerve conduction and somatosensory evoked potentials studies may show abnormality
            - Cardiomyopathy is seen in 50% and diabetes in 10%
            - Idebenone has been found to be useful for cardiac dysfunction
            - Diagnosis is confirmed by genetic testing showing GAA trinucleotide repeats in the range of 600–900 repeats

CLINICAL PEARL

- Deep tendon reflexes can be normal in 25% of patients with Friedreich's ataxia.

        - Ataxia telangiectasia:
            - Autosomal recessive disorder affecting nervous and immune system due to deficiency of ataxia-telangiectasia mutated (ATM) protein
            - Mutation in the large *ATM* gene linked to chromosome 11q22-23
            - Choreoathetosis followed by ataxia and dysarthria occur early
            - Oculomotor apraxia is seen in 90% of patients.
            - Telangiectasia:
                - Develops after 2–10 years of age
                - Seen in bulbar conjunctiva, upper ears, forearm, and face **(Fig. 1)**
                - Exacerbated by exposure to sunlight
                - Tends to grow with advancing age
            - Recurrent sinopulmonary infection and prone for lymphoma and leukemia (38%)
            - Serum α-fetoprotein and carcinoembryonic antigen are elevated
            - Serum IgG, IgA are reduced and IgM elevated

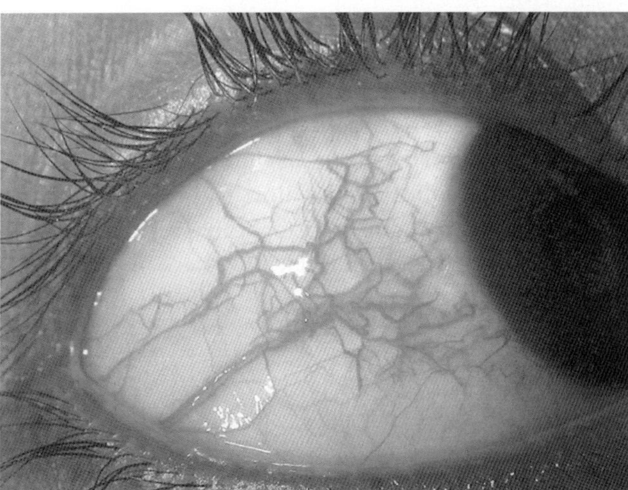

Fig. 1: Bulbar conjunctival telangiectasia. *(For color version, see Plate 8)*

- Betamethasone 0.1 mg/kg/day divided every 12 hours for 4 weeks has been found to be useful in some patients.

CLINICAL PEARLS

- Conjunctival telangiectasia develops later usually after 2 years of age.
- Telangiectasia tends to grow with age.
- Telangiectasia becomes more prominent after exposure to sunlight for some time.
- Oculomotor apraxia is seen in Joubert's syndrome, ataxia telangiectasia, ataxia with oculomotor apraxia without telangiectasia, and in Gaucher's disease.
- Serum albumin testing is important.

- Ataxia with oculomotor apraxia **(Table 4)**:
  - Autosomal recessive disorder often mistaken for ataxia telangiectasia
  - No conjunctival telangiectasia and linked to chromosome 9p14
  - Two types are described.
- Others:
  - GM2 Gangliosidosis—low α and β hexosaminidase A in fibroblasts
  - Ramsay-Hunt syndrome is characterized by progressive myoclonus and ataxia
  - Marinesco-Sjögren syndrome is characterized by congenital cataract, skeletal abnormalities, mental retardation, and ataxia
  - Dentato rubro-pallidoluysian atrophy seen mostly among Japanese.

- Metabolic disorders causing progressive ataxias:
  - Abetalipoproteinemia (Bassen-Kornzweig disease):
    - Autosomal recessive disorder
    - Due to absence of microsomal triglycerides transfer protein, linked to chromosome 4q22-q24 causing absence of apolipoprotein B which results in deficiency of vitamins A, D, E, and K
    - Failure to thrive, steatorrhea, vomiting, ataxia, areflexia, and proprioceptive disturbance are the common clinical features

TABLE 4: Types of ataxia with oculomotor apraxia.

Features	*Type I*	*Type II*
Age of onset	Early age	Adolescence
Gait ataxia	+	+
Oculomotor apraxia	Common and prominent	Less common
Serum albumin	Reduced	Normal

    - Retinitis pigmentosa is a constant feature usually seen before 10 years of age
    - Peripheral smear will reveal acanthocytosis
    - Plasma cholesterol and triglycerides are low (due to low apolipoprotein B)
    - Nerve conduction studies may show abnormalities
    - Treatment includes restriction of fat, and large doses of vitamin E (100 mg/kg/day).
  - Vitamin E deficiency:
    - Autosomal recessive disorder linked to chromosome 8q13
    - No malabsorption only isolated deficiency of vitamin E
    - Ataxia and peripheral neuropathy
    - Resembles Friedreich's ataxia
    - Diagnosed by low vitamin E level and normal vitamin E absorption
    - Treatment includes 800–900 IU of vitamin E.

CLINICAL PEARL

- Isolated vitamin E deficiency can resemble Friedreich's ataxia. Hence, when in doubt, it is always better to give a therapeutic trial with vitamin E.

  - Refsum disease:
    - Autosomal recessive disorder due to deficiency of phytanic acid oxidase
    - Clinical features include:
      - Cerebellar ataxia
      - Deafness
      - Retinitis pigmentosa
      - Thickened nerves
      - Chronic demyelinating sensory motor neuropathy
      - Increased CSF proteins
      - *Serum phytanic acid level increased:* Plasma exchange is useful apart from restriction of dietary phytanic acid.
  - Congenital disorder of glycosylation (carbohydrate deficient glycoprotein syndrome):
    - Autosomal recessive disorder linked to chromosome 16p13 affecting glycoprotein synthesis as a result of abnormal glycosylation
    - Clinically characterized by multisystem involvement:
      - *Neurological:* Psychomotor retardation, hypotonia ataxia, cerebellar hypoplasia, squint,

stroke-like-episodes, sometimes seizures, and peripheral nerve involvement
  - *Dysmorphism:* Almond shaped eyes, large forehead, and inverted nipples
  - *Lipocutaneous anomalies:* Peau d'orange skin, and infiltration with fat over the thighs and buttocks producing pads of fat
  - *Hepatodigestive:* Hepatic cytolysis, and hepatic fibrosis
  - *Cardiac:* Pericarditis and cardiomyopathy
- *Diagnosis:* Isoelectrofocusing of serum transferrin
- Treatment consists of use of ketogenic diet, mannose, aspirin, and bisphosphonates.

> **CLINICAL PEARL**
>
> Suspect congenital disorder of glycosylation in a child with ataxia with inverted nipples, supragluteal pads of fat and peau d' orange skin.

- Cerebellar tumors:
  - Medulloblastoma
  - Cerebellar astrocytoma
  - Ependymoma
  - Cerebellar hemangioblastoma (von Hippel-Lindau disease)
  - Brainstem glioma.

Flowchart 3: Summary of approach to ataxias in children.

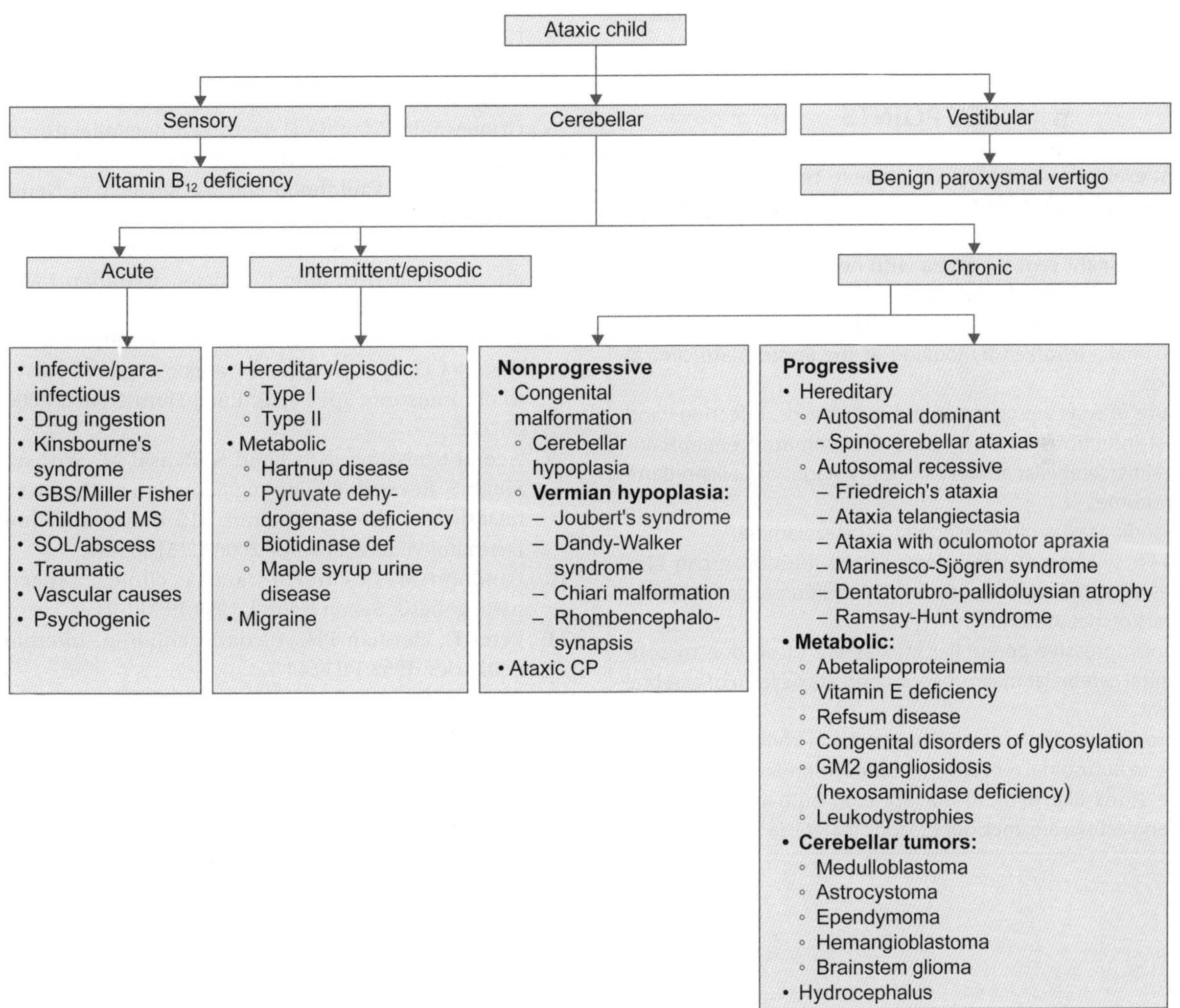

(CP: cerebral palsy; GBS: Guillain-Barré syndrome; MS: multiple sclerosis; SOL: space occupying lesion)

CLINICAL PEARLS

- Vomiting, nystagmus, truncal ataxia and torticollis in a preschool child suggest the possibility of medulloblastoma.
- Unilateral cerebellar signs with features of increased intracranial pressure (ICP) in a 5–10 years old child think of the possibility of cerebellar astrocytoma which has a good prognosis.
- Ependymoma of the floor of the fourth ventricle can present with only intractable vomiting.
- Presence of retinal angioma in an ataxic child suggests the possibility of von Hippel-Lindau disease.
- Ataxia with multiple lower cranial nerve palsies (6th and 7th) suggest the possibility of brainstem glioma where symptoms of ICP manifest late.

- *Hydrocephalus:* Hydrocephalus due to any cause can present with gait ataxia and symptoms of raised ICT.

Flowchart 3 gives the summary of approach to ataxias in children.

KEY POINTS

- First evaluate whether ataxia is due to cerebellar, vestibular or sensory involvement.
- Vitamin B_{12} deficiency should be suspected when there is predominant sensory ataxia with hyperpigmentation over the knuckles, interphalangeal joints.
- In cerebellar ataxias ascertain which part of cerebellum is maximally involved by looking at the appropriate clinical signs.
- Acute ataxias are commonly due to drugs, infectious and post-infectious causes, acute disseminated encephalomyelitis, cerebellar abscess and early stages of Guillain-Barré syndrome.
- Episodic ataxias often respond to acetazolamide.
- Down syndrome with atlantoaxial subluxation can also present with intermittent ataxia in addition to some inborn errors of metabolism.
- Nonprogressive cerebellar ataxias are often due to congenital cerebellar malformations and ataxic form of cerebral palsy.
- Chronic hereditary cerebellar ataxias in children are often due to autosomal recessively inherited conditions.
- Eye signs like oculomotor apraxia, bulbar conjunctival telangiectasia are important to look for (ataxia telangiectasia).
- Vitamin E deficiency induced ataxia may resemble Friedreich's ataxia. Hence a therapeutic trial of vitamin E is worth.
- Cerebellar tumors and hydrocephalus can present as chronic progressive cerebellar ataxia.
- Always look for treatable causes of cerebellar ataxia before making the diagnosis of cerebellar degeneration.

SUGGESTED READING

1. Brazis PW, Masdeu JC, Biller J. Localization in clinical Neurology, 5th edition. (Indian reprint). Philadelphia: Lippincott Williams & Wilkins; 2007. p. 374.
2. Buoni S, Zannolli R, Sorrentino L, Fois A. Betamethasone and improvement of neurological symptoms in ataxia-telangiectasia., Arch Neurol. 2006;63:1479-82.
3. Facchini SA, Jami MM, Neuberg RW, Sorrell AD. A treatable cause of ataxia in children. Pediatr Neurol. 2001; 24(2):135-8.
4. Ghezzi A, Deplano V, Faroni J, Grasso MG, Liguori M, Marrosu G, et al. Multiple sclerosis in childhood: clinical features of 149 cases. Mult Scler. 1997;3(1):43-6.
5. Grunewald S, Matthijs G, Jaeken J. Congenital disorders of glycosylation: a review. Pediatric Research. 2002;52:618-24.
6. Jayakumar V. Childhood ataxias. Reviews in Neurology. 2008;14:339-72.
7. Jayaram S, Soman A, Tarvade S, Londhe V. Cerebellar ataxia due to isolated vitamin E deficiency. Indian J Med Sci. 2005;59(1):20-3.
8. McHale DP, Jackson AP, Campbell, Levene MI, Corry P, Woods CG, et al. A gene for ataxic cerebral palsy maps to chromosome 9p12–q12. Eur J Hum Genet. 2000;8(4): 267-72.
9. Neeraj Srivastava N, Chand S, Bansal M, Srivastava K, Singh S. Reversible hyperpigmentation as the first manifestation of dietary vitamin B12 deficiency. Indian J Dermatol Venereol Leprol. 2006;72(5):389-90.
10. Pandolfo M. Friedreich's ataxia: clinical aspects and pathogenesis. Semin Neurol. 1999;19:311-21.
11. Peter H, Berman PH. Ataxia in children. International Pediatrics. 1999;14(1):44-7.
12. Schöls L, Bauer P, Schmidt T, Schulte T, Riess O. Autosomal dominant cerebellar ataxias; clinical features, genetics and pathogeneses. The Lancet Neurology. 2004;3:291-304.
13. Singhvi JP, Prabhakar S, Singh P. Episodic ataxia: a case report and review of literature. Neurol India. 2000;48: 78-80.

Acute Hemiplegia in Children: An Algorithm for Diagnosis and Treatment

Monika Chhajed

INTRODUCTION

Hemiplegia is defined as severe or complete loss of strength in the arm, leg, and sometimes face on one side of the body. Hemiparesis is defined as partial weakness of one-half of the body. The etiology of hemiplegia is vast and varied. It can be quite challenging to recognize acute hemiparesis in young children.

HEMIPLEGIA IN INFANTS

Infantile hemiplegia occurs due to brain injuries that happen before or at birth and lead to hemiplegia. Infantile hemiplegia can be because of prenatal and perinatal disorders, which may not be recognized until several months after birth, although the insult to the developing brain was sustained earlier. The most common cause is probably a vascular lesion occurring during birth. It can also be associated with viral and bacterial infections, trauma, systemic diseases, cerebral arteriovenous malformations, porencephaly, cardiac abnormalities, status epilepticus, and tumors and their related complications. Recently, COL4A1 mutations have been identified as a cause of infantile hemiplegia/quadriplegia, stroke, or epilepsy, in children. The presence of eye, kidney abnormalities, and white matter changes on magnetic resonance imaging (MRI) brain help point toward the diagnosis.

Perinatal Stroke

Perinatal ischemic stroke is a cerebrovascular disease that leads to ischemic and hemorrhagic injury around focal or multiple cerebral vessels. In 2006, perinatal ischemic stroke was defined as "a group of heterogeneous conditions in which there is focal disruption of cerebral blood flow secondary to arterial or cerebral venous embolization or thrombosis, between 20 weeks of fetal life and the 28th postnatal day, which can be confirmed by neuroimaging or neuropathological studies." Perinatal ischemic stroke can be divided into two main groups: Perinatal arterial ischemic stroke (PAIS) and cerebral sinovenous thrombosis (CSVT). The incidence of PAIS ranges from 1 in 2,300 to 1 in 5,000 births, while the incidence of CSVT is much lower, ranging from 0.6 to 12 per 100,000 live births. PAIS is associated with significant morbidity, including long-term neurological complications, such as epilepsy, cerebral palsy, and cognitive abnormalities. The risk factors for PAIS include intrapartum fever >38°C, pre-eclampsia, primiparity, forceps delivery, oligohydramnios, vacuum delivery, fetal heart rate abnormalities, abnormal cardiotocography tracing, cord abnormalities, birth asphyxia, emergency cesarean section, tight nuchal cord, meconium-stained amniotic fluid, umbilical arterial pH <7.10, Apgar score at 5 min <7, resuscitation at birth, hypoglycemia, male gender and small for gestational age, etc. **(Fig. 1)**.

> **CLINICAL PEARL**
>
> - Focal clonic seizure in the newborn period is the most common clinical symptom of perinatal arterial ischemic stroke.

Hemiconvulsion–Hemiplegia–Epilepsy Syndrome

Hemiconvulsion–hemiplegia–epilepsy syndrome is a rare outcome of prolonged focal status epilepticus in childhood. The prolonged focal motor seizure usually occurs during the course of a febrile illness and is followed by hemiplegia, ipsilateral to the side of convulsions. A prolonged febrile seizure leads to inflammation, which may worsen the level of cell injury. Inflammation and prolonged ictal activity act on blood-brain-barrier permeability. There may also be predisposing factors facilitating prolonged seizure such as focal epileptogenic lesion or genetic factors **(Fig. 2)**.

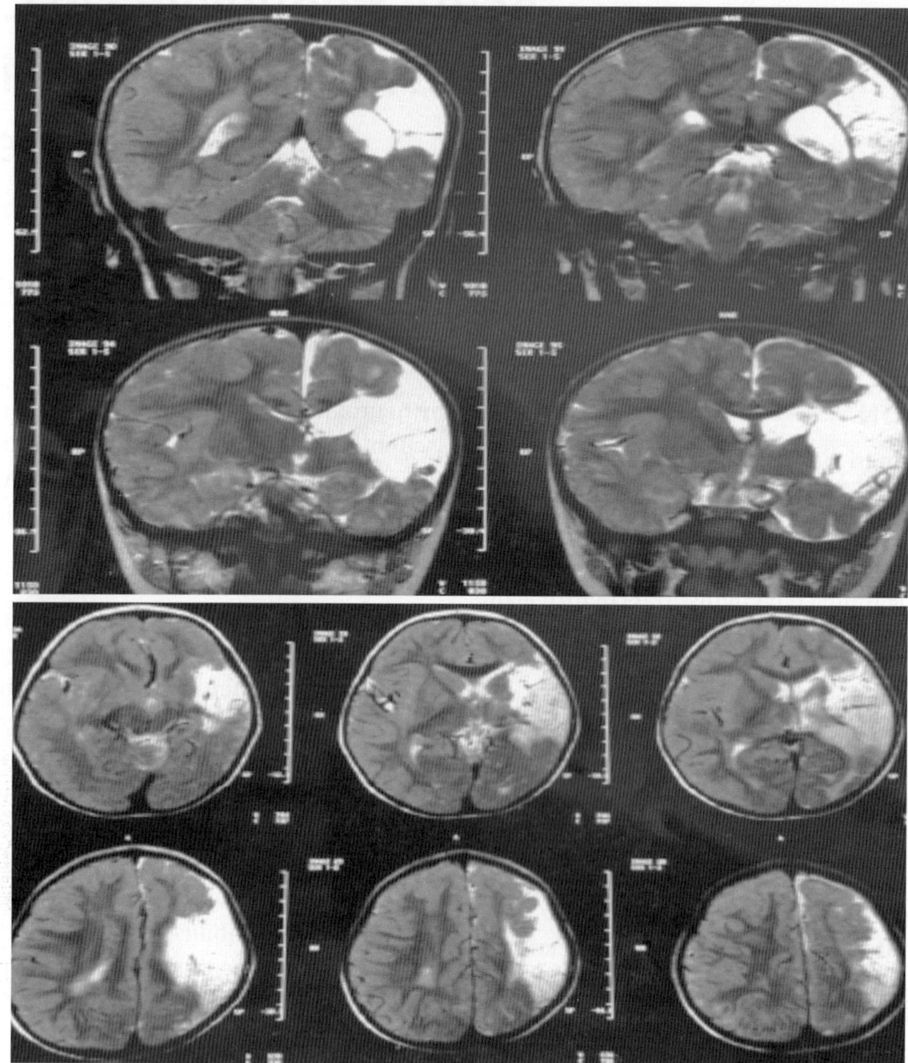

Fig. 1: *T2-weighted coronal and axial magnetic resonance imaging:* Large cystic encephalomalacia lesion in left hemisphere due to perinatal stroke.

HEMIPLEGIA IN OLDER CHILDREN

Acute hemiparesis is the most common presentation of the vascular stroke syndromes, particularly arterial ischemic stroke (AIS) and intraparenchymal hemorrhage. However, around one-fourth of children with acute hemiparesis will have a nonvascular diagnosis, collectively these conditions are termed "stroke mimics." **Table 1** lists some clinical features that may be helpful in differentiating between vascular stroke syndromes and stroke mimics; however, neuroimaging is essential to make an accurate diagnosis. Neuroimaging should be performed as soon as possible in any child with hemiplegia as this is crucial for further management.

Detailed clinical history and examination are very important in establishing the diagnosis in these patients. Headache can be a feature of AIS, sinovenous thrombosis, central nervous system (CNS) infection, or hemiplegic migraine. "Thunderclap" headache is classically a feature of subarachnoid hemorrhage; though it may also be seen in reversible cerebral vasoconstriction syndrome. A sudden onset of symptoms is suggestive of a vascular stroke syndrome. Intracranial hemorrhage can present with severe headache and rapid onset of coma. Acute encephalopathy is suggestive of acute disseminated encephalomyelitis (ADEM) or CNS infection. A reduced consciousness level is a danger sign in AIS, and it may be

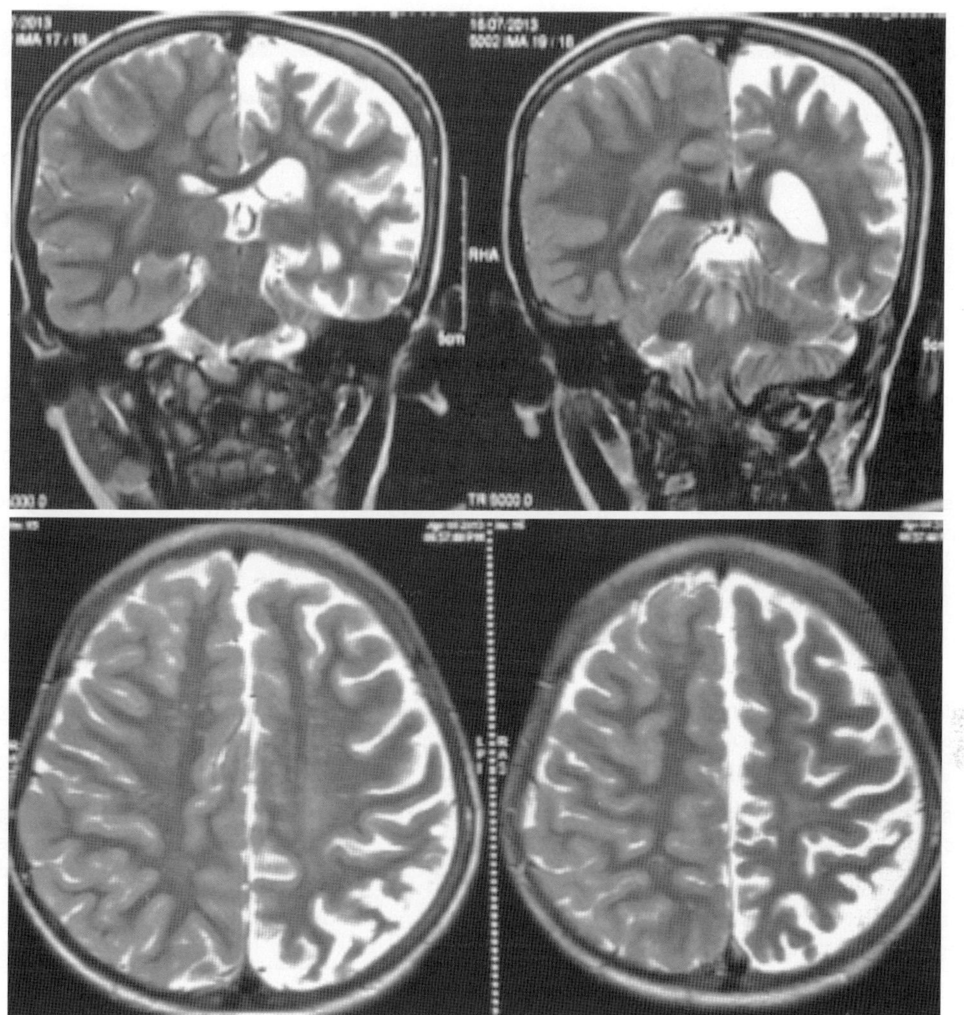

Fig. 2: T2-weighted magnetic resonance imaging of brain: left hemispheric atrophy in chronic stage of hemiconvulsion–hemiplegia–epilepsy syndrome.

due to significant raised intracranial pressure that can be secondary to middle cerebral artery (MCA) territory infarction or associated with brainstem or posterior fossa infarction. Seizures are commonly seen in meningitis, posterior reversible encephalopathy syndrome, and CSVT. The clinical assessment includes detailed cardiovascular examination, including careful evaluation of peripheral pulses and blood pressure, and systemic features of sepsis, endocarditic, or an underlying syndromic disorder.

Childhood Stroke

The major syndromes comprising ischemic stroke in childhood consist of AIS and sinovenous thrombosis (SVT). AISs constitute 80% of cases. AIS in children is a rare but important disorder with a high rate of morbidity and mortality. Nearly two-thirds of affected patients suffer from adverse outcomes including long-term cognitive, behavioral, and functional deficits. Reported incidence rate for AIS is between 2 and 13 in 100,000 children per year. The risk factors of AIS include congenital or acquired cardiac disease, large vessel arteriopathies, and prothrombotic abnormalities in children. Infection, hematologic disorders and coagulopathies, metabolic disorders, trauma, medications, iron deficiency, and migraine are other less common causes of AIS in children.

Cerebral arteriopathies are these days increasingly recognized as one of the major causes of childhood stroke, in otherwise healthy children. Some arteriopathies are due to well-recognized causes such as arterial dissection, moyamoya syndrome or disease, connective

TABLE 1: Causes of acute hemiparesis in children.

Etiology	*History*	*Clinical examination*	*Investigations*
Meningitis/ meningoencephalitis	Fever, headache, and vomiting	Neck rigidity, Kernig's sign, and Brudzinski sign encephalopathy	CSF biochemistry, cytology, latex agglutination, gram stain, culture studies, and neuroimaging
Arterial ischemic stroke	Onset may be stuttering, it may be preceded by febrile illness, chickenpox, head injury, and cardiac condition	Consciousness usually intact unless large MCA/brainstem infarct	Neuroimaging may reveal arteriopathy
Intracranial hemorrhage	Sudden onset, headache, and vomiting	Encephalopathy and rapid evolution of neurological findings	Neuroimaging may reveal etiology, e.g., arteriovenous malformation
Acute disseminated encephalomyelitis	Prodromal symptoms such as fever, headache, and subacute onset	Reduced level of consciousness, focal neurological deficits	Neuroimaging may show mainly patchy white matter involvement
Metabolic	History of acute deterioration with illness, developmental delay, vomiting, and encephalopathy	Seizures, movement disorder, rash, and specific odor	Abnormal biochemistry and neuroimaging
Posterior reversible encephalopathy syndrome	Seizures and headache drugs (tacrolimus and cyclophosphamide)	Hypertension and encephalopathy	Neuroimaging
Reversible cerebral vasoconstriction syndrome	History of thunderclap headache	Focal neurological deficit	Vascular imaging reveals diffuse segmental narrowing of intracranial arteries
CNS tumor associated with edema or bleeding	Chronic/subacute onset of symptoms with rapid deterioration	Focal neurological deficit	Neuroimaging

tissue disorders, and sickle-cell disease. Delayed effects of radiation to the head and neck in childhood cancer patients have also been associated with stroke due to cerebrovascular disease, and children with neurofibromatosis may have complications of a cerebral arteriopathy. However, in up to 30% of children presenting with a first AIS, a focal arterial stenosis is identified but none of the classic underlying causes are discovered.

Transient cerebral arteriopathy (TCA) is the most common type of arteriopathy seen in pediatric stroke. It is a monophasic arterial disease which is characterized by a unilateral segmental or focal stenosis involving the distal part of the internal carotid and the initial segments and branches of the anterior and/or MCA followed by complete or partial resolution. The pathophysiology of TCA is uncertain. 44% of TCA cases are associated with varicella zoster infection in 12 months prior to AIS, causing postvaricella arteriopathy. Varicella virus invades the arterial wall, causing an acute vasculitis. Other frequent infectious agents such as parvovirus B19, cytomegalovirus, *Mycoplasma pneumoniae*, *Borrelia burgdorferi*, enterovirus, human immunodeficiency virus, and *Helicobacter pylori* might be responsible for TCA **(Flowchart 1)**.

Toddlers with AIS more frequently present with abrupt onset of a hemiparesis, with facial droop, weakness of one hand, or dragging of one leg. In school age children, presentation may be with headache, speech or visual disturbance or focal sensory deficits in addition to hemiparesis. Seizures accompany the stroke in around 50% of children **(Box 1)**.

In SVT, a clinical picture indistinguishable from "pseudotumor cerebri" is the most frequent presentation, characterized by severe headache, papilledema and occasionally sixth nerve palsy. Visual disturbances including diplopia or an increased central scotoma are

Flowchart 1: Causes of stroke in children.

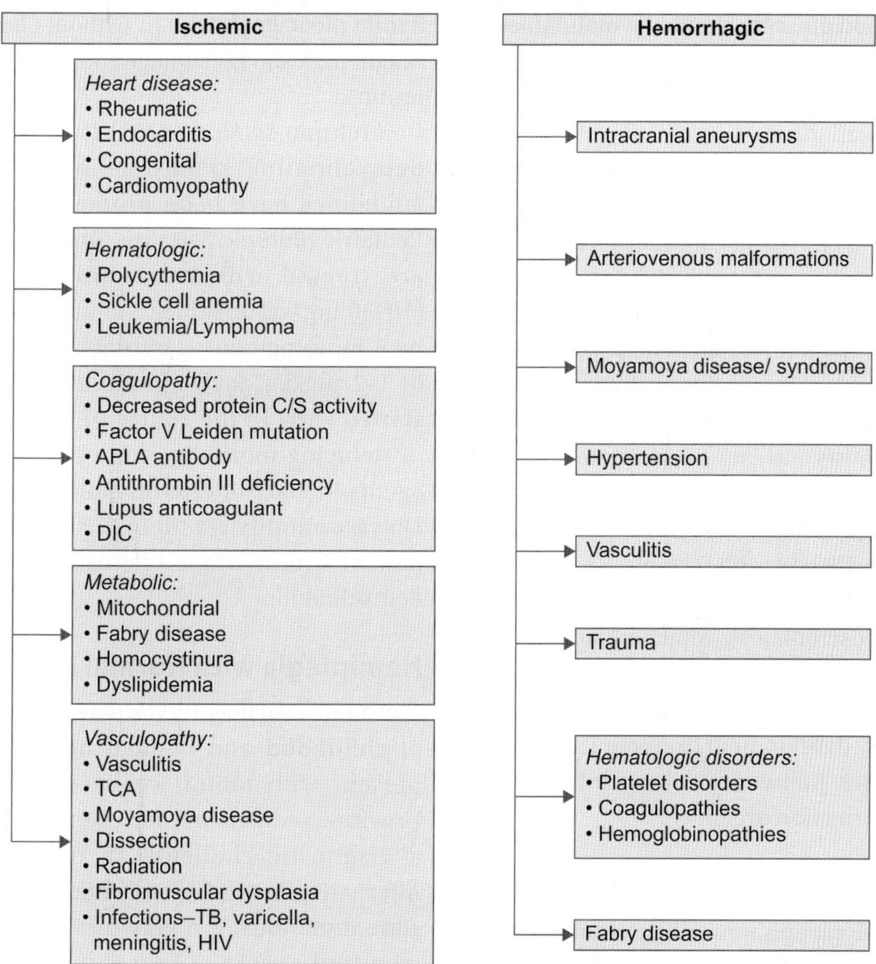

(APLA: antiphospholipid antibody; DIC: disseminated intravascular coagulation; HIV: human immunodeficiency virus; TB: tuberculosis; TCA: transient cerebral arteriopathy)

BOX 1: Clinical presentation of arterial ischemic stroke.

- *Toddlers:*
  - Facial droop
  - Difficulty using one hand
  - Dragging of one leg
- *Older children:*
  - Hemiparesis
  - Speech disturbances
  - Visual disturbances
  - Headache
  - Focal sensory deficits
  - Seizures

present in 18% of children with SVT. Hemiparesis and focal deficits are present in 35–45% cases. Seizures occur at the onset in 48% of older infants and children **(Box 2)**.

BOX 2: Clinical presentation of sinus venous thrombosis.

- Headache, papilledema, and sixth nerve palsy
- Hemiparesis
- Visual disturbances
- Seizures

Management

The initial management should focus on prompt resuscitation and establishment of homeostasis.

- *Acute treatment of children with stroke includes:*
  - Maintenance of respiratory and cardiovascular status
  - Aggressive management of infection, seizures, and fever

- Maintenance of euglycemia and normovolemia
- Adequate blood pressure should be maintained.
- Intracranial hypertension may require hypertonic saline, mannitol, and hyperventilation to prevent cerebral herniation.

Anticoagulation with heparin can be considered in some patients with AIS, particularly those with arterial dissection or progressive neurologic deficits thought to be a result of recurrent emboli or thrombosis. Anticoagulation in cardiac embolism is controversial. Aspirin is the most commonly used antiplatelet agent. The recommended dosage is 3–5 mg/kg/day. Treatment of children with AIS using tissue plasminogen activator (t-PA) is limited due to delay in the diagnosis and lack of adequate safety and efficacy studies and is not currently recommended as standard treatment protocol. Moyamoya disease can be managed surgically with revascularization.

In case of secondary deterioration, in the form of reduced level of consciousness, repeated seizures, any new neurological deficit, or recurrent "transient ischemic attacks", urgent repeat neuroimaging should be done. The aim is to identify development of cerebral edema and herniation syndromes, infarct extension, and secondary hemorrhagic transformation urgently.

Demyelination in Children

Acute disseminated encephalomyelitis is an immune-mediated, inflammatory demyelinating disease of the CNS that usually affects children and young adults commonly preceded by an infection or vaccination. ADEM typically has a monophasic course and is self-limiting, with regain of normal function within around 3 months after the onset of symptoms. Also, a subset of ADEM patients with relapsing disorders, including recurrent DEM (RDEM), multiphasic DEM (MDEM), multiple sclerosis, and neuromyelitis optica spectrum disorders (NMOSD) have been reported. The clinical presentation is variable. The prodromal symptoms are fever, headache, malaise, nausea, and vomiting. The acute phase occurs is characterized by altered behavior (e.g., irritability and confusion) and consciousness (lethargy, stupor, and coma) associated with focal or multifocal neurological deficits depending on the area involved in the demyelinating process. It mainly involves the white matter tracts of the cerebral hemispheres, optic nerves, brainstem, and spinal cord. Cerebrospinal fluid examination may be normal or show a mild pleocytosis with or without elevated protein levels. Magnetic resonance image shows multiple demyelinating lesions.

Multiple sclerosis (MS) is a chronic, inflammatory demyelinating syndrome of the CNS. Consensus guidelines have been proposed by the International Pediatric Multiple Sclerosis Study Group. Acute episodes are treated with intravenous methylprednisolone (10–30 mg/kg/dose) for 3–5 days. This may be followed by a tapering course of oral prednisone (starting dose of 1–2 mg/kg/day). Immunomodulatory therapies are started early in the course of disease with the purpose of reducing morbidity and cerebral atrophy. First-line agents include interferon alpha and glatiramer acetate. Disease-modifying therapy should be started in any patient with multiple sclerosis after a second attack of demyelination.

Hemiplegia with Normal Neuroimaging

Conditions such as Todd's paresis, alternating hemiplegia of childhood and familial hemiplegic migraine, can present with motor weakness and normal imaging. Unwitnessed seizure, for example, nocturnal can pose a diagnostic challenge in postictal Todd's paresis. Alternating hemiplegia of childhood, caused by *ATP1A3* gene mutations, is a very rare disease characterized by recurrent attacks of loss of muscular tone resulting in hypomobility of one side of the body along with epilepsy, developmental delay, and variable dystonia **(Flowchart 2)**. Familial hemiplegic migraine (FHM) comes in the category of migraine with aura. Though rare, it can be associated with motor weakness.

Recurrent Hemiplegia in Children

Few common causes of recurrent hemiplegia in children are:

- *Demyelination:* Relapsing ADEM, neuromyelitis optica, and MS
- *Ischemic stroke:* Cardioembolic, vasculitis, and moyamoya vasculopathy
- *Metabolic:* Mitochondrial
- Alternating hemiplegia of childhood
- Familial hemiplegic migraine
- Todd's paralysis

Flowchart 2: Management of acute hemiplegia in children.

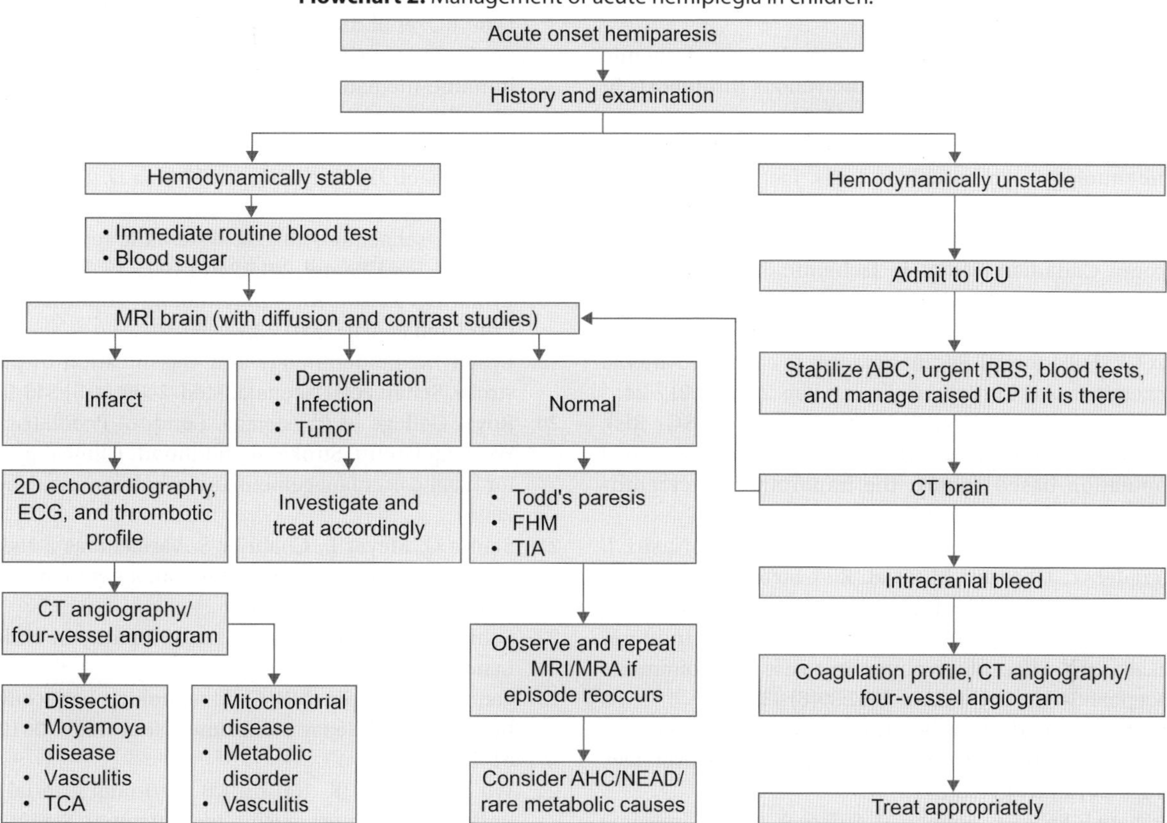

(ABC: airway, breathing, and circulation; AHC: alternating hemiplegia of childhood; CT: computed tomography; ECG: electrocardiogram; FHM: familial hemiplegic migraine; ICP: intracranial pressure; ICU: intensive care unit; MRA: magnetic resonance angiography; MRI: magnetic resonance imaging; NEAD: non-epileptic attack disorder; RBS: random blood sugar; TCA: transient cerebral arteriopathy; TIA: transient ischemic attack)

KEY POINTS

- Detailed clinical history and examination are vital in establishing a diagnosis.
- Focal clonic seizure in the newborn period is the most common presentation of perinatal arterial ischemic stroke.
- The most common etiology of infantile hemiplegia is perinatal stroke; the risk of recurrence is extremely low.
- Pediatric stroke Is not uncommon. The diagnosis is many a time delayed, and early recognition is essential.
- In previously normal children, the most common cause of stroke is arteriopathy. Imaging with CT angiography or conventional 4-vessel angiography is essential.
- Transient cerebral arteriopathy is an important cause of stroke in children. Preceding history of varicella infection (up to 12 months prior) must be asked for, as it is a major cause of transient cerebral arteriopathy.
- Acute episodes of demyelination must be treated with intravenous steroids. Differentiating ADEM from MDEM, NMOSD, MS in children using current criteria is essential for long-term therapy and prognosis.

SUGGESTED READING

1. Alper G. Acute disseminated encephalomyelitis. J Child Neurol. 2012;27(11):1408-25.
2. Amlie-Lefond C, Bernard TJ, Sebire G, Friedman NR, Heyer GL, Lerner NB, et al. Predictors of cerebral arteriopathy in children with arterial ischemic stroke: results of the International Pediatric Stroke Study. Circulation. 2009;119:1417-23.
3. Armstrong-Wells J, Ferriero DM. Diagnosis and acute management of perinatal arterial ischemic stroke. Neurol Clin Pract. 2014;4(5):378-85.
4. Auvin S, Bellavoine V, Merdariu D, Delanoë C, Elmaleh-Bergés M, Gressens P, et al. Hemi convulsion-hemiplegia-epilepsy syndrome: current understandings. Eur J Pediatric Neurol. 2012;16(5):413-21.
5. Bhate S, Ganesa V. A practical approach to acute hemiparesis in children. Developmental Medicine & Child Neurology. 2015;689-97.
6. Chabrier S, Husson B, Dinomais M, Landrieu P, Nguyen The Tich S. New insights (and new interrogations) in

perinatal arterial ischemic stroke. Thrombosis Research. 2011;127:13-22.

7. deVeber G, Andrew M; the Canadian Pediatric Ischemic Stroke Study Group. Cerebral Sino venous thrombosis in children. N Engl J Med. 2001;345:417-23.
8. deVeber G. Stroke and the child's brain: an overview of epidemiology, syndromes and risk factors. Curr Opin Neurol. 2002;15:133-8.
9. deVeber G. The Canadian Pediatric Ischemic Stroke Study Group. Canadian Pediatric Ischemic Stroke Registry: analysis of children with arterial ischemic stroke. Ann Neurol. 2000;48:526.
10. Fox CK, Fullerton HJ. Recent advances in childhood arterial ischemic stroke. Cur Atherosclerosis Rep. 2010;12:217-24.
11. Fullerton HJ, Wu YW, Sidney S, Johnston SC. Risk of recurrent childhood arterial ischemic stroke in a population-based cohort: the importance of cerebrovascular imaging. Pediatrics. 2007;119:495-501.
12. Ghofrani M, Tonekaboni H, Karimzadeh P, Nasiri J, Pirzadeh Z, Ghazzavi M, et al. Risk factors of pediatric arterial ischemic stroke. Int J Prev Med. 2018;9:69.
13. Hirano K, Ariba H, Yano M, Watanabe S, Okumura Y, Takahashi Y. Effect of tacrolimus in a case of autoimmune encephalitis. No To Hattatsu. 2007;39(6):436-9.
14. Johnston J, So TY. First-line disease-modifying therapies in pediatric multiple sclerosis: a comprehensive overview. Drugs. 2012;72(9):1195-211.
15. Kirkham F, Sebire G, Steinlin M, Sträter R. Arterial ischemic stroke in children. Thromb Haemost. 2004;92:697-706.
16. Krupp LB, Tardieu M, Amato MP, Banwell B, Chitnis T, Dale RC, et al. International Pediatric Multiple Sclerosis Study Group criteria for pediatric multiple sclerosis and immune-mediated central nervous system demyelinating disorders: revisions to the 2007 definitions. Mult Scler. 2013;19(10):1261-7.
17. Li C, Miaob JK, Xuc Y, Huaa YY, Maa Q, Zhoua LL, et al. Prenatal, perinatal and neonatal risk factors for perinatal arterial ischaemic stroke: a systematic review and meta-analysis. Eur J Neurol. 2017;24(8):1006-15.
18. Lynch JK, Nelson KB. Epidemiology of perinatal stroke. Curr Opin Pediatr. 2001;13(6):499-505.
19. Lynch JK. Epidemiology and classification of perinatal stroke. Semin Fetal Neonatal Med. 2009;14(5):245-9.
20. Royal College of Physicians, London. Paediatric Stroke Working Group. Stroke in childhood. Clinical guidelines for diagnosis, management and rehabilitation. November 2004.
21. Sebire G, Meyer L, Chabrier S. Varicella as a risk factor for cerebral infarction in childhood: a case-control study. Ann Neurol. 1999;45:679-80.
22. Sebire G. Transient cerebral arteriopathy in childhood. Lancet. 2006;368:8-10.
23. Tenney JR, Schapiro MB. Child neurology: hemiconvulsion-hemiplegia-epilepsy syndrome. Neurology. 2012;79(1):e1-4.
24. Wu YW, Lynch JK, Nelson KB. Perinatal arterial stroke: understanding mechanisms and outcomes. Semin Neurol. 2005;25(4):424-34.

Approach to a Child with Spastic Paraplegia

Arun G Roy, Vinayan KP

INTRODUCTION

Paraplegia is defined as partial or complete weakness of both legs sparing the upper limbs. This can be due to upper motor neuron (UMN) or lower motor neuron (LMN) pathology. The UMN lesion should be above L1 segment involving the pyramidal tract (thoracic or cervical) of spinal cord or rarely in cerebral cortex involving the leg area (parasagittal) or subcortical regions affecting the fibers to legs to cause spastic paraplegia. Lower motor neuron lesion of paraplegia is secondary to intramedullary lesion affecting the lumbar and sacral spinal segments of legs (L1–5 and S1–3), multiple root involvement (L1–5 and S1–3), multiple peripheral nerve involvement, and rarely anterior horn cell disease. In this chapter we are describing paraplegia secondary to spinal lesions. The most common cause of cerebral paraplegia in children is cerebral palsy, which is not discussed in this chapter.

CLINICAL PEARL

- The first step of diagnosis is to localize whether it is primarily upper motor neuron or lower motor neuron lesion as it helps to narrow down the localization and avoid over investigating the patient. Hence, a detailed history and examination is vital.

CLINICAL FEATURES OF UPPER MOTOR AND LOWER MOTOR NEURON LESIONS

A child refusing to stand or walk or bear weight is the most common complaint in acute causes, while dragging of legs, tripping of toes while walking may favor spasticity of legs in chronic disorders. Parents may describe the limb as flaccid or stiff on handling. In an acute UMN lesion, muscle tone is flaccid with hyporeflexia before the appearance of spasticity. The pyramidal distribution of weakness has specific pattern in limbs which is seen when weakness is not severe. In lower limbs, weakness is most marked in flexors and internal rotators of hip, knee flexors, and toe and ankle dorsiflexors. The spasticity is most marked in extensors of lower limbs which is best elicited on flexion movements of leg. Deep tendon reflexes (DTR) are exaggerated with extensor plantars in UMN lesion.

CLINICAL PEARL

- By rule, upper motor neuron (UMN) lesions cause spastic paraplegia and lower motor neuron lesions result in flaccid paraplegia with exemption of acute spinal shock where lesion is UMN but paraplegia is flaccid.

In LMN lesion, the weakness is in distribution of spinal segment, root, nerve, anterior horn cell, or muscle depending on site of involvement with hypotonia in weak muscles. Wasting of muscles is another feature noted. The DTRs are hyporeflexic with flexor plantars **(Table 1)**.

Primary sensations, pain, and temperature are carried by lateral spinothalamic tract while vibration, joint-position sensations, and fine touch are by posterior column and crude touch by anterior spinothalamic tract. An older child can complain of burning pain, tingling, numbness of legs, or loss of sensations which can indicate a sensory involvement. The distribution of sensory level depends on site of lesion. In spinal cord, there can be differential involvement of tracts and sensation will be lost

TABLE 1: Clinical features to differentiate upper motor neuron and lower motor neuron.

Features	*Upper motor neuron*	*Lower motor neuron*
Weakness	Pyramidal pattern	Depending on site of lesion
Atrophy	Late disuse atrophy	Prominent, early feature
Tone	Spasticity	Flaccid
DTR	Exaggerated	Sluggish/Absent
Plantar reflex	Extensor	Flexor

(DTR: deep tendon reflexes)

below the level of lesion. Since posterior column crosses at level of medulla, spinal cord lesion causes loss of sensation ipsilaterally, while spinothalamic tract crossing occurs at spinal level, hence, the loss of sensation will be contralateral to site of lesion while transection of cord will cause sensation loss of all tracts bilaterally **(Fig. 1)**. In cortex and subcortical region, sensory loss is contralateral to site of lesion **(Table 2)**.

Normal bladder and bowel control depends on segmental reflexes involving both autonomic and somatic motor neurons, as well as descending and ascending tracts of the spinal cord. Hence, bladder and bowel function may be impaired after an injury to any segmental level of the spinal cord. Bladder involvement can be retention of urine or incontinence of urine (urge or over flow). Urge incontinence is seen in UMN bladder, where lesion is above S2–S4 segments, while retention and overflow incontinence favors LMN bladder (S2–S4 segments or roots). A palpable bladder indicates retention of urine. Injuries to the spinal cord that result in paraplegia from a lesion above T6 may also impair autonomic control and result in episodes of severe hypertension or hypotension. This is due to excessive and uncontrolled sympathetic output from the spinal cord. Common triggers include bladder distension, constipation, rectal fissures, joint injury and urinary tract infection.

CLINICAL PEARLS

- *Cortical lesions:* Spastic paraparesis is usually accompanied by upper motor neuron (UMN) cranial nerve palsies, UMN bladder.
- *Brainstem lesions:* Spastic paraparesis is accompanied by cranial nerve palsies—UMN or lower motor neuron depending on the site of lesion (mid brain, pons, medulla), UMN bladder ± sensory tracts.
- *Spinal cord lesions:* Spastic paraparesis with sensory tract involvement, sensory level and UMN bladder, there is no cranial nerve involvement.

TYPES OF SPINAL CORD DISORDERS

Spinal cord disorders can be extramedullary or intramedullary **(Figs. 2 and 3)**. The clinical features can vary in extramedullary and intramedullary spinal disease **(Table 3)**. This is because of the lamination of tracts in the cord and type of compression of these tracts. Extramedullary means the lesion is outside the cord and can be intradural or extradural. Intradural lesions involve predominantly dura and root (examples: neurofibroma, meningioma), while extradural lesions are in vertebrae and surrounding structures (example: Pott's spine). Radicular pain, gibbus, vertebral pain, and spine tenderness are features of extramedullary disorders.

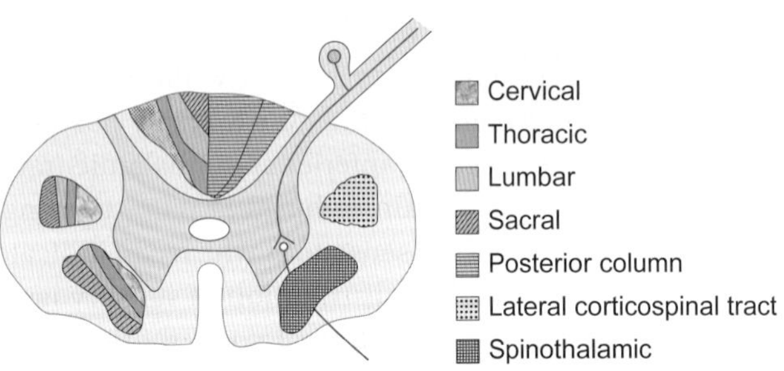

Fig. 1: Transection of spinal cord.

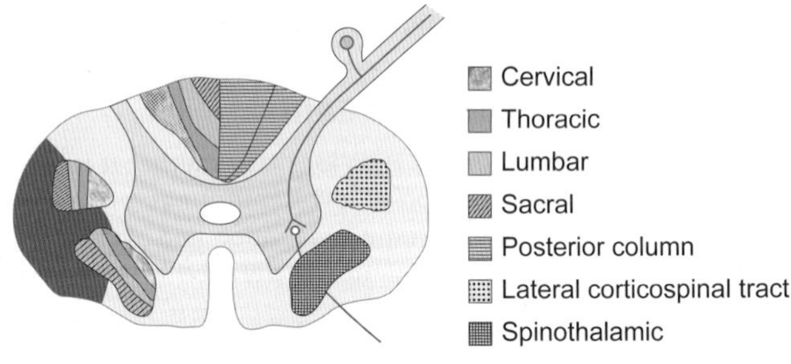

Fig. 2: Extramedullary compression.

TABLE 2: Major tracts of the spinal cord-location and functions.

Tracts	*Location in spinal segment*	*Function*
Posterior column	Posterior cord	Vibration, joint position, fine touch
Lateral spino-thalamic tract	Lateral cord	Pain and temperature
Anterior spino-thalamic ract	Anterior cord	Crude touch

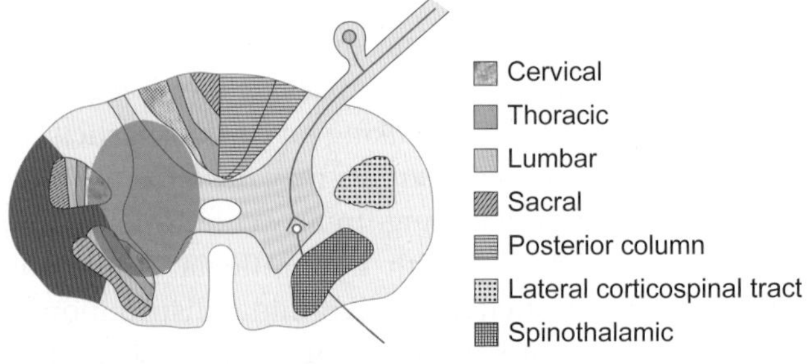

Fig. 3: Intramedullary compression.

Spinal Cord Syndromes (Table 4)

These depend on the extent of lesion: (1) Hemisection of the cord (Brown Sequard syndrome), (2) complete spinal cord syndrome, (3) central cord syndrome **(Box 1)**, (4) Combined posterior and lateral column disease, (5) anterior spinal artery disease.

At the site of lesion, there can be LMN weakness, band of hyperesthesia, and loss of all sensations due to radicular involvement.

CAUSES OF SPASTIC PARAPLEGIA

Depending on presentation and duration it can be acute or chronic. Etiology varies depending on presentation, hence onset is important. Family history should be asked regarding similar illness, which helps in diagnosing inherited causes of spastic paraplegia like hereditary spastic paraplegia and leukodystrophy. Etiology can be broadly classified into compressive and noncompressive myelopathy **(Tables 5 and 6)**. In compressive myelopathy, there is definite sensory level, radicular symptoms at site of compression with asymmetric involvement of tracts while in non compressive myelopathies, radicular symptoms and definite sensory level are not seen and there is selective sparing of tracts and findings are usually symmetric.

TABLE 3: Clinical features of extramedullary and intramedullary spinal cord disorders.

Clinical features	*Extramedullary*	*Intramedullary*
Radicular pain	Common	Rare
Funicular or tract pain	Rare	Common
Sensory loss	Ascending type	Descending type
Band of hyperesthesia	At the site of lesion	Rare
Lower motor neuron signs	At the site of compression	Depends on extent of lesion
Upper motor neuron signs	Below the level of lesion and early	Late and less severe

Pott's Spine

One of the leading causes of compressive myelopathy in children. This can have an acute or a chronic presentation and is due to cord compression secondary to vertebral destruction and wedging. Local spine tenderness and Gibbus are features of Pott's spine. Gentle tapping over vertebra with finger is best and safe way to elicit tenderness. Direct spinal cord involvement due to tuberculosis infection is seen but less compared to Pott's spine. Magnetic resonance imaging (MRI) is the investigation of choice as it shows involvement of disk, vertebra, and the extension of disease into soft tissues. Treatment is with antitubercular drugs and surgical intervention is indicated in acute and severe paraparesis secondary to compression and unstable spine.

Acute Transverse Myelitis

Transverse myelitis is a segmental spinal cord injury caused by acute inflammation. The inflammation of TM is generally restricted to one or two segments, usually in the thoracic cord. The deficits are usually bilateral, producing weakness and multimodality sensory disturbance below the level of the lesion. Majority of cases are idiopathic but other causes are infections, autoimmune disorders, demyelinating disorders like multiple sclerosis (MS) and neuromyelitis optica. Cerebrospinal fluid can be normal or may show a moderate lymphocytosis (typically $<100/mm^3$) and an elevated protein level (usually 100–120 mg/dL). Glucose levels are normal. Magnetic resonance imaging is the investigation of choice and can show local enlargement of the spinal cord and increased signal intensity on

TABLE 4: Clinical features of various spinal cord syndromes.

Spinal cord syndrome	*Motor deficit*	*Spinothalamic tract involvement*	*Posterior columns involvement*
Brown Sequard syndrome (hemisection of cord)	Ipsilateral UMN weakness below the lesion	Contralateral loss of pain and temperature sensation	Ipsilateral loss of touch, position, and vibratory sensation
Complete transection of cord	Bilateral UMN weakness below lesion	Bilateral loss of pain and temperature	Bilateral loss of touch, position, and vibratory sensation
Anterior cord syndrome	Bilateral UMN weakness	Bilateral loss of pain and temperature	Sparing of touch, position, and vibration sensation
Posterior lateral column syndrome	UMN weakness	Sparing of pain and temperature sensation	Loss of touch, position, and vibratory sensation

(LMN: lower motor neuron; UMN: upper motor neuron)

BOX 1: Central cord syndrome.

This is not a classical cause for paraplegia. Lesion in cervical cord resulting in upper limb weakness more than leg weakness. Another classical feature is suspended sensory loss for pain and temperature due to involvement of decussating fibers carrying these sensations

TABLE 5: Causes of acute myelopathy.

Compressive myelopathy	
Traumatic	Vertebral body fracture, or direct injury
Hemorrhage	Epidural or subdural hematoma
Infective	Epidural or subdural abscess, Pott's spine
Noncompressive myelopathy	
Vascular	Embolism, dural arteriovenous fistula, APLA syndrome
Inflammatory	Demyelinating disorders (MS, ADEM, NMO)
Infective	Viral, bacterial, tuberculosis

(ADEM: acute disseminated encephalomyelitis; APLA: antiphospholipid antibody; MS: multiple sclerosis; NMO: neuromyelitis optica)

TABLE 6: Causes of chronic myelopathy.

Compressive myelopathy	
Neoplasm	Neurofibroma, meningioma
Infective	Pott's spine
Congenital disorders	Dermoid cyst, arachnoid cyst
Noncompressive myelopathy	
Demyelinating disorders	MS, NMO
Infections	HIV, neurosyphilis, TB
Vascular	Ischemia due to AVM
Nutritional	Vitamin B_{12} deficiency
Toxic	Radiation and chemotherapeutic agents
Congenital disorders	Tethered cord syndrome

(AVM: arteriovenous malformation; HIV: human immunodeficiency virus; MS: multiple sclerosis; NMO: neuromyelitis optica; TB: tuberculosis)

T2 weighted images which can extend few segments of cord. In MS, the extent is two or less than two segments. Contrast enhancement may or may not be there.

Intramedullary Spinal Arteriovenous Malformations

Twenty percent of the lesions are diagnosed in children under 16 years of age. Myelopathy is produced by the mass effect of the lesion or by ischemia or hemorrhage into the cord.

Adrenomyeloneuropathy

A variant of adrenoleukodystrophy, an X-linked recessive disorder, is characterized by a slowly progressive spastic paraparesis and mild polyneuropathy. Sensory and sphincter disturbances are typically absent. There may be mild adrenal insufficiency.

Hereditary Spastic Paraplegia

Inherited disorders, in which the prominent feature is a progressive spastic paraparesis. Hereditary spastic paraplegia is classified according to the mode of inheritance, and the spastic paraplegia syndrome occurs alone or is accompanied by additional neurologic or systemic abnormalities ("pure" versus "complicated"). Hereditary spastic paraplegia is a clinical diagnosis, based in large part on the family history. Magnetic resonance imaging spine may be normal or show cord atrophy.

Spinal Cord Tumors

This is a rare diagnosis in the pediatric population. The types of tumors seen in children tend to be different than the adult types. Intramedullary tumors are most common type in children. In children with intramedullary tumors, astrocytomas represent around 60% of tumors, ependymomas 30%, developmental tumors 4%, and then a group of other less frequently identified types.

Deficiency of Vitamin B_{12}

Deficiency of vitamin B_{12} leads to degeneration of the dorsal and lateral white matter of the spinal cord, producing a slowly progressive weakness, sensory ataxia, and paresthesias, and ultimately spasticity, paraplegia, and incontinence.

Tethered Cord Syndrome

Classically tethered cord syndrome has been defined as a spectrum of congenital anomalies resulting in an abnormally low position of the conus medullaris. Motor deficits are due to UMN and LMN features, since there is involvement of pyramidal tracts and lumbosacral roots. Children can present with delayed gait development, spasticity, hyperreflexia, hyporeflexia, and muscular atrophy. Sensory deficits, when present, are due to tract or

Flowchart 1: Approach to paraplegia.

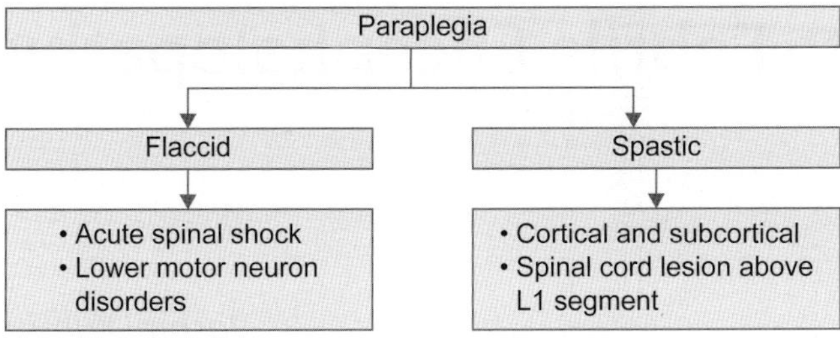

root involvement and children can present with painless ulcers in leg. Neurogenic bladder dysfunction can be incontinence, urgency, or with recurrent urinary tract infections. Magnetic resonance imaging is the modality of choice in visualizing the level of the conus medullaris and for identifying terminal filum.

KEY POINTS

- Paraplegia is weakness of lower limb sparing upper limbs; it can be flaccid or spastic.
- Involvement of sensory tracts and bladder with sparing of the cranial nerves and cognition localizes the lesion to spinal cord.
- The causes can be compressive and noncompressive, extramedullary and intramedullary which can be differentiated by history and clinical findings.
- History of systemic illness, family history, trauma, onset and progression of disease can give clue to etiology **(Flowchart 1)**.

SUGGESTED READING

1. Blackmer J. Rehabilitation medicine: 1. autonomic dysreflexia. CMAJ. 2003;169(9):931-5.
2. Brinar VV, Habek M, Brinar M, Malojcić B, Boban M. The differential diagnosis of acute transverse myelitis. Clin Neurol Neurosurg. 2006;108:278-83.
3. Bui CJ, Tubbs RS, Oakes WJ. Tethered cord syndrome in children: a review. Neurosurg Focus. 2007;23(2):E2.
4. Fowler CJ, Griffiths D, de Groat WC. The neural control of micturition. Nat Rev Neurosci. 2008;9(6)453-66.
5. Lindenbaum J, Healton EB, Savage DG, Brust JC, Garrett TJ, Podell ER, et al. Neuropsychiatric disorders caused by cobalamin deficiency in the absence of anemia or macrocytosis. N Engl J Med. 1988;318:1720-8.
6. Moser HW, Mahmood A, Raymond GV. X-linked adrenoleukodystrophy. Nat Clin Pract Neurol. 2007;3:140-51.
7. Pidcock FS, Krishnan C, Crawford TO, Salorio CF, Trovato M, Kerr DA. Acute transverse myelitis in childhood: center-based analysis of 47 cases. Neurology. 2007;68:1474-80.
8. Raghavan N, Barkovich AJ, Edwards M, Norman D. MR imaging in the tethered spinal cord syndrome. AJR Am J Roentgenol. 1989;152(4):843-52.
9. Salinas S, Proukakis C, Crosby A, Warner TT. Hereditary spastic paraplegia: clinical features and pathogenetic mechanisms. Lancet Neurol. 2008;7:1127-38.
10. Schick U, Marquardt G. Pediatric spinal tumors. Pediatr Neurosurg. 2001;35: 120-7.
11. Yasargil MG, Symon L, Teddy PG. Arteriovenous malformations of the spinal cord. In: Symon L (Ed). Advances and Technical Standards in Neurosurgery. Wien: Springer; 1984. p. 61.

Acute Febrile Encephalopathy

Rashmi Kumar

INTRODUCTION

The term acute febrile encephalopathy (AFE) literally means acute onset of fever with encephalopathy (or altered consciousness). This presentation is a very important cause of hospital admissions in children in India. In 2006, World Health Organization coined the term acute encephalitis syndrome (AES) to include "a person of any age at any time of year with the acute onset of fever and a change in mental status (including symptoms such as confusion, disorientation, coma, or inability to talk) and/or new onset of seizures (excluding simple febrile seizures)". Basically these two terms mean the same thing and for the sake of uniformity the term "acute encephalitis syndrome" is used.

CAUSES

Causes of AFE/AES are varied. Most commonly this presentation is caused by actual invasion of the brain by an infectious agent. The important causes of AFE are given in **Box 1**.

History and examination should be focused as shown in **Box 2**.

Although the etiology is varied, common causes may predominate depending on the region. For example, Japanese encephalitis (JE) is very common in large parts of east and south India. Cerebral malaria is important in areas endemic for *Plasmodium falciparum*. Dengue encephalopathy, rickettsiae, leptospirosis, etc. are also reported from different parts of India. The age, seasonal and rural-urban distribution, and other epidemiologic clues may be helpful in suspecting specific infections. **Box 3** gives some epidemiological and clinical clues to etiology.

In practice, the diagnosis of encephalitis is presumptive, based on clinical assessment and exclusion of other possibilities. Specific virological investigations are complex, time consuming, and expensive. Even in advanced centers, etiological diagnosis is possible in only a small proportion of clinically suspected cases **(Flowchart 1)**.

WORKUP

A pragmatic investigative workup can be planned according to common etiology of the region **(Box 4)**.

> **CLINICAL PEARL**
>
> - Acute febrile encephalopathy/acute encephalopathy syndrome can be divided into illnesses which are purely neurological as in Japanese encephalitis, herpes simplex virus and rabies; or into neurological plus systemic type as in dengue, malaria, enteric and other non-viral agents like leptospirosis and rickettsioses.

Encephalopathies versus Meningoencephalitis

The term encephalopathy, besides meaning altered sensorium also refers to a diffuse disturbance of cerebral function due to a noninflammatory cause. Metabolic or toxic encephalopathy can produce a picture of AFE. Examples of such metabolic/toxic causes include Reye's syndrome, dyselectrolytemia, diabetic, uremic or hepatic coma, poisoning, and heat stroke. Clues must be sought to differentiate encephalopathy from encephalitis, but the distinction is not always possible on clinical grounds. General features of encephalopathies are shown in **Box 5**.

TREATMENT (BOX 6)

Supportive treatment is the mainstay of therapy. A severe case should be managed in an intensive care unit. Measures include maintenance of airways, breathing, and circulation; hydration; electrolyte status; and control of pyrexia and convulsions. It is prudent to use appropriate parenteral antibiotics to cover for meningitis. Raised intracranial tension should be controlled with mannitol infusion (0.25–1.0 g/kg every 4–6 hours),

BOX 1: Causes of acute febrile encephalopathy/acute encephalopathy syndrome (AFE/AES).

Neuroinfections
- Viruses
  - Arbo or "arthropod borne" viruses: examples, Western equine, Eastern equine, Venezuelan equine, Japanese, St Louis, West Nile, Dengue, Murray valley encephalitis viruses. These viruses are naturally transmitted between insects and vertebrate animals that decide the geographical habitat and seasonal occurrence of the infection
  - Herpesviruses: Herpes simplex 1 and 2, Varicella zoster, Epstein-Barr, *Cytomegalovirus*, *Human Herpesvirus-6*, B virus
  - Enteroviruses: Polioviruses, Coxsackie, Echo, Enteroviruses 70 and 71
  - Orthomyxoviruses: Influenza viruses
  - Paramyxoviruses: Measles, Mumps, parainfluenza, Nipah virus
  - Adenoviruses
  - Rhabdoviruses: Rabies, chandipura
  - Parvoviruses
- Nonviral agents
  - Bacteria:
    - Pyogenic and tuberculous meningitis
    - *Mycoplasma pneumoniae*
    - *Listeria monocytogenes*
    - Spirochetes: Syphilis, Leptospirosis, Lyme disease
    - Brucellosis
    - Legionella
    - *Salmonella typhi*
    - Cat scratch disease (Bartonellosis)
  - Rickettsia
  - Fungi: Cryptococcus, histoplasma, *Aspergillus*, mucormycosis, *Candida*, coccidioidomycosis
  - Protozoa: *Plasmodium*, *Trypanosoma*, *Naegleria*, *Acanthamoeba*, *Toxoplasma gondii*, schistosomiasis, *Echinococcus granulosus*
  - Metazoa: Trichinosis, *Echinococcus*, cysticercus, *Schistosoma*

Noninfectious inflammation
- Acute disseminated encephalomyelitis
- Autoimmune encephalitis

Infectious encephalopathy
- Cerebral malaria
- Dengue encephalopathy
- Virus associated encephalopathy, e.g., influenza
- Enteric encephalopathy
- Sepsis
- Shigella encephalopathy

Structural coma with fever due to another cause
- Structural causes of coma like tumors, vascular events, etc. if associated with fever due to any other cause may present as AFE/AES

Functional coma with fever due to another cause
- Many causes of coma such as toxic and metabolic disorders, poisoning, inborn errors, etc. if associated with fever due to another cause may present as AFE/AES

BOX 2: Clinical assessment.

Epidemiology
- Age
- Location
- Rural/urban
- Season of year

History
- Fever
- Headache
- Vomiting
- Seizures
- Altered sensorium
- Altered behavior
- Personality changes
- Prodromal flu-like symptoms
- Rash, bleeding from any site
- Animal contact or dog bite
- Drug or toxin exposure
- Recent travel or immunization
- Trauma
- Recurrent episodes of encephalopathy
- Jaundice
- Premorbid medical condition such as diabetes or renal impairment

Examination
- Depth of coma
- Bleeding manifestations
- Features of shock
- Hepatosplenomegaly
- Rash
- Signs of raised intracranial tension
- Meningeal signs
- Focal neurological deficits
- Muscle tone
- Extrapyramidal features
- If in deep coma, signs of brainstem death

BOX 3: Epidemiological and clinical clues.

- Monsoon and postmonsoon season, rural, older child, endemic area—Japanese encephalitis
- *Plasmodium falciparum* endemic area—cerebral malaria
- Prominent extrapyramidal features—Japanese encephalitis
- Sudden onset high fever with chills and rigors, multisystem involvement with anemia, acidosis, blackwater fever, and bilateral upper motor neuron signs—cerebral malaria
- Rash, bleeding, hepatic involvement, nonpitting edema—dengue encephalopathy
- History of exposure to animal urine, and liver and kidney involvement—leptospirosis
- Prominent meningeal signs—bacterial meningitis
- Focal neurological deficits, personality change, fulminant course—herpes encephalitis
- History of animal bite, fatal course—rabies
- Rash, eschar

Flowchart 1: Approach to diagnosis in acute febrile encephalopathy.

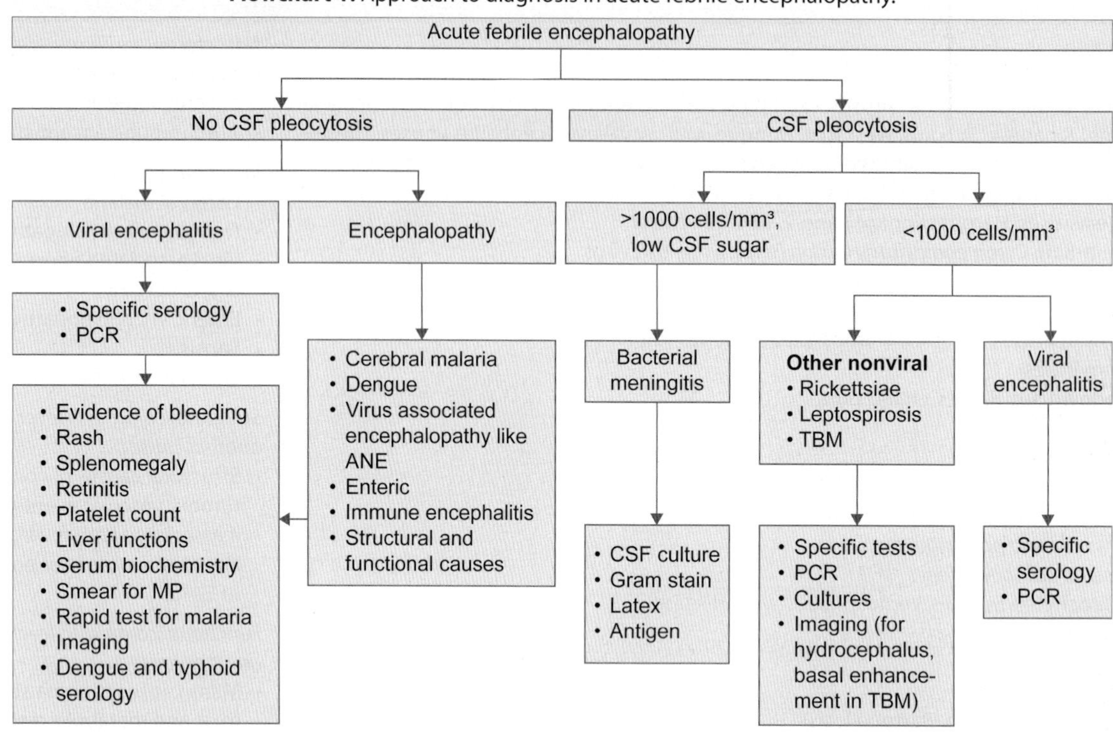

(ANE: acute necrotizing encephalopathy; CSF: cerebrospinal fluid; MP: malarial parasite; PCR: polymerase chain reaction; TBM: tuberculous meningitis)

BOX 4: Suggested workup for acute febrile encephalopathy/acute encephalopathy syndrome.

Workup

- Blood counts including platelets and packed cell volume
- Rapid malaria test and smear for malarial parasite/dengue
- *Cerebrospinal fluid (CSF) examination:* This is an essential investigation but should be done only when considered safe. CSF should be examined for total and differential cell count, protein and sugar, bacterial culture and Gram stain; viral PCRs and serology
- *Virology:* Samples for viral culture from respiratory secretions, throat swab, CSF, blood, urine, and stool taken as early as possible in the illness should be collected in appropriate transport media and sent to the reference laboratory
- Serological investigations in acute serum for specific immunoglobulin M (IgM) antibody level. JE is commonly diagnosed by the antibody capture ELISA for IgM antibody in acute phase serum and CSF, NS1 antigen for dengue
- Polymerase chain reaction is being developed to provide a rapid, and accurate diagnostic tool for a host of pathogens and is the mainstay of diagnosis. This is widely used for diagnosis of HSE with high sensitivity (>90%) and specificity (100%)
- Neuroimaging should be done whenever possible. As far as possible, magnetic resonance imaging should be insisted on. It can show nonspecific features of encephalitis or specific features suggestive of JE, Herpes simplex encephalitis or acute disseminated encephalomyelitis. Imaging may also occasionally reveal structural cause of coma **(Figs. 1 and 2)**
- *Blood chemistry:* A routine blood chemistry may reveal a metabolic cause of encephalopathy. Blood glucose, urea, creatinine, electrolytes and liver function tests should be done
- *Blood culture:* Should be done in every case
- Other investigations may be done according to clinical clues

(ELISA: enzyme-linked immunosorbent assay; HSE: herpes simplex encephalitis; JE: Japanese encephalitis; PCR: polymerase chain reaction)

hypertonic saline infusion, intravenous furosemide or intermittent positive pressure ventilation to keep arterial CO_2 tension between 25–30 mm Hg. Proper nursing care must be given. The role of steroids in acute viral encephalitis is debatable. Theoretic arguments exist for and against their use. A study that evaluated high-dose dexamethasone in JE found no benefit of steroid therapy.

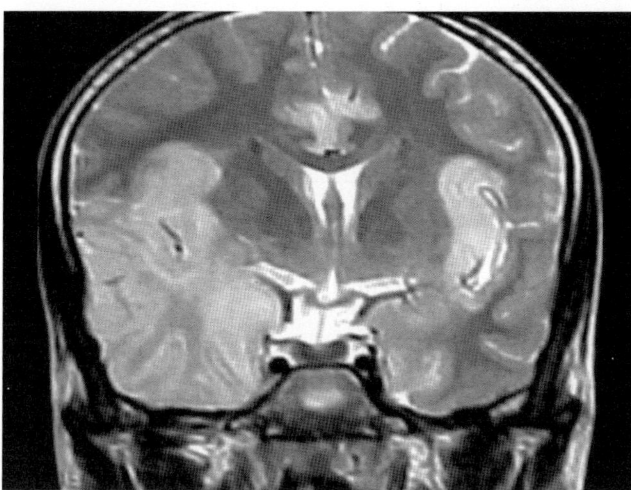

Fig. 1: Magnetic resonance imaging brain showing temporal lobe changes in herpes encephalitis.

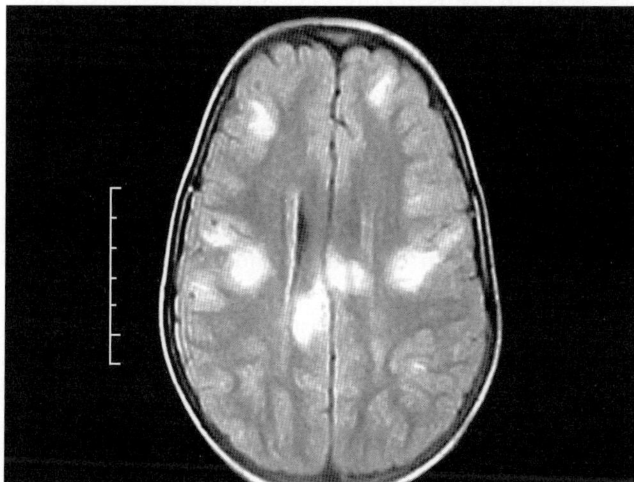

Fig. 2: Magnetic resonance imaging brain showing changes of acute disseminated encephalomyelitis.

BOX 5: Features of encephalopathies (diffuse cerebral disturbance without inflammation).

Features of encephalopathies
- Absence of fever or meningeal signs
- Absence of focal neurologic signs or focal seizures
- No peripheral leukocytosis
- Normal cerebrospinal fluid
- Diffuse slowing on electroencephalography
- Normal imaging studies

Specific therapy is recommended in encephalitis caused by herpes group of viruses. Acyclovir in a dose of 10 mg/kg administered as an intravenous infusion over 1 hour every 8 hours for 14 days (21 days in immunocompromised) is indicated in herpes simplex encephalitis. Success of antiviral therapy depends on early institution of therapy. Acyclovir is also recommended for varicella-zoster encephalitis. Oseltamivir can be considered for influenza encephalitis. Trials with α-interferon and nasogastric ribavirin in JE in children have revealed no benefit. Specific antimalarial therapy may also be indicated if suspicion of cerebral malaria exists.

BOX 6: Treatment of AFE/AES.

Initial rapid assessment and stabilization
- *Establish and maintain airway:* Intubate if GCS ≤8, impaired airway reflexes, abnormal respiratory pattern, signs of raised ICP, oxygen saturation <92% despite high flow oxygen, fluid refractory shock
- Ventilation, oxygenation
- *Circulation:*
  - Establish IV access, take samples (CBC, Blood sugar, KFT, LFT, electrolytes, blood gas, lactate, PS and RDT for malarial parasite, serology for viruses),
  - Fluid bolus if in circulatory failure (20 mL/kg NS), inotropes if required
- Identify signs of cerebral herniation or raised intracranial pressure
- Temperature: treat fever and hypothermia
- Treat ongoing Seizures: Benzodiazepine, followed by phenytoin loading

Empirical treatment must be started if CSF examination cannot be done or report will take time and patient is sick:
- Ceftriaxone
- Acyclovir (treat in all suspected sporadic viral encephalitis)
- Artesunate (stop if peripheral smear and rapid malaria test are negative)

Supportive care and treatment
- Maintain euglycemia, control fever, maintain hydration
- Treat raised intracranial pressure, mild head end elevation—15–30°
- Treat seizures. Give anticonvulsant if history of seizures or if GCS <8, or child has features of raised ICT
- Steroids—Pulse steroids (methylprednisolone or dexamethasone) must be given in children with suspected ADEM

Prevention/treatment of complications and rehabilitation
- Physiotherapy, posture change, prevent bed sores and exposure keratitis
- Complications—aspiration pneumonia, nosocomial infections, coagulation disturbances
- Nutrition—early feeding
- Psychological support to patient and family

(ADEM: acute disseminated encephalomyelitis; CBC: complete blood count; CSF: cerebrospinal fluid; GCS: glasgow coma scale; ICP: intracranial pressure; ICT: intracranial tension; IV: intravenous; KFT: kidney function test; LFT: liver function test; PS: peripheral smear; RDT: rapid diagnostic test)

Minocycline is a semisynthetic penicillin which has neuroprotective properties. It has excellent penetration in the cerebrospinal fluid. Besides its direct effects on non-viral pathogens like rickettsiae. It has been shown to have antiviral, anti-apoptotic and anti-inflammatory actions with significant benefit in animal models of viral encephalitis. There may be some role of minocycline in AES even of undetermined etiology as shown in human trials.

CLINICAL PEARL

- Tuberculous meningitis (TMB) usually has a subacute onset. Here the prodromal stage with nonspecific symptoms will be longer than a week. If the child is comatose and computed tomography scan does not show hydrocephalus it is unlikely to be TBM; presence of basal exudates and/or granulomas is suggestive of TBM while subdural collections are suggestive of bacterial meningitis. Cerebral malaria is a multisystem illness with acute onset of high fever, chills and rigors, bilateral upper motor neurone signs, anemia, hemoglobinuria and normal cerebrospinal fluid.

KEY POINTS

- Acute febrile encephalopathy is a common cause of intensive care admissions in pediatrics.
- Etiology is varied with both infectious and non infectious causes.
- A good history along with targetted investigations like Magnetic resonance imaging brain, infection screen and Cerebrospinal fluid analysis help in reaching diagnosis in majority.
- Pending investigations, empirical ceftriaxone, acyclovir and artesunate could be started in Indian scenario.
- A subset of patients may be undiagnosed despite extensive investigations. Autoimmune or inflammatory causes should be suspected in these.

SUGGESTED READING

1. Bale JF. Viral encephalitis. Med Clin North America. 1993;77(1):25-41.
2. Cherry JD. Encephalitis. In: Behrman RE, Kleigman RM (Eds). Nelson Textbook of Pediatrics, 14th edition. Pennsylvania: WB Saunders Co; 1993. pp. 666-9.
3. Glaser CA, Honarmand S, Anderson LJ, Schnurr DP, Forghani B, Cossen CK, et al. Beyond viruses: clinical profiles and etiologies associated with encephalitis. Clinical Infect Dis. 2006;43:1565-77.
4. Kalra V. Acute febrile encephalopathy. In: Gupta V, Gupta D (Eds). Practical Paediatric Neurology, 2nd edition. Avichal Publishing Co. (Arya Publication). 2008. p. 112.
5. Kumar R. Viral encephalitis and encephalopathies in Medical Emergencies in Children Ed M Singh.
6. Sharma S, Mishra D, Aneja S, Kumar R, Jain A, Vashishth VM. Evaluation and Management of Suspected Acute Viral Encephalitis in Children in India. Indian Pediatrics. 2012;49:897-903.
7. Rashmi Kumar, Anirban Basu, S Sinha, M Das, P Tripathi, A Jain, et al. Role of oral Minocycline in acute encephalitis syndrome in India—a randomized controlled trial. BMC Infectious Diseases 2016;16:67.

CHAPTER 97

Approach to Pediatric Movement Disorders

PAM Kunju, Anoop K Verma

INTRODUCTION

Movement disorders are characterized by abnormal or excessive involuntary movements that may result in abnormalities in posture, tone, balance, or fine motor control. It is often used synonymously with basal ganglia or extrapyramidal disease but it does not adequately describe all the movement disorders.

Basically movement disorders are characterized as akinetic rigid syndrome and hyperkinetic or dyskinetic syndrome. In akinetic syndrome, there is slowness or paucity of movement, e.g., parkinsonism (this particular disorder is rare in pediatric age group). In dyskinetic syndrome, there is excessive movement, e.g., chorea, athetosis, ballismus, tremor, dystonia, tics, and other stereotypic behavior.

HOW THEY DIFFER IN CHILDREN?

Movement disorders in childhood are a heterogeneous group of diseases with presentations that vary according to etiopathogenesis and age of onset. Involuntary movements can represent the sole disease manifestation, or they may be one of many symptoms and signs of other systemic disorder. While sharing certain characteristics with the conditions that affect adults, they also have unique features that are determined by the metabolic, physiological, and environmental distinctiveness of the developing brain. So they show some particular characteristics:

- An increased occurrence of hyperkinetic movements, rather than bradykinesia or rigidity
- A higher frequency of transient motor phenomena in the first year of life
- A higher prevalence of paroxysmal movement disorders
- A major primary etiology for chronic motor dysfunction being residue of static encephalopathy
- A greater likelihood that symptoms are secondary to hereditary metabolic disorders
- An evolving pattern of movements associated with metabolic disorders

Some of the common benign movement disorders that have to be ruled out in infancy are:

- Benign neonatal sleep myoclonus
- Benign myoclonus of infancy
- Jitteriness
- Shuddering attacks
- Paroxysmal tonic upgaze of infancy
- Spasmus nutans
- Benign paroxysmal torticollis
- Benign idiopathic dystonia of infancy

CATEGORIZATION OF MOVEMENT DISORDER

If we categorize the movement disorder according to the level of involvement at the brain, it can be summarized as per the following **Flowchart 1**.

The structures responsible for motor control are upper motor neuron (UMN), lower motor neuron (LMN), cerebellar circuitry, basal ganglia circuitry, motor activation cortex, and sensory cortex. Virtually the entire nervous system is engaged in motor control.

The basal ganglia consist of five large subcortical nuclei that are the caudate nucleus, putamen, globus pallidus, substantia nigra, and subthalamic nuclei. Bradykinesia is related to insult at substantia nigra, ballismus to subthalamic nucleus, dystonia to putamen, and chorea to caudate nucleus, but overlaps are also seen.

Flowchart 1: Categorization of movement disorders.

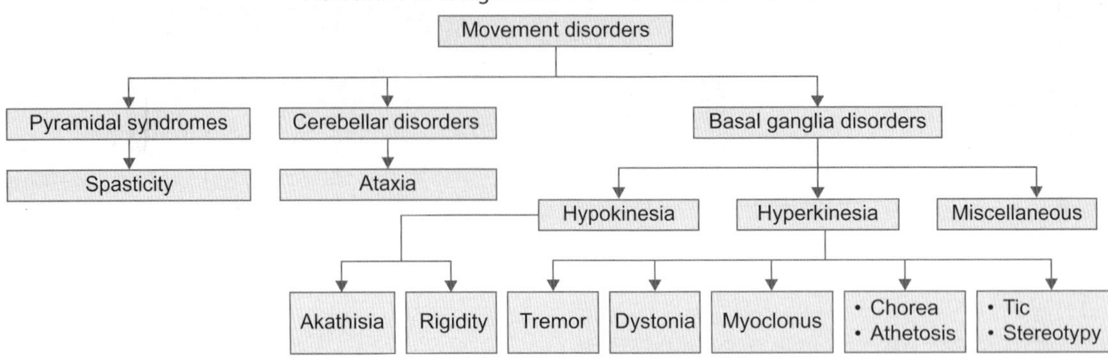

CLINICAL PEARLS

- Movement disorder can be differentiated from seizures by the preservation of consciousness.
- Except ballism movement disorders stop during sleep.
- Video recording using mobile phones will help in identifying the type of abnormal movements.

PHENOMENOLOGY OF MOVEMENT DISORDERS

Phenomenology refers to the clinically observable aspects of movement disorder, and one must be able to identify, the characteristic of each movement disorder as each of them has a different character **(Table 1)**.

CLINICAL PEARLS

- Movement disorders can be grouped according to the speed of movement.
- Fastest being myoclonus, slightly slower will be ballism, then chorea, then athetosis, and slowest dystonia.

GENERAL APPROACH TO MOVEMENT DISORDERS

Evaluation of movement disorders, like all neurologic symptoms, begins with a comprehensive history:

- Patient's gestation, detailed birth history, early development, previous illnesses, drug history, exposure to potential toxins, and social and family history, are often essential for proper classification
- The key questions to be asked are as follows:
  - What is the distribution? (e.g., orofacial—chorea)
  - Is it unilateral or generalized? (e.g., hemidystonia associated with structural lesion and generalized idiopathic/genetic)

TABLE 1: Characteristics of movement disorders.

Movement disorder	***Brief description***
Chorea	Chorea is rapid jerky, large amplitude involuntary movements of proximal more than distal muscles
Athetosis	Slower writhing irregular movements predominantly in the hands and wrist
Dyskinesia	General term for abnormal movement; however, commonly denotes movements of mouth and face, usually drug induced (orofacial dyskinesia)
Dystonia	Co-contraction of agonist and antagonist, which lead to an intermittent or persistent maintenance of abnormal posture and or twisting
Hemiballismus	Violent flinging movements, which are irregular affecting one side
Myoclonus	Sudden shock-like contraction of a muscle or a group of muscle leading to involuntary purposeless jerk of limbs or trunk
Ataxia	Ataxia is inability to control movements and typically is caused by cerebellar dysfunction
Tics	Tics are rapid, complex, nonvoluntary, repetitive segmental movements. Simple tics last <6 months. Chronic tics last longer than 6 months
Tourette syndrome	There are motor tics and vocalizations lasting longer than 12 months, start between 2 and 10 years of age, and may fluctuate in severity over time
Tremor	Regular rhythmic repetitive to and fro oscillation about a certain point or position involving one or more body part
Stereotypies	Stereotypies are repetitive, patterned involuntary movements that have no apparent function
Akathisia	An inability to remain still; an intense sensation of unease or an inner restlessness that usually involves the lower extremities

- What is the speed of movement—fast (excessive movement and hyperkinetic) or slow (paucity of movement and hypokinetic)?
- Is it rhythmic or is it jerky? (e.g., rhythmic—tremor; palatal myoclonus)
- Is it present at rest? With action? Is there any relation to certain postures or positions? (e.g., rest tremor—parkinsonism; action tremor—familial essential tremor)
- Is there any task specificity? (e.g., kinesigenic choreoathetosis)
- Is patient able to suppress it? (e.g., tics)
- Is it stereotyped? (e.g., tics/stereotypy)
- Is movement disorder continuous or intermittent or occurring in discrete episodes? (e.g., paroxysmal dyskinesia)
- Is there an association with an urge? (e.g., tics)
- Is it related to sleep? (e.g., hemiballism/restless leg syndrome; seizure)
- Is it associated with functional motor impairment?
- Are there any aggravating/alleviating factors?

CLINICAL PEARLS

- Video of abnormal movement is important. It can supplement witnessing the real-time abnormal movement of the patient.
- General examination is further required for properly defining the movement and identifying clues indicating a systemic problem.

A critical feature is determining whether the presenting signs/symptoms are an isolated disorder, associated with other neurologic findings, part of a static condition, or appearing in conjunction with a loss of other previously acquired skills.

A comprehensive general examination is further required for properly defining the movement and identifying clues indicating a systemic problem. The category of movement assists in localizing the pathologic process, whereas the onset, age, and degree of abnormal motor activity and associated neurologic findings help organize the investigation. Correct classification of the type of movement disorder forms the basis for the subsequent diagnostic process.

The features of movement disorders are discussed in **Table 2**.

Thus, compiling the important pieces of information from history and examination, the strategy is to reach the diagnosis from recognizing the patterns based on phenomenology and then focus on the causes as possible etiologies for acute, subacute onset and acquired causes.

CAUSES OF MOVEMENT DISORDERS

The causes of movement disorders can be summarized as in **Flowchart 2**.

CLINICAL PEARL

- Hemidystonia may indicate a structural abnormality and generalized dystonia may indicate a possible idiopathic disorder.

DRUG-INDUCED MOVEMENT DISORDERS

There are various movement disorders which are caused due to adverse effects of medications or drugs. They are summarized in **Table 3**.

Before discussing the individual movement disorders, it would be prudent to take a look at the inherited disorders causing movement disorders **(Table 4)**.

TABLE 2: Features of movement disorders.

Features	***Category***	***Examples***
Speed	• Hyperkinetic • Hypokinetic	• Tremor, chorea, myoclonus, tics, restless legs syndrome, and dystonia • Apraxia and Parkinson bradykinesia
Region	• Whole body • Hemibody • Segmental • Multifocal • Focal • Proximal • Distal • Oral	• Generalized dystonia • Hemidystonia and hemichorea • Segmental myoclonus • Polyminimyoclonus • Writer's cramp • Rubral tremor • Athetosis • Tardive dyskinesia

Contd...

Contd…

Features	***Category***	***Examples***
Character	*Rhythm*	
	Rhythmic	Tremor, dystonic tremor, and periodic movements in sleep
	Arrhythmic	Akathitic movements, athetosis, ballism, chorea, dystonia, hemifacial spasm, hyperekplexia, arrhythmic myoclonus, stereotypy, and tics
	Frequency	
	• Fast • Slow	• Chorea, tics, and minipolymyoclonus • Ballism
	Amplitude	
	• Large • Fine	• Ballism • Tremor and minipolymyoclonus
	At rest	
	• At rest and continues with action • With action	• Ballism, chorea, dystonia, and postural tremor • Action tremor and ataxia
	Force	
	Powerful	Stiff-man syndrome
Trigger	• Action • Position	• Writer's cramp • Orthostatic tremor
Intentionality	• Voluntary • Involuntary	• Tics • Tardive dyskinesia
Relieving factor	Sleep	Dystonia and tremor
Psychiatric		Huntington disease

Flowchart 2: Causes of movement disorders.

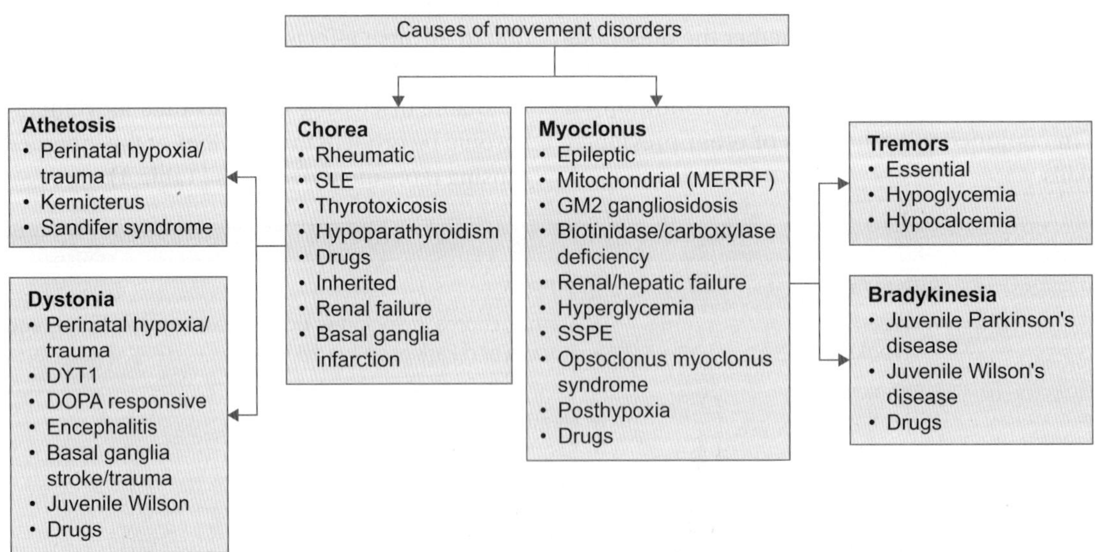

(DOPA: dopamine; MERRF: myoclonic epilepsy with ragged red fibers; SLE: systemic lupus erythematosus; SSPE: subacute sclerosing panencephalitis)

TABLE 3: Drug-induced movement disorders.

Type of movement disorder	***Drugs***	***Presence in sleep***
Bradykinesia	Typical neuroleptics and atypical antipsychotic	No
Chorea/athetosis	Phenytoin, carbamazepine, valproic acid, dopamine receptor blocking agent, tricyclic antidepressant, theophylline, oral contraceptives, steroids, and stimulants	No
Dystonia	Typical neuroleptics, antipsychotics, and metoclopramide	No
Myoclonus	Epileptic myoclonus can be aggravated by some antiepileptics	Yes
Tremor	Tricyclic antidepressant, valproic acid, phenytoin, carbamazepine, and theophylline	No
Tics	Lamotrigine, stimulants, levodopa, and neuroleptics	Yes
Akathisia	Due to antipsychotics blocking dopamine type-2 receptors., e.g., haloperidol	No

TABLE 4: Some inherited condition causing movement disorders.

Etiology	***Age at onset***	***Clinical signs***	***EEG and imaging***	***Laboratory finding and genetic testing***
Glutaric aciduria type 1	5–10 months	Acute encephalopathy followed by dystonia, motor impairment, and macrocephaly	*CT/MRI:* Frontotemporal atrophy, bat wing appearance of Sylvian fissure **(Fig. 1)**	Organic acid in urine and enzyme assay
Glucose transporter 1 deficiency syndrome	Infancy	Seizures, developmental delay, complex movement disorder; alternating hemiplegia of child hood	EEG improves postprandially	Low-glucose concentration in CSF
Lesch–Nyhan syndrome	3–13 months	Self-mutilation, facial grimacing, and involuntary writhing repetitive movement of arm	Development of kidney stone	Hyperuricemia
Leigh's disease	Birth to first year	Diffuse encephalopathy, dysphagia, dystonia, myoclonus, and hypotonia central respiratory insufficiency	*MRI:* PVL, hyperintense T2 signal in the basal ganglia and thalami	High serum/CSF lactate
PKAN	1st decade	Delayed motor and language, later choreoathetosis, dystonia, dysarthria, dysphasia, and spasticity retinopathy	*MRI:* Eye of the tiger sign	Genetic testing
Wilson's disease	1st and 2nd decade	Dysarthria, gait disturbances, risus sardonicus, dystonia, rigidity, tremor, and dysphagia	*MRI:* High signal in basal ganglia, dentate nuclei, and cerebellum on T2	KF ring and low-serum ceruloplasmin
Huntington's disease	2nd decade	Neurological and psychiatric symptoms, chorea, rigidity, and hypokinesia	*MRI:* Nonspecific generalized or striatal atrophy	Gene-CGG repeat testing
Early-onset torsion dystonia	Between 3 and 26 years	Ashkenazi Jews, dystonia affecting first one arm or leg progressing to generalized or multifocal	Noncontributing	*DYT* gene mutations

(CSF: cerebrospinal fluid; CT, computed tomography; EEG: electroencephalography; KF ring: Kayser–Fleischer ring; MRI: magnetic resonance imaging; PKAN: pantothenate kinase-associated neurodegeneration; PVL: periventricular leukomalacia)

CLINICAL PEARL

- Three generations pedigree, including cousins and siblings of parents and grandparents can give a clue to the hereditary causes of movement disorders.

The category of movement assists in localizing the pathologic process, whereas the onset, age, and degree of abnormal motor activity and associated neurologic findings help to organize the investigation.

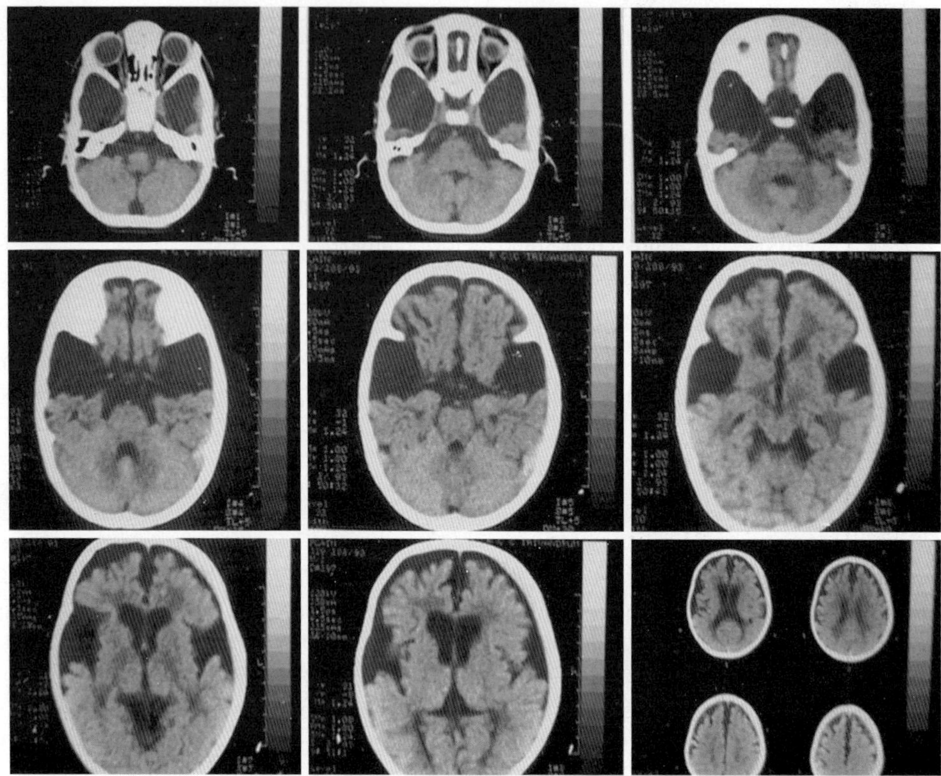

Fig. 1: CT scan showing bat wing appearance of Sylvian fissure and expanded subarachnoid space in frontal region.

Correct classification of the type of movement disorder forms the basis for the subsequent diagnostic process.

No specific biological marker is available:
- Many diagnostic tests are available but these are often expensive, time-consuming or invasive; however, the reduction in cost of genetic testing has improved the diagnosis and thus offering specific treatment.
- The diagnostic value of these tests is often limited, especially in early stages of the disease.

The investigational workup can be greatly simplified once the type of movement disorder has been defined properly.

Investigations

The investigations in movement disorders can be divided under different headings of neuroimaging, hematological, immunological, or other investigations as applicable. Magnetic resonance imaging (MRI) brain is the neuroimaging modality of choice in pediatric movement disorders and proves a good guide to diagnosis **(Flowchart 3)**.

> **CLINICAL PEARL**
>
> MRI will help in identifying various disorders. Basal ganglia calcification can be due to Fahr syndrome or pseudo-hypoparathyroidism and basal ganglia hyperintensity can be commonly due to Wilson disease (caudate) and kernicterus (globus pallidus).

Treatment

Although the treatment of movement disorders is varied and multidisciplinary according to the type, the common drugs used to treat and their dosages are given in **Table 5**. The drugs are thereafter mentioned briefly when describing the individual movement disorders.

INDIVIDUAL MOVEMENT DISORDERS

Following is a short discussion of movement disorders.

Dystonia

Though dystonia is a common symptom in neurology, it is being recognized less frequently by pediatricians.

Flowchart 3: Brain MRI changes in movement disorders.

MRI brain in movement disorders

Basal Ganglia T1 hyperintensities
Related to deposition of T1-intense elements within the basal ganglia
- Methemoglobin in intracranial hemorrhage
- Calcium
- Hepatic failure
- Hyperalimentation or long-term parenteral nutrition (manganese)
- Carbon monoxide
- Hemorrhagic infarct
- Japanese encephalitis

Basal Ganglia T2 hyperintensities
- Lymphoma
- Ischemia
- Hypoxia
- Venous infarction (internal cerebral vein thrombosis)
- Neurodegenerative/metabolic
  - *Wilson disease:* Putamen + face of panda sign on axial section of midbrain
  - *Huntington disease:* Caudate heads
- Mitochondrial diseases, e.g., Leigh's disease
- Extrapontine myelinolysis
- Hypoglycemia
- Toxins
- CO exposure
- Methanol
- Methyl malonicacidurias
- Creatine deficiency
- Kernicterus

(Methyl malonicacidurias, Creatine deficiency, Kernicterus: Globus pallidus)

Basal Ganglia Calcification
- Fahr disease
- CNS tuberculosis
- AIDS
- Neurocysticercosis
- CNS toxoplasmosis
- Hypoparathyroidism
- Pseudohypoparathyroidism
- Pseudo-pseudohypoparathyroidism
- Mitochondrial diseases, e.g., MELAS
- Cockayne syndrome
- Radiation therapy

(AIDS: acquired immunodeficiency syndrome; CNS: central nervous system; CO: carbon monoxide; MELAS: mitochondrial encephalomyopathy, lactic acidosis, and stroke-like episodes; MRI: magnetic resonance imaging)

TABLE 5: Drugs used in movement disorders.

Drugs	*Doses*	*Precautions*	*Indications in movement disorders*
Pimozide	1–2 mg/day (2–6 mg, if required)	Prolong QT interval Cardiac arrhythmias	Gilles de la Tourette syndrome
Haloperidol	20–50 µg/kg initially; maximum to 10 mg/day	Liver and kidney disease, epilepsy, and thyrotoxicosis	• Choreiform movement, rheumatic chorea, and hemiballismus • Gilles de la Tourette syndrome
Tetrabenazine	12.5 mg BID; increment of 12.5 mg every 3–4 day to a maximum of 3 mg/kg/day	Pregnancy, lactation depression, patient on levodopa, and reserpine	Chorea, hemiballismus, myoclonus, buccolingual dyskinesia, and in certain dystonia
Trihexyphenidyl	1 mg first day, 2 mg second day, then increase to 2 mg every 3–5 day; maintenance usually 6–16 mg/day	Glaucoma, sick sinus syndrome, cardiac failure, and tachycardia	Dystonia, myoclonus, drug-induced movement disorders, and torticollis
Levodopa–carbidopa	Up to 5 mg/kg/day	Levodopa-induced dyskinesia	Dopa-responsive dystonia, dystonia, and Parkinson state
Carbamazepine	• *<6 years:* 5 mg/kg/24 hours orally; may increase every 5–7 day by 5 mg/kg/day • *6–12 years:* Initially 10 mg/kg/day; increase by 5/mg/day at weekly intervals Usual dose—800–1200 mg/24 h	Porphyria, hepatic failure, and MAO inhibitors	Chorea, athetosis, ballismus, and paroxysmal kinesigenic dyskinesia

Contd...

Contd...

Drugs	**Doses**	**Precautions**	**Indications in movement disorders**
Sodium valproate	• *Below 20 kg:* 20 mg/kg/day • *Above 20 kg:* 400 mg/day	Liver disease, SLE, and porphyria	Chorea
Clonazepam	Initial 0.01–0.03 mg/kg/24 h in 2–3 divided doses; increase 0.25–0.5 mg/24 h every 3–5 days; maximum dose 0.3 mg/kg/24 h	Hypersensitivity to benzodiazepine	Dystonia, torticollis, myoclonus, and startle syndrome

(BID twice a day; MAO: monoamine oxidase; SLE: systemic lupus erythematosus)

Definition

Dystonia is a hyperkinetic movement disorder characterized by sustained or intermittent muscle contractions causing abnormal (often repetitive) movements, postures, or both. The factor which distinguishes myoclonus, chorea, athetosis, and dystonia would be the variable speed of movement; fastest being myoclonus, 50–100 ms and slowest one being dystonia, which may last at least a second.

Dystonia evolves in a focal manner and during voluntary activity—"action dystonia".

Pathophysiology

Dystonia is a circuit disorder, historically thought to arise from basal ganglia but now recognized to result from injury or malfunction in any of the several nodes within the motor cortex.

Classification

The dystonias are classified according to their distribution, age of onset, type of onset, and etiology.

Distribution

- *Focal:*
  - When dystonia is confined to anyone single region:
    - *Ocular muscles:* Blepharospasm
    - *Tongue:* Lingual dystonia
    - *Vocal cord:* Dystonic dysphonia
    - *Mouth:* Oromandibular dystonia
    - *Neck:* Torticollis
    - *Hand:* Writer's cramp **(Figs. 2A and B)**
- *Segmental:*
  - When focal dystonia spreads to contiguous area:
    - *Cranial:* Face and neck
    - *Axial:* Neck and trunk
    - *Brachial:* Arm and trunk

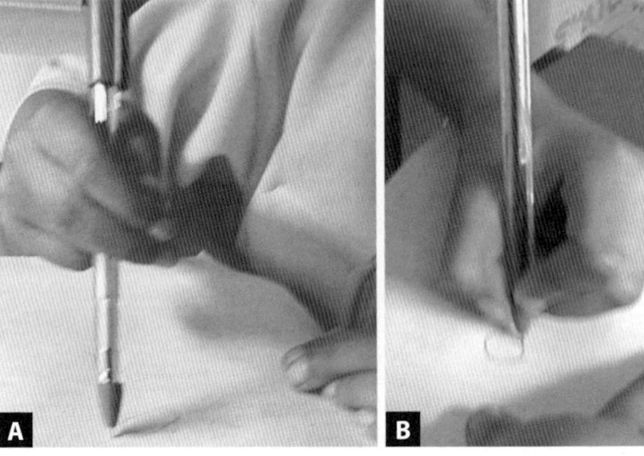

Figs. 2A and B: Writers cramps—before and after Botox injection.

    - *Crural:* One leg and trunk; both legs with or without trunk
- *Generalized—Crural:*
  - With any other segmental involvement
  - Focal or segmental dystonia may progress and become generalized if:
    - Childhood or adolescent onset
    - Beginning in the lower limbs
- *Hemidystonia:* When one side of the body is involved.

Type of Onset

It is broadly divided in to four groups:
1. Acute dystonia
2. Tardive dystonia
3. Paroxysmal dystonia
4. Chronic nonprogressive/progressive dystonia.

Acute dystonia: Acute dystonia arise from neuroleptic drugs, exposure to toxins, infections, and certain familial disorders. Acute reactions can appear soon after starting treatment with phenothiazine, or even promethazine. Manifestations include bizarre postures of face (sustained grimacing), eyes (oculogyric crisis), jaw (trismus and mandibular dystonia), tongue (lingual dystonia), neck (torticollis), trunk (scoliosis, lordosis, kyphosis, and opisthotonos), and limbs (torsion spasm). These may be confused with seizure, tetany, or encephalitis if a proper history of drug ingestion is not obtained.

The acute dystonic reactions may be the result of excess dopaminergic activity. Response to treatment of acute dystonia is often dramatic. Anticholinergic drugs like diphenhydramine or promethazine will reverse the acute dystonia within minutes. We have seen transient dyskinesia in asthmatic patients receiving theophylline. Interaction of theophylline and hypoxemia with other factors may induce this.

CLINICAL PEARLS

Acute dystonias can be remembered by VITS:
- V—Vascular (infarct; hemorrhage, etc.)
- I—Infection and postinfectious, e.g., Japanese encephalitis; autoimmune encephalitis
- T—Toxin (drugs like phenothiazine toxicity)
- S—Space occupying lesion (subacute)

Tardive dystonia: It is a separate entity from acute dystonic reactions in that it is persistent, does not show response to intravenous diphenhydramine or anticholinergics. Another striking feature is the distribution of dystonic movement. Generalized dystonia is more in younger individuals whereas in older subjects it has a more restricted distribution.

Paroxysmal dystonia: A group of interesting disorders which may be confused with seizures:
- *Familial paroxysmal dystonic choreoathetosis:* This rare bizarre paroxysmal movements occurring in an autosomal dominant manner. Each attack is characterized by (1) painful spasm of affected musculature, (2) choreoathetosis, and (3) return to normality.
- *Paroxysmal kinesigenic dystonia:* Sudden movement or startle and stress will precipitate an attack. These patients can avert an attack by avoiding abrupt movement and sensory stimuli. *Proline-rich transmembrane protein 2 (PRRT2)* gene (16p11.2) is believed to be the major causative gene.
- *Paroxysmal nonkinesigenic dystonia (PNKD):* Attacks are typically precipitated by coffee, tea, or alcohol; they can also be triggered by excitement, stress, or fatigue, or can be spontaneous. Caused by mutations in the *PNKD* gene.
- *Exercise-induced paroxysmal dystonia:* A paroxysmal dystonic choreoathetosis, which is seen after continued exercise or by sensory stimuli but not after a sudden movement
- *Paroxysmal hypnogenic dystonia:* Certain varieties of dystonia may be brought on by sleep. Now considered as autosomal dominant nocturnal frontal lobe epilepsy
- In addition to the idiopathic variety, we have seen paroxysmal dystonias due to intracranial tumor, hyperthyroidism and transient ischemic attacks.

Recently following genetic associations are found with paroxysmal movement disorders. Paroxysmal kinesigenic dyskinesia due to *PRRT2* mutations (DYT10); paroxysmal nonkinesigenic dyskinesias (DYT8) with mutations in the *PNKD* (also known as *MR-1*) gene; and exertion-induced dyskinesia (DYT18) with *SLC2A1* mutations.

CLINICAL PEARL

- Paroxysmal movement disorders [paroxysmal dyskinesias (PD)] may resemble seizures but will respond to antiepileptic drugs such as phenytoin, carbamazepine (kinesigenic PD), or clonazepam (nonkinesigenic PD).

Treatment: Paroxysmal *kinesigenic choreoathetosis* responds to phenytoin. Other varieties may respond to clonazepam, L-tryptophan and carbamazepine.

Chronic nonprogressive/progressive dystonias: Chronic nonprogressive disorder is cerebral palsy. Mostly due to Kernicterus or hypoxia (status marmoratus) **(Fig. 3)**. Approach to dystonia is given in **Flowchart 4**.

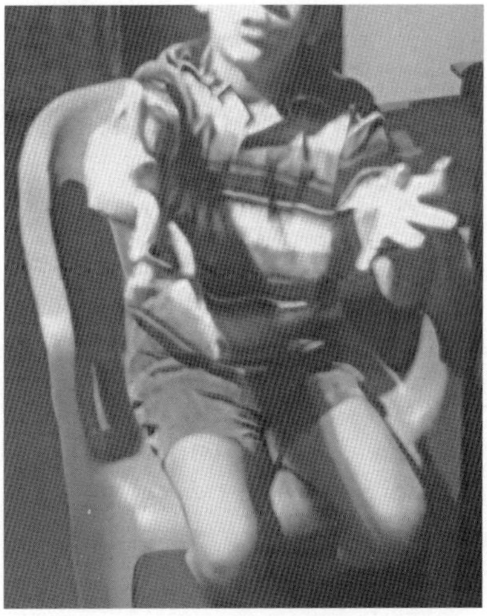

Fig. 3: A child with dystonic choreoathetosis.

Flowchart 4: Clinical approach to diagnosis of dystonia in children.

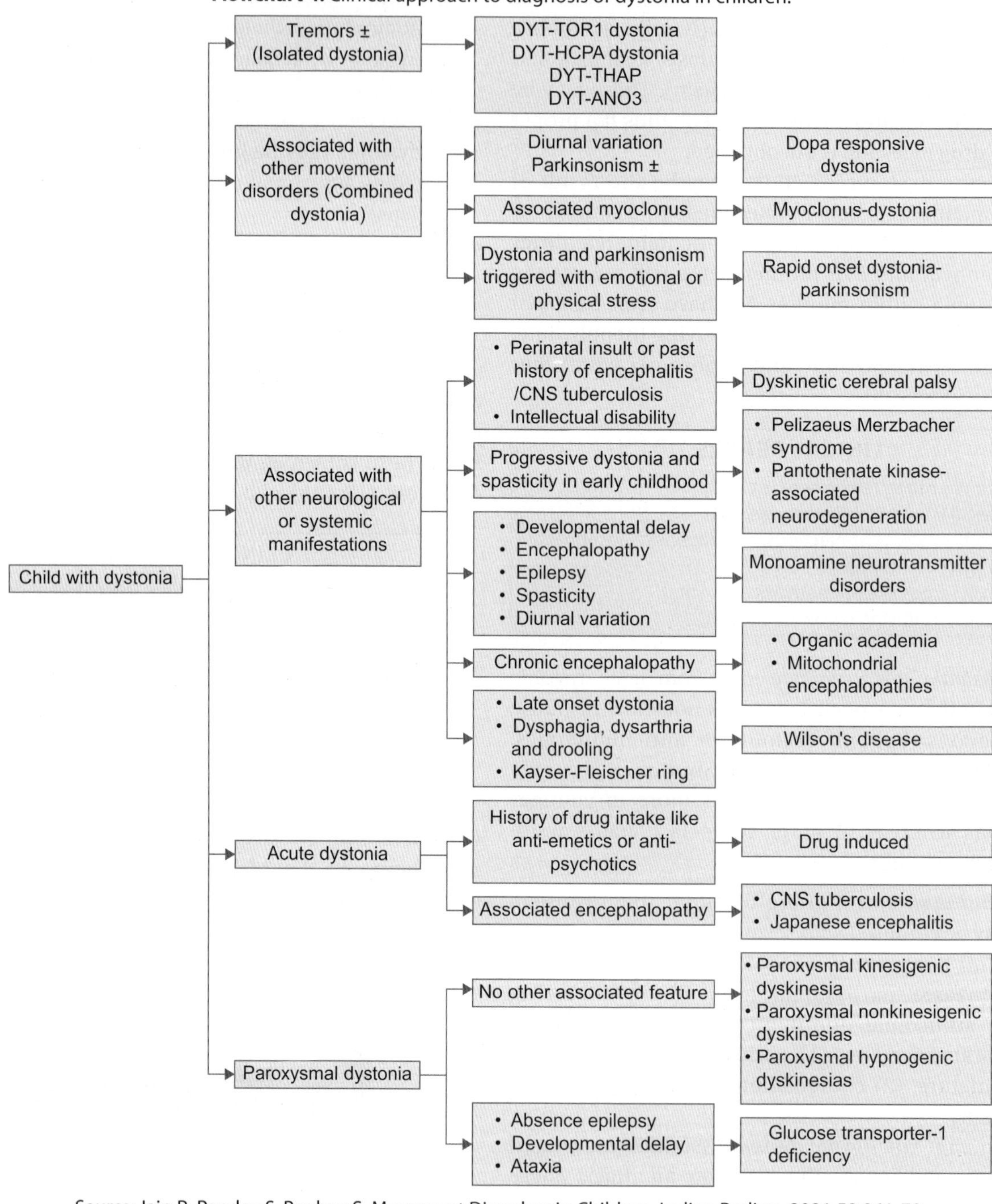

Source: Jain R, Pandey S, Raghav S. Movement Disorders in Children. Indian Pediatr. 2021;58:861-70.

Progressive dystonias:

Etiology: Dystonias are divided into two types on the basis of etiology as follows:

1. Primary dystonia
2. Secondary dystonia

Primary dystonia: Algorithm to dystonia is given in **Flowchart 4**. In the past 20 years, monogenic defects have been found to underlie many forms of dystonia. Monogenic forms of isolated dystonia are referred to as DYTs.

- *Idiopathic torsion dystonia (ITD)/dystonia musculorum deformans (DMD):* Autosomal dominant dystonia gene is found to be located on chromosome 9q34. The usual age of onset is 5–15 years with dystonia of legs and within 5–10 years disease reach to maximum level of disability. At that time they are twisted axially with contorted oromandibular, neck, trunk, and limb musculature.
- *Dopa-responsive dystonia:* This group of patients with dystonia responds dramatically to a very low dosage of levodopa. Features include onset of dystonia before the age of 16, onset in the legs or with gait, and often having features of parkinsonism. Inheritance is autosomal dominant. Since the demonstration of dopa-sensitive dystonic states, levodopa has been tried in some of the cases of the congenital cerebral palsy where choreoathetotic rigidity is seen.
- *Diurnal dystonia (Segawa syndrome):* Relatively free of dystonic movements and postures in the morning and be afflicted severely in the late afternoon. Segawa had described this type of dystonia and we have seen many with similar involvement and who showed dramatic response to levodopa. The disease is caused by a GTP cyclohydrolase 1 (GCH) deficiency. Genetic mutations in the tetrahydrobiopterin synthetic pathway, specifically the *GCH1* gene (DYT 5) in the autosomal-dominant variant, and the *TH* gene in the autosomal recessive form, are responsible for the condition.

CLINICAL PEARLS

- Common cause of nonprogressive dystonia is dyskinetic cerebral palsy due to kernicterus or birth asphyxia **(Fig. 3)**
- However, in such cases a dose of levodopamine must be tried to rule-out diurnal dystonia (Segawa syndrome), which is an eminently treatable condition.

Secondary dystonias: Secondary dystonia can be due to congenital, hereditary, metabolic, vascular, infection, degeneration, demyelination, tumor, drugs, toxins, etc.

Useful clinical pointers to suggest a secondary dystonia:

- History to suggest involvement of other organ systems, e.g., liver (Wilson's disease) and multiple system (systemic lupus erythematosus)
- Coexistent neurological signs indicating involvement of higher mental, retinal, pyramidal, or LMN function
- History of exposure to antipsychotic drugs, toxins, injury, or cerebrovascular disorders.

Treatment

Treatable dystonic conditions such as Wilson's disease and tardive dystonias have to be considered first.

- *Drugs:* Trihexyphenidyl, dopamine agonists, baclofen, clonazepam, carbamazepine, and clonidine
- Local administration of botulinum toxin for focal dystonias
- Surgical methods
- Psychological methods

CLINICAL PEARL

- Dopa-responsive dystonia (DYT5 and Segawa disease) is the most important cause of primary dystonia with childhood onset, responds dramatically to low doses of levodopa.

Chorea

Involuntary, purposeless/quasi purposive, jerky, and dance-like movements.

Athetosis: Now described as a slow and writhing form of chorea.

Ballism: Forceful and flinging form of chorea; proximal more than distal, typically unilateral, and often coexistent with chorea.

Pathophysiology of Chorea

Injury to basal ganglia, especially the striatal indirect pathway, is a common anatomic precipitant for many forms. The neurophysiology underlying chorea is still poorly understood.

Causes of Chorea

- *Structural:*
  - Ischemic stroke—acute/subacute—unilateral chorea; localizing neurologic signs
  - Tumor—subacute—symptoms of raised intracranial pressure
  - Moyamoya disease—subacute and multifocal seizures
- *Metabolic/endocrine:*
  - Hypernatremia/hyponatremia; hypomagnesemia—altered biochemical status
  - Hyperparathyroidism/hypoparathyroidism, pseudohypoparathyroidism—basal ganglia calcification.
- *Autoimmune:*
  - Autoimmune encephalitis—underlying ovarian teratoma/positive N-methyl-D-aspartate receptor antibody

- Systemic lupus erythematosus—signs of systemic erythematosus
- Sydenham's chorea—preceding streptococcal infection
- Antiphospholipid antibody syndrome—focal signs stroke; hypercoagulable state

- *Genetic:*
  - Chorea-acanthocytosis syndrome—obsessive compulsive behaviors, orolingual dystonia, peripheral neuropathy, and seizures
  - Wilson's disease—tremor, dystonia typical, and psychiatric features
  - Huntington's disease—in children more of rigid dystonia
  - Ataxia-telangiectasia—ataxia, oculomotor apraxia, and increased sinopulmonary infection
  - Spinocerebellar ataxia 1, 2, 3, 17—ataxia, peripheral neuropathy, and abnormal movements
  - Lesch-Nyhan syndrome—self mutilation
  - Leigh's syndrome—dystonia, spasticity, myoclonus, and lactic acidosis
  - Pantothenate kinase-associated neurodegeneration—progressive dystonia, dysarthria, rigidity, ballism, choreoathetosis, spasticity, dementia, and pigmentary retinal degeneration; MRI shows the characteristic "eye of the tiger" sign within globus pallidus interna **(Figs. 4 and 5)**
  - Fahr's disease—second decade of life, microcephaly, hypertonia, and choreoathetosis. Basal ganglia and cerebellar nuclei calcification and also punctate calcifications in thalamus **(Fig. 6)**.

Approach to chorea is given in **Flowchart 5**

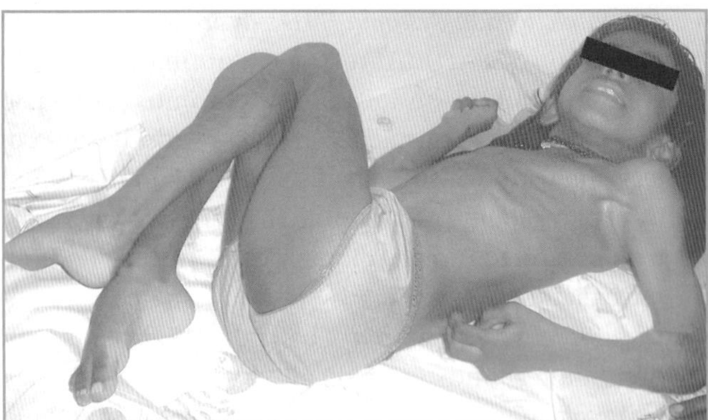

Fig. 4: Pantothenate kinase-associated neurodegeneration—severe dystonia.

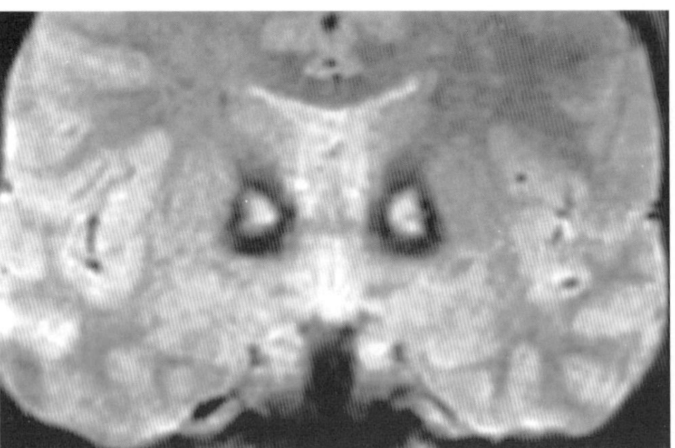

Fig. 5: Eye of the tiger sign in coronal magnetic resonance imaging.

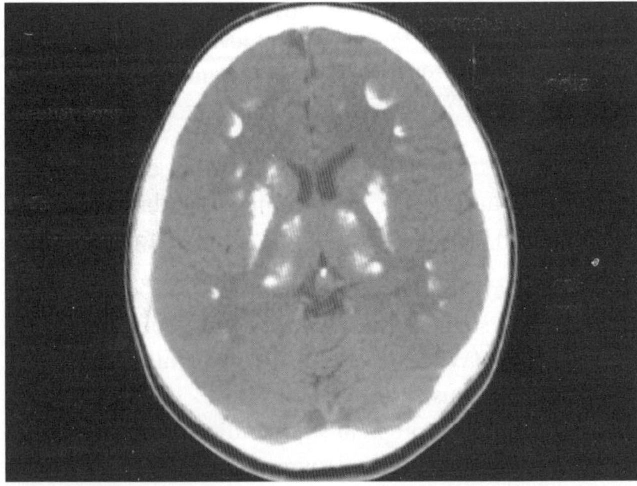

Fig. 6: Computer tomography scan—basal ganglia calcification—pseudohypoparathyroidism.

Tremor

Definition

Tremor is defined as regular rhythmic repetitive to and fro oscillatory movements.

Pathophysiology

Can arise from cortex, basal ganglia, brainstem, cerebellum, or periphery—each location associated with distinct tremor characteristics.

Types

- Resting tremor—decreases or resolves with movement. Worsens with agitation or inattention

Flowchart 5: Clinical approach to diagnosis of chorea in children.

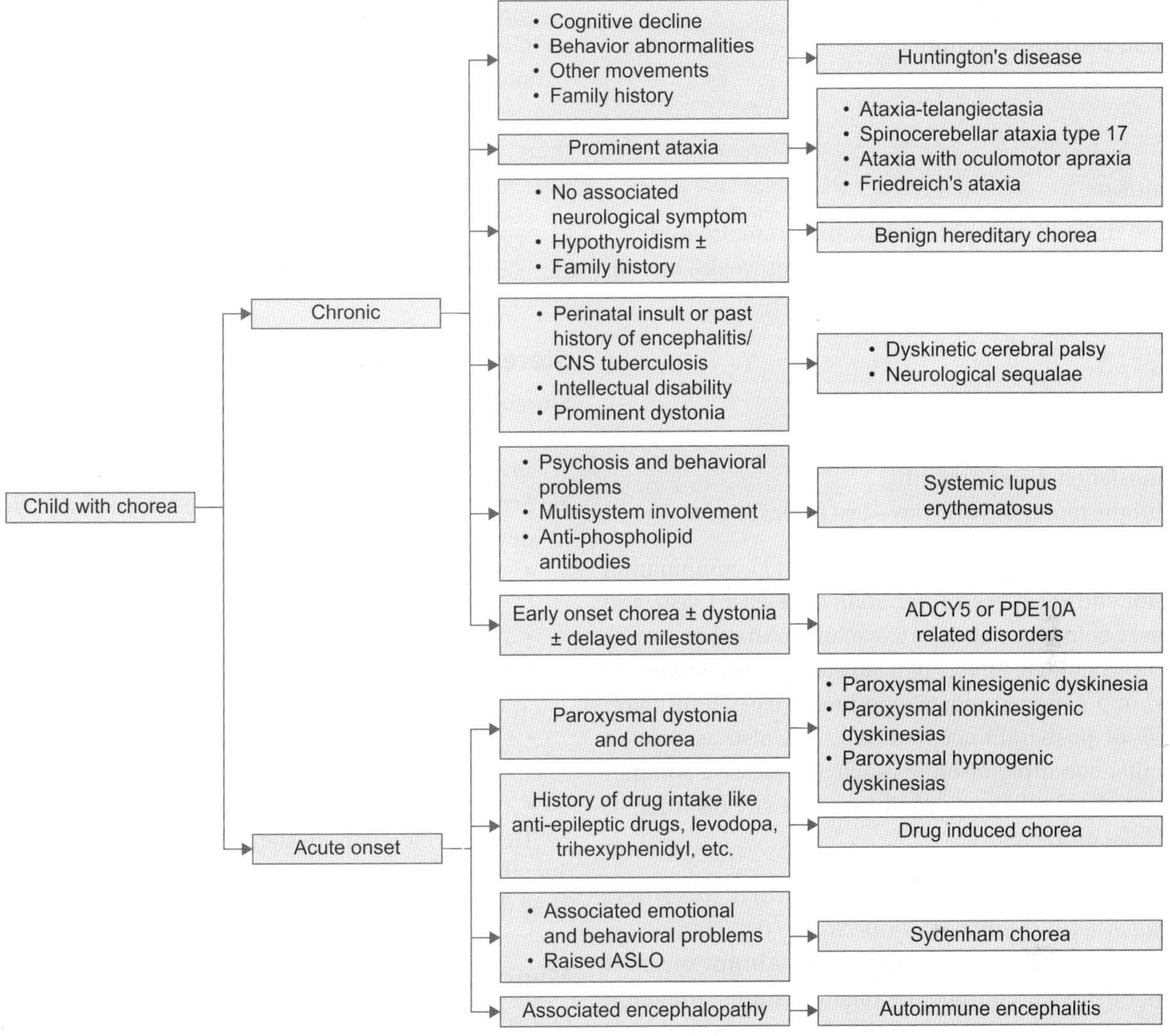

- Action tremor—elicited by initiating movement or increasing force generated. Four subtypes can be postural tremor, intention tremor kinetic, or isometric tremor
- Physiologic tremor—seen with particular situational challenges, e.g., stress, caffeine, and fatigue
- Rubral tremor—coarse, jerky, irregular, large amplitude, and low frequency (Holmes tremor or midbrain tumor)
- Psychogenic tremor—variability in tremor frequency, amplitude, distribution, and direction. Usually acute in onset but non progressive
- Drug-induced tremors—seen with medications (bronchodilators, thyroid hormone, stimulants, steroids, etc.)
- Orthostatic tremor, sometimes known as "shaky legs syndrome", is a disorder characterized by feelings of unsteadiness in the legs and a fear of falling when standing. A subtype of essential tremor.

Rigidity

A form of hypertonia in which resistance to passive movement is present at low speeds, does not depend on the speed and does not exhibit a speed or threshold angle.

Hallmarks of Rigidity

Associated with diseases with a primary failure of dopamine production:

- Juvenile Parkinson's disease—rigidity and bradykinesia (no tremor in children)
- Dopa-responsive dystonia
- Dystonic cerebral palsy

Tics

Definition

Tics are defined as rapid, arrhythmic, repetitive movements, or sounds that wax and wane over weeks/months to involve other body parts and actions.

Types

- Simple—e.g., blinking or sniffing
- Complex—e.g., gesticulating or uttering
- Transient tics—<12 months
- Chronic motor or vocal tics—last at least 1 year

Tourette syndrome: Criteria require the (1) combination of motor and vocal tics, (2) duration of at least 1 year, and (3) onset before the age of 18; exclusion of other causes [direct physiologic effects of a substance (e.g., stimulant drugs) or a general medical condition (e.g., Huntington disease or postviral encephalitis)]. It is also associated with other comorbid disorders such as obsessive compulsive disorders, attention deficit hyperactivity disorder, or behavioral problems.

Pediatric autoimmune neuropsychiatric disorders associated with streptococcal infections (PANDAS): Now regarded as a controversial diagnosis. Abrupt onset of tics or obsessive compulsive disorders after infection with group A β-hemolytic streptococcus in prepubertal children, with motoric hyperactivity and adventitious movements but not frank chorea. PANDAS-related disorders, including pediatric acute-onset neuropsychiatric syndrome (PANS), childhood acute neuropsychiatric symptoms (CANS), and pediatric infection triggered autoimmune neuropsychiatric disorders (PITANDs), have also been described. PANS is characterized by an abrupt onset of OCD and/or severe eating restrictions along with at least other concomitant cognitive, motor, behavioral, or affective symptoms

Treatment of Tics

- *1st tier drugs:* α2-agonists (clonidine and guanfacine)
- *2nd tier drugs:* Atypical antipsychotics (risperidone, olanzapine, etc.)
- *3rd tier drugs:* Typical antipsychotics (haloperidol, pimozide, and fluphenazine)
- *Others:* Tetrabenazine and botulinum toxin (for single site bothersome tics)

CLINICAL PEARLS

Tics "rule of three":
- One-third disappears
- One-third are better
- One-third continue

Stereotypy

Stereotypy is described as repeated and purposeless movements. It is divided into two groups:

1. *Primary,* indicating a physiologic basis, and
2. *Secondary,* for those associated with other neurodevelopmental problems such as:
   - Pervasive developmental disability—autism spectrum disorders and Rett syndrome
   - Intellectual disability
   - Sensory deprivation—congenital blindness/deafness
   - Inborn errors of metabolism—Lesch-Nyhan syndrome
   - Genetic—neuroacanthocytosis

Tics are different from stereotypies which can be reproduced voluntarily and the patient has partial control. They do not interfere with voluntary activity.

Myoclonus

Definition

It is an involuntary muscle jerk which cannot be suppressed and generally with no premonitory features. It can be isolated though uncommon in children or a symptom of other disorders. In children it should be evaluated for epileptic myoclonus.

Types

Myoclonus can be subdivided according to the anatomic origin:

- *Cortical:* Originates from the sensorimotor cortex. Seen as focal, distal and arrhythmic movement usually seen in the arms or trunk. It can be spontaneous or induced by action. Examples: Progressive myoclonic epilepsies, Angelman syndrome, Huntington's disease, Rett syndrome, etc.

- *Subcortical:* Seen with injury to thalamus or brainstem. Examples: Palatal myoclonus, hyperekplexia, etc.
- *Spinal:* Duration is longer and more variable than cortical or subcortical myoclonus. Examples: Post-trauma, ischemic myelopathy, etc.
- *Peripheral:* Peripheral nerves lesions where sensory input is affected. They are typically arrhythmic and nonstimulus sensitive. Example: Hemifacial spasm.

Physiological myoclonus is much more common and should be differentiated from pathological causes. The common types of physiological myoclonus include benign neonatal sleep myoclonus and benign myoclonus of infancy.

Opsoclonus-myoclonus-ataxia Syndrome (Dancing Eyes and Dancing Feet)

It is a rare but a dramatic, autoimmune disorder most commonly seen between 1 and 5 years.

Etiology

In children, 50% are associated with neuroblastoma and majority of nonneoplastic remain idiopathic but presumed postinfectious.

Clinical Presentation

Presents with robust myoclonus and opsoclonus seen as multidirectional, darting, chaotic, and conjugate eye movements. Excessive irritability, sleep disturbances, and mutism are common.

Diagnosis

It is essentially a clinical diagnosis but neuroblastoma screening is mandatory.

Prognosis and Treatment

Neurologic outcome is unfavorable and a significant affected are left with motor and cognitive sequelae. Treatment includes immunosuppression and supportive medication for sleep and behavior disruption.

FUNCTIONAL (PSYCHOGENIC) MOVEMENT DISORDERS

It refers to movements that result from abnormal mental state or condition, and are incompatible with recognized neurological conditions. Most common presentations are tremor, dystonia, myoclonus, or gait disturbances (astasia-abasia). Many children have identifiable precipitating factors such as school examination, bullying, injury, illness, sexual abuse of the child or family member, parental discord or domestic violence, and death of a close relative.

The diagnosis is suggested by a history of sudden onset, marked variability of symptoms, and sustained spontaneous remissions. Examination often shows symptom variation, incongruous movements, distraction during spontaneous speech and behavior, the appearance of symptoms, or worsening during attention and production or suppression of symptoms on examiner's suggestion. In psychogenic tremor, entrainment or alteration with rhythmic tapping of another body part is seen. For management, behavior therapy and relaxation techniques are usually employed.

KEY POINTS

- Establishing phenomenology is the key to diagnosis to movement disorder.
- Every type of MD has its own characteristic, and combinations of them are also not rare, try to find the dominant one and existence of others also.
- Presence of neurological and non-neurological causes of abnormal movements, epilepsy, and epilepsy mimics should be also considered.
- After having reached to clinical based movement disorder type, proceed for diagnostic workup to locate the cause behind and accordingly plan for treatment.
- Keep your camcorder ready; patient never gives you second chance.

SUGGESTED READING

1. Albanese A, Bhatia K, Bressman S, Delong MR, Fahn S, Fung VS, et al. Phenomenology and classification of dystonia: a consensus update. Mov Disord. 2013;28(7): 863-73.
2. Delgado MR, Albright AL. Movement disorders in children: definitions, classifications, and grading systems. J Child Neurol. 2003;18:S1-8.
3. Fenichel GM. Movement disorders. In: Fenichel GM (Ed). Clinical Pediatric Neurology: A Signs and Symptoms Approach, 4th edition. Philadelphia: W. B. Saunders; 2001. pp. 281.
4. Fuchs T, Ozelius LJ. Genetics of dystonia. Semin Neurol. 2011;31:(5):441-8.
5. Grosset KA, Grosset DG. Prescribed drugs and neurological complication. J Neurol Neurosurg Psychiatry. 2004;75(Suppl 3):iii2-8.

6. Harris SR. Psychogenic movement disorders in children and adolescents: an update. Eur J Pediatr. 2019;178: 581-5.
7. Jain R, Pandey S, Raghav S. Movement Disorders in Children. Indian Pediatr. 2021;58:861-70.
8. Jarman PR, Wood NW. Genetics of movement disorders and ataxia. J Neurol Neurosurg Psychiatry. 2002;73: ii22.
9. Korn-Lubetzki I, Stelner I. Common movement disorders in children: diagnosis, pathogenesis and management. Neurosci Med. 2012;3:90-100.
10. Kunju PAM. Extrapyramidal disorders. In: Gupte S (Ed). Recent Advances in Pediatrics. New Delhi: Jaypee Brothers Medical Publishers (P) Ltd.; 1994. pp. 140-66.
11. Lees AJ. Odd and unusual movement disorders. J Neurol Neurosurg Psychiatry. 2002;72:i17-21.
12. Maas RPPWM, Wassenberg T, Lin JP, van de Warrenburg BPC, Willemsen MAAP. l-Dopa in dystonia: A modern perspective. Neurology. 2017;88:1865-71.
13. Pandey S, Koul A. Psychogenic movement disorders in adults and children: A clinical and video profile of 58 Indian patients. Mov Disord Clin Pract. 2017;4:763-67.
14. Powis Z, Towne MC, Hagman KDF, Blanco K, Palmaer E, Castro A, et al. Clinical diagnostic exome sequencing in dystonia: Genetic testing challenges for complex conditions. Clin Genet. 2020;97:305-11.
15. Prato A, Gulisano M, Scerbo M, Barone R, Vicario CM, Rizzo R. Diagnostic Approach to Pediatric Autoimmune Neuropsychiatric Disorders Associated With Streptococcal Infections (PANDAS): A Narrative Review of Literature Data. Front Pediatr. 2021;9:746639.
16. Rojahn J. Self-injurious and stereotypic behavior of non-institutionalized mentally retarded people: prevalence and classification. Am J Ment Defic. 1986;91(3):268-76.
17. Singer HS, Mink JW, Gilbert DL, Jankovik J. Movement Disorders in Childhood, 1st edition. Philadelphia: Elsevier; 2010.
18. Wichmann T. Pathophysiologic Basis of Movement Disorders. Prog Neurol Surg. 2018;33:13-24.

Afebrile Encephalopathy: Bedside Approach to Diagnosis and Management

Lokesh Lingappa, Ramya Bandi, Nihaal Reddy

INTRODUCTION

Encephalopathy [encephalo (in the brain) and pathos (suffering)] refers to an alteration in mental status affecting the patient's cognition or level of arousal.

While it can occur due to diffuse or focal brain insults, it commonly refers to diffuse involvement of the brain.

It is divided into hyperacute (presenting over a few seconds to minutes), acute (few hours to days), subacute (weeks to months), and chronic.

Approach to a child with afebrile encephalopathy with hyperacute, acute, and subacute causes will be discussed in this chapter.

Few important conditions are also outlined.

ETIOLOGY

The causes are variable including both neurological causes and non-neurological causes. They can be broadly classified depending on onset **(Table 1)**.

TABLE 1: For hyperacute/acute and subacute and causes (nonexhaustive).

Categories	*Hyperacute/acute causes*	*Subacute causes*
Infective	• CNS infections (streptococcal—**Figs. 1A to E**) • Meningoencephalitis (HSV—**Figs. 2A to E**, Japanese encephalitis, dengue encephalitis, etc.) • Acute necrotizing encephalopathy **(Figs. 3A to D)** • Sepsis-related encephalopathy • Systemic inflammatory response syndrome (viral/bacterial pathogens) • Acute hypoxia	Subacute infections [tubercular **(Figs. 11A to D)**/HSV/atypical bacterial/fungal/SSPE/(HIV related)]
Vascular	• Hemorrhagic **(Figs. 4A to D)** and ischemic stroke **(Figs. 5A to F)** • Vasculitis • Hypertensive emergencies including PRES **(Figs. 6A and B)**	• Vasculitis • Autoimmune disorders-related vasculitis (SLE)
Inflammatory	• Demyelinating disorders [ADEM, MOGAD **(Figs. 7A to E)**/NMOSD] • Infection—triggered encephalopathy syndrome **(Figs. 3 and 8)** • Bickerstaff encephalitis	Demyelinating disorders
Metabolic	• Hypoglycemia • Electrolyte disturbances (calcium and sodium) • Hyperammonemia, hyperuricemia • Inborn errors of metabolism with decompensation [UCD, organic acidemias **(Figs. 9A and B)**, FAOD, mitochondrial disorders]	• Hepatic or renal failure • Acquired thiamine deficiency **(Fig. 9A)** • Inherited (mitochondrial disorders) **(Figs. 12A to C)**

Contd...

Contd...

Categories	*Hyperacute/acute causes*	*Subacute causes*
Autoimmune	Anti-NMDAR encephalitis and autoimmune encephalitis	Autoimmune pathologies (NMDAR/Hashimoto's encephalopathy)
Trauma	Accidental and nonaccidental trauma	Nonaccidental trauma
Toxin	• Accidental and nonaccidental drug poisoning/ herbal medication overdose • Drug abuse • Envenomation (snake/scorpion)	• Drug overdose • Drug-induced toxic leukoencephalopathy (e.g., methotrexate) • Drug abuse
Others	Acute raised intracranial pressure **(Figs. 10A to C)**	Raised intracranial pressure (tumor/hydrocephalus/bleed)

(SSPE: subacute sclerosing panencephalitis; NMDAR: N-methyl-D-aspartate receptor; HIV: human immunodeficiency virus; SLE: systemic lupus erythematosus)

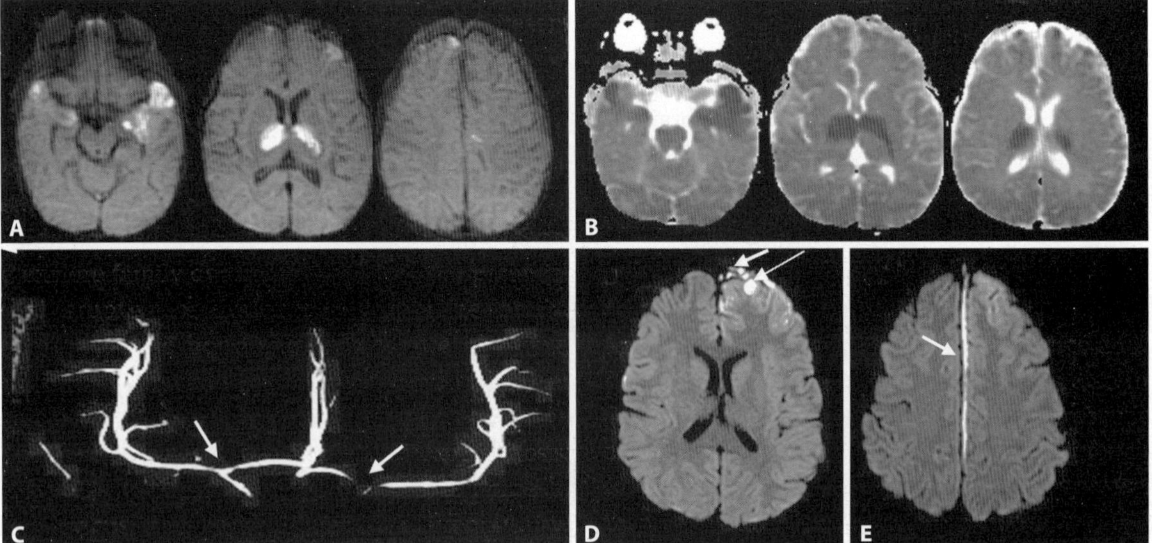

Figs. 1A to E: Group B streptococcus. *Case 1 (A to C):* Axial DWI and ADC brain MRI (A and B) demonstrates multifocal areas of restricted diffusion-cytotoxic edema—infarcts in the bilateral globus pallidus, frontal and temporal lobes. Angiography MIP image (C) demonstrates focal arteriopathy in the proximal segments of the anterior cerebral arteries (arrows). *Case 2 (D and E):* Axial DWI demonstrates subdural empyemas in the left frontal and parafalcine regions (arrows) and focal parenchymal areas of restricted diffusion in the left frontal lobe—like small abscesses (long arrow).

Approximately, 30–70% of acute encephalopathies do not receive etiologic diagnoses. A study by the California Encephalitis Project on epidemiology and etiology of encephalitis found that 63% of the patients remained without an etiology after a battery of tests for 16 potential infectious agents.

CLINICAL PEARL

- Absence of fever does not negate the presence of infection, 10% of herpes simplex encephalitis children may not have fever as presenting manifestation.

HISTORY

History from parents/caregiver at onset of encephalopathy is very important to generate appropriate differential diagnoses (80% of diagnoses are suspected based on history). History of trauma, accidental drug/substance ingestion, past history of any illness, and medication history should always be asked for.

CLINICAL PEARL

- Suspect nonaccidental injury (battered child syndrome) when an inconsistent history from different family members and varied stage of injuries or unexplained fractures are present.

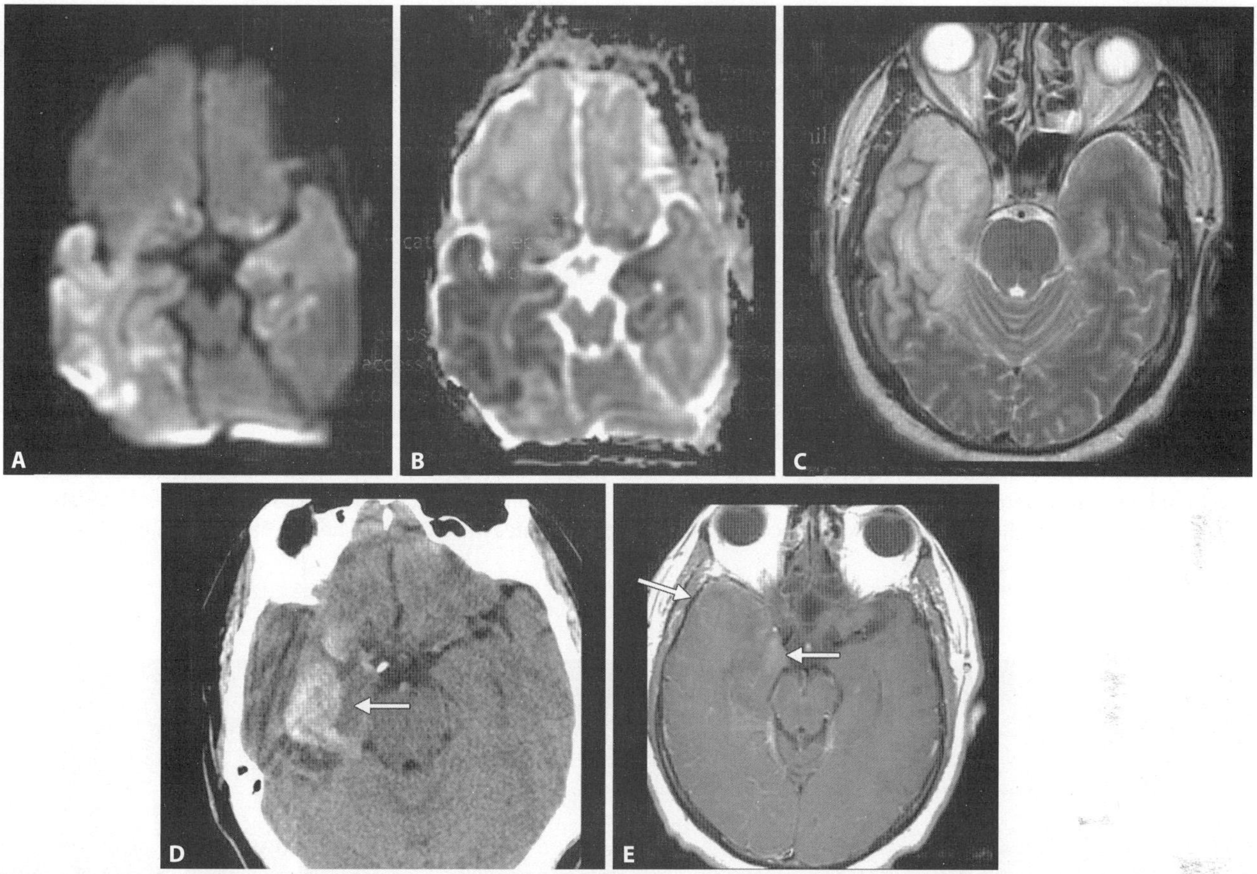

Figs. 2A to E: *Herpes simplex virus type 2 (HSV-2):* Axial DWI and ADC (A and B) demonstrates restricted diffusion—cytotoxic edema in the distributed in an asymmetrical manner in the bilateral temporal and basifrontal lobes. *Herpes simplex virus type 1 (HSV-1):* Axial T2 (C) demonstrates edematous changes in the right temporal lobe. Axial noncontrast CT (D) demonstrates hemorrhagic changes (arrow) within the right temporal lobe abnormality. Axial T1 contrast (E) demonstrates minimal enhancement along the cortical regions of the anterior and medial temporal lobes (arrows).

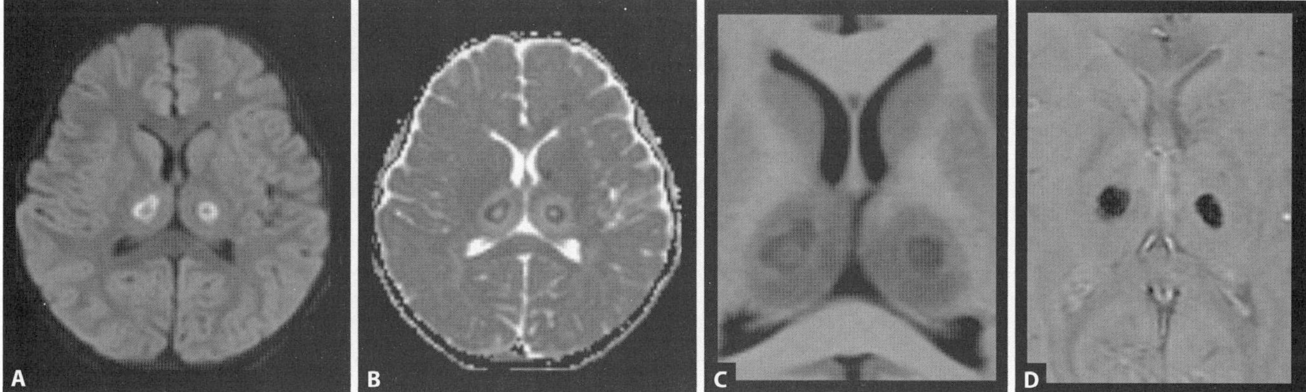

Figs. 3A to D: Acute necrotizing encephalopathy of childhood (ANEC). Axial brain DWI and ADC (A and B) demonstrates bilateral thalamic lesions with facilitated diffusion in the center and restricted diffusion in the periphery with mild perilesional edema. Axial T1 and SWI (C and D) demonstrates hemorrhagic changes.

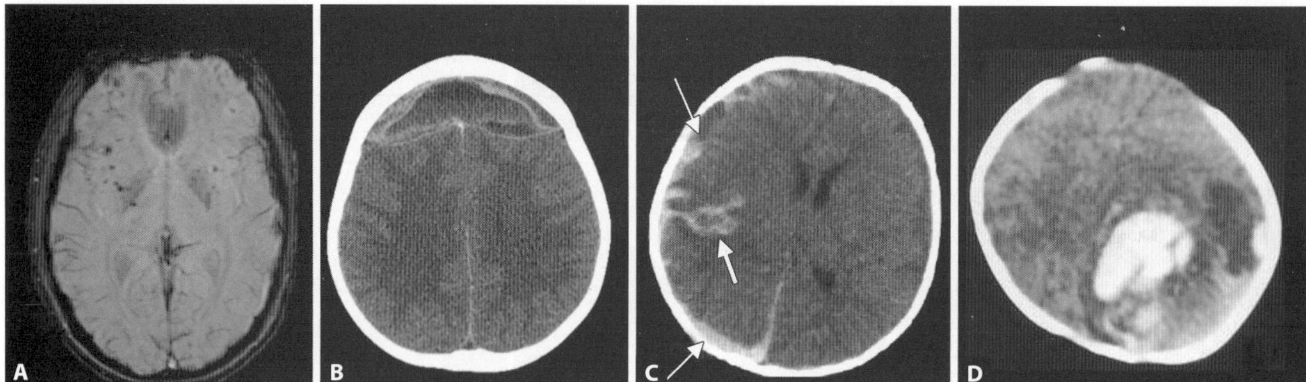

Figs. 4A to D: Intracranial hemorrhage. DAI: Axial SWI (A) demonstrates multiple small foci of blooming (low signal) changes in the bilateral frontal lobes, basal ganglia suggestive of hemorrhage—diffuse axonal injury. EDH: Axial noncontrast CT (B) demonstrates extradural hemorrhage in the frontal regions. SAH and SDH: Axial noncontrast CT (C) demonstrates hyperdense changes in the subarachnoid perisylvian regions (arrow) and subdural hemorrhage in the frontal, parietal lobes and along the posterior falx cerebri (long arrows). Parenchymal hemorrhage—axial noncontrast CT (D) demonstrates mixed density hemorrhagic lesion in the left parietal lobe.

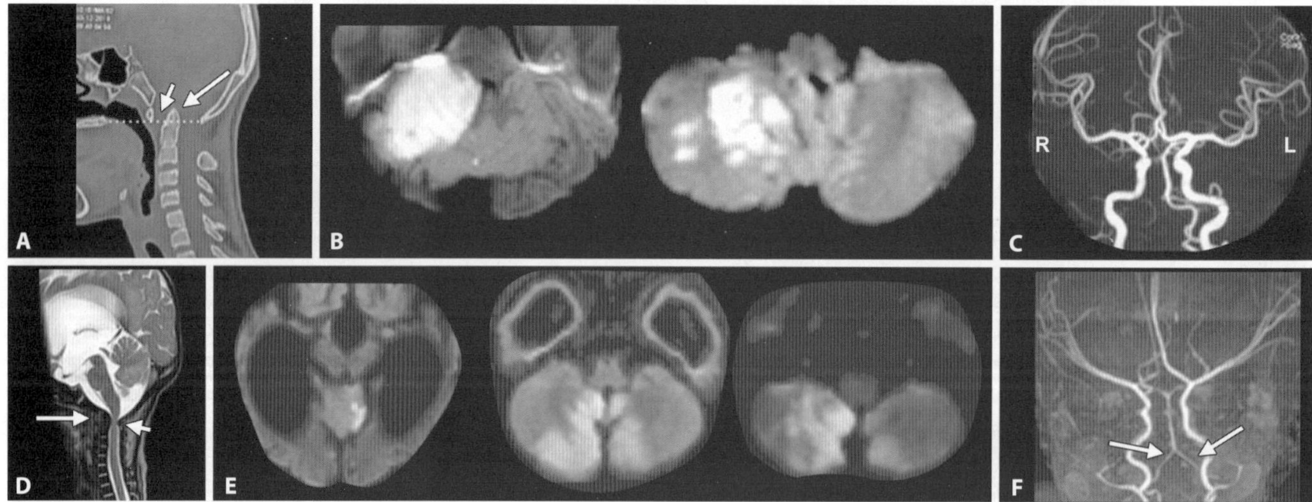

Figs. 5A to F: Posterior circulation strokes. *Case 1 (A to C):* (A) Sagittal CT image demonstrates CVJ abnormality with basilar invagination (arrow), atlantoaxial dissociation (arrowhead) and absence of posterior arch of atlas; (B and C) Diffusion-weighted images (DWI) demonstrates infarcts in the right side of the vermis and cerebellar hemisphere; (C) MR angiography of the brain demonstrates nonvisualization of the V4 segment of the right vertebral artery and anterior–inferior cerebellar artery. *Case 2 (D to F):* (D) Sagittal T2 image demonstrates CVJ abnormality and narrowing with basilar impression (arrow), overgrowth of the opisthion (arrowhead); (E) DWI demonstrates infarcts in the left half of superior vermis, bilateral cerebellar hemisphere; (F) MR angiography of the brain demonstrates hypoplasia of the posterior circulation arteries including V4 segments of the bilateral vertebral arteries, basilar artery, and proximal posterior cerebral arteries.

INITIAL STABILIZATION AND EXAMINATION

A quick focused examination should be done to assess the level of encephalopathy and to reach diagnosis **(Table 2)**. Pupil examination, breathing pattern, motor examination, and eye movements are important in assessing the level of encephalopathy.

Initial stabilization should be done as per standard protocol.

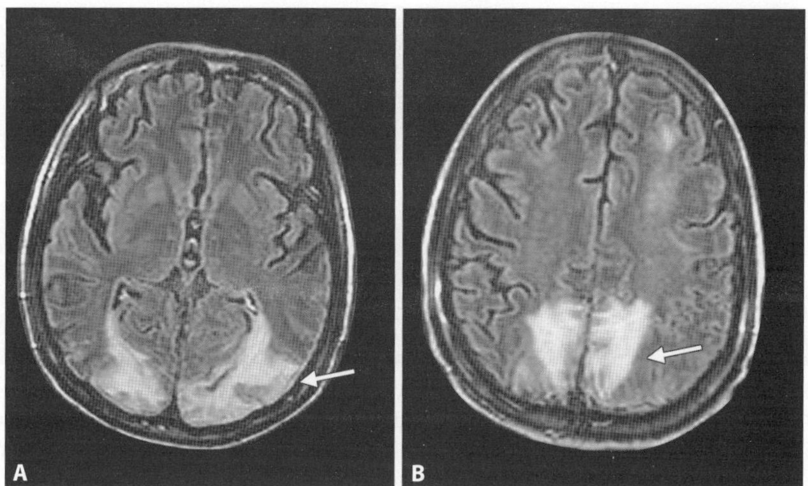

Figs. 6A and B: Acute hypertensive encephalopathy—PRES. (A and B) Axial FLAIR brain MRI demonstrating hyperintense edematous changes (arrows) in the periventricular, deep, subcortical white matter and cortical regions on the parietal, occipital and left frontal lobes.

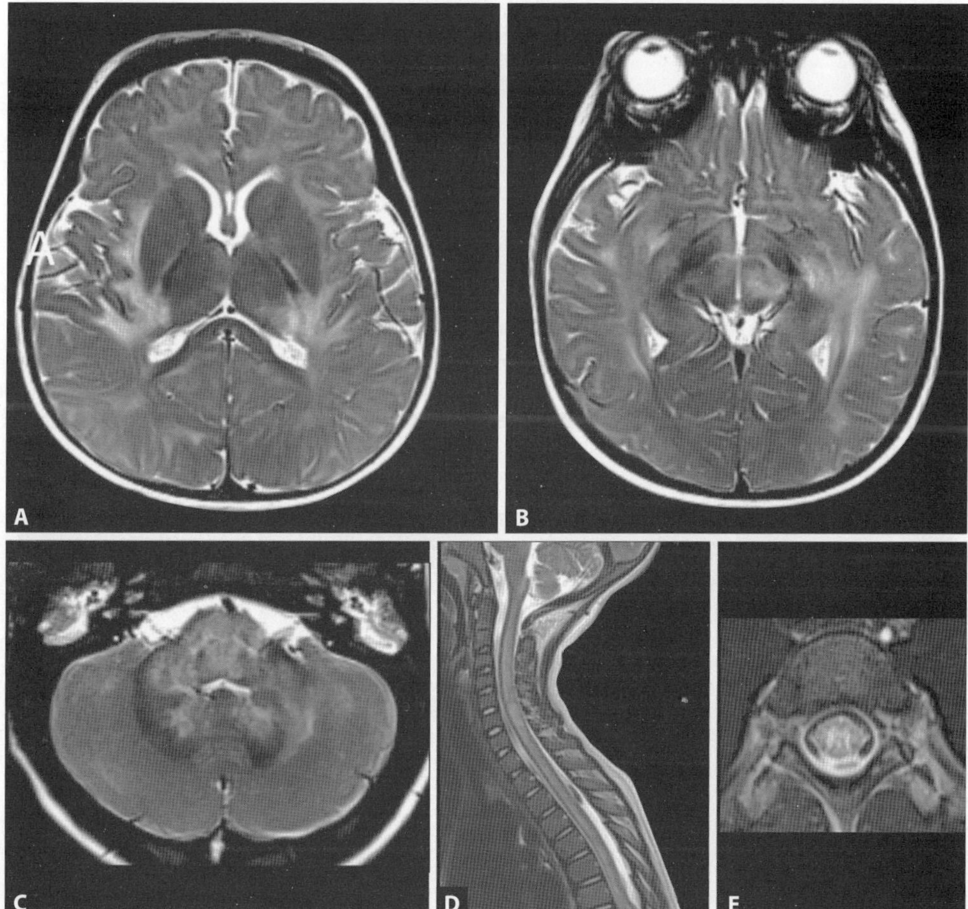

Figs. 7A to E: Demyelination—MOGAD. Axial T2 Brain MRI (A to C) demonstrates edematous changes in the bilateral subinsular, lateral and posterior thalamic nuclei, posterior limb of internal capsule, left globus pallidus, temporal lobes, brainstem and cerebellum. Sagittal T2 spine (D) demonstrates long segment cord myelopathy, (E) axial spine at level of cervical card demonstrates central gray matter (H-shaped) hyperintensities.

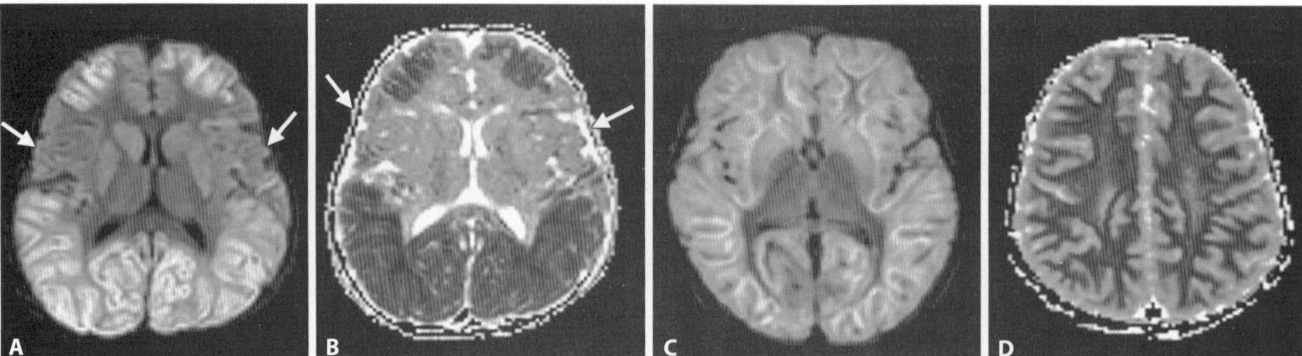

Figs. 8A to D: Acute leukoencephalopathy with restricted diffusion (ALERD). Axial brain MRI demonstrating restricted diffusion—cytotoxic edema on DWI (A) and corresponding low signals on ADC (B) in the bilateral cerebral hemispheres, with sparing of the central— perisylvian regions (arrows). Axial brain MRI demonstrating diffuse restricted diffusion—cytotoxic edema on DWI (C) and corresponding low signals on ADC (D) in the bilateral cerebral hemispheres.

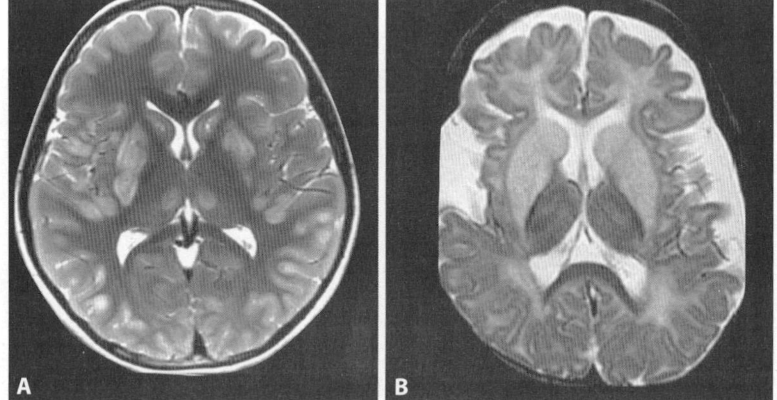

Figs. 9A and B: (A) Biotin-thiamine deficiency. Axial T2 demonstrates symmetrical hyperintense changes in the bilateral dorsal striatum, median thalamic nuclei and subcortical—cortical regions in the bilateral cerebral hemispheres; (B) Glutaric aciduria. Axial T2 demonstrates symmetrical hyperintense changes in the bilateral basal ganglia, widened underopercularized Sylvian fissures, periventricular hyperintense changes.

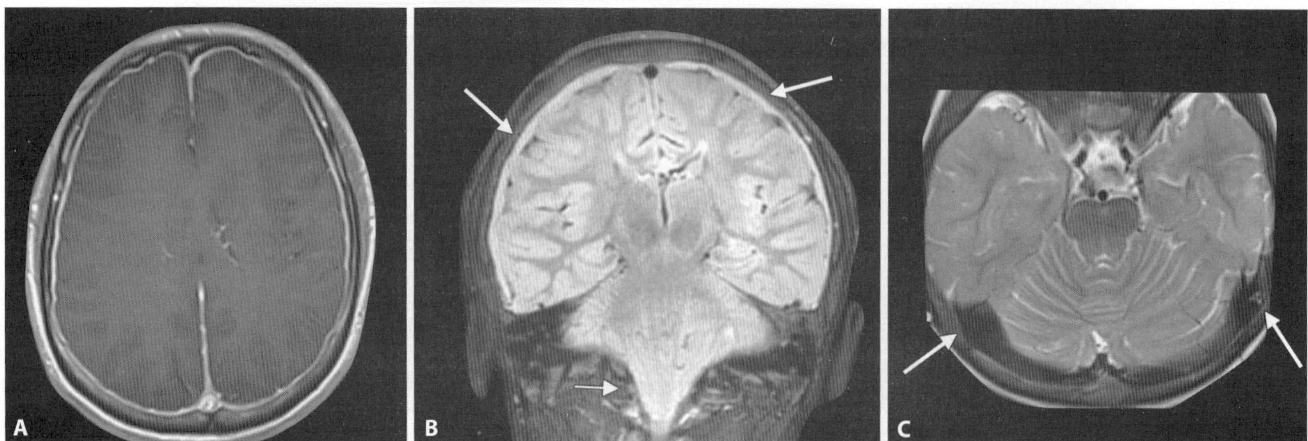

Figs. 10A to C: Intracranial hypotension. Axial T1 contrast brain MRI (A) demonstrating diffuse pachymeningeal enhancement. Coronal FLAIR (B) demonstrates subdural collections (arrows) and inferior tonsillar ectopia (small arrows). Axial T2 (C) demonstrates distended transverse sinuses (arrows).

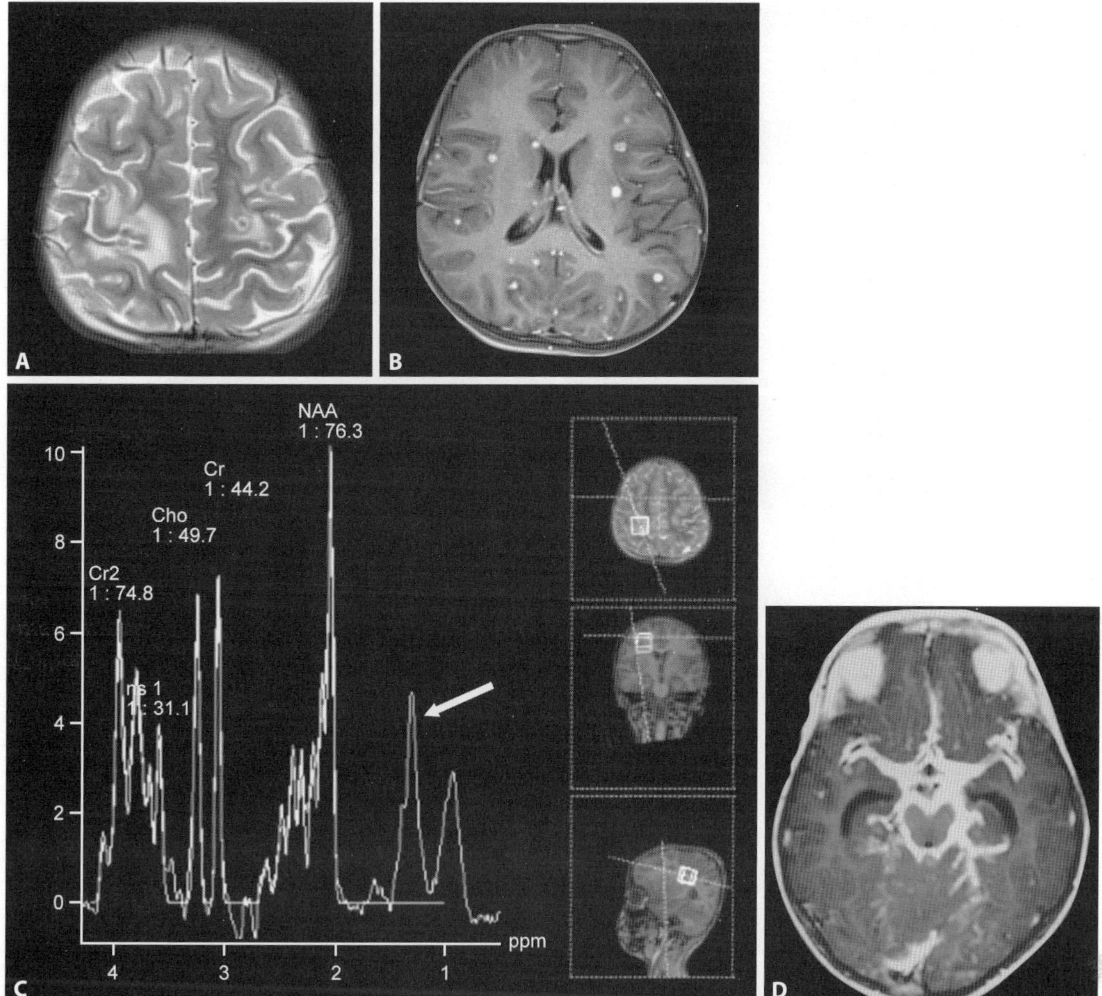

Figs. 11A to D: Tuberculomas and tuberculous meningitis (TBM). Axial T2 brain MRI (A) demonstrates multiple subcentimetric granulomatous lesions with perilesional edema. The lesions demonstrate central hypointensity and periphery capsular hyperintensity. Axial T1 contrast (B) nodular enhancing lesions. Spectroscopy (C) demonstrates elevated lipid-lactate peaks at 0.9 and 1.3 ppm. Axial T1 contrast (D) of another child demonstrates diffuse leptomeningeal enhancement in the basal cisterns, Sylvian fissures, basifrontal regions, and vermis.

CLINICAL PEARLS

- Documentation of anthropometry, blood pressure, heart rate, and breathing pattern are important clues to etiologic diagnosis.
- Detailed eye examination—pupils, eye movements, and fundus examination has localizing and diagnostic value.

INVESTIGATIONS

Clinical history and examination should guide the investigations and further management **(Table 3)**.

Blood glucose should be done bedside in all children and should be corrected when low.

TREATMENT

Written hospital protocols should be tailor made depending on the epidemiology and experience. On a broader perspective, treatment should include appropriate antibiotics and antiviral medications with symptomatic treatment of seizures and management of raised intracranial pressure. Ongoing monitoring on vital parameters and end-organ functions is essential in treating a child with encephalopathy. Once accurate etiology is established, more definitive treatment should be initiated and unwarranted medications can be withdrawn.

Few conditions are outlined along with treatment.

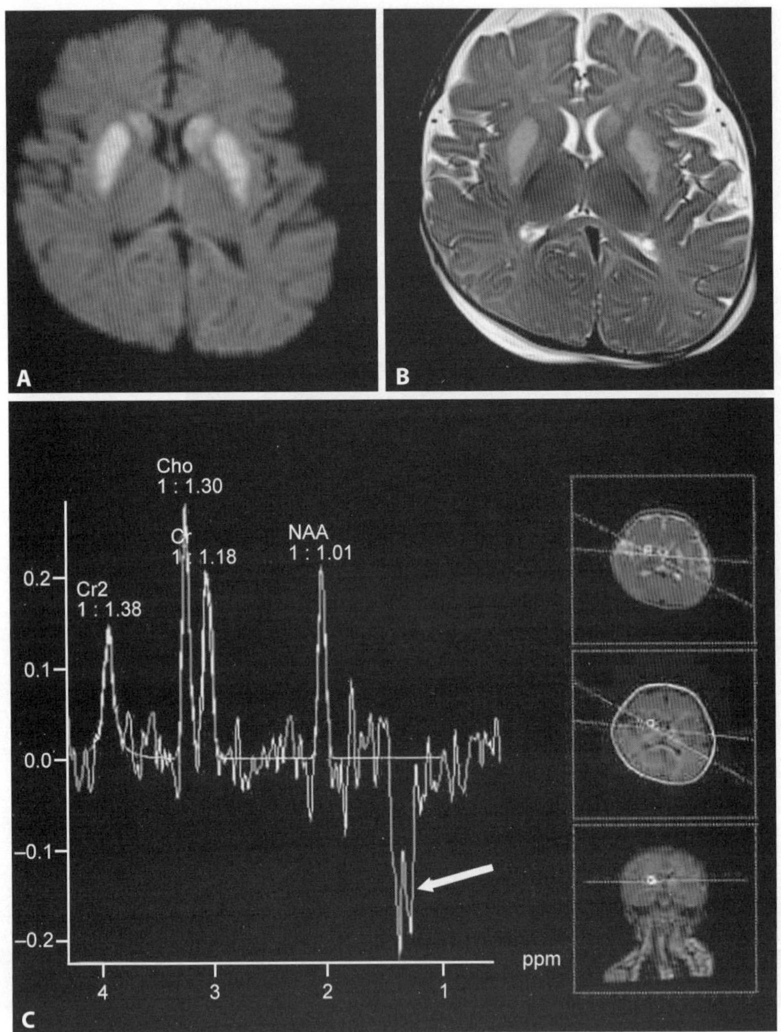

Figs. 12A to C: Leigh disease. Axial brain DWI and T2 (A and B) demonstrates bilateral symmetrical edematous changes in the dorsal striatum. Spectroscopy (C) demonstrates inverted lactate peak at 1.33 ppm (arrow).

Acquired Non-neurological Conditions

Hypertensive Encephalopathy and Posterior Reversible Encephalopathy Syndrome

Malignant hypertension due to any cause can lead to encephalopathy in children. Cardiac causes (coarctation of aorta), acute glomerulonephritis, and hemolytic uremic syndrome are common causes. Posterior reversible encephalopathy syndrome (PRES) etiology includes autoimmune, hematological, renal, and drug-related causes **(Figs. 13A to C)**.

Fundus examination and imaging can aid in diagnosis.

Typical neuroimaging findings include symmetric vasogenic edematous changes in the subcortical-cortical regions of the posterior portions of the cerebral hemispheres **(Figs. 6A and B)**. Imaging findings in atypical PRES include involvement of the frontal lobes, watershed zones, basal ganglia and/or thalami, brainstem, cerebellum, and even the spinal cord. Cytotoxic edema and microhemorrhagic foci are also known to be present in atypical forms of PRES.

Blood pressure control, aggressive seizure management, and treating underlying causes usually reverse the encephalopathy.

CLINICAL PEARL

- Early central visual impairment before losing consciousness would be a pointer toward hypertensive emergency causing posterior reversible leukoencephalopathy syndrome **(Figs. 6A and B)**

TABLE 2: Clinical clues to diagnosis.

General physical examination	• Short stature—chronic renal failure, primary immune deficiencies • Icterus—hepatic encephalopathy, rarely in FAOD • Hypertension—hypertensive encephalopathy, raised ICP • Skin-rash—vasculitis, HSP • Joint swelling—HSP, rachitic features in chronic renal failure
Large head	Hydrocephalus, glutaric aciduria type I (6–18 months)
Neurocutaneous markers	• Multiple café-au-lait spots—moyamoya syndrome with stroke • Hypopigmented macules—TSC complex with nonconvulsive status epilepticus • Facial angioma—stroke-like episodes, status epilepticus in Sturge–Weber syndrome
Abdomen	• Hepatosplenomegaly—hemophagocytic lymphohistiocytosis • Splenomegaly—malaria, subacute bacterial endocarditis with stroke, young sickler with stroke

(FAOD: fatty acid oxidation disorder; ICP: intracranial pressure; HSP: Henoch-Schönlein purpura; TSC: tuberous sclerosis complex)

TABLE 3: Investigations.

Blood investigations	• CBC, CRP, serum electrolytes, LFT, RFT, procalcitonin, blood, and urine cultures • Store one sample for toxicology tests • PS for MP, mycoplasma antibodies, Weil–Felix test • ESR—elevation >100 mm/1st hour usually indicates either active systemic vasculitis/chronic infection or a malignancy • Viral markers in appropriate setting—bilateral thalamic/basal ganglia lesions (Dengue/Japanese encephalitis, mumps, mycoplasma, etc.) • MOG/NMO antibodies guided by MRI brain studies • ANA, APLA, ANCA antibody studies • Thyroid function, antithyroid antibodies • Toxicology screen • IEM workup—blood lactate, ammonia, tandem mass spectroscopy, and urine GCMS • HIV testing • 3 mL EDTA and 3 mL heparinized blood sample storage in acutely ill child for genetic testing in case of untimely death without a diagnosis
Neuroimaging	• CT brain—done in acute situation to rule out acute bleeding, head injuries, and space-occupying lesion • MRI brain with or without contrast is the imaging of choice • Caveat—normal MRI brain is seen in significant proportion of NMDAR encephalitis/ADEM in first week of illness • MR angiogram and venogram in appropriate clinical setting
EEG	EEG monitoring will help to diagnose nonconvulsive status epilepticus and pattern of encephalopathy
Cerebrospinal fluid	• Opening pressure, cell count, protein, paired sugar and lactate, cultures • PCR testing for appropriate organisms • Anti-N-methyl-D-aspartate receptor antibodies and anti-voltage-gated potassium channel antibodies • Store extra samples
Ophthalmological opinion	• Retinal hemorrhages—consider nonaccidental injury/severe raised ICP • Papilledema—sinovenous thrombosis/acute hydrocephalus • Hypertensive changes • Whitening of vessels, papilledema, and cotton wool spots in malaria
Urine	Cultures, toxicology screen
Respiratory secretions	For viral panel (adenovirus/influenzae/enterovirus)

(ADEM: acute disseminated encephalomyelitis; ANA: antinuclear antibodies; ANCA: anti-neutrophil cytoplasmic antibody; APLA: antiphospholipid antibodies; CBC: complete blood count; CRP: C-reactive protein; CT: computed tomography; ESR: erythrocyte sedimentation rate; GCMS: gas chromatography and mass spectrometry; IEM: inborn error of metabolism; LFT: liver function tests; MP: malarial parasite; MRI: magnetic resonance imaging; NMDAR: N-methyl-D-aspartate receptor; PS: peripheral smear; RFT: renal function tests)

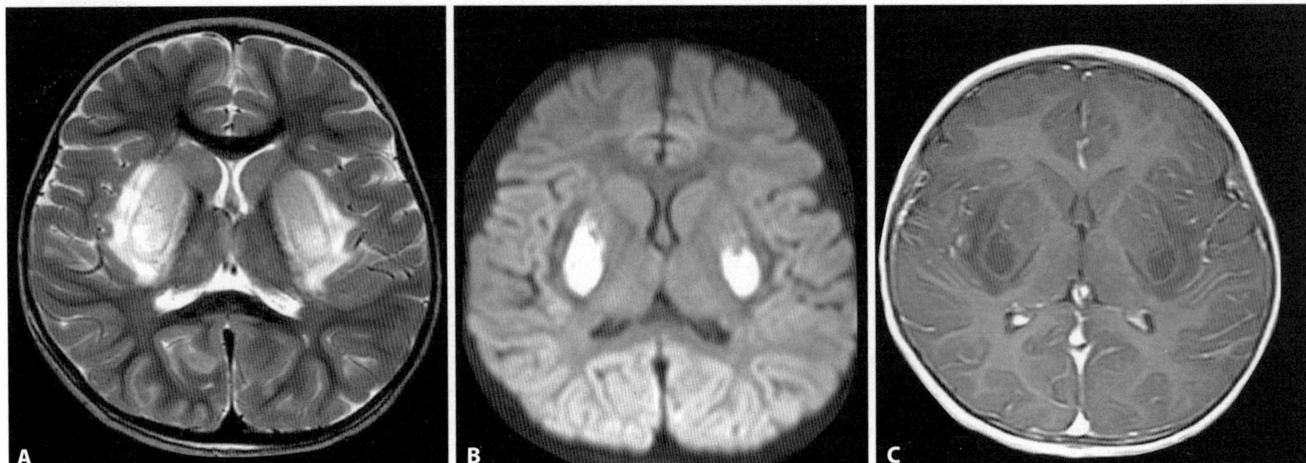

Figs. 13A to C: Hemolytic uremic syndrome. Axial T2 brain MRI (A) demonstrates symmetrical edematous changes in the bilateral lentiform nuclei, internal and external capsules. Axial DWI (B) demonstrates restricted diffusion (cytotoxic edema) in the mid and posterior putamen. Axial T1 contrast (C) demonstrates no abnormal enhancement.

Electrolyte Disturbances/Hyperglycemia/Hypoglycemia

Metabolic derangements in children due to any cause could lead to encephalopathy and should be included in the first tier investigations. Sodium abnormalities (hypo-/hypernatremia) are common with acute gastroenteritis, adrenal insufficiency, acute kidney injury, and excessive or decreased water intake. Correction of sodium should be done slowly to prevent rapid osmolar shifts. Pontine/extrapontine myelinolysis is a serious complication with rapid correction of hyponatremia.

Hypocalcemia can occur due to vitamin D deficiency, parathyroid metabolism defects, and rapid acidosis correction. Hypomagnesemia can coexist with hypocalcemia and should be corrected.

Diabetic ketoacidosis as first presentation or poor control of insulin-dependent diabetes mellitus can be associated with encephalopathic presentation.

Hepatic and Uremic Encephalopathy

Spectrum of neuropsychiatric abnormalities in patients with liver dysfunction is characterized by personality changes, intellectual impairment, and depressed level of consciousness. The diagnosis is usually straightforward by presence of icterus, significant elevation of liver enzymes, and in few children with history of preexisting liver disease.

Uremic encephalopathy may be more challenging to diagnose. Hypertension would be an independent risk factor for encephalopathy. Short stature, anemia, hypertension, and features of rickets would be the systemic clues to chronic kidney disorders.

CLINICAL PEARL

- Normal magnetic resonance imaging brain with symmetrical encephalopathy (encephalopathy with preserved eye movement without lateralizing neurological findings) points toward metabolic encephalopathy, systemic inflammatory response syndrome, and toxins.

Parainfectious/Postinfectious Demyelination

Acute disseminated encephalomyelitis (ADEM) is the most important condition among this group. Children present with biphasic illness, neurological worsening with polyfocal symptoms, and encephalopathy. In all children with ADEM, myelin oligodendrocyte glycoprotein antibody-associated disease (MOGAD) should also be considered and testing should be done. Bilateral optic neuritis, seizures, mild encephalopathy, and recurrent presentations are common with MOGAD. Magnetic resonance imaging brain performed early into the illness may be normal; usually demonstrates bilateral lesions mostly affecting the subcortical and deep white matter and the deep gray matter **(Figs. 7A to E)**. Lesions are T2-hyperintense, large (>2 cm in size), blurred, and poorly demarcated. In the acute stage, lesions may demonstrate restricted diffusion.

Neuromyelitis optica spectrum disorder (NMOSD) is another group of demyelinating disorder which occurs in older children and can be associated with encephalopathy, seizures in addition to optic neuritis and vomiting.

Intravenous methylprednisolone at 30 mg/kg/day for 3–5 days is the initial treatment of choice. Intravenous immunoglobulins can be administered as guided by the clinical picture.

Inflammatory and Cytokine Storm Syndromes

Children with acute worsening of symptoms after initial brief febrile seizures and recovery. They can present with recurrent seizures with worsening encephalopathy. MRI brain demonstrates features of ALERD (acute leukoencephalopathy with restricted diffusion).

- *ANEC:* Children with acute febrile illness with rapid worsening of encephalopathy within 6–24 hours of neurological onset with high mortality rate. The neuroimaging demonstrates bilateral thalamic, basal ganglia, white matter, dorsal pontine, and cerebellar white matter with trilaminar sign in thalamus due to necrosis.
- *MERS:* Fever followed by mild encephalopathy with reversible splenial lesion has the best outcome.
- *FIRES:* Refractory seizures persisting beyond 24 hours even after using anesthetic agents, MRI brain can be normal or can show signal changes in the perisylvian regions including the claustrum.

Autoimmune Pathologies

Children present with neurological syndromes associated with serum and/or cerebrospinal fluid (CSF) antibodies directed against ion channels, receptors, and associated proteins are diagnosed as antibody-mediated encephalopathies, best example being anti-NMDAR encephalitis. Some others include voltage-gated potassium channel (VGKC) complex proteins, glutamic acid decarboxylase, and CASPR2—contactin-associated protein-like 2 receptors.

In some children, they can be part of paraneoplastic syndrome. Majority of children do not have detectable tumors, except in adolescent girls who can have ovarian teratoma.

The clinical features of these disorders overlap and, in many cases, the etiology may not be apparent at presentation. Many patients present as subacute encephalopathy with fever, seizures, amnesia, sleep disturbances, confusion, psychiatric features, and with movement disorder. The clinical phenotypes are increasingly recognized but some patients are negative for the available antibody tests.

For autoimmune encephalitis, immunomodulation with steroids and/or intravenous immunoglobulins is the first line of treatment. For anti-NMDAR encephalitis, if there is no response to the first line, rituximab can be given as second-line treatment (once a week for 4 weeks). It is imperative to monitor CD19 levels during therapy. In this condition, even the severe motor disability improves significantly with treatment.

> **CLINICAL PEARL**
>
> Presence of characteristic movement disorder with perioral dyskinesia and dystonia with encephalopathy with or without psychiatric disturbances is the cardinal feature and clue for diagnosis of N-methyl-D-aspartate encephalitis even with nondiagnostic cerebrospinal fluid or magnetic resonance imaging brain findings.

Vasculitis/Vascular Etiologies

Vasculitis can be a primary disorder or occurs as a part of multisystem autoimmune disorder like lupus. Vasculitis should be considered in adolescent age group especially in girls presenting with multisystem involvement and/or focal neurological presentation or diffuse encephalopathy.

Antinuclear antibodies/autoimmune antibody panel, complement levels, and erythrocyte sedimentation rate (ESR) are few of the initial investigations.

Moyamoya disease/syndrome is one of the important vasculopathy of childhood. Neuroimaging and vessel wall imaging can provide clues to the etiology.

Treatment depends on the underlying etiology. Multidisciplinary approach is recommended for these conditions.

Metabolic

Inborn Errors of Metabolism

In infants and young children presenting with encephalopathy, this is an important etiological group that should be considered especially in children born to consanguineous parents.

In metabolic disorders, small molecule diseases present with acute encephalopathy (aminoacidopathies, fatty acid oxidation and carnitine disorders, organic acidemias and urea cycle disorders, and mitochondrial disorders), usually triggered by infection, fasting state, or other stressors. Most present before the age of 2 years, with few exceptions. They can be readily detectable with biochemical signatures in blood and urine.

Disorders of cerebral energy metabolism (mitochondrial disorders and pyruvate metabolic defects) have a chronic progressive course, often with acute exacerbations.

As the diagnosis is based on laboratory testing, care should be taken to minimize the errors with the collection techniques, storage, and transport of the samples. Hemodynamic instability and intervention before the sample collection can alter the values and hence the categorization. Samples that need to be collected in a suspected case include arterial/venous blood gas, blood lactate, urine/blood ketones, TMS sample, and urine for gas chromatography and mass spectrometry (GCMS). Urine samples should be frozen or transported readily under 25°C as the organic acids are volatile.

Few clinical presentations that can point out to certain disorders include:

- Presence of metabolic acidosis with variable lactic acidosis and hypoglycemia and ketosis would point toward organic acidurias.
- Evidence of bone marrow suppression with bicytopenia and hypocalcemia is manifestation of organic acidurias.
- Newborn presentation with progressive encephalopathy and abnormalities on magnetic resonance imaging (MRI) brain with restricted diffusion of myelinated white matter is suggestive of maple syrup urine disease.
- Children presenting with nonketotic hypoglycemia especially in early morning hours with or without hepatomegaly and anicteric hepatitis would strongly point toward the presence of underlying fatty acid oxidation disorder. Medium-chain acyl-CoA dehydrogenase deficiency is the most common followed by carnitine palmitoyl 1A deficiency (CPT1A).

CLINICAL PEARL

- In fatty acid oxidation disorder, hepatomegaly and elevation of liver enzymes may evolve over initial days and may not be seen at presentation.

- Urea cycle disorder will have variable presentations including encephalopathy and recurrent vomiting in association with hyperammonemia.

CLINICAL PEARL

- Ammonia levels need to be processed immediately and to be transported on ice to the laboratory for accurate results. Borderline elevation of ammonia is usually due to delayed processing of samples.

- Stepwise decompensation in infancy with presence of breathing difficulty and lactic acidosis needs consideration of mitochondrial disorder.
- Neuroimaging demonstrating bilateral basal ganglia hypodensities on computed tomography of the brain along with involvement of periaqueductal gray matter suggests Leigh's disease **(Figs. 12A to C)**. Magnetic resonance imaging with MRI spectroscopy with elevated lactate and elevated CSF lactate further confirms the diagnoses **(Figs. 12A to C)**.
- An eminently treatable condition with similar presentation especially in developing countries is acquired thiamine deficiency presenting in infants of 1–6 months age. Dramatic response is seen with thiamine supplementation.

CLINICAL PEARL

- It is imperative that in an infant or young child <3 years with unexplained encephalopathy with or without acidosis and hypoglycemia, samples (tandem mass spectroscopy, lactate and ammonia, and urine for organic acids) should be taken before starting vitamin cocktails.

For metabolic conditions, appropriate cofactors can be added to enhance the residual enzyme activity. If metabolic condition is strongly suspected and pending the results, metabolic cocktail can be added. This includes carnitine, riboflavin, thiamine, coenzyme Q, and biotin supplementation. Hydroxycobalamin can be given if MMA/PA is suspected. Sodium benzoate and L arginine are used to treat hyperammonemia. Sodium bicarbonate infusion can be given in case of severe acidosis.

Outcomes depend upon etiology and severity of the pathology. Ongoing counseling of family and involving them in important decision making will help to reduce the stress on the treating team and the family.

A 3-mL EDTA and heparinized blood sample should be stored (to be sent for DNA/extraction as soon as possible) in case of sudden death of the child. Genetic testing of the index child will help in counseling the family in further pregnancies. It also gives a closure to the child's condition which has a huge impact on the parent's emotional health.

KEY POINTS

- Acute febrile/afebrile encephalopathy is a common clinical problem of varied etiologies and presentations.
- Accurate history and comprehensive examination will provide clue to the etiologic diagnosis in many children.
- Investigations are to be performed as per individual patient including appropriate neuroimaging.
- Early identification of etiologic diagnosis helps in appropriate management and improved outcome.

SUGGESTED READING

1. Imataka G, Kuwashima S, Yoshihara S. A Comprehensive Review of Pediatric Acute Encephalopathy. J Clin Med. 2022;11(19):5921.
2. Lim YXJ, Kwek SY, How CH, Chan WSD. A clinical approach to encephalopathy in children. Singapore Med J. 2020;61(12):626-32.
3. Mizuguchi M, Ichiyama T, Imataka G, Okumura A, Goto T, Sakuma H, et al. Guidelines for the diagnosis and treatment of acute encephalopathy in childhood. Brain Dev-Jpn. 2021;43(1):2-31
4. Nosadini M, Thomas T, Eyre M, Anlar B, Armangue T, Benseler SM, et al. International Consensus Recommendations for the Treatment of Pediatric NMDAR Antibody Encephalitis. Neurol Neuroimmunol Neuroinflamm. 2021;8(5):e1052.
5. Sugiyama Y, Murayama K. Acute Encephalopathy Caused by Inherited Metabolic Diseases. J Clin Med. 2023;12(11):3797.
6. Yoganathan S, Umakanth BS. Metabolic encephalopathies. Indian Journal of Practical Pediatrics2020;22(1):26-35.

KEY POINTS

SUGGESTED READING

SECTION 12

Nephrology

Section Editors: *Anand S Vasudev, Pankaj V Deshpande*

CHAPTER 99

Algorithmic Approach to Rickets

Sabharitha G, S Thangavelu

INTRODUCTION

Rickets is a commonly encountered metabolic bone disease. Causative factors are many like nutritional, renal, hepatic, gastrointestinal, and metabolic disorders. Though clinical manifestations of rickets are similar, because of the diverse etiological factors, symptoms and signs of underlying diseases are different. Majority of the time, underlying etiology can be identified only by basic investigations.

DIAGNOSIS OF RICKETS

Rickets is diagnosed by clinical features, radiological findings, biochemical and genetic tests. Approach to rickets is based on three components **(Figs. 1A to D)**:

1. *Clinical features:* Common clinical features are divided as skeletal and extraskeletal features.
   - *Presence of bony deformities and delayed bony growth:* From head to foot, they are delayed closure of anterior fontanelle, large head, tooth abnormalities (delayed eruption of primary teeth, enamel defects, and caries teeth), chest deformities such as Harrison's sulcus and rachitic rosary, widened bony ends around wrist and ankles, bowing of legs, knock knees, double malleoli.
   - Delayed motor milestones particularly delayed walking, hypocalcemic seizures, and rarely hypocalcemic cardiomyopathy.

   Differential diagnosis for skeletal deformities: Metaphyseal dysplasia, type IV mucopolysaccharidosis (Morquio disease) and hypophosphatasia.
2. *Radiological features:* Radiological evidence is seen in the ends of growing bones which are cupping, fraying of the metaphysis and widening of the growth cartilage. Generalized osteopenia and sometimes pathological fractures are additional radiological signs. Best site is wrist or knee, but sometimes the same features are identified in the upper end of humerus, widening of anterior ends of the ribs in a cheat X-ray AP view taken for respiratory illness **(Figs. 2A to C)**.
3. *Other laboratory features:* Depending on the underlying causative features, laboratory features change. They are categorized into Tier 1 and Tier 2 investigations.

Tier One Investigations

These are available in general pediatric hospital, can be ordered and interpreted by a general pediatrician. These are not sophisticated investigations, which are reliably done only in tertiary care center. Once the clinician identifies signs of rickets, do the following investigations **(Box 1)**.

Tier Two Investigations

These are available or done perfectly only in specialist laboratories or tertiary care hospitals. They can be ordered by specialists, interpreted or done under the supervision or advice of specialists. Then only reliability is acceptable. These are done after the tier one investigations or clinical categorization points to a non-nutritional rickets **(Box 2)**.

How to choose tier one or tier two?

If there are no signs of non-nutritional rickets, start with tier one alone, and based on the diagnosis, decide about the need for tier two investigations.

If there are clues to suggest non-nutritional rickets **(Box 3)**, do the first tier. Tier two will be definitely needed, but should be done in specialty laboratory under the advice and supervision of specialists (nephrologists, gastroenterologist, endocrinologists, or hepatologists). Or else, refer to a multispecialty center. If the tier two investigations are done in a smaller laboratory, it may not be reliable or the specialist will like to repeat in a specialty laboratory.

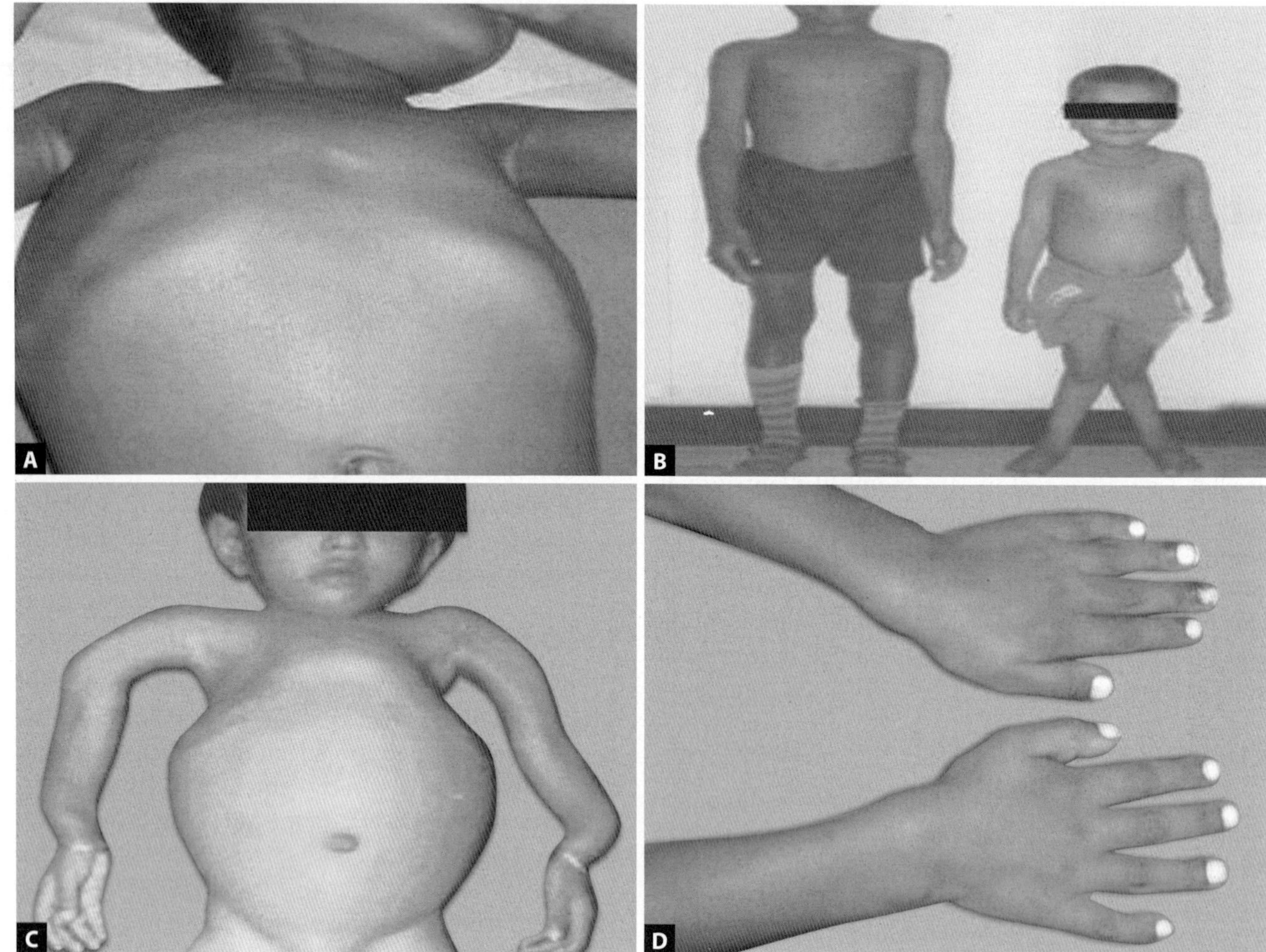

Figs. 1A to D: Clinical features of rickets. (A) Rachitic rosary; (B) Normal child and child of same age with short stature and bow legs; (C) Pot belly; (D) Widening of wrist.

EVALUATION FOR ETIOLOGY OF RICKETS

Once the diagnosis of rickets is strongly considered, next step is to find out the underlying etiology to initiate specific management. They are grouped under clinical classification and laboratory classification. Clinical classification is comprised of (1) nutritional and (2) non-nutritional **(Table 1)** and biochemical classification includes (1) calcipenic rickets and (2) phosphopenic rickets.

- *Nutritional:* Due to inadequate intake of vitamin D in diet or poor exposure to sun light.
- Non-nutritional includes renal, gastrointestinal, hepatic, and metabolic causes.
- *Biochemical classification:* Based on the main biochemical disturbance, rickets is classified into calcipenic and phosphopenic rickets **(Table 2)**.

EXPLANATORY NOTES FOR ALGORITHM (FLOWCHART 1)

1. *Rickets mimics:* There are few conditions which closely mimic the clinical features of rickets and their features favoring their diagnosis are given below.
   - *Metaphyseal dysplasia:* All bones will not be uniformly affected, and the biochemical features will be absent. Serum calcium, phosphorous, alkaline phosphate, and vitamin D levels will be normal.
   - *Morquio's disease* (type 4 mucopolysaccharidosis): Here, serum calcium, phosphorous, serum alkaline phosphate (SAP), and vitamin D levels are normal.
   - *Hypophosphatasia:* Rare disorder in infancy, presents with clinical and radiological features of rickets and bent bones. Laboratory features

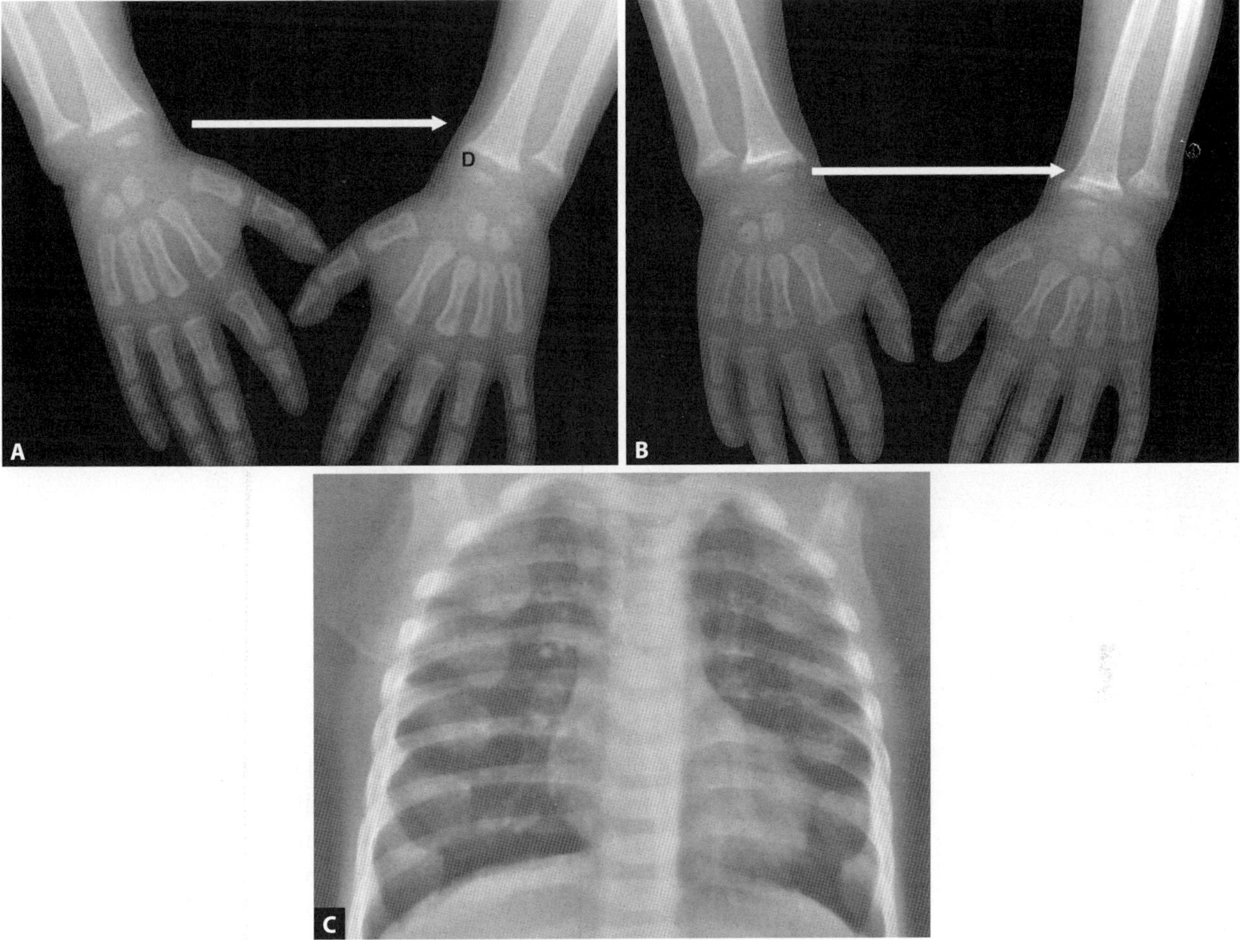

Figs. 2A to C: (A) Active rickets (before vitamin D); (B) Healing rickets—line of preparatory calcification (after vitamin D); (C) Widening of anterior end of ribs.

BOX 1: Tier one investigations.

- X-ray of both wrist AP view
- Urine routine for glycosuria, proteinuria
- Serum 25-OH vitamin D, calcium, phosphorous, and alkaline phosphatase
- *Electrolytes:* Sodium, potassium, chloride, and bicarbonate
- Urea and creatinine
- Serum albumin, total bilirubin, direct and indirect bilirubin
- Arterial or venous blood gas
- USG abdomen

(USG: ultrasound)

are—high calcium, low serum alkaline phosphatase. *X-ray:* Moth-eaten appearance at the ends of the long bones, and marked shortening. *Treatment:* Bone marrow transplantation, recombinant alkaline phosphate (ALP).

BOX 2: Tier two investigations.

- Simultaneous estimation of 25-OH and 1,25-OH vitamin D levels
- Serum PTH level
- Tubular reabsorption of phosphate
- Urinary electrolytes, bicarbonate, chloride, and calcium
- Plasma FGF-23 level
- Ophthalmological examination for cataract, cystine crystals in cornea, KF ring
- USG examination for chronic liver disease and neonatal cholestasis
- Bone mineral profile
- Genetic studies

(FGF: fibroblast growth factor; PTH: parathyroid hormone; USG: ultrasound)

2. *Nutritional or non-nutritional:* Once rickets diagnosis is confirmed after excluding mimics, next step is to identify whether it is nutritional or non-nutritional cause.

BOX 3: Clinical and laboratory clues to suggest non-nutritional rickets.

- Age of onset <6 months or beyond 2 years
- Presence of family history
- When associated with failure to thrive or global developmental delay
- Presence of specific clinical clues such as jaundice, recurrent diarrhea, hypertension, alopecia, and hepatosplenomegaly
- Presence of biochemical abnormalities such as raised urea, creatinine, acidosis, hypokalemia, urine glycosuria or proteinuria, abnormal liver function, or hypoalbuminemia
- Normal vitamin D level
- Inadequate response to vitamin D therapy

TABLE 1: Clinical classification.

Nutritional rickets	*Non-nutritional rickets*
• Reduced intake of vitamin D either as enriched food items or supplements • Reduced intake of calcium • Reduced exposure to sunlight due to cultural or behavioral reasons • Others—skin pigmentation, atmospheric pollution	• *Renal rickets:* – Renal tubular acidosis – Fanconi syndrome – Chronic kidney disease • *Gastrointestinal:* – Malabsorption syndrome • *Hepatic:* – Neonatal cholestasis – Wilson's disease • *Metabolic:* – Vitamin D-dependent rickets type 1 (one alpha hydroxylase defect) – Vitamin D (resistant)-dependent rickets type 2 (receptor defect) – Drug induced—anticonvulsants by stimulating vitamin D metabolism – Lowe's syndrome • *Others:* – Oncogenic rickets – Rickets of prematurity

Nutritional etiology is still common. When will you consider the possibility of non-nutritional rickets?

- Nutritional rickets is common between the age group 6 months and 2 years. Rickets presenting outside this age group (either below or above)
- Rickets associated with failure to thrive
- Presence of family history
- When the serum vitamin D level is normal
- When there is no response to vitamin D therapy

TABLE 2: Biochemical classification of rickets.

Characteristics	*Calcipenic rickets*	*Phosphopenic rickets*
Clinical conditions	Nutritional, vitamin D-dependent rickets, chronic kidney disease, GI causes	• Conditions with phosphate loss • Hypophosphatemic rickets • Proximal RTA
Limbs involved	Both upper and lower limbs	Lower limbs
Bone pain, muscle weakness	Present	Absent
Tetany	Present	Absent
Serum calcium	Normal/low	Normal
Serum phosphate	Normal	Low
SAP	Elevated	Mildly elevated
PTH	Elevated	Normal

(GI: gastrointestinal; PTH: parathyroid hormone; SAP: serum alkaline phosphate)

- Presence of clinical clues such as global developmental delay, jaundice, recurrent diarrhea, hypertension, cataract, and alopecia
- When there are obvious laboratory clues such as raised urea, creatinine, high phosphate, metabolic acidosis, hypokalemia, features of chronic liver disease

3. If non-nutritional, what is the etiological group? Renal or gastrointestinal or hepatic or metabolic etiology?
   At this stage, underlying etiology is identified by both clinical features and laboratory evaluation. Renal causes are more common next to nutritional rickets **(Table 3)**.
4. Next is gastrointestinal (GI) and hepatic causes, clinical clues and laboratory abnormalities point to this group. Further investigations should be done to confirm individual diseases **(Table 4)**.
5. Third group is vitamin D metabolic disorders which are anticonvulsant therapy interfering with vitamin D metabolism, vitamin D-dependent rickets (VDDR) type 1 [one alpha-hydroxylase deficiency and VDDR type 2 (receptor defect)]
   Anticonvulsant therapy: Anticonvulsants particularly phenobarbitone and phenytoin cause rickets by increased catabolism and excretion of vitamin D and its products, direct inhibition of calcium absorption,

Flowchart 1: Algorithmic approach to rickets.

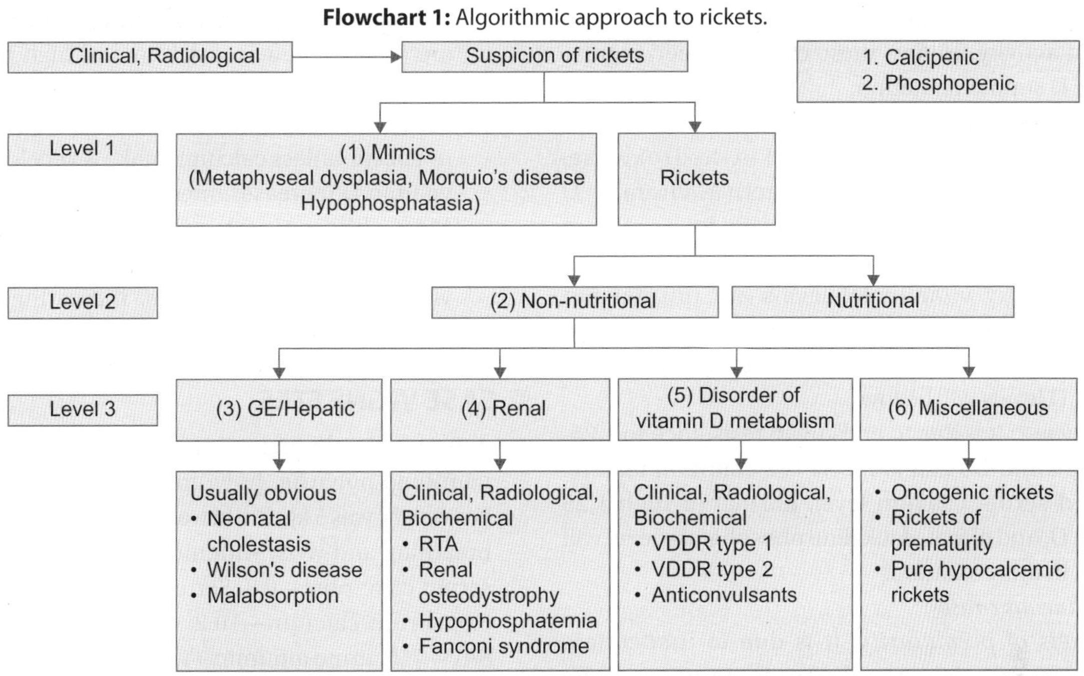

TABLE 3: Renal causes of rickets.

	Clinical features	*Laboratory features*
RTA	Failure to thrive, frequent admissions with dehydration, weakness due to hypokalemia, fast breathing	Normal anion gap metabolic acidosis, hypokalemia, normal urea and creatinine, USG—nephrocalcinosis
CKD	Features of obstructive uropathy, chronic renal failure—hypertension, anemia, short stature	Raised renal parameters, anemia, high phosphate, low calcium, high PTH
HPR	Family history present, lower limbs involved more than the upper limbs	• Low serum phosphate • Normal urea and creatinine
Fanconi syndrome	Severe failure to thrive, features of systemic diseases—cataract, mental retardation, hepatosplenomegaly	• Multiple electrolyte disturbances—hypokalemia, hypophosphatemia, NAGMA • Normal urea and creatinine

(CKD: chronic kidney disease; HPR: hypophosphatemic rickets; NAGMA: normal anion gap metabolic acidosis; PTH: parathyroid hormone; RTA: renal tubular acidosis; USG: ultrasound)

TABLE 4: GI and hepatic causes.

Individual disease	*Clinical features*	*Laboratory abnormalities*
Malabsorption syndrome	Recurrent diarrhea, oily stools, failure to gain weight, multiple deficiencies—anemia, vitamin A, D, and B12, protein	Low serum albumin, low Hb, microcytic or macrocytic
Neonatal cholestasis	Jaundice, pale stools, features of cirrhosis liver and portal hypertension	Conjugated hyperbilirubinemia, low serum albumin
Wilson's disease	Jaundice, personality changes, movement disorder, features of cirrhosis, KF ring	Low serum ceruloplasmin level, increased urinary copper level

(GI: gastrointestinal)

patient factors like poor exposure to sunlight, and reduced activity. Hence, these children need regular vitamin D supplementation.

VDDR type 1: It is a genetic disease associated with defect in the enzyme 1-α-hydroxylase, hence they respond only to active vitamin D (1,25-hydroxycholecalciferol) and fails to respond to regular vitamin D. In these children, serum vitamin D (25-hydroxy vitamin D) levels are normal but 1,25-hydroxy vitamin D levels are decreased, in contrast to nutritional rickets where serum 25-hydroxy vitamin D levels will be low.

VDDR type 2: It is due to end-organ resistance to 1,25-$(OH)_2$ vitamin D3 and alopecia is a common feature. Reduced serum calcium level, normal or high 1,25 vitamin D, and elevated alkaline phosphatase level will be seen in this condition.

6. *Miscellaneous causes:*
   - *Rickets of prematurity:* It is due to inadequate transfer of calcium and phosphate to meet the requirements. In the third trimester, fetus receives approximately 120–140 mg/kg of calcium and 70–80 mg/kg of phosphorus. A preterm baby is devoid of this transfer and vitamin D deficiency may be an additional risk factor.

     Contributing factors are prolonged parenteral nutrition, vitamin D and calcium malabsorption, diuretics causing urinary calcium losses.

     Clinical features are progressive osteopenia, demineralized bones, and, occasionally, pathologic fractures.

     Laboratory features: The SAP may be raised to 1,000 U/L and useful for monitoring. Therapeutic targets are: serum PO_4—4–5 mg and vitamin D >20 ng. SAP should decrease.

     Treatment: Additional oral supplements of Ca and PO_4, vitamin D (400–1,000 IU/day unless severe cholestasis or vitamin D resistance is present).
   - *Oncogenic rickets:* It is a rare disease, where phosphate loss in the urine is associated with mesenchymal tumors like hemangioendothelioma or neurofibroma. Sometimes, they may be small and undetectable and rickets develops years before tumor is apparent. Phosphate loss is due to secretion of fibroblast growth factor. Phosphate replacement along with 1,25-dihydroxy vitamin D and tumor removal are the steps in the management.
   - *Hypocalcemic rickets:* In Indian children, diets are typically low in calcium and high in phytate. Despite adequate vitamin D levels, rickets can occur if the calcium intake is very low. This does not occur unless calcium intake is very low because vitamin D increases intestinal calcium absorption. Most children with calcium deficiency rickets have normal 25(OH) vitamin D and high 1,25(OH) vitamin D concentrations, indicating adequate intake of vitamin D.

CASE VIGNETTES

1. A 9-month-old male infant with recurrent fever, vomiting, polyuria, polydipsia, and failure to thrive. His weight was 5 kg. Child was dehydrated with acidotic breathing and wrist widening. Investigations showed serum creatinine—0.8, Serum K^+—2.2, serum HCO_3—8.0, serum calcium—10.2, serum phosphorus—3.0, SAP—750, urine albumin ++, urine reducing sustances present, sugar +, TRP—78%, and aminoaciduria +
   Diagnosis: Fanconi syndrome
2. A 2-year-old male child with delayed motor milestones, not walking and also had hypocalcemic seizures. Child had clinical and radiological features of rickets. Investigations showed serum calcium—7.0, serum phosphorus—5.2, and SAP—1525. Surprisingly 25-OH vitamin D3 levels are normal but low levels of 1,25-$(OH)_2$ vitamin D3.
   Diagnosis: VDDR-1
3. An 8-year-old male child with posterior urethral valve/valve fulguration done and is conservatively managed. Child is brought with bony deformities, breathlessness, acidosis, hypertension, anemia, and volume overload. Investigations showed serum creatinine—6.8, serum potassium—6.0, serum HCO_3—8.0, serum calcium—7.0, serum phosphorus—8.2, and Hb—5.6. USG abdomen: Bilateral small kidneys.
   Diagnosis: CKD-MBD (chronic kidney disease-mineral and bone disorder)
4. A 6-year-old girl child with swelling of hand following fall, generalized bony changes, more in lower limbs. Investigations showed serum calcium—9.4, serum phosphorus—2.3, SAP—2100, serum creatinine and electrolytes—normal, urine routine—normal, TRP—80%.
   Diagnosis: Hypophosphatemic rickets

KEY POINTS

- Vitamin D deficiency still commonest cause of rickets in a pediatric hospitals.
- If vitamin D level is low IAP guidelines have to be followed by giving oral vitamin D biweekly therapy in children beyond one year and daily therapy in infants.
- If there are features to suggest non nutritional rickets, investigations are to be planned with the joint care pediatric nephrologists and endocrinologists.
- Genetic tests play a great role in the diagnosis of non nutritional rickets.

SUGGESTED READING

1. Chanchlani R, Nemer P, Sinha R, Nemer L, Krishnappa V, Sochett E, et al. An Overview of Rickets in Children. Kidney Int Rep. 2020;5(7):980-90.
2. Dhull RS, Jain R, Deepthi B, Cheong HI, Saha A, Mehndiratta M, et al. Vitamin D-dependent rickets (VDDR) type 1: Case series of two siblings with a CYP27B1 mutation and review of the literature. J Bras Nefrol. 2020; 42(4):494-7.
3. Haffner D, Leifheit-Nestler M, Grund A, Schnabel D. Rickets guidance: part I-diagnostic workup. Pediatr Nephrol. 2022;37(9):2013-36.
4. Iyengar A, Thangavelu S. Renal rickets. In: Iyenger AA, Uthup S, Ekambaram S (Eds). Nammalwar's Principles and Practice of Pediatric Nephrology. New Delhi: Jaypee Brothers Medical Publisher; 2022. pp. 470-9.
5. Sahay M, Sahay R. Rickets-vitamin D deficiency and dependency. Indian J Endocrinol Metab. 2012;16(2):164-76.

Disorders of Sodium and Potassium

Sushmita Banerjee

INTRODUCTION

Sodium (Na) is the major extracellular cation in the body, whereas potassium (K) is the main intracellular cation. Their location across the cell membrane is maintained by the Na-K-ATPase pump which by an active process extrudes Na from the cell and pushes K into the cell.

The mechanisms of Na and K balance are closely interlinked, and both are dependent on renal function. In health, the kidney tubules help maintain sodium and potassium homeostasis by reabsorbing these electrolytes from the glomerular filtrate, and with fine-tuning under the influence of the renin-angiotensin-aldosterone system (RAAS) in the distal nephron. Sodium balance occurs in close conjunction with water balance, with the RAAS causing parallel changes in sodium and water. In addition, the action of antidiuretic hormone (ADH) influences renal water reabsorption. **Boxes 1 and 2** list the common causes of Na and K imbalance in children.

CLINICAL FEATURES

Electrolyte abnormalities are commonly seen in children with vomiting, diarrhea, and dehydration. They also occur when patients are otherwise ill and dependent on extraneous fluid therapy to maintain balances. This is particularly seen in PICU patients who may also have disorders of different organs and altered homeostatic mechanisms. More rarely electrolyte abnormalities occur due to chronic diseases which may be genetically acquired.

The symptoms of sodium imbalance are nonspecific and can include lethargy, irritability, drowsiness, confusion, convulsions, and coma. There is often associated abnormalities in water balance, with history of vomiting or diarrhea and clinical features of dehydration, hypo- or hypervolemia. Hyponatremic symptoms are more marked if the disorder develops acutely and occurs due to fluid shift from extracellular fluid (ECF) compartment to intracellular fluid (ICF) compartment causing brain edema. On the other hand, acute hypernatremia causes brain cell shrinkage due to fluid shifts from ICF to ECF, and in severe cases can cause intracerebral hemorrhage, venous sinus thrombosis, or rhabdomyolysis.

Abnormalities in K balance may present as an emergency and significant hyperkalemia can cause ventricular arrhythmias and death. Acute severe hypokalemia can cause acute profound weakness, cardiac arrhythmias,

BOX 1: Etiology of Na imbalances.

Causes of hyponatremia:

- Associated with reduced or normal total body water:
  - Excess Na loss compared to water loss, from:
    - GIT (diarrhea, vomiting, fistulae, ileostomies)
    - Skin (burns, cystic fibrosis)
    - Kidney (tubular diseases—Bartter syndrome, Fanconi syndrome, hypoaldosteronism, diuretics, cerebral salt wasting)
  - Administration of hyponatremic fluids in sick patients or hyponatremic feeds in infants
- Associated with increased total body water:
  - Increased levels of antidiuretic hormone (SIADH, systemic illness)
  - Fluid overload (oliguric renal failure, excessive fluid administration) ±intravascular volume depletion (nephrotic syndrome, hepatic cirrhosis, congenital heart failure)

Causes of hypernatremia:

- Associated with normal or increased total body water:
  - Administration of hypernatremic fluids to sick patients or hypernatremic feeds to infants
  - Hyperaldosteronism
- Associated with decreased total body water:
  - Inadequate fluid administration to sick patients
  - Fluid losses (excess water loss compared to Na loss)—GIT/renal (diabetes insipidus, osmotic diuresis in diabetes mellitus)/skin (burns)

(GIT: gastrointestinal tract; Na: sodium; SIADH: syndrome of inappropriate antidiuretic hormone secretion)

BOX 2: Etiology of K imbalances.

Causes of hyperkalemia:
- *Increased total body K (TBK):*
  - *Reduced excretion:* Renal failure, mineralocorticoid deficiency, type 4 RTA, potassium-sparing diuretics, RAAS inhibitors
  - *Increased intake:* Iatrogenic K administration, large blood transfusion
- *Increased cell breakdown:* Hemolysis, tumor lysis (also increased TBK), rhabdomyolysis
- Increased catabolism—sepsis and burns
- Redistribution from ICF to ECF—acidosis, insulin deficiency

Causes of hypokalemia:
- *Reduced total body potassium:*
  - Inadequate intake, iatrogenic
  - Renal loss—renal artery stenosis, tubular diseases, mineralocorticoid excess, diuretics, and other drugs
  - GIT loss—diarrhea, vomiting, fistulae, stomas, and laxatives
- *Redistribution from ECF to ICF:*
  - Alkalosis
  - β_2 agonists
  - Insulin
  - Periodic paralysis

(ECF: extracellular fluid; ICF: intracellular fluid; K: potassium; RAAS: renin-angiotensin-aldosterone system; RTA: renal tubular acidosis)

ileus, myopathy, and respiratory failure. Characteristic ECG changes are used in monitoring of severity and treatment. Hypokalemia is associated with appearance of U wave, flattening of T wave and ST depression. In hyperkalemia, there is appearance of tallT waves, widening of QRS complex, and disappearance of P waves.

Chronic disorders, most commonly the renal tubular diseases, present with chronic weakness, recurrent dehydration and fever, failure to thrive, short stature, rickets, and polyuria. Hypertension may be associated with conditions like Liddle's syndrome and hyperaldosteronism. Ultimately, the diagnosis of the specific etiology is necessary for directing specific treatment, and for predicting long-term outcome.

DIAGNOSTIC TESTS

Patients who are at risk of having electrolyte abnormalities, as discussed above should have biochemical tests including serum Na, K, chloride as well as urea and creatinine levels checked at presentation, and regularly thereafter until resolution. Further investigations are directed according to the specific etiology suspected.

The defining values of Na and K abnormalities are given in **Table 1**.

TABLE 1: Definitions.

Hyponatremia	Na <135 mmol/L
Hypernatremia	Na >145 mmol/L
Hypokalemia	K <3.5 mmol/L
Hyperkalemia	K >5.5 mmol/L (>6.5 in neonates)

[*Note*: Hyperglycemia causes 1.6 mmol/L fall in serum Na for every 100 mg/dL rise in blood glucose concentration. Spurious hyponatremia (due to high serum lipids or proteins) is unusual nowadays due to technical improvements in sodium assay. Spuriously high potassium levels can occur due to hemolysis during sampling or passage of K outside cells in the drawn sample]

USEFUL BIOCHEMICAL INDICES IN INVESTIGATION OF NA AND K ABNORMALITIES

Several biochemical parameters that are easily obtained can help to narrow down and differentiate between underlying etiologies. However, these should be used along with clinical and other clues, as they are not always foolproof.

- *Renal sodium excretion* can be measured as a *spot urinary sodium* or the *fractional excretion of sodium* (FeNa):

  FeNa = [Urinary Na × plasma creatinine/urinary creatinine × serum sodium] × 100

  The spot urinary sodium concentration may be unreliable and variable as it would depend on the volume and concentration of the urine sample. The FeNa measurement is more reliable, fairly easy to perform, and requires a random spot urine sample with a simultaneous blood sample.
  - Urinary sodium is low (<5–10 mg/dL in a spot sample or FeNa <1%) in intravascular hypovolemia, or extrarenal sodium losses
  - Urinary sodium is high (>20 mg/dL in a spot sample or FeNa >1%) in intrinsic renal injury, excessive sodium intake, renal sodium loss, hypervolemia, or syndrome of inappropriate antidiuretic hormone secretion (SIADH).
- *Plasma (P) and urine (U) osmolality*: The normal threshold for ADH release ranges from 275 to 290 mOsm/kg H_2O. Patients, who are in an antidiuretic mode due to intravascular volume depletion or increased plasma osmolality, will normally concentrate their urine and will have U:P osmolality ratio >1. Conversely in the diuretic mode, due to the presence

of hypervolemia or hyponatremia, dilute urine will be produced and U:P osmolality will be <1. If the serum Na is below 130 mmol/L, or if the serum osmolality is <270 mOsm/kg H_2O, the urine should be maximally dilute.
- Urine osmolality is high in intravascular volume depletion, osmotic diuresis, renal salt loss, or SIADH.
- Urine osmolality is low in hypervolemia and diabetes insipidus (DI).

- *Urinary potassium* levels of >20 mg/dL or potassium/creatinine ratio of >15 mmol/g in a spot sample, in the presence of hypokalemia, are an indication of renal K loss, while low levels suggest extrarenal K loss.
- *Transtubular potassium gradient (TTKG):* In the presence of normal renal function, this assesses the response of the distal tubule and collecting duct to aldosterone which is influenced by serum potassium. (This test requires that urinary Na >25 mmol/L and urine osmolality > plasma osmolality.)

  TTKG = Urinary K × Plasma osmolality/plasma K × Urinary osmolality

  Normal value being 8–9. A high TTKG in the presence of hypokalemia indicates renal potassium loss. A low TTKG in the presence of hyperkalemia indicates inability of the kidneys to excrete K, due to mineralocorticoid deficiency or inactivity.
- *Renin and aldosterone levels:* Raised levels of both renin and aldosterone levels occur in diseases with primary renal Na and water loss, and contribute to the development of hypokalemia (e.g., Bartter's syndrome, renal tubular acidosis, and pseudohypoaldosteronism). Both these levels are suppressed in Liddle's syndrome. Primary diseases of the adrenals associated with reduced or increased levels of aldosterone will be associated with conversely increased or decreased renin, respectively. The titers of these hormones are affected by body position and stress, therefore, standard levels are described according to body position in which sample is taken (e.g., on 2-hour supine samples).

MANAGEMENT

Sodium abnormalities in particular are often associated with abnormalities in water balance, and the correction of overt hypo- or hypervolemia takes precedence. Subsequent correction should mimic assessed rate of development of the dysnatremia.

Flowcharts 1A and B: Management of Na imbalances.

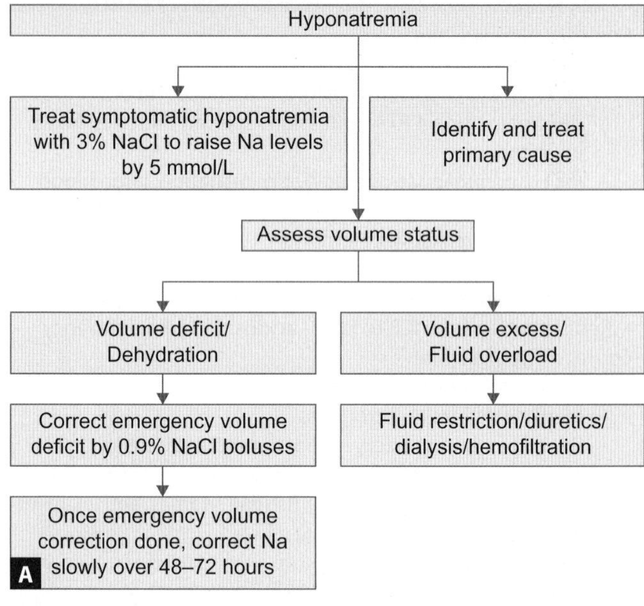

Notes:
- The total sodium correction is calculated as: deficit + assessed ongoing losses, where deficit (mmol) = (desired Na – present Na) × 0.6 × Weight (kg)
- The change in serum Na should not exceed 0.5 mmol/L/h, and aim for correction by 10–20 mmol/L in first 48 hours.

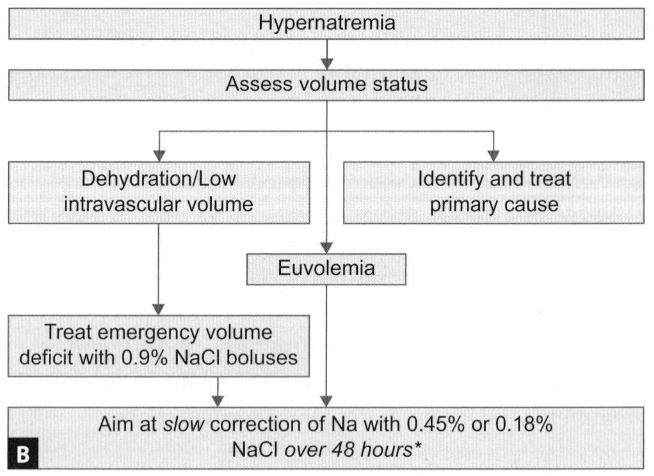

Notes:
- Free water deficit (liters) is calculated by: 0.6 × lean body weight (kg) × [(serum Na/140) – 1] to be added to ongoing maintenance fluid requirement and ongoing losses
- *To calculate decrease in serum Na with 1 liter of infusate: Change in serum Na = [Infusate Na – Serum Na]/[Total body water (0.6 × Weight) +1]
- The change in serum Na should not exceed 0.5 mmol/L/h
- Correction should be limited to 8 mmol/L in the first 24 hours and 18 mmol/L in the first 48 hours

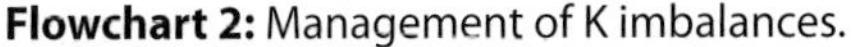

Flowchart 2: Management of K imbalances.

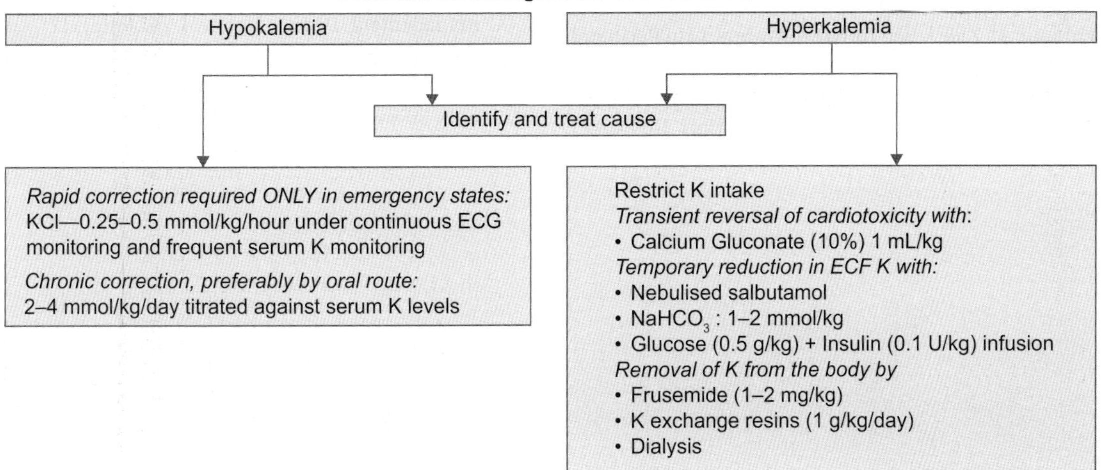

Acute symptomatic hyponatremia is corrected on an emergency basis with hypertonic saline. However, generally, abnormal Na levels are corrected slowly over 48-72 hours, particularly in conditions of chronic hyponatremia, to prevent rapid reversal of fluid shifts from the brain cells to the ECF which can cause a CNS demyelinating disorder known as central pontine myelinosis **(Flowcharts 1A and B)**. Antagonists of type 2 vasopressin receptor (AVPR2) (e.g., Tolvaptan) and oral urea supplements are recently available for management of hyponatremia; however, their use is not yet routine in children.

Hypernatremia may be associated with severe dehydration and volume depletion which needs emergency correction. However, further Na correction should be slow to prevent rapid fall in ECF osmolality which may cause reverse fluid shift into brain cells and cerebral edema.

Severe abnormalities in K balance may need to be treated on an emergency basis, since significant hyperkalemia can cause cardiac arrhythmias and death and severe hypokalemia can cause weakness, muscular paralysis, and respiratory failure. Once the acute stage is corrected, determination of etiology allows planning of a long-term corrective therapy. Approach to treatment is given in **Flowchart 2**.

CLINICAL PEARLS

- Sodium abnormalities are often associated with anomalies of water balance.
- In such cases, restoration of intravascular volume to normal takes precedence.

CLINICAL PEARLS

- In hyperkalemia, methods to shift K to intracellular spaces are quick acting and should be instituted first for rapid effect.
- Methods to remove K from the body take time but are effective in the long term.

SUMMARY

Sodium and K abnormalities occur in a large number of acute and chronic conditions. The imbalances may be acute and severe and need emergency treatment. Occasionally, the etiology is chronic and requires prolonged specific and supportive treatment with long-term monitoring and follow-up. A systematic clinical and biochemical work-up will usually indicate the cause and guide directed therapy once the acute situation is controlled.

KEY POINTS

- Sodium and K imbalances are common in acutely ill children, and in some renal and endocrine diseases.
- Abnormalities of intravascular volume often coexist with Na imbalances and take precedence in management.
- After emergency management, further correction of Na levels should match the duration of evolution of the abnormality: Acutely occurring Na imbalances can be treated rapidly, while chronic imbalances of Na require slow correction to prevent complications.
- Potassium imbalances can present as major emergencies, and need rapid recognition and correction.
- Once the emergency electrolyte imbalances are corrected, a diagnostic work-up and specific management of the cause are instituted.

SUGGESTED READING

1. Bockenhauer D, Zieg J. Electrolyte disorders. Clin Perinatol. 2014;41(3):575-90.
2. Brown DH, Paloian NJ. Hypokalemia/Hyperkalemia and Hyponatremia/Hypernatremia. Pediatr Rev 2023; 44(7):349-62.
3. Moritz ML. Sodium and water disorders: evaluation and management. Pediatr Nephrol. 2021;46:1-17.
4. Suarez-Rivera M, Stalin LM, Bonilla-Felix M. Potassium Disorders: evaluation and management. Pediatr Nephrol. 2022;47:1123-43.

Acute Glomerulonephritis

Abhijeet Saha, Rupal Gupta

INTRODUCTION

The term "glomerulonephritis" encompasses a subset of renal diseases characterized by immune-mediated damage to the basement membrane, mesangium, or capillary endothelium, leading to hematuria, proteinuria, and azotemia. The term acute glomerulonephritis (AGN) defines a pathological process that may present clinically as acute nephritic syndrome, nephrotic syndrome, or rapidly progressive glomerulonephritis (RPGN). Nephritic syndrome is a clinical syndrome defined by the association of hematuria, proteinuria, and often arterial hypertension and kidney failure.

A widely accepted way to classify glomerulonephritis is to divide it into five forms based on underlying immune processes. **Box 1** consists the classification of glomerulonephritis, including pathogenic type and the disease entity associated with it.

Acute postinfectious glomerulonephritis (APIGN) includes a large apportionment of AGN resulting from a variety of infectious agents, most common being streptococci. The common infectious agents leading to the causation of APIGN have been enumerated in **Box 2**. Acute poststreptococcal glomerulonephritis (APSGN) is the prototype of APIGN occurring due to immune complex deposition. Recently, novel entities have been reported, including COVID-19-associated nephropathy (COVAN).

BOX 1: Classification of glomerulonephritis.

Immune-complex GN:
- IgA nephropathy
- IgA vasculitis
- Infection-related GN
- Lupus nephritis
- Fibrillary GN with polyclonal Ig deposits

Pauci-immune:
- PR3-ANCA (C-ANCA) GN
- MPO-ANCA (P-ANCA) GN
- ANCA-negative GN

Antiglomerular basement membrane (GBM) GN:

C3 glomerulopathy:
- C3 glomerulonephritis
- Dense deposit disease

BOX 2: Etiology of postinfectious glomerulonephritis (GN).

Bacteria:
- Gram-positive bacteria (*streptococci, staphylococci, pneumococci, enterococci, Listeria monocytogenes*)
- Gram-negative cocci (*meningococcus, Neisseria gonorrhoeae*)
- Gram-negative coccobacilli (*Haemophilus*)
- Gram-negative bacilli (*Salmonella, Klebsiella, Serratia, Yersinia, Proteus, Pseudomonas*)
- Other infections (*Legionellosis, brucellosis, bartonellosis*)

Mycobacteria, Rickettsia, Mycoplasma, Chlamydia, and Spirochetes:
- Tuberculosis and nontuberculous *mycobacteria*
- Syphilis (*Treponema pallidum*)
- Leptospirosis (*Leptospira interrogans*)
- Rickettsial diseases (*Coxiella burnetii*)
- *Mycoplasma pneumoniae*
- *Chlamydia pneumoniae*

Viruses:

DNA viruses:
- Hepatitis B
- Varicella zoster
- Epstein-Barr
- Cytomegalovirus
- Parvovirus B19
- Adenovirus

RNA viruses:
- HIV
- Coxsackie, enteric cytopathic human orphan (ECHO) virus
- Hepatitis A, hepatitis C
- Dengue virus
- Mumps and measles
- Hantavirus and rotavirus

Contd...

Contd...

Fungi:
- *Candida albicans*
- *Histoplasma capsulatum*
- *Coccidioides immitis*

Parasitic infestations:
- *Plasmodium falciparum, P. malariae*
- *Schistosoma haematobium, S. mansoni*
- *Toxoplasma gondii*
- Filariasis, trichinosis, and hydatid disease
- Amebiasis (*Entamoeba histolytica*)

EPIDEMIOLOGY

Group A streptococci are most commonly typed by their surface M proteins, which are virulence factors. They can also be divided into two groups based on the presence or absence of lipoproteins that causes serum to become opaque (serum opacity factor). Each of these two groups contains a characteristic group of M proteins. The opacity factor-positive group contains the "nephritogenic" strains. Nephritogenic strains are further subdivided into those primarily associated with pyoderma (M47, M49, M55, M56, M57, and M 60), and those that most often cause pharyngitis (M1, M4, M25, and some M12 strains).

Acute poststreptococcal glomerulonephritis is one of the most common causes of acute kidney injury (AKI) in children of developing countries. Poor hygiene and lack of access to medical care increases the risk in these countries.

PATHOGENESIS

Immune complex accumulation within glomerular tufts is thought to be the primary pathogenic mechanism of postinfectious GN. Molecular mimicry, which involves evoking an autoimmune response in response to both streptococcal and renal components, and modifications to a normal renal antigen that trigger autoimmune reactivity are other pathways that have been suggested.

Much of the early work on the pathogenesis of APSGN focused on the group A-specific streptococcal M proteins but it has now been discounted as the nephritogenic antigen because, in addition to the increasing number of M-serotype strains that are nephritogenic (M serotypes 1, 2, 4, 12, 18, 42, 49, 56, 57, and 60), some M-type strains are non-nephritogenic.

Nephritogenic Streptococcal Antigens

A cationic cysteine proteinase called streptococcal pyrogenic exotoxin B, which is produced by proteolysis of a zymogen precursor, and the nephritis-associated plasmin receptor, also known as glyceraldehyde-3-phosphate dehydrogenase, are the two potential antigens under investigation as the possible cause of APSGN at this time. It is possible to activate the complement system's alternative pathway using either of these fractions.

Glomerular binding and plasmin activation are considered key pathogenic properties of these proteins. When deposited in glomeruli, glyceraldehyde 3-phosphate dehydrogenase, streptococcal cationic proteinase exotoxin B (speB), or zymogen (whether bound by specific antibody or not), can interact with plasmin or plasminogen to cause glomerular damage by degrading the glomerular basement membrane (GBM) through the activation of latent metalloproteinases or collagenases **(Fig. 1)**. The circulating or in situ immune complexes can then move across the altered GBM and accumulate as "humps" in the subepithelial space.

Immune Complex Deposition and Complement Activation

Rodriguez-Iturbe suspected the crucial role played by an in situ immunological reaction resulting from the antibody meeting free antigen deposited in the glomeruli. The difficulties of generating GN and the near impossibility of generating subepithelial immune deposits (humps), the APSGN prototype lesion, using premade immune complexes highlighted this possibility. Gene negativity (GN) can be produced by huge numbers of premade complexes; however, this is leukocyte-mediated, with the immune deposits primarily located subendothelium.

A key component of APSGN is complement activation. The immunofluorescence pattern, which usually consists of immunoglobulin G (IgG), C3, and C5, and the serum complement profiles (low C3 and normal C4) indicate that the alternative route is preferably activated. The elements C1q and C4 of the traditional route are hardly ever present in these deposits.

Cellular Immune Mechanisms

The glomeruli are invaded by immune-competent cells such as T helper cells and macrophages. Monocytic chemotactic protein-1, tumor necrosis factor-α, IL-6, and IL-8 are all more prevalent in the blood. The inflammatory process and its intensity are significantly influenced by the immune cells that infiltrate the body.

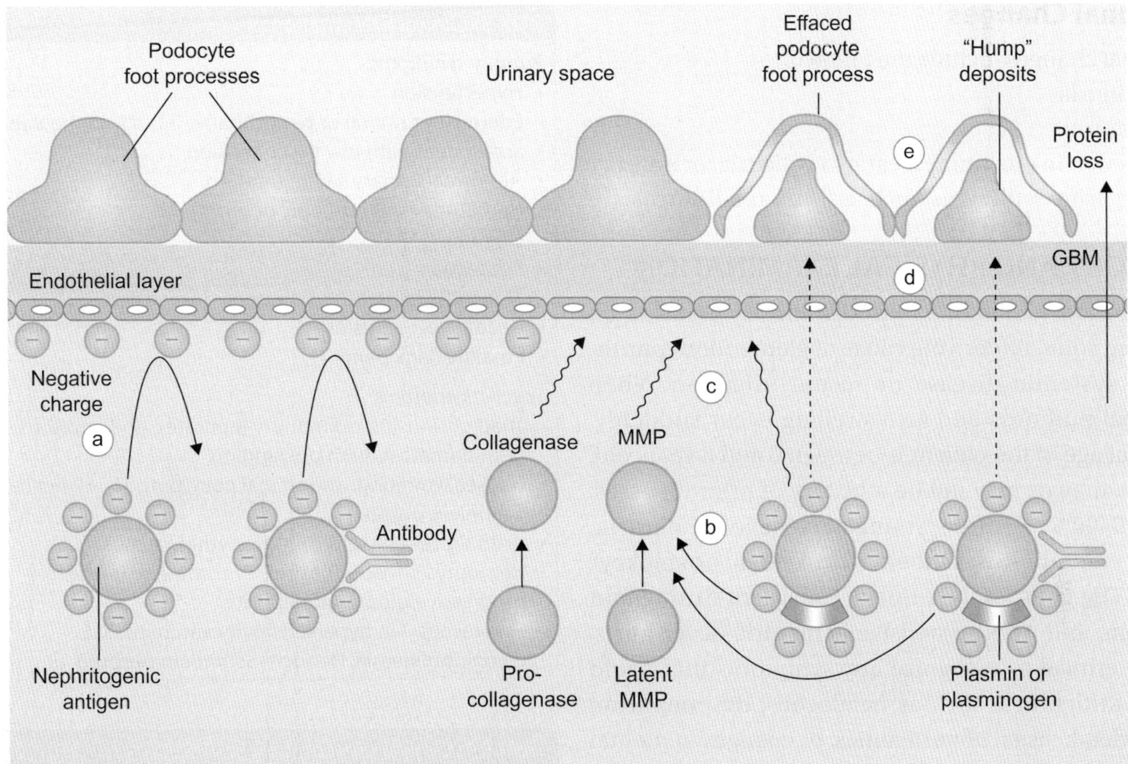

Fig. 1: Possible pathogenic mechanism causing glomerulonephritis after streptococcal infection. The putative nephritogenic antigens, namely streptococcal cationic proteinase exotoxin B (speB) or zymogen and glyceraldehyde 3-phosphate dehydrogenase, are typically repelled by the negatively charged glomerular basement membrane (GBM) in both their free and antibody-bound forms; (b) Nevertheless, these antigens can interact with plasmin or plasminogen to activate procollagenase and latent matrix metalloproteinase; (c) The active enzymes break down the GBM and eliminate its negative charge; (d) The nephritogenic antigen and immune complexes can then pass through the damaged GBM and form the distinctive "hump"-like deposits under the podocyte processes; (e) Damage to the GBM also causes effacement of podocyte foot processes, which leads to loss of protein in the urine. (GBM: glomerular basement membrane; MMP: matrix metalloproteinase; speB: streptococcal cationic proteinase exotoxin B)

Autoimmune Reactivity

Even though APSGN has documented a number of autoimmune findings, these results are epiphenomena rather than definitive clinical courses of the disease. Anti-IgG antibodies are commonly observed in glomerular deposits and serum. The course of APSGN may be modulated by this immunological reaction.

PATHOPHYSIOLOGY

Structural Changes

Structurally, cellular proliferation causes an increase in the cellularity of the glomerular tuft due to the excess of endothelial, mesangial, and epithelial cells. The proliferation may be of two types:

1. *Endocapillary*—within the glomerular capillary tufts
2. *Extracapillary*—in the Bowman space, including the epithelial cells

In extracapillary proliferation, parietal epithelial cells proliferate to cause the formation of crescents, characteristic of some forms of RPGN.

Thickening of glomerular basement membrane appears as thickened capillary walls on light microscopy. However, on electron microscopy, this may look like a consequence of the thickening of the basement membrane proper, for instance, electron-dense deposits either on the epithelial or endothelial side of the basement membrane. There can be various types of electron-dense deposits corresponding to an area of immune complex deposition, such as subendothelial, subepithelial, intramembranous, and mesangial.

Features of irreversible injury include hyalinization or sclerosis that can be focal, diffuse, segmental, or global.

Functional Changes

Functional changes include the following:

- Proteinuria
- Hematuria
- Reduction in creatinine clearance, oliguria, or anuria
- Active urine sediments, such as RBCs and RBC casts

HISTORY AND PHYSICAL EXAMINATION

It is important to obtain a thorough history focusing on identifying some underlying cause of glomerulonephritis, such as systemic disease or recent infection When periorbital puffiness and face swelling occur suddenly, the typical age of the patient is between 6 and 8 years old, and there may or may not be a history of prior illnesses. About 25–60% of these youngsters have hematuria, which is commonly described as "coke, tea, or smokey" colored. The color of the urine is consistent throughout the stream, and AGN's extensive hematuria never hurts. It is also critical to recognize any symptoms that could indicate difficulties, such as headaches, dyspnea from fluid overload, visual abnormalities, or changes in mental status from hypertension. Searching for alternate reasons should be prompted by the presence of rash, arthritis, hepatosplenomegaly, recent weight change, or recent medication exposure. Pharyngitis or pyoderma caused by group A β-hemolytic streptococcal bacteria often occurs prior to it. In cases of sore throat, the latency period between the streptococcal infection and the start of the clinical illness is 7–14 days, whereas in cases of pyoderma, it is 2–4 weeks. Minor pharyngitis sometimes goes unreported, but healed scars from prior pyoderma can be used to identify it.

CLINICAL PRESENTATION OF ACUTE GLOMERULONEPHRITIS

Acute glomerulonephritis is most commonly present as edema along with hematuria (can be microscopic or gross) and oliguria. Clinical examination may reveal hypertension. **Box 3** comprises primary and specific presentations of AGN.

BOX 3: Clinical presentation of AGN.

Primary symptoms:

- Hypertension
- Edema (peripheral or periorbital)—initially in the dependent areas/areas with low tissue tension
- Abnormal urinary sedimentation
- Hematuria—microscopic or gross
- Oliguria
- Azotemia
- Shortness of breath or dyspnea on exertion
- Headache, confusion
- Possible flank pain

Specific symptoms:

- Triad of sinusitis, pulmonary infiltrates, and nephritis—granulomatosis with polyangiitis
- Nausea, vomiting, abdominal pain, purpura: Henoch–Schönlein purpura
- Arthralgias—systemic lupus erythematosus (SLE)
- Hemoptysis—Goodpasture syndrome or idiopathic progressive glomerulonephritis
- Skin rashes—in hypersensitivity vasculitis, SLE, cryoglobulinemia, Henoch–Schönlein purpura

Acute poststreptococcal glomerulonephritis is classically present as triad of acute onset gross hematuria, and hypertension, but it can have variable presentations also. **Table 1** summarizes certain presentations.

TABLE 1: Clinical presentation of APSGN.

Acute nephritic syndrome (most common)	Active urinary sediment (red cell casts, white blood cells, and dysmorphic red blood cells); proteinuria (usually <1 g/m²/day); gross hematuria/cola colored urine in 30–70%; variable degrees of hypertension in 60–80% and acute kidney injury (AKI)
Subclinical disease (during epidemics)	Asymptomatic microscopic hematuria (>3 red blood cells per high-power field of centrifuged urine specimen), or proteinuria (<40 mg/m²/hour); blood pressure may be normal or transiently increased; normal kidney function
Atypical presentation	Acute pulmonary edema, hypertensive encephalopathy, nephrotic syndrome (proteinuria >1 g/m²/day, serum albumin <3g/dL, edema), anuric AKI, rapidly progressive renal failure (acute GN with rapid decline in kidney function within 7–10 days)

(APSGN: acute poststreptococcal glomerulonephritis; GN: glomerulonephritis)

Acute poststreptococcal glomerulonephritis has to be differentiated from features that are suggestive of nephrotic syndrome. **Table 2** enumerated few features specific of nephrotic syndrome.

The three stages of disease manifestation are latent, acute, and recovery **(Fig. 2)**. Following the resolution of fluid overload with diuresis, blood pressure normalization, and the resolution of proteinuria and gross hematuria, the

TABLE 2: Difference between nephrotic and nephritic syndrome.

	Nephrotic syndrome	Nephritic syndrome
Edema	Gross	Mild to moderate
Hematuria	Absent/minimal	Marked/gross
Hypertension	Absent/minimal	Common
Urine output	Normal/ decreased	Decreased
Serum cholesterol	Elevated	Mildly elevated/ normal
Proteinuria	Gross	Moderate
Glomerular filtration rate	Normal	Decreased

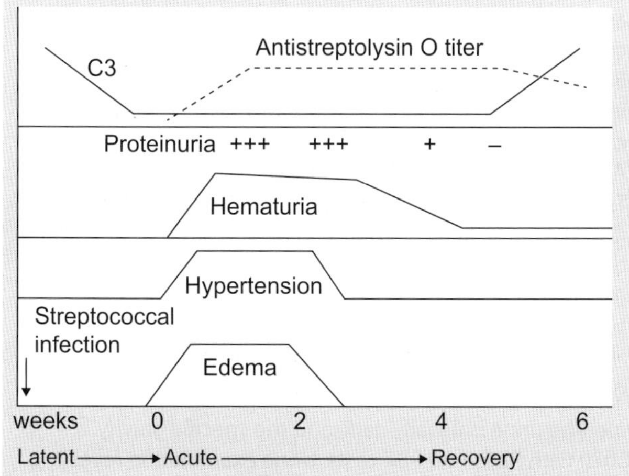

Fig. 2: Summary of the typical clinical course of poststreptococcal acute glomerulonephritis.

recovery phase begins. 4–7 days after being admitted to the hospital, urine production usually increases. The edema quickly goes away and blood pressure quickly returns to normal after this increase. Microscopic hematuria can persist for a year from the commencement of the disease and takes many months to eradicate.

Acute poststreptococcal glomerulonephritis can have varying severity, mild cases may just present with microscopic hematuria with mild proteinuria, while those at the other end of the spectrum may have anuria and severe hypertension. Unlike nephrotic syndrome, where edema is flaccid and can increase across the entire body with unlimited fluid intake, turgid edema occurs. Proteinuria is usually mild and not in the nephrotic range. Massive proteinuria may be found in about 2–4% of cases and its persistence is a risk factor for progression to RPGN.

CLINICAL PEARLS

Indications for hospitalization:
- Severe edema
- Severe azotemia
- Hypertension
- Respiratory distress

CLINICAL PEARLS

When to suspect rapidly progressive glomerulonephritis?
- Persistent oliguria
- Severe azotemia
- Nephrotic range proteinuria

Up to 80% of children with APSGN experience hypertension as a result of extracellular space expansion brought on by sodium and water retention. About 30–35% of children experience cerebral consequences from hypertension, such as headache, sleepiness, seizure, mental status, and visual alterations. Pulmonary edema symptoms can manifest clinically and radiologically in patients. Nearly half of these kids may have congestive heart failure symptoms. Blood pressure is high at first, but as heart failure and shock take over, hypotension sets in later. The clinical pearl below has a list of a few unusual APSGN appearances.

Rapidly increasing azotemia and persistent oliguria should raise a dubiety of RPGN.

CLINICAL PEARLS

Atypical presentations of APSGN:
- Subclinical disease
- Seizures
- Acute hypertensive crisis
- Acute pulmonary edema
- Acute kidney injury
- Reversible posterior leukoencephalopathy syndrome
- Autoimmune hemolytic anemia
- Rash similar to Henoch–Schönlein purpura

INVESTIGATIONS

In 60–65% of patients, blood urea is elevated, and in 20% of cases, estimated creatinine clearance is reduced to <90 mL/min/1.73 m^2. During the acute phase of the disease, the glomerular filtration rate (GFR) frequently decreases. Due to volume overload, a moderate case of normocytic normochromic anemia is also observed. Patients with nephrotic range proteinuria may have hypoalbuminemia.

In suspected instances of APSGN, serologic evidence of a recent streptococcal infection should be investigated since positive streptococcal serology has a higher diagnostic sensitivity (94.6%) than positive cultures (24.3%) or the history of a recent infection (75.7%). The antistreptolysin O (ASO) titer is the most significant serological marker. Pharyngitis-associated APSGN is associated with greater ASO titers, while cases that follow pyoderma are more likely to have raised anti-deoxyribonuclease (DNase) B titers. 80% of the samples tested positive for the streptozyme test, which consists of four antigens (DNase B, streptolysin O, hyaluronidase, and streptokinase). The most crucial diagnostic indicator for APSGN is an acute drop in serum C3 levels, which typically returns to normal levels 6 weeks after beginning. A little drop in C4 may happen momentarily.

Upon examination, the urine exhibits an acidic pH, dysmorphic red blood cells, granular casts, red cell casts, and neutrophils that may indicate inflammation in the glomerulus. It is typical to see mild to moderate (1-2+) proteinuria.

Box 4 provides an overview of the necessary investigations in the event of an AGN.

BOX 4: Workup for AGN.

Blood:
- *Complete blood count:* A decreased hematocrit may suggest a dilutional type of anemia. With history of infection, leukocytosis may be present
- *Serum electrolytes:* Potassium levels may be raised in patients with AKI
- *Renal function tests:* BUN and creatinine levels are raised, demonstrating a degree of renal impairment. In addition, the glomerular filtration rate (GFR) may be low
- *Liver function tests:* May point toward the underlying etiology
- C-reactive protein (CRP)
- *Complement (C3, C4 levels):* Low complement levels indicate the following diseases: APSGN, cryoglobulinemia, systemic lupus erythematosus, infective (bacterial) endocarditis, shunt nephritis, and membranoproliferative GN
- Autoantibodies, such as antinuclear antibodies (ANA), anti-neutrophil cytoplasmic antibodies (ANCA), and anti-ds-DNA, anti-glomerular basement membrane (GBM) to rule out collagenopathy as the underlying cause of AGN
- *Blood culture:* Blood culture is indicated when there is a fever, immunosuppression, intravenous drug abuse, indwelling catheters, or shunts
- Antistreptolysin O (ASO) titer increases in 60–80% of cases. The rise begins in 1–3 weeks, peaks in 3–5 weeks, and returns to baseline in 6 months. It is unrelated to the severity, duration, and prognosis of renal disease
- *Anti-DNase B:* Often elevated preceding streptococcal pharyngitis and skin infections
- *Hepatitis serology:* As infectious hepatitis can lead to glomerulonephritis of various types

Urine: The urine is usually dark, and the specific gravity is >1.020 with RBCs and RBC casts. Urine examination revealing acidic pH, dysmorphic red blood cells, red cell casts, granular casts, and neutrophils suggestive of glomerular inflammation. Mild-to-moderate (1–2+) proteinuria is commonly seen. The 24-hour urinary protein excretion and creatinine clearance may help establish the degree of renal impairment and proteinuria. The following parameters are usually helpful:
- Microscopy, culture, and sensitivity
- Albumin-to-creatinine or protein-to-creatinine ratio
- RBC casts

Imaging:
- Chest X-ray (helps to see for evidence of pulmonary hemorrhage, if any)
- Renal ultrasound (helps in assessing the size and anatomy for biopsy)

(AGN: acute glomerulonephritis; AKI: acute kidney injury; BUN: blood urea nitrogen)

Renal Biopsy Findings

A renal biopsy is not indicated for diagnosis of APSGN but is usually performed when atypical clinical manifestations are present or the healing is delayed. Conditions which need renal biopsy in the course of APSGN are listed in **Box 5**.

Light Microscopy

Under light microscopy, polymorphonuclear cells infiltrate the glomerular tuft, obliterating the capillary lumina, while endothelial and mesangial cells exhibit pervasive hypercellularity. There is little to no sign of tubular or vascular damage, and GBM is normal **(Fig. 3)**. Rarely, crescent formation in >50% of glomeruli may be present in APSGN patients, resulting in the clinical presentation of rapidly progressing GN.

Immunofluorescence

Discrete granular deposits of IgG and C3 are visible in the immunofluorescence pattern, which is commonly observed during the acute phase of APSGN in the mesangium and capillary loops **(Figs. 4 and 5)**. **Box 2** describes three patterns of the deposits. A poorer long-term prognosis and high proteinuria are linked to the garland pattern. The search for c-ANCA and p-ANCA antibodies should begin when immunofluorescence (IF) deposits are absent **(Box 6)**.

BOX 5: Indication of renal biopsy.

Early stage:
- Severe anuria
- Rapid progressive course
- Hypertension >2 weeks
- Decreased GFR >2 weeks
- Normal complement levels
- Extrarenal manifestation

Recovery phase:
- Depressed GFR >4 weeks
- Hypocomplementemia >12 weeks
- Persistent proteinuria >6 months

(GFR: glomerular filtration rate)

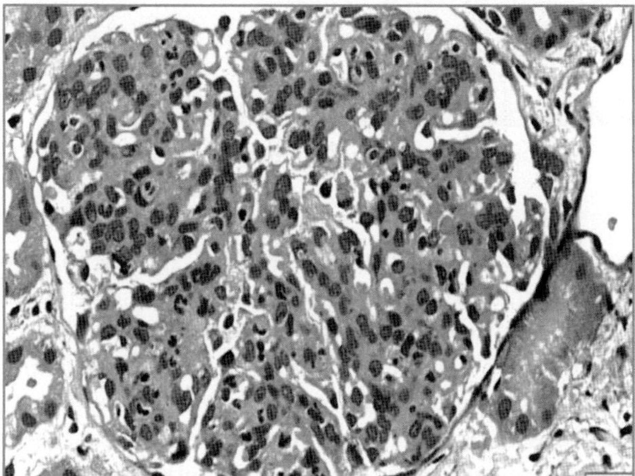

Fig. 3: Acute postinfectious glomerulonephritis. Glomerulus showing cellular proliferation obstructing capillaries and there are abundant polymorphs (hematoxylin and eosin). *(For color version, see Plate 8)*

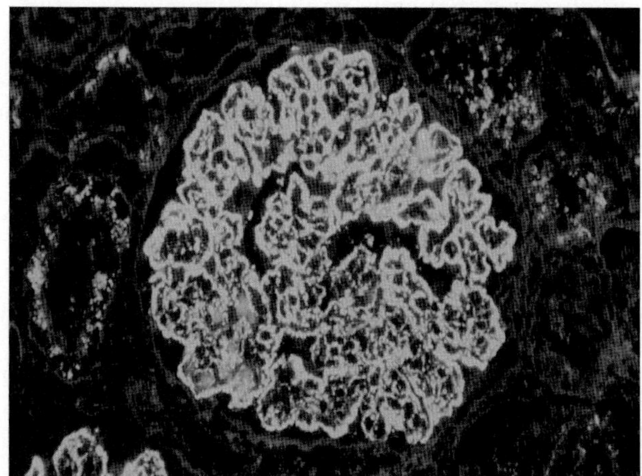

Fig. 4: Acute postinfectious glomerulonephritis. Immunofluorescence for immunoglobulin G showing smaller and spaced parietal granular deposits giving a "starry sky" appearance. *(For color version, see Plate 8)*

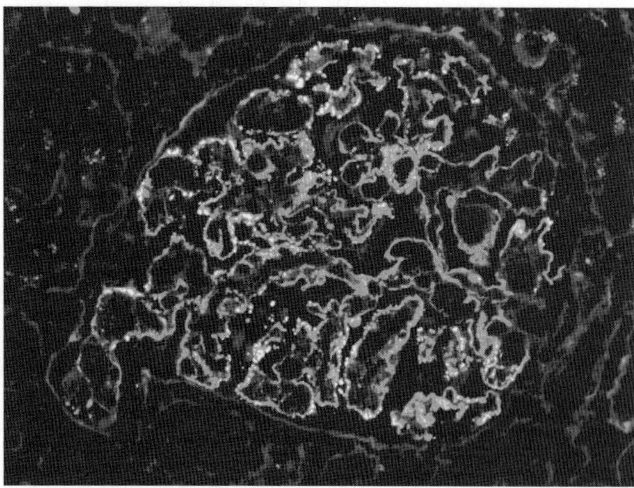

Fig. 5: Acute postinfectious glomerulonephritis. Immunofluorescence for C3 showing extensive granular deposits in the capillary walls giving it a garland appearance. *(For color version, see Plate 8)*

BOX 6: Immunofluorescence patterns in acute poststreptococcal glomerulonephritis.

- Starry sky appearance (discrete mesangial and basement membrane deposits, usually of complement)
- Mesangial pattern (thick deposits in the mesangium)
- Garland pattern (heavy garland-like deposits in the basement membrane)

Electron Microscopy

The subepithelial "hump" that denotes the deposition of subepithelial immune complex is the classic pathologic observation in electron microscopy. Using immunoelectron microscopy, it is now possible to see IgG, C3, and SPEB inside the subepithelial humps **(Figs. 6A and B)**.

DIFFERENTIAL DIAGNOSIS

For the most part, APSGN is an easy diagnosis to make. A number of glomerulonephritis associated with persistent infection, infectious glomerulonephritis devoid of an immune-mediated etiology, and more primary and secondary glomerular disorders are included in the differential diagnosis. It needs to be distinguished from the following conditions: Henoch- Schönlein purpura (normal C3), endocarditis-associated nephritis, shunt nephritis, membranoproliferative GN (persistent hypocomplementemia, unresolving nephritic syndrome),

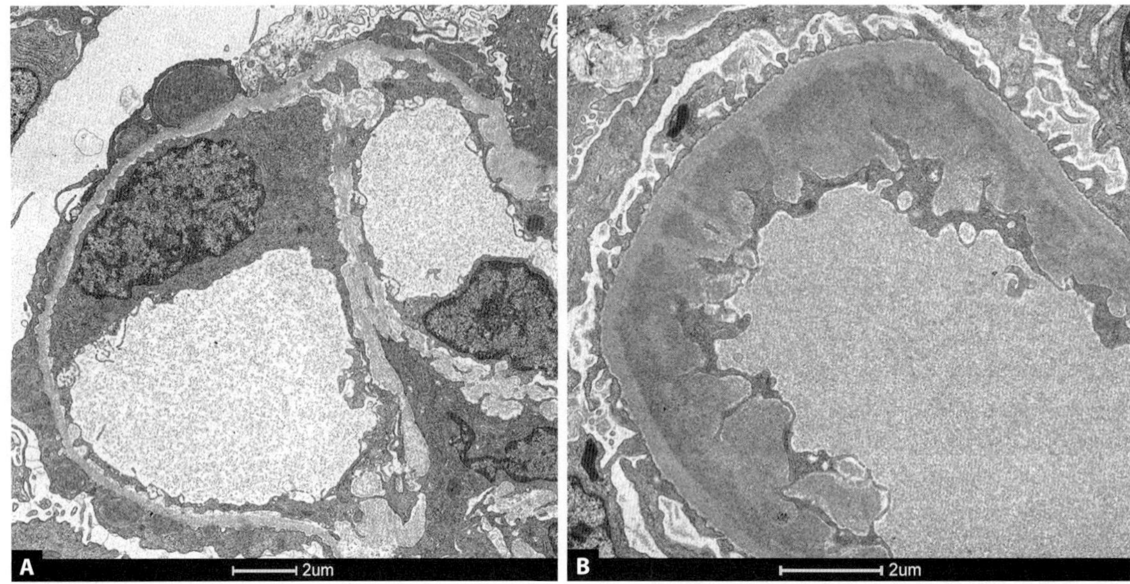

Figs. 6A and B: EM showing subepithelial humps and subendothelial deposits respectively. (EM: electron microscopy)

lupus nephritis (persistent hypocomplementemia, systemic manifestation), vasculitis (polyarteritis nodosa), hemolytic uremic syndrome (hemolysis, thrombocytopenia), hemolytic uremic purpura (hemolysis), and Henoch–Schönlein purpura (short latent period). **Flowchart 1** depicts the approach to acute glomerulonephritis.

MANAGEMENT

The mainstay of treatment for APSGN is supportive care, with an emphasis on managing fluid excess and hypertension. It is advised to limit sodium and fluid intake while consuming enough calories. Fluid restriction and the administration of loop diuretics, such as furosemide, are used to treat hypertension. One or more calcium-channel blockers and other antihypertensive medications may be required. It has been demonstrated that captopril lowers blood pressure and increases GFR in individuals with APSGN; nevertheless, angiotensin-converting enzyme inhibitors should be taken cautiously because of the potential for renal failure and hyperkalemia. Vasodilators (hydralazine) or sodium nitroprusside infusion may be necessary in cases of severe hypertension.

Although pulmonary edema is rare, when it does occur, oxygen and loop diuretics should be used for treatment. Because digitalis is ineffective and can produce drunkenness, it is not recommended. On rare occasions, the clinical course may be complicated by pulmonary *edema* and overt heart failure. AKI, significant fluid retention that is not relieved by diuretics, pulmonary *edema,* and uncontrollably high potassium levels can sometimes require continuous kidney replacement therapy or hemodialysis. Standard protocols must be followed while managing hypertensive situations, acute pulmonary *edema,* AKI, and severe hyperkalemia.

Early antibiotic treatment for streptococcal infections can prevent APSGN, and treating at-risk persons prophylactically with antibiotics can stop the spread of streptococcal infections linked to nephritis. It has been observed that early penicillin therapy can stop or lessen the severity of AGN. It is advised to administer a single injectable dosage of benzathine penicillin G, or alternatively, oral penicillin V for 10 days. Patients who are allergic to penicillin are treated with erythromycin or azithromycin.

CLINICAL PEARLS

Antibiotic therapy in APSGN:
- Children <27 kg: Benzathine penicillin G single dose 600,000 units intramuscularly
- Children >27 kg: Benzathine penicillin G single dose 1.2 million units intramuscularly
- Oral penicillin V 250 mg 2–3 times per day for 10 days

Allergic to penicillin:
- Erythromycin 40 mg/kg/day for 10 days
- Azithromycin for 5 days

Management of APSGN is summarized in **Box 7**.

Flowchart 1: Approach to the patient with acute glomerulonephritis.

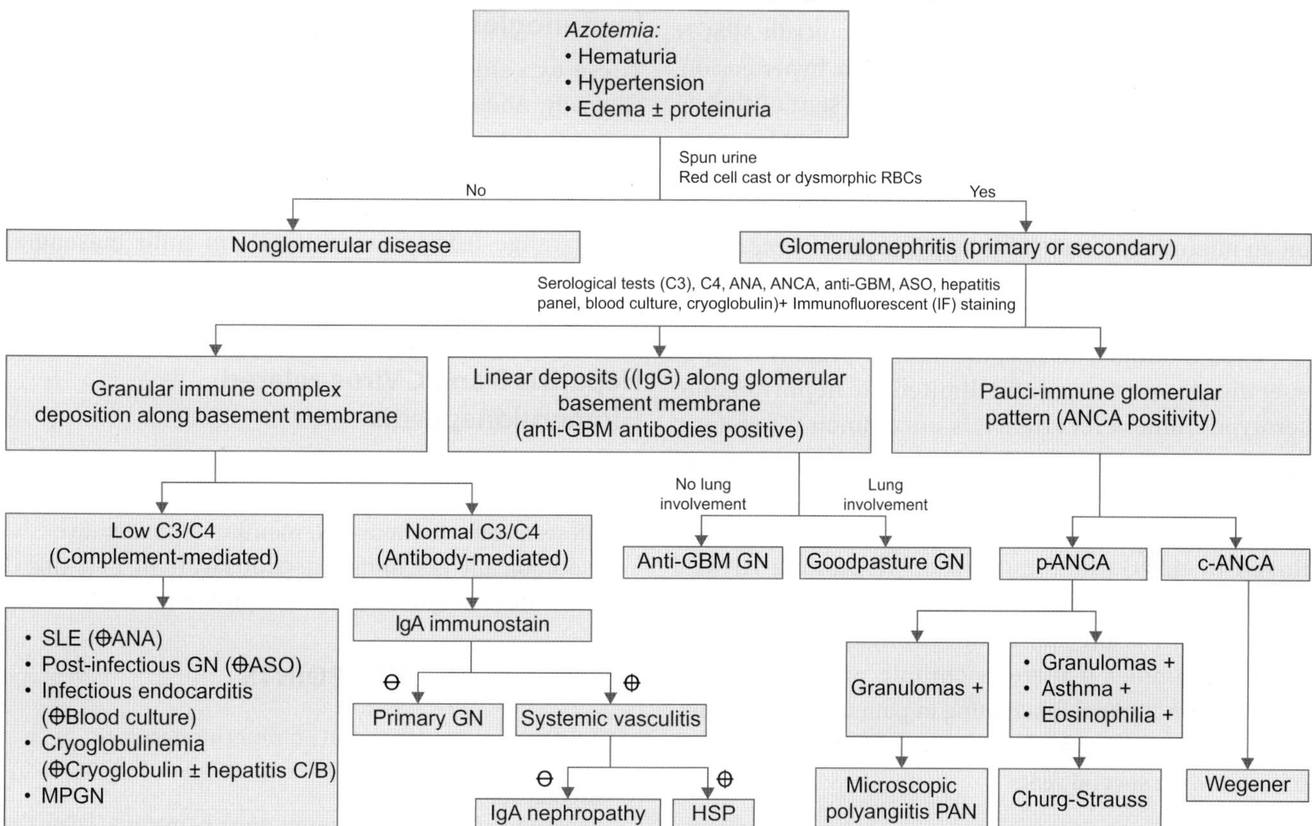

(ANCA: anti-neutrophil cytoplasm antibody; GBM: glomerular basement membrane; GN: glomerulonephritis; HSP: Henoch-Schönlein purpura; MPGN: membranoproliferative glomerulonephritis; PAN; polyarteritis nodosa)

BOX 7: Management of APSGN.

Pharmacological therapy:
- *Antimicrobials:* Patients with evidence of a streptococcal infection should receive a course of antibiotic therapy and they may not prevent the development of PSGN
- *Diuretics:* Loop diuretics (furosemide) are preferred over thiazides (hydrochlorothiazide or chlorthalidone). The efficacy of thiazide diuretics is very minimal when GFR <30 mL/min
- *Antihypertensive medications:* Blood pressure can be managed by restricting salt and fluid intake along with diuretics in presence of fluid overload. In cases with uncontrolled blood pressure, the use of calcium channel blockers is recommended. The use of angiotensin-converting enzyme inhibitors (ACEI) and angiotensin receptor blockers (ARBs) is recommended in patients with stable GFR and with normal potassium levels
- *Immunosuppressive therapy:* Use of immunosuppressant is not recommended. Patients with progressive kidney failure or the presence of crescents on the renal biopsy may warrant the use of corticosteroids
- *Dialysis:* Dialysis is done in case of dyselectrolemia, acid–base disbalance, and fluid overload

General measures:
- Salt and water restriction to treat the edema
- Bed rest and immobilization are recommendations in the first few days of the disease
- Throat cultures on the patient and family members are important
- All affected members need to be treated with penicillin or erythromycin

(APSGN: acute poststreptococcal glomerulonephritis; GFR: glomerular filtration rate)

PROGNOSIS

Prognosis is usually good and resolution is quick in APSGN cases. A 4–6 day period of decreased edema, hypertension, and increased urine production marks the start of clinical improvement. Microscopic hematuria can last for up to 6–12 months, but gross hematuria goes away in the first week. It is not significant if moderate proteinuria persists on an intermittent basis. Although it happens very rarely, pulmonary edema or severe hyperkalemia may be the cause of death.

Since immunity to streptococcal M protein is type-specific, long-lasting, and limited to nephritogenic serotypes, illness recurrence is uncommon. Therefore, long-term antibiotic prophylaxis is not advised. A bad prognosis could be predicted by specific histologic findings. Heavy proteinuria and unfavorable results have been linked to the Garland pattern on IF. Among APSGN histopathological findings extracapillary crescent development is the most concerning. A renal biopsy is recommended if there is chronic proteinuria or a deterioration in renal functioning in patients with APSGN. Patients should have blood pressure and proteinuria monitored for several years.

Endocarditis Associated Kidney Disease

In children suffering from infective endocarditis, microscopic hematuria and proteinuria are suggestive of a renal lesion. Although it can occur, azotemia is usually moderate unless crescentic GN develops. Decreased C3 and C4 are among the serological results. Treatment with antibiotics must be administered for 4–6 weeks.

Shunt Nephritis

The development of postinfectious GN can complicate ventriculoatrial shunts, and less frequently, ventriculoperitoneal shunts. About 75% of instances of shunt infections are caused by *S. epidermidis*, whereas *S. aureus* is less common. Proteinuria (nephrotic range), hematuria, and hypertension are signs of renal involvement. Reduced C3 and C4 levels were observed in the laboratory when the organism was isolated from blood or shunt fluid cultures. The majority of renal biopsies reveal membranoproliferative GN. Antibiotics administered intravenously and shunt removal are two treatments for shunt nephritis.

Henoch–Schönlein Purpura and Immunoglobulin A Nephropathy

These two entities have the same histology but differ clinically. Abdominal pain, arthritis, purpura, *edema*, and extensive hematuria are the usual symptoms of Henoch–Schönlein purpura. The hallmark of IgA nephropathy is recurrent gross hematuria. The histology of the kidney might range from crescentic GN to mild mesangial proliferation. One hallmark is the presence of prominent IgA deposition in the mesangium.

Hepatitis B and C Virus-related Glomerulonephritis

Hepatitis B is especially common in East Asian nations and South Africa to involve the kidneys. This infection typically manifests as membranous GN, membranoproliferative GN, and sporadically vasculitis. Infections with the hepatitis C virus are more frequently linked to proliferative GN.

KEY POINTS

- Acute poststreptococcal glomerulonephritis is a nonsuppurative complication of group A β-hemolytic streptococci.
- Clinical triad of abrupt onset of gross hematuria, edema, and hypertension
- Acute reduction in serum C3 levels with return to normal levels within 6 weeks is characteristic.
- Treatment is largely supportive.
- Prevention of glomerulonephritis is by early administration of penicillin after streptococcal infection.

ACKNOWLEDGMENT

We are thankful to Professor Vinta Batra, Department of Pathology, GBPIMER, Delhi for giving pictures for the chapter.

SUGGESTED READING

1. Ahn SY, Ingulli E. Acute poststreptococcal glomerulonephritis: an update. Curr Opin Pediatr. 2008;20(2):157-62.
2. American Academy of Pediatrics, Committee on infectious diseases. Group A streptococcal infections. Red Book, CBS Paediatric series, 27th edition. Itasca, Illinois, US: American Academy of Pediatrics; 2006. pp. 610-20.
3. Carapetis JR, Steer AC, Mulholland EK, Weber M. The global burden of group A streptococcal diseases. Lancet Infect Dis. 2005;5(11):685-94.

4. Chauvet S, Berthaud R, Devriese M, Mignotet M, Vieira Martins P, Robe-Rybkine T, et al. Anti-Factor B Antibodies and Acute Postinfectious GN in Children. J Am Soc Nephrol. 2020;31(4):829-40.
5. Eison TM, Ault BH, Jones DP, Chesney RW, Wyatt RJ. Poststreptococcal acute glomerulonephritis in children: Clinical features and pathogenesis. Pediatr Nephrol. 2011;26(2):165-80.
6. Kanjanabuch T, Kittikowit W, Eiam-Oug S. An update on acute postinfectious glomerulonephritis worldwide. Nat Rev Nephrol. 2009;5(5):259-64.
7. Kasahara T, Hayakawa H, Okubo S, Okugawa T, Kabuki N, Tomizawa S, et al. Prognosis acute of poststreptococcal glomerulonephritis (APSGN) is excellent in children, when adequately diagnosed. Pediatr Int. 2001;43(4):364-67.
8. Rodriguez-Iturbe B, Batsford S. Pathogenesis of post-streptococcal glomerulonephritis a century after Clemens von Pirquet. Kidney Int. 2007;71(11):1094-104.
9. Rodriguez-Iturbe B, Musser JM. The current state of poststreptococcal glomerulonephritis. J Am Soc Nephrol. 2008;19(10):1855-64.
10. Sethi S, Fervenza FC. Standardized classification and reporting of glomerulonephritis. Nephrol Dial Transplant. 2019;34(2):193-9.
11. Srivastava RN. Acute glomerulonephritis. Indian J Pediatr. 1999;66:199-205.
12. Vijayakumar M. Acute and crescentic glomerulonephritis. Indian J Pediatr. 2002;69:1071-74.
13. Wang SY, Bu R, Zhang Q, Liang S, Wu J, Liu XZS, et al. Clinical, Pathological, and Prognostic Characteristics of Glomerulonephritis Related to Staphylococcal Infection. Medicine (Baltimore). 2016;95(15):e3386.
14. Wen YK, Chen ML. The significance of atypical morphology in the changes of spectrum of postinfectious glomerulonephritis. Clin Nephrol. 2010;73(3):173-9.

Approach to Hematuria in Children

Mukta Mantan, Anand S Vasudev

INTRODUCTION

Hematuria is an uncommon condition in childhood. Yet, it is frightening to the parents and results in an almost immediate referral to a pediatrician. An approach to this entity will be discussed in this chapter. The incidence of gross hematuria in children is estimated to be around 0.13%. Asymptomatic microscopic hematuria is common in unselected populations of children, with a prevalence that ranges from 0.4 to 4.1%. However, on repeated evaluations, the prevalence of persistent microscopic hematuria is about 0.5% based on the surveys of schoolgoing children.

DEFINITION

Hematuria is defined as the presence of five or more red blood cells (RBCs) per high-power field in multiple centrifuged urine examinations (at least 3; 1 week apart). Children are referred for presence of gross hematuria, persistent isolated microscopic hematuria, and microscopic hematuria with clinical symptoms or with proteinuria.

GROSS HEMATURIA

Gross hematuria is visible blood in urine and must be confirmed by microscopic demonstration of RBCs. If no RBCs are seen on microscopy, a dipstick test is done to look for other causes of red-colored urine. If the dipstick is positive, it is indicative of hemoglobinuria (usually caused by severe intravascular hemolysis) or myoglobinuria from rhabdomyolysis (due to muscle trauma or strenuous exercise). A negative dipstick test would point toward the discoloration due to porphyria, drugs such as rifampicin, pigments in foods, ingestion of beetroot and urates **(Box 1)**.

BOX 1: Causes of red-colored urine.

- *Food items:* Ingestion of beetroot, blackberries, and food-coloring agents
- *Drugs:* Nitrofurantoin, phenolphthalein, pyridium, rifampicin, phenothiazines, and sulfasalazine
- *Metabolites:* Homogentisic acid, melanin, methemoglobin, porphyrins, urates, and tyrosinosis

GLOMERULAR AND EXTRAGLOMERULAR HEMATURIA

Bright-red urine, visible clots or crystals with normal-looking eumorphic RBCs **(Fig. 1)** suggest bleeding from the urinary tract (extraglomerular). Cola-colored urine, presence of RBC casts, and deformed (dysmorphic) RBCs suggest glomerular bleeding. Phase contrast microscope or staining with special stains (Wright stain) is required for detection of dysmorphic RBCs **(Fig. 2)**. Presence of >20% dysmorphic RBCs suggests glomerular hematuria **(Table 1)**. The causes of hematuria are listed in **Table 2**.

HISTORY AND PHYSICAL EXAMINATION

Some clinical pointers in history and examinations may indicate the cause for hematuria **(Table 3)**.

INVESTIGATIONS

An episode of gross hematuria needs evaluation. After confirming hematuria, **Flowchart 1** can be followed. If the onset is acute and proteinuria is present, the likelihood of an episode of postinfective glomerulonephritis (PIGN) is high. The relevant investigations like anti-streptolysin O (ASLO) titers, complement C3 levels, and kidney function tests (KFTs) should be done. An elevated ASLO (>200 IU/L) and low C3 levels with normal or deranged KFT are confirmative of poststreptococcal glomerulonephritis (PSGN). If the history is of prolonged (3–4 weeks) duration, other causes like immunoglobulin A (IgA) nephropathy, membranous or membranoproliferative disease are more likely. Patients with IgA nephropathy are likely to have recurrent episodes of gross hematuria, especially with episodes of upper respiratory tract infections (synpharyngitic). Presence of fever, joint pains, and photosensitive rash points toward a diagnosis of

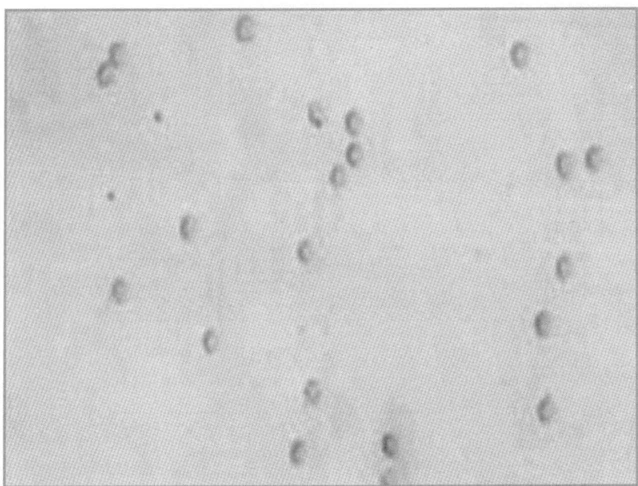

Fig. 1: Urine microscopy showing normal red blood cell.

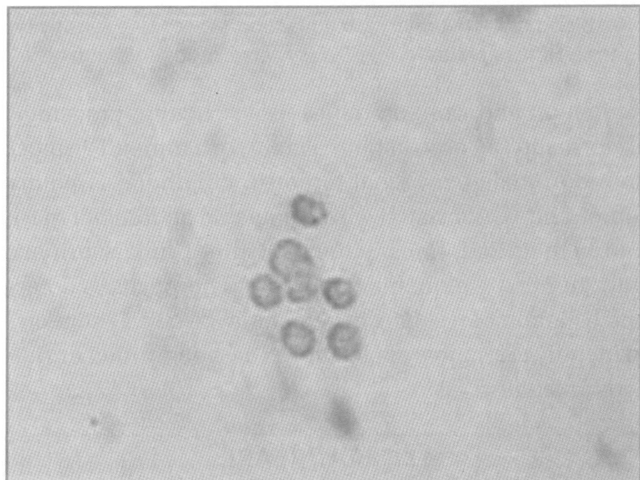

Fig. 2: Urine examination with phase contrast microscopy showing dysmorphic red blood cell.

TABLE 1: Differentiation of glomerular and extraglomerular hematuria.

Glomerular hematuria	*Extraglomerular hematuria*
Color red or brown	Bright red usually
Clots absent	Clots present
Proteinuria (2 + or more)	No proteinuria; trace to 1 +
Red cell casts	Absent cellular casts
Dysmorphic RBC >20%	Dysmorphic RBC <20%

(RBC: red blood cells)

TABLE 2: Causes of hematuria.

Glomerular	*Extraglomerular*
Acute onset:	
• Acute glomerulonephritis (PIGN, others*) • Rapidly progressive glomerulonephritis • Hemolytic uremic syndrome *Chronic glomerulonephritis:* • Membranous, membranoproliferative GN, IgA nephropathy • Thin basement membrane disease • Alport syndrome • Focal segmental glomerulosclerosis • Goodpasture's syndrome *Multisystem disease:* • SLE, IGAV, vasculitis • Hepatitis B and hepatitis C related GN	• Urinary tract infections • Urolithiasis; hypercalciuria • Cystic kidney disease • Vascular malformations (kidney or bladder) • Wilms tumor • Renal vein thrombosis • Trauma • Bleeding and clotting disorders • Drugs (NSAIDs)

Note: *Typhoid, pneumococcal pneumonia, meningococcemia, shunt nephritis, bacterial endocarditis, varicella, and mumps associated

(PIGN: postinfectious glomerulonephritis most commonly poststreptococcal; GN: glomerulonephritis; IgA: immunoglobulin A; SLE: systemic lupus erythematosus; IGAV: immunoglobulin A related vasculitis formerly known as HSP or Henoch-Schönlein purpura; NSAIDs: nonsteroidal anti-inflammatory drugs)

TABLE 3: Clinical pointers in history to identify the causes of hematuria.

Clinical signs/symptoms	*Likely diagnosis*
Edema, hypertension	Glomerulonephritis
Dysuria, loin pain, colic	Calculi, hypercalciuria
Joint pains, rash, edema	SLE, IGAV, vasculitis
Positive family history, deafness	Alport syndrome, thin basement membrane disease
Renal lump	Polycystic kidney disease, Wilms tumor, hydronephrosis
Bleeding tendency	Coagulation and bleeding disorders

(IGAV: immunoglobulin A related vasculitis; SLE: systemic lupus erythematosus)

systemic lupus erythematosus. Most of these conditions can be identified on a renal biopsy specimen which should include light microscopy, immunofluorescence, and electron microscopy (if available). Serological tests that help in identification of the underlying cause are hepatitis B surface antigen (HBsAg) and anti-hepatitis C virus (HCV) for related nephropathy [membranous and membranoproliferative glomerulonephritis (MPGN)].

Flowchart 1: Approach to gross hematuria.

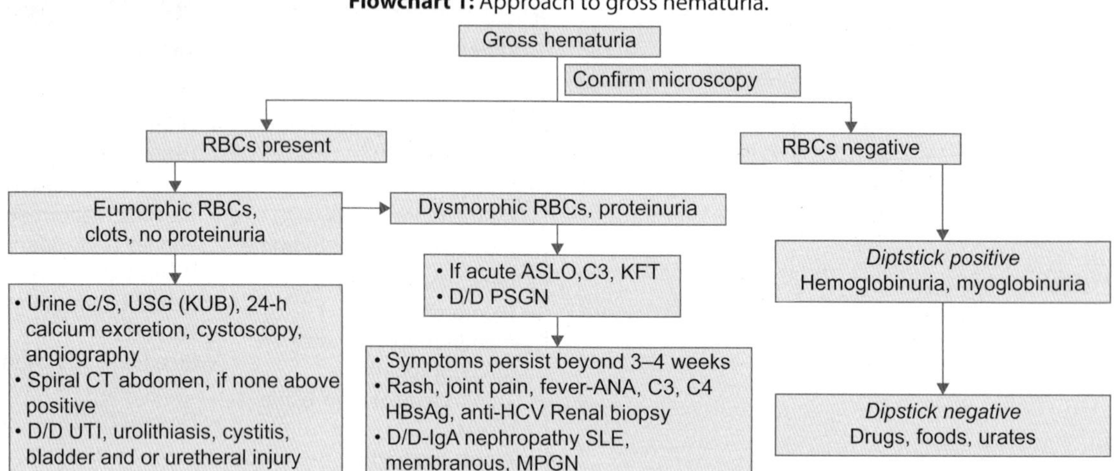

(ANA: antinuclear antibodies; ANCA: antineutrophilic cytoplasmic antibodies; ASLO: antistreptolysin O; HBsAg: hepatitis B surface antigen; IgA: immunoglobulin A; KUB: kidney, ureter, bladder; KFT: kidney function tests; MPGN: membranoproliferative glomerulonephritis; PSGN: poststreptococcal glomerulonephritis; RBC: red blood cell; UTI: urinary tract infection; C/S: culture sensitivity; USG: ultrasonography; CT: computed tomography; D/D: differential diagnosis; HCV: hepatitis C virus; SLE: systemic lupus erythematosus)

Antinuclear antibodies (ANAs) and anti-dsDNA for lupus nephritis; antineutrophilic cytoplasmic antibodies (P-ANCA and C-ANCA; both these are immunofluorescence based tests) for identification of vasculitis (microscopic polyangiitis, Wegener's and Churg–Strauss disease). Identification of ANCA can also be done by enzyme-linked immunosorbent assay (ELISA)-based tests (antimyeloperoxidase-anti-MPO corresponding to P-ANCA; antiproteinase-3-antiPR3 corresponding to C-ANCA) which are more sensitive and yield faster results.

Presence of extraglomerular hematuria points toward local causes, polycystic kidneys, hydronephrosis, urolithiasis, and hypercalciuria. Vascular abnormalities of urinary bladder can also cause hematuria rarely. An ultrasound kidney, ureter, bladder (KUB) would identify any structural abnormalities and/or stones in kidney. Ureteric stones are usually not identified with ultrasound and require a radiograph of KUB region or a noncontrast CT scan of the abdomen. If calculi are identified, a complete urinary biochemistry needs to be done (24-h urinary excretion of calcium, oxalates and urates). If there is a difficulty in collecting 24-hour sample, spot urine sample can be used for determining urinary calcium/creatinine ratio and oxalate/creatinine ratio. Hypercalciuria is defined as urine calcium to creatinine ratio greater than 0.2 (under 6 months of age: >0.8; 6–12 months: >0.6) or a 24-hour calcium excretion exceeding 4 mg/kg/day. Referral to a pediatric surgeon/urologist will be required when clinical evaluation and work-up indicates a structural urogenital abnormality, an obstructing calculus, or a tumor. The most common malignant renal tumor in childhood is Wilms tumor and is associated with a palpable abdominal mass and hematuria in most patients. Other primary urinary tract tumors, e.g., hemangiomas, rhabdomyosarcomas, and lymphomas resulting in hematuria are rare. Cystoscopy to identify the source of bleeding is best performed during active bleeding.

CLINICAL PEARL

- Neither visual description nor the dipstick alone is sufficient to diagnose gross hematuria; urine microscopy is essential to confirm.

MICROSCOPIC HEMATURIA

Isolated microscopic hematuria is benign on most occasions. However, it needs to be evaluated if it is symptomatic, i.e., associated with edema, hypertension, rash, fever, joint pains or deranged KFT. Also, persistent microscopic hematuria (>1–2 years duration) needs an evaluation. The approach for evaluation is given in **Flowchart 2**. If the hematuria is associated with proteinuria, chronic glomerulonephritis is the chief suspect, hence investigations as suggested for gross hematuria should be performed (C3, ANA, ANCA, and renal biopsy). Other causes of asymptomatic isolated microscopic hematuria are benign familial hematuria, IgA nephropathy, MPGN, and Alport syndrome. If the hematuria is nonglomerular, investigations should be done to identify hypercalciuria and urolithiasis. Invasive investigations, like cystoscopy and angiography, would be required if no cause is found on other investigations.

INDICATIONS FOR RENAL BIOPSY

Glomerular hematuria persisting for >4 weeks and without features of PSGN merits a renal biopsy. Also, decreased complement levels beyond 3 months indicate a need for renal biopsy to rule out other causes like IgA nephropathy, membranous, or MPGN nephropathy. Patients with deranged renal functions (urea and creatinine) and/or presence of proteinuria also need a renal biopsy to detect the presence of chronic glomerulonephritis. Patients with rapid worsening of renal functions presenting like RPGN should have an early biopsy to detect crescentic glomerulonephritis. Presence of ANA, HBsAg, anti-HCV, or ANCA positivity is an indication for renal biopsy.

MANAGEMENT

The definitive management of hematuria is based on the underlying etiology. Briefly the management of the two most common causes of hematuria, i.e., postinfective glomerulonephritis and idiopathic hypercalciuria is discussed here.

Postinfective Glomerulonephritis

The investigations useful in confirming the diagnosis are a urinalysis, complete blood count, antistreptolysin O (ASLO) titers, blood urea, serum creatinine, and complement C3 levels. Most patients with PSGN would have elevated ASLO titers (>200 IU/L), low complement levels (<60 mg/dL), and mildly deranged KFT. Urinalysis always shows glomerular hematuria, presence of RBC casts, and leukocyturia. Proteinuria is usually less than 2+. If these tests are negative and there is resolution of symptoms, a presumptive diagnosis of postinfectious glomerulonephritis can be made. Most patients with an acute PIGN would resolve of their hematuria and edema within 10–14 days. The kidney functions also normalize by this time. Persistence of gross hematuria or proteinuria beyond 4 weeks is unusual and often becomes an indication for kidney biopsy in these patients. Hypertension and fluid overload can be managed by use of diuretics like furosemide in doses of 2–4 mg/kg/day in two or three divided doses. If hypertension persists, it can be controlled with calcium channel blockers or use of β-blockers. Amlodipine in doses of 0.2–0.5 mg/kg/day and atenolol in doses of 0.5–2 mg/kg/day are often sufficient in controlling elevated blood pressure. Use of angiotensin-converting enzyme inhibitors and angiotensin receptor blockers in postinfective glomerulonephritis is not recommended as most patients

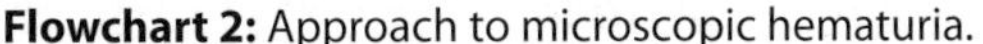

Flowchart 2: Approach to microscopic hematuria.

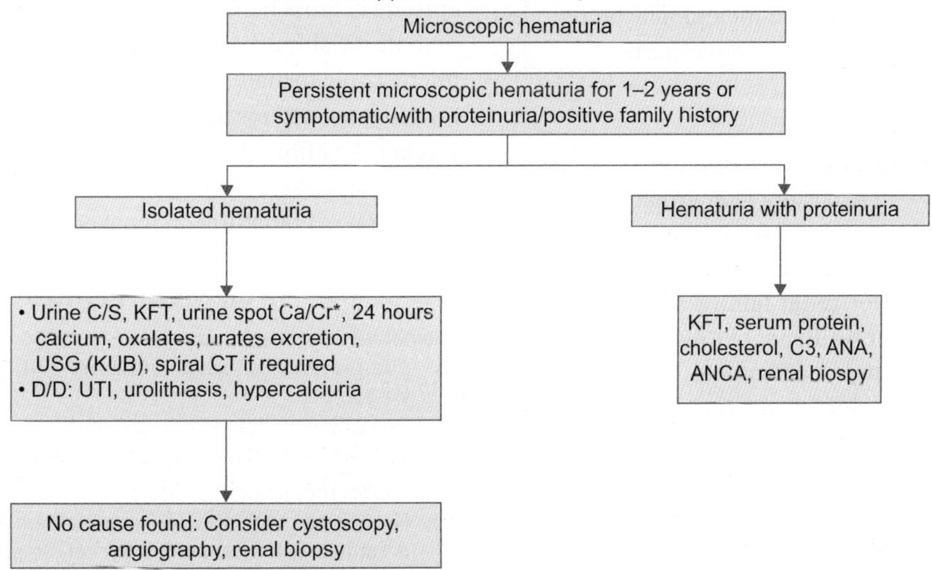

Note: *Urine spot calcium/creatinine ratio (>0.2 mg/mg abnormal)

(ANA: antinuclear antibodies; ANCA: antineutrophilic cytoplasmic antibodies; KFT: kidney function tests; KUB: kidney, ureter, bladder; UTI: urinary tract infection; USG: ultrasonography; CT: computed tomography; D/D: differential diagnosis; C/S: culture sensitivity)

with acute glomerulonephritis have a transient reduction in their glomerular filtration rate. The duration for use of diuretics and antihypertensives is usually <2 weeks. Patients with severe fluid overload and acute renal kidney injury may require kidney replacement therapy in the form of peritoneal or hemodialysis. This is however needed in <10% patients of acute glomerulonephritis.

Patients having persistence of gross hematuria or heavy proteinuria beyond 4 weeks duration need a renal biopsy to determine the underlying cause. Presence of rapidly progressive renal failure is an urgent indication for biopsy. Persistence of hypocomplementenemia (beyond 12 weeks) or absence of it is also an indication for kidney biopsy.

Immunoglobulin A Nephropathy

The condition is typically associated with gross hematuria but, at times, may present with microscopic hematuria. Often, the episodes of hematuria are synpharyngitic, i.e., occur along with an episode of upper respiratory tract infection. It is caused by the deposition of IgA immune complexes in the glomeruli of the kidneys which triggers a cascade of inflammatory events that lead to kidney damage. The diagnosis of IgA nephropathy is confirmed on renal biopsy that shows predominantly immunoglobulin IgA deposits in the mesangium on immunofluorescence. While ACE inhibitors are given to all patients with IgA nephropathy, immunosuppressants like steroids, azathioprine, or mycophenolate mofetil may be required in patients having nephrotic range proteinuria.

Alport Syndrome

Alport syndrome should be suspected in patients (especially males) with persistent glomerular microscopic hematuria once structural abnormalities of the kidney and urinary tract have been ruled out. A positive family history of hematuria or renal failure and hearing loss may suggest the diagnosis. Renal biopsy changes are less marked in children compared to adults. Light microscopy shows variable thickening of the glomerular basement membrane. Electron microscopy shows thinning of the glomerular basement membrane in early stages, that later changes to basket weaving. The diagnosis of Alport syndrome is confirmed if there is a lamellated glomerular basement membrane or a pathogenic mutation in *COL4A5* gene or two pathogenic *COL4A3* or *COL4A4* mutations. Genetic testing has a sensitivity of >90% for the diagnosis of X-linked disease; >700 variants are described. Early treatment with ACE inhibitors has been shown to slow down the progression to end-stage kidney disease in children.

Idiopathic Hypercalciuria

It is found to be a common cause of gross as well as microscopic hematuria. A family history of renal calculi may be present. A spot urinary calcium to creatinine ratio of >0.2 or a 24-hour urinary calcium excretion of over 4 mg/kg is abnormal. The condition is managed with a high fluid and low salt intake, and use of potassium citrate supplements; hydrochlorothiazide is sparingly used if these measures fail. Dietary calcium is not usually restricted. These measures reduce urinary calcium excretion, stop hematuria, and prevent further stone formation.

Benign Familial Hematuria

It is characterized by persistent, isolated microscopic hematuria. Other family members may also have microscopic hematuria. Glomerular capillary basement membrane thinning is seen on electron microscopy. Though the condition is usually benign but these children need a long-term follow-up.

CONCLUSION

Hematuria is an uncommon condition in childhood. An episode of gross hematuria and symptomatic microscopic hematuria should always be evaluated. Asymptomatic microscopic hematuria needs evaluation only if it persists on repeated microscopic examination of urine (beyond 1 year). An effort should be made to identify the underlying cause of hematuria. Treatment of the cause results in resolution of hematuria on most occasions.

CLINICAL PEARLS

Hematuria and proteinuria:

- The presence of both hematuria and proteinuria needs evaluation.
- Renal biopsy should be considered whenever glomerular or tubulointerstitial lesions are suspected.

What to tell the parents?

- For children with only microscopic hematuria, reassurance is sufficient. They should, however, be instructed to notify as and when gross hematuria occurs. These children should have an annual urine examination to detect any proteinuria for identification of a glomerular disease.

KEY POINTS

- Hematuria is defined as the presence of five or more red blood cells (RBCs) per high-power field in multiple centrifuged urine examinations.
- Visible clots and bright red color suggest extraglomerular hematuria while cola colored urine is a pointer towards glomerular cause.
- An episode of gross hematuria should always be confirmed on microscopy and needs an evaluation.
- Isolated microscopic hematuria is benign on most occasions however symptomatic microscopic hematuria needs evaluation.
- Management of hematuria is based on the underlying cause.

SUGGESTED READING

1. Brown DD, Reidy KJ. Approach to the child with hematuria. Pediatr Clin North Am. 2019;66(1):15-30.
2. Crompton CH, Ward PB, Hewitt IK. The use of urinary red cell morphology to detect the source of hematuria in children. Clin Nephrol. 1993;39:44-47.
3. Diven SC, Travis LB. A practical primary care approach to hematuria in children. Pediatr Nephrol. 2000;14:65-72.
4. Kashton CE. Familial hematuria. Pediatr Nephrol. 2009;24:1951-8.
5. Kashton CE. Familial hematuria: What we know and what we don't. Pediatr Nephrol. 2005;20:1027-35.
6. Stapleton FB. Hematuria associated with hypercalciuria and hyperuricosuria: a practical approach. Pediatr Nephrol. 1994;8:756-61.
7. Vehaskari VM. Asymptomatic hematuria: a cause for concern? Pediatr Nephrol. 1989;3:240-41.
8. Wood EG. Asymptomatic hematuria in childhood: a practical approach to evaluation. Indian J Pediatr. 1999;66:207-14.
9. Youn T, Trachtman H, Gauthier B. Clinical spectrum of gross hematuria in pediatric patients. Clin Pediatr (Phila). 2006;45(2):135-41.

CHAPTER 103

Approach to Urinary Tract Infection

Pankaj V Deshpande

INTRODUCTION

Urinary tract infections (UTIs) in children generate the strongest emotions across the pediatric field! There has been literature ad *nauseam* about UTIs in children and I do not intend to add to that volume. Let us look at the practical aspect of approaching a child with UTI **(Flowchart 1)**.

In the first year of life, both boys and girls have the same rate of developing a UTI (certainly in the first 6 months). Thereafter, the incidence in girls is higher than boys.

DEFINITION

Urinary tract infection in children is based on the presence of a positive urine culture in a symptomatic child. There are several parts to this statement. Firstly, the child has to be symptomatic, either in the form of urinary symptoms or have a fever without an identifiable source. Secondly, urine culture being positive would vary according to the method of collection of urine (clean catch, catheter, suprapubic, etc.).

As you will realize, the common test used for diagnosing UTI is not included in the pure definition of UTI. Pyuria (presence of leukocytes in the urine) is only an indicator of inflammation and not always the sign of an UTI in children.

CLINICAL FEATURES (WHEN TO SUSPECT)

The first major task is to be aware of UTIs in children but also that only appropriate tests done at the appropriate times will help you in diagnosing but not over or underdiagnosing UTIs! Unfortunately, both are common!

In infants and children up to 2 years of age, the symptoms may be subtle. Fever without a focus is an important feature to be aware of! Let us be clear that this means that on clinical examination, you cannot identify a source of the fever. All of us are pretty good clinicians and hence, let us use our clinical skills well! There is no point in sending tests in a child with fever and a severe cough or cold!! You have identified a cause of fever and doing tests at this stage will only serve to confuse you as urine tests are likely to reveal pyuria commonly. More importantly, in infants having fever without focus, the incidence of UTIs is quite low (about 5%) with most infants having a viral infection. As **Flowchart 2** shows below, leukocyturia and positive urine culture in an infant having fever without focus may not always indicate a UTI!

Apart from this, in the presence of urinary symptoms; like if the infant is obviously crying persistently (not an occasional episode in 2 days) while voiding, has turbid/discolored urine, or has a poor stream of urine (in a boy), an UTI should be thought of. Persistent jaundice in a neonate beyond 2 weeks of age is also an indication.

In older children, the symptoms are more likely to be related to the urinary tract as they will be able to communicate their ailment better. Presence of frequency of voiding, dysuria (pain while voiding), and urgency with daytime wetting may be seen more commonly here. They may also have fever, loin pain, vomiting, and, in some cases, may actually have diarrhea as the presenting symptom. Fever without focus should also prompt a thought about UTI though it will be less common than in infants.

DIAGNOSIS OF URINARY TRACT INFECTION

I am not going to quote all literature about this aspect but let us get our basic concepts right before embarking on other thought provoking aspects of diagnosis.

As explained above, once a UTI is suspected, urine tests will be required to diagnose or rule out a UTI. Those who have sat patiently beside their child (boy or girl) waiting for him/her to pee (void) will realize the eureka moment when the child pees (voids)! The two tests that are used commonly are a routine examination of urine with microscopy and a urine culture.

Flowchart 1: Diagnosis of urinary tract infection.

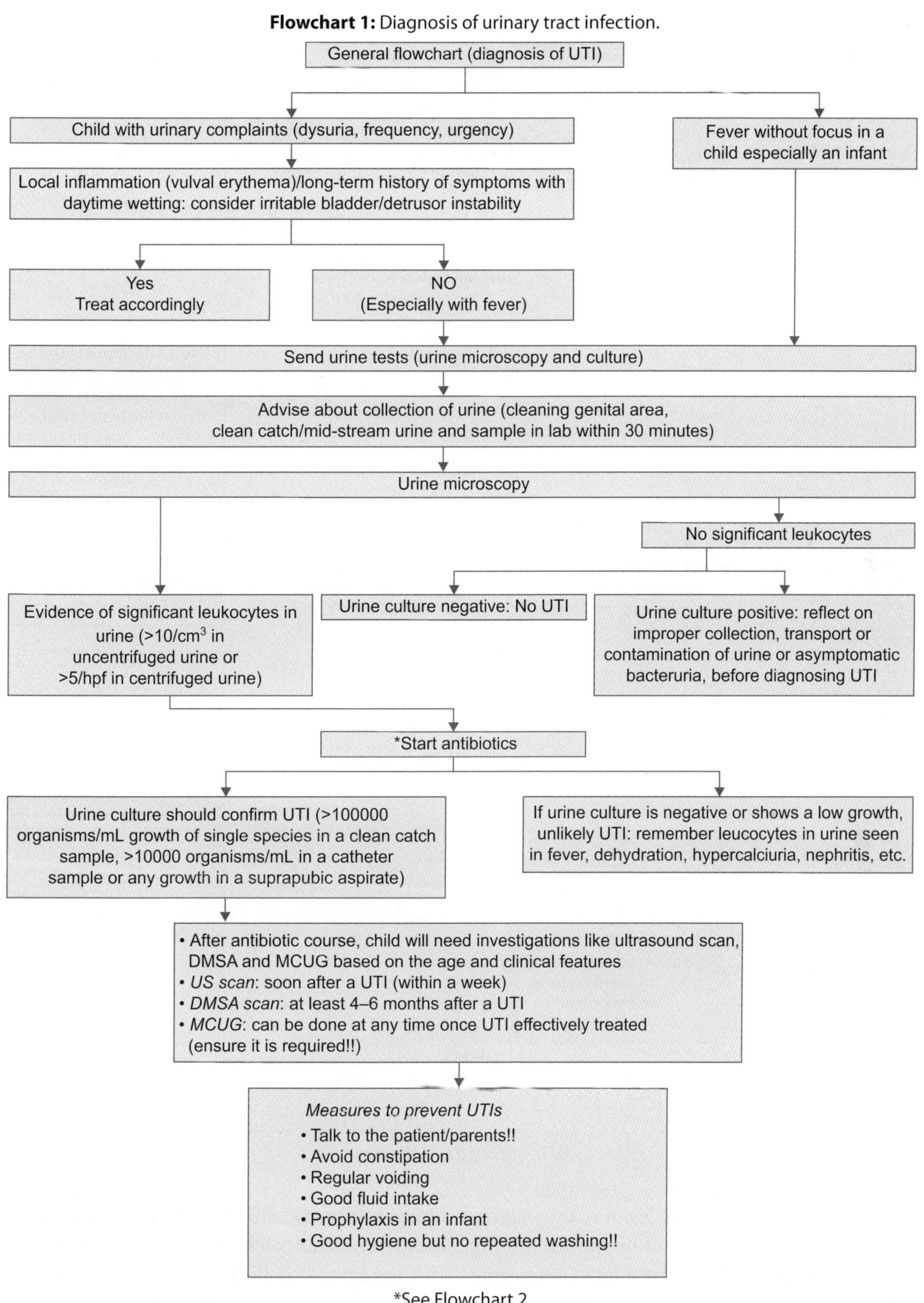

*See Flowchart 2

(DMSA: dimercaptosuccinic acid; MCUG: micturating cystourethrogram; US: ultrasound; UTI: urinary tract infection)

Flowchart 2: Interpretation of urine reports based on appearance of the child.

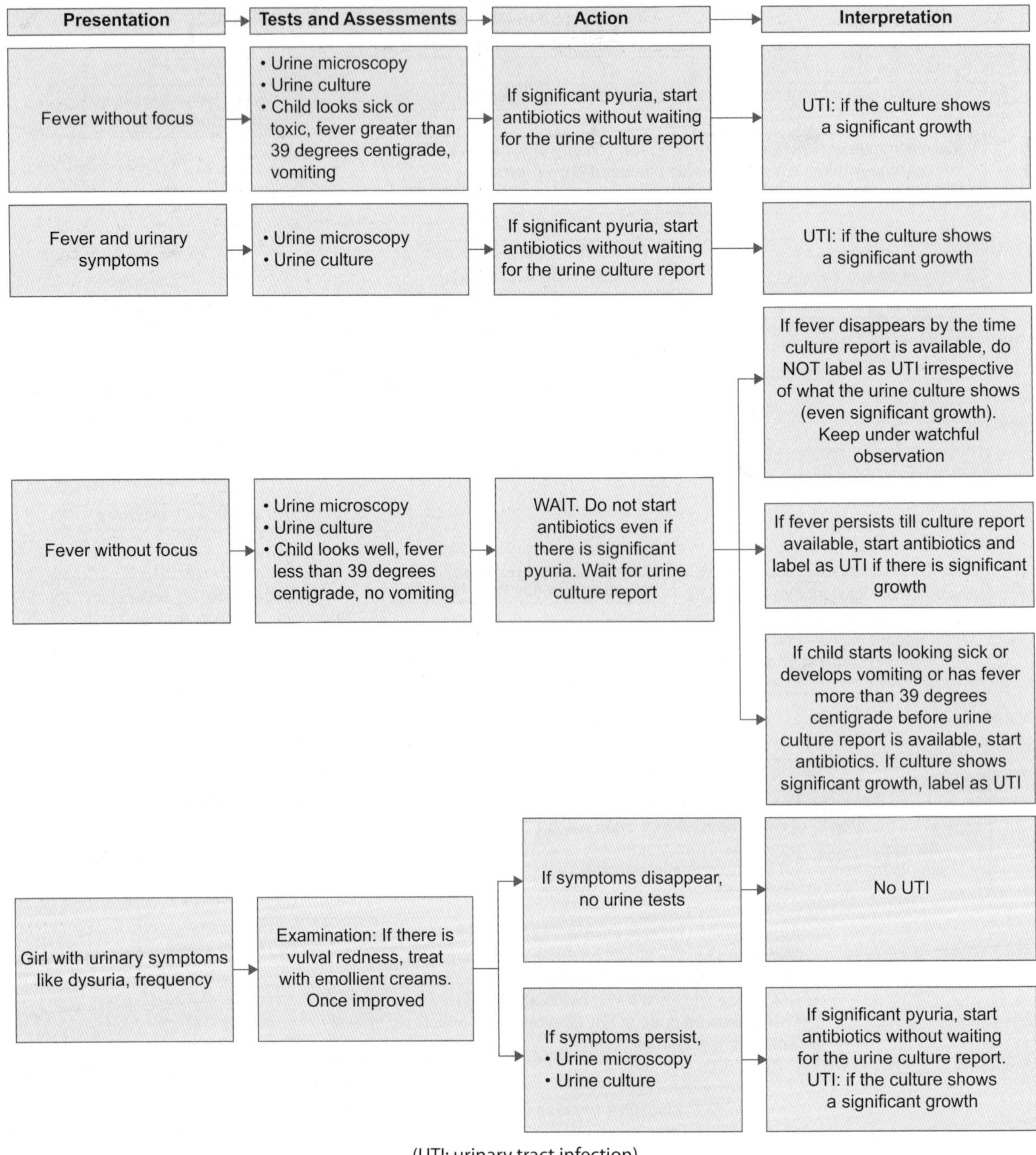

(UTI: urinary tract infection)

Unfortunately, there is no advice given to the parents in most places which causes a lot of heartburn among doctors regarding results as they cause a lot of confusion! Sample collection is crucial to the diagnosis of UTI.

For a clean catch/mid-stream urine sample, the genital area is cleaned with normal soap and water and dried. In an older child, a mid-stream sample can be attempted but in an infant, a clean catch sample is good enough. This implies that the urine is collected straight into the container and not on a plastic sheet, "dabba" or cotton! Once collected, it needs to be transported to the microbiology laboratory immediately and plated within 30–60 minutes. If a delay is anticipated, the sample should be stored in the refrigerator at 4°C (to a maximum of 24 hours). This implies that the urine sample will not be left on the table for 2 hours before being given in the laboratory. This is because it will allow the growth of contaminant organisms.

If the urine is collected appropriately as described above, a pure growth of >100,000 (1 lakh) organisms/mL is considered as significant and positive. Recent literature would even suggest that a count of 50,000 may also be significant. Recent guidelines suggest a growth of 10000 organisms/mL may also be significant. However, lower counts are more likely to represent contamination and efforts should be made to collect the urine appropriately, unless the child is completely asymptomatic in which case doing the urine sample is pointless.

If the urine is collected by using a urinary catheter, the cleaning and strict asepsis should be maintained or you may be the cause of the child's subsequent UTI! If this is done, a colony count of >10,000 organisms/mL will be considered significant and positive.

Suprapubic aspiration of urine (using a syringe and needle to aspirate urine directly from the bladder) is possible in young children as the bladder is an abdominal organ till 5 years of age. In this case, the trick lies in knowing when to do the aspiration. If one waits till about half to one hour after the last void, the chances of obtaining urine increase. In this case, any growth of organisms is considered significant and implies a UTI. Recent guidelines suggest that there should be a growth of 1000 organisms/ml even in a suprapubic aspirate.

It is important to note that bag urine samples have a high contamination rate and are not recommended for urine collection in children. In any case, bag urine is often collected in an inappropriate manner (as the child needs to be upright before collection and the bag removed soon after voiding) and hence should not be used in children.

EXAMINATION OF URINE

Microscopy of the urine may reveal the presence of leukocytes. There is ample literature about what constitutes significant pyuria, but it is very important to note that leukocytes may be present in the urine for varied other reasons and do not always imply a UTI. They may be seen in any fever, dehydration, hypercalciuria, urolithiasis, inflammatory conditions like interstitial nephritis, glomerulonephritis, and in fact in any inflammatory condition in the body (even a severe respiratory infection!). For the purpose of diagnosing UTI, presence of >5 leukocytes/hpf in fresh centrifuged sample or >10 leukocytes per mm^3 in an uncentrifuged sample is considered significant.

Presence of a positive urine culture in the absence of leukocytes in the urine, especially in an older child, should be a cue for a thoughtful consideration about whether it is really a UTI. Though significant leukocyturia by itself is not diagnostic of a UTI, merely a positive urine culture in the absence of leukocyturia is very unlikely to represent a UTI. Here, the symptoms of a child play an important role. Positive cultures may be due to many reasons, the chief being improper collection and contamination and no test is 100% accurate. Recent literature and a review also indicate that the bladder is not a completely sterile organ as was previously believed. Asymptomatic bacteriuria is far more common than what was believed earlier.

Urine dipstick can also be used to screen for UTI. Presence of leukocytes is detected by the presence of leukocyte esterase and the conversion of nitrate to nitrite is detected by the nitrite test. When both are positive, the predictive value for a UTI is very high (UTI very likely). Again, it is important to emphasize that the symptoms of the child are of paramount importance. If the urine is not checked freshly or done in an asymptomatic child, they may be fallaciously abnormal. It should be remembered that false positives for both leukocytes and nitrites can occur (especially in exposed sticks, medications, etc.).

Dipslide has been used to plate the urine immediately after it is collected with good results.

URINARY TRACT INFECTION MIMICS

It is extremely important to realize that every "positive" urine test is not a UTI. As explained above, urine routine showing "significant" number of leukocytes when the child is asymptomatic carries no meaning in the general population of children! Similarly, one of the biggest problems with a positive urine culture is contamination as the collection is not ideal in children and several authors have addressed this issue suggesting that a fair number of children/adults receive antibiotic therapy when they do not have a UTI. Also as alluded to earlier, the bladder is not a completely sterile organ as was believed earlier and asymptomatic bacteriuria is common. The most important message is that in the absence of symptoms suggesting UTIs, urine tests are not required and do not indicate a UTI!!

Similarly, there are several conditions in children that mimic a UTI and unfortunately all these children keep on receiving antibiotics for suspected UTIs! I will mention a couple of them. One of the common causes of dysuria, frequency, and urgency in girls is vulval erythema! Remember, this is not a bacterial or fungal infection! They will present with exactly the same symptoms as a UTI and unless local examination is done properly, they will all have urine tests done. The typical history is of vulval pain, itching even when the child is not voiding (and not only dysuria) and the child splashing water on the vulva after voiding. Often, the urine tests are abnormal as they reflect local inflammation rather than a UTI and they get treated with antibiotics and have many unnecessary tests done! It is an extremely common condition in OPD practice, more so in the tropical countries and the common causes of worsening this condition are repeated washing of the genital area and use of antifungal creams. These children do not have a UTI and do not need antibiotics!

Another condition that gets treated with multiple courses of antibiotics is detrusor instability in children that presents with frequency, urgency, and dysuria. They also will have daytime wetting, the information usually not being volunteered. Again, stimulant drinks worsen this condition and no amount of antibiotic therapy will alleviate the symptoms.

Another "mimic" of a different category is a positive tests for urine routine and/or urine culture when the child is asymptomatic. This is usually contamination and needs no treatment!!

When interpreting a urine test, all the above factors need to be borne in mind.

COMMON ORGANISMS

Briefly, gram-negative organisms usually cause UTIs. They include *Escherichia coli*, *Klebsiella*, *Proteus*, and, in some cases, *Pseudomonas*. Enterococci may be seen in infants and some older children. UTIs due to gram-positive cocci like *Staphylococcus* should raise suspicion of obstructive pathology in the urinary tract. Atypical infections with fungi like *Candida* are also seen especially in children exposed to many antibiotics.

TREATMENT

Once a suspicion of UTI has been confirmed on the urine tests, an antibiotic course has to be started **(Flowchart 1)**.

Something New

An interesting observation is the presence of significant pyuria in a child having fever without focus but the fever disappearing without antibiotics before the urine culture report is available. **Flowchart 2** suggests a way out of this problem. As has been clearly indicated in many papers, the incidence of UTIs in children having fever without focus is diminishing because of proper definition of UTI. At present, it is believed to be about 5% and most of the children have viral infections. Pyuria may be seen in any fever. Attempts have been made to refine the indications for sending a urine test in such children (fever >39°C, previous proven UTI, young age, persistent high grade fever, etc.). It has also been suggested to look at the clinical appearance of the child and not do a urine sample at all in those looking well and follow them up carefully.

Flowchart 2 suggests labeling a child as having a UTI if there is fever along with urinary symptoms or the child looks sick in the presence of significant pyuria. In such cases, antibiotics can be started without waiting for the culture report (but culture has to be sent!). However, if the child looks well (happy, nontoxic, no vomiting, especially with lower grades of fever), it is recommended to not start antibiotics even if there is significant pyuria. If the child appears sick in the next 2 days or fever continues till culture report is available, antibiotics can be started. However, if the fever settles down without antibiotics, it should not be labeled as a UTI even if the urine culture shows a significant growth. A study looking at simultaneous urine cultures done by clean catch and suprapubic growth showed that less than half of the positive cultures on clean catch samples were confirmed on suprapubic aspirates while the rest were clearly contaminants. At the same time, it has been shown conclusively that 0.7% of infants with no symptoms have a positive urine culture even when it is repeated 3 times.

Thus, it is important to diagnose UTI appropriately. Clearly with local symptoms secondary to vulval redness, UTI should not be diagnosed unless the local redness is treated irrespective of the urine reports of pyuria or a positive culture.

What to do once UTI is "diagnosed"?

Remember, urine culture reports become available after 24–48 hours and hence, antibiotics have to be started based on local practice. **Tables 1 and 2** suggest the antibiotics that can be used.

A single antibiotic is adequate to clear a UTI. Following would be the indications for parenteral (intravenous) antibiotics:

- Inability to tolerate oral antibiotics
- Persistent vomiting

TABLE 1: Oral antibiotics.

Cefixime	10 mg/kg/day in 2 doses
Co-amoxiclav	35 mg of amoxicillin in 2 doses
Ciprofloxacin	10–20 mg/kg/day in 2 doses
Ofloxacin	15–20 mg/kg/day in 2 doses
Cephalexin	50 mg/kg/day in 3 doses

TABLE 2: Intravenous antibiotics.

Ceftriaxone	75–100 mg/kg/day in 1–2 doses
Amikacin	10–15 mg/kg single dose
Gentamicin	5–6 mg/kg/day single dose
Co-amoxiclav	35 mg/kg/day of amoxicillin in 2 doses

- Sick looking/"toxic" child
- Very young infants (<3 months of age) with high-grade fever.

In case of an "office" UTI (OPD treatment), antibiotic course of 7–10 days is sufficient. In children needing parenteral antibiotics, a total duration of 14 days would be required. However, once the fever and symptoms settle in 48–72 hours, the antibiotic can be changed to an appropriate oral antibiotic. Recent literature suggests that the duration could be curtailed to 10 days for someone who looks sick and 5–7 days for an "office" UTI.

There is no need to repeat the urine culture after the treatment is complete. Urine culture may need to be done again only if there is no symptomatic improvement suggesting that UTI persists.

One of the common queries that crop up is regarding the antibiotic sensitivity pattern. It usually becomes available after about 48–72 hours of starting therapy. Unless the child has not responded in terms of symptoms, there is usually no need to change antibiotics. In vitro and in vivo sensitivities are quite different and an antibiotic that is perceived as resistant often works well in eliminating a UTI.

Other/Nonpharmacologic Therapy

Often the most forgotten part, one needs to make an effort to try and decipher the reason for developing the UTI. This not mean jumping to radiological investigations, but talking to the child and parents!! Local factors, especially bladder bowel dysfunction is a major risk factor for UTI. Addressing constipation, voiding regularly, ensuring an adequate fluid intake, and keeping the post void residue to a minimum are some factors that go a long way in preventing UTIs. Using a cotton underwear and clean hygienic practice should also be advised.

Follow-up and Subsequent Care

Once the antibiotic course is completed, one of the dilemmas is about prophylaxis, especially in view of recent literature that is suggesting that prophylaxis is not always indicated in children with UTI. The recommendation here is that prophylaxis is advocated for all infants who have a UTI till all radiological investigations are complete or till 1 year of age. For older children, the role of prophylaxis looks less clear and if used, should be till all investigations are complete or factors that are believed to be a risk factor for recurrent UTIs are addressed (e.g., constipation). There certainly seems no role for long-term prophylaxis for years together. The commonly used prophylactic agents are:

- Co-trimoxazole (to give trimethoprim in the dose of 1–2 mg/kg) once a day
- Nitrofurantoin 1 mg/kg once a day
- Cephalexin 15 mg/kg once a day.

The ideal prophylactic agent should not change the normal periurethral flora. Hence, co-trimoxazole and nitrofurantoin are better agents than cephalexin. There is no need to rotate prophylactic agents. If the urine culture shows resistance to the preventive agent, there is usually no need to change the agent after the treatment of the UTI.

There is no role for checking urine regularly (once a week/fortnight/month) for reasons made very clear above. If the child has symptoms, he/she should have urine tests done.

Radiological Investigations

There are recommended guidelines about the investigations required after a child develops a UTI. They are listed in **Table 3**. Recent guidelines have tried to reduce the radiological investigations. MCUG is recommended only if the ultrasound scan is abnormal, non E.coli UTI in an infant or the child has recurrent UTIs.

These are the minimum investigations suggested for the particular age group. Additional investigations are recommended in the presence of recurrent UTIs, pyelonephritis, or abnormal investigations like an US scan. Again, recent literature would suggest that micturating cystourethrogram (MCUG) is not really indicated in all infants with a UTI and should be reserved for infants with an abnormal ultrasound, UTI with atypical organisms,

TABLE 3: Recommended guidelines about the investigations required after a child develops a UTI.

Age	*Investigations recommended*
Less than 1 year	US scan, DMSA, and MCUG
1–6 years	US scan, DMSA
More than 6 years	US scan

(DMSA: dimercaptosuccinic acid; MCUG: micturating cystourethrogram; US: ultrasound; UTI: urinary tract infection)

repeated UTIs, etc. Suffice to say, in the coming years, it is very likely that the number of MCUG tests done will decrease significantly. Recent guideline suggest that MCUG should be done in a child with UTI only if the ultrasound scan shows dilatation, in the presence of recurrent UTIs or UTI with atypical organisms.

Unfortunately, the recommended tests get done at the wrong time and are liable to wrong interpretation.

An ultrasound scan of the kidneys and bladder should be done as soon as possible in a child with UTI. For an inpatient, it should be when the child is admitted and for an outpatient, it should be soon and certainly within a week. Please be careful about interpreting the evidence of cystitis on the ultrasound scan as a mildly thickened bladder wall. Unless the bladder is full, thickness cannot be interpreted with accuracy and will look "thickened"! One needs to look at the scan and not the report.

The dimercaptosuccinic acid (DMSA) scan is useful in showing up nonfunctioning areas of the kidneys. Acute changes secondary to a UTI can last for as long as 4–6 months!! The DMSA scan is used to determine changes that may need to long-term monitoring. Hence, it is pointless to do a DMSA scan soon after a UTI! Please remember that a DMSA scan should be done at least 4–6 months after an episode of UTI (the later, the better).

One should also realize that all changes seen on a DMSA scan do not indicate scarring secondary to a UTI (though the report may say so!). One presumes that the DMSA scan would have shown normal kidneys before the episode of UTI to be able to confidently report scarring. That is a very big presumption. There are many children who are born with abnormal kidneys/imperfect embryogenesis/dysplasia and changes seen on a DMSA scan are similar to those reported as scarring. Note that the ultrasound scan may actually show normal kidneys in these children. Hence, abnormalities on a DMSA scan have to be interpreted with caution. Clinical interpretation is more important rather than what is printed on the report (e.g., a single UTI is unlikely to cause a small kidney with very poor function!).

Finally, an MCUG is not indicated in all children with UTIs. Far too many MCUGs are done for weak indications. In children <1 year of age with a UTI or when bladder outlet obstruction is suspected, it is definitely indicated. Symptoms suggesting bladder outlet obstruction:

- Poor urine stream
- Dribbling of urine
- Abdominal swelling (bladder)
- Voiding by pressing the abdomen
- Bilateral hydronephrosis and hydroureter on ultrasound scan
- Large thick-walled trabeculated bladder on ultrasound
- Antenatal scans with bilateral hydronephrosis/hydroureter or large bladder.

Please remember to give antibiotics to the child when the MCUG is being done. A 7-day course of antibiotics (2 days before and 5 days after MCUG) is a fair practice. One could also use IV antibiotics before MCUG or follow any other local practice guideline for the purpose. I have seen several children who have developed a UTI after an MCUG when antibiotics have not been used and that is not acceptable.

It would be impossible to start commenting on actions required for various abnormalities seen on various scans as that would take up too much space. It should be remembered that an IVP (intravenous pyelogram) is an extremely poor test for renal scarring and is not recommended.

CONCLUSION

Last but not the least, do not forget to check the renal function of the child. As explained above, the only way to detect children with abnormal DMSA scans (abnormality existing before the UTI) is looking at the renal parameters. Ensure a serum creatinine is done at least 2 weeks after the episode of UTI and interpret appropriately to calculate the eGFR (estimated GFR). Also ensure a urine protein/creatinine ratio is done to look for proteinuria at the same time.

Urinary tract infection is a fairly common condition in children and instead of alarming everyone including ourselves, let us analyze the situation correctly and take appropriate steps so that management of a child with UTI is kept simple. Let us also realize that recent literature is suggesting that long-term outcome for the kidneys is good in the face of an occasional UTI also! In fact, the question of diagnosis of UTI is called upon if there are no symptoms suggestive of a UTI, especially so in a young child having fever without focus. Let us all start diagnosing UTI appropriately looking at the child and not the laboratory reports. It is not all doom and gloom!

KEY POINTS

- Presence of significant number of leukocytes in urine can be due to many reasons, UTI being one of them. Unless associated with suggestive symptoms and a positive urine culture, it does not represent a UTI.
- DMSA scan for detecting long-term changes should be done at least 4–6 months after a UTI.
- US scan soon after a UTI.
- MCUG, if required, after the UTI is adequately treated.

SUGGESTED READING

1. Bachur R, harper MB. Reliability of urinalysis for predicting UTI in young febrile children. Arch Pediatr Adolesc Med. 2001;155(1):60-5.
2. Deshpande PV. Dilemmas in Diagnosis of Urinary Tract Infection (UTI)in Fever without focus and other conditions. Pediatr Inf Dis. 2022;4(4):138-142.
3. Fischer GD, Rogers M. Vulval diseases in children: a clinical audit of 130 cases. Pediatr Dermatol. 2000;17:1-6.
4. Fischer GD. Vulval disease in prepubertal girls. Australian J Dermat. 2001;42:225-36.
5. Hannula A, Perhomaa M, Venhola M, Pokka T, Renko M, Uhari M. Long term follow-up of patients after childhood UTI. Arch Pediatr Adolesc Med. 2012;166(12):1117-22.
6. Indian Society of Pediatric Nephrology; Vijayakumar M, Kanitkar M, Nammalwar BR, Bagga A. Revised Statement on management of Urinary Tract Infection. Indian Pediatr. 2011;48(9):709-17.
7. Luco M, Lizame M, Reichhard C, Hirsch F. Urine microscopy as a screen for urinary tract infection in a pediatric emergency unit in Chile. Pediatr Emerg Care. 2006;22(10):705-9.
8. Meena J, Bagga A, Hari P. Management of urinary tract infections and vesicoureteric reflux: Key updates from the revised Indian Society of Pediatric Nephrology Guidelines 2023. Indian Pediatr. 2024;61(4):363-9.
9. Silver SA, Baillie L, Simor A. Positive urine cultures: A major cause of inappropriate antimicrobial use in hospitals? Can J Inf Dis Med Microbiol. 2009;20(4):107-11.
10. Subcommittee on Urinary Tract Infection, Steering Committee on Quality Improvement and Management; Roberts KB. Urinary Tract Infection: Clinical Practice Guideline for the Diagnosis and Management of the Initial UTI in Febrile Infants and Children 2 to 24 Months. Pediatrics. 2011; 128(3):595-610.
11. Tosif S, baker A, Oakley E, Donath S, Babl FE. Contamination rates of different urine collection methods for the diagnosis of urinary tract infections in young children: observational cohort study. J Pediatr Child Health. 2012; 48(8):659-64.

Antenatal Renal Anomalies: Outcome and Postnatal Management

Mehul A Shah

INTRODUCTION

Antenatal renal anomalies detected by ultrasound were first reported by Garrett et al. in 1970. Data from the past three decades indicate a higher incidence of renal anomalies especially fetal HN in up to 4.5% of pregnant women. The management of antenatal renal anomalies has undergone a two stage paradigm shift over the past three decades. The initial enthusiasm was to operate on a number of these asymptomatic infants to minimize long-term morbidity. However, it has now become apparent over the past 20 years that several of these anomalies [such as pelviureteric junction obstruction (PUJO), vesicoureteral junction obstruction (VUR), megaureter, and multicystic dysplastic kidney (MCDK)] can resolve spontaneously over time reducing the number of surgical or medical interventions to a select few infants.

The renal anomalies present at birth have been referred to as congenital anomalies of the kidney and urinary tract (CAKUT), a term introduced in 1998 by the group of Ishikawa, and used extensively in literature. CAKUT refers to a spectrum of structural abnormalities resulting from disturbance in the embryonic development of the kidney and urinary tract. It is the most diagnosed antenatal condition, and comprises ~20–30% of all congenital anomalies. CAKUT can range from mild transient HN to dysplasia and severe urinary tract obstruction and is associated with varying prognoses including completely normal kidney function to end stage renal disease (ESRD) in children as well as later adult life. CAKUT is noted in ~40% of children reaching ESRD making CAKUT spectrum the most frequent cause of kidney failure in children and up to 7% of adults with ESRD.

The CAKUT could be renal limited or associated with multiorgan dysgenesis (especially with brain and eyes), or part of syndromic association. Early insults during first and early second trimester often lead to renal parenchymal defects whereas third trimester insults often cause urinary tract abnormalities. These insults could be due to monogenic, epigenetic factors, or maternal disease, or environmental factors/drugs/toxins.

Transient fetal hydronephrosis (HN) is common and can be due to a delay in the maturation of renal system, absence of peripelvic fat, or due to the effect of bladder filling. The early diagnosis of renal anomalies allows the obstetrician to plan delivery especially in those women with associated oligohydramnios. Early neonatal evaluation and management helps in prevention of long-term complications such as recurrent urinary tract infections (UTIs), hypertension, and chronic kidney disease (CKD). On the other side, the disadvantages of early detection of renal anomalies include over work-up and also excessive parental anxiety since ~70% of these anomalies are benign and known to resolve spontaneously.

Two risks should be avoided when managing antenatal detected renal anomalies—(1) delayed therapy, and (2) excessive treatment. Hence, knowledge about the correlation of fetal renal ultrasonography (USG) abnormalities and the final outcome is important for proper counseling. The challenge, within the babies with antenatal detected renal anomalies, is to identify the small (<25%) number of babies who have significant nephron-uropathies or urinary tract anomalies (UTA) requiring later surgery or long term follow-up without subjecting the majority (~75% of those detected antenatally) to unnecessary investigations, antibiotic prophylaxis, or surgery. These significant nephrouropathies/UTA include bilateral dysplastic kidneys, posterior urethral valves (PUV), pelviureteric junction obstruction (PUJO), vesicoureteral reflux (VUR), vesicoureteral junction obstruction (VUJO), multicystic dysplastic kidneys (MCDK), polycystic kidney disease, renal agenesis, and duplex systems with ureterocele.

EMBRYOLOGY OF THE RENAL SYSTEM

The development of the mammalian kidney is a multistage synchronized process involving the ureteric bud (UB) and the metanephric mesenchyme (MM). It begins at 35–37 days of gestation in humans with the induction of the ureteric bud from the nephric duct, followed by mesenchymal to epithelial transition (MET) and branching morphogenesis, and terminates with nephron patterning and elongation. Majority of the nephrons (~60%) are formed in the second half of gestation. Nephrogenesis is a time-limited event during development that is completed by 36 weeks in humans and after birth, it is not reactivated post injury to the kidneys.

These embryologic events require a tight regulation at the deoxyribonucleic acid (DNA) level (mediated by transcriptional factors) and the post-transcriptional level. Bone morphogenetic proteins (BMP) are growth factors/cytokines and their modifiers are invaluable to the formation of the kidney, especially BMP4, expressed in the mesenchyme surrounding the nephric duct, and BMP7 expressed in the metanephric mesenchyme and ureteric buds. The ureteric bud expresses Hoxb, and the metanephric mesenchyma expresses the transcription factors Six2, fibroblast growth factor (FGF2), and BMP7 that are essential for the proliferation of metanephric mesenchyma and the production of Wilms tumor protein (WT1).

The major signaling pathways in the kidney development in metanephric mesenchyma are WT1, hepatocyte growth factor (HGF), mesenchymal epithelial transition factors (MET), glial cell-line derived neurotrophic factor (GDNF) and rearranged during transfection (RET, a receptor for GDNF family). WT1 is expressed in the metanephric mesenchymal (MM) and as the differentiation proceeds, its expression is lost in the tubular cells and retained only in the podocytes. Bone morphogenetic protein (BMP), fibroblast growth factor (FGF), paired box gene 2 (*PAX-2*), hepatocyte nuclear factor 1B (HNF1B), and WNT-4 are important signaling pathways from the ureteric bud. PAX-2 and WNT-4 cause mesenchyme to epithelialize for tubule differentiation as well as production of laminin and type IV collagen of basement membrane.

As mentioned earlier, perturbation in each of these steps, due to exposure to environmental risk factors or to the dysfunction of genes that direct this process, can lead to CAKUT. Moreover, the interdependence between distinct developmental pathways explains why defects in different genes result in similar phenotypes, why a mutation in a single gene can have pleiotropic effects and, therefore, why a morphologic classification alone cannot predict the primary genetic defect.

NORMAL FETAL URINARY TRACT

The fetal kidneys can be identified in utero by the 15th gestational week but visualization of internal renal architecture is usually not possible until after the 20th week. The pelvicalyceal system and capsule are highly echogenic while the medulla is almost anechoic. The urine filled pelvis may appear prominent without obstruction. The fetal bladder can also be identified in the early second trimester. Hourly fetal urine production increases from 12 mL/hour at 32 weeks to 26 mL/hour at term. The ureters are not seen unless they are dilated.

The amniotic fluid volume reflects renal function and patency of the genitourinary tract. The total volume of amniotic fluid, which ranges from 500 to 2,000 mL, is also an important factor in a fetus with hydronephrosis (HN). In early gestation, the source of amniotic fluid is a transudate of maternal plasma. Fetal urine contributes to the amniotic fluid from 14 weeks and by 20 weeks, 90% of the amniotic fluid is fetal urine. The volume increases until the end of the second trimester at a relative constant rate, then it remains steady, and subsequently decreases shortly before term. The reference range for amniotic fluid index is between 8 and 20 cm.

Decreased amniotic fluid volume, called oligohydramnios (amniotic fluid index (AFI) <8 cm], often indicates decreased fetal kidney function (dysplasia). Oligohydramnios can also be associated with intrauterine growth retardation, placental insufficiency, and use of nonsteroidal anti-inflammatory drugs/angiotensin-converting enzyme inhibitors (ACEI) or angiotensin II receptor blockers (ARB) by the mother. Oligohydramnios not only affects lung development causing pulmonary hypoplasia and resultant poor postnatal respiratory outcome but is the single most important predictor of postnatal kidney outcome. The amniotic fluid (AF) volume will play a significant role in prenatal counseling. On the contrary, polyhydramnios (AFI >20 cm) is most often associated with renal tubulopathy (such as Bartter's syndrome) indicating fetal polyuria, and occasionally, due to upper gastrointestinal (GI) tract obstruction, central nervous system (CNS) malformation, and maternal diabetes mellitus.

ETIOLOGY OF CONGENITAL ANOMALIES OF THE KIDNEY AND URINARY TRACT

The CAKUT is multifactorial in origin with complex etiological landscape and incompletely understood. It is hypothesized that genes essential for kidney development are subject to mutations, epigenetic modifications, and environmental factors that disrupt their regulation and contributes to CAKUT. Familial clustering of CAKUT suggests an important genetic contribution to its etiology. In 1995, the first gene defect described as being causative of CAKUT was a frameshift deletion in PAired boX2 gene (*PAX-2*) in a family with optic nerve coloboma, renal hypoplasia, and VUR. This was followed by identification of mutation in hepatocyte nuclear factor 1β (HNF1β) gene that encodes a transcription factor involved in the embryogenesis of the pancreas and liver and expressed in the Wolffian duct from a very early stage of kidney development. These "monogenic" forms of CAKUT are mostly explained by pathogenic single gene variants in 10–15% of cases and besides *PAX-2, HNF1β*, and *EYA1* genes are most frequently affected. Mutations of PAX-2 seem to be more frequently associated with renal hypoplasia, while mutations in HNF1β are more frequently associated with cystic kidneys. PAX2, EYA1, and SALL1 all belong to the GDNF-RET signaling pathway, which is required for the normal growth and morphogenesis of the ureteric bud during kidney development.

Since *PAX-2* gene is expressed in multiple tissues including optical disc, cap mesenchyma, and podocytes, mutations in PAX-2 may cause syndromic CAKUT with ocular anomalies, such as optic nerve coloboma as well as steroid resistant nephrotic syndrome due to podocytopathy. Hence, physician should carefully search for eye involvement and consider genetic testing for PAX-2 mutations in patients with CAKUT and early albuminuria.

The most recognized example for monogenic CAKUT in human patients is HNF1β nephrouropathy. Deleterious heterozygous variants in HNF1β (expressed in epithelial cells in the liver, pancreas, and in kidney tubules), such as the frequently reported whole gene deletion (about 50% of cases), lead to heterogeneous malformations of the kidney and/or the urinary tract (small, or normal sized echogenic kidneys, with or without cysts), and/or diabetes mellitus. In developing kidney tubules, HNF1β promotes SOCS3 expression, which plays an important role in tubulogenesis. Tubular dysgenesis in patients with deleterious variants in HNF1β is appreciated by the clinical term "HNF1β associated autosomal dominant tubular kidney disease (HNF1β-ADTKD)," which is characterized by CKD including hyperuricemia with or without gout, hypokalemia, hypomagnesemia, and polyuria.

Mutations in the genes encoding several components of the renin–angiotensin system such as angiotensinogen (AGT), renin (REN), ACE, and angiotensin II receptor type 1 (AGTR1) have been linked to renal tubular dysgenesis. The Uromodulin (UMOD) gene encodes the Tamm–Horsfall protein (which is the most abundant physiological urinary protein in humans produced by renal tubular cells of the distal loop of Henle) and its mutations have been linked to the pathogenesis of familial juvenile hyperuricemic nephropathy (FJHN), glomerulocystic kidney disease (GCKD) and autosomal dominant medullary cystic kidney disease 2 (MCKD2).

Pathogenic copy number variants (CNVs) are a second important cause of monogenic CAKUT in 5–10%. CNVs are structural variations in the genome of an individual in the form of gains (duplications) or losses (deletions) of DNA fragments. 22q11 microdeletion and the 17q12 microdeletion are two common types of CAKUT due to copy number variations.

Studies on the influence of epigenetics in the etiology of CAKUT are in an early phase. Epigenetic modifications are molecular "switches" capable of turning genes on and off or of fine-tuning gene expression, which can result in a change in phenotype without a change in genotype. The main mechanisms involved are DNA methylation, histone modifications, chromatin remodeling, and non-coding RNA-based gene regulation

Several environmental risk factors that can disturb normal nephrogenesis include maternal diabetes, overweight, vitamin A deficiency, and intrauterine exposure to toxins and medications such as ACEI/ARB/NSAIDs.

Finally, mutations in TBX18, NRIP1, and genes associated with various transcription factors (GDNF, SLIT2-ROBO2, etc.) as well as extracellular matrix proteins (Fraser syndrome genes *FRAS1, FREM2*, and *GRIP1*) have also been implicated in development of CAKUT.

From a clinical point of view, monogenic CAKUT may be undistinguishable from multifactorial CAKUT. A careful evaluation of family members and thorough screening for involvement of other organs may indicate a monogenic form of CAKUT that could be confirmed by next generation sequencing (NGS)-based genetic testing. Physicians caring for families with CAKUT need to be aware that different individuals from the same family may have different CAKUT phenotypes ("variable expressivity") and that variant carriers may not be affected ("reduced or incomplete penetrance"), which further complicates the identification of familial cases and counseling of families.

ANTENATAL RENAL MALFORMATIONS

Renal anomalies detected antenatally, referred to as CAKUT, can be broadly classified into four groups:

1. *Dysgenesis:* Unilateral agenesis, multicystic dysplastic kidney (MCDK), polycystic kidney disease [AR and autosomal dominant polycystic kidney disease (ADPKD)], cystic dysplasia, and proximal tubular dysgenesis (PTD).
2. *Upper tract dilatation* with and without ureteric dilatation and without bladder abnormalities [antenatal hydronephrosis (ANH), most common].
3. *Bladder outlet obstruction* (PUV).
4. *Disorders of position, and shape of kidney:* Ectopic kidney and horseshoe kidney.

Of all these antenatal detected renal anomalies, only autosomal recessive polycystic kidney disease (ARPKD), PUV in ~30% boys (those with associated oligohydramnios suggestive of in utero renal dysplasia), bilateral cystic kidneys, and bilateral small/normal sized/enlarged echogenic kidneys have the worst long-term renal outcomes with progressive CKD and need for dialysis and kidney transplantation. The remaining anomalies usually have a benign course with only ~10–20% requiring surgery (severe PUJO, high grade VUR, and some cases of megaureters).

Fetuses with multicystic dysplastic kidney (unilateral nonfunctioning kidney), ectopic, congenital absence of one kidney, or horse-shoe kidney have excellent long-term outcome and should not be a cause of worry.

We shall first focus on ANH/urinary tract dilation (UTD), one of the most common types of CAKUT. Despite the common nature of ANH, there is as yet no consensus on management especially with regards to mild-moderate HN. It is important to note that dilatation is not synonymous with obstruction as dilatation could be due to obstruction, VUR or benign. *Also, presence of dilatation does not specify abnormality of the kidney.*

ANTENATAL HYDRONEPHROSIS OR URINARY TRACT DILATION

As with the grading system for postnatal HN, there is no uniformly accepted definition of AH. In general, most authors would define AH when the anteroposterior renal pelvis diameter (APRPD) is >5 mm at 20 weeks of gestation and >7 mm at 32 weeks. The APRPD ≥ gestational age (GA) in months is considered significant (for e.g., at 6 months, 6 mm or greater dilatation of pelvis is significant). Of importance to note is that presence of calyceal dilatation at any stage is significant. The afore mentioned data is based on the work done by Corteville et al. In their report, the minimum threshold for significant HN was >4 mm in second trimester and >7 mm in third trimester. Renal pelvis anteroposterior (AP) diameter of >10 mm in second trimester or >15 mm in third trimester had an almost 100% sensitivity for identification of babies that required intervention postnatally. Despite accounting for expected increases in GA to accommodate for renal growth, these thresholds are arbitrary and not evidence-based. Siemens et al. demonstrated prenatal renal pelvis APD thresholds of <6 mm (<20 weeks GA), <8 mm (20–30 weeks GA), and <10 mm (>30 weeks GA) to be predictive of those patients that did not manifest postnatal urologic disease. Hence, the severity of ANH can be graded in to three categories based on renal pelvis anterior-posterior diameter (RPAPD) and GA as mentioned in **Table 1**.

TABLE 1: Antenatal hydronephrosis.

Classification	*Second trimester (APRPD mm)*	*Third trimester (APRPD mm)*
Mild	4–6	7–9
Moderate	7–10	10–15
Severe	>10	>15

(APRPD: Antero-posterior renal pelvis diameter)

Prenatal USG examination is important not only in mid pregnancy (~20–22 weeks) to look for anomalies but also in the third trimester to detect ~two-thirds of upper tract anomalies that can be missed in early scans. Hence, it is recommended that three antenatal scans should be performed—one during each trimester—to detect significant number of renal anomalies. Third trimester scan can also reveal resolution of some earlier UTD that may not need further post-natal evaluation.

HYDRONEPHROSIS GRADING SYSTEMS (TABLE 2)

Two main grading systems that are accepted include (1) Qualitative change in pelvicalyceal dilatation (Society for Fetal Urology system), and (2) Measurement of the APRPD.

TABLE 2: Hydronephrosis grading systems.

Grades	***Society for Fetal Urology Grading System (Qualitative)***	***Blachar's Grading System (Quantitative)***
Grade 0: Normal	No hydronephrosis, Intact central renal complex	Pelvis APD* <4 mm
Grade 1: Mild	Dilated renal pelvis	Pelvis APD 5–9 mm
Grade 2: Moderate	Dilated renal pelvis (>Grade 1)	Pelvis APD 10–15 mm
Grade 3: Severe	Dilated renal pelvis + Dilated calyces	Pelvis APD >15 mm + Cortical thinning
Grade 4: Severe	Dilated renal pelvis + Dilated calyces + Cortical thinning	—

(APD: Antero-posterior diameter)

Society for Fetal Urology Grading System (1993)

This is one of the early scoring systems published in 1993 and is still popular among the pediatric urologist. The main drawback is that it is a subjective (qualitative) system and the reporting depends upon the performer. The major advantage is that it includes calyceal dilatation as well as parenchymal changes in the description.

Blachar's Grading System for Hydronephrosis (1994)

This is based on APRPD. Although the grading is a quantitative system, and more likely to be reproducible, APD measurements are not ideal because they are dynamic—dependent on gestational age, maternal and fetal hydration, and effect of full bladder. The other limitation of this classification is that it does not consider calyceal dilatation and parenchymal changes that reflects severe HN.

Urinary Tract Dilation Classification System (UTD 2014)

Urinary tract dilation affects 1–2% of fetuses and reflects a spectrum of possible uropathies. The grading of ANH remains an ongoing challenge with different classification systems reported. Unfortunately, there is no consensus between different disciplines. Also, there is variability in clinical management, and lack of correlation between prenatal US and final urologic diagnosis. AP diameter is a very dynamic parameter and is affected by many factors (hydration, bladder filling, position, respiration, and as well as the operator). Also, its measurement is variable and misleading due to different renal pelvic configurations. More importantly, the different grading systems do not take in to account the ureter dilation, bladder abnormalities, and amniotic fluid adequacy—all important parameters that would indicate lower urinary tract obstruction and fetal kidney function. Therefore, there was a need for unified classification system and standard terminology for diagnosis and management of prenatal and postnatal UTD.

Dr Hiep Nguyen et al. published the multidisciplinary consensus classification on UTD in 2014 (based on current literature as well as expert opinions of members from eight societies) **(Table 3)**. It incorporates three broad categories of sonographic findings—degree of UTD, parenchymal quality, and associated ureter or bladder abnormality.

The classification is based on six categories in US findings:
1. APRPD
2. Calyceal dilatation
3. Renal parenchymal thickness
4. Renal parenchymal appearance
5. Ureteral abnormalities
6. Bladder abnormalities

It is stratified based on GA, and whether UTD is detected prenatally or postnatally. Based on literature and clinical experience, it is difficult to differentiate between central and peripheral calyceal systems on antenatal scans. Hence, intermediate and high risk groups are combined together in one category (A2–3).

ANTENATAL HYDRONEPHROSIS–POSTNATAL OUTCOME

One of the first report by Kitagawa et al. showed that 73% babies with antenatal renal anomalies had benign or transient HN and 27% had significant nephrouropathy.

TABLE 3: Urinary tract dilation (UTD) classification. (APRPD: anteroposterior renal pelvis diameter; RPAPD: renal pelvis anterior-posterior diameter.

	Antenatal		*Postnatal (>48 hours)*		
	UTD A1	*UTD A2–3*	*UTD P1*	*UTD P2*	*UTD P3*
Antero-posterior renal pelvis diameter (APRPD)	4–6 mm (<28 weeks) 7–9 mm (>28 weeks)	≥7 mm (<28 weeks) ≥10 mm (>28 weeks)	10–14 mm	≥15 mm	≥10 mm
Calyceal dilation		Any dilation	Central	Peripheral	Any dilation
Parenchymal abnormalities, bladder abnormalities, oligohydramnios		Yes (with RPAPD >4 mm or calyceal dilation)			YES
Ureter dilation		Yes (with RPAPD >4 mm or calyceal dilation)		≥ 4 mm (with APRPD ≥10 mm or calyceal dilation)	

Parenchymal abnormalities: Echogenicity, cystic dysplasia, cortical thinning, loss of CM differentiation.
Bladder abnormalities: Thickened wall, dilated posterior urethra, ureterocele
Oligohydramnios: Amniotic fluid index (AFI) <8 cm

Based on this and several other reports, the following observations can be made:

- ~65% with AH are isolated, transient, and benign (resolve spontaneously over first 2–3 years).
- 15–20% have VUR (irrespective of severity of HN)
- 8–10% have PUJO (severe HN)
- 5–10% have other urinary tract anomalies (PUV, VUJO, duplex, etc.)

In our own unpublished observation of records over 2 years at a tertiary center between 2009 and 2010, the incidence of antenatal renal anomalies was 1.7% (160 of 9,500 deliveries). The distribution of renal anomalies was as follows:

- *Isolated benign HN:* 60%
- *PUJO:* 18%
- *PUV:* 10%
- *VUR:* 10%
- *MCDK,* ectopic kidney: 2%
- *Others:* (1%)

IS THERE A CO-RELATION BETWEEN URINARY TRACT DILATION CLASSIFICATION AND POSTNATAL OUTCOME?

According to a recent study from Turkey, Cakici et al. in 2019 reported the outcome of postnatal HN based on UTD classification in 260 infants with prenatal detected UTD. In infants with UTD-P1 (APRPD <10 mm), the possibility of transient dilation (TD) or isolated HN was ~70% whereas ~30% had urinary tract anomaly (UTA)/significant nephrouropathy (VUR, PUJO, and VUJO). In contrast, of the infants with APRPD ≥10 mm (P2–P3), 20% had TD, and 80% had UTA [35% had VUR, 30% PUJO, and 15% VUJO, and 33% of UTA group (53 of 160) required surgery]. The slope of decrease in APRPD was significantly lower in UTA compared with the TD group. In the TD group, the difference between 1 and 3 month postnatal APRPD was—2.72 ± 3.3 mm, while in the UTA group this difference was—0.24 ± 3.5 mm (p <0.001). APRPD >10 mm at 1 month USG increased the risk of UTA by 7.2 fold. However, this cutoff of 10 mm does not exclude the diagnosis of UTA, since 17 units (12%) were diagnosed to have VUR, 14 renal units (10%) as PUJO, and 12 (9%) as VUJO (total 31%). Important to note that all the 43 units with UTA in those with APRPD <10 mm also had ureter dilation and calyceal dilation, important clues to the diagnosis of UTA. Patients with PUJO who required surgery were classified as P2 and P3, an independent risk factor for surgery.

ANTENATAL RENAL ANOMALIES: WHEN TO WORRY? (~5–10% OF ALL ANTENATAL RENAL ANOMALIES)

- Oligohydramnios (indicates renal dysplasia/decreased renal function)
- Bilateral hydro-uretero-nephrosis (boys)—PUV

- Bilateral persistent echogenic kidneys (ARPKD, renal tubular dysgenesis, infantile nephronophthisis, and cystic dysplasia)
- Other organ anomalies

ANTENATAL RENAL ANOMALIES: WHEN NOT TO WORRY? (~90% OF ALL ANTENATAL RENAL ANOMALIES)

- Unilateral HN or hydro-uretero-nephrosis of any severity
- Bilateral mild-moderate HN
- Bilateral severe HN with adequate AF
- Unilateral multicystic dysplastic kidney
- Congenital absence of one kidney, ectopia, horse-shoe kidney.

POSTNATAL EVALUATION (TABLE 4)

The main objective of postnatal management of antenatal renal anomalies is to attempt to segregate babies into two groups—those with significant nephrouropathies or UTA (~25% of the total group) and those with benign conditions (75%). Significant nephrouropathies could be considered in those babies with antenatal severe HN (RPAPD >15 mm), unilateral or bilateral hydro-uretero-nephrosis, enlarged and echogenic kidneys, and if there is associated oligohydramnios. According to Lee et al.'s large systematic review, the risk of any postnatal significant pathology is 11.9% for mild, 45.1% for moderate, and 88.3% for severe ANH. This demonstrates that there is an association between increasing severity of HN and increased incidence of postnatal pathology. There are two main exceptions to this association—VUR and distal ureteral obstruction. The incidence of VUR between groups of children with mild, moderate, and severe ANH is not significantly different ($p = 0.10$). In the study by Barbosa et al., the incidence of reflux was not statistically different between groups with mild (38/165, 23%), moderate (10/34, 29%), and severe (5/17, 29%) postnatal HN who had a VCUG ($p = 0.61$). *This implies that the presence or severity of ANH may have no reflection upon the presence of VUR, and further belies the efficacy of renal US in screening for VUR.* Distal ureteral obstruction especially type 1 and type 2 megaureters may have only ureteral dilatation without significant HN.

Certainly, babies with severe HN (renal pelvis APD >15 mm) would need detailed postnatal evaluation. However, no universal guidelines exist for the management of patients with mild-to-moderate ANH (5–15 mm). Since VUR can be noted in ~15% of all babies with HN, a micturating cystourethrography (MCUG) should be first performed in these babies with persistent mild-to-moderate HN between 3 and 6 months of age. If there is no VUR, possibility of either isolated/benign HN (90%) or PUJO (<10%) can be considered. PUJO is less likely to be observed in these babies and also, since a significant number of babies with PUJO will have spontaneous improvement with time, a diuretic renogram [EC or diethylene-triamine-penta-acetic acid (DTPA) renal scan] can be deferred unless there is an increasing trend in the HN along with parenchymal thinning (noticed with PUJO associated with intrarenal pelvis).

Despite a large number of reports on postnatal management of antenatal HN, there is as yet no uniform recommendations. A universal classification system and

TABLE 4: Postnatal evaluation of antenatal hydronephrosis—timing of imaging studies.

Hydronephrosis	*USG*	*MCUG*	*DTPA/EC/MAG3 Renal scan*
Unilateral hydronephrosis	*1st:* 7–14 days *2nd:* 1–2 months[#]	3–6 months age* If HN persisting (*See* **Figs. 2A and B**)	2–3 months age If HN >15 mm (*See* **Figs. 2A and B**)
Bilateral moderate-to-severe[^] hydronephrosis or unilateral/bilateral hydro-uretero-nephrosis	1st: 1–3 days *2nd:* 1–2 months	*Boys:* 2-4 days (Before discharge) to rule out PUV *Girls:* 2–3 months	2–3 months age
Severe hydronephrosis in a solitary kidney	*1st:* 1–3 days *2nd:* 1–2 months	*Boys:* 2–4 days *Girls:* 2–3 months	2–3 months or may be earlier if serum creatinine is increasing, or urosepsis

*Perform micturating cystourethrography (MCUG) in first week of life if there is any suspicion of posterior urethral valves (PUV) (in boys)
[#]Always perform second ultrasonography (USG) at 1–2 months even if first USG was normal
[^]*Hydronephrosis (HN):* Mild—pelvis APD 5–9 mm, Moderate—pelvis APD 10–15 mm, Severe—pelvis APD >15 mm

nomenclature are needed to best identify patients at risk of renal deterioration, UTI, and need for surgical intervention. Most reports recommend step wise approach to investigations and judicious use of chemoprophylaxis in high risk babies. One such recent protocol published by Timberlake et al. proposes three groups—low risk (postnatal RPAPD <20 mm), intermediate risk (RPAPD 20–30 mm), and high risk (RPAPD >30 mm). For low risk group (RPAPD <20 mm), they recommend only serial USG without any further imaging (MCUG or renogram) or chemoprophylaxis. The other two groups would need both chemoprophylaxis and further imaging. Based on our own experience at following a large number of babies with antenatal renal anomalies and low incidence of febrile UTIs 1.5% at 2 years of follow-up, unpublished data), we present our own protocol regarding serial USG schedule, prophylactic antibiotics, voiding cystourethrogram, and renal scintigraphy **(Flowchart 1)**. Based on the second USG obtained at 1–2 months age, we suggest to continue observation with serial USGs if there is mild HN (RPAPD 5–9 mm), obtain MCUG to rule out VUR if renal pelvis is between 10 and 15 mm (moderate HN), and a diuretic renal scan at 2–3 months for severe HN (RPAPD >15 mm).

Based on the recent UTD classification system's risk stratification of UTD A1 and UTD A2–3, antenatal scan has to be repeated after 32 weeks and after 4–6 weeks, respectively. For UTDA1 category, postnatal, 2 USG examination has to be performed at 7–14 days and 1–6 months. In contrast, babies with UTD A2–3 severity need to have first USG at first week along with additional investigations (MCUG and DTPA renal scan) and specialist consultation. MCUG should be done in first week of life in baby boys with clinical and USG suspicion of PUV.

Postnatal Management (Table 4 and Flowchart 1)

- Reassure the family.
- One of the objective is Not to miss PUV in early neonatal period. All the remaining renal anomalies can be evaluated safely between 1-2 weeks and 3 months age.
- PUV in a baby boy should be evaluated by:
  - Clinical exam (urinary stream, renal and bladder mass, and respiratory distress).
  - Serial serum creatinine estimation (at least two reports 1–2 days apart).
  - Renal USG on day 1–2 and MCUG.
- *Prevent UTI:* Cephalexin drops (5 mg/kg/dose Bid) in select high risk babies.
- Obtain two renal USGs in first 2 months of life before ruling out significant nephrouropathy—first between 1 and 2 weeks and second at 1and 2 months age.
- If renal USG is performed on day 1–3 of life, repeat renal USG is mandatory between 2 and 4 weeks of age (since in first few days, because of physiological

Flowchart 1: Approach to a newborn with antenatal hydronephrosis.

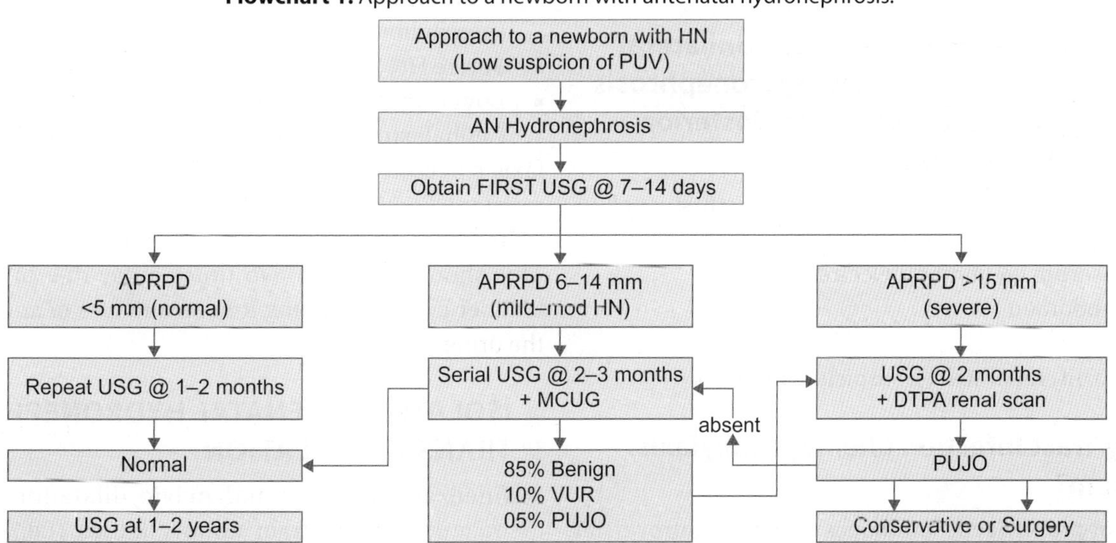

(AN: antenatal; APRPD: antero-posterior renal pelvis diameter; HN: hydronephrosis; IAHN: isolated antenatal hydronephrosis/benign HN; PUJO: pelvi-ureteric junction obstruction; PUV: posterior urethral valves; VUR: vesico-ureteric reflux)

oliguria and reduced breast milk quantity, HN may not be evident).

- The two main imaging modalities to evaluate renal anomalies further are MCUG and diuretic renogram (DTPA or EC or MAG3 renal scan). Timing of these tests are detailed in **Table 2**.

Management schema based on UTD classification system risk stratification suggests that for babies with UTD P1 and P2 (low and intermediate group, respectively), two USG examinations between 2 days–1 month and 1–3 months should be obtained. As there is still ongoing controversy regarding clinical importance of diagnosing VUR and the effectiveness of prophylactic antibiotics, recommendations for performing MCUG and use of prophylactic antibiotic are left to the physician's discretion. Similarly, the need for DTPA or EC scan to rule out PUJO in a baby with UTD P2 or P3 is also left to the physician's discretion. Certainly, babies with UTD P3 or ureteric dilation (high risk group) need to be initiated on prophylaxis and MCUG performed to rule out VUR. If there is no VUR, DTPA or EC scan should be performed at 2–3 months to rule out PUJO.

Unilateral Hydronephrosis (Any Severity) (Flowchart 1)

- 10–14 days and 4–8 weeks of age—renal USG.
- 8–12 weeks—DTPA renal scan to rule out PUJO if APRPD >15 mm.
- 3–6 months—MCUG if APRPD persisting above 10 mm, increasing or fluctuating.

Bilateral Severe Hydronephrosis, Unilateral Or Bilateral Hydronephrosis, Hydronephrosis in Solitary Kidney, or Suspected Posterior Urethral Valve (Table 4)

Investigations have to be performed in the first week of age before the neonate is discharged from the nursery.

- Serial serum creatinine + electrolytes
- USG abdomen
- MCUG
- MAG 3/EC renal scan, if suspicion for PUJO.

Urinary Tract Infection Chemoprophylaxis: For Whom?

The use of prophylactic antibiotics remains controversial because no uniform guidelines exist. This controversy stems from a number of factors including the fact that most babies with high grade VUR are boys and have dysplasia or congenital scarring (i.e., scarring in absence of febrile UTI), there are contrasting results of efficacy of antibiotics in prevention of UTI, concern about bacterial resistance to drugs used for prophylaxis, and also, the importance of early diagnosis and treatment of febrile UTI in reducing risk of scar formation.

A systematic review of the available literature identified limited data to support the proposed protective effect of antibiotic prophylaxis. Pooled UTI rates in patients with low-grade HN (SFU grades 1–2 or RPAPD 4–14 mm) were similar regardless of continuous antibiotic prophylaxis (CAP) status: 2.2% on prophylaxis versus 2.8% not receiving prophylaxis. In children with high-grade HN (SFU grades 3–4 or RPAPD >15 mm), patients receiving CAP had a significantly lower UTI rate versus those not receiving CAP [14.6% (*95% confidence interval:* 9.3–22.0] versus 28.9% [*95% confidence interval:* 24.6–33.6, $p < .01$). The estimated number needed to treat to prevent 1 UTI in patients with high-grade HN was 7. This systematic review suggests value in offering CAP to infants with high-grade HN.

In our experience of prospective follow-up of 160 babies with antenatal renal anomalies, the incidence of UTI was only 1.7% (all with PUV). Hence, we do not routinely initiate chemoprophylaxis for all babies with antenatal renal anomalies.

High risk babies that would benefit from chemoprophylaxis include:

- Unilateral or bilateral hydro-uretero-nephrosis (possibility of VUR or VUJO)
- Severe HN (RPAPD > 15 mm or SFU Grades 3–4)
- Boys with PUV.

Cephalexin is generally accepted for chemoprophylaxis since there is increasing incidence of Amoxicillin resistant *Escherichia coli* organisms. Dose is 25–30% of therapeutic dose (5 mg per kg per dose 2 times a day). This should be given two times a day due to frequent bladder cycling in young infants and loss of antibiotic in the urine.

ISOLATED ANTENATAL HYDRONEPHROSIS/ TRANSIENT DILATION

Defined as isolated renal pelvic dilatation without associated urinary tract abnormalities (i.e., absence of calyceal dilatation, cortical thinning, hydroureter, vesicoureteric reflux, PUJO, and bladder anomalies).

This is confirmed when both MCUG and diuretic renogram study are negative for VUR/PUV and PUJO, respectively.

In a systematic analysis of papers on ANH, Sidhu et al. from the Hospital for Sick Children, Canada, had the following observations:

- *APRPD <12 mm, SFU grade 1–2:* Benign condition, most improve (95%).
- *Presence of cortical thinning:* Marker of deterioration.
- *Severe grades:* Variable rates of stabilization (60%).

The authors concluded that there is sufficient evidence to suggest that mild HN (APRPD <12 mm) is a self-limited condition and that clarification is required for moderate-severe HN.

This entity, benign HN or TD, is the most common cause of antenatal detected HN noted in neonates with RPAPD between 5 and 15 mm. MCUG should be done in this group of neonates to rule out VUR/PUV before labeling as benign HN.

VESICOURETERIC REFLUX

After isolated (benign) HN, VUR is the next common urinary tract abnormality detected though antenatal screening.

Through antenatal screening, VUR is suggested by:

- APRPD <15 mm (10–20% incidence)
- APRPD >15 mm and PUJO is ruled out on DTPA scan
- Fluctuating renal pelvis AP diameter on serial USGs
- Hydro-uretero-nephrosis.

The VUR is associated with long-term complications related to recurrent urinary tract infections, renal scarring, and hypertension as well as dysplasia associated with high-grade reflux (congenital scarring).

Diagnosis

MCUG under antibiotic cover (1 day before and 2 days after MCUG).

Treatment

- Long-term chemoprophylaxis (in select few children) with:
  - Cephalexin drops (100 mg/1 mL) 5 mg/kg/dose Bid
  - Nitrofurantoin 2–3 mg/kg/dose HS (infants >1 year age)
  - Bactrim 2–3 mg/kg/day HS (infants >9–12 months age)
  - Cefaclor 5 mg/kg/dose Bid (if recurrent UTI on above medicines)
- Circumcision, especially in boys in infancy, with breakthrough UTIs or high-grade VUR.
- Surgery in select group usually after 1 year of age (ureteric reimplantation) or temporary procedures such as Deflux injection/unilateral ureterostomy in younger infants with high grade VUR and recurrent breakthrough UTIs—where definitive surgery is not feasible).

PELVIURETERIC JUNCTION OBSTRUCTION

The PUJO is often due to lack of or decreased ganglion cells with resultant decreased peristalsis. It is suggested by APRPD greater than 15 mm and diagnosis is confirmed by DTPA (or EC or MAG3) renal scan at 2–3 months of age. This renal scan is delayed until 2 months of age since there is a natural maturation of renal function and GFR usually triples that of newborn period at 2 months (~60 mL/min/1.73 m^2) that permits better visualization of the kidneys. Occasionally, EC or MAG3 renal scan may be performed in the first few weeks of life especially if there is bilateral severe HN or HN in a solitary kidney. IVP essentially does not have a role in diagnosis of PUJO. Since the natural history of PUJO is that of spontaneous resolution in a significant number of cases, majority of children with PUJO can be managed conservatively. The most compelling data to support an initial interval of observation are the long-term follow-up by Koff et al. In this study, 104 newborn with unilateral severe HN were managed expectantly. A deterioration of renal function was the indication for surgical repair. A total of 23 patients required intervention and a return of function was appreciated in all of these patients. In addition, HN resolved in 69% and improved in 31%. The average time to this resolution was 2.5 years.

Conservative management includes 3–6 monthly USG and DTPA renal scan until 1 year of age and then 6–12 monthly for another 2 years. Improvement is usually noted in most children by 2–3 years age. A small percentage of children the PUJO due to aberrant lower pole vessel can have fluctuating pelvis AP diameter and present between 5 and 10 years. Hence, a follow-up USG is suggested every 2–3 years up to 15 years age. Early detection and prompt treatment of UTI is very important.

Surgery for PUJO is indicated if:

- Palpable renal mass
- Presence of cortical thinning
- APRPD >25 mm
- Split renal function <40% on DTPA renal scan

Ross et al. demonstrated that SFU system could be used to identify patients most likely to require surgical intervention. In their study, 125 patients with SFU grade 3 or 4 HN (assessed neonatally) were included and *followed-up* with serial diuretic renography. Utilizing their algorithm, 11 (15%) of 71 kidneys with Grade 3 and 37 (69%) of 54 kidneys with grade 4 HN underwent pyeloplasty. Patients with SFU grade 4 HN were more likely to require surgical intervention for decreased drainage or impaired renal function than their counterparts with grade 3 HN.

Management of infants with severe PUJO associated poorly functioning kidney (especially split function <10%) remains controversial. Options include pyeloplasty, or trial of stent/percutaneous nephrostomy placement followed by repeat DTPA scan or primary nephrectomy. In majority of infants, there is no significant improvement in renal function postpyeloplasty and these children do carry risk of long-term hypertension due to irreversible changes that have occurred in the poorly functioning kidneys. Hence, it is preferable to perform nephrectomy if the function is <10% and in those who have undergone pyeloplasty, long-term monitoring of blood pressure is mandatory.

MULTICYSTIC DYSPLASTIC KIDNEY

The MCDK is the most common cystic renal anomaly and occurs in ~1 in 2,000 births. The MCDK is a nonfunctioning kidney characterized by multiple noncommunicating cysts and absence of identifiable renal parenchyma **(Fig. 1)**. It results from disturbance in ureteric bud development during early pregnancy. The differential diagnosis of MCDK includes severe PUJO (dilated pelvicalyceal system appears as "cysts"), ADPKD, and simple cysts (usually single). DTPA renal scan is useful to differentiate MCDK from these conditions since by definition MCDK is nonfunctional and hence, will not be seen on the dynamic renal scan. There is a 15–25% incidence of renal anomalies on the contralateral side (i.e., the normal kidney). Of these, VUR (reflux) is the most common followed by PUJO, VUJO, and duplex system.

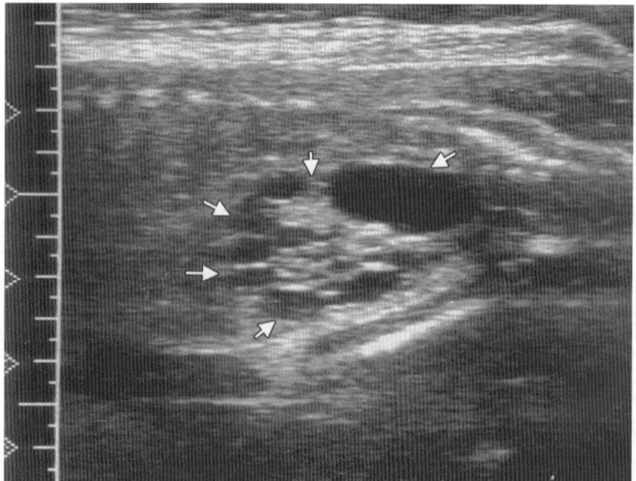

Fig. 1: Antenatal scan at 34 weeks showing unilateral multicystic kidney (arrows) confirmed postnatally to have multicystic dysplastic kidney (MCDK).

The natural history of MCDK includes spontaneous involution/regression in 75% cases and decrease in size by 6 years of age in majority. The outcome of children with MCDK is benign. In a systematic review of 29 published articles, Narchi found only 6 children out of 1,115 eligible children with MCDK to have hypertension giving a probability of 0.5% that is lower than the risk in general population (1–4%). Also, they did not find any reported cases of Wilms tumor in 1,041 eligible cases.

Evaluation of a neonate with antenatal suspicion of MCDK includes:

- Renal USG once in 1–2 years until 15 years.
- DTPA renal scan at 3 months of age especially if there is confusion between MCDK and severe PUJO on USG.
- MCUG at 3–6 months of age to rule out VUR on the normal side if there is HN or hydroureter.
- Management of MCDK is conservative. Until mid-1980s, infants were subjected to surgery (nephrectomy) that is now reserved only for infants with huge renal mass. Most children are followed conservatively with:
  - Renal USG once in 1–2 years until 15 years.
  - Assessment of growth, and blood pressure (BP) once a year (routine).
- Moderate salt and nonvegetarian (meat) protein reduction in family's diet to decrease the risk of hypertension and proteinuria in later life (due to hyperfiltration injury to contralateral glomeruli).
- Surgery (nephrectomy) if there is no spontaneous regression of MCDK by 10–15 years (no solid data).

POSTERIOR URETHRAL VALVE

The PUV are the most serious and fortunately less common of the antenatal renal anomalies. During the antenatal period, PUV can be suggested by bilateral hydro-uretero-nephrosis/bilateral HN **(Fig. 2A)**, echogenic renal cortex, distended bladder, and decreased

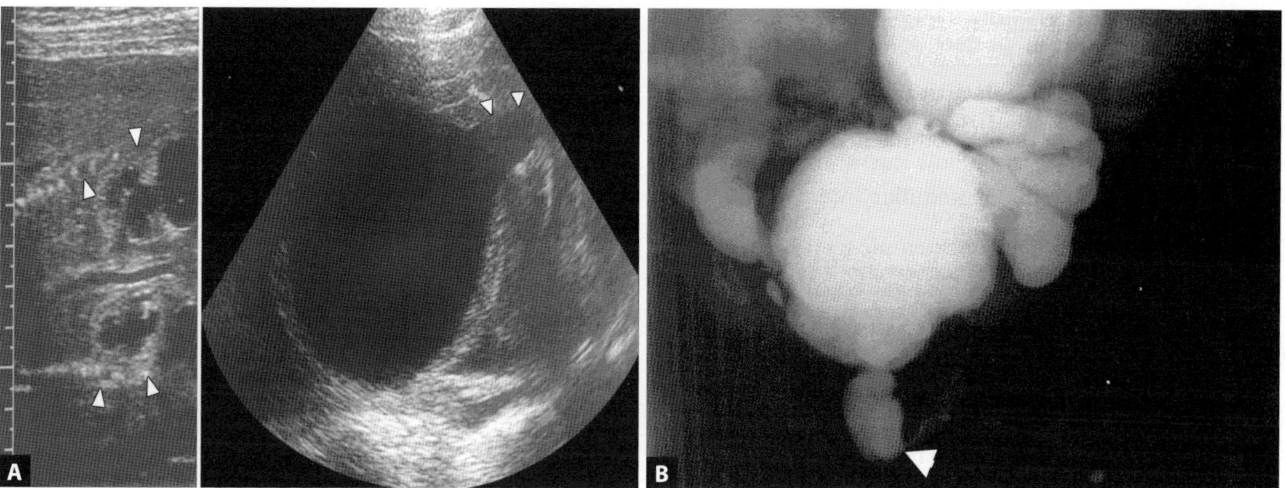

Figs. 2A and B: (A) Antenatal ultrasonography (USG) showing bilateral severe hydronephrosis (with dilated calyces) on the left side (arrowheads), and distended, thick walled bladder with dilated posterior urethra on the right side (arrowheads); (B) Postnatal micturating cystourethrography (MCUG) confirming posterior urethral valves (PUV) (with arrowhead), trabeculated bladder, and bilateral grade V vesicoureteral junction obstruction (VUR).

amniotic fluid. Of all the available fetal renal functional parameters including amniotic fluid adequacy, amniotic fluid electrolytes and β2 microglobulin, and cortical echogenicity, adequate amniotic fluid index is one of the most important predictors of long-term renal outcome in PUVs. As reported by Zaccara et al., 12 of 18 fetuses with bilateral obstructive uropathy and associated oligohydramnios survived. Of these 12 surviving neonates, 3 died in first month of life due to severe lung hypoplasia and the remaining 9 had renal failure with a mean serum creatinine of 1.3 ± 0.2 mg/dL at 1 year of age. In contrast, all the 10 babies with adequate amniotic fluid (25–75th percentile) had near normal serum creatinine of 0.6 ± 0.1 mg/dL. They demonstrated that amniotic fluid index remains a reproducible and inexpensive method to predict renal function in cases of bilateral obstructive uropathy of any origin. It retained its validity not only in severe but also milder reduction. Conversely, intact amniotic fluid most invariably predicts normal renal function at long-term evaluation.

Postnatal evaluation includes observation of urinary stream, presence of renal and bladder mass, and respiratory status (distress, oxygen requirement, and lung expansion on X-ray). Renal USG is to be performed on day 2–3 followed by MCUG under antibiotic cover **(Fig. 2B)**. Serial monitoring of renal parameters and serum electrolytes including bicarbonate is very important. In most cases, cystoscopy and primary fulguration of valves can be performed in the neonatal period. Occasionally, some neonates or infants may initially need urinary diversion in the form of vesicostomy or ureterostomy followed by fulguration at a later date. Postfulguration, infants need to be maintained on cephalexin prophylaxis (until at least 6 months or longer duration in presence of VUR). Long-term follow-up for growth, metabolic acidosis [type IV renal tubular acidosis (RTA)], blood pressures, renal and bladder function is required (several decades).

Approximately 25–30% of children with PUVs can progress to end-stage renal disease. Poor prognostic markers include oligohydramnios, bilateral high grade VUR, and echogenic kidneys. Appropriate and timely postnatal intervention can decrease the morbidity associated with PUVs. Antenatal interventions like vesico-amniotic shunt makes no significant difference to the outcome and long-term results of patients with PUV and debate about its efficacy on renal outcome continues.

ECHOGENIC FETAL KIDNEYS

The normal echogenicity of the fetal kidney is equal to that of the liver. Generally, fetal renal echogenicity refers to the appearance of the entire kidney rather than to an isolated component of the kidney, i.e., the cortex, medulla, or pyramids. The glomeruli and tubules in the renal cortex provide the interfaces that contribute to renal echogenicity. The absence of glomeruli in the medulla, as well as the radial arrangement of the tubules results in the lower echogenicity of the renal medulla and the normal corticomedullary differentiation. Occasionally, the renal medulla may appear echogenic on postnatal scans usually due to reduced urine flow rate and deposition of Tamn-Horsfall protein in the medullary renal tubules.

There are various reasons for echogenic fetal kidneys:

- Polycystic kidney disease (Autosomal recessive and autosomal dominant), usually with enlarged kidneys
- Renal dysplasia either primary due to HNF1β (Hepatocyte Nuclear Factor) gene mutation or associated with obstructive uropathy.
- Renal tubular dysgenesis (RTD)—either primary due to mutations in genes encoding the renin-angiotensin System (RAS) or secondary to fetal exposure to RAS blockade drugs such as ACE inhibitors & ARB's and NSAIDs, donor twin of severe twin-to-twin transfusion syndrome, and in fetuses with congenital hemochromatosis. Renal tubular dysgenesis (RTD) is a severe fetal disorder characterized by the absence or poor development of proximal tubules, early onset and persistent fetal oligo-anuria (leading to oligohydramnios and the Potter sequence) and ossification defects of the skull. In most cases, early death occurs from pulmonary hypoplasia, anuria and refractory arterial hypotension. Survivors will have progressive kidney failure with need for renal replacement therapy.
- Infantile nephronopthisis
- Congenital nephrotic syndrome
- Associated with syndromes such as Beckwith-Wiedemann syndrome and Trisomy 13 and 18.
- Transient fetal hyperechogenicity is a usually benign condition when the amniotic fluid remains adequate. Majority of these fetuses will show resolution of hyperechogenicity on postnatal USG and normal renal function by 3 years age. The etiology of hyperechogenicity is not known but some may have associated genetic etiology (as in ARPKD), or associated VUR. Fetuses with ARPKD or ADPKD will have enlarged and echogenic kidneys whereas other causes are associated with normal kidney size.

DISORDERS OF NUMBER, SIZE, AND POSITION

Babies with unilateral congenital absence, ectopic, dysplastic, or horse-shoe kidney usually have excellent long-term outcome as long as the other kidney is normal. Postnatally, these babies should have an USG at 2–3 months age and then at 1 year age. If there is kidney size discrepancy or ectopic smaller kidney, MCUG should be performed at 3–6 months age to rule out VUR and a DMSA renal scan for split renal function. Long term, low salt, low fat vegetarian diet for family, and annual check-up for BP and urinalysis is recommended.

INDIAN PERSPECTIVE

There are very few studies from India describing the postnatal outcome of infants with antenatal detected renal anomalies. One of the first studies reported by Sanghvi et al. found 0.2% incidence of congenital renal anomalies (65 of 31,217 pregnant women over 3 year period). Of these 65, urinary tract dilatation was the most common renal anomaly and found in 39 neonates. Saha et al., reported antenatal renal malformations in 35 of 6,682 antenatal scans (0.4%) with 50% showing HN, 30% with unilateral empty fossa, 10% MCDK, and 10% had other various anomalies. In our own unpublished observations, the incidence of antenatal renal anomalies was ~1.7% (160/9,500 deliveries over 2 years from Jan 2008 to Dec 2009) with most ANH being transient/isolated (60%). Significant nephrouropathies were found in 40% babies with PUJO in 18%, VUR in ~10%, PUV in 10%, and MCDK in 2%. The Indian Society of Pediatric Nephrology had published a revised statement on management of ANH in 2013 to aid practicing pediatrician in appropriate management of these babies. We follow a slightly different protocol in management of babies with antenatal renal anomalies **(Flowchart 1)**. This is based on the reports over the past one decade about the benign nature of isolated HN and low incidence of UTI in this group. Our objective is not to miss a baby boy with PUV before discharge from the nursery and also to detect significant nephrouropathies such as VUR, PUJO, VUJO, etc., during the serial follow-up.

PRENATAL COUNSELING

Obviously, presence of fetal kidney dilatation causes parental anxiety and raises a number of doubts regarding the immediate and long-term outcome of the baby specifically regarding the kidney function. Since, most studies report lower incidence of significant nephrouropathies or UTA (PUV, PUJO, VUR, etc), first thing to do is to reassure the family regarding the common nature and usually benign course of most conditions. Most unilateral HN, unilateral cystic kidneys (MCDK), and unilateral renal agenesis have a good long-term outcome as long as the other kidney is normal. These children will have adequate physical and mental growth, and normal life expectancy. When dealing with unilateral HN, the family can be counseled regarding the step-wise work up of the baby between birth and 3 months of age. Unilateral HN of any severity does not need any fetal intervention or early delivery.

With bilateral severe HN, possibilities of PUV, VUR, PUJO, and other uropathies are discussed. Of all the nephrouropathies, PUV is the only one that is more likely to be associated with progressive CKD in ~30% children. Adequacy of amniotic fluid in the 2nd and 3rd trimester is an important prognostic marker for future/long-term renal function. If amniotic fluid is decreased (AFI <5 cm) in presence of bilateral HN, the risk of postnatal renal failure requiring dialysis and transplantation is very high (~90%). In case of VUR or PUJO, even if surgery is required, the timing of surgery is usually between 2 months (PUJO) and 24 months (for high grade VUR) of age and not immediately after birth.

The indication for early delivery is usually based on obstetric factors. The only fetal factor that may necessitate early delivery is when there is worsening oligohydramnios usually seen in boys with PUV. After inducing lung maturation with steroids, early delivery can then be planned.

Finally, there are only few antenatal renal anomalies where family may opt for medical termination of pregnancy due to high risk of progressive CKD and need for dialysis and kidney transplantation—ARPKD—enlarged and echogenic fetal kidneys with oligohydramnios, bilateral cystic dysplasia, PUV in male fetus associated with oligohydramnios, and multiorgan dysgenesis (syndromic association). The prognosis of other fetal renal anomalies is generally good and does not warrant termination of pregnancy.

PRENATAL INTERVENTIONS

Interventions for congenital kidney anomalies vary from conservative management to fetal intervention and surgery. Fetal lower urinary tract obstruction has been managed with antenatal vesico-amniotic shunting (VAS) or serial amnioinfusion by many fetal medicine specialists over the last three decades, but the literature for these interventions remains controversial. Although pulmonary function may improve with fetal procedures, there is no convincing evidence that relieving the urinary tract obstruction improves postnatal kidney outcomes as it is likely that kidney dysplasia occurred early in fetal development. It is also important to note the risks associated with VAS, including risks of miscarriage along with other risks such as dislodgement of shunt and bladder rupture following shunt insertion. Fetal cystoscopy for the diagnosis and treatment of lower urinary tract obstruction with prenatal laser ablation of the PUV has also been studied. A meta-analysis in 2011 concluded that there was very little evidence at present to support routine use of fetal cystoscopy, and further studies are required.

Long-term Outcome: Is There Risk of Chronic Kidney Disease in Infants with Congenital Anomalies of Kidney and Urinary Tract?

The major goal of management of infants with antenatal renal anomalies is to identify those who are at risk of hypertension, proteinuria, and progressive CKD. Infants with echogenic kidneys, bilateral cystic, or hypodysplastic kidneys, and boys with PUV associated oligohydramnios are certainly going to progress to CKD. Oligohydramnios in itself is a poor prognostic marker for future need of renal replacement therapy.

The challenge is to identify infants with UTD who will have CKD at follow-up. One of the few studies to address this question was reported from Brazil, who analyzed a cohort of 447 children with isolated antenatal APRPD >5 mm in the third trimester. 5% children experienced hypertension, proteinuria, and/or reduced GFR at median follow-up of 6.4 years and all these children had HN of SFU grade 3–4. Conversely, none of the children with mild UTD developed CKD during the study period. In another study from Sweden, Herthelius et al. showed that among children with postnatal APRPD >7 mm and/or calyceal, ureteric, or bladder pathology in the neonatal period, 39% had signs of permanent kidney damage (based on USG or DMSA findings) at 12–15 year follow-up. In these 39% children, all but 1 (93%) had moderate-or-severe antenatal UTD (UTD A2–3). In contrast, among children without these postnatal findings, only one boy (5%) had signs of CKD.

SUMMARY

Most renal anomalies are benign with excellent long-term prognosis and can be evaluated in a step wise manner after delivery. Fetuses with bilateral hydro-uretero-nephrosis and echogenic cortex (suggestive of PUV), echogenic kidneys (suggestive of ARPKD, renal tubular dysgenesis, and dysplasia), and oligohydramnios (suggestive of decreased fetal renal function) are likely to have poor postnatal outcome in terms of renal failure and pulmonary hypoplasia. Most others (90%) have a good postnatal outcome including those with disorders of number, size, and position. The objective of postnatal management is to identify significant nephrouropathies (such as PUJO, VUR, PUV, and megaureter), with timely management to minimize long-term complications of UTI, hypertension, and CKD.

The risk increases with increasing degree of the antenatal dilatation for all CAKUT conditions except vesicoureteral reflux (VUR), which is diagnosed in approximately 7–24% of all cases regardless of the degree of antenatal dilatation. A meta-analysis published in 2006 found that 12% of infants with mild dilatation, 45% with moderate dilatation, and 88% with severe fetal dilatation were postnatally diagnosed with CAKUT.

Postnatal evaluation begins with obtaining two USGs in first week of life and 1–2 months of age. Based on the renal pelvis APD on the second USG at 2 months, decision regarding further imaging is taken. If renal pelvis APD is between 5 and 15 mm, MCUG is performed to rule out VUR and if the RPAPD is greater than 15 mm, diuretic renal scan (DTPA or EC) is performed first to rule out PUJO. The only exception is in boys with suspected PUV where USG and MCUG are performed in first few days of life. With two consecutive postnatal USG showing normal anatomy (RPAPD <5 mm), 95% of significant nephrouropathies can be ruled out (VUR is the only possibility with normal USG).

Infants with PUJO and VUR can be managed conservatively with only a select few who would need surgery. Babies with unilateral multicystic kidney (MCDK), unilateral renal agenesis, and ectopic kidney/s usually have excellent long-term outcome as long as the other kidney is normal.

KEY POINTS

- 75% of renal anomalies are going to be benign or transient and ~ 25% will be significant nephro-uropathies that will require further evaluation.
- Of these 25% fetuses, only those with bilateral echogenic kidneys (suggestive of ARPKD, HNF1B mutation, infantile nephronophthisis, syndromic), and severe HUN associated oligohydramnios (suggestive of PUV) are associated with progressive CKD postnatally.
- Other conditions associated with significant nephro-uropathies include PUJO, VUR, VUJO, unilateral MCDK, duplex system, bilateral renal cysts.
- Possibility of significant nephro-uropathies is suggested by fetal echogenic kidneys, unilateral or bilateral hydro-ureteronephrosis, moderate to severe hydronephrosis and oligohydramnios.
- First post-natal USG should be delayed until end of first week after increase in urine volume and second USG should always be repeated at 4-6 weeks.
- Boys with unilateral or bilateral hydroureteronephrosis should have USG, MCUG, and renal function tests performed before discharge to rule out PUV.
- Other babies can be evaluated between 2-4 months with DTPA scan if renal pelvis AP diameter is more than 15 mm to rule out PUJO and MCUG if there is persistent hydronephrosis (renal pelvis between 6-14 mm) to rule out VUR.
- Babies with single functioning kidney status, unilateral multicystic dysplastic kidney, ectopic kidney, and unilateral severe hydronephrosis (PUJO) have excellent long-term outcome.
- Chemoprophylaxis is not indicated in all babies but should be reserved for those with unilateral or bilateral hydro-ureteronephrosis (VUR, VUJO or PUV).

SUGGESTED READING

1. Barbosa JA, Chow JS, Benson CB, Yorioka MA, Bull AS, Retik AB, Nguyen HT. Postnatal longitudinal evaluation of children diagnosed with prenatal hydronephrosis: insights in natural history and referral pattern. Prenatal Diagnosis. 2012;32:1242-9.
2. Blachar A, Blachar Y, Livne PM, Zurkowski L, Pelet D, Mogilner B, et al. Clinical outcome and follow-up of prenatal hydronephrosis. Pediatr Nephrol. 1994;8(1): 30-5.
3. Braga LH, Mijovic H, Farrokhyar F, Pemberton J, DeMaria J, Lorenzo AJ. Antibiotic prophylaxis for urinary tract infections in antenatal hydronephrosis. Pediatrics. 2013;131: e251-61.
4. Brophy MM, Austin PF, Yan Y, Coplen DE. Vesicoureteral reflux and clinical outcomes in infants with prenatally detected hydronephrosis. J Urol. 2002;168:1716-9.
5. Brunisholz Y, Vial Y, Maillard Brignon C, et al. Prenatal diagnosis of urinary malformations: results in a series of 93 consecutive cases. Swiss Med Weekly 2001;131:95-8.
6. Cakici EK, Aydog O, Eroglu FK, Yazilitas F, Ozlu SG, Uner C, et al. Value of renal pelvic diameter and urinary tract dilation classification in the prediction of urinary tract anomaly. Pediatr Int. 2019;61:271-7.
7. Capone VP, Morello W, Taroni F, Montini G. Genetics of congenital anomalies of the kidney and urinary tract: The current state of play. Int. J. Mol. Sci. 2017;18(4): 796-809.

8. Carr MC, Benacerraf BR, Estroff JA, Mandell J. Prenatally diagnosed bilateral hyperechoic kidneys with normal amniotic fluid: postnatal outcome. J Urol. 1995;153(2): 442-4.
9. Chandrasekharam VVS, Shah MA, Padua M, et al. Results of temporary drainage of poorly functioning kidneys with ureteropelvic junction obstruction: Does the histology of persistent poor functioning kidneys indicate an increased risk of hypertension? Urology. 2023. In press. https://doi.org/10.1016/j.urology.2023.10.011
10. Corteville J, Gray D, Crane J. Congenital hydronephrosis: correlation of fetal ultrasonographic findings with infant outcome. Am. J. Obstet. Gynecol. 1991;165(2):384-8.
11. Costa FP, Simoes E, Silva AC, Ix JH, Vasconcelos MA, Dias CS, et al. A clinical predictive model of renal injury in children with isolated antenatal hydronephrosis. Clin Kidney J. 2019;13(5):834-41.
12. Emma YXW, Winyard P, Marlais M. Congenital anomalies of the kidney and urinary tract: antenatal diagnosis, management and counselling of families. Pediatr Nephrol. 2024;39:1065-75.
13. Farhat W, McLorie G, Geary D, Capolichhio G, Bagli D, Merguerian P, et al. The natural history of neonatal vesico-ureteral reflux associated with antenatal hydronephrosis. J of Urol. 2000;164(3):1057-60.
14. Fernbach SK. USG grading of hydronephrosis: Introduction to the system used by the Society of Fetal Urology. Pediatric Radiology. 1993;23(6):478-80.
15. Garrett W J, Grunwald G, Robinson DE. Prenatal diagnosis of fetal polycystic kidney by ultrasound. Aust NZ J Obstet Gynaecol. 1970;10(1):7-9.
16. Gubler MC. Renal tubular dysgenesis. Pediatr Nephrol. 2014;29(1):51-9.
17. Gunn TR, Mora JD, Pease P. Antenatal diagnosis of urinary tract abnormalities by ultrasonography after 28 weeks gestation: incidence and outcome. Am J Obstet Gynaecol. 1995;172:479-86.
18. Gupta DK, Bajpai M, Chandrasekharam VVSS, Srinivas M. Antenatally detected pelviureteric junction obstruction: Safety of conservative management by our protocol. Indian J Urol. 2000;17(1):24-7.
19. Hadlock FP, Deter RL, Carpenter R, Gonzalez ET, Park SK. Sonography of fetal urinary tract anomalies. Am J Radiology. 1981;137(2):261-7.
20. Herthelius M, Axelsson R, Lidefelt KJ. Antenatally detected urinary tract dilatation: a 12–15-year follow-up. Pediatr Nephrol. 2020;35:2129-35.
21. Herthelius M. Antenatally detected urinary tract dilatation: long-term outcome. Pediatr Nephrol. 2023;38:3221-7.
22. Ismaili K, Avni FE, Alexando M. Routine VCUG is of no value in neonates with unilateral MCDK. J Pediatr. 2005;146(6):759-63.
23. Ismaili K, Hall M, Piepsz A, Wissing KM, Collier F, Schulman C, et al. Primary vesico-ureteral reflux detected in neonates with a history of fetal renal pelvis dilatation: A prospective clinical and imaging study. J of Pediatr. 2006;148(2):222-7.
24. Ismaili Khalid, Fred EA, Wissing M, Hall M; Brussels Free University Perinatal Nephrology Study Group. Long-term clinical outcome of infants with mild and moderate fetal pyelectasis: Validation of neonatal ultrasound as a screening tool to detect significant nephro-uropathies. J of Pediatr. 2004;144(6):759-65.
25. Jawson MS, Dibble L, Puri S, Davis J, Young J, Dave R. Prospective study of outcome in antenatally diagnosed renal pelvis dilatation. Arch Dis Child. 1999;80:F 135-F 138.
26. Kaneyama K, Yamataka A, Satake S, Yanai T, Lane GJ, Kaneko K, et al. Associated urologic anomalies in children with solitary kidney. J Pediatr Surg. 2004;39(1): 85-7.
27. Karmarkar SJ. Long-term results for posterior urethral valves: A review. Pediatr Surg Int. 2001;17(1):8-10.
28. Kitagawa H, Pringle KC, Stone P, Flower J, Murakami N, Robinson R, et al. Postnatal follow-up of hydronephrosis detected by prenatal ultrasound: the natural history. Fetal Diagn Ther. 1998;13(1):19-25.
29. Kohl S, Habbig S, Weber LT, Liebau MC. Molecular causes of congenital anomalies of the kidney and urinary tract (CAKUT). Mol Cell Pediatr. 2021;8(1):2-7.
30. Kuwertz-Broeking E, Brinkman OA, Von-Lengerke H-J, Sciuk J, Fruend S, Bulla M, et al. Unilateral Muliti-cystic dysplastic kidney: Experience in children. BJU Int. 2004; 93(3):388-92.
31. Lee RS, Cendron M, Kinnamon DD, Nguyen HT. Antenatal hydronephrosis as a predictor of postnatal outcome: a meta-analysis. Pediatrics. 2006;118(2):586-93.
32. Lidefelt KJ, Hertherlius M. Antenatal hydronephrosis: Infants with minor postnatal dilatation do not need prophylaxis. Pediatr Nephrol. 2008;23(11):2021-2024.
33. Moorthy I, Joshi N, Cook JV, Warren M. Antenatal hydronephrosis: negative predictive value of normal postnatal ultrasound: a 5 year study. Clin Radiol. 2003;58(12): 964-70.
34. Narchi H. Risk of hypertension with multicystic kidney disease: A systematic review. Arch Dis Child. 2005;90(9):921-4.
35. Narchi H. Risk of Wilm's tumour with multicystic kidney disease: A systematic review. Arch Dis Child. 2005;90(2):147-9.
36. Nguyen HT, Benson CB, Bromley B, Campbell JB, Chow J, Coleman B, et al. Multidisciplinary consensus on the classification of prenatal and postnatal urinary tract dilation (UTD classification system). J Pediatr Urol. 2014; 10(6):982-99.
37. Ross, SS. Kardos S, Krill A, Bourland J, Sprague B, Majid M, et al. Observation of infants with SFU grades 3–4 hydronephrosis: worsening drainage with serial diuresis renography indicates surgical intervention

and helps prevent loss of renal function. J Pediatr Urol. 2011;7(3):266-71.

38. Saha A, Batra P, Chaturvedi P, Mehera B, Tayade A. Antenatal detection of renal malformations. Indian Pediatr. 2009;1-3.
39. Salam MA. Posterior urethral valve: Outcome of antenatal intervention. Int J Urol. 2006;13(10):1317-22.
40. Sanghvi KP, Merchant RH, Gondhalekar A, Lulla CP, Mehta AA, Mehta KP. Antenatal diagnosis of congenital renal malformations using ultrasound. J Trop Ped. 1998; 44(4):235-40.
41. Sidhu G, Beyene J, Rosenblum ND. Outcome of isolated antenatal hydronephrosis: a systematic review and meta-analysis. Pediatr Nephrol. 2006;21(2):218-24.
42. Siemens D, Prouse K, MacNeily A, Sauerbrei EE. Antenatal hydronephrosis: thresholds of renal pelvic diameter to predict insignificant postnatal pelviectasis. Tech. Urol. 1998;4(4):198-201.
43. Sinha A, Bagga A., Krishna A, Bajpai M, Srinivas M, Uppal R, et al. Revised guidelines on management of antenatal hydronphrosis. Indian Pediatr. 2013;50(2): 215-31.
44. Timberlake MD, Herndon, CD. Mild to moderate postnatal hydronephrosis -grading systems and management. Nat Rev Urol. 2013;10(11):649-56.
45. Ulman I, Jayanthi V, Koff S. The long-term follow-up of newborns with severe unilateral hydronephrosis managed nonoperatively. J Urol. 2000;164:1101-5.
46. VAM Knoers N. The term CAKUT has outlived its usefulness: the case for the defense. Pediatric Nephrology. 2022;37(11):2793-8.
47. Yerkes E, Nishimura H, Ichikawa I, Miyazaki Y, Ma J, Hunley TE, et al. Role of angiotensin in the congenital anomalies of the kidney and urinary tract in the mouse and the human. Kidney Int Suppl. 1998;67: S75-77.
48. Zaccara A, Giorlandino C, Mobili L, Brizzi C, Bilancioni E, Capolupo I, et al. Amniotic fluid index and fetal bladder outlet obstruction. Do we really need more? J Urol. 2005; 174(4 Pt. 2):1657-60.

Acute Kidney Injury in Children

PK Pruthi

INTRODUCTION

Acute kidney injury (AKI) is characterized by an abrupt deterioration of renal function, and it is a common clinical condition in pediatric intensive care unit (PICU). The term AKI has largely replaced acute renal failure and it more clearly defines kidney dysfunction as a continuing process rather than a single parameter of failed kidney function.

The incidence of AKI in children appears to be increasing and the etiology has shifted from primary renal diseases to multifactorial causes. Despite advances in therapy, the mortality due to AKI is still high (30–40%) and a proportion of patients may progress to chronic kidney disease (CKD) and dialysis dependency.

DEFINITION

An accepted definition of AKI is an increase in serum creatinine by ≥0.3 mg/dL or an increase of ≥1.5 times baseline, known to have occurred within last 7 days or a urine volume of <0.5 mL/kg/h for 6 hours [kidney disease: improving global outcomes (KDIGO) classification].

INCIDENCE

Acute kidney injury is common in PICU, with an incidence of 10–35%. The rate is higher in children who have been ventilated or have undergone cardiac surgery. The AWARE study showed that 26.9% children had AKI, while severe AKI was observed in 11.6% of children within 7 days of ICU admission. Another study, AWAKEN, revealed that AKI was occurring in 30% of newborns with a higher incidence in preterm infants. It has been observed that very low birth weight (<15,00 g), a low Apgar score, and patent ductus arteriosus compromising heart function are associated with higher probability of development of AKI.

STAGING OF ACUTE KIDNEY INJURY

In 2002, the acute Dialysis Quality Initiative Group proposed the RIFLE criteria for staging AKI and this was followed by another classification proposed by Acute Kidney Injury Network (AKIN) **(Table 1)**.

In 2007, Arikan et al. came out with a pediatric patient-modified RIFLE criteria and termed it pRIFLE **(Table 2)**. These criteria are based on estimated creatinine clearance calculated by means of Schwartz formula. To determine the severity and progress of AKI, Basu et al. in 2012, proposed a method termed pediatric renal angina criteria **(Table 3)**.

For neonates, a slightly different classification known as "modified AKI classification for neonates" has been proposed by KDIGO **(Table 4)**.

ETIOLOGY

There are many causes of AKI, the more common ones are listed in **Table 5**.

The etiology of AKI has traditionally been classified as prerenal, renal (or intrinsic renal), and postrenal **(Flowchart 1 and Table 5)**. Prerenal AKI occurs due to inadequate systemic or renal circulation, the cause of which could be either hypovolemia or renal hypoperfusion. Both prerenal and postrenal categories can get converted to intrinsic AKI.

CLINICAL FEATURES

Children who have prerenal AKI may present with features of fluid loss, sepsis, and dehydration. Those having acute intrinsic AKI may present with oliguria, edema, hematuria, proteinuria, dysuria, hypertension, pallor, dark urine, or jaundice. Interrupted urinary stream and palpable bladder suggest postrenal AKI **(Table 6)**.

It is important to note the volume status of a patient and different methods for its assessment have been proposed.

TABLE 1: RIFLE and Acute Kidney Injury Network (AKIN) staging criteria for acute kidney injury.

RIFLE[a] stage	*AKIN stage*	*Serum creatinine criteria*	*Urine output criteria*
Risk	1	Increase in serum creatinine of 1.5–2-fold from baseline (RIFLE and AKIN) or increase in serum creatinine of ≥0.3 mg/dL (AKIN)	<0.5 mL/kg/h for 6 hours
Injury	2	Increase in serum creatinine of two to threefold from baseline	<0.5 mL/kg/h for 12 hours
Failure	3	Increase in serum creatinine of more than threefold from baseline or a scrum creatinine of >4 mg/dL with an acute rise of ≥0.5 mg/dL	<0.3 mL/kg/h for 24 hours or anuria for 12 hours
Loss		Persistent renal failure for >4 weeks	
End-stage renal disease		Persistent renal failure for >3 months	

[a]RIFLE defines three grades of increasing severity of acute renal dysfunction (risk, injury, and failure; respectively R, I, and F) on the basis of graded changes in serum creatinine or urine output and two outcomes variables (loss and end-stage kidney disease, L and E, respectively) based on the duration of loss of kidney function.

TABLE 2: pRIFLE criteria.

pRIFLE criteria		*Estimated CrCl (Schwartz)*	*Urine output*
Early	R (risk)	Decrease by 25%	<0.5 mL/kg/h × 8 hours
	I (injury)	Decrease by 50%	<0.5 mL/kg/h × 16 hours
	F (failure)	Decrease by 75% or <35 mL/min/1.73 m^2	<0.5 mL/kg/h × 24 hours or anuria for 12 hours
Late	L (loss)	Renal failure >4 weeks	
	E (end-stage)	Renal failure >3 months	

(CrCl: creatinine clearance)

TABLE 3: Pediatric renal angina criteria.

Level of risk based on clinical status	*Renal angina threshold*
Moderate-risk patients	
Patients admitted to PICU	• Doubling of serum Cr OR • eCrCl decrease >50% OR • ICU fluid overload >15%
High-risk patients	
Acute decompensated heart failure Stem cell transplant recipient	• Serum Cr increase ≥ 0.3 mg/dL OR • eCrCl decrease 25–50% OR • ICU fluid overload >10%
Very-high-risk patients	
Receiving mechanical ventilation and one or more vasoactive medications	• Any serum Cr increase OR • eCrCl decrease >25% OR • ICU fluid overload >5%

(Cr: creatinine; eCrCl: estimated creatinine clearance; ICU: intensive care unit; PICU: pediatric intensive care unit)

TABLE 4: Modified KDIGO AKI definition for neonates.

Stage	*Serum creatinine (SCr)*	*Urine output (UOP)[a]*
0	No change in SCr or rise <0.3 mg/dL	>1 mL/kg/h
1	• *SCr rise:* >0.3 mg/dL within 48 hours or • *SCr rise:* ≥1.5–1.9 × rise from baseline (previous lowest value) within 7 days	>0.5 and ≤1 mL/kg/h
2	*SCr rise:* ≥2–2.9 × rise from baseline	>0.3 and ≤0.5 mL/kg/h
3	• *SCr rise:* ≥3 × rise from baseline or • *SCr* ≥2.5 mg/dL or • KRT initiation	≤0.3 mL/kg/h

(AKI: acute kidney injury; KRT: kidney replacement therapy; KDIGO: kidney disease improving global outcomes)
[a]For 24-hour period

- Fluid overload percentage = Daily fluid intake (liters) – fluid output (liters) × 100/weight (in kg)
- In units that perform daily weight measurement, an alternative weight-based formula for calculating fluid may be used.

TABLE 5: Categories and causes of acute kidney injury in children.

Prerenal	*Intrinsic renal*	*Postrenal*
Intravascular volume depletion: • Dehydration • Gastroenteritis • Hemorrhage • Diabetes insipidus • Burns • Diuretics *Redistribution of fluid/vasodilatation*: • Sepsis • Pancreatitis • Intestinal obstruction • Peritonitis • Nephrotic syndrome • Hepatic failure *Decreased cardiac output:* • Congestive heart failure • Cardiogenic shock • Myocarditis • Cardiac tamponade	*Acute tubular necrosis (ATN):* *Ischemic injury:* Prerenal causes *Exogenous toxins:* • Nephrotoxic antibiotics • Chemotherapeutic agents • Nonsteroidal anti-inflammatory drugs (NSAIDs) • Angiotensin-converting enzyme (ACE) inhibitors • Angiotensin II receptor blocker (ARBs) • Radiographic contrast agents • Venoms • Heavy metals • Ethylene glycol *Endogenous toxins:* • Myoglobinuria/hemoglobinuria • Tumor lysis syndrome *Acute interstitial nephritis:* • Drug-induced or idiopathic *Acute glomerulonephritis:* • Postinfectious (streptococcal) – Henoch-Schönlein purpura (HSP) – Systemic lupus erythematosus (SLE) – Goodpasture syndrome *Vascular pathology:* • Renal artery/vein thrombosis • Hemolytic uremic syndrome (HUS)/thrombotic thrombocytopenic purpura (TTP) • Cortical necrosis *Congenital*: Renal dysplasia/hypoplasia polycystic kidney disease	• Posterior urethral valves • Obstruction of a solitary kidney • Bilateral ureteral obstruction neurogenic bladder, and • Trauma

Flowchart 1: Classification of acute kidney injury.

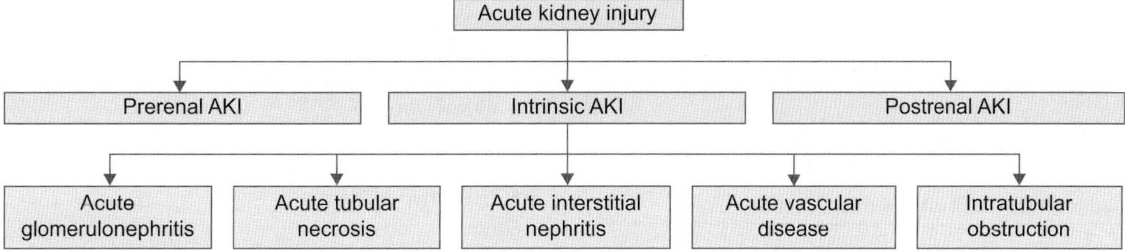

Fluid overload percentage = Current weight (kg) – ICU admit weight (kg) × 100/Admit weight (kg)

INVESTIGATIONS

The clinical evaluation of a patient who has AKI begins with assessing whether the patient has prerenal, postrenal or intrinsic disease.

Few blood and urine tests help to determine whether AKI is prerenal or acute intrinsic AKI **(Table 7)**.

Appropriate investigations are performed to establish a diagnosis. **Box 1** depicts the plan of common investigations required in a child who has AKI.

Kidney Biopsy

In some cases, when the cause of AKI cannot be identified, then a kidney biopsy is undertaken generally at 2 weeks but early if indicated. The indications of renal biopsy are shown in **Box 2**.

TABLE 6: Clinical features with probable diagnosis.

Clinical features	*Probable diagnosis*
History of vomiting, diarrhea, blood loss, sepsis, burns, and diabetes insipidus	Prerenal AKI
Nephrotic syndrome, hepatic failure, pancreatitis, and peritonitis	Prerenal AKI
Congestive heart failure, cardiogenic shock, and myocarditis	Prerenal AKI
Dysentery anemia, bleeding tendency (low platelet count), hypertension, hematuria, proteinuria, and oliguria	Hemolytic uremic syndrome (HUS)
Hypertension, hematuria, proteinuria, and oliguria	Poststreptococcal glomerulonephritis (PSGN)/ infection-associated glomerulonephritis (GMN)
History of drugs and toxins • Chemotherapeutic agents • Nonsteroidal anti-inflammatory drugs (NSAIDs) • Angiotensin-converting enzyme (ACE) inhibitors • Angiotensin II receptor blocker (ARBs) • Radiographic contrast media • Venoms • Heavy metals • Antibiotics/penicillin group sulfonamides • Diuretics • Cimetidine	Acute intrinsic AKI (ATN) Interstitial nephritis
Colicky abdominal pain, hematuria, UTI	Urinary calculi
Urinary stream problems and palpable bladder	Obstructive uropathy (post-renal AKI)

(AKI: acute kidney injury; UTI: urinary tract infection)

TABLE 7: Reduced renal perfusion (prerenal) versus acute tubular necrosis (intrinsic renal).

	Prerenal		***Intrinsic renal***	
	Child	***Neonate***	***Child***	***Neonate***
U_{Na}(mEq/L)	<20	<20	>40	>40
FeNa (%)	<1	<2	>1	>3
U_{osm} (mOsm/kg)	>500	>400	<300	<300
U_{osm}/P_{osm}	>1.5	>2	<0.8–1.2	<1
BU/creat	>20:1	>20:1	<20:1	<20:1
Fluid push	Urine ↑	Urine ↑	No response	No response

Note: Fractional excretion of sodium (FeNa) = [(urine sodium × serum creatinine)/(serum sodium × urine creatinine)] × 100%

(BU: blood urea; Creat: serum creatinine; P_{osm}: plasma osmolality; U_{Na}: urinary sodium; U_{osm}: urinary osmolality)

BOX 1: Recommended investigations.

- *Blood*
  - Complete blood counts with peripheral smear, ESR, reticulocyte count, and schistocyte index
  - Blood urea, creatinine, serum sodium, potassium, calcium, and phosphate
  - Blood gases
  - Lactate dehydrogenase (LDH), direct Coombs test (DCT)
  - Blood antistreptolysin O (ASO), serum complement C3 level, antinuclear antibody (ANA), antineutrophil cytoplasmic antibodies (ANCAs)
- *Urine:*
  - Urine routine exam and culture
  - Fractional excretion of sodium (FeNa)
  - Osmolality
  - Urine sodium and potassium
- *Radiology:*
  - X-ray chest
  - Ultrasound kidney and bladder
  - Renal Doppler
  - Micturating cystourethrogram (MCU)
  - Diethylenetriamine pentaacetate (DTPA) scan
- *ECG:* For hyperkalemia
- *Others*
  - Renal biopsy
  - AKI biomarkers

(AKI: acute kidney injury; ESR: erythrocyte sedimentation rate)

Biomarkers of Acute Kidney Injury

Serum creatinine at present is commonly used as a biomarker of AKI, but it has some limitations. It does not change until up to 50% of kidney function has been lost [50% reduction of glomerular filtration rate (GFR)] and it rises to 72 hours after an injury event. Also, its value is affected by age, sex, muscle mass, and volume status. Cystatin C, neutrophil gelatinase-associated lipocalin (NGAL), kidney injury molecule-1 (KIM-1). Interleukin 18 (IL-18), N-acetyl-beta-D-glucosaminidase (NAG), and liver-type fatty acid-binding protein (L-FABP), are some of the biomarkers that can be used to detect AKI at an early stage. NGAL and KIM-1 are specific for hypoxic and nephrotoxin-mediated kidney injury, whereas IL-18 is specific for hypoxic and ischemic renal damage. These biomarkers help in early detection of AKI, approximately 1–2 days prior to the rise in serum creatinine values.

MANAGEMENT

Many children would require a fluid bolus to differentiate prerenal from intrinsic renal AKI. One or more fluid challenges of 20 mL/kg of 0.9% saline or ringer lactate are given over 30–60 minutes. Furosemide may be tried if the bolus has shown no effect. A good urine output indicates prerenal AKI.

BOX 2: Indications of renal biopsy in acute kidney injury.

- Rapidly progressive glomerulonephritis
- AKI in transplanted kidney
- Unremitting AKI lasting for >2 weeks
- AKI in children on nephrotoxic drugs
- Prognostication in hemolytic uremic syndrome
- AKI of unknown etiology

(AKI: acute kidney injury)

Management includes handling fluid overload, electrolyte imbalance, hypertension, metabolic acidosis, and other complications of AKI **(Table 8)**. Management of AKI in context to type of AKI is shown in **Table 9**.

Renal Replacement Therapy

There are various modalities of renal replacement therapy (RRT) available to the pediatric nephrologists today to support the renal system, giving it the much-needed time to recover from injury. The usual indications are shown in **Table 10**.

Assessment Before Initiating Renal Replacement Therapy

Before starting RRT, identification of patient characteristics is required as the major goal is to obtain good results **(Box 3)**.

TABLE 8: Management of AKI and its complications.

Complication	*Treatment*	*Assessment*
Pulmonary edema	• IV furosemide 3–4 mg/kg. Respiratory support, e.g., highflow nasal cannula (HFNC) and ventilation • Dialysis	• Chest X-ray • Ultrasound • Inferior vena cava (IVC) assessment • Central venous pressure (CVP) line monitoring
Fluid overload	• Restricted fluids (in 24 hours) = 400 mL/m^2 + urine output of last 24 hours • In general, fluid calculated can be given as 10% glucose. Composition can be changed according to the electrolyte report • Any other loss (like gastric aspirate) to be replaced	Assess for dialysis
Hyperkalemia	• No potassium-containing fluids, foods, or medicines • Salbutamol nebulization, repeat if needed • Sodium polystyrene sulfonate resin (kayexalate) 1 g/kg orally or by retention enema can be given with 20% sorbitol 2 mL/kg. If required repeat after 2 hours. In case of ECG, changes or serum K above 7 mEq/L. • IV calcium gluconate (10%) 0.5–1 mL/kg, IV over 10 minutes with heart rate monitoring • Stop infusion if heart rate falls by >20/min • Sodium bicarbonate (7.5%) 2 mL/kg over 20 minutes • Glucose 50% solution 1 mL/kg with regular insulin, 1 unit/5 g of glucose IV over 1 hour	Treatment should start when serum K rises above 5.5 mEq/L
Metabolic acidosis	• Sodium bicarbonate 2 mL/kg over 20 minutes or correction formula HCO_3 = 0.3 × BW (kg) × 12 serum HCO_3 level mEq/L • Remainder correction by oral administration of bicarbonate or citrate solution	If fluid overload, consider dialysis

Contd...

Contd...

Complication	*Treatment*	*Assessment*
Hypertension	• Labetalol 0.25–1 mg/kg/h • Nitroprusside 1–8 µg/kg/min infusion • Inj. furosemide 2–4 mg/kg/IV • *Nifedipine:* Sublingual 0.3–0.5 mg/kg/dose oral	Monitor BP by monitor or if in ICU, intra-arterial BP
Anemia	Packed cell transfusion 3–5 mL/kg	
High serum phosphate (*Normal:* 4–7 mg/dL)	• Calcium carbonate (30–50 mg/kg/day of calcium) • If S calcium is high, then sevelamer 50 mg/kg/day	Assess for hypercalcemia
Hyponatremia	*Fluid restriction:* • If abnormal sensorium or seizures with serum Na <120 mEq/L, give 3% saline 6–10 mL/kg over 60–90 minutes	
Diet	• *Protein:* 0.8–1.2 g/kg/day • *Calories:* Minimum 60 calories/kg/day • Increase carbohydrate intake	Once dialysis is initiated, protein, fluid, and electrolyte intake can be increased
Infection	All procedures are to be done with aseptic precautions. Treat infection if present	Frequent examination to detect infection
Medication	Depending on severity of AKI, doses to be modified	

TABLE 9: Management in context to type of AKI.

Prerenal AKI		• Administer crystalloids • Bolus 10–15 mL/kg/ normal saline in 30–60 minutes • Stop NSAIDs, ACE inhibitors, and diuretics • Antibiotics for sepsis • Blood transfusion for blood loss • Inotropes if needed
Intrinsic AKI		
	ATN	• Discontinue offending drug or toxin • Supportive care
	HUS	Plasma infusion/exchange
	Vasculitis	Immunosuppression and plasma exchange
	Interstitial nephritis	Steroid therapy, discontinue offending drug/agents
	Renal artery occlusion	Angioplasty and anticoagulation
	Glomerulonephritis	Supportive care
Obstructive AKI (postrenal)		
	Bladder catheter or nephrostomy, surgical treatment if obstruction	

(ATN: acute tubular necrosis; HUS: hemolytic uremic syndrome)

TABLE 10: Indications of renal replacement therapy (RRT).

Renal indications	*Nonrenal indications*
Oliguria (nonresponsive to diuretics and fluid challenge)	Fluid overload 15% or greater
Anuria (nonobstructive)	Anticipated blood transfusion in trauma
Severe metabolic acidosis (pH <7.2, despite bicarbonate treatment)	Sepsis
Severe or persistent hyperkalemia: K >6.5 mEq/L or K = 5.5–6.5 mEq/L with ECG changes	Inborn errors of metabolism
Azotemia, encephalopathy, seizures, and pericarditis	Drug overdose
Hyponatremia, Na <120–125 mEq/L	Postcardiopulmonary bypass surgery
Hypercatabolic state	
Need to give large amounts of fluid, e.g., shock, medications, and blood products	Systemic inflammatory response syndrome

Choice of Renal Replacement Therapy Modality

Choice of RRT modality depends upon the age, condition, hemodynamic stability, abdominal surgery, and availability of vascular access, or hemodialysis/continuous RRT machine. A comparison between various modalities of RRT is shown in **Table 11**.

BOX 3: Assessment before initiating renal replacement therapy (RRT).

- *Identification of major goal:* Solute clearance or fluid removal
- *Identification of patient characteristics:*
  - Size of patient
  - Hemodynamic instability
  - Abdominal or diaphragmatic pathology (usually excludes use of PD)
  - Lack of vascular access
  - Anticipated duration of RRT

(PD: peritoneal dialysis)

TABLE 11: Comparison between the three techniques of renal replacement therapy (RRT).

	PD	*HDi*	*CRRT*
Method specificities			
Vascular access (ECC)	No	Yes	Yes
Complex method with specific expertise	Low	Moderate	High
Systemic anticoagulation	No	Frequent	Frequent
Dialysis dose			
Efficacy to remove a toxin	Moderate	High	High
Efficacy to remove fluid	Moderate	Moderate	High
Clinical situation indication			
Hemodynamic instability	Yes	No	Yes
Intracranial hypertension	Yes	±	Yes
ARDS	±	Yes	Yes
Abdominal surgery	±	Yes	Yes

(ARDS: acute respiratory distress syndrome; CRRT: continuous renal replacement therapy; ECC: extracorporeal circulation; HDi: intermittent hemodialysis; PD: peritoneal dialysis)

OUTCOMES

Despite all advances in RRT, the morbidity and mortality due to AKI remains high (30–40%). The recovery of AKI depends upon the underlying condition, need for inotropes, degree of fluid overload at initiating of RRT, associated sepsis, multiorgan dysfunction, and delay in onset of appropriate therapy.

A prospective two-center study of 250 children showed that stage 2 or worse AKI during ICU admission was associated with a sixfold increase in risk of CKD or prehypertension at 6 years follow-up. In non-ICU hospitalized children, one study showed that 70% of children exposed to nephrotoxins had evidence of CKD at 6 months follow-up.

PREVENTION

General measure to help prevent AKI include use and close monitoring of levels of nephrotoxic drugs, adequate fluid repletion in hypovolemia, adequate hydration before administration of contrast media, and proper fluid administration with alkalization of urine before chemotherapy. Mannitol, furosemide, and low-dose dopamine have been evaluated with either inconclusive results or no evidence of benefit.

For primary prevention, those children who have CKD, past AKI history, cardiac or liver disease, hypotension, hypertension, fluid overload, sepsis, oliguria, signs of urinary obstruction, and vasculitis should be observed very closely in the hospital and should be diagnosed at early stage if they develop AKI. For secondary prevention, the goal should be for survival with recovery to baseline kidney function in the shortest time possible and with few or no complications.

CONCLUSION

Acute kidney injury is an important problem in children especially in the PICU or cardiac surgery PICU, with resultant mortality, CKD, and end-stage renal disease (ESRD).

Long-term complications can be avoided by identifying high-risk patients and by diagnosing AKI at an early stage. The mortality in patients on RRT occurs due to the inherent disease and not due to the RRT procedures.

KEY POINTS

- AKI is a common clinical condition encountered in PICU with an incidence of 10–35%.
- The staging criteria are based on serum creatinine/creatinine clearance and urine output values.
- pRIFLE criteria are based on estimated creatinine clearance and are suitable for pediatric population.
- KDIGO has proposed a modified AKI classification for neonates.
- Kidney biopsy is generally indicated in rapidly progressive glomerulonephritis or when cause is not clearly known by end of two weeks.
- Prevention includes:
  a. Early recognition and treatment of at risk children.
  b. Monitoring during high risk situations (ICU, Postsurgery).
  c. Prompt management of pre-renal AKI as prognosis is very good in this category.
- Long term follow up is needed to detect and manage the sequelae.

SUGGESTED READING

1. Agras PI, Tarcan A, Baskin E, Cengiz N, Gürakan B, Saatci U. Acute renal failure in the neonatal period. Ren Fail. 2004;26(3):305-9.
2. Akcan-Arikan, Zappitelli M, Loftis LL, Washburn KK, Jefferson LS, Goldstein SL. Modified RIFLE criteria in critically ill children with acute kidney injury. Kidney Int. 2007;71(10):1028-35.
3. Alkandari O, Eddington KA, Hyder A, Gauvin F, Ducruet T, Gottesman R, et al. Acute kidney injury is an independent risk factor or pediatric intensive care unit mortality, longer length of stay and prolonged mechanical ventilation in critically ill children: A two-center retrospective cohort study. Crit Care. 2011;15(3):R146.
4. Andreoli SP. Acute kidney injury in children. Pediatr Nephrol. 2009;24(2):253-63.
5. Anigilaje EA, Adebayo AI, Ocheni SA. Acute kidney injury in children: A study of etiology, clinical profile, and short-term outcomes at the University of Abuja Teaching Hospital, Gwagwalada, Abuja, Nigeria. Saudi J Kidney Dis Transpl. 2019;30(2):421-39.
6. Askenazi DJ, Ambalavanan N, Goldstein SL. Acute kidney injury in critically ill newborns: What do we know? What do we need to learn? Pediatr Nephrol. 2009;24(2): 265-74.
7. Bagga A, Srivastava RN (Eds). Acute kidney injury. Pediatric Nephrology, 6th edition. New Delhi: Jaypee Brothers Medical Publishers (P) Ltd; 2016. pp. 236, 247, 248-50, 256.
8. Basu RK, Chawla LS, Wheeler DS, Goldstein SL. Renal angina: An emerging paradigm to identify children at risk for acute kidney injury. Pediatr Nephrol. 2012;27(7): 1067-78.
9. Bellomo R, Ronco C, Kellum JA, Mehta RL, Palevsky P; Acute Dialysis Quality Initiative workgroup. Acute renal failure-definition, outcome measures, animal models, fluid therapy and information technology needs: The Second International Consensus Conference of the Acute Dialysis Quality Initiative (ADQI) group. Crit Care. 2004;8(4):R204-12.
10. Benisty K, Morgan C, Hessy E, Huynh L, Joffe AR, Garros D, et al. Kidney and blood pressure abnormalities 6 years after AKI in critically ill children: A prospective cohort study. Ped Res. 2020;88(2):271-8.
11. Blinder JJ, Goldstein SL, Lee VV, Baycroft A, Fraser CD, Nelson D, et al. Congenital heart surgery in infants: Effects of acute kidney injury on outcomes. J Thorac Cardiovasc Surg. 2012;143(2):368-74.
12. Cho MH. Pediatric Acute Kidney Injury: Focusing on Diagnosis and Management. Child Kidney Disease. 2020; 24(1):19-26.
13. de Galasso L, Picca S, Guzzo I. Dialysis modalities for the management of pediatric acute kidney injury. Pediatr Nephrol. 2020;35(5):753-65.
14. Jetton JG, Boohaker Ij, Sethi SK, Wazir S, Rohatgi S, Soranno DE, et al. Incidence and outcome of neonatal AKI (AWAKEN): A multicenter, multinational cohort study. Lancet Child Adolesc Health. 2017;1(3):184-94.
15. Kaddourah A, Basu RK, Bagshaw SM, Goldstein SL; AWARE Investigators. Epidemiology of acute kidney injury in critically ill children and young adults. N Engl J Med. 2017;376(1):11-20.
16. Kavaz A, Ozçakar ZB, Kendirli T, Oztürk BB, Ekim M, Yalçinkaya F, et al. Acute kidney injury in a paediatric intensive care unit: Comparison of the pRIFLE and AKIN criteria. Acta Paediatr. 2012;101(3):e126-9.
17. KDIGO. KDIGO Clinical Practice Guideline for Acute Kidney Injury. Kidney international supplements. Int J Nephrol. 2012;2(1):19-36.
18. Krishnamurthy S, Mondal N, Narayanan P, Biswal N, Srinivasan S, Soundravally R. Incidence and etiology of acute kidney injury in southern India. Indian J Pediatr. 2013;80(3):183-9.
19. Menon S, Kikendall ES, Aguyen H, Goldstein SL. AKI associated with high nephrotoxin medication exposure leads to CKD after 6 months. J Pediatr. 2014;165(3) 522-7
20. Schneider J, Khemani R, Grushkin C, Bart R. Serum creatinine as stratified in the RIFLE score for acute kidney injury is associated with mortality and length of stay for children in the pediatric intensive care unit. Crit Care Med. 2010;38(3):933-9.
21. Sethi SK, Bunchman T, Chakraborty R, Raina R. Pediatric acute kidney injury: New advances in the last decade. Kidney Res Clin Pract. 2021;40(1):40-51.
22. Tóth R, Breuer T, Cserép Z, Lex D, Fazekas L, Sápi E, et al. Acute kidney injury is associated with higher morbidity and resource utilization in pediatric patients undergoing heart surgery. Ann Thorac Surg. 2012;93(6):1984-90.
23. Zapitelli M, Ambalavanam N, Askenazi DJ, Moxey-Mims MM, Kimmel PL, Star RA, et al. Developing a neonatal AKI research definition: A report from the NIDDK neonatal AKI workshop. Pediatr Res. 2017;82(4):569-73
24. Zappitelli M, Goldstein SL, Ricci Z. Evaluation and management of AKI in children. Emma P, Goldstein SL, Bagga A, Bates CL, Shroff R (Eds). Pediatric Nephrology, 8th edition. Berlin, Germany: Springer; 2022. pp. 1624, 1626, 1632.

CHAPTER 106

Enuresis

Jyoti Sharma

INTRODUCTION

Enuresis refers to intermittent incontinence in discrete episodes while asleep; sometimes called nocturnal enuresis (NE) to add extra clarity. The International Children's Continence Society recommends therapy for these children once they are 6 years old.

It is essential to subgroup these children as having monosymptomatic (MNE) and nonmonosymptomatic enuresis (NMNE). The latter refers to children who have concomitant symptoms of lower urinary tract (LUT) dysfunction, identified by increased (>8 times) or decreased (<3 times) voiding frequency, daytime incontinence, urgency, hesitancy, straining, a weak stream, intermittency, voiding postponement (holding maneuvers), a feeling of incomplete emptying, post-micturition dribble, and genital or LUT pain.

CLINICAL PEARLS

- Nonmonosymptomatic enuresis is more common; when a detailed history is obtained, most children have daytime symptoms.
- Perceptions of daytime voiding symptoms seem to differ; hence, careful questioning of the child is recommended.

The term secondary enuresis is used to describe children who have had a previous dry period of at least 6 months. A cause for secondary enuresis can usually be identified and management should be directed toward this **(Table 1)**.

The focus of this chapter is primary enuresis and does not address pathological conditions causing enuresis e.g., neurogenic bladder; or when enuresis is a manifestation of polyuria e.g. in chronic kidney disease (tubulointerstitial), diabetes mellitus.

PATHOGENESIS

The three factors presumed to play a role in the pathogenesis and also targeted for management are:

TABLE 1: Conditions that may precipitate secondary enuresis.

Condition	*Possible mechanism*
Cystitis	Bladder overactivity
Diabetes mellitus	Polyuria
Diabetes insipidus	Polyuria
Chronic kidney disease (tubulointerstitial disease)	Polyuria
Neurogenic bladder	Reduced bladder capacity
Psychological stress	—

BOX 1: Important bladder volumes.

- *Expected bladder capacity (EBC):* For children >1 year of age = [Age (years) + 1] × 30 mL
- Maximum bladder capacity is too small if <65% or too large if >150% EBC
- *Nocturnal polyuria:* Volume of urine voided during the night (diaper weight) + volume of 1st morning void >130%

1. *A disorder of sleep arousal:* Children do not wake up to the sensation of a full or contracting bladder.
2. A reduced bladder capacity as recorded on a voiding diary [maximum voided volume (MVV) of the child <65% expected bladder capacity (EBC)]. EBC = (age + 1) × 30 mL **(Box 1)**. Younger children have a small normal functional bladder capacity.
3. Nocturnal polyuria due to inadequate secretion of antidiuretic hormone; the amount of urine produced during the night exceeds EBC by 130%. Additional factors that may contribute to nocturnal polyuria include a low fluid intake during the school hours, *large intakes in the evening,* and a high solute intake (dinner) close to the bedtime.

In addition, there may be certain *comorbid conditions* associated with enuresis that need to be addressed either concomitantly or prior to the management of enuresis.

Flowchart 1: Evaluation of a child with enuresis.

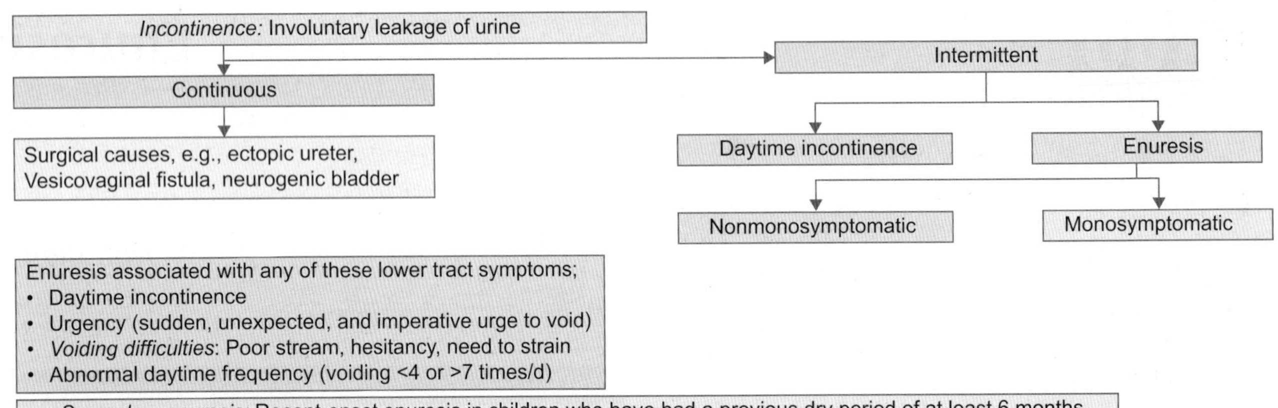

Neuropsychiatric disorders, such as attention deficit hyperactivity disorder (ADHD), *obesity*, and *constipation* must be managed concurrently. The bladder, which lies in the narrowest dependent portion of the funnel formed by the pelvic bones, is impinged upon by the impacted mass of stool in the small pelvis of a child who suffers from constipation; nocturnal colonic movement may stimulate detrusor contractions causing enuresis. *Adenotonsillar hypertrophy* is also associated with enuresis and surgery ameliorates sleep-disordered breathing as well as enuresis in some children.

HISTORY

History taking for evaluation of enuresis is given in **Flowchart 1.**

The most important aspect of evaluation of a child with enuresis is a meticulous history, which can establish whether enuresis is primary or secondary. If primary is it monosymptomatic or nonmonosymptomatic and to identify any associated comorbidities, most children do not need investigations.

CLINICAL PEARLS

Usefulness of a voiding diary:
- Provides objective data that may support the history.
- Helps detect children with NMNE.
- Detects children who require extra evaluation.
- *Detects families with low adherence to instructions:* If they are unable to keep a diary, they are unlikely to comply with the support required for the use of the alarm.

Parents are requested to maintain a record over 2–3 days of a frequency–volume chart and a record of bowel movements during a week. Points to be noted are details of fluid intake, daytime voiding pattern, and number and time of episodes of bedwetting. Other details required are a sleep history, which should include the time the child goes to bed, falls asleep, and awakens in the morning, and the presence of snoring. Presence of an overactive bladder, i.e., frequency, urgency, maneuvers to suppress the urge to void (squatting behavior), daytime incontinence, and nighttime wetting including the amount and number of times of wetting should be noted. The history should carefully rule out a pathological cause of polyuria that may manifest as enuresis for example, weight loss, and decreased activity as may be seen in a child with chronic kidney disease or diabetes mellitus.

PHYSICAL EXAMINATION

The examination should be carried out to exclude pathological causes of incontinence, i.e., measurement of blood pressure, inspection of external genitalia and of the lumbosacral spine, palpation in the renal and suprapubic areas to look for enlarged kidneys or bladder, and a thorough neurologic examination of the lower extremities. Abnormal physical findings are absent in children when enuresis is the sole symptom.

LABORATORY TESTING AND IMAGING STUDIES

A urine examination by dipstick is warranted in children to rule out a urinary tract infection and glycosuria only where there is a clinical suspicion. Ultrasonography (USG) of the pelvis, performed occasionally, is helpful in confirming the presence of constipation which is identified as a rectal diameter of greater than 30 mm. It may also be used to rule out a suspected pathological condition by ruling out hydroureteronephrosis, increased bladder wall thickness, and a postvoid residue.

MANAGEMENT

Enuresis that occurs as infrequently as once a month is associated with reduced self-esteem and treatment has been reported to improve self-esteem. Management should be instituted as soon as the child is motivated to be dry, and the parents are supportive. An explanation of the probable cause of the enuresis is important. Motivation of the child needs to be sustained by providing emotional support and an attempt to remove any feelings of guilt. *Efforts of the child to remain dry* need to be rewarded with praise.

Behavioral Therapy or Urotherapy

Behavioral modification or urotherapy directed at good bladder and bowel health offers the potential to alleviate daytime symptoms **(Box 2)**. It also increases the success rate of the alarm or pharmacological therapy when enuresis is accompanied by daytime symptoms. Clinical experience suggests that the ability to establish a rapport with the child and to induce and sustain motivation is important for successful behavioral therapy. Specific therapy for enuresis should be initiated simultaneously as given in **Flowchart 2**.

BOX 2: Behavioral therapy—good bladder and bowel habits.

- Advise regarding timed voiding during the day, i.e., every 3–4 hours, frequent enough to avoid urgency/incontinence, including during school hours, and before going to bed
- Voiding should be unhurried and complete
- Instruct to drink liberal amounts of fluids during the day (50–75 mL/kg/ day), not to drink excess with the evening meal, and to minimize fluid intake afterward
- Encourage good bowel health, characterized by a soft-bowel movement passed without discomfort every morning before the child leaves for school
- Strategies to improve bowel emptying include the intake of foods that soften stool, use of a stool softener, and patient and parent education about optimal posture to relax the pelvic floor muscles. Children should be counseled not to rush or push

CLINICAL PEARLS

Training programs that involve either "holding on" and waiting before voiding or stopping the flow of urine have not been shown to be effective, and hence, have no role in management.

Alarm Therapy

Alarm therapy is presumed to cure enuresis by the conditioning effects on arousal and by increasing nocturnal bladder capacity. The device consists of a sensor and is attached to the child's underwear or to a mat placed below the child, which is activated when the child begins to wet the bed. It works on the principle that sustained use causes conditioned wakening to a full bladder. Success rate with alarm therapy is 50–75% and is dependent on the motivation of the child and that of the parents who must participate in the therapy. It requires a minimum 3-month trial. A relapse can be minimized by close follow-up during therapy and by "overlearning", which involves slowly increasing the evening fluid intake in successfully treated patients while continuing to wear the alarm.

Desmopressin Acetate

Desmopressin acetate (DDAVP) is a synthetic vasopressin (ADH) analog recommended when nocturnal polyuria is present or when alarm therapy alone fails or when alarm is not acceptable. It is also a useful therapy for short-term

Flowchart 2: Management of enuresis.

- Educate child and parents about the condition
- Normalize fluid intake
- Advise about good voiding and bowel habits

↓

- If nocturnal urine output is normal
- Low max daytime voided volumes
alarm is the 1st choice

- Nocturnal polyuria present
- Normal daytime voided volume
desmopressin is tried first

↓

- Regardless of the strategy—if the first choice of therapy (alarm or desmopressin) did not make the child dry then the other alternative should be offered.
- If both fail as monotherapy a combination of the two can be considered

use on special occasions, for example, for stayovers and camps. It is available as a *melt* tablet (120–240 µg), to be taken 1 hour before bedtime. The patient is advised to restrict evening fluid intake to <200 mL and the last drink to be taken 1 hour before the tablet to avoid the risk of hyponatremia. DDAVP may need to be used for months to years and has a high relapse rate. A slow stepwise dose reduction over 6–7 months is recommended when a decision to discontinue therapy has been made.

Patients with therapy-resistant enuresis should be managed by a specialist. Anticholinergics (oxybutynin or tolterodine) can be considered as a second-line antienuretic therapy in combination with desmopressin when bladder overactivity is suspected to contribute to enuresis. Presence of residual urine should be excluded and there should be no constipation.

The International Children's Continence Society recommends that imipramine should be used only when all other therapies have failed, only after assessment by a healthcare professional who specializes in the management of bedwetting. Its use is limited by its potential to cause cardiotoxicity.

CONCLUSION

Nocturnal enuresis is very common and has the potential to cause appreciable negative emotional impact on affected children. It is important to take history to differentiate between MNE and NMNE. Urotherapy, alarm, and desmopressin are the initial measures of management. Treatment for comorbid conditions, like constipation and ADHD, must be offered simultaneously.

KEY POINTS

- A detailed history regarding enuresis, associated daytime symptoms, and comorbid conditions should be substantiated with a voiding diary.
- Constipation, daytime incontinence, and adenotonsillar hypertrophy if present, should be treated.
- The mainstay of management of primary MNE is the enuresis alarm and desmopressin.
- Second-line therapy is best used in consultation with a specialist.

SUGGESTED READING

1. Kosilov KV, Geltser BI, Loparev SA, Kuzina IG, Shakirova OV, Zhuravskaya NS, et al. The optimal duration of alarm therapy use in children with primary monosymptomatic nocturnal enuresis. J Pediatr Urol. 2018;14(5):447.e1-6.
2. Nevéus T, Fonseca E, Franco I, Kawauchi A, Kovacevic L, Nieuwhof-Leppink A, et al. Management and treatment of nocturnal enuresis-an updated standardization document from the International Children's Continence Society. J Pediatr Urol. 2020;16(1):10-9.
3. Nevéus T. Pathogenesis of enuresis: Towards a new understanding. Int J Urol. 2017;24(3):174-82.
4. Vande Walle J, Rittig S, Tekgül S, Austin P, Yang SS, Lopez PJ, et al. Enuresis: Practical guidelines for primary care. Br J Gen Pract. 2017;67(660):328-9.

Approach to Renal Tubular Disorders in Children

Manoj G Matnani

INTRODUCTION

Renal tubules are the real brains of the kidney. They reabsorb most of the glomerular ultrafiltrate and fine-tune the remainder of urine by the processes of concentration, dilution, acidification, and secretion in order to maintain an intact homeostatic milieu on a continuous basis.

Hence, it is obvious that disorders of the renal tubules will lead to serious fluid-electrolyte and acid–base disturbances, affecting the growth and development of the child, and sometimes even posing a serious threat to survival.

PATHOPHYSIOLOGY

Pathophysiology of renal tubular disorders is given in **Table 1**.

Functionally, various diseases affecting a particular segment of the kidney lead to the following pathophysiological features:

- Disorders affecting the proximal tubule, which is the main site of reabsorption of multiple solutes, for example, Fanconi's syndrome.
- Disorders affecting the loop of Henle and the early parts of the distal tubule, which fine-tune the sodium chloride reabsorption and potassium secretion, for example, Bartter syndrome and its variants.
- Disorders affecting the α-intercalated cells of the cortical collecting ducts, which are the main site for hydrogen ion secretion (aldosterone-sensitive segment), for example, distal renal tubular acidosis (RTA), type 4 RTA, and pseudohypoaldosteronism.
- Disorders affecting the medullary collecting ducts, which is the antidiuretic hormone (ADH)-sensitive segment (responsible for water reabsorption through aquaporin channels), for example, nephrogenic diabetes insipidus (DI).
- Disorders affecting primarily the phosphate (PO_4) reabsorption by the proximal tubule, for example, X-linked hereditary hypophosphatemic rickets (XLHHR)

CLINICAL FEATURES

The clinical features are given in **Figure 1**.

TABLE 1: Clinicophysiologic correlation of renal tubular disorders.

Segment	*Function*	*Disorder*
Proximal tubule	Phosphate transport	Hypophosphatemic rickets
	Glucose transport	Renal glucosuria
	Amino-acid transport	Isolated, generalized aminoaciduria
	Bicarbonate transport	Proximal renal tubular acidosis
Ascending limb of loop of Henle	Sodium–potassium chloride transport (NKCC-2 and others)	Bartter syndrome and variants
Distal tubule	Proton secretion	Distal RTA
	Sodium chloride transport (sodium chloride cotransporter)	Gitelman syndrome
Collecting duct	Sodium-potassium transport	Pseudohypoaldosteronism
	Sodium transport (epithelial sodium channel)	Liddle's syndrome
	Water transport	Nephrogenic diabetes insipidus

(RTA: renal tubular acidosis)

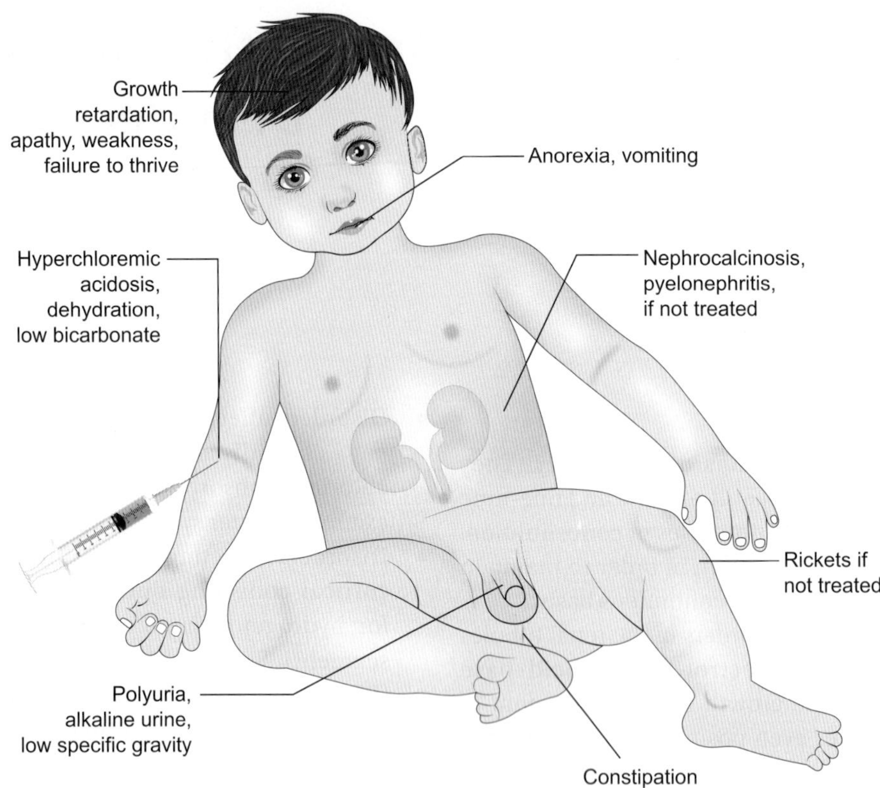

Fig. 1: Features suggestive of renal tubular disorders.

Clinical Features

- Recurrent episodes of dehydration, vomiting, and fever causing growth retardation and failure to thrive
- Polyuria, polydipsia causing constipation and preference for savory foods and salt craving
- Refractory rickets, bone pains, and muscle weakness causing delayed gross motor milestones
- Renal calculi and nephrocalcinosis, if untreated for prolonged periods
- Hypertension seen in monogenic disorders, for example, Liddle's syndrome/pseudohypoaldosteronism

Laboratory Features

- Hyperchloremic metabolic acidosis
- Metabolic alkalosis with or without hypokalemia
- Hyponatremia with hyperkalemia
- Hypercalciuria with normal serum calcium

The clinical phenotypes can be classified into following four groups:

1. *Hyperchloremic normal anion gap metabolic acidosis:* RTA, Fanconi's syndrome
2. *Hypokalemic metabolic alkalosis:* Bartter syndrome and its variants
3. *Polyuria with/without hypernatremic dehydration with normal acid-base status*: Nephrogenic diabetes insipidus (DI)
4. *Rickets with phosphate wasting*: Fanconi's syndrome, XLHHR.

CLINICAL PEARLS

Suspect renal tubular disorder in a child with gastroenteritis if:

- The amount of dehydration is out of proportion to the number of loose stools
- Fairly preserved urine output despite severe dehydration

EVALUATION OF RENAL TUBULAR DISORDERS

Evaluation of renal tubule disorders is given in **Flowcharts 1 and 2**.

- Estimate acid-base status—metabolic acidosis or metabolic alkalosis
  - If metabolic acidosis, determine

$$\text{Plasma anion gap} = Na^+ - (Cl^- + HCO_3^-)$$

Flowchart 1: Approach to metabolic acidosis.

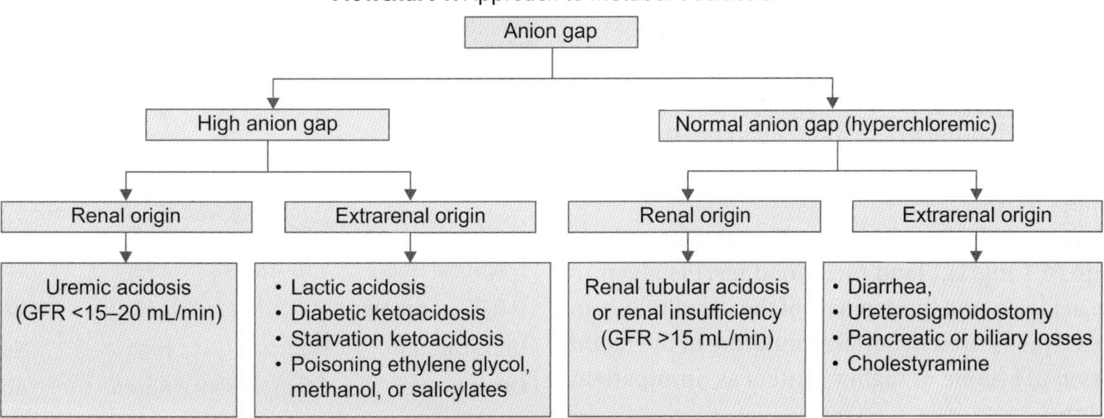

(GFR: glomerular filtration rate)

Flowchart 2: Evaluation of a patient with renal tubular acidosis.

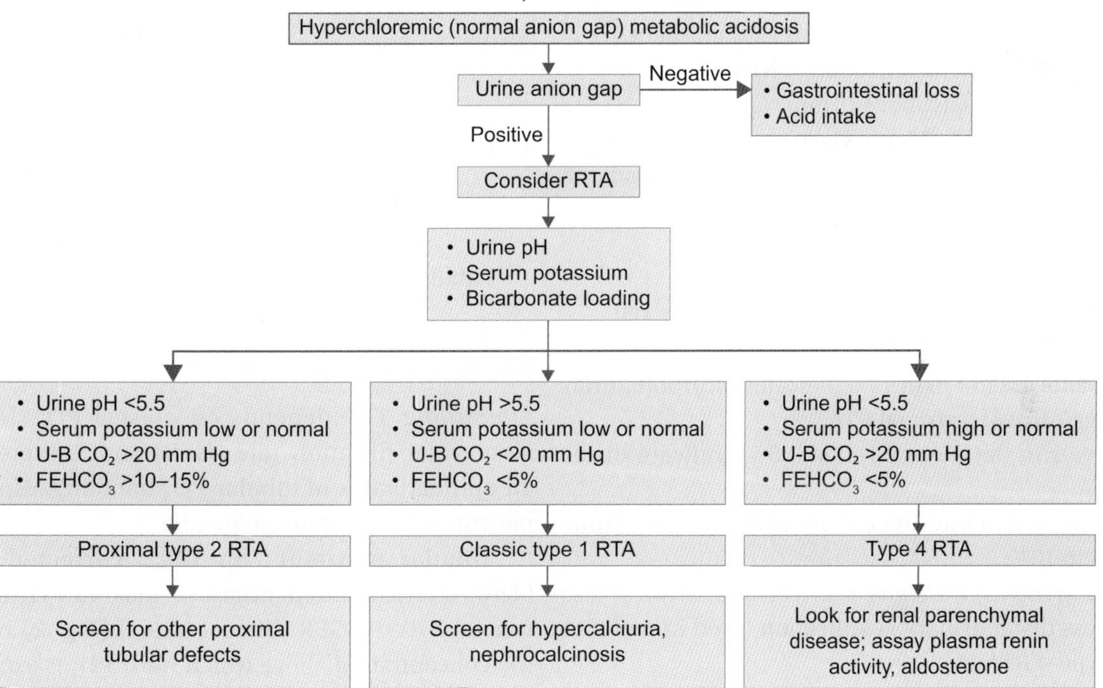

($FEHCO_3$: fractional excretion of bicarbonate; RTA: renal tubular acidosis; U-B CO_2: urine to blood CO_2 gradient)

- Normal plasma anion gap is 8–12 mEq/L. Normal anion gap is seen in RTA (renal loss of HCO_3^-) and diarrhea (gastrointestinal loss of HCO_3^-)

- *Estimate urine anion gap (UAG):* The UAG (urine net charge) is useful for estimating NH_4^+ excretion in patients with hyperchloremic metabolic acidosis.

$$Na^+ + K^+ + \text{Unmeasured cations} = Cl^- + \text{Unmeasured anions}$$

- Since the sum of charges on cations and anions is equal, the difference between unmeasured anions (sulfates, phosphates, and organic anions) and cations (calcium and magnesium) is relatively constant (about 80 mEq/L), hence,

$$Na^+ + K^+ + NH_4^+ = Cl^- + 80$$

- The UAG is the difference between the sum of urinary Na^+, K^+, and Cl^-, hence UAG gives an approximate estimate of urinary NH_4^+ excretion.

$$UAG = 80 - NH_4^+$$

A positive UAG indicates inappropriately low renal NH_4^+ excretion, as seen in RTA.

- *Determine the urine pH:* It is useful for assessing the integrity of distal urinary acidification.
    - Presence of urine pH >5.5 during metabolic acidosis suggests defective distal secretion of H^+ (distal RTA); urine pH <5.5 is seen in proximal RTA or in patients with selective aldosterone deficiency (type-4 RTA)
- If systemic acidosis is absent, an oral ammonium chloride (0.1 mg/kg) load (acid load test) is given to induce acidosis, and the capacity of the distal tubule to secrete H^+ is assessed by serial monitoring of the blood and urine pH (done at higher centers as an inpatient procedure).
- To characterize the type of RTA, bicarbonate loading test is done:
    - Measurement of fractional excretion of bicarbonate ($FEHCO_3$) and urine to blood CO_2 gradient (U-B CO_2) allows characterization of RTA.
    - The urine PCO_2 is above 70 mm Hg and the U-B CO_2 gradient is above 20 mm Hg in normal individuals.
    - Urine PCO_2 below 50 mm Hg and U-B CO_2 gradient below 10 mm Hg suggests distal RTA.
- $FEHCO_3$ (%) =

$$\frac{\text{Urine bicarnbonate} \times \text{plasma creatinine}}{\text{Plasma bicarbonate} \times \text{urine creatinine}} \times 100$$

- A value greater than 15% indicates bicarbonaturia, suggestive of proximal RTA.
- Levels in the normal range (<5%) indicate distal RTA.
- In hyperkalemic (type 4 RTA), levels vary from 5% to 10%.
- *Fludrocortisone furosemide test:* This is a sensitive test to assess distal urinary acidification, used in patients with type-4 RTA.

Additional Tests for Renal Tubular Acidosis

Additional tests for renal tubular acidosis are given in **Table 2 and Flowchart 3**.

Proximal Renal Tubular Acidosis (Type 2)

Proximal RTA (type 2) needs evaluation for other proximal tubular functions.

- Evaluation of aminoaciduria, glucosuria, and low-molecular-weight proteinuria (if available)
- Assessment of phosphate excretion to assess phosphaturia

TABLE 2: Investigations to differentiate types of renal tubular acidosis (RTA).

	Proximal RTA	*Distal RTA*	*Type 4 RTA*
Plasma K^+	Normal/low	Normal/low	High
Urine pH	<5.5	>5.5	<5.5
Urine anion gap	Positive	Positive	Positive
Urine NH_4^+	Low	Low	Low
Fractional HCO_3^-	>10–15%	<5%	>5–10%
U-B PCO_2 mm Hg	>20	<20	>20
Urine calcium	Normal	High	Normal/low
Other tubular defects	Often present	Absent	Absent
Nephrocalcinosis	Absent	Present	Absent
Bone diseases	Common	Often present	Absent

(U-B PCO_2: urine-to-blood PCO_2 gradient)

- Fractional excretion of phosphate ($FEPO_4$) =

$$\frac{\text{Urine phosphate} \times \text{plasma creatinine}}{\text{Plasma phosphate} \times \text{urine creatinine}} \times 100$$

Tubular reabsorption of PO_4^{3-} (TRP) = 100 – $FEPO_4$.

Normally, 5–15% of the filtered PO_4^{3-} is excreted and the tubular reabsorption is 85–95%

Limitation: TRP depends on plasma PO_4^{3-} levels and glomerular filtration rate (GFR) and is therefore, not an optimal index of tubular PO_4 handling, especially in patients with hypophosphatemia.

Tubular maximum for PO_4^{3-}, corrected for GFR (TmP/GFR) is independent of plasma PO_4 and renal function. TmP/ GFR (Bijvoet index) **(Fig. 2)** represents the concentration above which most PO_4 is excreted and below which most is reabsorbed. The normal value is 2.8–4.4 mg/dL with lower values for older children and can be calculated from **Figure 2**.

Distal Renal Tubular Acidosis (Type 1)

All patients should undergo:

- Hearing evaluation to diagnose proton adenosine triphosphatase channel defects causing distal RTA.
- Renal ultrasound for medullary nephrocalcinosis **(Fig. 3)** and renal calculi
- Measurement of urinary calcium and citrate excretion to assess hypercalciuria and hypocitraturia

Flowchart 3: Diagnostic approach to hypokalemic metabolic alkalosis with/without hypertension.

- Hypokalemic metabolic acidosis
  - Hypertension
    - No
      - Age of onset
        - Neonatal/infancy
          - Hypermagnesemia → HELIX syndrome
          - Hypomagnesemia → EAST syndrome (neurological extrarenal manifestations)
          - Normomagnesemia (or mild hypomagnesemia) → Bartter syndrome (Type III/IV associated with mild hypomagnesemia)
        - Early childhood/ adolescence → Gitelman syndrome
    - Yes
      - • ↓ Aldosterone • ↓Renin → Liddle syndrome or Apparent mineralocorticoid excess
      - • ↑ Aldosterone • ↓ Renin → Primary hyperaldosteronism

(EAST: Epilepsy, Ataxia, Sensorineural deafness, and (a renal salt-wasting) Tubulopathy. HELIX: Hypohidrosis, Electrolyte imbalance, Lacrimal gland dysfunction, Ichthyosis, Xerostomia)

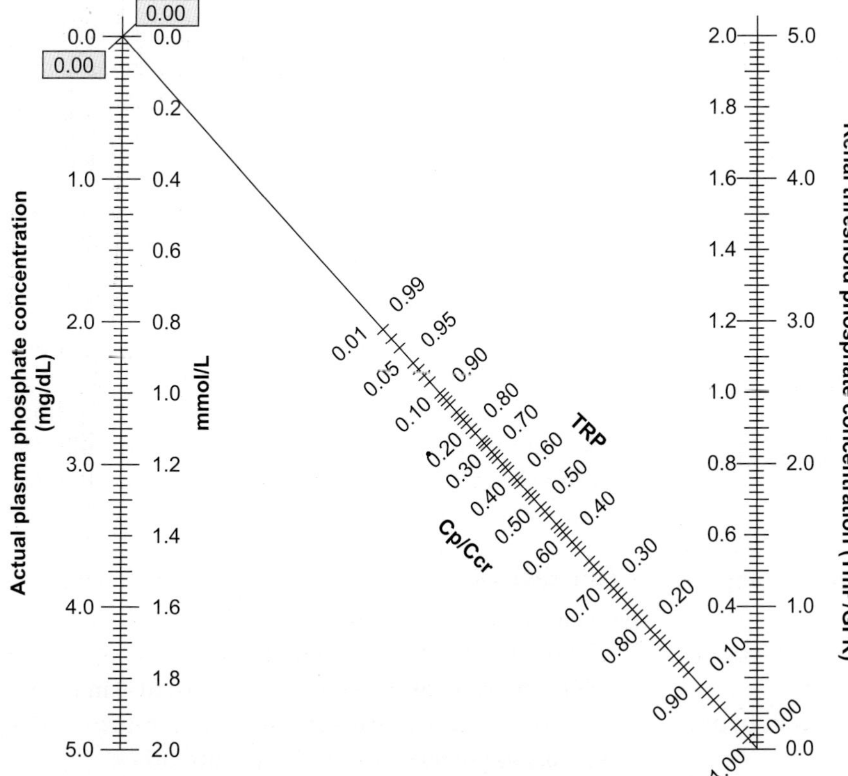

Fig. 2: Bijvoet nomogram for estimation of renal threshold phosphate concentration (TmP/GFR). (Cp: renal phosphate clearance; Ccr: creatinine clearance; GFR: glomerular filtration rate; TRP: tubular reabsorption of phosphate; TmP/GFR: tubular maximum for phosphate, corrected GFR)

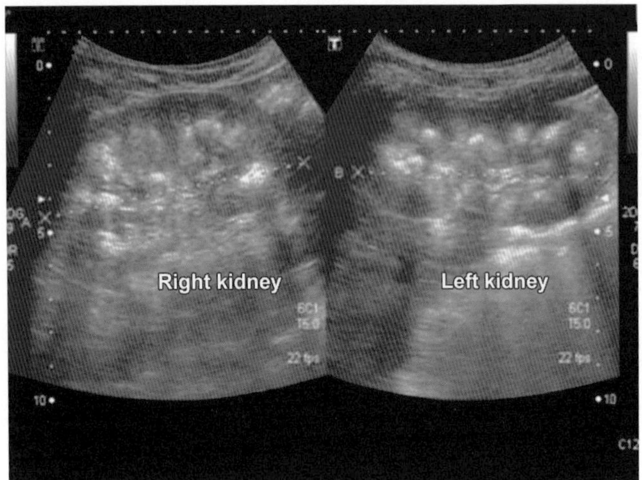

Fig. 3: Medullary nephrocalcinosis in a child with distal renal tubular acidosis (RTA).

- Hypercalciuria (*see* **Appendix** for normal values) and hyperphosphaturia occur due to:
  - The release of calcium phosphate from bone in order to buffer excess H^+ during acidosis
  - The direct effects of acidosis on tubular reabsorption of these ions
- Hypocitraturia results from:
  - Citrate utilization in proximal tubular cells
  - Due to high luminal pH favoring conversion of $citrate^{3-}$ to the readily absorbable $citrate^{2-}$

Hyperkalemic Renal Tubular Acidosis (Type 4)

In children, aldosterone unresponsiveness is more common than aldosterone deficiency and is commonly associated with obstructive uropathy.

Transtubular potassium gradient (TTKG): This provides an accurate estimate of aldosterone effect on late distal and cortical collecting tubules.

$$\text{TTKG} = \text{Urine } K^+ \times \text{Plasma osmolality/Plasma } K^+ \times \text{Urine osmolality}$$

It is an index of K^+ gradient in the distal tubular lumen and interstitial blood capillaries. Normal range is 6–12.

- Hypokalemia from extrarenal causes results in renal K^+ conservation and TTKG<2.
- Higher TTKG suggests renal losses, as seen in hyperaldosteronism.
- During hyperkalemia, the expected TTKG should be greater than 10, an inappropriately low level suggests hypoaldosteronism or tubular resistance to aldosterone.

EVALUATION OF METABOLIC ALKALOSIS

Algorithmic approach to evaluation of metabolic alkalosis is given in **Flowchart 4**).

- Rule out common causes first, namely, vomiting, nasogastric suction, diuretic usage, or drugs like bicarbonate and steroids.
- Examine for presence of dehydration/hypovolemia and hypertension.
- Clinical features like failure to thrive and triangular facies suggest Bartter syndrome.
- Laboratory investigations needed serum electrolytes (Na^+, K^+, and Cl^-), urine electrolytes (Na^+, K^+, and Cl^-), plasma renin activity, and aldosterone levels in patients with hypertension.
- Rare monogenic disorders (Liddle's syndrome and 11β-hydroxysteroid dehydrogenase deficiency) present with hypertension, mild metabolic alkalosis, and hypokalemia and can be evaluated through the algorithmic approach mentioned in **Flowchart 5**.

TREATMENT GUIDELINES

- *Alkali supplements:* Bicarbonate solutions **(Table 3)** and tablets to correct acidosis are given. The requirement in distal RTA is around 2–5 mEq/kg/day, and higher, around 5–20 mEq/kg/day, in proximal RTA/Fanconi's syndrome.
- Phosphate supplements with vitamin D are needed in Fanconi's syndrome and hypophosphatemic rickets.
- Electrolyte solutions to correct hypokalemia and hyponatremia are needed in salt-losing tubulopathies like Fanconi's syndrome, Bartter's syndrome, etc.
- Thiazides and sometimes prostaglandin inhibitors like indomethacin are used to decrease polyuria **(Flowchart 6)** (to augment growth) in Bartter syndrome and nephrogenic DI.

APPENDIX

Hypercalciuria is defined as:

- 24-hour urine calcium >4 mg/kg/day
- *Spot urine calcium*: Creatinine ratio >0.8 (0–6 months)
  - >0.6 (6 months–2 years)
  - >0.2 (>2 years).

Flowchart 4: Evaluation of a patient with metabolic alkalosis and hypokalemia.

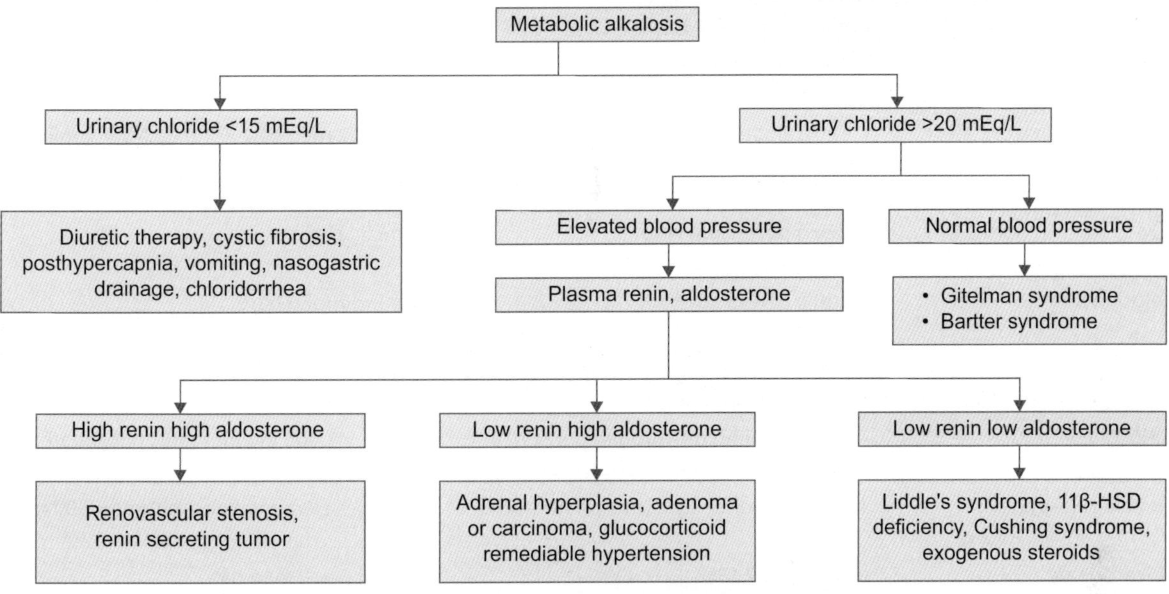

(11 β-HSD: 11b-hydroxysteroid dehydrogenase deficiency)

Flowchart 5: Diagnostic approach to hypokalemic metabolic acidosis with/without low-molecular-weight proteinuria and aminoaciduria.

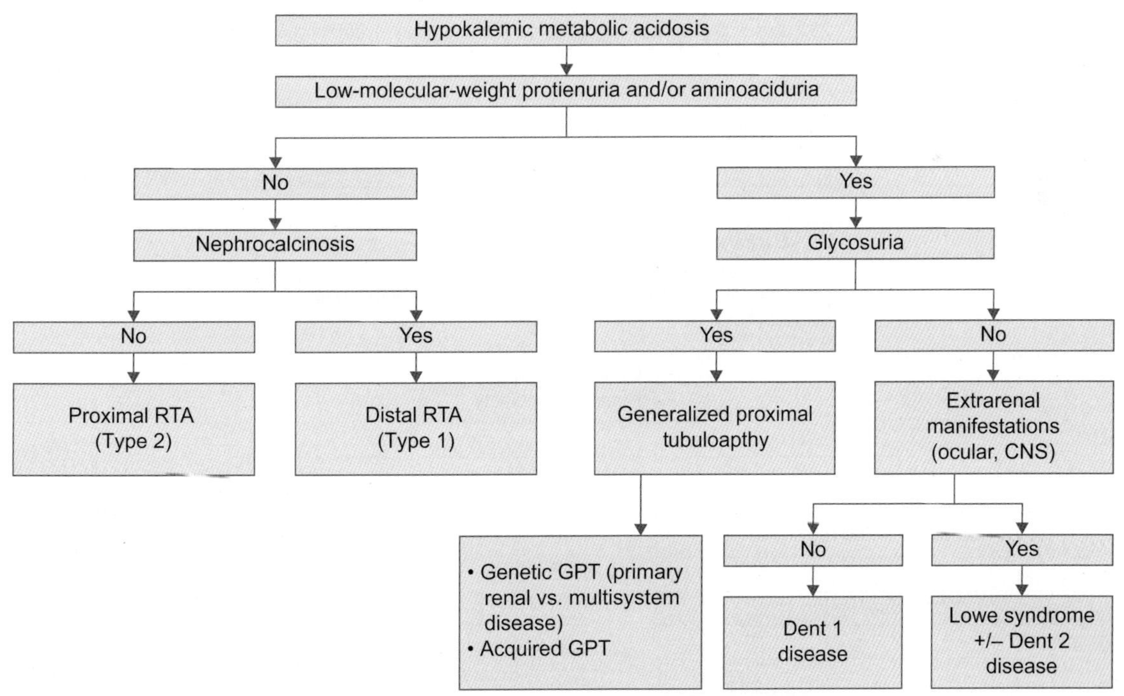

(GPT: generalized proximal tubulopathy; RTA: renal tubular acidosis)

CONCLUSION

It is important to make a prompt and accurate diagnosis of tubulopathies in children and young adults. This allows timely and appropriate management, including disease-specific therapies, and avoids complications such as growth failure. Tubulopathies can present with a variety of nonspecific clinical features that can be diagnostically challenging.

TABLE 3: Commonly available alkali and phosphate supplements.

Preparation	*Composition (per 1,000 mL)*	*Remarks*
Bicitra	• 100 g sodium citrate • 60 g citric acid	1 mL = 1 mEq base
Polycitra	• 110 g potassium citrate • 100 g sodium citrate • 66.8 g citric acid	1 mL = 2 mEq base = 1 mEq Na^+= 1 mEq K^+
Polycitra K	• 220 g potassium citrate • 66.8 g citric acid	1 mL = 2 mEq base
Shohl's solution	• 140 g citric acid • 90 g sodium citrate	1 mL = 1 mEq base
Joulie solution	• 136 g dibasic sodium phosphate • 58.8 g phosphoric acid	1 mL = 30 mg inorganic phosphorous
Neutral phosphate	• 18.2 g sodium dihydrogen phosphate • 145 g dibasic sodium phosphate	60 mL = 1,000 mg inorganic phosphate
• Sodium acid phosphate • (ADDPHOS granules – 3.2 g)	1.936 gm sodium acid phosphate sachet	Provides elemental phosphorus = 500 mg
Sodium bicarbonate	• Solution (7.5%) • 325 and 650 mg tab	• 1 mL = 0.9 mEq base • 325 mg = 4 mEq base
• Sodium bicarbonate • (NODOSIS/SOBISIS) • NODOSIS solution	• 500, 1,000 mg tab • 1000 mg/15 mL solution	• 500 mg = 6 mEq base • 1,000 mg = 12 mEq base • 1,000 mg/15 mL = 12 mEq base
Calcium carbonate	250 and 500 mg tab	1,000 mg = 22.3 mEq base

Flowchart 6: Approach to a patient with polyuria.

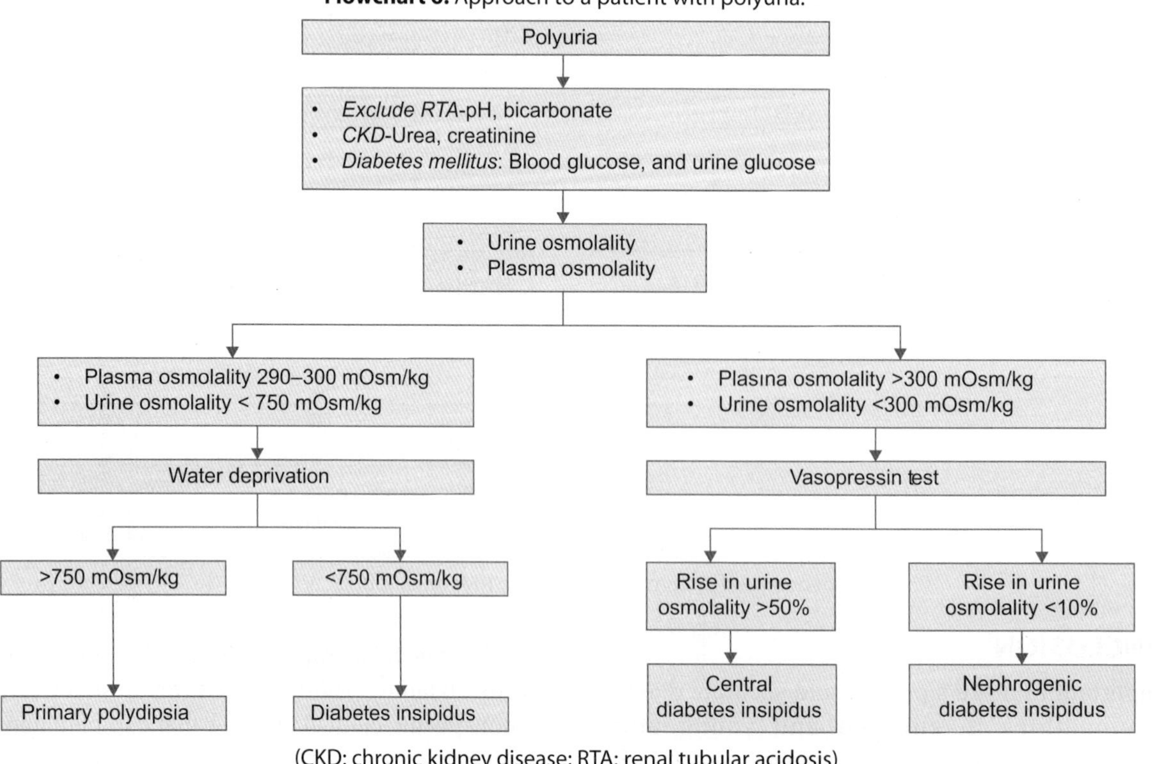

(CKD: chronic kidney disease; RTA: renal tubular acidosis)

KEY POINTS

- Early diagnosis of renal tubular disorders is of paramount importance as most of them present with recurrent life-threatening episodes of vomiting and dehydration.
- Early treatment is essential as it prevents growth failure, stunting, and wasting along with metabolic bone complications like recurrent pathological fractures, osteopenia, etc.
- Early treatment of distal RTA prevents grave consequences like medullary nephrocalcinosis and end-stage renal disease (ESRD), hence it is a preventable cause of ESRD.
- Early treatment of distal RTA leads to good catch-up growth in children. It is important to rule out renal tubular disorder in patients presenting with recurrent dehydration as the blood gas and electrolyte abnormalities frequently overlap in both the conditions (e.g., metabolic acidosis and hypokalemia in gastroenteritis and RTA and metabolic alkalosis and hypokalemia in vomiting and Bartter's syndrome)
- Children with obstructive uropathy should undergo a detailed renal tubular evaluation to categorize the tubulopathy.

SUGGESTED READING

1. Ali U. Renal tubular disorders. IAP: Specialty Series on Pediatric Nephrology. New Delhi: Jaypee Brothers Medical Publishers; 2019. pp. 212-23.
2. Bagga A, Bajpai A, Menon S. Approach to renal tubular disorders. Indian J Pediatr. 2005;72(9):771-6.
3. Bagga A, Sinha A, Gulati A. Metabolic alkalosis. Protocols in Pediatric Nephrology. New Delhi: CBS Publishers and Distributers; 2012. pp. 66-72.
4. Bagga A, Sinha A, Gulati A. Renal tubular acidosis. Protocols in Pediatric Nephrology. New Delhi: CBS Publishers and Distributers; 2012. pp. 55-65.
5. Kermond R, Mallett A, McCarthy H. A clinical approach to tubulopathies in children and young adults. Pediatr Nephrol. 2023;38(3):651-62
6. Sobh M. Renal tubular disorders. Essentials of Clinical Nephrology. Cairo, Egypt: Dar El Shorouk; 2000. pp. 197-211.

CHAPTER 108

Nephrotic Syndrome in Children

Mukta Mantan, Anand S Vasudev

INTRODUCTION

Nephrotic syndrome is a common chronic disorder in children, characterized by heavy proteinuria (>40 mg/m²/h in timed urine sample), hypoalbuminemia, and edema. The proteinuria in nephrotic syndrome is relatively selective and constitutes primarily of albumin. The peak incidence of the disease is in between 2 and 6 years of age. 90% of the children with minimal change disease respond to treatment with steroids. Majority of these relapse and about 50–60% become steroid-dependent or frequent relapsers. Frequency of relapses is higher in first 10 years after the diagnosis. By puberty, the relapse rate decreases and most children show sustained remission.

Some common definitions to describe the course of nephrotic syndrome are listed in **Table 1**.

The most common etiology of childhood nephrotic syndrome is minimal change disease. The other glomerular etiologies causing nephrotic syndrome are focal segmental glomerular sclerosis, mesangioproliferative glomerulonephritis, membranoproliferative glomerulonephritis, and membranous nephropathy.

TABLE 1: Definitions.

Terms	*Definitions*
Nephrotic syndrome	Presence of edema, serum albumin <3.0 g/dL and proteinuria >40 mg/m²/h in timed urine sample or urine spot (mg/mg) Up/Uc >2
Relapse	Urine protein ≥3 by dipstick or Up/Uc >2 mg/mg for 3 consecutive early morning samples having been in remission previously
Remission	Urine protein nil or trace by dipstick or Up/Uc <0.2 mg/mg for 3 consecutive early morning samples
Frequent relapses	Two or more relapses in 6 months of initial response or > 3 in 6 months or >4 in any 12-month period
Steroid dependence	Occurrence of 2 consecutive relapses during steroid therapy or within 2 weeks of its cessation in absence of infections
Steroid-resistance	Failure to achieve remission after 6 weeks of daily therapy of steroids (prednisolone oral) 2 mg/kg/day
Initial resistance	Failure to achieve complete remission after 6-week initial therapy with prednisolone
Late resistance	Initially, steroid-sensitive and develops steroid resistance in any subsequent relapse
Calcineurin (CNI)-resistant nephrotic syndrome	Nonresponse to cyclosporine or tacrolimus, given in adequate doses and titrated to optimal blood trough levels, for 6-month
Complicated relapse	Relapse associated with life-threatening complications like hypovolemia requiring admission, serious infection (peritonitis, cellulitis, and meningitis) or thrombosis

(Up/Uc: urinary protein or creatinine ratio)

EVALUATION

The primary evaluation of a child with suspected nephrotic syndrome includes estimation of serum total proteins, albumin, globulin, cholesterol, urea, and creatinine concentrations. Urinary proteins can be estimated with dipsticks. Values of >+3 proteins are indicative of nephrotic range proteinuria. Urinary spot samples can be used for determining the urinary protein or creatinine ratio. Values beyond 2 are suggestive of nephrotic range proteinuria. Hepatitis B status should be determined if the child is unimmunized. Serum complement (C3) levels are recommended if persistent hematuria or hypertension occurs. Acute infections should be ruled out; latent or active tuberculosis too should be identified before starting prednisolone. Investigations at first and subsequent relapses are provided in **Box 1**. Urine culture and sensitivity is indicated only if clinical features of urinary tract infection are there.

BOX 1: Investigations at first episode of nephrotic syndrome.

- Investigations
  - Urinalysis
  - Blood counts
  - KFT, serum proteins, albumin, globulin, and total cholesterol
  - CXR and tuberculin test

  Additional investigations
  - C3, C4, ASLO, if hematuria and hypertension
  - HBSAg, anti HCV—if history of jaundice, liver disease
  - Usg (KUB), only if hematuria and renal vein thrombosis is suspected or planning renal biopsy

  Subsequent relapses
  - KFT, serum albumin, total cholesterol
  - CBC if infection suspected

(ASLO: antistreptolysin O; CBC: complete blood count; CXR: chest X-ray; HBSAg: hepatitis B surface antigen; HCV: hepatitis C virus; KFT: kidney function test; KUB: kidney, ureter, and bladder X-ray)

INDICATIONS FOR RENAL BIOPSY

Renal biopsy is indicated for children with steroid-resistant nephrotic syndrome, gross or persistent microscopic hematuria, or persistent hypertension. Children with features suggestive of systemic lupus erythematosus, other secondary causes of nephrotic syndrome, or before starting calcineurin inhibitors should also be biopsied. Prolonged (>30–36 months) therapy with calcineurin inhibitors (CNI) or reduced kidney function during their use is also an indication.

MANAGEMENT

Management of nephrotic syndrome includes specific and supportive management **(Table 2)**.

Specific Management

Treatment of the Initial Episode

Indian Society of Pediatric Nephrology currently recommends that initial episode of nephrotic syndrome be treated with prednisolone at 2 mg/kg (maximum 60 mg) or 60 mg/m^2 in single or divided dose for 6 weeks followed by 1.5 mg/kg (maximum 40 mg) or 40 mg/m^2 single-morning dose on alternate days for next 6 weeks.

Management of Relapse

Identify and treat any infections present. Prednisolone is administered at a dose of 2 mg/kg/day until protein is nil or trace for 3 consecutive days followed by 1.5 mg/kg/day on alternate days for 4 weeks and then discontinued abruptly.

Frequent Relapser and Steroid-dependent

Long-term alternate day oral prednisolone is the initial strategy. Prednisolone, initially at doses of 0.5–0.7 mg/kg on alternate days is administered followed by slow tapering to 0.2–0.3 mg/kg; these doses are given for prolonged periods of 6–12 months. Requirement of steroids at doses more than 0.7 mg/kg/day or having features of steroid toxicity need alternative agents. The commonly used steroid-sparing drugs are levamisole, mycophenolate mofetil (MMF), and alkylating agents (cyclophosphamide and chlorambucil). Calcineurin inhibitors like cyclosporine and tacrolimus are used sparingly for steroid-sensitive disease **(Flowchart 1)**. Specific drug usage is given in **Table 2.**

Steroid-resistant Disease

All patients with minimal change disease, focal segmental glomerulosclerosis, or mesangioproliferative changes on renal biopsy are treated with calcineurin inhibitors like cyclosporine and tacrolimus. The duration of treatment is at least 2–3 years for steroid-resistant disease. The response rate to these agents is about 70–80%. Intravenous steroids like methylprednisolone and dexamethasone have been used for prolonged periods in the past, but due to their poor response rates and high toxicity, their use is discouraged. Intravenous cyclophosphamide monthly pulses in doses of 500 mg/m^2 for 6 doses along with low-dose alternate day steroids have a response rate of about 50%. This drug can be used if the cost of calcineurin inhibitors is a constraint.

Supportive Management

Diet

A balanced diet adequate in protein (1.5–2 g/kg) and calories is recommended. Fats should provide <30% calories, and saturated fats should be avoided. Salt restriction is advised only for patients with persistent edema or hypertension.

The initial strategy is to administer prednisolone at a dose of 0.5–0.7 mg/kg on alternate days. In patients with stable remission (sustained remission or infrequent relapses), therapy may be tapered to 0.2–0.3 mg kg on alternate days for 6–12 months. Daily therapy at the same dose for 5–7 days, during minor infections, prevents infection-associated relapses. Patients who relapse at steroid threshold >0.7 mg/kg or show steroid toxicity require therapy with steroid-sparing medications **(Flowchart 1)**. The choice of agents is based on disease

TABLE 2: Drugs used for treatment of steroid-sensitive nephrotic syndrome.

	Dosage and side effects
Levamisole	Immunomodulatory drug. Doses of 2–2.5 mg/kg/day on alternate days for 2–3 years. Low-dose alternate day prednisolone is coadministered. Side effects include neutropenia, rashes, cutaneous vasculitis, and gastrointestinal symptoms. Monitoring of total leukocyte counts recommended every 3–4 months. Available 50 mg/150 mg tablets
Cyclophosphamide	It is administered at a dose of 2–2.5 mg/kg/day for 8–12 weeks. Prednisolone is coadministered at a dose of 1.5 mg/kg on alternate days for 4 weeks, followed by 1 mg/kg the following 8 weeks; steroid therapy tapered and stopped in 2–3 months. The drug should be started once child is in remission. Side effects include bone marrow suppression with leukopenia, hemorrhagic cystitis, alopecia, vomiting, and gonadal toxicity. Monitoring of total leukocyte counts is recommended every 2 weeks. Discontinue during infections and maintain hydration during therapy. Available as a 50 mg tablet
Mycophenolate mofetil	It is a purine antagonist. It is a prodrug that is rapidly hydrolyzed to its active metabolite mycophenolic acid in the liver. It is given in doses of 25–35 mg/kg/day in 2 doses (12 hourly) for prolonged periods (1–2 years). Side effects include gastrointestinal intolerance. The drug can also cause lymphopenia. Monitoring of counts and LFT should be done. Available as 250 mg/500 mg tablets
Cyclosporine	It inhibits interleukin-2-driven T-cell activation. In SSNS, it is used in doses of 3–5 mg/kg (100–150 mg/m^2) in 2 divided doses for 1–2 years. For SRNS, duration of therapy is 2–3 years. Coadministration of low-dose corticosteroids is often required. Side effects includes nephrotoxicity, hypertension, and hypertrichosis. Monitor KFTs every 2–3 months. Kidney biopsy is recommended after 2–3 years of use to identify nephrotoxicity. While drug levels are recommended to monitor toxicity, finances often becomes a limitation. It is available as syrup (100 mg/mL) and capsules (25, 50, and100 mg)
Tacrolimus	It is given in doses of 0.1–0.2 mg/kg/day and available as 0.5 mg/1.0 mg/2.0 mg tablets. Side effects are nephrotoxicity, hyperglycemia, neurotoxicity, diarrhea. Cosmetic side effects are less with tacrolimus compared to cyclosporine. Monitoring od Hb1AC, lipid profile, uric acid, serum magnesium should be done every 3 months. It is available as 0.5, 1.0, and 2 mg capsules
Rituximab	It is a chimeric monoclonal antibody that inhibits CD20-mediated B lymphocyte proliferation and differentiation. It is used in severe steroid dependency. It is given at doses of 375 mg/m^2 as weekly infusion for 2–4 doses. Available in 100 mg/500 mg vials.

(KFT: kidney function test; LFT: liver function tests; SRNS: steroid-resistant nephrotic syndrome; SSNS: steroid-sensitive nephrotic syndrome)

Flowchart 1: Management protocol for childhood nephrotic syndrome.

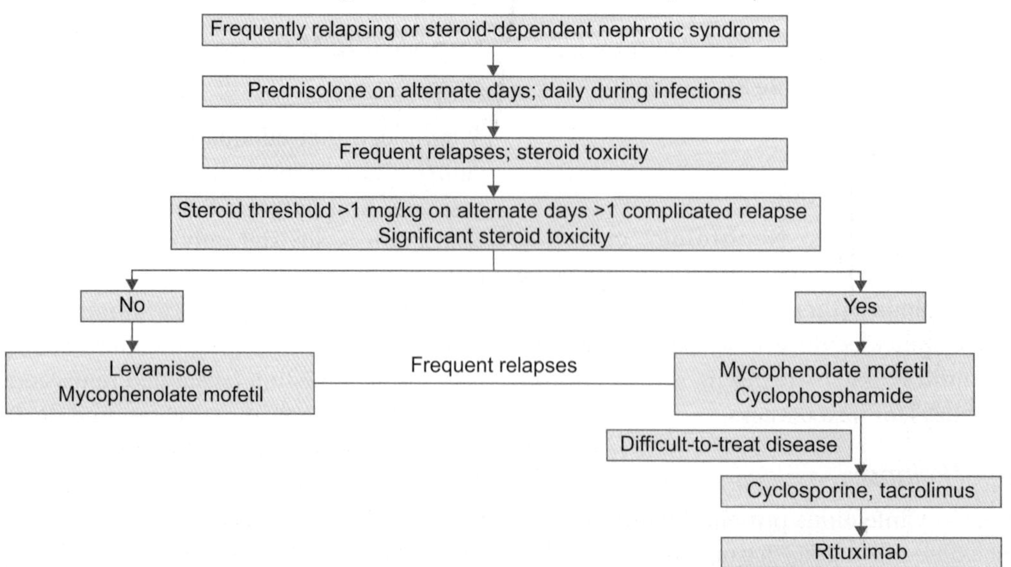

Source: Sinha A, Bagga A, Banerjee S, Mishra K, Mehta A, Agarwal I, et al; Expert Group of Indian Society of Pediatric Nephrology. Steroid Sensitive Nephrotic Syndrome: Revised Guidelines. Indian Pediatr. 2021;58(5):461-81.

severity, adverse effects, patient age, cost of therapy, and parental preference. Levamisole or MMF are preferred medications for mild disease. Patients with high steroid threshold (>1 mg/kg on alternate days), complicated relapses, and those with significant steroid toxicity may be treated with MMF at higher doses (1,000–1,200 mg/m/day) or cyclophosphamide. The use of cyclophosphamide is avoided in children <5-7-year-old and in peripubertal boys due to reduced efficacy and risk of gonadal toxicity, respectively. Patients who relapse despite therapy with two or more steroid-sparing agents (difficult-to-treat steroid sensitive disease) are considered for therapy with calcineurin inhibitors, and failing that, rituximab. The use of rituximab is avoided in young children due to the risk of hypogammaglobulinemia.

Edema

Judicious use of diuretics helps in controlling edema. A protocol of edema management is given in **Table 3**. Rapid diuresis can occur with synergistic therapy, resulting in hypovolemia and hypokalemia. Monitoring of electrolytes is recommended during diuretic therapy.

TABLE 3: Management of edema in nephrotic syndrome.

Step 1	Assess volume status*
Step 2a	If hypovolemia, give 5 or 20% albumin infusion**
Step 2b	If normovolemia or hypervolemia, use furosemide 2–8 mg/kg/day. Add spironolactone 2–3 mg/kg/day at high doses of furosemide. Restrict sodium intake. If inadequate response, add metol zone (0.1–0.3 mg/kg/ day) or hydrochlorothiazide 2–3 mg/kg/day
In cases of ill-sustained response to above measures:	
Step 3	Administer intravenous furosemide 2–3 mg/kg/day every 12 hours
Step 4	Consider intravenous furosemide infusion 0.1–1.0 mg/kg/h if the intravenous bolus effect not sustained
Step 5	If significant edema persists, give 20% albumin infusion with intravenous furosemide over 4 hours

*Assess volume status clinically—monitor pulse and blood pressure. In patients with hypovolemia, blood urea may be elevated, fractional excretion of sodium <0.2%.
**20% albumin may be diluted in normal saline or 5% dextrose to prepare 5% albumin if preparation unavailable
Source: Vasudevan A, Mantan M, Bagga A. Management of edema in nephrotic syndrome. Indian Pediatr. 2004;41(8):787-95

TABLE 4: Complications of nephrotic syndrome and their management.

Complication	***Management***
Infections	• Most common being peritonitis, cellulitis, and pneumonias • Penicillin most effective • Injectable third-generation cephalosporins and aminoglycosides are used in serious cases • Duration of therapy is 7–10 days, more prolonged up to 14 days in sepsis
Thromboembolism	• Ultrasound Doppler for diagnosis of deep vein thrombosis is useful • Ventilation–perfusion scan helps in identification of pulmonary embolism • Low molecular weight heparin + oral warfarin for 3 months duration or till relapse persists is used • Aim INR between 2.5–3.0 when on warfarin therapy
Hyperlipidemia	• Dietary management with fat restriction • No clear guidelines for use of statins in children • Simvastatin and atorvastatin can be used in children with persistent hypercholesterolemia in steroid-resistant disease
Hypertension	• ACE inhibitors and ARBs are preferred drugs • Beta-blockers and calcium channel blockers can be used additionally if not controlled • Use diuretics if edema is present
Steroid toxicity	• Short stature, cataract, glaucoma, and hypertension features of toxicity • Use alkylating and steroid-sparing agents like cyclophosphamide, levamisole, cyclosporine, and mycophenolate mofetil

(ACE: angiotensin-converting enzyme; ARB: angiotensin receptor blockers; INR, international normalized ratio)

The new ISPN guidelines recommend use of diuretics if the weight gain due to edema is moderate to severe (>7% body weight). Minimal edema does not need any treatment and once prednisolone is started most patients will go into remission within 5–7 days.

The complications of nephrotic syndrome and their management is given in **Table 4**.

Vaccination

Most live and killed vaccines can be given to children with nephrotic syndrome if they are off steroids for >1 month. For patients on low-dose alternate-day steroids, live and killed vaccines can be administered. However, live vaccines are to be avoided for those on doses of steroids >1 mg/kg on alternate days. For patients on cyclophosphamide, live vaccines should be avoided for 3 months after therapy while for those on MMF, levamisole, or calcineurin inhibitors, the waiting is usually 1 month after stopping therapy. For patients who have received rituximab live vaccines should be administered after B-cell recovery (6–9 months). All routine vaccination should be done as per national schedule and varicella vaccine should be given to all children with nephrotic syndrome.

KEY POINTS

- Treatment with daily steroids for 6 weeks distinguishes steroid-sensitive from steroid-resistant nephrotic syndrome.
- Edema needs to be treated only if there is significant ascites, respiratory distress due to ascites or effusions, excoriation, and extrusion of fluid from the skin.
- Intravenous albumin is indicated for treatment of hypovolemia in nephrotic syndrome.
- Alternative agents like cyclophosphamide, levamisole, and MMF are used in patients having a frequently relapsing or dependent course.
- Calcineurin inhibitors along with low-dose alternate-day steroids are the first-line drugs for treatment of steroid-resistant disease.

SUGGESTED READING

1. Bagga A, Mantan M. Nephrotic syndrome in children. Indian J Med Res. 2005;122(1):13-28.
2. Boyer O, Saleem MA, Feltran L, Müller-Deile J, Becker JU, Cano F, et al; International Pediatric Nephrology Association. IPNA clinical practice recommendations for the diagnosis and management of children with steroid-resistant nephrotic syndrome. Pediatr Nephrol. 2020;35(8):1529-61.
3. Sinha A, Bagga A, Banerjee S, Mishra K, Mehta A, Agarwal I, et al; Expert Group of Indian Society of Pediatric Nephrology. Steroid Sensitive Nephrotic Syndrome: Revised Guidelines. Indian Pediatr. 2021;58(5):461-81.
4. Trautmann A, Boyer O, Hodson E, Bagga A, Gipson DS, Samuel S, et al; International Pediatric Nephrology Association. IPNA clinical practice recommendations for the diagnosis and management of children with steroid-sensitive nephrotic syndrome. Pediatr Nephrol. 2023;38(3):877-919.
5. Vasudevan A, Thergaonkar R, Mantan M, Sharma J, Khandelwal P, Hari P, et al; Expert Group Of The Indian Society Of Pediatric Nephrology. Consensus Guidelines on Management of Steroid-Resistant Nephrotic Syndrome. Indian Pediatr. 2021;58(7):650-66.

Endocrinology

Section Editors: *Vaman V Khadilkar, Anju Virmani*

CHAPTER 109

Approach to Short Stature

Vaman V Khadilkar, Supriya Phanse Gupte

INTRODUCTION

Short stature is a common referral to pediatric endocrinologists and a systematic approach is needed to reach the diagnosis. Short stature is a symptom and not a diagnosis; a variety of general pediatric and pediatric endocrine conditions can cause short stature. Growth monitoring provides invaluable information toward diagnosis and management of short children, and can prevent reduced adult height due to a delayed or missed diagnosis. The growth trajectory gives invaluable insights into the diagnosis of growth disorders, and is therefore much more useful than a single reading. Therefore, it is very important to monitor the growth of every child on a regular basis. Parents often bring their child with the complaint of short stature because they compare the height of their child with his/her peers at school. This can be misleading and needs to be confirmed by use of appropriate growth charts.

When a short child is referred, the following important points need to be considered:

- Define whether the child is actually short, taking midparental height (MPH) into account, and using appropriate growth charts
- Differentiate a short normal child from a child with an organic cause for short stature
- Decide whether a child can be monitored or needs immediate referral.

DEFINITION

A child is short if the height is less than 2 standard deviations (SDs) below the mean for age and gender for country-specific updated population standards (i.e., below the 3rd centile on country-specific growth charts). However, a child falling below his midparental (target) range percentile by 1.5 SD (2 major percentile lines) and a child having a poor growth velocity (<25th percentile) also needs to be investigated.

ETIOLOGY

Most children presenting with short stature have physiological causes, namely familial short stature (FSS) and constitutional delay in growth and puberty (CDGP). Among the pathological causes, chronic illnesses and malnutrition are major contributors in a developing country like India. Relatively small numbers have an endocrinopathy, genetic disorder, syndrome, bone disease, or skeletal dysplasia causing the short stature.

In many cases, short stature may be the only presentation of a disease and therefore, investigating the cause of short stature is important.

Familial Short Stature

These are usually normal short children born to short parents. Their height falls below the 3rd percentile of population standards, but is within the MPH range. They do not need any treatment, just careful monitoring of growth velocity to ensure growth is normal, and detect growth faltering, if any, well in time. Rarely, short stature in both or either parent is caused by a genetic condition manifesting in a mild form, while the child has a more severe manifestation, with severe short stature. In consanguineous marriages, the parents may be carriers for a gene that manifests in the child, with the homozygous form causing severe short stature, such as in growth hormone deficiency (GHD). In dominantly inherited conditions such as hypochondroplasia, the affected parent is short and transmits the mutated gene to the offspring, resulting in short stature in the child. Treatment of these children is warranted.

Constitutional Delay in Growth and Puberty

This is usually seen in boys. These children grow well in infancy and early childhood. Thereafter, their height begins to falter on growth charts and usually lies just below the 3rd percentile as well as below the MPH. It cruises parallel to the 3rd percentile from thereon. They also may have delayed puberty, further worsening the growth pattern at puberty. Family history of short stature in childhood and adolescence, late pubertal spurt, and achievement of final height as per genetic potential usually exists, mostly if the father is affected. These children usually follow the same trend and will achieve their final height as per their genetic potential. If the puberty is delayed beyond the age of 15 years, it may require treatment in the form of small dose of sex steroids.

Malnutrition and Chronic Illness

Chronic malnutrition leads to stunting of growth due to lack of nutrient supply, associated illnesses leading to a state of catabolism, anemia, and micronutrient deficiency. Chronic illnesses, such as chronic anemia, chronic kidney disease, liver disease, and heart and respiratory disease including asthma, are catabolic states. In addition, poor appetite, electrolyte imbalance, and congestive heart failure further worsen the condition. Malabsorption syndromes, including celiac disease, also cause stunting.

Hypothyroidism

Short stature can be the presenting complaint of children with acquired hypothyroidism; other symptoms may be constipation, anemia, cold intolerance, delayed puberty, and drop in academic performance, though the latter is often not much affected. They may have puffy, coarse facies, dry skin, and mental slowing. Rarely, a girl with very high thyroid-stimulating hormone (TSH) levels may present with pseudoprecocious puberty, ovarian cysts, and even menarche. This is due to molecular mimicry of the TSH receptor with the beta-subunit of follicle-stimulating hormone (FSH) and luteinizing hormone (LH) receptors (specificity spillover). Boys may present with macroorchidism due to the earlier-mentioned mechanism. A child with precocious puberty but short stature is most likely to have hypothyroidism. Sometimes children are referred for a "pituitary mass" which is actually a massively enlarged pituitary gland secondary to pituitary thyrotroph hyperplasia. Occasionally, a child with less severe congenital hypothyroidism (e.g., dyshormonogenesis) may present in childhood for the first time. Children with hypothyroidism (autoimmune thyroid disease/dyshormonogenesis) who present with goiter may thus be diagnosed early. Thyroxine replacement leads to improvement of clinical symptoms as well as dramatic catch-up growth. However, in long-standing cases, the final height may remain well below the target height, so early diagnosis is important.

Growth Hormone Deficiency

These children usually have normal weight and height at birth. They grow normally in the first year of life as growth in this phase is influenced by nutrition and is mediated by thyroid hormones, insulin, and related growth factors. Growth falters in early childhood, leading to severe stunting. They can have immature facies, childlike voice, and small hands and feet. Body proportions are preserved. Obesity is uncommon in Indian children, unlike their counterparts in Western countries. They may have low values of the screening tests, insulin-like growth factor 1 (IGF-1) and insulin-like growth factor binding protein 3 (IGF BP3). Diagnosis is based on low stimulated growth hormone (GH) levels; a single value of GH has no significance and should not be done. All these tests should only be done after ruling out or normalizing other conditions which may cause short stature, such as hypothyroidism, chronic illnesses, and malabsorption **(Box 1)**. Children with GHD respond well to GH therapy. Rare exceptions are conditions with GH antibodies and GH insensitivity syndromes.

With the recent advances in molecular genetics, we now know much more about the GH-IGF-1 axis. Genetic mutations in the pathway beyond GH secretion can lead to a spectrum of short stature disorders. Thus, many conditions initially classified as idiopathic short stature (ISS) may actually have a genetic etiology. Clinical exome sequencing has helped us to understand these lesser known conditions. Newer therapies such as IGF-1 (Increlex) are useful for patients with IGF-1 deficiency disorders.

Cushing Syndrome

In childhood, it is usually the result of exogenous steroid administration or adrenal tumors. Rarely, in older children, a pituitary lesion or a carcinoid tumor may be the cause. These children are short and obese. Other stigmata, such as purplish striae, muscular weakness, and buffalo hump,

BOX 1: Causes of short stature.

- *Physiological short stature:*
  - Idiopathic short stature:
    - Familial
    - Nonfamilial
  - Constitutional delay in growth and puberty
- *Pathological short stature:*
  - Malnutrition
  - *Chronic illness:*
    - Chronic anemia
    - Chronic renal disease and renal tubular acidosis
    - Chronic liver disease
    - Chronic pulmonary disease including asthma
    - Celiac disease and giardiasis
    - Hematological disorders, e.g., thalassemia
  - *Endocrinopathies:*
    - Growth hormone deficiency
    - Hypothyroidism
    - Cushing syndrome
    - Pseudohypoparathyroidism
  - *Syndromes:*
    - Turner syndrome
    - Down syndrome
    - Noonan syndrome
    - Other syndromes, e.g., Edward syndrome and Patau syndrome
  - *Small for gestational age:*
    - Nonsyndromic
    - Syndromic with primordial short stature: Russell–Silver syndrome and Seckel syndrome
  - Nutritional rickets and hypophosphatemic rickets
  - Skeletal dysplasia and osteogenesis imperfecta
  - Intracranial tumors, trauma, surgery, and irradiation
  - Psychosocial short stature
  - *Medications:* Prolonged steroid intake and methylphenidate

are not commonly seen in children. Hypertension is an important indicator of this disorder in children. Treatment consists of omission of exogenous steroids and excision of tumors.

Turner Syndrome

Short stature is a consistent feature of Turner syndrome (TS), especially as the child grows older. The other stigmata, including webbing of neck, low posterior hair line, antimongoloid slant, widely spaced nipples, wide carrying angle, Madelung deformity, and short 4th/5th metacarpals or metatarsals. Girls with TS develop ovarian failure early in life and so have no/delayed puberty and infertility. They are predisposed to autoimmune disorders such as autoimmune thyroid disease and celiac disease. Higher incidence of hearing loss, coarctation of aorta, left-sided heart disease, renal disorders, and pigmented nevi have been noted in these children. All features may not be present in most children and short stature may be the only indicator of the disorder. GH is a licensed indication for treatment of short stature in TS.

Psychosocial Short Stature

Emotionally deprived children do not grow well. They do not respond to nutritional supplementation or any other form of treatment. However, it is a reversible condition and these children grow well once placed in a loving environment as their pituitary hypothalamic function reverts to normal when they live in a stress-free environment.

Small for Gestational Age Sequelae

Most small for gestational age (SGA) children catch-up by 2–4 years of age. However, up to 30% do not catch-up. In addition, girls (and less commonly boys) born SGA tend to enter puberty early, and progress rapidly, with early menarche. Hence, height predictions based on bone age are often unreliable. Those who fail to catch-up and remain below –2.5 SD score for the population by 2 years of age and <–2 SD by 4 years of age are candidates for GH therapy.

Skeletal dysplasias, hypophosphatemic rickets, and pseudohypoparathyroidism are other rare causes of short stature and should be looked for.

MANAGEMENT

Measurement of Height/Length

It is important to accurately measure height with a stadiometer, to avoid errors in measurement. For children <2 years of age, the length is measured with the child in supine position, with the help of an infantometer.

Calculate the Midparental Height (Target Height) and the Target Range

Midparental height (MPH) = (father's height + mother's height + 13)/2 for boys and
= (father's height + mother's height – 13)/2 for girls.
Target range = MPH ± 6 cm

Plot the child's height and target height (with target range) on country-specific contemporary growth charts. For children under the age of 5 years, use of the World Health Organization (WHO) 2006 growth standards is recommended.

If previous height records are available, plot previous height readings to observe the pattern of the growth.

Calculate the annual growth velocity as change in height divided by change in time. For example, if a child grows 3 cm in 6 months, the annualized growth velocity is 3 divided by half year which is 6 cm.

Normal Growth Velocity

- *In first year:* 25 cm/year (or 50% of the birth length)
- *In second year:* 12 cm/year (or 25% of the birth length)
- *In third year:* 6 cm/year
- *From fourth year till pubertal spurt:* 5 cm/year
- *During puberty:* 6–8 cm/year in girls and 10–12 cm/year in boys.

Growth velocity can be plotted on growth velocity curves. Growth velocity <25th percentile is abnormal and needs investigations.

If previous height records are not available, assess the height of the child in relation to the MPH.

If the height of the child is >3rd percentile and within target range, it is a normal child. No investigations are needed. Serial height measurements need to be plotted on growth charts at 6 monthly-yearly intervals. Monitor growth velocity annually.

If height of the child is <3rd percentile but within target range, it is a short normal child with FSS. Continue annual plotting on growth chart and monitor growth velocity. A high index of suspicion is needed to suspect and diagnose a subtle growth disorder in parents, such as hypochondroplasia, which may be inherited by the child.

Indications for Further Workup

- Height <–2.5 SD of population standard for age and gender
- Height <–1.5 SD below the MPH
- Growth velocity has deteriorated and dropped below 25th percentile

CLINICAL PEARL

- A child with height plot above the 3rd percentile may still be abnormal if he falls below the target range or has a growth velocity <25th percentile.

Preliminary Workup (Box 2)

History (Table 1)

A detailed history of duration of apparent short stature, history of pubertal delay in adolescent boys and girls should be noted. Evidence of chronic illnesses, such as renal, liver, malabsorption, respiratory illness including asthma, and tuberculosis, should be looked for.

BOX 2: Causes of proportionate and disproportionate short stature.

Proportionate short stature:
- Growth hormone deficiency
- Malnutrition
- Rickets
- Chronic illness
- Syndromic short stature
- Small for gestational age sequelae

Disproportionate short stature:
- *Short upper segment:*
  - Mucopolysaccharidosis
  - Spondyloepimetaphyseal dysplasia
- *Short lower segment:*
  - Achondroplasia, hypochondroplasia
  - Osteogenesis imperfecta
  - Hypophosphatemic rickets

History of severe headache, vomiting suggestive of intracranial space-occupying lesions, intracranial surgeries, craniospinal irradiation, head trauma, history of other malignancies, bone disorders, and prolonged steroid intake would add valuable information.

Birth history including birth weight (SGA), birth length, history of breech delivery, birth trauma, neonatal hypoglycemia, and neonatal jaundice should be asked for. Family history of consanguinity, short stature, delayed puberty, sterile uncle/aunts, and tuberculosis should be reviewed.

Developmental history suggestive of delayed milestones, and visual disturbances (r/o anatomical causes such as corpus callosum agenesis and septo-optic dystrophy associated with multiple pituitary hormone deficiency) could be pointers toward an anatomical brain abnormality and congenital hypothyroidism.

A proper assessment of dietary intake helps to ensure adequate calorie intake and assess for malnutrition. Social history to assess for signs of child abuse and neglect should be looked for.

Anthropometry

Interpreting the severity of height and weight deficit can be very useful to reach the diagnosis. This can be assessed by calculating child's height age and weight age.

Height age is assessed by drawing a horizontal line from the present height plot to the 50th percentile and drawing

TABLE 1: Pointers toward diagnosis from history.

Small for gestational age (SGA)	*SGA sequelae, Russell–Silver syndrome, and Seckel syndrome*
Breech delivery	Growth hormone deficiency (GHD) and multiple pituitary hormone deficiency (MPHD)
Neonatal hypoglycemia and jaundice	GHD and MPHD
Family history of consanguinity	Genetic causes
Family history of delayed puberty with short stature with normal final height	Constitutional delay in growth and puberty
Family history of short stature	Familial short stature, parents with heterozygote state for conditions such as achondroplasia and hypochondroplasia
Short stature in infancy	Syndromic short stature and skeletal dysplasia
Short stature in childhood	GHD, hypothyroidism, MPHD, chronic illness, and Turner syndrome
Intracranial tumors, irradiation, trauma, and surgery	MPHD
Headache, vomiting, and visual disturbances	Intracranial tumor
Persistent diarrhea and abdominal distension	Celiac disease
History of asthma, liver, and renal disease	Pointers of chronic disease

a perpendicular on the X-axis (age in years) on the growth chart. The point on the X-axis where the perpendicular meets, gives the height age. Weight age is calculated in a similar way. If the weight age is more retarded than the height age, it is a case of malnutrition, chronic disease, or syndrome. The height age is more retarded than the weight age in endocrinopathies as weight is usually preserved.

In addition to height and weight, the upper segment/lower segment ratio (US/LS ratio) provides useful information and helps in establishing a definite etiology. The LS is measured from the superior border of pubic rami till the feet with the child standing upright. The US (vertex-pubic symphysis) is calculated by subtracting the LS from the total height. Another method of assessing US/LS ratio is by measuring the sitting height and subtracting it from the standing height to get the subischial limb length.

This can be plotted on sitting height and subischial leg length combined charts.

The US/LS ratio is 1.7:1 at birth. It gradually decreases, reaching a ratio of 1:2 at around 7 years and 1.1:1 at 10 years. It remains so till puberty when it further dips to 0.98:1 due to an earlier spurt in limb height as compared to the spine growth. Toward the end of puberty with an increase in spine height with a nearly stabilized limb length, the ratio again rises to 1:1, or 0.9:1, which persists thereafter.

Disproportionate short stature is seen in conditions wherein the growth of either the limbs or spine is more affected. In skeletal dysplasias, the limbs are more affected and the spine is spared. An exception is spondyloepiphyseal dysplasia wherein both the spine and limbs are affected. Spinal shortening is seen in storage disease such as mucopolysaccharidosis.

CLINICAL PEARLS

- A short and thin child with weight most severely affected: think of chronic illness, syndromic short stature, and malnutrition
- A short and overweight child: think of endocrinopathy—hypothyroidism, GHD, and Cushing syndrome.

Clinical Examination (Table 2)

It includes a thorough examination to look for any pointers of a specific etiology of short stature. Facial dysmorphism adds important information. Few of these are listed here.

Evidence of anemia, cyanosis, jaundice, signs of chronic illness such as renal, liver, pulmonary disorders including asthma, and nutritional deficiency, including features of malabsorption syndrome. Bony deformities including bow legs, knock knees, kyphosis, and scoliosis would indicate involvement of the skeletal system. A detailed systemic examination would add to the information.

CLINICAL PEARL

- Short stature with anemia should raise suspicion of celiac disease.

TABLE 2: Clinical signs indicating etiology.

Clinical signs	*Etiology*
Immature facies with frontal bossing, depressed nasal bridge, midfacial hypoplasia, and high-pitched voice	Growth hormone deficiency
Mental slowing, coarse facies, puffy appearance, and goiter	Hypothyroidism
Antimongoloid slant, low posterior hairline, webbed neck, short 4th/5th metacarpals, metatarsals, wide carrying angle, pigmented nevi, and difference in upper limb lower limb blood pressure	Turner syndrome
Beak-headed dwarfism, height <–7 SD, and developmental delay	Seckel syndrome
Small triangular facies with hemiatrophy	Russell–Silver syndrome
Almond-shaped eyes, hypogonadism, obesity, behavioral problems, and hyperphagia	Prader–Willi syndrome
Coarse facies, macrocephaly, short stubby fingers, and rhizomelia	Skeletal dysplasia
Short 4th/5th metacarpal or metatarsal	*SHOX* gene defect, pseudo-pseudohypoparathyroidism, and Turner syndrome

1sttier investigations:

- Hemogram
- *Biochemical investigations*:
  - Serum creatinine (renal function)
  - Serum glutamic pyruvic transaminase (liver function)
  - Venous blood gas (if evidence of rickets to rule out renal tubular acidosis in case of rickets)
  - Thyroid function test: T4 and TSH
  - Anti-tissue transglutaminase (TTG) immunoglobulin A (IgA) (anti-TTG antibody, if low, get total IgA done to look for IgA deficiency, and confirm with immunoglobulin G antibody)
  - FSH, karyotype in a girl with unexplained short stature
- *Radiological investigations:* Bone age [using Greulich and Pyle, Tanner Whitehouse 3 (TW 3), or Gilsanz and Ratib methods].

Bone age is a useful, cheap, and invaluable investigation in the assessment of short children. In Greulich and Pyle atlas, comparison of a radiograph of the left hand is done with that of standard age and gender specific radiographs. The age at which the radiograph in the atlas matches closest to the actual one of the patients in terms of maturity of ossification centers of bones, is the bone age of the patient. This is a fairly reliable method that can be used in day-to-day practice.

The TW 3 atlas is more exhaustive method, wherein 20 ossification centers in the hand are scored. The summation of these is then looked up in a table to give the final bone age. This is more precise, less subjective, but more time consuming.

Gilsanz and Ratib have recently released their own atlas of bone age assessment which is very similar to Greulich and Pyle method, with an added advantage of digital processing.

CLINICAL PEARL

- Karyotype to rule out TS is needed in all short girls even in the absence of stigmata.

Interpretation of Growth Velocity

A child who has normal growth velocity with growth curve cruising below the 3rd percentile is a short normal child and needs continued monitoring. He/she may need second level of investigations to rule out all-causes before diagnosing as ISS. GH has been used to treat short normal children who are below –2.5 SD and who are not likely to achieve normal adult stature.

Low Growth Velocity (Faltering Growth Curve)

Consider second-tier investigations:

- *GH stimulation test*: Two provocation tests using clonidine, glucagon, insulin, dopamine, arginine, and GH-releasing hormone (in India, clonidine, glucagon, arginine, and insulin are available)
- *Magnetic resonance imaging brain:* Pituitary size and congenital malformations of the brain
- Molecular testing for syndromes
  Idiopathic short stature if all tests are negative.

Management Strategies

Treatment of the underlying condition usually leads to improvement in the growth velocity and catch-up growth.

Growth Hormone (Table 3)

The GH therapy is licensed to be used in the following conditions:

- GHD
- SGA sequelae
- TS
- Prader–Willi syndrome
- ISS
- Chronic renal failure prior to renal transplant
- Glucocorticoid-induced short stature

Conditions with doubtful benefit (under research at present):

- Hypochondroplasia
- Chronic inflammatory disorders like rheumatoid arthritis
- Noonan syndrome
- Other skeletal dysplasia.

Recombinant human GH is given in the form of subcutaneous injections daily at bedtime for a period of at least 2 years, ideally till the final height is achieved. GH therapy is not useful once there is complete bony fusion. Response depends on the indication for which it is used, age of starting therapy, duration of therapy, dose used, MPH, and bone age at onset.

Although adverse effects are rare, they may include benign intracranial hypertension, hyperglycemia, worsening of scoliosis, slipped capital femoral epiphyses, gynecomastia, rash, and hives. Increased predisposition for neoplasia in those with increased chromosomal breakage syndromes has also been reported and is a contraindication to GH therapy.

TABLE 3: Growth hormone dose.

Underlying condition	*Dose*
Growth hormone deficiency	25–35 μg/kg/day
Turner syndrome	45–68 μg/kg/day
Small for gestational age sequelae	35–70 μg/kg/day
Prader–Willi syndrome	20–40 μg/kg/day, in obese: 0.5–1 mg/m²/day
Idiopathic short stature	25–50 μg/kg/day

Androgens

Depot testosterone in small doses of 50 mg monthly for 3–6 months has been used in boys with CDGP. It is used to trigger the onset of pubertal spurt without advancing bone age, and usually results in attainment of satisfactory final height. In some conditions wherein the predicted adult height is less, it may be combined with GH. The disadvantage of testosterone is that it aromatizes to estrogen and thus higher doses result in rapid bone maturation and fusion. Oxandrolone, a nonaromatizable

Flowchart 1: Short stature.

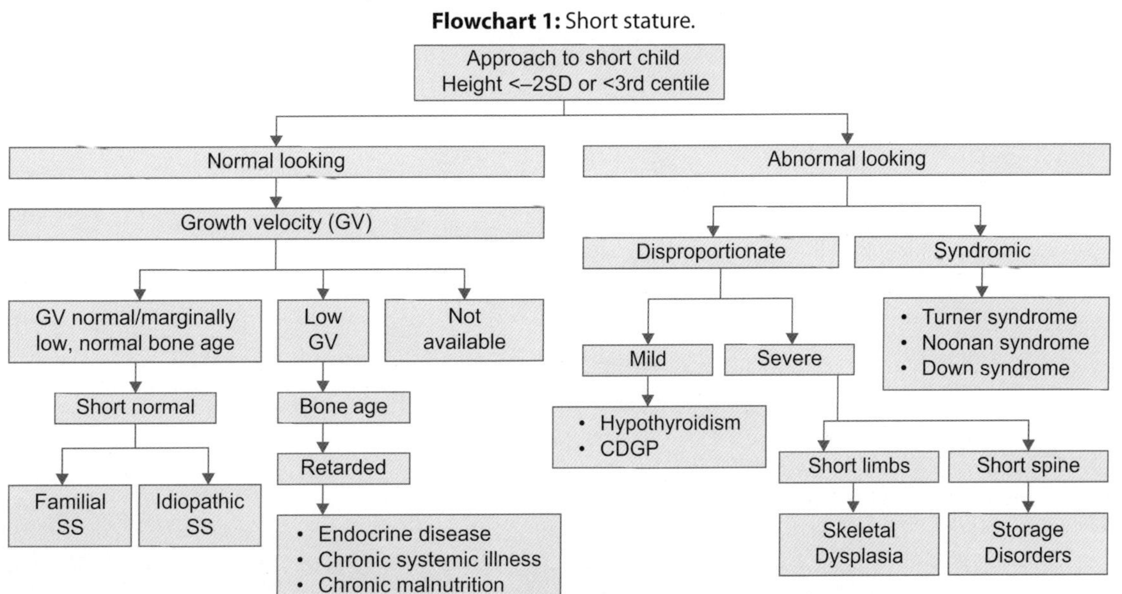

(BA: bone age; CDGP: constitutional delay in growth and puberty; GV: growth velocity; SD: standard deviation; SS: short stature)

androgen is a better alternative as it does not lead to early bony fusion.

Limb lengthening using Ilizarov technique may be offered for children with achondroplasia.

CONCLUSION

It is necessary to differentiate a short normal child from a short child with pathology. Treatment of only pathological short stature is warranted. GH therapy is indicated for special conditions, and is usually for the long term. The therapy aims at achieving genetic potential and depends on many factors, such as age at onset of therapy, etiology, degree of short stature, and duration of therapy, which may be contrary to unrealistic expectations of most parents **(Flowchart 1)**.

KEY POINTS

- Anthropometry and plotting of growth chart remain the most powerful tool for the diagnosis of short stature.
- Longitudinal assessment of growth and growth velocity is much more important than a single one-time evaluation, as it gives an idea of the growth pattern.
- Bone age beyond 2 years of actual age on either side is considered abnormal and points toward an endocrine disease.
- Adjusting height for midparental target height often reduces unnecessary investigations in the short child.
- A short and fat child has an endocrine disease, skeletal dysplasia, or a syndrome; whereas a tall and fat child has nutritional obesity.

SUGGESTED READING

1. Bull RK, Edwards PD, Kemp PM, Fry S, Hughes IA. Bone age assessment: a large scale comparison of the Greulich and Pyle, and Tanner and Whitehouse (TW2) methods. Arch Dis Child. 1999;81:172-3.
2. Cohen P, Rogol AD, Deal CL, Saenger P, Reiter EO, Ross JL, et al. Consensus statement on the diagnosis and treatment of children with idiopathic short stature: a summary of the Growth Hormone Research Society, the Lawson Wilkins Pediatric Endocrine Society, and the European Society for Paediatric Endocrinology Workshop. J Clin Endocrinol Metab. 2008;93(11):4210-7.
3. Gilsanz V, Ratib O. Hand Bone Age: A Digital Atlas of Skeletal Maturity. Berlin, Heidelberg: Springer-Verlag; 2005.
4. Indian Academy of Pediatrics Growth Charts Committee; Khadilkar V, Yadav S, Agrawal KK, Tamboli S, Banerjee M, Cherian A, Goyal JP, Khadilkar A, Kumaravel V, Mohan V, Narayanappa D, Ray I, Yewale V. Revised IAP growth charts for height, weight and body mass index for 5- to 18-year-old Indian children. Indian Pediatr. 2015;52(1):47-55.
5. Khadilkar V, Khadilkar A. Growth charts: a diagnostic tool. Indian J Endocr Metab. 2011;15(Suppl 3):S166-71.
6. Khadilkar V, Phanse S. Growth charts from controversy to consensus. Indian J Endocrinol Metab. 2012;(16):S185-7.
7. World Health Organization. WHO Multicentre Growth Reference Study standards. [online] Available from https://www.who.int/tools/child-growth-standards/who-multicentre-growth-reference-study. [last accessed December, 2024].
8. Wilson TA, Rose SR, Cohen P, Rogol AD, Backeljauw P, Brown R, et al. Update of guidelines for the use of growth hormone in children: the Lawson Wilkins Pediatric Endocrinology Society Drug and Therapeutics Committee. J Pediatr. 2003;143(4):415-21.

Childhood Obesity

Alapan Mahapatra, Anurag Bajpai

INTRODUCTION

Childhood obesity has emerged as a global epidemic with a doubling of prevalence over the last two decades. India is in the middle of an escalating epidemic of metabolic disorders associated with childhood obesity. This has led to an increased prevalence of obesity complications, imposing a significant burden on society, making timely evaluation and management essential.

CRITERIA

Obesity represents increased body fat and not just increased weight. Body fat can be estimated by several methods, such as dual-energy X-ray absorptiometry (DEXA), bioelectrical impedance assay (BIA), computed tomography (CT), and magnetic resonance imaging (MRI) of the abdomen. However, these methods are time-consuming, costly, and prone to radiation risk. So, in practice, surrogate markers of adiposity using a combination of height and weight are used.

Body Mass Index

Body mass index (BMI) is used for diagnosing obesity after 5 years of age. It takes into account the weight and height of the individual.

$$BMI = \frac{\text{Weight (kg)}}{\text{Height (m)}^2}$$

Body mass index correlates with body fat and complications in children; however, it may incorrectly diagnose obesity in muscular individuals while underestimating adiposity in sedentary children with reduced muscle mass. Asian Indians have more central fat distribution compared to peripheral, leading to a lower cutoff value for the diagnosis of obesity and its complications. The use of World Health Organization (WHO) criteria underestimates the prevalence of obesity while missing obesity complications in Indian children. BMI levels above 23 kg/m^2 and 27 kg/m^2 adult equivalent, as per Indian Academy of Pediatrics (IAP) 2015 criteria, indicate overweight and obesity, respectively.

Weight-for-Height

Weight-for-height should be used before 5 years of age. Weight for height above +2 and +3 standard deviation scores suggest overweight and obesity, respectively.

Waist Circumference

Waist circumference is a marker of abdominal obesity, a predictor of metabolic syndrome. Levels above 70th percentile for age and gender increase the risk of metabolic syndromes.

ETIOLOGY

Most children with obesity do not have an underlying cause (exogenous obesity 95–98%) **(Flowchart 1)**. This makes the identification of exogenous obesity due to lifestyle issues important. Earlier onset, delayed development or puberty, short stature, syndromic features, and abnormal facies suggest a pathological cause of obesity.

Constitutional/Exogenous Obesity

Constitutional obesity results from an imbalance between energy intake and expenditure. Both low birth weight and high birth weight, maternal history of diabetes, obesity, and smoking are associated with an increased risk of obesity later in life. Dietary habits associated with childhood obesity include missing meals (especially breakfast), higher portion size, energy-dense and nutrient-poor food, refined packaged food, frequent snacking and eating out, watching television while eating, and reduced

Flowchart 1: Etiology of obesity.

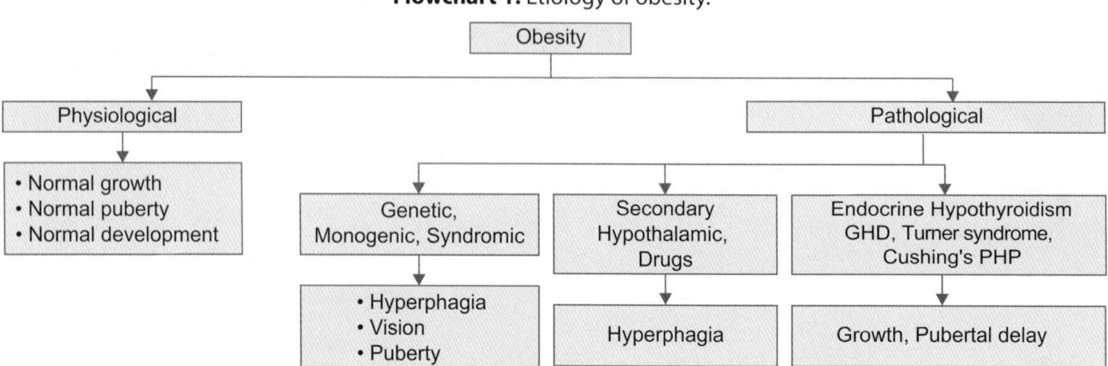

(GHD: growth hormone deficiency; PHP: pseudohypoparathyroidism)

Source: Bajpai A, Dave C. Obesity. MedEClasses Online Course in Pediatric Endocrinology, October 2023. (https://learning.growsociety.in/unit/obesity)

TABLE 1: Syndromic causes of obesity.

Disease	*Pointers*	*Diagnosis*
Prader–Willi	Infantile hypotonia and failure to thrive followed by rapid weight gain after two years, almond-shaped eyes and prominent philtrum, acromicria and hypogonadism, hyperphagia, and behavioral abnormalities	Methylation-sensitive polymerase chain reaction (PCR) for chromosome 15 (imprinting disorder)
Bardet–Biedl	Polydactyly and retinitis pigmentosa, developmental delay and polyphagia, and renal abnormalities	Next generation sequencing (NGS)
Alström	Dilated cardiomyopathy, type 2 diabetes, progressive loss of vision and hearing	NGS (*ALMS1* gene mutation)
Beckwith–Wiedemann	Organomegaly, ear lobe creases, and hemihypertrophy	MLPA imprinting 11p15.4

physical activity. Breastfeeding in infancy has a protective effect. Reduced sleep and increased screen time of over 1 hour a day are also associated with obesity.

CLINICAL PEARL

Childhood obesity is most commonly due to lifestyle factors.

Endocrine Causes

Endocrine diseases are rare but treatable causes of childhood obesity. They should be considered in the presence of clinical pointers—mainly, growth failure and delayed puberty. Cushing's syndrome presents with central obesity, high blood pressure, growth failure, violaceous striae, and proximal myopathy. Hypothyroidism is a rare cause of isolated obesity, usually associated with growth failure and developmental delay. In growth hormone (GH) deficiency, children typically present with short stature, micropenis, and mild truncal obesity. In pseudohypoparathyroidism, growth retardation, ectopic calcification, brachymetacarpia, and hypocalcemia are dominant clinical features.

Dysmorphic Syndromes

Obesity is often a manifestation of dysmorphic syndromes **(Table 1)**. Many of these syndromes are associated with hyperphagia, hypogonadism, hypotonia, or finger abnormalities (syndactyly and polydactyly) such as Prader–Willi, Carpenter, Lawrence–Moon–Biedl–Bardet syndromes, and Alström.

Hypothalamic Obesity

Hypothalamic obesity is caused by increased appetite due to a central nervous system (CNS) insult by surgery, radiation, tumors, and trauma. Destruction of the central processing unit causes functional leptin resistance. These disorders are associated with excessive appetite, signs and symptoms of CNS involvement, and other hypothalamic-pituitary defects. Neuroimaging is done to identify these lesions.

Monogenic Obesity

Single gene defects are a rare cause of obesity and should be suspected with early onset obesity, rapid weight gain, syndromic features, and family history.Inefficient leptin action (deficiency or resistance) results in uncontrolled appetite and obesity. Abnormalities in mineralocorticoid receptor and proconvertase have also been associated with obesity. Melanocortin 4 (MC4) receptor defects are the most common monogenic obesity associated with growth acceleration and insulin resistance.

Drugs

Commonly used drugs associated with obesity include corticosteroids, antipsychotics (olanzapine and risperidone), antidepressants (paroxetine), and antiepileptics (valproate and lamotrigine) **(Table 2)**.

COMPLICATIONS

Childhood obesity predicts several short- and long-term complications **(Table 3)**. Endocrine complications are the most significant adverse effects of childhood obesity. Central to this is insulin resistance, caused by an overspill of fat and its deposition in the liver and skeletal muscle. Insulin resistance predisposes to the development of type 2 diabetes mellitus (T2DM), polycystic ovarian syndrome (PCOS), and nonalcoholic fatty liver disease (NAFLD). Hyperandrogenism is common in obese girls, as is accelerated growth, skeletal maturation, and early puberty.

- *Cardiovascular:* Obese children have a higher prevalence of dyslipidemia, hypertension, atherosclerosis, and an increased risk of adult coronary disease. Significantly, hypertension may be masked, warranting repeated blood pressure measurements.
- *Central nervous system:* Benign intracranial hypertension is common in children with obesity and presents with headache and vomiting.
- *Orthopedic:* These children have a higher risk of flat foot, Blount's disease, fractures, genu valgum, and osteoarthritis. The most debilitating complication is slipped capital femoral epiphysis, which presents with dull, aching pain in the knee, hip, or groin, with abnormal gait. Blount's disease (tibia vara) presents with progressive bowing of legs and knee pain. X-rays of the knee and hip should be done in obese children with pain in the hip or knee or abnormal gait.
- *Respiratory:* Obese children are at increased risk of respiratory distress and restrictive pattern of respiratory symptoms. Obesity predisposes to the development of sleep-disordered breathing and hypoventilation syndrome.
- *Gastrointestinal:* Obesity is associated with gastroesophageal reflux and NAFLD. Fatty liver is present in 40%, elevated transaminases in 25%, and gallstones in 2%. Rapid weight fluctuations are associated with gallstone disease, which should be suspected in an obese child with abdominal pain, jaundice, nausea, and intolerance to fatty foods.
- *Psychological:* Obesity is associated with an increased prevalence of mood disorders. This represents the

TABLE 2: Drugs causing obesity.

Drugs	*Agents*	*Alternatives*
Glucocorticoids	Prednisolone	Local route, low dose, and sparing agent
Antipsychotics	Risperidone and olanzapine	Ziprasidone
Antiepileptics	Valproate and carbamazepine	Topiramate
SSRI	Paroxetine and amitriptyline	Fluoxetine and sertraline

(SSRI: selective serotonin reuptake inhibitors)

TABLE 3: Complications of obesity

Category	*Complications*
Metabolic	Insulin resistance, type 2 diabetes mellitus, metabolic syndrome, and hyperandrogenism
Cardiovascular	Hypertension, dyslipidemia, and atherosclerosis
Gastrointestinal	Nonalcoholic fatty liver disease, gall stones, and gastroesophageal reflux
Skeletal	Blount's disease, slipped capital femoral epiphysis, and fractures
Respiratory	Obstructive sleep apnea and hypoventilation syndrome
Neurological	Benign intracranial hypertension

Flowchart 2: Approach to a child with obesity.

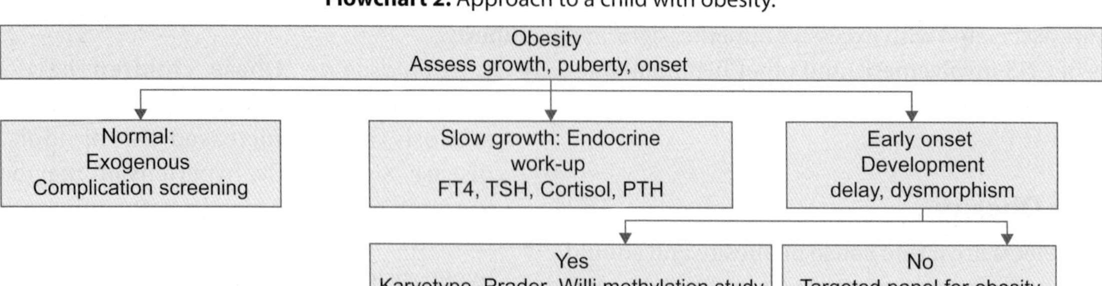

(FT4: free thyroxine; PTH: parathyroid hormone; TSH: thyroid-stimulating hormone)
Source: Bajpai A, Dave C. Obesity. MedEClasses Online Course in Pediatric Endocrinology, October 2023. (https://learning.growsociety.in/unit/obesity)

intrinsic effects of obesity on one hand and the psychological effects of bullying on the other. It is essential to assess the impact on an obese child, as depression increases the risk of obesity.

CLINICAL PEARL

- Obesity causes several short- and long-term complications, including insulin resistance, T2DM, PCOS, NAFLD, dyslipidemia, hypertension, atherosclerosis, orthopedic problems, obstructive sleep apnea, and mood disorders.

ASSESSMENT

Assessment is given in **Flowchart 2**.

Clinical

The clinical evaluation should include a detailed history and examination. Pathological obesity should be considered with early onset of obesity, rapid weight gain, growth failure, dysmorphism, developmental delay, and pubertal delay. Pointers to specific disorders should be evaluated **(Table 4)**. Detailed dietary history, including duration of breastfeeding, age at weaning, meal pattern, calorie intake, snacking, consumption of junk food, and features of feeding disorders, should be taken. Duration of activity and inactivity should be looked into. Family history of consanguinity, T2DM, ischemic heart disease, and dyslipidemia should be inquired. Drug history should assess intake of steroids, valproate, antipsychotics, and any other drugs. History of CNS infection, trauma, radiation, tumor, or surgery indicates hypothalamic obesity.

Examination should include assessment of growth parameters, pubertal status, and clues to diagnosis. Parents of obese girls are often concerned about premature thelarche. While this may reflect true precocious puberty caused by obesity, it is most likely due to increased fat and not true thelarche. To distinguish these conditions, approximate the thumb and index finger around the nipple: Lack of resistance indicates lipomastia; breast nodule can be felt as an area of resistance. Obese boys frequently present with concerns of small penile size, which is usually due to the penis being buried in the suprapubic pad. Stretched penile length should be measured after pressing the suprapubic pad of fat to ascertain the actual size of the penis.

TABLE 4: Pointers to etiology of obesity.

Pointers	*Disorders*
Delayed puberty	Bardet–Biedl and Prader–Willi
Retinitis pigmentosa and polydactyly	Bardet–Biedl and Alström
Short hand and feet	Prader–Willi
Buffalo hump and striae	Cushing's syndrome
Short fourth metacarpal	PHP and Turner syndrome
Developmental delay	Hypothyroidism, parathyroid hormone (PHP), and Prader–Willi

Investigations

No diagnostic workup is required in children with normal growth, facies, and pubertal development. Thyroid profile and evaluation for Cushing's (serum cortisol at 8 am after dexamethasone at 11 pm) should be done in the presence of growth failure and characteristic clinical features. The effect of obesity on endocrine function should be considered while assessing endocrine functions. Mildly elevated thyroid-stimulating hormone (TSH) levels with normal free thyroxine are typical in obesity and should not be treated unless TSH is persistently and significantly

TABLE 5: Cutoffs for investigations for assessment of obesity complications.

Investigation	*Normal*	*Borderline*	*Abnormal*
Blood sugar fasting	<100 mg/dL	100–125 mg/dL	>126 mg/dL
Blood sugar 2 hours after glucose load	<140 mg/dL	140–199 mg/dL	>200 mg/dL
Total cholesterol	<170 mg/dL	170–199 mg/dL	>200 mg/dL
LDL cholesterol	<110 mg/dL	110–129 mg/dL	>130 mg/dL
Triglyceride	<90 mg/dL	90–129 mg/dL	>139 mg/dL
HDL cholesterol	>45 mg/dL	40–45 mg/dL	<40 mg/dL
AST	• <22 in Girls • <26 in Boys	• 22–43 in Girls • 26–51 in boys	• >44 in Girls • >56 in Boys

(AST: aspartate aminotransferase; HDL: high-density lipoprotein; LDL: low-density lipoprotein)

elevated (>10 IU/mL). Similarly, cortisol levels may be mildly elevated and should not be mistakenly diagnosed as Cushing's syndrome. Genetic testing for Prader–Willi syndrome should be done in the presence of facial features, a history of infantile hypotonia, and growth failure. Monogenic causes of obesity should be considered only in the presence of clinical features or pointers to diagnosis.

Complication Assessment

Investigations should include an oral glucose tolerance test (fasting blood sugar and 2 hours after 1.75 g/kg glucose; maximum of 75 g), lipid profile, and liver function tests. Age-appropriate cutoffs should be used for interpretation **(Table 5)**. These tests should be repeated every 3 years if normal. Fasting insulin has a limited role and is not recommended. Mildly elevated liver transaminases are common in obesity; elevation two times above the upper limit indicates nonalcoholic steatohepatitis. Children with elevated transaminases should undergo an ultrasound of the abdomen and workup for other causes of hepatic dysfunction (hepatitis B and C, Wilson disease, and autoimmune hepatitis). Sleep studies may be required in the presence of snoring, daytime sleepiness, or lethargy.

MANAGEMENT

Management of pediatric obesity is a big challenge, requiring a multidisciplinary approach involving physicians, nutritionists, and physical trainers, with changes made by the entire family.

- *Goal:* The goal is to bring BMI as close to the normal range for age and gender as possible. Normalization may be problematic; excessive and rapid weight loss adversely affects the child's growth and should be avoided. In most cases, weight stabilization is the initial aim. Weight loss should not exceed 1 kg monthly to reduce BMI standard deviation scores (SDS) by 5% over 6 months. The key focus is on changing the lifestyle of the child and family with the use of drugs and surgery in refractory cases.
- *Lifestyle measures:* This is the cornerstone of management. The whole family is encouraged to follow a healthy lifestyle—focusing on the child alone is counterproductive. The child should be advised to eat regular meals. Skipping meals and snacking between meals should be discouraged. The caloric intake should be reduced by 20%. Overzealous restriction and fad diets are not recommended. Food pyramid and traffic light approach for diet may be used to highlight healthy eating patterns, with particular emphasis on fixed portion size, decreased junk food consumption, avoiding television viewing while eating, and increased fruit consumption. Periods of inactivity should be reduced and increased physical activity should be planned. Screen time (television, computer, and mobile devices) should be restricted to less than 1 hour daily. Increased routine activities (e.g., household chores and walking to school) should be encouraged. A minimum of 30 minutes daily of enjoyable activities like dancing, sports, and running should be ensured, avoiding weight-bearing exercises and over-regimented schedules.

CLINICAL PEARL

- Lifestyle measures should be adopted by the entire family, not just the child.

TABLE 6: Drugs used for the treatment of childhood obesity.

Drugs	*Action*	*Dose*	*Status*
Orlistat	Gastric lipase inhibitor	120 mg with meals	After 12 years
Liraglutide	GLP1 analog	3 mg daily injection	After 12 years
Semaglutide	GLP1 analog	2.4 mg weekly	After 12 years
Metformin	Insulin sensitizer	500–2,000 mg daily	T2DM and NAFLD
Topiramate	Increased satiety	7.5/46 mg daily	After 12 years
Octreotide	Central	Experimental	Hypothalamic obesity
Growth hormone	Increased metabolism	20–30 µg/kg/day	PWS
Metreleptin	Leptin effect	Experimental	Leptin deficiency
Setmelanotide	MC4R agonist	Experimental	POMC and PCK defect

(GLP1: glucagon-like peptide 1; NAFLD: nonalcoholic fatty liver disease; PWC: Prader–Willi syndrome; POMC: Proopiomelanocortin; T2DM: type 2 diabetes mellitus)

- *Specific management:* Specific treatment is needed for hypothyroidism, GH deficiency, and Cushing's syndrome. Mild elevations of TSH do not require treatment. Obese children with Prader–Willi Syndrome and growth failure may benefit from GH therapy.
- *Treatment of complications:* Complications should be treated early to avoid long-term adverse effects. Metformin is indicated for T2DM, NAFLD, and PCOS; statins are for persistent dyslipidemia. Treatment of NAFLD includes metformin, ursodeoxycholic acid (UDCA), and vitamin E. Girls with PCOS benefit from lifestyle modification, metformin, oral contraceptives, and antiandrogens. Continuous positive airway pressure is needed in obstructive sleep apnea.
- *Medical treatment* ***(Table 6)****:* Orlistat is the only drug approved for use in children with obesity. It inhibits gastric lipase, resulting in reduced fat absorption with modest weight loss. Significant side effects include abdominal pain, bloating, steatorrhea, and anal leakage of oil. It has to be combined with fat-soluble vitamins. Recently, glucagon-like peptide-1 (GLP1) receptor agonists semaglutide and liraglutide have been approved for the treatment of adolescents with obesity. Other therapeutic options include metformin for T2DM and antipsychotic-induced obesity, leptin for leptin deficiency, and MC4 receptor analog setmelanotide for proopiomelanocortin (POMC), MC4 receptor, or proconvertase defect.
- *Surgical management:* Bariatric surgery is a major undertaking and should be considered only with morbid obesity (BMI above 40 kg/m^2 or 35 kg/m^2 with comorbidity) after achievement of final height. Patients need to adhere to strict dietary restrictions for life. In children, laparoscopic adjustable banding is recommended; malabsorptive procedures and gastric sleeve should be avoided.

CLINICAL PEARL

- Medical and surgical treatment of childhood obesity should be considered only in severe cases associated with complications.

PREVENTION

Given the difficulties in management, prevention is the desirable goal. Key measures include prevention and treatment of adult obesity (due to intergenerational effects of obesity), early identification and treatment of gestational diabetes mellitus, and increased consumption of healthy food. Exclusive breastfeeding should be done till 6 months, on a demand basis, not according to a schedule. Infants should be free to decide the frequency and amount of feeds. Saturated fats (e.g., full-fat milk) should be restricted after 2 years. Changes in dietary habits, including eating food with family regularly, avoiding snacking, avoiding television while eating, and fixed portion size, should be advised. The child is encouraged to play (moderate physical activity) for at least 60 minutes daily. The screen time should be limited to <2 hours daily. Television should be removed from children's bedrooms and avoided in children under 2 years.

KEY POINTS

- Childhood obesity is now a global epidemic mainly due to lifestyle changes; pathologic causes are rare.
- BMI after the age of 5 years according to IAP guidelines 2024, and weight-for-height in infants, and waist circumference, are used for routine diagnosis.
- In constitutional obesity, the child is usually tall for age. Pathologic causes should be suspected in a child with growth retardation (i.e., short and fat) and/or delayed puberty.
- Obesity leads to several health problems, therefore, it should be taken seriously.
- Most obese children require investigations not for the cause, but for the consequences of obesity.
- Management involves lifestyle changes for the entire family and treatment of consequences.
- Management is difficult. Prevention is critical, at all levels, from individual to societal.
- Lipomastia and buried penis require weight loss and no other treatment.

SUGGESTED READING

1. Bajpai A, Dave C. Obesity. In: Bajpai A (Ed). Practical Pediatric Endocrinology. New Delhi: Indian Journal of Pediatrics; 2020. pp. 65-73.
2. Bajpai A, Shenoy MT, Karia P. IAP Standard Treatment Guidelines Childhood Obesity. [online]. Available from https://iapindia.org/pdf/Ch-026-Childhood-Obesity.pdf [Last accessed December, 2024].
3. Dave C, Agarwal N, Patel R, Shukla R, Bajpai A. Comparison of the predictive value of IAP 2015 and WHO body mass index criteria for hypertension in Indian children and adolescents. Indian J Pediatr. 2022;89(12):1175-9.
4. Dave C, Agarwal N, Patel R, Shukla R, Bajpai A. Determinants and predictors of body fat in Indian children and adolescents. Indian J Pediatr. 2022;89(5):473-6.
5. Dave C, Agarwal N, Patel R, Shukla R, Bajpai A. Predictors of metabolic complications in obese Indian children and adolescents. Indian J Pediatr. 2021;88(3):252-6.
6. Hampl SE, Hassink SG, Skinner AC, Armstrong SC, Barlow SE, Bolling CF, et al. Clinical practice guideline for the evaluation and treatment of children and adolescents with obesity. Pediatrics. 2023;151(2):e2022060640.
7. Patel R, Dave C, Mehta S, Mendpara H, Shukla R, Bajpai A. Metabolic impact of subclinical hypothyroidism in obese children and adolescents. Indian J Pediatr. 2021;88(5):437-40.
8. Styne DM, Arslanian SA, Connor EL, Farooqi IS, Murad MH, Silverstein JH, et al. Pediatric obesity-assessment, treatment, and prevention: An endocrine society clinical practice guideline. J Clin Endocrinol Metab. 2017;102(3):709-57.

An Approach to Hyperglycemia

Aspi J Irani

INTRODUCTION

Normoglycemia is defined as fasting venous plasma glucose between 70 and 100 mg/dL and a 2-hour post-prandial or post-glucose-load value less than 140 mg/dL. Corresponding values more than 126 and 200 mg/dL are used to define diabetes mellitus (DM).

Hyperglycemia is encountered by the pediatrician/neonatologist in five different settings:

1. Child or adolescent with typical symptoms of DM
2. Hyperglycemia as an incidental pick up (or during screening) in an obese (but asymptomatic) adolescent
3. Neonate or infant (below 6 months) with symptoms of hyperglycemia
4. Hyperglycemia during an acute illness in a child/adolescent [stress hyperglycemia (SH)]
5. Hyperglycemia in a sick neonate in the neonatal intensive care unit (NICU).

Hyperglycemia is due to a disturbed balance between insulin on one hand and the counter-regulatory hormones (adrenaline, glucagon, cortisol, and growth hormone) on the other. While insulin promotes utilization or storage of glucose entering the body, and promotes protein and fat anabolism, the counter-regulatory hormones promote catabolism of protein and fat and favor movement of glucose into the blood stream from storage sites (chiefly liver, muscle, and kidneys) by promoting gluconeogenesis and glycogenolysis.

Adverse effects of hyperglycemia include:

- Osmotic diuresis with dehydration and electrolyte derangements once the renal threshold has been exceeded
- Hyperosmolarity (An 18 mg/dL rise in blood glucose (BG) raises osmolarity by 1 mOsm/L) and osmotic shifts with brain cell dehydration and risk of intracranial bleeds
- Glucose overload in insulin independent endothelial cells (hepatic, immune, and nerve cells) with generation of oxygen free radicals and resultant mitochondrial dysfunction and enhanced apoptosis
- Impaired leukocyte phagocytic function predisposing to infections and leading to delayed clearing of infections
- In the NICU, an increased risk of severe retinopathy of prematurity, necrotizing enterocolitis (NEC), bronchopulmonary dysplasia, septicemia, with longer duration of NICU stay, and a higher mortality
- In the long-term, persistent hyperglycemia can affect many organs by glycosylation of proteins/collagen.

CHILD OR ADOLESCENT WITH TYPICAL SYMPTOMS OF DIABETES MELLITUS

Polyuria, polydipsia, polyphagia, weight loss, and weakness (with or without a history of ants around the urine and of vaginal candidiasis) are typical symptoms due to hyperglycemia.

If ketosis has set in, there would be anorexia, vomiting, abdominal pain and distension, followed by dehydration and acidotic breathing, with a peculiar "acetone" odor to the breath, and eventually, drowsiness and coma. Shock can occur but is uncommon.

In the presence of typical symptoms of hyperglycemia with ketosis, single random BG over 200 mg/dL is sufficient to clinch the diagnosis of DM. In this situation, an oral glucose tolerance test (OGTT) is not only unnecessary but can also be dangerous.

In an asymptomatic or mildly symptomatic child, a fasting BG (done after 8 h of no calorie intake) of 126 mg/dL or above, with 2-hour postprandial value of 200 mg/dL or more on two occasions is diagnostic of DM. The OGTT should never be done if DM can be diagnosed from the fasting, random, or postprandial BG values.

A fasting BG glucose between 100 and 125 mg/dL is referred to as "impaired fasting glucose" while a post glucose reading between 140 and 199 mg/dL is labeled as "impaired glucose tolerance"; both these are considered as prediabetic states.

Having made the diagnosis of DM, the next step is to ascertain the type of DM. Type 1, is, by far, the commonest variety encountered in childhood. Presence of detectable pancreatic autoantibodies (common antibodies tested are to glutamic acid decarboxylase (GAD 65), insulin, islet cell, and tyrosine phosphatase or IAA2, and zinc transporter 8) with low or inappropriately low C-peptide values ('normal' value of C-peptide in the presence of hyperglycemia) in a child with acute onset of symptoms of DM is highly suggestive of a diagnosis of T1DM. However, in Indian studies, absence of antibodies has been reported in over 25% of individuals who behave clinically just like those who are antibody positive. C-peptide values in a child with acute onset of symptoms of DM confirms the diagnosis of T1DM. However, absence of antibodies does not rule out T1DM, as Indian studies have reported over 25% of antibody negative T1DM. One should look for associated autoimmune disorders, both endocrine (thyroid dysfunction, adrenal disease, and hypoparathyroidism) and nonendocrine (celiac disease, alopecia areata, vitiligo, autoimmune hepatitis, mucocutaneous candidiasis, and pernicious anemia).

Type 2 DM (T2DM) is becoming commoner because of the increasing incidence of increasing incidence of childhood and adolescent obesity. It must be suspected in any obese adolescent with a family history of T2DM, especially if there are associated features indicating insulin resistance [acanthosis nigricans, hypertension, hyperlipidemia, evidence of polycystic ovarian syndrome (PCOS)]. It must be emphasized that diabetic ketoacidosis (DKA) at presentation does not exclude T2DM: 6-33% of T2DM present in DKA. Absence of pancreatic antibodies or long periods of low or no insulin requirements initially, is suggestive of T2DM. Initially c-peptide levels may be low due to glucotoxicity; normal or high levels of C-peptide after initial control of hyperglycemia is suggestive of T2DM. In such cases, absence of antibodies typical of T1DM with high C-peptide levels would confirm T2DM. It must be emphasized that diabetic ketoacidosis (DKA) at presentation does not exclude T2DM; 6–33% of T2DM present in DKA.

A nonobese adolescent with mild diabetes and a family history of DM in three generations, possibly has one of the varieties of maturity onset diabetes of the young (MODY), usually a form of monegenic diabetes. If there is optic atrophy or associated deafness or persistent polyuria despite good control of DM (pointing to an associated diabetes insipidus), the diagnosis would be "Wolfram syndrome". In a child with recurrent abdominal pain, the development of DM should initiate a search for pancreatic calculi (fibrocalculus pancreatic diabetes). Diabetes associated with sensorineural deafness and thiamine responsive megaloblastic anemia is referred to as "Roger syndrome". The clinician needs to look for any syndromic features in a child with DM as Down syndrome, Turner syndrome, Prader-Willi, and Klinefelter syndromes (besides many others) can be associated with DM with a higher frequency than in the general population. Adolescents with thalassemia major tend to develop DM in the second decade of life due to iron deposits in the pancreas (causing insulin deficiency) and in the liver (leading to insulin resistance). **Flowchart 1** outlines the approach to a pediatric patient with typical symptoms of hyperglycemia with or without ketonuria.

Insulin is the mainstay of treatment for T1DM, and initial treatment of any diabetes with severe hyperglycemia, including T2DM. Metformin was till recently the only approved oral drug, but in the last 5 years, liraglutide and empagliflozin have also been approved as add-on therapy for T2DM in adolescents (age 10 years and above) not controlled adequately with metformin alone. Oral drugs are not approved for T1DM at present. All varieties of DM also require lifestyle change, medical nutrition therapy, regular physical activity, regular BG monitoring, and attention to comorbidities and mental health. All patients with DM must receive intensive and ongoing education in diabetes self-management.

HYPERGLYCEMIA DETECTED ON SCREENING IN AN OBESE ASYMPTOMATIC ADOLESCENT

Children above the age of 10 years who have attained puberty must be screened for DM if they have any two of the following risk factors

- Obesity
- Family history of DM in a 1st or 2nd degree relative
- Evidence of insulin resistance (hypertension, acanthosis nigricans, dyslipidemia, fatty liver, and PCOS)
- Gestational or pre-existing diabetes in the mother.

In these adolescents, a fasting and preferably also a 2-hour post glucose (1.75 g/kg to a maximum of 75 g)

Flowchart 1: Approach to a pediatric patient with typical symptoms of hyperglycemia with or without ketonuria.

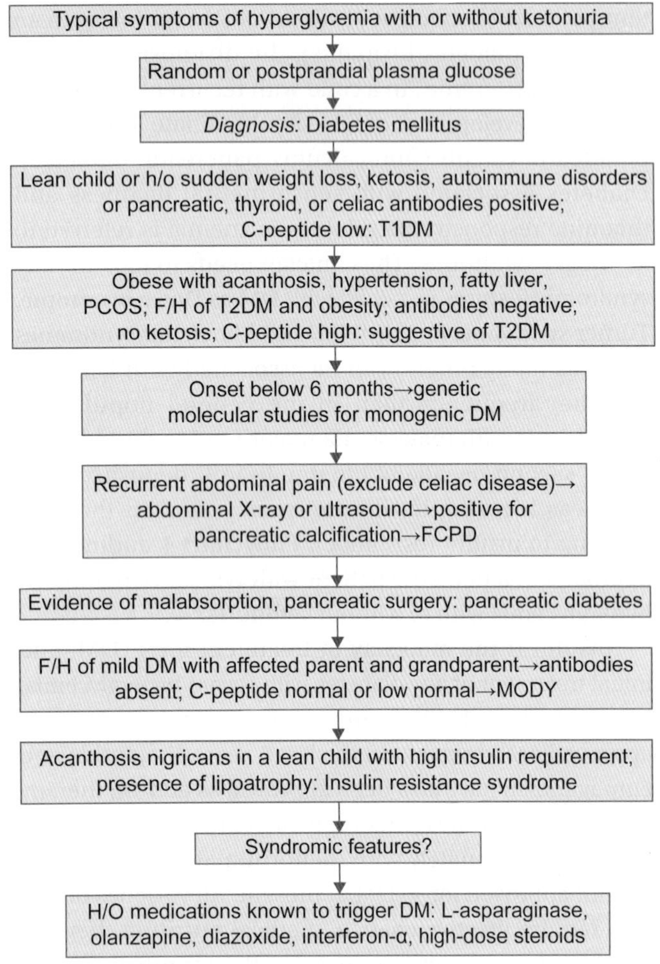

(F/H: family history; FCPD: fibrocalculous pancreatic diabetes; H/O: history of; MODY: maturity onset diabetes of the young; PCOS: polycystic ovarian syndrome; T1DM: type 1 diabetes mellitus; T2DM: type 2 diabetes mellitus)

BG should be checked once in every 3 years, annually if previous tests were borderline, or whenever there are symptoms suggestive of hyperglycemia. **Flowchart 2** outlines the diagnostic approach and classification of deranged glucose metabolism in these cases.

CLINICAL PEARL

- Obese adolescents with evidence of insulin resistance or a family history of diabetes mellitus (DM) or with *in-utero* exposure to DM must have a fasting blood glucose test every 3 years to screen for DM.

Early detection and treatment with lifestyle changes, tight glycemic control (metformin, incretins like liraglutide, gliflozins), and careful control of comorbidities (hypertension, dyslipidemia, fatty liver, sleep apnea) are very important as T2DM may remain asymptomatic and escape detection for a prolonged period of time. Some patients with T2DM may test positive for autoantibodies characteristic of T1DM; they are classified as having "latent autoimmune diabetes" and are likely to need insulin in the near future (usually in next 3 years).

Flowchart 2: Approach to an adolescent with mild symptoms suggestive of hypergnlycemia, or clinical setting suggestive of type 2 diabetes mellitus.

Mild symptoms suggestive of hyperglycemia but nondiagnostic random plasma glucose Or Asymptomatic pubertal adolescent with any two of:
- Obesity
- T2DM in a 1st or 2nd degree relative
- Evidence of insulin resistance
- *In utero* exposure to DM

↓

Fasting and 2-hours post-glucose plasma glucose (1.75 g glucose/kg: maximum of 75 g)

↓

- Fasting plasma glucose <100 mg/dL and 2-hours post-glucose value <140 mg/dL →normoglycemia
- Fasting plasma glucose 100–125 mg/dL and 2-hours post-glucose value <140 mg/dL →impaired fasting glucose
- Fasting plasma glucose <100 mg/dL and 2-hours post-glucose value 140–199 mg/dL →impaired glucose tolerance
- Fasting plasma glucose ≥126 mg/dL and 2-hours post-glucose value ≥200 mg/dL →DM

(DM: diabetes mellitus; T2DM: type 2 diabetes mellitus)

NEONATE/INFANT (BELOW 6 MONTHS) WITH SYMPTOMS OF HYPERGLYCEMIA

The neonate/infant with diabetic hyperglycemia would present with irritability, polyuria, weight loss, failure to thrive, and dehydration with or without acidotic breathing and occasionally with candidiasis in the genital region. Important differentials include diabetes insipidus, renal tubular acidosis, diluted feeds, and hyperthyroidism. In patients presenting with hyperglycemia and metabolic acidosis, if there is lack of improvement with appropriate treatment of DKA, the possibility of certain inborn errors of metabolism must be kept in mind: these include methylmalonic acidemia, propionic acidemia, isovaleric acidemia, biotinidase deficiency, and cobolamine metabolism defects. If the diagnosis of DM is confirmed (as above), the two broad possibilities are: (1) transient neonatal diabetes mellitus (TNDM) and (2) permanent neonatal diabetes mellitus (PNDM).

Transient Neonatal Diabetes Mellitus

The presentation is soon after birth (median age 3 days). Most infants are below the 3rd percentile in weight (average weight 2 kg). Associated congenital anomalies reported include macroglossia in 20% and umbilical hernia in 10%. They show remarkable improvement with insulin therapy. This is a self-limited condition and resolves by 18 months (median age 12 weeks).

Abnormalities of chromosome 6q24 with overexpression of paternally expressed genes are seen in 65% of cases. The defect may be paternal uniparental isodisomy of chromosome 6, paternally inherited duplications within the long arm of chromosome 6, or loss of methylation within the TNDM critical region of chromosome 6 on the paternally inherited chromosome. Three novel heterozygous mutations in the KCNJ11 gene (G53S, G53R, and I182V) have been shown to result in TNDM in some patients who do not have abnormalities of chromosome 6q24. Some mutations in the ABCC8 gene and the HNF1b gene are also associated with this transient variety of DM.

Although these patients grow out of their insulin dependence by 18 months of age (usually earlier), 50–60% will have a recurrence of DM later in life (average age 14 years with a range of 4–25 years). On recurrence, most would require insulin though the dose is small or the requirement may be intermittent; some may be controlled with sulfonylureas. A few may display hyperglycemia only during intercurrent illnesses.

Thus, what is referred to as TNDM may actually be a permanent defect in b-cell insulin release with variable expression at different stages of development.

Permanent Neonatal Diabetes Mellitus

Permanent neonatal diabetes mellitus is a genetically heterogeneous disorder with at least nine different genetic etiologies reported till date. These genetic defects may be associated with either deranged b-cell function or reduced pancreatic mass with or without syndromic features. Thyroid, pancreas, liver, heart, brain, kidney, and skeletal abnormalities may be associated.

Approximately 95% of patients with monogenic causes of neonatal DM present within the first 6 months of life, with around 3% diagnosed between 6 and 12 months of age.

CLINICAL PEARL

- All patients diagnosed with diabetes mellitus before 6 months of age, as well as those patients diagnosed between 6 and 12 months of age, who have no detectable pancreatic autoantibodies, should undergo molecular genetic testing.

There are five genes known to be associated with nonsyndromic PNDM. The first two listed below have important therapeutic significance as they can be managed on sulfonylurea group of drugs and do not require insulin for treatment:

1. Heterogeneous activating mutations of the KCNJ11 gene which encodes one of the two protein subunits (Kir6.2) of the adenosine triphosphate sensitive K^+ (KATP) channel in the b-cells account for 30% of cases of PNDM. Low birth weight (LBW) is a consistent phenotypic marker but after insulin treatment, there is marked catch up growth followed by normal growth. Twenty percent have developmental delay and muscle weakness and 5% have epilepsy in association with neonatal diabetes (the so-called DEND syndrome)
2. Mutation in the ABCC8 gene which encodes the other protein subunit (the SUR1 subunit) of the KATP channel constitutes another genetic etiology and is the cause in 19% of all PNDM.
3. Mutations of the gene encoding insulin (INS gene) accounts for a further 20% of cases of PNDM: these babies are born at full term, have a better birth weight (median 2.86 kg in one study), and are diagnosed later (3–6 months of age), vs. those with ABCC8 or KCNJ11 defects (median age 9 weeks).
4. Homozygous inactivating mutations of the gene encoding glucokinase must be suspected in PNDM with history of consanguinity, especially if both parents have mild hyperglycemia. These infants present at birth with severe LBW. As a first test in any LBW baby born with neonatal diabetes, parents' BG should be checked.
5. Rarely, neonatal diabetes may be due to inactivating mutations of the PDX1 (IPF1) gene. This is associated with pancreatic agenesis or hypoplasia and hence with exocrine pancreatic insufficiency. These patients have the severest insulin deficiency and present early with significant LBW. Carrier parents would have mild adult onset diabetes.

CLINICAL PEARL

- Neonatal diabetes mellitus due to mutations of the KCNJ11 and ABCC8 genes do not require insulin therapy; these can be controlled with sulfonylurea group of drugs.

There are at least four syndromes associated with neonatal DM which can be suspected in a given case from their associated features:

1. *GLIS3* gene mutation has PNDM due to pancreatic hypoplasia with severe congenital hypothyroidism, glaucoma, hepatic fibrosis, and cystic renal disease.
2. *PTF1α* gene mutation causes severe PNDM with pancreatic agenesis or hypoplasia with associated exocrine pancreatic insufficiency, dysmorphic facies, microcephaly, and impaired cerebellar development with severe developmental delay and occasionally, gall bladder agenesis.
3. *FOXP3* gene mutation (the "IPEX syndrome") is a X-linked disorder of autoimmunity that occurs in males who present with neonatal diabetes, immune dysregulation, autoimmune thyroid disease, intractable diarrhea, exfoliative dermatitis, eczematous skin rash, and very high serum immunoglobulin E. Most die of overwhelming sepsis in the first months or years of life.
4. Mutations of the *EIF2AK3* gene lead to persistent neonatal diabetes and either multiple epiphyseal or spondyloepiphyseal dysplasia (Wolcott-Rallison syndrome). Transmission is autosomal recessive. Some may have progressive renal failure from glomerulonephritis. One-fourth patients have exocrine pancreatic insufficiency. They may also have recurrent hepatitis and intellectual disability.

Newer mutations are being reported, e.g. mutations in trascription factors, GATS6 and GATS4 (pancreatic hypoplasia and agenesis, congenital heart disease and various dysmorphic features).

While it may be difficult clinically to distinguish TNDM from PNDM, genetic studies, which are mandatory in infants with diabetes, often give the answer.

MANAGEMENT OF NEONATAL DIABETES MELLITUS

Molecular genetic studies must be done in all infants presenting below 6–12 months of age with diabetes. A search for the KCNJ11 and ABCC8 mutations should be urgently undertaken as it has important therapeutic implications. An ultrasound or preferably computed tomography or magnetic resonance imaging scan of the abdomen should be obtained to look for hypoplastic/absent pancreas. Appropriate tests to detect associated hypothyroidism, cerebellar hypoplasia, renal cysts, skeletal defects, agenesis of the gall bladder, or deranged liver function should be undertaken in selected cases. Screening of the parents for undiagnosed diabetes and gene mutations is essential.

At presentation, if the infant is dehydrated, with or without ketoacidosis, intravenous fluids and insulin infusion would be required as per the DKA protocol.

For long-term management, insulin, coupled with a high calorie intake, is crucial to achieve normal growth and sustained weight gain. Insulin therapy is guided by continuous glucose monitoring (CGM) using sensors applied on the thigh or the abdomen. It may be given by insulin pump, using rapi acting analogs, or by multiple subcutaneous injections, using either short-acting ('Regular' or soluble) insulin, or neutral protamine Hagedorn (NPH) insulin, carefully resuspended before injecting. The average dose is 0.3-1 unit/kg/day, adjusted on basis of CGM patterns. Insulin pump giving 30% of the dose as basal and rest 70% divided into boluses to cover the feeds is successful, but has several issues.

In the first 6 months, the infant needs to be exclusively breastfed every 3 hours or so. If the mother is not in a position to breastfeed, a milk formula may be offered. Frequent small feeds are preferred in order to prevent swings in blood glucose. When weaning foods are introduced, one should prefer foods with a low glycemic index.

BG should be maintained between 100–200 mg/dL with use of CGM. Prevention of both hypoglycemia and hyperglycemia is an important priority in the first 3 years of life to prevent detrimental effects on brain development. If CGM is not possible, regular BG monitoring using glucometer before and 2–3 hours after every feed should be done.

Patients with NDM owing to KCNJ11 and ABCC8 mutations can be successfully shifted to oral treatment with sulfonylureas after initial stabilization with insulin. Glibenclamide appears to be more effective than other sulfonylureas. Doses required are usually higher than those used in adult patients with T2DM (0.33 mg/kg/day for a 60 kg adult). The median dose in NDM is 0.45 mg/kg/day (range 0.1–1.5 mg/kg/day). Glycemic control tends to improve with time, and the dose of sulfonylurea can subsequently be decreased. Transient diarrhea and yellow or grayish staining of deciduous teeth may occur, but other adverse effects are rare.

Pancreatic enzyme replacement therapy is required for those with exocrine deficiency.

STRESS HYPERGLYCEMIA

Stress hyperglycemia refers to transiently elevated BG during an illness. The American Diabetes Association has defined SH as any BG more than 140 mg/dL in a hospitalized nondiabetic patient. About 3.8% of children presenting to the emergency department would have SH. Fever more than 39.5°C, febrile seizures, traumatic brain injuries, burns, sepsis, pancreatitis, and dehydration are the most common acute situations associated with SH. The more severe the illness, the greater is the likelihood of SH. A glycosylated hemoglobin test would help in excluding the possibility of hitherto undetected DM as the cause for hyperglycemia.

SH is caused by changes in glucose metabolism, due to increase in counter-regulatory hormones, leading to increased glycogenolysis, neoglucogenesis, and development of insulin resistance both central (in the liver) and peripheral (in muscle and fat). Proinflammatory cytokines tumor necrosis factor-α [increased free fatty acid (FFA) causing insulin resistance], interleukin (IL)-1 (increased gluconeogenesis), and IL-6 (increased glycogenolysis) also contribute. Interleukin-10 and transforming growth factor-β may also be involved. Intensive care unit (ICU) procedures (particularly, mechanical ventilation), use of vasoactive agents, prolonged immobilization, and nutritional practices in the ICU further add to SH.

Modest hyperglycemia (<180 mg/dL) may be beneficial (an adaptive response) by providing additional energy to meet the increased metabolic demand of the brain, red blood cells, and other cells; but if prolonged or severe, it has been associated with higher morbidity and mortality. Both the peak and the duration of hyperglycemia affect prognosis. SH is more dangerous than hyperglycemia without stress. In the former, the glucose transporters are over-expressed. Hence, more glucose enters the cells. This leads to altered cell metabolism with increased reactive oxygen species generation which causes altered mitochondrial function and apoptosis. SH also impairs macrophage and neutrophil function and complement activity.

Does SH need to be treated and if so, what is the best approach? There is no conclusive answer to this question in adult and in pediatric studies conducted till date. Trials concluded so far in the pediatric population using insulin infusion to achieve tight BG control have given conflicting results. The duration of hospital stay may be reduced with tight BG control but the incidence of hypoglycemia also goes up significantly. Thus, it may be reasonable to try and maintain the BG at levels of 140–180 mg/dL rather than aggressively controlling BG to lower levels. When insulin is used, it should be given as a continuous infusion of regular human insulin with close monitoring of BG.

CLINICAL PEARL

- Stress hyperglycemia needs treatment with insulin infusion, only if blood glucose is more than 180 mg/dL with glycosuria; the target blood glucose should be 140–180 mg/dL, with all efforts to prevent hypoglycemia.

Are children with SH more likely to develop DM in future? Studies have reported an incidence of later diabetes ranging from 0–33% in patients with a history of SH. In one detailed study only 2.1% developed T1DM during 42 months of follow-up; all of these had human leukocyte antigen types or autoimmune markers known to be associated with T1DM, or an abnormal OGTT on recovery from the acute illness. Those with hyperglycemia during relatively minor illnesses, or a family history of T1DM or other autoimmune disorders have a higher risk than those who develop SH during major illnesses.

HYPERGLYCEMIA IN NEONATAL INTENSIVE CARE UNIT

Hyperglycemia in neonates, defined historically as a whole blood glucose more than 125 mg/dL or serum glucose more than 150 mg/dL, is common in critically ill neonates and in the very low birth weight (VLBW) premature babies. Its occurrence is inversely related to gestational age and birth weight and directly related to the severity of any accompanying illnesses.

Pathophysiology and Causes

Lower and delayed insulin production in response to glucose load is reported in the VLBW neonates, due to smaller beta cell mass, preferential release of inactive proinsulin instead of insulin, and lack of enteral feeding which eliminates the boosting effect of gut incretins on insulin release. Glucose utilization is further limited because of their small mass of insulin dependent tissues: fat and muscle. Sick preterm babies have increased insulin resistance due to increased inflammatory markers, cytokines, and catecholamines.

Hyperglycemia could result from:

- Excess/rapid exogenous glucose delivery (iatrogenic)
- Stress (serious illness especially septicemia, respiratory distress, or NEC; pain; surgical procedures)
- Therapy with certain drugs (corticosteroids, theophylline, caffeine, phenytoin, or use of diazoxide in mother)

- Cerebral pathology with large damaged areas having reduced metabolism and thus, decreased glucose utilization (trauma, hypoxemic-ischemic lesions, hemorrhage, meningitis, and encephalitis)
- Total parenteral nutrition can also affect BG status.

Intralipid infusion raises BG as it stimulates gluconeogenesis by supplying FFA and glycerol. Intralipid supplies nearly three times more energy than glucose, hence when a neonate is started on intralipid, there is no need to give glucose at higher than physiological rate of 6–8 mg/kg/min. Aminoacids also support gluconeogenesis but to a lesser extent than intralipid. High amounts of aminoacid infusion, however, may help by increasing insulin secretion and glucose utilization.

Management

- *Anticipate and monitor for hyperglycemia:* All susceptible neonates must have blood glucose screening. Heel prick or fingers prick BG at bedside though inaccurate is very useful in screening for hyperglycemia. The results must be confirmed with laboratory estimation of plasma glucose. The CGM system measures interstitial tissue glucose level every 5 minutes; it has been successfully used in the NICU. Urine should be checked for glycosuria as this is likely to be accompanied with changes in serum osmolarity.
- Any underlying cause of hyperglycemia must be sought out and addressed first (such as sepsis, TNDM and PNDM, specific illnesses, or hyperglycemia inducing drugs).
- Consider limited reduction of glucose infusion rate: When hyperglycemia is detected, the first intervention is to reduce the glucose infusion rate to 6–12 mg/kg/min; stable preterms need a glucose supply of 6 mg/kg/min, an ill preterm would require more glucose. A lower rate would not meet the basic glucose requirement. A higher rate than 12 mg/kg/min would be detrimental as the maximal glucose oxidative capacity is exceeded and beyond this level, conversion to fat occurs. Further, high glucose rates increase carbon dioxide production which is undesirable in respiratory compromised infants. Dextrose solutions with concentration less than 5% should never be used as these would be hypo-osmolar and can cause hemolysis and hyperkalemia. Total parenteral nutrition should be started as soon as possible in LBW babies; certain aminoacids can stimulate insulin release.
- *Insulin therapy:* It should be started when the BG exceeds 250 mg/dL or when there is glycosuria despite above measures. BG should be brought down slowly to avoid rapid fluid shifts. Insulin is given as an infusion at a rate of 0.02–0.1 units/kg/h. At the outset, it is important to run off about 50 mL of the insulin infusion to saturate binding sites on the tubing. The infusion should be changed every 24 hours. Large inter-subject variation in response is common, thus BG must be checked every 30–60 minutes initially till it has stabilized and thereafter every 4 hours for titration of insulin dose. Some studies have shown insulin to be safe and beneficial, while others report risks and problems. A threefold increased lactate concentration and significant acidosis is reported when insulin is given with high glucose infusion rate. Careful monitoring is required to minimize risks of hypokalemia and hypoglycemia which are known complications of insulin therapy. **Flowchart 3** outlines the approach to a neonate with symptoms of hyperglycemia or who is susceptible to hyperglycemia.

Flowchart 3: Approach to a neonate with suspected hyperglycemia or susceptible to hyperglycemia.

- Any neonate/infant with dehydration and polyuria
- All preterm babies and critically ill babies

↓

Test/screen for hyperglycemia:
Whole blood glucose >125 mg/dL or serum glucose >150 mg/dL

↓

- Baby with dehydration and polyuria→check serum insulin/C-peptide→if low→neonatal diabetes mellitus→start insulin therapy→obtain genetic molecular test for monogenic diabetes→if positive for *KCNJ11* or *ABCC8* gene mutations →switch to sulfonylurea
- Preterm and sick babies→treat underlying illness (sepsis/NEC/RDS)/eliminate causative drugs (if possible) or modify dosage

↓

If hyperglycemia persists: Lower glucose infusion rate to 6–12 mg/kg/min (do not use <5% dextrose)

↓

If blood glucose continues to be >250 mg/dL or in presence of glycosuria: Start insulin infusion

↓

Adjust infusion rate (0.02–0.10 units/kg/h) to achieve gradual reduction without hypoglycemia/hypokalemia (check blood glucose every 30 min till stable, then 4 hourly)

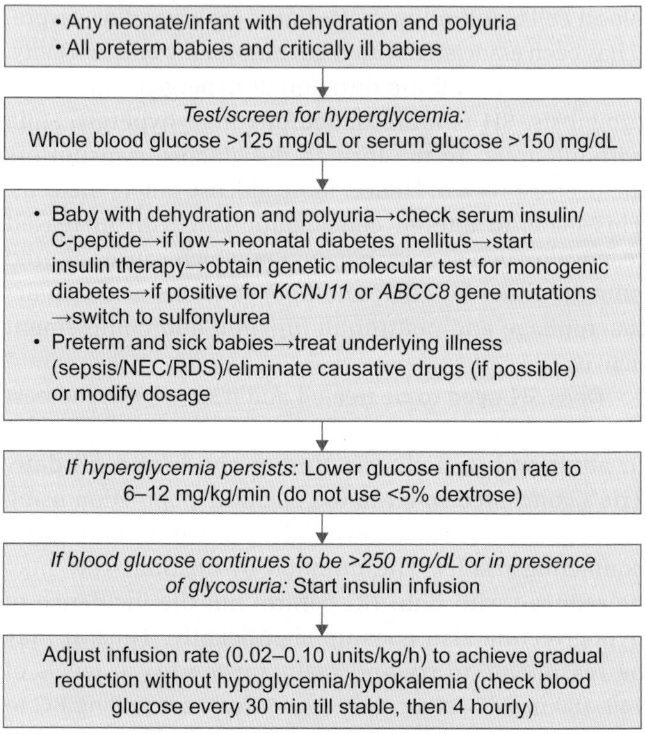

(NEC: necrotizing enterocolitis; RDS: respiratory distress syndrome)

KEY POINTS

- Diabetes mellitus (DM) must be considered in any child presenting with polyuria, polydipsia, polyphagia, weight loss, and weakness or with secondary enuresis, ants around the urine, or recurrent vaginal candidiasis.
- All pubertal adolescents with obesity and a family history of type 2 diabetes mellitus or evidence of insulin resistance or with history of *in utero* exposure to DM must be screened for DM every 3 years.
- Neonates/infants with irritability, polyuria, weight loss, failure to thrive, and dehydration with or without acidotic breathing or genital candidiasis must have a blood glucose test; if diagnosed to have diabetes, they should undergo genetic molecular testing for monogenic diabetes.
- Preterm babies, very low birth weight babies, and critically ill neonates must be screened for hyperglycemia and measures should be instituted to keep the blood glucose below a level at which there is significant glycosuria.

SUGGESTED READING

1. Aguilar-Bryan L, Bryan J. Neonatal diabetes mellitus. Endocr Rev. 2008;29(3): 265-91.
2. Chen L, Li T, Fang F, Zhang Y, Faramand A. Tight glycemic control in critically ill pediatric patients: a systematic review and meta-analysis. Crit Care. 2018;22(1):57.
3. Guven A, Cebeci N, Dursun A, Aktekin E, Baumgartner M, Fowler B. Methylmalonic acidemia mimicking diabetic ketoacidosis in an infant. Pediatr Diabetes. 2012;13(6): e22-5.
4. Honarmand K, Sirimaturos M, Hirshberg E, et al. Society of Critical Care Medicine guidelines on glycemic control for critically ill children and adults 2024. Crit Care Med. Online special article. January 19, 2024.
5. ISPAD Clinical Practice Consensus Guidelines 2009 Compendium. [online] Available from: www.ispad.org.
6. Khadilkar VV, Khadilkar AV, Kapoor RR, Hussain K, Hattersley AT, Ellard S. KCNJ11 activating mutation in an Indian family with remitting and relapsing diabetes. Indian J Pediatr. 2010;77(5):551-4.
7. Pati NK, Maheshwari R, Chellani H, Salhan RN. Transient neonatal hyperglycemia. Indian Pediatr. 2001;38(8): 898-901.
8. Pearson ER, Flechtner I, Njølstad PR. Switching from insulin to oral sulfonylureas in patients with diabetes due to Kir6.2 mutations. N Engl J Med. 2006;355:467-77.
9. Preissig CM, Hansen I, Roerig P, Rigby MR. A protocolized approach to identify and manage hyperglycemia in a pediatric critical care unit. Pediatr Crit Care Med. 2008;9: 581-8.
10. Preissig CM, Rigby MR. Pediatric critical illness hyperglycemia: risk factors associated with development and severity of hyperglycemia in critically ill children. J Pediatr. 2009;155(5):734-9.
11. Rafiq M, Flanagan SE, Patch AM, Shields BM, Ellard S, Hattersley AT. Effective treatment with oral sulfonylurea in patients with diabetes due to sulfonylurea receptor 1 (SUR1) mutations. Diabetes Care. 2008;31(2):204-9.
12. Sellers EAC, Moore K, Dean HJ. Clinical management of type 2 diabetes in indigenous youth. Pediatr Clin North Am. 2009;56(6):1441-59.

Gynecomastia in Children

Raghupathy Palany

INTRODUCTION

Gynecomastia is a benign enlargement of the male breast due to proliferation of the glandular component. It can develop in males of any age or weight, but often arises around puberty, as breast development is affected by hormonal changes. The condition may occur in one or both breasts and begin as a small firm lump beneath the nipple, which may be tender and later extend concentrically. If the breast enlargement is soft in consistency and does not contain true breast tissue, then it indicates fat deposition which is termed as pseudogynecomastia (lipomastia or adipomastia), and there is no glandular proliferation. The degree of gynecomastia in such cases is directly related to body mass index (BMI).

Physiologic gynecomastia is seen in newborns and in pubescent males. In newborns, breast enlargement in *both sexes* seen as a waning effect of transplacentally acquired maternal estrogen and usually lasts for a couple of weeks, but in rare cases may last until the child is 2 years old. This condition may even be associated with milk flow (galactorrhea).

Pubertal (also considered physiologic) gynecomastia is quite common and occurs in nearly two-thirds of pubertal boys. It appears around 12 years, more so during mid puberty and regresses without treatment in around 18 to 24 months. Obese boys appear to be more affected and may improve when adipose tissue becomes less on weight reduction. Gynecomastia is stated to be caused by relatively increased aromatization or higher than normal adult values of estrogen : testosterone ratio in this period, or through episodic elevations of estrogen, although many studies failed to document these changes conclusively. Increased sensitivity of the breast tissue to estrogens may be operative.

The histology of the male and female breast tissue being similar, exposure to estrogen in both sexes induces ductal epithelial hyperplasia, ductal elongation and branching, proliferation of the periductal fibroblasts, and an increase in vascularity.

Increased estrogen production and/or action can occur at the testicular level or at the periphery and is characterized as follows:

- *From peripheral conversion:* This can be due to increased substrate or increased activity of aromatase, as in chronic liver disease, malnutrition, hyperthyroidism, adrenal hyperplasia, when poorly controlled, adrenal tumors, and familial gynecomastia.
- *From the testes:* This can be due to testicular tumors or to ectopic production of human chorionic gonadotropin (hCG), as is reported with carcinoma of lung, kidney, gastrointestinal (GI) tract, and extragonadal germ cell tumors.

Pathologic gynecomastia should be distinguished carefully **(Flowchart 1)** as they require to be treated appropriately and can be caused by

- Increase in the production and/or action of estrogen,
  - Increased aromatization of androgens to estrogens
  - Increased androgenic precursors (dehydroepiandrosterone [DHEA] and androstenedione)
  - Increased SHBG – binds testosterone > estrogen favoring greater peripheral estrogen action
  - Estrogen receptor agonism
- Decrease in the production and/or action of testosterone
  - Decreased production
    - Primary hypogonadism
      - Klinefelter syndrome
      - Congenital anorchia
      - Enzymatic defect in testosterone biosynthesis
      - Infection (viral orchitis)
      - Infiltrative disorders
      - Testicular trauma

Flowchart 1: Approach to gynecomastia (estrogen excess, androgen deficiency, or androgen/estrogen imbalance).

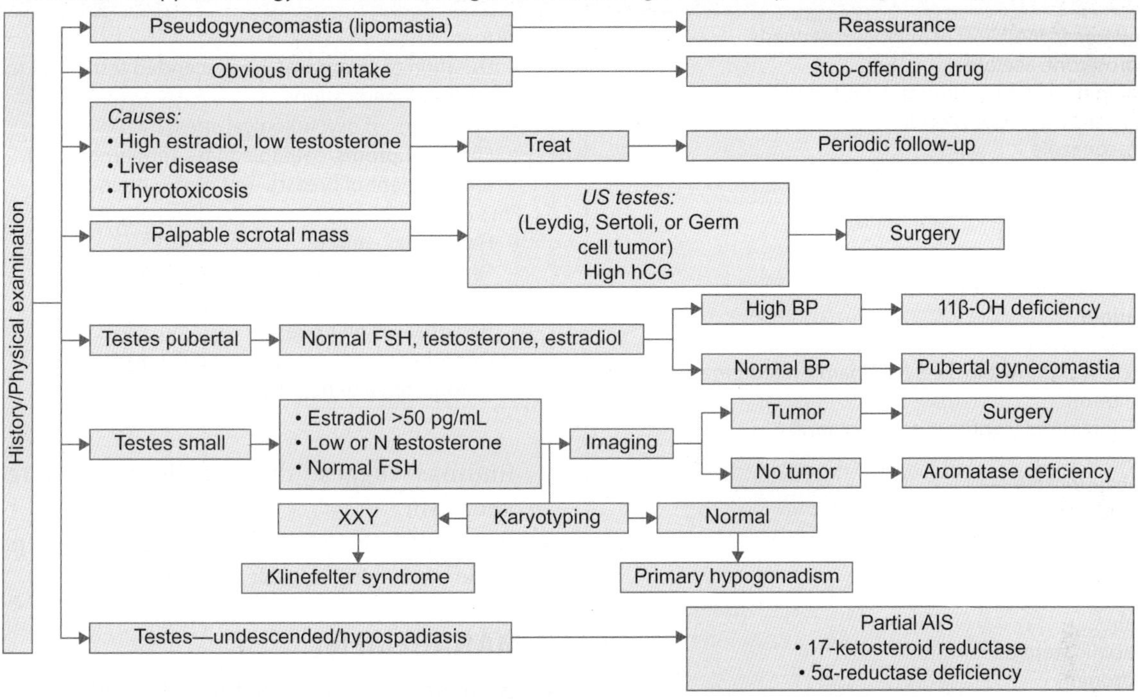

(AIS: androgen insensitivity syndrome; BP: blood pressure; FSH: follicle-stimulating hormone; hCG: human chorionic gonadotropin; US: ultrasound)

- Secondary hypogonadism
  - Hypothalamic or pituitary disorder (low testicular production of testosterone/estriol-adrenal androgens are aromatized - estrogen/androgen imbalance)
  - Kallmann syndrome with anosmia
- Androgen insensitivity syndrome
- Increased sex-hormone binding globulin (SHBG) - binds testosterone > estrogen favoring greater peripheral estrogen action
- Androgen receptor antagonism

- Idiopathic
- Drug use **(Box 1)**

SIGNS AND SYMPTOMS

- History of mumps, testicular trauma or drug use should be obtained.
- Thorough examination of the size and consistency of the breasts and to differentiate from lipomastia is essential.
- Examination of the testes, with attention to size and consistency, as well as nodules or asymmetry.
- Dimpling of the skin, nipple retraction and discharge, axillary lymphadenopathy are suggestive of breast carcinoma (rare).

DIAGNOSIS (BOX 2)

Patients with physiologic, asymptomatic and pubertal gynecomastia do not require further evaluation and should be reevaluated in 6 months. Further evaluation is necessary in the following situations:

- Breast size greater than 5 cm (macromastia)
- A lump that is tender, of recent onset, progressive, or of unknown duration
- Signs of malignancy (e.g., hard or fixed lymph nodes or positive lymph node findings)

Laboratory tests:

- Free or total testosterone, luteinizing hormone (LH), estradiol, dehydroepiandrosterone levels
- Thyroid-stimulating hormone (TSH) and free thyroxine levels

Imaging studies:

- Mammography is done, if one or more features of breast cancer are apparent upon clinical examination, followed by fine-needle aspiration or breast biopsy as appropriate.
- Testicular ultrasonography: Indicated if the serum estradiol level is elevated and the clinical examination

BOX 1: Drugs known to cause gynecomastia.

- *Antiandrogens/inhibitors of androgen synthesis*:
  - Cyproterone acetate
  - Flutamide, bicalutamide, and nilutamide
  - Finasteride and dutasteride
  - Ketoconazole
  - Spironolactone
- *Chemotherapeutic drugs:*
  - Alkylating agents
  - Methotrexate
  - Vinca alkaloids
  - Imatinib
- *Cardiac drugs and antihypertensives:*
  - Calcium channel blockers (verapamil, nifedipine, and diltiazem)
  - ACE inhibitors (captopril and enalapril)
  - Digoxin
  - Alpha-blockers
  - Amiodarone
  - Methyldopa
  - Reserpine
  - Nitrates
- *Hormones:*
  - Anabolic steroids
  - Androgens
  - Estrogens
  - Chorionic gonadotropin
- *Psychoactive drugs:*
  - Haloperidol
  - Diazepam
  - Tricyclic antidepressants
  - Phenothiazines
- *Anti-infective agents:*
  - Antiretroviral therapy for HIV/AIDS (e.g., indinavir)
  - Isoniazid
  - Ethionamide
  - Griseofulvin
  - Minocycline
  - Metronidazole
  - Ketoconazole
- *Drugs of abuse:*
  - Amphetamines
  - Heroin
  - Methadone
  - Alcohol
  - Marijuana
- *Miscellaneous:*
  - Theophylline
  - Omeprazole
  - Auranofin
  - Diethylpropion
  - Heparin
  - Domperidone
  - Penicillamine
  - Sulindac
  - Heparin

(AIDS: acquired immunodeficiency syndrome; HIV: human immunodeficiency virus)

BOX 2: Clinical evaluation of gynecomastia.

- *History:*
  - Duration of symptoms, undescended testis, and mumps
  - Intake of medications
  - Symptoms of psychological stress
  - Local symptoms, palpable mass, tenderness and enlargement of breasts, and nipple discharge
- *Physical examination:*
  - Height and weight
  - Feminizing signs and Tanner staging
  - Breast and overlying skin
  - Regional lymph nodes
  - Undescended testes and testicular mass
  - Chronic renal or hepatic disease

findings suggest the possibility of a testicular neoplasm.

- Breast ultrasonography (though the positive predictive value of imaging in males is low).

MANAGEMENT

- No treatment is required for physiologic gynecomastia.
- Pubertal gynecomastia resolves spontaneously within several weeks to 2 years in most patients; therapy must be considered if remission has not occurred in 2 years.
- Breasts larger than 4 cm in diameter may not regress completely.
- Identifying and managing an underlying primary disorder often alleviates breast enlargement.
- For patients with idiopathic gynecomastia or with residual gynecomastia after treatment of the primary cause, medical or surgical treatment may be considered.
- In pathologic causes of gynecomastia, medical therapies should be tried early after onset.

Medical therapy of persistent adolescent gynecomastia is effective only when given early in the course of the disease and usually more successful in cases with small or moderate breast enlargement. The following drugs are often used and involve three possible pathways:

1. By blocking the effects of estrogens on the breast (e.g., clomiphene, tamoxifen, raloxifene),
2. Administering androgens (e.g., danazol), and
3. Inhibiting estrogen production (e.g., anastrozole, testolactone)

With only a few small case series and case reports without control groups, lack of data on risks, benefits and efficacy, there is no approved medical treatment for gynecomastia in children and adolescents. Surgical approach may be needed under special conditions, viz., macromastia, failed medical therapy, if no regression is observed after a period of observation of at least one year, or for cosmetic reasons, such as embarrassment or significant emotional distress in adolescents. Surgical excision of glandular and adipose tissues by circumareolar approach leaving minimal scarring by an experienced plastic surgeon is the best form of treatment for those requiring surgery. Liposuction may not be as safe and successful.

PATIENT EDUCATION

Patients with physiologic gynecomastia should be reassured regarding the benign nature of their condition, and informed that most cases spontaneously resolve.

PROGNOSIS

In approximately 90% of cases, pubertal gynecomastia resolves completely or partially within a period of months to several years. However, macromastia seldom resolves completely and often requires surgery.

Gynecomastia that occurs secondary to an underlying, treatable cause (e.g., drug-induced gynecomastia) usually responds to treatment or removal of the primary cause. Men with Klinefelter syndrome have a 10- to 20-fold increased risk for breast cancer.

KEY POINTS

- Gynecomastia is a benign proliferation of glandular tissue of the breast in males.
- Breast enlargement in infancy is a common condition due to the effect of maternal estrogen level from intrauterine life.
- It usually resolves spontaneously, typically within the first year of life.
- GM of puberty is a common condition, affecting approximately 50% of mid-pubertal boys; in more than 90% of cases, it resolves spontaneously within 24 months.

SUGGESTED READING

1. Kanakis GA, Nordkap L, Bang AK, Calogero AE, Bártfai G, Corona G, et al. EAA clinical practice guidelines-gynecomastia evaluation and management. Andrology. 2019;7:778-93.
2. Metwalley KA, Farghaly HS. Gynecomastia in adolescent males: current understanding of its etiology, pathophysiology, diagnosis, and treatment, Ann Pediatr Endocrinol Metab. 2024;29:75-81.
3. Soliman AT, De Sanctis V, Yassin M. Management of adolescent gynecomastia: an update. Acta Biomed. 2017; 88:204-13.

Precocious Puberty

PSN Menon, Madhava Vijayakumar

INTRODUCTION

Precocious puberty (PP) is characterized by the appearance of markers of pubertal development at an age earlier than the usual pattern for that population. PP represents a significant diagnostic, psychosocial, and therapeutic challenge for the pediatrician. Most cases in girls are an exaggeration of the normal physiological process, whereas in boys *approximately half of the cases are pathological.* In general, younger the age, more is t he chance of an underlying organic pathology. Early diagnosis and treatment is pivotal since, if left untreated, PP leads to eventual short stature and also causes psychological stress in the affected children. Some of the underlying causes (e.g., tumors) may even be fatal.

PHYSIOLOGY OF PUBERTY

The pulsatile release of gonadotropin-releasing hormone (GnRH) from the hypothalamus stimulates the pituitary gland to secrete the gonadotropins—luteinizing hormone (LH) and follicle-stimulating hormone (FSH). LH stimulates the Leydig cells of testes which secrete testosterone, initiating the pubertal changes in boys. FSH stimulates spermatogenesis by the seminiferous tubules. LH and FSH stimulate the ovaries to secrete estrogen which initiates the onset of puberty in girls and leads to the development of secondary sexual characters as well.

The secretion of GnRH is regulated by the "hypothalamic pulse generator" constituted by the neurons in the arcuate nucleus of the hypothalamus, which expresses several neurotransmitters, including kisspeptin and neurokinin B. The gonadal sex steroids exert a negative feedback regulation of gonadotropin secretion through the hypothalamic neurons.

Adrenarche is the increased production of the adrenal androgens—dehydroepiandrosterone (DHEA), associated with the development of the zona reticularis of the adrenal cortex and is independent of gonadal maturation.

NORMAL PUBERTY

Testicular enlargement from 3 to 4 mL is the first sign of puberty in boys, followed by enlargement of penis, pigmentation of scrotum, and growth of pubic and axillary hair. The various stages of puberty in boys are graded as Tanner stages 1–5 (sexual maturity rating; **Table 1**). Peak growth velocity occurs in the later stages of puberty in boys (Tanner stage 3–4) but earlier in girls (Tanner stage 2–3) **(Table 2)**. Onset of puberty is closely related to skeletal maturation.

Breast development is the first sign of puberty in girls, followed by growth acceleration, pubic hair development, and menarche **(Tables 3 and 4)**. Onset of breast development usually occurs at a bone age of 10 years and menarche at 12.5 years, irrespective of the chronological age. Peak growth velocity occurs in the initial 2 years, before menarche.

DEFINITION OF PRECOCIOUS PUBERTY

Puberty is considered precocious when signs of puberty appear before the age of 9 years in boys and 8 years in girls. The onset of menarche before 9.5 years is also termed as precocious.

TYPES OF PRECOCIOUS PUBERTY

Central precocious puberty (CPP) or gonadotropin-dependent PP is caused by early release of gonadotropins (FSH and LH) from the pituitary, which in turn stimulate the testes to produce testosterone, or ovaries to produce estrogen. In CPP, the sequence of pubertal changes mimics normal puberty, but begins at an earlier age.

Peripheral precocious puberty (PPP) or gonadotropin-independent PP is caused by secretion of sex steroids from any organ which is outside the hypothalamic–pituitary–gonadal (HPG) axis and independent of the hypothalamic pulse generator. Here, the sequence of puberty does not follow the normal pubertal pattern.

TABLE 1: Classification of sexual maturity rating (Tanner's staging) in boys.

Pubertal stage	*Genital development*	*Pubic hair development*	*Axillary hair development*
1	*Prepubertal:* Testes size 1–3 mL	Nil	Nil
2	• Testes size >4 mL in volume or >2.5 cm in length • Early penile growth • Scrotal skin thin and pink	Minimally pigmented hair at base of penis	Few axillary hair
3	• Testes enlarge to 10–15 mL in volume or >3.3–4 cm in length • Penis grows in length • Scrotal thickening and pigmentation	Darker, coarser, and curled hair extending to mons pubis	Adult pattern
4	• Testes enlarge to 15–20 mL in volume or >4–4.5 cm in length • Penis grows in breadth; glans increases in size	Thicker adult pattern of hair not yet extending to medial surface of thighs	
5	Adult genitalia; testes 25 mL in volume or >4.5 cm in length	Adult distribution spreading to medial side of thighs	

TABLE 2: Normal pubertal development in boys.

Onset of pubertal changes	*Mean age (years)*	*Range (years)*
Testicular enlargement begins	11–12	9–14
Penile enlargement begins	12	9–14
Pigmentation of scrotum	12	9–14
Pubic hair appears	12–13	11–14
Acceleration of growth	13–14	12–16
Axillary hair appears	14	12–16

Premature thelarche is the early development of breasts, without other signs of puberty such as rapid linear growth or pubic hair development. *Premature adrenarche* is the early development of pubic hair without other pubertal changes. Both are normal physiologic variants.

CAUSES OF PRECOCIOUS PUBERTY

Box 1 lists the common causes of PP. Idiopathic precocity is rare in boys. Organic causes account for a majority of cases in younger girls, whereas idiopathic causes are more common after the age of 6 years.

APPROACH TO DIAGNOSIS

History

Note the age at onset of the first signs of puberty and its progress over time. The growth spurt or peak growth velocity is important, as the acceleration of linear growth results in tall stature initially, but eventually the affected children become short adults since fusion of bones occur early. Onset of puberty in early childhood (below age 6 years) is highly suggestive of an organic central nervous system (CNS) pathology, particularly hypothalamic hamartoma, or McCune-Albright syndrome (MAS). Inquire about details of childbirth, perinatal insults, head trauma, CNS infections, tumors, and craniospinal radiation. History of headache, vomiting, and visual disturbances suggests an intracranial tumor. Gelastic epilepsy is a characteristic feature of hypothalamic hamartoma. Prematurity, intrauterine growth retardation, and adoption may be associated with PP. Developmental delay and behavioral disturbances are associated with CNS involvement as in cerebral palsy, hamartoma, and CNS malformations **(Fig. 1)**. A detailed family history of early puberty and consanguinity is helpful to diagnose constitutional forms, familial male-limited precocious puberty (FMPP or testotoxicosis) and congenital adrenal hyperplasia (CAH). Carefully elicit the history of drugs or creams consumed/applied by the child or parents/other family members, including illicit drug use (anabolic steroids, estrogen creams, androgen, and phytoestrogens). Possibility of sexual abuse, foreign body, or vaginal infection must be probed in girls with isolated vaginal bleeding. Ask for any previous height measurements (pediatrician/school).

CLINICAL PEARL

- Onset of puberty in early childhood (below age 6 years) is highly suggestive of an organic CNS pathology, particularly hypothalamic hamartoma, or MAS.

TABLE 3: Classification of sexual maturity rating (Tanner's staging) in girls.

Pubertal stage	*Breast development*	*Pubic hair development*	*Axillary hair development*
1	Prepubertal	Nil	Nil
2	Appearance of breast buds and slight areolar enlargement	Minimally pigmented hair on labia	Few axillary hair
3	Further enlargement of breast and areola	Darker, coarser, and curled hair extending to mons pubis	Adult pattern
4	Areola and nipple (papilla) form a secondary mound above the level of the breast	Thicker but not yet adult pattern	
5	Areola part of breast contour, projection of nippl e only	Adult distribution extending to medial surface of thighs	

TABLE 4: Normal pubertal development in girls.

Onset of pubertal changes	*Mean age (years)*	*Range (years)*
Breast development (thelarche)	10–11	8–15
Acceleration of growth	10–11	8–15
Pubic hair appears (pubarche)	11–12	9–15
Menarche	12–13	10–16

Physical Examination

The height, weight, span, and body proportions should be measured carefully and plotted on growth charts. It is important to measure the height of father and mother to calculate the midparental height, which is plotted on the right side of the growth chart. Compare with previous height measurements to assess growth velocity. Note the development of acne, pubic, axillary, and facial hair, as well as appearance of hair in unusual areas. Look for voice change and muscle development. Skin should be checked for texture (hypothyroidism), macules (neurocutaneous syndromes), neurofibromas, and cafe-au-lait spots (neurocutaneous disorders and MAS; **Fig. 2**). It is important to look for skeletal deformities (e.g., MAS). Hyperpigmentation of mucosa and skin is a common feature of CAH. Check for other clinical stigmata of hypothyroidism, e.g., weight gain with decreased linear growth, puffiness, lethargy, constipation, or coarse skin. PP is characterized by rapid growth rate, deepening of voice (in boys), and enlargement of genitalia. However, PP associated with hypothyroidism is characterized by growth faltering and absence of pubarche.

Pubertal development should be assessed according to Tanner's stages. In boys, assess testicular volume using an orchidometer and measure the stretched penile length (from the base of the shaft of the penis to the tip, excluding the foreskin). In children with CPP (e.g., hypothalamic hamartoma), penile enlargement is associated with increase in testicular volume (>4 mL, or diameter >2.5 cm). In PPP (e.g., CAH), testicular volume remains prepubertal (<4 mL). In testotoxicosis and human chorionic gonadotropin (hCG)-secreting tumors, testes are modestly and symmetrically enlarged (3–4 mL). Asymmetrical or unilateral enlargement of testis is seen in Leydig cell tumors or adrenal rests.

CLINICAL PEARL

- Measuring testicular volume carefully narrows down the possibilities, thus reducing the cost and number of investigations and the time taken for establishing the etiology of PP in boys.

In girls, evaluation of the breast as well as genital examination in an appropriate position is important. Vaginal mucosa should be examined in good light for signs of estrogen effect (e.g., pale pink color instead of glistening red prepubertal mucosa). Presence of vaginal secretions and menstruation should be noted. Clitoral size should be evaluated. Vaginal bleeding without breast development may indicate sexual abuse: Marks of injury should be looked for. Virilization without signs of estrogen effect indicates androgens from the adrenal or rarely, the ovary or an androgen-secreting tumor. Rapid virilization may suggest androgen-secreting tumors of adrenal gland or ovary. Breasts should be carefully examined for nodules and galactorrhea.

In a boy with CPP, an organic cause is far more likely, unlike in girls older than 6 years, where most investigations

BOX 1: Etiology of precocious puberty.

Central isosexual precocious puberty in girls and boys

- *Idiopathic (common in girls):* Sporadic and familial
- *Genetic: KISS1, GPR54,* and *MKRN3* mutations
- *Neurogenic:*
  - Hypothalamic hamartoma (common)
  - *Central nervous system tumors:* Glioma, astrocytoma, ependymoma, pineal tumors, and craniopharyngioma
  - *Central nervous system infections:* Neurotuberculosis and post-meningitis/encephalitis
  - *Central nervous system insults:* Trauma, neurosurgery, cranial irradiation, and perinatal asphyxiation
  - *Central nervous system malformations:* Arachnoid cyst, hydrocephalus, septo-optic dysplasia, neurofibromatosis, neural tube defects, and cerebral dysgenesis
- *Miscellaneous:* Adoption, intrauterine growth retardation, Russell–Silver syndrome, and endocrine disruptor syndrome

Peripheral precocious puberty in girls

- Hypothyroidism
- Ovarian causes
  - McCune–Albright syndrome (more common in girls)
  - Benign follicular cysts
  - *Tumors:* Granulosa-theca cell tumors, arrhenoblastoma, and teratoma
- *Adrenal causes:* Feminizing adrenal neoplasia
- *Exogenous estrogen exposure:* Medications and phytoestrogens

Peripheral precocious puberty in boys

- *Adrenal causes:*
  - *Congenital adrenal hyperplasia (CAH):* 21-hydroxylase and 11β-hydroxylase deficiency
  - *Adrenal tumors:* Virilizing adenoma and carcinoma
- *Testicular causes:*
  - *Tumors:* Leydig cell tumor and adrenal rest tumor
  - *Apparent LH excess:* Familial male-limited precocious puberty (FMPP or testotoxicosis)
- *Human chorionic gonadotropin-secreting tumors:* Intracranial (germinoma or teratoma) and ectopic (hepatoblastoma, teratoma, and choriocarcinoma)
- *Exogenous androgen/testosterone exposure:* Testosterone creams and medications

Combined peripheral and central precocious puberty

- Prolonged undertreated precocious puberty (CAH, McCune–Albright syndrome, and FMPP)

Heterosexual precocity

- *Virilization in girls:* CAH, virilizing ovarian/adrenal neoplasia, and polycystic ovarian syndrome
- *Feminization in boys:* Estrogen secreting adrenal tumor and exogenous estrogens/drugs

Variations in pubertal development

- Premature thelarche
- Premature pubarche/adrenarche
- Premature menarche

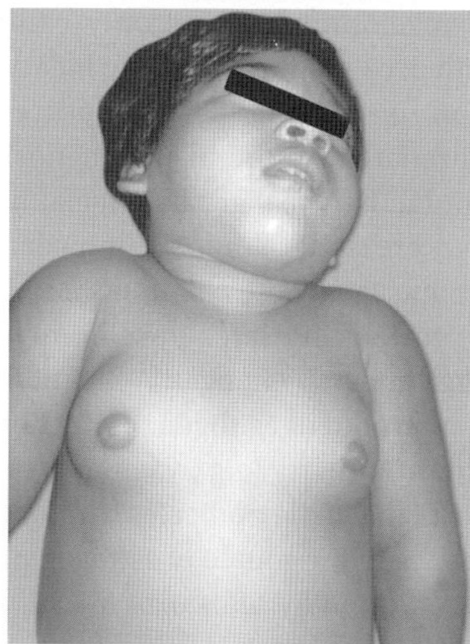

Fig. 1: Premature thelarche due to gonadotropin-dependent precocious puberty in a 4-year-old girl with spastic quadriplegia with seizures on anticonvulsant therapy. *(For color version, see Plate 9)*

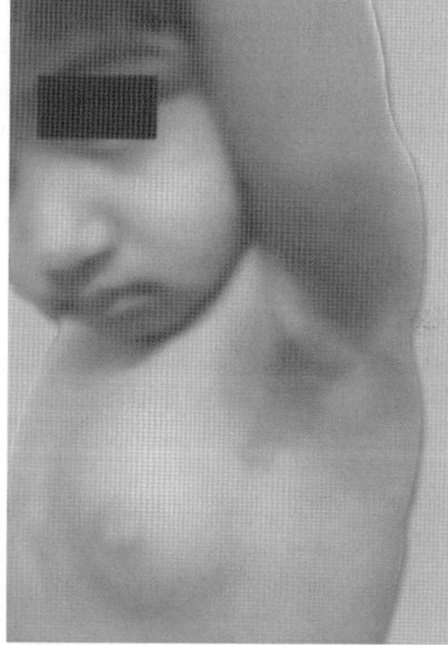

Fig. 2: McCune–Albright syndrome in a 4-year-old girl. Note the premature thelarche and the large cafe-au-lait pigmented macule in the axilla. *(For color version, see Plate 9)*

are likely to be normal. All young children with PP should be evaluated for an underlying CNS disorder. This should include the signs of raised intracranial pressure and examination of optic fundi. Blood pressure may be high in children with 11β-hydroxylase deficiency or adrenal tumor. Abdominal examination may reveal adrenal or ovarian mass as well as enlarged uterus. Firm hepatomegaly may be a manifestation of hCG-secreting tumors such as hepatoblastoma.

If breast development is the only clinical feature, without growth acceleration and pubic hair development, the condition is labeled as premature thelarche. Premature adrenarche is the likely diagnosis if signs of virilization (pubic hair, axillary hair, facial hair, or acne) appear without breast development, growth acceleration, or advanced bone age. These children should be followed up regularly, to look for later development of growth spurt and other pubertal changes. A fluctuating course is suggestive of intermittent estrogen production by ovarian cysts. Discordant puberty (e.g., vaginal bleeding within short duration of thelarche) indicates withdrawal bleeding following removal of the source of estrogen production as with ovarian cyst, hypothyroidism, or MAS.

Investigations

Bone Age

Investigations should be directed to confirm PP and find out the etiology. Bone age should be assessed accurately, using a Greulich–Pyle or Tanner–Whitehouse atlas. PP is associated with advanced bone age except in hypothyroidism. If the bone age advancement is appropriate for the height age, it is likely that the precocity is benign, probably a normal variant that needs only careful follow-up and no treatment. In girls, an advanced bone age, coupled with pubertal changes on pelvic ultrasound, suggests the need for an endocrine evaluation.

CLINICAL PEARL

- Precocious puberty is associated with advanced bone age except in hypothyroidism.

Hormones

Hormonal investigations are recommended in very young children with advancing puberty—if more than one sign of puberty is present; if a new sign of puberty appears during follow-up; if the growth rate is accelerated; or if bone age is advancing rapidly. Serum estradiol in girls and testosterone in boys in early morning samples confirm the diagnosis. Serum levels of testosterone <25 ng/dL rule out CPP in boys. Testosterone levels are very high in tumors. Pubertal testosterone levels with suppressed gonadotropins are seen in FMPP (testotoxicosis). Estimation of serum total testosterone is useful in girls to differentiate between premature adrenarche and virilization, and in polycystic ovarian syndrome.

Serum estradiol concentration >10 pg/mL is suggestive of pubertal onset in girls. Circulating estradiol concentration increases gradually as pubertal stages advances. Estradiol level >75 pg/mL is abnormal and suggestive of ovarian or adrenal tumors and require prompt workup. Presence of clearly detectable sex steroids with undetectable LH values indicate PPP. However interpretation of the results, especially for serum estradiol, might be difficult as the sensitivity of most available assays is much above these levels.

Basal level of LH is the best screening test to diagnose CPP. Basal FSH has less predictive value because of considerable overlap between prepubertal and pubertal values. With the currently available ultrasensitive immunoassay methods, LH level >0.3 IU/L is considered as the marker of pubertal onset. In PPP, LH levels are suppressed.

Gonadotropin-releasing Hormone Agonist Analog Test

Gonadotropin-releasing hormone stimulation test or GnRH agonist analog stimulation test is required if baseline gonadotropin levels are inconclusive in spite of high clinical suspicion of CPP. Gonadotropin-releasing hormone agonist analog (GnRHa) test is the preferred test now due to the limited availability of GnRH. A single sample is taken 60 minutes after a subcutaneous injection of leuprolide acetate 10–20 μg/kg (maximum of 500 μg) or of triptorelin 0.1 mg. A stimulated LH level of >5 IU/L is consistent with CPP.

CLINICAL PEARL

- LH level is the best screening test for CPP; GnRH agonist analog stimulation test is confirmatory.

Other Hormones

Pubertal levels of DHEAS characterize premature adrenarche, while greatly elevated level of DHEAS is seen in virilizing adrenal tumors.

Elevated unstimulated plasma 17-hydroxyprogesterone (17-OHP) levels are seen in CAH. If the levels are inconclusive, an adrenocorticotropic hormone (ACTH) stimulation test is performed.

Human chorionic gonadotropin and often alpha-fetoprotein (AFP) are elevated in patients with hCG-secreting tumors. In girls, increased estrogen with suppressed gonadotropins is seen in conditions causing autonomous secretion of estrogen such as functional ovarian cysts, ovarian tumor, or MAS.

Serum thyroid-stimulating hormone (TSH) and free thyroxine (FT4) levels should be checked if the bone age is delayed, especially with slow height velocity. Serum prolactin levels should be estimated in the presence of galactorrhea.

Hormonal markers such as anti-Müllerian hormone (AMH), inhibin B, and MKRN3 have only theoretical importance as of now. Boys with CPP have lower AMH levels compared to normal boys of that age because of suppressing effect of intratesticular testosterone on AMH production. In both sexes, inhibin B levels show gradual increase as pubertal stages progress. This represents a reliable marker during follow-up of puberty. Serum levels of insulin-like factor 3 (INSL3) increase as puberty advances whereas levels of MKRN3 shows a declining trend.

Imaging

Plain X-rays of the Skull and Skeletal Survey

They may show enlargement of sella, calcification, and evidence of raised intracranial pressure, but are almost always of limited utility. A skeletal survey should be done if clinical features suggest fibrous dysplasia (MAS).

Pelvic Ultrasound

It helps in girls to arrive at a diagnosis by visualizing the uterus, adrenals, and ovaries. Ovarian volume >1–2 mL, with multiple cysts (>6 cysts and >4 mm diameter) is characteristic of a peripubertal state. The pubertal ovarian volume is usually above 3 mL. Large ovarian cysts are often seen in girls with hypothyroidism (Van Wyk–Grumbach syndrome): These regress with thyroxine replacement, and do not require surgery. Persistent cysts are seen in MAS and tumors.

In the uterus, the earliest feature of estrogenization is a change in the shape from prepubertal tubular shape (diameters of fundus and cervix are equal) to pubertal pear shape (diameter of the fundus is more than that of cervix >2:1). Uterine length >3.5–4 cm and endometrial thickness >3 mm are suggestive of pubertal changes. Endometrial thickness of 6–8 mm indicates menarche is imminent.

Abdominal Imaging

It is useful in diagnosing adrenal tumors and ultrasound of testes is used to diagnose adrenal rests and testicular tumors. Computed tomography (CT) or magnetic resonance imaging (MRI) of abdomen may be confirmatory in adrenal tumors. Testicular ultrasonography (USG) helps to rule out testicular tumors, especially indicated if the testicular sizes are not equal on both sides.

Neuroimaging

High resolution MRI of hypothalamus and pituitary helps to detect lesions such as hypothalamic hamartoma, glioma, astrocytoma, and structural malformations like septo-optic dysplasia. MRI should be done in all boys, and in girls below 6 years, since the chance of finding an organic cause is high. In girls above 6 years, since most will be idiopathic, MRI should be individualized, e.g., it should be done if the pubertal progression is very rapid or there is other evidence of a CNS pathology. Further hormonal evaluation of the hypothalamic–pituitary axis may be indicated if an abnormality is detected. Chance of getting an organic pathology is less if there is a genetic origin for CPP like mutations in *MKRN3, DLK1, KISS1, KISSR*, or in familial *CPP*.

CLINICAL PEARL

- An organic etiology is more likely in a young boy with CPP, unlike an older girl where most investigations are likely to be normal.

Flowchart 1 summarizes the approach to the diagnosis of PP in girls whereas **Flowchart 2** details the approach to the diagnosis of PP in boys.

MANAGEMENT

Untreated PP leads to early pubertal maturation with advancement of bone age and early epiphyseal fusion, leading to tall stature in childhood, but short stature in adulthood, and psychological problems. Treatment is aimed at arresting the progression of puberty, identifying and managing the underlying cause, increasing the prospects for better adult height, and providing psychosocial support to affected children and their families.

Tumors of the brain, gonads, adrenals, or ectopic sites may require surgery, radiotherapy, or chemotherapy. Ovarian cysts >3 cm in diameter, which are persistent or have a solid component, may need exploration and excision. Smaller cysts are monitored by frequent estrogen estimations and ultrasounds. CAH is managed with hydrocortisone (15–20 mg/m^2) and fludrocortisone. Hypothyroidism is managed with thyroxine replacement.

Flowchart 1: Approach to the diagnosis in a girl with precocious puberty.

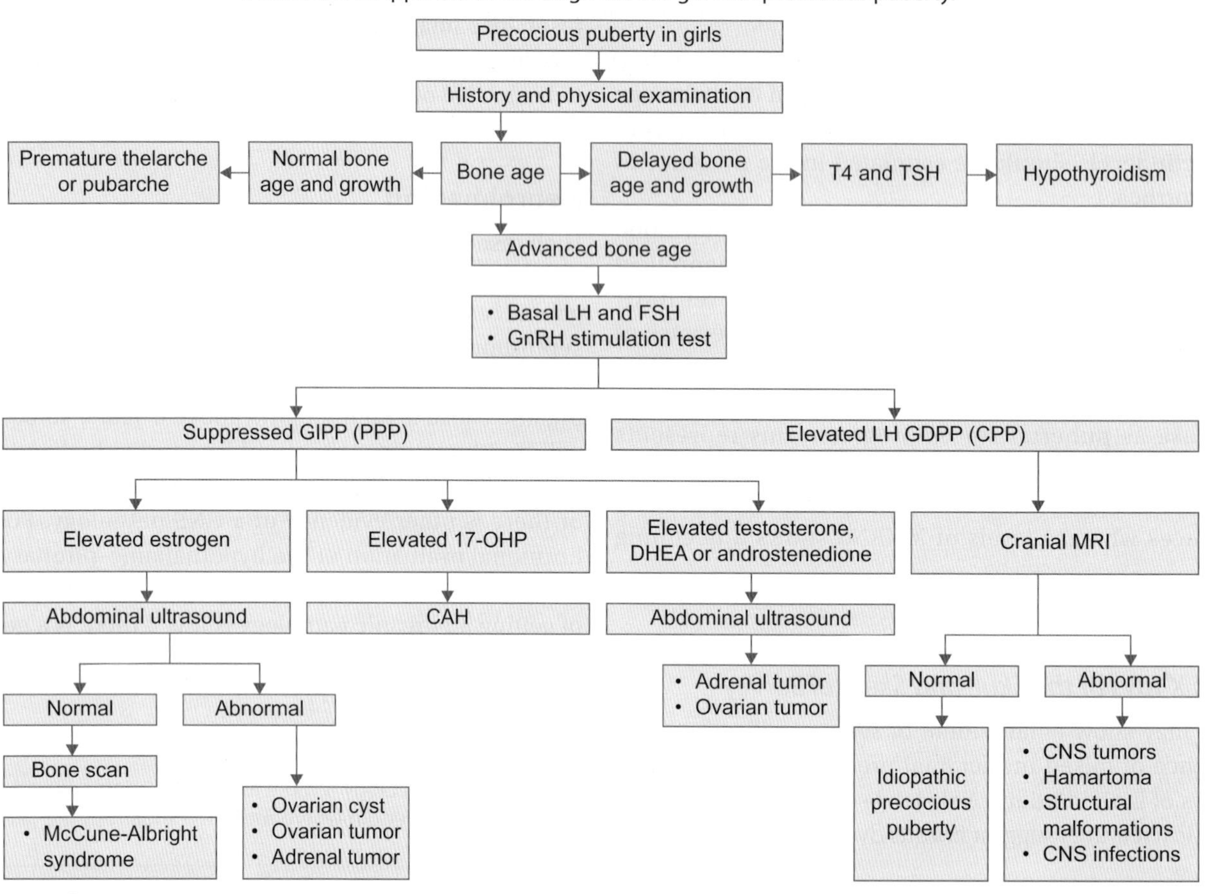

(CNS: central nervous system; CPP: central precocious puberty; DHEA: dehydroepiandrosterone; FSH: follicle-stimulating hormone; GDPP: gonadotropin-dependent precocious puberty; GIPP: gonadotropin-independent precocious puberty; GnRH: gonadotropin-releasing hormone; LH: luteinizing hormone; PPP: peripheral precocious puberty; T4: thyroxine; TSH: thyroid-stimulating hormone; 17-OHP: 17-hydroxyprogesterone)

In CPP, long-acting GnRH analogs are the mainstay of treatment. They decrease the episodic release of GnRH due to their continued high levels, causing desensitization of gonadotropin-producing cells of the pituitary. They slow down rapid skeletal maturation and linear growth, which remain unaffected by other forms of therapy. Depot preparations are preferred. These include leuprolide (3.75 and 11.25 mg), triptorelin (3.75 and 11.25 mg), and goserelin (3.6 mg). Treatment should be continued till the child reaches the normal pubertal age (10–11 years). The effectiveness of therapy is monitored by clinical evaluation of puberty, growth, and hormone evaluation. The sex steroids should revert to normal prepubertal levels for age. An effective dose is one where the gonadotropin response to exogenous GnRH is obliterated. This can be done by testing serum LH 60 minutes after the depot injection. GnRH analog treatment in girls with CPP has no long-term deleterious effects on reproductive function or bone mineralization.

In patients with autonomous gonadal steroid production such as MAS and FMPP, therapy is aimed at reducing sex steroid production or its effects, thereby arresting acceleration of growth and progression of puberty. Medroxyprogesterone acetate and cyproterone acetate interfere with sex steroid synthesis, but have no beneficial effect on final height outcome. Aromatase inhibitors prevent testosterone conversion to estrogens or block the receptors for testosterone and dihydrotestosterone. Medical management of peripheral precocity has not been generally successful, in contrast to the success of GnRH analogs for CPP.

Flowchart 2: Approach to the diagnosis of precocious puberty in boys.

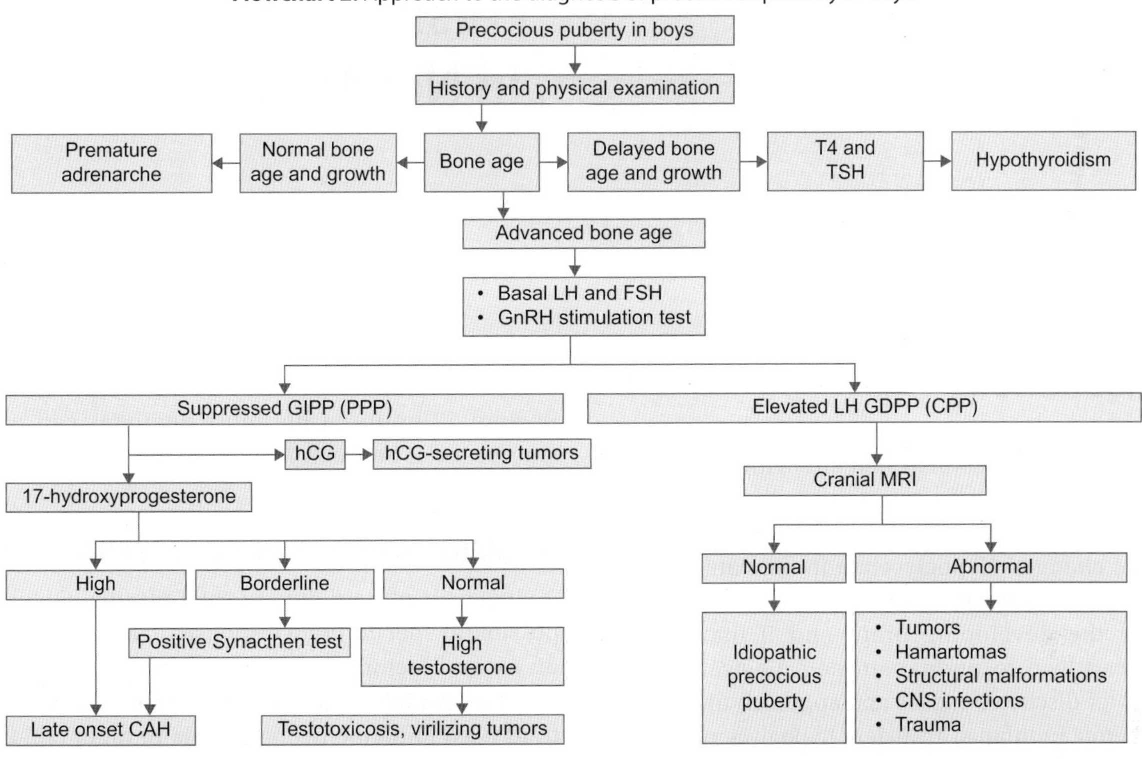

(CAH: congenital adrenal hyperplasia; CNS: central nervous system; CPP: central precocious puberty; FSH: follicle-stimulating hormone; GDPP: gonadotropin-dependent precocious puberty; GIPP: gonadotropin-independent precocious puberty; GnRH: gonadotropin-releasing hormone; hCG: human chorionic gonadotropin; LH: luteinizing hormone; MRI: magnetic resonance imaging; PPP: peripheral precocious puberty; T4: thyroxine; TSH: thyroid-stimulating hormone)

KEY POINTS

- CPP is idiopathic in 90% girls, but only 10% boys. Hence, careful search for a cause, including neurological imaging, is warranted in boys and girls <6 years of age.
- Genital maturation without testicular enlargement rules out CPP in boys serum LH level (pooled sample) is the best screening test for CPP; GnRH stimulation test is confirmatory untreated PP is associated with short final height.
- GnRH analog is the treatment of choice for CPP.
- Hypothyroidism is the only condition which causes PP associated with growth delay and retarded bone age.

SUGGESTED READING

1. Aguirre RS, Eugster EA. Central precocious puberty: from genetics to treatment. Best Pract Res Clin Endocrinol Metab. 2018;32:343-54.
2. Bajpai A, Menon PS. Contemporary issues in precocious puberty. Indian J Endocrinol Metab. 2011;15:S172-9.
3. Bangalore Krishna K, Fuqua JS, Rogol AD, Klein KO, Popovic J, Houk CP, et al. Use of gonadotropin-releasing hormone analogs in children: Update by an international consortium. Horm Res Paediatr. 2018;90:1-7.
4. Haddad NG, Eugster EA. Peripheral precocious puberty including congenital adrenal hyperplasia: causes, consequences, management and outcomes. Best Pract Res Clin Endocrinol Metab. 2019;33:101273.
5. Latronico AC, Brito VN, Carel JC. Causes, diagnosis and treatment of central precocious puberty. Lancet Diabetes Endocrinol. 2016;4:265-74.
6. Menon PSN, Paulose A. Precocious puberty. In: Desai MP, Menon PSN, Bhatia V, Seth A (Eds). Pediatric Endocrine Disorders, 4th edition. Hyderabad, Telangana: Orient Blackswan Pvt Ltd; 2022. pp. 153-69.
7. Palmert MR, Chan Y-M, Dunkel L. Puberty and its disorders in the male. In: Sperling MA (Ed). Sperling Pediatric Endocrinology, 5th edition. Amsterdam: Elsevier; 2020. pp. 661-94.
8. Rosenfield RL, Cooke DW, Radovick S. Puberty in the female and its disorders. In: Sperling MA (Ed). Pediatric Endocrinology, 3rd edition. Philadelphia: Saunders Elsevier; 2020. pp. 528-626.
9. Soriano-Guillén L, Argente J. Central precocious puberty, functional and tumor-related. Best Pract Clin Endocrinol Metab. 2019;33:101262.
10. Vijayakumar M, Menon PS. Precocious puberty—Perspectives in diagnosis and management. Indian J Pediatr. 2014;81:76-83.

Persistent Hypoglycemia in Newborns and Infants

Ganesh S Jevalikar

INTRODUCTION

At birth, there is a transition of continuous supply of glucose as the energy fuel from maternal circulation in utero to interrupted availability in extrauterine life. Adaption to this change is possible secondary to several hormonal and metabolic changes. Hypoglycemia in neonate is often a result of abnormalities in this adaptation. It is a significant threat to the developing brain and if inadequately treated, can lead to permanent neurological damage. This chapter discusses causes and approach to persistent hypoglycemia in infants. Transient hypoglycemia is more common, particularly in preterm, low birth weight, and sick newborns and is discussed in the later section.

GLUCOSE METABOLISM IN FETUS AND NEWBORN

In fetal life, glucose is continuously supplied from maternal circulation through facilitated diffusion across placenta. Hence, maternal hypoglycemia can have adverse fetal neurological outcomes. Fetal glucose values are maintained approximately 80% of the maternal values. Fetal insulin is responsive to glucose concentrations but is primarily responsible for growth rather than controlling glucose levels.

At birth, cord clamping leads to interruption of the continuous glucose supply, which now depends on intermittent feeds. As a result of this, glucose values drop to a nadir by about 2 hours of life with as many as 30% normal newborns having glucose value <50 mg/dL. Adaptive mechanisms to this include suppression of insulin secretion and activation of glucagon and epinephrine as immediate defenses and growth hormone (GH) and cortisol as delayed responses. This leads to increased glucose levels derived from glycogenolysis, gluconeogenesis, and ketogenesis. This drop of glucose is referred to as transitional hypoglycemia. Biochemical changes in this phase include low free fatty acids (FFAs) and ketones indicative of metabolic footprint of insulin. Beyond 72 hours of life most neonates can maintain glucose levels between 70 and 100 mg/dL similar to older children.

DEFINITION OF HYPOGLYCEMIA

A single cut-off to define normal plasma glucose is not possible as specific brain responses to low glucose depend on several factors such as the duration of low glucose and the availability of alternative fuels. The Whipple's triad used to define hypoglycemia in older children and adults cannot be used in infants, due to the inability to communicate symptoms and the nonspecific nature of the symptoms. Recognition of hypoglycemia may therefore require confirmation by repeated measurements of plasma glucose.

Due to the possible risks of hypoglycemia to the developing brain, evaluation and management is recommended in infants whose plasma glucose concentrations are documented by laboratory quality assays to be below the normal threshold for neurogenic responses (<60 mg/dL). This is especially applicable beyond the first 2–3 hours of life. Plasma glucose values are 10–15% higher than whole blood values and appropriate corrections should be made before interpreting the values.

Low values obtained on capillary testing should be confirmed by laboratory assessment, since capillary assessments are not accurate enough, particularly in the low range. Samples for blood glucose must be analyzed immediately as delayed processing decreases values.

CLINICAL PEARLS

- Diagnosis of hypoglycemia should be based on a level in a venous sample, not capillary glucose by finger stick.
- Plasma glucose values are 10–15% higher than whole blood.
- Delay in processing of sample causes drop in measured glucose.

GLUCOSE HOMEOSTASIS IN FETUS AND NEWBORN

Fetal blood glucose remains around 54 mg/dL over most of gestation, especially after 20 weeks of pregnancy. In the first 1–2 hours after birth, blood glucose drops to as low as 30 mg/dL. This stimulates glycogenolysis, gluconeogenesis, and ketogenesis, mediated by hormonal changes (suppression of insulin and release of counter-regulatory hormones: Catecholamines, glucagon, and GH), changes in hormone receptors, and expression of key enzymes of glucose production, which increase the blood glucose to >45 mg/dL by 12 hours of birth. Initiation of feeding after birth maintains ongoing supply of energy substrates. Breastfed newborns have lower blood glucose and higher ketone concentrations (principal alternative fuel for brain) compared to formula-fed newborns.

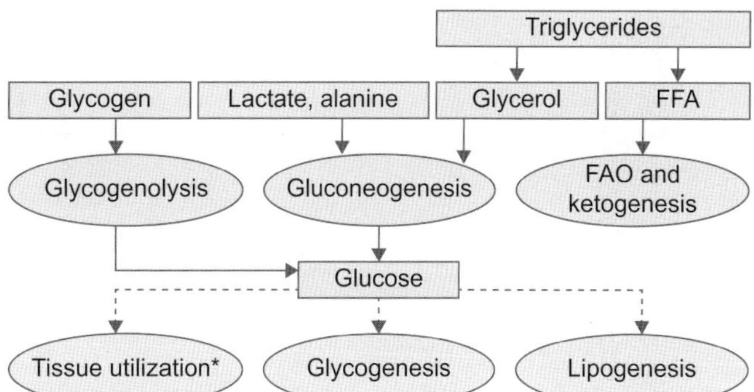

Fig. 1: Glucose homeostasis in fasting state. The dashed arrows indicate actions mediated by insulin which are inhibited in a fasting state, whereas weighted arrows indicate actions which maintain plasma glucose level or provide alternate fuel in fasting state. These are mediated by counter-regulatory hormones. Insulin is inhibitory to fatty acid breakdown and ketogenesis. *Important reactions involved in glucose homeostasis.
(FFAs: free fatty acids; FAO: fatty acid oxidation)

GLUCOSE HOMEOSTASIS IN OLDER CHILDREN

Understanding glucose homeostasis in the fed and fasting states is important to understand the causes of hypoglycemia. Although the mechanisms of control are analogous to adults, children have lesser tolerance to fasting due to lesser glycogen stores and lesser muscle mass. In the fed state, insulin promotes glucose utilization by insulin-dependent tissues (utilization by brain is insulin independent) and promotes glycogenesis and lipogenesis, the storage forms of energy. In the fasting state, a drop in blood glucose is prevented by suppression of insulin and release of counter-regulatory hormones (catecholamines, glucagon, GH, and corticosteroids) which mediate glycogenolysis, gluconeogenesis, and lipolysis. Lipolysis generates alternative fuels through fatty acid oxidation (FAO) and formation of ketone bodies. These mechanisms come into play at different intervals of fasting, with glycogenolysis being the immediate mechanism and gluconeogenesis the principal mechanism after depletion of glycogen stores. Insulin has an inhibitory effect on fatty acid breakdown and ketogenesis. **Figure 1** illustrates glucose homeostasis in the fasting state in a simplified way.

Interruption of normal homeostatic mechanisms maintaining blood glucose levels causes hypoglycemia.

Glucose entry into β-cells through glucose transporter 2 initiates the process of insulin secretion **(Fig. 2)**. Upon entry, glucose is metabolized to glucose-6-phosphate by glucokinase which is further metabolized, leading to generation of adenosine triphosphate (ATP). Increase in intracellular ATP/adenosine diphosphate ratio closes ATP sensitive potassium (KATP) channels [which consist of inward rectifying K^+ channel Kir6.2, surrounded by sulfonylurea receptor (SUR)]. This causes depolarization and opening of voltage-gated calcium channels. Increased intracellular calcium causes exocytosis of insulin vesicles. Glutamate dehydrogenase (GDH) catalyzes glutamate oxidation leading to formation of ATP and further cascade of reactions leading to insulin release. Leucine is an allosteric activator of GDH action.

TRANSIENT HYPOGLYCEMIA OF NEWBORN

As noted earlier, blood glucose <45 mg/dL may be observed in 5–15% healthy term newborns. Some newborns are at risk for transient hypoglycemia **(Box 1)**. In some of these conditions, hypoglycemia may be recurrent or persistent over first few weeks (e.g., in small for gestational age babies), therefore needing evaluation as for persistent hypoglycemia.

PERSISTENT HYPOGLYCEMIA IN NEWBORNS, INFANTS, AND CHILDREN

Persistent hypoglycemia can result from conditions **(Box 2)** which interfere in normal glucose homeostasis **(Fig. 1)** including alterations in hormones, or deficiencies of enzymes of glycogenolysis, gluconeogenesis, and FAO.

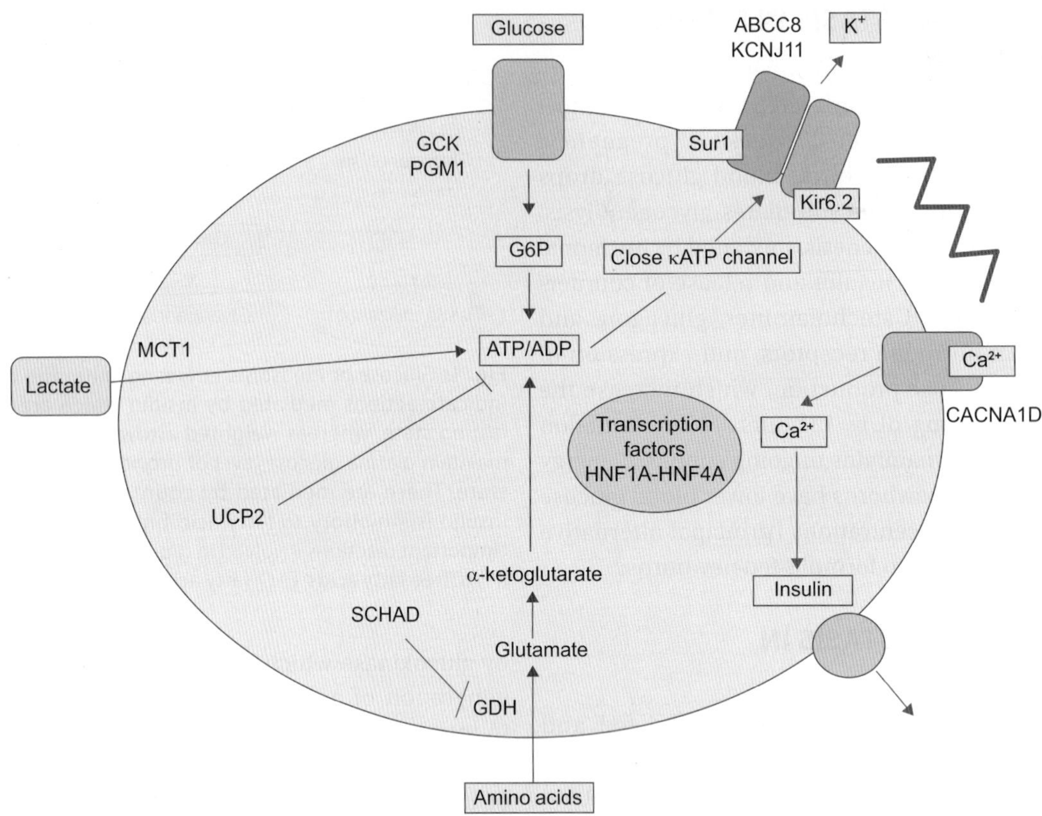

Fig. 2: Schematic diagram of pancreatic B-cell showing mechanism of insulin secretion and important genes involved. (Ca^{2+}: calcium; HNF1A and 4A: hepatocyte nuclear factor 1A and 4A; G6P: glucose 6 phosphate; Kir6.2: inwardly rectifying potassium channel 6.2; MCT1: monocarboxylate transporter 1; PGM1: phosphoglucomutase 1; SCHAD: short-chain L-3-hydroxyacyl-CoA dehydrogenase; SUR1: sulfonylurea receptor 1; UCP2: mitochondrial uncoupling protein 2)

BOX 1: Causes of transient hypoglycemia in neonatal period.

- Preterm appropriate for gestational age
- Small for gestational age (term or preterm)
- Birth asphyxia
- Neonatal sepsis
- *Systemic diseases:* Liver disease and cardiac failure/cyanotic heart disease
- Polycythemia
- Cold injury
- Transient hyperinsulinism:
  - Infant of diabetic mother
  - Small for gestational age
  - Birth asphyxia
  - Rh incompatibility
  - Exchange transfusion
  - *Syndromic causes:* Beckwith–Wiedemann, Turner, Kabuki, and trisomy 13 syndromes

Congenital Hyperinsulinism

Congenital hyperinsulinism (CHI) [previously called nesidioblastosis, persistent hyperinsulinemic hypoglycemia of infancy (PHHI), or leucine sensitive hypoglycemia] is the most common cause of persistent hypoglycemia in neonates and infants. Insulin secretion is inappropriate (rather than excessive) at the time of hypoglycemia (normally with low blood glucose, insulin gets totally suppressed). It poses more risk to the brain than other causes, as unsuppressed insulin also prevents ketogenesis (alternative fuel for the brain). In spite of significant recent advances in molecular genetics, in nearly 40% of cases of CHI, precise genetic mechanisms remain unknown. Mutations causing CHI generally increase intracellular ATP, leading to persistent closure of KATP channels and uninhibited insulin release. Most commonly, these are mutations in subunits of KATP channels (SUR1 receptor coded by *ABCC8* gene and Kir6.2 channel coded by *KCNJ11* gene). Autosomal recessive (AR) mutations present earlier, are associated with macrosomia, and are more commonly unresponsive to diazoxide. Autosomal dominant (AD) mutations are generally milder and diazoxide responsive. Other types include

BOX 2: Etiology of persistent hypoglycemia in newborns, infants, and children.

Hyperinsulinism:
- Congenital hyperinsulinism:
  - *ABCC8, KCNJ11, GDH, GCK, HADH, HNF4a, HNF1a, SLC16A1, UCP2, PGM, FOXA2*, and *HK1*
  - *Syndromic:* Beckwith–Wiedemann, trisomy 13, Kabuki, and Costello syndromes
- Insulinoma (sporadic or MEN1 associated)
- Dumping syndrome
- Exogenous insulin administration
- Sulfonylurea ingestion

Hormone deficiencies:
- Adrenocorticotropic hormone/cortisol deficiency
- Growth hormone deficiency
- Catecholamine deficiency (rare as isolated entity)

Carbohydrate disorders:
- Glycogen storage diseases
- Galactosemia
- Hereditary fructose intolerance
- Other disorders of gluconeogenesis

Fatty acid disorders:
- Carnitine transporter deficiency
- Carnitine palmitoyltransferase-1/2 deficiency
- Carnitine translocase deficiency
- Very long/long/medium/short chain acyl-coenzyme A dehydrogenase deficiency

Amino acid disorders:
- Methylmalonic acidemia
- 3-hydroxy-3-methylglutaric aciduria
- Maple syrup urine disease
- Tyrosinemia type 1

Increased utilization:
- Sepsis
- *Systemic diseases:* Liver disease, heart failure, and falciparum malaria

Miscellaneous:
- Ketotic hypoglycemia
- Congenital disorders of glycosylation
- Insulin antibodies
- *Drugs*:* Quinine, pentamidine, salicylates, and alcohol

*Except insulin and sulfonylurea

activating mutations of glucokinase, *GDH* (characterized by hyperammonemia and leucine sensitivity, macrosomia is unusual), short chain hydroxyacyl-coenzyme A (CoA) dehydrogenase, *SLC16A1* (characterized by exercise-induced hyperinsulinism), and recently described mutations in several newer genes **(Box 2)**.

Histologically, focal and diffuse types are seen. Focal forms are due to paternally inherited recessive mutations of KATP channel and somatic loss of heterozygosity in maternal chromosome 11, and can be completely cured by selective pancreatectomy.

Clinically, CHI can be divided into diazoxide responsive and unresponsive. Genetic studies can be helpful in predicting response to treatment and need for surgical management, and must be attempted in all cases presenting with CHI.

CLINICAL PEARLS
- CHI is the most common cause of persistent neonatal hypoglycemia.
- Insulin secretion is inappropriate rather than excessive.
- Genetic analysis is helpful in deciding the line of treatment and must be attempted in all cases.

Counter-regulatory Hormone Deficiencies

Growth hormone and/or adrenocorticotropic hormone (ACTH) deficiency can present as neonatal hypoglycemia. It is more common with multiple pituitary hormone deficiencies than with isolated hormone deficiencies. Microphallus, conjugated hyperbilirubinemia, and midline defects are clinical clues to these deficiencies. Low serum free thyroxine can be suggestive. The diagnosis is suspected if GH and/or cortisol levels are low in a hypoglycemic blood sample, keeping in mind that persistent or recurrent hypoglycemia per se can impair GH and cortisol responses. Primary adrenal insufficiency can cause hypoglycemia, e.g., neonates with congenital adrenal hyperplasia, but usually other clinical features dominate (genital ambiguity and salt wasting crisis). Hypoglycemia due to hormone deficiencies responds to appropriate hormone replacement.

Disorders of Carbohydrate Metabolism

Glycogen storage disorders (GSDs) are AR enzyme deficiencies of glycogen metabolism. Ketotic hypoglycemia is commonly seen in types I, III, VI, and IX GSD. Although they can present in the newborn period, more often they manifest when the interval between feeding and the duration of fasting increases. Failure to thrive, short stature, hepatomegaly, and doll-like facies are clinical clues. In some, skeletal or cardiac muscle involvement may be present but is usually asymptomatic in childhood. Renal tubular dysfunction can be seen in type 1 GSD, and hypophosphatemic rickets in Fanconi–Bickel syndrome. Biochemical evaluation shows elevated lactate, uric acid, triglycerides, and hepatic transaminases (serum glutamic oxaloacetic transaminase and serum glutamic pyruvic transaminase). Lactate and uric acid are usually elevated in type 1 GSD. Glycemic response to glucagon tends to be absent or poor. Definitive diagnosis can be established by genetic analysis or enzyme studies in liver biopsy specimen. Treatment of hypoglycemia usually consists of frequent carbohydrate feeding and supplementation with uncooked cornstarch.

Defects in gluconeogenesis (phosphoenolpyruvate carboxykinase deficiency and fructose-1,6-bisphosphatase deficiency) present with fasting hypoglycemia, high lactate and alanine levels, and fatty infiltration of liver and other organs. Hereditary fructose intolerance presents on exposure to fructose containing food (sucrose, fruits, and juices), with hypoglycemia, vomiting, failure to thrive, hepatomegaly, and renal tubular dysfunction.

Classic galactosemia [galactose-1-phosphate uridyltransferase (GALT) deficiency] presents in neonates and infants with hypoglycemia, cholestatic jaundice, vomiting, and *Escherichia coli* sepsis. Urine tests positive for nonglucose reducing substances and diagnosis is confirmed by GALT assay.

Fatty Acid Oxidation Disorders

Hereditary or acquired defects of FAO impair ketogenesis and produce nonketotic hypoglycemia, liver dysfunction, cardiomyopathy, and encephalopathy. Manifestations can be of variable severity, including risk of sudden death. Episodes of decompensation are usually triggered by fasting or intercurrent illnesses. Treatment includes avoidance of fasting, frequent feeding, high carbohydrate (up to 70% of energy intake)-low fat diet, use of cornstarch, and carnitine supplementation (not useful in long chain hydroxyacyl CoA dehydrogenase).

Aminoacidopathies

Aminoacidopathies **(Box 2)** present with ketotic hypoglycemia, repeated vomiting, and developmental delay. Seizures, encephalopathy, and hepatomegaly can be present. Hyperammonemia is seen in organic acid disorders. Diagnosis depends on finding of specific organic acids in urine and analysis of liver biopsy or cultured fibroblasts.

Insulinoma

Islet cell adenoma (insulinoma) is a rare cause of hypoglycemia in older children. Diagnosis is based on magnetic resonance imaging or functional scanning of pancreas. If present, it should prompt evaluation for features of MEN1 in the child.

Accelerated Hypoglycemia (Ketotic Hypoglycemia)

This condition usually presents at 1.5–5 years of age, typically as early morning lethargy and difficulty in getting up in the morning, associated with ketonemia/ketonuria. These children have relatively lesser concentrations of alanine and less tolerance to fasting. Spontaneous improvement is seen after 8–9 years of age.

SYMPTOMS OF HYPOGLYCEMIA

Symptoms of hypoglycemia in neonates **(Box 3)** can be nonspecific and caused by other etiologies such as sepsis, asphyxia, and electrolyte disturbances.

Symptoms are usually divided into those resulting from autonomic system activation and those resulting from neuroglucopenia **(Table 1)**. However, in newborns, in poorly controlled type 1 diabetes mellitus, and in those with autonomic dysfunction, autonomic symptoms may be absent. The threshold blood glucose value at which symptoms appear can be variable.

CLINICAL EVALUATION

Careful history and examination is the first step in diagnosis. Clues to diagnosis on history and examination are listed in **Tables 2 and 3**, respectively.

Diagnostic Algorithm

Evaluation of the hypoglycemic infant starts with an accurate blood glucose, obtained by laboratory analysis. Plasma blood glucose <50 mg/dL during infancy, and <60 mg/dL beyond infancy is consistent with the diagnosis,

BOX 3: Symptoms of hypoglycemia in newborns.

- Seizures
- Jitteriness
- Apathy
- Cyanosis
- Apnea or tachypnea
- Hypothermia
- Limpness
- Lethargy
- Poor suck/feeding
- Eye rolling
- Sudden pallor, mottling
- Cardiac arrest

TABLE 1: Symptoms of hypoglycemia in children.

Autonomic symptoms	*Neuroglycopenic symptoms*
Tremors	Headache
Palpitations and tachycardia	Lightheadedness
Anxiety	Sensation of warmth
Restlessness	Fatigue and weakness
Sweating	Inability to think and inappropriate behavior
Hunger	Emotional lability
Paresthesias	Blurring of vision
Pallor	Seizures
Increased systolic blood pressure	Transient focal neurological deficits (diplopia, hemiparesis, etc.), unconsciousness, brain damage, and death if prolonged untreated episode

TABLE 2: Clues to diagnosis of persistent hypoglycemia in children.

Points in history	*Diagnostic clues*
Age of onset	• Early onset in hyperinsulinism (severe forms) • Onset after gaps between feeds increase (GSD)
Gestational age and birth weight	• Transient hyperinsulinism in SGA • Macrosomia (infant of diabetic mother and hyperinsulinism) • Prematurity
Relation of hypoglycemia to feeding	• In fed and fasting state—hyperinsulinism • In early hours of fasting—defects in glycogen metabolism • In later hours of fasting—defects in gluconeogenesis and FAO disorders
Relation of specific feeds	• Protein (leucine) exposure—hyperinsulinism • Fruits—hereditary fructose intolerance • Milk—galactosemia
Antenatal history	• Gestational diabetes (infant of diabetic mother, HNF4A and HNF1A mutations) • Medications (tocolytics in mother) • Blood group (Rh incompatibility)
Perinatal history	• Prolonged labor in macrosomia • Birth asphyxia
Family history	• Consanguinity (autosomal recessive disorders) • Affected siblings • Neonatal/sudden deaths (hyperinsulinism and FAO disorders)
Associated symptoms	• Jaundice (hypopituitarism, galactosemia, and other inborn errors of metabolism) • Features of sepsis/cardiac failure or other systemic disease • Recurrent vomiting (metabolic disease and adrenal insufficiency) • Abnormal odors (aminoacidopathies) • Genital ambiguity (congenital adrenal hyperplasia)
Drug history	Potential exposure to insulin/sulfonylurea

(FAO: fatty acid oxidation; GSD: glycogen storage disorder; SGA: small for gestational age)

especially when associated with symptoms. At all ages, cases with persistent hypoglycemia must be referred urgently to centers having expertise in managing CHI. Prolonged fruitless attempts at making diagnosis can lead to irreversible brain damage. Diagnostic sampling at the time of hypoglycemia is most important; this critical sample taken before administering medication, of blood and urine (passed after the hypoglycemic episode) needs

TABLE 3: Clues to diagnosis of persistent hypoglycemia on physical examination.

Clinical feature	***Possible diagnosis***
Short stature	GSDs and hypopituitarism
Macrosomia	Infant of diabetic mother and hyperinsulinism
Hepatomegaly	GSDs, FAO disorders*, galactosemia, and other metabolic diseases
Midline defects (midline cleft lip and single central incisor), micropenis, and nystagmus	Hypopituitarism
Hyperpigmentation	Adrenal insufficiency
Hyperventilation	Metabolic acidosis (inborn errors of metabolism)
Gallop rhythm	Cardiomyopathy in FAO disorders
Dysmorphism	Beckwith–Wiedemann and other syndromes

*Hepatomegaly may be present only in decompensated stage.
(FAO: fatty acid oxidation; GSDs: glycogen storage disorders)

TABLE 4: Tests to be done on critical sample collected during hypoglycemia.

Blood	***Urine***
• Glucose (fluoride vial) • Insulin • C-peptide • Cortisol • Growth hormone • β-hydroxybutyrate • Plasma acylcarnitine profile • Ammonia (heparinized sample on ice) • Lactate (fluoride vial)	• Ketones • Urinary organic acids • Urine acylglycines

to be analyzed for tests mentioned in **Table 4**. In any sick neonate/child, a sample of blood should be taken and stored, so further tests can be decided depending on further clues and detecting the cause of the seizure/coma (e.g., hypoglycemia/hypocalcemia/hyponatremia/other). Alongside diagnosis, hypoglycemia has to be managed, especially if neuroglycopenic symptoms (like seizures) are present. High intravenous (IV) glucose requirement (>8 mg/kg/min) is a strong pointer in favor of CHI. Criteria for diagnosis of hyperinsulinism are mentioned in **Box 4**.

Growth hormone levels >20 ng/mL in neonates (>10 ng/mL in children) and cortisol >20 μg/dL in the critical sample rule out GH and cortisol deficiency, respectively. Lower values in the hypoglycemic sample need confirmation by definitive testing unless hypopituitarism/adrenal insufficiency is obvious clinically. High insulin with low C-peptide indicates exogenous insulin administration.

A commonly used algorithm for diagnosis of persistent hypoglycemia is given in **Flowchart 1**.

BOX 4: Criteria for diagnosis of hyperinsulinism.

Evidence of excessive insulin action at the time of hypoglycemia:
- Suppressed plasma β-hydroxybutyrate (<1.8 mmol/L)/absent or low urinary ketones
- Suppressed plasma free fatty acids (<1.7 mmol/L)
- Inappropriately large glycemic response to glucagon (≥30 mg/dL)
- Increased glucose infusion rate required to maintain euglycemia above normal for age
  - >8 mg/kg/min for neonates
  - >3 mg/kg/min for adults

Evidence of excessive insulin secretion/inadequate suppression of insulin secretion at the time of hypoglycemia (these are less definitive than evidence of excessive insulin action)
- Plasma insulin >1.25 μU/mL (8.7 pmol/L)
- C-peptide >0.5 ng/mL (>0.17 nmol/L)

A serum and urine sample is preserved for subsequent analysis.

A fasting challenge may be occasionally required for diagnosis, but should be done only at experienced centers under careful supervision of pediatric endocrinologists. It may be particularly risky for infants with FAO disorders.

MANAGEMENT

Acute symptomatic hypoglycemia should be treated with a 2 mL/kg IV 10% dextrose bolus, followed by continuous infusion of 10% dextrose at the rate of 6–8 mg/kg/min. The goal of treatment is to maintain blood glucose >70 mg/dL; however, this may need to be individualized. Real-time continuous glucose monitoring can be a useful tool. Efforts

Flowchart 1: Diagnostic algorithm for persistent hypoglycemia.

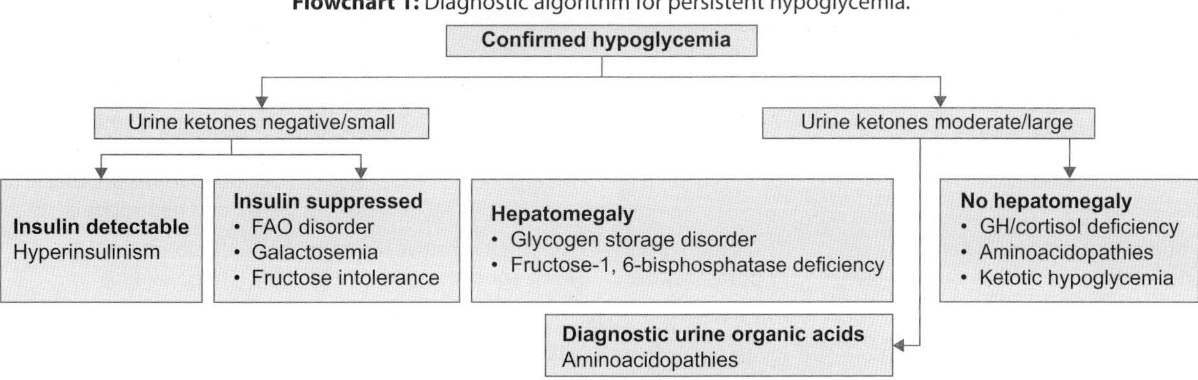

(FAO: fatty acid oxidation; GH: growth hormone)

to start and maintain enteral feeds can then be done, and if successful, IV glucose tapered gradually. Breastfeeding should be encouraged, as it favors ketogenesis. Frequent feeding, including at night, is important, and may require tube feeding. Raw cornstarch (1–2 g/kg/day) can be added to feeds for children older than 1 year of age. It can be given at bedtime to prevent morning hypoglycemia. Glucose polymers (polyjoule, maxijoule, etc.) can be useful for infants as a source of complex carbohydrates, but are not easily available in India. Higher concentrations should be avoided as they increase the risk of necrotizing enterocolitis.

Inability to start or maintain enteral feeds/persistent hypoglycemia is managed with increasing the concentration of IV glucose. Glucose infusion rates >8 mg/kg/min should prompt consultation with a pediatric endocrinologist to rule out CHI (such infants often require rates >10–15 mg/kg/min). Glucose boluses reflexly stimulate insulin secretion and should be avoided after the initial bolus. A patent IV access must always be ensured and higher concentrations of glucose (>10–12%) given through central vascular access.

All families with persistent hypoglycemic disorder should receive comprehensive education on symptoms of hypoglycemia, glucose monitoring, use of CGMS, and management of hypoglycemia and importance of regular follow-up.

Specific Treatment for Congenital Hyperinsulinism

After confirming hyperinsulinemia hypoglycemia, a trial of diazoxide is given for infants with proven or suspected CHI, usually started at 7–10 mg/kg/day in three divided doses orally, and increased up to 20 mg/kg/day. A trial of at least 5–7 days is needed before labeling a patient diazoxide unresponsive. Common side effects include fluid retention, tachycardia, and hypertrichosis (reversible on stopping). If being given for preterm, low birth weight or those with underlying heart disease, starting dose can be as low as 2–3 mg/kg/day. Fluid restriction and/or addition of thiazide diuretic along with echocardiogram are needed to rule out fluid overload. Diazoxide is not freely available and costs up to INR 50–60 per tablet. IV glucagon infusion (2.5–20 µg/kg/h) can be useful to avoid fluid overload in those requiring high concentration of IV dextrose. Diazoxide unresponsive hypoglycemia can be medically managed with injection octreotide or glucagon. Nifedipine and chlorothiazide may help as add-on oral agents but should not be used alone **(Table 5)**. There is no role for hydrocortisone in the absence of primary or secondary adrenal insufficiency in hypoglycemia management.

Genetic testing is recommended for all diazoxide unresponsive patients as well as diazoxide responsive hyperinsulinism persistent beyond 3 months of life. Rapid genetic testing for *ABCC8* and *KCNJ11* genes is very useful in diazoxide unresponsive cases. A paternally inherited pathogenic variant in these indicates possibility of focal HI with high sensitivity. The presence of focal HI can be confirmed by 6-fluoro-(18F)-L-3,4-dihydroxyphenylalanine positron emission tomography (18F-DOPA PET scan) in combination with CT or MRI. The gold standard for focal HI continues to be intraoperative frozen sections. Recently, 68Gallium-NOGADA-exendin-4-PET/CT has been reported as a beta-cell-specific tracer. Conventional imaging such as ultrasound, CT, or MRI alone is not indicated. In patients where the genetic

TABLE 5: Medications used in management of hyperinsulinism.

Medication	*Route*	*Dose*	*Mechanism*	*Side effects*
Diazoxide	Oral	5–20 mg/kg/day 3 doses/day	ATP sensitive K^+ channel agonist	*Common:* Fluid retention Hypertrichosis *Rare:* Pulmonary hypertension, coarse facies, and neutropenia
Chlorothiazide (used with diazoxide)	Oral	7–10 mg/kg/day 2 doses/day	ATP sensitive K^+ channel agonist	Hyponatremia Hypokalemia
Nifedipine	Oral	0.25–0.5 mg/kg/day	Calcium channel blockade	Hypotension (uncommon)
Glucagon	SC/IV infusion	1–20 µg/kg/h or 20 µg/kg/dose	Gluconeogenesis and glycogenolysis	Vomiting, rebound hypoglycemia, skin rash, and necrolytic migratory erythema
Octreotide	SC/IV infusion or 6–8 hourly divided	5–25 pg/kg/day	Multiple actions	GI side effects, cholelithiasis, tachyphylaxis, NEC, and suppression of pituitary hormones
Long-acting octreotide/ lanreotide	Deep SC	Dose calculated using cumulative dose of octreotide and given 4 weekly, usually 15–60 mg 4 weekly	Similar to octreotide	Similar to octreotide and long-term studies awaited

(GI: gastrointestinal; IV: intravenous; SC: subcutaneous)

analysis is consistent with diffuse form of HI, 18F-DOPA-PET is not necessary. Selective pancreatectomy can be curative in cases with the focal form. The diffuse form can be managed with long-term medical management with somatostatin analogues. Long-acting somatostatin analogs are helpful for this purpose. Patients' refractory to medical management or where medical management is logistically becoming difficult, subtotal or near-total pancreatectomy may be necessary. This is associated with development of diabetes mellitus in the postoperative period. At present use of sirolimus is not advised beyond research settings due to high incidence of serious side effects.

Specific Treatment of Other Causes of Persistent Hypoglycemia

General principles of management of persistent hypoglycemia are described in **Box 5**.

Growth hormone/cortisol deficiencies are treated with specific hormone replacement. Galactosemia and fructose intolerance require avoidance of milk or lactose-containing substances/fruits, honey, and sucrose-containing foods, respectively. Frequent feeds, nocturnal cornstarch, and avoidance of fasting are the treatment for many of the metabolic diseases. Carnitine supplementation can be useful in some FAO disorders.

BOX 5: Principles of management of persistent hypoglycemia.

- Early recognition and aggressive treatment of hypoglycemia
- Frequent/continuous glucose monitoring
- Early referral to pediatric endocrinologist
- Intravenous glucose treatment through patent central/ peripheral line
- Regular enteral feeds and addition of glucose polymer/ cornstarch, if necessary
- Specific treatment of underlying cause

PROGNOSIS

Persistent hypoglycemia, especially hyperinsulinism, is a major risk for neurologic damage, resulting in sequelae such as psychomotor retardation and epilepsy. Regular follow-up by a multidisciplinary team involving pediatrician, pediatric neurologist, pediatric endocrinologist, dietitian, nurse educator, physiotherapist, and occupational therapist is needed. All children should have periodic neurodevelopmental evaluation and neuroimaging if necessary. MRI is the best imaging modality to diagnosed hypoglycemic brain injury. Early referral to experienced centers, aggressive treatment of hypoglycemia, and timely decision of surgery in diazoxide unresponsive cases can help prevent brain damage in hyperinsulinism. Surgical treatment for diffuse hyperinsulinism results in diabetes mellitus.

KEY POINTS

- Persistent hypoglycemia, especially in the newborn/infant, can permanently damage the developing brain.
- Early diagnosis and aggressive management are important to prevent brain damage.
- Neonatal hypoglycemia is usually defined as <47 to <50 mg/dL beyond the first 2–3 hours of life. Low values obtained on capillary testing should be confirmed by laboratory assessment.
- A critical sample of blood and urine must be collected in any sick baby before starting medication.
- CHI is the most common cause of persistent nonketotic hypoglycemia in neonates and infants. Genetic analysis must be done to look for mutations.
- In CHI of focal type, selective pancreatectomy is curative.
- Diazoxide and other drugs may give long-term control of hypoglycemia. In diazoxide unresponsive babies, near-total pancreatectomy may be needed, and results in diabetes.
- Hormone deficiencies (GH and/or ACTH deficiency) and inborn errors of metabolism need specific treatment.

SUGGESTED READING

1. Brar PC, Heksch R, Cossen K, De Leon DD, Kamboj MK, Marks SD, et al. Management and Appropriate Use of Diazoxide in Infants and Children with Hyperinsulinism. J Clin Endocrinol Metab. 2020;105(12):3750-61.
2. Committee on Fetus and Newborn; Adamkin DH. Postnatal glucose homeostasis in late-preterm and term infants. Pediatrics. 2011;127:575-9.
3. De Leon DD, Thornton PS, Stanley CA, Sperling M. Hypoglycemia in the newborn and infant. In: Sperling M, Majzoub J, Menon R, Stratakis C (Eds). Sperling Pediatric Endocrinology, 5th edition. Philadelphia, PA: Elsevier; 2021. pp. 175-201.
4. Demirbilek H, Hussain K. Congenital Hyperinsulinism: Diagnosis and Treatment Update. J Clin Res Pediatr Endocrinol. 2017;9(Suppl 2):69-87.
5. Hewat TI, Johnson MB, Flanagan SE. Congenital Hyperinsulinism: Current Laboratory-Based Approaches to the Genetic Diagnosis of a Heterogeneous Disease. Front Endocrinol. 2022;13:873254.
6. Thornton PS, Stanley CA, De Leon DD, Harris D, Haymond MW, Hussain K, et al.; Pediatric Endocrine Society. Recommendations from the Pediatric Endocrine Society for Evaluation and Management of Persistent Hypoglycemia in Neonates, Infants, and Children. J Pediatr. 2015;167:238-45.
7. Win M, Beckett R, Thomson L, Thankamony A, Beardsall K. Continuous Glucose Monitoring in the Management of Neonates With Persistent Hypoglycemia and Congenital Hyperinsulinism. J Clin Endocrinol Metab. 2022;107(1):e246-53.

Approach to a Child with Disorders of Sex Development

Vijaya Sarathi

INTRODUCTION

Disorders of sex development (DSDs) are defined as congenital conditions in which the development of chromosomal, gonadal, or anatomical sex is atypical. A 2006 Consensus Conference suggested that the potentially pejorative terms "pseudohermaphroditism" and "intersex" be replaced by the diagnostic category "DSDs". The most common presentation of DSDs is abnormalities of the external genitalia (atypical genitalia), usually detected at birth. Abnormalities of the external genitalia sufficient to prompt evaluation **(Box 1)** occur in approximately 1 in 4,500 live births. Early evaluation of a child with atypical genitalia is of utmost importance due to their association with life-threatening disorders such as congenital adrenal hyperplasia (CAH) and to facilitate the early sex assignment with the most appropriate one. Some DSDs are not characterized by atypical genitalia (e.g., Turner syndrome and Klinefelter syndrome). Others may have apparently normal genitalia at birth and get diagnosed at an older age. Presentation in older individuals may include atypical genitalia unrecognized at birth, inguinal hernia, delayed or incomplete puberty, primary amenorrhea, virilization in an apparent female, breast development, or gross hematuria in an apparent male.

BOX 1: Problems in newborns that merit evaluation for disorders of sex development.

- Ambiguous genitalia
- Apparent female genitalia with:
  - Enlarged clitoris
  - Posterior labial fusion
  - Inguinal/labial mass
- Apparent male genitalia with:
  - Nonpalpable testes
  - Isolated perineoscrotal hypospadias
  - Severe hypospadias, undescended testis, and micropenis
- Family history of DSD, such as complete AIS
- Discordance between genital appearance and prenatal karyotype

(AIS: androgen insensitivity syndrome; DSD: disorders of sex development)

CLINICAL PEARL

- Isolated penile hypospadias or micropenis does not warrant evaluation for DSDs.

CAUSES AND CLASSIFICATION

Evaluation of a Child with Atypical Genitalia

Atypical genitalia usually results from the virilization of a female fetus (XX DSD), the undervirilization of a male fetus (XY DSD), or mixed sex chromosome disorders. An example of the classification of DSDs is shown in **Table 1**.

Virilization of a female fetus occurs due to androgen exposure during the critical period of external genitalia development. Fetal androgen exposure between 8 and 12 weeks of fetal life leads to the formation of a urogenital sinus (a single opening at the introitus) and labioscrotal fusion. Androgen exposure after 12 weeks of gestation leads to isolated clitoromegaly. Significant undervirilization of a male fetus occurs due to low or absent fetal androgen exposure during the critical period. Low or absent androgen exposure after this critical developmental period will cause isolated micropenis.

Evaluating an infant or a child with atypical genitalia presents significant challenges. While most virilized 46,XX infants are diagnosed with CAH, only about 50% of undervirilized 46,XY patients receive a definitive diagnosis.

HISTORY

A detailed history and thorough physical examination play a vital role in the evaluation of a child with atypical genitalia. The history should include a family history of DSD,

TABLE 1: An example of classification of disorders of sex development.

Sex chromosome DSD	*46,XY DSD*	*46,XX DSD*
• 45,XO (Turner syndrome and variants) • 47,XXY (Klinefelter syndrome and variants) • 45,XO/46,XY (mixed gonadal dysgenesis) • 46,XX/46,XY (Chimeric ovotesticular DSD)	• *Disorders of gonadal development:* – Gonadal dysgenesis – Ovotesticular DSD • *Disorders of androgen synthesis or action:* – Androgen biosynthesis defect (e.g., 17α-hydroxylase deficiency, 3β-hydroxysteroid dehydrogenase deficiency, 5αRD2 deficiency and star mutations) – Defect in androgen action (e.g., CAIS and PAIS) – Luteinizing hormone receptor defects (e.g., Leydig cell hypoplasia, aplasia) • Disorders of anti-Müllerian hormone and anti-Müllerian hormone receptors (persistent Müllerian duct syndrome)	• *Disorders of gonadal (ovarian) development:* – Ovotesticular DSD – Testicular DSD (e.g., SRY, duplicate SOX9) – Gonadal dysgenesis • *Androgen excess:* – Fetal (e.g., 21-hydroxylase deficiency, 11-hydroxylase deficiency) – Fetoplacental (aromatase deficiency, P450 oxidoreductase deficiency); and – Maternal (luteoma, exogenous, etc.) • *Others:* – Cloacal exstrophy – Vaginal atresia – MURCS (Müllerian, renal, and cervicothoracic somite abnormalities) – Other syndromes

(CAIS: complete androgen insensitivity syndrome; DSD: disorders of sex development; PAIS: partial androgen insensitivity syndrome; StAR: steroidogenic acute regulatory protein; 5αRD2: 5-alpha-reductase type 2)

any previous perinatal or neonatal deaths among siblings or other family members, consanguinity, maternal intake of drugs (such as androgens, alcohol, or progesterone) during pregnancy, and any maternal history of virilization during pregnancy. For an infant, it is important to ask about symptoms such as vomiting, dehydration, inadequate weight gain, and dark pigmentation of the oral and/or genital mucosa. In a newborn boy with marked pigmentation of the scrotum, CAH should be considered and ruled out. For an older child, the history should also focus on the postnatal progression of virilization (e.g., increasing clitoral size, premature pubarche, or precocious puberty), pubertal events (such as virilization of an apparent girl at puberty, gynecomastia, delayed, or absent puberty), gross or cyclical hematuria in a boy, and the response to hormonal therapy, especially testosterone in boys. Certain key pointers from the history and physical examination can provide useful clues toward the etiological diagnosis and are listed in **Table 2**.

PHYSICAL EXAMINATION

The physical examination should include the measurement of blood pressure using an appropriately sized cuff, an accurate and objective assessment of the genitalia, and an evaluation for any dysmorphic features. While 21-hydroxylase deficiency is characterized by hypotension, dyselectrolytemia, and hypoglycemia due to adrenal insufficiency, the presence of hypertension raises the possibility of 11β-hydroxylase deficiency or 17α-hydroxylase deficiency.

Dysmorphic Features

A comprehensive evaluation should be conducted for all children presenting with atypical genitalia to ensure that if it is indicative of a syndrome, an accurate diagnosis can be established.

CLINICAL PEARL

- All infants presenting with atypical genitalia and nonpalpable gonads should be presumed to have CAH and closely monitored until the diagnosis is conclusively ruled out.

Gonads

The scrotum, labia majora, and inguinal area should be carefully palpated to identify the presence, position, size, and consistency of the gonads. Palpable gonads in the scrotum or inguinal canal are almost always testes, or more rarely, ovotestes; this suggests a 46,XY DSD or ovotesticular DSD. The pigmentation and rugae of the labioscrotal folds and the presence of the epididymis should also be evaluated. Nonpalpable gonads may indicate either an XX DSD (most likely CAH) or an XY DSD with gonadal dysgenesis or cryptorchidism.

TABLE 2: Clinical pointers towards etiology of disorders of sex development.

Clinical pointer	Etiology
Maternal virilization during pregnancy	Placental aromatase deficiency, P450 oxidoreductase deficiency, luteoma of pregnancy, maternal androgen secreting tumors, and maternal androgen intake
Early sibling death	CAH with salt wasting
Failure to thrive, hypotension, hyperkalemia, and/or hyperpigmentation	CAH with salt wasting, SF1-deficiency, and Smith–Lemli–Opitz syndrome
Hypertension and hypokalemia	11β-hydroxylase deficiency, 17α-hydroxylase deficiency, and glucocorticoid resistance syndrome
Peripheral precocity	21-hydroxylase deficiency, 11β-hydroxylase deficiency, 3β-hydroxysteroid dehydrogenase 2 deficiency, and gonadal dysgenesis with gonadoblastoma
Inguinal hernia in a baby girl	Complete androgen insensitivity, severe testosterone synthetic defects, and Leydig cell aplasia
Bilateral well palpable gonads with atypical genitalia	Androgen insensitivity syndrome, 5α reductase deficiency, testosterone synthetic defects, and Leydig cell hypoplasia
Asymmetric genitalia	Mixed gonadal dysgenesis, ovotesticular DSD, and 46,XY DSD
Apparent male external genitalia with no palpable gonads	Severely virilized CAH female, hypogonadotropic hypogonadism, and testicular regression syndrome
Cyclical hematuria	Ovotesticular DSD, late presenting classic CAH
Virilization at puberty	Partial androgen insensitivity syndrome, 5a-reductase deficiency, 17β-hydroxysteroid dehydrogenase deficiency, and partial gonadal dysgenesis
Gynecomastia	Partial androgen insensitivity syndrome, partial gonadal dysgenesis, and 17β-hydroxysteroid dehydrogenase deficiency
Progressive postnatal virilization	CAH (except POR deficiency) and aromatase deficiency (at puberty)
Primary amenorrhea, severe oligohypomenorrhea	Complete androgen insensitivity, pure gonadal dysgenesis, severe testosterone synthetic defects, Leydig cell aplasia, and aromatase deficiency

(CAH: congenital adrenal hyperplasia; DSD: disorders of sex development)

Phallic Length

The penile or clitoral length is measured from the pubic ramus to the tip of the glans (excluding any excess foreskin) after stretching the penis or clitoris to the point of increased resistance. The ruler should be pressed down against the ramus to completely depress the suprapubic fat pad. Normal values for stretched penile length and clitoral size are available and vary among different ethnic populations. In general, a penile length of <2.5 cm suggests a micropenis, whereas a clitoral length of 1 cm or more suggests clitoromegaly in term infants.

CLINICAL PEARL

- Normal preterm female infants may appear to have clitoromegaly since they have larger clitoral breadth compared to body size.

Anogenital Ratio

In cases where the external genitalia appear female but show a mild degree of virilization, such as posterior labial fusion, evaluation can be done through the measurement of the anogenital ratio. This ratio compares the distance from the anus to the posterior fourchette with the distance from the anus to the base of the clitoris. A ratio >0.5 indicates antenatal virilization (8–12 weeks of gestation) and suggests some degree of posterior labial fusion.

Urethral Opening

The urethral opening can be located anywhere from the tip of the phallus down to the perineum. It is essential to carefully examine the ventral aspect of the phallus for any grooves, as this can provide insights into the urethral opening's location. A solitary opening at the base of the phallus might represent either an incompletely fused penile urethra, known as hypospadias, or a virilized urogenital sinus, which could indicate an internal connection between the vagina and urethra. To accurately determine the nature of these findings, confirmation through cystoscopy/vaginoscopy or radiographic imaging

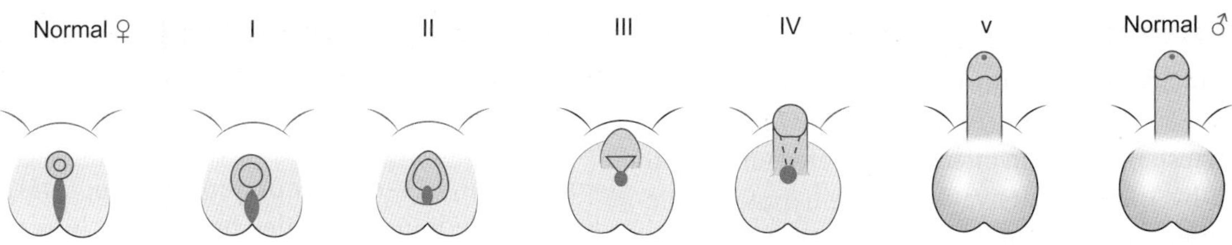

Fig. 1: Prader's staging to describe the degree of virilization in female infant.

is necessary since physical examination findings can sometimes be misleading.

Prader Stages

Degree of genital ambiguity does not differentiate between 46,XX DSD and 46,XY DSD. It merely provides information about the extent of abnormality once the karyotype is known. Prader staging is commonly used to describe the degree of virilization in 46,XX DSDs. Different Prader stages are depicted in **Figure 1**. Stage 1 is otherwise normal looking female genitalia with isolated phallic enlargement, stage 2 is further phallic enlargement and posterior labial fusion without urogenital sinus, stage 3 is significant phallic enlargement with almost complete fusion of labioscrotal folds and urogenital sinus with single perineal opening, stage 4 is phallus with penile appearance with complete labioscrotal fusion and urogenital sinus opening at the base or ventral surface of the phallus, and stage 5 is phallus with the appearance of well-developed penis with completely fused labioscrotal folds and urogenital sinus opening at the body or glans of the phallus.

LABORATORY EVALUATION

First-line laboratory testing, especially in newborns, includes karyotyping with SRY detection (even when prenatal karyotype is available), imaging (abdominopelvic ultrasound), and measurement of 17-hydroxyprogesterone (17-OHP), testosterone, gonadotropins, anti-Müllerian hormone, and electrolytes. The results of these investigations are generally available within 48 hours and will be sufficient for making a working diagnosis. To minimize psychological distress during evaluation, the patient/family should be informed exactly what will be done and why. CAH is always a possibility in an infant with ambiguous genitalia. Hence, throughout the evaluation period, careful monitoring of the infant for weight, vitals, and blood chemistry (blood glucose, sodium, and potassium) should be carried out to start early treatment if the findings suggest CAH.

Karyotype

Karyotype is performed, usually using peripheral leukocytes. Because of the possibility of mosaicism, it is suggested that at least 200 cells should be examined. The results of the karyotype permit classification of the infant into one of three diagnostic categories (XX DSD, XY DSD, and mixed sex chromosome DSD) that guide further evaluation.

Fluorescence *In Situ* Hybridization

Fluorescence *in situ* hybridization (FISH) using Y specific (SRY) and X specific probes will provide results within hours compared to conventional karyotype which takes days to provide results.

Adrenal Steroids

Measurement of 17-OHP should be done promptly in all infants presenting with atypical genitalia or marked genital pigmentation, to exclude CAH due to 21-hydroxylase deficiency. It should be measured on or after day 3–4 of life since maternal steroids in neonatal circulation may result in spuriously high values if determined during days 1–2. Levels of 17-OHP should be interpreted using gestational age-matched reference ranges to avoid spurious diagnosis of CAH. It should also be noted that stress responses like sepsis may falsely elevate 17-OHP levels. In 46,XX children with atypical genitalia but normal/marginally elevated 17-OHP, measurement, measurement of other adrenal steroids including cortisol, 11-dexoycortisol, progesterone, 11-dexocorticosterone, corticosterone, dehydroepiandrosterone (DHEAS), androstenedione, and testosterone using blood steroid panel help to diagnose rarer forms of DSD.

CLINICAL PEARLS

- Measurement of 17-OHP should be avoided during the first 2 days of life.
- Levels of 17-OHP may be falsely elevated in infants with sepsis and prematurity, so interpretation should be done with caution.

Gonadal Steroids

Assessing gonadal steroids during the prepubertal period necessitates a human chorionic gonadotropin (hCG) stimulation test. However, in infants aged between 1 month and 6 months, transient activation of the hypothalamic-pituitary-adrenal axis may offer an opportunity for gonadal steroid assessment without the need for hCG stimulation.

Human Chorionic Gonadotropin Stimulation Test

Several protocols exist for the hCG stimulation test, with the short hCG stimulation test being the most widely used. hCG (500–1,500 IU/day) is administered intramuscularly for 3 consecutive days. 24 hours after the final dose, a blood sample is collected and analyzed for testosterone, dihydrotestosterone, and androstenedione.

High testosterone levels suggest androgen insensitivity, or 5α-reductase deficiency whereas normal testosterone levels indicate either of these two conditions or 17β-hydroxysteroid dehydrogenase 3 (17β-HSD3) deficiency. An elevated (>20) testosterone to dihydrotestosterone ratio (T/DHT) indicates 5α-reductase deficiency whereas a low (<0.8) testosterone to androstenedione ratio (T/A) indicates 17β-HSD3 deficiency. However, recent studies have indicated that T/DHT and T/A ratios have low accuracy for diagnosing 5α-reductase deficiency and 17β-HSD3 deficiency, respectively. Therefore, molecular studies are essential for the accurate diagnosis of these conditions.

Low testosterone values suggest gonadal dysgenesis, Leydig cell hypoplasia, or testosterone biosynthetic defects. A low anti-Müllerian hormone helps distinguishing gonadal dysgenesis from the latter two conditions. In patients with normal AMH, measurement of adrenal steroid levels in blood (cortisol, progesterone, corticosterone, 11-deoxycorticosterone, DHEAS and androstenedione) provides hormonal clues toward the defective enzymes in the synthesis of androgens.

Imaging

Ultrasonography of the abdomen and pelvis by an experienced pediatric sonologist is crucial to determine the presence of gonads, a uterus, and/or a vagina. While a retrograde urethrogram may be necessary, most surgeons prefer direct visualization through cystoscopy/vaginoscopy under general anesthesia as the optimal method for assessing urethral and vaginal anatomy. In complicated cases, especially those involving both male and female gonads/internal reproductive structures, laparoscopic visualization may be ultimately required to fully delineate reproductive anatomy, allowing for simultaneous gonadal biopsy for histologic/genetic evaluation.

Given the spectrum of findings and diagnoses, there is no specific, one-size-fits-all evaluation protocol. Evaluation for each case must be individualized. In this chapter, the author provides a practical decision-making algorithm based on physical examination and pelvic/inguinoscrotal ultrasound **(Flowchart 1)**, which is typically useful in decision making during the early postnatal period. However, facilities to obtain karyotype using FISH encourage the use of karyotype-based algorithms **(Flowcharts 2 to 4)**.

Flowchart 1: A simplified practical algorithmic approach to a neonate with atypical genitalia.

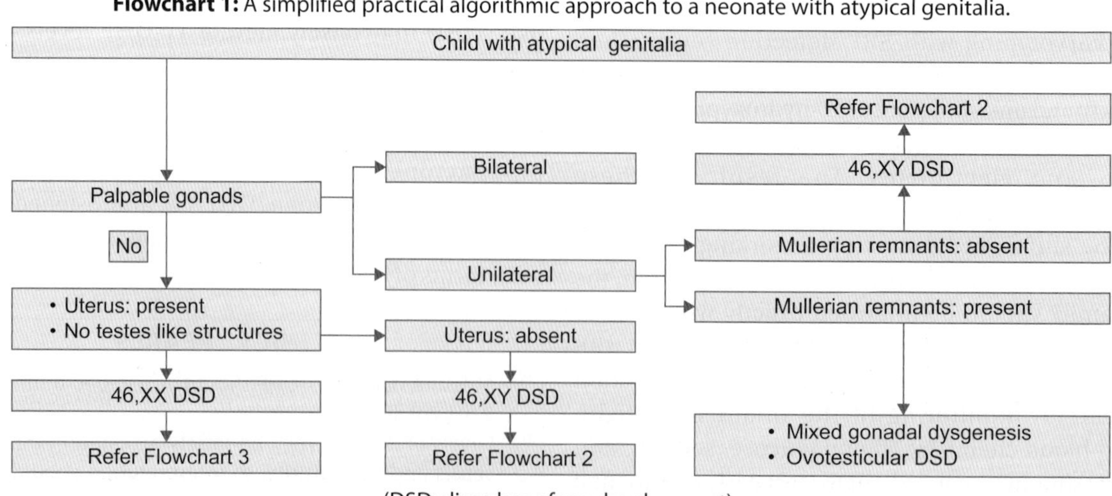

(DSD: disorders of sex development)

Flowchart 2: Karyotype-based algorithm to approach a child with atypical genitalia.

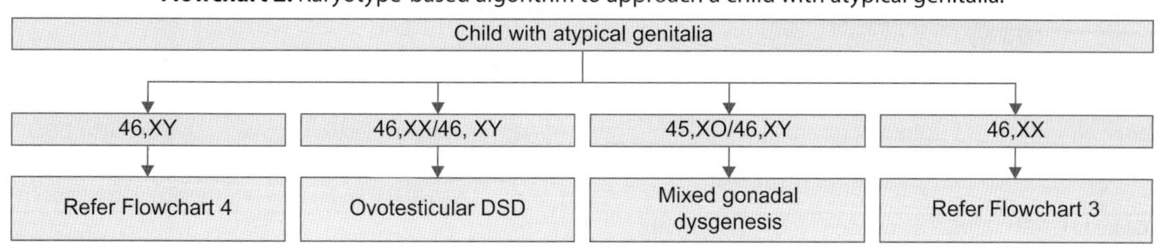

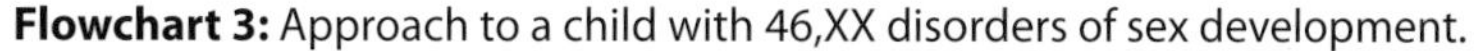

(DSD: disorders of sex development)

Flowchart 3: Approach to a child with 46,XX disorders of sex development.

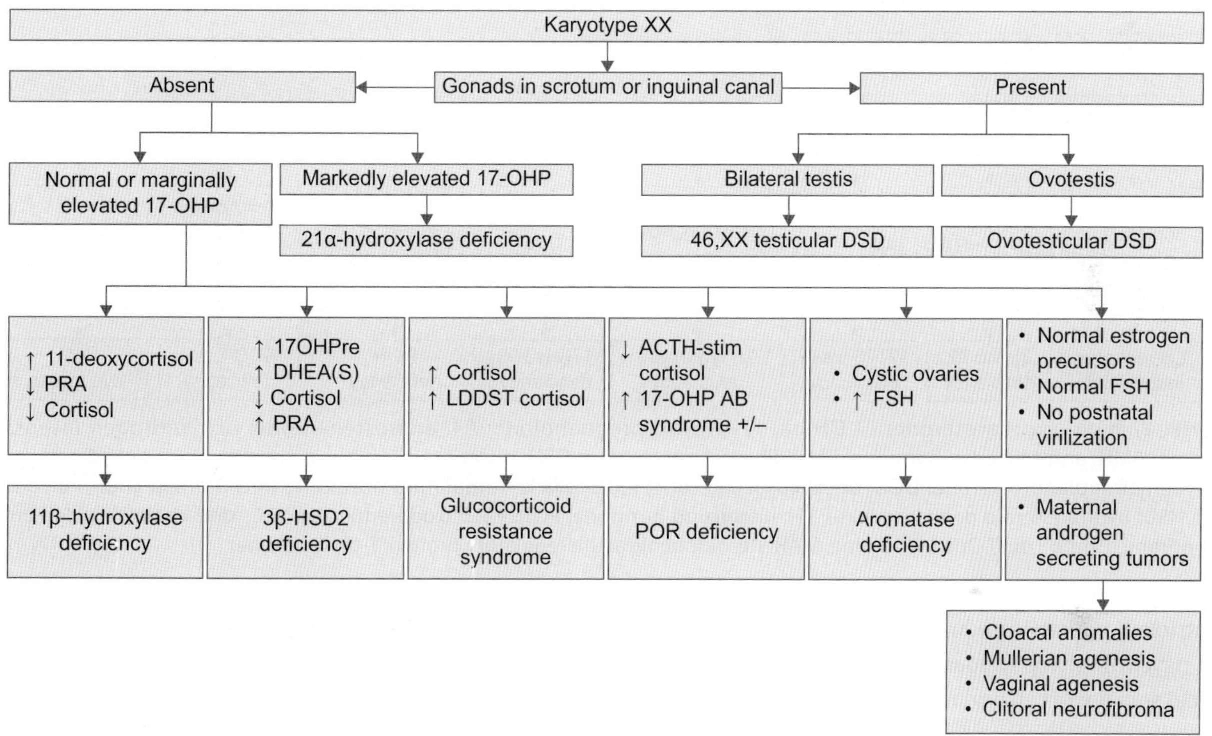

(17-OHP: 17-hydroxyprogesterone; 3β-HSD: 3β-hydroxysteroid dehydrogenase; AB: Antley-Bixler; ACTH: adrenocorticotrophic hormone; DHEA: dehydroepiandrosterone; DSD: disorders of sex development; FSH: follicle-stimulating hormone; LDDST: low-dose dexamethasone suppression test; POR: P450 oxidoreductase; PRA: plasma renin activity)

Genetic Testing

Although the diagnosis of a few common DSD such as 21α-hydroxylase deficiency and 11β-hydroxylase deficiency is most often diagnostic on hormonal parameters, the diagnosis of other forms of DSD requires molecular testing for the accurate diagnosis. Clinical exome or whole exome sequencing is the most preferred test. It is noteworthy that the genetic diagnosis of 21α-hydroxylase deficiency may be missed on exome sequencing and additional testing using multiple ligation-dependent probe amplification (MLPA) is recommended. Among 46,XY DSD, the diagnostic yield of molecular testing is low (30–50%), particularly in patients with clinical/hormonal diagnosis of gonadal dysgenesis or partial androgen insensitivity syndrome (PAIS) (type 2).

MANAGEMENT

The primary goal in managing an infant with DSD should be to swiftly establish a diagnosis, determine sex of rearing, and formulate a management plan. Achieving this requires the collaboration of an experienced multidisciplinary team. Ideally, the team includes a neonatologist/

Flowchart 4: Approach to a child with 46,XY disorders of sex development.

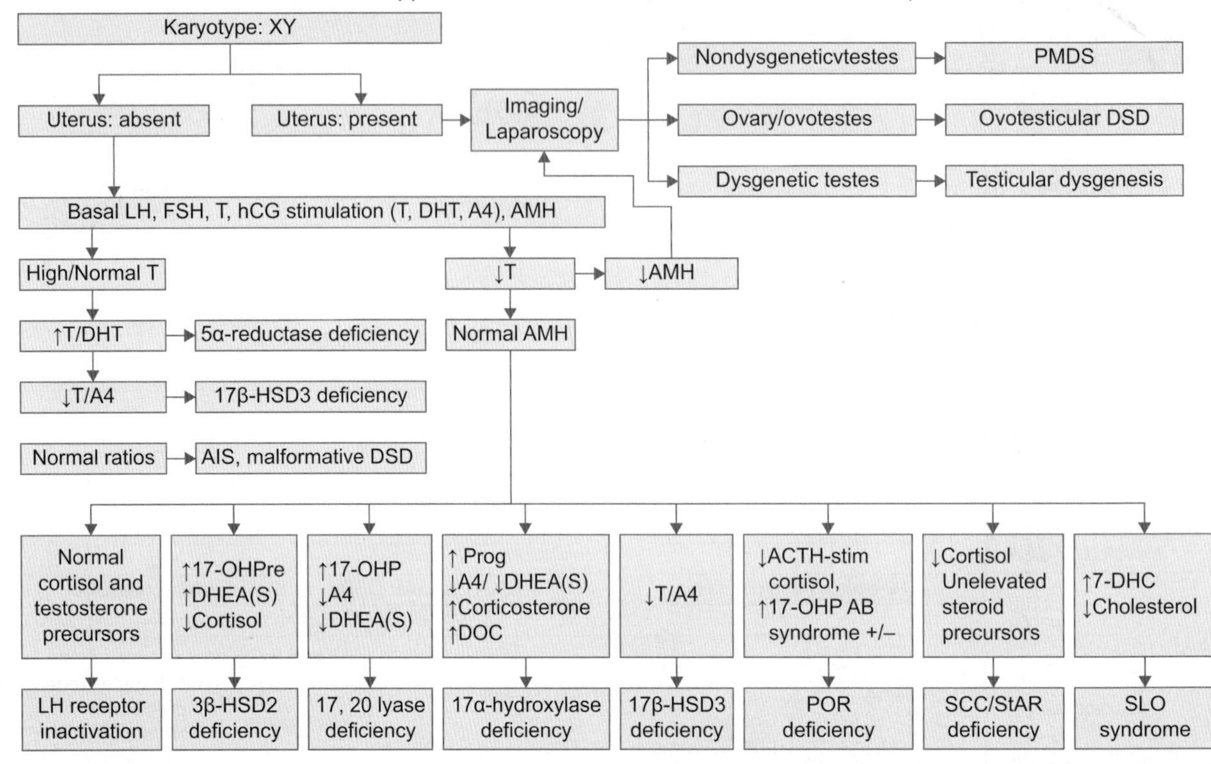

(17-OHP: 17-hydroxyprogesterone; 17-OHPre: 17-hydroxypregnenolone; A4: androstenedione; AIS: androgen insensitivity syndrome; AMH: anti-Müllerian hormone; DHT: dihydrotestosterone; DSD: disorders of sex development; DHC: dehydrocholesterol; DHEA: dehydroepiandrosterone; DOC: deoxycorticosterone; FSH: follicle-stimulating hormone; hCG: human chorionic gonadotropin; HSD: hydroxysteroid dehydrogenase; LH: luteinizing hormone; POR: P450 oxidoreductase; SCC: side-chain cleavage enzyme; SLO syndrome: Smith-Lemli-Opitz syndrome; StAR: steroidogenic acute regulatory protein; T: testosterone)

pediatrician, pediatric endocrinologist, pediatric surgeon, child psychologist/psychiatrist, gynecologist, geneticist, medical social worker, and medical ethics specialist.

Newborn Gender Assignment

Management of Gender Assignment and Genital Surgery

Infants with 46,XY complete androgen insensitivity syndrome (CAIS) or complete gonadal dysgenesis and 46,XX CAH with mild-moderate virilization should be reared as females. Conversely, for those with 5α-reductase deficiency or 17β-HSD3 deficiency, a male assignment may be favored, as gender role change is often noted around puberty. However, the decision regarding the sex of rearing is a significant one and should be based on the following factors—the most probable gender identity in adulthood, as indicated by clinical outcomes for the specific DSD type (when available); the potential for psychosocial and psychosexual functioning in adulthood, including fertility potential; the degree of virilization as a marker of prenatal androgen exposure; and the family's preferences and expectations, which may be influenced by their sociocultural background.

Feminizing Genital Surgery

Feminizing genital surgery involves external genitalia reconstruction and vaginal exteriorization, with separation of the vagina and urethra. Clitoral reduction is considered in cases of severe virilization (Prader III-V) and is preferably performed in conjunction with common urogenital sinus repair. Early surgical correction may be considered to derive the benefits of estrogen on tissues during early infancy and avoid infections due to communication between urinary tract and peritoneum via fallopian tubes. Procedures should prioritize functional cosmetic appearance, designed to preserve erectile function and innervation. Vaginal dilatation should be avoided before puberty and vaginoplasty is typically performed during adolescence.

Masculinizing Genital Surgery

Masculinizing genital surgery involves more procedures and urologic challenges compared to feminizing genitoplasty. Standard surgical repair for hypospadias includes chordee correction, urethral reconstruction, and judicious testosterone supplementation. If necessary, adult-sized testicular prostheses should be inserted after sufficient pubertal scrotal development.

For XY DSD individuals (except for CAIS) assigned female gender, gonadectomy should be performed before puberty. Patients with Y chromosome and gonadal dysgenesis have a high risk of germ cell malignancy and should undergo gonadectomy in the first decade.

Hypogonadism Management

Hypogonadism is common in patients with dysgenetic gonads, defects in sex-steroid biosynthesis, and resistance to androgens. Intramuscular depot injections of testosterone esters are commonly used in males. Other options include oral testosterone undecanoate and transdermal preparations. For optimal effect, patients with PAIS may require supraphysiologic doses of testosterone. Females with hypogonadism require estrogen supplementation to induce pubertal changes and menses. For women with a uterus, a progestin is usually added after breakthrough bleeding develops or within 1–2 years of continuous estrogen.

Congenital Adrenal Hyperplasia

Among all causes of DSD, CAH is the most critical condition that needs prompt diagnosis and treatment. Typically manifesting with a salt-wasting crisis during the second week of life, untreated CAH can lead to death. In infancy, the initial reduction of markedly elevated adrenal sex hormones may require hydrocortisone up to 25 mg/m^2 per day, but typical dosing is 10–15 mg/m^2 per day divided three times daily. Mineralocorticoid replacement should be administered in the form of fludrocortisone (100–200 µg/day). Sodium chloride supplements are often needed in infancy (1–3 g/day), distributed in several feedings. During periods of sickness or surgery, stress doses of hydrocortisone should be supplemented.

KEY POINTS

- The most common presentation of DSD is with abnormalities of the external genitalia (ambiguous genitalia), usually detected at birth (1 in 4,500 live births).
- Most virilized 46,XX infants have CAH, which may lead to death if untreated.
- <50% of under virilized 46,XY patients receive a definitive diagnosis. Common diagnoses include androgen insensitivity syndrome, 5α-reductase deficiency, gonadal dysgenesis, and testosterone biosynthetic defects.
- The degree of atypical genitalia (Prader staging) does not differentiate between 46,XX DSD and 46,XY DSD. It merely provides information about the extent of abnormality once the karyotype is known.
- First-line investigations of an infant with atypical genitalia should include FISH karyotyping for sex chromosomes, pelvic ultrasound, and measurement of 17-OHP (day 3 onward).
- All infants with suspected CAH should be closely monitored for weight, serum electrolytes, and blood glucose.
- The management of an infant with atypical genitalia requires the involvement of an experienced multidisciplinary team. Ideally, the team includes a pediatric endocrinologist, pediatric surgeon/urologist, child psychologist/psychiatrist, gynecologist, geneticist, neonatologist, medical social worker, and medical ethics specialist.
- Infants with 46,XY CAIS or complete gonadal dysgenesis and 46,XX CAH should be reared as females, whereas for those with 5α-reductase deficiency or 17β-HSD3 deficiency, a male assignment should be strongly considered.
- Patients with Y chromosome and gonadal dysgenesis should undergo gonadectomy during the first decade of life.

SUGGESTED READING

1. Ahmed SF, Achermann JC, Arlt W, Balen A, Conway G, Edwards Z, et al. Society for Endocrinology UK guidance on the initial evaluation of an infant or an adolescent with a suspected disorder of sex development (Revised 2015). Clin Endocrinol (Oxf). 2016;84(5):771-88.
2. Carillo AA, Damian M, Bercovitz G. Disorders of sexual differentiation. In: Lifshitz F (Ed). Pediatric Endocrinology, Vol 2. 5th edition. London: Informa Healthcare; 2007. pp. 365-413.
3. Houk CP, Hughes IA, Ahmed SF, Lee PA; Writing Committee for the International Intersex Consensus Conference Participants. Summary of consensus statement on intersex disorders and their management. International Intersex Consensus Conference. Pediatrics. 2006;118(2):753-7.

Approach to Thyroid Disorders in Newborns, Children, and Adolescents

Anju Virmani

INTRODUCTION

Thyroid disorders are common in childhood, and can cause significant morbidity. Symptoms may be confusing or misleading. The widespread availability of reliable thyroid hormone (TH) and other tests, has made diagnosis and treatment easier; but it has also increased needless treatment and testing, more so because thyroid medications are inexpensive and also easily and widely available. This increases the responsibility of the pediatrician to take timely and correct decisions. This chapter will discuss the approach to the following:

- Universal thyroid screening
- Hypothyroidism
- Hyperthyroidism
- Hyperthyroidism
- Goiter, thyroid nodules

CONGENITAL HYPOTHYROIDISM

Congenital hypothyroidism (CH) is the most common cause of preventable intellectual disability (ID), with normal brain development if diagnosis is made and adequate thyroxin replacement started within 2 weeks of birth. However, over 90% of affected newborns look normal, and by the time signs and symptoms appear brain damage is usually permanent. So, ensuring normal development and preventing ID is feasible only with screening every newborn at birth. The cost-effectiveness of screening *each and every newborn* is undoubted. Therefore, CH is the most important thyroid disorder, and ensuring universal screening for CH is the responsibility of all healthcare personnel involved in childbirth and newborn care. While the worldwide incidence of CH is reported as 1 in 3,000–4,000 newborns, a multicentric Indian Council for Medical Research (ICMR) study found a prevalence of 1 in 722 births, underlining the urgency to provide nation-wide, universal screening. Several hospitals in the private sector now screen all newborns, and some States are also conducting universal screening in government hospitals.

> **CLINICAL PEARL**
>
> - All newborns must get thyroid function tested, not just those whose mothers have thyroid disorders. If not done at birth, it should be done as early as possible whenever the baby is first seen (e.g., for jaundice or for vaccination).

International recommendations for universal newborn screening advise taking a heel prick sample on special filter papers on day 3–5 of age (or at time of discharge). This timing reduces the impact of the neonatal thyroid surge, in which the thyroid-stimulating hormone (TSH) rises sharply within 30 minutes of delivery, followed by a rise in T4 and T3, falling gradually by day 3–4 of life. It also allows screening of disorders like phenylketonuria (PKU) which cannot be done in cord blood. Other advantages of this approach are that only 1–2 persons need to be trained in collecting the sample; posting the filter paper sample to a central laboratory or storing it are much easier. However, considerable expertise is needed to collect the samples correctly and sensitive assays are necessary to handle such tiny sample volumes, so the filter papers must be sent to central laboratories. In India [and most Low- and middle-income countries (LMIC)], this approach has several other major disadvantages. Ensuring *universal* screening is near-impossible—mothers get discharged early; communicating with parents after discharge for recall is difficult and expensive, especially in remote areas and with low literacy. The multicentric ICMR study collected heel prick samples, and could test only 73% of the babies. Thus, affected newborns may be detected late, or not at all, negating the whole purpose of universal screening. One practical way to ensure near 100% thyroid screening is to emulate the early studies in the 1970s, by training labor room staff to collect cord blood for testing TSH, and getting the test done locally. This is achievable in all deliveries, the baby does not get a needle prick, problems due to early discharge of mothers are avoided, "sample insufficient" is not an issue, and communication gaps can easily be avoided. Since the report is usually available before the baby is discharged, venous sampling for confirmation can be considered for all newborns with suspect values while they are still in hospital, enabling starting of timely replacement in affected babies with minimal logistics involved. A meta-analysis found that though screen positivity rates were higher for cord blood screening, compliance with confirmatory testing was also higher. Testing for other conditions such as PKU or congenital adrenal hyperplasia can be offered in the first week of life **(Flowchart 1)**.

What should be screened? TSH alone, T4 alone, or both? Primary TSH testing is most widely used across the world, with some centers preferring to combine TSH and T4 screening. Testing both marginally increases the cost of testing, but greatly reduces the need for recall and confirmation, and therefore related costs and inconvenience. Cord blood TSH up to 20 mIU/L is considered normal; values of 20–40 needs a second screen at age 7–10 days; values >40 mIU/L need immediate confirmation by testing venous blood for T4 and TSH, so that if replacement is needed, it can be started early. Replacement should start only after confirming, but latest by age 2 weeks, to ensure normal brain development. After confirming the diagnosis, a Tc-99m thyroid scan (if conveniently possible), and an ultrasound of the thyroid gland (if experienced radiologist available) should be done, for information about structure and function. This could help in diagnosing dysgenesis (agenesis, hypoplasia, or ectopia, i.e., lingual thyroid), or suspecting dyshormonogenesis. However, if the Tc scan would take time to organize, treatment should not be delayed, as it can be done at time of confirming permanency (vide infra). Preterm, sick, and very low birthweight babies should be retested at age 2 weeks, as the cord blood screen may be unreliable.

The initial dose of thyroxine should be 10–15 pg/kg, i.e., usually 25–37.5 μg, given orally as a once-daily dose, so serum T4 can be rapidly normalized. Close monitoring to ensure individualization of the dose is needed, with repeat T4 done after 2 weeks of starting. TSH levels take 4–5 weeks to stabilize, and can be misleading if tested at shorter intervals. T4 should be maintained in the upper half of the normal range in the sample taken before the morning thyroxin is given. Subsequent dose titration is based on serum T4 and TSH, done every 1–2 months for the first 6 months, then every 3 months till age 3 years. Administration of iron, calcium, or soy should be spaced a few hours away, as they interfere with absorption of thyroxin.

CLINICAL PEARL

- Congenital hypothyroidism confirmation should be done urgently, so that thyroxine can be started as soon as possible, certainly before age 2 weeks, to ensure normal brain development.

Flowchart 1: Approach to thyroid function at birth.

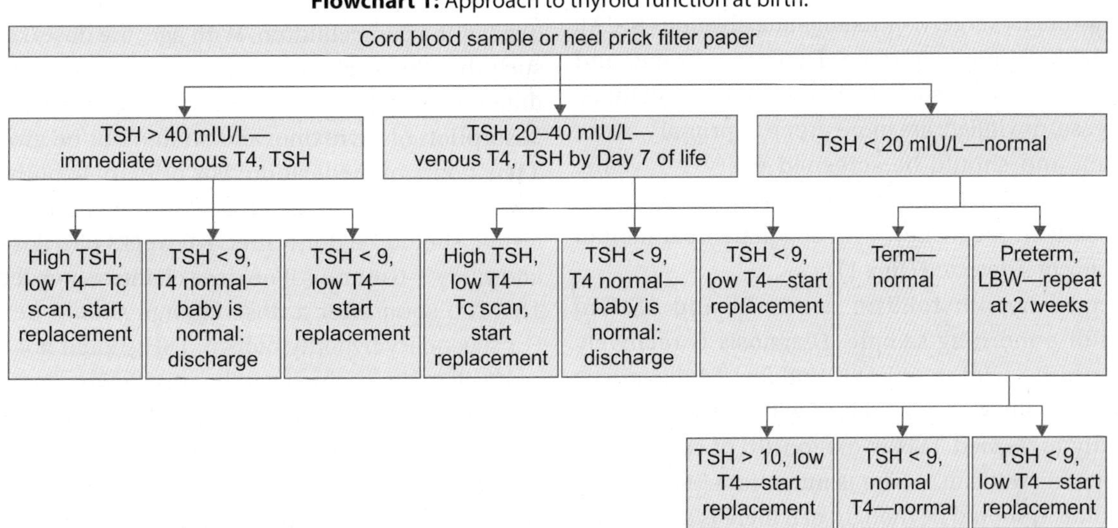

(LBW: low birthweight; TSH: thyroid-stimulating hormone)

Not all CH is permanent. If a cause of permanent CH is documented, e.g., lingual thyroid, parents are explained that treatment is needed lifelong. Otherwise, to confirm if permanent or transient, then at the age when brain development is complete, i.e., 2.5–3 years, thyroxine is discontinued for 5–6 weeks, and T4, TSH repeated. If the TSH rises > 10 mIU/L, or the T4 is low, replacement should be restarted. If the thyroid scan had not been done at birth, it can be done at this time, before restarting thyroxine. The family is explained the need for lifelong replacement, with dose titration based on monitoring T4 and TSH every 6–12 months.

HYPOTHYROIDISM IN THE OLDER CHILD AND ADOLESCENT

Acquired hypothyroidism, unlike CH, is much more common in girls. Symptoms and signs are variable and may be subtle, so the index of suspicion should be high. The child may have slow height gain, unexplained weight gain, decreased academic performance, dullness, fatigue, lethargy, increased sleep, cold intolerance, constipation, delayed or rarely precocious puberty, irregular and/or heavy periods, puffy pale face, goiter, dry skin and hair, bradycardia, hoarse voice, and thinning of sides of eyebrows. Decreased growth velocity is characteristic; any child with a growth disorder merits testing of thyroid function. In the rare event of presentation with precocious puberty, the short stature and delayed bone age are a give away. The most common cause is chronic lymphocytic thyroiditis. Iodine deficiency is now rare with universal salt iodization; other, rarer causes include CH (diagnosed late), pituitary disorders, surgery, or radioiodine ablation (RAIA). Children with Turner syndrome, Down syndrome, and autoimmune disorders such as type 1 diabetes mellitus, celiac disease, or vitiligo, are more prone to primary hypothyroidism, and should be screened every 1–2 years. If cost is not a constraint, universal TSH screening is desirable early in pregnancy, with adequate treatment of hypothyroidism if detected **(Box 1)**.

Suspected hypothyroidism needs T4 and TSH to be tested in a morning sample. Diagnosis is relatively straightforward—with raised TSH and low T4 diagnostic of primary hypothyroidism. Low T4 with normal, low, or even mildly increased TSH is diagnostic of secondary/tertiary hypothyroidism, which is much rarer. Secondary hypothyroidism should be thought of if there is any reason to suspect pituitary or hypothalamic disorders and poor growth. Sampling should be done in the morning, as TSH levels decrease by the afternoon. Serum triiodothyronine (T3) hardly ever contributes to the diagnosis or later monitoring. Thyroid antibody testing is expensive, and does not alter the management except if pregnancy may occur. In addition, antibodies may be present in 5–10% of the normal population—raised antibodies by themselves do not justify any medication. Indian normative data for THs is comparable with that elsewhere. Bone age is delayed, and usually corresponds to the height age. In the rare event of a thyroid nodule being palpable, ultrasound and fine needle aspiration cytology (FNAC) are required.

BOX 1: Thyroid function in hypothyroidism.

- *High thyroid-stimulating hormone (TSH), low T4:* Primary hypothyroidism
- *High TSH, high T4:* Primary hypothyroidism with poor compliance (likely), thyroid hormone resistance (rare)
- *Normal/borderline high TSH or low TSH, low T4:* Central (secondary/tertiary) hypothyroidism
- *Borderline TSH, normal T4:* Subclinical or Biochemical hypothyroidism

CLINICAL PEARL

- Hypothyroidism must be confirmed by laboratory testing. Treatment started on clinical suspicion alone is not justified.

Replacement is usually straightforward, with oral thyroxine, started as a once daily, early morning, dose of 2–10 pg/kg/day, given 15–20 minutes before food. Consistency of timing is important: a shorter gap between food is acceptable if it is consistent. Higher doses are needed in young children. With age, the dose/kg reduces, such that the total daily dose is not very different across different ages. Iron, soya, and calcium can interfere with absorption of thyroxine, and should not be given within a few hours of medication. For primary hypothyroidism, doses are titrated on the basis of serum TSH and T4. Thus, testing should be done after 4–6 weeks of a dose change, and every 3–6 months if no dose change is needed. Testing TSH too soon after a dose change should be avoided. For secondary hypothyroidism, TSH should not be tested, as it will be low, which can be misleading. Paradoxically, school performance may drop for a while, as the child changes from being passive and lethargic, to a normally "naughty" one. Growth velocity, bone age, and puberty should be monitored. After initial catchup growth, it should proceed normally if replacement is adequate.

However, if treatment has been very delayed, there may not be enough time for catch up growth, and final height may be less than that predicted by midparental height (MPH). Once growth is complete, a trial of stopping thyroxine can be offered: thyroxine is stopped for 4–5 weeks and then TSH and T4 tested. If the TSH rises, the family is counseled that replacement would be needed lifelong, and thyroxine is restarted, the dose being titrated with T4 and TSH monitored every 6–12 months. If iodine deficiency is suspected or proven, treatment should be with thyroxine, not iodine.

CLINICAL PEARL

- TSH takes 4–6 weeks to change. Testing too soon after a dose change may be misleading.

If the TSH is < 10 mIU/L with normal T4 (free T4 or total T4), this is considered *subclinical* or *compensated* or *biochemical hypothyroidism*, and ordinarily does not merit thyroxine replacement. Obese children may have mildly raised TSH, and are not considered hypothyroid unless they are short (cf. age and MPH), growing slowly, or have low T4. Lifestyle measures are needed, rather than thyroxine. In a child with slow height gain, T4 and TSH are among the primary tests, and should be normalized before doing any further evaluation, e.g., for growth hormone status.

CLINICAL PEARL

- Obese children with a TSH < 10 mIU/L and normal T4, are not hypothyroid. Start treatment only if TSH is >10, and/or T4 is low, in a child who is short for age and midparental height, or growing slowly.

HYPERTHYROIDISM

Thyrotoxicosis is a hypermetabolic state due to high levels of TH. It could be due to hyperthyroidism (increased TH production, as in Graves' disease (GD), toxic benign or malignant nodule, McCune Albright syndrome), thyroiditis (increased TH release due to destruction in thyroiditis due to any reason), or iatrogenic (increased ingestion of thyroxin, iodine, radiocontrast agents, or amiodarone). It is uncommon in children, increasing with age, and found more often in girls. Symptoms and signs are variable and could be confusing, so a high index of suspicion is needed. The child may have unexplained weight loss (often in spite of increased appetite), decreased academic performance, irritability, increased stool frequency, palpitations, sweating, nervousness, fatigue, poor sleep, and heat intolerance. A small, smooth goiter is almost always present. Other signs include nervousness, fine tremors, warm sweaty palms, tachycardia, staring look due to lid lag, and/or exophthalmos. The most common causes are GD, the initial stages of thyroiditis, or an autonomous thyroid nodule. Serum T4 and T3 are high, and TSH is suppressed; antibodies may be positive. Rarely, T3 may be raised with normal T4 (T3 toxicosis). A thyroid scan is useful to distinguish *GD*, which shows increased uptake, from *thyroiditis*, which will show decreased, patchy uptake, or from a *nodule*, which shows up as a discrete lesion. Before starting treatment, baseline liver function, and white blood cell (WBC) counts should be tested, as they could be affected by GD itself.

CLINICAL PEARL

- Tc thyroid scan is useful in distinguishing the cause of hyperthyroidism, and in guiding which treatment is appropriate.

Treatment of GD can be with drugs, radioiodine ablation (RAIA), or surgery. Thyroiditis merely needs symptomatic relief with beta-blockers till hypothyroidism sets in. An autonomous nodule needs surgical excision **(Box 2)**.

Usually, GD is initially treated with antithyroid drugs (ATDs), usually neomercazole (NMZ) given once or twice daily, along with beta-blockers initially for symptomatic relief. Propyl thiouracil has fallen into disfavor as it was shown to have higher risk of hepatic failure. NMZ is started in a dose of 0.5–1 mg/kg/day, and then titrated every 2–4 weeks on the basis of serum TSH and T4. Remissions are less common in children, and relapses

BOX 2: Treatment of hyperthyroidism.

- *Graves' disease:*
  - *Medical:* Neomercazole + beta-blockers
  - Definitive treatment followed by lifelong thyroxin replacement:
    - *Radioiodine ablation:* No anesthesia/scar. Slow response. Not appropriate if nodular or large goiter, or ophthalmopathy
    - *Surgical:* Thyroidectomy: Immediate relief, no worsening of ophthalmopathy. Risk of hypoparathyroidism or injury to recurrent laryngeal nerve
- *Thyroiditis:* Symptomatic relief with beta blockers
- *Thyroid nodule:* Surgical excision

after discontinuation of medicine are common, so medication may be needed for several years. The major side effects of ATD are agranulocytosis (which may reverse on stopping the drug) and fulminant hepatic failure. Therefore, the patient should be advised if ever fever or sore throat occurs, to stop NMZ and review urgently with total leukocyte count. In a thyrotoxic crisis, iodine may provide urgent, short-lived relief. RAIA or surgery was advised in those with allergy to ATDs, large or multinodular goiters, or prolonged therapy (no remission, or relapse).

However, increasingly, RAIA is being preferred as it avoids long periods of ATD therapy and their side effects. It works slowly, and beta-blockers are needed for the initial few weeks. There is no risk of anesthesia or scarring as with surgery. However, RAIA is contraindicated if the patient is possibly pregnant (rule out pregnancy); less appropriate if ophthalmopathy is present (may get aggravated); and does not work well if the thyroid is large or has multiple nodules. In these circumstances, surgery (thyroidectomy) is preferable. It gives immediate relief, but common complications include transient or permanent hypoparathyroidism and injury to the recurrent laryngeal nerve. Risks are lower in experienced hands, so it should be done in centers with considerable experience.

GOITER AND THYROID NODULE

Thyromegaly may be caused by thyroiditis, iodine deficiency or excessive intake of goitrogens, dyshormonogenesis, and malignancy; or it may be idiopathic. It may be diffuse or nodular. Diffuse thyromegaly is defined as simple goiter if thyroid function is normal, and hardly ever needs intervention. Autoimmune thyroiditis or iodine deficiency with hypothyroidism respond well to thyroxin replacement. Nodular goiter could be multinodular (MNG) or unimodular. MNG, usually due to thyroiditis and/or iodine deficiency, and almost always benign, take several years to develop, so they are rarely seen in the pediatric age group. In the setting of an MNG, a nodule turning toxic (overproduction of TH) or malignant is even rarer.

Solitary thyroid nodules (STN) are rare in children, usually picked up incidentally by family or physician, or on radiologic examination. They could be a dominant nodule in an MNG, focal thyroiditis, simple cyst, adenoma, or even a thyroglossal duct cyst. However, if solitary, a nodule is more likely to be malignant, so the concern is to determine whether it is malignant or benign, though thyroid cancer, uncommon in general, is even rarer in children. A history of previous thyroid disease or radiation to the head/neck region, or family history of thyroid disease is important. During work-up, along with TSH and T4, a Tc scan and a careful ultrasound should look at the size of the gland, the number, size, and appearance of nodules (and cervical lymph nodes on the US). A "hot" autonomously functioning nodule on the Tc scan is less likely to be malignant. An US-guided FNAC is needed if STN is larger than 1 cm, or suspicious looking, or increasing in size. If the cells are follicular, the entire nodule would have to be surgically removed (lobectomy) since adenoma and carcinoma cannot be distinguished on FNAC. If a papillary carcinoma is detected, or FNAC is suspicious for malignancy, a total thyroidectomy should be done **(Flowchart 2)**.

Flowchart 2: Approach to goiter.

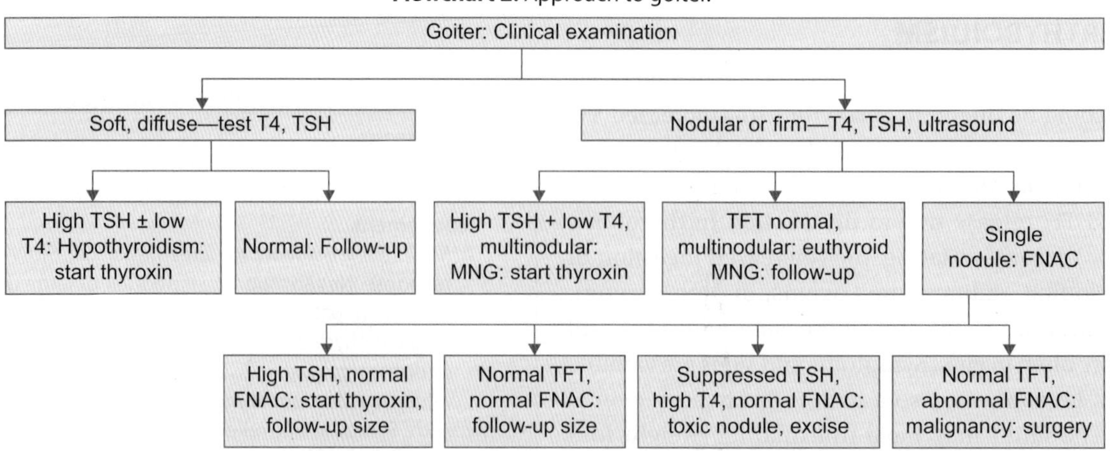

(FNAC: fine needle aspiration cytology; TFT: thyroid function test; TSH: thyroid-stimulating hormone)

KEY POINTS

- Screening for congenital hypothyroidism (CH) must be offered to every single newborn, since it is the most common cause of preventable intellectual disability.
- Screening for CH can be done in cord blood, or in a filter paper heel prick sample on day 3–5 of age.
- Primary TSH method is most widely used worldwide for screening.
- High levels should be urgently confirmed, and replacement started within 7-14 days of birth.
- Initial treatment is with high doses of oral thyroxine (10–15 μg/kg/day), titrated with T4 and TSH.
- In older children, a high index of suspicion is needed. High TSH and low T4 confirm hypothyroidism.
- Children at risk of primary hypothyroidism should be screened every 1–2 years.
- Treatment is with oral thyroxine, doses to be titrated with TSH, and T4 levels every 3-6 months.
- Compensated or biochemical hypothyroidism (TSH < 10 mIU/L, normal T4) may not need treatment, just follow-up.
- Hyperthyroidism is characterized by suppressed TSH, and raised triiodothyronine (T3) and T4 (rarely only T3). A thyroid scan helps decide treatment.
- Treatment of GD is with drugs, or radioactive iodine ablation, or surgery. Thyroiditis needs only symptomatic treatment.
- Malignancy should be ruled out in STNs.

SUGGESTED READING

1. American Academy of Pediatrics, Rose SR; Section on Endocrinology and Committee on Genetics, American Thyroid Association, Brown RS; Public Health Committee, et al. Update of newborn screening and therapy for congenital hypothyroidism. Pediatrics. 2006;117(6):2290-303.
2. Anne RP, Rahiman EA. Congenital hypothyroidism in India: A systematic review and meta-analysis of prevalence, screen positivity rates, and etiology. Lancet Reg Health Southeast Asia. 2022;5:100040.
3. Desai MP, Sharma R, Riaz I, Sudhanshu S, Parikh R, Bhatia V. Newborn screening guidelines for congenital hypothyroidism in India: Recommendations of the Indian Society for Pediatric and Adolescent Endocrinology (ISPAE)—Part I: Screening and confirmation of diagnosis. Indian J Pediatr. 2018;85(6):440–7.
4. Dhabhai N, Chowdhury R, Virmani A, Chaudhary R, Taneja S, Mittal P, et al. Burden, risk factors and outcomes associated with adequately treated hypothyroidism in a population-based cohort of pregnant women from North India. PLoS One. 2023;18(9):e0282381.
5. ICMR Task Force on Inherited Metabolic Disorders. Newborn Screening for Congenital Hypothyroidism and Congenital Adrenal Hyperplasia. Indian J Pediatr. 2018; 85(11):935-40.
6. Marwaha RK, Tandon N, Karak AK, Gupta N, Verma K, Kochupillai N. Hashimoto's thyroiditis: countrywide screening of goitrous healthy young girls in postiodization phase in India. J Clin Endocrinol Metab. 2000;85(10): 3798-802.
7. Sudhanshu S, Riaz I, Sharma R, Desai MP, Parikh R, Bhatia V. Newborn Screening Guidelines for Congenital Hypothyroidism in India: Recommendations of the Indian Society for Pediatric and Adolescent Endocrinology (ISPAE) - Part II: Imaging, Treatment and Follow-up. Indian J Pediatr. 2018;85(6):448-53.

Endocrine Hypertension in Children

Sudha R Chandrashekhar

INTRODUCTION

Systemic hypertension is a leading cause of morbidity and mortality in adults and is an emerging public health concern. Hypertension in childhood and adolescence tracks into adulthood. The prevalence of hypertension increases with age from 15% in young adults to 60% in persons older than 65 years of age. The reported prevalence of hypertension in children is around 5% and hence, routine measurement of blood pressure (BP) in children is recommended to pick up this silent killer disease. In infants and younger children, systemic hypertension is almost always secondary to an underlying disease process and hence, careful and thorough evaluation is essential. Endocrine hypertension in children is less common than renovascular or cardiovascular causes.

Diagnosis of hypertension depends on accurate measurement of BP which is a difficult and time-consuming part of clinical examination. Blood pressure is measured in a calm and quite child, may be in parent's lap, with a cuff size completely encircling upper part of the arm and an inflatable bladder covering two-thirds of upper arm length and encircling at least three-fourths of the circumference. Although Doppler or oscillometric methods are useful, sphygmomanometry happens to be the gold standard and the time of appearance of the first sound and complete disappearance of Korotkoff sound is taken as systolic and diastolic BP, respectively. Mean of at least three BP readings is taken as the representative value. Interpretation of BP is dependent on age, gender, height, and population-specific reference standards.

Hypertension, defined as either systolic or diastolic BP more than 95th percentile of the reference standard, can be primary or essential where cause is not known or secondary to cardiac, renal, or endocrine disturbances.

Multiple endocrine systems can lead to hypertension—the renin-angiotensin-aldosterone system (RAAS), mineralocorticoid and mineralocorticoid receptors, catecholamine and sympathetic nervous system, the kinin system, vasopressin, insulin and insulin receptors, endogenous ouabain and cardiotonic steroids, nitric oxide, etc. **(Box 1)**.

BOX 1: Endocrine causes of hypertension.

- Hyperthyroidism
- Hyperparathyroidism
- Congenital adrenal hyperplasia
  - 11β-hydroxylase defect
  - 17α-hydroxylase defect
- Cushing syndrome
- Pheochromocytoma
- Neuroblastoma and other neural crest tumors
- Primary aldosteronism
- Apparent mineralocorticoid excess
- Dexamethasone suppressible hyperaldosteronism
- Liddle syndrome
- Gordon syndrome
- Mineralocorticoid receptor mutation
- Diabetic nephropathy

CLINICAL APPROACH TO ENDOCRINE HYPERTENSION

Primary hypertension in children and adolescents is incidentally detected as they are silent and chronic. Secondary hypertension that is sustained or is rising rapidly is always symptomatic and mode of presentation depends on age of the child.

Symptoms in infants could vary from irritability, poor feeding, lethargy, vomiting to convulsions, altered sensorium, paresis/paralysis, or congestive cardiac failure. Older children may complain of headache, behavioral changes, epistaxis, dizziness, and visual disturbances. Intense headache, vomiting, ataxia, hyperthermia, altered consciousness, and seizures suggest hypertensive encephalopathy and is a medical emergency.

To rule out cardiac causes, palpation of all peripheral pulses, four limb BP measurements, and auscultation of abdominal bruit is essential. Renal cause of hypertension is either renovascular or glomerular and hence, presence of urinary symptoms like oliguria, dysuria, gross hematuria, anasarca, pallor, failure to thrive, rickets must be looked for. Signs of systemic diseases like vasculitis syndrome, collagen vascular disorder, neurocutaneous syndrome should be examined.

Features of stigmata of endocrine disturbances like Cushing syndrome (centripetal fat distribution, pink striae, buffalo hump, etc.), hyperthyroidism (tachycardia, palpitation, flushes, loss of weight, etc.), pheochromocytoma (episodes of palpitation, sweating, flushes, etc.), palpable abdominal mass (Wilms' tumor, pheochromocytoma, adrenal tumor, etc.), features of atypical genitalia [congenital adrenal hyperplasia (CAH) 11β-hydroxylase and 17α-hydroxylase deficiency] are clues to underlying diagnosis **(Table 1)**.

High body mass index, presence of acanthosis nigricans, and normal stature suggest metabolic syndrome and the hypertension is often essential or primary where a cause is not known. A family history for hypertension, stroke, myocardial infarction, and dyslipidemia needs to be elicited in the first-degree relatives.

In comparison to essential hypertension where the typical presentation is an adolescent, who is obese with positive family history and has mildly elevated BP without signs and symptoms of underlying disease, secondary hypertension is seen in younger children, with moderate-to-severe elevation of BP with symptoms and signs pertaining to organ system affection.

Transient hypertension is seen in children with acute illnesses like glomerulonephritis, rapid colloid infusion,

TABLE 1: Clinical clues to underlying cause.

Endocrine hypertension	***Features***	***Causes***
Hyperthyroidism	Weight loss, goiter, tremors, excessive sweating	Increased sympathetic activity mediated by high thyroid hormone levels
Hyperparathyroidism	Muscle weakness, seizures, failure to thrive, polyuria, fever	Hypercalcemia
Congenital adrenal hyperplasia 11β-hydroxylase defect	• Hypokalemic metabolic alkalosis • In females—virilization, atypical genitalia • In males—precocious puberty • May present in metabolic crisis of salt waste, shock, hypoglycemia	• Excess androgens, low cortisol, • Low aldosterone, high deoxycorticosterone
17α-hydroxylase defect	• In females—sexual infantilism • In males—undervirilization	• Low gonadal steroids, • High 17-deoxy-steroids
Cushing syndrome	Obesity, poor linear growth, striae, hyperglycemia, hypertrichosis, abdominal mass	Hypercortisolism with/without mineralocorticoid excess
Primary aldosteronism	Edema, muscle weakness, failure to thrive, polyuria, familial hypokalemic metabolic alkalosis	Hyperaldosteronism
Dexamethasone suppressible hyperaldosteronism	Autosomal dominant trait	11β-hydroxylase gene, aldosterone synthase gene defect
Liddle syndrome	• Autosomal dominant • Low renin, low aldosterone	Gain of function mutation in epithelial sodium channel
Apparent mineralocorticoid excess	Low birth weight, failure to thrive, polyuria, nephrogenic diabetes insipidus, nephrocalcinosis, severe hypertension, end-organ damage, renal failure	11β-hydroxysteroid dehydrogenase type 2 mutation
Mineralocorticoid receptor activating mutation	• Rare autosomal dominant • Hypokalemic metabolic alkalosis • Low renin, low aldosterone	Mineralocorticoid receptor activating mutation
Pheochromocytoma	Features of catecholamine excess, tachycardia, flushing, abdominal mass, excessive sweating, weight loss	Increased adrenergic hormones
Neuroblastoma and other neural crest tumors	• Similar to pheochromocytoma • Abdominal mass	Increased sympathetic activity mediated by adrenergic hormones
Diabetic nephropathy	Poorly controlled diabetes	Persistent hyperglycemia, glomerular injury due to ultrafiltration

drugs (catecholamines), and autonomic disturbances. Although hypertension is transient, these children need to be monitored and treated as other causes.

INVESTIGATIVE APPROACH

Investigations are guided by the underlying diagnosis suspected and are not only for ascertaining the etiology but also to find out the degree of end organ damage.

Initial test would include screening for renal and cardiac disorders. Thus, serum creatinine, blood urea nitrogen, serum electrolytes, routine urine analysis, testing for presence of hematuria, proteinuria, and calciuria would be required in all cases. Renal sonography for sizes of the kidneys, collecting system defects besides renal Doppler and renal scan should be done to rule out renal/renovascular cause of hypertension.

Echocardiography to rule out coarctation of aorta and end-organ changes like hypertrophic cardiomyopathy, diastolic dysfunction, and carotid intimal thickness are advised.

Hypokalemia with metabolic alkalosis is seen in primary or secondary hyperaldosteronism.

Plasma renin activity helps in differentiating the high renin (renal/renovascular hypertension) from low renin (hyperaldosteronism, Gordon syndrome, hypercortisolism) or normal renin (often seen in essential hypertension) forms of hypertension.

Plasma aldosterone concentration (PAC) to plasma renin activity (PRA) ratio helps in differentiating primary hyperaldosteronism wherein the PAC/PRA ratio is greater than 20 from secondary hyperaldosteronism (renovascular disease, renin producing tumors, coarctation of aorta) where it is less than 10. These ratios are very high in aldosterone producing adrenal adenoma. Both PAC and PRA are low in hypercortisolism and thus the ratio is less than 10. Saline loading test, fludrocortisone suppression, or captopril challenge tests are other confirmatory tests for primary hyperaldosteronism.

Urinary vanillylmandelic acid (sensitivity 63%, specificity 94%), urinary catecholamine (sensitivity 73%, specificity 94%), plasma epinephrine/metanephrine (sensitivity 85%, specificity 80%), urinary total metanephrine (sensitivity 76%, specificity 94%), plasma-free metanephrine (sensitivity 99%, specificity 92%) levels are useful in children suspected to have pheochromocytoma.

Urinary and plasma steroid profile in CAH, hypercortisolism; thyroid profile in suspected hyperthyroidism; serum calcium, parathyroid hormone, and serum 25-hydroxyvitamin D levels in hypercalcemia; are some of the other tests which provide diagnostic clue.

Radiographic imaging of the adrenals, ^{123}I-metaiodobenzylguanidine (MIBG) scan in suspected pheochromocytoma, positron emission tomography radiotracers like fluorine-18 L-3,4-dihydroxyphenylalanine (18F-DOPA), 18-fluoro-2-deoxyglucose (18F-FDG), etc. help localizing tumors as cause of hypertension.

Detailed ophthalmological evaluation for hypertensive retinopathy and urine for microalbuminuria for hypertensive nephropathy should also be checked to rule out end-organ effects.

TREATMENT

Therapy is provided to children with persistent hypertension and the goal is to decrease BP to less than 95th percentile of the target for age, gender, and height.

In mild cases as also in adolescents with primary hypertension, this could be achieved by nonpharmacological means like dietary modifications, weight reduction, regular exercise, and stress reduction. Sodium intake restricted to less than 1.2 g per day by avoiding added salt in the diet, pickles, baked, canned, and processed foods help decrease BP. Fruits and nuts beneficial in lowering BP should be included in the diet. Regular exercise schedule helps and outdoor activities like swimming, running, sports should be promoted. Weight reduction is an important therapeutic aspect of BP control in obese children.

Children with persistent hypertension require long-term therapy and the drug of choice depends on the underlying pathophysiology.

Angiotensin converting enzyme inhibitors are used in high renin hypertension (renovascular, essential). Angiotensin receptor blockers (ARBs) like losartan are useful in high renin hypertension wherein they block angiotensin II receptors. Aldosterone antagonist (spironolactone) or ARB (eplerenone) is used in hyperaldosterone states. Adrenergic blockers (labetalol, phenoxybenzamine, propranolol) are indicated in increased catecholamine states (pheochromocytoma, neural crest tumors). Diuretics are indicated in high volume output states.

Calcium channel blockers are often used as first line antihypertensives.

In hypertensive crisis, gradual drop in BP over 24–48 hours should be aimed with a drop of not more than 25% every hour as acute drop in BP leads to ischemic damage to brain, myocardium, retina, and kidneys. Controlled drop in BP is best achieved with nitroprusside infusion drip. Sublingual nifedipine can be used where facilities for infusion or monitoring for cyanide toxicity

Flowchart 1: Approach to endocrine hypertension.

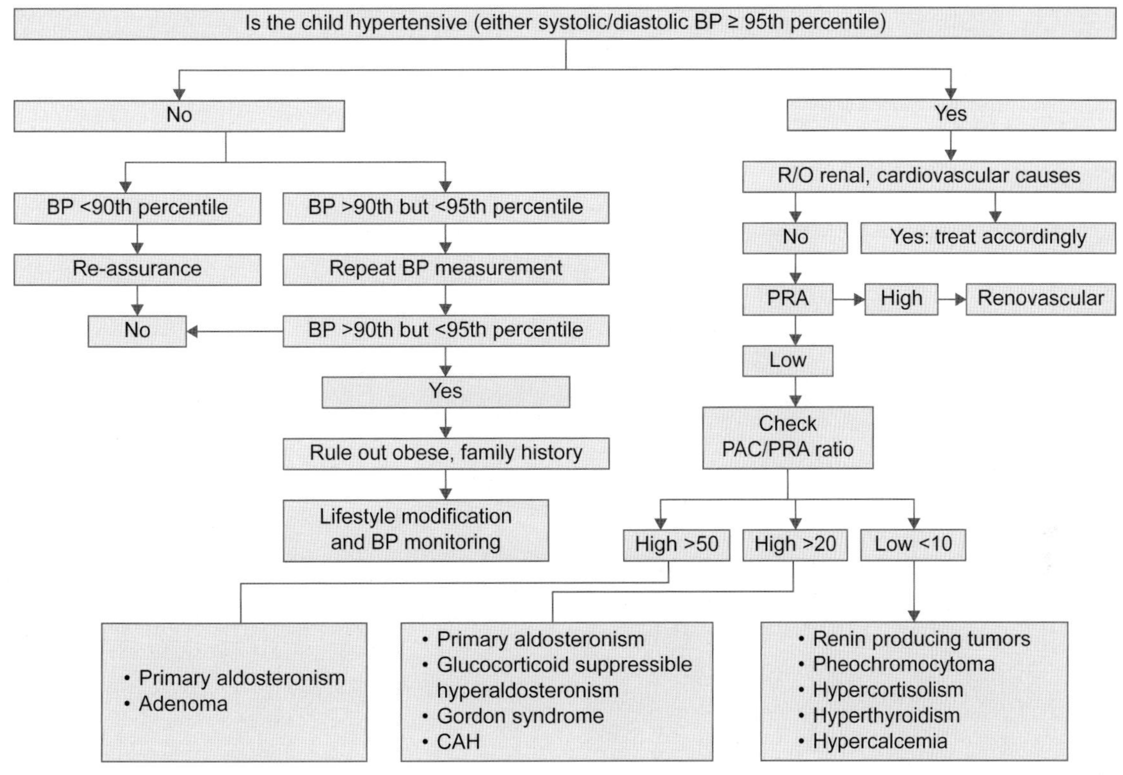

(BP: blood pressure; CAH: congenital adrenal hyperplasia; PAC: plasma aldosterone concentration; PRA: plasma renin activity)

are not available. Labetalol and nicardipine infusions can also be used **(Flowchart 1)**.

CLINICAL PEARLS

- Hypertension in children is often due to an organic cause.
- Measurement of blood pressure should always be done annually in children as a screening parameter.
- Blood pressure measurement should be done with appropriate cuff size and interpreted in relation to age gender and height.
- Both systolic and diastolic blood pressure should be recorded.
- Investigations depend on clinical clues to underlying etiology.
- Therapy is tailored to the underlying pathophysiology.

KEY POINTS

- Endocrine causes of hypertension are rare in children and are often chronic, persistent, and symptomatic.
- Etiological investigations are based on clinical clues.

SUGGESTED READING

1. Ali US. Systemic hypertension in children. In: Kumar K, Prabhu S, et al. (Eds). IAP Textbook of Pediatric Cardiology, 1st edition. Jaypee Brothers Medical Publishers; 2009. pp. 143-62.
2. Bernstein D. Systemic hypertension. In: Behrman RE, Kliegman RM, Jenson HB (Eds). Nelson Textbook of Pediatrics, 17th edition. Elsevier Saunders; 2004. pp. 1592-8.
3. Carey RM. Overview of endocrine systems in primary hypertension. Endocrinol Metab Clin North Am. 2011; 40(2):265-77.
4. National High Blood Pressure Education Program Working Group on High Blood Pressure in Children and Adolescents. The fourth report on the diagnosis, evaluation and treatment of high blood pressure in children and adolescents. Pediatrics. 2004;114 (2 Suppl):555-76.
5. Sahay M, Sahay R. Low renin hypertension. IJEM. 2012; 16(5):733-9.
6. Sorof JM, Lai D, Turner J, Poffenbarger T, Portman RJ. Overweight, ethnicity and the prevalence of hypertension in school aged children. Pediatrics. 2004;113(3):475-82.

SECTION 14

Rheumatology

Section Editor: *Priyankar Pal*

CHAPTER 118

Approach to Oligoarthritis

Vijay Viswanathan

INTRODUCTION

Arthritis in childhood is not that uncommon. Depending on the number of joints involved, it could either be oligoarticular (≤4 joints) or polyarticular (≥5 joints). Formerly known as pauciarticular, the oligoarticular variant can be a single joint (monoarthritis) or more than a single but <4 joints. It could be acute or chronic. A detailed history with regards to the onset, pattern of involvement, presentation, and duration of arthritis help differentiate between the various possible diagnoses. This, coupled with a meticulous clinical examination and supported by relevant investigations, helps in nailing the diagnosis. In this chapter, a clinical approach to decipher oligoarticular presentation in a child is discussed.

DEFINITION

Acute monoarthritis suggests inflammation of one joint only, characterized by pain, swelling, redness, and/or restriction of movement with duration of <1–2 weeks.

Chronic monoarthritis: Arthritis in the single joint lasting for at least 6 weeks is said to be chronic **(Box 1)**.

BOX 1: Causes of monoarthritis in children.

Acute:
- Septic arthritis
- Reactive
- Hemarthrosis
- Traumatic joint effusion/mechanical causes
- Bone tumors and acute leukemia
- Juvenile arthritis (systemic onset or enthesitis)/collagen vascular disease

Chronic:
- Juvenile arthritis (systemic onset, oligoarticular, and the enthesitis-related arthritis subcategories)
- Chronic hemarthrosis
- Malignancies/bone tumors
- Infections such as tuberculosis
- Miscellaneous disorders, e.g., sarcoidosis and pigmented villonodular synovitis

SOME COMMON SCENARIOS OF ACUTE ARTHRITIS

Scenario 1: Reactive/Postinfectious Arthritis

Many viral illnesses may be followed by onset of inflammation at the joints after an incubation period. Most of them are self-limiting and do not leave any long-term deformities. A few-specific types of the same with some salient features are shown in **Box 2**.

BOX 2: Specific causes of postinfectious/reactive arthritis.

Postinfectious/viral:
- Immediately/weeks to months
- Pauci/polyarticular
- Lower limb joints knees/ankles
- Flu virus, parvovirus B19, C
- Coxsackie, chikungunya, arbovirus, HIV, hepatitis A, and HBsAg

Poststreptococcal RA:
- Short incubation period
- Large and small joints
- Additive involvement (nonfleeting)
- Poor response to NSAIDs
- Echocardiography/penicillin prophylaxis

Reactive (Reiter syndrome) arthritis:
- Arthritis, conjunctivitis, and urethritis
- Time to evolve 2–4 weeks
- Lower limb joints knees/ankles
- Occasionally dactylitis
- *Shigella*, *Salmonella*, *Yersinia*, *Campylobacter*, *Chlamydia*, and *Mycoplasma*
- HLA B27

Transient synovitis of hip:
- Up to 8 years
- Differentiate from septic arthritis
- Nonweight bearing, leukocytosis, ESR, and CRP
- Always aspirate when in doubt

(CRP: C-reactive protein; ESR: erythrocyte sedimentation rate; HbsAG: hepatitis B surface antigen; HIV: human immunodeficiency virus; HLA: human leukocyte antigen; NSAIDs: nonsteroidal anti-inflammatory drugs; RA: reactive arthritis)

CLINICAL PEARLS

- Most cases of postinfectious/reactive arthritis (RA) are self-limiting.
- Anti-inflammatory agents/intra-articular steroids form the main line of therapy.
- Poststreptococcal RA necessitates a two dimensional echocardiography and occasionally penicillin prophylaxis.
- Transient synovitis can recur in 4–17% (first 6 months); differentiation from infection is mandatory.

Scenario 2: Septic Arthritis

Septic arthritis in infancy and childhood is a true clinical emergency. Delay in the diagnosis and treatment of septic arthritis can result in disastrous complications including complete destruction of the articular cartilage and epiphysis, loss of the growth plate, and joint dislocation.

CLINICAL PEARLS

- Fever, malaise, along with erythema, local warmth, and significant pain.
- Pain on passive motion (many times position of pseudoparalysis) highly suggestive of septic arthritis.
- Joint aspiration is a must in all doubtful scenarios (occasionally fluid may be sterile).
- Imaging is not the primary means of diagnosing septic arthritis.
- Ensure complete therapy for 4–6 weeks.

Scenario 3: Malignancies

Hematological malignancies (leukemia and lymphoma) as well as localized osseous, malignancy (osteosarcoma/Ewing's sarcoma) can present with musculoskeletal complaints. Symptoms of arthritis, sometimes with a migratory pattern can precede hematological feature of malignancy by months.

CLINICAL PEARLS

- Sick child with nocturnal pains (bone pains)
- Periarticular pain
- Pallor
- Lymphadenopathy
- Organomegaly
- High lymphocytes, elevated erythrocyte sedimentation rate with low platelets
- Whenever in doubt, order a marrow prior to starting steroids.

Scenario 4: Mechanical Causes

Acute pain and limitation of movement may be due to mechanical causes such as Osgood-Schlatter syndrome (osteochondritis), which is a painful condition caused by irritation and sometimes fragmentation at the tibial tuberosity. It is an apophysitis of the immature skeleton subjected to too much physical strain causing pull on the tibial tubercle that sits adjacent to a growth plate. Slipped upper femoral epiphyses occurring in adolescent/preadolescent boys can present with hip pain/knee pain (due to radiation from hip). Perthes disease or avascular necrosis of head of femur is classically seen in toddlers and early childhood. It affects boys more than girls, and presents as a painful limp. In addition, children who have excess ligament laxity (hypermobile) do complain aches and pains and also benign joint effusions.

A detailed history and clinical examination reveal that the problem is mechanical and there is no/mild arthritis on examination.

CHRONIC OLIGOARTICULAR PRESENTATION

History

Inquire about systemic symptoms such as fever, weight loss, and night sweats.

Detailed history of morning stiffness, night pains, and restriction of activities are important. History of a recent sore throat, gastroenteritis, red and painful eyes, and chronic skin disease such as psoriasis or significant trauma should be asked for. A past history of tuberculosis (TB) or contact with an open case of TB is important in India, where monoarticular disease in a child is often considered to be TB unless proved otherwise. It is also important to check for the history of recent travel to an area endemic for Lyme disease, brucellosis, or a history of tick bite.

Examination

Detailed general, systemic, and local examination as previously outlined above including skin examination, formal ophthalmology evaluation by slit lamp for uveitis, and musculoskeletal examination are a must in all children who present with a single swollen joint.

Chronic Oligoarticular Juvenile Idiopathic Arthritis

Oligoarticular juvenile idiopathic arthritis (JIA) can present with less than four joints (oligo persistent) or can involve more than four joints after 6 months (oligo extended).

CLINICAL PEARLS

- Systemically well
- Present with a painless limp with swollen joint
- Blood tests are usually normal with magnetic resonance imaging revealing effusion and synovitis.
- Antinuclear antibody positivity associated with uveitis
- Intra-articular steroids form first-line therapy
- Good prognosis except in extended oligovariant
- Rule out mimics such as TB, pigmented villonodular synovitis, and associated collagen disorder.

APPROACH TO ACUTE ONSET OLIGOARTICULAR ARTHRITIS

The following approach may assist in finding out the etiology behind the articular involvement. These are generalized guidelines and there may be the odd exception to the rule, however, this could serve as a starting approach.

History

- *Number of joints:*
  - Monoarthritis—reactive, septic/osteomyelitis, malignancies, trauma/mechanical, and other collagen diseases
  - More than one joint-reactive, leukemia, sickle cell disease, systemic (metastatic) infections, e.g., infective endocarditis and meningococcemia
- *Nature of onset:*
  - Acute/in minutes to hours—reactive, septic arthritis, trauma, and coagulopathy/sickle cell disease
  - Hours to days—reactive, systemic infections, hemarthrosis, and leukemia
- *Diurnal variation:*
  - Morning stiffness/pain—inflammatory arthritis
  - Nocturnal pains—malignancies and mechanical (growing pains)
- Trauma—important only when considering coagulopathies
- *Pattern of involvement:*
  - Migratory—acute rheumatic fever and leukemia
  - Additive or simultaneous—reactive/poststreptococcal reactive arthritis (PSRA), collagen vascular disease, systemic infections, and evolving JIA.
- *Associated features:*
  - Fever—infection. Inflammation [other collagen disorders, e.g., systemic lupus erythematosus (SLE)], malignancy, systemic disease and infective endocarditis/meningococcemia
  - Bleeding tendency/fly—hemophilias
  - Septic focus—septic arthritis and osteomyelitis
  - Systemic features—systemic-onset JIA, SLE, juvenile dermatomyositis (JDM), reactive, and infection
  - Eye—conjunctivitis—reactive (Reiter's syndrome)
  - Uveitis—evolving JIA
  - Episcleritis/scleritis—collagen vascular disease, e.g., vasculitis.

Physical Examination

- *Appearance:*
  - Sick—malignancy, infection, and systemic disease
  - Well—reactive arthritis and mechanical
- *Gait/posture:* Antalgic/pain on passive motion/pseudoparalysis—septic arthritis
- *Nature of joint swelling:*
  - Articular—septic arthritis (erythematous and warm joint), acute rheumatic fever, and other arthritis
  - Periarticular/focal tenderness—leukemia and osteomyelitis
- *Pattern of pain:*
  - Pain throughout range of movement—septic arthritis and reactive arthritis
  - Pain experienced as the joint is gently forced (i.e., stressed) toward its limitation of range—synovitis (transient synovitis, evolving JIA)
  - Pain not present throughout the entire range of motion—mechanical and tendinitis.
- Skin—petechiae, purpura, Gottron's papules (JDM), rashes (e.g., Butterfly rash in SLE < vasculitis rashes, etc.).

Laboratory Investigations (As Guided by History and Examination)

- Complete blood count, erythrocyte sedimentation rate, C-reactive protein, viral titers, and blood culture
- Antistreptolysin O titer
- Throat swab
- Coagulation studies
- Tuberculin test
- Joint aspiration (always whenever in doubt to rule out septic arthritis specially hip joint)
- *Imaging:*
  - X-rays—trauma and malignancy
  - Bone scan—infections

Flowchart 1: Algorithmic approach to acute arthritis.

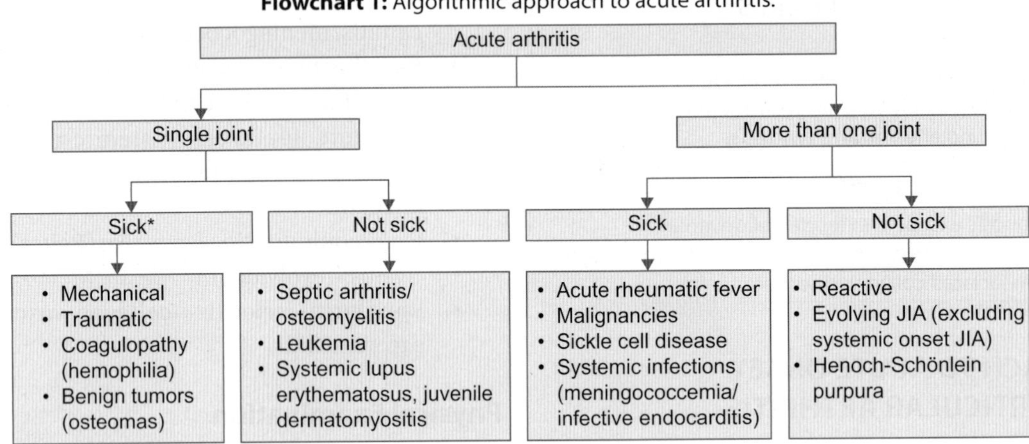

Note: *Appearance, constitutional.
(HSP: Henoch–Schönlein purpura; IE: infective endocarditis; JDM: juvenile dermatomyositis; JIA: juvenile idiopathic arthritis; SLE: systemic lupus erythematosus)

- Magnetic resonance imaging—synovitis, tumors, and infections
- Two dimensional echocardiography—PSRA and Kawasaki disease
- Antinuclear antibody (suspected juvenile oligo-arthritis), HLA B27 (suspected enthesitis)

KEY POINTS

- More than one joint involvement almost always rules out an infective arthritis (more likely to be reactive).
- Morning stiffness suggests inflammatory etiology, while nocturnal limb pains are always suggestive of a malignancy.
- Always aspirate a joint when in doubt.
- Recognizing patterns through a good history, clinical examination, and less reliance on costly investigations is paramount.

SUGGESTED READING

1. Cabral DA, Tucker LB. Malignancies in children who initially present with rheumatic complaints. J Pediatr. 1999; 134:53-7.
2. Cassidy JT, Petty RE. Textbook of pediatric rheumatology. 4th ed. Philadelphia: WB Saunders; 2001. pp. 726-79.
3. Kocher MS, Zurakowski D, Kasser JR. Differentiating between septic arthritis and transient synovitis of the hip in children: an evidence based clinical prediction algorithm. J Bone Joint Surg Am. 1999;811662-70.
4. Prabhu AS, Balan S. Approach to a child with monoarthritis. Indian J Pediatr. 2010;77(9):997-1004.
5. Roberton DM, South MJ. Arthritis and connective tissue disorders. In: Roberton DM, Robinson MJ (Eds). Practical Pediatrics, 5th edition. London: Churchill Livingstone; 1994. pp. 457.

Approach to Polyarthritis

Rashna D Hazarika, Pratap Kumar Patra

INTRODUCTION

Children often have joint diseases that originate from a wide array of clinical conditions. The leading causes are infections, trauma, and hematological disorders like hemophilia, leukemia, and several inflammatory and non-inflammatory arthritis. It often becomes a cause of concern for parents and caregivers, especially if the etiology is chronic. Herein, an approach to polyarthritis in children has been described.

Arthritis is inflammation of the joints and can be monoarticular or polyarticular. Usually, acute-onset monoarthritis, due to septic arthritis, prompts urgent medical attention. Similarly, patients with polyarthritis require detailed evaluation and investigation as it may lead to adverse consequences if not treated appropriately. Polyarthritis in children has a multifactorial etiology. It may present as a sequelae of acute self-limiting viral illness or the beginning of a chronic sinister disease. The "pattern recognition" is one of the most important aspects of approaching children with polyarthritis. Most of the viral infections cause transient arthritis, whereas reactive arthritis is caused by a distinct group of microorganisms, i.e., *Chlamydia, Gonococci, Salmonella,* and *Shigella.* At times, it is very difficult to ascertain the underlying cause of arthritis, as it precedes the systemic manifestation by months to years. An algorithmic approach to polyarthritis in children has been elucidated in this chapter.

DEFINITIONS OF ARTHRITIS

- *Arthritis:* Swelling of the joints or swelling with pain and limitation of movements.
- *Polyarthritis:* Involvement of more than four joints is known as polyarthritis.
- *Acute polyarthritis:* Arthritis for <6 weeks
- *Chronic polyarthritis:* Persistent arthritis for >6 weeks

ETIOLOGY

The etiology of polyarthritis is varied and depicted in **Table 1**.

TABLE 1: Etiology of polyarthritis.

Viral	Parvovirus B19, mumps, rubella, varicella, hepatitis B, coxsackie virus, cytomegalovirus, EBV, HIV, enteroviruses, and adenoviruses
Bacterial	Neisseria meningitidis, gonococci, bacterial endocarditis, staphylococci, streptococci, and *Haemophilus*
Other infectious agents	Mycobacteria, fungal infections, and leptospirosis
Reactive arthritis	*Chlamydia, Yersinia, Mycoplasma, Campylobacter, Salmonella, Shigella,* tuberculosis (Poncet's arthritis), and HIV
Rheumatological	Juvenile idiopathic arthritis, systemic lupus erythematosus, juvenile dermatomyositis, Behcet's disease
Vasculitides	Kawasaki disease, Henoch–Schönlein purpura, and polyarteritis nodosa
Spondyloarthropathy	Juvenile ankylosing spondylitis, psoriatic arthritis, and enteropathic arthritis
Miscellaneous	Drug reactions, leukemia, sickle cell crisis, neuroblastoma, metabolic conditions (Fabry's, Gaucher's), mechanical problems (Ehlers–Danlos syndrome and benign joint hypermobility syndrome), skeletal dysplasias, inflammatory bowel disease

(EBV: Epstein–Barr virus; HIV: human immunodeficiency virus)

IMPORTANT POINTS IN HISTORY

It is a widely believed aphorism that a physician should "listen to the patient and he or she will tell you the diagnosis". The history is the key to the appropriate management of children with joint pains. Considering the differentials, a structured history will generally point to one or a few diagnoses, which can be confirmed on examination or simple investigations.

Age

Juvenile idiopathic arthritis (JIA), juvenile psoriatic arthritis, Kawasaki disease (KD), and reactive arthritis are the leading causes of polyarthritis in early childhood (1–4 years of age). Polyarticular JIA, Juvenile dermatomyositis, Henoch–Schönlein purpura, and polyarteritis nodosa are primarily seen in the mid-childhood (7–11 years). On the other hand, enthesitis-related arthritis (ERA) and systemic lupus erythematosus (SLE) are predominantly seen during late childhood. Rheumatoid factor—positive polyarthritis, which mimics adult rheumatoid arthritis, usually occurs after the age of 10 years. Diseases like gout, calcium pyrophosphate deposition disease, polymyalgia rheumatica, and primary osteoarthritis are almost rare in childhood.

Sex

Polyarticular JIA and SLE have a propensity for girls, whereas ERA, KD, and systemic JIA are common in boys. However, many of these clinical conditions can occur in both sexes.

Onset and Duration

Conditions like septic arthritis, trauma, and arthritis due to hemophilia present within hours to days. Likewise, arthritis related to viral infection, acute rheumatic fever, vasculitides, leukemia, reactive arthritis, and JIA evolves over days to weeks. Polyarticular JIA, tubercular arthritis, sarcoidosis, and fungal arthritis run through an indolent course and present in weeks to months. However, many of these conditions may be in the evolution phase in the initial weeks; hence, giving a diagnostic label at this stage may not be possible.

Pattern

In inflammatory arthritis, early morning stiffness is a prominent feature noticed after a period of inactivity. This is attributed to the jelling phenomenon due to chronic inflammation. Pain at night causing sleep disturbance should always be looked upon with caution, may indicate an underlying malignancy.

Past History

History of recent diarrhea, acute conjunctivitis, urethritis, and fever with or without rash is a pointer toward reactive arthritis. Similarly, history of heel pain, back pain, or transient redness of eyes in a boy above 6 years can indicate the beginning of ERA. A history of repeated swelling in the same joint after a trivial trauma may indicate a previously undiagnosed bleeding disorder.

Family History

Diseases such as JIA, inflammatory bowel disease (IBD), and psoriasis may have a familial predilection.

EXAMINATION

The diagnosis of inflammatory arthritis can be made based on examination alone. Key features include joint swelling with or without effusion, warmth, joint line tenderness, pain and/or restriction of movement, although not all may be present. Children often deny pain verbally when examined; therefore, the physician should pay close attention to the child's face to detect grimaces and note involuntary flinching when a joint is passively moved. Young people with hip inflammation often localize pain to the groin, although it may be referred to the thigh or knee. Arthritis tends to affect certain movements before others, and the following features are most sensitive: loss of internal rotation at the hip, hyperextension of the knee, and extension of the cervical spine. It is also important to note the extraarticular manifestation, which helps to reach a conclusive diagnosis.

Articular Involvement

Synovium, synovial fluid, articular cartilage, intra-articular ligaments, joint capsule, and juxta-articular bone form a part of the articular structures. Presence of pain, joint line tenderness and limitation of both active and passive movements, instability, locking of the joint, crepitus, and joint deformity signify articular involvement. In addition, swelling may be there due to synovial thickening, joint effusion, or joint enlargement. In nonarticular involvement, findings are away from the joint, and pain may be noticed only on active movement.

Inflammatory Versus Noninflammatory Arthritis

Signs of local inflammation are erythema, tenderness, and redness of the joint. Systemic inflammatory signs include fever, weight loss, and fatigue. An effusion and pain at the end of the range of movement indicates active arthritis. Morning stiffness is uncommon in noninflammatory arthritis and inflammatory parameters, synovial fluid analysis remains within normal limit.

Pattern of Joint Involvement

The pattern of joint involvement often provides important clues about the underlying disease conditions.

- *Evolution of the joint pain:*
  - Migratory joint involvement is seen in acute rheumatic fever and gonococcal arthritis. In acute rheumatic fever, the joint can swell up in hours, whereas in gonococcal arthritis, it develops over days.
  - Additive joint involvement, where new joints are involved when the previously affected ones are still painful, seen in post-streptococcal reactive arthritis, SLE, JIA, and psoriasis.
  - Intermittent arthritis, where the symptoms can appear and disappear, is a characteristic of reactive arthritis.
- *Topography:* The involvement of the axial or peripheral joints is an important clue to diagnosis. Axial skeleton includes the spine, sacroiliac joints, sternoclavicular joints, and the manubriosternal joints. ERA has predilection for sacroiliac, lower spine, and knee. Other conditions, like JIA and SLE, have peripheral joint involvement, though rarely they may have both axial and peripheral joint involvement.
- *Symmetry:* Symmetric joint involvement is seen in rheumatoid factor positive polyarthritis, SLE, whereas asymmetric joint involvement is common in reactive arthritis and ERA.
- *Specific joint involvement:* Some diseases involving specific joints, like dactylitis and distal interphalangeal joint involvement, indicate psoriatic arthritis. Similarly, temporomandibular joint involvement indicates rheumatoid factor positive polyarthritis. Reactive arthritis and ERA have a propensity to have a lower limb joint involvement.
- *Presence of joint deformity:* Joint deformity usually follows long-standing undiagnosed or untreated arthritis and commonly seen with JIA or hemophilia. Joint deformities are also common in noninflammatory arthropathies. Arthritis associated with SLE and IBD is usually nondeforming.

Extra-articular Manifestations

Diseases like SLE, IBD, malignancies, and systemic onset JIA have dominant extra-articular manifestations **(Table 2)**.

Pattern Recognition

A good history and clinical examination can help the astute and observant clinician recognize some typical patterns of joint disease. Some examples are:

- Polyarthritis in a young girl may suggest SLE or polyarticular JIA.
- Scattered small distal interphalangeal joint involvement indicates psoriatic arthritis.
- Hip and lower back involvement may point toward ERA.
- Inflammatory tarsitis and enthesopathy may be a distinguishing feature between ERA and JIA in the absence of axial disease.

An algorithmic approach to polyarthritis is shown in **Flowchart 1**.

LABORATORY TESTS

More than 95% of the cases of polyarthritis can be diagnosed based on a good history and examination. However, tests like complete blood count and peripheral smear examination can reveal malignant processes like leukemia. Thrombocytopenia is commonly seen in SLE and leukemia, whereas in KD, thrombocytosis along with raised acute phase reactants, like ESR and CRP, is commonly seen. Likewise, antinuclear antibodies are commonly found in SLE. Rheumatoid factor positivity is found in polyarticular JIA. Human leukocyte antigen B27 (HLAB27) is commonly associated with ERA and antineutrophil cytoplasmic antibodies are associated with small-vessels vasculitis. Other investigations, like ASO and echocardiography, are useful in acute rheumatic fever. Synovial fluid analysis is helpful in differentiating infective and an inflammatory process.

TREATMENT

Treatment of polyarthritis depends on the underlying etiology. Pending the final diagnosis, one must focus on providing symptomatic relief by using nonsteroidal

TABLE 2: Extra-articular features in a patient with polyarthritis.

Site	*Manifestations*	*Diseases*
Eye	• Nonpurulent conjunctivitis • Anterior uveitis • Posterior uveitis	• KD • JIA • Psoriasis
Mouth	• Fissures in lips, strawberry tongue • Oral ulcers • Red gums at tooth line	• KD • SLE, Behçet's disease • JDMS
Head and neck	• Alopecia/hair loss • Malar/discoid rash • Heliotrope rash • Psoriasis	• SLE • SLE • JDMS • Psoriatic arthritis
Hands	• Raynaud's phenomenon • Nail pitting, onycholysis • Nail fold infarct • Periungual desquamation • Digital infarct • Gottron's papules • Subcutaneous calcinosis	• SLE, JDMS, scleroderma • Psoriasis • Connective tissue disease • KD • PAN • JDMS • JDMS
Trunk and arms	• Erythema marginatum • Subcutaneous nodules • Urticaria	• ARF • ARF, RF +ve JIA • CTD
Muscles	• Wasted muscles • Tender muscles, proximal muscles weakness	• JIA • JDMS
Hematological	• Lymphadenopathy • Petechiae • Pallor	• TB, SLE, malignancy, KD • Malignancy, SLE • Malignancy, SLE, SOJIA
Gastrointestinal	• Dysphagia • Abdominal pain • Diarrhea • Malabsorption • Hepatic involvement • Organomegaly	• JDMS, scleroderma • SLE, PAN • IBD, reactive arthritis • Scleroderma • SLE • SLE, malignancy
Respiratory	• Upper airway symptoms • Pleuritis, pleural effusion	• Wegener's granulomatosis • SLE, SJIA
Cardiovascular	• Pericarditis • Myocarditis • Valvular disease • Coronary artery dilatation	• SLE, SJIA, ARF • ARF, SJIA, polymyositis • ARF, SLE, ERA, hypermobility • KD
Genitourinary	• Urethritis • Genital ulcers • Proteinuria • Renal failure, hematuria	• Reactive arthritis, Reiter's syndrome • Behcet's syndrome • SLE, amyloidosis, NSAIDs • SLE, NSAIDs, amyloidosis, systemic vasculitides
Central nervous system	• Chorea • Convulsions, coma, psychosis, headache • Neuropathies	• ARF, SLE • SLE • PAN

(KD: Kawasaki disease; TB: tuberculosis; ARF: acute rheumatic fever; JIA: juvenile idiopathic arthritis; SLE: systemic lupus erythematosus; IBD: inflammatory bowel disease; JDMS: juvenile dermatomyositis; SJIA: systemic JIA; ERA: enthesitis-related arthritis; PAN: polyarteritis nodosa; CTD: connective tissue disease; NSAIDs: nonsteroidal anti-inflammatory drugs)

Flowchart 1: Algorithmic approach to polyarthritis.

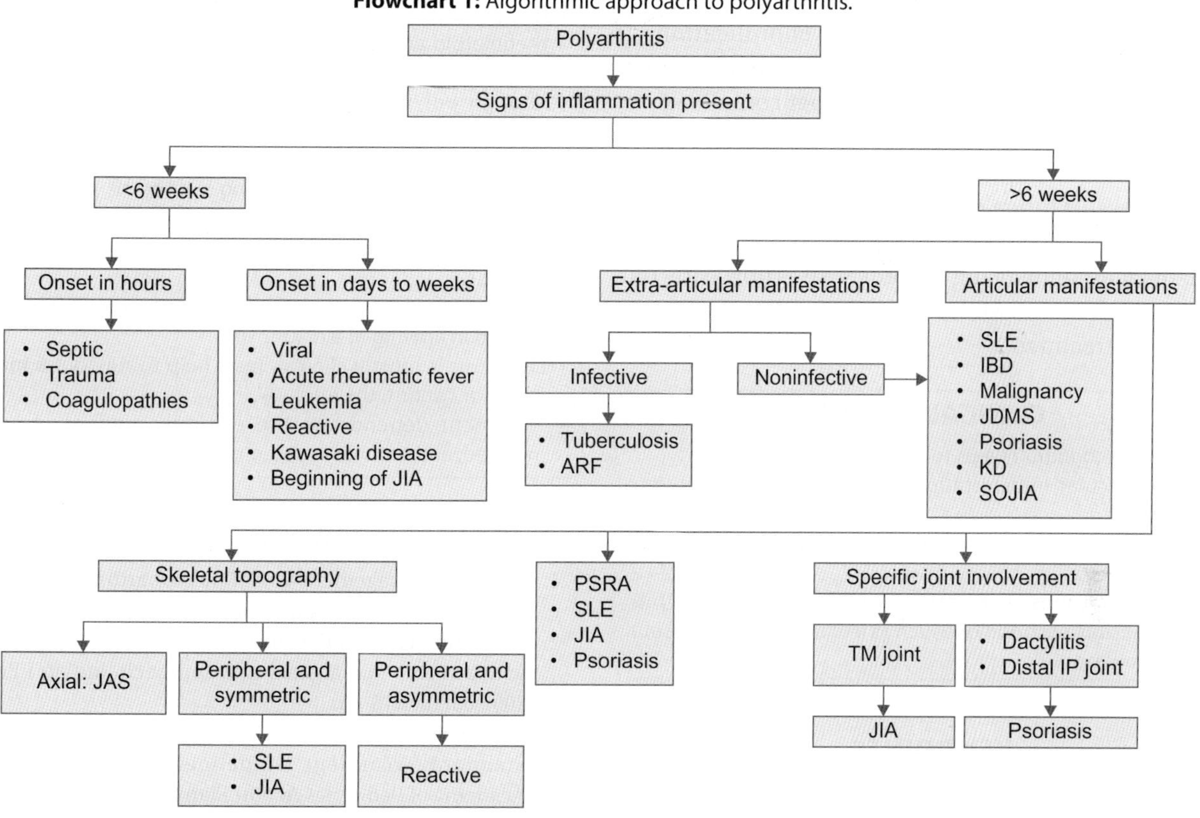

(KD: Kawasaki disease; ARF: acute rheumatic fever; JIA: juvenile idiopathic arthritis; SLE: systemic lupus erythematosus; IBD: inflammatory bowel disease; JDMS: juvenile dermatomyositis; SOJIA: systemic onset juvenile idiopathic arthritis; JAS: juvenile ankylosing spondylitis; PSRA: poststreptococcal reactive arthritis; TM: temporomandibular; IP: interphalangeal)

TABLE 3: Outline of treatment of polyarthritis.

Etiology	*Specific treatment*	*Supportive treatment*
Viral arthritis	NSAIDs	Self-limiting illness—counseling and reassurance
Bacterial arthritis	Specific antibiotics. NSAIDs if needed	Long-term penicillin prophylaxis for patients with rheumatic fever
Reactive arthritis	NSAIDs	Specific treatment for bacterial etiology if any such as gonococcal infection
Rheumatological arthritis	NSAIDs/steroids depending on specific etiology	Physiotherapy, counseling, and occupational therapy
Systemic vasculitides	Intravenous immunoglobulin for Kawasaki disease, NSAIDs, or steroids in Henoch–Schönlein purpura and other vasculitides	Appropriate and prompt treatment in Kawasaki disease with intravenous immunoglobulin prevents long-term cardiac morbidity and steroids in lupus may be life-saving

(NSAIDs: nonsteroidal anti-inflammatory drugs)

anti-inflammatory agents, rest to the affected part, and physiotherapy if possible. A brief outline of the management has been documented in **Table 3**. However, many diseases may require extensive and long-term management for remission and morbidity prevention.

PROGNOSIS

Prognosis depends on the diagnosis, time to diagnosis, presence of complications, and how management has been done. For example, reactive arthritis would have an excellent prognosis with supportive management, intravenous immunoglobulin in Kawasaki disease would lead to a possible cure and prevent complications if treated early. Early diagnosis and aggressive management of arthritis prevent joint damage and other complications. Acute rheumatic fever responds well to nonsteroidal anti-inflammatory drugs, and initiating penicillin prophylaxis prevents future recurrences and valvular damage. Institution of glucocorticoids in SLE is life-saving. However, the main factor influencing the prognosis is how early one has identified the possible etiology of polyarthritis and initiated the treatment.

CLINICAL PEARLS

- Pattern recognition helps to arrive at a diagnosis.
- Extra-articular manifestations form an important clue to diagnosis.
- Early morning stiffness characteristic of inflammatory arthritis
- Diagnosis is mostly clinical. Laboratory tests only help to rule out sinister conditions such as leukemia, and also useful for follow-up.

KEY POINTS

- Polyarthritis has multifactorial etiology.
- Pattern recognition is very important.
- Rheumatoid factor positive arthritis mimicking adult onset rheumatoid arthritis usually occurs after 10 years of age. It has no diagnostic significance but helps in prognostication.
- Though polyarthritis can occur in both the sexes, it is important to remember that juvenile idiopathic arthritis and systemic lupus erythematosus are more common in girls whereas juvenile ankylosing spondylitis and Kawasaki disease are more common in boys.
- Inflammatory arthritis is characterized by early morning stiffness.
- Prominent extra-articular manifestations must be looked for and aid in arriving at a diagnosis.
- Diagnosis is mostly clinical. Tests help to rule out a malignancy or confirm the etiology.
- Treatment depends on the etiology, number of joints involved, and other associated manifestations.

SUGGESTED READING

1. Hull RG. Management guidelines for arthritis in children. Rheumatology. 2001;40:1308.
2. Khubchnadani RP, D'Souza S. Initial evaluation of a child with arthritis—an algorithmic approach. Indian J Pediatr. 2002;69(10):875-80.
3. Kumar S, Bagri N, Bhat C. Juvenile Idiopathic Arthritis. Standard Treatment Guidelines, Chapter 51, Indian Academy of Pediatrics Action Plan 2022.
4. Singh S, Mehra S. Approach to polyarthritis. Indian J Pediatr. 2010;77:1005-10.

Fever with Arthritis: An Algorithmic Approach

T Sathish Kumar

INTRODUCTION

"When an arthritis patient walked in the front door I wanted to walk out the back one"—Sir William Osler (1849–1919) Principles and Practice of Medicine, 1892

When a child presents with fever with arthritis, a broad differential diagnosis might represent a diagnostic challenge for the pediatrician who first approaches the patient. This chapter is focused on algorithmic approach to a child who presents with fever and arthritis.

All joint pains are not arthritis. Arthritis is defined as a swollen joint or a joint having at least two of the following conditions: tenderness, limited range of motion, pain on movement, or warmth overlying the joint.

The first step in initial screening is to establish whether a single joint or multiple joints are involved. The second important step is to determine whether or not there is associated fever **(Flowchart 1)**. For practical purposes, this initial screening should lead to the following four possible groups of diagnoses:

1. Single joint involvement with associated fever
2. Single joint involvement without fever
3. Multiple joint involvement with associated fever
4. Multiple joint involvement without fever

ALGORITHMIC APPROACH TO MONOARTHRITIS (SINGLE JOINT)

A carefully conducted history taking and physical examination are the initial and most important steps in narrowing the differential diagnosis and guiding the diagnostic evaluation **(Flowchart 2)**.

Flowchart 1: Approach to the child with joint pain.

The child with joint pain

- Single joint involvement
  - *With fever:*
    - Septic arthritis/osteomyelitis
    - Sympathetic arthritis
    - Foreign body infection
    - Traumatic arthritis
    - Soft tissue infection
    - Rheumatic diseases
    - Reactive arthritis
    - Toxic synovitis
    - Diskitis
    - Sarcoidosis
    - Hemoglobinopathy
    - Malignancies
  - *Without fever:*
    - Trauma
    - Mechanical derangement
    - Rheumatic diseases
    - Toxic synovitis
    - Avascular necrosis
    - Subacute osteomyelitis
    - Diskitis
    - Hemoglobinopathy
    - Reflex sympathetic dystrophy
    - Malignancies
    - Psychogenic pain
- Multiple joint involvement
  - *With fever:*
    - Bacterial infections
    - Sepsis
    - Viral infections
    - Lyme disease
    - Reactive arthritis
    - Rheumatic diseases
    - Postimmunization
    - Immune deficiencies
    - Serum sickness
    - Sarcoidosis
    - Familial Mediterranean fever
    - Malignancies
  - *Without fever:*
    - Malignancies
    - Joint hypermobility
    - Growing pains
    - Postimmunization
    - Immune deficiencies
    - Guillain-Barre syndrome
    - Lyme disease
    - Fibromyalgia syndrome
    - Chronic fatigue syndrome
    - Psychogenic pain
    - Malignancies

Flowchart 2: Approach to fever with monoarthritis.

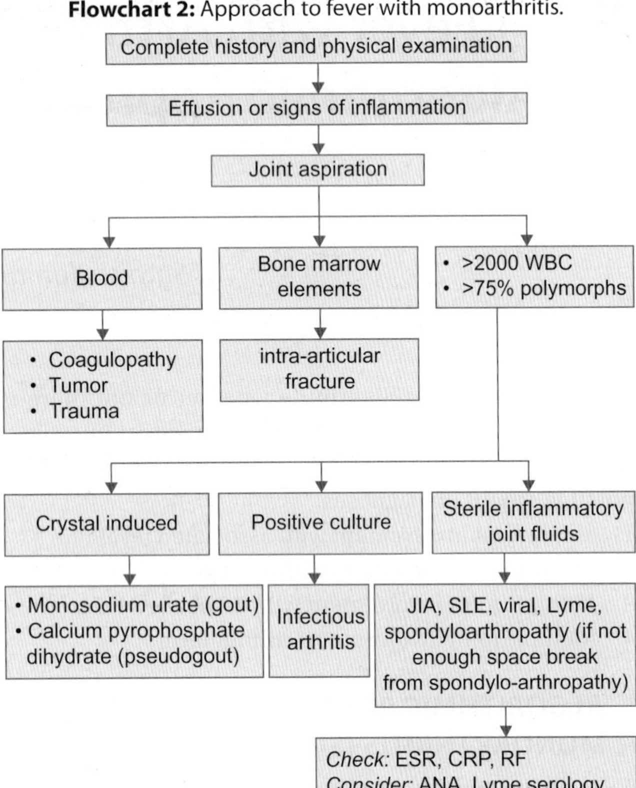

(WBC: white blood cell; JIA: juvenile idiopathic arthritis; SLE: systemic lupus erythematosus; ESR: erythrocyte sedimentation rate; CRP: C-reactive protein; RF: rheumatoid factor; ANA: antinuclear antibody)

History Taking

Important aspects to be considered in the history taking are as follows:

- Characteristics of the pain and/or stiffness (site, number of joints, severity, frequency, duration, pattern, and association of warmth or discoloration). Morning stiffness is a characteristic feature of inflammatory arthritis. Night pain should alert the clinician to a malignancy or an osteoid osteoma.
- Review of systems focused on the presence of fever or other constitutional symptoms (e.g., weight loss, anorexia, night sweats, or nocturnal pain).
- *Precipitating factors:* Traumas, infections (streptococcal, enteric), travel to Lyme disease or tuberculosis (TB) endemic areas or other risk factors for TB (exposure to a person with TB; close contact with a person with a positive TB skin test result).
- Presence of extra-articular features (diarrhea, urethral discharge, ocular symptoms, and rash).
- Personal or family history of a bleeding diathesis or human leukocyte antigen (HLA) B27-associated diseases like inflammatory bowel disease (IBD), acute anterior uveitis, psoriasis, and ankylosing spondylitis.

Physical Examination

The presence of fever should alert the clinician to the potential for more severe conditions requiring urgent treatment (e.g., septic arthritis). On general examination, clues to underlying diagnosis include rash (psoriasis, viral exanthems, systemic arthritis, and Kawasaki disease), iritis (ANA+ oligo JIA, IBD, or enthesitis-related arthritis), and hepatosplenomegaly/lymphadenopathy suggestive of malignancy.

The focused examination of the affected joint should include inspection of the skin for warmth, redness, swelling, and soft tissue involvement, using the contralateral side for comparison. Palpation of the surrounding bone is important because the presence of pinpoint bony tenderness is suggestive of fracture, osteomyelitis, or malignancy. An exquisite pain in the joint on range of motion or a joint that is severely restricted in its range of motion suggests an etiology other than inflammatory arthritis (e.g., septic joint and malignancy).

The differential diagnosis of monoarthritis includes entities in the broad categories of infection, postinfection, inflammation, and malignancy and trauma related to a systemic illness **(Box 1)**.

Preliminary investigations that are to be considered for the evaluation of monoarthritis are presented in **Box 2**. Laboratory investigations of acute or chronic monoarthritis are performed to confirm the clinician's impression regarding the suspected diagnosis or to exclude conditions.

Laboratory Investigations

Complete blood count (CBC) and differential white blood cell count, inflammatory markers, and liver and renal functions should be considered in any child with monoarthritis.

If the presentation is acute (<72 hours), a joint aspiration must be performed if the clinician suspects a septic joint, with the fluid sent for blood cell count, Gram stain, and culture. In addition, culture of the throat, blood, stool, and/or urine should be considered to identify

BOX 1: Differential diagnosis of monoarthritis.

Infection-related:
- Septic arthritis
- Osteomyelitis
- Transient synovitis
- Reactive arthritis
- Lyme disease
- Tuberculosis

Trauma:
- *Fracture:* Accidental and nonaccidental
- *Internal derangement:* Ligament rupture
- *Foreign body:* Synovitis

Malignancy:
- Leukemia
- Neuroblastoma

Inflammation:
- Juvenile idiopathic arthritis
- Inflammatory bowel disease
- Familial Mediterranean fever

Hemarthrosis:
- Hemophilia
- Pigmented villonodular synovitis
- Synovial hemangioma

BOX 2: Preliminary investigations to be considered for the evaluation of monoarthritis.

Basic screening:
- Complete blood count and differential white blood cell count
- Erythrocyte sedimentation rate
- C-reactive protein
- Renal function and liver enzyme
- Serum lactate dehydrogenase
- Radiographs

Further investigations:
- Cultures of throat, blood, joint fluid, stool, and/or urine
- Partial thromboplastin time
- Antinuclear antibody titer
- Serologic testing for Lyme disease
- Antistreptolysin O titer
- Urinalysis
- Tuberculin skin test
- Further imaging (ultrasonography and magnetic resonance imaging)
- Bone marrow aspiration
- Slit lamp examination of the eyes

a potential organism in the case of reactive arthritis. An acute presentation is also observed with hematologic and malignant diseases (e.g., hemophilia and leukemia), highlighting the importance of CBC and coagulation studies. Antistreptolysin O (ASO) and antideoxyribonuclease B (anti-DNaseB) titers are useful to identify a recent streptococcal infection.

In chronic monoarthritis, antinuclear antibody (ANA) and human leukocyte antigen B27 testing is most relevant in chronic arthritis when the child is suspected of having a specific category of juvenile idiopathic arthritis (JIA) (enthesitis-related arthritis), which is generally seen in boys older than 6 years and often associated with enthesitis, lumbosacral back pain, and a family history of HLA-B27-associated diseases (e.g., IBD and ankylosing spondylitis).

The presence of ANA or RF is neither necessary nor sufficient to make a diagnosis of JIA. Antinuclear antibody should not be used as a screening test for rheumatic illness in a primary care setting, because it may be positive in up to 5–10% of healthy children. In the context of JIA, a positive ANA titer is associated with a significantly increased risk of developing chronic anterior uveitis.

Rheumatoid factor has been associated with aging (>60 years), infections (bacterial endocarditis, hepatitis B or C, parasitic disease, and viral infection), pulmonary disease (sarcoidosis and interstitial pulmonary fibrosis), malignancy, and primary biliary cirrhosis and thus is not a specific test for the diagnosis of rheumatic disease.

Only 5–10% of patients with JIA have a positive RF, highlighting the lack of sensitivity for the diagnosis of JIA.

A joint aspiration must be performed when a septic joint (bacterial) is suspected but is also recommended for the diagnosis of TB arthritis. The presence of hemarthrosis suggests coagulation disorder, trauma, or rare causes, including synovial hemangioma or pigmented villonodular synovitis. The more common and/or serious causes of monoarthritis are addressed here.

- *Septic arthritis:* This condition classically presents with a severely painful, swollen, warm, and red joint in a febrile child. The join must be aspirated for Gram stain, cultures and examination of the synovial fluid, and cell count. In the absence of Gram stain or culture, a cell count of 40,000/mm^3 is regarded as evidence of bacterial infection.
- *Osteomyelitis:* With reactive arthritis or sympathetic arthritis, this is arthritis with effusion in a nearby joint as a reaction to osteomyelitis. A technetium or gallium joint bone scan often reveals an osteomyelitis in the adjacent bone.
- *Traumatic arthritis:* Traumatic serosanguineous effusion can cause fever secondary to blood within the joint. There is almost always a history of trauma.

Aspiration usually reveals sterile surgery will reveal the nature of this condition. In addition, clotting abnormalities must be ruled out.

- *Rheumatic diseases:* Oligoarticular onset of juvenile idiopathic arthritis may present with single joint disease. Usually, one of the large joints is affected, and the patient is either afebrile or has a low-grade fever. Very rarely, children with systemic onset JIA may also present initially with monoarticular disease, usually in the knee or hip. In that case, look for other manifestations of the disease such as rheumatoid rash, hepatosplenomegaly, lymphadenopathy, pericarditis, and, in rare instances, iritis. A diagnosis of JIA is made based on history taking and physical examination and after exclusion of other causes.

  It is unusual for children with systemic lupus erythematosus to present with single joint involvement. Occasionally, rheumatic fever, Kawasaki disease, juvenile dermatomyositis, and certain viral infections may begin with arthritis affecting one joint.
- *Postinfectious reactive arthritis:* This includes postviral or postbacterial diseases such as poststreptococcal reactive arthritis and post-*Salmonella*, *Shigella*, and *Yersinia* reactive arthritis. These postviral or postbacterial conditions have a benign, self-limited course that may require symptomatic and supportive therapy.
- *Toxic synovitis:* If the hip joint is affected, toxic synovitis must be taken into account. It is also called transient synovitis and occurs in children aged 8 ± 10. Most of the patients are boys, and there is often a history of respiratory infection. Within a few weeks, a limp and pain referred to the knee develop along with a low-grade fever. The erythrocyte sedimentation rate may be mildly elevated. The disease usually subsides after 1 ± 2 weeks and does not commonly recur. However, Legg–Calve–Perthes disease is occasionally a sequela.
- *Hemoglobinopathy:* In a child, sickle cell anemia must be ruled out by hemoglobin electrophoresis. In the very young child, it causes a dactylitis that may mimic true arthritis; in older children, it causes microinfarcts that give rise to periostitis and periarthritis which are responsible for the pain crises in this disease.
- *Malignancies:* Leukemia is the most common malignancy in childhood. However, it rarely presents with single joint involvement. Tumors, such as synovial cell sarcoma or bone tumors like osteosarcoma and Ewing's sarcoma, can rarely present as single joint involvement with fever. In any malignancy, bone pain is usually prominent, and other features, such as weight loss and fatigue, are commonly present.

ALGORITHMIC APPROACH TO POLYARTHRITIS (MULTIPLE JOINTS)

Differential diagnosis of polyarthritis essentially includes infectious, inflammatory, and malignant causes **(Box 3)**.

Reviewing systems and physical examination **(Flowchart 3)** is critical to establishing a diagnosis. For post-infectious etiology (ASO and anti-DNAase B titers), cardiac evaluation (electrocardiography and echocardiography), chest radiography, ANA titer, and other autoantibodies (in case of connective tissue disorder) often provide the correct diagnosis **(Table 1)**.

When polyarthritis is the presenting complaint, in addition to the investigations outlined in **Box 2**, additional investigations may include serum C3 and C4 complement levels, serum levels of quantitative immunoglobulins, urinalysis, serologic testing for viral pathogens, swabs for gonococcal anti-La, anti-Smith, anti-ribonucleoprotein, anti-Scl 70, and antineutrophil cytoplasmic antibody.

BOX 3: Differential diagnosis of polyarthritis.

- *Infection-related:*
- *Neisseria gonorrhoeae* infection
- Viral infections (e.g., parvovirus B19, rubella virus/vaccine)
- Infective endocarditis
- Acute rheumatic fever
- Poststreptococcal reactive arthritis
- Reactive arthritis

Inflammatory:
- Juvenile idiopathic arthritis
- Systemic lupus erythematosus
- Juvenile dermatomyositis
- Systemic vasculitides (Henoch–Schonlein purpura, Kawasaki disease)
- Hereditary autoinflammatory syndromes
- Sarcoidosis
- IBD-related arthritis

Malignancy:
- Leukemia
- Neuroblastoma

Mechanical:
- Hypermobility
- Skeletal dysplasia

Other systemic illness:
- Immunodeficiency-associated arthritis
- Serum sickness

(IBD: inflammatory bowel disease)

Flowchart 3: Approach to fever with polyarthritis.

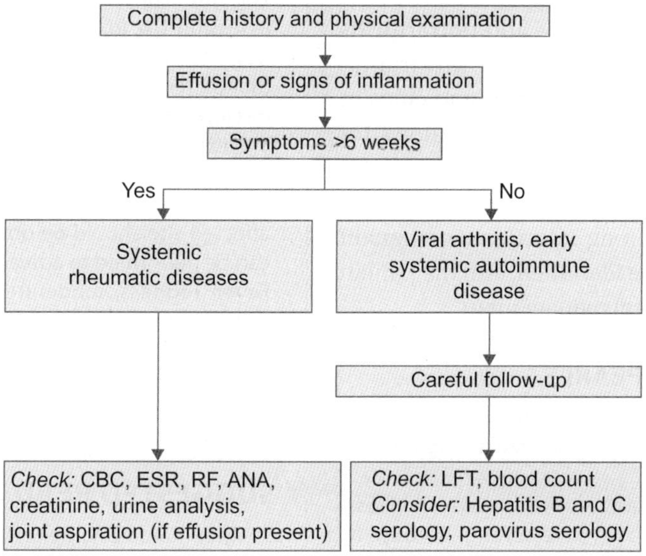

(ESR: erythrocyte sedimentation rate; RF: rheumatoid factor; ANA: antinuclear antibody; LFT: liver function test)

TABLE 1: Review of systems in the differential diagnosis of polyarthritis.

System involved	*Review of system or physical finding*	*Diagnosis*
Ophthalmologic	• Uveitis • Conjunctival injection without exudate	• JIA • KD
Dermatologic	• Malar rash, alopecia • Heliotrope rash, Gottron's papules • Polymorphous rash, perianal desquamation, edema, and erythema of hands • Evanescent salmon-colored rash • Palpable purpura • Nail pitting or onycholysis • Oral ulcers	• SLE • JDM • KD • SJIA • HSP, SLE • JIA (psoriatic) • SLE
Cardiovascular	• New heart murmur • Pericarditis • Raynaud phenomenon	• ARF, IE • SJIA, SLE, ARF • SLE, MCTD, scleroderma
Respiratory tract	• Pleuritis • Acute or chronic sinusitis, pulmonary nodules, or hemorrhage • Interstitial lung disease	• SJIA, SLE • GPA • SLE or scleroderma
Gastrointestinal/ genitourinary tract	• Weight loss or poor growth • Diarrhea/hematochezia, colicky abdominal pain • History of gastroenteritis • History of urethritis or cervicitis	• IBD, malignancy, SLE • IBD, HSP • Reactive arthritis • Reactive arthritis, gonococcal arthritis
Neurologic	• Seizures, psychosis, mood disorder, decline in school performance • Stroke • Proximal muscle weakness	• SLE • SLE, vasculitis • JDM, MCTD

(JIA: juvenile idiopathic arthritis; KD: Kawasaki disease; SLE: systemic lupus erythematosus; JDM: juvenile dermatomyositis; SJIA: systemic juvenile idiopathic arthritis; HSP: Henoch–Schonlein purpura; ARF: acute rheumatic fever; IE: infective endocarditis; MCTD: mixed connective tissue disease; GPA: granulomatosis with polyangiitis; IBD: inflammatory bowel disease)

CONCLUSION

Differential diagnosis for monoarthritis and polyarthritis is broad. An organized approach within the framework presented, including carefully attending to clues in the history taking and physical examination, allows for correct diagnosis in most cases. Laboratory evaluation is performed to support the clinician's impression. Serious and/or potentially life-threatening infections, malignant or orthopedic causes need to be identified, and the patient is referred for surgical or medical management.

CLINICAL PEARLS

- Presence of antinuclear antibody or rheumatoid factor is neither necessary nor sufficient to make a diagnosis of juvenile idiopathic arthritis.
- Antinuclear antibody should not be used as a screening test for rheumatic illness in a primary care setting, because it may be positive in 5–10% of healthy children.
- High ASO titer with arthralgia does not warrant penicillin prophylaxis.

KEY POINTS

- A detailed history and physical examination are critical in the initial assessment, with attention paid to the nature of the pain, presence of limp, weight-bearing status, morning stiffness, systemic symptoms (fever, rash, weight loss, and fatigue), history of past medical illnesses, and travel or positive family history (arthritis, bleeding disorders, sickle cell anemia, inflammatory bowel disease, and psoriasis).
- The important aspects of physical examination include assessing the joints (swelling, erythema, warmth, tenderness, deformity, and range of motion), adjacent structures (bones, tendons, muscles, and skin), and gait and leg length discrepancy.
- The extent of investigations is determined from the information gained through the history and physical examination.
- Basic screening laboratory tests and radiographs of the affected site should be obtained. Additional investigations can be performed to arrive at a clinical diagnosis.
- Fever, redness, moderate-to-severe pain, pinpoint pain or tenderness, and weight loss are clues to more serious causes of limb pain that require additional investigations and referrals to specialists (rheumatologists, orthopedic surgeons, neurologists, and hematologist/oncologists).

SUGGESTED READING

1. Alpay-Kanıtez N, Çelik S, Bes C. Polyarthritis and its differential diagnosis. Eur J Rheumatol. 2018;6(4):167-73.
2. Berard R. Approach to the child with joint inflammation. Pediatr Clin North Am. 2012;59(2):245-62.
3. Gamalero L, Ferrara G, Giani T, Cimaz R. Acute Arthritis in Children: How to Discern between Septic and Non-Septic Arthritis? *Children*. 2021;8(10):912.
4. Prabhu AS, Balan S. Approach to a Child with Monoarthritis. Indian J Pediatr. 2010;77:997-1004.
5. Singh S, Mehra S. Approach to polyarthritis. Indian J Pediatr. 2010;77(9):1005-10.
6. Thomas M, Bonacorsi S, Simon AL, Mallet C, Lorrot M, Faye A, et al. Acute monoarthritis in young children: comparing the characteristics of patients with juvenile idiopathic arthritis versus septic and undifferentiated arthritis. Sci Rep. 2021;11:3422.

CHAPTER 121

Childhood Vasculitis

Sikha Agarwal

INTRODUCTION

Vasculitis is characterized by inflammation of blood vessel wall with resultant tissue ischemia and necrosis. The first case was described by Adolf Kussmaul and Rudolf Maier more than 150 years ago, when they described a patient with what is today known as polyarteritis nodosa (PAN). Since then, many more in these categories have been described. Most pediatric vasculitic disorders need individual specific classification criteria for their identification.

EPIDEMIOLOGY

Estimated overall annual incidence of new cases of pediatric vasculitis is 53.3 per 100,000 children under 17 years of age. The two most common vasculitides are IgA vasculitis and Kawasaki disease, with estimated annual incidences of 20.4 and 5.5 per 100,000 in children <17 years of age, respectively. Reported geographical variations in vasculitis may reflect an environmental influence, like infections, drugs, allergy, vaccination, and desensitization procedures.

PATHOGENESIS

The exact pathogenesis of pediatric vasculitis is not known. The proposed mechanisms are vascular injury caused by inflammation of vascular wall. The triggers for injury can be genetic, environmental, infective, and immune factors.

Irrespective of the initial insult, inflicted injury to the vessel wall results in healing of vascular wall by fibrosis. It causes narrowing of vascular lumen and ischemic injury to target organ. Abnormal healing of the vascular wall leads to aneurysm formation with disorganized blood flow which can lead to ischemic target organ damage with or without thrombus formation **(Fig. 1)**.

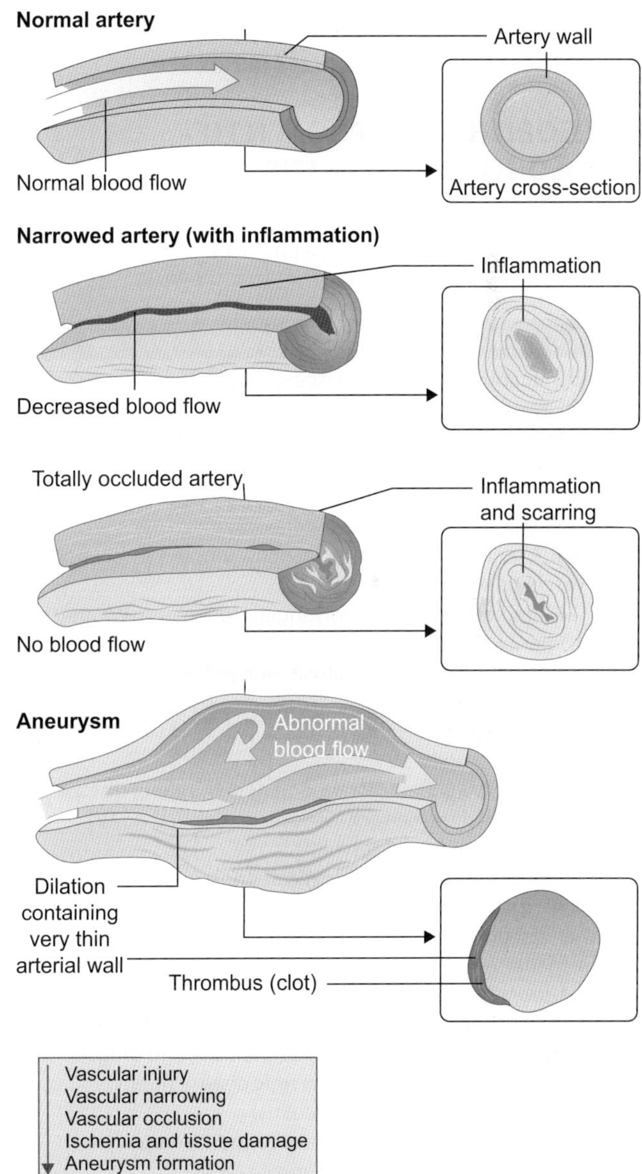

Fig. 1: Schematic diagram showing vascular injury causing different changes including aneurysm formation.

CLASSIFICATION

International Consensus Conference in Vienna (June 2005) under the Pediatric Rheumatology European Society resulted in a new proposal for childhood vasculitis classification which was validated and given the final form at the 2008 Ankara Consensus Conference with support from the European League Against Rheumatism (EULAR) and the Pediatric Rheumatology International Trials Organization. There has been trend for use of vasculitic disorders names that reflect increased pathophysiologic understanding of these conditions. The 2012 International Chapel Hill Consensus Conference (CHCC) on nomenclature of vasculitides is summarized in **Box 1**.

ALGORITHMIC APPROACH TO CHILDHOOD VASCULITIS

Diagnosis and treatment of childhood vasculitis are explained in detail below **(Flowchart 1)**.

BOX 1: Classification of childhood vasculitis.

- Predominantly large-vessel vasculitis (LVV):
  - Takayasu arteritis
- Predominantly medium-vessel vasculitis (MVV):
  - Polyarteritis nodosa (PAN)
  - Kawasaki disease (KD)
- Predominantly small-vessel vasculitis (SVV):
  - ANCA (antineutrophil cytoplasmic antibody)-associated vasculitis (AAV):
    - Granulomatosis with polyangiitis (previously Wegner's granulomatosis)
    - Eosinophilic granulomatosis with polyangiitis (Churg–Strauss)
    - Microscopic polyangiitis (MPA)
  - Immune complex SVV
    - Anti GBM (glomerular basement membrane) disease
    - IgA vasculitis (Henoch–Schönlein purpura) (IgAV)
    - Cryoglobulinemic vasculitis
    - Hypocomplementemic urticarial vasculitis (HUV, anti-C1q vasculitis)
- Other vasculitides:
  - Variable vessel vasculitis (Behçet's disease, Cogan's syndrome)
  - Vasculitis secondary to probable etiology (including hepatitis B-associated PAN, malignancies, and drugs)
  - Vasculitis associated with systemic disease (lupus, rheumatoid, and sarcoid vasculitis)
  - Single organ vasculitis (primary central nervous system, isolated cutaneous, isolated aortitis, etc.)
  - Unclassified

Source: Adapted from 2012 ICHCC.

Suspect Childhood Vasculitis

Common symptoms suggestive of childhood vasculitis include:

- Fever, weight loss, and fatigue
- *Skin manifestation:* Ranges from palpable purpura to urticaria, livedo reticularis, nodules, ulcers, even gangrenes
- Hypertension
- *Organ-specific involvement:* This depends on the size of the vessel involved, degree of collateral circulation, and the organ involved:
  - *Musculoskeletal:* Arthritis and myositis
  - *Serous cavities:* Serositis
  - *Cardiac:* Myocarditis and cardiomyopathy
  - *Pulmonary:* Infiltrates, infarct, and/or hemorrhage
  - *Neurologic:* Mono- or polyneuritis, focal central nervous system lesions

Support from Laboratory Findings

- *Raised inflammatory markers:* Erythrocyte sedimentation rates and C-reactive protein
- Polymorphonuclear leukocytosis or eosinophilia, thrombocytosis
- Presence of hematuria, proteinuria, red blood cell cast, and azotemia
- Circulating immune complexes
- Antineutrophil cytoplasmic antibodies

Categorize the Involved Vessel Type

Typical clinical findings according to vessel involvement are given in **Table 1**.

Predominantly Large-vessel Vasculitis

Large-vessel vasculitis (LVV) mainly affects aorta and its major branches. Takayasu arteritis (TA) is the primary LVV in childhood. It is characterized by granulomatous vasculitis of aorta and/or its main branches, also can involve coronary and pulmonary arteries. Clinical presentation may be mild with hypertension or weak peripheral pulses or severe with cardiac or respiratory failure. Diagnosis is mainly based on imaging findings—angiographic abnormalities (mandatory criterion). The treatment is systemic immunosuppression and is guided by organ involvement.

Flowchart 1: Approach to childhood vasculitis.

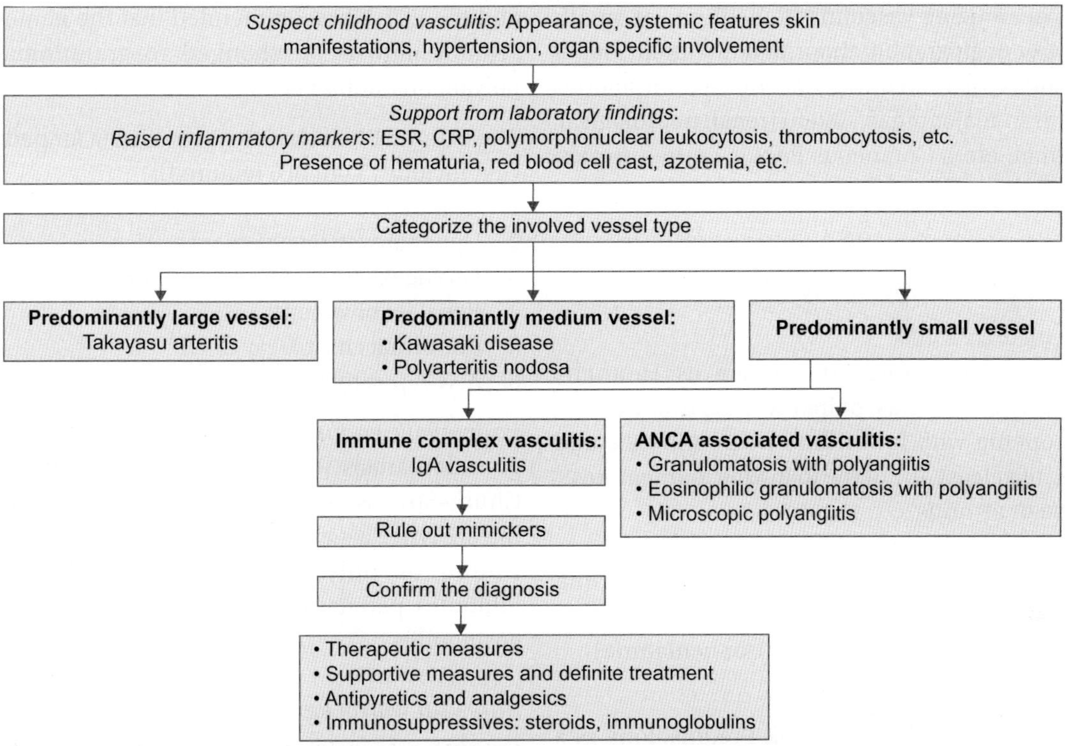

Suspect childhood vasculitis: Appearance, systemic features skin manifestations, hypertension, organ specific involvement

↓

Support from laboratory findings:
Raised inflammatory markers: ESR, CRP, polymorphonuclear leukocytosis, thrombocytosis, etc.
Presence of hematuria, red blood cell cast, azotemia, etc.

↓

Categorize the involved vessel type

↓

- **Predominantly large vessel:** Takayasu arteritis
- **Predominantly medium vessel:**
  - Kawasaki disease
  - Polyarteritis nodosa
- **Predominantly small vessel**
  - **Immune complex vasculitis:** IgA vasculitis
  - **ANCA associated vasculitis:**
    - Granulomatosis with polyangiitis
    - Eosinophilic granulomatosis with polyangiitis
    - Microscopic polyangiitis

Immune complex vasculitis → Rule out mimickers → Confirm the diagnosis →

- Therapeutic measures
- Supportive measures and definite treatment
- Antipyretics and analgesics
- Immunosuppressives: steroids, immunoglobulins

(ANCA: antineutrophil cytoplasmic antibody; CRP: C-reactive protein; ESR: erythrocyte sedimentation rate)

TABLE 1: Clinical findings according to vessel involvement.

Large vessel	*Medium vessel*	*Small vessel*
• Limb claudication • Asymmetric blood pressure • Absent pulses • Bruits • Aortic dilation	• Cutaneous nodules • Ulcers • Livedo reticularis • Digital gangrene • Mononeuritis multiplex • Microaneurysms	• Purpura • Vesiculobullous nodules • Urticaria • Glomerulonephritis • Alveolar hemorrhage • Cutaneous granulomas • Splinter hemorrhages • Uveitis/episcleritis/scleritis

CLINICAL PEARLS

- Severe constitutional symptoms, skin rash, and hypertension are important clues for suspicion of vasculitides in children.
- Raised inflammatory parameters, e.g., raised C-reactive protein, erythrocyte sedimentation rate, polymorphonuclear leukocytosis, and thrombocytosis add as diagnostic clues.

Predominantly Medium-sized Vessel Vasculitis

Kawasaki disease: It is an acute febrile illness of childhood with medium-sized vessel vasculitis (MVV). Fever for 5 days or longer and at least four of the following five signs:

1. Bilateral nonpurulent conjunctivitis
2. Rash (polymorphous exanthem)
3. Hyperemic lips and/or mucous membranes, strawberry tongue
4. Changes in the extremities (peripheral edema, peripheral erythema, and periungual desquamation in subacute phase)
5. Cervical lymphadenopathy (>1.5 cm, usually unilateral)

Complication: Coronary artery aneurysm

The mainstay of treatment is intravenous immunoglobulin (infusion of 2 g/kg) along with aspirin—initially 30–50 mg/kg till afebrile for 48 hours and then antiplatelet dose of 3–5 mg/kg/day for at least 6–8 weeks (total duration is dependent on the 2D echo findings).

Childhood polyarteritis nodosa: It has histological evidence of necrotizing vasculitis in medium- or small-sized arteries or angiographic abnormalities (aneurysm or occlusion) and is associated with systemic manifestations with vasculitis in major organ system (renal, neurological, gastrointestinal, etc.). Cutaneous PAN is limited to skin with possible manifestations in the musculoskeletal system.

Predominantly Small Vessel Vasculitis

Immune complex vasculitis:

IgA vasculitis: It was formerly known as Henoch-Schönlein purpura. It has palpable purpura without thrombocytopenia with lower limb predominance and the presence of at least one of the following four features:

1. Arthralgia or arthritis
2. Diffuse abdominal pain
3. Skin biopsy showing leukocytoclastic vasculitis and predominant immunoglobulin A deposition
4. Renal involvement (proteinuria and/or hematuria)

Complication: Mainly nephritis

It is usually mild and self-limited. Prednisolone in a tapering dose over 4–6 weeks is used only in select cases.

Antineutrophil Cytoplasmic Antibody-associated Vasculitis

Antineutrophil cytoplasmic antibody-associated vasculitis (AAV) has pauci-immune complex deposition in the tissues. Cytoplasmic antineutrophil cytoplasmic antibody (cANCA) can be positive in granulomatosis with polyangiitis (GPA) and eosinophilic granulomatosis with polyangiitis (EGPA) and perinuclear ANCA (pANCA) can be positive in microscopic polyangiitis (MPA), inflammatory bowel disease, and sclerosing cholangitis.

Microscopic polyangiitis: Microscopic polyangiitis is characterized by necrotizing vasculitis with few or no immune deposits affecting small vessels. Clinical features of MPA include disease involving the kidneys, lungs, joints, skin, gastrointestinal tract, and peripheral nerves. The cardinal features of MPA include glomerulonephritis, pulmonary hemorrhage, fever, and mononeuritis multiplex. Necrotizing glomerulonephritis is very common. Pulmonary capillaritis often occurs, but no granulomatous lesions of the respiratory tract are seen.

Granulomatosis with polyangiitis: In January 2011, the Board of Directors of the American College of Rheumatology, the American Society of Nephrology, and the EULAR recommended that the name Wegener's granulomatosis be changed to granulomatosis with polyangiitis, abbreviated as GPA.

The EULAR/PReS classification criteria for pediatric onset GPA include (3 out of 6 required):

1. Granulomatous inflammation on biopsy
2. Upper airway involvement
3. Laryngeal, tracheal, or endobronchial stenosis
4. Renal involvement
5. Abnormal chest X-ray or CT
6. ANCA positivity

Eosinophilic granulomatosis with polyangiitis: Eosinophilic granulomatosis with polyangiitis previously known as Churg-Strauss syndrome requires any four or more of the six criteria—asthma, eosinophilia >10%, neuropathy (mono or polyneuropathy), nonfixed pulmonary infiltrates, paranasal sinus abnormality, and extravascular eosinophils.

Rule Out Mimickers

Mimickers for vasculitis include following:

- Infections such as pneumococcal, mycobacterial, and rickettsial
- Connective tissue disorders
- Bacterial endocarditis
- Atrial myxoma
- Vasoconstrictive drugs
- Malignancy such as lymphomas
- Disorders associated with antiphospholipid antibody syndrome

Confirm the Diagnosis

The clinical diagnosis is confirmed by some specific tests in association with supportive indicators and specific pattern of clinical involvement such as:

- Tissue biopsy (PAN)
- X-rays of the sinuses and chest
- Angiographic studies of the vessels (PAN and Takayasu arteritis)
- Nerve conduction studies
- *Assessment of autoantibodies such as antinuclear antibody (ANA) and ANCA:* ANA would be positive in lupus-associated vasculitis.
- Rheumatoid factor positivity is seen in hepatitis B-associated cryoglobulinemia.

Therapeutic Measures

Medical Management

- *Supportive care:* Nonsteroidal anti-inflammatory drugs and analgesics—ibuprofen and naproxen
- *Steroids:* Reduce pain and inflammation of severe joint disease, skin lesions, eye disease, or central nervous system. It is mostly used as a bridge therapy. Depending on the diagnosis and severity, pulse methylprednisolone may be required. Routine follow-up is needed to detect features of steroid toxicity.
- *Other immunosuppressants:* The immunosuppressants choice depends on the diagnosis. The conventional disease-modifying antirheumatic drugs (DMARDs) commonly used are methotrexate, azathioprine, and cyclophosphamide.
- *Biologic DMARD:* It can be used in patients not responding to initial first-line and conventional treatment. For example, tocilizumab (humanized monoclonal antibody, targeting both membrane bound and soluble IL-6 receptors) is used in Takayasu arteritis, rituximab (chimeric monoclonal antibody against CD20, targeting B cells) in GPA, and infliximab (chimeric monoclonal antibody against tumor necrosis factor-α) in resistant Kawasaki disease.
- *Other:* Aspirin, clopidogrel, and intravenous immunoglobulin in Kawasaki disease.

Surgical Management

- Amputation of nonsalvageable gangrenous part
- Repair of aneurysm

INDIAN SCENARIO

Large studies with uniform comprehensive data are not available from Asia. Indian data that included adult population is not a true representation of pediatric vasculitides from all over the country.

A pediatric study was done from Eastern India over a period of 7 years (2004–2010), on prospectively followed up children (under 12 years) with vasculitis from a tertiary care hospital from Kolkata. The study revealed 10.2% children (n = 158) had vasculitis among all rheumatological cases (n = 1,544). IgA vasculitis (56.9%) and Kawasaki disease (24%) were major groups. The study revealed that primary vasculitides were diagnosed in 135 patients (male:female ratio was 1.9:1 and the mean age of onset was 5.5 years). Among the 38 cases of Kawasaki disease, 20 had coronary artery involvement, 5 had persistent aneurysms, 29 received IVIG, and none required angioplasty. Other vasculitides included PAN (n = 4), granulomatosis with polyangiitis (n = 2), and Takayasu arteritis (n = 1). Secondary vasculitis accounted for 23 cases.

CONCLUSION

Pediatric vasculitis is a challenging disease for diagnosis as well as treatment. It should be considered whenever there is unexplained multisystem disease with evidence of vascular involvement. Fever, extreme irritability, hypertension, hematuria, and skin lesions are some of the important clues for diagnosis. Other organs, such as the eye, peripheral nervous system, and the kidneys, must be examined to pick up asymptomatic involvement. Prompt and aggressive treatment can prevent complications and decrease the morbidity and mortality in pediatric populations.

KEY POINTS

- Vasculitis is inflammation of the vessel wall which can be active or chronic.
- Classification is based on vessel size involved.
- Kawasaki disease and IgA vasculitis are the commonest pediatric vasculitis.
- Timely diagnosis and treatment with immunosuppressants is required to prevent long-term complications.

SUGGESTED READING

1. Bosch X, Guilabert A, Font J. Antineutrophil cytoplasmic antibodies. Lancet. 2006;368:404-18.
2. Firestein GS, Budd RC, Harris ED, McInnes IB, Ruddy S, Sergent JS. Kelley's TB of Rheumatology, 8th edition. Philadelphia: WB Saunders & Co.; 2008.
3. Gardner-Medwin JM, Dolezalova P, Cummins C, Southwood TR. Incidence of Henoch-Schönlein purpura, Kawasaki disease, and rare vasculitides in children of different ethnic origins. Lancet. 2002;360:1197-202.
4. Jennette JC, Falk RJ, Bacon PA, Basu N, Cid MC, Ferrario F, et al. 2012 Revised International Chapel Hill Consensus Conference Nomenclature of Vasculitides. Arthritis Rheum. 2013;65:1-11.
5. Joshi VR, Mittal G. Vasculitis—Indian perspective. JAPI. 2006;54:12-4.
6. Khasnis A, Langford CA. Update on vasculitis. J Allergy Clin Immunol. 2009;123:1226-36.
7. Maksimowicz-McKinnon K, Clark TM, Hoffman GS. Limitations of therapy and a guarded prognosis in an

American cohort of Takayasu arteritis patients. Arthritis Rheum. 2007;56:1000-9.
8. Morishita K, Brown K, Cabral D. Pediatric vasculitis: advances in treatment. Curr Opin Rheumatol. 2015;27(5): 493-9.
9. Ozen S, Pistorio A, Iusan SM, Bakkaloglu A, Herlin T, Brik R, et al. EULAR/PRINTO/PRES criteria for Henoch-Schönlein purpura, childhood polyarteritis nodosa, childhood Wegener granulomatosis and childhood Takayasu arteritis: Ankara 2008. Part II: Final classification criteria. Ann Rheum Dis. 2010;69:798-806.
10. Ozen S, Ruperto N, Dillon MJ, Bagga A, Barron K, Davin JC, et al. EULAR/PRES endorsed consensus criteria for the classification of childhood vasculitides. Ann Rheum Dis. 2006;65:936-41.
11. Peru H, Soylemezoglu O, Bakkaloglu SA, Elmas S, Bozkaya D, Elmaci AM, et al. Henoch-Schönlein purpura in childhood: clinical analysis of 254 cases over a 3-year period. Clin Rheumatol. 2008;27:1087-92.
12. Sarkar S, Mondal R, Nandi M, Ghosh A. Trends of childhood vasculitides in eastern India. Indian Pediatr. 2011; 48:814.
13. Saulsbury FT. Henoch-Schönlein purpura in children. Report of 100 patients and review of the literature. Medicine (Baltimore). 1999;78:395-409.
14. Schnabel A, Hedrich CM. Childhood Vasculitis. Front Pediatr. 2019;6:421.
15. Tse SM, Silverman ED, McCrindle BW, Yeung RS. Early treatment with intravenous immunoglobulin in patients with Kawasaki disease. J Pediatr. 2002;140:450-5.

CHAPTER 122

Kawasaki Disease

Anju Gupta, Aaqib Zaffar Banday

INTRODUCTION

Kawasaki disease (KD) is an acute systemic medium-vessel vasculitis with a strong predilection to occur in early childhood. Since its first description in the 1960s by Dr Tomisaku Kawasaki, this disease continues to remain enigmatic due to lack of understanding about etiologic agent and pathophysiology, lack of specific diagnostic test in acute phase, and unpredictable long-term complications. Clinical features may be transient and the examining physician may not be able to see all the characteristic clinical features at presentation, further leading to a delay in diagnosis.

EPIDEMIOLOGY

Japan has the maximum incidence of KD with rates of 359/100,000 children <5 years in 2018. South Korea and Taiwan have reported the next high incidences (191/100,000 in 2017 and 90/100,000 in 2013 among under-five children, respectively). In India, incidence of KD in under-five children has been estimated to be about 11/100,000 in 2019. A distinct seasonal predilection exists with maximum cases seen in December–January in Japan, and April–June in Taiwan.

ETIOLOGY

The precise etiology of KD remains elusive; however, it likely involves an environmental agent in presence of certain genetic factors. Distinct seasonality, occurrence of epidemics, occurrence of rash similar to toxin mediated diseases, highest incidence in children <5 years old, and efficacy of intravenous immunoglobulins (IVIg) suggest a possibility of an environmental agent. The potential list of environmental triggers includes viruses, bacteria (especially superantigen producing), gut dysbiosis, and tropospheric winds. Genetic factors have been implicated because of strong racial predilection (highest incidence in children of Japanese descent even outside of Japan).

PATHOGENESIS

Kawasaki disease is characterized by activation of adaptive and innate arms of the immune system encompassing intense T-cell stimulation, IgA-secreting plasma cell response, proinflammatory cytokinemia (interferons, tumor necrosis factor-α, etc.), and leukocyte recruitment. Besides, upregulation of metalloproteinase expression occurs which increases the vessel wall damage and elastin degradation resulting in characteristic coronary lesions seen in this disease.

CLINICAL FEATURES

Characteristic clinical features of KD include fever, polymorphous exanthem, bilateral conjunctival injection, changes in extremities, changes in lips and oral cavity, and cervical adenopathy.

- *Fever:* Fever is typically high grade (>39°C) with an abrupt onset and responds transiently to antipyretics. Usually, fever lasts for 1–2 weeks and can persist for >3 weeks, if not treated.
- *Skin changes:* A diffuse erythematous maculopapular rash often appears within the first 5 days of illness. Changes in extremities include diffuse erythema or nonpitting edema on the dorsum of hands and feet in the acute phase and characteristic periungual desquamation starting in late second or third week of illness **(Figs. 1 and 2)**. Perianal desquamation is also characteristic and usually precedes periungual desquamation **(Fig. 3)**.
- *Mucosal changes:* Conjunctival injection is typically bilateral, nonexudative, and spares limbus **(Fig. 4)**. Changes in lips and oral cavity include strawberry tongue **(Fig. 5)**, erythema/cracking of lips, and congestion of the oropharyngeal mucosa.

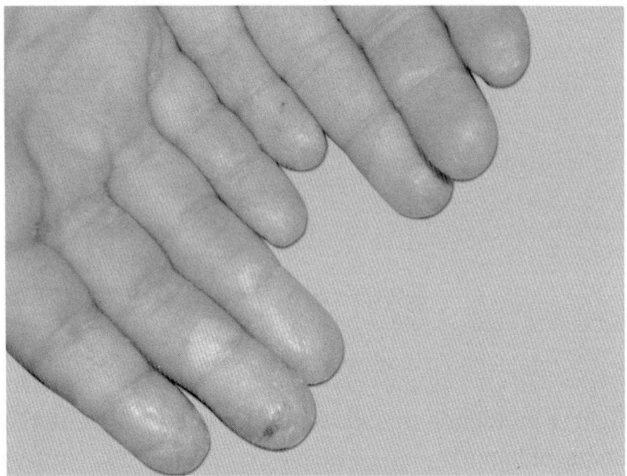

Fig. 1: Periungual desquamation in hands. *(For color version, see Plate 9)*

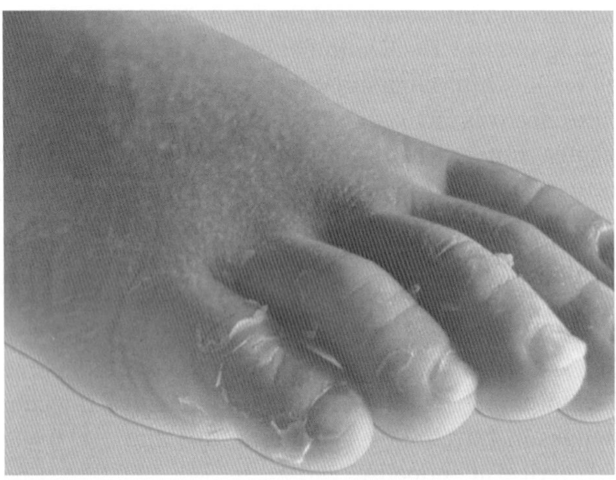

Fig. 2: Periungual desquamation in feet, which usually follows similar findings in hands. *(For color version, see Plate 9)*

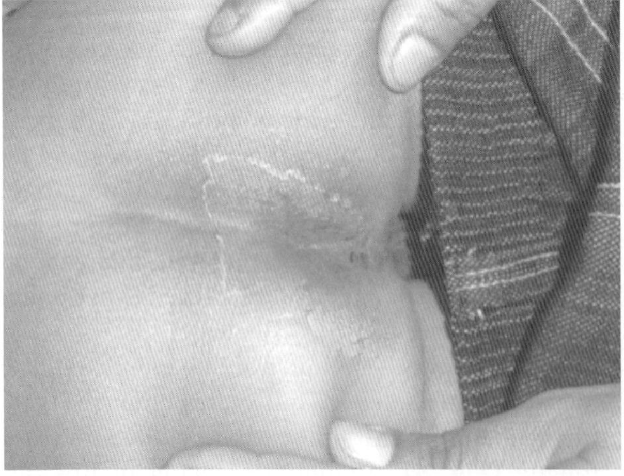

Fig. 3: Perianal desquamation. *(For color version, see Plate 9)*

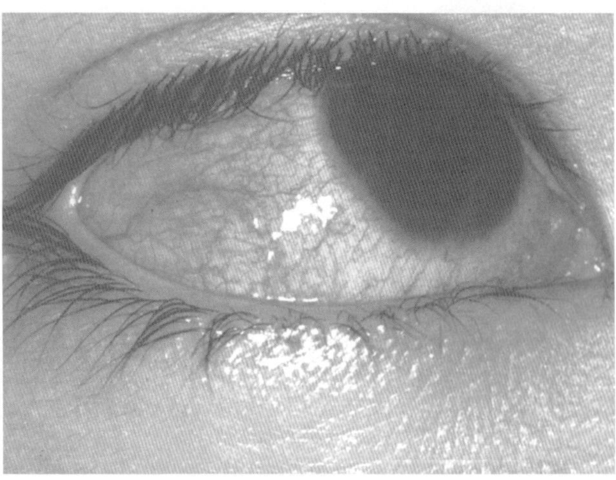

Fig. 4: Nonexudative conjunctivitis. *(For color version, see Plate 9)*

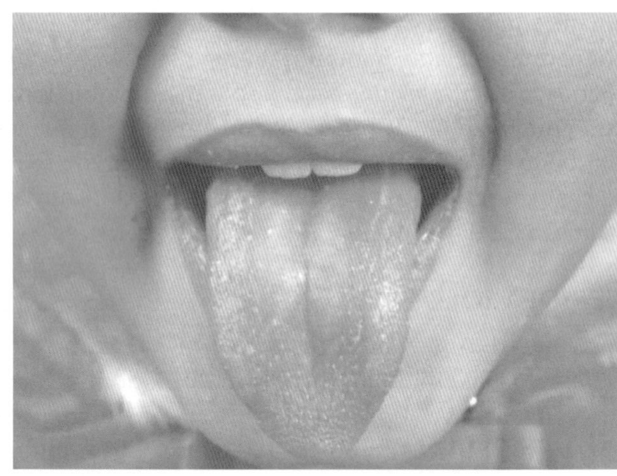

Fig. 5: Strawberry tongue. *(For color version, see Plate 10)*

- *Adenopathy:* Cervical adenopathy is usually single, unilateral, and nontender involving anterior cervical chain.

Whether noted by the clinician at presentation or elicited on prudent history taking, these clinical features must be considered significant in children suspected to have KD. Besides the above-mentioned features described in the American Heart Association diagnostic criteria **(Box 1)**, many other clinical features may be present and may help the treating physician in diagnosis or result in furthering the diagnostic dilemma! It is imperative to note that occasionally nonspecific gastrointestinal (pain abdomen and diarrhea) and respiratory (cough and chest congestion) complaints may be noted before onset of fever in KD **(Fig. 6)**. Other features of KD include:

- Irritability is usually extreme in infants and may lead the clinician to think of pyogenic meningitis. It occurs due to aseptic meningitis and responds briskly to IVIg.
- Arthralgia and arthritis involving large and/or small joints may also be present.
- Significant right hypochondriac pain can occur due to hydrops of gallbladder. Hepatic dysfunction with conjugated jaundice and transaminitis can occur in KD leading to a diagnosis of infectious hepatitis.

BOX 1: Diagnostic criteria for Kawasaki disease.

Fever for at least 5 days plus at least four of the following five diagnostic features:

1. Polymorphous exanthem
2. Bilateral bulbar conjunctival injection without exudate
3. Changes in lips and oral cavity: Erythema, fissured cracked lips, strawberry tongue, or diffuse injection of oral and pharyngeal mucosae
4. Cervical lymphadenopathy (>1.5 cm diameter), usually unilateral
5. Changes in extremities:
   - *Acute:* Erythema/edema of hands and feet
   - *Subacute:* Periungual peeling of fingers and toes

- Reactivation of BCG site with erythema and induration, especially in young children, can be a helpful sign to recognize KD.
- Rarely, respiratory complications in the form of pulmonary nodules, interstitial infiltrates, pleural effusions, and pneumothorax can occur.
- Cranial nerve palsies, anterior uveitis, myocarditis [even leading to shock (KD shock syndrome)], valvular regurgitation, and peripheral gangrene are other rarely described manifestations.
- Beau's lines are frequently seen in convalescent phase **(Fig. 7)**. They occur due to arrest of nail growth during the illness.

INVESTIGATIONS

None of the investigations are diagnostic in KD. Acute phase is associated with various markers of inflammation which include neutrophilia, high erythrocyte sedimentation rate (ESR), high C-reactive protein (CRP), high procalcitonin, high fibrinogen and D-dimer levels. Other abnormalities include anemia, hyponatremia, hypoalbuminemia, sterile pyuria (due to urethritis),

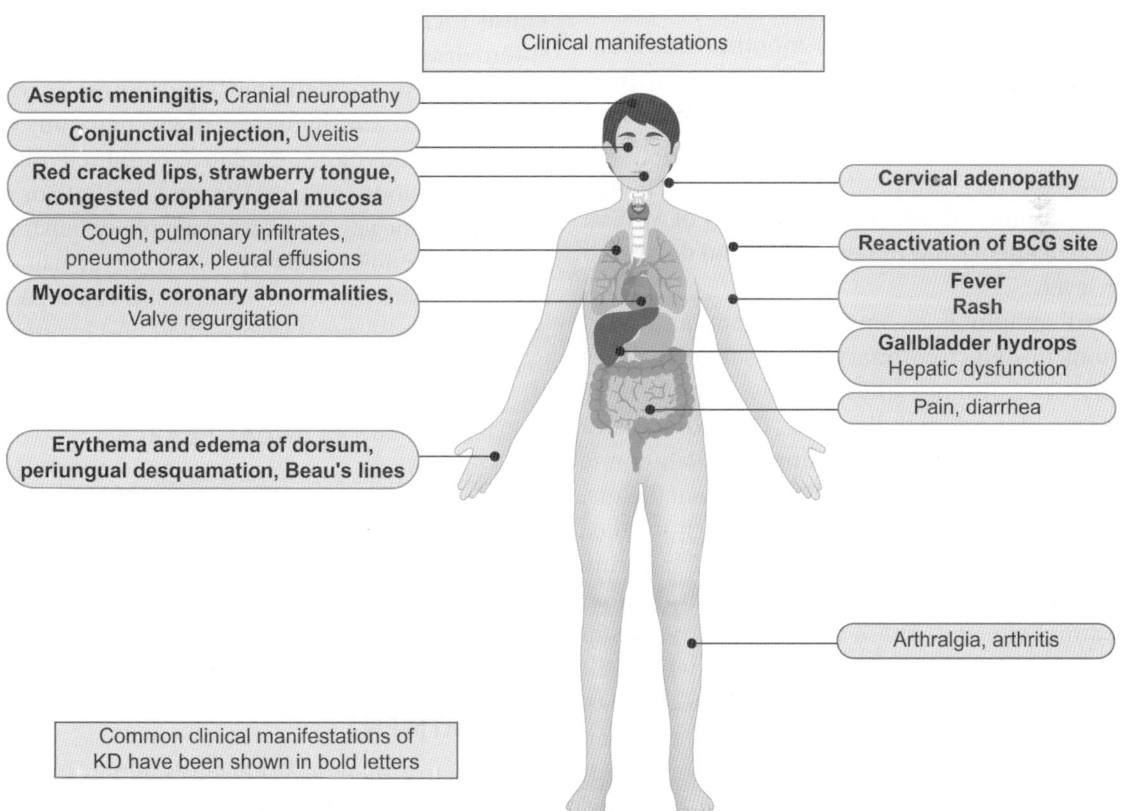

Fig. 6: Clinical features of KD. (KD: Kawasaki disease)

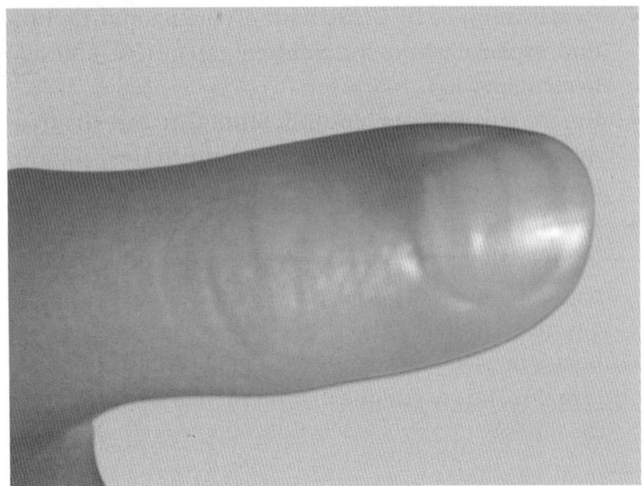

Fig. 7: Prominent Beau's lines. *(For color version, see Plate 10)*

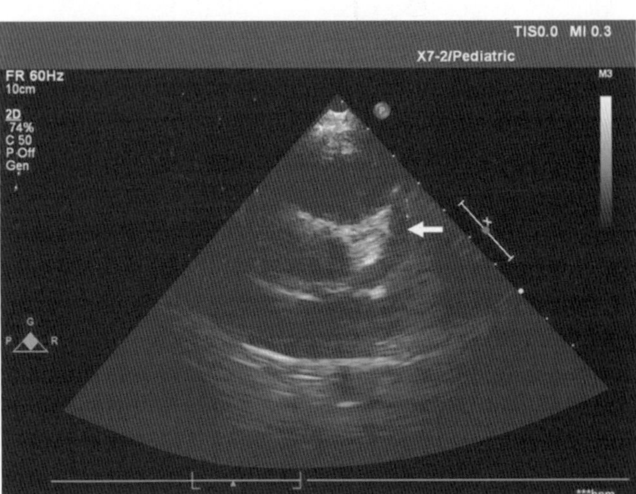

Fig. 8: Coronary aneurysms on echocardiography.

and transaminitis. Cerebrospinal fluid analysis may reveal pleocytosis. In children with arthritis, there may be synovial fluid pleocytosis. Thrombocytosis, which is described as a characteristic feature of KD, is often not seen in the first week of the illness and hence, is not useful in making a decision regarding treatment. Besides, platelet counts may continue to increase even after defervescence and last for several months. Thrombocytopenia has been described in a small minority of patients at onset and has been attributed to increased adherence of platelets to activated endothelium, disseminated intravascular coagulation, and macrophage activation syndrome (MAS). Other indicators of MAS in KD include leukopenia, low or falling ESR, and decreased fibrinogen levels.

Echocardiography is an important, safe, and noninvasive tool to detect coronary artery abnormalities (CAAs) in KD. Coronary aneurysm is described as Z scores of ≥2.5 for internal diameters for both left and right coronary arteries. However, coronary dilatation is usually not seen in the first week of illness. Nonetheless, there could be other suggestive findings in echocardiography like perivascular brightness, lack of tapering of vessels, low ejection fraction, mitral regurgitation, and pericardial effusion. These findings may be useful in diagnosis especially in those children where all the clinical features are not present (incomplete KD). Echocardiography is usually done at baseline and then after 6–8 weeks of illness **(Fig. 8)**. Another echocardiography may be needed in the second week of illness to detect CAAs especially in "at risk" cases and guide further treatment. Other imaging modalities to evaluate the coronaries are not currently recommended to be performed routinely in children with KD.

DIFFERENTIAL DIAGNOSIS

Since most of the clinical features are relatively nonspecific, there are many differential diagnoses of KD **(Box 2)**. These include viral infections (measles, adenovirus, enterovirus, and Epstein–Barr virus), Stevens–Johnson syndrome, toxin-mediated syndromes, scarlet fever, leptospirosis, and hypersensitivity reactions to drugs. Exudative pharyngitis, exudative conjunctivitis, discrete intraoral lesions (e.g., oral ulcers), bullous or vesicular rash, splenomegaly, and diffuse lymphadenopathy suggest another diagnosis **(Box 3)**. Scarlet fever usually is not associated with conjunctivitis and shows a brisk response to antibiotics. Visceral involvement and hypotension are frequent in toxin-mediated syndromes.

CLINICAL PEARLS

Think of another diagnosis in presence of:
- Exudative pharyngitis
- Exudative conjunctivitis
- Discrete intraoral lesions (e.g., oral ulcers)
- Bullous or vesicular rash
- Diffuse lymphadenopathy
- Splenomegaly

TREATMENT

Standard treatment of KD involves administration of IVIg and aspirin **(Flowchart 1)**. It is better to wait for a day or two if one is seeing the child for the first time on day 4 or 5 of illness and clinical features are not clear-cut.

This helps to see evolution of signs and symptoms as well as to evaluate response to empirical antibiotics.

Intravenous immunoglobulin is usually given at a dose of 2 g/kg as a single-dose infusion. Single-dose infusion has been found to be more effective than divided dose infusions. Most patients show a brisk response to IVIg with defervescence and improvement in general well-being. Inflammatory parameters (except ESR which remains elevated due to IVIg administration) also show gradual improvement. IVIg therapy has been shown to reduce the risk of coronary abnormalities from 25 to 3–5%, if given within the first 10 days of illness. Beyond the first 10 days, the benefit is not so great; however, most clinicians would give IVIg even beyond 10 days if the child is febrile and

BOX 2: Differential diagnosis.

- Viral infections (measles, adenovirus, enterovirus, and Epstein–Barr virus)
- Stevens–Johnson syndrome
- Toxin-mediated syndromes
- Scarlet fever
- Leptospirosis

BOX 3: Risk factors for coronary abnormalities.

- Infants, especially aged <6 months
- Adolescent age-group
- Male sex
- Specific ethnicities
- Markers of severe inflammation (high neutrophils, low platelets, low sodium, high C-reactive protein, and transaminitis)
- IVIg resistance
- Delayed treatment

(IVIg: intravenous immunoglobulin)

Flowchart 1: Algorithm for management of KD.

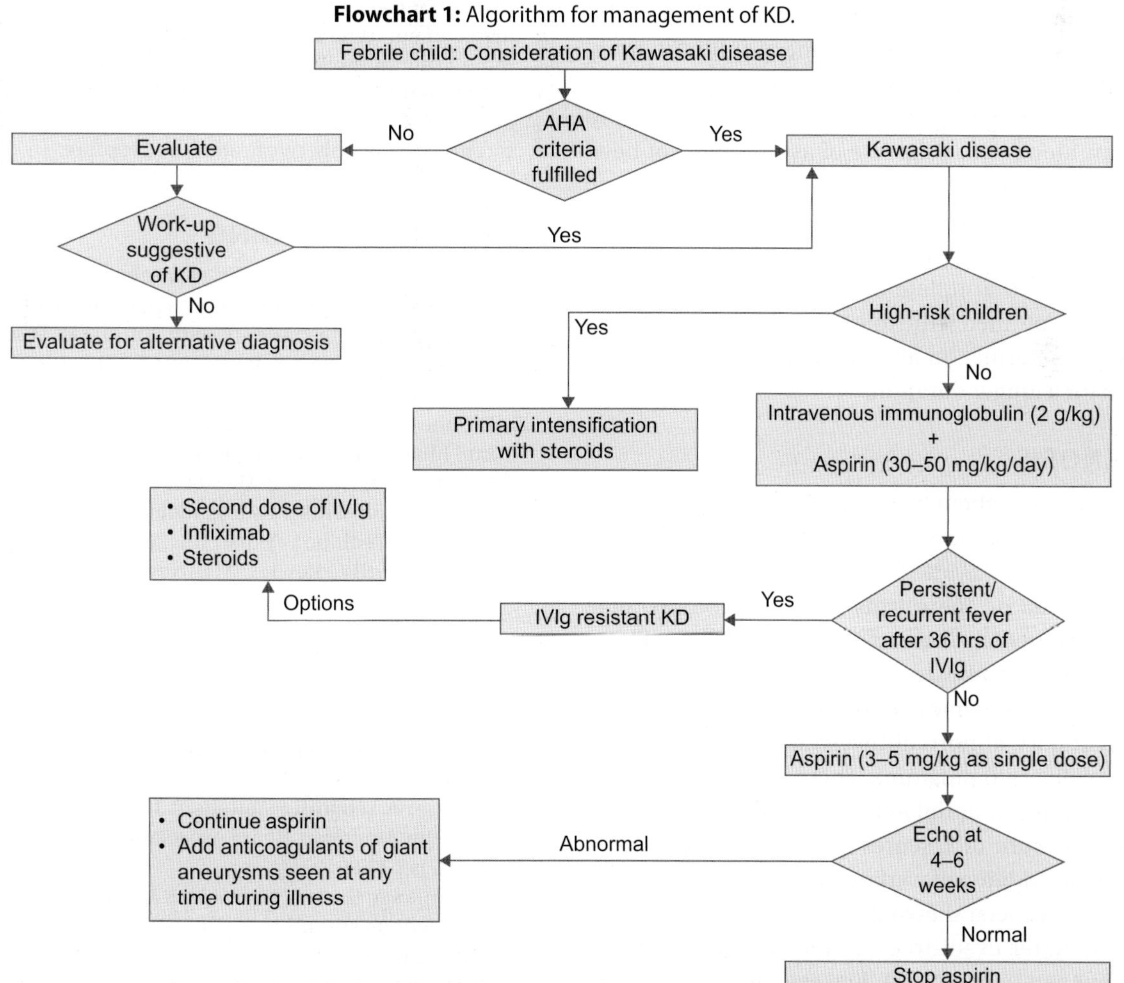

(IVIg: intravenous immunoglobulin; KD: Kawasaki disease)

continues to have high inflammatory parameters. It has also been seen that the children who are diagnosed with KD and receive IVIg within the first 5 days of illness are more likely to need additional therapy. Whether this is due to more inflammation per se and hence, more severe disease is not very clear.

However, 10–15% patients show IVIg resistance which is described as persistence or recrudescence of fever after 36 hours of completion of IVIg infusion. IVIg resistance is an important clinical feature associated with high risk of coronary abnormalities **(Box 3)**. One or two fever spikes during or immediately after IVIg infusion are common and should not be labeled as IVIg resistance. Treatment of IVIg-resistant KD includes a second dose of IVIg, oral/intravenous steroids, and tumor necrosis factor-α (TNF-α) inhibitors.

In children with KD who are at high risk of developing CAAs **(Box 3)** or present with significant CAAs during acute or subacute phase, it may be prudent to intensify treatment with steroids, TNF-α inhibitors, and/or cyclosporine to prevent or reduce coronary inflammation, respectively.

Aspirin (30–50 mg/kg/day) is routinely used as first-line therapy along with IVIg. Use of aspirin has not been shown either to reduce the coronary risk or the time to defervescence. Once the child is afebrile and inflammatory parameters (CRP) show declining trend, dose of aspirin can be reduced to antiplatelet doses (1–5 mg/kg/day). Aspirin is discontinued if the follow-up echocardiography at 6–8 weeks is normal. In all other children, aspirin may be needed for a longer duration.

PROGNOSIS

In the pre-IVIg era, about 25% of children with KD would go on to develop coronary abnormalities. Use of IVIg has reduced this risk to 3–5%. Coronary abnormalities can persist as ectasia or aneurysms which can be saccular, fusiform, or segmental. These aneurysms carry a significant risk of rupture, thrombosis, and stenosis, and predispose the individual to ischemic events. Hence, all patients who develop coronary abnormalities should continue to be on lifelong follow-up programs. These children also need long-term aspirin in antiplatelet doses. Those with giant aneurysms (>8 mm or Z scores >10) have higher risk of complications. Addition of warfarin or heparin to aspirin in such patients has been shown to reduce risk of thrombosis and lead to better event-free survival. Peripheral artery involvement can occur in KD; however, it is uncommon in the absence of coronary artery involvement.

CONCLUSION

Kawasaki disease is an acute systemic vasculitis which can mimic a myriad of childhood illnesses. Importance of timely recognition and management is important as it reduces the risk of coronary complications to a significant extent. No single diagnostic test is useful in the acute phase. Intravenous immunoglobulin along with aspirin is the standard of care, and most patients respond briskly to this treatment.

KEY POINTS

- Diagnosis of Kawasaki disease in the acute phase is based on clinical findings and supportive investigations. No single investigation helps in clinching the diagnosis in this phase.
- Coronary involvement is the most sinister long-term complication and seen more frequently in infancy.
- Intravenous immunoglobulin therapy is the standard of care and has been shown to reduce the risk of coronary complications.
- Despite timely intravenous immunoglobulin therapy within 10 days, 3–5% children would develop coronary involvement. Whereas, coronary dilatation and ectasia is more likely to show anatomical regression by remodeling in the long-term, the same is not frequently seen in giant aneurysms. These aneurysms carry a high likelihood of thrombosis, stenosis, calcification, and rupture.

SUGGESTED READING

1. Ae R, Makino N, Kosami K, Kuwabara M, Matsubara Y, Nakamura Y. Epidemiology, Treatments and cardiac complications in patients with Kawasaki Disease: The Nationwide Survey in Japan, 2017-2018. J Pediatr. 2020; 225:23-9.e2.
2. Dionne A, Dahdah N. Myocarditis and Kawasaki disease. Int J Rheum Dis. 2018;21(1):45-9.
3. Kobayashi T, Ayusawa M, Suzuki H, Abe J, Ito S, Kato T, et al. Revision of diagnostic guidelines for Kawasaki disease (6th revised edition). Pediatr Int. 2020;62(10):1135-8.
4. McCrindle BW, Rowley AH, Newburger JW, Burns JC, Bolger AF, Gewitz M, et al.; American Heart Association Rheumatic Fever, Endocarditis, and Kawasaki Disease Committee of the Council on Cardiovascular Disease in the Young; Council on Cardiovascular and Stroke Nursing; Council on Cardiovascular Surgery and Anesthesia; and Council on Epidemiology and Prevention. Diagnosis, treatment, and long-term management of Kawasaki Disease: A scientific statement for health professionals from the American Heart Association. Circulation. 2017; 135(17):e927-99.
5. Nakamura A, Ikeda K, Hamaoka K. Aetiological significance of infectious stimuli in Kawasaki Disease. Front Pediatr. 2019;7:244.
6. Onouchi Y. The genetics of Kawasaki disease. Int J Rheum Dis. 2018;21(1):26-30.

CHAPTER 123

Henoch-Schönlein Purpura

Anand P Rao

INTRODUCTION

Henoch-Schönlein purpura (HSP) is the most common childhood vasculitis with an annual incidence of 20.4 per 100,000 population less than 17 years. It is characterized by leukocytoclastic vasculitis histopathologically. It commonly affects children between 5 and 15 years of age. About 50% cases are reported in less than 5 years and 75% cases in less than 10 years of age. It occurs most frequently between the ages of 3 and 15 years and is slightly more common in boys than in girls (1.5:1).

It commonly affects the small vessels of the skin, joints, gastrointestinal tract, and kidneys. It is generally a self-limited condition, but rarely can be associated with complicated chronic course.

ETIOPATHOGENESIS

Henoch-Schönlein purpura is thought to be an immunoglobulin A (IgA) mediated dysregulated immune process with probable involvement of alternate complement pathway caused by as yet unknown etiological agent.

CLINICAL MANIFESTATIONS

Constitutional: It may be associated with low grade fever and malaise.

Cutaneous: Predominant lower limb purpura with involvement of buttocks, upper limbs, face, and very rarely, the trunk is the classical feature of this condition. The rashes can range from petechiae to ecchymosis to hemorrhagic bullae. Edema of the dorsal surfaces of feet, hands, scrotum, scalp, and face may sometimes be seen. Presence of palpable purpura is a sine qua non for the diagnosis of HSP **(Fig. 1)**.

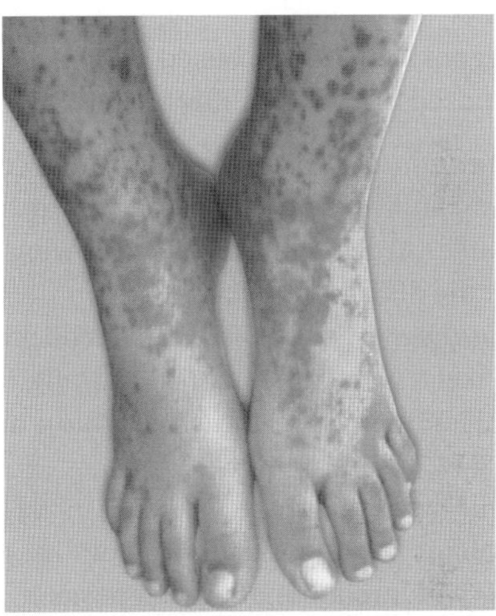

Fig. 1: Predominant lower purpura in an adolescent girl.
(For color version, see Plate 10)

Gastrointestinal manifestations: it is seen in about 70% of patients. It can precede the purpura in about 14–46% of the patients but mostly happens in the first week of the onset of the disease. Vasculitis of the bowel wall can lead to intussusception, gangrene, and perforation of the bowel wall.

> **CLINICAL PEARL**
>
> - Please keep in mind Henoch-Schönlein purpura in any child who presents with acute abdominal pain and look for rashes over the lower limbs before involving the surgeon.

Genitourinary involvement: It more often than not determines the outcome of the disease. The manifestations can range from microscopic hematuria and mild proteinuria to nephrotic syndrome, acute nephritic syndrome, hypertension, or renal failure. The renal manifestations have been reported to be seen in about 40% of patients and about 1–3% of the patient's progress to an end-stage renal disease (ESRD). Acute pain in the scrotum can sometimes bring the child to medical attention and might indicate testicular ischemia.

CLINICAL PEARL

> The nephritis in Henoch-Schönlein purpura can be silent. It is important to look for it by checking the blood pressure, urine routine, and microscopy weekly for at least 3 months from onset of disease. Serum creatinine should be checked at baseline.

Arthritis: Large joints like knee, ankle, wrist, and elbow seem to be involved in this condition. It may precede the rashes occasionally. It tends to be transient and may last from a few days to a few weeks. Arthritis rarely goes on for months.

The diagnosis of HSP is based on the classification criteria proposed by EULAR/PRINTO/PRES.

Purpura (mandatory criterion): Purpura (commonly palpable and in crops) or petechiae, with lower limb predominance. At least one of the following criteria is required for the diagnosis of HSP:

- *Abdominal pain:* Diffuse abdominal colicky pain with acute onset assessed by history and physical examination. It may include intussusception and gastrointestinal bleeding
- *Histopathology:* Typically, leukocytoclastic vasculitis with predominant IgA deposits or proliferative glomerulonephritis with predominant IgA deposits
- *Arthritis or arthralgia:* Arthritis of acute onset defined as joint swelling or joint pain with limitation of motion. Arthralgia of acute onset defined as joint pain without joint swelling or limitation of motion
- *Renal involvement:* Proteinuria more than 0.3 g/24 hours or more than 20 mg/mmol of urine albumin/creatinine ratio on a spot morning sample. Hematuria or red blood cell casts: more than 5 red blood cells/high power field or red blood cells.

The following factors that are thought to be associated with severe renal disease:

- Age more than 7 years of age
- Severe gastrointestinal disease as manifested by severe abdominal pain or bloody stools
- Persistent or recurrent skin disease.

The cumulative proportion of patients with HSP developing HSP nephritis by 1 month is 85%, by 2 months is 90%, and by 6 months is 97%, respectively. It has been suggested that all patients should have urine routine microscopy examination once a week for 3 months and for 6 months in those with evidence of nephritis or recurrent purpura.

INVESTIGATIONS

- Complete blood count might reveal mild leukocytosis and thrombocytosis.
- Mild elevation of erythrocyte sedimentation rate is expected.
- Urine routine microscopy might reveal hematuria/proteinuria.
- Serum creatinine might be increased in cases of nephritis.
- Skin biopsy is indicated in incomplete or atypical HSP. It reveals leukocytoclastic vasculitis involving dermal capillaries and postcapillary venules with IgA deposition.
- Imaging like ultrasonography might be required in patients with severe abdominal pain to rule out intussusception.

CLINICAL PEARL

> Serum immunoglobulin A levels are not useful for the diagnosis of Henoch-Schönlein purpura (HSP) as they are elevated only in 50% of patients with HSP.

TREATMENT

- Rest
- Hydration
- Paracetamol/nonsteroidal anti-inflammatory drugs for analgesia
- Steroids indicated in the following conditions:
    - Orchitis
    - Severe gastrointestinal disease and hemorrhage
    - Henoch-Schönlein purpura nephritis (prophylactic steroid therapy has no role in preventing onset of nephritis).

The steroid regimen recommended for severe extrarenal manifestations and renal manifestations of HSP is 1 mg/kg for 2 weeks followed by gradual taper over the subsequent 2 weeks time. The diagnosis and management of HSP has been outlined in **Flowchart 1**.

COURSE

Two-thirds of patients get better by 4 weeks. But, one-third of patients can have recurrences, commonly manifesting as rash and abdominal pain and tends to be milder than the previous one. Prognostic features which portend poor outcome are:

- Severe gastrointestinal manifestations
- Frequent skin rashes
- Severe renal manifestation at onset.

Flowchart 1: Diagnosis and management of Henoch-Schönlein purpura.

Predominant lower limb palpable purpura

If other features are absent, then it would be prudent to wait and watch and consider other differential diagnosis like systemic lupus erythematosus, granulomatosis with polyangiitis

Diagnosis of Henoch-Schönlein purpura confirmed if there is presence of one of the following manifestations:
- Abdominal pain
- Arthritis/arthralgia
- Skin biopsy showing leukocytoclastic vasculitis with IgA deposits
- Renal involvement showing proteinuria/hematuria/combination

Investigations:
- Complete blood count
- Erythrocyte sedimentation rate
- Serum creatinine
- Urine routine and microscopy
- USG abdomen if suspicion of intussusception

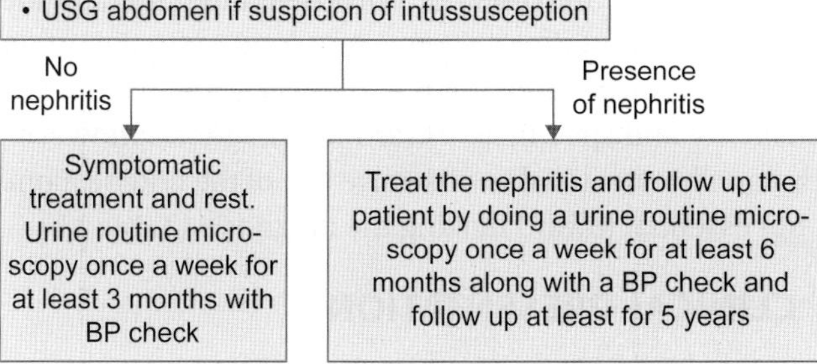

(BP: blood pressure; IgA: immunoglobulin A; USG: ultrasonography)

Less than 5% of patients progress to ESRD. Those with clinical nephritis should be closely followed up for at least 5 years.

KEY POINTS

- Henoch-Schönlein purpura is a usually benign small vessel vasculitis involving skin, joint, and kidneys.
- The presence of severe gastrointestinal and renal involvement would indicate worse prognosis.
- Skin biopsy is indicated when the diagnosis is in doubt.
- Steroids are recommended when there is evidence of gastrointestinal or genitourinary involvement.
- Weekly urine dipstick for the first 3 months useful to pick up patients with indolent nephritis.

SUGGESTED READING

1. Jauhola O, Ronkainen J, Koskimies O, Ala-Houhala M, Arikoski P, Hölttä T, et al. Clinical course of extrarenal symptoms in Henoch-Schönlein purpura: a 6-month prospective study. Arch Dis Child. 2010;95:871-6.
2. Jauhola O, Ronkainen J, Koskimies O, Ala-Houhala M, Arikoski P, Hölttä T, et al. Renal manifestations of Henoch-Schönlein purpura in a 6-month prospective study of 223 children. Arch Dis Child. 2010;95:877-82.
3. Narchi H. Risk of long term renal impairment and duration of follow up recommended for Henoch-Schonlein purpura with normal or minimal urinary findings: a systematic review. Arch Dis Child. 2005;90:916-20.
4. Ozen S, Pistorio A, Iusan SM, et al. EULAR/PRINTO/PRES criteria for Henoch-Schönlein purpura, childhood polyarteritis nodosa, childhood Wegener granulomatosis and childhood Takayasu arteritis: Ankara; 2008. Part II: Final classification criteria.
5. Saulsbury FT. Henoch-Schonlein purpura in children. Report of 100 patients and review of the literature. Medicine (Baltimore). 1999;78:395-409.

Systemic Lupus Erythematosus

Suma Balan

INTRODUCTION

Acquired connective tissue disorders in children are a group of conditions among which the most common is systemic lupus erythematosus (SLE). This is a disease of immune dysregulation where the immune system appears to be activated with the formation of autoantibodies to a wide variety of antinuclear antigens and the formation of immune complexes which can affect any organ, thus, creating a multisystem illness which can damage any organ in the body if left untreated long term.

EPIDEMIOLOGY

Worldwide SLE has an incidence between 20 and 150/100,000. Most prevalence studies come from developed world literature where comparing the incidence between various ethnic minorities shows a significantly higher incidence in Asian/Afro-Caribbean and Oriental population compared to the white/Caucasian population. The incidence in children has been quoted between 4 and 250/100,000 depending upon race and location.

Approximately 20% of SLE commences in childhood, before 18 years of age. The most common age of onset is during teenage coinciding with puberty; however, it can occur at any age. It is very uncommon to present below 5 years of age. In prepubertal children, the boy:girl ratio is almost equal (4:3), but postpubertal children show a significant girl to boy dominance of 4:1. In a patient with early onset SLE prior to the age of 5 years, strong consideration to the possibility of monogenic causes must be considered.

There are no clear described prevalence figures for SLE in the Indian population.

DIAGNOSIS OF SYSTEMIC LUPUS ERYTHEMATOSUS

Like tuberculosis (TB) and syphilis, SLE is considered as one of the great mimics in medicine owing to its widely variable presentation, multisystem involvement, and the diagnosis, especially in the absence of the classic malar rash can be very confusing. A series of clinical and laboratory criteria have been set out with mainly toward standardization for research purposes, but generally the presence in four criteria even over a longitudinal manner contribute toward making a diagnosis. They have >95% sensitivity and specificity toward the diagnosis; however, it is equally essential that obsessive use of the criteria alone is not essential toward making the diagnosis **(Table 1)**.

CLINICAL PRESENTATION

Systemic lupus erythematosus can present as a chronic slowly progressing low grade illness with troublesome skin, joint and constitutional symptoms, as a subacute illness with internal organ involvement or even as an acute florid illness with catastrophic presentations such as renal failure, strokes, and major thrombosis.

As it is capable of involving every organ, the clinical features are myriad and difficult to outline all possible presentations. There are several children who are initially diagnosed as Henoch-Schönlein purpura or idiopathic thrombocytopenic purpura who turn out to have SLE. Again, children with existing autoimmune disease as in autoimmune hypothyroidism or autoimmune hemolytic anemia might over the course of time develop a second autoimmune illness like SLE **(Table 2)**.

WORKUP

Once SLE is suspected, the following multisystem assessment should be carried out:

- *Skin:* A biopsy can often be confirmatory, especially if a second sample is also sent for immunofluorescence.
- *Eyes:* Retinopathy and vasculitis of the retina can be frequently associated and a professional ophthalmological examination must be undertaken in all children.

TABLE 1: Updated revised criteria for classification of SLE.

Criterion	*Definition*
Malar rash	Flat or raised erythema over the malar eminences, spares the nasolabial folds **(Fig. 1)**
Discoid rash	Erythematosus raised patches with adherent keratotic scaling and follicular plugging; atrophic scarring may occur
Photosensitivity	Skin rash following sunlight exposure, by history or physician observation
Oral ulcers	Oral or nasopharyngeal ulceration, usually painless **(Fig. 2)**
Arthritis	Nonerosive arthritis involving two or more peripheral joints, characterized by tenderness, swelling, or effusion
Serositis	Pleuritis—convincing history of pleuritic pain or rub on auscultation or evidence of pleural effusion or pericarditis—documented by electrocardiogram, echocardiogram, or rub
Renal disorder	Persistent proteinuria >0.5 g/day or cellular casts—may be red cell, hemoglobin, granular, tubular, or mixed
Neurological disorder	Seizures in the absence of offending drugs or metabolic derangements or psychosis in the absence of offending drugs or metabolic derangements
Hematological disorder	Hemolytic anemia with reticulocytosis or leukopenia <4,000/mm^3 on two or more occasions, or lymphopenia <1,500/mm^3 on two or more occasions, or thrombocytopenia <100,000/mm^3
Immunological disorder	Antibody to native deoxyribonucleic acid, or antibody to Sm protein, or antiphospholipid antibodies—either anticardiolipin antibodies, presence of the lupus anticoagulant, or false-positive serological test for syphilis
Antinuclear antibody	Presence of antinuclear antibody by immunofluorescence or an equivalent assay

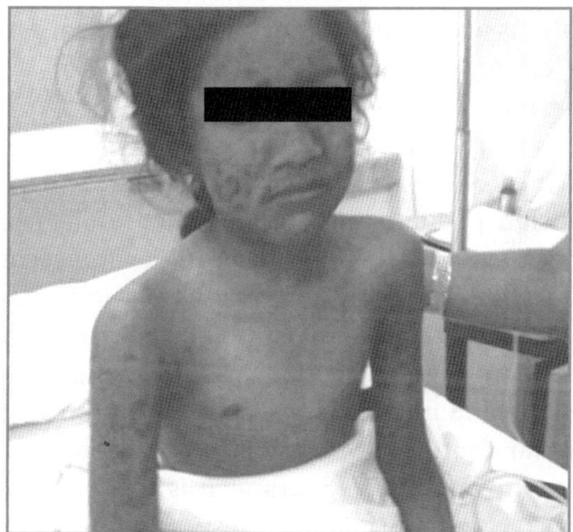

Fig. 1: Extensive rash malar and on extremities in a child with systemic lupus erythematosus. *(For color version, see Plate 10)*

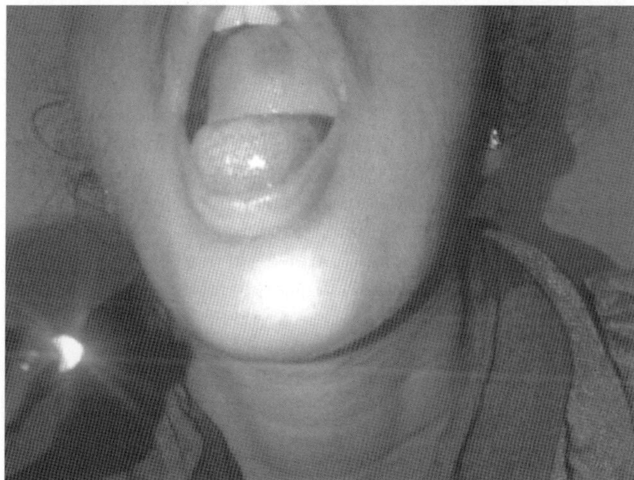

Fig. 2: Oral ulcer on hard palate in systemic lupus erythematosus. *(For color version, see Plate 10)*

- *Blood:* Check for hematological manifestations. Baseline clotting tests with prolongation of activated partial thromboplastin time (aPTT) are strongly suggestive of the presence of antiphospholipid antibodies. A differential diagnosis for a child presenting with constitutional symptoms and pancytopenia/bicytopenia is SLE and the presence of lymphopenia on the white blood cell count is a clue as opposed to neutropenia in childhood hematological malignancies.
- *Renal:* Check serum albumin and a routine urine examination in all children—the presence of active urinary sediment is indicative of nephritis. If edema, hypertension, oliguria, etc., are present, be alert to a proliferative nephritis and workup has to be prioritized toward a biopsy to aid early treatment.
- *Musculoskeletal system:* Often more symptoms and signs and rarely erosive arthritis. Muscle enzymes may be elevated.

TABLE 2: The varied clinical manifestations of SLE.

System	*Clinical feature*
Constitutional	• Fever—low grade/high grade • Weight loss • Malaise
Cutaneous	• Rashes—malar/discoid/vasculitis • Photosensitivity • Oral ulcers (oral and nasal) • Alopecia
Musculoskeletal	• Polyarthralgia/arthritis (nonerosive) • Tenosynovitis • Myopathy • Avascular necrosis
Vascular	• Lupus crisis • Raynaud's • Livedo reticularis
Cardiac	• Pericarditis • Myocarditis • Endocarditis • Coronary arteritis
Pulmonary	• Pleuritis/effusion • Pneumonitis • Pulmonary hemorrhage
GI manifestations	• Esophagus—dysphagia/reflux • Stomach—gastritis and pernicious anemia (rare) • Small bowel—mesenteric vasculitis • Intestinal pseudo—obstruction (enteric nervous system dysfunction) • Malabsorption—antigliadin antibodies • Peritonitis/ascites • Large bowel—enteritis • Vasculitic ulcers of rectum • Liver—deranged LFTs • Autoimmune hepatitis • Hepatic vein thrombosis • Biliary tract—sclerosing cholangitis • Acalculous cholecystitis • Autoimmune cholangiopathy • Pancreatitis—rare, but can be fulminant
Immunological—increased susceptibility to infection	• Functional asplenia • Multiple defects—macrophage/neutrophil/T cell/B cell/complement
Renal	• Nephritis classified as per WHO/ISKDC classification • Renal vein thrombosis
Neuropsychiatric	• Aseptic meningitis • Headache • Seizures • Cerebrovascular disease • Movement disorder • Acute confusional state • Anxiety disorder • Mood disorder • Psychosis • Guillain–Barré syndrome • Acute transverse myelitis • Mono/poly/cranial neuropathy • Plexopathy
Hematological	• Anemia—hemolytic/macrocytic • Leukopenia—often lymphopenia • Occasionally neutropenia • Thrombocytopenia • Antiphospholipid antibodies

(ISKDC: International Study of Kidney Disease of Children; LFTs: liver function tests; SLE: systemic lupus erythematosus; WHO: World Health Organization)

- *Central nervous system:* Observe mood and sleep patterns and be alert to cognitive changes or seizures. Baseline scans and electroencephalogram are not warranted unless clinical concern exists.
- *Pulmonary:* Observe clinical changes
- A chest X-ray will reveal the presence of pleural effusion/pneumonitis, etc. One needs to be cautious to distinguish between active disease and secondary infection that can present with similar signs. A serum C-reactive protein is rarely elevated in active SLE and is often a good marker to distinguish active disease and intercurrent sepsis. TB can present with similar features and prior to commencement of immunosuppressive therapy, it is recommended to check a Mantoux and other tests as required—lymph node biopsy if significant lymphadenopathy, etc., to rule out the presence of latent or active TB.
- In the presence of significant pneumonitis or pulmonary vasculitis, a high-resolution computed tomography scan of the chest may be required to delineate the detailed changes present. Children can present with acute respiratory deterioration, hypoxia, and diffuse alveolar hemorrhage must be suspected if ground-glass picture of lungs noted. Hemoptysis may not be present externally and the child can develop acute pallor in this setting. Equally, a pulmonary embolism can also cause acute respiratory deterioration and hypoxia.

- *Cardiovascular system:* Pericardial effusion at presentation is not uncommon. Myocarditis due to SLE carries a grave prognosis if not recognized early and treated with aggressive immunosuppression. Endocarditis with large valve deposits (traditionally known as Libman-Sacks endocarditis) is rare. The author has seen two children with coronary arterial dilatations and aneurysms akin to the picture in Kawasaki who presented with cardiac failure at presentation.
- *Abdomen:* SLE can present with a picture of hepatitis, hepatosplenomegaly and ascites, abdominal lymphadenopathy, etc. Acute abdominal pain in SLE needs attention as can be rarely due to pancreatitis, mesenteric vasculitis, or mesenteric thrombosis or even renal vein thrombosis and these conditions need to be addressed very urgently.

> **CLINICAL PEARL**
>
> Along with making the diagnosis, describing the extent of involvement is also important.

INVESTIGATIONS

- *Complete blood count:* Anemia—usually direct Coombs test/cold agglutinin positive
- *White blood cell:* Leukopenia with lymphopenia
- A child with SLE presenting with fever and a neutrophilic count must be assessed for the presence of secondary infection
- Platelet counts (often reduced)
- When significant pancytopenia is present with high fever, always consider the possibility of macrophage activation syndrome due to uncontrolled inflammation from active disease and look for the necessary parameters in biochemical testing and bone marrow examination may be helpful
- *Inflammatory markers:* Erythrocyte sedimentation rate often elevated significantly in disease activity. C-reactive protein is rarely elevated in active lupus disease—unless in presence of active pleural and pericardial effusions or synovitis with effusions. C-reactive protein can be considered a good marker for detecting secondary bacterial infection in a child with SLE, a condition that needs to be addressed urgently.
- *Baseline renal function tests:* Liver function tests must be done in every patient. A low serum albumin can be part of active inflammation as well as indicate proliferative nephritis or hepatic disease.
- A detailed urine routine examination with examination of the urinary sediment has to be done for every patient. The presence of proteinuria/active sediment should lead to quantification of proteinuria by 24 hours urinary protein estimation or a random spot urinary protein/creatinine ratio.
- Serum complement levels, both C3 and C4 are reduced in SLE.

Immunological Testing

Antinuclear Antibody Test

The antinuclear antibody (ANA) screening is advised by immunofluorescence rather than the more commonly or cheaper mode of enzyme-linked immunosorbent assay (ELISA) testing. Immunofluorescence yields a titer and has both qualitative and quantitative enumeration with less false positivity and greater reliability than the ELISA test. It is important to know that presence of ANA positivity **(Flowchart 1)** does not imply SLE—the ANA

Flowchart 1: How to interpret ANA positivity.

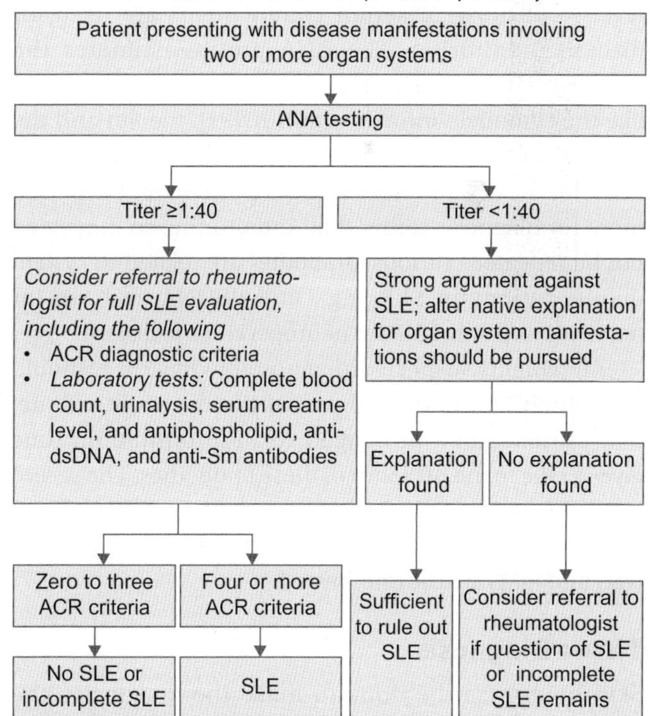

(ACR: American College of Radiology; ANA: antinuclear antibody; dsDNA: double-stranded deoxyribonucleic acid; SLE: systemic lupus erythematosus)

can be falsely positive in normal individuals, common infective, and other inflammatory conditions as well as other autoimmune diseases. The clinical strength of a suspicion of SLE or the pretest probability of a patient to have lupus makes the positive ANA more diagnostic. However, a negative ANA (by immunofluorescence) with today's techniques is more than enough to rule out a diagnosis of lupus in the vast majority of patients. No single titer is diagnostic though titers of 1:1,280 or greater are less associated with false positives.

> **CLINICAL PEARLS**
> - All that is ANA positive is not SLE.
> - The pretest probability (clinical suspicion) increases the diagnostic yield of the immunological testing.
> - ANA screen is for diagnosis and does not need repeating.

If ANA is positive, the serum complements have to be estimated as hypocomplementemia is a feature of disease activity. The antidouble-stranded deoxyribonucleic acid (anti-dsDNA) is the most common antibody associated with SLE and can be estimated qualitatively by immunofluorescence and quantitatively by ELISA. A quantitative estimation is recommended since these levels and those of serum complements are used for disease monitoring. The ANA profile estimates the presence of other extractable antinuclear antibodies like the ribonucleoproteins (anti-RNPs), the Sm and the Ro (anti-SSA), and La (anti-SSB) and antihistone levels. Many of these antibodies remain positive and are used more for diagnosis rather than monitoring, so they need not be repeated. Various antibodies are related to system manifestations in SLE, e.g., anti-dSDNA and Sm for nephritis and anti-RNP for neuropsychiatric disease.

All patients suspected/diagnosed to have SLE should have their antiphospholipid antibody testing done. The presence of a prolonged APTT/prothrombin time gives a clue to the presence of these antibodies. The serum levels of anticardiolipin-immunoglobulin G (IgG) and IgM, the lupus anticoagulant and the anti-lipoprotein 1 (IgG and IgM) are the ones tested.

Tissue Diagnosis

Skin biopsy can be done to make the diagnosis—the histopathological appearances are characteristic as well as immunofluorescence showing "full-house" deposition of IgG/IgM/IgA/C3/C1q.

Lymph node biopsy may pick up Kikuchi-like changes or a paracortical hyperplasia. Depending on the clinical presentation, the presentation of a significant lymphadenopathy in the background of a pyrexia of unknown origin presentation may necessitate a lymph node biopsy to rule out differentials like TB or lymphoma.

Renal Biopsy

A renal biopsy with histologic, immunofluorescent, and electron micrographic analysis (where available) is necessary to classify the histologic type of renal disease. In our country, electron microscopy is very expensive with very limited availability, hence, not routinely requested.

Renal biopsy is rarely done to make a diagnosis of SLE or lupus nephritis which is often already decided by this time; however, it is to ascertain the class of nephritis which can then guide the level of treatment.

The International Society of Nephrology and the Renal Pathology Society have revised the original World Health Organization classification of renal biopsy findings in SLE into six different classes:

- Class 1 is generally considered minimal change and needs no treatment.
- Class 2 is mesangioproliferative and needs no additional treatment to steroids for a few months as would likely be used for background systemic disease.
- Class 3 (focal proliferative) and 4 (diffuse proliferative) are proliferative and the most common presentations. This class of patients commonly present with proteinuria/nephritis, hematuria, hypertension, and some azotemia. Patients may change from one class to another either before or during treatment. These classes of patients are meant to be treated aggressively to recruit back as many nephrons to normal activity and degree of reversibility makes timely and appropriately aggressive therapy very important in these patients.
- Class 5 is called membranous nephropathy and often presents as a nephrotic syndrome with the ongoing issues of anasarca. It can also be associated with proliferation which indicates aggressive management compared to pure membranous change which is controlled by antiedema measures and lower levels of immunosuppression.
- Class 6 or advanced glomerular sclerosis when >90% of glomeruli are sclerosed, dictates poor renal prognosis and need for renal replacement therapy and a transplant.

TREATMENT OF SYSTEMIC LUPUS ERYTHEMATOSUS

The treatment of SLE can be divided into:

- General measures
- Specific measures

General Measures

- Use of sunscreen of sun protection factor 30+ to exposed body areas when going out in sun
- Ensuring activity and exercise and preventative measures toward good cardiovascular health
- Maintenance of weight and body mass index in healthy zone
- Intake of nutritious healthy varied diet unless specific restriction advised
- Medication compliance
- Regular follow-up as advised
- Hydroxychloroquine is now recommended to be continued indefinitely for all children with SLE to improve cardiovascular health and stabilization of antiphospholipid antibodies.

Specific Measures

The pharmacological management depends on level of disease activity and severity of internal organ involvement.

Mild lupus: Largely characterized by musculoskeletal symptoms, and signs, mild systemic symptoms and mild hematological manifestations. A combination of low dose steroids and hydroxychloroquine (up to 6 mg/kg/day) may be all that is required.

Moderate lupus: Some systemic symptoms, moderate degree of hematological, and some internal organ affectation. Moderate dose of steroids 0.5–1 g/kg/day weaned slowly over 3–6 months with hydroxychloroquine and often second-line agents like methotrexate/azathioprine may be needed.

Severe lupus: With severe internal organ involvement, lupus nephritis, neuropsychiatric manifestations, macrophage activation syndrome, etc., are seen. High dose pulsed intravenous steroids (30 mg/kg methylprednisolone to a maximum dose of 1 g/day for 3 days) followed by high dose oral steroids—1–2 mg/kg/day initially in divided doses moving to single dose over 2 weeks and then a very slow wean is essential in the management of these patients. After appropriate assessment, there is a need for early consideration of a secondary agent in the form of mycofenolate mofetil or intravenous cyclophosphamide (intravenous pulse/month for 6 months). In nonrenal systemic severe lupus like neuropsychiatric/lung, cyclophosphamide has better results than mycophenolate mofetil.

Catastrophic lupus, e.g., pancreatitis, diffuse alveolar hemorrhage, severe neuropsychiatric manifestation, gangrene, etc.—high dose steroids intravenous cyclophosphamide have to be commenced early. Intravenous immunoglobulin 2 g/kg over 1 day, 2 days in divided doses or divided over 5 days has also been very helpful in serious emergencies with SLE.

Overall, the management is targeted toward seriousness of disease manifestations and balanced between controlling active disease, preventing organ damage due to disease, and damage, and morbidity due to treatment itself. All medications used in SLE have significant potential toxicity and administration and care should be under the supervision of a rheumatologist. Currently, the management of SLE solely with long duration of systemic steroids alone is discouraged due to problems with long-term steroid usage. Rituximab, an anti-CD20, monoclonal antibody is gaining preference in the management of refractory or resistant manifestations of SLE and may become part of the primary protocol for the management of proliferative lupus nephritis in the future.

Counseling

Counseling the family and the patient about the diagnosis of SLE is very important. The family and patient need to understand that it is a chronic lifelong disease. However, there can be periods of activity and inactivity and inactive periods can often last very long durations. Hydroxychloroquine is now recommended for indefinite use (and 6–12 monthly eye assessments with Humphrey Field Analyzer assessments are very important). Along with the medication, the need for regular follow-up and disease monitoring is very important. Pregnancy and fertility are specific areas that need very careful counseling and a rheumatologist has to remain part of the loop from the advice of planning pregnancy through the pregnancy and delivery. Medications have to be explained with awareness of potential side effects. The relationship between the rheumatologist and the patient and family is very important to the patients overall improvement and well-being.

KEY POINTS

- Between 15 and 20% of SLE commences in childhood
- High clinical suspicion in a child with a multisystem illness
- Investigations only when there are clinical pointers because false-positive ANA screen can cause much concern
- A detailed multisystem assessment at diagnosis needs to be done
- Treatment is tailored according to disease manifestations
- Appropriate disease-related counseling is essential
- Long-term follow-up and management is necessary for these patients

SUGGESTED READING

1. Habibi S, Saleem MA, Ramanan AV. Juvenile systemic lupus erythematosus: review of clinical features and management. Indian Pediatrics. 2011;48(11):879-87.
2. Morgan TA, Watson L, McCann LJ, Beresford MW. Children and adolescents with SLE: not just little adults. Lupus. 2013;22(12):1309-19.
3. Vachvanichsanong P, McNeil E. Pediatric lupus nephritis: more options, more chances? Lupus. 2013;22(6):545-53.
4. Weiss JE. Pediatric Systemic Lupus Erythematosus: More Than a Positive Antinuclear Antibody Weiss. Pediatr Rev. 2012;33:62-73.

CHAPTER 125

Approach to Juvenile Dermatomyositis

Ridhima Aggarwal, Sagar Bhattad, Deepti Suri

INTRODUCTION

Juvenile dermatomyositis (JDM) is an uncommon inflammatory myositis, characterized by a proximal muscle weakness, a heliotrope rash, and Gottron papules over the knuckles and elbows. It can involve several other organ systems such as the gastrointestinal tract, lungs, and heart. Lipodystrophy with insulin resistant diabetes is also a well-known association with this condition.

The primary lesion in JDM is a small vessel vasculopathy of varying severity. Unlike adults, in whom polymyositis (PM), inclusion body myositis, and cancer-associated myositis are common causes of inflammatory myopathy; JDM is the most common inflammatory myopathy in children. In the presteroid era, one-third children died, one-third recovered, and one-third of those who survived had significant residual problems of contractures and muscle atrophy. Over the last few decades, survival and outcome has improved considerably with aggressive immunosuppressive therapies. Mortality rate in children in the West is reported to be <3%. However, JDM is still associated with significant morbidity and mortality in our setting.

DEFINITION

The diagnosis is essentially clinical and with the advent of muscle magnetic resonance imaging (MRI), very few rheumatologists obtain electromyographs, or muscle biopsies unless the diagnosis is in doubt.

EPIDEMIOLOGY

Incidence of JDM is reported to be 3.2 children/million/year and girls are more commonly affected than the boys. Onset is between 4 and 10 years, with average age at onset being 7 years. However, 25% of children have onset before 4 years of age.

CLINICAL MANIFESTATIONS

Classical JDM, as the name suggests, involves skin along with proximal muscle weakness. Characteristic cutaneous abnormalities are seen in 75% of patients. These include erythematous violaceous heliotrope rash seen over the upper eyelids **(Fig. 1)** and Gottron papules which are symmetrical shiny, erythematous, scaly papules noted over extensor surfaces of small joints, and wrist and elbows **(Fig. 2)**. Nailfold capillaroscopy reveals periungual erythema and capillary loop abnormalities which are pathognomonic and correlates with the disease severity.

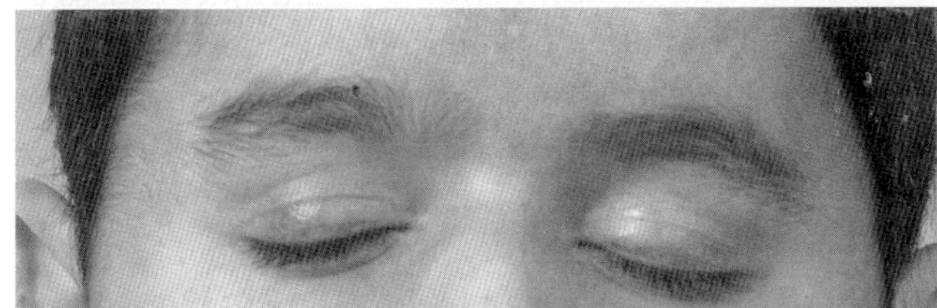

Fig. 1: Erythematous violaceous heliotrope rash seen over the upper eyelids. *(For color version, see Plate 10)*

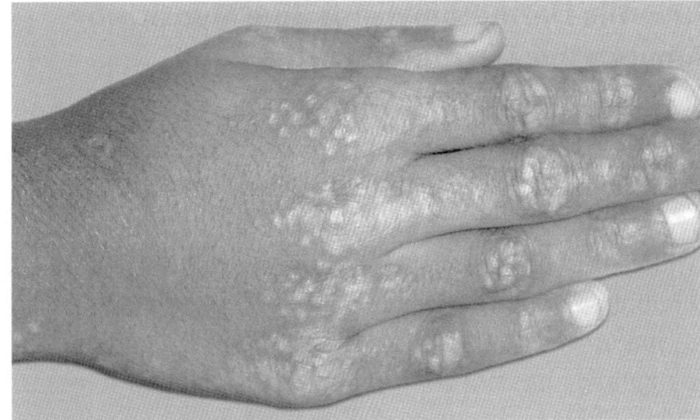

Fig. 2: Juvenile dermatomyositis. Erythematous, scaly papules noted over extensor surfaces of small joints, and wrist and elbows. *(For color version, see Plate 11)*

Classical JDM presents with insidious progression of malaise, easy fatigue, muscle weakness, fever, and rash that may predate diagnosis by 3–6 months. Muscle weakness at onset is predominantly proximal and children most commonly present with involvement of musculature of hip girdle. Involvement of anterior neck flexors leads to inability to hold head upright and is an important finding pointing toward the diagnosis of JDM. Pharyngeal, hypopharyngeal, and palatal muscles are frequently affected, resulting in difficulty in swallowing, nasal regurgitation of feeds, and nasal twang to the voice. Weak gag reflex increases the risks of aspiration pneumonias. Although, muscle weakness may be impressive, the deep tendon reflexes are usually preserved.

CLINICAL PEARL

- Weakness of anterior flexor muscles of the neck is important early indicator of inflammatory myositis.

Diagnosis is rather clinical and certain in presence of pathognomonic dermatological findings and proximal muscle weakness. However, some children present with atypical features like subcutaneous tissue edema and can be confused with nephritic syndrome and other causes of anasarca. Some children demonstrate exquisite muscle tenderness and refusal to walk or bear weight. Close looks for the dermatological features help differentiate it from viral myositis. Transient nondeforming arthritis may also occasionally occur. However, presence of significant and persistent arthritis in a child with JDM should suggest the possibility of an overlap syndrome such as mixed connective tissue disorder.

Juvenile Dermatomyositis Sine Myositis or Amyopathic Dermatomyositis

It is characterized by only the skin manifestations and paucity of muscle involvement and is relatively rare in childhood. Whether these children develop clinical overt myositis at follow-up is unclear, although some studies report up to 26% of children do, when followed for about 4 or more years. In contrast to adult amyopathic dermatomyositis, interstitial lung disease (ILD) or internal malignancy has not been reported from pediatric cases, and thus this subgroup carries good prognosis in children. MRI is said to be a sensitive modality for detection of muscle abnormalities in patients with amyopathic dermatomyositis.

Juvenile Dermatomyositis with Associated Rheumatic Diseases

A subset of children with JDM may have features of other rheumatic diseases as well. If children present with features of any two of the following diseases—juvenile rheumatoid arthritis, systemic lupus erythematosus (SLE), systemic scleroderma, and JDM—one should consider mixed connective tissue disease. Manifestations develop sequentially, but not in any predictable order, although majority would have the rash of SLE or JDM at the onset. Anti-U1 small nuclear ribonucleoproteins antibodies are characteristically elevated.

COMPLICATIONS

Vasculopathy results in many systemic complications in JDM. Gastrointestinal vasculitis and mesenteric ischemia can lead to acute gastrointestinal hemorrhages, intestinal perforation, and even mortality. Abdominal pain, therefore, must never be neglected in patients with JDM as this could be the earliest clue to gastrointestinal vasculitis.

CLINICAL PEARL

- Abdominal pain in patients with JDM may be the earliest clue to intestinal vasculopathy.

Pulmonary involvement can occur in the form of ILD, bronchiolitis obliterans organizing pneumonias, and rarely pneumothorax and other air leak syndromes.

During the convalescence phase late complications such as calcinosis and lipodystrophy are recognized. They have been linked to poor management of the disease at the initial presentation and also corroborate well with the severity of the first presentation. Calcinosis occurs in 10–40% of JDM patients and are extremely disfiguring. Calcinosis affecting subcutaneous tissues may result in cellulitis and painful superficial ulceration of overlying skin. Flexion contractures may occur when these occur across joints.

Lipodystrophy is usually associated with series of metabolic derangements such as insulin resistance, glucose intolerance and hypertriglyceridemia, and lipid abnormalities. Hirsutism and prominent dilated peripheral veins are also seen in some patients.

CLINICAL PEARL

- Calcinosis is a late complication seen in patient with poor initial immunosuppressive therapy.

INVESTIGATIONS

Indicators of inflammation (thrombocytosis, elevated erythrocyte sedimentation rate, and C-reactive protein) correlate with the degree of inflammation and help to differentiate inflammatory myopathies from noninflammatory disorders like muscular dystrophy **(Flowchart 1)**.

Muscle Enzymes

Serum levels of muscle enzymes are important for diagnosis and for monitoring patients of JDM on therapy. Aspartate aminotransferase, creatinine kinase (CK), lactate dehydrogenase (LDH), and aldolase should be measured at baseline. Aspartate aminotransferase or CK may be elevated 20–40 times normal. However, it is to be noted that occasionally, CK levels may be normal, particularly with a longer duration of untreated disease. LDH appears to correlate best with measures of disease activity. Serum levels of all muscle enzymes usually decrease 3–4 weeks before improvement in muscle strength and rise 5–6 weeks before clinical relapse. As a general rule, CK levels return to normal first (usually several weeks after instituting therapy); and aldolase and LDH levels return to normal the last.

Flowchart 1: Basic diagnostic algorithm for diagnosis of juvenile dermatomyositis (JDMs).

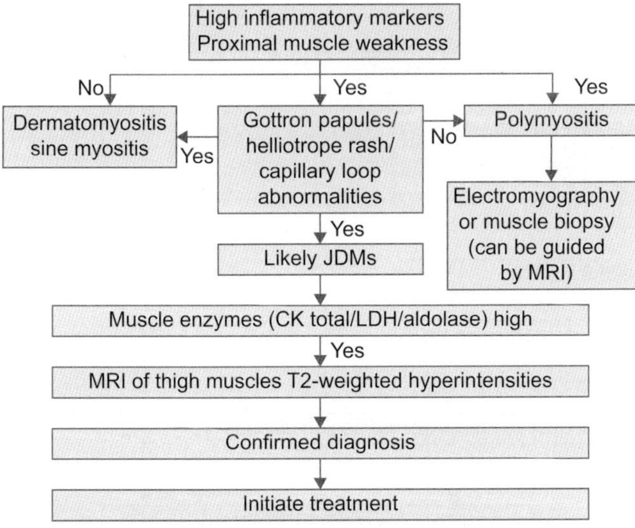

(CK: creatinine kinase; LDH: lactate dehydrogenase; MRI: magnetic resonance imaging)

Autoantibodies

Antinuclear antibodies may be positive in 10–85% and is neither specific, prognostic, nor diagnostic in patients with JDMs. Myositis antibodies are of two types: Myositis-specific antibodies (MSAs) and myositis-associated antibodies (MAAs). MSAs are present specifically in patients with inflammatory myopathies, whereas MAAs occur in conditions wherein myositis is associated with other autoimmune conditions such as in overlap syndromes. MSAs are not diagnostic, but in the background of suggestive clinical features, their positivity often supports the diagnosis. An important role of MSA positivity is in predicting clinical phenotype, complications, and outcomes in JDM, and may also determine the treatment intensity in these patients. Commonly isolated MSAs are:

- *Antitranscription intermediary factor 1 gamma (anti-TIF-1 gamma):* In adult dermatomyositis, these have a strong association with malignancy; however, in pediatric disease this antibody is strongly associated with presence of typical skin features (Gottron papules and shawl sign). Small, discrete subcutaneous nodules of calcification develop in prolonged disease.
- *Antinuclear matrix protein 2 (anti-NXP2) antibodies:* These children tend to develop severe degree of calcinosis as a complication (calcinosis universalis or tumoral calcinosis causing restriction of movement). They also have a greater degree of muscle weakness and a prolonged disease course.
- *Antibodies directed against MDA5 (Anti-MDA5):* These children tend to have less severe muscle disease, however are at high risk of developing ILD. Development of vasculitis and large skin ulcers are also associated with this antibody.
- *Anti-Mi2 antibodies:* These present with severe muscle weakness and typical skin signs.
- *Anti-signal recognition peptide (Anti-SRP):* These patients may present with immune-mediated necrotizing myopathy and severe muscle weakness. These patients should be screened for cardiac muscle involvement resulting in cardiomyopathy by cardiac enzyme, electrocardiogram, or echocardiogram.

Magnetic Resonance Imaging

Magnetic resonance imaging has dramatically replaced the need for muscle biopsy for the diagnosis of JDM. The T2-weighted magnetic resonance image with fat suppression demonstrates muscle edema and inflammatory changes by a hyperintense signal. Magnetic resonance also helps in guiding the extent of disease and also helps in selecting a site for muscle biopsy.

Electromyography

Electromyography findings that suggest inflammatory myopathy include a combination of changes of myopathy and denervation.

Muscle Biopsy

Muscle biopsy is largely performed when the diagnosis is in doubt if there are no skin findings and sometimes to evaluate the disease activity. It may occasionally help in making alternative diagnosis in children who fail trial of immunosuppression.

Biopsy usually is performed from quadriceps or deltoid, although the best specimen may be chosen based on electromyography or MRI. Muscle biopsy reveals perifascicular atrophy and variations in fiber size, as an outcome to ongoing degeneration and regeneration. Areas of focal necrosis would be noted, and inflammatory exudates are often presented.

TREATMENT

Morbidity and mortality have greatly reduced over the decades as a result of effective immunosuppressive therapies. Use of high dose corticosteroids early in the disease course has dramatically improved prognosis. Decision on treatment protocol is dependent on the clinical features present:

- *Severe disease:* Major organ involvement (JDM-associated cardiac disease and ILD), severe muscle weakness (pharyngeal muscle weakness and respiratory muscle weakness), gastrointestinal involvement, and skin ulceration. Patients with MDA5 antibody positivity must be screened for ILD via contrast-enhanced computed tomography. Treatment regimen advised is—as summarized as **Flowchart 2**.
    - Injection cyclophosphamide (500 mg/m^2 per month for 6 months)
    - Pulse methylprednisolone (30 mg/kg/day for 5 days) followed by initiation of oral steroids

Flowchart 2: Basic management algorithm for juvenile dermatomyositis (JDMs).

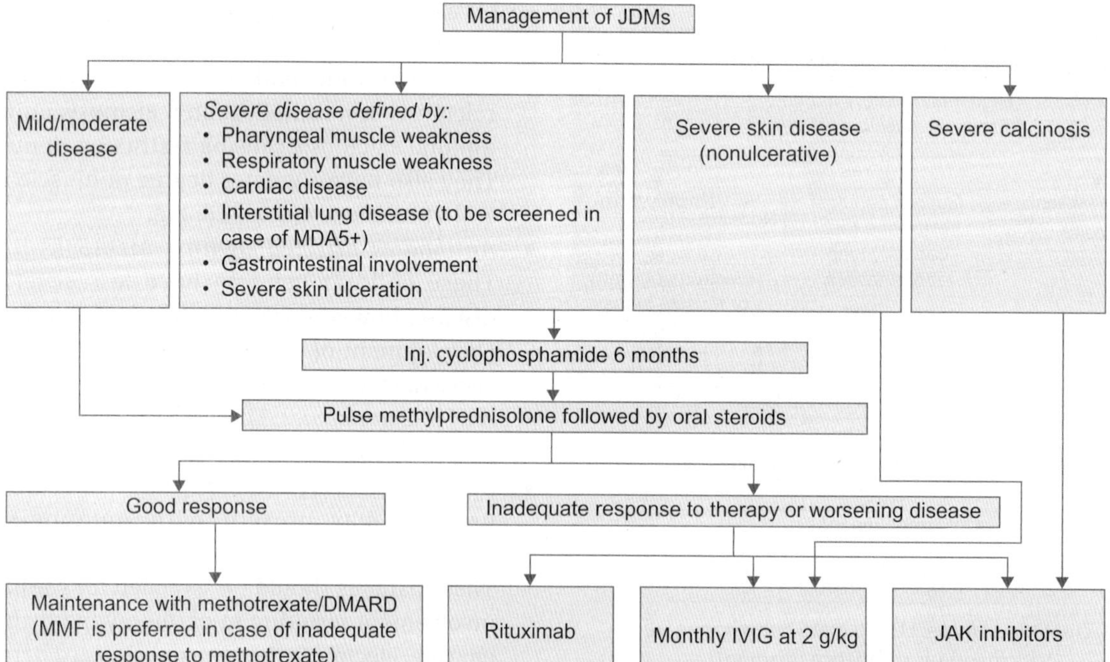

(DMARD: disease-modifying antirheumatic drug; IVIG: intravenous immunoglobulin; JAK: Janus kinase; MMF: mycophenolate mofetil)

(2 mg/kg/day) that should be tapered slowly over the next 9–10 months.
    - Add methotrexate (15 mg/m^2 subcutaneous weekly) with folic acid 5 mg weekly
    - After 6 months of cyclophosphamide, maintenance may be continued with methotrexate. Alternate disease-modifying antirheumatic drug (DMARD) such as mycophenolate mofetil can also be tried in case of inadequate response.
- *Mild/moderate disease*: Treatment regimen advised is:
    - Pulse methylprednisolone (30 mg/kg/day for 5 days) followed by initiation of oral steroids (2 mg/kg/day) that should be tapered slowly over the next 9–10 months
    - In addition, steroid sparing agent—methotrexate is advised (15 mg/m^2 subcutaneous weekly) with folic acid 5 mg weekly.

Regular review of muscle disease, skin disease, and major organ involvement must be done. If there is no significant improvement, revision of treatment protocol must be considered. In case of severe disease and nonresponse to cyclophosphamide, intensification of therapy by addition of intravenous immunoglobulin therapy with monthly doses at 1 g/kg or other biologicals (infliximab or rituximab) may be considered. Recently, the role of Janus kinase inhibitor (JAK-i) therapy has been described in treatment refractory patients with JDMs, especially those with difficult to treat calcinosis. In cases of severe skin disease, intravenous immunoglobulin therapy is advised early in the treatment protocol in case of nonresponse to standard therapy.

KEY POINTS

- Juvenile dermatomyositis is the most common inflammatory myopathy of childhood.
- Serum muscle enzymes correlate with disease activity, although normal CK level does not exclude JDM.
- MRI is a good modality to demonstrate muscle inflammation and is investigation of choice.
- Muscle biopsy/electromyography is less commonly used and has a role in cases with diagnostic difficulties.
- MSAs and MAAs help classify the disease phenotype.
- Corticosteroids and methotrexate form the cornerstone of therapy for the majority of patients with JDM.

SUGGESTED READING

1. Bellutti Enders F, Bader-Meunier B, Baildam E, Constantin T, Dolezalova P, Feldman BM, et al. Consensus-based recommendations for the management of juvenile dermatomyositis. Ann Rheum Dis. 2017;76(2):329-40.
2. Halilu F, Christopher-Stine L. Myositis-specific antibodies: Overview and clinical utilization. Rheumatol Immunol Res. 2022;3(1):1-10.
3. Martin N, Krol P, Smith S, Murray K, Pilkington CA, Davidson JE, et al.; Juvenile Dermatomyositis Research Group. A national registry for juvenile dermatomyositis and other paediatric idiopathic inflammatory myopathies: 10 years' experience; the Juvenile Dermatomyositis National (UK and Ireland) Cohort Biomarker Study and Repository for Idiopathic Inflammatory Myopathies. Rheumatology (Oxford). 2011;50(1):137-45.
4. Wu JQ, Lu MP, Reed AM. Juvenile dermatomyositis: advances in clinical presentation, myositis-specific antibodies and treatment. World J Pediatr. 2020;16:31-43.

Acute Osteoarticular Infections

Jasodhara Chaudhuri, Tapas K Sabui

INTRODUCTION

Acute osteoarticular infections (AOIs) are prominent areas of bacterial infection in infancy and childhood with variable clinical features that are often nonspecific. They may cause significant mortality and morbidity. Major clinical entities that are seen in children are septic arthritis, classic long bone osteomyelitis, skeletal tuberculosis, discitis, and osteochondritis complicating puncture wounds to the foot. Early diagnosis and treatment of musculoskeletal infection are critical to prevent sequelae. In children, these mean impaired growth with restricting lifelong deformity. However, children show a high potential for healing and remodeling and less comorbidity than adults. Childhood bone infection generally has good outcome provided appropriate treatment with antibiotics and surgical intervention are offered in timely manner.

The patterns of bone infection in children are changing in terms of both clinical syndrome (fewer acute presentation) and of microbiology (e.g., increased bacterial resistance among community-acquired *Staphylococcus aureus*). A greater understanding of pathogenesis and the varied manifestations of osteomyelitis and septic arthritis is thus required. There is also a need of clear guidelines with respect to treatment strategy, particularly the role of surgery and choice of antibiotic agents.

CLINICAL PEARLS

- AOIs are prominent areas of bacterial infection in infancy and childhood.
- Joint space infection in children usually arises as a complication of bacteremia.
- Virus, fungal, and tuberculous infections are rare.

SEPTIC ARTHRITIS AND OSTEOMYELITIS

Joint space infection in children usually arises as a complication of bacteremia. Virus, fungal, and tuberculous infections are rare. Bacterial infection elsewhere in the body may also give rise to reactive arthritis.

Acute hematogenous osteomyelitis (AHOM) is most common in childhood with a peak incidence in neonates. The reported incidence has been falling around the world but remains high in developing nations.

Osteomyelitis often is categorized into three different types:

- AHOM
- Osteomyelitis secondary to contiguous spread of infection after trauma, puncture wounds, surgery, or joint replacement
- Osteomyelitis secondary to vascular insufficiency

Acute hematogenous osteomyelitis is seen most often in children. Osteomyelitis caused by contiguous spread of infection is less common in children, and infection secondary to vascular insufficiency is rare in children.

CLINICAL PEARLS

- Osteomyelitis is most common in neonates.
- Osteomyelitis is most common at metaphysis of long bones.
- The history of trauma is common.

PATHOGENESIS

Pyogenic arthritis usually occurs as a result of infection of the vascular synovium by means of hematogenous dissemination of bacteria followed by an acute inflammatory response, resulting in migration of polymorphonuclear white blood cells (WBCs), production of proteolytic enzymes, and cytokine secretion by chondrocytes. Degradation of articular cartilage begins 8 hours after onset of infection. In children younger than 18 months of age, pyogenic arthritis can result from extension of a metaphyseal bone infection through transphyseal blood vessels. The growth plate, the epiphysis, and eventually the joint space may be infected.

On the other hand, osteomyelitis occurs mostly by hematogenous colonization of the bones by bacteria. The metaphysis of long bones is the most common site. Theories supporting this fact include decreased blood flow in sinusoidal vessels in this area along with relative lack of phagocytic cells. Although many children give a history of minor trauma, it is very rare to see osteomyelitis complicating a closed fracture treated by nonoperative means. Other notable features of epidemiology including the male preponderance and peak incidence remain to be explained. The pathological response to osteomyelitis is one of acute inflammation in the intramedullary cavity of the metaphysis of the long bone. After 48 hours, pus accumulates subperiosteally and then portions of the cortex may die as a result of the loss of blood supply forming a sequestrum and the abscess may rupture. Occasionally, osteomyelitis can involve the epiphysis of a long bone and then is usually subacute although acute epiphyseal osteomyelitis has been reported.

EPIDEMIOLOGY

Most cases of AOI occur in children 3 years old or younger. Boys are more frequently affected. The lower extremities (hips and knees) are most commonly affected.

CLINICAL PEARLS

- AOI is most common under 3 years of life.
- The most common agent is *Staphylococcus aureus.*

MICROBIOLOGY

The most common agent is *Staphylococcus aureus*, followed by respiratory pathogens *Streptococcus pyogenes, Streptococcus pneumoniae* (pneumococcus), and *Haemophilus influenzae* type b (Hib). *Kingella kingae* is a common cause of osteomyelitis and septic arthritis in some areas and requires special culture techniques or real-time polymerase chain reaction for diagnosis.

CLINICAL MANIFESTATIONS

The classical presentation of AOI is a locally swollen, warm limb, or joint combined with high fever with no or minor prior history of trauma. Pyrexia of unknown origin may be initial mode of presentation.

Generally, children with septic arthritis are clinically more ill than those with osteomyelitis, which has a more insidious onset. Plenty of useful information may be obtained from the disease history and mere observation of the patient. Limping, pseudoparalysis, refusal to use particular limb, and focal tenderness are the common mode of presentation. Whenever a previously well child presents with monoarthritis of acute origin, the possibility of septic arthritis should be considered. Pelvic osteomyelitis is well known to mimic a number of other diseases including appendicitis, lumbar disk prolapse, and septic arthritis of the hip **(Fig. 1 and Flowchart 1)**.

CLINICAL PEARLS

- The classical presentation of AOI is a locally swollen, warm limb, or joint combined with high fever.
- Children with septic arthritis are clinically more ill than those with osteomyelitis.
- Whenever a previously well child presents with monoarthritis of acute origin, think of AOI.

DIFFERENTIAL DIAGNOSIS

The most common cause of hip pain in childhood is transient synovitis. Transient synovitis is predominantly seen in children 5–10 years old. Pain is usually unilateral. Pain ranges from mild to severe enough to wake the child up. Physical examination generally reveals a nonill-appearing

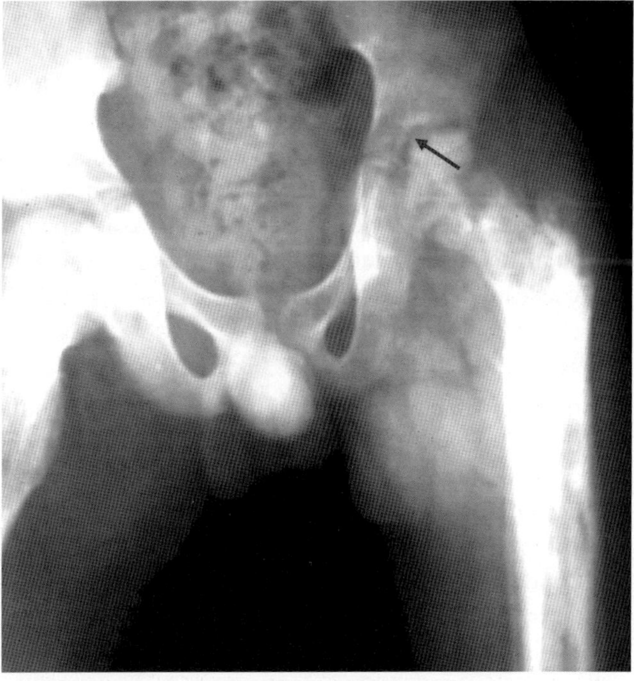

Fig. 1: X-ray of hip joint in a case of septic arthritis. The arrow sign shows the affected hip joint showing decreased and eroded joint space. Periosteal reaction in adjoining femur.

Flowchart 1: Algorithmic approach to monoarticular joint pain and arthritis.

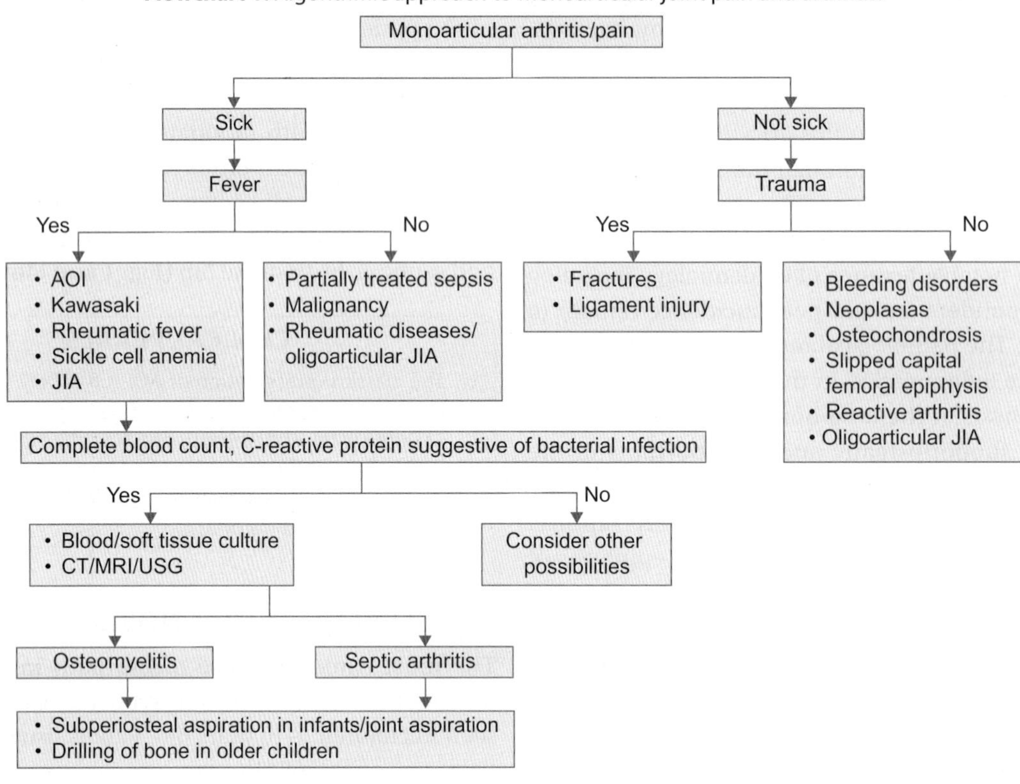

(AOI: acute osteoarticular infection; CT: computed tomography; JIA: juvenile idiopathic arthritis; MRI: magnetic resonance imaging; USG: ultrasonography)

child with decreased range of motion of the hip joint. Other common causes of joint pain and swelling include reactive arthritis, rheumatic fever, juvenile rheumatoid arthritis, trauma, and malignancy. Malignancy often turns out to be the most important differential diagnosis for osteomyelitis. Legg–Calvé–Perthes disease is an idiopathic avascular necrosis of the capital femoral epiphysis and may cause mild pain and limp in boys.

DIAGNOSIS

A sample for bacteriology may be obtained by needle aspiration of soft tissue in neonates, subperiosteal aspiration in infants, or drilling of bone in older children. Blood and joint fluid should be obtained for aerobic and anaerobic cultures.

Blood tests, namely hemogram and acute phase reactants, are used to assess the extent of inflammation. Blood leukocyte count (WBC) is nonspecific and elevated only in 20% of cases. Out of all acute phase reactants, C-reactive protein (CRP) here is extremely helpful in diagnosis and monitoring of AOI. Procalcitonin (PCT) level is usually found raised. However, the specific optimal cutoff value of PCT is not well established.

The initial diagnostic approach when AHOM is suspected is the imaging as it helps to differentiate between traumatic or noninfectious lesions.

Traditional radiographs have minimum or no value in diagnosis of it as the changes appear late. Ultrasound is extremely helpful for detection of joint effusion, soft tissue abscess, and subperiosteal collection.

However, magnetic resonance imaging (MRI) and computed tomography are the investigations of choice for early diagnosis. MRI is the gold standard in the diagnosis of osteomyelitis, due to its higher sensitivity and specificity (respectively of 82–100% and 75–99%. MRI is also able to document bone edema, the first nonspecific sign of osteomyelitis, within 24–48 hours from the infection onset. MRI is also increasingly used in evaluating multifocality. It has almost completely replaced bone scintigraphy, being more sensitive and avoiding exposure to radiations.

Bone scans in AHOM have a sensitivity of 84–100% and a specificity of 40–96%. The sensitivity of bone scans is least in the first 48 hours due to the transitional period between decreased and increased activity. Scintigraphy is most helpful in detecting multiple foci of disease and in the assessment of the young child, where localization is difficult.

Although cultures frequently fail to disclose the causative agent, every attempt should be made for isolation of causative agent from the site of infection. The only indication of joint aspiration in pediatric age group nowadays is septic arthritis, even though the chance of getting positive culture is only 30%. Aspirated fluid should be inoculated directly into blood culture bottles. Gram stain and cell count should also be performed on joint fluid. A WBC count of 50,000/mm^3 or greater with a predominance of polymorphonuclear cells is consistent with bacterial infection.

CLINICAL PEARLS

- Every attempt should be made to find out the etiological agent from infected tissue.
- CRP here is extremely helpful in diagnosis and monitoring of AOIs.
- Traditional radiographs have minimum or no value in diagnosis.
- MRI and computed tomography are the investigations of choice for the early diagnosis.

TREATMENT

A local antibiogram would be of paramount importance in these situations. As *Staphylococcus aureus* is a major player in AOIs, its local sensitivity pattern and bone penetration influences the choice of the initial antibiotic. The empiric antibiotic treatment of AOI in primary methicillin-sensitive and methicillin-resistant *Staphylococcus aureus* (MRSA) infections is first or second-generation cephalosporins (150 mg/kg/day four times a day)/cloxacillin (200 mg/kg/day four times a day) and vancomycin (40 mg/kg/day four times a day)/trimethoprim/sulfamethoxazole (TMP-SMX) (TMP 16 mg/kg/day twice a day), respectively. Linezolid (30 mg/kg/day three times a day) is the drug of choice in areas where the organism is resistant to vancomycin/TMP-SMX. A Hib unvaccinated child from Hib endemic area should receive concomitant ampicillin or amoxicillin (200 mg/kg/day divided in four equal doses) until the agent is identified. There is no consensus about the route or duration for antibiotic treatment of acute osteomyelitis in children. Until recently, the standard therapy was a long intravenous therapy and a long duration of 4–6 weeks. However, the short antibiotic courses tested in recent trials on osteomyelitis and septic arthritis. The entire course of antibiotic was approximately 3 weeks for uncomplicated osteomyelitis and 10–14 days for septic arthritis. A high dose of well absorbed first/second-generation cephalosporins or clindamycin in equal doses four times a day was used. These antibiotics penetrate bone and soft tissue well in intravenous and oral administration. In absence of definite laboratory or clinical parameters that would determine the decision to switch to oral therapy, there is no clear guideline of when to switch from intravenous to oral therapy. The drugs were given in recent trials intravenously for first 2–4 days except in newborns and thereafter it was given orally, provided the first signs of recovery including disappearance of fever, taking oral fluids were observed, and the level of CRP began to descend. However, this protocol is not applicable in the case for the management of complex infections including those with multifocal disease, significant bone destruction, resistant or unusual pathogens, sepsis, or in immunosuppressed children, and in neonates. The intravenous therapy to be continued for 14–21 days in complex situations and switched over to oral medication provided the baby is afebrile, pain free for at least 24 hours, and CRP descended by two-thirds of highest value. The total antibiotic therapy here will be 6 weeks both in septic arthritis and osteomyelitis. In most studies, oral therapy is done with high-dose cephalosporin, clindamycin, linezolid or amoxicillin–clavulanic acid, alone or in combination with rifampicin.

The role of surgery in the treatment of septic arthritis is in fact poorly defined except in relation to the hip, where prompt surgical drainage is absolutely necessary. Aspiration, irrigation, and intravenous antibiotic therapy is the preferred first line of treatment of septic arthritis except in hip joint. No consensus prevails in the timing, procedures, extent, or even the overall need for surgical intervention in osteomyelitis **(Fig. 2)**. Surgical drainage is mandatory in osteomyelitis if pus is obtained from the subperiosteal space or metaphysic in nature. The abscess should be decompressed, evacuated, and washed-out under general anesthesia. A suction drain should be left in place for 48 hours.

Though further studies are needed in this field, a placebo controlled randomized controlled trial examined the use of 4 days of intravenous dexamethasone (0.2 mg/kg/dose intravenously 8 hourly) and it significantly reduced the duration of acute phase and morbidity.

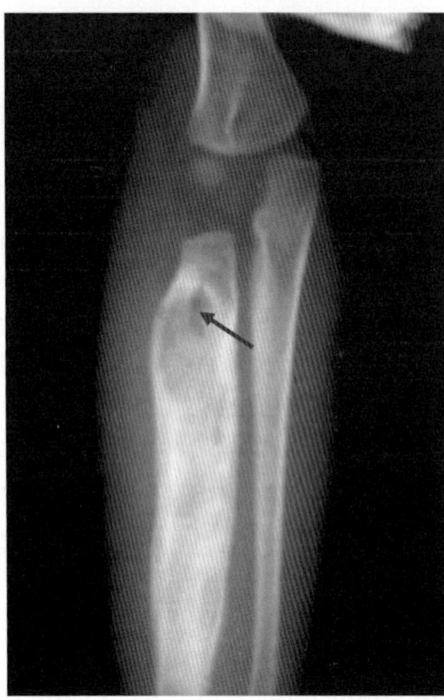

Fig. 2: X-ray showing osteomyelitis. The arrow symbol shows the visible osteolytic changes of osteomyelitis and sequestrum.

PROGNOSIS

Complications of AOI include abnormal bone growth, limp, unstable articulation of the affected joint, and decreased range of motion. Complications are reported in approximately 10–25% of all cases. Risk factors for squeal include delay in time to diagnosis of >4 or 5 days, onset of disease in infancy, infection with *Staphylococcus aureus* or gram-negative bacteria, and infection of adjacent bone.

CLINICAL PEARLS

- A local antibiogram would be of paramount help.
- The empiric antibiotic treatment depends on nature of etiological agent.
- No consensus about the route or duration for antibiotic treatment of acute osteomyelitis in children.
- Complications are reported in approximately 10–25% of all cases.

CONCLUSION

The number of bone and joint infections resulting from vaccine preventable pathogens such as *Haemophilus influenzae* and *Streptococcus pneumoniae* are on the decline. *Staphylococcus aureus* is the most common pathogen causing septic arthritis and osteomyelitis in children all over the world. The incidence of community acquired MRSA is increasing and is a cause of concern for pediatricians. Early diagnosis and prompt and appropriate treatment consisting of antibiotic therapy and surgical intervention when required is the mainstay of treatment and is extremely rewarding in majority of the occasions.

KEY POINTS

- AOIs are common in infancy and childhood under 3 years of age.
- Joint space infection in children usually arises as a complication of bacteremia and the most common agent is *Staphylococcus aureus*.
- High fever and painful warm swollen limb or joint are the most common mode of presentation.
- Children with septic arthritis are clinically more ill than those with osteomyelitis.
- Whenever a previously well child presents with monoarthritis of acute origin, think of AOI.
- MRI and computed tomography is the investigation of choice for the early diagnosis.
- Identification of etiological agent and local antibiogram are of paramount help.
- There is no consensus about the route or duration for antibiotic treatment of acute osteomyelitis in children.
- Treatment is rewarding.

SUGGESTED READING

1. Disch K, Hill DA, Snow H, Dehority W. Clinical outcomes of pediatric osteomyelitis. BMC Pediatr. 2023;23:54.
2. Faust SN, Clark J, Pallett A, Clarke NM. Managing bone and joint infection in children. Arch Dis Child. 2012;97:545-53.
3. Grammatico-Guillon L. Paediatric bone and joint infections are more common in boys and toddlers: a national epidemiology study. Acta Paediatrica. 2012;11:1-6.
4. Grimprel E, Lorrot M, Haas H, Pinquier D, Parez N, Ferroni A, et al. Bone and joint infections: treatment proposals from the Group of Pediatricians Specialised in Infectious Diseases (GPIP) French Pediatrics Society. Arch Pediatr. 2008;15:S74-80.
5. Gutierrez K. Bone and joint infections in children. Pediatr Clin North Am. 2005;52:779-94.
6. Musso P, Parigi S, Bossi G, Marseglia GL, Galli L, Chiappini E. Epidemiology and Management of Acute Hematogenous Osteomyelitis, Neonatal Osteomyelitis and Spondylodiscitis in a Third Level Paediatric Center. Children. 2021;8:616.
7. Peltola H, Pääkkönen M, Kallio P, Kallio MJ; Osteomyelitis-Septic Arthritis Study Group. Short-versus long-term antimicrobial treatment for acute hematogenous osteomyelitis of childhood: prospective, randomized trial on 131 culture-positive cases. Pediatr Infect Dis J. 2010;29:1123-8.
8. Susan S. Review article: paediatric bone and joint infection. J Orthop Surg. 2001;9:83-90.

CHAPTER 127

Eye Involvement: Beyond Infections

Manjari Agarwal

INTRODUCTION

Eyes are a window to systemic disease and can help a clinician reach an elusive diagnosis, by simply doing a proper detailed ophthalmological examination. Eyes are involved in a multitude of rheumatological illnesses and every incidence of eye problem is not due to infection. For the sake of this review, infectious etiologies would not be discussed. This review aims at stressing upon the eye involvement in various rheumatological/immunoinflammatory diseases. For ease of explanation, involvement of each layer of the eye is discussed separately **(Fig. 1)**.

CONJUNCTIVITIS

Redness of eyes with photophobia is seen in about 85% children with Kawasaki disease. Bilateral, nonexudative, and bulbar conjunctivitis is the hallmark of the disease. Perilimbal sparing of the conjunctiva is usually seen. Uveitis may or may not be present in Kawasaki disease. Presence of purulent conjunctivitis usually rules out Kawasaki disease.

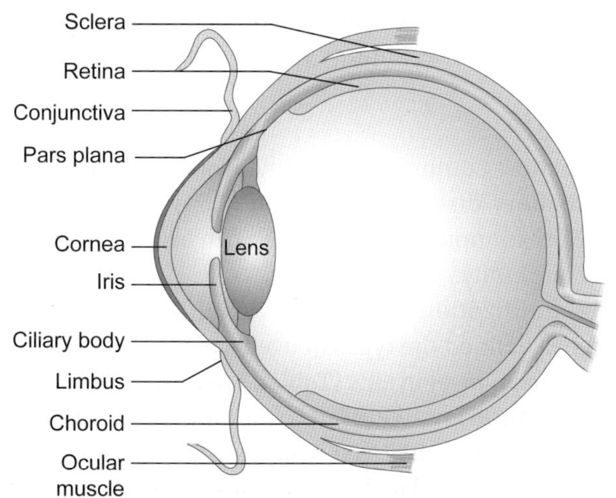

Fig. 1: Schematic representation of eye.

SCLERITIS

Sclera is the outer protective layer of the eye, begins at the limbus and is continuous with the cornea and ends at the optic canal in continuity with the dura.

Episcleritis is usually more painful and is often self-limiting.

Scleritis usually affects the adult population between 30 and 50 years of age. The most common association of scleritis in this age group is with Granulomatous polyangiitis and rheumatoid arthritis **(Table 1)**.

DIAGNOSIS

Detailed history, and physical examination is a must. Investigations pertaining to the system involved must be carried out. Specific serologic testing should include

TABLE 1: Etiology of scleritis.

Infections	*Autoimmune diseases*	*Others*
Viruses (varicella zoster, herpes simplex, hepatitis C)	Rheumatoid arthritis	Trauma
Bacteria	Granulomatous polyangiitis	Drug induced pamidronate
Mycobacteria	Inflammatory bowel disease	35–45
Fungi	Systemic lupus erythematosus	–
Amebae	Sarcoidosis	–
Parasites	• Takayasu's arteritis • Cogan's syndrome • Spondyloarthropathies • Polyarteritis nodosa • Vasculitis	

antinuclear antibodies (ANA), antineutrophil cytoplasmic antibodies (ANCA), rheumatoid factor, and anticyclic citrullinated peptide antibodies.

Other investigations like Mantoux test can be done after history and physical examination.

TREATMENT

Treatment of scleritis can be divided on the type of scleritis and has been detailed in **Table 2**.

INTERSTITIAL KERATITIS

Interstitial keratitis is characterized by a nonsuppurative inflammation, with vascularization of the cornea. It is commonly seen with Cogan syndrome. It usually presents with pain, lacrimation, photophobia, and conjunctival injection. This usually responds to topical corticosteroid therapy.

CLINICAL PEARLS

- Eyes can be involved in a myriad of immunoinflammatory conditions.
- Redness of eyes with photophobia, with or without diminution of vision might be a red flag and should be appropriately evaluated.

RETINAL VASCULITIS

Retinal vascular inflammatory diseases are termed retinal vasculitis even in the absence of true vasculitis. It can be defined as inflammation of the retinal vessels accompanied by intraocular inflammation and retinal vessel occlusion. Retinal vasculitis may involve retinal arteries, veins, or capillaries.

A common cause of retinal vasculitis leading to significant ocular morbidity is Behçet's disease. Both retinal veins as well as arteries can be involved in Behçet's disease and may lead to arterial occlusion.

Systemic vasculitides can also cause retinal vasculitis although these are uncommon.

Systemic lupus erythematosus can also cause retinal vasculitis even in the absence of antiphospholipid antibodies. The retinal vessels can be involved causing cotton-wool spots or microinfarcts of the nerve fiber layer of retina.

Therapy

Systemic glucocorticoids usually pulse methylprednisolone (10–30 mg/kg/day) for 3–5 days followed by oral glucocorticoids are needed. Steroid sparing agents like methotrexate and mycophenolate mofetil might be required for maintenance therapy.

TABLE 2: Therapy of scleritis.

Type of scleritis	*Systemic therapy*
Nodular anterior scleritis	NSAIDs
Necrotizing anterior scleritis	• Systemic glucocorticoids • Systemic Immunosuppression: – *First line agents:* - Cyclophosphamide - Methotrexate - Azathioprine - Mycophenolate mofetil – *Second line agents:* - Cyclosporine - Tacrolimus – *Third line/experimental* - Infliximab - Rituximab
Posterior scleritis	• Systemic glucocorticoids • Systemic immunosuppression

ORBITAL DISEASE

Primary inflammation of the orbital tissue, e.g., orbital pseudotumor or orbital myositis due to inflammation of the extraocular muscles is usually seen. Secondary involvement occurs most commonly due to contiguous spread of inflammation from the sinuses seen typically in ANCA associated vasculitis.

Therapy

Control of underlying disease with systemic corticosteroids or immunosuppressive drug therapy, decreases associated symptoms, as well as improves visual acuity.

UVEITIS

It is the most common ocular involvement of immunoinflammatory diseases in childhood. Usually uveitis in children is asymptomatic and hence can lead to significant ocular morbidity.

Standardization of Uveitis Nomenclature working group has defined the types of uveitis along with descriptors for each type of uveitis **(Tables 3 to 5)**.

Acute anterior uveitis is characteristic of human leukocyte antigen B27 (HLA-B27)-associated diseases such as enthesitis-related arthritis. Patient presents with a red, painful, and photophobic eye. The anterior chamber

TABLE 3: Standardization of Uveitis Nomenclature Working Group classification of uveitis.

Type	*Primary site of inflammation*	*Lesions*
Anterior uveitis	Anterior chamber	• Iritis • Iridocyclitis • Anterior cyclitis
Intermediate uveitis	Vitreous	• Pars planitis • Posterior cyclitis • Hyalitis
Posterior uveitis	Retina/choroid	• Chorioretinitis • Neuroretinitis • Retinochoroiditis • Focal, multifocal, diffuse choroiditis • Retinitis

TABLE 4: Standardization of Uveitis Nomenclature Working Group descriptors of uveitis.

Category	*Description*	*Comment*
Onset	Sudden insidious	–
Duration	Limited persistent	≤3 months >3 months
Course	Acute	Episodes of sudden onset and limited duration
	Recurrent	Repeated episodes separated by periods of inactivity without treatment >3 months in duration
	Chronic	Persistent uveitis with relapses in <3 months after discontinuing therapy

TABLE 5: Guidelines for the ophthalmological screening of children with juvenile idiopathic arthritis.

JIA onset type	*ANA*	*Onset <7 years of age*	*Onset >7 years of age*
Oligoarticular	Positive	Every 3–4 months	Every 4–6 months
Oligoarticular	Negative	Every 4–6 months	Every 4–6 months
Polyarthritis	Positive	Every 3–4 months	Every 4–6 months
Polyarthritis	Negative	Every 4–6 months	Every 4–6 months
Systemic onset	Negative/ positive	Every 12 months	Every 12 months

(ANA: antinuclear antibodies; JIA: juvenile idiopathic arthritis)

is best visualized by the help of a slit lamp. The presence of cells in the anterior chamber indicates disease activity. At times, the cells might aggregate in the lower part of the anterior chamber due to gravity and produce a hypopyon. If left untreated, there is a tendency to form adhesions between the posterior part of iris and lens; these are termed as posterior synechiae.

CLINICAL PEARL

- Acute anterior uveitis might often be the first presentation of disorders like juvenile spondyloarthropathy and inflammatory bowel disease.

Similar adhesions between peripheral iris and posterior cornea are called anterior synechiae. Chronic uveitis is the most common ocular complication of oligoarticular juvenile idiopathic arthritis (JIA). It is initially asymptomatic and is picked up on routine screening. It is predominantly insidious in onset, anterior, nongranulomatous inflammation affecting the iris and ciliary body.

Few children, especially older than 7–8 years of age can complain of pain, redness, headache, photophobia, or blurring of vision.

Slit lamp examination is mandatory to diagnose uveitis. Presence of inflammatory cells and increased protein concentration (flare) in the aqueous humor of the anterior chamber are the classic hallmark.

Keratic precipitates (deposition of inflammatory cells on the inner surface of the cornea) may be detected at onset or may develop later.

Band keratopathy occurs due to deposition of calcium in the corneal epithelium and is also a late feature.

Presence of posterior synechiae is also a feature of late disease. Untreated synechiae might occasionally cause obstruction to aqueous outflow and cause increased intraocular pressure.

Since chronic uveitis might lead to significant visual morbidity, it is prudent to electively screen children with JIA. **Table 5** gives a guideline for screening of children depending upon the risk involved. Uveitis may also be associated with other inflammatory disorders in children like inflammatory bowel disease and reactive arthritis. Uveitis can also in occur in chronic infantile neurological cutaneous and articular syndrome, sarcoidosis, Blau syndrome, Bechet's disease and Kawasaki disease. **Flowchart 1** gives provides an outline of the diagnostic possibilities for children presenting with uveitis.

Management

Uveitis associated without arthritis needs to be evaluated and infections like tuberculosis need to be ruled out. Angiotensin converting enzyme levels for sarcoidosis,

Flowchart 1: Approach to a child with uveitis.

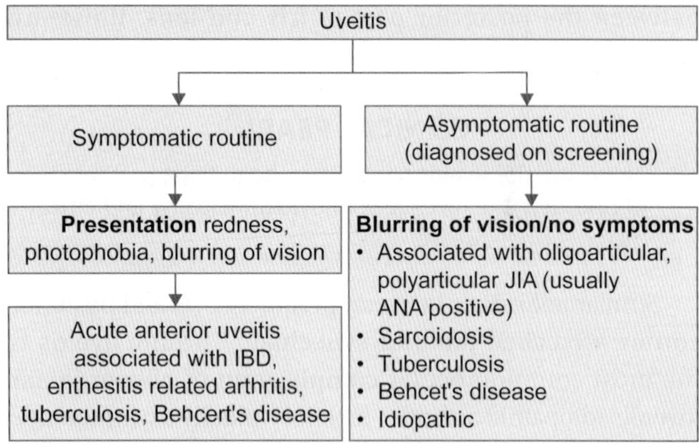

(ANA: antinuclear antibodies; IBD: inflammatory bowel disease; JIA: juvenile idiopathic arthritis)

HLA B51 for Behçet's disease, ANA need to be done if child does not have arthritis. Human leukocyte antigen B27 associated uveitis is usually acute symptomatic but rarely may be chronic persistent. Rheumatoid factor positivity generally has a protective role for uveitis.

Treatment

The management of uveitis is done by ophthalmology and rheumatology teams jointly.

Topical glucocorticoid drops with or without mydriatics are the first line agents. Topical therapy for prolonged period is associated with severe ocular complications like cataract and glaucoma.

Second line agent for uveitis unresponsive to topical therapy is methotrexate. It can also be used as a steroid sparing agent with excellent results.

Mycophenolate mofetil, cyclosporine, and tacrolimus are the next line of management.

Severe, unresponsive disease can be managed by tumor necrosis factor alpha blocker, infliximab.

There is also some role of costimulatory blockade, abatacept for resistant uveitis though large trials are still required.

CLINICAL PEARLS

- In children with diagnosed juvenile idiopathic arthritis, routine screening for chronic anterior uveitis is a mandate.
- Topical therapy for prolonged period of time can cause significant morbidity and must be avoided.

KEY POINTS

- Acute anterior uveitis might often be the first presentation of disorders like juvenile spondyloarthropathy and inflammatory bowel disease (IBD).
- Detailed ophthalmic examination is necessary in every child with juvenile idiopathic arthritis (JIA).
- Chronic anterior uveitis is asymptomatic and a young child might not be able to complain of blurring of vision.
- In a child with uveitis, diseases like tuberculosis, sarcoidosis, Behçet's, IBD, and JIA must be ruled out.
- Disease-modifying antirheumatic drugs are essential early in the disease course to prevent side effects of topical/oral steroids.

SUGGESTED READING

1. Galor A, Thorne JE. Scleritis and periplheral ulcerative keratitis. Rheum Dis Clin N Am. 2007;33:835-54.
2. Jabs DA, Nussenblatt RB, Rosenbaum JT. Standardization of uveitis nomenclature for reporting clinical data: results of the First International Workshop. Amer J Ophthalmol. 2005;140:509-16.
3. Nguyen QD, Foster CS. Systemic lupus erythematosus and the eye. Int Ophthalmol Clin. 1998;38:33-60.
4. Okhravi N, Mc Cluskey P. Scleritis. Surv Ophthalmol. 2005; 50(4):351-63.
5. Yancey C, White P, Magilavy D, Gewanter H, Lowe B, Passo M, et al. The Guidelines of the Rheumatology and Ophthalmology sections of the American Academy of Pediatrics. Pediatrics. 1993;92:295-6.

SECTION 15

Pediatric Surgery

Section Editors: *Anurag Krishna, Rasiklal S Shah*

Empyema Thoracis: Management Algorithm

Rasiklal S Shah, Suyodhan A Reddy, Manika Boipai

INTRODUCTION

Empyema thoracis (ET) is collection of purulent fluid in the pleural cavity, which is either free or localized. Pneumonic infection and the associated inflammation of the pleural lining lead to an exudative parapneumonic pleural effusion, which upon invasion by bacteria becomes empyema. The term "empyema" is derived from the Greek words *pyon*, meaning pus and *empyein*, meaning pus producing. The optimal time and the manner of drainage of empyema was a matter of concern since the times of Hippocrates and Fabricius. In the last two decades, many pediatric surgical centers are increasingly using minimal access techniques in management of ET patients.

EPIDEMIOLOGY

Childhood empyema occurs in 0.7–3.3 per 100,000 worldwide. There is gradual decrease in the incidence. The pattern of use of antibiotics and incorporation of polyvalent pneumococcal vaccine (13vPVC) into immunization programs has led to an increase in invasive pneumococcal empyema by nonvaccine serotypes.

ETIOPATHOGENESIS

Empyema thoracis most often occurs as a sequel of bacterial pneumonia; however, it can also occur following pulmonary tuberculosis, trauma, perforation of intrathoracic esophageal, or operations on chest. Lower respiratory tract infection in children may get complicated by parapneumonic fluid collections in 50% of patients. Progression to an established ET occurs in 1 of every 155 cases of pneumonia according to one large pediatric series.

In India, *Staphylococcus aureus* is still the most common isolate from the children of ET. This is followed by *Streptococcus pneumoniae* and *Streptococcus pyogenes*. Although *S. pneumoniae* produces large effusion in 40% of the cases, only 5% eventually progress to frank ET. Tubercular empyema is rare and occurs only in 2% of the cases of tubercular pleural infections. Anaerobes are common in older children who often have predisposing factors such as aspiration pneumonia, lung abscess, and poor dental hygiene. *Aspergillus* and *Candida albicans* also have been isolated. Rarely, *Entamoeba histolytica* abscess in the liver may rupture in the pleural cavity and produce ET with *Entamoeba histolytica*.

PATHOPHYSIOLOGY

The smooth and synchronized expansion of the lung in consonance with the expansion of the chest wall is facilitated by a small amount of intrapleural fluid (0.3 mL/kg). This is maintained in a dynamic equilibrium in visceral and parietal pleura by unidirectional flow created by lymphatics. These lymphatics generate a negative pressure of about 7 mm Hg and are capable of absorbing large volumes of clear low solute fluids in the pleural space. However, a secondary infection in the pleural space triggers an inflammatory process, which makes the pleural vasculature to become more permeable to inflammatory cells and bacteria. The pleural fluid now transforms into exudates of frank pus, resulting in the classical empyema. This influx is mediated by proinflammatory cytokines, such as tumor necrosis factor, interleukin (IL)-1, and IL-6, secreted from mesothelial cells. The activation of the coagulation cascade and disruption of enzymes of the fibrinolytic system, such as tissue type plasminogen activator and plasminogen activator inhibitor type 1, results in fibrin deposition and blockage of lymphatic pores leading to further accumulation of fluid. This imbalance of the fibrin produces multiple loculations and formations of fibrinopurulent peel as seen in the later stages of empyema.

TABLE 1: Stages of empyema.

Stage	*Duration*	*Cellular content*	*Glucose ratio fluid/ plasma*	*pH*	*LDH*	*Pleural space*
Exudative	1–3 days	Low	>60 mg (>0.5)	>7.30	<1,000	Thin sterile and low sediment fluid
Fibrinopurulent	4–14 days	Neutrophilia and fibrin	<60 mg (<0.5)	<7.10	>1,000	• Purulent, viscous fluid, loculations, and limiting membranes • Organisms isolated
Organized	>14 days	Fibroblasts proliferation leads to thick peel, which encases the lung. The pleural space contains very thick exudates				

(LDH: lactate dehydrogenase)

Empyema thoracis is classified into three stages, i.e., exudative, fibrinopurulent, and organizing stage by the American Thoracic Society. The pathological response is divided in three phases that are not sharply distinct but gradually one phase merges into another **(Table 1)**.

Hamm and light described a stage that proceeds to the stage of exudation, which they termed "pleuritis sicca stage"; this is characterized by the presence of pleuritic chest pain and pleural rub. This does not proceed to exudative stage.

CLINICAL FEATURES

Empyema is more common in the poor socioeconomic group. The incidence peaks between 6 months and 3 years of age. Clinical signs vary depending on the type of organism isolated, age of the patient, stage of the effusion, and type of prior antibiotic therapy.

The bacterial pneumonia in children usually presents with cough and fever, development of pleuritic chest pain, and dyspnea heralds complication of ET. Children may lie on the affected side in attempt to splint the chest. The breath sounds and respiratory movements' decreases on the side of empyema. There may be shift of the mediastinum. Often scoliosis is seen toward the affected side on both clinical examination and chest X-ray. This occurs initially in an attempt to reduce the pleural pain and later on due to the result of fibrosis of the parietal pleura. In late stages of ET, the ipsilateral chest is collapsed with crowding of ribs leading to obliteration of intercostal space, pulling of mediastinum, and diaphragm on the side of ET and scoliosis. The patients can develop pyopneumothorax due to air leak either from lung parenchyma [parenchymo-pleural fistula (PPF)] or by erosion of bronchus [bronchopleural fistula (BPF)].

INVESTIGATIONS

Investigations are performed to determine quantity and quality of fluid present in the pleural space and its effect on the cardiorespiratory system.

Chest Radiograph

All children with symptoms suggestive of febrile respiratory illness should have a chest X-ray posteroanterior view. Blunting of costophrenic angle and pleural shadowing suggests presence of free fluid in the pleural space. Massive fluid accumulation in the chest may show opacified hemithorax with or without mediastinal shift. Presence of air fluid level suggests either anaerobic infection, or BPF or PPF. Advanced stage of the disease may show fibrosis where the mediastinum is pulled toward the fibrosed pleura. The chest X-ray is not helpful in monitoring the progress of the disease and radiological features lag behind the physiological changes.

Ultrasonography of Chest

The ultrasonography of chest is the most useful investigation; it is noninvasive, does not use ionizing radiation, provides a dynamic assessment of the chest, and can be done repeatedly without fear of any adverse effect. It can differentiate between consolidated lungs from fluid in pleural space. It also detects presence of loculations and fibrin strands, and volume of the fluid in the pleural space. The sonologist can mark the spot for the aspiration of fluid and/or chest-tube insertion. The aspiration of fluid differentiates between sympneumonic effusion and ET. Though ultrasound is useful to stage the ET in children, it is not helpful in predicting its outcome.

Computed Tomography Scan

The role of routine computed tomography (CT) is controversial. The CT scan often requires general anesthesia or sedation, which may be a limiting factor in some very small and sick child. CT scan also gives lot of radiation. Its role is limited in patients, who are not responding to the treatment. The CT scan precisely shows site of fluid collection, thickness of fibrotic peel, its location, and whether it is on visceral surface of lung or on diaphragm or chest-wall. This information is useful to endoscopic surgeons for the port placement to avoid trauma to the lung and subsequent PPF or BPF. Though the CT scan can demonstrate the lung parenchyma and it pathologies accurately, it is unable to identify the presence of thin fibrinous strands in pleural fluid. Coren et al. reviewed the use of CT scanning in preoperative assessment and found that CT scans were least useful in the preoperative assessment of empyema complicating community-acquired pneumonia.

CLINICAL PEARLS

- X-ray chest posteroanterior view should be done in all children in whom an empyema is suspected.
- Ultrasound is the most informative investigation.
- Computed tomography scan is reserved for patients who are not responding to treatment or as a preoperative investigation.

Hematological Investigations

The total blood count may reveal anemia, leukocytosis with polymorphonuclear predominance, and thrombocytosis and raised C-reactive protein. The falling levels of white blood cell count and C-reactive protein are indicative of clinical improvement. Thrombocytosis is common in many chronic inflammatory conditions including empyema. However, low platelet count with low hemoglobin in a child with empyema should alert the physician about possibility of the hemolytic uremic syndrome, which often develops secondary to neuraminidase release by *Streptococcus pneumoniae*.

The coagulation studies are usually normal in healthy children with normal liver. However, children with impaired liver and chronic malnutrition may have abnormal blood coagulation. Single screening of coagulation should suffice at the time of initial venous cannulation.

CLINICAL PEARL

- Resolution of fever, falling levels of total leukocyte counts, and C-reactive protein are favorable indicators.

Pleural Fluid Analysis

Pleural fluid tapping is highly informative; however, the procedure is challenging as it might require sedation in a sick child. Small collections are best left alone. The fluid is examined for Gram staining, aerobic and anaerobic culture, pH, specific gravity, protein content, glucose estimation, and lactate dehydrogenase (LDH) levels. The specimen should be sent for microscopy and culture. The reported rate of isolating a pathogen varies and depends on the prior antibiotic usage. If facilities permit 16s ribosomal ribonucleic acid (RNA) polymerase chain reaction (PCR) should be done and suitable antibiotics should be instituted. The fluid should also be cultured for *Mycobacterium tuberculosis*.

CLINICAL PEARLS

- Pleural fluid is sent for microscopy, cytology, and culture.
- PCR, if available, should be used.
- There is no role of biochemical markers in children.

MANAGEMENT

The broad principles in management of empyema include treatment to stop ongoing sepsis, restoring the normal lung volume, and reestablish the physiological pleural fluid circulation. The child's hemodynamic status should be stabilized with oxygen therapy, parenteral fluids, antipyretics, and analgesia.

CLINICAL PEARL

- Sterilize and evacuate the thorax at the earliest.

Antibiotics

Antibiotics alone have a role in small effusions in which the child has no respiratory compromise. The choice of antibiotic should be based on local policy on pneumonia guidelines and knowledge of both community- and hospital-acquired pathogens. The antibiotics are selected empirically and changed according to the Gram staining and culture sensitivity of the aspirated pus. Broad-spectrum antibiotics are used to ensure adequate cover for *S. pneumoniae*, and consideration should be given to antistaphylococcal cover, particularly if pneumatoceles are present. Adequate anaerobic cover should be given when there is a clinical suspicion for aspiration pneumonia. Once the child is afebrile then child can be shifted to oral therapy, which can extend up to 6 weeks.

Modalities for the Drainage of Empyema

CLINICAL PEARLS

Modalities for drainage:
- Multiple needle thoracocentesis
- Tube drainage of chest with or without fibrinolytics
- Video-assisted thoracic surgery
- Open thoracotomy

Timing of Drainage

The timing of pleural cavity drainage should be individualized depending upon the local expertise and the balance of noninvasive monitoring and expectant management. The decision to intervene and drain the fluid is taken when the fluid analysis is suggestive of empyema and/or if child develops respiratory distress **(Flowchart 1)**.

Options for Drainage

Aspiration is done under local anesthesia with sedation at the most dependent site or in the fifth intercostal space in midaxillary line. In the exudative stage, it may be possible to aspirate ET completely; however, as the pus becomes thicker and flakes of fibrinopurulent material starts forming, it is not possible to aspirate the ET completely. Some studies have compared the efficacy of repeated thoracocentesis to that of chest tube drainage and found both comparable. These studies concluded that repeated needle aspirations are more traumatic; require multiple anesthesia and ultrasonography assistance. These studies recommend early chest tube insertion.

Chest tube drainage along with parenteral antibiotic is the standard management in the exudative stage and in fibrinopurulent stage. Addition of fibrinolytics shortens the duration of the chest drainage and improves the clinical outcome. Recent studies have shown addition of streptodornase and D Plasma Thrombin Activation DTPA shortens the hospital stay. Adequate chest drainage and good broad-spectrum antibiotics resolve the fever and leukocytosis, with almost complete lung reexpansion as seen on X-ray and/or sonography. The chest drainage should be continued till drainage decrease to less than 10–15 mL/day, which usually takes 7–14 days. The successful resolution with conservative management has been reported in 65–82% of the patients, and rest will require surgical therapy.

Flowchart 1: Management algorithm for empyema in children.

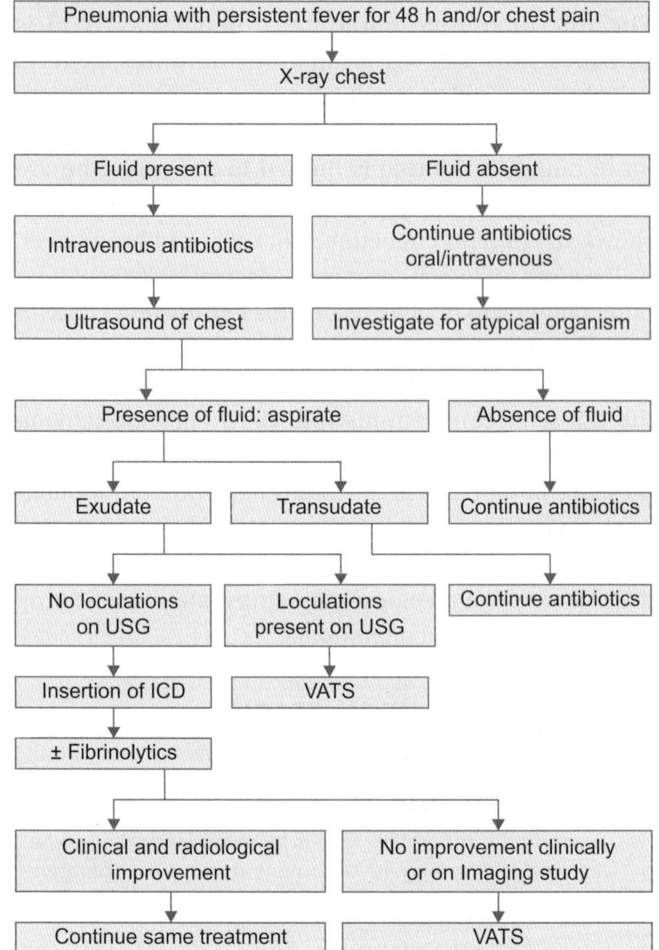

(ICD: intercostal drainage; USG: ultrasonography; VATS: video-assisted thoracoscopic surgery)

CLINICAL PEARL

- More than two-thirds of early empyema can resolve with standard management of antibiotics and chest tube drainage. Remaining needs surgical intervention.

Pepperpoint et al. compared and reviewed the outcomes in terms of length of hospital stay and the need for further intervention in children with empyema treated either with a stiff large bore tube or with small bore pig tail catheter. The outcomes were significantly better in children who received small bored catheter. It has been observed that the most of the patients in India presents late and they do better with large bore chest drain then pigtail catheter.

Satish et al. in their study conducted in the secondary referral center on 14 children concluded that chest drainage along with antibiotics is sufficient to treat empyema. They also suggested there is no need for surgical decortications in children. However, in this study, the physiological and radiological resolution was obtained up to 16 months. The prolonged hospital stay, coupled with the extraordinarily long recovery of lung has significant economic, social, and academic implications of a growing child. Spencer in his editorial comment observed, "it is not time to put the knife down".

As the duration of the empyema advances, there is increased fibrin formation and this result in loculated pus pockets. Use of fibrinolytics in pleura is to lyse the fibrin strands, clear the lymphatics, and liquefy the pus. The literature is replete with case series describing the management using streptokinase, urokinase, alteplase, or tissue plasminogen activator in various different protocols.

In fibrinopurulent stage with loculations and in organizing stage, the simple chest drain or cyclical irrigation is unlikely to work and they would need either formal decortication or video-assisted thoracoscopic surgery (VATS). In fibrinopurulent stage, it is more of pleural debridement and breaking up of the loculations, which ensures adequate drainage. This can be safely accomplished by VATS. Open decortication is required in a miniscule number of advanced cases of empyema. The term decortication refers to the removal of the thick fibrotic parietal and visceral pleural peel found in the late chronic disease is accomplished with open thoracotomy either with or without rib resection.

CLINICAL PEARL

- Early surgical intervention allows faster recovery and rapid lung expansion.

The term primary and secondary VATS is used for the procedures performed before or after the trial of standard management, respectively. VATS offsets many disadvantages of open thoracotomy and provides excellent vision of the entire hemithorax. The primary VATS allows determination of the stage of the disease, breaking of all loculi with complete evacuation of thick pus, and fibrinopurulent material. In early stage, it may reduce the bacterial load and chest drain is inserted in the proper dependent position. In addition, VATS gives visual impression of condition of underlying lung, its capacity to expand, and presence, site, and size of PPF or BPF. The near complete removal of thick pus and fibrinopurulent material results in early resolution of fever, chest drain is required for shorter duration. VATS causes minimal disturbance in the anatomy of nerves, muscles, and ribs. Kyphoscoliosis is avoided in children who undergo VATS. The aesthetic appearance and the normal anatomy of the spine and the rib cage improve the child's posture and self-esteem.

Open thoracotomy and decortication involves opening of the thorax posterolaterally and excision of the thickened pleural encasing the lung. Lung pathologies such as lung abscesses, necrotic lung, and BPF, if any, can be addressed simultaneously. Alexiou et al. reviewed their data of 44 children and concluded that open decortications are an excellent option for treating of advanced empyema. Fibrinolysis and VATS should be considered on their own merits, and should not be based on the adverse outcomes of open thoracotomy.

In the past, VATS was used after the failure of medical therapy, but now it is increasingly used as primary therapy. Cohen et al. compared results of primary VATS with chest drainage alone and found significant reduction in the hospital stay (7.4 vs. 15.4 days) and removal of chest drain (4.0 vs. 10.2 days) in VATS group. In an study from Dallas on 139 children, Doski et al. demonstrated that children who underwent primary VATS significantly reduced hospital stay compared to those who had secondary VATS or open decortications for failed medical treatment. Subramanium et al. demonstrated reduced hospital stay in VATS group of children in comparison to the open thoracotomy group in children who were referred for the failure of medical treatment. VATS in combination with bronchoalveolar lavage significantly improves the outcomes in pediatric empyema.

Gates et al. carried out a systematic review of 44 retrospective studies to assess the superiority of VATS over chest drainage alone, fibrinolysis, or thoracotomy. They concluded VATS and open decortication led to early recovery in children. The study also identifies the lack of properly designed study to answer the question of superiority of VATS over the other available modalities of treatment.

CLINICAL PEARL

- Multiple studies throughout the world have confirmed the safety, efficacy, and cost effectiveness of video-assisted thoracoscopic surgery in the treatment of empyema in children.

KEY POINTS

- ET is a complex pediatric surgical disease and the best standard of care involve pediatric surgeon as soon as it is suspected.
- Management needs to be individualized depending upon the presentation and stage of disease.
- For patient presents early (<7 days of symptoms), standard management can be offered in the form of intravenous antibiotics and intercostal drainage.
- Patients presenting late (>7 days of symptoms), or having loculations on imaging studies (X-ray or ultrasonography of chest) should be offered primary VATS.
- Patients who fails to respond to standard management clinically and radiologically in 48–72 hours should be offered secondary VATS.
- Patients having chronic disease with crowding of ribs should be offered an open surgery.
- VATS in treatment of empyema has decreased morbidity and mortality of the disease.
- In India, due to limited availability of resources and the endoscopic surgical expertise, many patients who fails to receive standard care may need either referral to higher center or an open surgery at appropriate time.

SUGGESTED READING

1. Alexiou C, Goyal A, Firmin RK, Hickey MS. Is open thoracotomy still a good treatment option for the management of empyema in children? Ann Thorac Surg. 2003;76:1854-8.
2. Balfour-Lynn IM, Abrahamson E, Cohen G, Hartley J, King S, Parikh D, et al. BTS guidelines for the management of pleural infection in children. Thorax. 2005;60(1):1-21.
3. Chiu CY, Wong KS, Huang JL Tasi MH, Lin TY, Hsieh SY. Proinflammatory cytokines, fibrinolytic system enzymes, and biochemical indices in children with infectious parapneumonic effusions. Pediatr Infect Dis J. 2008;27(8):699-703.
4. Cohen G, Hjortdal V, Ricci M, Jaffé A, Wallis C, Dinwiddie R, et al. Primary thoracoscopic treatment of empyema in children. J Thorac Cardiovasc Surg. 2003;125:79-84.
5. Coren ME, Ng M, Rubens M, Rosenthal M, Bush A. The value of ultrafast computed tomography in the investigation of pediatric chest disease. Pediatr Pulmonol. 1998;26:389-95.
6. Doski JJ, Lou D, Hicks BA, Megison SM, Sanchez P, Contidor M, et al. Management of parapneumonic collections in infants and children. J Pediatr Surg. 2000;35:265-8.
7. Gates RL, Hogan M, Weinstein S, Arca MJ. Drainage, fibrinolytics, or surgery: a comparison of treatment options in pediatric empyema. J Pediatr Surg. 2004;39:1638-42.
8. Hamm H, Light RW. Parapneumonic effusion and empyema. Eur Respir J. 1997;10(5):1150-6.
9. Hoff SJ, Noblett WW, Heller RM, Pietsch JB, Holcomb GW Jr, Sheller JR, et al. Post pneumonic empyema in childhood: selecting appropriate therapy. J Pediatr Surg. 1989;24:659-64.
10. Livingston MH, Mahant S, Ratjen F, Connolly BL, Thorpe K, Mamdani M, et al. Intrapleural Dornase and Tissue Plasminogen Activator in pediatric empyema (DTPA): a study protocol for a randomized controlled trial. Trials. 2017;18(1):293.
11. Hull J, Thomson A. Empyema thoracis: a role for open thoracotomy and decortication. Arch Dis Child. 1999;80:581.
12. Jaffe A, Balfour-Lynn IM. Management of empyema in children. Pediatr Pulmonol. 2005;40(2):148-56.
13. Jaffe A, Calder AD, Owens CM, Stanojevic S, Sonnappa S. Role of routine computed tomography in paediatric pleural empyema. Thorax. 2008;63(10):897-902.
14. Jaffé A, Cohen G. Thoracic empyema. Arch Dis Child. 2003;88:839-41.
15. Merry CM, Bufo AJ, Shah RS, Schropp KP, Lobe TE. Early definitive Intervention by thoracoscopy in pediatric empyema. J Pediatr Surg. 1999;34:178-80.
16. Mitri RK, Brown SD, Zurakowski D, Chung KY, Konez O, Burrows PE, et al. Outcomes of primary image-guided drainage of parapneumonic effusions in children. Pediatrics. 2002;110:e37.
17. Pierrepoint MJ, Evans A, Morris SJ, Harrison SK, Doull IJ. Pigtail catheter drain in the treatment of empyema thoracis. Arch Dis Child. 2002;87:331-2.
18. Satish B, Bunker M, Seddon P. Management of thoracic empyema in childhood: does the pleural thickening matter? Arch Dis Child. 2003;88:918-21.
19. Shoseyov D, Bibi H, Shatzberg G, Klar A, Akerman J, Hurvitz H, et al. Short-term course and outcome of treatments of pleural empyema in pediatric patients: repeated ultrasound guided needle thoracocentesis vs. chest tube drainage. Chest. 2002;121:836-40.
20. Singh M, Singh SK, Chowdhary SK. Management of empyema thoracic in children. Indian Pediatrics. 2002;39:145-57.
21. Sonnappa S, Cohen G, Owens CM, van Doorn C, Cairns J, Stanojevic S, et al. Comparison of urokinase and video-assisted thoracoscopic surgery for treatment of childhood empyema. Am J Respir Crit Care Med. 2006;174(2):221-7.
22. Sonnappa S, Jaffe A. Treatment approaches for empyema in children. Paediatr Respir Rev. 2007;8:164-70.
23. Spencer D. Empyema thoracis: not time to put down the knife. Arch Dis Child. 2003;88:842-3.
24. Subramaniam R, Joseph VT, Tan GM, Goh A, Chay OM. Experience with video- assisted thoracoscopic surgery in the management of complicated pneumonia in children. J Pediatr Surg. 2001;36:316-9.
25. Yim AP, Wan S, Lee TW, Arifi AA. VATS lobectomy reduces cytokine responses compared with conventional surgery. Ann Thorac Surg. 2000;70:243-7.
26. Wiese AD, Griffin MR, Zhu Y, Mitchel EF Jr, Grijalva CG. Changes in empyema among U.S. children in the pneumococcal conjugate vaccine era. Vaccine. 2016;34(50): 6243-9.
27. Yue F, Yang Z, Yang F, Liu Y, Zhao L, Chen Z, et al. Clinical observation of bronchoscopy alveolar lavage combined with thoracoscopy in the treatment of empyema in children. Medicine (Baltimore). 2019;98(52):e18528.

Evaluation of Acute Abdominal Pain in Children

Amar Shah, Anirudh Shah

INTRODUCTION

Acute abdominal pain is one of the most common reasons for the child visiting a pediatrician or a pediatric surgeon. It poses a diagnostic challenge owing to the nonspecific nature of symptoms, difficulty in the assessment, and physical examination. The history, physical examination, laboratory tests, and imaging studies should initially be directed at differentiating surgical versus nonsurgical conditions; both categorized as urgent versus nonurgent. The goal of every clinician is to identify children who have uncommon or potentially life-threatening conditions so that appropriate treatment can be initiated without any diagnostic delays. An accurate and timely diagnosis is the key to preventing significant morbidity and mortality.

Acute abdominal pain in some children may sometimes be so elusive that it may cause for it being labeled as functional or psychogenic. However, it needs to be emphasized that labeling of pain as psychogenic should be an opinion of exhaustive exclusion rather than a default assumption.

TERMINOLOGY

- Acute abdominal pain is defined as pain of a nontraumatic origin with a maximum duration of 5 days.
- Acute abdomen is defined as onset of sudden and severe abdominal pain due to some intra-abdominal or extra-abdominal pathology and often requires surgical intervention.

TYPES OF ABDOMINAL PAIN

- Visceral
- Parietal
- Referred

PATHOPHYSIOLOGY

- *Visceral pain:*
  - *Innervation:* Sympathetic autonomic nervous system ending in T6-T12 and L1-L2 segments of the spinal cord
  - *Character:* Results from stimulation of a viscous such as distention, ischemia, squeezing, or torsion. It is dull, cramping, poorly localized, and experienced in the midline. It is insensitive to heat, cutting, or electrical shock.
  - *Localization:* Pain arising from the foregut structures (from oropharynx to second part of duodenum including liver, biliary tree, pancreas, and spleen) is felt in the epigastrium. Pain from the midgut structures (from second part of duodenum to proximal two-thirds of the transverse colon) is felt in the umbilical area. Pain from the hindgut structures (from distal one-third of transverse colon to the anal canal above the dentate line, genitourinary organs) is felt in the hypogastrium.
- *Parietal pain:*
  - *Innervation:* Somatic nerve distribution (T7–L2 and umbilicus at T10). Exception is the diaphragm (C3–C5). It is sensitive to mechanical stimuli (stretching, pinprick, and pinch), heat, electrical shock, and chemical stimulus.
  - *Character:* Results from infection/inflammation of the parietal peritoneum. It is sharp, discrete, and localized. It aggravates on coughing and movements.
  - *Localization:* This pain is due to irritation of the parietal peritoneum and is well localized to the site of the organ, e.g., right iliac fossa pain of late appendicitis. The peritoneum has a higher number of sensitive nerve fibers and so the pain is generally more severe and easier to localize.

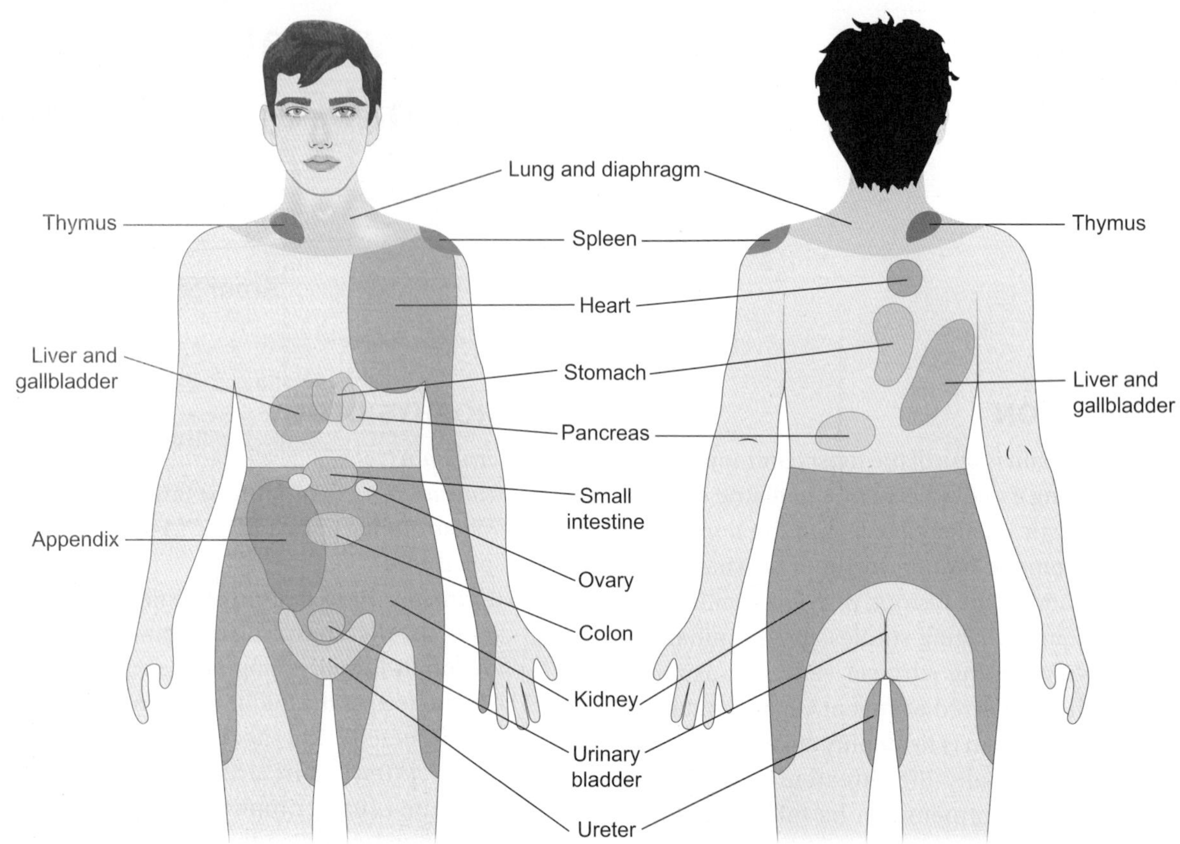

Fig. 1: Common location for referred pain.

- *Referred pain:*
  - *Innervation:* Results from convergence of nerve fibers at the spinal cord
  - *Character:* The characteristics are the same as parietal pain, but it is felt in remote areas. It produces symptoms and not signs, e.g., tenderness.
  - *Localization:* Localized to the dermatome above the site of the stimulus (e.g., abdominal pain due to supra diaphragmatic irritation of the pleura due to lobar pneumonia) **(Fig. 1)**

EVALUATION OF A CHILD WITH ABDOMINAL PAIN

Approach to abdominal pain comprises a thorough history, physical examination and often laboratory tests, and/or imaging studies.

History

History is obtained keeping in mind three components—(1) pain itself; (2) associated symptoms; and (3) predisposing conditions.

1. *Pain:* A classic PQRST mnemonic has been suggested to obtain a thorough pain history.
   - P3—*P*ositional, *P*alliating, and *P*rovoking factors for pain
   - Q—*Q*uality of pain
   - R3—*R*egion, *R*adiation, and *R*eferral of pain
   - S—*S*everity of pain
   - T—*T*emporal factors (such as time and mode of onset of pain, its progression and previous episodes)

   Key questions while evaluating abdominal pain: Location, character, onset, intensity, radiation, aggravating and relieving factors, progress, and past episodes

   Progress of pain (intensity/time) ***(Figs. 2A to C)****:*
   - *Neonates and infants:* Excessive crying, transient apneic spells and grunting
   - *Preadolescents:* They have a poor sense of onset or location of pain. Children who cannot verbalize may present in the second stage of visceral pain.
2. Associated symptoms **(Table 1)**
3. Predisposing conditions **(Table 2)**

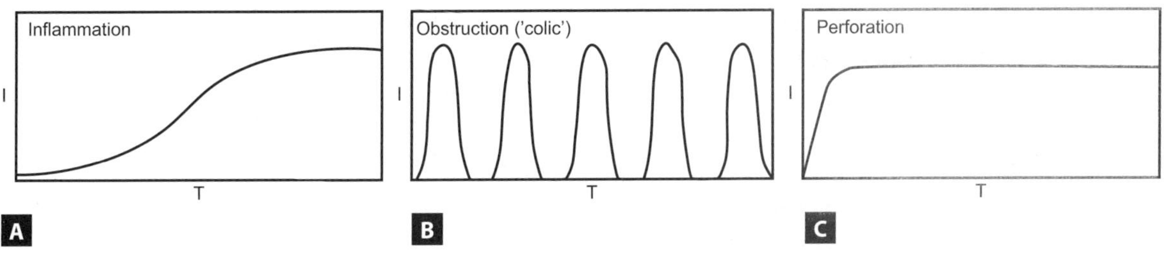

Figs. 2A to C: Progress of pain (I—Intensity, T—Time)

TABLE 1: Associated symptoms with possible cause of acute abdominal pain in children.

Associated symptoms		***Possible cause of abdominal pain***
Vomiting	Before onset of pain	Medical cause likely
	After onset of pain	Surgical cause likely, e.g., appendicitis/intestinal obstruction
	Bilious	Surgical cause likely, e.g., intestinal obstruction
	Nonbilious	Either medical condition (gastritis/hepatitis, etc.) or early surgical cause
Abdominal distension	After excessive crying especially in a small child	Aerophagia
	With acute constipation	Surgical cause likely, e.g., intestinal obstruction
	Upper abdominal distension	Upper abdominal obstruction likely
	With diarrhea	Severe watery—possibly enterocolitis Persistent but small quantity—possibly peritonitis
Constipation	Absolute (feces + flatus)	Intestinal obstruction
	Passing more flatus	Aerophagia (possibly supradiaphragmatic cause)
Fever	Following 1 or 2 days of abdominal pain	Surgical cause likely, e.g., appendicitis/peritonitis, etc.
	Precedes abdominal pain	Inflammatory cause likely, e.g., enterocolitis
Loose motions	If feculent	Enterocolitis
	Mainly mucus/blood	Intussusception/peritonitis/high intestinal obstruction
Dysuria	Abnormal ultrasonography	May be renal colic urinary tract infection (UTI)
	Normal ultrasonography	Maybe appendicitis especially if pain is right sided, UTI
Gait	Walking with stoop on one side	Appendicitis/psoas irritation
Abdominal movements	Restricted	? Peritonitis
Cough/shortness of breath	—	Pleural pathology
Joint pains/purpura	—	? Henoch–Schönlein purpura

TABLE 2: Predisposing conditions which may be a cause of acute abdominal pain.

Predisposing/underlying conditions	***Causes of acute abdominal pain***
Hirschsprung's disease, cystic fibrosis	Enterocolitis
Nephrotic syndrome, liver disease, Ventriculoperitoneal shunt, splenectomy	Primary bacterial peritonitis
Chemotherapy, immunosuppressants	Pancreatitis
Inflammatory bowel disease, immunocompromised patient	Toxic Megacolon
Sickle cell disease	Vaso occlusive crisis

CHALLENGES OF INTERPRETATION OF ABDOMINAL PAIN IN A CHILD

The presence or persistence of pain in children is consistently underestimated by parents and professionals alike, largely because of the young child's inability to voice his symptoms adequately and partly because of the unrealistic expectation that pain must of dramatic severity before it can have any surgical significance. The pain of an unobstructive appendicitis is usually undramatic and a child may even rupture a gangrenous appendix during play. Children may provide exceptions to the classic descriptions of specific sites on the anterior abdominal wall to which pain from particular viscera is referred. Pain arising in the kidney or ureter may be referred to the midline or even to the opposite site, whereas pain of appendicitis is often felt to commence not in the midline but directly over the appendix itself. Contradictory or misleading answers are often given by children to the standard questions beloved of medical writers or examiners concerning the quality, periodicity, and radiation of the pain. In a young child, the observation of unnatural immobility or of sudden spasms even during sleep are more helpful than questioning in determining the persistence of pain. It is of greater practical importance to establish whether pain is still present, becoming worse or subsiding. If the pain is present, observation must be continued and reexamination repeated until there are definite signs which indicate surgical intervention or until the pain has subsided.

The age- and system-wise classification of different conditions that may cause acute abdominal pain in children are listed below **(Tables 3 and 4)**.

PHYSICAL EXAMINATION

General Examination

The physical examination of a child with acute abdominal pain should begin with an overall assessment of the

TABLE 3: Age-wise classification of conditions causing acute abdominal pain in children.

Age	***Surgical conditions***	***Medical conditions***
Neonates and infants	• Incarcerated inguinal hernia • Malrotation and volvulus • Intestinal obstruction • Intussusception • Hypertrophic pyloric stenosis • Hirschsprung's disease	• Infantile colic • Gastroenteritis • Urinary tract infection • GERD • Constipation • Sepsis
Children	• Appendicitis • Malrotation and volvulus • Intussusception • Meckel's diverticulum • Hirschsprung's disease • Trauma	• Diabetic ketoacidosis • Ureteric colic • Pancreatitis • Pneumonitis • Tonsillitis • Gastroenteritis • Hepatitis • UTI • Constipation • Mesenteric lymphadenitis • Viral infective gastroenteritis/colitis
Adolescents	• Appendicitis • Cholecystitis • Testicular/ovarian torsion • Small bowel obstruction • Obstructed inguinal hernia • Pancreatitis • Ectopic pregnancy	• Diabetic ketoacidosis • Pancreatitis • Constipation • Gastroenteritis • Inflammatory bowel disease • Pneumonitis • Hepatitis • UTI • Pelvic inflammatory disease

(GERD: gastroesophageal reflux disease; UTI: urinary tract infection)

TABLE 4: System-wise classification of conditions causing acute abdominal pain in children.

System	*Conditions*
Gastrointestinal	Appendicitis, abdominal trauma, obstructed hernia, intussusception, volvulus, Meckel's diverticulum, necrotizing enterocolitis, bowel perforation, inflammatory bowel disease, gastroenteritis, constipation, mesenteric lymphadenitis, and peritonitis
Genitourinary	Urinary tract infection, nephrolithiasis, ovarian/testicular torsion, dysmenorrhea, pelvic inflammatory disease, and ectopic pregnancy
Hepatobiliary, spleen, and pancreas	Hepatitis, liver abscess, cholecystitis, cholelithiasis, splenic abscess/infarct, and pancreatitis
Cardiac	Myocarditis, pericarditis, endocarditis, and congestive heart failure
Metabolic	Diabetic ketoacidosis, hypoglycemia, acute adrenal insufficiency, and acute porphyria
Pulmonary	Lower lobe pneumonia, pneumothorax, and diaphragmatic pleurisy
Neurology	Abdominal epilepsy, abdominal migraine, herpes zoster, and nerve root compression
Hematology	Sickle cell anemia, hemolytic uremic syndrome, acute leukemia, Henoch-Schönlein purpura, and vaso-occlusive crisis
Drugs and toxins	Lead poisoning, venoms, erythromycin, and salicylates
Miscellaneous	Infantile colic, pharyngitis, functional pain, and angioneurotic edema

child's appearance (interactive, lethargic, establishes eye contact, and comforted by a family member), hydration status, activity level, and vital signs. Children with peritoneal irritation remain still or resist movement, while children with visceral pain change position frequently, often writhing with discomfort. Fever suggests infection; however, its absence does not rule it out, especially in patients who are immunocompromised. High fever with chills is typical of pyelonephritis and pneumonia. Tachycardia and hypotension suggest hypovolemia. If a postmenarcheal girl is in shock, ectopic pregnancy or toxic shock syndrome should be suspected. Hypertension may be associated with renal disease, Henoch–Schönlein purpura (HSP), or hemolytic-uremic syndrome. Deep labored respiration may indicate diabetic ketoacidosis. Infections in the ear, tonsils, and respiratory passages may be accompanied by abdominal pain and vomiting. The enanthem of measles or chicken pox may also produce abdominal signs.

Abdominal Examination

A young child is best examined in a parent's arms or lap. Abdominal examination should be performed gently with careful hands-off inspection being the first step. Distracting the child while palpating the abdomen is very helpful. Palpation should gradually proceed toward the area of maximal tenderness. A more urgent surgical diagnosis is likely if there is distension, peritoneal signs, and abnormal bowel sounds. Abdominal distension may be absent in patients with gastric outlet or proximal small bowel obstructions. It may also happen in patients who have recently vomited as they may decompress the gastrointestinal tract proximal to the obstruction.

Peritoneal signs including localized tenderness, rebound tenderness, and involuntary or voluntary guarding are indicative of an acute surgical abdomen. The presence of these features demands careful evaluation, surgical consultation, hospitalization, and repeated active observation. It is suggested that positive palpatory findings such as rigidity and guarding are helpful diagnostic indicators for surgical conditions, whereas negative palpatory findings have little value in excluding surgical conditions entirely **(Figs. 3 and 4)**.

Examination of the groins and genitals is mandatory for any child with acute abdominal pain. By doing so, additional surgical conditions such as incarcerated hernia and testicular torsions that need immediate attention can be uncovered. Diagnostic delay in such conditions can result in significant morbidity **(Figs. 5 and 6)**.

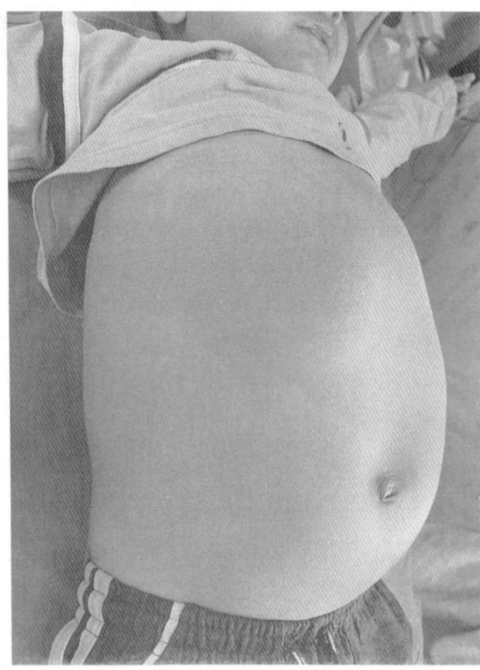

Fig. 3: Generalized abdominal distention with visible dilated bowel loops—intestinal obstruction. *(For color version, see Plate 11)*

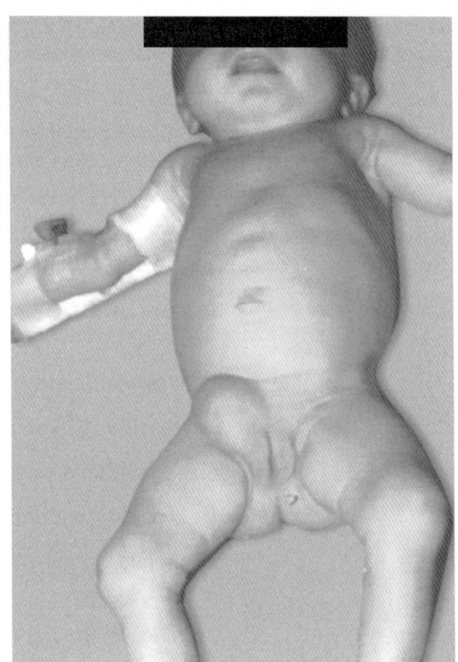

Fig. 5: Incarcerated right inguinal hernia causing intestinal obstruction. *(For color version, see Plate 11)*

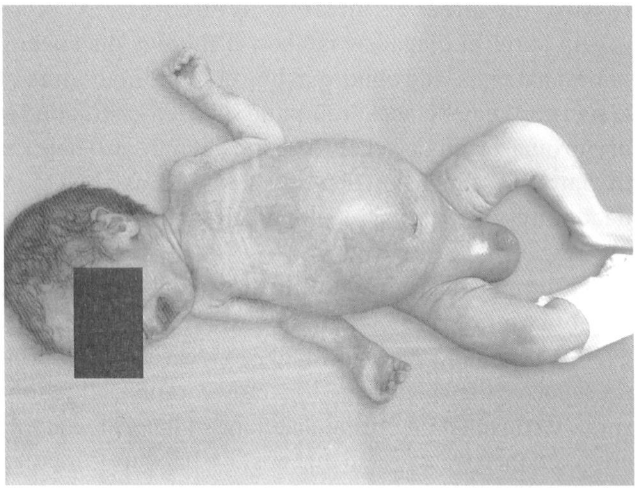

Fig. 4: Distended shiny abdomen—peritonitis. *(For color version, see Plate 11)*

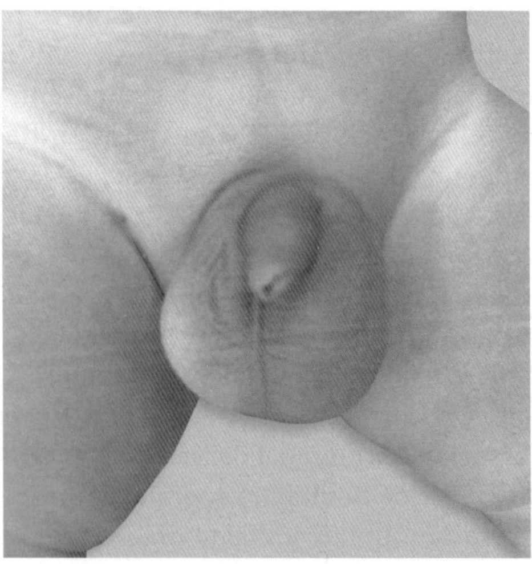

Fig. 6: Acute left scrotum (tender and red scrotum on the left)—left testicular torsion. *(For color version, see Plate 11)*

Rectal examination may be necessary to identify a perianal lesion, rectal polyp, presacral mass, blood in the stool, and possibly help for fecal disimpaction. However, routine rectal examination is of little value for diagnosing appendicitis, peritonitis, or small bowel obstruction.

INVESTIGATIONS

Laboratory Testing

It is important to be aware that there are no laboratory tests that sufficiently differentiate between surgical and nonsurgical conditions and more definitive testing should not be delayed while awaiting routine test results. Although a complete blood count (CBC) is appropriate if a serious infection or blood loss is suspected, CBC, erythrocyte sedimentation rate (ESR), or C-reactive protein (CRP) alone do not appear to differentiate between urgent and nonurgent diseases. Leukocytosis alone is not predictive of a surgical disease as the white blood cell (WBC) count lacks sufficient sensitivity or specificity to be a good predictor of an acute surgical abdomen. Clinical predictive tools for diagnosis of acute appendicitis such as the Pediatric Appendicitis Score and Alvarado score use leukocytosis and elevated polymorphonuclear cells >75% as parameters in order to reduce uncertainty and improve diagnostic accuracy. However, neither meet the current performance requirements. When a clinically nonurgent condition is suspected but the CRP is above 100 mg/L or the WBC count is above 15×10^9/L, the possibility of an urgent surgical condition should be reconsidered, and additional imaging may be warranted. While in general laboratory tests do not sufficiently differentiate between surgical and nonsurgical cases, they may be helpful in identifying associated morbidity. For example, in the setting of a possible bowel obstruction, electrolytes should be obtained as acidosis may indicate impending decompensation or sepsis. Also, laboratory tests may be helpful in identifying urgent medical conditions that may mimic surgical diseases such as severe pancreatitis or pyelonephritis. A urinalysis should be obtained in all patients with hematuria, dysuria, or flank pain. In absence of any other source of fever, a urinary tract infection is most likely in any febrile female patient or in a patient younger than 6 months old with a WBC count >15,000/mm^3. A blood glucose check is recommended if acute abdominal pain is associated with polyuria or polydipsia or with changes in sensorium to rule out diabetic ketoacidosis, an urgent medical condition. In cases of right upper quadrant pain with jaundice, signs of chronic liver disease (e.g., spider angiomas) or changes in mental status, a prompt chemistry panel, albumin, and liver function tests should be obtained. Obtaining laboratory tests for clinical suspicion of acute cholecystitis is not indicated because there are no clinical findings or laboratory tests sufficient to establish or exclude cholecystitis without further imaging.

In summary, laboratory tests can narrow a differential diagnosis or can help confirm or exclude the clinical suspicion of a disease process. However, they can be confounding if factors are not adequate to differentiate surgical from nonsurgical conditions. Therefore, it is suggested that laboratory testing should generally be obtained to answer a focused clinical question.

Imaging

The accuracy of clinical evaluation is often insufficient for arriving at a correct and specific diagnosis and the clinician may have to resort to additional imaging modalities for diagnostic certainty.

- *X-rays:* Abdominal X-rays are not routinely helpful for evaluation of a child with acute abdominal pain. However, when the child has abdominal distention, signs of peritonitis, and bilious vomiting or has a history of previous surgery, abdominal X-rays may help to diagnose intestinal obstruction or intestinal perforation. Plain X-rays may also help to identify radio-opaque objects such as a renal, ureteric or bladder calculus, an ingested foreign body or even severe constipation **(Figs. 7 and 8)**.

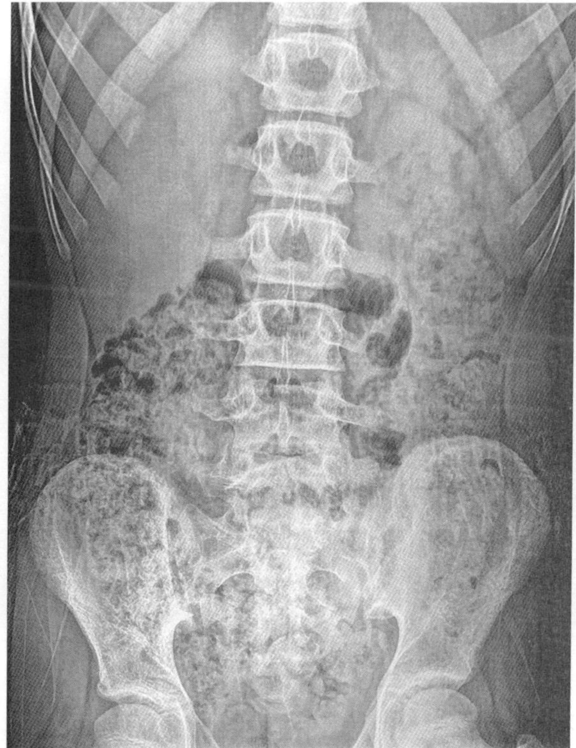

Fig. 7: X-ray abdomen showing severe constipation.

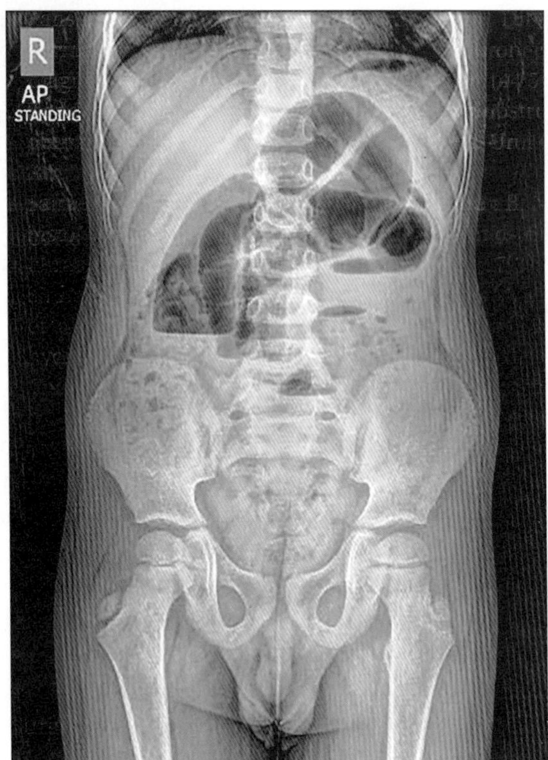

Fig. 8: X-ray abdomen showing intestinal obstruction.

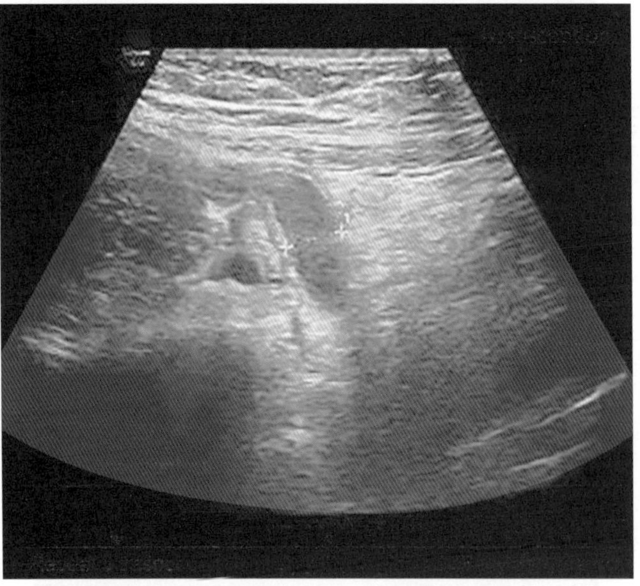

Fig. 9: Ultrasound scan showing acute appendicitis.

- *Ultrasound scan:* Ultrasound scan is the preferred initial imaging in children with acute abdominal pain. It has a sensitivity of 90–96%, specificity of 94–96%, and accuracy of 94% in diagnosing acute appendicitis in pediatric patients **(Fig. 9)**. It is the imaging of choice for children for suspected acute conditions such as pancreatitis, cholecystitis, ovarian cyst, ovarian torsion, and intussusception **(Figs. 10 to 12)**. However, the accuracy varies depending upon the experience of the radiologist and other factors such as obesity and bowel distention.

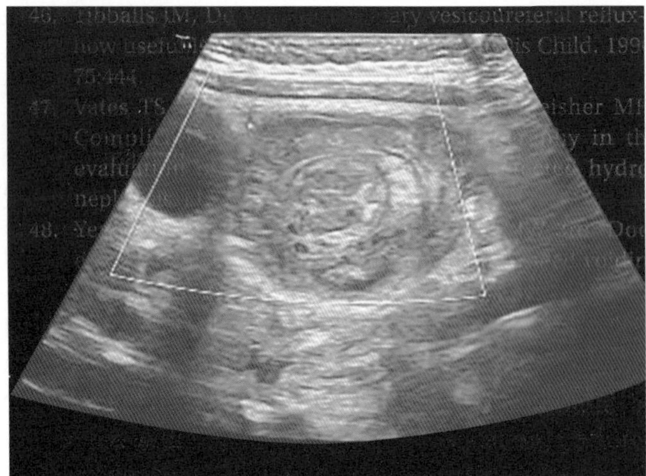

Fig. 10: Ultrasound scan showing intussusception.

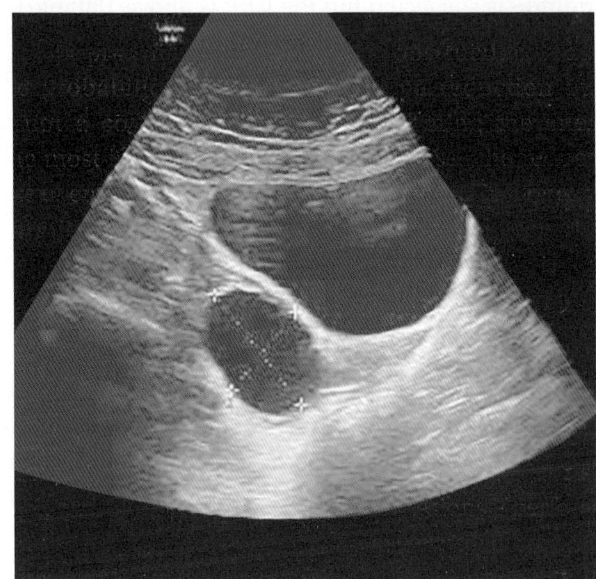

Fig. 11: Ultrasound scan showing ovarian cyst.

- *Computed tomography (CT):* CT is the most sensitive imaging investigation for detecting urgent conditions in children with acute abdominal pain. However, ultrasound remains the primary investigation of choice and only in critically ill patients CT scan may

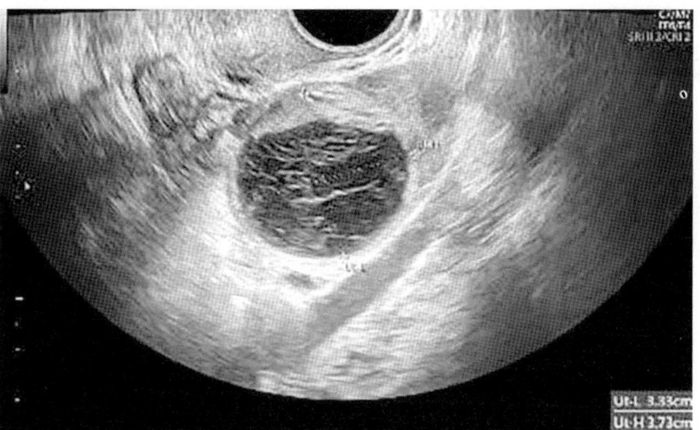

Fig. 12: Ultrasound scan showing a hemorrhagic ovarian cyst.

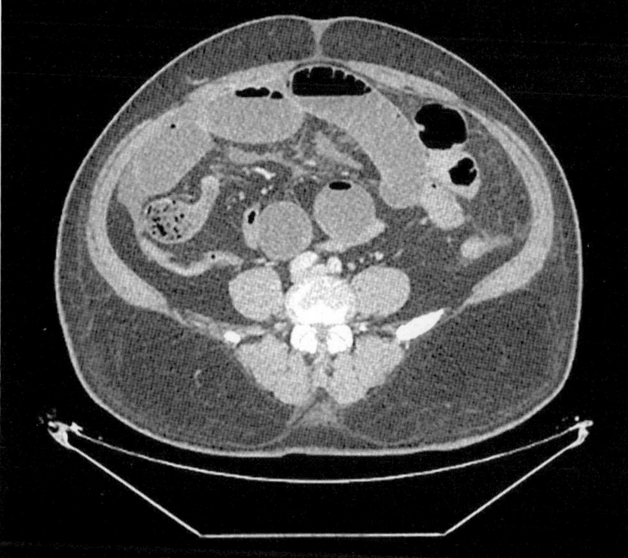

Fig. 13: CT scan abdomen showing intestinal obstruction.

be performed without a prior ultrasound. Because of radiation exposure, routine use of CT scan for suspected appendicitis or similar intra-abdominal pathologies should be discouraged until ultrasound is inconclusive or negative in children with a strong clinical suspicion **(Fig. 13)**.

- *Magnetic resonance imaging (MRI):* MRI would be an ideal imaging tool for diagnosis of acute abdominal pain in children because of no radiation exposure and high sensitivity and specificity for many intra-abdominal pathologies. It also carries an advantage that no administration of contrast media is mandatory. The disadvantages are that it is time consuming, expensive, may require sedation in children and lacks ease of availability **(Table 5)**.

TABLE 5: Investigations for suspected nonurgent problems of acute abdominal pain.

Symptoms	***Work up***
Upper abdominal pain ± vomiting	*Serology:* CBC, liver function tests, S. Amylase, S. lipase *Imaging:* Ultrasound abdomen
Periumbilical pain	*Serology:* CBC, electrolytes, RBS, and urine examination *Imaging:* Ultrasound abdomen
Lower abdominal pain	*Serology:* CBC, ESR, CRP, and urine examination *Imaging:* Ultrasound abdomen
Flank pain	*Serology:* CBC, urine examination, and urine culture *Imaging:* Ultrasound abdomen
Genital or scrotal pain/vaginal discharge	*Serology:* CBC and urine examination *Imaging:* Ultrasound abdomen
Hematemesis	*Serology:* CBC, Liver function tests, S. Amylase, and S. Lipase *Imaging:* Ultrasound abdomen
Hematochezia	*Serology:* CBC, ESR, CRP, BUN, S. creatinine, stool calprotectin, and stool culture *Imaging:* Ultrasound abdomen
Hematuria	*Serology:* CBC, urine examination, and urine culture *Imaging:* Ultrasound abdomen ± CT scan abdomen
Polyuria	*Serology:* S. electrolytes, RBS, and urine examination
Failure to thrive or weight loss	*Serology:* CBC, ESR, CRP, stool calprotectin, and celiac serology
Diarrhea	Stool examination

(CBC: complete blood count; CRP: C-reactive protein; CT: computed tomography; ESR: erythrocyte sedimentation rate; RBS: random blood sugar)

MANAGEMENT

Treatment of the child should be directed at the underlying cause when it can be identified. While the treatment of each specific condition is beyond the scope of the current chapter, some general points need to be highlighted **(Flowchart 1)**.

In patients with a high suspicion of a surgical condition, urgent consultation with a pediatric surgeon is mandated while the patient is getting stabilized with adequate hydration and pain control. If an acute surgical or medical condition has been satisfactorily excluded, the child can

Flowchart 1: Management of acute abdominal pain.

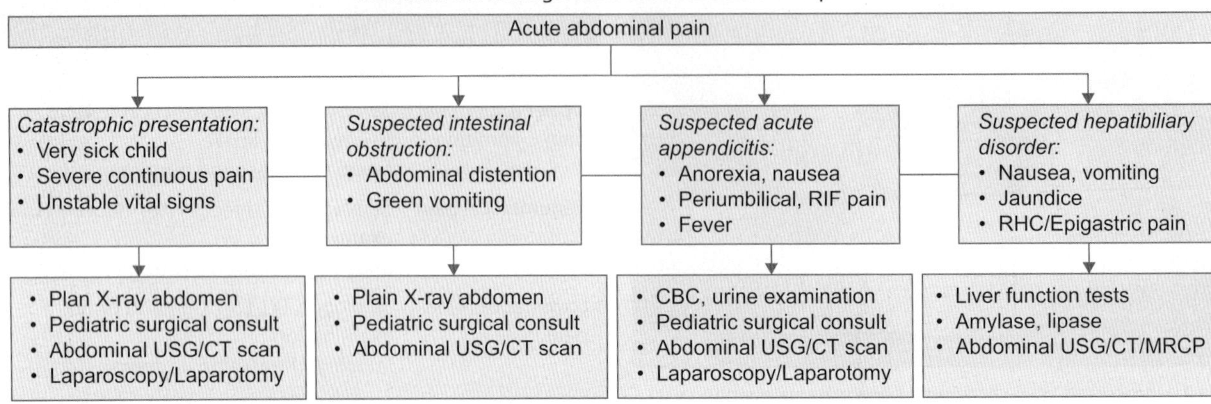

(CT: computed tomography; MRCP: magnetic resonance cholangiopancreatography; USG: ultrasonography)

TABLE 6: Criteria for hospitalization in children with acute abdominal pain.

Indication for hospitalization	*Indication for follow-up*
• Intractable nausea, vomiting, abdominal pain • Appears ill with unclear diagnosis • Intolerable oral intake • Abnormal vital signs • Abnormal physical examination (signs of peritonitis) • Immunocompromised • Poor social support/home care	• Asymptomatic • No abnormal clinical features • Normal vital signs • Tolerate oral intake • Adequate social support/ home care

be discharged if in a stable condition. In case of any doubt, the child should be hospitalized for clinical evaluation, reevaluation, and further investigations if necessary.

Pediatric patients in general are at risk for receiving less than optimal analgesia as clinicians are often concerned that strong analgesia may mask the symptoms and result in complications and increased morbidity. Several prospective randomized studies have shown that judicious use of analgesia may enhance diagnostic accuracy by permitting a more thorough physical examination. As a general rule, adequate pain control should be a therapeutic goal, and this appears safe especially if there is need for a frequent reevaluation of the patient's condition.

In patients identified as having nonurgent medical conditions, initial empiric therapy based on symptoms may be initiated in the absence of an established diagnosis. Close follow-up and reevaluation of response are required in all patients treated symptomatically **(Table 6)**.

KEY POINTS

- Acute abdominal pain can be a diagnostic challenge due to its nonspecific symptoms.
- Diagnosis involves differentiating surgical versus nonsurgical conditions with the goal to identify life-threatening conditions early to prevent morbidity and mortality.
- Pain may be subtle, and children may not clearly identify its origin. Unnatural immobility or sudden spasms are key signs in younger children.
- Pain should not be prematurely labeled as psychogenic; exhaustive exclusion is essential before this assumption.
- Accurate diagnosis of acute abdominal pain in children requires a structured approach, including detailed history, thorough physical examination, and selective use of investigations.
- Examination of the groins and genitals is mandatory for any child with acute abdominal pain.
- Management should be tailored to the underlying cause, with particular attention to urgent surgical conditions and appropriate pain control.

SUGGESTED READING

1. Böhner H, Yang Q, Franke C, Verreet PR, Ohmann C. Simple data from history and physical examination help to exclude bowel obstruction and to avoid radiographic studies in patients with acute abdominal pain. Eur J Surg. 1998;164(10):777-84.
2. Carty HM. Paediatric emergencies: non-traumatic abdominal emergencies. Eur Radiol. 2002;12(12):2835-48.
3. Couture E, Labbé V, Cyr C. Clinical predictors of positive urine cultures in young children at risk for urinary tract infection. Paediatr Child Health. 2003;8(3):145-9.
4. Davies AH, Mastorakou I, Cobb R, Rogers C, Lindsell D, Mortensen NJ. Ultrasonography in the acute abdomen. Br J Surg. 1991;78(10):1178-80.

5. Gans SL, Atema JJ, Stoker J, Toorenvliet BR, Laurell H, Boermeester MA. C-reactive protein and white blood cell count as triage test between urgent and nonurgent conditions in 2961 patients with acute abdominal pain. Medicine (Baltimore). 2015;94(9):e569.
6. Gans SL, Pols MA, Stoker J, Boermeester MA; expert steering group. Guideline for the diagnostic pathway in patients with acute abdominal pain. Dig Surg. 2015;32(1):23-31.
7. Hayes R. Abdominal pain: general imaging strategies. Eur Radiol. 2004;14(Suppl 4):L123-37.
8. Hijaz NM, Friesen CA. Managing acute abdominal pain in pediatric patients: current perspectives. Pediatric Health Med Ther. 2017;8:83-91.
9. Kulik DM, Uleryk EM, Maguire JL. Does this child have appendicitis? A systematic review of clinical prediction rules for children with acute abdominal pain. J Clin Epidemiol. 2013;66(1):95-104.
10. Laméris W, van Randen A, van Es HW, van Heesewijk JP, van Ramshorst B, Bouma WH, et al. Imaging strategies for detection of urgent conditions in patients with acute abdominal pain: diagnostic accuracy study. BMJ. 2009;338:b2431.
11. Laurell H, Hansson LE, Gunnarsson U. Diagnostic pitfalls and accuracy of diagnosis in acute abdominal pain. Scand J Gastroenterol. 2006;41(10):1126-31.
12. Leung AK, Robson WL. Urinary tract infection in infancy and childhood. Adv Pediatr. 1991;38:257-85.
13. Macaluso CR, McNamara RM. Evaluation and management of acute abdominal pain in the emergency department. Int J Gen Med. 2012;5:789-97.
14. Manterola C, Vial M, Moraga J, Astudillo P. Analgesia in patients with acute abdominal pain. Cochrane Database Syst Rev. 2011;(1):CD005660.
15. Moll van Charante E, de Jongh TO. Onderzoek bij patiënten met een acute buik [Physical examination of patients with acute abdominal pain]. Ned Tijdschr Geneeskd. 2011;155:A2658.
16. Nauta RJ, Magnant C. Observation versus operation for abdominal pain in the right lower quadrant. Roles of the clinical examination and the leukocyte count. Am J Surg. 1986;151(6):746-8.
17. Nosaka S, Hayakawa M, Miyazaki O, Kawaguchi H, Watanabe T, Tani I, et al. Ultrasonography of pediatric right lower abdominal pain: correlation with clinical and pathological results. Nihon Igaku Hoshasen Gakkai Zasshi. 1995;55(12):855-60.
18. Patrick GL, Stewart RJ, Isbister WH. Patients with acute abdominal pain: white cell and neutrophil counts as predictors of the surgical acute abdomen. N Z Med J. 1985;98(778):324-6.
19. Poonai N, Paskar D, Konrad SL, Rieder M, Joubert G, Lim R, et al. Opioid analgesia for acute abdominal pain in children: a systematic review and meta-analysis. Academic Emerg Med. 2014;21(11):1183-92.
20. Rothrock SG, Green SM, Hummel CB. Plain abdominal radiography in the detection of major disease in children: a prospective analysis. Ann Emerg Med. 1992;21(12): 1423-9.
21. Saito JM. Beyond appendicitis: evaluation and surgical treatment of pediatric acute abdominal pain. Curr Opin Pediatr. 2012;24(3):357-64.
22. Shaikh N, Morone NE, Lopez J, et al. Does this child have a urinary tract infection? JAMA. 2007;298(24):2895-904.
23. Toorenvliet BR, Bakker RF, Flu HC, Merkus JW, Hamming JF, Breslau PJ. Standard outpatient re-evaluation for patients not admitted to the hospital after emergency department evaluation for acute abdominal pain. World J Surg. 2010;34(3):480-6.
24. Trowbridge RL, Rutkowski NK, Shojania KG. Does this patient have acute cholecystitis? JAMA. 2003;289(1):80-6.
25. Wang PY, Chang HC, Lei RL, Kao JK, Wu CL, Lee CH, et al. Personal History and Physical Examination in judgment of urinary tract infection in children aged 3 months to 2 years. Pediatr Neonatol. 2016;57(4):274-9.

Management of Undescended Testis: Cryptorchidism

Rasiklal S Shah, Suyodhan A Reddy, Manika Boipai

INTRODUCTION

Undescended testis (UDT) or cryptorchidism is the most common congenital abnormality of the genitourinary tract. It comprises of true cryptorchid or UDT, ectopic testis, absent testis, atrophic testis, retractile testis, and ascended testis. It is important to differentiate the aforementioned conditions, as their individual management is different.

TERMINOLOGY

- *Cryptorchidism:* Cryptorchidism, by definition, means absence of one or both testis in the scrotum.
- *True UDT:* The testis, which has failed to descend along its normal pathway from the retroperitoneum to the scrotum, is known as true UDT. If the testis remains in abdominal cavity, then it is known as abdominal UDT; if it comes out of internal ring and goes back to the abdomen, then it is known as emergent UDT; if it is in inguinal canal, then it is known as intracanalicular UDT; if it is just outside the external ring, then it is known as suprascrotal UDT.
- *Ectopic testis:* The testis, which has normally descended from retroperitoneum up to the external ring subsequently gets deviated to an aberrant position, is known as ectopic testis. It may be palpable in the superficial inguinal pouch (most common), suprapubic region, femoral triangle, or perineum. Rarely, testis travels via opposite internal ring into contralateral scrotal compartment and then it is known as transverse testicular ectopia **(Fig. 1)**.
- *Absent testis:* Testis which embryologically has failed to develop is known as absent testis.
- *Atrophic testis:* The testis was developed normally and at some stage, it has undergone atrophy secondary to vascular compromise. If it occurs in the prenatal period, then it is also known as the vanishing testis syndrome or testicular regression syndrome.
- *Retractile testis:* The testis normally descends to the scrotum at birth; however, the hyperactive cremasteric reflex pulls the testis into suprascrotal position. This testis can be manipulated into a dependent scrotal position, by making the patient relax his cremasteric muscle. The testis will remain there as long as the cremasteric muscles are relaxed.
- *Ascended testis:* The testis, which has been documented to be in the scrotum in neonatal period, is found to be at higher position in later childhood and is known as the ascended testicle.
- *Acquired UDT:* It may also be iatrogenic, after inguinal surgery (commonly repair of inguinal hernia), a previously descended testis gets trapped in scar tissue cephalad to the scrotum.
- Congenital Anorchia (also known as vanishing testis syndrome) is a rare condition in which one (monorchia) or both testes are absent in a phenotypically and genotypically normal male.

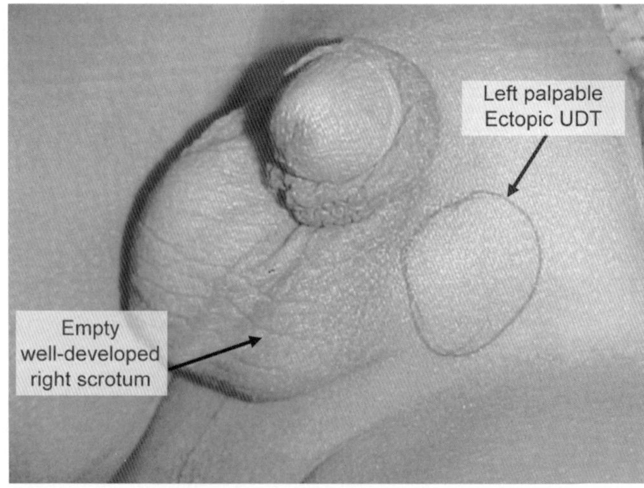

Fig. 1: Left ectopic testis—testis noted to be in ectopic site, different from the normal path of testicular descent. *(For color version, see Plate 11)*

PATHOGENESIS

The factors responsible for normal testicular descent are not well understood. The intra-abdominal phase of descent is thought to be androgen-independent and is mediated by a polypeptide "descending". The testis passes through the inguinal canal in 28th week of gestation; it is believed to be the combined result of interactions between mechanical, hormonal, and neurotransmitters. Changes in abdominal pressure, patency of the processus vaginalis, gubernacular regression, androgens, gonadotropins, Müllerian inhibiting substance (MIS), insulin-like factor 3 (INSL3), and calcitonin gene-related peptide are all thought to play a role.

The pathogenesis of UDT is less understood than that of normal testicular descent. Alterations in any of the factors that contribute to normal testicular descent may theoretically result in UDT. Gonadotropin deficiencies *in utero*, decreased MIS, and increased expression of estradiol in the placenta have been proposed as contributing factors. Cryptorchidism is related to defects in hypothalamic-pituitary-testicular-end organ axis and can be considered as an endocrinopathy.

EPIDEMIOLOGY AND RISK FACTORS

At birth, 2–5% of full-term and 25–30% of premature male infants are born with an UDT. Of these, in approximately 70%, the testis descends spontaneously within first 2–3 months of life and is unlikely to descend after 3 months. At 1 year of age, the prevalence of UDT is around 0.8–1%, which is similar to that in adults.

Maternal risk factors such as advanced maternal age, maternal obesity, breech presentation, and cesarean section have been suggested.

The prevalence of UDT varies geographically, which may be due to genetics or environmental factors. Prematurity, being small for gestational age at birth, and birth weight <2.5 kg are common risk factor. Prenatal exposure to endocrine disruptors (e.g., diethylstilbestrol and pesticides) also has been associated with cryptorchidism in some studies.

The UDT has a familial preponderance, with prevalence of UDT in 4.0% of fathers and 6.2–9.8% of their brothers.

Associated Conditions

Cryptorchidism usually is an isolated finding. However, it may occur in association with endocrine disorders, genetic syndromes, and morphologic abnormalities, especially if it is bilateral. Associated conditions are shown in **Box 1**.

BOX 1: Associated conditions.

- Prune belly syndrome
- Abdominal wall defects—gastroschisis, omphalocele, and bladder exstrophy
- Myelomeningocele
- Cerebral palsy
- Disorders of sexual development
- Genetic disorders with diminished testosterone production:
  - Kallmann syndrome
  - Klinefelter syndrome
  - Prader–Willi syndrome
  - Androgen insensitivity syndrome
- *Genetic disorders:* Noonan's syndrome
- *Primary hypogonadism with increased gonadotropin levels:* Laurence–Moon syndrome
- *Other genetic disorders:* Trisomy 18
- *With no effect on testosterone and gonadotropin levels:*
  - Trisomy 13
  - 22q11.2 deletion syndrome
  - 1p36 deletion syndrome
  - Beckwith–Wiedemann syndrome Smith–Lemli–Opitz syndrome, Cornelia de Lange syndrome, etc.

CLINICAL PEARL

- Patients having UDT and hypospadias have high incidence of underlying disorders of sexual development.

CLINICAL FEATURES

Clinical features of cryptorchidism include an empty, hypoplastic, hypopigmented, and poorly developed rugae of scrotum or hemiscrotum. Inguinal fullness may be present **(Figs. 2 and 3)**.

The first maneuver to locate the testis is to walk the fingers from the iliac crest along the inguinal canal toward the scrotum, pushing subcutaneous structures toward the scrotum. The scrotum should not be palpated prior to this as it may activate the cremasteric reflex, thus retracting the testis.

In approximately 10%, it is a bilateral condition. Bilateral UDT are more commonly associated with other conditions. Unilateral UDT is more common on right side.

The most common location for an UDT is just outside the external ring (superficial inguinal pouch), followed by the inguinal canal (intracanalicular), and finally intra-abdominal. The testis is not palpable in 20% of patients with UDT.

The growth of unilateral UDT is impaired compared with the normally descended contralateral testis, whether it descends spontaneously or it is surgically brought

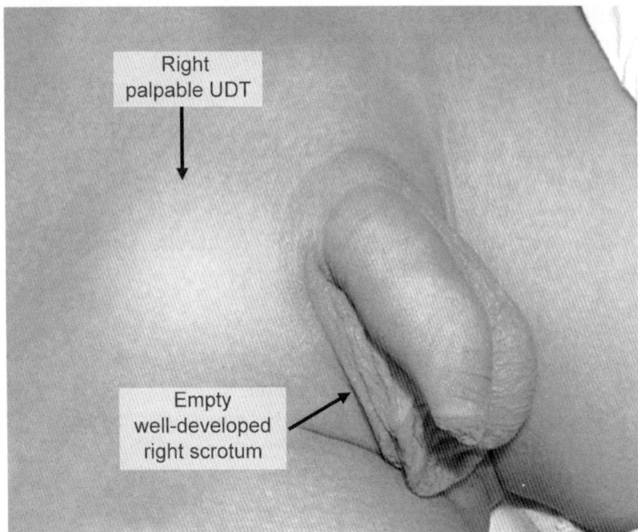

Fig. 2: Right palpable undescended testis—testis palpable in inguinal region and scrotal sac is empty but well developed. *(For color version, see Plate 12)*

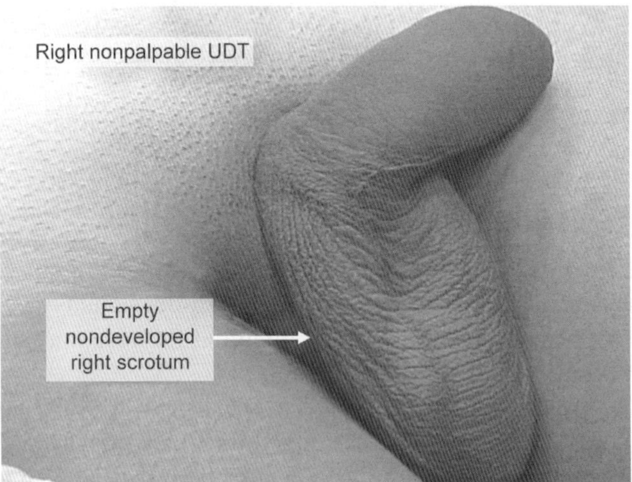

Fig. 3: Right nonpalpable undescended testis—scrotal sac is empty and underdeveloped. Further evaluation is needed to rule out intra-abdominal position, atrophy, or absence of testis. *(For color version, see Plate 12)*

in scrotum. Treatment before 1 year of age is associated with partial catch-up of growth.

COMPLICATIONS AND SEQUELS

Complications and sequels of UDT include inguinal hernia, testicular torsion, testicular trauma, subfertility, and testicular cancer. The potential seriousness of these complications and sequels demands early referral for definitive treatment **(Box 2)**.

BOX 2: Complications and sequels of undescended testes.

- Hernia
- Torsion
- Trauma
- Subfertility
- Testicular cancer with late detection

Inguinal Hernia

The UDTs have an associated patent processus vaginalis in about 60% cases. Inguinal hernia in UDT can present at any age with the typical symptoms or complications, including incarceration.

Testicular Torsion

Testicular torsion is approximately 10 times more common in UDT than in normal scrotal testis, but the true relative risk is not known. The rate of salvage of torsion in cryptorchid testis is decreased compared to that in normally descended testis, perhaps related to delay in diagnosis.

If patient with inguinal testis develops the torsion, then he will present with local swelling and tenderness with an empty ipsilateral hemiscrotum. If patient with intra-abdominal testis develops torsion, then he will present as an acute abdomen with empty one side of scrotum and usually diagnosis of torsion is made only at the time of abdominal exploration.

TESTICULAR TRAUMA

Testis located in the inguinal canal is at increased risk of blunt traumatic injury from compression against the pubic bone.

Subfertility

Men with a history of UDT have lower sperm counts, sperms of poorer quality, and lower fertility rates than men with normally descended testis. Impaired spermatogenesis is probably related to underlying genetic, hormonal, and developmental abnormalities, some of which may be partially reversible through early surgical intervention. Sperm counts in adulthood are directly related to prepubertal germ cell counts and type of cell (gonocyte versus adult dark spermatogonia) at the time of orchidopexy. The local milieu reduces the number of Leydig cells, which produce testosterone. Testosterone plays an important role in maturation of gonocyte to dark adult spermatogonia. This affects both quality and quantity of the mature germ cells in the testis.

The degree of germ cell dysfunction increases with bilateral involvement and with increasing duration of suprascrotal location. Intra-abdominal and intracanalicular UDT are affected similarly, probably related to the damaging effect of higher temperatures outside the scrotum on spermatogenesis.

Elevated serum gonadotropin [follicle stimulating hormone (FSH) and luteinizing hormone (LH)] concentration and decreased serum inhibin B concentration are endocrinologic markers of testicular dysfunction.

Testicular Cancer

Men with a history of UDT have an increased risk of developing testicular cancer compared with men in the general population in whom the age adjusted incidence is approximately 5.4 per 100,000. The epidemiological data points toward a definite relationship between the intrauterine, perinatal development, and UDT.

Seminomas (74%) are commonly seen in intraabdominal testes, whereas malignancies arising after successful orchidopexy, are most frequently nonseminomatous germ cell tumors (63%). In patients with a UDT, the normally descended contralateral testis still carries a possibility of testicular tumors (increased relative risk of 1.7).

The risk of developing testicular cancer is further increased in men with bilateral cryptorchidism (which may be associated with endocrinologic abnormalities or abnormal karyotype) and intra-abdominal UDT.

A history of cryptorchidism is also a risk factor for developing intratubular germ cell neoplasia of unclassified type, a premalignant condition, which is also called carcinoma in situ, or testicular intraepithelial neoplasia.

Surgical repositioning of the testis (orchidopexy) before puberty appears to decrease the risk of testicular cancer, but does not completely eliminate it. Testicular malposition is not the only factor in the development of testicular cancer in men with a history of cryptorchidism because surgical repositioning does not completely eliminate the risk.

CLINICAL PEARL

- Children who have been operated for orchidopexy should be taught self-examination for early detection of testicular carcinoma.

MANAGEMENT (FLOWCHART 1)

The patients of UDT should be worked up for anesthesia fitness preoperatively. Other hormonal investigations are optional and may be performed depending upon

Flowchart 1: An overview of management of undescended testis.

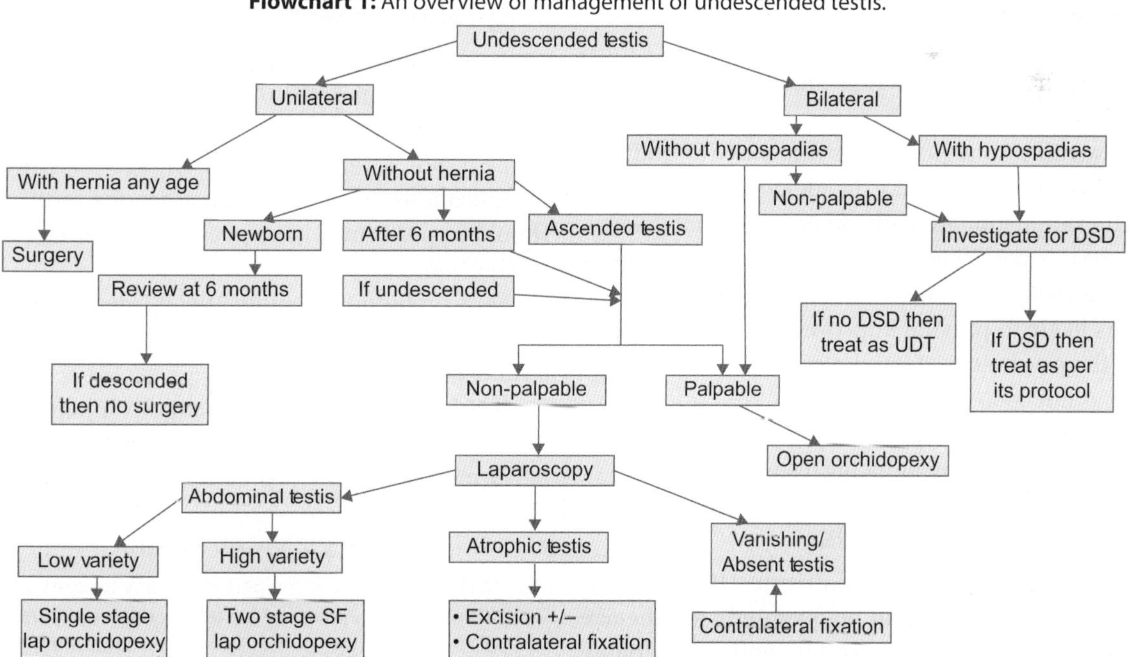

(DSD: disorders of sex differentiation; UDT: Undescended testis)

local institutional policy. However, if the testosterone level does not increase appropriately (in case of hCG stimulation test), exploration should still be performed as nonfunctional testicular tissue may still be present. This test does not distinguish between normal nonpalpable testes and functioning testicular remnants.

Imaging studies for locating testis are not required, as they have limited specificity and sensitivity. The sensitivity of imaging is poor in detection of soft tissue masses <1 cm. MRI with gadolinium may be useful in bilateral nonpalpable testes for detecting abdominal testes because testicular tissue is particularly bright on MRI. However, negative imaging is not confirmatory of testicular absence. In addition, these investigations induce confusion in minds of parents. On imaging, if the testis is not visualized and surgeon recommends surgery, then family start thinking although the testis is not seen and even then, the surgeon still wishes to operate. If the surgeon explains why surgery is essential, then the parents might raise the query that if the surgeon has already decided to operate upon then what was the need to do imaging studies. In order to avoid confusion, it is safer not to order investigations for locating testis.

The goal is to bring the apparently normal looking testis into the scrotum from its abnormal position and to prevent the complications. Treatment is based on the assumption that secondary degeneration of the testes caused by high temperature will be prevented by early intervention. It is essential to pex testes into scrotum to prevent postoperative ascent. Small atrophic testes should be removed.

The testis in scrotal position is less likely to undergo torsion or blunt traumatic injury. In addition, it also permits easier self-examination for early detection of malignancy. If orchidopexy is performed early, it may reduce the risk of infertility and testicular cancer. The testis in normal scrotal position is likely to provide improved body satisfaction, although the psychological impact of abnormal testicular position has not been studied.

Hormonal therapy has been tried in past, but it has not proven to be efficacious in inducing testicular descent.

Bilateral Undescended Testis

If the patients have bilateral palpable UDT without hypospadias, then they should be operated after the age of 6 months. If the patients have bilateral nonpalpable UDT or if UDT is associated with hypospadias, then they should be investigated for disorders of sex differentiation (DSD). If investigations are in line of a normal boy, then the orchidopexy should be performed after the age of 6 months. Authors operate on both sides in the same sitting even when they are nonpalpable **(Fig. 4)**, though some institutes have protocol of operating on one side first and then on other side. If investigations are suggestive of DSD, then one should follow DSD protocol **(Flowchart 2)**.

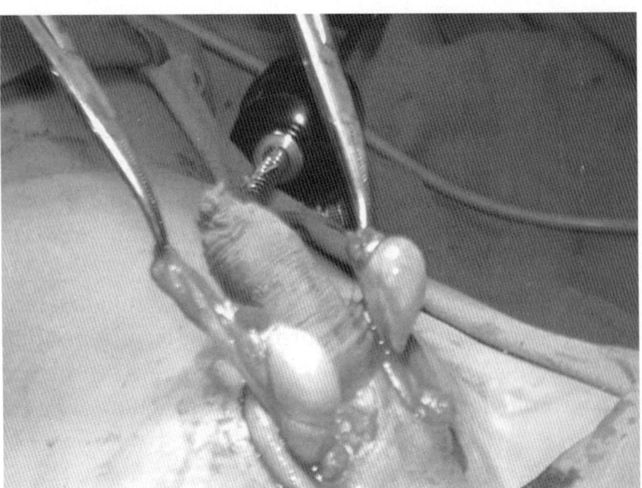

Fig. 4: Laparoscopic bilateral orchidopexy.
(For color version, see Plate 12)

Surgical Treatment

Timing of surgery—the spontaneous descent is less likely to occur after 3 months of age and it has recommended that children with UDT should be operated as soon as possible after 6 months of age to prevent the complications. In children with ascended testicle, surgery should be performed as soon as possible after diagnosis is established.

Early orchidopexy before 2 years (ideally before 1 year) of age is associated with improved testicular growth and fertility potential.

If a patient with UDT presents with inguinal hernia, then orchidopexy with repair of inguinal hernia should be performed at the time of presentation **(Flowchart 3)**.

CLINICAL PEARL

- Orchidopexy should be performed any time after the age of 6 months, the earlier the better to prevent its complications. UDT presenting with inguinal hernia should be operated at the time of diagnosis.

Flowchart 2: Management algorithm for bilateral undescended testis.

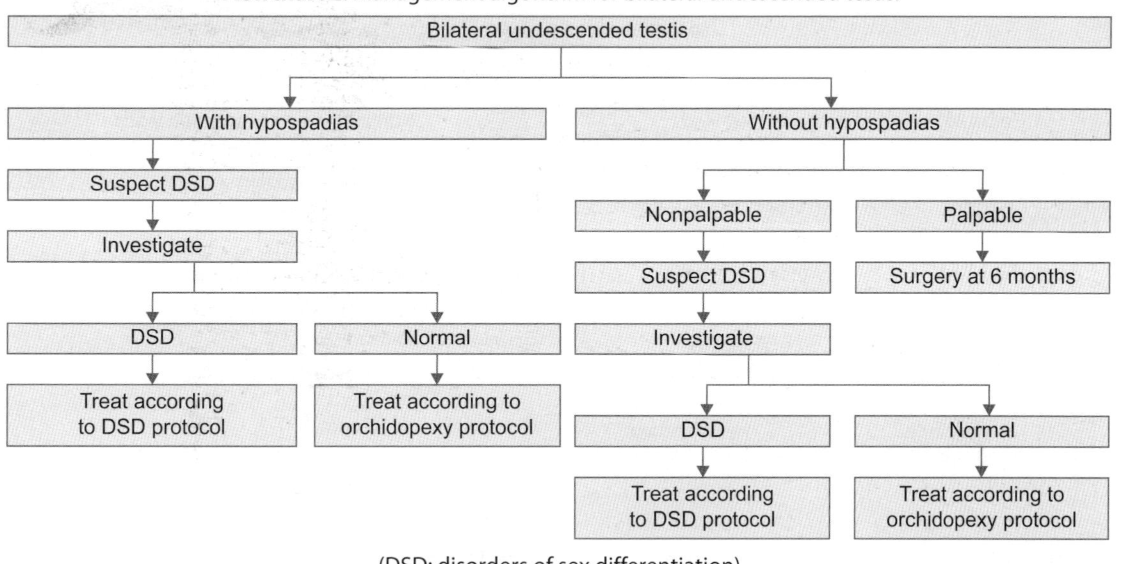

(DSD: disorders of sex differentiation)

Flowchart 3: Timeline for surgery in undescended testis.

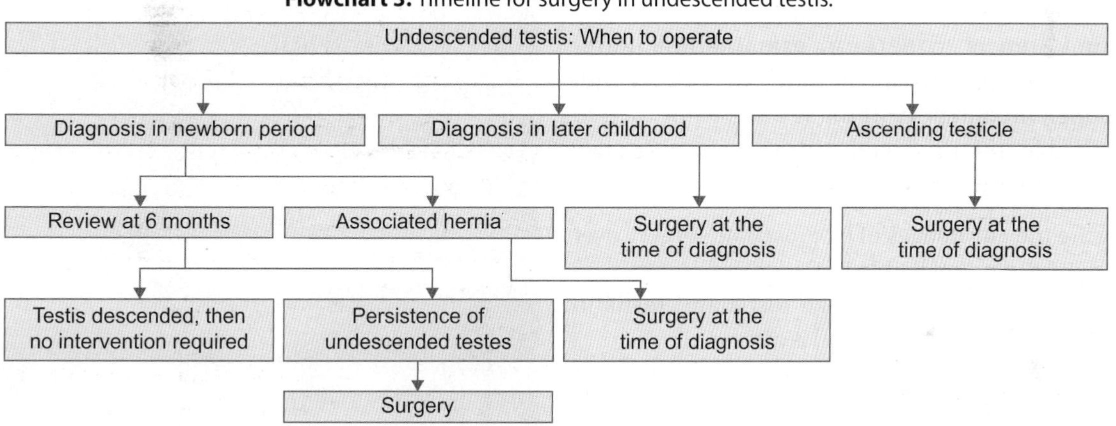

Palpable Testis

Patients with palpable UDT should undergo open orchidopexy. The surgery is usually carried out as a day care procedure under laryngeal mask and caudal anesthesia. An incision is taken in the lower skin crease in the groin. The testis along with the cord structures are mobilized, herniotomy (if hernial sac is present) is performed and testis is manipulated into the scrotum and sutured in place. Usually, palpable testis can be brought down to the scrotum as the cord structures have adequate length. Sometimes, even palpable (especially emergent) UDT has short cord and they may not come down to scrotum without tension and can ascend post-operatively into higher position needing second surgery. The exact incidence of such a scenario has not been reported, but it is likely to be in range of 2–3% (personal experience).

CLINICAL PEARL

- Palpable UDT should undergo open surgery and nonpalpable UDT should undergo laparoscopic surgery.

Nonpalpable Testis

The nonpalpable testis can be abdominal, atrophic, or absent. It is difficult to differentiate between these conditions preoperatively and parents of these patients should be explained about possible outcome of surgery, i.e., single stage orchidopexy, two-stage orchidopexy,

Flowchart 4: Treatment algorithm for undescended testis.

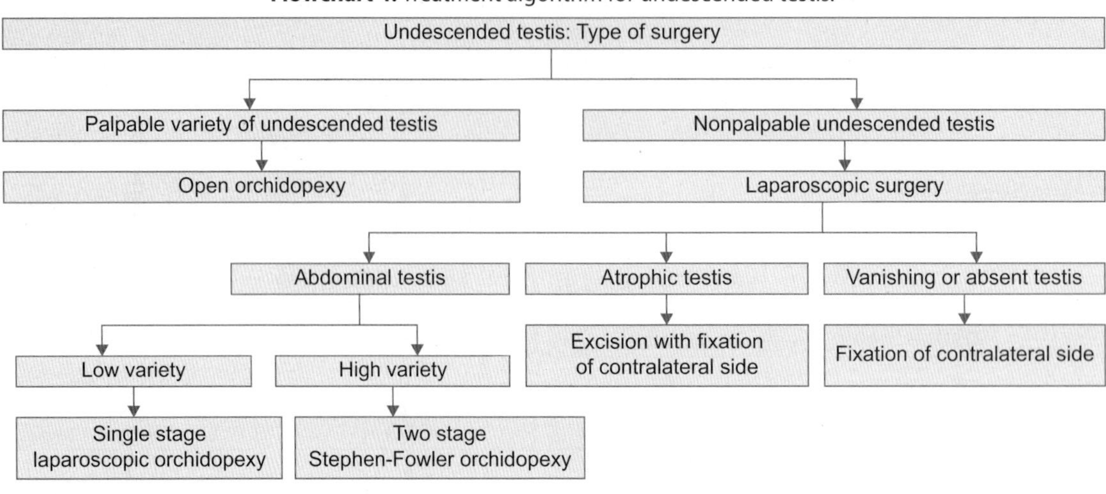

or orchiectomy depending upon the operative findings. Even patients with nonpalpable UDT can be operated as a day care surgery, but they need to be preferably scheduled as first case in the morning.

The first step is to perform examination under anesthesia and if testis is palpable, then to proceed with standard open orchidopexy. If the testis is confirmed to be not palpable, then proceed with the next step, i.e., laparoscopic surgery.

Following are the advantages of laparoscopic surgery over open procedure in nonpalpable UDT:

- Probability of missing the high testis and testis in abnormal position (retrovesical) is almost nil.
- Laparoscopic mobilization of testicular vessels is far superior as compared to open mobilization. The incidence of postoperative ascent and atrophy is less common compare to open surgery.

In a place, where option of laparoscopic pediatric surgery is not available, surgeon may proceed with open surgery by lower inguinal crease incision. If the testis is not found in the groin, then the peritoneal exploration may be performed by extending the groin incision laterally or to reverse the patient from anesthesia and refer the patient to the higher center. If cord structures or testicular remnants are found, they are removed and the procedure is terminated.

The diagnostic laparoscopy is a safe procedure in experienced hands. The laparoscope is placed via the umbilicus and following observations are carried out, patency of the processus vaginalis, location of testis, testicular vessels, vas deferens, gubernaculum, and presence of Müllerian structures. The findings on laparoscopy decide the further plan of action **(Flowchart 4)**.

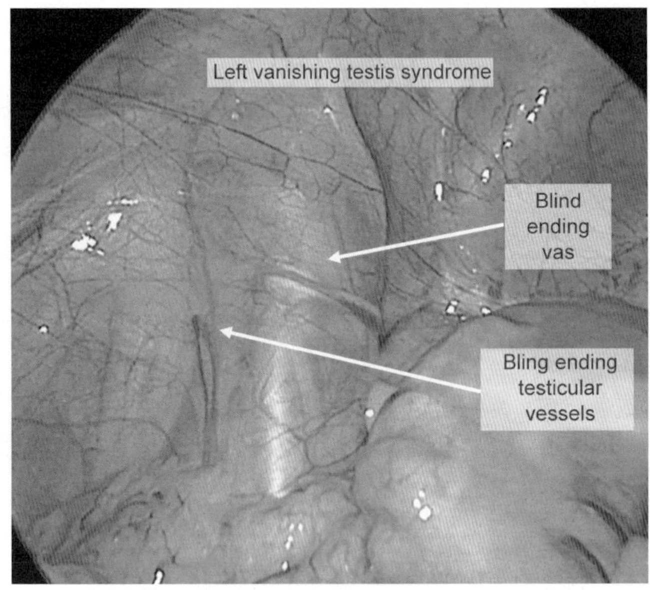

Fig. 5: Blind ending vas and vessels in left vanishing testis syndrome. *(For color version, see Plate 12)*

The presence of blind ending vas and vessels in the retroperitoneum (usually 2–3 cm proximal to the internal ring) is suggestive of vanishing testis syndrome **(Fig. 5)**. In this situation, nothing further needs to be done for the UDT, though fixation of contralateral testis to prevent torsion and loss of only testicular tissue remains controversial at present. Authors routinely fix the contralateral testis in such a scenario. In addition, if facilities are available, then surgeon can insert the testicular prosthesis on the ipsilateral side at the time of surgery or later on at puberty. If the prosthesis is inserted in a young child, then it may need to be revised at the time of puberty to match the normal contralateral testicular size. The psychological assessment of these young adults with or without prosthesis has not been performed, but logically the person with normal feel of scrotum is likely to have better self-esteem.

Orchiectomy should be performed if the UDT is abnormally soft and small (atrophic). Laparoscopic orchidopexy or orchiectomy is also the treatment of choice for the postpubertal, unilateral intra-abdominal UDT because of increased cancer risk. If the testis is brought and fixed in the scrotum then the diagnosis of cancer can be established early before it spreads to retroperitoneum. It is duty of treating doctors to teach the self-examination to these children when they reach puberty and understands the possibilities of cancer.

On laparoscopy, if vas and vessels are entering internal ring, then patient is likely to have atrophic testis either in the inguinal canal or in the scrotum. This patient should undergo excision of atrophic testicle either laparoscopically (if hernial sac is open and atrophic testis is visualized) or by an open inguinal incision along with fixation of contralateral testis by scrotal incision to prevent torsion and loss of only testicular tissue.

On laparoscopy, if apparently normal looking testis is seen, then surgeon needs to decide whether to bring the testis to scrotum in one or two operations. This decision is based on following factors:

- Age of patient
- Distance of testis from the internal ring
- Mobility of testicular vessels.

In infants, length of the inguinal canal is much shorter than the older children and it is easy to bring the testis in scrotum. The term low abdominal testis is used when the distance of testis from the internal ring is <2.5 cm **(Fig. 6)**. The term high abdominal testis is used when the distance of testis from internal ring is >2.5 cm. In children who are <5 years old with low abdominal testis and mobile vessels, usually the testis can be brought down in single operation. The success rate of single stage orchidopexy is >95%.

The children with high abdominal testis, age >5 years, and short testicular vessels usually needs two-stage Stephen–Fowler (SF) orchidopexy **(Fig.7)**. In the first stage, the testicular vessels are controlled either using bipolar diathermy, clipped or with an ultrasonic scalpel and then transected. This is performed approximately 2.5 cm away from the testis. This allows the development of collaterals between artery to vas deferens and testicular vessels **(Fig. 8)**. The second-stage SF orchidopexy is usually performed after 6 months, wherein the testis is brought down to scrotum on the pedicle of vas. The two-stage orchidopexy has success rate of >80%.

In past for high abdominal testis, microvascular surgery was performed by anastomosis of testicular artery with inferior epigastric artery but has limited success and is not popular.

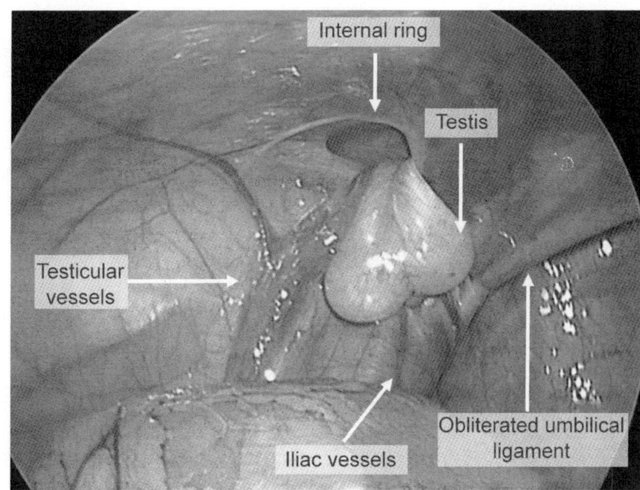

Fig. 6: Laparoscopic findings in the low abdominal testis near the internal ring. *(For color version, see Plate 12)*

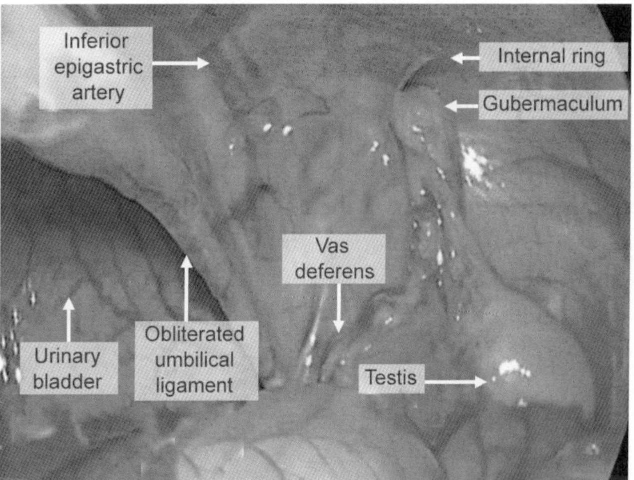

Fig. 7: Laparoscopic findings in the high abdominal testis—usually need two-stage orchidopexy. *(For color version, see Plate 12)*

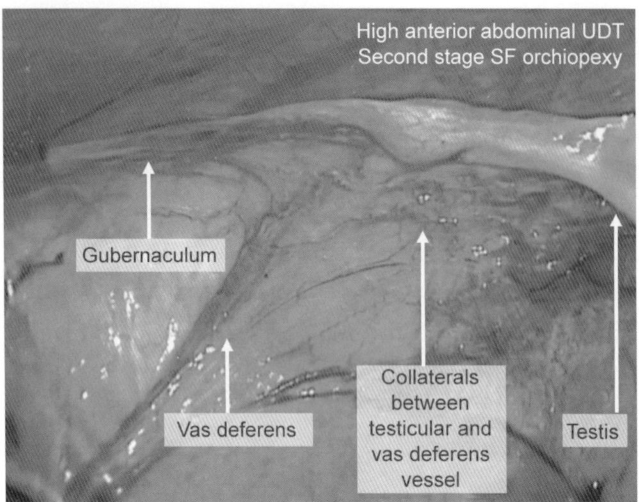

Fig. 8: Laparoscopic findings during second stage of Stephen–Fowler orchidopexy showing collaterals between artery to vas deferens and testicular artery. *(For color version, see Plate 13)*

Retractile Testis

A retractile testis should be under careful surveillance. The probability of spontaneous descent is 58 % in boys older than 7 years and 21% in boys younger than 7 years. It has 32% risk of becoming an ascending UDT. Surgical repositioning of the testis should be done if the testes become ascended testes (acquired cryptorchidism) or if there is significant loss of testicular volume in comparison to contralateral testes.

> **CLINICAL PEARL**
>
> - Retractile testis needs a close supervision and 32% becomes ascended testicle needing surgery.

Ascended Testicle

Ascended testicle should be surgically positioned at the time of presentation. Ascended testes are seen in mid-childhood, are usually unilateral, and are present in distal inguinal canal. Ascended testis is prone to the same germ cell maldevelopment seen in congenital cryptorchidism.

Long-term Outcome of The Orchidopexy

When assessed with color Doppler ultrasonography, the volume of the operated unilateral testes was seen to be smaller than the normal nonoperated side. The smaller testicular volume was observed despite maintained blood supply to the testes. In cases of bilateral UDT, both testes were smaller in size but were comparable to each other (personal experience).

Testicular Atrophy

Testicular atrophy is a serious negative outcome of the orchidopexy. It is reported in 1% in ectopic testis, up to 5% of the distal testis, and in up to 9% of cases in intra-abdominal testis. The preoperative location of testes, torsion, and anomalies of vas deferens determines the occurrence of postorchidopexy testicular atrophy. Inadvertent trauma to the testicular vessels, postoperative edema, and local infections may also play a role in testicular atrophy. The resultant postoperative ischemia leads to complete or partial atrophy of the testis.

Fertility

Adults with bilateral UDT have azoospermia in almost 100% of cases, while >20% adults will have normal sperm counts when their orchidopexy was done in early childhood. Adults who underwent orchidopexy generally have low sperm count and have poor semen quality. This subfertility is not completely compensated by the contralateral descended testis. The fertility is further compromised if both testes are undescended and if the treatment is delayed. In bilateral UDT, the studies quote normal sperm counts in up to 76% of cases when the orchidopexy was done between 10 months and 4 years of age and in up to 26% of cases who underwent orchidopexy in the age group 4–14 years of age. The timing of the surgery does not influence fertility in unilateral cryptorchidism. Though the fertility is not impaired, there are distinct benefits of early surgical orchidopexy.

Malignancy

Adult men with history of UDT have higher probability of developing a testicular malignancy. The risk increases to 32-fold in comparison to the general population. The intra-abdominal testis has the highest risk of developing malignancy, which is five times higher than that of inguinal UDT. The risk of malignancy is higher in bilateral UDT. The children who undergo orchidopexy after puberty are twice at the risk of developing the malignancy than those who undergo orchidopexy before puberty. The incidence of malignant degeneration in contralateral descended testis is about 8–15%.

KEY POINTS

- 1% of male child suffers from UDT at the age of 1 year.
- Imaging studies are not reliable and are not advocated to locate UDT.
- Surgery is performed to prevent the complications, e.g., hernia, torsion, trauma, subfertility, and malignancy.
- Clinically, UDT should be classified as palpable and nonpalpable variety.
- Surgery should be performed after the age of 6 months.
- UDT presenting with hernia should be operated at the time of diagnosis.
- Retractile testis needs a close supervision.
- In 32% of patients diagnosed to have retractile testis, becomes ascended testicle and needs surgery.
- Palpable UDT should undergo an open surgery.
- Nonpalpable UDT should undergo laparoscopic surgery.
- There is no role of hormonal treatment.
- Insertion of testicular prosthesis should be considered in patients with absent or atrophic type of UDT to prevent psychological issues and to improve the self-body image.
- All children undergoing orchidopexy should be taught self-examination for early detection of malignancy.

SUGGESTED READINGS

1. Abaci A, Catli G, Anik A, Bober G. Epidemiology, classification and management of undescended testes: does medication have any value in its treatment? J Clin Res Pediatr Endocrinology. 2013;5(2):65-72.
2. Agarwal PK, Diaz M, Elder JS. Retractile testis—is it a normal variant? J Urol. 2006:175(4):1496-9.
3. Akre O, Pettersson A, Richiardi L. Risk of contralateral testicular cancer among men with unilaterally undescended testis: A meta-analysis. Int J Cancer 2009;1(124):687–9.
4. Alagaratnam S, Nathaniel C, Cuckow P, Duffy P, Mushtaq I, Cherian A, et al. Testicular outcome following laparoscopic second stage Fowler-Stephens orchidopexy. J Pediatr Urol. 2014;10(1):186-92.
5. Al-Zahem A, Shun A. Routine contralateral orchidopexy for children with a vanished testis. Eur J Pediatr Surg. 2006;16(5):334-6.
6. Baker LA, Docimo SG, Surer I, Peters C, Cicek L, Diamond DA, et al. A multi-institutional analysis of laparoscopic orchidopexy. BJU Int. 2001;87:484-9.
7. Barthold JS, González R. The epidemiology of congenital cryptorchidism, testicular ascent and orchidopexy. J Urol. 2003;170:2396-401.
8. Belkar AM. Urologic microsurgery—current perspectives: II. Orchiopexy and testicular homotransplantation. Urology. 1980;15(2):103-7.
9. Berkowitz GS, Lapinski RH, Dolgin SE, Gazella JG, Bodian CA, Holzman IR. Prevalence and natural history of cryptorchidism. Pediatrics. 1993;92(1):4.
10. Biers SM, Malone PS. A critical appraisal of the evidence for improved fertility indices in undescended testes after gonadotrophin-releasing hormone therapy and orchidopexy. J Pediatr Urol. 2010;6(3):239-46.
11. De Filippo RE, Barthold JS, González R. The application of magnetic resonance imaging for the preoperative localization of nonpalpable testis in obese children: An alternative to laparoscopy. J Urol 2000; 164:154–5.
12. Ein SH, Nasr A, Wales PW, Ein H. Testicular atrophy after attempted pediatric orchidopexy for true undescended testis. J Pediatr Surg. 2014;49(2):317-22.
13. Esposito C, Damiano R, Gonzalez Sabin MA, et al. Laparoscopy assisted orchidopexy: An ideal treatment for children with intraabdominal testes. J Endourol 2002; 16:659–62.
14. Favorito LA, Costa WS, Sampaio FJ. Relationship between the persistence of the processus vaginalis and age in patients with cryptorchidism; International. Braz J Urol. 2005; 31(1):57-61.
15. Fedder J. History of cryptorchidism and ejaculate volume as simple predictors for the presence of testicular sperm. Syst Biol Reprod Med. 2011;57(3): 154-61.
16. Giwercman A, Bruun E, Frimodt-Møller C, Skakkebaek NE. Prevalence of carcinoma in situ and other histopathological abnormalities in testes of men with a history of cryptorchidism. J Urol. 1989;142:998-1001.
17. Giwercman A, Grindsted J, Hansen B, Jensen OM, Skakkebæk NE. Testicular cancer risk in boys with maldescended testis: A cohort study. J Urol. 1987;138:1214-6.
18. Jarow JP, Berkovitz GD, Migeon CJ, Gearhart JP, Walsh PC. Elevation of serum gonadotropins establishes the diagnosis of anorchism in prepubertal boys with bilateral cryptorchidism. J Urol. 1986;136:277-9.
19. Joshi NC, Shah RS. Long term outcome of laparoscopic surgery for Non-Palpable Undescended Testis. J Indian Assoc Pediatr Surg. 2024;29(1):39-42.
20. Lee PA, Coughlin MT, Bellinger MF. Inhibin B: Comparison with indexes of fertility among formerly cryptorchid and control men. J Clin Endocrinol Metab. 2001;86(6): 2576-84.
21. Lee PA, Coughlin MT. Fertility after bilateral cryptorchidism. Evaluation by paternity, hormone, and semen data. Horm Res. 2001;55:28-32.
22. Lee PA. Fertility in cryptorchidism. Does treatment make a difference. Endocrinol Metab Clin North Am. 1993;22(3):479-90.
23. Lip SZ, Murchison LE, Cullis PS, Govan L, Carachi R. A meta-analysis of the risk of boys with isolated cryptorchidism developing testicular cancer in later life. Arch Dis Children. 2013;98(1):20-6.
24. Ludwikowski B, GonzálezR. The controversy regarding the need for hormonal treatment in boys with unilateral cryptorchidism goes on: a review of the literature. Eur J Pediatr. 2013;172(1):5-8.

25. Mano R, Livne PM, Nevo A, Sivan B, Ben-Meir D. Testicular torsion in the first year of life—characteristics and treatment outcome. Urology. 2013;82(5):1132-7.
26. Mathers MJ, Sperling H, Rubben H, Roth S. The undescended testis: diagnosis, treatment and long-term consequences. Dtsch Artzbel Int. 2009;106(33):527-32.
27. McAleer IM, Packer MG, Kaplan GW, Scherz HC, Krous HF, Billman GF. Fertility index analysis in cryptorchidism. J Urol. 1995;153:1255-8.
28. Miller KD, Coughlin MT, Lee PA. Fertility after unilateral cryptorchidism. Paternity, time to conception, pretreatment testicular location and size, hormone and sperm parameters. Horm Res. 2001;55:249-53.
29. Osifo DO, Osaigbovo EO. The prevalence, postnatal descent, and complications of undescended testes among children who underwent neonatal circumcision in Benin City, Nigeria. J Pediatr Surg. 2009;44(4):791-6.
30. Osime O, Momoh M, Elusoji S. Torsed intraabdominal testis: a rarely considered diagnosis. Cal J Emerg Med. 2006;7(2):31-3.
31. Pettersson A, Richiardi L, Nordenskjoid A, Kaijser M, Akre O. Age at surgery for undescended testis and risk of testicular cancer. N Engl J Med. 2007;356(18):1835-41.
32. Virtanen HE, Bjerknes R, Cortes D, Jørgensen N, Rajpert-De Meyts E, Thorsson AV, et al. Cryptorchidism: classification, prevalence and long-term consequences. Acta Paediatr. 2007;96(5):611-6.
33. Weir HK, Marrett LD, Kreiger N, Darlington GA, Sugar L. Pre-natal and peri-natal exposures and risk of testicular germ-cell cancer. Int J Cancer. 2000;87:438-43.
34. Wood HM, Elder JS. Cryptorchidism and testicular cancer: Separating fact from fiction. J Urol. 2009;181:452.
35. Zilberman D, Inbar Y, Heyman Z, Shinhar D, Bilik R, Avigad I, et al. Torsion of the cryptorchid testis—can it be salvaged? J Urol. 2006;175(6):2287-9; discussion 2289.

Acute Scrotum in Children

Anand Alladi

INTRODUCTION

Acute scrotum is the presentation of a group of diseases, involving the scrotum or its contents, with sudden onset symptoms and/or signs, which are related to the scrotum.

The two important pathologies presenting with acute scrotum are acute epididymo-orchitis and torsion testes, one requiring medical management while the other is a surgical emergency, needing immediate intervention. There are a few other pathologies, albeit rarer, to complete the list, but are not of serious consequence as torsion of the testes.

BODY TEXT

Children with acute scrotum generally have sudden-onset symptoms such as pain, swelling, or redness of usually one, rarely, both sides of the scrotum. Some may have systemic symptoms also like nausea or vomiting.

The list of pathologies presenting as acute scrotum, other than the mentioned two, namely torsion and epididymo-orchitis, include, torsion of appendage of testes, acute idiopathic edema, testicular trauma, and rare causes such as Henoch–Schonlein purpura and fat necrosis.

Briefly, discussing the more dangerous entity testicular torsion, it can be intra- or extravaginal, depending on the investment of the tunica vaginalis and the age group affected. Torsion occurring in neonates are usually extravaginal wherein, the tunica and spermatic cord gets twisted, while those occurring in older children are, in general, due to high investment of the tunica vaginalis, the "bell clapper" deformity, where a mobile testes gets torted. Though the exact inciting factor is not clear, some predispositions including cold temperature, peripubertal age, undescended or retractile testes, and family history of torsion, with a final common pathway of acute hyperactive cremasteric reflex.

A typical presentation of intravaginal torsion is a peripubertal boy with sudden-onset scrotal pain with or without associated symptoms of abdominal referred pain, nausea, or vomiting.

Clinical findings include any or all of the following—redness and/or edema of scrotum, testicular tenderness, abnormal position or lie of testes, and absent cremasteric reflex. The duration and degree of torsion determine the chances of salvageability of the testes. Though many modalities of investigation continue to evolve, to differentiate between torsion and other acute scrotal pathologies, as well as predict salvageability of testes, ultrasound with Doppler is presently the tool used. Findings of reduced or absent blood flow, parenchymal heterogeneity, "*snail sign*" on high resolution ultrasound, all suggest testicular torsion. However, this should not be done at a cost of time to surgical exploration. The long-term effects of torsion is still not clear, though some degree of impact on fertility are generally reported, even those in whom testes has been salvaged.

Perinatal torsion occurs usually in infants, are usually extravaginal, presenting as vanishing testes or a hard fixed neonatal testis, depending on when the torsion occurred. They can be bilateral, which can be synchronous or metachronous.

Intermittent testicular torsion with spontaneous detorsion is known to occur in the peripubertal age group. It can be recurrent and clinical and ultrasound findings of torsion at time of pain may confirm the diagnosis. In others, a high index of suspicion is necessary to detect the same and bilateral prophylactic orchidopexy offered to prevent torsion.

Torsion testes is a surgical emergency requiring immediate exploration, without wasting time on evaluation, especially when that's going to delay surgery. In cases where the duration of pain is >24 hours, time may be spent on evaluation and then plan exploration semielectively.

Surgical exploration, detorsion, assessment of viability, and additional procedures such as tunica albuginea incision with tunica vaginalis flap and orchidopexy if viable, else orchidectomy is done. Contralateral orchidopexy is prophylactically done. Ipsilateral prosthesis at a later date is an option offered if orchidectomy is carried out, while some do it simultaneously.

Counseling regarding and follow-up is essential as some testes undergo atrophy later, even though they appear viable at surgery. In addition, there may be chances of subfertility.

Torsion of the appendage of the testes is the *most common cause of acute scrotum* in peripubertal age. They usually present as acute scrotum but differ clinically from torsion of testes in having localized tender nodule and not completely tender testes, normal cremasteric reflex, normal position, and lie of testes and the *"blue dot sign"*—a discolored area on upper pole of testes, seen through stretched scrotal skin. All these, however, in later stages due to increased inflammation and edema, make it difficult to differentiate from torsion of the testes.

Treatment of torsion of appendage is usually symptomatic with anti-inflammatory medications. However, if there is difficulty in differentiating from torsion of the testes, exploration is recommended.

Epididymitis is an inflammatory pathology of the epididymis presenting with acute scrotal symptoms, but more insidiously than torsion. There are two peaks of presentation—(1) infants and (2) peripubertal. There may be history suggestive of predisposing anomalies such as recurrent urinary infections, dysfunctional voiding, and hematuria. Clinically there is a continuum of signs starting from tender swollen epididymis to completely indurated, tender scrotum.

Recommendations to evaluate further, after diagnosis has been variable, and include ultrasound, voiding cystourethrography, and cystoscopy, depending on the history, recurrent episodes, or abnormal findings on preliminary investigations.

Treatment of epididymitis includes anti-inflammatory analgesics, scrotal elevation, and antibiotics, if pyuria coexists.

Idiopathic scrotal edema usually presents with scrotal edema without pain, with edema sometimes extending onto penis, perineum, and inguinal region. Testes are normal. It may be allergic in origin. The condition is usually self-limiting and treatment is symptomatic with antihistamines. Transverse scrotal ultrasound with Doppler demonstrates the characteristic *"Fountain sign"* due to hypervascularity of the scrotum.

Vasculitis due to Henoch–Schonlein purpura may involve the scrotum in up to one-third of the patients, with acute scrotal symptoms and signs. Typical purpuric rashes on the body, usually suggest the diagnosis.

Flowchart 1: Patient presenting with acute scrotal symptoms.

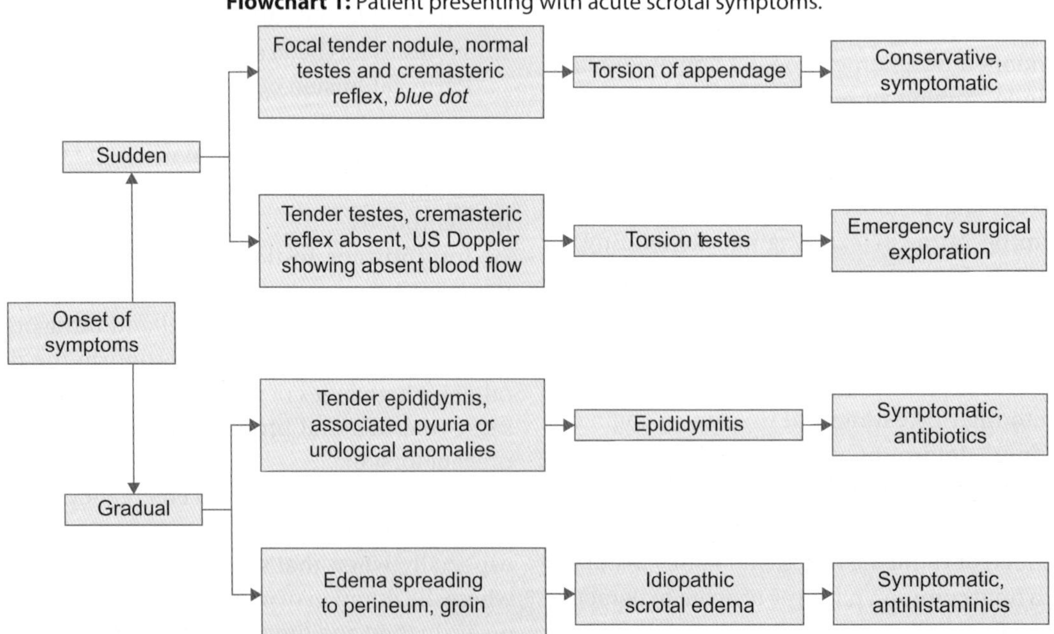

Sudden-onset tender bilateral scrotal lumps in obese children on exposure to cold water is a typical presentation of rare condition of acute fat necrosis **(Flowchart 1)**.

KEY POINTS

- Testicular torsion is an emergency requiring immediate surgical intervention.
- While ultrasound with Doppler is useful in confirming or ruling out torsion, it should not be done at the cost of delaying the surgery.
- Intermittent torsion should be kept in mind and addressed by fixation, in recurrent acute testicular pain.
- Children presenting with epididymo-orchitis should be evaluated further for associated, predisposing urological anomalies.

SUGGESTED READING

1. ICMR. (2024). Acute Scrotum in Children: Standard Treatment Workflow. [online] Available from https://www.icmr.gov.in/icmrobject/uploads/STWs/1726569369_acute_scrotum_in_children.pdf [Last accessed December, 2024].
2. Partin AW, Dmochowski RR, Kavoussi LR, Peters CA. Acute Scrotum. Campbell Walsh Wein Urology, 12th edition. Philadelphia: Elsevier; 2020. pp. 3950-67.
3. Radmayr C, Bogaert G, Burgu B, Castagnetti MS, Dogan HS, O'Kelly F, et al. Acute Scrotum. EAU guidelines on Pediatric Urology. Netherlands: European Association of Urology; 2023. pp. 24-7.
4. Shenoy V, Saha S. Testicular torsion. Standard treatment Guidelines of Indian Association of Paediatric Surgeons in Paediatric Urology. India: Indian Association of Paediatric Surgeons; 2018. pp. 40-1.

Inguinal Hernia

Vikesh Agrawal, Himanshu Acharya, Rasiklal S Shah

INTRODUCTION

Inguinoscrotal swellings in children are a common reason for pediatric consultation. This chapter aims to enable a pediatrician to understand the anatomy and pathology of inguinal hernia and other patent processus vaginalis-related anomalies. The reader should be able to make a correct diagnosis, decide on the management of the patient, and make timely surgical referrals to avoid complications. The topic shall cover inguinal hernia, hydrocele, and their associated presentation. A brief description of available surgical techniques is also given.

The testis descends into the scrotum during the seventh month of gestation pushing a diverticulum of the peritoneum (processus vaginalis) ahead of it. This processus begins to obliterate in a caudal-cranial fashion once the testis descends to the scrotal base. The closure of processus vaginalis starts shortly before birth and patency obliterates by birth, while anatomical closure occurs during the first year of life, leaving only the tunica vaginalis surrounding the testis. The obliterated processus vaginalis lies alongside the vas and vessels within the spermatic cord. Failure of obliteration results in patent processus vaginalis—the underlying abnormality in all hernias, hydroceles, and encysted hydroceles of the cord **(Table 1)**. Nearly all inguinal hernias in children are indirect, with patent processus vaginalis being the underlying abnormality. It travels from the deep inguinal ring across the inguinal canal, comes out of the superficial ring, and travels along the spermatic cord to the scrotum. Direct inguinal hernia results from a weakness in the posterior wall of the inguinal canal, which is rare in children.

EPIDEMIOLOGY AND ETIOLOGY

The incidence in full-term babies is estimated at 1–5% of live births, and it is six times more common in boys with male-to-female ratio of 3–10:1. Preterm babies accordingly have the highest incidence varying from 16% to 25%. Right-sided hernias are more common (60%), attributable to the late descent of the right testis compared to the left, hence a higher probability of patent processus vaginalis on the right. The incidence of right-sided hernias is more than three times that of left-sided hernias. Bilateral hernias are more common in premature infants and are found in about 10% of children. The incidence of bilateral hernia is higher if the first presentation is on the left side. In girls, the canal of Nuck undergoes the same obliteration as the processus vaginalis in boys. The obliteration is more likely to be complete, hence a lower overall incidence of hernias, but there is a higher incidence of bilateral hernias. The small intestines are the most herniated intra-abdominal content in boys. In female infants, the ovaries have the most herniated content; however, after 1 year of age, the bowel becomes more common, and a herniated ovary in an adolescent would be extremely unlikely. In a female full-term infant, bilateral inguinal hernias that may contain ovaries should prompt investigation for a possible androgen insensitivity syndrome (AIS).

Risk factors for pediatric inguinal hernia are poorly understood, but family history in 10% of cases points toward unknown genetic cause. Generally, there is no predisposing factor in a full-term child for the development of inguinal hernia; however, predisposing factors such as prematurity, cryptorchidism, connective tissue disorders, mucopolysaccharidoses, congenital hip dislocation, cystic fibrosis, ascites, ventriculoperitoneal (VP) shunt, peritoneal dialysis, abdominal wall defects, meningomyelocele, and exstrophy bladder are variably found.

CLINICAL PRESENTATION AND EXAMINATION

The typical presentation of inguinal hernia in boys is a smooth painless swelling in the groin, which bulges

TABLE 1: Various commonly used definition in clinical practice for inguinal hernia and hydrocele.

Term	*Definition*
Hernia	A hernia is the protrusion of a portion of an organ or tissue through an abnormal opening in the wall that normally contains it
Incarceration	Implies a hernia that cannot be reduced by manipulation
Obstructed hernia	Implies a hernia which is incarcerated and has led to intestinal obstruction
Strangulated hernia	Implies an incarceration leading to vascular compromise of the bowel
Hernia uteri inguinale	Implies an inguinal hernia in a male, where Müllerian structures have persisted and forms the content of hernia sac
Amyand's hernia	Implies hernia with appendix as its content
Littre's hernia	Implies hernia with Meckel's diverticulum as its content
Hydrocele (in children)	A hydrocele is a fluid-filled collection that can occur anywhere along the path of descent of the testis or ovary between parietal and visceral layer of tunica vaginalis as a result of patent processus vaginalis.
Vaginal hydrocele	Implies hydrocele extending up to the base of scrotum
Encysted hydrocele	Implies localized cystic collection of fluid along the path of processus vaginalis
Abdominoscrotal hydrocele	Implies hydrocele extending from to the base of scrotum distally to intra-abdominal proximally. It may give rise to abdominal lump.

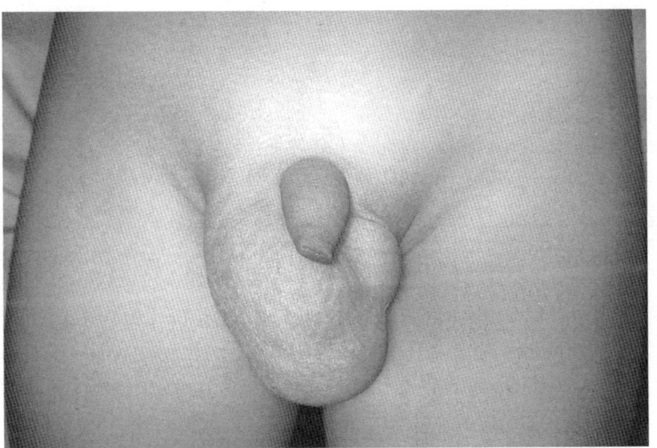

Fig. 1: Clinical picture of inguinal hernia.
(For color version, see Plate 13)

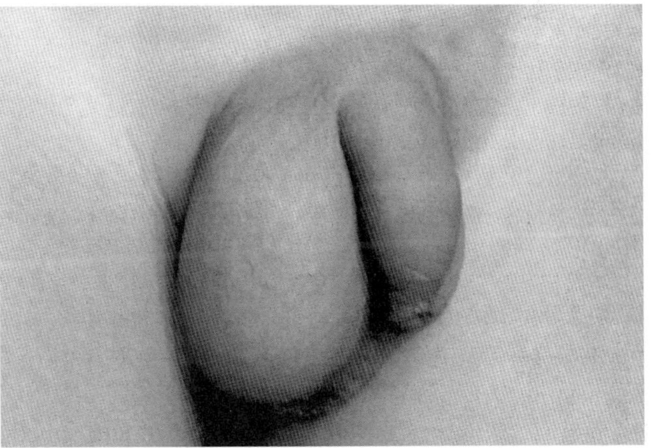

Fig. 2: Clinical picture of hydrocele.
(For color version, see Plate 13)

on crying or straining. The swelling may extend to the scrotum as seen in **Fig. 1**. It reduces in the abdomen either spontaneously when the child is quiet and relaxed, or by gentle manual pressure—a maneuver to elicit "reducibility" of a hernia. Older children often complain of groin or inguinal pain during exercise.

When the processus vaginalis is patent with a small lumen, it allows some peritoneal fluid to seep down along the cord producing a soft, fluid-filled swelling **(Fig. 2)**. The swelling usually is very mild in the morning when the child wakes up; it gradually fills up during the day as the child remains active. When sleeping, some fluid recedes gradually making the swelling smaller. But this swelling is not reducible manually because of the very small size of the patent processus (ink well effect). The swelling is painless; it is situated around the testis, is brightly translucent, and cannot be emptied by pressure. Uncommonly, an acute hydrocele develops secondary to epididymo-orchitis, torsion, trauma, or tumor—these hydroceles resolve spontaneously. The operation for hydrocele is the same as that for hernia.

The various tests for clinical examination and signs are depicted in **Table 2**.

TABLE 2: A brief tabulation of various tests and signs noticeable during clinical examination.

Test or sign	*Description*	*Hint**
Inguinoscrotal swelling on straining	• Swelling noticed while a baby strains or cry, or in older kids if asked to stand and perform valsalva maneuver or blow a balloon • Any swelling noticed by parents at home and not recognized during clinical examination should not be disregarded	Inguinal hernia
Reducibility	Spontaneous or manual reduction of content which does not reappear unless a strained by the child (cry/cough)	Inguinal hernia
One cannot get above the swelling	One cannot appreciate the upper edge of the swelling and it appears to extend into deep inguinal ring.	Inguinal hernia
Impulse on cry/cough	After reduction, the transmission of impulse is felt if cord is held between index finger and thumb.	Inguinal hernia
Silk glove sign	The index finger is rolled transversely across the spermatic cord over the pubic bone; if there is a hernial sac, the "rustle" of contiguous layers of peritoneum represents the empty hernial sac is felt.	Inguinal hernia
Mobile testes	Testes can be moved freely between scrotum and the inguinal canal and does not come back to the scrotum unless milked down.	Inguinal hernia with mobile/ undescended testes
Swelling present during most of the day and increases by the end of the day, and reduces on waking up in the morning	Elicited during history taking	Hydrocele
One can get above the swelling	One can appreciate the upper edge of the swelling	
Transillumination	Brilliant glowing of light across the swelling when a torch is placed on one side of the swelling, with a negative shadow of the testes	Hydrocele

*Opposite side should always be examined as inguinal hernia or hydrocele are found bilaterally in about 10% of cases.

MANAGEMENT

Flowcharts 1 and 2 show a suggested approach to the management of hernia and hydrocele and include all key areas such as timing, anesthesia, technique, and special scenarios.

An inguinal hernia will not resolve spontaneously, so surgery is always indicated. Most full-term infants and older children undergo an elective herniotomy soon after diagnosis. It is a daycare operation performed under anesthesia either through an open or laparoscopic approach. The hernia sac is gently dissected from the cord structures (vas and vessels) and transected and ligated at the deep inguinal ring. The distal sac is left *in situ* but opened widely. The testis is confirmed in the scrotum before closing. Repair of the inguinal arch is indicated in special situations as mentioned in **Flowchart 1**.

Most hydroceles resolve spontaneously as the processus obliterates by the age of 1 year, and surgery is only required if the hydrocele persists beyond 1 year. Unusual situations that may warrant an early surgery are very tense hydrocele, causing discomfort to the child and possible compression of testicular vessels, abdominoscrotal hydroceles, hydroceles associated with VP shunts, and when a hernia cannot be excluded with certainty. An encysted hydrocele of the cord is a loculus of fluid located above and separate from the tunica vaginalis. Clinically, the swelling is separate from the testis, and one can get both above and below the swelling. As it is in line with the processus, it moves when the testis is pulled down. Uncommonly, an acute hydrocele develops secondary to epididymo-orchitis, torsion, trauma, or tumor—these hydroceles resolve spontaneously. The operation for hydrocele is the same as that for hernia.

Special Scenarios

Preterm Babies

Low birth weight babies, who are admitted to neonatal units with prematurity-related issues, often develop a hernia.

Flowchart 1: Algorithm depicting clinical approach toward management of hernia and hydrocele.

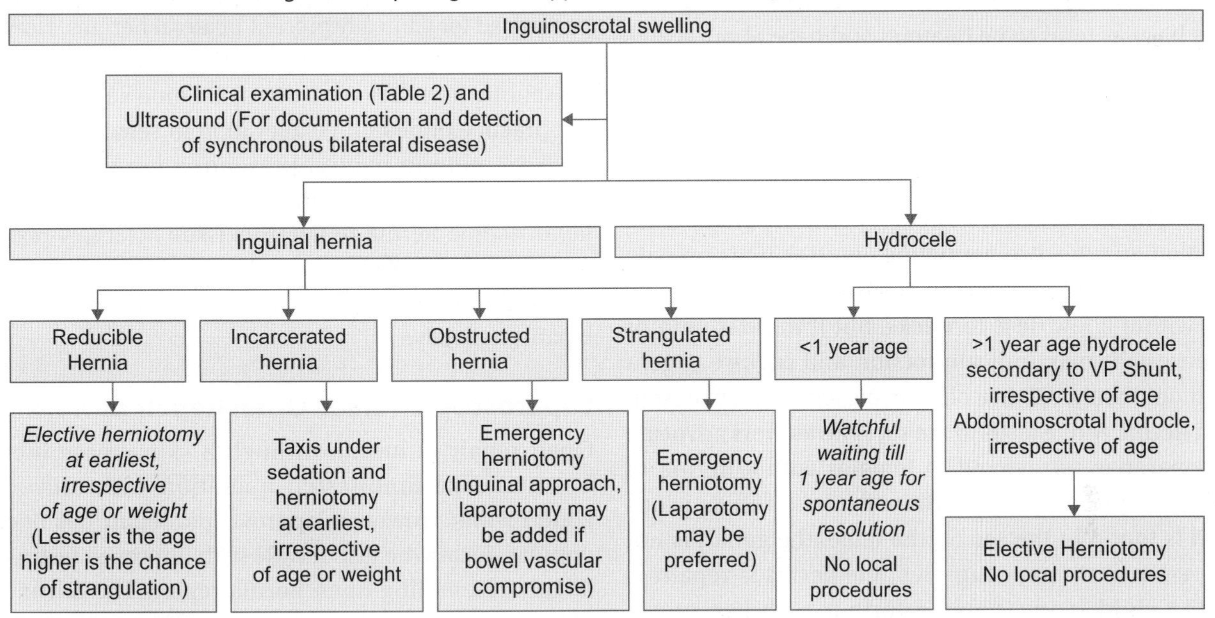

The author's practice is to operate on them once the medical issues are over, and the child is otherwise ready to be sent home. However, there is an increased risk of anesthesia and postoperative apnea risk. They may require postoperative monitoring and ventilation for about 24 hours. Contralateral synchronous (clinically evident or not evident) and metachronous (future risk) hernia is very common in preterm infants; therefore, many clinicians advocate contralateral open exploration or taking advantage of laparoscopic repair to detect and repair contralateral hernia. Preoperative ultrasound is useful for detecting synchronous hernias.

Obstructed and Strangulated Hernias

An incarcerated hernia does not reduce spontaneously and is not reducible by gentle pressure. If left untreated, it soon becomes obstructed, causing symptoms of intestinal obstruction which may progress quite rapidly to strangulation. Strangulation may cause intestinal and testicular ischemia—the swelling becomes tense and tender and there are features of intestinal obstruction. Strangulated hernia requires emergency surgery to relieve intestinal obstruction and save the gut and the testis. If the hernia is incarcerated but not strangulated, the child may be mildly irritable with groin pain, but there is no abdominal distension and no features of intestinal obstruction or hemodynamic instability. Such a child should be admitted for monitoring and sedated. Often the hernia will reduce spontaneously within about 30 minutes of the child becoming quiet. If not, "taxis" is applied—the surgeon stands on the side of the hernia and pushes the contents toward the inguinal canal across the superficial ring with the fingers of the right hand, simultaneously aligning the sac to the superficial ring by the fingers of the left hand on the top of the sac. Simply pushing the contents is not successful because the sac turns on itself as it comes out of the superficial ring. If taxis are successful, the hernia should be repaired in 24–48 hours after the tissue edema subsides. If taxis are unsuccessful, an urgent operation should be carried out. The risk of incarceration is highest in infancy, reaching an incidence of up to 30%. Therefore, surgery should be performed soon after the diagnosis in this subset of patients to avoid the risk of incarceration and strangulation. An obstructed or strangulated hernia is operated only after adequate resuscitation.

Hernia with Undescended Testis

Undescended testis is always accompanied by a hernial sac but is at low risk of incarceration. They can be safely repaired at the time of orchidopexy (generally at 6 months). However, the parents are warned about the danger signs of obstruction. If a symptomatic hernia develops, an early repair of the hernia and undescended testis is performed.

Hernia with Ventriculoperitoneal Shunts

These hernias tend to be bilateral and have about a 20% risk of incarceration. Bilateral early repair is in order.

Hernia in a Female Child

The incidence of bilaterality is high in females. The ovary may be content, and it is difficult to reduce. Often, there is a fallopian tube also herniating out. If there is no pain or tenderness in the ovary, an elective operation may be done within a few days to weeks, but if there is pain or tenderness, it may indicate torsion and require urgent operation. Rarely, AIS in a phenotypic female may present with a hernia with a testis in the sac. The authors advocate a preoperative ultrasound in females with a hernia to confirm the presence of a uterus and tubes. If a suspicious gonad is found in the sac on the table, the gonad is not removed; parents are counseled, the hernia is repaired, and the child is investigated further with karyotype. Laparoscopy is a good tool to confirm internal genital anatomy and repair hernias, which are often bilateral. Routine use of karyotype to pick up a rare case of AIS is not warranted. AIS requires the removal of both testes and life-long replacement with estrogens.

Bilateral Hernia

Ten-twenty percent of hernias are bilateral. A contralateral hernia may also develop later after the repair of the ipsilateral hernia. It is more common in infancy and girls, and when the presenting hernia is on the left, especially when the hernia is large. Bilateral repair should be performed for clinically present bilateral hernias. However, routine contralateral exploration for a unilaterally presenting hernia is controversial. Some surgeons follow the practice of bilateral exploration in selected situations such as preterm babies, presenting hernia on the left side, and infants, and female hernia. With the advent of laparoscopic hernia repair, this issue is largely resolved as both the deep rings are clearly visible and without any additional ports, bilateral repair can be performed laparoscopically.

Laparoscopic versus Open Repair of Hernia

Open repair of hernia through a skin crease incision is a standard time-tested operation with universally good results. However, laparoscopic repair has become popular during the last decade with improved techniques largely resembling open hernia repair. The advantages of laparoscopic hernia repair is magnified view of vas and vessels **(Figs. 3A and B)** avoiding injury, no need of streching or opening of spermatic cord and ability to do biletral herniotomy if needed. The disadvantages are the need to go transperitoneally, more cost, and a slightly higher recurrence rate of 1–3%. The various techniques of laparoscopic repair which are effective are mentioned in **Flowchart 2**. The most preferred techniques are the incision, dissection, excision and suturing (IDES) technique and percutaneous internal ring suturing (PIRS) technique. The choice of technique varies among various surgeons.

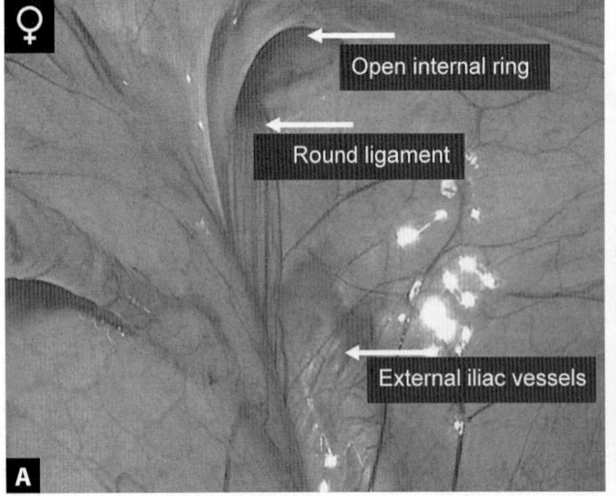

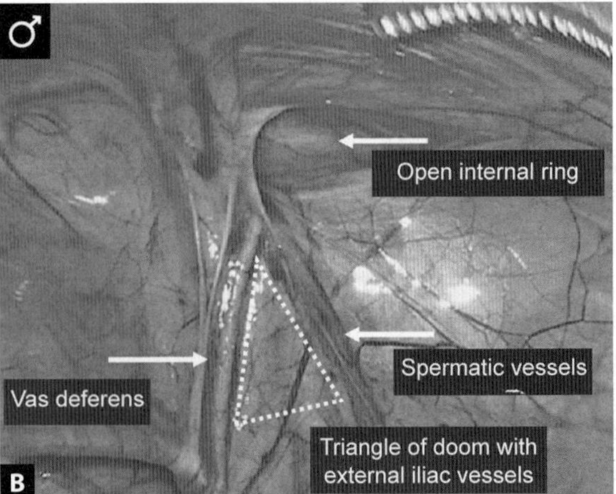

Figs. 3A and B: Laparoscopic internal view of inguinal hernia in a girl (A) and a boy (B).
(For color version, see Plate 13)

Flowchart 2: Algorithm depicting surgical approach toward management of hernia and hydrocele.

Herniotomy procedure is grossly similar for both hernia and hydrocele

- Under sedation
- Caudal block (open) under general anesthesia ± caudal block (Laparoscopic)
- Day care surgery

Hernia

- Open inguinal crease approach*
  - Infant → Mitchelbank's technique without opening inginal canal as canal is short
  - >1 year → Fergusson's technique with opening of inguinal canal
- Laparoscopic approach*# preferred for bilateral hernias no co-morbid illness
  - Incision, dissection, excision and suturing technique (IDES), three port → Most effective with <3% rcurrence rate
  - Percutaneous internal ring suturing (PIRS), single port →
    - Equally effective
    - Avoided for large hernias with wide deep ring
    - Preferred for female hernias

Hydrocele†

- Open inguinal crease approach →
  - Fergusson's technique with opening of inguinal canal
  - Aspiration of hydrocele fluid is added to give immediate relief
- Laparoscopic approach; Preferred for bilateral hydrocele →
  - Incision, dissection, excision and suturing technique (IDES) is standard approach
  - PIRS/nonsuturing techniques can be used
  - Aspiration of hydrocele fluid is added to give immediate relief

*When IR diameter is >2.5 cm or in recurrent cases, the interrupted muscular arch repair after sac disconnection is equivocally recommended in both open and laparoscopic hernia repair.

#Diagnostic laparoscopy is indicated in females where gonads are palpable in inguinal region to rule out androgen insensitivity syndrome along with karyotyping and ultrasound for visualization of Müllerian structures, and if its AIS, gonadal biopsy, gonadectomy, and herniotomy is done.

†In abdominoscrotal hydrocele, sac excision has to be performed.

KEY POINTS

- Congenital hernia and hydroceles develop from patent processus vaginalis.
- Hydrocele contains fluid, and hernia contains bowel or omentum.
- Hernia is inguinoscrotal, while hydrocele is scrotal.
- Incidence of hernia is high in infants. The probability of complications—obstruction and strangulation—is also higher in them.
- Surgery should be performed soon after diagnosis to prevent complications in hernias.
- Obstructed or strangulated hernia requires an emergency operation.
- Hydroceles usually resolve spontaneously in the first year of life, and surgery is performed if it fails to resolve by 1 year of age.

SUGGESTED READINGS

1. Acharya H, Agrawal R, Agrawal V, Tiwari A, Chanchlani R. Management of inguinal hernia in children: A single center experience of 490 patients. Int Surg J. 2016;3(1): 345-8.
2. Barthold JS. Abnormalities of the testis and scrotum and their surgical management. In: Wein AJ, Kavoussi LR, Partin AW (Eds). Campbell Walsh Urology, 10th edition. Elsevier-Saunders; 2012. pp. 3556-96.
3. Glick PL, Boulanger SC. Inguinal hernias and hydroceles. In: Coran G, Adzick NS, Krummel TM (Eds). Pediatric Surgery, 7th edition. Elsevier-Saunders; 2012. pp. 985-1001.
4. Hutson JM, Brien MO, Woodward AA (Eds). Inguinal Region and Acute Scrotum in Children. Jones' Clinical Paediatric Surgery Diagnosis and Management, 6th edition. Blackwell Publishing; 2008. pp. 168-71.

5. Morini F, Dreuning KMA, Janssen Lok MJH, Wester T, Derikx JPM, Friedmacher F, et al. Surgical Management of Pediatric Inguinal Hernia: A Systematic Review and Guideline from the European Pediatric Surgeons' Association Evidence and Guideline Committee. Eur J Pediatr Surg. 2022;32(3): 219-32.
6. Parelkar SV, Oak S, Gupta R, Sanghvi B, Shimoga PH, Kaltari D, et al. Laparoscopic inguinal hernia repair in the pediatric age group—experience with 437 children. J Pediatr Surg. 2010;45(4):789-92.
7. Schier F, Montupet P, Esposito C. Laparoscopic inguinal herniorrhaphy in children: A three-center experience with 933 repairs. J Pediatr Surg. 2002;37(3):395-7.
8. Shah R, Arlikar J, Dhende N. Incise, dissect, excise and suture technique of laparoscopic repair of pediatric male inguinal hernia. J Minim Access Surg. 2013;9(2): 72-5.
9. Shehata SM, Attia MA, Attar AAE, Ebid AE, Shalaby MM, ElBatarny AM. Algorithm of Laparoscopic Technique in Pediatric Inguinal Hernia: Results from Experience of 10 Years. J Laparoendosc Adv Surg Tech A. 2018;28(6): 755-9.
10. Verma S, Agrawal V, Acharya H, Sharma D. Laparoscopic suture-less herniotomy using tissue-sealing device for paediatric hydrocele. J Minim Access Surg. 2020;16(2): 111-4.

Antenatal Hydronephrosis

Anurag Krishna

INTRODUCTION

Antenatal ultrasonography has focused our attention on urological abnormalities that occur in babies. Ultrasonologists routinely use terms such as pelvicaliectasis, caliectasis, and hydronephrosis, leading to confusion in the minds of the obstetrician, the neonatologist, and the pediatric surgeon as to the precise significance of this finding. This chapter aims to outline a logical approach to this problem through the gestational period into the neonatal period, emphasizing what needs to be done and when, and more importantly, what need not be done.

MAGNITUDE OF THE PROBLEM

It is estimated that some degree of dilatation of the fetal renal collecting system is identified in 1–5% of all pregnancies, but in only one-fifth of these, dilatation is significant. The term hydronephrosis simply denotes dilatation of the upper urinary tract and does not necessarily imply the presence of an obstruction or a significant functional abnormality of any kind. In fact, only 3% of babies with a renal pelvis diameter <10 mm had a significant abnormality needing surgery. Antenatal hydronephrosis (ANH) could occur because of:

- *Functional dilatation:* Minor degree of dilatation that usually spontaneously resolves or stabilizes later in gestation or early infancy
- *Obstruction:* Usually at the pelviureteric junction, at the ureterovesical junction, or in the urethra [as in posterior urethral valves (PUV)]
- Vesicoureteral reflux (VUR)
- Renal dysplasia including multicystic dysplastic kidneys
- Uncommon conditions such as duplex collecting system or prune belly syndrome.

More recently, it has been suggested that the term "antenatal hydronephrosis", which focuses only on the kidney, be replaced with "antenatal urinary tract dilatation (UTD)", which emphasizes the importance of the entire urinary tract.

What is Significant Dilatation?

The Society of Fetal Urology (SFU) has recommended a grading system for hydronephrosis **(Table 1)**. An alternate method is to measure the renal pelvis anteroposterior diameter (APD).

A renal pelvis APD of >10 mm after 24–26 weeks of gestation is generally accepted as a reasonable criterion to denote significant dilatation. The presence of caliectasis or calyceal dilatation is considered an additional factor indicative of significant hydronephrosis. More recently, there is evidence to suggest that milder degrees of dilatation may also be significant in such babies, who may have VUR rather than obstruction. Currently, a renal pelvis diameter of at least 4 mm before 33 weeks and 7 mm after 33 weeks is considered significant. ANH can be classified as mild, moderate, or severe for prognostic purposes **(Table 2)**. A large systematic review suggests that the risk of significant postnatal pathology is 11.9% for mild, 45.1% for moderate, and 88.3% for severe hydronephrosis.

TABLE 1: Grading of hydronephrosis.

Grade	*Pattern of renal sinus splitting*
0	No splitting
1	Urine in pelvis barely splits sinus
2a	Urine fills intrarenal pelvis
2b	Urine fills extrarenal pelvis, major calyces dilated
3	SFU grade 2 and minor calyces dilated and parenchyma preserved
4	SFU grade 3 and parenchyma thin

(SFU: Society of Fetal Urology)

TABLE 2: Definition of antenatal hydronephrosis by anteroposterior diameter.

Degree of ANH	Second trimester	Third trimester
Mild	4–<7 mm	7–<9 mm
Moderate	7–≤10 mm	9–≤15 mm
Severe	>10 mm	>15 mm

(ANH: antenatal hydronephrosis)

Information from a Good Antenatal Ultrasound Scan

While assessing the significance of the antenatal renal dilatation, particularly with a view to identify a possible cause and whether it is worth continuing pregnancy, the ultrasound must be done carefully and must give the following information:

- Estimated fetal size and weight and its comparison with normal for that gestational age
- Amniotic fluid volume (AFV)
- Whether dilatation is unilateral or bilateral, and whether ureters are dilated or not
- Degree of dilatation (SFU grading) and dilatation of calyces
- Bladder fullness, thickness, and emptying
- Appearance of external genitalia
- Any other associated malformation

The initial study is usually done at 16–20 weeks of gestation using an appropriate transducer. There are no specific guidelines on how frequently to image the fetus. It would be reasonable to do the ultrasound every 4 weeks till 32 weeks and 2 weekly thereafter, mainly to assess the AFV.

Current Status of Fetal Intervention

The rationale for fetal urinary decompression is that those with severe obstruction early in gestation have significant impairment of both renal and pulmonary development. It has been recognized that if the AFV is adequate up to 27 weeks of gestation, then severe pulmonary hypoplasia is unlikely to occur. Percutaneous shunting of the bladder into the amniotic space is technically feasible with some morbidity. However, its role is extremely limited.

There is no place for any fetal intervention in unilateral hydronephrosis. Even with bilateral pelviureteric junction obstruction (PUJO), if the AFV is normal, percutaneous drainage of the fetal kidneys or early delivery are not warranted.

Natural History of Antenatal Hydronephrosis

Spontaneous resolution of prenatally detected hydronephrosis occurs in 50–70% of all fetuses. Resolution occurs in 80–90% of mild dilatations, 45–70% of moderate, and 25–35% of severe. This regression may be noted on serial antenatal ultrasound scans or in the postnatal life up to 3 years. Furthermore, in a substantial number, even if the hydronephrosis does not resolve completely, the renal function does not deteriorate despite persistence of pelvic dilatation. On the other hand, 15–33% of patients show progressive renal deterioration during observation. It has been noted that increasing degrees of hydronephrosis correlated with increased risk of urological pathologies that may need surgical intervention. Current evidence suggests that the need for surgery is low (between 2% and 5%, overall).

POSTNATAL EVALUATION OF ANTENATAL HYDRONEPHROSIS

Immediately after birth, the following must be recorded:

- *Sex of the baby:* In males, PUV is an important diagnosis to be ruled out as it requires early surgical intervention.
- *Palpable kidney:* Common causes are PUJO (more commonly unilateral), multicystic dysplastic kidney (unilateral), and PUV.
- *Palpable bladder:* It is indicative of PUV in boys.

If the diagnosis of PUV is suspected, all further investigations need to be done urgently as the baby requires early surgical intervention. These babies need renal function tests, ultrasound scan, voiding cystourethrogram (VCUG) within a day or two after birth so that surgical ablation of the valves may be done at the earliest.

In all other situations, there is no haste to perform investigations **(Flowchart 1)**. The initial study to be done is the ultrasound scan that must preferably not be done in the first 2–3 days. However, if the mother is being discharged earlier, it is practical to send the baby with the ultrasound scan results.

Following the ultrasound scan, a VCUG is done. There is no doubt that the conventional VCUG is preferred to a direct radionuclide cystogram (DRCG) because the latter does not give a good delineation of the bladder and urethral anatomy and that reflux, if present, cannot be accurately graded. Controversy surrounds two aspects of VCUG:

- Should VCUG be done in all babies?
- When should it be done?

Flowchart 1: Scheme for postnatal evaluation in patients with antenatal hydronephrosis.

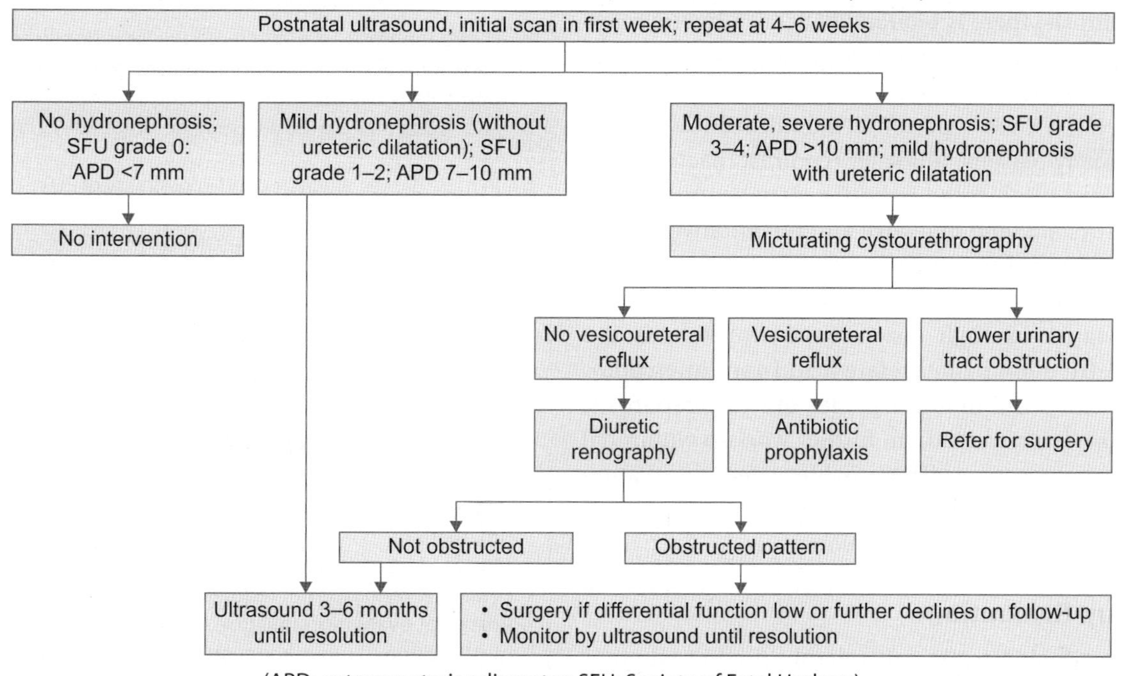

(APD: anteroposterior diameter; SFU: Society of Fetal Urology)

Should VCUG be done in all babies?

Voiding cystourethrogram is an invasive procedure, and some studies have quoted a 6% rate of urinary tract infection (UTI) following VCUG. This has made most clinicians reluctant to ask for a VCUG in newborn babies. However, if properly performed under antibiotic cover, the procedure is safe with minimal risk of UTI. This risk may be reduced by catheterizing with strict aseptic precautions and doing the procedure yourself, rather than leave it to the technician. There are some recent reports that claim that routine VCUGs may not be indicated in all babies with antenatally detected hydronephrosis. These studies recommend VCUG for those babies with:

- Bilateral hydronephrosis
- Dilated ureters
- Presence of UTI

This literature against routine use of VCUG is far from convincing. Most large centers recommend that this test must be done in all babies with ANH even if the postnatal ultrasound scan is normal. VUR has been recorded in 15–30% babies born with an antenatal diagnosis of hydronephrosis. Tibballs reported that among 255 renal units with reflux, the postnatal ultrasound was normal in 177 (70%). Furthermore, some studies have shown that the postnatal ultrasound may be normal even with the higher grades of VUR (12% of grade V and 31% with grade IV). The Indian Society of Pediatric Nephrology has recommended a middle path for performing VCUG if there is moderate-to-severe hydronephrosis, dilated ureters, or bladder or urethral abnormalities.

When should it be done?

Some authors recommend that a VCUG should be done at 4–6 weeks postnatal age. Though, again, it would be more practical to do it before the baby leaves hospital. Either way, till the VCUG has been done and VUR excluded the baby needs to be on low-dose antibiotics using amoxicillin (15 mg/kg/day) or cephalexin (50 mg/kg/day). Trimethoprim (2 mg/kg/day) may be used safely in babies after 4–6 weeks of age. Neonates who do not have VUR do not need further antibiotic chemoprophylaxis.

Role of Radionuclide Imaging Studies

In most babies, the ultrasound scan is repeated at 4–6 weeks of age. In most situations, a diuretic renogram is done at about 4 weeks of age to evaluate renal functional status and presence of obstruction. Renograms performed immediately after birth may be difficult to interpret due to the immature function of the kidneys and their handling of the radioisotope. Diuretic renogram is indicated in all kidneys with grade 3 or 4, and occasionally grade 2 hydronephrosis; there is bilateral PUJO or ureterovesical junction obstruction; if there is a solitary kidney; or, the kidney is palpable and tense.

The renal scan is superior to the introvenous pyelogram for many reasons. It is safer (contrast reactions and radiation are less), there is better visualization of the collecting system, and objective and quantitative assessment of relative function of each kidney is possible. The ideal radionuclide is mercaptoacetyltriglycine, but a cheaper, though less accurate option, is the diethylenetriamine pentaacetate acid (not dimercaptosuccinic acid) scan. In lower grades of hydronephrosis, if VUR has been excluded, no further workup with renal scans may be necessary. These babies need observation with 3-monthly ultrasound to ensure that the degree of hydronephrosis is static and not worsening.

Follow-up Evaluation

Currently, no single test can reliably predict whether a hydronephrotic kidney will improve or deteriorate. Most people agree that nearly all infants with unilateral PUJO are initially managed conservatively if the diuretic renogram shows at least 35–40% differential renal function. Exception are infants with renal infection, tense renal lump, or pelvis APD >50 mm. Follow-up ultrasound scan and diuretic renography are repeated at 3–6 months and if there is a deterioration in differential renal function, pyeloplasty is indicated. Nearly 20% infants will show deterioration on follow-up, requiring pyeloplasty. This usually happens in the first year of life.

Children with lesser degree of hydronephrosis (up to pelvis APD of <20 mm) need to be followed up with a ultrasound scan at 3 months, 1 year, then 2, 5, and 10 years. Radionuclide study is done at 3 months, 1 year, and if required at 2, 5, and 10 years. If the renal function or degree of dilatation improves, there is no further need for the isotope study.

Risk of Permanent Kidney Injury

In one study of children with APD >5 mm in the third trimester, 5% had hypertension, proteinuria, and/or reduced estimated glomerular filtration rate (eGFR) at a median follow-up of 6.5 years. In another study of children with APD >7 mm, 15% had persistent urinary tract dilatation and 39% had permanent renal damage at 12–15 years follow-up.

CLINICAL PEARLS

- Hydronephrosis >7 mm after 33 weeks is significant.
- Look for bladder emptying in fetuses with hydronephrosis, particularly bilateral.
- First postnatal ultrasound may be done 48–72 hours after birth.
- In male babies, always exclude possibility of PUVs by looking for bladder emptying.
- Till a VCUG is done, it may be safer to give low-dose antibiotic prophylaxis.
- Diethylenetriamine pentaacetate acid renogram should be done if obstruction is suspected. Dimercaptosuccinic acid renal scan is to be done in cases with vesicoureteral reflux.

KEY POINTS

- Antenatal hydronephrosis does not necessarily mean obstruction.
- Most such pregnancies can be carried to term.
- Fetal intervention is not required in majority of cases.
- Postnatal evaluation must be done in all such babies and must include a surgical opinion.
- A majority does not need surgical intervention, but those that do need require an early surgical evaluation.

SUGGESTED READING

1. Ansari MS, Ayyildiz HS, Jayanthi VR. Is voiding cystourethrogram necessary in all cases of antenatal hydronephrosis? Indian J Urol. 2009;25(4):545-6.
2. Becker AM. Postnatal evaluation of infants with an abnormal antenatal renal sonogram. Curr Opin Pediatr. 2009;21(2):207-13.
3. Blane CE, DiPietro MA, Zerin JM, Sedman AB, Bloom DA, et al. Renal sonography is not a reliable screening examination for vesicoureteral reflux. J Urol. 1993;150:752.
4. Coret A, Morag B, Katz M, Lotan D, Heyman Z, Hertz M. The impact of fetal screening on indications for cystourethrography in infants. Pediatr Radiol. 1994;24: 516-8.
5. Corteville JE, Gray DL, Crane JP. Congenital hydronephrosis: correlation of fetal ultrasonographic findings with infant outcome. Am J Obstet Gynecol. 1991;165:384.
6. Costa FP, Simoes E, Silva AC, Mak RH, Ix JH, Vasconcelos MA, et al. A clinical predictive model of renal injury in children with isolated antenatal hydronephrosis. Clin Kidney J. 2019;13:834-41.
7. De Kort EHM, Bambang Oetomo S, Zegers SH. The long term outcome of antenatal hydronephrosis up to 15 millimeters justifies a noninvasive postnatal follow-up. Acta Paediatrica. 2008;97;708-13.
8. Dhillon HK. Prenatally diagnosed hydronephrosis: the Great Ormond Street experience. Br J Urol. 1998;81(Suppl 2): 39-44.

9. DiSandro MJ, Kogan BA. Neonatal management. Role for early intervention. Urol Clin North Am. 1998;25(2): 187-97.
10. Dudley JA, Haworth JM, McGraw ME, Frank JD, Tizard EJ. Clinical relevance and implications of antenatal hydronephrosis. Arch Dis Child. 1997;76:F31.
11. Elder JS. Antenatal hydronephrosis. Fetal and neonatal management. Pediatr Clin North Am. 1997;44(5):1299-321.
12. Freedman ER, Rickwood AMK. Prenatally diagnosed pelviureteric junction obstruction: a benign condition? J Pediatr Surg. 1994;29:769-72.
13. Gloor JM, Ramsey PS, Ogburn Jr PL, Danilenko-Dixon DR, DiMarco CS, Ramin KD. The association of isolated mild fetal hydronephrosis with postnatal vesicoureteral reflux. J Matern Fetal Neonatal Med. 2002;12:196-200.
14. Green CA, Adams JC, Goodnight WH, Odibo AO, Bromley B, Jelovsek JE, et al. Frequency and prediction of persistent urinary tract dilation in third trimester and postnatal urinary tract dilation in infants following diagnosis in second trimester. Ultrasound Obstet Gynecol. 2022;59:522-31.
15. Grignon A, Filion R, Filiatrault D. Urinary dilatation in utero: classification and clinical applications. Radiology. 1986;160:645.
16. Herndon C, McKenna P, Kolon T, Gonzales ET, Baker LA, Docimo SG. A multicenter outcomes analysis of patients with neonatal reflux presenting with prenatal hydronephrosis. J Urol. 1999;162(3 Pt 2):1203-8.
17. Herndon CD. Antenatal hydronephrosis: differential diagnosis, evaluation, and treatment options. Scientific World J. 2006;6:2345-65.
18. Herthelius M, Axelsson R, Lidefelt KJ. Antenatally detected urinary tract dilatation: a 12–15-year follow-up. Pediatr Nephrol. 2020;35:2129-35.
19. Herthelius M. Antenatally detected urinary tract dilatation: long-term outcome Pediatr Nephrol. 2023;38(10):3221-7.
20. Homsy YL, Williot P, Danais S. Transitional neonatal hydronephrosis: fact or fantasy? J Urol. 1986;136:339.
21. Kitagawa H, Pringle KC, Stone P, Flower J, Murakami N, Robinson R. Postnatal follow-up of hydronephrosis detected by prenatal ultrasound: the natural history. Fetal Diagn Ther. 1998;13(1):19-25.
22. Kleiner B, Callen PW, Filly RA. Sonographic analysis of the fetus with ureteropelvic junction obstruction. AJR. 1987;148:359-63.
23. Koff SA, Campbell KD. The nonoperative management of unilateral neonatal hydronephrosis: natural history of poorly functioning kidneys. J Urol. 1994;152:593.
24. Koff SA, McDowell GC, Byard M. Diuretic radionuclide assessment of obstruction in infant: guidelines for successful interpretation. J Urol. 1988;140:1167-8.
25. Koff SA. Postnatal management of antenatal hydronephrosis using an observational approach. Urology. 2000;55: 609-11.
26. Lee RS, Cendron M, Kinnamon DD, Nguyen HT. Antenatal hydronephrosis as a predictor of postnatal outcome: a meta-analysis. Pediatrics. 2006;118:586.
27. Longpre M, Nguan A, Macneily AE, Afshar K. Prediction of the outcome of antenatally diagnosed hydronephrosis: a multivariate analysis. J Pediatr Urol. 2012;8(2):135-9.
28. Mandell J, Blyth BR, Peters CA, Retik AB, Estroff JA, Benacerraf BR. Structural genitourinary defects detected in utero. Radiology. 1991;178:193-6.
29. Mandell J, Lebowitz RL, Peters CA, Estroff JA, Retik AB, Benacerraf BR. Prenatal diagnosis of the megacystis-megaureter association. J Urol. 1992;148:1487-9.
30. Mandell J, Peters CA, Estroff JA, Benacerraf BR. Late onset severe oligohydramnios associated with genitourinary abnormalities. J Urol. 1992;148:515.
31. Marra G, Barbieri G, Moioli C, Assael BM, Grumieri G, Caccamo ML. Mild fetal hydronephrosis indicating vesicoureteric reflux. Arch Dis Child. 1994;70:F147-9.
32. Mears AL, Raza SA, Sinha AK, Misra D. Micturating cystourethrograms are not necessary for all cases of antenatally diagnosed hydronephrosis. J Pediatr Urol. 2007;3(4):264-7.
33. Moorthy I, Joshi N, Cook JV, Warren M. Antenatal hydronephrosis: negative predictive value of normal postnatal ultrasound—a 5-year study. Clin Radiol. 2003;58: 964-70.
34. Nguyen HT, Herndon CD, Cooper C, Gatti J, Kirsch A, Kokorowski P, et al. The Society of Fetal Urology consensus statement on the evaluation and management of antenatal hydronephrosis. J Pediatr Urol. 2010;6(3):212-31.
35. Nguyen HT, Phelps A, Coley B, Darge K, Rhee A, Chow JS. 2021 update on the urinary tract dilation (UTD) classification system: clarifications, review of the literature, and practical suggestions. Pediatr Radiol. 2022;52:740-51.
36. Ouzounian JG, Castro MA, Fresquez M, al-Sulyman OM, Kovacs BW. Prognostic significance of antenatally detected fetal pyelectasis. Ultrasound Obstet Gynecol. 1996;7(6): 424-8.
37. Palmer LS, Maizels M, Cartwright PC, Fernbach SK, Conway JJ. Surgery versus observation for managing obstructive grade 3 to 4 unilateral hydronephrosis: a report from the Society for Fetal Urology. J Urol. 1998;159:222.
38. Passerotti CC, Kalish LA, Chow J, Passerotti AM, Recabal P, Cendron M, et al. The predictive value of the first postnatal ultrasound in children with antenatal hydronephrosis. J Pediatr Urol. 2011;7:128-36.
39. Persutte WH, Koyle M, Lenke RR, Klas J, Ryan C, Hobbins JC. Mild pyelectasis ascertained with prenatal ultrasonography is pediatrically significant. Ultrasound Obstet Gynecol. 1997;10(1):12-8.
40. Phan VR, Traubici J, Hershenfield B, Stephens D, Rosenblum ND, Geary DF. Vesicoureteral reflux in infants with isolated antenatal hydronephrosis. Pediatr Nephrol. 2003;18:1224-8.

41. Ransley PG, Dhillon HK, Gordon I, Duffy PG, Dillon MJ, Barratt TM. The postnatal management of hydronephrosis diagnosed by prenatal ultrasound. J Urol. 1990;144:584-7.
42. Reddy PP, Mandell J. Ureteropelvic junction obstruction: prenatal diagnosis, therapeutic implications. Urol Clin N Am. 1998;25(2):171-80.
43. Sairam S, Al-Habib A, Sasson S, Thilaganathan B. Natural history of fetal hydronephrosis diagnosed on mid-trimester ultrasound. Ultrasound Obstet. Gynecol. 2001;17(3):191-6.
44. Sinha A, Bagga A, Krishna A, Bajpai M, Srinivas M, Uppal R, et al. Revised guidelines on management of antenatl hydronephrosis. Indian Pediatr. 2013;50(2):215-31.
45. Thomas DFM, Madden NP, Irving HC, Arthur RJ, Smith SE. Mild dilatation of the fetal kidney: a follow-up study. Br J Urol. 1994;74:236-9.
46. Tibballs JM, De Bruyn R. Primary vesicoureteral reflux—how useful is postnatal ultrasound? Arch Dis Child. 1996; 75:444.
47. Vates TS, Shull MJ, Underberg-Davis SJ, Fleisher MH. Complications of voiding cystourethrography in the evaluation of infants with prenatally detected hydronephrosis. J Urol. 1999;162(3 Pt 2):1221-3.
48. Yerkes E, Adams M, Pope JC 4th, Brock JW 3rd. Does every patient with prenatal hydronephrosis need voiding cystourethrography? J Urol. 1999;162:1218-23.
49. Zerin JM, Ritchey ML, Chang AC. Incidental vesicoureteral reflux in neonates with antenatally detected hydronephrosis and other renal abnormalities. Radiology. 1993; 187:157-60.

Management of Vesicoureteric Reflux

Ramesh Babu, Geminiganesan Sangeetha

INTRODUCTION

Primary vesicoureteric reflux (VUR) is seen in around 30% of children and up to 50% of neonates who present with urinary tract infection (UTI). VUR refers to retrograde flow of urine into the ureters during the act of micturition. VUR may resolve spontaneously with increasing age. Median years to resolution are 2.7 years for grade I, 3.1 years for grade II, 4.5 years for grade III, and 9.5 years for grade IV–V reflux. Favorable factors for resolution of VUR include: Age <1 year; absence of renal scarring, unilateral VUR, absence of anatomical factors such as diverticulum, and grade 1–2 VUR seen only during voiding phase. Unfavorable factors for VUR resolution include: Age >5 years at diagnosis, presence of multiple scars at the time of diagnosis, bilateral grade 4–5 VUR noted even during filling phase, presence of anatomical factors such as paraureteric diverticulum, duplication, crossed ectopia, obstructed refluxing megaureter, bladder trabeculations, and presence of dysfunctional voiding.

WHEN AND HOW TO EVALUATE FOR VESICOURETERIC REFLUX?

- Prenatally detected urinary tract dilatation (UTD) and recurrent/febrile UTI are the two common presentations of VUR.
- While all patients with UTD may not have VUR, in the following situations a voiding cystourethrogram (VCUG) is indicated: UTD with hydroureter, shrunken kidney, elder sibling with VUR, or an episode of UTI.
- Conditions such as duplication anomalies or pelvic kidneys have a risk of ipsilateral VUR, while multicystic dysplastic kidney and renal agenesis have an increased incidence of contralateral VUR.
- In children presenting with febrile UTI/recurrent UTI, a stepwise approach is recommended for VUR **(Flowchart 1)**.
- An ultrasonogram (USG) is preferable in all children following a febrile UTI/recurrent UTI as it does not require special preparation, there is no risk of radiation exposure and it is cost effective.
- Although USG is not a very sensitive tool in evaluation of VUR, one can suspect VUR if there is transient fullness of collecting system, prominent lower ureters exhibiting frequent peristalsis, parenchymal thinning, pyelitis, and renal size discrepancy.
- USG aids in diagnosis of anatomical abnormalities such as ectopic kidney, horse shoe kidney, cystic kidney, duplication of renal collecting system, ureterocele, and other underlying causes of secondary VUR.
- If USG is abnormal a full evaluation is done; if USG is normal the evaluation for VUR depends on the age **(Flowchart 1)**.
- In infants with febrile UTI, a VCUG is performed 2–3 weeks after controlling UTI as the incidence of

Flowchart 1: Evaluation of a child following a febrile UTI or recurrent UTI.

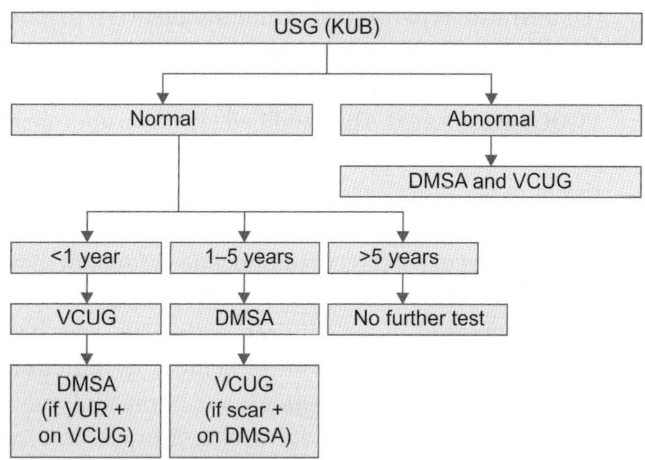

(DMSA: dimercaptosuccinic acid; KUB: kidneys, ureters, and bladder; USG: ultrasonogram; UTI: urinary tract infection; VCUG: voiding cystourethrogram; VUR: vesicoureteric reflux)

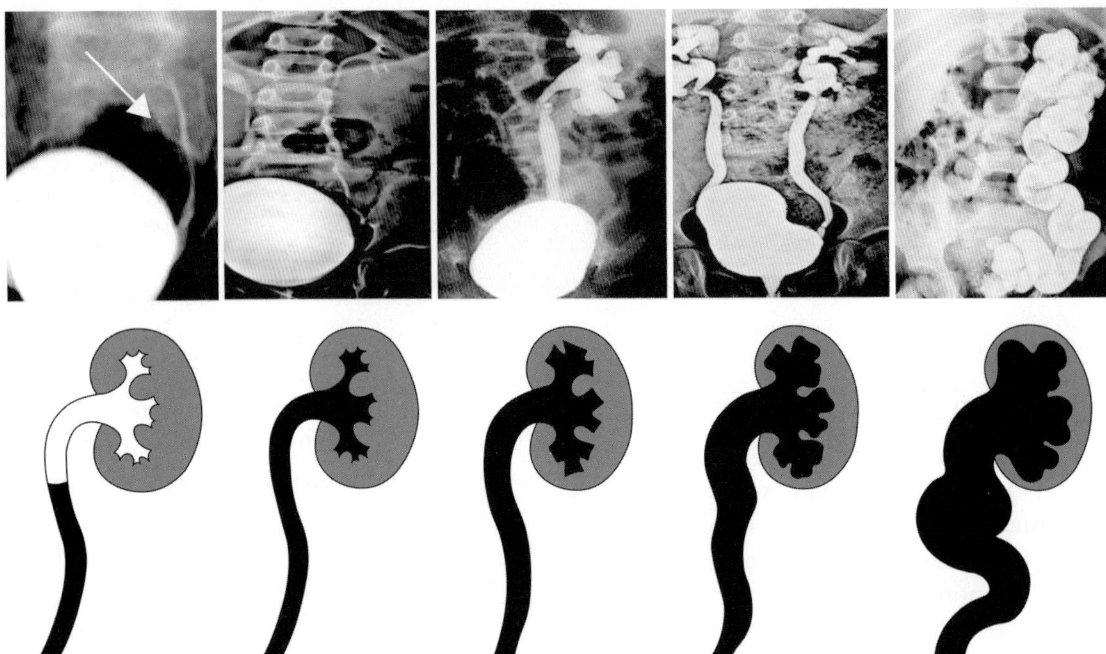

Fig. 1: International reflux grading system. *Grade 1:* Reflux into undilated distal ureter; *Grade 2:* Reflux into undilated pelvicalyceal system; *Grade 3:* Mild dilatation of ureter pelvis and calyces; *Grade 4:* Moderate dilatation/tortuosity; blunting of fornices; *Grade 5:* Gross dilatation and tortuosity of ureters with loss of papillary impressions.

VUR is as high as 30–50%. According to the International Reflux Grading System, there are 5 grades of reflux **(Fig. 1)**. VCUG also helps us to diagnose secondary causes of VUR such as paraureteric diverticulum, posterior urethral valve (PUV), neurogenic bladder, ectopic insertion of urethra, and voiding dysfunction (spinning top deformity).

- In children aged 1–5 years, a dimercaptosuccinic acid (DMSA) scan is performed, 3 months after UTI, to look for scarring. Acute phase DMSA for pyelonephritis is not recommended any more. If scars are present VCUG is performed. This modified top down approach reduces the number of invasive VCUG with radiation risk.
- In children >5 years, a normal USG is often sufficient. If the UTI recurs, a direct radionuclide cystogram may be performed to rule out VUR.
- In toddlers and older children with VUR, one has to carefully evaluate for bowel bladder dysfunction (BBD). USG for rectal diameter and X-ray abdomen looking for fecal loading are useful. A uroflowmetry is useful to diagnose voiding dysfunction. A routine urodynamic testing is not performed in all children with VUR; but preferred in those with bladder wall thickening, large postvoid residual volume, or irregular bladder outline on VCUG.

PRINCIPLES IN THE MANAGEMENT OF VESICOURETERIC REFLUX

- Although management of VUR is highly individualized, a few general consensus points about management are worth enumerating.
- During early childhood (first year of life), the kidneys are at a higher risk of developing new scars; hence, all patients diagnosed within the first year of life with dilating VUR should be treated initially with continuous antibiotic prophylaxis (CAP).
- Immediate antibiotic treatment should be initiated for febrile UTIs, especially breakthrough infections. Oral medication is as effective as parenteral treatment. Intravenous antibiotics are indicated in infants with constitutional symptoms and in children who are not capable of taking oral medications.
- In those who were diagnosed with low-grade VUR (grade I–II) following fetal UTD, in the absence of UTI no CAP is indicated as per latest AAP and AUA guidelines. In older children with BBD/recurrent UTI and low-grade VUR (grade I–II), CAP is preferred **(Flowchart 2)**.

- A detailed investigation for the presence of BBD should be performed in all children with VUR after toilet training. If BBD is detected, aggressive management must be initiated upfront.
- The management of VUR should be tailored according to risk groups. In high-risk groups, early surgical management to cure VUR may be indicated.
- The risk-grouping and hence the choice of management depends on the age, presence of renal scars, reflux grade, laterality (unilateral or bilateral), presence of BBD, associated anomalies of the urinary tract, compliance, breakthrough infections, and parental preference. Febrile UTI, high-grade reflux, bilaterality, cortical abnormalities, and BBD are considered to be risk factors for renal damage and new scar (high risk group).

Flowchart 2: Medical management of low-grade VUR (grade I–II).

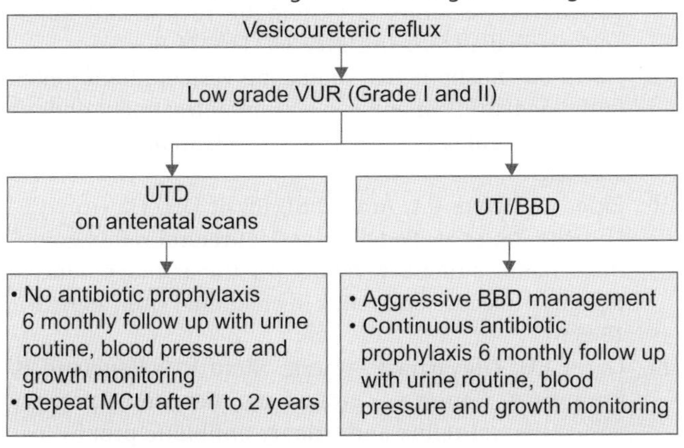

(BBD: bowel bladder dysfunction; UTD: urinary tract dilatation; UTI: urinary tract infection; VUR: vesicoureteric reflux)

- In those with high-grade VUR (grade III–IV) in the absence of recurrent UTI/BBD, CAP is continued and patient re-evaluated after a period of 1–2 years **(Flowchart 3)**.
- Breakthrough UTIs in infants with high-grade VUR (grade III–IV) can be challenging. Circumcision is known to reduce UTIs in male infants. Endoscopic treatment may be useful in grade III VUR. In grade IV–V VUR, endoscopic treatment may downgrade VUR. Diversion procedures are preferred in infants with high-grade VUR as reimplantation is generally not preferred in infants **(Flowchart 3)**.
- In chilldren >1 years age with breakthrough UTI and renal scarring intervention is indicated; endoscopic treatment can be a useful option in grade III–IV VUR while reimplantation in grade IV–V.

Endoscopic Treatment

Endoscopic treatment recreates the antireflux mechanism by injecting an inert material into the bladder wall at the ureteric orifice. While general anesthesia is required, it is generally performed as a day care procedure. Best success rates of 70–80% are reported for grade III VUR with single injection. For grades IV–V, two or more injections may be needed. Polyvinyl polyalcohol co-polymer (PPC) has slightly higher success rate than dextranomer/hyaluronic acid (DXHA).

Reimplantation—Open/Laparoscopic/Robotic

The aim of reimplantation of ureter is to stop VUR by restoring the antireflux mechanism. Success rates for open surgery are 98%, with few complications.

Flowchart 3: Role of interventions in high grade VUR (grade III–V).

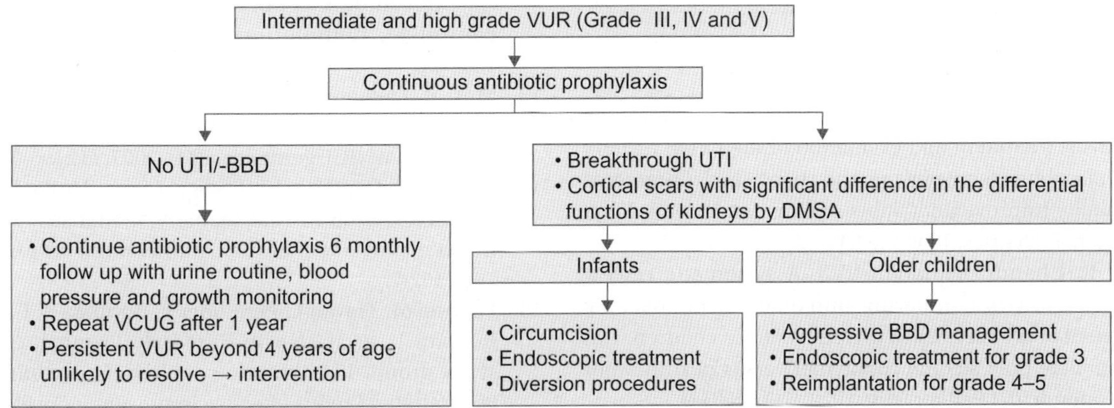

(BBD: bowel bladder dysfunction; DMSA: dimercaptosuccinic acid; VCUG: voiding cystourethrogram; UTI: urinary tract infection; VUR: vesicoureteric reflux)

- Open reimplantation is widely used option in the presence of breakthrough UTI, high-grade VUR, and new scars in DMSA scanning.
- Transvesicoscopic ureteric reimplantation (TVUR) is becoming a favorable minimally invasive option in grade IV–V bilateral VUR.
- Laparoscopic extravesical ureteric reimplantation (LEVUR) is an equally successful operation for unilateral VUR. For bilateral VUR, it has slightly higher rate of urinary retention.
- Robot-assisted laparoscopic ureteric reimplantation (RALUR) has added precision to suturing and has comparable success.
- All minimally invasive options ensure faster recovery and higher success rate than endoscopic treatment.
- After reimplantation, ultrasonography should be performed to rule out obstruction. Follow-up monitoring should be carried out for infections, new scarring, and somatic growth through adolescence.

KEY POINTS

- In a child with UTI and VUR, it is essential to look for features of BBD and treat it aggressively.
- Modified top down approach (late DMSA scans and VCUG only if scarring is detected) is preferred in the evaluation of 1–5-year-old children with febrile UTI.
- Continuous antibiotic prophylaxis is preferred for children with dilating reflux (grade III–V).
- High-risk group (older children with recurrent UTI and BBD, persistent grade 4–5 VUR, and multiple scars) benefit from interventions.
- Endoscopic treatment is preferred to open surgery by many in those with grade III reflux.
- Endoscopic/surgical interventions have an established role in reducing recurrent pyelonephritis.

SUGGESTED READING

1. American Academy of Pediatrics. Practice parameter: the diagnosis, treatment and evaluation of the initial urinary tract infection in febrile infants and young child. Committee on Quality Improvement Subcommittee on Urinary Tract Infection. Pediatrics. 1999;103:843-52.
2. Babu R, Chandrasekharam VVS. A systematic review & meta-analysis comparing outcomes of endoscopic treatment of primary vesico ureteric reflux in children with polyacrylate poly alcohol copolymer versus dextranomer hyaluranic acid. J Pediatr Surg. 2022;57(11):683-9.
3. Babu R, Chandrasekharam VVS. A systematic review and meta-analysis comparing outcomes of laparoscopic extravesical versus trans vesicoscopic ureteric reimplantation, J Pediatr Urol. 2020;16(6):783-9.
4. Babu R, Chowdhary S. Controversies Regarding Management of Vesico-ureteric Reflux. Indian J Pediatr. 2017l; 84(7):540-4.
5. Babu R, Sriram K. Extravesical (modified Gregoir Lich) versus intravesical (Cohen's) ureteric reimplantation for vesicoureteral reflux in children: a single center experience. Indian J Urol. 2016;32(4):306-9.
6. Bajpai M, Verma A, Panda SS. Endoscopic treatment of vesico-ureteral reflux: experience of 99 ureteric moieties. J Indian Assoc Pediatr Surg. 2013;18(4):133-5.
7. Chandrasekharam VVS, Babu R. A systematic review and metaanalysis of open, conventional laparoscopic and robot-assisted laparoscopic techniques for re-do pyeloplasty for recurrent uretero pelvic junction obstruction in children. J Pediatr Urol. 2022;18(5):642-9.
8. Chandrasekharam VVS, Babu R. Robot-assisted laparoscopic extravesical versus conventional laparoscopic extravesical ureteric reimplantation for pediatric primary vesicoureteric reflux: a systematic review and meta-analysis. Pediatr Surg Int. 2020;36(11):1371-8.
9. Davis TD, Rushton HG. Managing vesicoureteral reflux in the pediatric patient: a spectrum of treatment options for a spectrum of disease. Curr Treat Options Peds. 2016; 2:23-34.
10. Elder JS, Peters CA, Arant BSJ, Ewalt DH, Hawtrey CE, Hurwitz RS, et al. Pediatric vesicoureteral reflux guidelines panel summary report on the management of primary vesicoureteral reflux in children. J Urol. 1997;157: 1846-51.
11. Garin EH, Olavarria F, Garcia Nieto V, Valenciano B, Campos A, Young L. Clinical significance of primary vesicoureteral reflux and urinary antibiotic prophylaxis after acute pyelonephritis: a multicenter, randomized, controlled study. Pediatrics. 2006;117:626-32.
12. Montini G, Rigon L, Zucchetta P, Fregonese F, Toffolo A, Gobber D, et al. Prophylaxis after first febrile urinary tract infection in children? A multicenter, randomized, controlled, noninferiority trial. Pediatrics. 2008;122: 1064-71.
13. Mori R, Lakhanpaul M, Verrier-Jones K. Diagnosis and management of urinary tract infection in children: summary of NICE guidance. BMJ. 2007;335:395-7.
14. Nelson CP, Copp HL, Lai J, Saigal CS; the Urologic Diseases in America Project. Is availability of endoscopy changing initial management of vesicoureteral reflux? J Urol. 2009; 182:1152-7.
15. Pennesi M, Travan L, Peratoner L, Bordugo A, Cattaneo A, Ronfani L, et al.; North East Italy Prophylaxis in VUR study group. Is antibiotic prophylaxis in children with vesicoureteral reflux effective in preventing pyelonephritis and renal scars? A randomized, controlled trial. Pediatr. 2008;121:e1489-94.

16. Peters CA, Skoog SJ, Arant BS Jr, Copp HL, Elder JS, Hudson RG, et al. Summary of the AUA Guideline on Management of Primary Vesicoureteral Reflux in Children. J Urol. 2010;184(3):1134-44.
17. Riccabona M. Management of recurrent urinary tract infection and vesicoureteral reflux in children. Curr Opin Urol. 2000;10:25-8.
18. RIVUR Trial Investigators, Hoberman A, Greenfield SP, Mattoo TK, Keren R, Mathews R, et al. Antimicrobial prophylaxis for children with vesicoureteral reflux. N Engl J Med. 2014;370(25):2367-76.
19. Roussey-Kesler G, Gadjos V, Idres N, Horen B, Ichay L, Leclair MD, et al. Antibiotic prophylaxis for the prevention of recurrent urinary tract infection in children with low grade vesicoureteral reflux: results from a prospective randomized study. J Urol. 2008;179:674.
20. Schwab CW Jr, Wu HY, Selman H, Smith GH, Snyder HM 3rd, Canning DA. Spontaneous resolution of vesicoureteral reflux: a 15-year perspective. J Urol. 2002;168(6): 2594-9.
21. Sencan A, Carvas F, Hekimoglu IC, Caf N, Sencan A, Chow J, et al. Urinary tract infection and vesicoureteral reflux in children with mild antenatal hydronephrosis. J Pediatr Urol. 2014;10(6):1008-13.
22. Sjöström S1, Sillén U, Bachelard M, Hansson S, Stokland E. Spontaneous resolution of high grade infantile vesicoureteral reflux. J Urol. 2004;172(2):694-8; discussion 699.
23. Smellie JM, Prescod NP, Shaw PJ, Risdon RA, Bryant TN. Childhood reflux and urinary infection: a follow-up of 10–41 years in 226 adults. Pediatr Nephrol. 1998;12: 727-36.
24. Suson KD, Mathews R. Evaluation of children with urinary tract infection—impact of the 2011 AAP guidelines on the diagnosis of vesicoureteral reflux using a historical series. J Pediatr Urol. 2014;10(1):182-5.
25. Van Batavia JP, Nees SN, Fast AM, Combs AJ, Glassberg KI. Outcomes of vesicoureteral reflux in children with non-neurogenic lower urinary tract dysfunction treated with dextranomer/hyaluronic acid copolymer (Deflux). J Pediatr Urol. 2014;10(3):482-7.

Intussusception

Gautam S Agarwal, Anurag Krishna

INTRODUCTION

Intussusception is an acquired invagination of the bowel into itself, usually involving both small and large bowel **(Figs. 1 and 2)**. Ileocolic intussusception is the most common cause of small bowel obstruction in children. Intussusception is an emergency. There is often a delay in recognition and diagnosis. This may result in bowel obstruction, venous congestion, subsequent bowel necrosis, and perforation.

INCIDENCE AND CLINICAL FEATURES

The peak age for idiopathic intussusception is 5–10 months and typically ranges up to 3 years. The most common clinical presentation is of an infant with crampy abdominal pain and irritability, vomiting, and, later, bloody stools. The signs and symptoms vary considerably and overlap with other abdominal conditions. The clinical features of intussusception are given in **Table 1**.

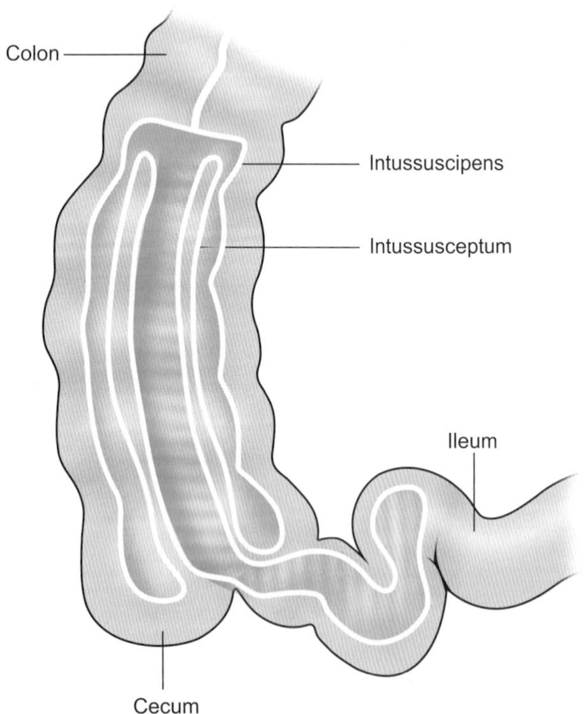

Fig. 1: Diagrammatic representation of intussusception.

DIAGNOSIS

Intussusception must be suspected in all infants who present with spasmodic abdominal pain and irritability.

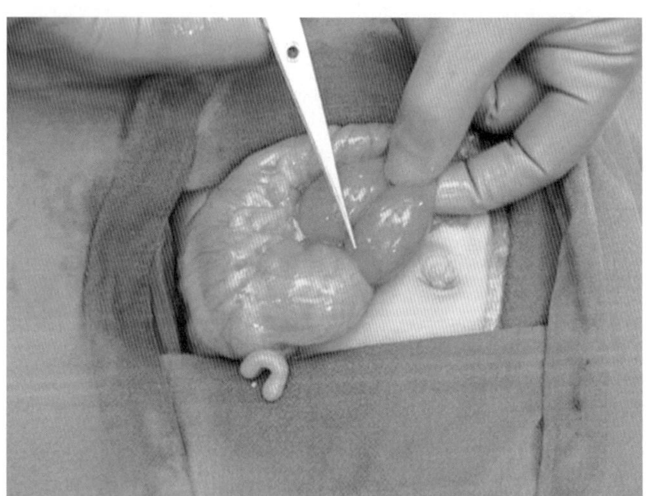

Fig. 2: Operative photograph showing the intussusception. *(For color version, see Plate 14)*

TABLE 1: Clinical features of intussusception.

Abdominal colic	65%
Lump	35–70%
Rectal bleeding	50–80%
Triad	7.5–50%
Vomiting	75–85%
Preceding respiratory/ gastrointestinal symptoms	<25%

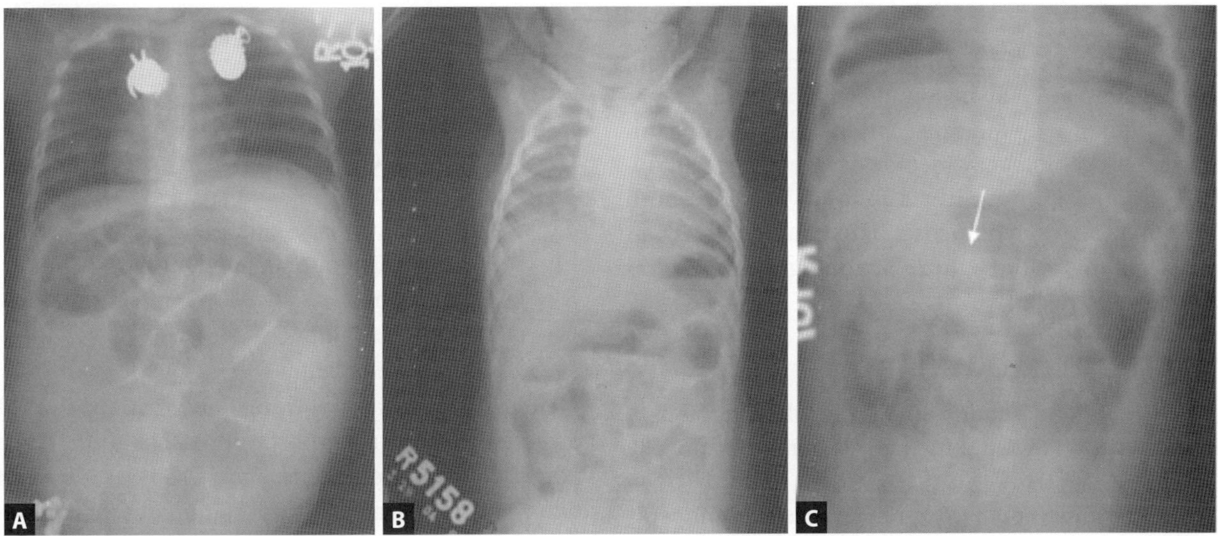

Figs. 3A to C: X-rays of abdomen: (A) Right iliac fossa empty; (B) Signs of intestinal obstruction; (C) Soft tissue mass (arrow). *Normal X-ray does not rule out intussusception.*

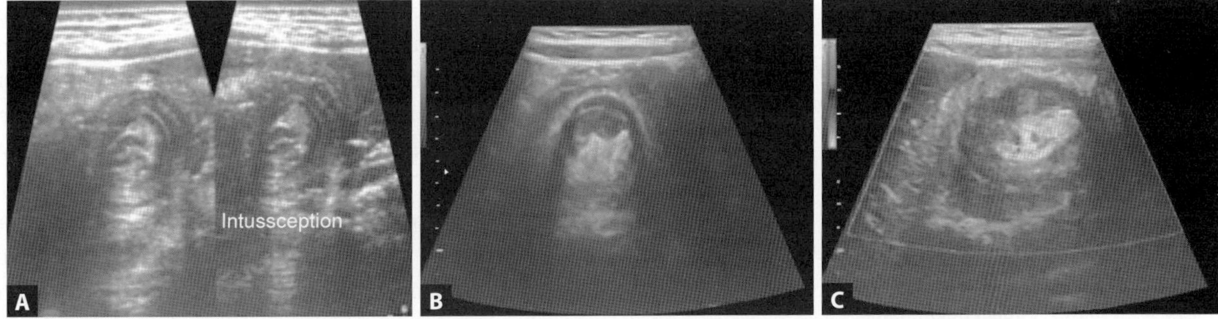

Figs. 4A to C: Ultrasound showing whorled appearance of intussusception.

Clinically, observation of the dance sign, a feeling of emptiness on palpation of the right lower quadrant of the abdomen, may be an indication of intussusception. A digital rectal examination is helpful, as a finger may feel the intussusceptum or may show blood on the fingertip.

Plain abdominal radiographs have poor sensitivity (45%) for the detection of intussusception but may serve to screen for other diagnoses in the differential diagnosis, such as constipation and free peritoneal air **(Figs. 3A to C)**.

The presence of a curvilinear mass within the course of the colon (the crescent sign), particularly in the transverse colon just beyond the hepatic flexure, is a nearly pathognomonic sign of intussusception. The absence of bowel gas in the ascending colon is one of the most specific signs of intussusception on radiographs.

Ultrasound is the investigation of choice for the diagnosis of intussusception. The image seen on transverse sonography or computed tomography is a doughnut shape, created by the hyperechoic central core of the bowel and mesentery surrounded by the hypoechoic outer edematous bowel. In longitudinal imaging, intussusception may resemble a sandwich.

There is no foolproof test that can accurately identify all patients with intussusception. The clinical triad of colicky abdominal pain, palpable abdominal mass, and currant jelly stools is present in <50% of cases but a high index of suspicion will help minimize delay in diagnosis and referral.

A computed tomography scan of the abdomen may help in diagnosis. However, the cost, radiation dose, and risk of sedation in these young children make it far less practical than sonography. Published sonography studies from single institutions suggest high accuracy, approaching 100% in experienced hands, with a sensitivity of 98–100% and specificity of 88–100% **(Figs. 4A to C)**.

Lead Points

In approximately 2–12% of children with intussusception, a surgical lead point may be found. Lead points are more likely in children with intussusception that present at an older age. Lead points may include Meckel diverticulum, polyps, enlarged mesenteric lymph nodes, small duplication cysts, or submucosal hematomas, which can occur in patients with Henoch-Schonlein purpura and coagulation dyscrasias.

TREATMENT (FLOWCHART 1)

Treatment of intussusception entails the following steps:

- Resuscitate first. Ensure the baby is hemodynamically stable.
- Nonsurgical preferred, except in few cases. Nonoperative reduction is contraindicated if:
  - Long-standing—intussusception present for >36–48 hours
  - Gross abdominal distension
  - Hemodynamic instability
- Surgery is absolutely indicated in:
  - Shock and sepsis
  - Perforation peritonitis
  - Failed reduction

Flowchart 1: Algorithm for management of intussusception.

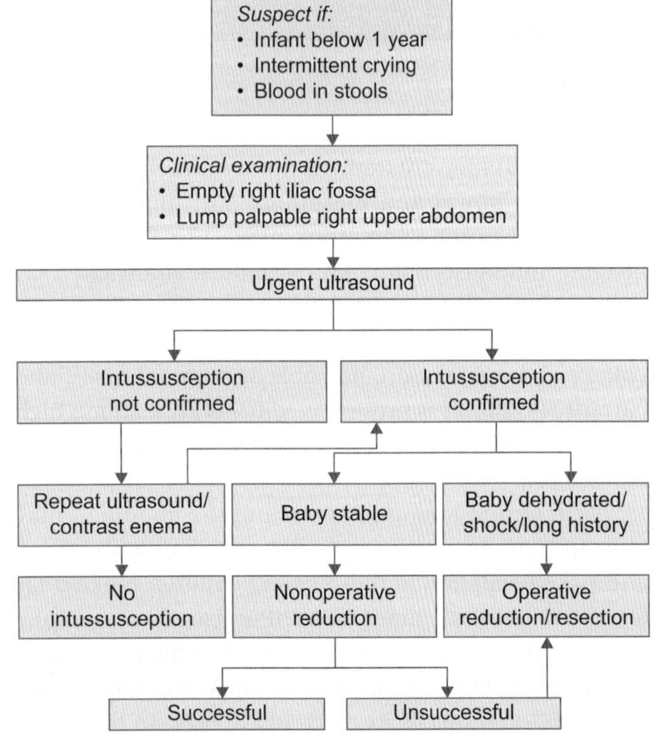

- *Nonsurgical:*
  - "Pushing" agent:
    - Air
    - Fluid—water, saline, and barium
  - Imaging modality:
    - Ultrasound:
      - *Pros:* Avoids radiation
      - *Cons:* Operator dependent
    - Fluoroscopy:
      - *Pros:* Confidence
      - *Cons:* Radiation

Before enema reduction, dehydration should be corrected with intravenous fluid resuscitation. Children with evidence of peritonitis, shock, sepsis, or free air on abdominal radiographs are not candidates for hydrostatic reduction. These children should be initially stabilized and treated operatively.

The presence of small-bowel obstruction reduces the probability of successful enema reduction but it is not a contraindication to performing the enema. The most important factor that decreases the reduction rate of enema is the duration of symptoms. The longer the duration of symptoms beyond 24 hours, the lower the likelihood of successful contrast enema reduction.

Age <3 months is associated with, both, a higher perforation rate and a lower rate of successful reduction, as is dehydration and small-bowel obstruction. These situations are less common.

Barium is no longer the liquid contrast medium of choice for reduction of intussusception due to risk of barium peritonitis, infection, and adhesions if perforation occurs during the enema. While iodinated contrast is considered a safer agent than barium, one should be aware that it may produce fluid and electrolyte shifts if perforation occurs.

An intussusception that reaches up to the rectum has only a 25% chance of reduction, but intussusceptions encountered elsewhere in the colon, including the hepatic flexure, can be expected to have a successful reduction rate of over 80%. The most common location to encounter idiopathic intussusception is at the hepatic flexure.

The most important potential complication of enema is bowel perforation. The most common site is at or just proximal to the intussusception in the transverse colon. Perforations with pneumatic reduction are smaller than those with liquid enema although the overall perforation rates are similar.

In a summary of the literature, there were 32 studies using air reduction and 39 using liquid (barium, iodinated contrast, saline, or water) reduction techniques. Air enema studies had significantly higher mean reduction rates compared with liquid enema studies (82 vs. 68%).

The air enema technique is well described in the literature. Briefly, the enema tip should be placed within the child's rectum and taped in place with abundant tape. The child is placed in a prone position to allow the radiologist or assistant to squeeze the buttocks closed and prevent air from leaking. Air is rapidly insufflated into the colon under fluoroscopic observation. One critical safety issue is to keep air pressure below a maximum limit of 120 mm Hg to avoid the risk of perforation. Once the intussusception is encountered, its reduction is followed fluoroscopically until it is completely reduced. Air should flow freely from the cecum into the distal small bowel loops to signify complete reduction.

The value of repeated attempts at nonoperative reduction has not been determined. Some clinicians recommend taking the patient to surgery if the first attempt fails. Other clinicians advocate 1 or 2 subsequent attempts within a few minutes to a few hours after the first attempt.

In case of failure of reduction and above-mentioned absolute indications, sometimes an operative reduction is required. At laparotomy, the mass is delivered and gentle manual reduction is done. The key to reduction is slow, constant milking, and squeezing in a retrograde manner. The intussusceptum is pushed rather than pulled. Infrequently, when the maneuver fails, or if the bowel is gangrenous, resection of the intestine with end-to-end anastomosis may be required.

RECURRENCE

Intussusception recurrence rates average 10% in large series, with a range of 5.4–15.4%, regardless of air versus liquid enema technique. The recurrence rates are ≤5% when surgical reduction is performed, presumably due to the development of adhesions.

Fifty percent of children who develop recurrent intussusception will present within 48 hours, although recurrences have been reported up to 18 months later. The risk of a pathologic lead point **(Fig. 5)** in children with recurrent intussusception is low. No predictive clinical factors have been identified for pathologic lead point in these children with recurrent intussusception. No clear risk factors are known for why some children have recurrences

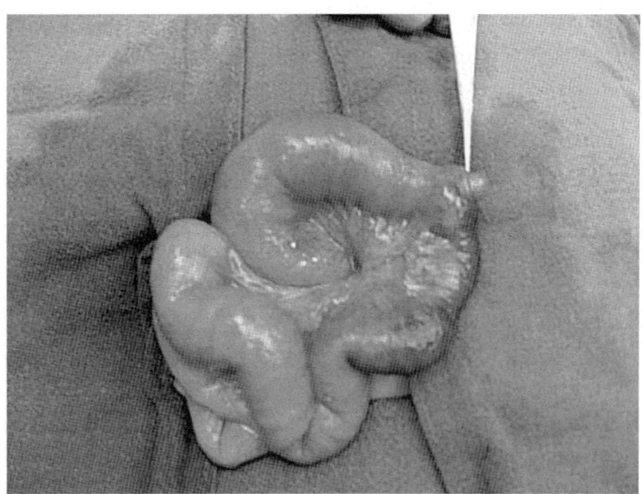

Fig. 5: Operative photograph showing a small Meckel's diverticulum as the lead point. *(For color version, see Plate 14)*

although some do have a focal pathologic lead point. Those with diffuse bowel abnormalities (diffuse pathologic lead points) and ileocolic intussusception, such as children with cystic fibrosis, Henoch–Schönlein purpura, or celiac disease, may be treated with enema reduction more aggressively than those with focal pathologic lead points to avoid surgery. Repeat enema is both safe and effective in recurrent intussusception as long as the child remains clinically stable.

KEY POINTS

- High index of suspicion
- Rapid initial resuscitation
- Attempt "safe" and "sure" reduction
- Operate if doubtful

SUGGESTED READING

1. Beasley SW, Glover J. Intussusception: prediction of outcome of gas enema. J Pediatr Surg. 1992;27:474-5.
2. Bratton SL, Haberkern CM, Waldhausen JH, Sawin RS, Allison JW. Intussusception: hospital size and risk of surgery. Pediatrics. 2001;107:299-303.
3. Burnett E, Parashar UD, Tate JE. Associations of Intussusception with Adenovirus, Rotavirus, and Other Pathogens: A Review of the Literature. Pediatr Infect Dis J. 2020;39:1127.
4. Daneman A, Alton DJ, Ein S, Wesson D, Superina R, Thorner P. Perforation during attempted intussusception reduction in children: a comparison of perforation with barium and air. Pediatr Radiol. 1995;25:81-8.

5. Daneman A, Navarro O. Intussusception part 1: a review of diagnostic approaches. Pediatr Radiol. 2003;33:79-85.
6. Daneman A, Navarro O. Intussusception part 2: an update on the evolution of management. Pediatr Radiol. 2004; 34:97-108.
7. Del-Pozo G, Gonzalez-Spinola J, Gomez-Anson B, Serrano C, Miralles M, González-deOrbe G, et al. Intussusception: trapped peritoneal fluid detected with US: relationship to reducibility and ischemia. Radiology. 1996;201:379-83.
8. Earl TM, Wellen JR, Anderson CD, Nadler M, Doyle MM, Shenoy SS, et al. Small bowel obstruction after pediatric liver transplantation: the unusual is the usual. J Am Coll Surg. 2011;212(1):62-7.
9. Ein SH. Leading points in childhood intussusception. J Pediatr Surg. 1976;11:209-11.
10. Ein SH. Recurrent intussusception in children. J Pediatr Surg. 1975;10:751-5.
11. Gu L, Alton D, Daneman A, Stringer DA, Liu P, Wilmot DM, et al. John Caffey award. Intussusception reduction in children by rectal insufflation of air. AJR. 1988;150: 1345-8.
12. Guo JZ, Ma XY, Zhou QH. Results of air pressure enema reduction of intussusception: 6396 cases in 13 years. J Pediatr Surg. 1986;21:1201-3.
13. Hernanz-Schulman M, Foster C, Maxa R, Battles G, Dutt P, Stratton C, et al. Experimental study of mortality and morbidity of contrast media and standardized fecal dose in the peritoneal cavity. Pediatr Radiol. 2000;30: 369-78.
14. Katz M, Phelan E, Carlin JB, Beasley SW. Gas enema for the reduction of intussusception: relationship between clinical signs and symptoms and outcome. AJR. 1993;160: 363-6.
15. Kirks DR. Diagnosis and treatment of pediatric intussusception: how far should we push our radiologic techniques? Radiology. 1994;191:622-3.
16. Ko HS, Schenk JP, Troger J, Rohrschneider WK. Current radiological management of Intussusception in children. Eur Radiol. 2007;17:2411.
17. Li XZ, Wang H, Song J, Liu Y, Lin YQ, Sun ZX. Ultrasonographic diagnosis of intussusception in children: a systematic review and meta-analysis. J Ultrasound Med. 2021;40:1077.
18. Mercer S, Carpenter B. Mechanism of perforation occurring in the intussuscipiens during hydrostatic reduction of intussusception. Can J Surg. 1982;25:481-3.
19. Milbrandt K, Sigalet D. Intussusception associated with a Meckel's diverticulum and a duplication cyst. J Pediatr Surg. 2008;43(12):e21-3.
20. Navarro O, Daneman A. Intussusception part 3: diagnosis and management of those with an identifiable or predisposing cause and those that reduce spontaneously. Pediatr Radiol. 2004;34:305-12.
21. Ntoulia A, Tharakan SJ, Reid JR, Mahboubi S. Failed intussusception reduction in children: correlation between radiologic, surgical, and pathologic findings. ARJ Am J Roentgenol. 2016;207:424.
22. Parashar UD, Holman RC, Cummings KC, Staggs NW, Curns AT, Zimmerman CM, et al. Trends in intussusception-associated hospitalizations and deaths among US infants. Pediatrics. 2000;106:1413-21.
23. Sandler AD, Ein SH, Connolly B, Daneman A, Filler RM. Unsuccessful air-enema reduction of intussusception: is a second attempt worthwhile? Pediatr Surg Int. 1999; 15(3-4):214-6.
24. Sanni RB, Nandiolo R, Coulibaly Diaoudia MT, Vodi L, Mobiot ML. Acute intussusception due to intestinal Kaposi's sarcoma in an infant. Afr J Paediatr Surg. 2009;6(2):131.
25. Shekherdimian S, Lee SL, Sydorak RM, Applebaum H. Contrast enema for pediatric intussusception: is reflux into the terminal ileum necessary for complete reduction? J Pediatr Surg. 2009;44(1):247-9; discussion 249-50.
26. Shiels WE II, Kirks DR, Keller GL, Ryckman FR, Daugherty CC, Specker BL, et al. John Caffey award. Colonic perforation by air and liquid enemas: comparison study in young pigs. AJR. 1993;160:931-5.
27. Shiels WE II, Maves CK, Hedlund GL, Kirks DR. Air enema for diagnosis and reduction of intussusception: clinical experience and pressure correlates. Radiology. 1991;181: 169-72.
28. Soccorso G, Puls F, Richards C, Pringle H, Nour S. A ganglioneuroma of the sigmoid colon presenting as leading point of intussusception in a child: a case report. J Pediatr Surg. 2009;44(1):e17-20.
29. Stringer MD, Pablot SM, Brereton RJ. Paediatric intussusception. Br J Surg. 1992;79:867-76.
30. West KW, Stephens B, Vane DW, Grosfeld JL. Intussusception: current management in infants and children. Surgery. 1987;102:704-10.
31. Yap Shiyi E, Ganapathy S. Intussusception in Children Presenting to the Emergency Department: An Asian perspective. Pediatr Emerg Care. 2017;33:409.

Neonatal Jaundice: Surgical Perspectives

Rajeev Redkar, Anant Bangar

INTRODUCTION

Jaundice is a most common neonatal condition requiring medical attention in newborn babies. Most of them have physiological jaundice or have pathological medical causes. Surgical causes are relatively uncommon and present with cholestatic jaundice. Pathological jaundice requires detailed investigations and management, with early consideration of extra-hepatic biliary atresia, as early surgical intervention leads to better outcomes. Most of the surgical jaundice is amenable to corrective surgical treatment and, if left untreated, rapid liver damage is a certain outcome in most of them. Even if curative surgical treatment is not available, early medical management and optimization of nutrition help infants with cholestasis by preventing complications. Criteria for pathological jaundice proposed by Maisels et al. in 1981 are as follows:

- Jaundice notice within first 24 hours of life
- Rate of bilirubin rise is >5 mg/dL/day
- Total serum bilirubin >12.9 mg/dL in a full-term or 15 mg/dL in a premature infant
- Direct serum bilirubin >1.5–2.0 mg/dL
- Jaundice persisting for >1 week in full-term or 2 weeks in a premature infant.

ETIOLOGY

Cholestatic jaundice affects approximately 1 in every 2,500 term infants and has conjugated hyperbilirubinemia due to bile flow obstruction (cholestasis) or hepatic cell injury **(Flowchart 1)**.

Extrahepatic causes of bile flow obstruction:

- Extrahepatic biliary atresia
- Choledochal cyst
- Bile plug syndrome

Flowchart 1: Causes of conjugated hyperbilirubinemia.

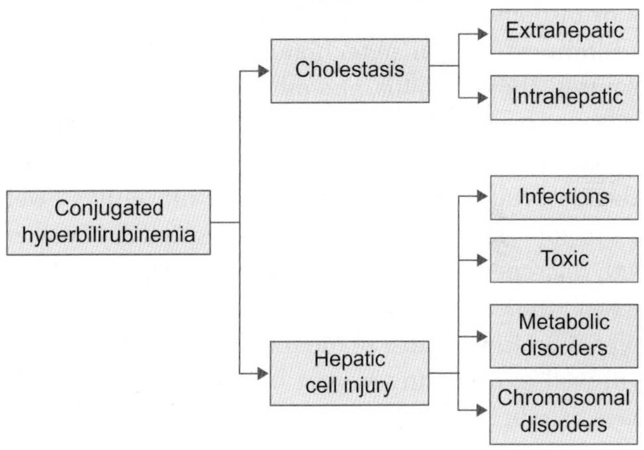

- Gallstones/biliary sludge
- Spontaneous perforation of bile duct
- Bile duct stenosis
- Sclerosing cholangitis

Intrahepatic causes of bile flow obstruction:

- Idiopathic neonatal hepatitis
- Alagille syndrome
- Biliary hypoplasia or nonsyndromic paucity of bile ducts
- Byler's disease
- Caroli's disease
- Congenital hepatic fibrosis

CLINICAL PRESENTATION

The typical presentation of cholestasis is prolonged jaundice, icterus, clay-colored stools, and dark yellow urine. Mostly it overlaps the physiological jaundice and gives false perception of decreasing jaundice when indirect bilirubin due to physiologic jaundice decreases.

Occasionally, cholestatic jaundice may present 2–3 weeks after birth once the physiological jaundice has completely resolved. Clay-colored stools in an infant should always prompt detailed evaluation.

Coagulopathy secondary to vitamin K malabsorption or end-stage liver disease may present with bleeding or bruising. Splenomegaly will suggest portal hypertension with cirrhosis, storage diseases, and hemolytic diseases. Lethargy, hypotonia, poor feeding, irritability, or seizures are indicative of sepsis, intracranial hemorrhage, hyperammonemia-encephalopathy, and metabolic disorders. Metabolic causes may present with a peculiar odor of body or urine. Low-birth weight, prematurity, thrombocytopenia, petechiae, purpura, dysmorphic features, chorioretinitis, and other congenital anomalies are associated with congenital infections. Alagille and chromosomal abnormalities will have facial dysmorphism. Alagille syndrome will have cardiac murmur as well. Panhypopituitarism and septo-optic dysplasia will present with micropenis and inability to fix and follow a moving object. Choledochal cyst will have palpable mass in right hypochondrium. Most of the infants with biliary atresia will well and healthy in first few weeks, but 20% will have extrahepatic congenital malformations like cardiac anomalies, situs inversus, polysplenia, asplenia, etc.

EVALUATION

Evaluation always begins with good history taking starting from antenatal period, followed by clinical examination and diagnostic tests **(Flowchart 2)**. Any infant presenting with jaundice at the age of 3 weeks or more needs fractionated bilirubin levels. Further detailed evaluation is required if there is conjugated hyperbilirubinemia, defined as serum conjugated bilirubin level >1.0 mg/dL.

Flowchart 2: Evaluation flowchart.

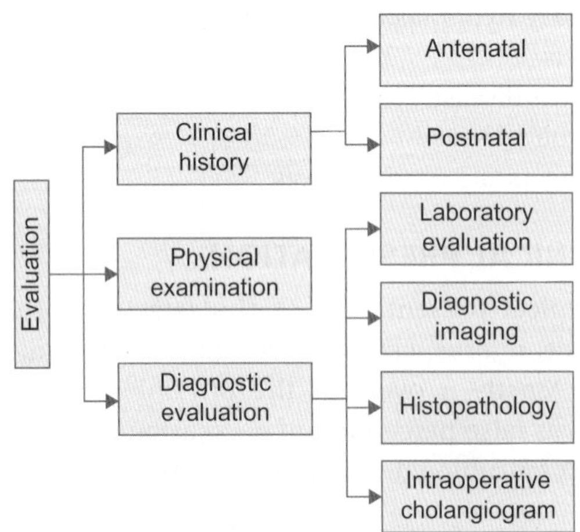

CLINICAL HISTORY

There are many conditions causing conjugated hyperbilirubinemia in an infant. Hence, detailed history is paramount for planning further evaluation. Parameters of clinical interest in the history of the cholestatic infant are enumerated in **Tables 1 to 3**.

PHYSICAL EXAMINATION

A comprehensive physical examination is necessary to plan for further evaluation. Important physical findings are enumerated in **Table 4**.

It is pertinent to know that differentiation between neonatal hepatitis and biliary atresia is usually not possible with clinical history and examination. Further laboratory and radiological investigations are a must and in some cases specific investigations are also required.

TABLE 1: Family history.

Family history	
Consanguinity	Increased risk of autosomal recessive disorders
Neonatal cholestasis in the parents or siblings	Cystic fibrosis, α-1-antitrypsin deficiency, progressive familial intrahepatic cholestasis, and Alagille syndrome are all genetic conditions causing neonatal cholestasis
History of repeated fetal loss or early demise	Gestational alloimmune liver disease
Spherocytosis and other hemolytic diseases	Known to aggravate conjugated hyperbilirubinemia

TABLE 2: Prenatal history.

Prenatal history	
Prenatal ultrasonography findings	• Choledochal cyst, cholelithiasis • Bowel anomalies • Syndromes
Cholestasis of pregnancy	• Heterozygotes for PFIC gene mutations • Mitochondrial disorder
Acute fatty liver of pregnancy	Gestational alloimmune liver disease
Maternal infections	TORCH infections

TABLE 3: Infant history.

Infant history	
Gestational age	Prematurity as a risk factor for neonatal hepatitis
SGA	• Increased risk of neonatal cholestasis • Congenital infections
Alloimmune hemolysis; glucose-6-phosphate-dehydrogenase deficiency; hydrops fetalis	Increased risk of neonatal cholestasis
Neonatal infection	Urinary tract infection, sepsis-related cholestasis, CMV, HIV, syphilis, etc.
Newborn screen	• Panhypopituitarism galactosemia • Fatty acid oxidation defects • Cystic fibrosis
Source of nutrition: Breast milk, formula, PN	Galactosemia, hereditary fructose intolerance, PN-associated liver disease
Growth	2 colors
Scissors	Genetic and metabolic disease
Vision	Septo-optic dysplasia
Hearing	PFIC1, TJP2
Vomiting	Metabolic disease, bowel obstruction, pyloric stenosis
Stooling	*Delayed stooling:* • CF • Panhypopituitarism *Diarrhea:* • Infection • Metabolic disease
Stool color	*Acholic stools:* Cholestasis, biliary obstruction
Urine characteristics: Smell and color	Dark urine (conjugated hyperbilirubinemia), metabolic disease
Excessive bleeding	May indicate coagulopathy, vitamin K deficiency
Disposition: Irritability, lethargy	Metabolic disease or sepsis, panhypopituitarism
Abdominal surgery	Necrotizing enterocolitis, intestinal atresia

(CMV: cytomegalovirus; HIV: human immunodeficiency virus; PN: parenteral nutrition; SGA: small for gestational age)

TABLE 4: Physical findings.

Physical findings	
Assessment of general health	Ill appearance may indicate infection or metabolic disease, infants with biliary atresia typically appear well
General appearance	*Dysmorphic features*: Alagille syndrome in the neonate rarely exhibits characteristic facial appearance with a broad nasal bridge, triangular facies, and deep-set eyes. Typical facial features may appear at around 6 months of age, but are often nonspecific
Vision/slit lamp examination *Hearing*	• Congenital infection, storage disease, septo-optic dysplasia, posterior embryotoxon, cataracts • Congenital infections, PFIC1, TJP2, mitochondrial
Ocular manifestations	Alagille syndrome, optic nerve hypoplasia in panhypopituitarism, chorioretinitis in congenital infections, cataract in intra-uterine infections or galactosemia, and ocular coloboma in cat eye syndrome
Cardiac examination: Murmur, signs of heart failure	*Congenital heart disease:* Alagille syndrome, biliary atresia splenic malformation syndrome

Contd...

Contd...

Physical findings	
Abdominal examination	Presence of ascites; abdominal wall veins, liver size and consistency, spleen size and consistency (or absence thereof), abdominal masses, umbilical hernia
Stool examination (crucial—the primary physician should make every effort to view stool pigment)	Acholic or hypopigmented stools suggest cholestasis or biliary obstruction
Neurologic	Note overall vigor and tone
A palpable mass in the right upper quadrant	May indicate a choledochal cyst

DIAGNOSTIC EVALUATION

Laboratory Evaluation: Diagnostic evaluation of infant involves laboratory evaluation (as detailed in **Table 5**) and diagnostic imaging.

TABLE 5: Investigations.

Investigation	***Salient features***
Fractionated bilirubin levels	Elevation of both the direct and indirect component is seen in neonatal hepatitis, whereas in extrahepatic obstruction, it is a late event
Alanine aminotransferase (ALT), aspartate amino-transferase (AST)	Nonspecific, rise more than twice suggestive of hepatocellular injury *Note:* AST is also present in red cells and myocytes
PT/aPTT and INR >3	Severity, liver failure
Alkaline phosphatase (less specific than GGT)	Hepatobiliary, kidney or bone disease, usually elevated in infants
γ-glutamyl transpeptidase (GGT) (Higher in neonates than older children)	• *Increased* in biliary atresia, α_1-antitrypsin deficiency, progressive familial intrahepatic cholestasis PFIC type 3, Alagille syndrome, and idiopathic neonatal hepatitis • *Normal or decreased* in progressive familial intrahepatic cholestasis (PFIC) type 1 and 2, bile acid synthesis disorders, and tight-junction protein type 2 deficiency
Sepsis screen, urine, blood, and CSF cultures	Helps identify underlying infections that can cause or exacerbate neonatal jaundice by triggering hemolysis, hepatic dysfunction, or cholestasis
Low serum albumin level	Liver synthetic failure, undernutrition, or protein loss from the kidney or intestine
Highlighter	2 colors
Scissors	1 pair

(aPTT: activated partial thromboplastin time; CSF: cerebrospinal fluid; PT: prothrombin time; INR: international normalized ratio)

Diagnostic Imaging

Fasting and Postfeeding USG Abdomen

It is readily available, noninvasive, and cheap initial investigation for evaluation of obstructive jaundice.

Role:
- Assess visible obstructing lesions of the biliary tree
- Identification of choledochal cyst
- To assess for signs of advanced liver disease or vascular and/or splenic abnormalities

Sonographic parameters suggestive of biliary atresia:
- Triangular cord sign (echogenic fibrous tissue anterior to the portal vein), abnormal gallbladder morphology
- Lack of gallbladder contraction after oral feeding
- Nonvisualization of the common bile duct
- Hepatic artery diameter >1.5 mm
- Hepatic artery diameter to portal vein diameter ratio >0.45
- Hepatic subcapsular blood flow sign-increased hepatic arterial flow in the peripheral regions of the liver. These signs cannot confirm diagnosis of biliary atresia.

Additional ultrasound findings increasing the biliary atresia with malformations:
- Abdominal heterotaxy
- Midline liver
- Polysplenia, asplenia
- Preduodenal portal

Note: Normal ultrasonography does not rule out non-syndromic BA.

One meta-analysis reported sensitivity and specificity of 0.85 (95% CI, 0.76–0.91) and 0.92 (95% CI, 0.81–0.97) of ultrasound for diagnosis of biliary atresia.

Tc99m-Hepatobiliary Scintigraphy

Among all the hepatobiliary radiotracers, Tc-99m disofenin (DISIDA) and mebrofenin (BrIDA) have the highest extraction and shortest transit time. After injection, the radiotracer is extracted by hepatocytes, secreted into the biliary ductal system, and eventually excreted into the intestines. In liver cell dysfunction, there is persistent cardiac pooling and nonvisualization of the liver. In bile duct obstruction or failure of secretion, the isotope is not visualized in intestines even up to 24 hours after injection. Pretreatment with phenobarbital (5 mg/kg/day for 5 days) stimulates liver enzymes enhancing biliary secretion. This decreases the false positive results and has some benefit for differentiation with neonatal hepatitis. Non-excreting hepatobiliary scintigraphy has around 70% specificity for biliary atresia and can show non-excretion in patients with bile duct paucity, neonatal hepatitis, low-birth weight, and parenteral nutrition-associated cholestasis. Recent meta-analysis showed sensitivity of 98.7% and specificity of 70.4% of nondrainage for excluding biliary atresia, suggesting false negatives are rare.

Endoscopic Retrograde Cholangiopancreatography

Endoscopic retrograde cholangiopancreatography (ERCP) has higher sensitivity and specificity as compared to scintigraphy, but its use is limited by need for general anesthesia, neonatal endoscopes, and experience endoscopist.

Magnetic Resonance Cholangiopancreatography

Magnetic resonance cholangiopancreatography (MRCP) may be helpful in cases where the diagnosis is elusive. This noninvasive modality is well established for visualization of biliary system up to first order branches of intrahepatic bile ducts. Biliary atresia will show incomplete visualization of the extrahepatic biliary system and periportal high-signal intensity on T2-weighted MRI scans. The 3-dimensional MRCP has shown better diagnostic yield in fewer studies. Still, utility of MRCP for neonatal cholestasis is not well established and higher costs with difficulty in conducting this test on neonates have resulted in its utilization in limited number of cases.

Liver Biopsy

Liver biopsy has sensitivity >95% and specificity >94% for biliary atresia.

Features suggestive of biliary atresia include:
- Bile duct proliferation
- Bile plugs
- Portal tract or perilobular edema and fibrosis
- Preservation of the basic hepatic lobular architecture

Liver biopsy is useful for following conditions:
- Biliary atresia
- α-1-antitrypsin deficiency
- Alagille syndrome
- Neonatal sclerosing cholangitis
- Cytomegalovirus
- Herpes simplex infections

To avoid false-negative results, biopsy should be avoided in early stage.

Conditions mimicking biliary atresia histologically are:
- PN-associated cholestasis
- Cystic fibrosis
- α-1-antitrypsin deficiency

Intraoperative Cholangiography

Cholangiography helps to assess the patency of the intrahepatic bile ducts and extrahepatic bile duct. Despite the advancements in noninvasive imaging of hepatobiliary anatomy, intraoperative cholangiography still is the gold standard for diagnosing biliary atresia. Cholangiography within these patients is performed by first placing a purse-string suture over gallbladder around the scalp vein needle or cholangiogram catheter placed within the lumen. Following placement, a contrast agent is introduced via the catheter, and the biliary anatomy is ascertained with the assistance of fluoroscopy **(Fig. 1)**. If contrast appears to freely flow into both the intrahepatic ducts and the duodenum, BA is excluded. In these cases, a liver biopsy is done to determine the underlying cause of cholestasis. If a whole biliary tree is not visualized, biliary-enteric continuity must be restored.

TREATMENT ALGORITHM

General approach in infant with cholestasis is to exclude biliary atresia and other treatable conditions, to ensure that there are no red flag findings from physical examination, family history, or imaging to suggest a specific diagnosis

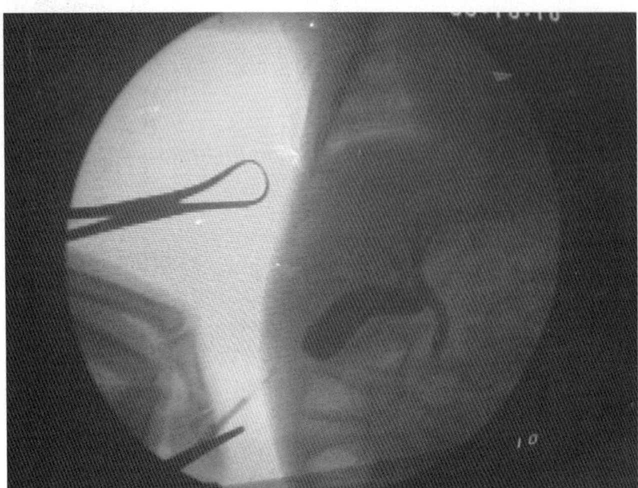

Fig. 1: Intraoperative cholangiogram.

Flowchart 3: Diagnosis and management—sick infants.

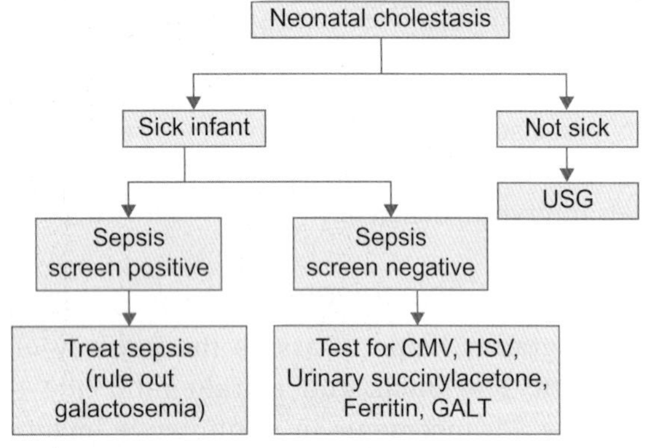

(CMV: cytomegalovirus; HSV: herpes simplex virus; USG: ultrasound)

and then to evaluate for common and finally rarer conditions. Initial treatment involves medical stabilization of the infant. Additionally, general medical care involves nutritional supplementation, fat-soluble vitamins, and symptomatic treatment for pruritus **(Flowcharts 3 and 4)**.

SURGICAL MANAGEMENT OF BILIARY ATRESIA: HOW WE DO? WHAT WE DO?

Preoperative Management

Nutrition

For formula-fed infants, medium chain triglyceride (MCT) is the predominant lipid source. For breast-fed infants, consider supplemental formula feeds employing an MCT-based feed while allowing the baby to continue the breastfeeding. An alternate choice would be to add MCT to expressed breast milk.

Flowchart 4: Diagnosis and management—not sick infants.

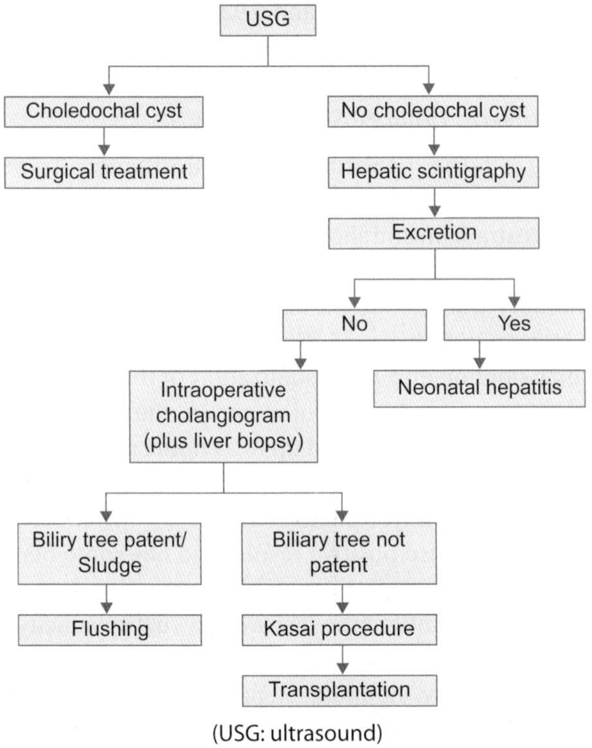

(USG: ultrasound)

Vitamin Supplementation

Children with BA are nearly always deficient in fat-soluble vitamins A, D, E, and K. Oral supplement should be commenced as soon as conjugated jaundice is detected and should continue throughout. Preoperatively, parenteral vitamin K is administered and correction of any coagulopathy is undertaken.

Surgical Preparation

Preoperative bowel preparation practices differ widely and depend on surgeons or institutional preference, but author recommends the patient should be on clear fluids 24 hours before surgery and polyethylene glycol (PEG) electrolyte solution should be administered at least 48 before the operation at dose of 25 mL/kg/dose with maximum dose of 100 mL/kg/day (not used in all institutes). Antibiotics should be administered before the operation for gut sterilization. Author recommends use of oral erythromycin and metronidazole combination for at least 3 days in two divided doses preoperatively.

Surgical Management

Surgery always begins with limited right-sided subcostal incision followed by visual inspection of liver, gallbladder, and surrounding structures. Direct cholangiogram is performed through this incision if deemed necessary.

In many cases, the diagnosis of BA is evident by visual inspection alone as the liver often appears cholestatic or fibrotic with a fibrotic and shrunken-appearing gallbladder. If the gallbladder is normal in appearance, or if there is a cyst within the hilum, the contents of the gallbladder or cyst could even be aspirated to assess whether further diagnostic workup is vital before proceeding with the HPE. If clear/white bile is aspirated, no further evaluation with cholangiogram is needed and one can proceed with KPE. If the fluid is darker appearing, it is recommended to perform a cholangiogram before proceeding to KPE.

Surgical Plan According to the Type of BA

The surgical plan proceeds according to the intraoperative findings about the type of biliary atresia as mentioned in **Table 6** (most of us always perform only portoenterostomy and never cystoenterostomy).

Kasai Portoenterostomy

First performed by Morio Kasai in 1959, the Roux-en-Y HPE (Kasai procedure) is the surgical intervention performed in the management of patients with BA. Recently, there was a trend favoring laparoscopic procedures, but meta-analyses have shown that the short-term outcomes following open surgery are comparable to laparoscopic HPE and are far superior to minimally invasive approaches when long-term outcomes like native liver survival were examined. Author prefers KPE by delivering and everting liver in the wound, which is achieved by division of the falciform ligament and triangular ligaments. During this procedure, the extrahepatic biliary tree is excised, and the fibrous portal plate at the hilum of the liver is transected **(Fig. 2)** and anastomosed to a Roux-en-Y limb **(Fig. 3)**, thus helping drainage of bile from the small ductules located within the portal plate.

The technical details of the HPE should not only seek to optimize the results of the HPE procedure itself, but should also aim to aid the subsequent liver transplant because some of the children will go on to liver transplantation in their lifetime.

TABLE 6: Surgical plan according to the type of biliary atresia.

Type	Surgical plan
Type I	Cholecystoenterostomy
Type II a	Hepatic portocholecystostomy
Type II b	Hepaticoenterostomy
Type II b (cystic)	Cystoenterostomy
Type III	Kasai portoenterostomy

Modifications of the traditional Kasai procedure:

Wide dissection:

- Hashimoto et al. proposed extension of the dissection to the left up to the umbilical point (segmental branches 1, 2, 3, and 4 on the left side of the hepatic hilum), and also to the right towards the dorsal aspect of the anterior portal branch over the bifurcation of the anterior and posterior segmental portal vein branches.
- In 1997, Ando et al. reported on their attempt to further expose the biliary remnant by dividing the ligamentum venosum; after a conventional approach to dissect the biliary remnant along the hilar vessels.

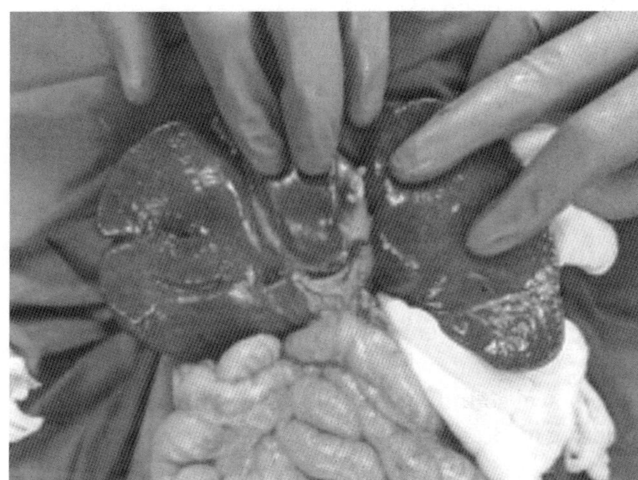

Fig. 2: Dissection of porta hepatis. *(For color version, see Plate 14)*

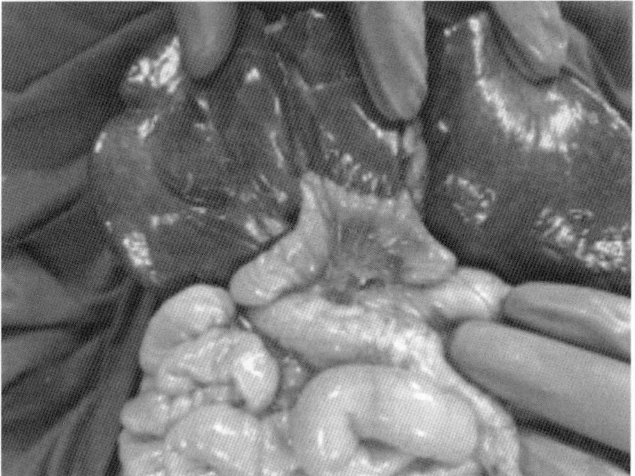

Fig. 3: Completed anastomosis. *(For color version, see Plate 14)*

- Suzuki modification is rimming of the segment 4 of the liver using the cavitational ultrasonic surgical aspirator (CUSA).

To prevent cholangitis, the use of an enteric conduit is rarely performed.

- Nakajo modification is creation of an approximate 2-cm long antireflux valve by invagination of the proximal intestinal portion of the Roux-en-Y limb into its denuded distal portion.
- *Kasai II-operation*: This is creation of a double-Y, wherein the proximal part of the Roux-en-Y limb is exteriorized on to the abdominal wall and the distal segment is an end-to-side anastomosis to the proximal segment for the continuity of bile flow.
- Sawaguchi modification is exteriorization of the entire Roux-en-Y limb as a jejunostomy.
- Suruga modification is creation of a double-barrel ostomy of the Roux-en-Y limb.
- *Endo modification*: This is done by anastomosis of an ileocolic conduit to the porta hepatis, and bringing the ascending colon as a colostomy including the ileocecal valve.

Postoperative Care

Postoperatively, patients are treated with antibiotics and analgesics (intravenously or through epidural). Child is started on orals with clear liquids early and escalated once bowel sounds resume. Drain removal is done after ensuring no drainage and starting of oral feeds. If findings suggestive of inflammation are present, then oral steroids (prednisolone) are started after day 5 of the surgery. After discharge from hospital, they closely followed for jaundice clearance and nutritional management.

All patients received prophylactic antibiotics (cotrimoxazole 2.5 mg/kg/day of trimethoprim component for 6 months), choleretics (ursodeoxycholic acid 15 mg/kg/day in 2 divided doses till bilirubin normalized or 1 year postoperatively), and fat-soluble vitamins during follow-up.

Complications

There are surgical and medical complications encountered postoperatively (early and late). Surgical complications are uncommon and they can be specific to Kasai procedure like bleeding from porta hepatis and anastomotic leak or the complications related to abdominal surgery like ileus, adhesive obstruction, wound dehiscence, etc. Various medical complications encountered commonly are cholangitis, portal hypertension, hepatopulmonary syndrome, intrahepatic bile lakes, and rarely malignancies.

In most patients with biliary atresia, bile drainage is achieved following Kasai portoenterostomy. However, in some cases, drainage stops due to cholangitis for unknown reasons. In such patients, redo Kasai portoenterostomy is indicated treatment for cholangitis, choleretics, or corticosteroids fail. However, liver transplantation should also be considered if indicated. We recommend redo Kasai portoenterostomy after carefully assessing the patient's condition, including the pattern of bile drainage, patient age, and the hepatic functional reserve.

Outcome

Kasai portoenterostomy has been accepted as an initial and standard treatment, with the widely successful jaundice-free outcomes. However, about 35–40% of patients who receive Kasai PE, unfortunately, fail to become jaundice-free even after the procedure. In these cases, medical therapies are administered to improve the bile flow after the Kasai operation. Various medical therapies described in literature for the postoperative medical therapy are prophylactic antibiotics to prevent cholangitis, barbiturate, cholestyramine, and ursodeoxycholic acid to enhance bile, and steroids to reduce inflammation.

CONCLUSION

Extrahepatic biliary atresia (EHBA), choledochal cysts, biliary sludge/gallstones, and inspissated bile are the common causes of surgically correctable neonatal jaundice, of which EHBA is the most common. USG, HIDA, and IOC should be undertaken early in the workup of direct hyperbilirubinemia to differentiate surgically correctable lesions from neonatal hepatitis. Surgical correction should be done as early as possible.

KEY POINTS

- Direct hyperbilirubinemia is always pathological.
- Intrahepatic or extrahepatic cholestasis causes direct hyperbilirubinemia.
- Extrahepatic cholestasis is amenable to surgical correction.
- Jaundice due to extrahepatic obstruction appears 5–7 days postnatally and may be waxing and waning.
- Infants with extrahepatic obstruction are better preserved than those with neonatal hepatitis.
- Intraoperative cholangiogram is the gold standard for diagnosing extrahepatic biliary obstruction.
- A nonexcretory Tc99mhepatobiliary iminodiacetic acid scan with suggestive ultrasonography mandates an intraoperative cholangiogram.

SUGGESTED READING

1. Bhatia V, Bavdekar A, Matthai J, Waikar Y, Sibal A. Management of neonatal cholestasis: consensus statement of the Pediatric Gastroenterology Chapter of Indian Academy of Pediatrics. Indian Pediatr. 2014;51(3):203-10.
2. Bhatnagar V, Sugandhi N. Neonatal Jaundice: Surgical Perspective. In: Vasudev AS, Shah NK (Eds). Algorithms in Pediatrics, 1st edition. New Delhi: Jaypee Brothers Medical Publisher; 2017.
3. Davenport M, Betalli P, D'Antiga L, Cheeseman P, Mieli-Vergani G, Howard ER. The spectrum of surgical jaundice in infancy. Pediatr Surg. 2003;38(10):1471-9.
4. Davenport M, Heaton N, Superina RA. Surgery of the liver, bile ducts and pancreas in children. Surgery of the Liver, Bile Ducts and Pancreas in Children, 3rd edition. Florida, United States: CRC Press; 2017. pp. 71-86.
5. Fawaz R, Baumann U, Ekong U, Fischler B, Hadzic N, Mack CL, et al. Guideline for the Evaluation of Cholestatic Jaundice in Infants: Joint Recommendations of the North American Society for Pediatric Gastroenterology, Hepatology, and Nutrition and the European Society for Pediatric Gastroenterology, Hepatology, and Nutrition. J Pediatr Gastroenterol Nutr. 2017;64(1):154-68.
6. Gupta R, Nagdeve NG, Sarin YK. Neonatal surgical jaundice revisited. Indian J Pediatr. 2005;72(5):415-23.
7. Redkar R, Karkera PJ, Raj V, Bangar A, Hathiramani V, Krishnan J. Outcome of Biliary Atresia After Kasai's Portoenterostomy: A 15-year Experience. Indian Pediatr. 2017;54(4):291-294.

Approach to Neonatal Intestinal Obstruction

Kanishka Das, Akash Bihari Pati

INTRODUCTION

Neonatal intestinal obstruction is a common clinical conundrum that must be quickly unraveled, and a working diagnosis made to initiate appropriate management. A brief description of the embryology, antenatal diagnosis, clinical presentation, and management of common causes of neonatal intestinal obstruction is attempted and clinical algorithms in differential diagnosis outlined.

Neonatal intestinal obstruction may be:

- *Congenital or acquired:*
  - *Congenital:* Bowel atresia—agenesis, stenosis, diverticulum, duplications, cystic fibrosis (CF)—meconium ileus complex, bowel aganglionosis, inguinal hernia
  - *Acquired:* Necrotizing enterocolitis (NEC), intussusception of Meckel's diverticulum
- *Structural, functional, or mixed:*
  - *Structural:*
    - *Complete obstruction:* Bowel atresia, agenesis
    - *Incomplete obstruction:* Stenosis, diverticulum, and duplications
  - *Functional:* Bowel aganglionosis
  - *Combination:* Cystic fibrosis—meconium ileus complex. The primary defect is functional, inspissated intestinal and exocrine glandular secretions, structural sequels and complicated forms include bowel obstructions, atresias, cysts, perforations, and adhesive bowel obstruction, etc.
- *Site of obstruction:*
  - *Small bowel:* Atresia, stenosis, duplication, persistent vitellointestinal duct (PVID), and meconium ileus
  - *Large bowel:* Hirschsprung disease (HD), anorectal malformation (ARM), and congenital short colon
  - *Both:* Necrotizing enterocolitis (NEC), total colonic aganglionosis (TCA), intussusception
- *Intrinsic or extrinsic:* Most causes are intrinsic, extrinsic causes include congenital bands, intestinal duplication, annular pancreas, tumors, adhesions, etc.

Antenatal diagnosis is possible occasionally in certain conditions, but most are discovered at birth. Antenatal imaging, commonly ultrasonography and selectively an MRI, may show one of more of the following—polyhydramnios, persistently visualized cystic structure with bowel signature, calcification, associated anomalies typical of certain entities (e.g., cardiac anomalies with duodenal obstruction, urogenital anomalies with anorectal malformations) and so on. Polyhydramnios is noted in gut obstructions till mid jejunum and less with distal obstructions. An earlier pregnancy with an index case may direct enquiry. Serial ultrasonographic findings at 4–6 weeks interval would strengthen the suspicion and facilitate counseling for select fetal investigations/intervention, in utero transfer and delivery.

At birth, a detailed history and physical examination is crucial. Precise information from history and physical examination **(Box 1; Figs. 1 and 2)** helps in planning laboratory and radiologic investigations **(Figs. 3 and 4)**, finally culminating in algorithms of differential diagnosis for small and large bowel obstruction **(Flowcharts 1 and 2)**. Medical conditions masquerading as intestinal obstruction are common and must be carefully excluded, similarly abdominal distension must not be considered synonymous with intestinal obstruction.

Certain specific and common surgical entities that are discussed in further detail are:

- *Duodenal obstruction:* Complete (atresia), incomplete (stenosis/web, malrotation of midgut)
- *Jejunoileal obstruction:* Atresia and stenosis, meconium ileus (MI), and persistent vitellointestinal duct (PVID) anomalies
- *Large gut obstruction:* ARM and HD
- Necrotizing enterocolitis

BOX 1: Neonatal intestinal obstruction (NIO)—history and physical examination.

NIO—History:
- Antenatal history, previous pregnancy and outcome, maternal medications
- Medical disorders (fetomaternal)—hypothyroidism, diabetes
- Birth history—prematurity, birth asphyxia—trauma, neonatal sepsis
- Meconium passage—yes/no, timing after birth, amount, consistency (fluid/tenacious), form (pellets/plug). Passage of stool/flatus in neonates on feeds and nature of stool (color/consistency/amount)
- Abdominal distension—born with a distended abdomen/insidious onset, static/progressive, localized/generalized. Visible lump/movement
- Vomitus—timing, frequency, color, odor
- Feeding practice—fed/not fed, if fed—breastfed/formulas/animal milk/others including native formulations, bottle feeding practice. Burping
- Voiding—timing, frequency, amount and color (hydration, renal status)
- Umbilical cord details—separation—usual/delayed separation, discharge, bulge
- Inguinoscrotal and inguinolabial bulges

NIO—Physical examination:

General examination:
- Weight, length, gestational maturity
- Dysmorphism
- Hypothermia, dehydration, hemodynamic status, tissue perfusion
- Sepsis
- Pallor, icterus
- NG tube insertion and aspirate details (volume, color, consistency)

Abdominal examination:
- Distended/unremarkable, generalized/localized (region) distension, static/progressive, associated skin changes—shiny, redness, edema, discoloration. Tenderness. Abdominal girth (mark level)
- Visible peristalsis, bowel patterning, visible or palpable bowel/mass
- Ascites, fluid thrill—shifting dullness
- Umbilicus and details—unremarkable/protrusion/hernia, clamp, discharge
- Inguinoscrotal/labial region—bulge, discoloration, tenderness
- Anus—orifice position and caliber, feeding tube insertable and stain thereof, response to rectal stimulation/PR

Perineum and spine

DUODENAL OBSTRUCTION

It is a common site of neonatal intestinal obstruction, the congenital etiology may be intrinsic (atresia, stenosis, diaphragm/web) or extrinsic (annular pancreas, malrotation of midgut) or combinations thereof.

Duodenal Atresia and Stenosis

Duodenal atresia is an error of recanalization of the embryonic gut and occurs in 1/6,000–10,000 live birth. More than half have associated congenital anomalies (Down's syndrome, annular pancreas, congenital heart disease, and malrotation of midgut) and a similar proportion are premature or have a low-birth weight. The common morphologic type (92%) is a mucosal and submucosal diaphragmatic membrane with an intact muscle wall. Other forms (fibrous cord connecting atretic ends, complete separation of the atretic ends with a mesenteric defect) are rare.

Antenatal ultrasonographic clues are maternal polyhydramnios with a "double bubble sign" (distended stomach and first part of duodenum); fetal echocardiography identifies typical cardiac anomalies (coarctation of aorta, septal defects) or trisomy 21 phenotype. Postnatally, the majority (85%) present with bilious vomiting within the first few hours of life or after an attempted feed as the obstruction is just distal to the ampulla (postampullary). The abdomen is scaphoid or mildly distended in the upper part. An erect abdominal X-ray with a "double bubble" gas shadow is diagnostic. Children with the rare preampullary form have nonbilious vomits and may be confused with gastric outlet obstruction.

Initial management includes nasogastric decompression, fluid-electrolyte resuscitation, and a preanaesthetic cardiac evaluation. A duodenoduodenostomy is performed and a short period of parenteral nutrition is useful till anastomotic transit resumes and feeds are established.

Duodenal stenosis due to a mucosal web/diaphragm is relatively less common rarer. The diaphragm has a small apical aperture and bellows antegrade (windsock). There is an abrupt transition of bowel diameters in the contrast study. It is associated with Trisomy 21 and is often identified late in evaluation.

Malrotation

This is a heterogeneous group of anomalies of midgut rotation and fixation of including nonrotation, incomplete rotation, and reverse rotation. The sine qua non of "incomplete rotation" is a duodenojejunal flexure fixed to the right of the midline/spine. Compressive bands that run from the mobile cecum/ascending colon to the right

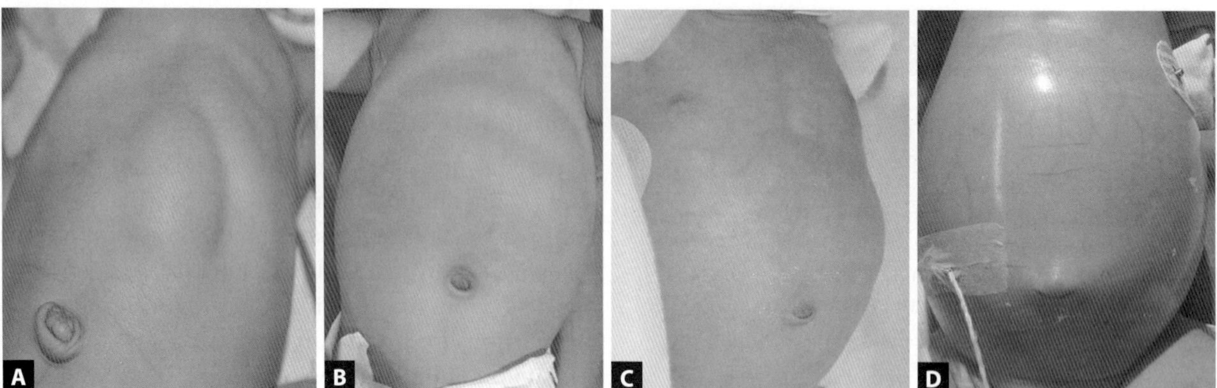

Figs. 1A to D: Spectrum of abdominal distension in neonatal intestinal obstruction. (A) Variably distended, peristaltic stomach/bowel in pyloroduodenal/upper jejunal obstruction; (B) Step-ladder bowel pattern in ileal obstruction; (C) Moderate, generalized distension and visible abdominal veins in necrotizing enterocolitis; (D) Shiny, grossly distended abdomen in Hirschsprung-associated enterocolitis. *(For color version, see Plate 14)*

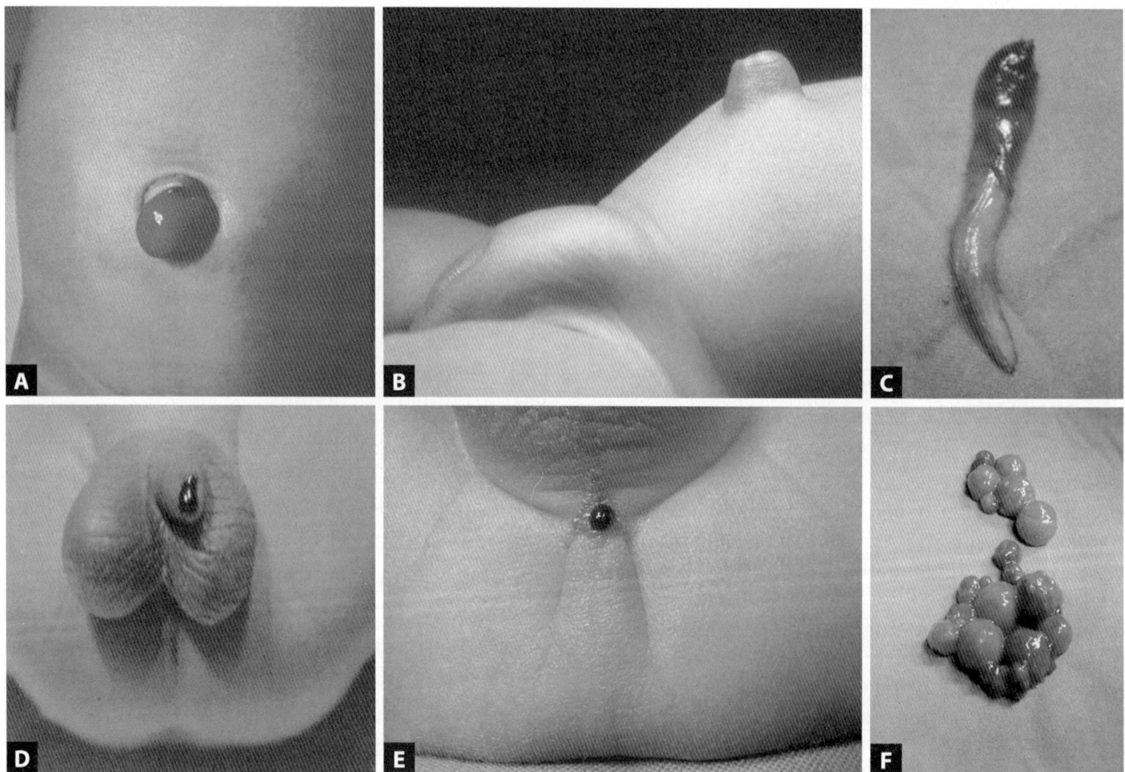

Figs. 2A to F: Typical physical signs lead to a diagnosis in neonatal intestinal obstruction. (A) Umbilical polyp in a PVID; (B) Umbilical and inguinal hernia in a neonate; (C) Meconium plug expelled by an infant of a diabetic mother; (D) Meconuria in a male, imperforate anus with high anorectal malformation; (E) Meconium extruding through perineal fistula in a male, low anorectal malformation; (F) Pale meconium pellets in distal ileal atresia. (PVID: persistent vitellointestinal duct) *(For color version, see Plate 15)*

parietes (Ladd's band) obstruct the second part of the duodenal and account for the bilious vomits. The narrow root of mesentery or duodenacolic isthmus through which the superior mesenteric artery (SMA) courses predisposes it to midgut volvulus and bowel ischemia. The incidence of malrotation is 1/6,000 live births and 80% present in the neonatal period. A sudden onset bilious vomiting with/without preceding normal feeding and bowel movement

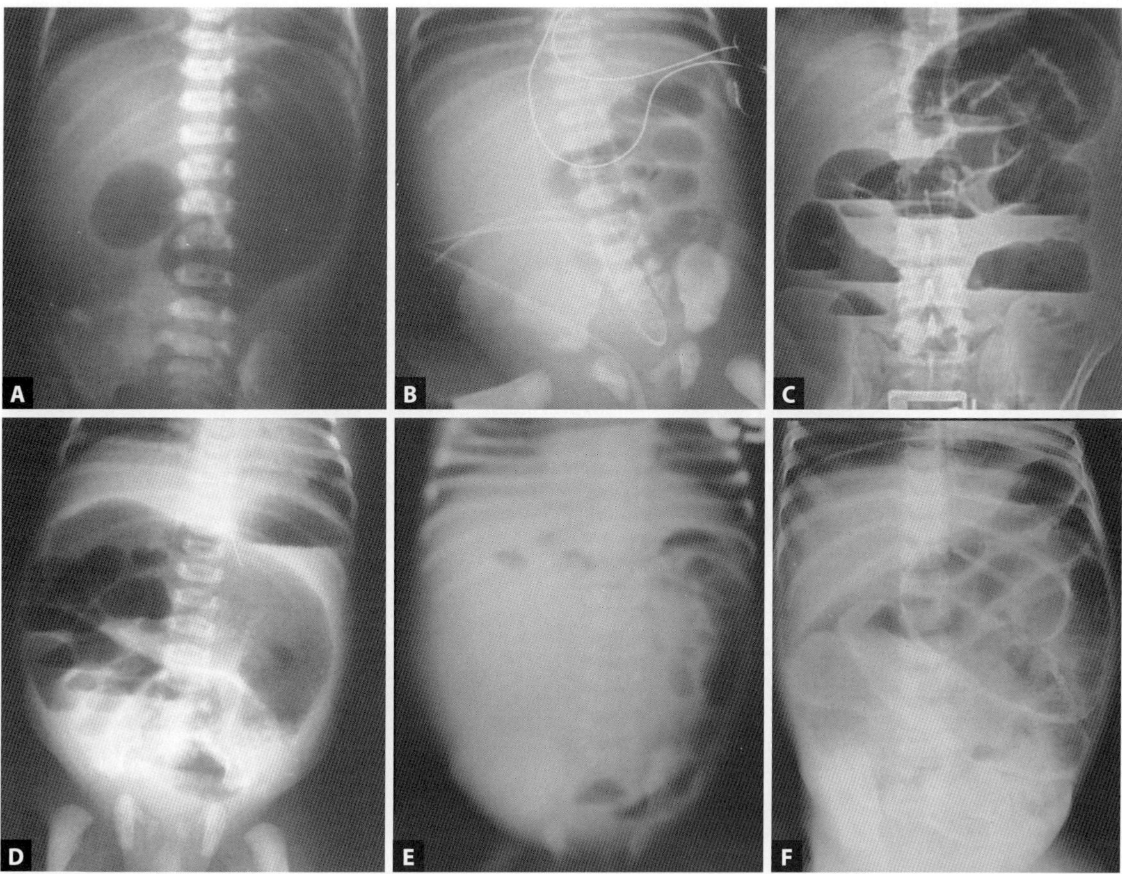

Figs. 3A to F: The plain abdominal X-ray, preferably erect, is a crucial preliminary investigation. (A) Double bubble of duodenal atresia; (B) Few left upper abdominal loops in jejunal obstruction (supine); (C) Multiple air fluid levels in ileal obstruction; (D) Small and large bowel dilatation, fecal shadows in peripherally placed large bowel and paucity of rectal gas shadow in classical Hirschsprung disease; (E) Right and mid abdomen opacity displacing bowel loops to the left, paucity of air fluid levels. Complicated meconium ileus; (F) Pneumoperitoneum with distended small bowel loops.

in a neonate is common. The bilious vomit may be intermittent, as is the obstruction. Initially, the abdomen is scaphoid/minimally distended. The neonate can rapidly lose weight to appear emaciated. The vascular catastrophe of midgut volvulus and ischemia in the superior mesenteric territory is associated with rapidly progressive abdominal distension, tender abdominal signs, malena, peritonitis, and shock.

Since clinical presentation is varied, a high index of suspicion leads to radiologic investigations. The plain abdominal skiagram shows paucity of bowel gas beyond the duodenum. With a midgut volvulus, vascular compromise, transmural ischemia, and exudative ascites, a plain X-ray becomes progressively "gasless". The upper GI contrast study under fluoroscopy shows a duodenojejunal junction located to the right of the midline/spine and the initial coil of small bowel on the right half of the abdomen. Volvulus with incomplete obstruction shows as a "coil spring" or "corkscrew" configuration of duodenal and upper jejunal loops as they wind around the SMA; with complete obstruction, only a "beak" is filled after the dilated duodenum. Careful assessment of the relative position of the superior mesenteric vein (SMV) and SMA on color Doppler ultrasonography can be conclusive. The normal SMV lies to the right of the SMA; in malrotation, this is reversed. Additionally, a "whirlpool" sign (SMV and mesentery wrapped around the SMA) implies a late midgut volvulus.

A midgut volvulus is a surgical emergency and must be expediently managed to salvage the neonate. After aggressive resuscitation and antibiotics for gut-associated sepsis, an exploration is scheduled. A "Ladd procedure" (detorsion of bowel, division of Ladd's band, broadening of small bowel mesentery, placement of small bowel to

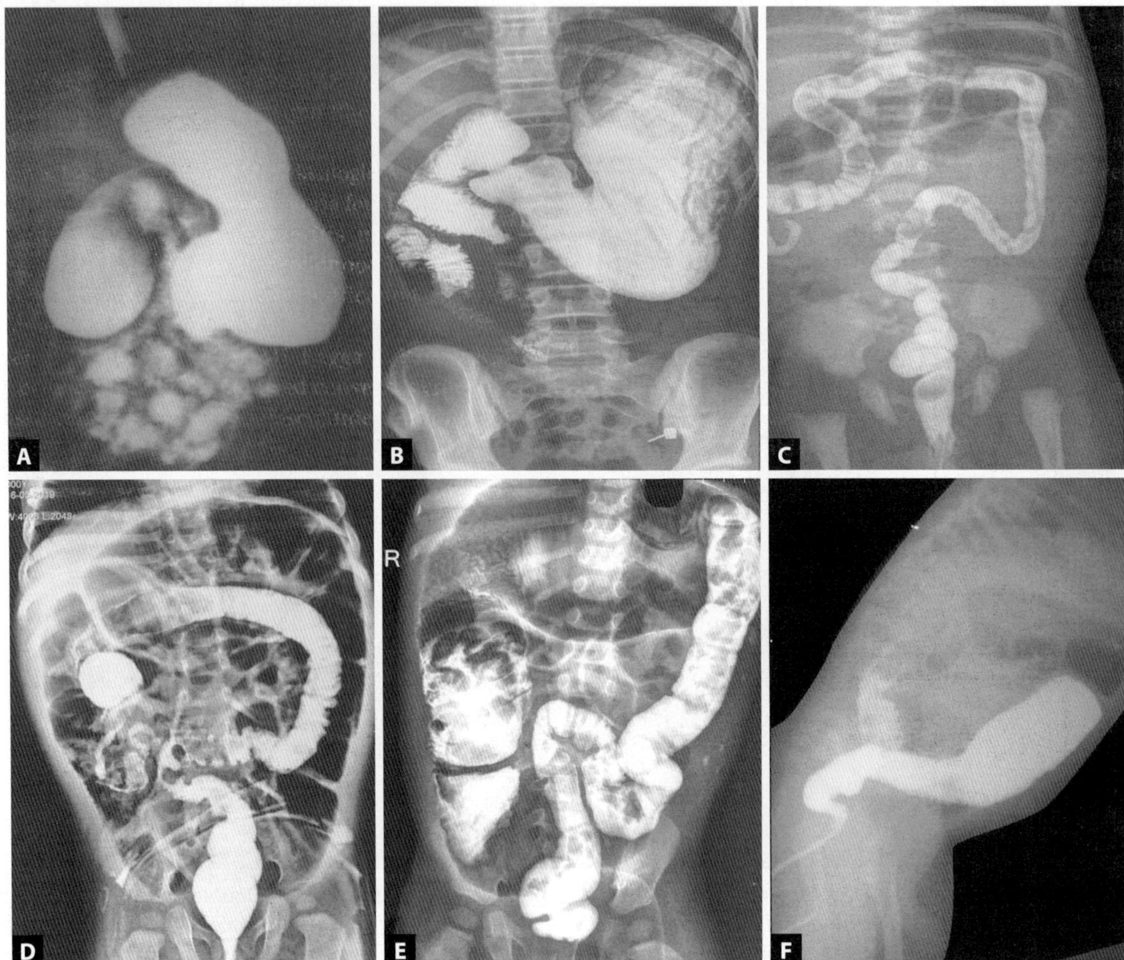

Figs. 4A to F: Contrast studies elucidate the differential diagnosis after plain X-rays in select few. Upper GI contrast studies. (A) Duodenal stenosis showing abrupt transition from a dilated duodenum to smaller caliber bowel distally; (B) Malrotation of midgut. Note the dilated stomach and proximal duodenum, duodenojejunal flexure to the right of the midline and the first coil of jejunum visualized in the right half of the abdomen. Contrast enema. (C) Microcolon with pellets of varying sizes in meconium ileus; (D) "Question mark" microcolon and gross small bowel dilatation in TCA; (E) Long-segment colonic HD with splenic flexure transition zone; (F) Rectosigmoid transition zone in classical HD. (HD: Hirschsprung disease)

the right half and colon to the left half of the abdomen, and elective appendectomy) that converts the midgut to an embryonic position of nonrotation is the definitive surgery. Postoperative ileus is significant and managed patiently.

JEJUNOILEAL OBSTRUCTION

Jejunoileal Atresia

At a frequency of roughly 1/1,000 live births, jejunal and ileal atresia is comparatively more prevalent than duodenal atresia. 60% of small bowel atresia are duodenal, and 20% of each are in the jejunum and ileum. The preferred sites are the proximal jejunum (30%) and distal ileum (35%); 6% have multiple atresia. Unlike duodenal atresia, few have associated congenital abnormalities **(Table 1)**.

Fetal vascular accidents are the cause of jejunoileal atresia, an early gestational incident results in a more proximal vascular disruption and a correspondingly severe atresia. They are categorized pathologically as follows:

- *Type 1:* Intestinal mucosal web with continuity of the muscular layer
- *Type 2:* A fibrous cord connecting the atretic segments, while the mesentery remains intact.
- *Type 3A:* Proximal and distal atretic intestines with an intervening V-shaped mesenteric defect—a sequel of necrosis and resorption

Flowchart 1: Algorithmic approach to upper small bowel obstruction.

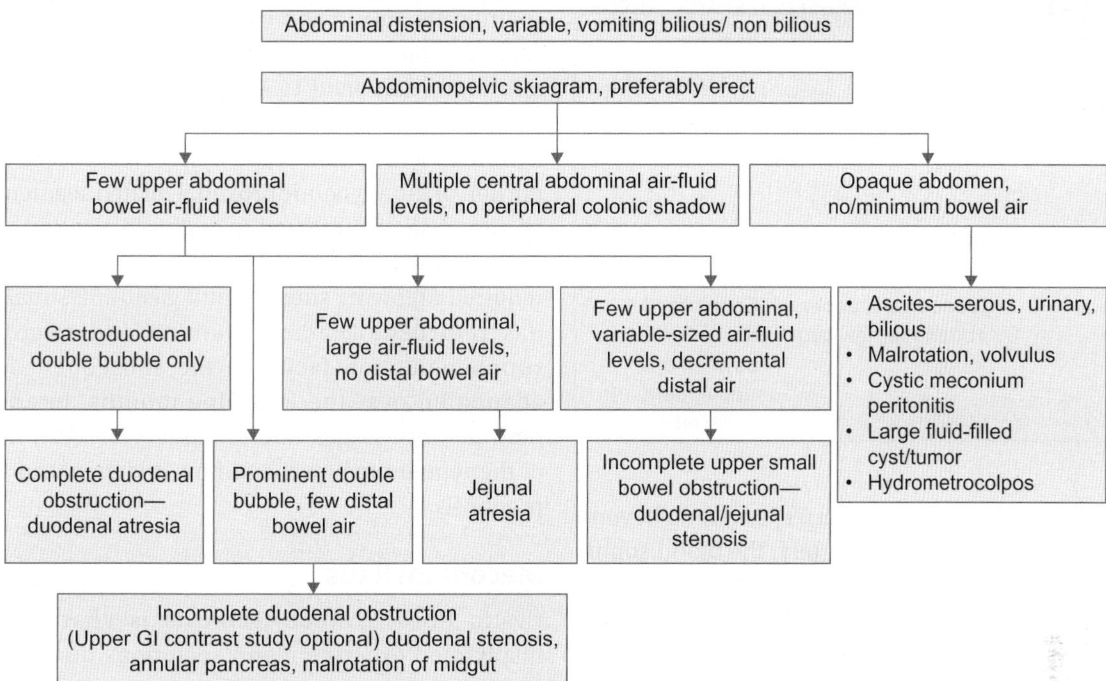

Flowchart 2: Algorithmic approach to distal small bowel and large bowel obstruction.

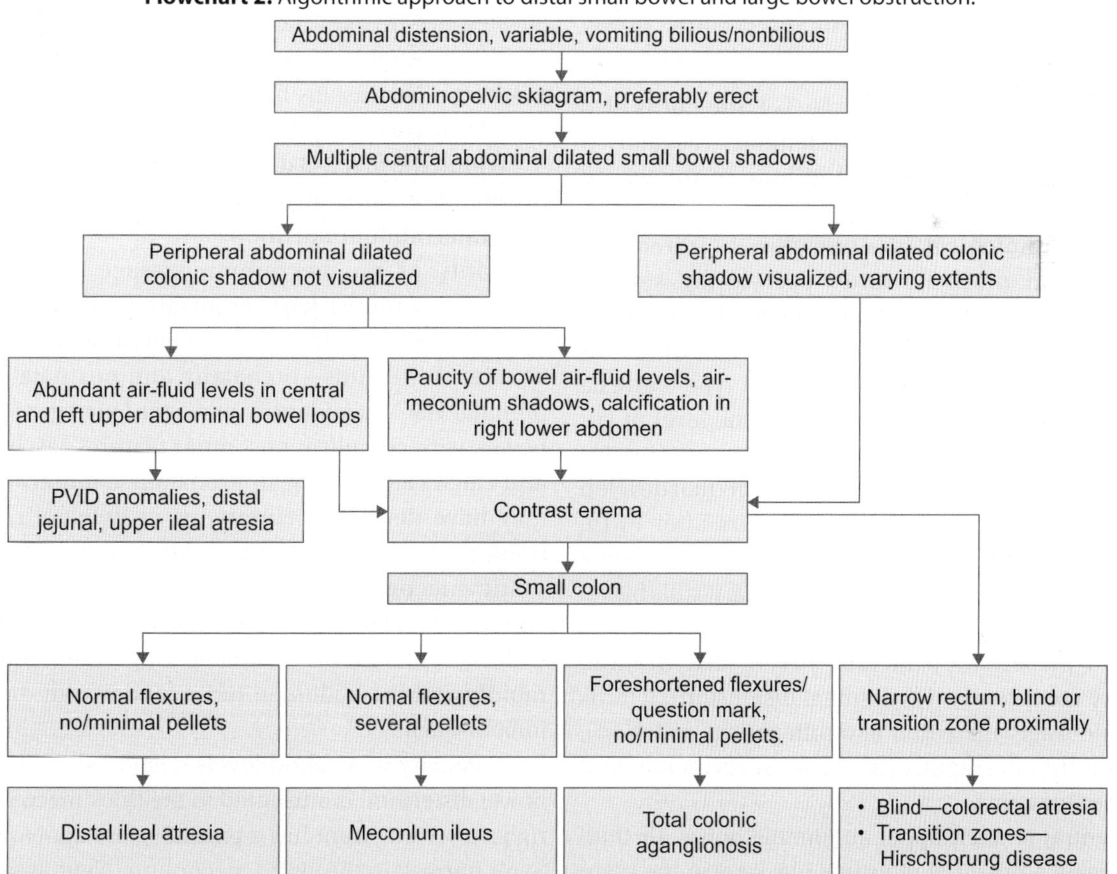

TABLE 1: Differentiating jejunal from ileal atresia.

Clinical picture	*Jejunal*	*Ileal*
Polyhydramnios, prematurity, low-birth weight, associated anomalies	More common	Less common
Vomiting	Appears early, bilious	Relatively bilious or feculent
Abdominal distension	Pronounced, upper abdominal, few large loops	Generalized distension, more bowel loops, stepladder patterning

- *Type 3B:* Superior mesenteric artery is atretic beyond the origin of the middle colic artery, the blood supply to the distal ileum is from a vulnerable retrograde collateral channel from the right colic artery. The distal ileum forms an "apple peel" around this axial artery and lacks a mesentery. The overall gut length is very short.
- *Type 4:* Multiple atresia with intervening bowel segments and fibrous cords, like a "chain of sausages"

In addition to being "short" in type 3–4, the gut is also dysfunctional; the lack of length, tenuous vascularity, and altered mucosal features contribute to the varied malabsorption in each type.

Prenatal sonological identification is infrequent and inapparent until the latter part of the second trimester. Polyhydramnios, ascites, dilated bowel loops, and echogenic bowel are indicative. Premature births frequently are associated with type 3 and type 4 atresia and probably hereditary. Depending on the level of gut blockage, bilious or feculent vomiting and progressive abdominal distension are the main symptoms that develop into a full-fledged picture by 36–48 hours after birth. A varying amount of meconium may be passed in some newborns and does not rule out bowel atresia. Visible bowel loops are seen in the central abdomen. Other symptoms of delayed presentation include severe dehydration, respiratory compromise (abdominal distension), icterus (enteric blockage, increased enterohepatic circulation), and perforation peritonitis (tenderness, erythema, and pneumoperitoneum).

Few central and left upper abdominal bowel air-fluid levels indicate a proximal intestinal blockage in the plain erect skiagram; a distal small bowel obstruction has more such levels and in some mandates a lower GI contrast examination to distinguish between distal ileal atresia, meconium ileus, and TCA in a stable infant.

The ideal surgical procedure following resuscitation is a primary anastomotic repair after resection of a variable portion of the adynamic proximal dilated segment. Several anastomoses are created in multiple atresia to avert an overall short bowel. Parenteral feeding is frequently required following surgery until gastrointestinal function has returned. Dietary vitamins and micronutrient supplementation facilitate the subsequent intestinal adaptation over the following months. In addition to perioperative issues due to surgery or TPN, the length of the remaining bowel and how it is managed affect the prognosis.

Meconium Ileus

Cystic fibrosis/mucoviscidosis is characterized by inspissated exocrine gland secretions due to a genetic defect. The tenacious meconium blocks the newborn bowel lumina in the mid and distal ileum. Approximately 80–90% of MI cases have CF; few occur in isolation in low-birth-weight infants. MI is uncommon in preterm newborns. Caucasians have a greater reported incidence (1 in 2,000 live births) than Asians (1 in 25,000 live births).

Within the first 2–3 days of life, simple/uncomplicated MI manifests as growing abdominal distension. Small intestinal abdominal loops are apparent, and there is scanty or no meconium passage (pellets, pale/sticky meconium) with associated bilious vomiting. Complicated states include bowel perforation, peritonitis, atresia, or volvulus—prenatally and postnatally. Serial prenatal USG may identify persistent echogenic, dilated bowel; with complications, other features (ascites, cysts, and calcification) appear. Prenatally complicated cases may have distended abdomens at delivery and show frank peritonitis soon. An abdominal lump at birth—cystic meconium peritonitis, comprises of densely adherent bowel loops surrounding a thick-walled cyst with meconium from perforated loop. These get infected rapidly and the abdomen turns tender with discolored, inflamed skin.

A paucity of air fluid levels despite significant small bowel distension is attributed to the thick meconium. The right lower quadrant has a ground-glass appearance due to air trapped in the viscid meconium (Neuhauser's sign).

After suitable hydration and antibiotics, a hyperosmolar diatrizoate contrast enema in uncomplicated cases shows a microcolon and narrow terminal ileum with filling defects (meconium pellets). After the procedure, gradual evacuation of the pellets and resolution of abdominal distension is often therapeutic in 20–40%. In "complicated" MI, combination of ascites, calcification, soft tissue densities, and pneumoperitoneum is noted. The cumbersome sweat test was earlier in vogue as a diagnostic tool, it has been replaced by DNA analysis for specific gene loci, but they are not always accurate.

Complicated cases and nonresponders to the hyperosmolar enema are explored. There are several surgical alternatives including enterotomy, lavage, diversion stomas (end, loop, chimney—Bishop Kopp, Santulli); occasionally, enterotomy closure/resection and anastomosis is opted for in stable newborns. N-acetylcysteine (NAC), a mucolytic, has been instilled into bowel to lyse and facilitate the ejection of the inspissated meconium at various phases of management.

Parenteral nutrition, broad-spectrum antibiotics, pulmonary function monitoring, and pancreatic enzyme supplements are adjuncts. The care of cystic fibrosis (CF) and its accompanying conditions continues. Ileostomy effluents are managed carefully, and stomas are closed after interim weight gain is ensured.

Umbilicus and Vitellointestinal Duct Anomalies

The umbilicus can be involved in various scenarios of neonatal intestinal obstruction—an obstructed umbilical hernia, an umbilical clamp that has crushed prolapsing bowel through a relatively wide umbilical defect/hernia of the umbilical cord/exomphalos minor; or a wet umbilicus announcing a vitellointestinal duct anomaly within.

As the amniotic cavity expands and the yolk sac regresses, the vitellointestinal duct (VID) is connecting the yolk sac to the gut obliterates by the 5th–7th week of intrauterine life. Persistence may assume various forms as enumerated here:

- Umbilical polyp—"cherry" like, glistening smooth surface, mucoid discharge
- Vitelline cyst—intraperitoneal cyst subjacent to abdominal wall, infected collection
- Patent VID—complete omphaloileal connection, bilious or feculent discharge—skin excoriation. The proximal and distal ileum may prolapse through the fistula—"stag horn».
- Fibrous tract from umbilicus to ileum, such bands can obstruct other bowel loops and serve as axis for volvulus.
- A true Meckel's diverticulum occurs at the antimesenteric ileal border within 40–100 cm proximal to the ileocecal junction.

Some forms are easily identifiable (wide umbilical fistula, stag horn ileal prolapse) while others (bowel incarcerated in the umbilical clamp) may be inapparent. In acute obstruction, an emergency exploratory laparotomy is in order; excision of VID remnant and bowel repair is performed, a "suspicious" diverticular base (indurated, wide, inflamed) is managed with a resection—anastomosis. Mild, persistent umbilical symptoms warrant a diagnostic laparoscopy/limited periumbilical exploration to confirm anatomy.

LARGE BOWEL OBSTRUCTIONS

These include the common anorectal malformations and HD and are associated with significant generalized abdominal distension.

Anorectal Malformations

The classical absence of a normally placed anal opening—"imperforate anus" is commoner in males while a small, malplaced fistulous perineal opening spewing out meconium is commoner in females. The former present at birth while the latter may present thereafter. Associated anomalies of the caudal hindgut, metanephric blastema, urogenital ducts, and adjacent mesodermal derivatives imply a "field defect." Sacral bony and spinal cord anomalies, deficient pelvic musculature, and innervation are evident to varying extents. The VACTERL association (10%) and chromosomal aberrations (Trisomy 21), renal tract (20–80%) and cardiac anomalies (10–30%) are common, and frequency depends on individual malformations.

- *Males:* The anomaly is high/supralevator when the rectum is superior to pelvic diaphragm/levator ani; it may terminate as a blind pouch or into the anterior urinary tract (bladder/urethra) by a fistula that explains the meconuria in some. The anal site is thus "imperforate." Low anomalies terminate caudal to the levator ani within 1–2 cm of a well-formed anal dimple, either as a blind pouch (imperforate), perineal tract filled with greenish meconium pearls, or as a perineal fistula discharging meconium at or anterior to an identifiable anal depression. Rectal atresia (normal appearing anus, short blind anal canal), H type malformation (H communication between normally coursing rectum and urethra), anal stenosis, anteriorly malplaced anus, and ectopic anus (anal orifice at different site from the anal sphincters) are other forms.

- *Females:* More commonly low anomalies that extend caudal to the levator ani, the rectum may open at varying points anterosuperiorly between the normal anal site and the upper vagina. The perineal openings of the anus, vagina, and urethra may be fused in various combinations—one (cloaca—urethra, vagina, and rectum altogether), two separate urethra, rectum and vagina as combined channel, or three (urethra and vagina normal, rectum opening as the common vestibular opening). As in the male, H type rectovestibular/vaginal fistula, anal stenosis, anteriorly placed anus, and ectopic anus opening posterior to the fourchette are also seen. Cloacas and other complex uterovaginal anomalies may present with obstructed, distended bladders, hydrometrocolpos, etc. Imaging (USG and MRI) and endoscopy will facilitate emergency and elective management.

Most ARMs are detected at birth, antenatal imaging may identify typical associated anomalies (renal and cardiac) or anatomy (hydrometrocolpos in cloaca) to suspect. The "low" malformations are often missed without a careful neonatal physical examination. Delayed presentation is associated with morbidity (severe dehydration, sepsis—meningitis, prerenal azotemia, urinary obstruction—infection, etc.) that is avoidable. Physical examination must test for esophageal patency and document perineal anatomy carefully.

A cross-table prone lateral skiagram has replaced the conventional invertogram to confirm a high/low malformation; other investigations (chest radiographs, abdominopelvic and spinal ultrasound, and ECHO) detect known associated anomalies. High anomalies in both sexes are managed with a diverting high sigmoid colostomy in most or a transverse colostomy in some (cloaca, complex malformations). A definitive repair by perineal/abdominoperineal route is scheduled for 4–5 months in most and the stoma closed a few months thereafter. Where feasible, stenotic low anomalies are managed with dilatations and treated with primary perineal surgery at birth or before weaning. The primary repair of high anomalies is also being done increasingly at birth in recent years.

Hirschsprung Disease

It is the most common cause of congenital and functional large gut pediatric obstruction, majority present in neonates (90%) or infancy. The western incidence of 1:5,000 LB is probably lower than Indian experience and most are term born and males (4:1). There is an embryonic failure of migration of the neural crest derived ganglion cells along the gut or a disturbance of their homing into the mural plexii thereafter. The loss of coordinated receptive relaxation in the aganglionic, spastic distal bowel to accommodate the luminal bolus from the ganglionic, propulsive, and proximal bowel segment leads to functional obstruction.

The disease extends across contiguous bowel proximally for variable distance from the anorectum; 80–85% is limited to sporadic rectosigmoid disease. Long-segment disease (colonic, total colonic and ileal) is commoner in females, familial and syndromic forms and genetic linked. Antenatal diagnosis is occasional and most present as neonates. Delayed meconium passage is classic (80–90%),but also seen in 30% without HD, 30% of premature births with colonic immaturity. An explosive expulsion (blast sign) of dammed up flatus/feces at withdrawal of finger at rectal examination or with negotiation of a rectal catheter across the spastic anorectum into the sigmoid colon is typical. Stigmata of neurocristopathies, ocular, cutaneous, visceral, etc., may be present. Hirschsprung-associated enterocolitis is a toxic, gut origin systemic sepsis with shock, peritoneal signs, and bloody diarrhea. A neonatal cecal–appendicular perforation may be the presentation.

Imaging (plain X-ray, contrast enema) suggests the diagnosis but a rectal biopsy (1–2 cm above the dentate line, mucosubmucosal/full thickness depending on the availability of histochemical modalities) is diagnostic. Further proximal bowel biopsies map the extent (leveling) of proximal, contiguous aganglionosis before resection. Surgical principles include excision of the ganglionic bowel and apposition of circumferentially normoganglionic bowel within a cm of the dentate line. The management may be single staged or staged with preliminary colostomy and later pull through. Primary neonatal single-stage management (transanal endorectal pull through/Duhamel) is dependent on robust intraoperative frozen section diagnostic support, technical feasibility, and availability of expertise. The outcome is excellent in the rectosigmoid form and relatively modest in the longer segment disease.

Hirschsprung-associated enterocolitis is managed like gut sepsis (intravenous fluids, antibiotics, bowel decompression—NG aspiration, and gentle rectal washes) and intensive care; in some, an emergency colostomy in the dilated and ganglionic segment may be necessary. Further management follows the general principles outlined earlier; however, these immune-mediated episodes may recur despite removal of aganglionic bowel entity even years later.

Total colonic aganglionosis is a long-segment disease that mimics a distal small bowel obstruction like ileal atresia and meconium ileus. It is commoner in females, twins, and low-birth weight than rectosigmoid disease. It is suggested by contrast enema features (foreshortened question mark microcolon, multiple proximal air-fluid levels, occasional colonic pellets) and operative findings (microcolon, terminal ileal transition zone, proximal dilated ileum) and confirmed by histology (rectal/leveling biopsy).

Necrotizing Enterocolitis

It is common in premature neonates with identifiable risk factors (birth asphyxia, sepsis, formula feeds, invasive umbilical lines, etc.). NEC presents with insidious to sudden onset and combination of several features—feeding intolerance, vomits (bilious/nonbilious), abdominal distension, gross melena, and variable hemodynamic instability. Fecal occult blood and unexplained hypoglycemia may be harbingers, advanced presentations include bowel necrosis, perforation, and frank peritonitis. The disease can mimic earlier described forms of intestinal obstruction at various stages and careful serial review of general and abdominal findings (distension, bowel sounds, edema, and tenderness), plain X-rays (bowel dilatation and wall edema, fixed bowel loops, intramural bowel air-pneumatosis, portal vein gas, and pneumoperitoneum), and ancillary laboratory investigations stages the entity, determines progression, and dictates management.

There are several less common anomalies of the bowel (intestinal duplications, congenital short colon, colonic atresia, and intestinal neuronal dysplasia) and variants of the entities described above that have not been elaborated on and warrant additional study.

BOX 2: Neonatal intestinal obstruction (NIO)—management.

Management of NIO—Investigations and treatment:

- Begin treatment, prioritize investigations simultaneously and sequentially
- Acute resuscitation—airway, breathing, circulation, decompression of gut, temperature maintenance
- Decompression of gut—nasogastric tube placement, gentle rectal stimulation
- Venous access—reliable bore line, secure. Collect samples—CBC, electrolytes, RBS, creatinine, blood gas, body fluid cultures
- Fluids—maintenance, replacement (nasogastric aspirates, fecal losses) qualitatively volume for volume. Titrate to urine output (bladder catheterization, if needed) and lab results
- Antibiotics—cover anaerobes (metronidazole), in addition to Gram-positive, Gram-negatives
- Radiological investigations—choice and timing, bedside/in radiology suite depending on hemodynamic stability
- Periodic physical review—hemodynamic status, abdominal signs, nasogastric aspirates, bowel movement
- Conservative management—IV fluids, crystalloid–colloid—blood product, antibiotics, other specific medications (e.g., IV antibiotics for sepsis, thyroxine for hypothyroidism)
- Emergency surgical procedure (laparotomy/-scopy, bowel resection/enteral stoma/bowel anastomosis, others, e.g., Ladd's procedure for malrotation of midgut—volvulus)
- Elective surgical procedure (laparotomy/-scopy, bowel resection/enteral stoma/bowel anastomosis, others, e.g., rectal biopsy, transanal endorectal pull through for rectosigmoid Hirschsprung disease)
- Follow-up—nutrition, growth, and development

The differential diagnosis and management run concurrently, especially in the acute setting; the principles are summarized in **Box 2**.

KEY POINTS

- The approach to diagnosis in a neonatal intestinal obstruction includes a review of antenatal details, a detailed birth & postnatal history, thorough clinical examination and directed, specific investigations.
- Medical entities may masquerade as or be associated with mechanical intestinal obstructions.
- Plain X-ray (erect, where feasible; else supine) is a crucial investigation that directs further imaging (contrast studies - upper/ lower GI) and specific tests (e.g. rectal biopsy in Hirschsprung disease) to clinch the final diagnosis.
- The treatment runs concurrently with investigations to resuscitate, establish a diagnosis and restore enteral nutrition at the earliest.

SUGGESTED READING

1. Das K, Pati AB, Mahalik SK. Neonatal intestinal obstruction and abdominal wall defects. In. Textbook of Clinical Neonatology. 1st edition, Ed. in Chief - Pejaver and Thakre, Jaypee Brothers Medical Publishers, New Delhi – 2020. ISBN 978-93-90595136. Pg. 908-16.
2. Hajivassiliou CA. Intestinal obstruction in neonatal/ pediatric surgery. Semin Pediatr Surg. 2003;12(4):241-53.
3. Pediatric Surgery. Part VII - Abdomen. 7th edition. Authors: Arnold G. Coran, N. Scott Adzick, Thomas M. Krummel, Jean-Martin Laberge, Robert Shamberger, Anthony Caldamone, Mosby, 2012. ISBN: 9780323072557
4. Ringer AS, Hansen AR, Mammen A. Surgical emergencies in the newborn. In. Cloherty and Stark's Manual of Neonatal Care. 9th edition. Editors-Anne R. Hansen, Ann R. Stark, Eric C Eichenwald, Camilia R. Martin,Wolters Kluver – 2022. ISBN/ISSN:9781975159528.

Approach to Neonate with Anorectal Malformation

Rajiv Chadha, Subhasis Roy Choudhury

INTRODUCTION

Anorectal malformations (ARMs), or "imperforate anus", have an incidence of around 1 in 5,000 live births with a slight male preponderance. ARM forms a significant proportion of neonates needing surgical evaluation and management. ARM can occur in association with several named syndromes, the most well-known being the VACTERL (vertebral defects, anal atresia, cardiac defects, tracheo-esophageal fistula, renal anomalies, and limb abnormalities) or VACTERL-H (VACTERL associated with hydrocephalus) association of defects. It is necessary to have a clear protocol for evaluation and subcategorization of newborns presenting with ARM so as to optimize initial management.

CLASSIFICATION OF ANORECTAL MALFORMATIONS

Anorectal malformations are classified as "High", "Intermediate", or "Low" depending on the termination of the gut above, within, or below the pelvic floor musculature. The terms high ARM (HARM), including both "high" and "intermediate" anomalies, and low ARM (LARM) are still widely used although the more recent Krickenbeck International classification **(Box 1)** has the advantage of being anatomically descriptive and more useful for therapeutic implications.

In males, the commonest defect is rectourethral fistula, and in females, it is a vestibular fistula. Imperforate anus without a fistula is rare in both sexes (5%), frequently occurring in association with Down syndrome. Rectal atresia or stenosis, in which the anal canal and a small length of distal-most rectum are patent, is rare (1–2%).

In India, an important regional variant is congenital pouch colon (CPC) in which a pouch-like dilatation of a shortened colon is associated with an ARM. About 90% of cases of CPC have been reported from India, especially northern India where it comprises around 15% of ARM. CPC is categorized into four subtypes based on the length of normal colon proximal to the colonic pouch. In the more severe subtypes, either the normal colon is absent with the ileum opening directly into the colonic pouch (Type I) or the ileum opens into a short segment of cecum, which then opens into the pouch (Type II) **(Fig. 1)**. The less severe subtypes have a longer length of normal colon proximal to the colonic pouch (Types III and IV CPC). CPC has also been classified into "*Incomplete*" (Types III–IV) or "*Complete*" CPC (Types I–II). In males, the colonic pouch usually ends in a colovesical fistula (CVF) opening just proximal to the bladder neck. The opening of the terminal fistula in girls is more variable but correlates with the "high" (cranial) opening in males.

BOX 1: Classification of anorectal malformations (ARM) (modified Krickenbeck).

Major clinical groups:
- Perineal (cutaneous) fistula
- Rectourethral fistula
  - Bulbar
  - Prostatic
- Rectovesical fistula
- Vestibular fistula
- Cloaca (≤3 cm common channel; >3 cm common channel)
- No fistula (imperforate anus without fistula)
- Anal stenosis

Rare/regional variants:
- Congenital pouch colon
- Rectal atresia/stenosis
- Rectovaginal fistula
- H-type fistula
- Others (including complex defects)

ASSOCIATED MALFORMATIONS

Associated abnormalities are present in 50–70% of cases and are more frequent with high or complex ARM. These include:

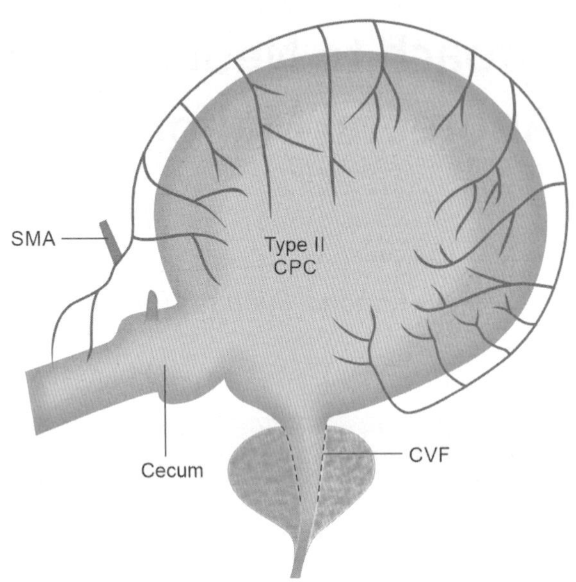

Fig. 1: Anatomy of a typical type II CPC in a male. (CPC: congenital pouch colon; CVF: colovesical fistula; SMA: superior mesenteric artery)

- *Cardiac anomalies (33% cases):* Atrial septal defect, patent ductus arteriosus, followed by tetralogy of Fallot and ventricular septal defect.
- About 10% ARM may have associated esophageal atresia with/without trachea-esophageal fistula (EA-TEF). Duodenal obstruction occurs in 1–2% patients.
- *Lumbosacral spinal anomalies (23%):* Hemivertebrae, scoliosis, and hemisacrum are common. A frequent spinal problem is tethered cord (25% cases).
- Genitourinary anomalies (33–50% patients) are more common with HARM or complex ARM. Vesicoureteral reflux (VUR) is the most common anomaly followed by unilateral renal agenesis or dysplasia. Cryptorchidism occurs in 20% and hypospadias in 5% of male ARM. Gynecologic anomalies, in about a third of female ARM, include uterine malformations (predominantly bicornuate uterus and uterus didelphys) and vaginal abnormalities such as a septate vagina or vaginal atresia.

In CPC, the sacrum is usually normal while there is a high incidence of VUR in males. All girls with CPC have a double vagina with a wide intervaginal bridge and a monocornuate uterus on each side of the pelvis.

CLINICAL EVALUATION AND MANAGEMENT IN MALE NEWBORN WITH ANORECTAL MALFORMATIONS

Flowchart 1 shows an algorithm for management of male ARM.

After initial *general clinical evaluation*, a thorough *perineal examination* is the mainstay to assess the type of ARM. In some babies, findings may be evident soon after birth. However, in many cases, the final decision regarding primary repair versus a colostomy may need to wait till the baby is 20–24 hours old as significant pressure may be required to force meconium through a fistula or gas to descend to the distal rectum. In practice, in India and other underdeveloped countries, newborns are often brought late, sometimes with features of advanced bowel obstruction, and delay in evaluation may not be necessary.

Initial stabilization is done with withdrawal of feeds, nasogastric aspiration, intravenous fluids, antibiotics, and thermoregulation. In the 20–24 hour-period after birth or at admission in newborns brought late, the newborn should undergo investigations to rule out associated malformations:

- An associated EA-TEF should be ruled out by passing an oro- or nasogastric tube.
- An echocardiogram, whenever possible, should be used to rule out congenital cardiac malformations.
- Ultrasound (US) abdomen to evaluate for associated urologic problems and a spinal US to screen for tethered cord and other intraspinal anomalies are crucial.
- A "babygram" or "infantogram" in the erect antero-posterior (AP) view is advisable as it can show skeletal anomalies, including lumbosacral spinal anomalies, cardiac enlargement, or any abnormal abdominal gas pattern. Especially in northern India, this should be mandatory because of the high incidence of CPC. A large air-fluid shadow occupying >50% width of abdomen, with usually a normal sacrum **(Fig. 2)** and meconuria (in males) suggests CPC.

Meconium on the perineum, a meconium-filled tract along the perineal raphé **(Fig. 3)**, and covered anus or a bucket-handle deformity signifies a perineal (cutaneous) fistula (low anomaly).

A flat-bottom perineum and/or a grossly abnormal sacrum usually signify a HARM. Meconuria confirms a rectourinary fistula or a colovesical fistula (in CPC).

If the baby has signs of a perineal fistula, a perineal cutback anoplasty or a minimal posterior sagittal anoplasty (PSAP) can be performed in the newborn period. If the baby is ill from associated problems and is very premature, the fistula can be gently dilated and anoplasty is delayed for 2–3 months.

If no meconium is seen on the perineum at 20–24 hours after birth, an invertogram or, preferably, a cross-table

Flowchart 1: Algorithm for the management of male ARM.

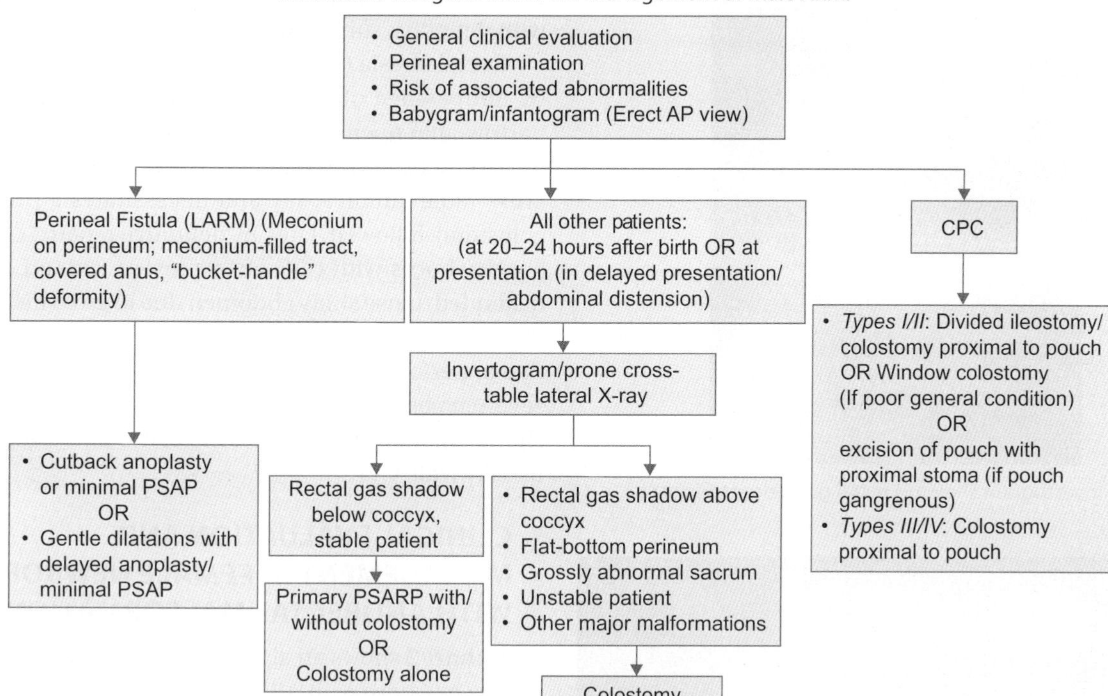

(ARM: anorectal malformations; CPC: congenital pouch colon; LARM: low anorectal malformations; PSAP: posterior sagittal anoplasty)

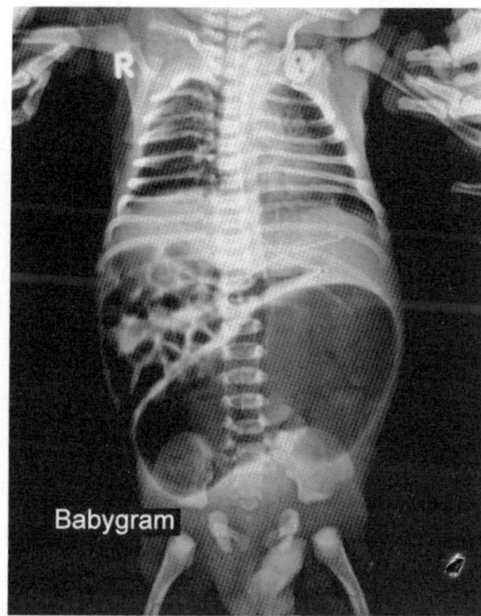

Fig. 2: "Babygram" of a neonate with type II congenital pouch colon (CPC) showing large air shadow in abdomen. Note the normal sacrum.

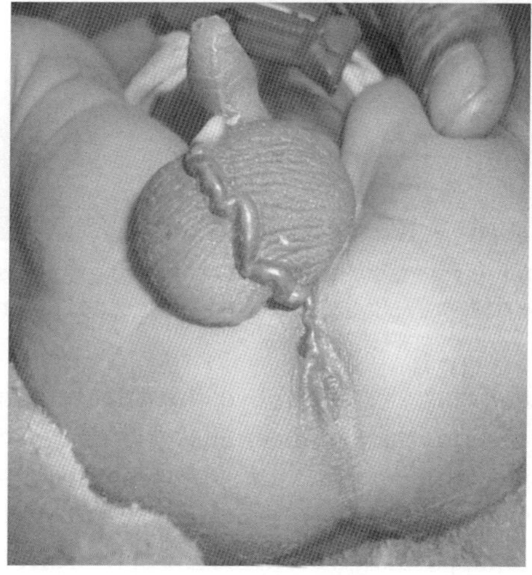

Fig. 3: Perineal fistula with meconium-filled tract along median raphé. *(For color version, see Plate 15)*

lateral X-ray with the baby in the prone position with the pelvis elevated should be obtained **(Figs. 4 and 5)**. If the rectal gas is located below the coccyx **(Fig. 4)** and the baby is in good condition with no significant associated defects, depending on the surgeon's experience, a posterior sagittal anorectoplasty (PSARP) with/without a protective colostomy can be considered. A more conservative, safer, and generally advisable approach is to perform a proximal sigmoid colostomy, with definitive repair 2–6 months later.

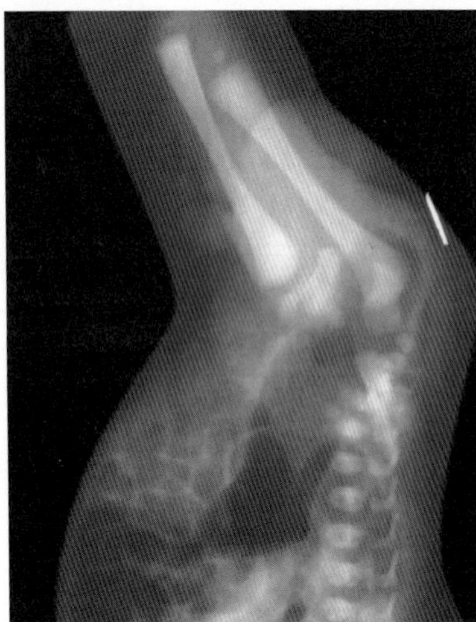

Fig. 4: Invertogram showing rectal gas below the coccyx.

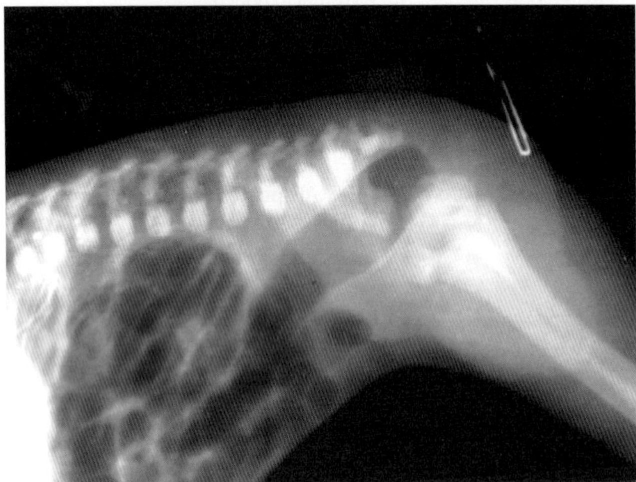

Fig. 5: Prone cross-table lateral X-ray showing rectal gas ending above the coccyx (HARM). (HARM: high anorectal malformations)

If rectal gas is seen above the coccyx **(Fig. 5)** or there is meconuria, significant associated defects, and/or an abnormal sacrum with a flat-bottom perineum, a preliminary colostomy is recommended. The definitive surgical repair, usually a PSARP alone or with an additional laparotomy (in male HARM with bladder-neck fistula) can be performed 2–6 months later following a distal colostogram to delineate the anatomy of the distal rectum and, if present, the terminal fistula.

In "imperforate anus without fistula" (5 % cases), a prone cross-table lateral radiograph shows a blind-ending rectal shadow suggestive of HARM. Almost 95% of patients with Down syndrome and ARM have this defect. Depending upon the surgeon's experience, surgery consists of a primary PSARP or a preliminary colostomy with definitive surgery later.

Rectal atresia (1–2 % ARM), in both sexes, is identified by nonpassage of meconium from a normal or slightly narrow anal opening, which allows passage of a catheter only for 1–2 cm. The condition can be confirmed by a prone cross-table lateral X-ray and necessitates a preliminary colostomy followed, later, by definitive repair.

Newborns with CPC often present with an extremely distended, tense shiny abdomen due to gross distension of the colonic pouch with, sometimes, pneumoperitoneum due to perforation of the pouch. In patients with the more severe types I–II CPC, initial management **(Flowchart 1)** should include, whenever feasible, division–ligation of the usually wide CVF.

CLINICAL EVALUATION AND MANAGEMENT IN FEMALE NEWBORN WITH ANORECTAL MALFORMATIONS

Flowchart 2 shows an algorithm for the management of a female newborn with ARM.

As in males, the most important step in diagnosis and decision-making is the perineal inspection.

Three openings in the perineum: The presence of three openings in the perineum (urethra, vagina, and the terminal rectal fistula) is the most common finding and is due to a vestibular fistula (most common) **(Fig. 6)** or a perineal fistula **(Fig. 7)**. These patients often present beyond the neonatal period because of decompression through the associated fistula. Around 6% cases with a vestibular fistula have a longitudinal vaginal septum. Rarely (1–2% of ARM), a rectal atresia may be present. For vestibular fistula/perineal fistula, definitive surgery in the form of limited PSARP or other options **(Flowchart 2)** can be performed during the neonatal period or, more usually, during early infancy without a protective colostomy if the baby is decompressing well, is of good weight, and does not have significant perineal/perianal excoriations and infection **(Flowchart 2)**. In the presence of any of these features, or even otherwise if the surgeon is not experienced, a preliminary colostomy to take care of the emergency situation followed by definitive surgery at 1–6 months of age is recommended. As in males, if the baby is ill from associated problems, is very premature, and is a poor-risk patient for anesthesia, the fistula can be gently dilated and colostomy or definitive surgery delayed for 2–6 months.

Flowchart 2: Management of a female newborn with ARM.

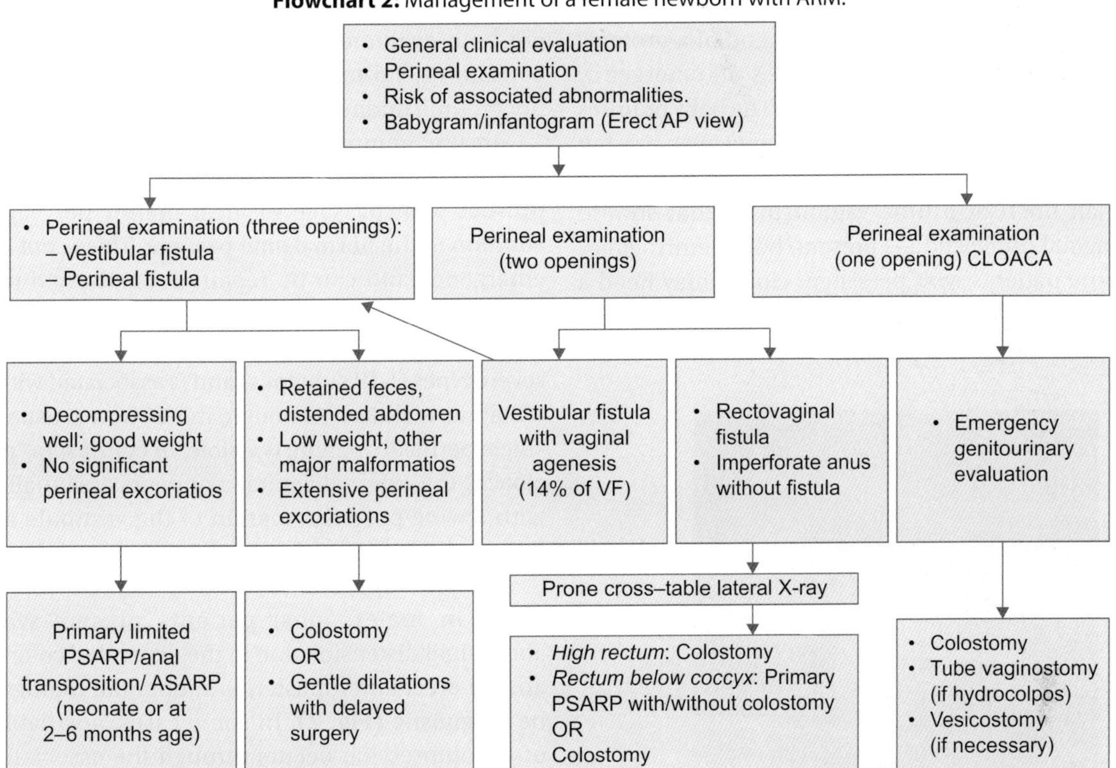

(AP: anteroposterior; ARM: anorectal malformations; ASARP: anterior sagittal anorectoplasty; PSARP: posterior sagittal anorectoplasty)

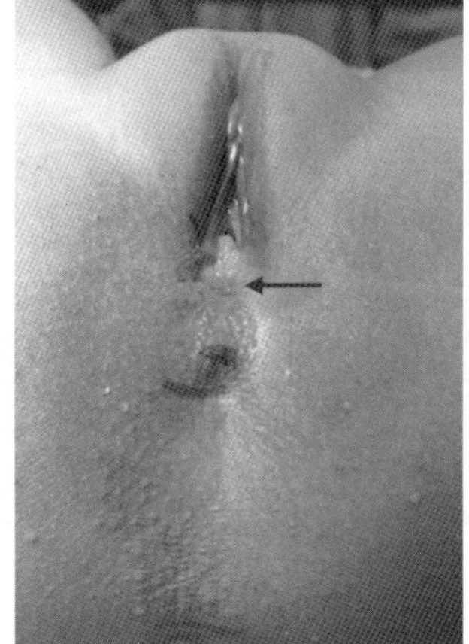

Fig. 6: Girl with vestibular fistula (arrow). *(For color version, see Plate 15)*

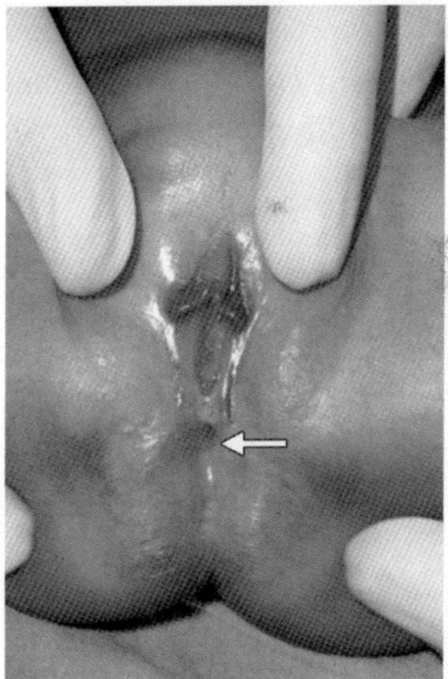

Fig. 7: Perineum of a girl with a perineal fistula (arrow). *(For color version, see Plate 16)*

In some cases of perineal fistula with a wide bridge of perineum between the fourchette and the fistulous opening, an anoplasty (as in males with perineal fistula) can be performed without a colostomy.

Two perineal openings: This may be due to a rectovaginal fistula, a vestibular fistula with vaginal agenesis (14% of cases), or imperforate anus without fistula. Rectovaginal fistula, although classified as "rare" (Krickenbeck classification) has been reported to have an incidence of 3.4–6 % in reports from Asia.

Single perineal opening: This finding, often with small-looking external genitalia **(Fig. 8)** and frequently, flat-bottom perineum is diagnostic of persistent cloaca (20% of female ARM) with a high likelihood of a urologic defect. Preliminary assessment includes an emergency genitourinary (GU) evaluation by the US. The baby requires a "high" colostomy. If present, a hydrocolpos may present with gross abdominal distension and should be drained by either an open or a tube vaginostomy that should drain, if vaginal duplication is present, both hemivaginas. Rarely, some patients with persistent cloaca may need a vesicostomy for urinary decompression. Definitive repair is usually performed at 6 months to 1 year of age.

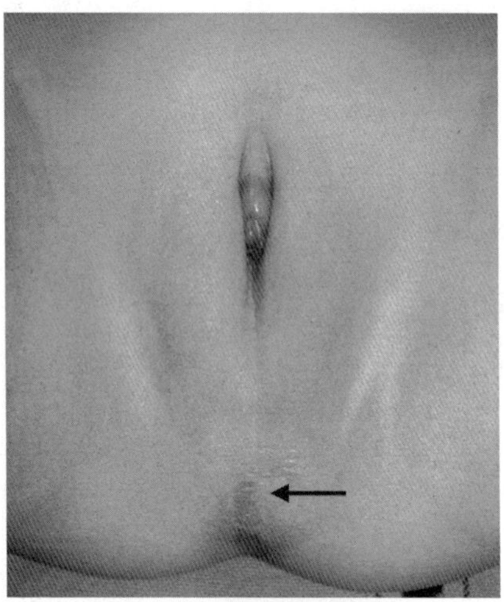

Fig. 8: Case of "persistent cloaca". Note small-looking external genitalia with a flat-bottom perineum (arrow). *(For color version, see Plate 16)*

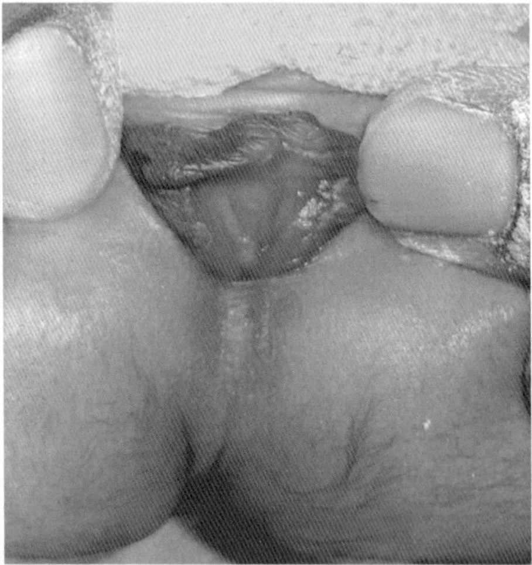

Fig. 9: Appearance of external genitalia in newborn girl with congenital pouch colon (CPC). Note wide margin of vestibule and folds radiating inward from margins of vestibule. *(For color version, see Plate 16)*

Imperforate anus without fistula and rectal atresia are both evaluated and managed as in males. In both conditions, failure to pass meconium after birth, an uncommon finding in female ARM, is a presenting feature.

An uncommon female ARM is a "perineal canal" or H-type rectovaginal or rectovestibular fistula. Patients present with passage of fecal matter per vaginum in addition to the normal anal passage. This is not a surgical emergency and can be repaired electively during later infancy.

Congenital pouch colon in girls is usually of the more severe types (I–III subtypes) and is associated with distinct GU abnormalities. Although, in newborns, usually only a single perineal opening is visible, in contrast to "persistent cloaca", the external genitalia appears essentially normal with a wide posterior margin of the vestibule and often folds radiating inward from the margins of the vestibule ("clover leaf" appearance) **(Fig. 9)**.

As in males, most patients present with gross abdominal distension due to the distended colonic pouch and an erect anteroposterior abdominal radiograph may be diagnostic **(Fig. 2)**. In some cases, a variable degree of decompression occurs through the associated fistula and the patients may present during infancy or later. The principles of management are similar to those of males.

KEY POINTS

- In males, the most common ARM is rectourethral fistula and in females, it is a vestibular fistula.
- Perineal examination is the key to assessing the type of ARM. Evaluation for associated major organ malformations (more common with HARM or complex ARM) is essential.
- *Sign of LARM:* Meconium-filled tract and meconium discharging perineal fistula are definite signs of LARM in males, usually manageable by cutback anoplasty.
- If no meconium is seen on the perineum by 20–24 hours after birth, findings on a prone cross-table lateral radiograph (rectal gas below/above the coccyx) can decide initial management in the form of a primary repair or, more usually, a colostomy.
- *Sign of HARM:* Meconium in urine (rectourinary fistula) in males and single perineal opening (cloaca) in females are diagnostic of HARM. Presence of flat bottom is suggestive of HARM.
- In girls, a vestibular fistula (most common) or a perineal fistula are common and present as three openings in the perineum. Late presentation due to decompression through the fistula is not infrequent. Around 14% girls with a vestibular fistula have vaginal agenesis. For both conditions, definitive surgery can be performed during the neonatal period or, more usually, within the first few months of life.

- Girls with a perineal canal or H-type rectovaginal/recto-vestibular fistula present with passage of fecal matter per vaginum in addition to the anal passage.
- A persistent cloaca needs urgent GU evaluation by US. The baby requires a "high" colostomy. If present, a hydrocolpos needs drainage by a vaginostomy and occasionally urinary diversion by a vesicostomy.
- Almost 95% of patients with Down syndrome and ARM have "imperforate anus without fistula" (5% of all ARM). Rectal atresia or stenosis is rare in both sexes (1–2% cases). In both conditions, preliminary colostomy is recommended.
- CPC usually presents with a grossly distended, tense shiny abdomen due to distension of the colonic pouch, and in males with meconuria. The diagnosis can be confirmed by an erect abdominal radiograph or an infantogram.

SUGGESTED READING

1. Chadha R, Khan NA. Congenital pouch colon. J Indian Assoc Pediatr Surg. 2017;22:69-78.
2. Choudhury SR, Khan NA, Debnath PR, Yadav PS, Shah S, Chadha R. Anorectal agenesis with rectovaginal fistula: A rare/regional variant. J Indian Assoc Pediatr Surg. 2017;22(2):79-82
3. Holschneider AM, Hutson JM (Eds). Anorectal malformations in children. Embryology, Diagnosis, Surgical Treatment, Follow-up. Heidelberg, Germany: Springer-Verlag; 2006.
4. King SK, Levitt MA. Advances in the management of the neonate born with an anorectal malformation. Clin Perinatol. 2022;49(4):965-79
5. Levitt MA, Pena A. Anorectal malformations. In: Coran AG, Caldamone A, Scott Adzich N, Krummel TM, Laberge JM (Eds). Pediatric Surgery, 7th edition. Oxford: Elsevier Limited; 2012. pp. 1289-309.
6. Oh C, Youn JK, Han JW, Yang HB, Kim HY, Jung SE, et al. Experiences of rectovaginal fistula in anorectal malformation. J Pediatr Surg. 2020;55(8):1495-8.
7. Son LT, Hung LT. Perineal canal: a special entity of anorectal malformation in Vietnam. Pediatr Surg Int. 2011;27(10):1105-10.
8. Van der Steeg HJ, Schmiedeke E, Bagolan P, Broens P, Demirogullari B, Garcia-Vasquez A, et al. European consensus meeting of ARM-Net members concerning diagnosis and early management of newborns with anorectal malformations. Tech Coloproctol. 2015;19(3):181-5.
9. Wood RJ, Levitt MA. Anorectal malformations. Clin Colon Rectal Surg. 2018;31(2):61-70.

Antenatally Detected Lung Anomalies

Avantika Tiwari, Zameer MM, Sanjay Rao

INTRODUCTION

The human respiratory system is a marvel of intricate design, essential for sustaining life by supplying our bodies with the oxygen needed for cellular functions. However, sometimes, this intricate system can develop abnormalities from birth, leading to a range of congenital lung lesions. These lesions, although rare, can profoundly impact an individual's health and well-being, making their understanding and management crucial in the field of medicine.

This chapter delves into the world of congenital lung lesions, offering a comprehensive exploration of their nature, classification, diagnosis, and treatment options. Through the pages that follow, we will examine the various types of congenital lung lesions, from the relatively common congenital pulmonary airway malformations (CPAMs) to rarer entities such as pulmonary sequestration and congenital lobar emphysema (CLE).

Moreover, this chapter will guide you through the principles of management and treatment strategies, ranging from conservative approaches to intricate surgical interventions.

CONGENITAL LUNG LESIONS

Congenital lung lesions or congenital thoracic malformations (CTMs) are a broad term that covers many disorders of lung development, including CLE, CPAMs, bronchopulmonary sequestrations (BPS), and bronchogenic cysts. The treatment of CTMs has evolved dramatically over the past several decades. These advancements have increased overall survival rates to around 95% from historical rates of 60%.

EPIDEMIOLOGY

The CTMs account for 5–18% of all congenital abnormalities, have a cumulative incidence of 30–42 cases per 100,000 individuals.

The true incidence of all CTMs is unclear. Historically, it was estimated to be between 1 in 20,000 and 1 in 35,000 live births. However, current estimates range between 1 in 2,500 and 1 in 8,000 live births. This rising incidence is likely due to the widespread availability of prenatal ultrasound combined with the improved resolution of ultrasound technology that enables the detection of smaller lung lesions. These lesions appear to be sporadic without any association with maternal factors such as ethnicity, parity, age, or other factors. They are not associated with karyotype anomalies.

Congenital Pulmonary Airway Malformation

These are the most common fetal lung lesions, accounting for 30–40% of all diagnosed CTMs. These are characterized by the abnormal proliferation of the terminal respiratory structures resulting in a mass of pulmonary tissue and abnormal development of alveoli. These lesions were previously known as congenital cystic adenomatoid malformations (CCAMs). These lesions were previously believed to contain cystic and adenomatoid components, hence, the historical name CCAM. This has been disproven leading to renaming these lesions as CPAMs.

The CPAMs may be found anywhere throughout the lung, but are generally unilateral and restricted to one lobe, though there are rare reports of multifocal and bilateral lesions. A defining characteristic of CPAMs is a connection to the tracheobronchial tree, although their abnormal alveoli make them generally incapable of normal gas exchange. Blood supply for CPAMs is derived from the normal pulmonary vasculature.

Stocker Classification System (Table 1)

Based on histopathology, it is classified by Dr Stocker as:

- *Type 0:* Acinar dysplasia associated with severe pulmonary hypoplasia

TABLE 1: Stocker classification of congenital pulmonary airway malformation lesions.

Type	Location	Characterization	%	Prognosis
Type 0	• Trachea • Bronchus	• Whole lung • Lungs small, solid, and firm	1–3%	Fatal
Type 1	• Distal bronchi • Proximal bronchioles	• One large dominant cyst • Late presentations • Most common	50–65%	Good
Type 2	Bronchiolar	• Multiple small cysts • Other anomalies	10–40%	Poor
Type 3	Alveolar	• Cystic with solid • Solid appearance	5–10%	Severe
Type 4	Acinar	Thin wall, fluid filled small cysts	10–15%	Good

Source: Stocker JT. Congenital pulmonary airway malformation—a new name for and an expanded classification of congenital cystic adenomatoid malformation of the lung. Histopathology. 2002;41:424.

- *Type 1:* Presence of one large cyst of 2–10 cm in diameter or multiple cysts which may compress other lobes. This is the most frequently occurring variety.
- *Type 2:* Presence of multiple smaller cysts with other associated congenital anomalies
- *Type 3:* Presence of multiple microscopic cysts
- *Type 4:* Presence of cysts of varying sizes lined by alveolar type I (ATI) and ATII cells

Stocker's pathological classification has been widely used to describe prenatal lung lesions, but this correlates poorly with postnatal diagnosis and has poor prognostic value. A more practical classification for fetal CPAMs was proposed by Adzick and is based on whether they are macrocystic (>0.5 cm) or microcystic (<0.5 cm) by ultrasound.

PATHOPHYSIOLOGY OF CONGENITAL PULMONARY AIRWAY MALFORMATIONS

One hypothesis states that there is persistent expression of early lung development markers leading to abnormal branching of bronchioles, thus disrupting normal pulmonary morphogenesis. The second proposed mechanism states that there is focal obstructive process of the tracheobronchial tree, such as bronchial atresia, resulting in pathological lung development.

The natural history of CPAMs during the prenatal period can vary from spontaneous regression to rapid growth and development of nonimmune hydrops fetalis and fetal demise. Microcystic CPAMs have a predictable growth, usually peaking at 25–26 weeks' gestation followed by regression with advancing gestation. Large macrocystic lesions can exhibit rapid growth, leading to hydrops. Once hydrops develops, mortality approaches 100% without interventions.

The CPAMs with associated extrapulmonary anomalies have a poor prognosis. In particular, Stocker type 2 CPAMs have a reported 60% incidence of associated anomalies, including cardiac, diaphragmatic, and renal abnormalities, many of which are life-threatening.

PRESENTATION

A large majority of fetal lung lesions are diagnosed based on routine prenatal ultrasound at 20 weeks' gestation. The cystic and/or solid lesion may progressively enlarge, with eventual mediastinal shift, or also regress totally or partially before birth. Antenatal complications of CPAMs include fetal hydrops, pleural effusion, or polyhydramnios secondary to failure of normal fetal swallowing because of esophageal compression. Hydrops, reported in 5–30% of all CPAMs, is the gravest complication, associated with high mortality.

The cystic pulmonary airway malformation volume ratio (CVR), calculated by ultrasound, helps us to predict the prognosis of a fetus with CPAM. This value is calculated by measuring three dimensions of the CPAM, calculating the elliptical volume of the mass, and dividing by the fetal head circumference to account for differences in gestational age [CVR = (length × height × width × 0.52)/head circumference]. A CVR >1.6 predicts an 80% increased risk of fetal hydrops, while a ratio <1.6 is associated with a survival rate of 94% and risk of hydrops < 3%. A CVR ≥0.84 is a good predictor of respiratory distress at birth.

Fetal Interventions

Fetal lung tissue on routine ultrasound seems similar in echogenicity to that of the liver or spleen. CPAMs can have variable echogenicity, either increased or decreased, depending on specific lesion characteristics. Mass effect may also be noted on ultrasound depending on the size of the lesion. Large lesions can cause compression of various thoracic structures, including the esophagus, which can result in polyhydramnios due to impaired swallowing. Larger abnormalities can also cause compression on adjacent areas of the lung resulting in the underdevelopment of normal lung tissue as well as shift of mediastinal structures due to mass effect. This mediastinal shift can not only cause lung compression but also affect cardiac function and decrease the amount of blood return due to venous compression. This venous compression leading to cardiac failure can progress to an entity referred to as nonimmune fetal hydrops, a poor prognostic indicator.

Current prenatal interventions for CPAM include medical therapy (namely systemic corticosteroid therapy), single-needle thoracocentesis, thoracoamniotic shunts, and open fetal surgery. These therapies are reserved for patients at risk for or having already developed hydrops. It is important to ensure the absence of relevant exclusion criteria, namely karyotype abnormalities or other major anatomic abnormalities.

Prenatal betamethasone therapy has been found to be effective for patients with microcystic CPAM at risk for hydrops fetalis. First round of steroids is administered at a mean gestational age of 22 weeks and the second is administered at 25 weeks after disease progression was noted. Betamethasone has not proven effective for large macrocystic lesions. In these cases, thoracentesis and shunting are available treatment options.

Fetal resection is indicated only when other fetal therapies have failed. Fetal lobectomy is usually performed at around 24 weeks' gestation, after which the fetus is placed back into the uterus for the pregnancy to continue. EXIT procedure allows for the resection of the lung malformation while the baby remains on placental bypass, after which the baby is then delivered.

At birth, clinical presentation of CPAMs is variable. Most neonates (>75%) are asymptomatic, with only a minority requiring any respiratory support. It has been reported that these complications occur in about 3.2% of nonoperated patients. The most common presentation postnatally is infection or other mass-related symptoms. They can cause a variety of symptoms including compression on trachea/bronchus, dysphagia, infections, and hemorrhage leading to the possible development of hemothorax.

X-ray images of CPAMs may visualize retained fluid within the lesion or increased aeration with visualization of air-filled cysts on imaging **(Figs. 1A and B)**. If symptomatic and deemed need for resection, further imaging is obtained to define the anatomy such as CT scan or MRI.

Neonatal resection is indicated for patients who develop respiratory distress at birth secondary to mass effect. Risk factors for the development of postnatal respiratory distress include prenatal evidence of ascites, polyhydramnios, and CVR > 0.84.

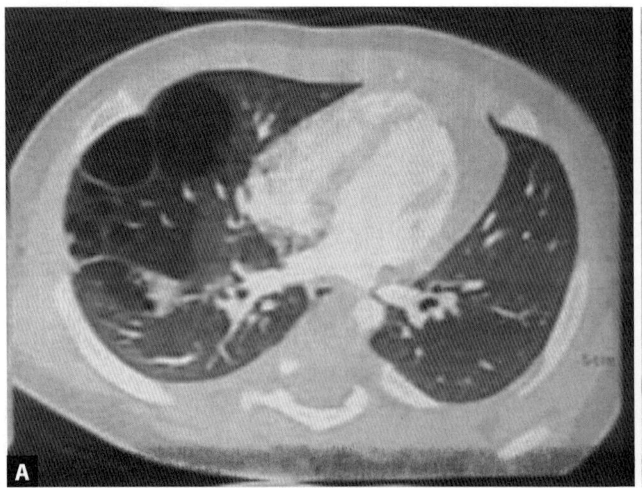

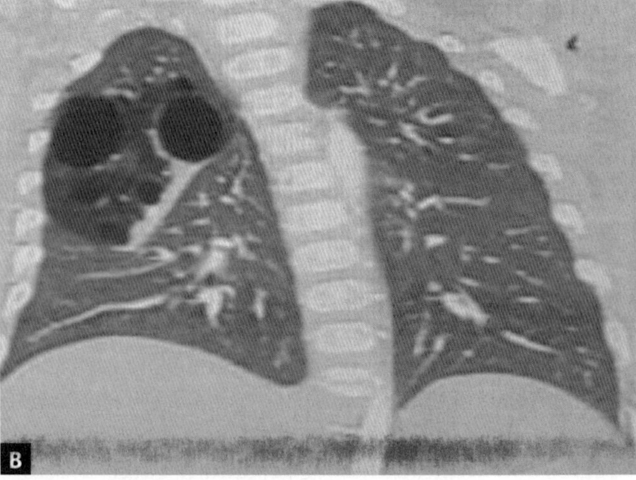

Figs. 1A and B: Congenital pulmonary airway malformations involving right upper and middle lobe.

For the remaining 75% of patients, who are initially asymptomatic at birth, the decision to offer resection remains controversial. The argument for expectant management for initially asymptomatic patients is a relatively low cited risk of infection over the first 5 years of life, typically reported between 3 and 10%. The possibility of spontaneous regression is believed to occur for approximately 6% of all lesions.

The accepted indications to operate on asymptomatic patients with CPAMs:

- Risk of malignancy (cumulative incidence rate of 4% of occult malignancy)
- Risk of complications, including infection and pneumothorax
- Potential for compensatory lung growth with earlier resection
- Reduction in postoperative complications following elective surgery

Arguments in favor of prophylactic resection include lower morbidity and mortality with elective procedures and lower thoracotomy rate. Higher incidence of conversion from thoracoscopic to thoracotomy had been reported in patients who had infection preoperatively.

The extent of resection is generally a formal lobectomy performed either via open thoracotomy, thoracoscopy or robot assisted. There is always the risk of missing additional lesions, which is possible even after contrast enhanced CT scan and occurs at an estimated rate of 15%. This risk is magnified given the potential for malignancy within missed lesions **(Figs. 2 and 3)**.

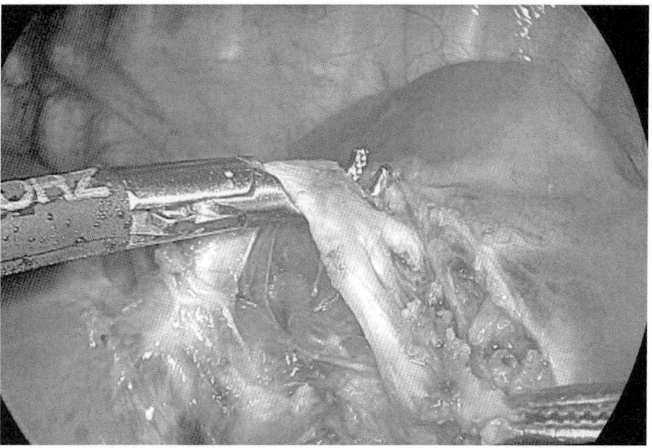

Fig. 2: Isolation of the lobar vessels prior to clamping and resection. *(For color version, see Plate 16)*

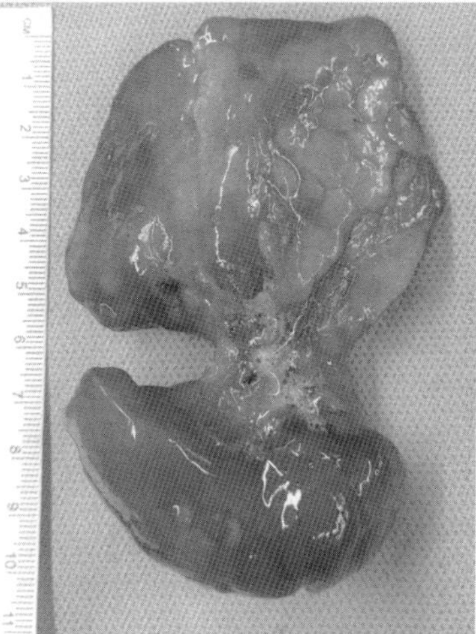

Fig. 3: Specimen of the lobe with multiple congenital pulmonary airway malformation lesions within. *(For color version, see Plate 16)*

Bronchopulmonary Sequestrations (BPSs)

After CPAMs, BPSs are the most frequent. The characteristic feature of all BPSs is that the lesion has no airway communication. It is comprised of nonfunctioning lung tissue. The abnormal lung tissue tends to be nonaerated although some collateral ventilation via the pores of Kohn from adjacent lung tissue is possible. The blood supply for a BPS arises from a systemic feeding vessel, generally originating from the thoracic aorta, although feeding vessels arising from the abdominal aorta, such as the celiac artery, have been seen.

It is hypothesized that during embryologic development, a supernumerary lung bud is formed posterior to the normal lung bud eventually becoming aberrant lung tissue. The intralobar versus extralobar distinction of BPS depends on the timing of the supernumerary lung bud development in relation to pleura. If lung bud develops before the pleura then the BPS will become intralobar, and if after the pleura, then it will become extralobar and develop its own pleura. These lesions are histologically similar, but differ based on venous drainage and location. Venous drainage of extralobar BPS is systemic, namely to the vena cava, azygous vein, and even directly into the right atrium. Drainage of intralobar BPS is via the pulmonary vasculature to the left atrium.

Also, the intralobar BPSs are invested within the visceral pleura of the normal lung. As such, they may develop abnormal connections to either the bronchi or the gastrointestinal tract, increasing the risk of infections such as pneumonia. In contrast, extralobar BPSs are completely separated from the normal lung parenchyma, so these anomalous connections do not occur. The most common location of intralobar BPS is the lower lobe, predominantly the posterior aspect of the left lower lobe. Similarly, extralobar BPSs also arise within the lower aspect of the left hemithorax, but may occasionally be located below the diaphragm, classically in the area of the adrenal gland, or rarely within the diaphragm musculature.

Hydrops associated with BPS is caused by fluid secreted from these lesions, rather than from the size of the lesions themselves, resulting in tension hydrothorax. When intervention is required, thoracentesis or thoracoamniotic shunting is the most common procedures selected and is largely effective in resolving symptoms.

The potential risk of infection with intralobar BPS is an indication for resection. Asymptomatic extralobar BPS may be monitored clinically without resection.

Removal of BPSs does require caution with ligation of their blood supply. Most arterial supply comes from the abdominal aorta and may cross the diaphragm. This makes careful ligation imperative due to concern that these vessels may retract into the abdominal cavity and lead to uncontrolled hemorrhage if not ligated adequately. An alternative to resection is postnatal arterial embolization of the sequestration feeding vessels by interventional radiology. Embolization is recommended for patients who may be poor candidates for surgical resection.

Congenital Lobar Emphysema

The CLE is a congenital lung malformation where one or more lobes of the lungs are congenitally emphysematous. Incidence of CLE is thought to be around 1 per 20,000–30,000 births. It is thought to originate from alterations in interactions between the endoderm and mesoderm of embryologic lung tissue that a cause increasing hyperinflation.

Mechanisms proposed to explain the air-trapping include dysplastic or deficient bronchial cartilage, thick mucus, extensive mucosal proliferation, bronchial torsion, bronchial atresia, and bronchial compression by cardiopulmonary vessels, lymph nodes, cysts, polyalveolar lung, or focal pulmonary hypoplasia.

The most common location of CLE is the left upper lobe. The overdistended lobes, the damaged alveoli are permanently ineffective for gas exchange. CLE lesions rarely grow large enough to cause intrauterine fetal demise and that a majority will regress significantly during gestation. Hence fetal intervention for CLE, such as lobectomy, is rarely indicated.

The CLE requiring intervention within the first week of life is <10%. Most neonatal patients with CLE will experience only mild respiratory distress at birth with a more insidious progression of symptoms as air-trapping worsens. CLE can seem as hyperinflated lung on X-ray **(Fig. 4)** or a radio-opaque mass due to delayed clearance of fluid from the overdistended lobe. If there are any diagnostic uncertainties, CT or ventilation/perfusion scans may be used to confirm the diagnosis. On CT scan, CLE lesions seem less attenuated or darker than normal lung tissue and will be visibly enlarged.

Resection may be completed by thoracoscopic or open techniques, although open thoracotomy is still the preferred method given the challenges in establishing sufficient working space around CLE lesions.

Bronchogenic Cysts

Bronchogenic cysts are unilocular, fluid, or mucus filled lesions, arising from the posterior membranous wall of the airway. They develop from abnormal buds of the primitive foregut. Cysts generally contain bronchial structural elements including cartilage, smooth muscle, mucous glands, and respiratory epithelium. Importantly, intrapulmonary bronchogenic cysts do not communicate with the airway.

Most commonly the cyst arises from the trachea or the mainstem bronchi. They may also occur in within the parenchyma of the lung or in other rarer sites such as the abdomen, tongue, and in the neck.

These cysts generally do not require any prenatal intervention. Thoracentesis or thoracoamniotic shunts are

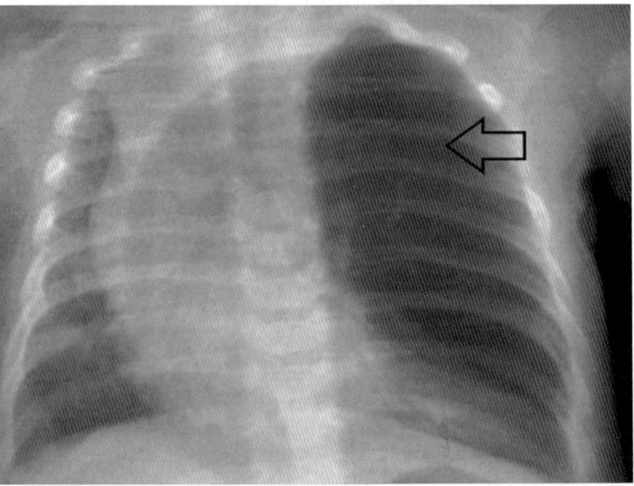

Fig. 4: CLE involving left upper lobe (with herniation) with collapsed lower lobe.

indicated in cases of very large cysts causing compressive symptoms and hydrops.

Given the risks of infection, respiratory distress from airway compression, and undiagnosed malignancy, resection of bronchogenic cyst is recommended for most patients. Treatment may consist of either enucleation (mediastinal cysts) versus wedge or anatomic resections (intrapulmonary cysts).

KEY POINTS

- CPAM is the most common congenital lung lesion.
- Fetal interventions are needed for complex CPAMs impending hydrops.
- Generally, CPAMs are unilateral and restricted to one lobe.
- CPAM has a blood supply from the pulmonary vasculature.
- Asymptomatic CPAMs need to be operated due to risk of complications (infection) and malignancy.
- Treatment for CPAM is lobectomy.
- BPS is of two type—(1) intralobar and (2) extralobar.
- BPS has no communication with the airway.
- BPS has blood supply from the systemic vessels.
- Intralobar sequestration drains into pulmonary veins whereas extralobar sequestration drains into systemic veins.
- Treatment for intralobar BPS is resection due to high risk of infection while extralobar asymptomatic BPS can be monitored.
- CLE generally asymptomatic at birth. Most common location is left upper lobe. They require lobectomy later.
- Bronchogenic cysts are mostly found in the posterior mediastinum. Treatment is resection.

SUGGESTED READING

1. Adzick NS, Harrison MR, Crombleholme TM, Flake AW HL. Fetal lung lesions: managemnt and outcome. Am J Obstet Gynecol. 1988;179(4):884-9.
2. Adzick NS, Harrison MR, Glick PL, Golbus MS, Anderson RL, Mahony BS, et al. Fetal cystic adenomatoid malformation: prenatal diagnosis and natural history. J Pediatr Surg. 1985;20(5):483-8.
3. Andrade CF, Ferreira HP, Fischer GB. Congenital lung malformations. J Bras Pneumol. 2011;37:259-71.
4. Ayloo SM, Addeo P, Buchs NC, Giulianotti P. Intralobar pulmonary sequestration with an aberrant artery arising from the celiac trunk. Eur J Cardiothorac Surg. 2011;39(3):418.
5. Azizkhan RG, Crombleholme TM. Congenital cystic lung disease: contemporary antenatal and postnatal management. Pediatr Surg Int. 2008;24(6):643-57.
6. Baird R, Puligandla PS, Laberge JM. Congenital lung malformations: Informing best practice. Semin Pediatr Surg. 2014;23(5):270-7.
7. Chetcuti PA, Crabbe DC. CAM lungs: The conservative approach. Arch Dis Child Fetal neonatal Ed. 2006;91(6): F463-4.
8. Conran RM, Stocker JT. Extraloabr sequestration with frequntly associated congenital adenomatoid malformation, type 2: report of 50 cases. Pediatr Dev Pathol. 1999;2:454-63.
9. Cook J, Chitty LS, De Coppi P, Ashworth M, Wallis C. The natural history of prenatally diagnosed congenital cystic lung lesions: long-term follow-up of 119 cases. Arch od Dis Child. 2017;102(9):798-803.
10. Correia-Pinto J, Gonzaga S, Huang Y, Rottier R. Congenital lung lesions—underlying molecular mechanisms. Semin Pediatr Surg. 2010;19(3):171-9.
11. Crombleholme TM, Coleman B, Hedrick H, Liechty K, Howell L, Flake AW, et al. Cystic adenomatoid malformation volume ratio predicts outcome in prenatally diagnosed cystic adenomatoid malformation of the lung. J Pediatr Surg. 2002;37(3):331-8.
12. Durell J, Lakhoo K. Congenital cystic lesions of the lung. Early Hum Dev. 2014;90(12):935-9.
13. Farrugia MK, Raza SA, Gould S, Lakhoo K. Congenital lung lesions: classification and concordance of radiological appearance and surgical pathology. Pediatric Surg Int. 2008;24(9):987-91.
14. Fowler DJ, Gould SJ. The pathology of congenital lung lesions. Semin Pediatr Surg. 2015;24(4):176-82.
15. Khalek N, Johnson MP. Management of prenatally diagnosed lung lesions. Semin Pediatr Surg. 2013;22(1):24-9.
16. Kini H, Sreeram S, Shukla S, Rao S, Sahu K, Adiga D, et al. Congenital Pulmonary Airway Malformation-19-Yera Experience from a Tertiary Care Center in India. Fetal Pediatr Pathol. 2019;38(6):449-59.
17. Kulaylat AN, Engbrecht BW, Hollenbeak CS, Safford SD, Cilley RE, Cilley RE, Dillon PW. Comparing 30-day outcomes between thoracoscopic and open approaches for resection of pediatric congenital lung malformations: Evidence from NSQIP. J Pediatr Surg. 2015;50(10):1716-21.
18. Laje P, Liechty KW. Postnatal management and outcome of prenatally diagnosed lung lesions. Prenat Diagn. 2008;28(7):612-8.
19. Laje P, Martinez-Ferro M, Grisosni E, Dudgeon D. Intrabdominal pulmonary sequatration. A case series and review of lietrature. J Pediatr Surg. 2006;41(7):1309-12.
20. Langston C. New concepts in the pathology of congenital lung maformations. Semin Pediatr Surg. 2003;12(1):17-37.
21. Leblanc C, Baron M, Desselas E, Phan MH, Rybak A, Thouvenin G, et al. Congenital pulmonary airway malformations: state-of-the art review for pediatrician's use. Eur J Pediatr. 2017;176(12):1559-71.
22. Lima JS, Camargos PA, Aguiar RA, Campos AS, Aguiar MJ. Pre and perinatal aspects of congenital cystic adenomatoid malformation of the lung. J Matern Fetal Neonatal Med. 2014;27(3):228-32.

23. Macardle CA, Ehrenberg-Buchner S, Smith EA, Dillman JR, Mychaliska GB, Treadwell MC, et al. Surveillance of fetal lung lesions using the congenital pulmonary airway malformation volume ratio: Natural history and outcomes. Prenat Diagn. 2016;36(3):282-9.
24. Markhardt BK, Farmer DL, Filly RA. Presumptive intrahepatic congenital cystic adenomatoid malformation. J Ultrasound Med. 2003;22(5):531-6.
25. Messinger YH, Stewart DR, Priest JR, Williams GM, Harris AK, Schultz KA, et al. Pleuropulmonary blastoma: A report on 350 central pathology-confirmed plueropulmonary blastoma cases by the International Pleuropulamonary Blastoma registry. Cancer. 2015;121(2):276-85.
26. Mon RA, Johnson KN, Ladino-Torres M, Heider A, Mychaliska GB, Treadwell MC, et al. Diagnostic accuracy of imaging studies in congenital lung malformations. Arch Dis Child Fetal neonatal Ed. 2018;104(4):F372-7.
27. Ng C, Stanwell J, Burge DM, Stanton MP. Conservative management of antenatally diagnosed cystic lung malformations. Arch Dis Child. 2014;99(5):432-7.
28. Niiagal A, Jelin E, Feldstein VA, et al. The diagnosis and management of intradiaphragmatic extralobar pulmonary sequestrations: a report of 4 cases. J Pediatr Surg. 2012;47(8):1501-5.
29. Palla J, Sockrider MM. Congenital Lung Malformations. Pediatr Ann. 2019;48(4):e169-74.
30. Papagiannopoulos KA, Sheppard M, Bush AP, Goldstraw P. Pleuropulmonary blastoma: is prophylactic resection of congenital lung cysts effective? Ann Thorac Surg. 2001;72(2):604-5.
31. Priest JR, Williams GM, Hill DA, Dehner LP, Jaffé A. Pulmonary cysts in early childhood and the risk of malignancy. Pediatr Pulmonol. 2009;44(1):14-30.
32. Riley JS, Urwin JW, Oliver ER, Coleman BG, Khalek N, Moldenhauer JS, et al. Prenatal growth characteristics and pre/postnatal management of bronchopulmonary sequestrations. J Pediatr Surg. 2018;53(2):265-9.
33. Rios LT, Araujo Junior E, Nardozza LM, Moron AF, Martins Mda G. Prenatal diagnosis and postnatal findings of bronchogenic cyst. Case Rep Pulmonol. 2013;2013:483864.
34. Ruchonnet-Metrailler I, Leroy-Terquem E, Stirnemann J, Stirnemann J, Cros P, Ducoin H, et al. Neonatal outcomes of prenatally diagnosed congenital pulmonary malformations. Pedaitrics. 2014;133(5):e1285-91.
35. Sacco A, Van der Veeken L, Bagshaw E, Ferguson C, Van Mieghem T, David AL, et al. Maternal complications following open and fetoscopic fetal surgery: A systematic review and meta-analysis. Prenat Diagn. 2019;39(4):251-68.
36. Stanton M. The argument for a non-operative approach to asymptomatic lung lesions. Semin Pediatr Surg. 2015;24(4):183-6.
37. Stocker LJ, Wellesley DG, Stantopn MP, Prasuraman R, Howe DT. The increasing incidence of foetal echogenic congenital lung malformations: an observational study. Prenat Diagn. 2015;35(2):148-53.
38. Thompson AJ, Sidebotham EL, Chetcuti PAJ, Crabbe DCG. Prenatally diagnosed congenital lung malformations-A long-term outcome study. Pedaitric Pulmonol. 2018;53(10):1442-6.
39. Usui N, Kamata S, Sawai T, Kamiyama M, Okuyama H, Kubota A, et al. Outcome predictors for infants with cystic lung diasease. J Pediatr Surg. 2004;39(4):603-6.
40. Vu LT, Farmer DL, Nobuhara KK, Miniati D, Lee H. Thoracoscopic versus open resection for congenital adenomatoid malformations of the lung. J Pediatr Surg. 2008;43(1):35-9.
41. Williams HJ, Johnson KJ. Imaging of congenital cystic lung lesions. Pediatr Respir Rev. 2002;3(2):120-7.
42. Yong PJ, Von Dadelszen P, Carpara D, Lim K, Kent N, Tessier F, et al. Prediction of pediatric outcome after prenatal diagnosis and expectant antenatal mangement of congenital cystic adenomatoid malformation. Fetal Diagn Ther. 2012;31(2):94-102.

SECTION 16

Dermatology

Section Editor: *Vibhu Mendiratta*

CHAPTER 140 Atopic Dermatitis

Vibhu Mendiratta

INTRODUCTION

Atopic dermatitis (AD), also known as atopic eczema, is the most common chronic inflammatory skin disorders of childhood and characterized by pruritus, dryness of skin, and scratching. It begins in infancy and continues up to adulthood. AD may be the first manifestation of "atopic march", which can be associated with development of asthma and allergic rhinitis at a later stage. The hallmark of this disease is eczematous, pruritic lesions that show distinct distribution in different pediatric age groups. It is a familial and chronic disease associated with episodes of clinical exacerbation called flares or flare ups.

EPIDEMIOLOGY

Atopic dermatitis most often begins in early childhood, 85% of cases are seen during the first 5 years of life and may persist into adulthood in small percentage of patients. For some, it flares periodically and then subsides for a time, even up to several years. AD can affect almost 5–20% of children. It is estimated that 75% of the cases of AD improve by the time children reach adolescence, whereas 25% continue to have difficulties with the condition through adulthood. Although, the frequency of AD is much higher in developed countries and urban areas, its prevalence is steadily rising in developing countries also. This increase has been attributed to change in lifestyle.

ETIOLOGY

Atopic dermatitis is multifactorial and heterogeneous skin disorder that results from close interaction between genetic predisposition, environmental factors, skin barrier defects, and immunological abnormalities **(Fig. 1)**.

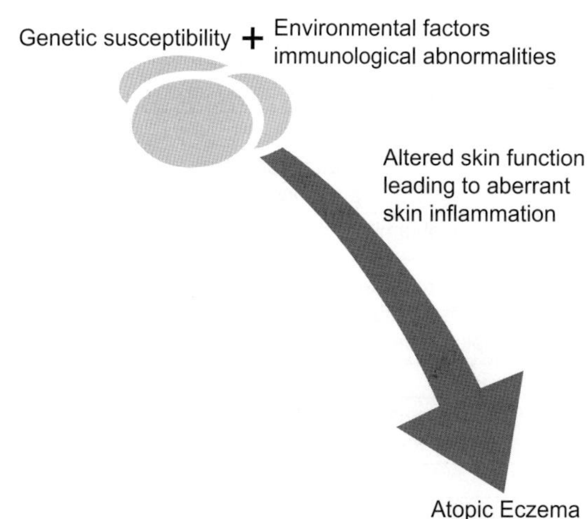

Fig. 1: Genetic predisposition.

APPROACH TO THE PATIENT (FLOWCHART 1)

Atopic dermatitis looks different in infants, children, and adults.

In infants, an erythematous oozy rash may develop by 2 or 3 months of age. It develops suddenly, predominantly affecting the scalp and face, especially on the cheeks. The extensors of the limbs such as elbows, knees, and ankles are more commonly involved. It is intensely itchy and interferes with the sleep of the child. The skin of the child in general is dry and xerotic. The diaper area being constantly moist and is never involved in AD. AD has to be differentiated from seborrheic dermatitis (SD) where in there are greasy scales over scalp (cradle cap), and face mostly over eyebrows, nasolabial folds, retroauricular grooves, and neck. Diaper area is classically involved unlike in AD. The rash in SD is nonpruritic, and the infants are totally undisturbed by it. Hair loss is rare in SD, but common in AD probably due to itching and rubbing.

CLINICAL PEARLS

- Pruritic exudative plaques over face and scalp: suspect atopic dermatitis.
- Diaper area is never involved in atopic dermatitis.

Flowchart 1: Approach to a patient with eczematous dermatitis.

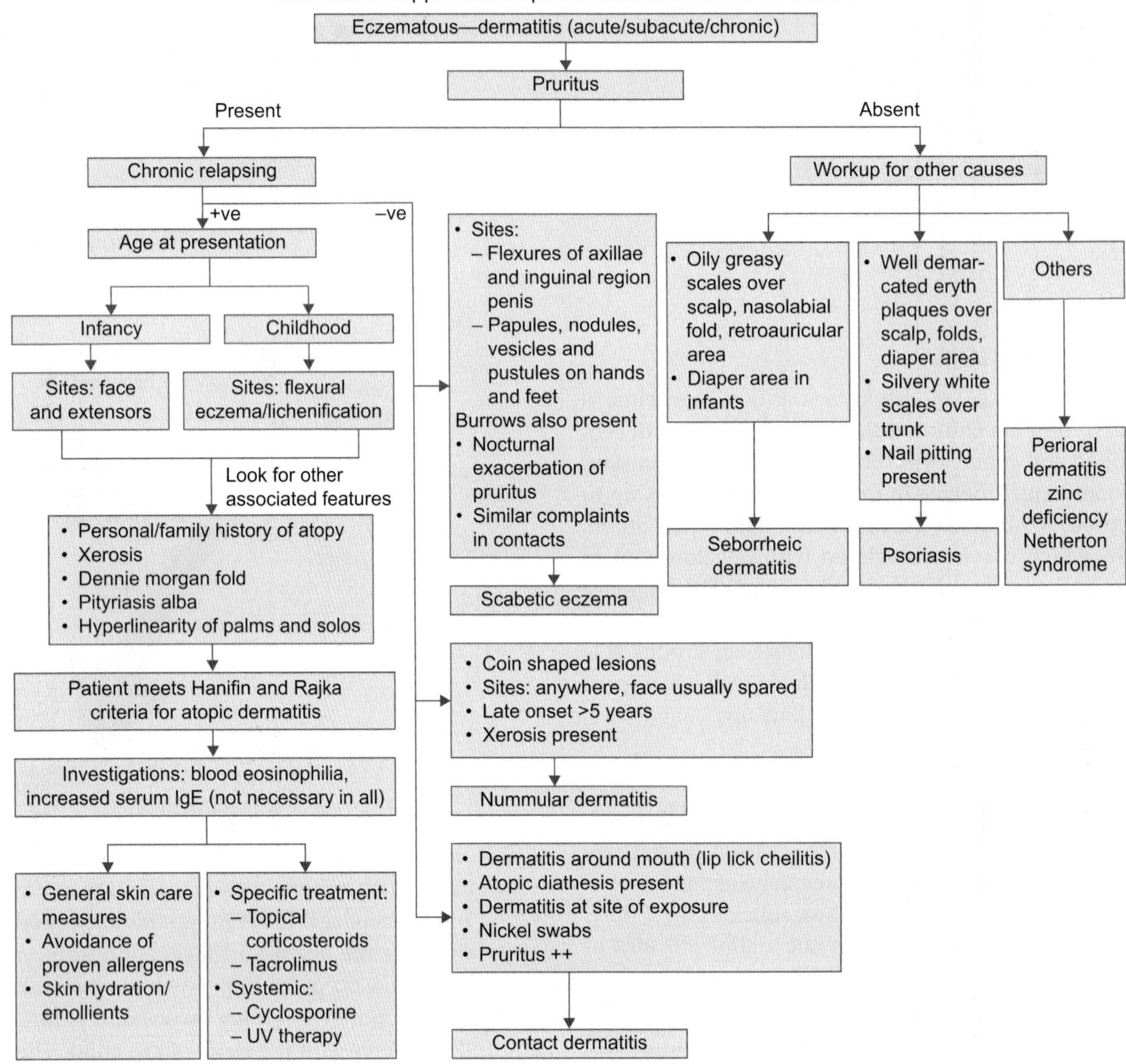

Psoriasis in infants is not uncommon and is often mistaken with AD. It often affects the scalp, folds, and diaper area. Lesions over trunk (if present) are well demarcated erythematous plaques surmounted by a thin white scale.

Atopic dermatitis in children beyond 2 years of age involves the flexures such as the cubital fossa, popliteal fossa, neck, groins, wrists, and ankles. The involved skin is erythematous and oozy, at places lichenification develops due to constant itching. Scabietic eczema should be ruled out where in lesions of varied morphology such as papules, pustules, and nodules along with burrows can be seen especially over hands and feet with relative sparing of face. History of nocturnal itching can be elicited in family members.

Flexural erythematous rash along with dry xerotic skin elsewhere is seen in Netherton syndrome, which makes it essential to differentiate it from AD. Here, examination of the hair will reveal trichorrhexis invaginata, with raised immunoglobulin E.

Zinc and biotin deficiency can present as an eczematous eruption or an erythroderma, and are often misdiagnosed as AD before other symptoms and signs become evident. The skin eruption consists of dermatitis on the face that has a typical horseshoe appearance on the cheeks and around the chin, with perianal involvement. However, there is no xerosis or pruritus. In older children the lesions are seen on the elbows and knees, whereas in AD the flexures are usually involved.

Other dermatitis such as nummular dermatitis, allergic, or irritant dermatitis can resemble AD and should be ruled out.

It is rare for adults to get AD. About half (50%) of people who get AD during childhood continue to have milder signs and symptoms of AD as an adult. When an adult has AD, it often looks different from the AD of childhood. They may continue to have a diffuse pattern of eczema but the skin is often more dry and lichenified than in children. Commonly, adults have persistent localized eczema, possibly confined to the hands, eyelids, flexures, nipples, or all of these areas. The skin is prone to secondary bacterial infections.

CLINICAL PEARL

- Always look for hyperlinearity of palms, Dennie–Morgan fold, and other features of atopy when suspecting atopic dermatitis.

Individuals with AD may show other associated features of atopy such as generalized xerosis, Dennie–Morgan fold, hyperlinearity of palms, pityriasis alba, keratosis pilaris, allergic shiners, and ichthyosis vulgaris.

MANAGEMENT

Treatment of AD is aimed at suppressing inflammation, eliminating triggers, reducing pruritus, and combating the development of xerosis, a major feature of AD. For this, conventional therapy is the first-line approach. It includes:

- Regular application of moisturizers, multiple times per day is very important. They are the mainstay of treatment, as they prevent dehydration, soften the skin, and increase water retention.
- Daily bathing with warm water is an extremely important step for hydration of skin, as well as removing allergens, irritants, crusts, and bacteria.
- *Antihistamines:* Itching is the most intolerable symptom of AD and has a devastating effect on social life and sleep. Due to their sedation property, first generation antihistaminics are used for severe case of pruritus and overcoming sleep disturbance.
- *Topical steroids (current mainstay of treatment; commonly used in conjunction with moisturizers):* Hydrocortisone, triamcinolone, or betamethasone; ointment bases are generally preferred, particularly in dry environments.
- *Immunomodulators:* Tacrolimus and pimecrolimus (calcineurin inhibitors) are considered second-line therapy.
- *Wet wrap:* It is application of topical agents over skin followed by a layer of wet tubular bandage and an outer layer of dry bandage. It intensifies the effect of moisturizers and topical agents by providing a smooth skin texture and preventing water loss.

Other treatments options available include the following:

- *Systemic therapy:* It is considered when the skin lesions do not ameliorate after usage of topical agents. It includes systemic corticosteroids, methotrexate, azathioprine, cyclosporine, and mycophenolate mofetil.
- *Phototherapy:* Ultraviolet A for acute exacerbations, narrowband ultraviolet B for chronic disease.
- *Biological agents and new treatment strategies*: JAK Kinase inhibitors such as, upadacitinib, abrocitinib, and topical ruxolitinib, tralokinumab, dupilumab, omalizumab. Lebrikizumab, and phosphodiesterase inhibitors.
- *Others:* Probiotics, antibiotics for clinical infections.

CLINICAL PEARLS

What to tell parents?

- Keep child in humid environment.
- Avoid pets, dust.
- Use lukewarm water for bathing.
- Apply adequate emollients immediately after bath.

KEY POINTS

- Atopic dermatitis is always itchy.
- It remits and relapses.
- It effects extensors and face in <2 years children, and flexures in children elder than 2 years and adults.
- Seborrheic dermatitis, flexural psoriasis, and zinc deficiency are great mimickers and should be excluded.

SUGGESTED READING

1. Arnacho-Saucedo G, Salido-Vallejo R, Moreno-Giménez JC. Actualización en dermatitis atópica. Propuesta de algoritmo de actuación. Actas Dermosifiliogr. 2013;104: 4-16.
2. Bhavani MN, Vandergriff T, Rasmussen H, Jacobe H. Phototherapy in the management of atopic dermatitis: a systematic review. Photodermatology, Photoimmunology & Photomedicine. 2007;23(4):106-12.
3. Çetinkaya PG, Şahiner ÜM. Childhood atopic dermatitis: current developments, treatment approaches, and future expectations. Turkish Journal of Med Sci. 2019;49(4): 963-84.
4. De Benedetto A, Agnihothri R, McGirt LY, Bankova LG, Beck LA. Atopic dermatitis: a disease caused by innate immune defects? The Journal of Investigative Dermatology. 2009;129(1):14-30.
5. McCollum AD, Paik A, Eichenfield LF. The safety and efficacy of tacrolimus ointment in pediatric patients with atopic dermatitis. Pediatr Dermatol. 2010;27:425-36.
6. Morris A, Rogers M, Fischer G, Williams K. Childhood psoriasis: a clinical review of 1262 cases. Pediatr Dermatol. 2001;18:188-98.
7. Torrelo A. Tacrolimus tópico en el tratamiento de la dermatitis atópica en ni˜nos. Actas Dermosifiliogr. 2008;99(Suppl 2):1428-9.

CHAPTER 141

Approach to a Child with Hypopigmented Macules

Vibhu Mendiratta, Bharati

INTRODUCTION

Hypopigmented macules in a child can be a cause of worry for the parents and physician alike. Hypopigmented macules may be present since birth or may appear later in childhood. This chapter briefly outlines the approach to such presentation **(Flowchart 1)**.

Various genetic, autoimmune, and infective diseases may manifest as hypopigmented lesions in children. Hypopigmented macules may present at birth or later in childhood. In most of the case the diagnosis is clinical, however in some atypical presentation we need to perform bedside tests such as wood lamps examination, diascopy, potassium hydroxide mount, etc., and even invasive test like skin biopsy. In children to avoid invasive test, dermoscopy can be used as an aid to support the diagnosis.

Localized hypopigmented lesions with forelocks may present at birth in patients with piebaldism or Waardenburg syndrome. Piebaldism presents as depigmented patches on the ventral or lateral trunk and/or the mid-extremities with the sparing of hand and feet. Poliosis is a common feature. It is not associated with systemic features. Waardenburg syndrome is associated with dystopia canthorum, broadening of the nasal root, presence of hypoplastic alae nasi, synophrys, poliosis, heterochromia iridis, congenital sensorineural hearing loss, musculoskeletal abnormalities such as limb contractures and hypoplasia of the limb musculature, and Hirschsprung disease.

Nevus depigmentosus presents as asymptomatic ill-defined hypopigmented macules with feathery margins. Similar cutaneous lesions along lines of blaschko with or without extracutaneous manifestations occur in hypomelanosis of Ito. Localized hypopigmented lesions without forelock may occur in vitiligo. Nevus anemicus presents as pale, ill-defined hypopigmented macules, which merges with surrounding skin on diascopy. Tuberous sclerosis may present as off white macules, which are oval at one end and taper to the other end, resembling ash leaf called as ash-leaf macules. They are often present at birth or appear within the first few years of life commonly over trunk and buttocks. Wood's lamp may be used to improve detection especially in light pigmented individuals. Three or more hypopigmented macules constitute a major feature for the diagnosis of tuberous sclerosis. A less common type of hypopigmentation is the "confetti" skin lesions involving the legs or forearms which are considered a minor feature for tuberous sclerosis.

Generalized hypopigmentation with hair and eye involvement occurs in albinism. It results either from enzymatic defects in the biosynthesis of melanin, from melanosomal defects that interfere with melanin formation, or from problems in the intracellular transport and localization of proteins essential for melanin biosynthesis. In oculocutaneous albinism (OCA) type 1A, or the classic tyrosinase negative OCA, there is a complete inability to synthesize melanin in skin, hair, and eyes, which results in the characteristic "albino phenotype". Affected individuals are born with white hair and skin. The phenotype OCA type 1B can range from minimal hair pigment to near normal skin and hair pigment. They have very little or no pigment at birth and develop varying amounts of melanin in the hair and skin in the first or second decade of life.

Localized well defined, slightly, scaly, hypopigmented macules involving the trunk, chest, back, and shoulders occur in pityriasis versicolor. However, extensive involvement has also been reported. It is caused by Malassezia species, which on potassium hydroxide microscopy show hyphae and blastospores in the typical "spaghetti and meatballs" appearance. A yellow-green fluorescence is visible using Wood's lamp examination.

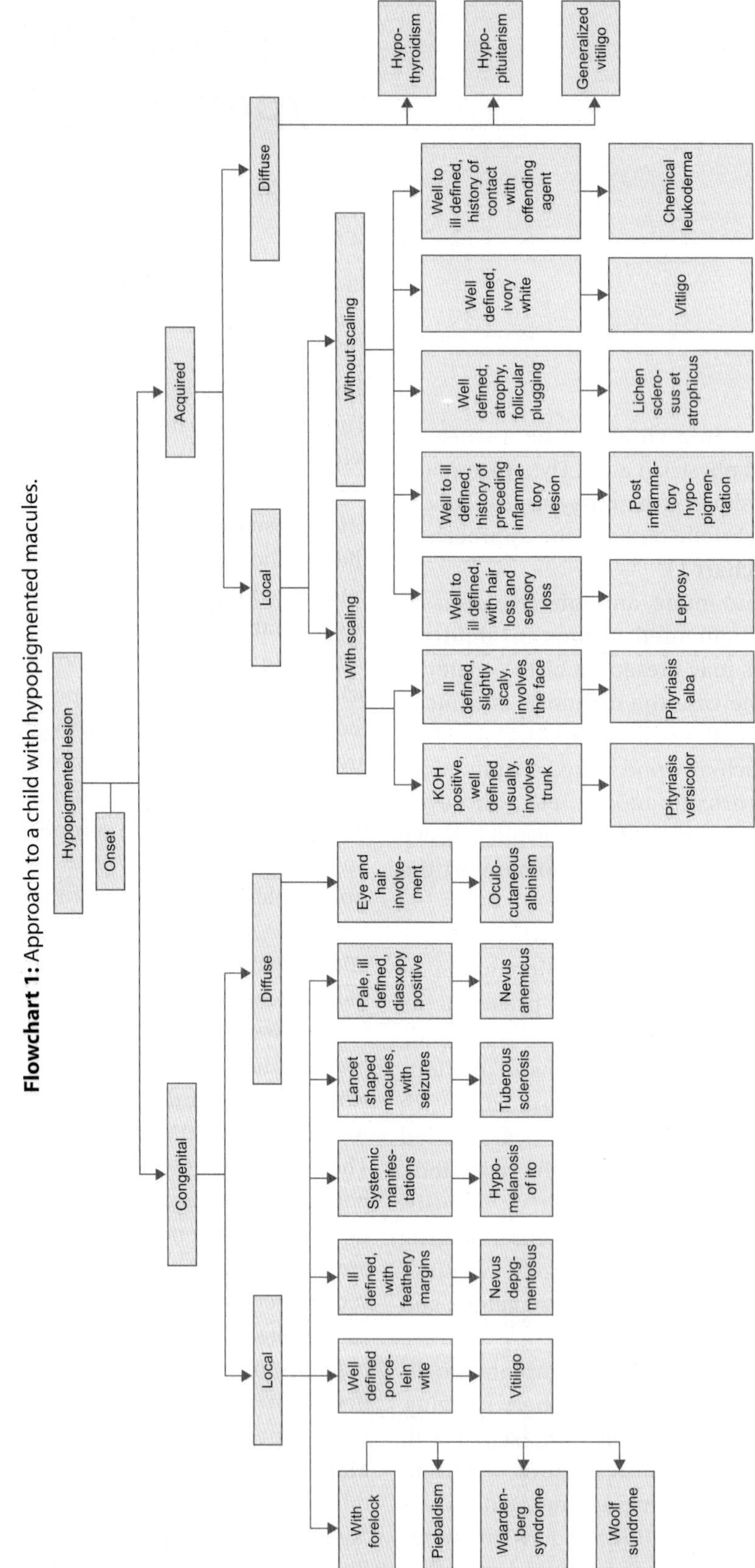

Flowchart 1: Approach to a child with hypopigmented macules.

Pityriasis alba typically presents as ill-defined localized powdery white scaly lesions involving the head and neck region, which may progress to nonscaly hypopigmented macules. It is commonly associated with atopy. Patients affected with leprosy presents with varied morphology based on the pole. Lesions in tuberculoid pole presents as single to a few xerotic hypopigmented macules with hair loss. Lesions in lepromatous pole present as multiple ill-defined, infiltrated hypopigmented macules, and hair loss may occur later on. Diagnosis of leprosy may be confirmed by slit skin smear or histopathological examination. Inflammatory lesions may lead to postinflammatory hypopigmentation which presents as well to ill-defined hypopigmented macules. Lichen sclerosus et atrophicus presents as a pruritic erythematous patch in the early stage, evolving into a well-defined porcelain hypopigmented plaques with epidermal atrophy and follicular atrophy. Vitiligo is a common disorder of depigmentation occurring in approximately 1% of the world's population. Various hypotheses have been proposed including autoimmune, neurogenic, etc. Vitiligo may be associated with other autoimmune disorders such as diabetes mellitus, thyroid diseases, etc. Histopathology shows absence of melanocytes and melanin in epidermis. Hypomelanotic macules present in a localized form or generalized form. Various morphological forms have been described such as acrofacial, segmental, etc. In children, segmental vitiligo is commonly seen. Hairs over the lesion may also turn gray. Spontaneous repigmentation may occur in some lesions. Exposure to chemicals may lead to ill- to well-defined hypopigmented macules of chemical leukoderma. Diffuse acquired hypopigmentation may occur in patients with hypothyroidism and hypopituitarism.

CLINICAL PEARLS

- Localized hypopigmented lesions with forelocks may present at birth in patients with piebaldism (without systemic features) or Waardenburg syndrome (with systemic features).
- Generalized congenital hypopigmentation with hair and eye involvement occurs in albinisim.
- Vitiligo may present in a localized form or generalized form at birth or later in life.

KEY POINTS

- Localized hypopigmentation without scaling at birth may be seen in nevus depigmentosus, nevus anemicus, vitiligo, piebaldism, or Waardenburg syndrome.
- Generalized hypopigmentation may be seen in albinism or vitiligo.
- Localized scaly acquired hypopigmentation may be seen in pityriasis versicolor, and pityriasis alba.
- Vitiligo presents as acquired depigmented, and nonscaly macules.
- Leprosy may present with hypopigmented lesions with loss of sensation.
- Dermoscopy can be used as an aid to diagnose hypopigmented macules in cases of dilemma.

SUGGESTED READING

1. Anstey AV. Disorders of skin colour. In: Burns T, Breathnach S, Griffiths C, Cox N (Eds). Rook's Textbook of Dermatology, 8th edition. India: Wiley-Blackwell; 2010. pp. 58.1-58.59.
2. Lapeere H, Boone B, Schepper SD, Verhaeghe E, Ongenae K, Geel NV, et al. Hypomelanoses and hypermelanoses. In: Wolff K, Goldsmith LA, Katz SI, Gilchrest BA, Pallar AS, Leffell DJ (Eds). Fitzpatrick's Dermatology in General Medicine, 7th edition. New Delhi: McGraw Hill; 2008. p. 622.

CHAPTER 142

Pediatric Acne

Vibhu Mendiratta, Amit Kumar Meena

INTRODUCTION

Acne vulgaris is a common inflammatory condition of the pilosebaceous unit with a peak incidence during adolescence. However, it may be found in all age groups including neonates and infants **(Flowchart 1)**.

NEONATAL ACNE

The onset of neonatal acne is usually before the first 6 weeks of life. It affects about 20% of the newborns. The papules typically occur across nasal bridge and cheeks. There are no comedones. This benign condition is hormonally mediated. Neonatal acne may be hard to distinguish from heterogeneous papulopustular acneiform conditions typically without comedones, such as neonatal cephalic pustulosis or transient neonatal pustular melanosis. Neonatal cephalic pustulosis pustules are usually confined to the cheeks, chin, eyelids, and forehead, but the scalp, neck, upper chest, and back may be involved. It has been attributed to overgrowth of Malassezia species. Newborns may present with or develop transient neonatal pustular melanosis, with pustules on the chin, neck, or trunk. Within 24 hours, these pustules rupture, leaving hyperpigmented macules with a rim of faint white scale. Most cases of neonatal acne resolve by 3 months of age but severe cases can be treated topically with 2% ketoconazole cream, benzoyl peroxide, or erythromycin.

INFANTILE ACNE

Infantile acne may begin approximately at 6 weeks of age and last for 6–12 months. It is more common in boys and presents with comedones as well as inflammatory lesions, which can include papules, pustules, or occasionally nodular lesions. Physical examination should include assessment of growth including height, weight, and growth curve; testicular growth and breast development; presence of hirsutism or pubic hair; clitoromegaly; and increased muscle mass. The etiology is postulated to be transient rise in dehydroepiandrosterone sulfate and luteinizing hormone levels. Most infantile acne is self-limited and not associated with underlying endocrine pathology. There is some evidence that infantile acne predisposes to more severe adolescent acne. Infantile acne may be treated with topical antimicrobial agents; topical retinoids; noncycline antibiotics, such as erythromycin; and, occasionally, isotretinoin.

CLINICAL PEARL

- Acne not responding to treatment or with unusual presentation should be further evaluated to look for underlying endocrine pathology.

MID-CHILDHOOD ACNE

Mid-childhood acne presents primarily on the face with a mixture of comedones and inflammatory lesions. Children between the ages of 1 and 7 years, however, do not normally produce significant levels of adrenal or gonadal androgens; hence, acne in this age group is rare. When it does occur, an endocrine abnormality should be suspected. In addition to treatments to address androgen-secreting tumors or congenital adrenal hyperplasia, the treatment of mid-childhood acne is similar to that of adolescent acne except that oral tetracyclines are usually not an option in children younger than 8 years of age because of the risk of damage to developing bones and tooth enamel. Hormonal therapy could be used if warranted by endocrinologic pathology.

CLINICAL PEARL

- Tetracyclines are contraindicated in children <8 years and oral isotretinoin is not recommended in children <12 years according to the Food and Drug Administration.

Flowchart 1: Approach to pediatric acne depending on age of onset.

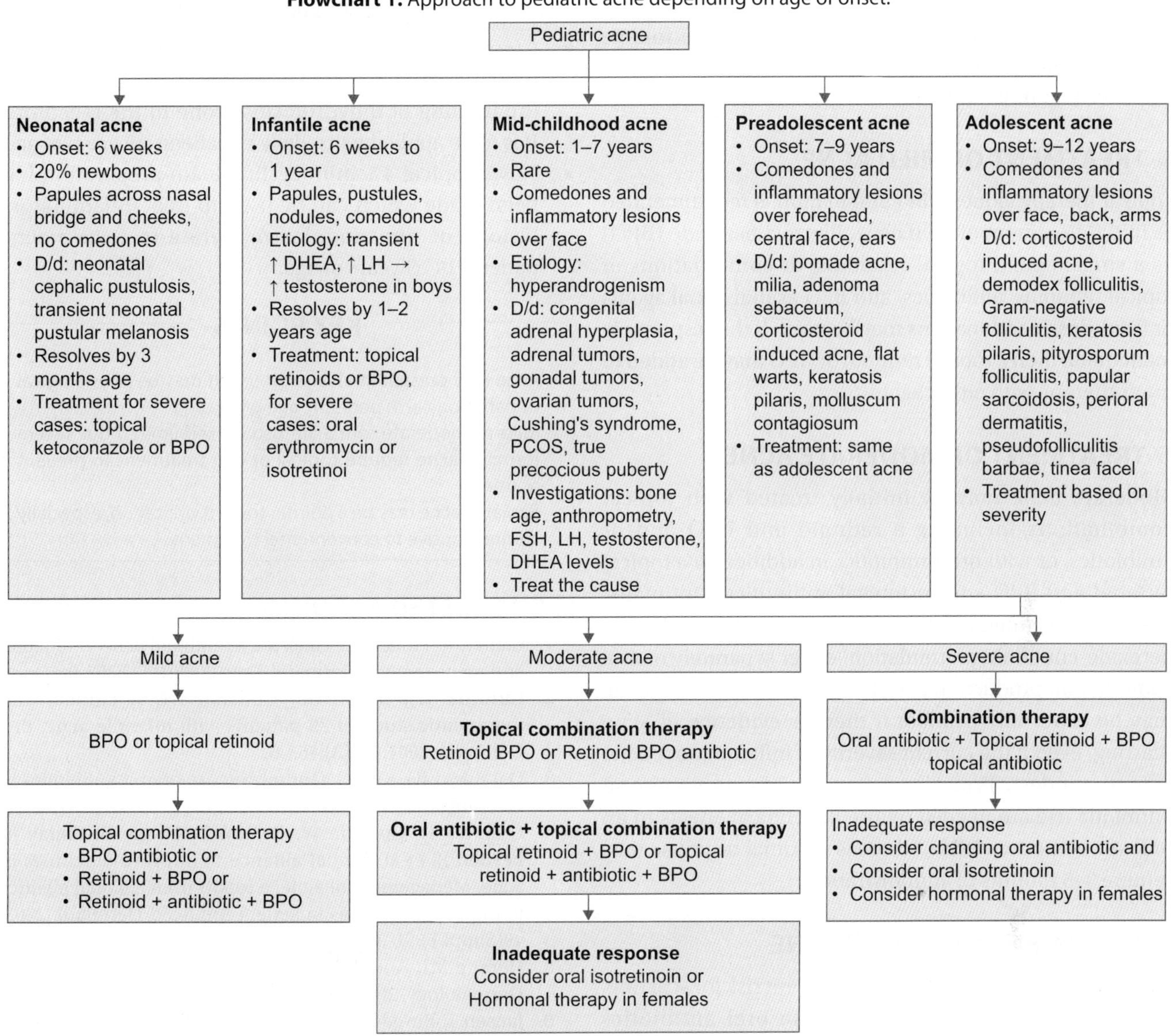

(BPO: benzoyl peroxide; DHEA: Dehydroepiandrosterone; FSH: follicle-stimulating hormone; LH: Luteinizing hormone)

PREADOLESCENT ACNE

Preadolescent (7-12 years) acne is common and may precede other signs of pubertal maturation. It is characterized by a predominance of comedones on the forehead and central face (the so-called "T-zone") with relatively few inflammatory lesions. Further workup is generally unnecessary unless there are signs of excess androgens. Treatment of uncomplicated preadolescent acne is comparable to that of acne in older age groups, as discussed later.

ADOLESCENT ACNE

Adolescent acne (12-19 years) is common and characterized by comedones and inflammatory lesions over face, back, and arms. Acne can be categorized as predominately comedonal, inflammatory, and/or mixed. Presence or absence of scarring, postinflammatory hyperpigmentation, or erythema should be assessed. Severity may be broadly categorized as mild, moderate, or severe. The pathogenesis of acne involves the interplay of four factors: sebaceous hyperplasia under the influence of increased androgen levels, alterations in follicular growth and differentiation, colonization of the follicle by Propionibacterium acnes, and consequent immune response and inflammation.

TREATMENT OF MILD ACNE

Topical therapy alone or in combination is recommended as initial treatment of mild acne. Benzoyl peroxide (BPO) as a single agent, topical retinoids, or combinations of topical retinoids, antibiotics, and BPO as individual agents or fixed-dose combinations may be used. If the response is inadequate then a topical retinoid or BPO may be added to monotherapy with either agent.

TREATMENT OF MODERATE ACNE

Moderate acne may be initially treated with topical combinations including a retinoid and BPO and/or antibiotics, or with oral antibiotics in addition to a topical retinoid and BPO and/or topical antibiotics. Optimally, the topical regimen would include a retinoid and a benzyl peroxide-containing formulation, either separately or as a combination product. In addition, use of an oral antibiotic may be especially prudent if there is evidence of acne scarring, even if the current severity of inflammatory acne is more modest. Typically, 4–8 weeks of compliant oral antibiotic use are needed before the clinical effects of an oral antibiotic are visible, whereas maximal response may require 3–6 months of administration.

TREATMENT OF SEVERE ACNE

Patients with severe acne are at significant risk for scarring. Severe acne should be treated with oral antibiotics and topical retinoids with BPO, with or without topical antibiotics, with consideration of hormonal therapy in pubertal females or oral isotretinoin. Patients unresponsive to these topical and oral therapies will benefit with oral isotretinoin.

CLINICAL PEARL

- Childhood acne may persist and raises the risk of development of severe scarring acne in adulthood.

NEWERS TREATMENTS IN ACNE

- *Clascoterone cream:* Clascoterone cream 1%, is a topical androgen receptor blocker. It acts by inhibiting the binding of dihydrotestosterone to the receptors. It is to be applied twice daily in patients ≥9 years of age.
- Novel topical 4% minocycline foam preparation has been made which can be used to treat inflammatory lesions of non-nodular moderate-to-severe acne patients of ≥9 years of age.

KEY POINTS

- Acne may present in all age groups. It may be physiological or pathological in pediatric age groups.
- Mild-to-moderate forms are usually self-limited but severe forms of acne require topical or oral treatment to prevent scarring.
- Pediatric acne may be a pointer toward virilization, especially if unresponsive to conventional treatment.

SUGGESTED READING

1. Cantatore-Francis JL, Glick SA. Childhood acne: evaluation and management. Dermatol Ther. 2006;19(4):202-9.
2. Cunliffe WJ, Baron SE, Coulson IH. A clinical and therapeutic study of 29 patients with infantile acne. Br J Dermatol. 2001;145(3):463-6.
3. Del Rosso JQ, Kim G. Optimizing use of oral antibiotics in acne vulgaris. Dermatol Clin. 2009;27(1):33-42.
4. Gollnick H, Cunliffe W, Berson D, Dreno B, Finlay A, Leyden JJ, et al. Global alliance to improve outcomes in acne. Management of acne: a report from a global alliance to improve outcomes in acne. J Am Acad Dermatol. 2003; 49(Suppl 1):S1-37.
5. Herane MI, Ando I. Acne in infancy and acne genetics. Dermatology. 2003;206(1):24-8.
6. Jansen T, Burgdorf WH, Plewig G. Pathogenesis and treatment of acne in childhood. Pediatr Dermatol. 1997;14(1): 17-21.
7. Krakowski AC, Eichenfield LF. Pediatric acne: clinical presentations, evaluation, and management. J Drugs Dermatol. 2007;6(6):589-93.
8. Niamba P, Weill FX, Sarlangue J, Labrèze C, Couprie B, Taïeh A. Is common neonatal cephalic pustulosis (neonatal acne) triggered by Malassezia sympodialis? Arch Dermatol. 1998;134(8):995-8.
9. Poli F. Acne on pigmented skin. Int J Dermatol. 2007; 46(Suppl 1):39-41.

Approach to Congenital Melanocytic Nevus

Vibhu Mendiratta, Vidya Yadav, Pravesh Yadav

INTRODUCTION

Congenital melanocytic nevus (CMN) are clusters of melanocytes found in the skin, with varying extensions to adipose tissue, muscles, and the adnexa. They are usually present at birth, however some occur after several months and can be found anywhere on the skin. The reported incidence of CMN of any size ranges from 1 to 31.7%. CMN represent a developmental abnormality of normal melanocytic development. This is probably due to mutation that occurs in a progenitor cell that results in the abnormal extensive accumulation of melanocytic cells along migration pathways during normal development. The events leading to the nevomelanocyte accumulation may also have effects on the surrounding tissue probably due to a change in the local cytokine environment of the nevomelanocytic cells. According to American National Institutes of Health consensus definition, CMN have been categorized according to size into small, under 1.5 cm in diameter, large as having a diameter between 1.5 and 20 cm and giant nevi as having a diameter of 20 cm or more **(Flowchart 1)**.

Congenital melanocytic nevi are usually obvious and deeply pigmented at birth. Majority of these nevi are macular at birth with smooth, regular, and sharply demarcated contour and distortion of the skin markings. As the child grows, the nevus usually grows in proportion. At some sites, such as the scalp, there is commonly a considerable increase in terminal hair. In other sites, an increase in terminal hair tends to occur more subtly over time and may be accompanied by the development of rugosity. As the infant grows, the surface of the nevus may become rugose or warty and nodules can develop within a large nevus. Congenital melanocytic nevi may develop a halo of depigmentation,

Flowchart 1: Approach to congenital melanocytic nevus.

Identify (diagnosis usually clinical)
- Usually deeply pigmented macular or popular lesions, may be large and extensive
- Grows proportionally to body size
- Pigmented terminal hair may grow and surface may develop rugosities

↓

Exclude differentials
CALM, nevus spilus, Becker's nevus, lentigo simplex, nevus sebaceous, smooth muscle hamartoma, epidermal nevi, dermal melanocytosis, solitary mastocytoma

↓

Measure the size (affects the risk of development of malignancy)
- Small under 1.5 cm diameter
- Large between 1.5 and 20 cm
- Giant nevi a diameter of 20 cm or more

↓

Look for the site
- Over the vertebral column or cranial large nevi-increased risk of leptomeningeal involvement; MRI indicated

↓

Dermatoscopy
- Reticular or globular pattern

↓

Parent counseling
- To keep the nevus under review
- To seek advice if it changes in shape, size, or color
- Photographs

↓

Genetic counseling
- Very low risk in subsequent pregnancies

↓

Aim of treatment
- Cosmetic and to reduce the risk of malignancy

↓

Treatment options
- Surgical, cryotherapy, laser, etc.

(CALM, café au lait macules; MRI: magnetic resonance imaging)

heralding a potential spontaneous resolution. Loss of pigmentation has been associated with regression of underlying melanocytes. Dermatoscopy can sometime prove to be helpful in the diagnosis showing a characteristic reticular or globular pattern. A significant proportion of nevi may become paler in the first 1–2 years of life, and at sites such as the scalp may fade to cosmetic insignificance.

There may be associated abnormalities such as meningeal involvement, spina bifida, or meningocele when the nevus is located over the vertebral column, or club-foot and hypertrophy or atrophy of the deeper structures of a limb. Absence of subcutaneous fat is the most common associated anomaly and may be symptomatic in sites such as over the sacrum. Melanoma and neural melanosis are both more likely in patients with CMN that have a projected adult size of >40 cm in diameter, multiple medium size CMN, numerous "satellite" nevi, and posterior axial location. Neurocutaneous melanosis may rarely produce raised intracranial pressure, hydrocephalus, or space-occupying spinal lesions. A variety of proliferative neoplasms may develop in CMN. Superficial spreading melanoma is the most significant complication of CMN but the level of risk is reasonably low. In giant nevi, there is a definite risk, with the age of onset of the melanoma being earlier than in the general population. A magnetic resonance imaging scan should be considered in babies with nevi over the cranium or spine to exclude significant leptomeningeal melanocytosis. Regular neurological examination, however, is clearly important. The location and characteristics of the nevus, the patient's age, parental concerns, and medical comorbidities all impact the frequency and timing of dermatology consultations. Palpate CMN with atypical characteristics and lymph nodes in high-risk individuals at each visit to rule out melanoma. When necessary, the clinical context, imaging, and biopsy are used to distinguish between benign and malignant lymph node enlargement. Because of the increased melanoma risk and need for family counselling, larger, multiple, and changing nevi should be closely monitored during infancy or times of expected nevus change, such as adolescence; visits every 3 months may be recommended.

Histopathology shows presence of nevomelanocytes in the epidermis as well ordered theques and/or nevomelanocytes in the dermis in the form of sheets, nests, cords, and/or single cells. Presence of nevomelanocytes in the lower two-thirds of the reticular dermis and association with appendageal and neurovascular structures is more commonly seen with CMN than acquired nevi. Nevomelanocytes may be prominent within and around the blood vessels showing an inflammatory appearance. Hair follicles are often quite large and associated with abundant melanin in the hair bulb.

Differentials of CMN include CALM (café au lait macules), nevus spilus, Becker's nevus, lentigo simplex, nevus sebaceous, smooth muscle hamartoma, epidermal nevi, dermal melanocytosis, and solitary mastocytoma.

Congenital melanocytic nevi are essentially considered to be developmental abnormalities of the skin, with a very low risk of recurrence in subsequent pregnancies, which is particularly important when reassuring parents who have a child with a giant melanocytic nevus. The aims of treatment are to improve the cosmetic effect of nevi and to reduce the risk of malignant transformation. General skin care includes bathing with water or a nonsoap cleaner at least twice a week, followed by the application of a mild emollient. The most common treatment is surgical, using a variety of plastic surgical techniques such as multistep surgery, the use of tissue expanders and grafting. Tissue expansion is usually used for the head and neck, but in other sites excision and grafting are more usual, with consequently poorer cosmetic results. Other ablative techniques have been tried such as cryotherapy and, more recently, the Q-switched ruby laser.

Parents of children with CMN left *in situ* should be advised to keep the nevus under review and to seek advice if it changes in shape, size, or color. Photographs of the child's nevus and images of melanomas may be useful tools. Even small nevi that are difficult to keep under review, such as those in the scalp or in the middle of the back may be prophylactically excised, particularly if they have any atypical features such as intense or irregular pigmentation which persists beyond infancy.

CLINICAL **PEARLS**

- *Nevus located over the vertebral column:* Rule out abnormalities such as meningeal involvement, spina bifida, or meningocele.
- *Giant nevi (diameter of 20 cm or more), multiple medium size nevi, satellite lesions:* Higher risk.

KEY POINTS

- Congenital melanocytic nevus (CMN) is a developmental abnormality of normal melanocytic development leading to an abnormal accumulation of melanocytic cells along migration pathways during normal development.
- Congenital melanocytic nevus are usually obvious and deeply pigmented macules at birth and grow in proportion to the body with age.
- Increase in terminal hair and rugosity are normal progression changes with age.
- Congenital melanocytic nevus may be associated with abnormalities such as meningeal involvement, spina bifida, or meningocele when the nevus is located over the vertebral column.
- A variety of proliferative neoplasms may develop in CMN, superficial spreading melanoma being the most significant.
- Treatment indications are mainly cosmetic.

SUGGESTED READING

1. Anon. Consensus conference: precursors to malignant melanoma. JAMA. 1984;251:1864-6.
2. Bishop JAN. Lentigos, melanocytic naevi and melanoma. In: Burns T, Breathnach S, Griffiths C, Cox N (Eds). Rook's Textbook of Dermatology, 8th edition. India: Wiley-Blackwell; 2010. pp. 54.1-54.57.
3. Goodman RM, Caren J, Ziprkowski M, Padeh B, Ziprkowski L, Cohen BE, et al. Genetic considerations in giant pigmented hairy naevus. Br J Dermatol. 1971;85:150-7.
4. Grichnile JM, Rhodes AR, Sober AJ. Benign neoplasias and hyperplasias of melanocytes. In: Wolff K, Goldsmith LA, Katz SI, Gilchrest BA, Pallar AS, Leffell DJ (Eds). Fitzpatrick's Dermatology in General Medicine, 7th edition. New Delhi: McGraw Hill; 2008. p. 1099.
5. Jahnke MN, O'Haver J, Gupta D, Hawryluk EB, Finelt N, Kruse L, et al. Care of congenital melanocytic nevi in newborns and infants: review and management recommendations. Pediatrics. 2021;148(6):2021051536.
6. Puig S, Guilabert A, Julià M, Romero D, Vicente A, González-Enseñat MA, et al. Prevalence study of nevi in children from Barcelona: dermoscopy, constitutional and environmental factors. Dermatology. 2009;218(3):203-14.
7. Strauss RM, Bishop JAN. Spontaneous involution of congenital melanocytic nevi of the scalp. J Am Acad Dermatol. 2008;58:508-11.

Seborrheic Dermatitis

Vibhu Mendiratta, Nikita Gandhi Sethi, Sarita Sanke, Apaopa Thekho

INTRODUCTION

Seborrheic dermatitis (SD) is a chronic papulosquamous inflammatory skin disorder affecting the sebaceous gland rich areas (scalp, face, and trunk). It is a benign self-limiting condition characterized by remissions and exacerbations. It occurs due to seborrhea, a pathologic overproduction of sebum, with subsequent infection and inflammation. It typically presents with yellowish-white greasy scales, red skin with or without itching. The severity ranges from mild dandruff to exfoliative erythroderma. It can occur in any age group; however, two age peaks are noted; in infants—during first 3 months of life and in adolescents or adults— during 4th to 7th decade of life. These age peaks correlate with the high activity of sebaceous glands.

EPIDEMIOLOGY

Seborrheic dermatitis affects individuals of any ethnicity, with no sex predilection. Estimates of SD prevalence and incidence are hindered by many cases being mild and poor case definition, so probably underestimate the true figure. Estimates are also limited due to absence of validated criteria for diagnosis. As per literature, SD affects approximately 11.6% of the general population. Up to 70% of newborns are affected by SD in their first 3 months of life. Dandruff, the mildest form of SD affects 15–20% of the population.

ETIOLOGY

The exact etiology remains uncertain. It involves a complex interaction between:

- Host factors
- Malassezia species
- Environmental factors
  - *Host factors:* Overactivity of sebaceous glands leads to excess production of sebum. SD is especially prevalent in immunocompromised individuals such as patients with malignancy, organ transplants, human immunodeficiency virus (HIV) infection, and chronic neurodegenerative disorders. Systemic drugs such as immunosuppressants, psoralen, PUVA (photochemotherapy), and lithium are also known to aggravate SD.

    In children, excessive vitamin A intake can cause seborrheic dermatitis. Lack of biotin, pyridoxine (vitamin B6), and riboflavin (vitamin B2) may also be a cause.
- *Malassezia species:* The most implicated species are *Malassezia globosa*, others being *Malassezia furfur* and *Malassezia restricta*. Infantile SD is more commonly associated with *Malassezia furfur*. Patients with seborrheic dermatitis appear to have a reduced resistance to the yeast. *Malassezia* hydrolyze human sebum releasing a mixture of saturated and unsaturated fatty acids (FAs). They take up the required saturated FAs, leaving behind unsaturated FAs. The unsaturated FAs penetrate the stratum corneum and because of their nonuniform structure breach the skin's barrier function. This barrier breach induces an irritation response, leading to seborrhea and dermatitis.
- *Environmental factors:* Worsening of SD occurs in winters with low ambient humidity and low ambient temperature. Remission can be seen in summers.

CLINICAL PRESENTATION AND APPROACH (FLOWCHART 1)

Infants

Cradle cap is the most common presentation in infants. It usually appears in the first few weeks of life and tends to last for 4–6 months. There are greasy, yellow scales and crusts that may eventually coalesce to a thick, scaly plaque with underlying mild-to-moderate erythema. The dermatitis is usually mild and self-limiting. Overall, scalp is the most commonly affected site, followed by face.

Flowchart 1: Seborrheic dermatitis and its differentials: Diagnostic approach.

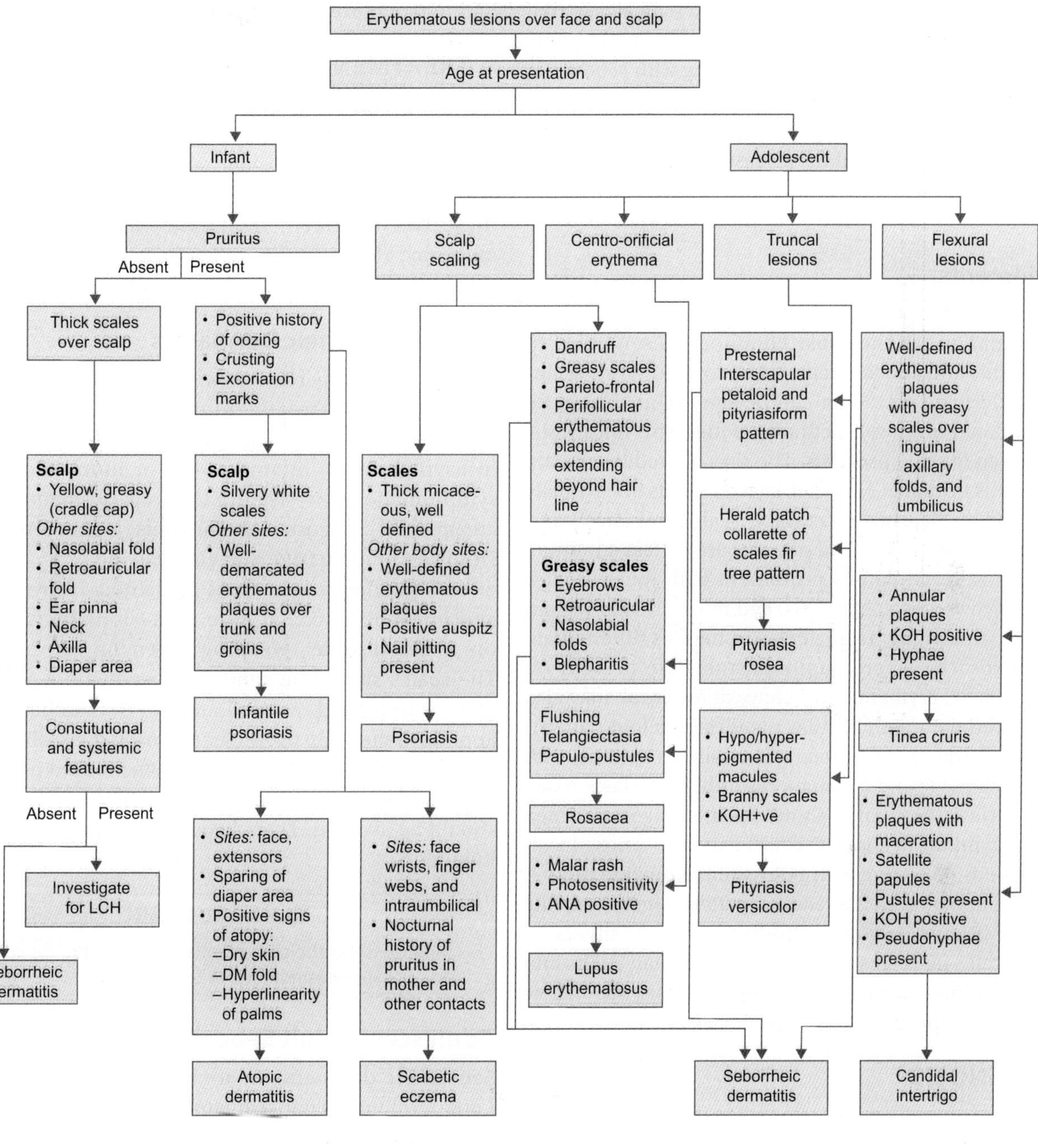

Areas of face commonly affected are forehead, eyebrows, nasolabial folds, and retroauricular areas. Seborrheic dermatitis can also involve the thorax, upper back, external genitalia, and skin creases. Involvement of perianal area in the form of diaper rash is also common. Leiner's disease (LD) is a rare generalized variant of seborrheic dermatitis in immunocompromised infants characterized by treatment resistant SD along with failure to thrive (FTT) and diarrhea.

CLINICAL PEARL

Seborrheic areas

- Scalp, retroauricular areas, medial eyebrows, nasolabial fold, anterior chest, interscapular area, axillae, groins, and diaper area.

On the other hand, patient with atopic dermatitis have scalp and facial involvement in the form of extremely pruritic oozy plaques. It first appears after 3 months of age with positive personal/family history of atopy. Extensors may also be involved. Diaper area is characteristically spared unlike infantile SD and psoriasis. If the infant exhibits systemic and constitutional features along with seborrheic dermatitis like lesions, he should be worked up for Langerhan's cell histiocytosis. Scabies with eczematization is also a close mimicker of the disease which presents with nocturnal exacerbation itching and lesions in contacts help differentiate from other conditions.

Adolescents

Seborrhea of scalp in the form of dandruff (mild desquamation) is the most common presentation in adolescents and adults. Greasy white to yellow, fine scales with underlying erythema can be seen. This should be differentiated from well-defined plaques with micaceous scales seen in scalp psoriasis. The sites of predilection are the same as in infants. However, in adolescents SD is usually worse in hair bearing areas (face, scalp, and chest) and involvement of flexures and perianal area is less common. Centrofacial erythema is prominent with greasy scales over eyebrows, nasolabial folds, and retroauricular region. Absence of flushing, telangiectasias help us differentiate it from rosacea where papulopustules are present on baseline facial erythema over convexities. Trunk may also be involved with perifollicular papules (petaloid pattern) and papulosquamous lesions (pityriasiform pattern) with greasy scales. Truncal lesions resemble pityriasis rosea and pityriasis versicolor. Candidal intertrigo and tinea cruris can mimic flexural SD which can be diagnosed with simple bedside testing with potassium hydroxide mount. Pityriasis amiantacea is a reaction pattern often occurring in older infants or young children as thick, silvery or yellow scales (asbestos-like) encircling the hair shafts into tufts which may occur due to scalp psoriasis, seborrheic dermatitis, atopic dermatitis, and tinea capitis.

DIAGNOSIS

Diagnosis is based on clinical presentation. Dermoscopy, a noninvasive tool can help in differentiating between SD and other dermatological disorders such as psoriasis or tinea capitis. SD shows dotty vessels in patchy distribution and yellowish-white fine scales, follicular plugs, orange yellow areas, whitish structureless areas, and linear branching vessels.

PROGNOSIS AND COMPLICATIONS

The SD runs a benign course. However, several complications may occur. They include secondary bacterial infections, overgrowth of *Candida*, and erythroderma in immunocompromised neonates.

TREATMENT

The symptoms of SD can be effectively controlled with a combination of self-care measures and drug therapy.

Topical antifungal agents and topical corticosteroids are the principal forms of management for SD. Of these two treatment modalities, antifungals are the mainstay. However, during acute exacerbations, topical corticosteroids are often used as first-line therapy.

Infant Seborrheic Dermatitis

Cradle cap usually resolves without treatment. However, it may require treatment in some cases. Regular emollients and mild nonmedicated baby shampoos in asymptomatic infantile SD. For more widespread, symptomatic or persistent SD, topical ketoconazole 2% cream, mild corticosteroid ointments (hydrocortisone 1%, Desowen lotion 0.05%, and clobetasone butyrate 0.05%) or combination preparations containing hydrocortisone and miconazole can also be used—initially twice daily on affected areas, weaning down on improvement. The scales should be gently removed with a soft brush after shampooing. A small amount of emollient can be applied to the scalp overnight to loosen the scaly plaques. Topical calcineurin inhibitors are effective but not USFDA approved for treatment of SD in <2 years of age, hence should be avoided. There is no role of oral antifungals in infantile SD.

CLINICAL PEARL

- Infantile seborrheic dermatitis is a physiological condition and usually does not require treatment.

Adolescent/Adult Seborrheic Dermatitis

Seborrheic dermatitis in adults is a chronic condition. Long-term maintenance treatment is often necessary.

Scalp Seborrheic Dermatitis

Dandruff (mild SD of the scalp) can be treated with antidandruff shampoos. Several types of antidandruff shampoos are available, with the main difference between them being the active ingredient. All of these treatments are equally effective when used daily or twice in a week. The main active ingredients are:

- Selenium sulfide
- Coal Tar

- Zinc pyrithione
- Ketoconazole

Shampoos containing corticosteroids, propylene glycol, and keratolytics such as coal tar and salicylic acid can also be used for additional benefits. For best results, the shampoo should be left in place for 5–10 minutes before rinsing. The shampoo should be rinsed out of the hair completely.

Nonscalp Seborrheic Dermatitis

Seborrheic dermatitis of the face, trunk, and skin folds generally is treated with topical corticosteroids or antifungal agents.

Low potency topical corticosteroids (e.g., hydrocortisone 1% cream) may be tried initially. The cream is applied once or twice a day until symptoms improve with gradual tapering. Topical antifungal agents (ketoconazole 2%, miconazole, ciclopirox 1%, and sertaconazole 2%) either alone or in combination with topical steroids can also be used. Long-term application of steroids should be avoided in view of side effects such as atrophy, striae, and telangiectasias.

Topical calcineurin inhibitors tacrolimus and pimecrolimus are effective in treating SD. Proactive treatment of adult facial SD to maintain remission with 0.1% tacrolimus ointment once or twice per week is also effective.

For refractory or widespread SD where topical therapy is impractical, oral antifungals such as terbinafine, fluconazole, and itraconazole should be used.

CLINICAL PEARLS

Cradle cap: What to tell parents

- Regular scalp wash with mild baby shampoo.
- Remove scales with a soft-bristled brush.
- Emollients can be used to loosen the scales.

KEY POINTS

- Seborrheic dermatitis (SD) is physiological in infants below 3 months of age.
- Cradle cap is the most common presentation.
- It is a nonitchy condition characterized by greasy yellow scales in seborrheic areas.
- Self-limiting course.
- Psoriasis, intertrigo, pityriasis rosea, and rosacea are close mimickers for adolescent SD.
- Antifungals and topical steroids form the main stay of treatment.

SUGGESTED READING

1. Bikowski J. Facial seborrheic dermatitis: a report on current status and therapeutic horizons. J Drugs Dermatol. 2009;8(2):125-33.
2. Dall'Oglio F, Nasca MR, Gerbino C, Micali G. An Overview of the Diagnosis and Management of Seborrheic Dermatitis. Clin Cosmet Investig Dermatol. 2022;15:1537-48.
3. Gaitanis G, Velegraki A, Alexopoulos EC, Chasapi V, Tsigonia A, Katsambas A. Distribution of malassezia species in pityriasis versicolor and seborrhoeic dermatitis in Greece. Typing of the major pityriasis versicolor isolate M. globosa. Br J Dermatol. 2006;154(4):854-9.
4. Gupta AK, Bluhm R. Seborrheic dermatitis. J Eur Acad Dermatol Venereol. 2004;18(1):13-26.
5. Hay RJ, Graham-Brown RAC. Dandruff and seborrhoeic dermatitis: causes and management. Clinical and Experimental Dermatology. 1997;22(1):3-6.
6. Sheffield RC, Crawford P, Wright ST, King VJ. Clinical inquiries. What's the best treatment for cradle cap? J Fam Pract. 2007;56(3):232-3.
7. Smoker AL. On top of cradle cap. J Fam Health Care. 2007;17(4):134-6.
8. Tucker D, Masood S. Seborrheic Dermatitis. In: StatPearls [Internet]. Treasure Island (FL): StatPearls Publishing; 2023.

Ophthalmology

Section Editor: *Shashi Vashisht*

Approach to Red Eye in Children

Mahrukh Bhat, Priyanka Arora

INTRODUCTION

Red eye is one of the most common reasons for acute eye-related visits to the pediatricians, while some causes are uncomplicated and resolve within a few days, many cases require prompt treatment to prevent the disease from worsening or spreading. The condition can be managed by pediatricians, but knowing when to refer the patient to an ophthalmologist is crucial. It can arise from a wide spectrum of pathologies and can involve various ocular structures.

CAUSES OF RED EYE IN CHILDREN

It is quite challenging to assess children with red eyes, owing to an unclear history and difficult examination. Conjunctivitis is the most common cause of red eye. It may be infectious (bacterial or viral) or noninfectious (allergic and chemical). Most cases of infectious conjunctivitis are self-limiting. Other common causes include blepharitis, corneal abrasion, foreign body, subconjunctival hemorrhage, keratitis, iritis, chemical burns, trauma, endophthalmitis, and severe dry eye. Some uncommon causes of red eye in children are iridocyclitis, episcleritis, contact lens related, chemical irritants such as chlorine in swimming pools, head lice if they spread to ocular area, and congenital glaucoma **(Table 1)**.

TABLE 1: Causes of red eye in children.

Most common	*Relatively common*	*Uncommon*
• *Conjunctivitis:* – *Infectious:* - Bacterial - Viral - Chlamydial – *Noninfectious:* - Allergic conjunctivitis - Chemical irritants • Foreign body • Blepharitis	• Mechanical trauma such as a foreign body or abrasion • Chemical trauma such as an acid or alkali burn • Subconjunctival hemorrhage due to vigorous coughing • Stye/hordeolum • Keratitis/corneal ulcer • Ocular fatigue	• Iridocyclitis or uveitis • Episcleritis • Scleritis • Contact lens related • Severe dry eye • Endophthalmitis • Glaucoma

HISTORY AND EXAMINATION

A thorough patient history and eye examination may provide clues toward etiology of red eye **(Table 2)**. Salient points in this history include whether the condition is unilateral or bilateral, duration and type of symptoms, presence of discharge and its nature, visual changes, pain, photophobia, itching, and any previous treatments.

Red flags for a pediatric red eye:

- Staining of the cornea
- Corneal haze/opacity
- Abnormal red reflex
- Photophobia or significant pain
- Lid swelling/blepharospasm
- Associated new-onset squint
- Reduced visual acuity
- Failure to improve by 2 weeks
- Contact lens use (older children)
- Abnormal pupillary reaction
- Difficulty in examination
- History of high-velocity injury

Tips for an Effective Patient History and Examination

When a child presents with red eye, one must be able to identify potentially serious ocular conditions that require immediate referral. Following questions can aid in differential diagnosis:

- When did the symptoms start?
- Are they in one eye or both?

TABLE 2: Clinical pointers in history and examination to identify the causes of red eye.

Signs	*Symptoms*	*Likely diagnosis*
Purulent discharge	Matting of eyelashes on waking up in morning (best predictor)	Bacterial conjunctivitis
Preauricular lymphadenopathy	• Watery or serous discharge • Recent history of upper respiratory tract infection	Viral conjunctivitis
• Larger cobble-stone papillae under upper eyelid • Eyelid swelling	• Bilateral eye involvement • Intense itching • Ropy discharge	Allergic conjunctivitis
• Lid vesicles • Decreased vision	• Painful red eye • Photophobia	Herpes simplex virus keratitis
• Dandruff-like flakes on eyelashes • Missing eyelashes • Swollen lids	• Red, irritated eye • Worse in morning • Itchy crusted eyelids	Blepharitis
• Corneal edema or haze • Blepharospasm • Profuse watering	• Unilateral foreign body sensation • Inability to open eyes • Profuse watering • Recent history of trauma (fingernail and paper)	Corneal abrasions
Halo vision (colored halos seen around light)	• Painful eye • Decreased vision	• Acute glaucoma • Uveitis

- Is there any discharge in the eye? If yes, what kind and how much?
- Is there any swelling or pain in eyes?
- Is there a history of similar complaints in any of the family member?
- *Any recent history of:*
  - Exposure to chemicals
  - Contact with another person with red eye
  - Injury to the eye
  - Upper respiratory tract infection (URI)
  - COVID-19 infection
- Is there a personal or family history of atopy, asthma, or eczema?
- Does the child wear any contact lens?
- Is there any history of ocular surgery?

During the examination, do not forget:
- To evert eyelids
- To examine periorbital skin for any lesions
- To palpate preauricular lymphnodes

In order of urgency, the conditions are:
- Chemical injury
- Angle-closure glaucoma
- Ocular foreign body
- Corneal abrasion
- Uveitis
- Conjunctivitis
- Ocular surface disease such as Stevens–Johnson syndrome
- Subconjunctival hemorrhage

CONJUNCTIVITIS

It is a nonspecific term that means inflammation of the conjunctiva, causing hyperemia, general discomfort, and other symptoms. Difference between bacterial and viral conjunctivitis has been provided in **Table 3**.
- Examination reveals diffuse conjunctival congestion, matted eyelashes, and normal visual acuity.
- Treatment includes topical antibiotics 2 hourly for 2 days and four times a day for a week.
- *Refer if:*
  - Decreased vision, photophobia, or pain at any stage
  - Does not improve in 2 weeks

CLINICAL PEARL

- Otitis media associated with conjunctivitis is most frequently caused by nontypeable *Haemophilus influenzae* and occasionally by *Streptococcus pneumoniae* and by other bacteria.

Allergic Conjunctivitis

- It is often associated with atopic diseases, such as allergic rhinitis, eczema, and asthma.
- Itching of the eyes is the most predominant symptom.
- Watery or mucoid discharge which is usually not copious
- Examination of eyes reveals diffuse redness in the eyes with severe papillary reaction, especially under the upper eyelids.

TABLE 3: Comparison of bacterial and viral conjunctivitis.

Parameters	***Bacterial***	***Viral***
Common organisms	• *Staphylococcus species (most common)* • *Haemophilus influenzae* • *Streptococcus pneumoniae* • *Moraxella Catarrhalis* • *Neisseria gonorrhoeae* • *Chlamydia trachomatis*	• Adenovirus type 8 and 19 • Herpes simplex virus
Incubation period	24–72 hours	1–14 days
Prevalent age group	Neonates to toddlers	School age to adults
Symptoms		
Photophobia	Mild	Moderate to severe
Blurred vision	Common due to discharge	Only if keratitis present
Foreign body sensation	Unusual	Yes
Signs		
Discharge	Purulent	Watery
Palpebral reaction	Papillary response	Follicular response
Preauricular	Unusual	Common
Chemosis	Moderate	Mild
Subconjunctival hemorrhage	Only with *Haemophilus*	Frequent
Associated disorders	Otitis media	• Pharyngitis • Upper respiratory tract infection • Fever • Generalized malaise
End of contagious period	24 hours after start of treatment	7 days after onset of symptoms

- It may be *seasonal or perennial acute allergic conjunctivitis*, which is a type 1 immediate hypersensitivity reaction mediated by immunoglobulin E (IgE).
- The reaction may be limited to the eye, or it may be part of a generalized allergic reaction with nasal and respiratory symptoms.
- *Vernal keratoconjunctivitis* is an allergic form of conjunctivitis occurring in children and young adults.
- It is bilateral and may be asymmetrical with recurrent episodes of inflammation of the conjunctiva.
- It is associated with intense pruritis, photophobia, tearing, and a thick ropy mucoid discharge.
- Treatment includes supportive measures such as avoidance of the common allergens and cold compresses.
- Drug treatment includes histamine receptor blockers, mast cell stabilizers, antihistamines with mast cell stabilizing activity, topical corticosteroids, oral antihistamines, and immunomodulators.
- Steroids and immunomodulators should not be used without ophthalmic supervision.

BLEPHARITIS

- Chronic inflammatory condition of eyelid margins
- Usually associated with seborrhea of scalp (dandruff) or can be due to chronic staphylococcal infection of the lid margin by coagulase positive strains
- Children present with complaints of deposition of whitish material at lid margins associated with irritation, redness, and occasionally watering. There is a history of falling of eye eyelashes.
- Treatment involves eyelid hygiene (cleansing with diluted baby shampoo), gentle lid massage, and water compresses. Associated seborrhea of the scalp should be adequately treated.

SUBCONJUNCTIVAL HEMORRHAGE

- Spontaneous appearance of bright red blood between the sclera and conjunctiva
- Looks scary and is worrisome to the patients, but is most of the times trivial
- *It can occur spontaneously (without any evident cause) or may be associated with:*
  - Severe coughing or straining
  - Enteroviral conjunctivitis
  - Trauma
  - Bleeding disorders such as purpura, hemophilia, and scurvy
  - Bleeding dyscrasias such as anemia and leukemia
  - Acute febrile systemic infections such as malaria, typhoid, diphtheria, meningococcal septicemia, measles, and scarlet fever
- Condition is often noticed incidentally and is asymptomatic.
- Reassure the parents about the benign nature of the disease.

- It could take 2 or more weeks for the redness to resolve.
- Refer if recurrent, persistent or severe

CORNEAL ABRASION

- Any break in the corneal surface is known as corneal abrasion.
- The patient presents with painful red eye with swollen eyelids, excessive watering, and blepharospasm.
- It can be associated with a corneal foreign body.
- The other eye is usually normal.
- Treatment includes topical antibiotics and frequent instillation of artificial tears eye drops.
- Referral to ophthalmologist is indicated if symptoms worsen or do not resolve within 48 hours.

CLINICAL PEARL

In patients with corneal abrasion, it is a good practice to check for retained foreign body under the upper eyelid.

RED EYE IN A NEWBORN (FLOWCHART 1)

- Red eye in a newborn can be an alarming sign to the pediatricians as well as parents.
- *The common causes could be:*
  - Ophthalmia neonatorum (neonatal conjunctivitis)
  - *Birth trauma:* Corneal injury during forceps delivery
  - Subconjunctival hemorrhage
  - Nasolacrimal duct obstruction/dacryocystitis

Flowchart 1: Approach to red eye in children.

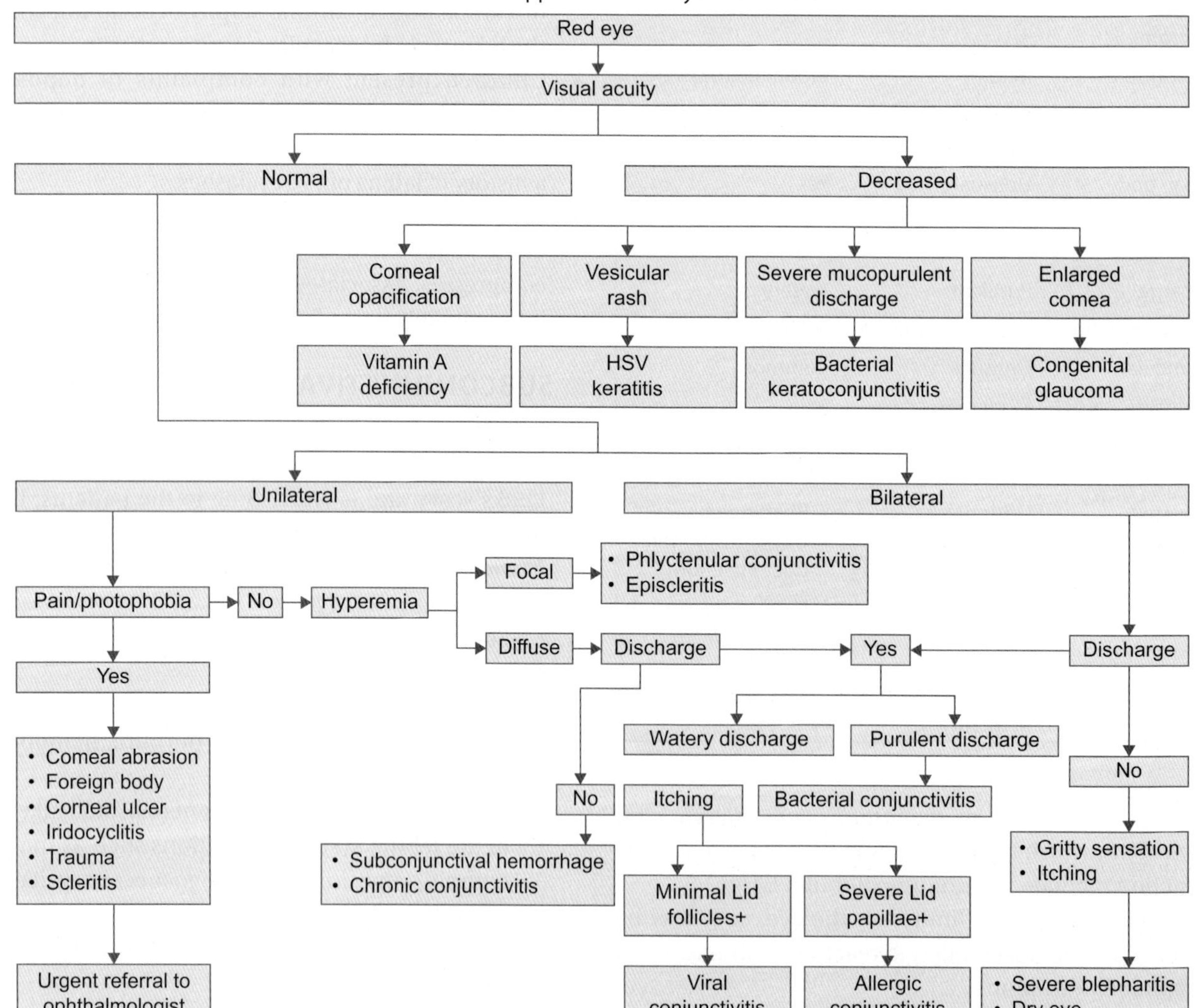

(HSV: herpes simplex virus)

Ophthalmia Neonatorum (Neonatal Conjunctivitis)

- The conjunctivitis may be bacterial, viral, or chlamydial or a toxic response to a topically applied chemicals.
- It is an extremely common form of conjunctivitis in the first month of life and is the most common infection i n the neonatal period.
- The incidence of neonatal conjunctivitis is significantly lowered by a good prenatal care and treatment of chlamydial, gonococcal, or herpetic infections during pregnancy.

Chemical Conjunctivitis

It occurs within first 24 hours of life:

- Watery discharge with mild redness of the eye
- Minimal swelling of eyelids
- Symptoms last for only 24–36 hours.

Gonococcal Conjunctivitis

- Gonococcal conjunctivitis is caused by *Neisseria gonorrhoeae.*
- There is development of a hyperacute form of conjunctivitis, 24–48 hours after birth.
- The clinical picture consists of marked lid edema, profound chemosis, and excessive purulent discharge. Conjunctival membrane formation may also occur.

Chlamydial Conjunctivitis

- Chlamydial conjunctivitis is caused by *Chlamydia trachomatis.*
- Mothers who have untreated chlamydial infections have their infants at risk of developing conjunctivitis as well as pneumonia.
- Symptoms typically develop 5–14 days after delivery.
- Lid edema, a papillary conjunctival response, and pseudo membrane formation are the signs seen.

CONCLUSION

With careful questioning and thorough examination, pediatricians can accurately differentiate among the various causes of red eye in children and address the common benign conditions. All newborns with conjunctivitis in first week of life should be evaluated with Gram staining and culture and, if gram-negative diplococci are seen, should be treated with systemic antibiotics. Older infants and toddlers usually have bacterial conjunctivitis associated with otitis media. So, their ears need to be evaluated for otitis and if present, should be treated with oral antibiotics. Viral conjunctivitis mostly affects older children or adolescents and is associated with pharyngitis and preauricular lymphadenopathy. It is a self-limiting disease and requires only conservative treatment. Allergic conjunctivitis is marked by presence of intense itching with associated rhinitis, asthma, or eczema. It is treated with antihistamines, decongestants, and mast-cell stabilizers. Referral to an ophthalmologist is necessary if child has visual loss, pain, copious purulent discharge, or corneal involvement.

KEY POINTS

- All cases of red eye with decreased vision, pain, or photophobia require urgent referral.
- Not every red eye is conjunctivitis.
- Never prescribe steroid eye drops without consulting an ophthalmologist.
- A newborn baby with red eyes and eye discharge has sight and life-threatening infections and requires urgent referral.

SUGGESTED READING

1. Bielory L, Friedlaender MH. Allergic conjunctivitis. Immunol Allergy Clin North Am. 2008;28(1):43-58.
2. Hammersmith KM, Cohen EJ, Blake TD, Laibson PR, Rapuano CJ. Blepharokeratoconjunctivitis in children. Arch Ophthalmol. 2005;123(12):1667-70.
3. Kleigman RM, Mar KJ, Jenson HB, Behrman RE. Nelson Essentials of Pediatrics, 5th edition. Philadelphia, PA, USA: Elsevier-Saunders; 2006.
4. Morrow GL, Abbott RL.Conjunctivitis. Am Fam Physician. 1998;57(4):735-46.
5. Teoh DL, Reynolds S. Diagnosis and management of pediatric conjunctivitis. Pediatric Emergency Care. 2003; 19(1):48-55.
6. Turner A, Rabiu M. Patching for corneal abrasion. Cochrane Database Syst Rev. 2006;(2):CD004764.
7. Wirbelauer C. Management of red eye for the primary care physician. Am J Med. 2006;119(4):302-6.
8. Rainsbury PG, Cambridge K, Selby S, Lochhead J. Red eyes in children: red flags and a case to learn from. Br J Gen Pract. 2016;66(653):633-34.
9. Yanoff M, Duker JS. Ophthalmology, 4th edition. 2014. pp. 183-88, 192-93.

Compensatory Head Posture

Manav Deep Singh, Digvijay Singh

INTRODUCTION

Head posture refers to the attitude of the head held by an individual and whilst it is dependent on various parameters, primarily it is dependent on the sensory inputs from the eyes, proprioceptive inputs from the neck, and sensory inputs from the vestibular system.

Anomalous or compensatory or abnormal head posture (AHP) is not an uncommon condition in childhood with estimated incidence of 1.3%. Mostly congenital, it may be an acquired finding, though the two may be difficult to differentiate in early childhood. Head posture can be orthopedic or neurologic or ocular in origin. In the current chapter, the focus is on head posture of ocular origin.

CAUSES FOR HEAD POSTURE

The various causes for compensatory head posture are depicted in **Table 1**.

CLINICAL PEARL

- Head posture is an adaptation of head and neck musculature to avoid diplopia and attain fusion and is mostly seen in congenital disorders.

COMPONENTS OF HEAD POSTURE

Observation of head posture is the first step in the examination of ophthalmic motor system. This should be done as soon as the patient enters the examination room before he becomes conscious of being examined. Compensatory head posture may be partially or totally lost by voluntary effort, and the examiner may miss important clinical cues. The AHP has three components **(Box 1)**.

Each of them is compensation at different joints of head and neck to correct respective ocular motility disorders in an effort to achieve fusion by minimizing ocular misalignment or deviation. If the deviation is too large to develop any level of fusion, no effort may be made for the purpose and no AHP may develop. If unable to fuse, head posture may also develop to reduce diplopia by

TABLE 1: Various causes of torticollis based on origin.

Origin/type of torticollis	*Subtype*	*Causes*
Orthopedic	Congenital muscular	• Congenital (tightness of the sternocleidomastoid muscle) • Klippel-Feil anomaly • Brachial plexus injury
	Noncongenital muscular	• Spasmodic torticollis • Grisel syndrome • Post-traumatic painful torticollis
Neurologic		• Visual disturbances (nystagmus, superior oblique, or lateral rectus paresis) • Dystonic drug reactions (phenothiazines, haloperidol, and metoclopramide) • Tumors (cervical cord tumor or posterior fossa brain tumor) • Syringomyelia • Wilson disease • Dystonia musculorum deformans
Ocular		• *Paralytic strabismus:* Abducens palsy, trochlear nerve palsy, and oculomotor palsy • *Restrictive strabismus:* Duane retraction syndrome, Brown syndrome, and thyroid eye disease • A or V pattern squint • Ptosis • Nystagmus

providing maximal deviation and subsequent separation of images, enabling patient to ignore the peripheral double image. It is also possible to develop AHP to permit fusion based on anomalous retinal correspondence (ARC) which entails having binocular vision in the presence of a squint. Occasionally, a patient with very poor vision in one eye may develop face turn in the direction of nonseeing eye in order to improve field of vision or to bring null point in straight gaze if he suffers from nystagmus **(Figs. 1A to C)**. Sometimes, presence of astigmatism or anisometropia may also stimulate head tilt and face turn, respectively. The component wise causes for head posture are listed in **Table 2**.

BOX 1: Components of abnormal head posture.

- *Chin:* Elevation or depression (vertical component)
- *Face turn:* To right or left (horizontal component)
- *Head tilt:* To right or left shoulder (torsional component)

Interpretation of Head posture

Face Turn

A face turn develops when the person prefers to keep his/her eyes in the direction opposite to the face turn due to

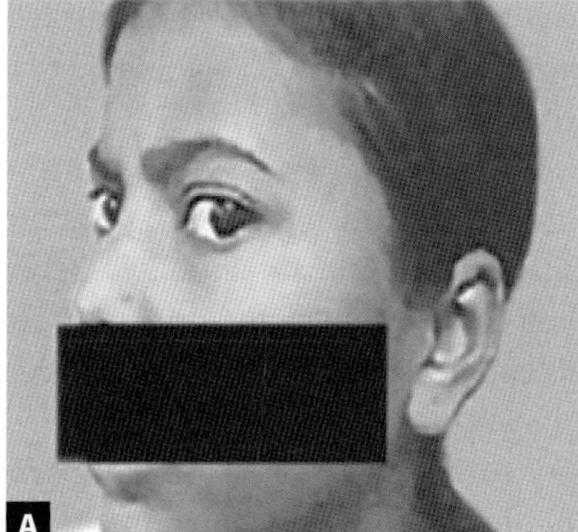

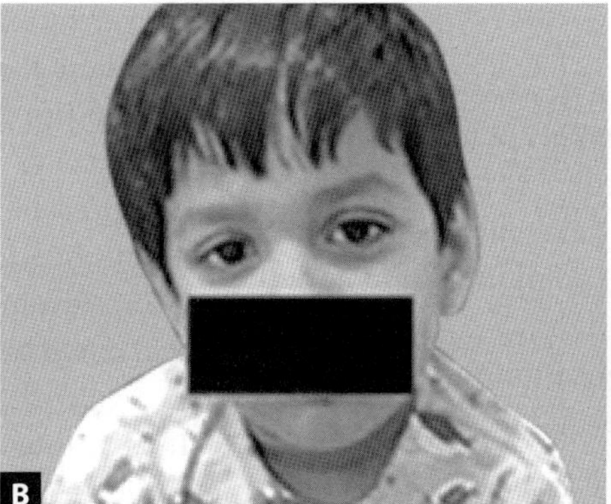

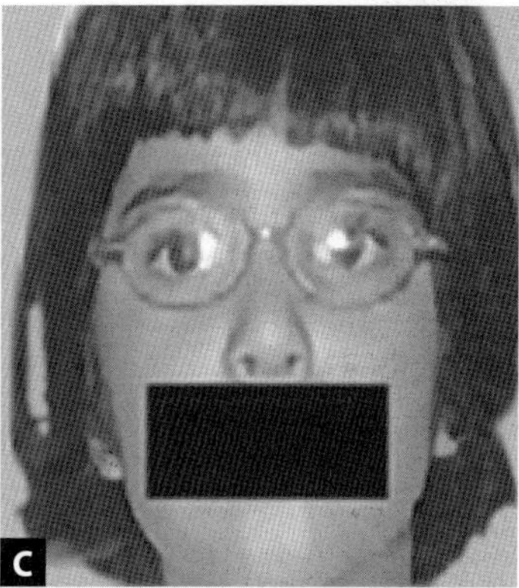

Figs. 1A to C: Various forms of ocular abnormal head posture. (A) Infantile nystagmus with null point in levoversion showing face turn to right; (B) A case of left superior oblique palsy showing a head tilt to right side; (C) A case of V pattern intermittent exotropia keeping a slight chin up posture. *(For color version, see Plate 17)*

TABLE 2: Differential diagnosis of ocular head posture based on component of head posture.

Face turn	• Sixth nerve palsy (the face is turned to the side of the paralyzed eye to maintain binocular single vision) • Duane's retraction syndrome (face turn is in direction of limitation of abduction of affected eye in order to maximize diplopia free gaze) • Congenital nystagmus (face turn may put the eyes in a particular position, which reduces the nystagmus and increases the visual acuity)
Head tilt	• Fourth nerve palsy or superior oblique muscle weakness (whatever cause) • Inferior oblique palsy (the face is turned to the uninvolved side with the head tilting to the affected side and the chin is elevated. Uncommon clinical case) • Superior rectus palsy (uncommon case; the tilt can be to either side) • Inferior rectus palsy (uncommon case; the tilt can be to either side) • Brown's syndrome (head tilt to the involved side, face turn to the normal side and chin elevation) • Dissociated vertical deviation (can be to either side)
Chin elevation	• A-pattern esotropia (more esotropia in up gaze than down gaze) • V-pattern exotropia (more exotropia in up gaze than down gaze) • Ptosis • Blow-out fracture with entrapment of inferior rectus • Brown's syndrome (bilateral case)
Chin depression	• V-pattern esotropia (more esotropia in down gaze than up gaze) • A-pattern exotropia (more exotropia in down gaze than up gaze) • Bilateral fourth nerve palsy

certain visual advantage of keeping eyes in that gaze. The face turn could be due to least ocular misalignment when eyes are in right of left gaze due to least effect of a paralytic muscle or due to least amount of nystagmus (null point) in that position of eyes **(Fig. 1A)**.

- *Face turn to right:* It keeps eyes in levoversion to avoid manifestation of weakness of right superior rectus, right inferior rectus, left inferior oblique, and left superior oblique.
- *Face turn to left:* It keeps eyes in dextroversion to avoid manifestation of weakness of right interior oblique, right superior oblique (RSO), left inferior rectus, and left superior rectus.

Head Tilt

A head tilt is a form of negating the impact or torsion of the globe, which may happen due to weakness of the oblique muscles of vertical recti muscles. It may also be seen in torsional nystagmus cases with null point in extorsion or intorsion **(Fig. 1B)**.

- *Head tilt to right:* It is a compensation for weakness of extorsion of right eye or/and intorsion of left eye.
- *Head tilt to left:* It is a compensation for weakness of intorsion of right eye or/and extorsion of left eye.

Chin elevation/depression

A chin elevation or depression posture is adopted when there is a binocular advantage in keeping the eyes in up gaze or down gaze. This may be seen in weakness of elevator or depressor muscles or in A or V pattern strabismus where the head posture is adopted to achieve least ocular deviation, i.e., chin up is preferred in V pattern exotropia and chin down in A pattern exotropia and vice versa for V or A esotropia **(Fig. 1C)**.

- *Chin up:* To compensate elevator weakness
- *Chin down:* To compensate depressor weakness

PHYSIOLOGICAL NEED FOR HEAD POSTURE OF OCULAR ORIGIN

- Ocular motor system has to respond to sensory inputs; head and neck musculature assist in the response.
- Need to maximize field of binocular vision
- Need to minimize field having double vision
- Need to enhance visual acuity

COMMON CAUSES OF OCULAR HEAD POSTURE

Incomitant Squint

Paralytic or restrictive musculofascial anomalies can lead to AHP. Most patients with paralytic strabismus habitually hold their head in a position so as to avoid the field of action of paretic muscle, thus eliminating diplopia. A classic example is congenital superior oblique (SO) palsy (ocular torticollis) in which patient maintains binocular vision with the help of compensatory head posture. In case of right SO palsy, the child will have chin depression, face turn to left and head tilt toward left shoulder. The head posture ensures that the SO muscle is always in the state of relaxation. Position of head is then so adjusted that the visual axes are directed straight forward. Thus, in case of right SO palsy, with its main action of SO as depression, chin depression develops and its secondary action as intorsion, head tilt toward opposite shoulder develops. Face turn toward left brings the eye in abduction, so that vertical movements can be executed exclusively by vertical recti.

It is important to distinguish, especially from a pediatrician's point of view, between congenital torticollis and ocular torticollis **(Table 3)**.

TABLE 3: Differences between congenital and ocular torticollis.

Feature	*Congenital torticollis*	*Ocular torticollis*
Age at onset	<6 months	>18 months
Restriction of passive movements	Present	Absent
Hardening of sternocleidomastoid muscle	Present	Absent
Visual disturbances	None	Diplopia on straightening or tilting of head to opposite side
Influence of occlusion	No effect of occlusion	None if normal eye occluded. Head straightens if eye with paretic muscle occluded unless secondary skeletal changes developed

Incomitance in Concomitant Squint (A or V Phenomenon)

Vertical incomitance is not uncommon in horizontal concomitant deviations (esotropia or exotropias). Here, strabismus is comitant in primary gaze but becomes incomitant in up or down gaze or both. They are called A or V patterns. The characters of common errors are given in **Table 2**.

Nystagmus

Nystagmus is a regular, rhythmic, to and fro movement of eyes. Two common types of nystagmus are pendular and jerk nystagmus. Pendular is smooth sinusoidal oscillations (commonly due to sensory deprivation) whereas jerk nystagmus has a slow and a fast component. In case of jerk nystagmus, there may be a gaze, where it cannot be elicited. This is called the null zone. Cases of nystagmus that have a null point may have a head posture which can have any of the three component(s) of head posture.

CLINICAL PEARLS

- Head posture is present only in jerk nystagmus with null point.
- The purpose of head posture is to bring null point in straight gaze for clear vision.
- It is the congenital motor nystagmus that responds best to surgery.

Other Causes

Some uncommon/atypical causes of AHP may also be seen in clinical situations:

- *Ptosis*, especially if bilateral, may lead to chin elevation to minimize restriction of superior field of vision
- *One eyed persons* or those with homonymous hemianopia **(Figs. 2A and B)** may assume a head posture to center their gaze to the available field.
- *Strabismus fixus* is an extremely large esotropic deviation of both eyes seen in patients with maximum contracture of medial rectus (MR) muscles secondary to replacement by fibrous tissue. A rarer variety may have fibrous band replacing lateral recti, leading to anchorage of both eyes in abduction **(Fig. 3A)**. Patient may adopt a head posture to center his/her gaze through the better seeing eye **(Fig. 3B)**.
- *Under corrected glasses* may result in head posture in an effort to take advantage of higher effective power in peripheral part of the lens.
- *Ocular/systemic syndromes* like Brown's (SO tendon sheath) syndrome or Duane syndrome, Mobius syndrome, progressive external ophthalmoplegia (alone or as part of Kearns–Sayre syndrome) may also lead to AHP.

WORKUP OF A CASE OF ABNORMAL HEAD POSTURE

The approach to a case of AHP is presented in **Flowchart 1**.

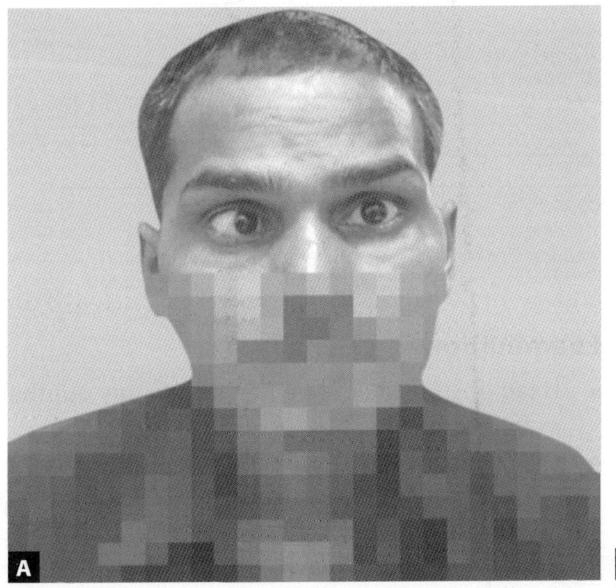

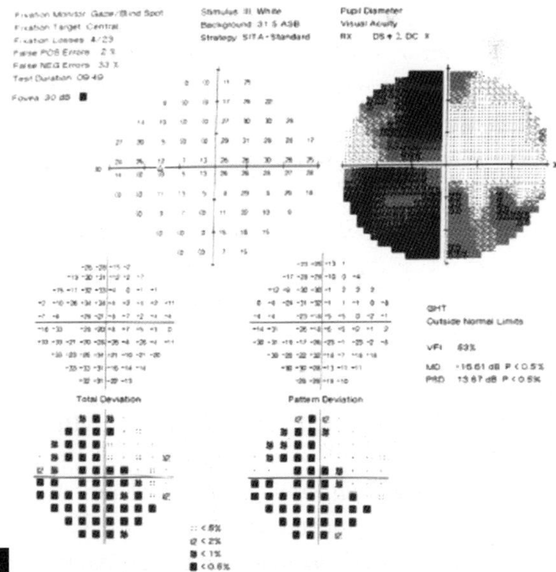

Figs. 2A and B: (A) A 34-year-old male with sellar tumor and right lateral rectus (RLR) palsy and face turn to left. Cause of face turn is not RLR palsy as this eye is blind but is hemianopic visual field defect of left eye; (B) Visual field of left eye showing temporal hemianopia.

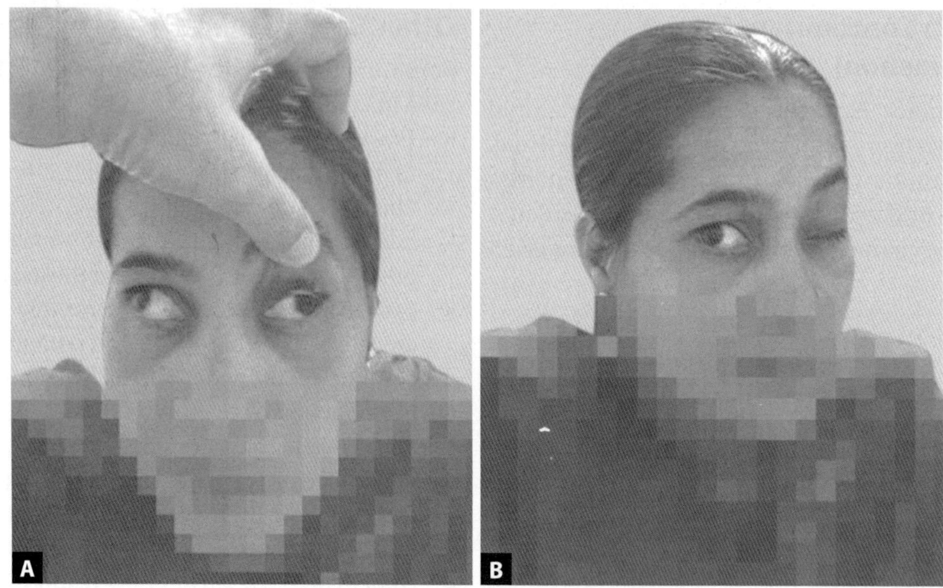

Figs. 3A and B: (A) A rare variety of strabismus fixus with both eyes anchored in abduction in a young lady; (B) Face turn toward left to get best possible vision in the central field.

Flowchart 1: Workup of a case with abnormal head posture.

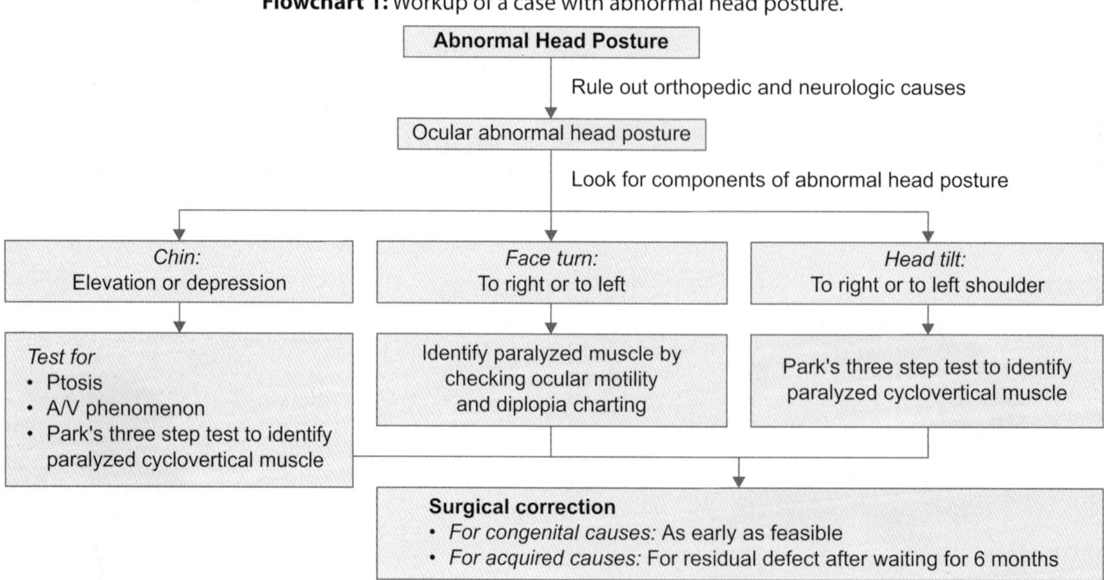

History

- Age of onset of head posture
- Is it congenital or acquired (confirm with old photographs)?
- *Ask for associated ocular problems*: Poor vision, double vision, abnormal eye movements, etc.
- *Ask for neurological history*: headache, vomiting, convulsions, or of infections such as meningitis and encephalitis are also important in relevant cases.

Examination

- Head posture should be first step in any ophthalmic examination
- Observe patient for head posture as soon as they enter room when they are not conscious of being observed.
- Look for components of head posture.
- Perform a comprehensive eye examination. Visual acuity, refraction, presence of any amblyopia, squint, restriction of ocular motility in any of the nine

directions of gaze, difference in ocular deviation in different directions of gaze and while separately fixing each eye, presence of nystagmus, effect of occlusion of individual eye on the head posture need to be assessed.
- *Special examination*: Bielschowsky sign (increase vertical squint on tilting head toward paretic SO), Park's three step test, and forced duction test
- Neurological examination

Investigations

The ocular system may be evaluated using sensory and motor testing apparatus such as synoptophore, cephalodeviometer, Hess's (or Lee's) chart, and diplopia charting. Imaging of brain using computed tomography (CT) or magnetic resonance imaging (MRI) scan may be required, especially in acquired cases to find out the cause or to plan the treatment. Certain electrophysiological investigations such as electromyography and electronystagmography may be invaluable in the management of certain case and also from academic point of view. Non-ocular causes of torticollis can be investigated using the ultrasonography for congenital torticollis or orthopedic causes or the MRI for neurological causes.

MANAGEMENT

Ocular Torticollis

Management depends on age at presentation and cause. Among congenital conditions, although no treatment is warranted in many cases, early treatment may be indicated in others before permanent secondary skeletal changes get established. However, in acquired cases, generally, a 6-month waiting period is given for the system to heal by itself **(Flowchart 1)**. Nonsurgical treatment such as prisms or occlusion may be temporarily prescribed to give relief to the patient from intractable diplopia. Indications of therapy are diplopia in the practical field of fixation and inability to maintain fusion without cosmetically acceptable head posture.

Nonsurgical Treatment

Correction of refractive error and amblyopia should be done in all cases. Prisms (in small ocular deviations) and occlusion may be indicated to avoid diplopia during acute phase or while waiting for surgery. Prisms are usually effective in correcting diplopia up to a deviation of 10 prism diopter. Chemodenervation with botulinum toxin may be helpful in cases of acute horizontal muscle paralysis, in dissociated vertical deviations and as postsurgical adjunct.

Surgical Treatment

The aim of treatment is to develop single binocular vision or provide clear vision without the presence of AHP. Type of preferred surgical technique depends on the cause and duration of problem.

Paralytic squint: In paralytic squint, general principle is to wait for 6 months for natural recovery and then to weaken the antagonist and to minimize innervations to the paretic muscle. Strengthening operations for paretic muscle are less effective. In case of paralysis of sixth nerve, surgery will generally consist of MR recession and lateral rectus (LR) resection or transposition of vertical recti lateral along with weakening of MR. Congenital superior rectus palsy with significant head posture should undergo surgery, as soon as diagnosis is confirmed, to prevent permanent torticollis, facial asymmetry, and scoliosis. For acquired fourth nerve paresis, after ruling out underlying disease and waiting for spontaneous recovery, recession of antagonist muscle or weakening of yoke muscle of paralyzed muscle may be done depending on presence or absence of contraction of antagonist. In congenital third nerve palsy, surgery is required for exotropia, hypotropia, and ptosis. Bell's phenomenon should be evaluated as there is significant risk of exposure keratitis following surgery. Acquired third nerve palsy in children is generally because of trauma, infections, tumors, aneurysm, or migraine. Treatment is of underlying cause. Residual diplopia and/or ptosis may require surgical correction depending on individual situation as the palsy is generally incomplete.

A and V Phenomenon: In cases with oblique over-action, oblique muscles should be weakened (inferior oblique for V patterns and SO for A patterns) in addition to recession-resection of horizontal recti. However, in the absence of this feature, 5–8 mm of vertical transposition of horizontal recti combined with their recession-resection may suffice. For the correction of A patterns, MR is shifted up and LR is shifted down. The opposite is done for patients with V patterns.

Nystagmus

Surgery for nystagmus is based on three principles:
1. To shift null point to primary position
2. To induce extra convergence innervations by weakening medial recti
3. To reduce muscle force by weakening all recti to dampen amplitude of nystagmus

Other Causes

Ptosis is generally corrected by resection of levator palpebrae superioris (LPS) muscle or by sling surgery. The choice of operation is generally dependent on amount of ptosis, LPS action present, Bell's phenomenon, and associated features. Causes of head posture other than these are treated by surgical/nonsurgical methods from case-to-case basis.

Nonocular Torticollis

Congenital muscular torticollis: The diagnosis can be confirmed with help of ultrasonography or MRI. Treatment involves passive stretching exercises by parents and active stretching exercises by physical therapist. In case of nonimprovement, surgical management is indicated with surgical options including unipolar or bipolar sternocleidomastoid muscle lengthening, Z lengthening, and radical resection of sternocleidomastoid muscle.

Neurologic torticollis: The investigation of choice is MRI when suspecting a physical lesion though the diagnosis is clinical in most cases. These cases require treatment of the primary cause and physical therapy apart from certain pharmacologic intervention.

Thus to conclude, "Abnormal Head Posture" can be ocular, orthopedic, or neurologic in origin. Ocular AHP is a compensatory mechanism and treatment is individualized based on the findings and the cause.

KEY POINTS

- Causes of abnormal head posture—ocular and non-ocular.
- Components of head posture.
- Physiological need for development of ocular head posture.
- Work-up of a case of abnormal head posture.
- Non-surgical and surgical management of a case of abnormal head posture.

SUGGESTED READING

1. Bagolini B, Campos EC, Chiesi C. Plagiocephaly causing superior oblique deficiency and ocular torticollis. A new clinical entity. Arch Ophthalmol.1982;100(7):1093-6.
2. Nucci P, Curiel B, Lembo A, Serafino M. Anomalous head posture related to visual problems. Int Ophthalmol. 2015;35(2):241-8.
3. Nucci P, Curiel B. Abnormal head posture due to ocular problems: a review. Curr Pediatr Rev. 2009;5(2):105.
4. Nucci P, Kushner BJ, Serafino M, Orzalezi N. A multidisciplinary study of the ocular, orthopedic, and neurologic causes of abnormal head postures in children. Am J Ophthalmol. 2005;140(1):65-8.
5. Pavan-Lagston D. Manual of Ocular Diagnosis and Therapy. 6th edition. Philadelphia: Lippincott Williams & Wilkins; 2008.
6. Teodorescu L. Anomalous head postures in strabismus and nystagmus diagnosis and management. Rom J Ophthalmol. 2015;59(3):137-40.
7. Von Noorden GK. Binocular Vision and Ocular Motility. 5th edition. St Louis: Mosby; 1996.

CHAPTER 147

Pediatric Epiphora

Shashi Vashisht, Mahrukh Bhat

INTRODUCTION

The ocular surface is covered by a thin tear film which provides a smooth optical surface for refraction, keeps the ocular surface moist, and plays an important role in the nutrition and protection of avascular cornea. Overflow of tears leads to watering from the eyes.

Tear film is heterogeneous and consists of three layers:

1. *Superficial lipid layer:* It is derived from secretions of meibomian, Zeiss, and Moll glands. The rate of evaporation of tears is delayed by this layer.
2. *Middle aqueous layer:* It is secreted by lacrimal and accessory lacrimal glands. The lubrication and protection of ocular surface are done by this layer.
3. *Deep mucus layer:* Secretions are principally from conjunctival goblet cells. It helps in stabilization of the aqueous layer by lowering the surface tension of the tear film. It also contains immunoglobulins, proteins, glucose, and salts.

OUTFLOW PATHWAY FOR TEARS

- *Lacrimal puncta:* A small oval opening near the inner canthus on upper and lower lids
- *Lacrimal canaliculi:* Two superior and inferior lacrimal canaliculi extending from superior and inferior lacrimal puncta, respectively, to lacrimal sac. The punctum leads to 2 mm vertical canaliculus, then about 8 mm of horizontal canaliculus and then the common canaliculus. This common canaliculus drains into the lacrimal sac. Valve of Rosenmuller is present at the junction of common canaliculus and the lacrimal sac, which prevents the reflux from lacrimal sac to the puncta.
- *Lacrimal sac:* It is located in lacrimal fossa in anterior part of medial orbital wall. The lacrimal sac is oval in form and measures from 12–15 mm in length.
- *Nasolacrimal duct (NLD):* It is a continuation of the lacrimal sac. It is about 12–18 mm long, directed downward, backward, and laterally and opens in the inferior meatus of nose. Valve of Hasner, a mucosal fold, covers the inferior nasal meatus partially.

DEVELOPMENT OF LACRIMAL DRAINAGE SYSTEM

The lacrimal sac develops as a solid cord of ectoderm which sends two columns to the lids which form the canaliculi. This solid cord descends down and starts canalizing around 3 months of intrauterine life to form the NLD. It is generally canalized by birth or few weeks before. However, in some cases, ectodermal debris or a membrane may remain at the nasal end of the NLD, resulting in congenital NLD block. Tear formation generally starts after second week of birth **(Fig. 1)**.

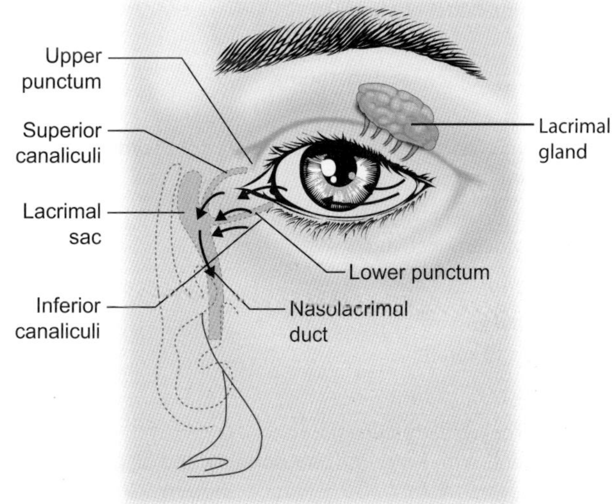

Fig. 1: Tear production and outflow pathway (lacrimal pathway).

CAUSES OF WATERING OF EYES IN RELATION TO LACRIMAL SYSTEM

Tear Reflex

- Afferent innervation is via ophthalmic division of trigeminal nerve.
- Efferent pathway is provided by parasympathetic fibers passing through the greater superficial petrosal branch of the fifth nerve via the sphenopalatine ganglion.

Hyperlacrimation

There is increased secretion of tears due to any of the following causes:

- *Primary:*
  - Due to direct stimulation from the lacrimal gland, rare
  - The causes are either pathology in the lacrimal gland or under the influence of drugs (parasympathomimetic).
- *Secondary:*
  - Due to stimulation of sensory branches of trigeminal nerve
  - Irritation of the ocular surface by problems such as trichiasis, conjunctivitis, blepharitis, corneal foreign body, corneal abrasions, and corneal ulcers
- *Neurological:*
  - Emotional
  - Stress induced
  - Supranuclear disorder
  - Aberrant innervation after facial nerve palsy

Epiphora

This is a condition that constitutes inadequate drainage of tears due to any of the following reasons:

- *Physiological:* Lacrimal pump failure secondarily to lower lid laxity or weakness of orbicularis muscle or seventh nerve palsy
- *Mechanical:* Obstruction in outflow pathway involving any of its components, i.e., punctum, canaliculus, lacrimal sac, or NLD. Treatment is discussed later. Causes and management of epiphora in infants and children are enlisted in **Table 1**.

Infective Causes

Depending on the causative organism suspected antimicrobial/antiviral eye drops/ointment started under ophthalmic supervision.

TABLE 1: Causes and management of epiphora in infants and children.

Causes	*Management*
Lacrimal drainage related: • Agenesis or stenosis of punctum • Canalicular obstruction • Mucocele • Encysted mucocele • Nasolacrimal duct obstruction	 • Punctoplasty • Conjunctivodacryocystorhinostomy • Dacryocystorhinostomy (DCR) • Dacryocystectomy • Discussed later
Lid related: Entropion, ectropion, and coloboma	Surgical intervention
Infections: Conjunctivitis (bacterial, viral, chlamydial), ophthalmia neonatorum	Treat with appropriate antibiotics or antivirals
Allergic: Vernal keratoconjunctivitis	Medical management
Refractive errors	Good cycloplegic refraction
Corneal problems: Abrasions and keratitis	Medical/surgical management
Foreign body	Removal and medical management
Congenital or juvenile glaucoma: Child presents with watering, photophobia, and blepharospasm	Ophthalmic referral
Other causes: Uveitis, episcleritis, scleritis, injuries. Some eye drops, such as pilocarpine, echothiophate, and epinephrine, can cause watering	Ophthalmic referral; treat the cause

Allergic Conjunctivitis

Vernal Keratoconjunctivitis

Vernal keratoconjunctivitis (VKC) or spring catarrh is seen in children of 4–20 years of age, more common in boys. It is an immunoglobulin E-mediated hypersensitivity reaction to exogenous allergens. Recurrent bilateral redness, itching, photophobia, and watering occur with onset of summer season. The term "spring catarrh" is a misnomer. Condition subsides in cooler months. About 95% of cases undergo remission in late teens. Pharmacological treatment constitutes following:

- *H1 receptor agonists:* Levocabastine
- *Mast cell stabilizers:* Sodium cromoglycate, lodoxamide, and nedocromil sodium
- *Antihistamines with mast cell stabilizing activity:* Olopatadine, azelastine, and bepotastine
- *Antihistamines with vasoconstrictor activity:* Antazoline and xylometazoline
- *Topical corticosteroids:* Loteprednol, fluorometholone, and rimexolone. These drops give quick relief, but their use should be minimized and monitored as an indiscriminate use may lead to steroid-induced glaucoma or cataract.
- *Immunomodulators:* Cyclosporine and tacrolimus

CLINICAL PEARL

- In a child complaining of recurrent redness, itching, and watering in both the eyes with onset of summer season, most common cause is VKC.

Ophthalmia Neonatorum

Ophthalmia neonatorum (ON) is any conjunctivitis that occurs in the first month of life. It may be bacterial, viral or chlamydial infection, or a toxic response to any chemicals applied topically. There is copious discharge, swollen lids, and watering without regurgitation. Conjunctival swab should be sent for Gram's stain and culture **(Table 2)**.

CLINICAL PEARL

- Watering and discharge from eyes in first week after birth, diagnosis should be ophthalmia neonatorum.

WORKUP

History

Complete history should be taken including time of onset and duration of watering, unilateral/bilateral, any contributory cause, associated symptoms, seasonal variation, and previous treatment taken.

TABLE 2: Ophthalmia neonatorum.

Etiology	*Causative factor*	*Incubation period*	*Treatment*
Gonococcal	• *Neisseria gonorrhoeae* • *Neisseria meningitidis (less common)*	2–4 days	• Erythromycin eye ointment QID • Bacitracin eye ointment QID • Aqueous penicillin G10,000–20,000 IU/mL eye drops • Systemic therapy with intravenous or intramuscular ceftriaxone 25–50 mg/kg (single dose) • Treatment of mother and her sexual partner with intramuscular ceftriaxone 250 mg (single dose)
Bacterial (other than gonococci)	• *Staphylococcus aureus* • *Streptococcus haemolyticus* • *Streptococcus pneumoniae* • *Pseudomonas aeruginosa*	2–5 days	• For gram-positive organisms erythromycin 0.5% ointment 4 times a day • For gram-negative organisms gentamycin, tobramycin or fluoroquinolone drops or ointment 4 times a day
Neonatal inclusion conjunctivitis	*Chlamydia trachomatis* serotype D to K	5–14 days	• Tetracycline 1% eye ointment QID • Erythromycin eye ointment 0.5% QID • Oral erythromycin syrup 50 mg/kg/day in 4 divided doses for 14 days • Treatment of the mother and her sexual partner with oral azithromycin 1 gram in a single dose
Herpes simplex	Herpes simplex II virus (more common than herpes simplex type I)	5–7 days	• Trifluorothymidine 1% drops every 2 hours for 7 days • Topical acyclovir ointment or ganciclovir drops 5 times a day

Clinical Examination with Torch Light

- Examine the lacrimal sac area for fullness, redness, or fistula.
- *Regurgitation test:* Reflux of mucoid or mucopurulent material from the punctum on pressure over the lacrimal sac area suggests blocked NLD or mucocele.
- Inspect lacrimal puncta for eversion or stenosis.
- Examine eyelids for any skin lesions, entropion, ectropion, trichiasis, stye, blepharitis.
- Examination of the conjunctiva for congestion, discharge, foreign body, tear, cyst, discoloration, chemosis, follicles, papillae (VKC), concretions, pterygium, pinguecula, tumors, or any other abnormality.
- Further examination should be done by an ophthalmologist.

Features of Congenital Obstruction of Nasolacrimal Duct

- The lacrimal gland starts secreting around 2–3 weeks after birth. Therefore, effect of NLD block is not seen at birth. This is seen in around 4–8% of newborns. It is more common in premature children. It may be uni- or bilateral and has no sex predilection. A membranous block at the lower end of NLD (valve of Hasner) is common, as this portion of NLD is last to canalize. Spontaneous resolution usually occurs in 90% of cases in first year. Other causes could be stenosis of opening of NLD or a hypertrophied inferior nasal turbinate.
- Watering with or without mucoid/mucopurulent discharge and/or matting of lashes is seen.
- It may be constant or intermittent. Severity of signs and symptoms can vary with upper respiratory tract infection (URI), exposure to cold and wind. Pressure over the sac may result in positive regurgitation from the puncta. Gradually, secretions start stagnating in the sac and can give rise to recurrent infection.
- Congenital block can involve any other part of the drainage system.
- *Complications of NLD obstruction are*:
  - Acute dacryocystitis
  - Chronic dacryocystitis
  - Lower-lid eczema or ectropion (constant rubbing)
  - Lacrimal sac mucocele/pyocele
  - Lacrimal sac fistula
  - Preseptal cellulitis and orbital cellulitis
  - Osteomyelitis of the underlying lacrimal bone

CLINICAL PEARL

- Blocked nasolacrimal duct is the most common cause of watering in infants.

Tests to Check for Nasolacrimal Duct Block

Sac Syringing

It is done to know patency of lacrimal drainage system. Under local/limited general anesthesia, lower punctum is dilated with a punctum dilator. A blunt tipped lacrimal cannula on a 2 mL syringe filled with saline is inserted into lower punctum and canaliculus and the plunger is pushed slowly. Management is done as per observations after syringing.

- Jones dye test
- *Jones dye test I:* Test for lacrimal outflow function
- *Jones dye test II:* Done when Test I is negative
- *Fluorescein dye disappearance test:* Fluorescein 2% drops are instilled in both conjunctival fornices. Normally, no dye remains after 3 minutes. Prolonged retention is inferred as inadequate lacrimal drainage.

There are multiple other tests, such as nasal endoscopy, dacryocystography (DCG), computed tomography DCG, magnetic resonance DCG, and nuclear scintigraphy. Other tests such as tear film breakup time and Schirmer's test, tests to check tear film and ocular surface, but they are all done at an ophthalmic setup.

CLINICAL PEARL

- When cause of watering is in doubt, ophthalmology reference is mandatory.

MANAGEMENT OF CONGENITAL BLOCKAGE OF NASOLACRIMAL DUCT

Sac massage is the mainstay, as spontaneous resolution occurs in 90% of cases within first year. Management of congenital blockage of NLD has been outlined in **Flowchart 1**.

- *Sac massage:* The child's head should be held firmly. Mother is instructed to compress the sac area by applying firm, gentle pressure with the pulp of index finger such that finger blocks the common canalicular opening. This finger is then firmly moved down the side of nose. Procedure is repeated 3–4 times a day (4–5 times every sitting) and it is followed by instillation of antibiotic (tobramycin or chloramphenicol eye drops). By doing this massage, hydrostatic pressure in the lacrimal sac increases, and it may rupture membranous obstructions and/or displace the debris.

Flowchart 1: Management of congenital nasolacrimal duct block.

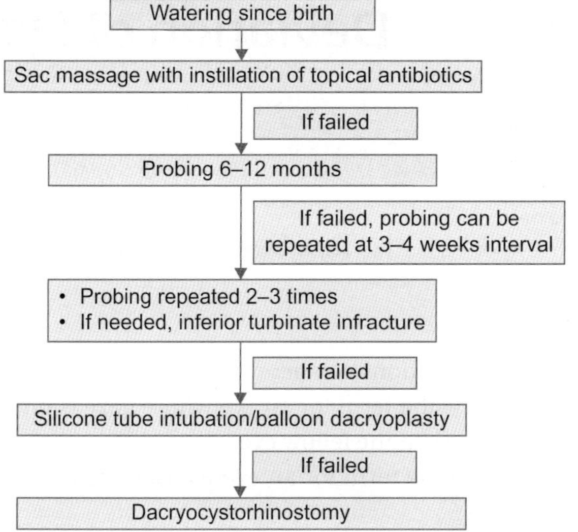

- *Probing:* If sac massage fails, probing and syringing are done under general anesthesia. Age at which massage should be discontinued and probing done is controversial. Early intervention at 6–8 months of age has advantage of high success rate and prevents longstanding infections. Late intervention at about 12 months has an advantage as many cases show spontaneous resolution by a year. This obviates the need of surgical intervention. Probing should be avoided if the child has URI. Sac massage should be continued after probing.

  In case of failure, probing can be repeated after 3–4 weeks. If need be, inferior turbinate infracture can be done at the same time.
- *In case of failed probing:*
  - Intubation with silicone tube can be done.
  - Balloon dacryoplasty can be done.
  - *Dacryocystorhinostomy (DCR):* If child presents late, after 3 years of age or if repeated probing fails, then DCR is done. In this procedure, NLD is bypassed by surgically creating anastomosis between the sac and nasal mucosa. This procedure can be performed by external approach or nasal approach.

CONCLUSION

Watering from eyes in childhood is a fairly common complaint. The cause needs to be diagnosed before starting treatment.

KEY POINT

- Proper history taking and examination are important to come to a diagnosis. NLD obstruction is the most common cause of epiphora in infants. In most of the cases, it can be treated conservatively. It is imperative that the proper procedure of sac massage be explained to the attendant and reassurance given. When in doubt, ophthalmic referral must be done.

SUGGESTED READING

1. Abdu L, Salisu AD. Pattern and outcome of surgical management of nasolacrimal duct obstruction in children: A five-year review. Ann Afr Med. 2014;13(3):130-3.
2. Balasubramaniam SM, Kumar DS, Kumaran SE, Ramani KK. Factors affecting eye care-seeking behavior of parents for their children. Optom Vis Sci. 2013;90(10):1138-42.
3. Bremond-Gignac D, Chiambaretta F, Milazzo S. A European perspective on topical ophthalmic antibiotics: current and evolving options. Ophthalmol Eye Dis. 2011;3:29-43.
4. Bremond-Gignac D, Nezzar H, Bianchi PE, Messaoud R, Lazreg S, Voinea L, et al. Efficacy and safety of azithromycin 1.5% eye drops in paediatric population with purulent bacterial conjunctivitis. Br J Ophthalmol. 2014;98(6):739-45.
5. Chirinos-Saldaña P, Bautista de Lucio VM, Hernandez-Camarena JC, Navas A, Ramirez-Miranda A, Vizuet-GarciaL, et al. Clinical and microbiological profile of infectious keratitis in children. BMC Ophthalmol. 2013;13:54.
6. Davey J, Billson FA. Watering eyes: an important sign of congenital glaucoma. Med J Aust. 1974;2(14):531-2.
7. Kumar R, Mehra M, Dabas P, Kamlesh, Raha R. A study of ocular infections amongst primary school children in Delhi. J Commun Dis. 2004;36(2):121-6.
8. Nemet AY, Fung A, Martin PA, Benger R, Kourt G, Danks JJ, et al. Lacrimal drainage obstruction and dacryocystorhinostomy in children. Eye (Lond). 2008;22(7):918-24.
9. Saboo US, Jain M, Reddy JC, Sangwan VS. Demographic and clinical profile of vernal keratoconjunctivitis at a tertiary eye care center in India. Indian J Ophthalmol. 2013;61(9):486-9.
10. Sielicka D, Mrugacz M, Bakunowicz-Lazarczyka A. [Nasolacrimal duct disorders in children. Part I. Anatomy, physiology and clinical signs]. Klin Oczna. 2010;112(10-12):342-5.
11. Stepankova J, Odehnal M, Malec J, Dotrelova D. [Corneal foreign bodies in children]. Cesk Slov Oftalmol. 2012;68(4):142-5.
12. Vichyanond P, Pacharn P, Pleyer U, Leonardi A. Vernal keratoconjunctivitis: a severe allergic eye disease with remodeling changes. Pediatr Allergy Immunol. 2014;25(4):314-22.
13. Yanoff M, Duker JS. Ophthalmology, 4th edition. 2014; pp. 187-88, 193.

CHAPTER 148

Deviation of Eyes

Taru Dewan, Harshika Chawla

INTRODUCTION

Early and accurate detection of ocular motility disorders in children can present a challenge for family physicians. Children may not be willing to participate in the screening process, and interesting fixation devices are often not available in the office. In addition, some of the diagnoses are complex. The involvement of pediatric ophthalmologists with specialized training, expertise, and examination equipment is, therefore, often required. Despite these difficulties, most significant eye problems in children can be identified with effective screening techniques.

STRABISMUS

Strabismus may result from a variety of ocular or systemic conditions. On the other hand, it can lead to severe visually disabling consequences (amblyopia, abnormal head posture, loss of binocularity, etc.).

The term "strabismus" is derived from the Greek word *strabismos*, to squint/to look obliquely/askance. Strabismus means ocular misalignment. The image is, therefore, not in corresponding areas of both eyes, which may result in eventual amblyopia in childhood or diplopia in adulthood.

CLASSIFICATION

There are several classifications that are used for strabismus.

Based on Direction

- Horizontal deviations are classified into two varieties:
  1. Eso—describes inward **(Fig. 1A)**
  2. Exo—describes outward misalignment **(Fig. 1B)**
- Vertical deviations can be:
  - Hyper—the term for an eye whose gaze is directed higher than the fellow eye
  - Hypo—the term for an eye whose gaze is directed lower
- *Torsional strabismus:* Occurs when the eyes rotate around the anterior-posterior axis to become misaligned, viz., incyclotorsion and excyclotorsion.
- *Combined:* Can be horizontal, vertical, torsional, or any combination thereof

Based on Latency

- *Latent squint (heterophoria):* It is present only when binocularity is disrupted, e.g., when covering an eye. Such a patient has normal fusion mechanisms. Latent strabismus is precipitated in conditions of ocular fatigue, general debility, etc.

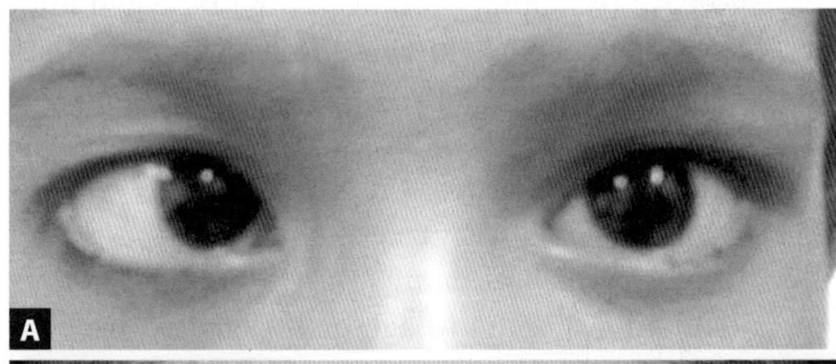

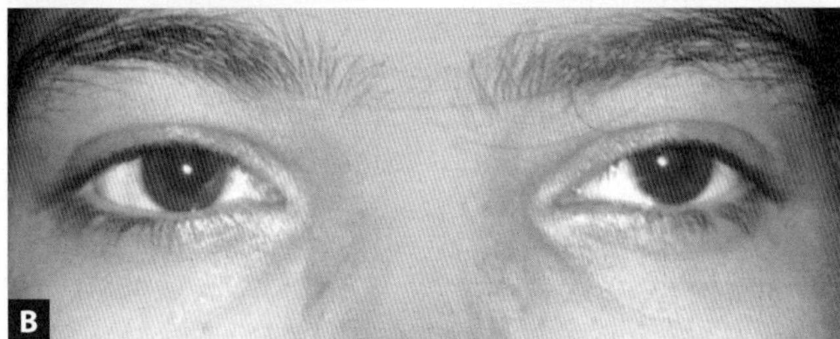

Figs. 1A and B: Horizontal deviations in strabismus. (A) Esodeviation; (B) Exodeviation. *(For color version, see Plate 17)*

- *Manifest squint (heterotropia):* It is present even when patient views binocularly, i.e., even without occluding an eye. Such patients cannot align gaze to achieve fusion and children with manifest squint usually develop amblyopia and adults present with diplopia.

Based on Onset

- *Infantile:* Deviation documented at birth or before 6 months of age, presumably related to a defect present at birth
- *Acquired:* A deviation with later onset, after a period of apparently normal visual development

Based on Constancy

- *Constant:* When one eye consistently deviates.
- *Intermittent:* When the deviation is not present all the time and may be noticeable for limited time during the day.

Based on Comitance

- *Comitant strabismus:* The size of deviation does not vary significantly with the gaze or eye used for fixating.
- *Noncomitant (incomitant) strabismus:* The deviation varies in size significantly with the gaze or eye used for fixating.

Based on Etiology

- *Paretic strabismus:* Due to paralysis of one or several extraocular muscles
- *Nonparetic strabismus:* Due to causes other than paralysis of extraocular muscles.

CLINICAL PEARL

- Pseudostrabismus is the false appearance of strabismus. It generally occurs in infants and toddlers whose bridge of the nose is wide and flat, causing the appearance of esotropia. With age, the bridge of the child's nose narrows and the folds in the corner of the eyes become less prominent. Pseudoexotropia occurs with a wide interpupillary distance or a positive angle kappa.

ETIOLOGY

Etiology of strabismus is generally presumptive, especially in congenital and nonparalytic cases. Development of nonparalytic squint is a result of factors which affect development of normal binocularity. Binocular vision and coordination of ocular movements is an acquired process which completely develops by the age of 5–6 years.

Factors, which hinder normal binocular development, can be:

- *Sensory:* Uncorrected refractive error, corneal opacity or cataract, optic atrophy, macular disorder, etc.
- *Motor:* Abnormal extraocular muscles or fascia, abnormal accommodation or convergence
- *Central:* Abnormal cortical control of ocular movements

Heredity does play a major role but a distinct genetic pattern for strabismus has not been completely identified.

Syndromes:

- *Down syndrome:* 33% cases have associated strabismus.
- *Partial trisomy 7q, 10p, and duplication 13q:* Children with intellectual disability are 5 times more likely to have strabismus.

CLINICAL PEARL

- The type of squint and the response to treatment in other family members may be similar.

CLINICAL FEATURES

- Patient may present with any of the following features:
  - Parental concern due to the presence of a manifest squint
  - Asthenopia
  - Detection at a preschool screening clinic
  - Compensatory abnormal head posture
- Special points in history:
  - Age of onset of deviation
  - Whether it was preceded by trauma or illness?
  - Constant or intermittent?
  - Unilateral or alternating?
  - Does the child close one eye?
  - History of double vision or abnormal tilting of head?
  - Family history of strabismus or amblyopia, the type of squint and the response to treatment
  - Prematurity, birth weight; neonatal history
  - Development milestones
  - Treatment history such as amblyopia treatment, squint surgery, and spectacle corrections

CLINICAL PEARL

- Increased prevalence of strabismus has been reported in association with assisted delivery (forceps or cesarean section), low-birth-weight (including premature infants) and maternal drug abuse.

TABLE 1: Techniques to assess visual acuity in different age groups.

Infants	*Preschool children*	*School-aged children*
Fixation behavior tests	Marble game test	Snellen's test chart
Preferential looking test	Hand figure test	Landolt's broken C chart
Optokinetic nystagmus	Sheridan–Gardiner HOTV test	E chart
Visually evoked potential	Pictorial vision tests	–

EXAMINATION

- *Visual acuity:* Special tests can be used depending on the age of the child to determine visual acuity for near and distance **(Table 1)**.
- *Inspection:* Make a note of—
  - Large angle squint
  - Facial asymmetry/presence of epicanthal folds/ ptosis or proptosis to rule out pseudostrabismus
  - Abnormal head posture
  - Red flags such as drooping of upper lid
- *Pupillary reactions:* Light reflex may be abnormal in diseases of optic nerve or retina; presence of white reflex is a red flag sign.
- *Hirschberg's reflex test:* It gives a rough estimate on the degree of manifest squint. Shine a pen torch into the patient's eyes at an arm's length away and ask them to look at the light (babies will tend to look toward it). Observe where the reflection of the pen torch lies with respect to the cornea. Normally, it should be central bilaterally. One millimeter of decentration of reflex corresponds to about 7° of deviation. When the reflection is at the margin of the pupil, there is approximately 15° deviation and, if it lies at the edge of the cornea, there is approximately 45° deviation.
- *Cover tests:* Perform the cover/uncover test; if this appears to be normal, try the alternate cover test:
  - *Cover/uncover test:* It confirms the presence of heterophoria. Patient is asked to focus on a target held in front of him (at 33 cm). One eye is completely occluded for several seconds and the uncovered eye is observed for movement as it focuses on the object. This eye is then covered, and the other eye is observed for movement. Movement of the eye outwards confirms that there is an esodeviation (i.e., the eye was turned inwards initially) and vice versa for exodeviation. The test is repeated for objects at 6 m.

Flowchart 1: Prism bar cover test.

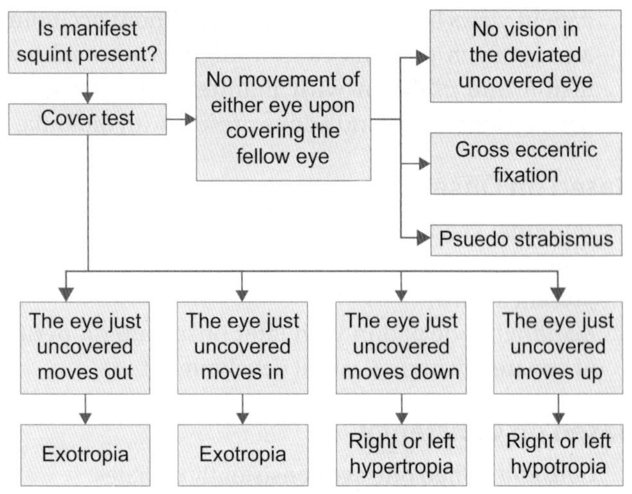

  - *Alternate cover test:* It differentiates comitant from noncomitant variety and it also tells us about the fixation behavior. The occluder is rapidly switched from one eye to the other. Observing the eye movement as the occluder is removed, depending on whether it moves inwards (i.e., there is an exophoria and the eye has to move in to see again) or outwards (revealing an esophoria), confirms the type of strabismus.
  - *Prism bar cover test* ***(Flowchart 1)****:* It is the most popular and informative method to estimate the amount of squint objectively. Prisms of increasing strength with apex toward the direction of deviation are placed over one eye and patient is asked to fixate a target with the other eye. Alternate cover test is done till there is no recovery movement of the deviating eye under the prism bar.
  - *Krimsky prism bar reflex test (PBRT):* In cases with poor vision in one eye, when patient cannot focus on fixation target, use of PBRT comes into play.

MANAGEMENT

- *Referral:*
  - A neonate with a constant squint or with a squint that is worsening should be referred to an ophthalmologist. The earlier the referral, the better chance the child has of avoiding the possibility of amblyopia.
  - Any new-onset squint in all pediatric age groups must be evaluated within weeks to rule out causes such as retinoblastoma, oculomotor, or abducens palsy.

- *Assessment:* There will be both an orthoptic assessment (to assess the visual acuity and ascertain the presence and nature of the squint) and a medical review to ensure that the eye is otherwise healthy.
- Detailed neurological assessment may be required only in cases of paretic squints.

CLINICAL PEARL

- Possible indications for neuro-imaging are: Headaches, cranial nerve palsies, afferent pupil defect, optic nerve pathology, neurological abnormality, unexplained visual loss or sudden onset strabismus.

- *General approaches* ***(Flowcharts 2 and 3)****:*
    - Treatment is guided by the exact nature of the squint and by the patient's age.
    - Correction of refractive errors will be the first step. In the subset of accommodative esotropia, appropriate refractive correction might be the only thing required. The true amount of surgically correctable deviation is assessed only after refractive correction.
    - Treatment of any concurrent amblyopia must be started as the next step, with occlusion or atropine penalization of the better seeing eye.
    - Practical considerations include using plastic instead of glass lenses for spectacles made for children and ensuring that the lenses are large enough to prevent the child from looking over them.
    - Frequent refractions under full cycloplegia may be required at short time intervals.
    - Some patients are treated with prisms (placed on spectacle lenses), miotics, or other methods of nonsurgical management.
    - Most patients may require surgical alignment which may be done using muscle recession (it is moved backwards on the globe and so its action is weakened) and/or antagonistic muscle resection (a segment of muscle is removed, so strengthening its action). Sometimes, it takes more than one procedure to get the satisfactory result.

CLINICAL PEARL

- Infantile esotropia is best managed with early surgical intervention to optimize outcome. There is evidence that early surgery is associated with better binocular outcome.

PROGNOSIS

This depends on the nature and degree of the squint and level of sensory development. Generally, early intervention

Flowchart 2: Algorithmic approach to esodeviation.

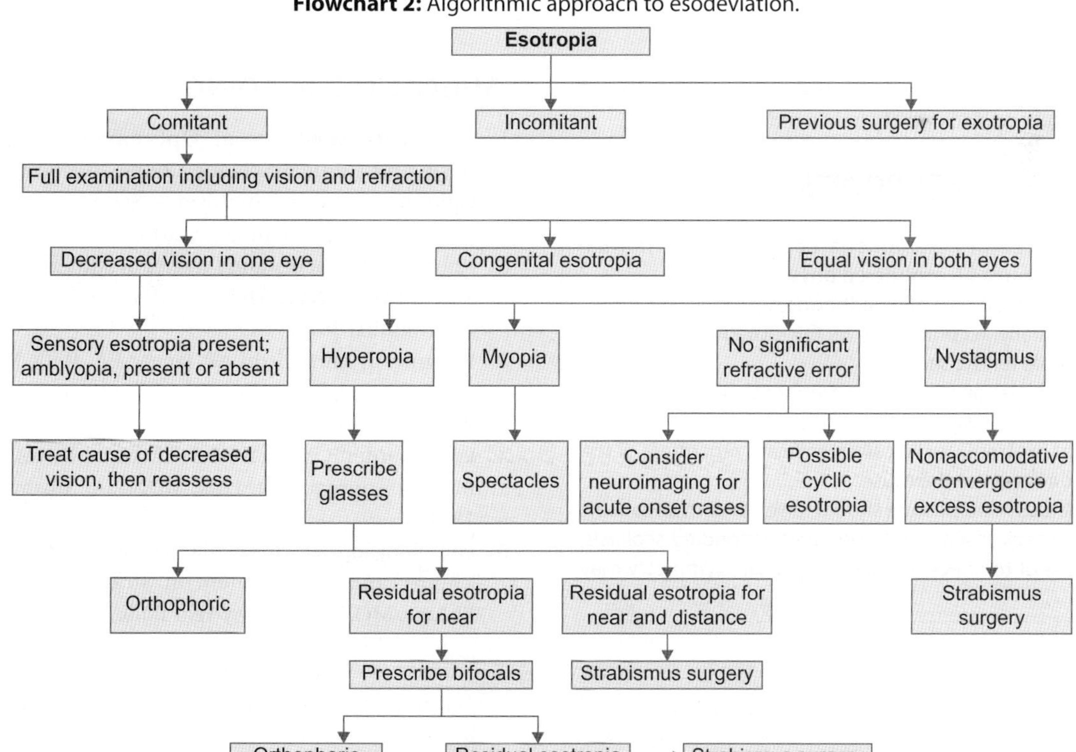

Flowchart 3: Algorithmic approach to exodeviations.

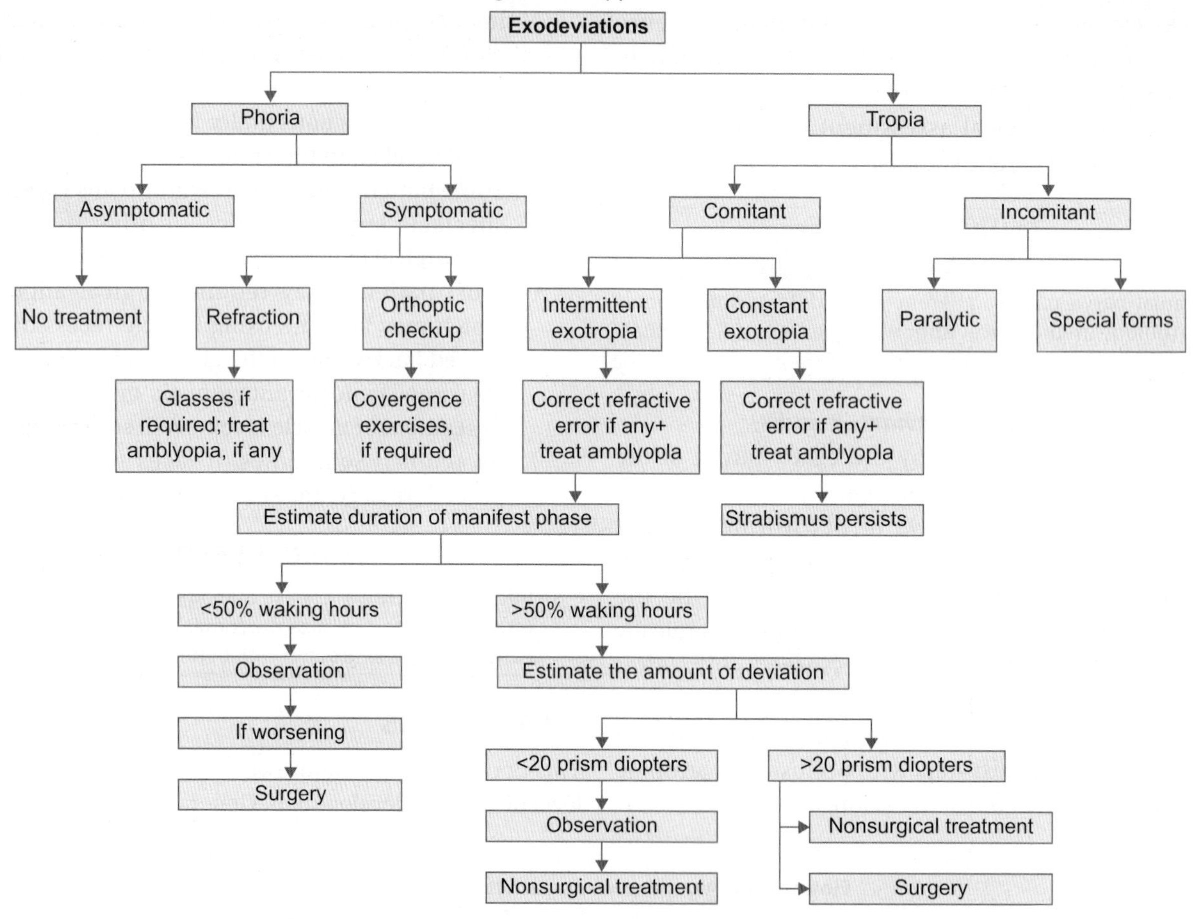

should produce good alignment and limit any amblyopia, but perfect stereopsis is rarely achieved.

KEY POINTS

- A small degree of heterophoria occurs in most normal subjects and must be considered physiologic.
- Approximately 50% of all childhood esotropias are either fully or partially accommodative. Cycloplegic refraction is indispensable for the same.
- Unlike exodeviations, which are frequently intermittent or latent, most esodeviations are manifest.
- A constant exotropia is clinically significant regardless of the angle of deviation or the cause.
- An anomalous head posture should raise concern because it may cause neck strain; if left untreated, secondary scoliosis, contracture of the neck muscles, and facial asymmetry may occur.

SUGGESTED READING

1. American Academy of Ophthalmology. 2013-2014 Basic and Clinical Science Course, Section 6: Pediatric Ophthalmology and Strabismus. San Francisco: American Academy of Ophthalmology; 2013.
2. Khurana AK. Theory and Practice of Squint and Orthoptics, 2nd edition. New Delhi, India: CBS Publishers and Distributors; 2013.
3. Maguire JI, Murchison AP, Jaeger EA. Wills Eye Institute 5-Minute Ophthalmology Consult. Philadelphia, PA, USA: Wolters Kluwer; 2012.
4. von Noorden GK, Helveston EM. Strabismus: A Decision Making Approach. St. Luis, MO, USA: Mosby-Year Book; 1994.
5. von Noorden GK. Binocular Vision and Ocular Motility: Theory and Management of Strabismus, 6th edition. St. Luis, MO, USA: Mosby-Year Book; 2002.

Decreased Vision in Children

Shikha Jain

INTRODUCTION

Decreased vision in children should be a cause of concern for all ophthalmologists, as well as nonophthalmologists; because if not corrected appropriately in time, it can cause amblyopia leading to permanent vision loss.

NORMAL VISUAL DEVELOPMENT

Visual development is a highly complex maturation process. Visual system is immature at birth. Myelination of optic nerve, development of visual cortex, and growth of lateral geniculate body occur over the first 2 years of life.

Visual Milestones

Pupillary light reflex is usually present after 31 weeks of gestation but it can be difficult to evaluate due to miosis in newborn. A blink reflex to light is usually present several days after birth. At 6 weeks of age, baby should be able to make and maintain eye contact and react with facial expressions. At 2–3 months of age, a child is usually interested in bright lights although premature infants may reach these landmarks later. Disconjugate eye movements may be noted initially but should not persist beyond 4 months.

Signs of Poor Visual Development

Some of the findings which should point to the examining pediatrician for a need for detailed examination and referral to an ophthalmologist are:

- Wandering eye movements
- No response to familiar faces and objects
- Nystagmus
- Staring at bright light and forceful rubbing of eyes in a visually disinterested infant (oculodigital reflex).

The common causes of decreased or blurred vision in children are given in **Table 1**.

TABLE 1: Common causes of decreased or blurred vision in children.

<2 years	*>2 years*
• Cataract • Congenital glaucoma • Strabismus • Corneal opacity/corneal ulcer • Orbital cellulitis	• Refractive errors • Trauma • Trachoma • Hyphema/hypopyon • Iridocyclitis • Retinoblastoma • Xerophthalmia

APPROACH TO AN INFANT WITH DECREASED VISION (FLOWCHART 1)

History

A careful history is essential. Antenatal history should include maternal infection, radiation, drugs, or any history of trauma. Perinatal history should include prematurity, birth weight, intrauterine growth retardation, fetal distress, meconium staining, forceps delivery, and any history of supplemental oxygen therapy in immediate postpartum period.

Examination

For a pediatrician, a thorough torch light examination can yield rewarding results. Following points should be carefully documented:

- *Ptosis:* Normally the upper lid covers one-sixth of the cornea and the lower drooping lid rests at the inferior margin of cornea. Any drooping of lids more than this can be classified as ptosis. In severe ptosis, the lower margin of the lid may cover the pupil resulting in decreased vision.
- Visual fixation of the child should be noted. This is done by shining a torch light and noting the corneal reflex. The reflex should be in the center of the pupil

Flowchart 1: Decreased vision in children.

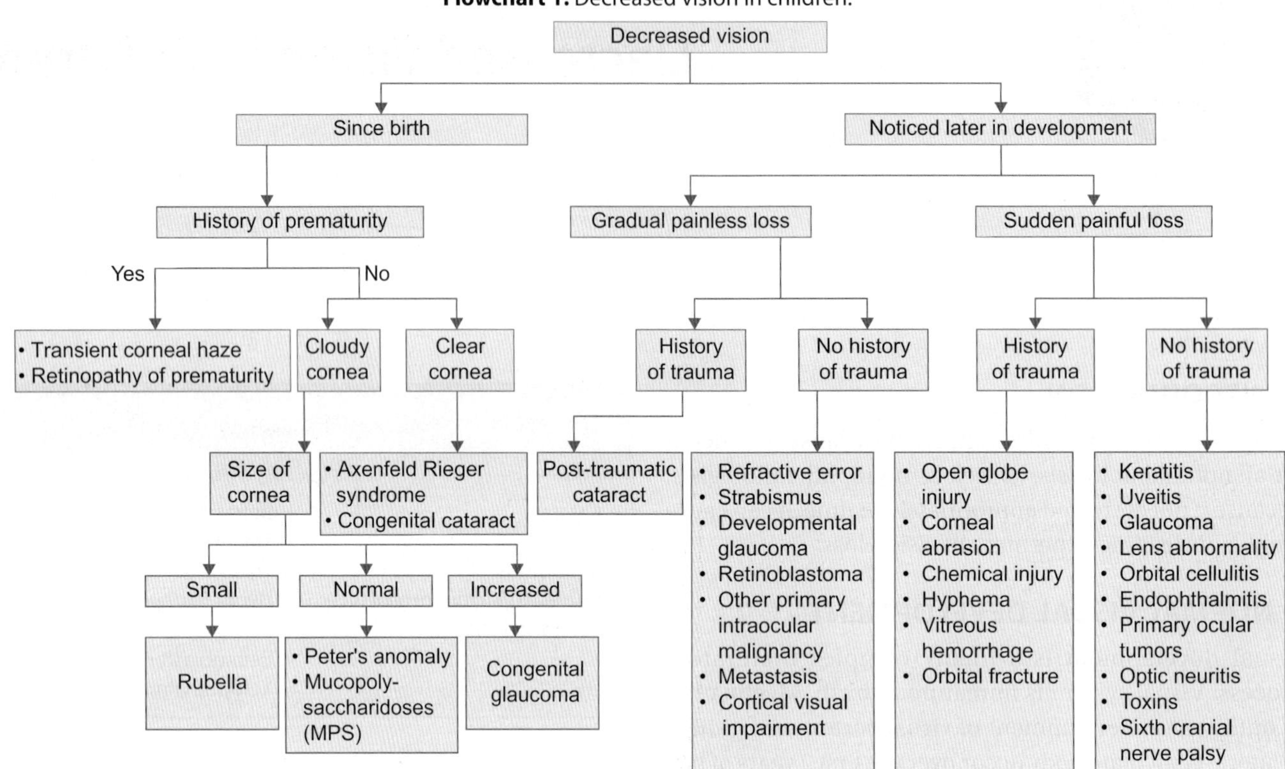

and the child should follow the light as it is moved to and fro.

- Ocular alignment, motility, and the presence of nystagmus or roving eye movements are important to be documented. Monocular cover-uncover test is the most important test for detecting the presence of manifest strabismus. As one eye is covered, the examiner watches for any movement in opposite noncovered eye, such movement indicates the presence of a tropia. Movement of covered eye in opposite direction as the cover is removed indicates a phoria that becomes manifest when binocularity is interrupted.
- *Cornea:* Any obvious corneal haze or opacity should be documented. It can be an indicator of glaucoma, Peters anomaly, sclerocornea, and mucopolysaccharide storage disorders among other causes.
- *Pupil:* It is normally grayish black in color. White reflex of the pupil is known as leukocoria.

Causes of leukocoria are:

- Cataract
- Retinoblastoma
- Retinopathy of prematurity
- Chorioretinal colobomas
- Uveitis
- Toxocariasis
- Tumors, e.g., hamartomas, choroidal hemangiomas.

Size of the normal pupil is 3–4 cm. A dilated or a miosed pupil may indicate some pathology, e.g., optic nerve lesion may have a dilated pupil while Horner's syndrome and some poisoning present with miosed pupil

- *Pupillary reflex:* A note should be made of the equality and briskness of pupillary responses.

ASSESSMENT OF VISUAL ACUITY

Infants

In infants it can be assessed by various methods:

- *Fixation behavior:* It has three components—central, steady, and maintained (CSM) fixation.
  - *C:* After covering one eye of the patient corneal light reflex is noted as the patient fixates the examiner's light. The light reflex should be near the center of cornea.

- *S:* Steadiness of fixation as the light is held motionless and then moved slowly.
- *M:* Ability to maintain alignment with both eyes as the other eye is uncovered.

- *Optokinetic nystagmus:* The patient follows a moving object, which then moves out of the field of vision at which point the eyes move back to the original position. The reflex develops at about 6 months of age.
- *Preferential looking:* The child is presented with two stimulus fields, one with alternating stripes and the other with a homogeneous gray area of the same average luminance as the striped field. It is based on the concept that the child will prefer to look at the more interesting stripes if he/she can detect them.
- *Visual evoked potential:* It measures acuity by assessing the response of the brain to alternating black and whites stripes or checks. Three small electrodes are placed on the child's head which are connected to a computer. When the child looks at the stripes, the signal is picked up by the electrodes.

Toddlers

Allen's picture cards are used which consist of familiar objects, e.g., cake, car, horse, duck, etc. **(Fig. 1)**.

Preschoolers

Matching cards are used, e.g., HOTV cards, where the child has to pick a matching card to that shown from a group of cards **(Fig. 2)**. Other useful tests include Landolt Rings (C) test or Tumbling "E" test **(Fig. 3)**.

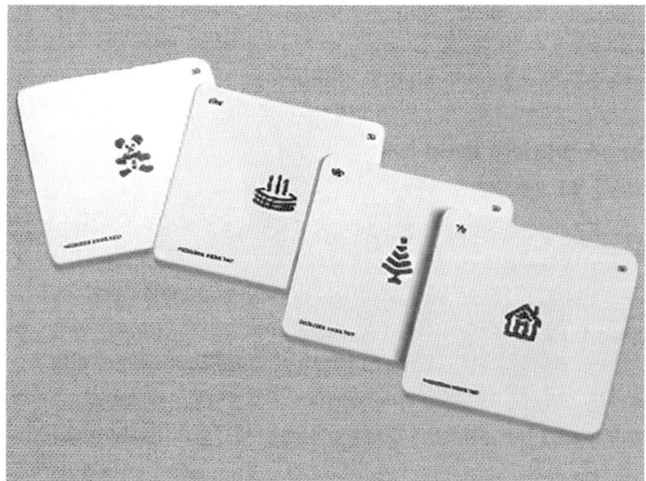

Fig. 1: Allen picture cards.

School-aged Children

In school-aged children, Snellen's visual acuity is usually done **(Fig. 4)**.

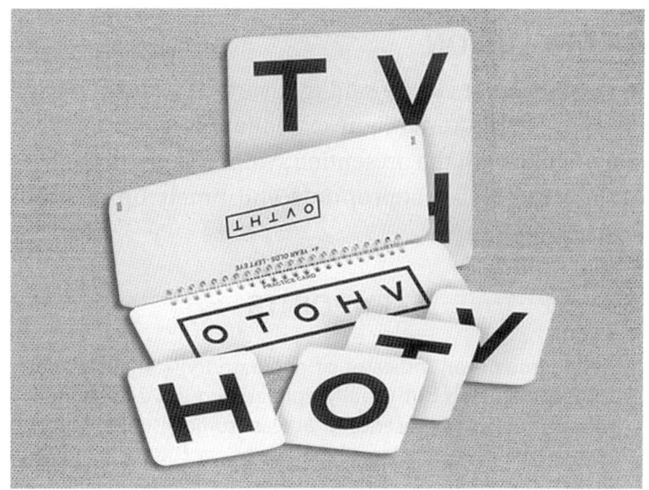

Fig. 2: HOTV cards.

Tumbling E's

Landolt C's

Fig. 3: Tumbling E's and Landolt C's.

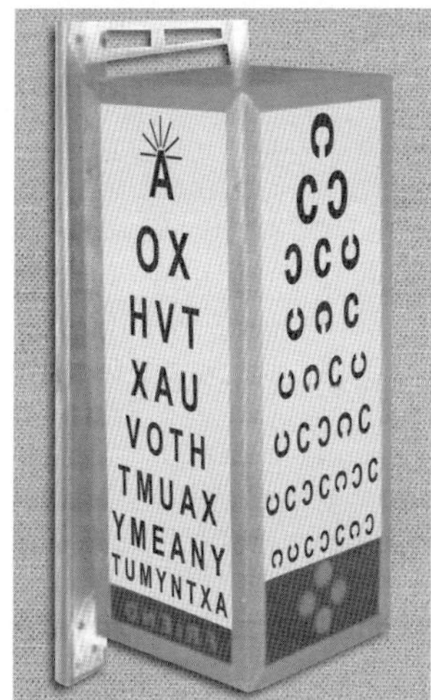

Fig. 4: Snellen's chart.

CLINICAL PEARL

- Use of pinhole helps to give us an estimate of best corrected visual acuity though it can be cumbersome in children.

CONCLUSION

In conclusion, it can be said that various features picked up on a simple torch light examination when taken in conjunction with the presenting symptoms give a fair idea of the need for an appropriate and timely ophthalmological reference.

KEY POINTS

- Nystagmus is an indicator of decreased vision and is not present at birth but usually appears around 2–3 months of age. It implies presence of at least some visual function. On the contrary, roving eye movements suggest total or near total blindness.
- In infants exotropia is more common as a form of abnormal binocular alignment whereas after 1 year of age esotropia becomes more common.
- Both direct and consensual pupillary responses are important. If direct response is defective, it indicates lesion in optic nerve while consensual indicates the motor pathway (oculomotor nerve) is defective.
- Pupillary response is normal in cortical visual impairment.

SUGGESTED READING

1. American Academy of Ophthalmology. Pediatric Ophthalmology and Strabismus: Basic and Clinical Science Course. Section 6. 2007-2008.
2. Atkinson J. Human visual development over the first 6 months of life. A review and a hypothesis. Hum Neurobiol. 1984;3(2):61-74.
3. Nelson LB, Olitsky SE, Harley RD (Eds). Harley's Pediatric Ophthalmology, 5th edition. Philadelphia, PA, USA: Lippincott Williams & Wilkins; 2005.
4. Taylor D. Pediatric Ophthalmology, 2nd edition. Cambridge, MA, USA: Blackwell Science; 1997.

CHAPTER 150

Headache in Children

Taru Dewan, Himanshu Garkoti

INTRODUCTION

Clinically, pain above the orbitomeatal line is defined as headache. It is commonly experienced by children of schoolgoing age. Children with headache face challenges like comorbid depression, anxiety, obesity, and attention-deficit disorder leading to a higher risk of suicide attempts. It is the most common neurological disorder with its lifetime prevalence in the pediatric population around 88% causing significant distress and disabilities.

Headaches in children may be due to primary or secondary etiologies. Secondary headaches are far more common than primary headaches due to migraine in children. But headaches seen in adults and primary headaches are also experienced in childhood. In this article, we will discuss regarding the secondary headache attributed to disorders of the eyes.

- *Primary headache syndromes:* Primary headaches in children are similar as those found in adults. Migraine headaches, tension-type headaches, and cluster headaches are most common causes.
- *Secondary headaches:* Its causes include infections, trauma, vascular disorders, substance use/withdrawal, psychiatric conditions, hunger, tiredness, and sinister causes such as brain tumors. It also includes headache related to ophthalmological cause.

HEADACHE ATTRIBUTED TO DISORDER OF THE EYES (BOX 1)

- *Headache attributed to acute angle-closure glaucoma*: Symptoms are eye and/or periorbital pain, visual acuity loss (blurring), conjunctival injection and edema, nausea and vomiting.
- Raised intraocular pressure causes risk of permanent visual loss, which is important to make early diagnosis.

BOX 1: The International Classification of Headache Disorders, 3rd edition (ICHD-3).

The International Classification of Headache Disorders, 3rd edition (ICHD-3) has four broad categories for headache due to ophthalmologic causes:

1. Headache attributed to acute angle-closure glaucoma
2. Trochlear headache
3. Headache attributed to ocular inflammatory disorder
4. Headache attributed to refractive error

- *Diagnostic criteria:* Evidence of causation demonstrated by at least two of the following:
  1. Headache has developed in temporal relation to the onset of the glaucoma.
  2. Headache has significantly worsened in parallel with progression of the glaucoma.
  3. Headache has significantly improved or resolved in parallel with improvement in or resolution of the glaucoma.
  4. Pain location includes the affected eye.
- *Headache attributed to refractive error:* Symptoms increase with prolonged visual tasks.
  Diagnostic criteria:
  - Uncorrected or miscorrected refractive error(s) in one or both eyes
  - Evidence of causation demonstrated by at least two of the following:
    1. Headache has developed and/or significantly worsened in temporal relation to the onset or worsening of the refractive error(s).
    2. Headache has significantly improved after correction of the refractive error(s).
    3. Headache is aggravated by prolonged visual tasks at an angle or distance at which vision is impaired.
    4. Headache significantly improves when the visual task is discontinued.

- *Headache attributed to ocular inflammatory disorder:* Causes are iritis, uveitis, scleritis or conjunctivitis, and other inflammatory diseases.
  Diagnostic criteria:
  - Clinical, laboratory, and/or imaging evidence of an ocular inflammatory disease known to be able to cause headache.
  - Evidence of causation demonstrated by at least two of the following:
    1. Headache has developed in temporal relation to the onset of the ocular disorder.
    2. Either or both of the following:
       i. Headache has significantly worsened in parallel with worsening of the ocular inflammatory disease.
       ii. Headache has significantly improved or resolved in parallel with improvement in or resolution of the ocular inflammatory disease.
    3. Either or both of the following:
       i. Headache significantly improves with topical application of local anesthetic agent to the eye.
       ii. Headache is aggravated by pressure applied to the eye.
    4. In the case of a unilateral ocular inflammatory disease, headache is localized and ipsilateral to it.
- *Trochlear headache:* A noninflammatory disorder associated with trochlear dysfunction, termed primary trochlear headache, produces pain in the trochlear and temporoparietal regions that worsens with supraduction of the eye (sheath of the superior oblique muscle). It can be provoked by reading.
  Diagnostic criteria:
  - Clinical and/or imaging evidence of trochlear inflammation or dysfunction including tenderness upon palpation of the trochlea in the superomedial orbit
  - Evidence of causation demonstrated by at least two of the following:
    1. Unilateral ocular pain
    2. Headache is exacerbated by movements of the eye.
    3. Headache is significantly improved by injection of local anesthetic or steroid agent into the peritrochlear region.
    4. Headache is localized and ipsilateral to the implicated trochlea.

CLINICALLY SIGNIFICANT CAUSES

Some clinically important causes of headache are due to refractive error (HARE), convergence insufficiency (CI), and accommodative spasm (AS).

Headache associated with refractive error (HARE) is more severe in patients with a high amount of refractive error.

Diplopia and strabismus are seen in CI or AS.

Head trauma or other systemic disorders are associated with both CI and AS.

Headaches due to ocular causes are frontally localized occurring near the end of the day and are associated with increased amount of near work.

Ophthalmologists regularly see children with complaints of headache. These complaints may or may not be genuinely related or de novo ophthalmologic in origin.

It becomes important for ophthalmologist to see the red flag signs **(Box 2)** to properly guide and refer the patient to the concerned department.

MANAGEMENT

A detailed ophthalmologic evaluation is important to diagnose, address health-related concerns, ensure proper treatment, and reduce anxiety. Evaluation and diagnosis starts with a thorough headache and medical history, family and social history, and identification of risk factors.

Predisposing, precipitating, and perpetuating factors are identified.

BOX 2: Red flags signs in secondary headache.

- Acute onset (<3 months)
- Severe vomiting
- High-risk underlying comorbidities
- Fever
- Focal motor abnormality
- Changes in mood or personality over days or weeks
- Altered conscious state
- Seizures
- Abnormal ocular movements, squint, pathological pupillary responses
- Increase in severity or characteristics of the headache
- Pain that wakes the child from sleep or occurs on waking
- Ataxia, gait abnormalities, and impaired coordination
- Meningism
- Occipital headache

Headache associated with refractive error is treated with glasses while CI or AS may need other therapies such as prism, eye drops, surgery, or orthoptic exercises.

Headache symptom diary: Prospective record keeping of description of the pain, location, severity (including pain score, for older children), duration, timing, precipitating and relieving factors, and associated features of the headaches. It can reveal specific pattern of certain type of headache. It is important for documentation and also to record the progress of treatment.

A stepwise approach is mandatory to avoid missing secondary headaches. A thorough physical and neurologic examination is important, with focus on features suggesting secondary headache. Identification of any red flag symptoms is necessary for appropriate referral to the concerned specialty. Neuroimaging and other testing should only be performed if there is concern for secondary headache.

KEY POINTS

- Refractive error, convergence insufficiency or accommodative spasm can be important causes of headache.
- It is important for ophthalmologist to see the red flag signs to properly guide and refer the patient to the concerned department.
- Headache symptom diary can reveal specific pattern of headache and is also important to record progress of treatment.

SUGGESTED READING

1. Akinci A, Güven A, Degerliyurt A, Kibar E, Mutlu M, Citirik M. The correlation between headache and refractive errors. J AAPOS. 2008;12(3):290-3.
2. Al Khalili Y, Asuncion RM, Chopra P. (2023). Migraine Headache in Childhood. [online] Available from https://www.ncbi.nlm.nih.gov/books/NBK557813/. [Last accessed December, 2024]
3. Dao JM, Qubty W. Headache diagnosis in children and adolescents. Curr Pain Headache Rep. 2018;22(3):17.
4. Greenbaum T, Emodi-Perlman A. Headache and orofacial pain: A traffic-light prognosis-based management approach for the musculoskeletal practice. Front Neurol. 2023;14:1146427.
5. Headache Classification Committee of the International Headache Society (IHS). The International Classification of Headache Disorders, 3rd edition. Cephalalgia. 2018; 38(1):152-3.
6. How CH, Chan WS. Headaches in children. Singapore Med J. 2014;55(3):128-30.
7. Kim S. Pediatric headache: a narrative review. J Yeungnam Med Sci. 2022;39(4):278-84.
8. Langdon R, DiSabella MT. Pediatric headache: an overview. Curr Probl Pediatr Adolesc Health Care. 2017;47(3): 44-65.
9. Nguyen E, Inger H, Jordan C, Rogers D. Ocular causes for headache. Semin Pediatr Neurol. 2021;40:100925.
10. Suh ES. Recent advances in pediatric headaches. J Korean Med Assoc. 2017;60(2):109-11.
11. Torelli P, Jensen R. Headache diaries and calendars. Handb Clin Neurol. 2010;97:137-46.

Amblyopia: An Iceberg for Vision Loss

Aakanksha Raghuvanshi

INTRODUCTION

Amblyopia is clinically defined as reduction of visual acuity in one or both eyes. It is caused by abnormal binocular interaction during the critical period of visual development, that cannot be attributed to any ocular or visual system abnormality. It is the difference of two or more lines on the Snellen's chart in best corrected visual acuity (BCVA) between the normal and amblyopic eye in the case of unilateral amblyopia. For bilateral amblyopia, BCVA should be <6/12.

The prevalence of amblyopia is reported to be 1–6% in children and 1.43–5.64% in adults.

It is to be diagnosed before 7 years of age, i.e., during the critical period, as visual neurodevelopment is most vulnerable during this period with high chances of good response to treatment. These patients have reduced stereoacuity and fine motor skills too. It is a common cause of low vision when there is delay in diagnosing and treating amblyopia. Amblyopia is either associated with strabismus or significant refractive error or sensory deprivation **(Fig. 1)**.

CLASSIFICATION OF AMBLYOPIA

On the basis of etiology, the types of amblyopia are:

- *Anisometropic amblyopia* occurs when there is a significant difference in refractive error in both eyes (>1.5D in hypermetropia, 2.0D in astigmatism, and 3D in myopia).
- *Isoametropic amblyopia* occurs when both eyes have similar and significant refractive error leading to amblyopia.
- *Meridional amblyopia* is caused by significant astigmatism.
- *Stimulus deprivation amblyopia* occurs when eye diseases prevent the light stimulus from reaching the retina, thus hindering the normal visual process.
- *Strabismic amblyopia* occurs when the squinting eye does not receive stimulus for a very long time leading to amblyopia.

For practical and clinical purposes, amblyopia is graded depending on visual acuity as given in **Table 1**.

How to screen amblyopia in preschool children?

CLINICAL PEARL

- Physicians should rule out amblyopia if they see a unilateral squint or congenital cataract or any child with occlusion of the visual axis of one eye due to any reason and is at risk of developing amblyopia.

In infants, amblyopia is presumed if he has fixation preference, more apparent in the presence of strabismus. If one eye of a child is occluded and he resists occlusion,

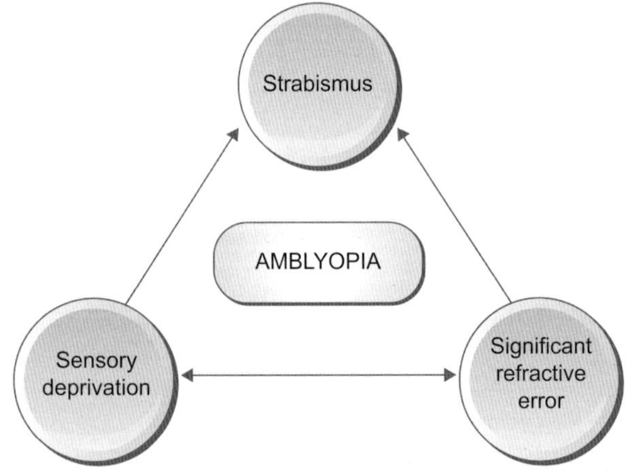

Fig. 1: Amblyopia X1.

TABLE 1: Types of amblyopia according to the severity.

Type of amblyopia	*Initial best-corrected visual acuity*
Mild	6/9–6/12
Moderate	6/12–6/36
Severe	<6/36

Flowchart 1: Diagnostic algorithm for amblyopia.

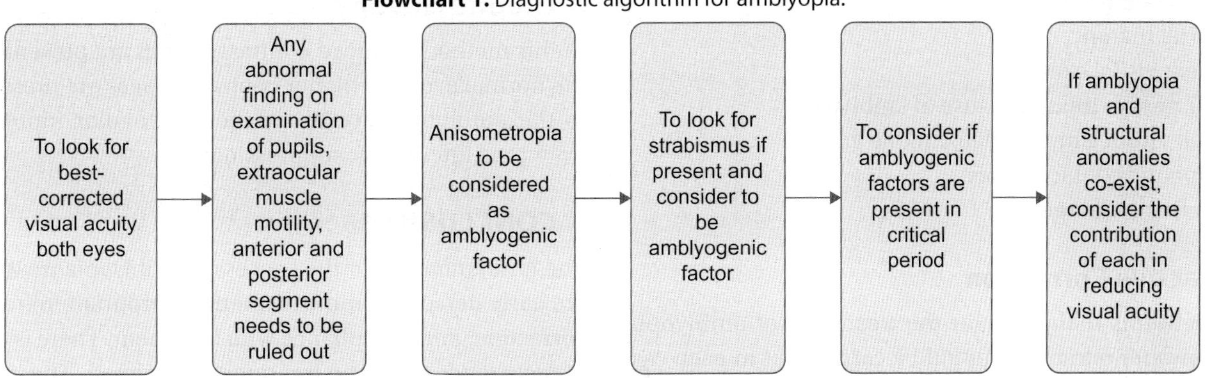

Flowchart 2: Management approach for treatment of amblyopia.

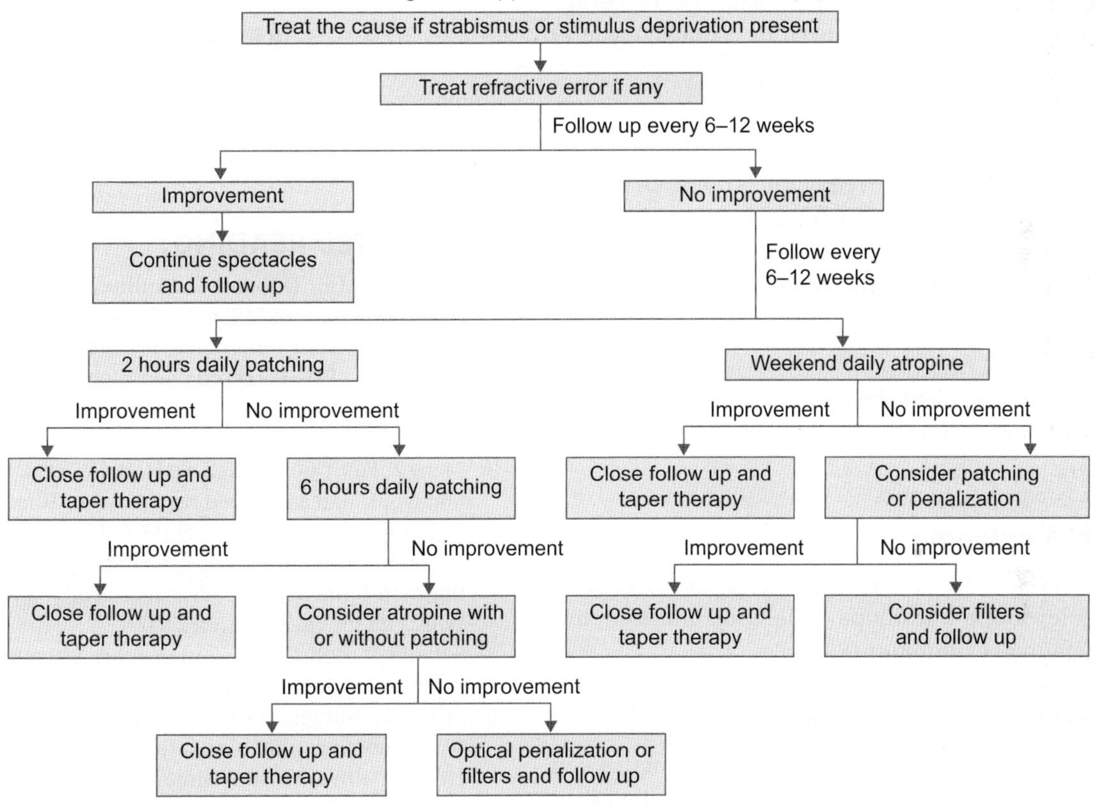

there are high chances of that eye to be amblyopic. The diagnostic algorithm of amblyopia is given in **Flowchart 1**.

MANAGEMENT OPTIONS

In amblyopia, structural integrity is maintained with decreased functional integrity. Early diagnosis and treatment of amblyopia in children can help improve visual acuity. Hence, amblyopia screening should be done at schoolgoing age, i.e., in the critical period. The management approach for amblyopia is given in **Flowchart 2**.

The goal of amblyopia management is to reduce the interocular difference in visual acuity preferably at an early age.

The treatment options for amblyopia are listed below:

- Refractive correction
- Occlusion

- Penalization
- Drug therapy
- Near visual exercises
- Surgery to treat the cause of amblyopia
- Television games/video/mobile games
- Opaque contact lenses
- Refractive surgeries

Refractive Correction

Refraction is main part for the treatment of amblyopia. So, a proper refraction should be carried out in each case with full cycloplegia. In younger children with atropine ointment of 1% thrice a day for 3 days before their visit and in older children (>8 years), cyclopentolate (1%, two drops at 15 min intervals) is used followed by retinoscopy after 30–40 minutes of instillation.

Occlusion

This method is used after the refraction is done. Occlusion of the better eye is done in which the patient is forced to use the amblyopic eye for a certain period in the day. The preferable patch is a direct skin patch.

Penalization

Penalization means obstructing the vision of the normal eye by cycloplegics most commonly with atropine drops or ointment.

Drugs in Amblyopia

Various drugs are tried in amblyopia treatment in recent years like levodopa–carbidopa, citicoline, and selective serotonin reuptake inhibitors (SSRIs).

Video Games and Television

It is based on the mechanism that repeated practice can influence neural plasticity by improving performance on sensory tasks. Perceptual learning has shown improvement in vision even in adult amblyopes in various studies.

Dichoptic Therapy

In this method, reduced contrast images are presented to the normal eye, and higher contrast images are presented to the amblyopic eye to balance the ocular input and overcome interocular suppression.

CONCLUSION

The fundamentals for the success of amblyopia treatment are early detection and treatment, appropriate refractive correction, and compliance with treatment. There is a risk of recurrence once the treatment is stopped. The earlier the amblyopes are treated, the better the chances of improvement.

KEY POINTS

- Amblyopia
- Refractive error
- Visual acuity

SUGGESTED READING

1. Hartmann EE, Dobson V, Hailine L, Marsh Tootle W, Quinn GE, Ruttum MS, et al. Preschool vision screening: Summary of a task force report. Pediatrics. 2000;106:1105-16.
2. Levi DM, Li RW. Perceptual learning as a potential treatment for amblyopia: A mini-review. Vision Res. 2009;49:2535-49.
3. Meng Z, Fu J, Chen W, Li L, Su H, Dai W, et al. Prevalence of amblyopia and associated risk factors in Tibetan grade one children. Ophthalmic Res. 2021;64:280-9.
4. O'Connor A, Birch E, Anderson S, Draper H. Relationship between binocular vision, visual acuity, and fine motor skills. Optom Vis Sci. 2010;87:942-7.
5. Saladin JJ, Bohman CE. Anaglyphic T.V. ping pong antisuppression trainer. J Am Optom Assoc. 1977;48:929-32.
6. Stifter E, Burggasser G, Hirmann E, Thaler A, Radner W. Monocular and binocular reading performance in children with microstrabismic amblyopia. Br J Ophthalmol. 2005;89:1324-9.
7. Von Noorden G, Campos E. Binocular Vision and Ocular Motility, 6th edition. St. Louis, Missouri: Mosby, Inc; 2002.

CHAPTER 152

Leukocoria

Shachi Srivastava

INTRODUCTION

Leukocoria means "white pupil". It has origin from the Greek words "leukos" meaning white and "kore" meaning pupil **(Fig. 1)**.

There can be multiple causes of leukocoria in pediatric age group, the most ominous being ocular malignancies. Hence, prompt diagnosis and early treatment is needed.

The abnormal white reflex is first noticed by the family members in most cases. Sometimes, pediatricians may be the first to be consulted.

A detailed history along with local and systemic examination is essential to find the cause.

CLINICAL PEARL

- The white pupillary reflex should alarm the treating pediatrician as it can be the first sign of retinoblastoma.

Common causes are:

- Congenital cataract
- Retinoblastoma
- Retinopathy of prematurity (ROP)
- Coats disease
- Persistent fetal vasculature
- Familial exudative vitreoretinopathy (FEVR)
- Coloboma
- Vitreous hemorrhage
- Retinal detachment
- Astrocytic hamartoma
- Ocular toxocariasis
- Endogenous endophthalmitis

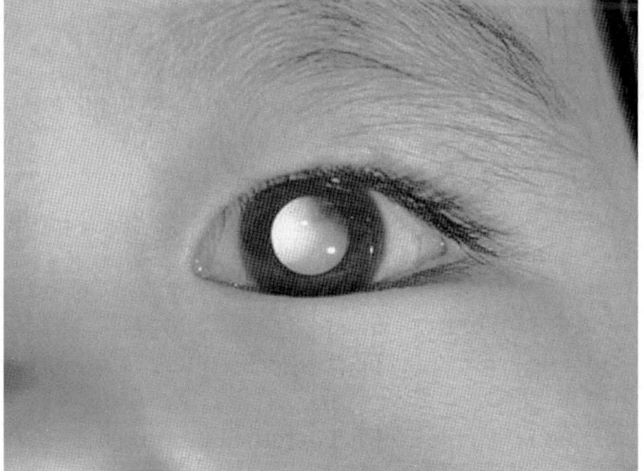

Fig. 1: White reflex in the pupillary area.
(For color version, see Plate 17)

CLINICAL PEARL

- It is very important to differentiate retinoblastoma from pseudoretinoblastoma conditions, as the treatment modality changes immensely.

A stepwise approach should be followed to arrive at the cause of the "white reflex" **(Flowchart 1)**.

HISTORY

A detailed history from the parents could be very helpful in the diagnosis.

- *History of present illness: Age* at onset is important. Retinoblastoma usually presents at 18 months, cataract can be present at birth, and Coats disease presents after 5 years.

  Duration of the white reflex should be asked. In congenital etiologies, white reflex may be present since birth, but in acquired causes, it presents some time after the birth of the child.

  Associated symptoms like pain, photophobia, redness, decreased vision, bulging of the eyeballs, squint, etc. should be inquired.
- *Past history:* Ocular trauma can cause retinal detachment, vitreous hemorrhage, or traumatic cataract and hence white pupillary reflex.

Flowchart 1: Flowchart depicting how to diagnose the causes of leukocoria and their management.

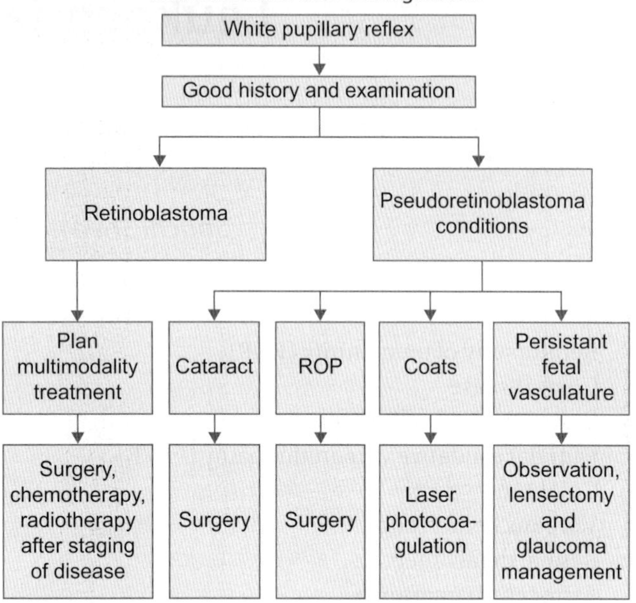

(ROP: retinopathy of prematurity)

- *Medical history:* It is important to take history regarding prematurity, perinatal infections (for TORCH), exposure to pets (toxocariasis in case of puppies, toxoplasmosis in case of pets), arthritis (for JIA which cause severe anterior uveitis with cyclitic membrane, which mimics leukocoria), skin lesions (incontinentia pigmenti is associated with skin lesions along with RD), systemic diseases like tuberous sclerosis (retinal astrocytomas), immunocompromised state, and infectious endocarditis (endogenous endophthalmitis).
- *Family history:* Several conditions causing leukocoria have hereditary components—
  - Congenital cataracts
  - Retinoblastomas
  - Familial exudative vitreoretinopathy
  - Colobomas
  - Familial retinal detachments

CLINICAL EXAMINATION

A good clinical examination along with history can contribute significantly to find the cause of the white pupillary reflex.

CLINICAL PEARL

Always ascertain if the white reflex is unilateral or bilateral.

Unilateral white reflex is most commonly seen in—cataracts, retinal detachment, retinoblastoma, vitreous hemorrhage, Coats disease, toxocariasis, and PFV

Bilateral: Bilateral cataracts, retinoblastoma, ROP, FEVR, etc.

- It is important to assess visual acuity in both preverbal and verbal child by various methods such as OKN, VEP, Teller's acuity cards, and Snellen's charts.
- Squint be may be seen in cases of retinoblastoma and cataract.
- Intraocular pressure may be elevated in retinoblastoma, Coats disease, and JIA.
- Anterior segment examination—for cataract, uveitis, iris, and lens colobomas, pseudohypopyon (in retinoblastoma), and iris neovascularization with secondary glaucoma.
- Fundus examination—to see for endophytic and exophytic growth (in retinoblastoma), retinal detachments, colobomas and optic disk anomalies, macular exudation, vitritis and vitreous exudation.

IMAGING AND OTHER TESTS

- *Ultrasonography*—should be performed in all cases of leukocoria as it is noninvasive and very specific for calcification which is seen in retinoblastoma (90%). Retinoblastoma presents as a solid mass which has high intensity internal echoes (due to calcification).

  It is also helpful in diagnosing RD, PFV, subretinal fluid in Coats disease and ocular toxocariasis.
- *Fundus fluorescein angiography* is especially helpful in ROP (in conjugation with RET CAM), Coats disease, FEVR, and also retinoblastoma
- *Optical coherence tomography* can be used to see subretinal fluid in Coats disease and FEVR.
- *MRI*—is specially recommended in retinoblastoma to see the involvement of the optic nerve and other structures.
- *Blood tests*—complete blood counts, TORCH titers, and ELISA for toxocariasis
- Genetic testing may be needed for retinoblastoma and FEVR.
- Biopsy is usually avoided in retinoblastoma.

In any case of white pupillary reflex, the pediatricians should refer the patient urgently to an ophthalmologist so that prompt clinical diagnosis can be made and treatment can be started as early as possible.

KEY POINTS

- Leukocoria
- White reflex
- Retinopathy of prematurity
- Retinoblastoma
- Coats
- Cataract

SUGGESTED READING

1. Balmer A, Munier F. Differential diagnosis of leukocoria and strabismus, first presenting signs of retinoblastoma. Clin Ophthalmol. 2007;1(4):431-9.
2. Kanukollu VM, Tripathy K. (2023). Leukocoria. Available from https://www.ncbi.nlm.nih.gov/books/NBK560794/. [Last accessed December, 2024]
3. Syed R, Ramasubramanian A. (2016). Ophthalmic Pearls: A Stepwise Approach to Leukocoria. EyeNet Magazine. Available from https://www.aao.org/eyenet/article/stepwise-approach-to-leukocoria. [Last accessed December, 2024]

Preseptal and Orbital Cellulitis in Children

Hina Kauser, Naushin Ahmad

INTRODUCTION

The infection of soft tissues anterior to orbital septum is known as preseptal cellulitis and infection posterior to orbital septum is known as orbital cellulitis. It is very important to distinguish preseptal cellulitis from orbital cellulitis because the treatment and the complications of these two entities are entirely different.

PRESEPTAL CELLULITIS

Preseptal cellulitis is more common and less aggressive as compared to orbital cellulitis and usually seen in children younger than 5 years of age.

Etiology

It usually occurs secondary to lid infections like acute hordeolum, cutaneous infections, lid trauma, acute dacryocystitis, dental abscess, or an insect bite.

Examination

Symptoms: Child presents with swelling and pain around the eye. Fever may or may not be present.

Signs: Upper and lower lid edema usually tense in nature with local rise of temperature, chemosis may be present.

> *Note:*
> - Other causes of lid swelling should be ruled out prior to establishing a diagnosis of preseptal cellulitis (e.g., adenoviral conjunctivitis, atopic conjunctivitis, etc.)
> - There will be no proptosis and extraocular movements along with optic nerve functions will be normal (visual acuity, color vision, and pupillary reaction).

ORBITAL CELLULITIS

Orbital cellulitis is mostly seen in children over 5 years of age with an average age being 8.3 years.

Etiology

- The most commonest source of infection leading to orbital cellulitis is through direct extension from the paranasal sinuses. In the first 5 years of life, ethmoidal sinusitis is exclusively responsible for the development of orbital cellulitis. Maxillary and frontal sinusitis leading to orbital cellulitis is seen in children over 7 years of age because they develop later on.
- Other causes include infections of adjacent structures such as acute dacryocystitis, lid and dental infections.
- Periocular trauma
- Postsurgical after strabismus, retinal detachment, lacrimal sac, lid, orbital or paranasal surgeries
- Hematogenous spread

Symptoms: Sick febrile child with red, painful, and swollen eye

Signs: Upper and lower lid edema, chemosis, proptosis, diplopia, defective optic nerve functions (decreased vision, color vision, pupillary reaction), pain, and restriction on extraocular movements **(Fig. 1)**.

> *Red flag signs for orbital cellulitis:*
> - Reduced visual acuity
> - Diplopia
> - Restricted and painful eye movements
> - Relative afferent pupillary defect
> - Proptosis

MICROBIOLOGY

Micro-organisms responsible for preseptal and orbital cellulitis are described in **Table 1**.

INVESTIGATIONS

- Complete blood counts and C-reactive protein (CRP)
- Cultures from nasal and throat swabs, blood culture, the cultures from the orbital abscesses and sinus aspirates

- *Imaging*: CT of the orbits and sinuses is the preferred imaging modality. MRI is more sensitive as compared to CT in detecting intracranial complications and in delineating the extent of fungal sinus disease. MRI has an advantage of having no radiation exposure but the need for sedation and anesthesia and the long time required in children makes it a second choice.

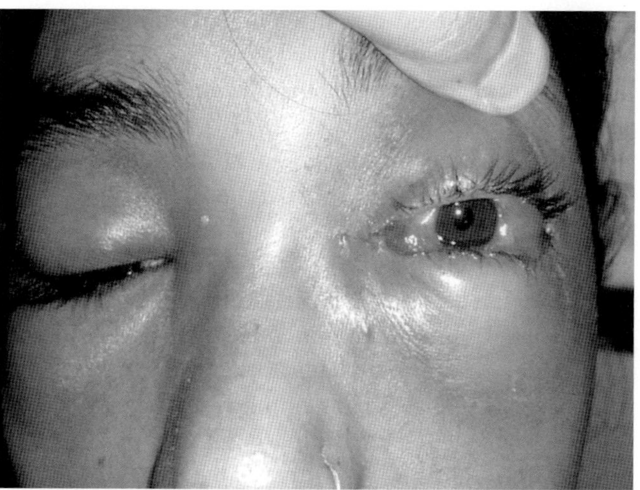

Fig. 1: Orbital cellulitis. *(For color version, see Plate 17)*

Indications of Imaging

- Severe orbital cellulitis—when there is clinical evidence of optic nerve involvement or intracranial extension on presentation
- When the patient is not responding to IV antibiotics or there is worsening of signs and symptoms

Note: No investigations are required in mild-to-moderate preseptal cellulitis. For severe type of preseptal cellulitis and immunocompromised patients, complete blood count and blood culture should be advised.

TREATMENT

- The nonsevere type of preseptal cellulitis can be treated on outpatient basis with oral antibiotics for a minimum period of 7–10 days.
- Patients with severe type of preseptal cellulitis and orbital cellulitis should be admitted under a

TABLE 1: Micro-organisms responsible for preseptal and orbital cellulitis.

Common bacteria	*Uncommon bacteria*	*Fungi*
Staphylococcus aureus, Staphylococcus epidermidis, methicillin-resistant *Staphylococcus aureus*	*Aeromonas hydrophila*	*Mucor*
Streptococcus pneumoniae, Streptococcus pyogenes, Streptococcus sanguinis	*Pseudomonas aeruginosa*	*Aspergillus*
Haemophilus influenzae (before the advent of HiB vaccine)	*Eikenella corrodens*	
	Bacillus anthracis	

TABLE 2: Summary of antibiotic treatment for preseptal and orbital cellulitis.

Stage	*Treatment*
Orbital cellulitis and severe preseptal cellulitis	IV 3rd generation cephalosporins Cefotaxime 50 mg/kg, 6 hourly (maximum—2 g) *Or* Ceftriaxone 50 mg/kg, 6 hourly (maximum—2 g) + Flucloxacillin 50 mg/kg, 6 hourly (maximum—2g) Or Amoxicillin + Clavulanic acid 30 mg/kg TDS (maximum—1.2 g) or Clindamycin (mixed aerobic and anaerobic infections) IV vancomycin—MRSA *Duration based on clinical severity and improvement, followed by a course of oral antibiotic therapy*
Mild-to-moderate preseptal cellulitis	Oral cefuroxime 100–150 mg/kg daily Or Amoxicillin + clavulanic acid 50–100 mg/kg, daily for a duration of 7–10 days

(MRSA: methicillin-resistant *Staphylococcus aureus*)

team of pediatricians with close follow-ups from ophthalmologists and otorhinolaryngologists.

- Intravenous antibiotic therapy should be targeted against the most common sinus pathogens followed by a course of oral antibiotic therapy for 1–3 weeks **(Table 2)**.
- Intravenous metronidazole can be added if there is clinical suspicion of anaerobic organisms.
- Antifungal therapy is only indicated when there is evidence of fungal disease.
- Nasal decongestants such as otrivin or ephedrine and saline washes should be given for drainage of infected sinuses.
- Analgesics such as NSAIDs and acetaminophen can be used to achieve effective pain control.
- The initial treatment may be modified according to the culture results obtained.

FOLLOW-UP

Child should be monitored closely for any deterioration of ocular and systemic signs. 6 hourly monitoring should be done by recording:

- Temperature
- Visual acuity, color vision, pupillary reaction
- Extraocular motility
- Degree of proptosis
- Corneal examination for exposure keratitis

If the condition of the child is improving, continue IV antibiotics followed by oral antibiotics. But if the clinical deterioration is noted after an adequate antibiotic therapy, *imaging should be repeated.*

If orbital abscess is noted in imaging, surgical drainage should be done.

The treatment of subperiosteal abscess is controversial. If there is no improvement on IV therapy, then surgical approach should be taken to drain the subperiosteal abscess. Majority of small subperiosteal abscesses can be treated successfully with IV antibiotics and surgical approach should be considered in case of clinical worsening. Treatment of preseptal and orbital cellulitis has been summarized in **Flowchart 1**. Approximately, 31% of the patients required surgical intervention. Orbital cellulitis is an emergency and if not treated properly, it can lead to various sight and life-threatening complications **(Box 1)**. Difference between

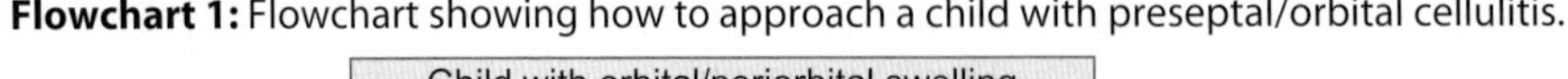
Flowchart 1: Flowchart showing how to approach a child with preseptal/orbital cellulitis.

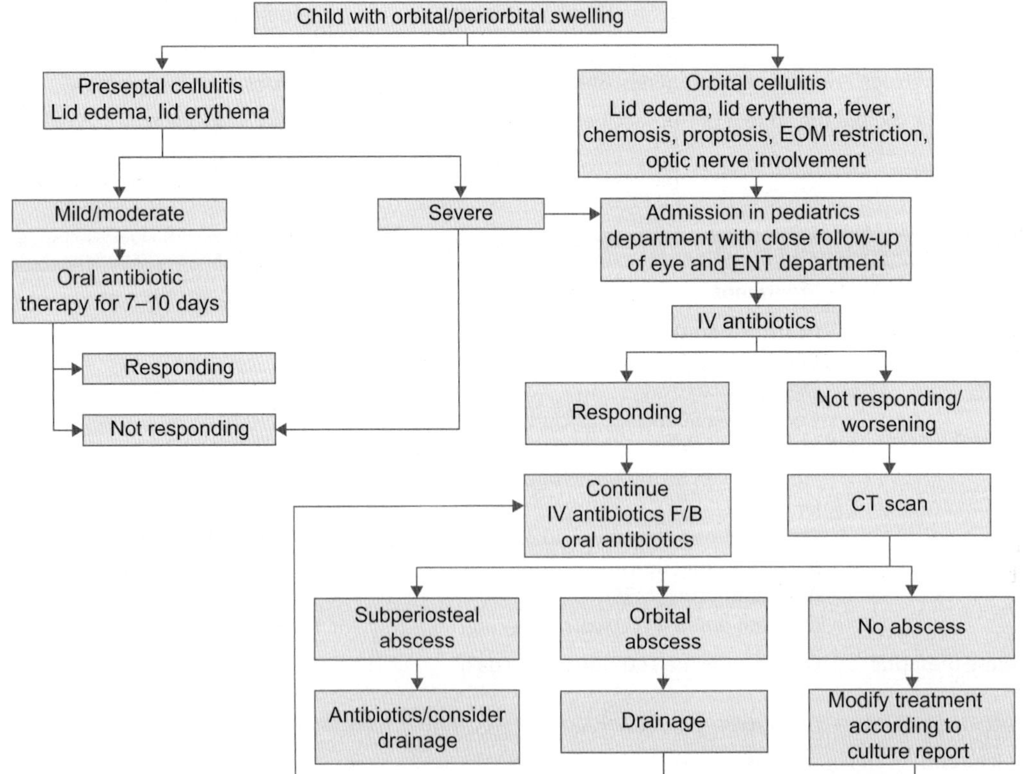

BOX 1: Complications if not treated promptly.

- Exposure keratitis
- Subperiosteal abscess
- Orbital abscess
- Brain abscess
- Cavernous sinus thrombosis
- Meningitis
- Septicemia
- Blindness due to central retinal artery and vein occlusion, optic nerve damage
- Death

TABLE 3: Summarizing the differences between preseptal and orbital cellulitis.

Features	*Preseptal cellulitis*	*Orbital cellulitis*
Definition	Infection anterior to orbital septum	Infection posterior to orbital septum
Etiology	Most common is lid infection	Most common is sinusitis
Symptoms	Sick child with painful swollen eye, fever ±	Sick, febrile child with painful swollen eye
Signs	Acute-onset edema and erythema of eyelids	Edema of eyelids, chemosis, proptosis, painful/restricted extraocular movements, diplopia, optic nerve involvement
Investigations	CBC and blood culture in severe and immunocompromised patient	CBC, blood culture, cultures from nose, throat, sinus aspirates, orbital abscess CT scan orbit and brain in severe orbital cellulitis and when not responding to treatment
Treatment	Oral antibiotic for a period of 7–10 days	Hospitalization and start IV antibiotics followed by oral antibiotics
Complications	Can progress to orbital cellulitis	Rapid progression can be seen leading to vision loss, meningitis, cavernous sinus thrombosis, subperiosteal abscess, orbital abscess, septicemia, and death

preseptal and orbital cellulitis are summarised in **Table 3**.

CONCLUSION

Orbital cellulitis is an ocular emergency and requires prompt treatment, failure of which can lead to loss of vision, meningitis, cavernous sinus thrombosis, brain abscesses, septicemia, and even death. Children are at a greater risk of development of these sequelae.

SUGGESTED READING

1. Daoudi A, Ajdakar S, Rada N, Draiss G, Hajji I, Bouskraoui M. Orbital and periorbital cellulitis in children. Epidemiological, clinical, therapeutic aspects and course. J Françaisd'Ophtalmologie. 2016;39(7):609-14.
2. Fuglsang M, Petersen KB, Bille J. Diagnosis and treatment of subperiosteal orbital abscess. Ugeskr Laeger. 2022;184(17): V11210856.
3. Hytönen M, Atula T, Pitkäranta A. Complications of acute sinusitis in children. Acta Otolaryngol Suppl. 2000;120(545): 154-7.
4. Ryan JT, Preciado DA, Bauman N, Pena M, Bose S, Zalzal GH, et al. Management of pediatric orbital cellulitis in patients with radiographic findings of subperiosteal abscess. Otolaryngol Head Neck Surg. 2009;140(6): 907-11.
5. Shoaei SD, Tehrani S, Arab-Mazar Z. Frequency of preseptal cellulitis and its risk factors in patients admitted to two educational hospitals in Tehran, Iran, during 2014-2015. Int J Infect. 2017;4(2):e42112.
6. Watts P. Preseptal and orbital cellulitis in children: a review. Paediatr Child Health. 2012;22(1):1-8.

Retinopathy of Prematurity

Deepa Sharma

INTRODUCTION

The term retinopathy of prematurity (ROP), originally called as retrolental fibroplasia, was first introduced by Terry in 1942. It is a disease of retinal vasculature in immature retina of a premature neonate. Normal vascularization starts from optic disc and progresses toward ora with nasally being completed at 36 weeks and temporally at 41 weeks **(Fig. 1)**. ROP results from interruption of normal vascularization process and is characterized by vaso-obliteration/vaso-cessation followed by abnormal neovascularization and ultimately cicatrization.

Initially rare, the disease has now become common due to improved neonatal care and improved survival of low birth weight and preterm babies. In India the annual incidence is about 38–51.9% in low birth weight infants.

Let us try to understand the disease by answering these simple questions one by one.

- Which babies have high chances of ROP?
- How ROP develops?
- Can ROP be prevented?
- How to prevent ROP?
- Is it treatable/available treatment options?

WHICH BABIES HAVE HIGH CHANCES OF RETINOPATHY OF PREMATURITY?

Certain risk factors increase the chances of ROP in a neonate.

Major risk factors:

- Preterm birth (<30 weeks gestational age)
- Low birth weight (<1,500 g)
- Excessive supplemental oxygen therapy

Other risk factors:

- Mechanical ventilation
- Hemodynamic instability
- Multiple births
- Blood transfusions
- Intrauterine growth retardation (IUGR)
- Respiratory distress (RDS)
- Sepsis
- Intraventricular hemorrhage
- Anemia

HOW RETINOPATHY OF PREMATURITY DEVELOPS?

The retinal vascularization begins at 16 weeks and occurs in two phases. Phase 1 vasculogenesis, which begins at posterior pole and is completed at 21–22 weeks and phase 2 angiogenesis progresses to ora serrata with nasal ora completed at term pregnancy of 37 weeks postmenstrual age (PMA) and temporal ora at 38 weeks PMA. During this critical period an inadvertent exposure of oxygen on immature retinal vessels can lead to development of ROP **(Fig. 1)**. This can be described in two stages:

1. Primary or vasoconstrictive stage (22–30 weeks)
   The retina at this stage is exposed to hyperoxic state → decreased vascular endothelial growth factor (VEGF) → arrest of growth of normal vessels.
2. Secondary or vasoproliferative stage (31–44 weeks)
   This occurs when infant is shifted from oxygen to room air. Avascular retina is hypoxic → Increased VEGF → New vessels grow

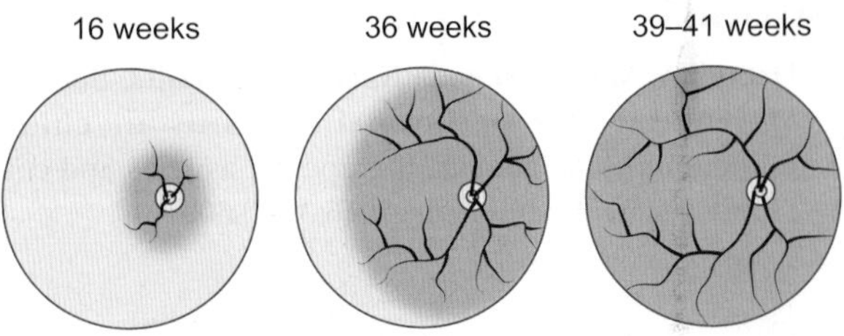

Fig. 1: Normal retinal angiogenesis.

CAN RETINOPATHY OF PREMATURITY BE PREVENTED? IF YES THEN HOW?

- Appropriate referral by the neonatologist of all at risk babies.
- Timely screening and management by trained ophthalmologist, preferably a retina specialist.

Whom to Screen?

Developed World

- Birth weight <1,500 g
- Gestational age <30 weeks
- Infants with birth weight between 1,500 and 2,000 gms or gestational age >30 weeks with unstable clinical course

Indian Scenario

- Birth weight <2,000 g
- Gestational age at birth 34 weeks or less
- Born at >34 weeks with associated risk factors such as cardiorespiratory support, prolonged oxygen therapy, respiratory distress, blood transfusion, sepsis, poor postnatal weight gain, and apnea.
- Other preterm infants based on the discretion of neonatologist or pediatrician.

Timing of First Screening

- Within 30 days (4 weeks) of life or before discharge from SNCU/NICU
- Earlier (within 2–3 weeks of life) if gestational age is <28 weeks or birth weight is <1,200 gms for early identification

Screening Protocol?

- Trained ophthalmologist
- Neonatal intensive care unit (NICU) setting/outpatient department (OPD)/clinic
- Asepsis
- Well fed, warm
- Systemic parameters to be monitored.
- *Communication with the parents and documentation is mandatory*

Check List

- Pupillary dilatation (2.5% phenylephrine and 5% tropicamide) twice 15 minutes apart
- Infant wire speculum (topical anesthetic eyedrops)
- Indirect ophthalmoscope (20 D/30D lens)
- Scleral depressor
- *Plus disease should always be looked for.*

Screening Method

- First examine the anterior segment.
- Posterior pole and the optic disc.
- Sequential examination of the peripheral retina.
- Indentation
- *Record the findings in the chart or card* **(Fig. 2)**.
- *Clearly state the date of follow-up.*

Retinal images can be obtained for documentation using wide angle fundus camera such as RetCam or 3Nethra neo followed by telescreening for opinion regarding management **(Figs. 3A to C)**.

RetCam

- Wide field fundus camera with a view of 130°.
- Overcomes logistics of screening.
- Can be used easily by nurses/technicians for tele-screening consultation.
- Eliminates interobserver variability.
- Great screening and teaching tool.

In India, as most of the children live in remote areas with limited access to tertiary level neonatal care, telescreening can bring more children into the screening program.

The model has been successfully used by Vinekar et al. in KIDROP program (Karnataka Internet Assisted Diagnosis of Retinopathy of Prematurity).

- India's first tele-ROP program and is currently one of the largest single-center ROP programs in the world.
- 127 NICUs across the state of Karnataka (Government and Private) are covered each week.
- Over 150,000 screening sessions have been completed and over 2,500 babies treated thus far.
- This program is a public-private partnership with the Government of Karnataka.
- KIDROP has received several awards nationally and internationally for its innovations, including Public-Private Partnership of the Year in 2012, National Award for Excellence in HealthCare in 2016, K R Datta Award for Community Outreach in 2017, and BIRAC Innovator Award for HealthCare in 2018.

ROP RECORDING FORM:

Neonatal Ophthalmology Examination Record for ROP									SNCU Data base:
Identification	**Name: Baby of**	**Date of birth**	**Birth weight**	/–/–/–gm	**Gestational age at time of birth**	**–/–/–/ weeks and days**	**Estimated day of delivery (by LMP/USG)**	**MM/DD/YYYY**	
Risk factor	Oxygen supplementation Y/N□□ □□ hrs. Sepsis Y/N. Clinical/screening proven/culture proven Blood transfusion Y/N No of unit □□ Multiple births Y/Order □□ NEC.Y/N Apnea, Y/N: no of episodes □□				RDS.Y/N □□ Anemia Y/N Hb g% □□ Thrombocytopenia Y/N Intra-ventricular hemorrhage Y/N, grade □ Cardiovascular defect other than PDA Y/N. PDA Y/N Maternal factor—H/o hypertension/anemia/assisted conception/premature rupture of AM				

Name of the Hospital: Dr RML HOSPITAL NEW DELHI

Current Date: __/__/____	Right eye: Zone 3, Zone 2, Zone 1 — Left eye: Zone 1, Zone 2, Zone 3
EDD: ____/____/____ (40 w)	
Current Gestational Age: (wk + days)	
Follow Up No.:	
Any Comments On: Cornea, Iris, lens, Pupil Vitreous, optic nerve	

Report DATE: ↓		Zone: 1–3	Stage: 1–5	Preplus: Y/N	Plus Disease: Y/N	Total Clock hours	APROP: Y/N	NEXT F/U DATE	Remarks/ DOCTOR SIGNATURE
	Right eye								
	Left eye								
	Right eye								
	Left eye								
	Right eye								
	Left eye								
	Right eye								
	Left eye								
	Right eye								
	Left eye								
	Right eye								
	Left eye								

Any other ocular abnormality detected	1. LIDS 3. CORNEA 5. ANTERIOR CHAMBER 7. VITREOUS 2. CONJUCTIVA 4. IRIS 6. LENS 8. OPTIC NERVE	
Recommendation	Follow Up/Laser ablation/referral to tertiary center, for surgical intervention:	
Next follow-up		

Fig. 2: Retinopathy of prematurity (ROP) recording form.
Courtesy: Format of the ROP form: Dr Ram Manohar Lohia Hospital.

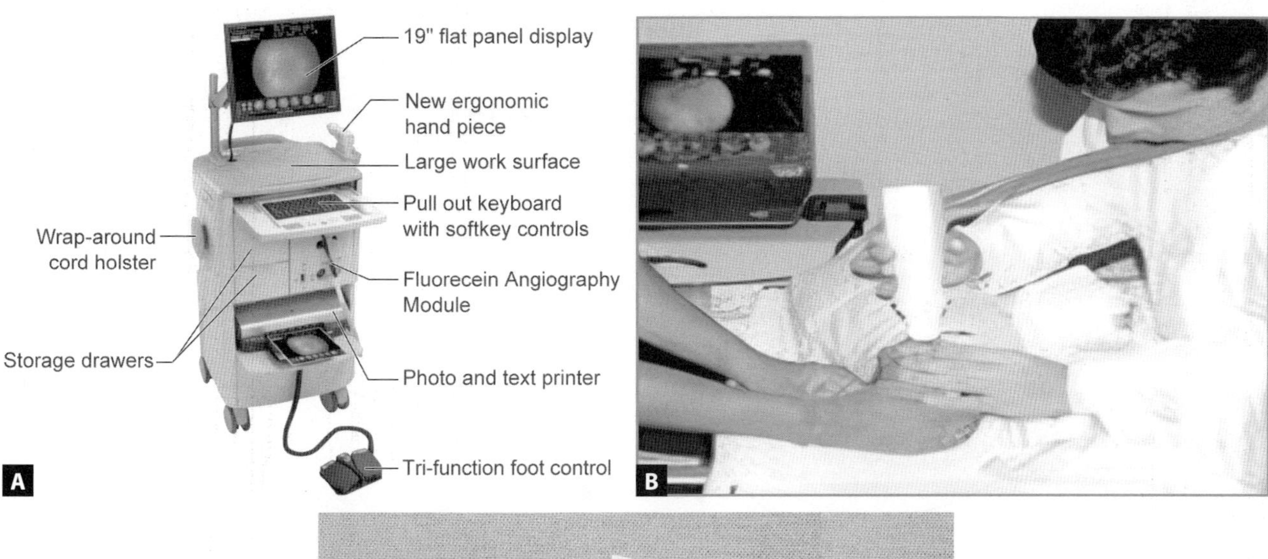

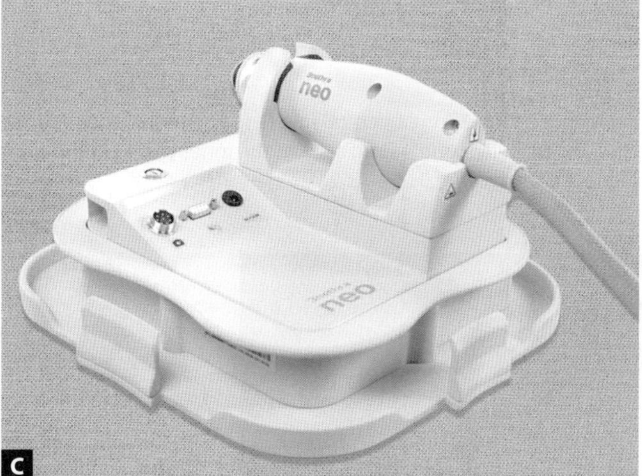

Figs. 3A to C: Wide field Fundus Camera for ROP Screening and Documentation—Retcam (A); 3Nethra (B); and 3Nethra neo (C).

What to Look for While Screening?

- Is there an ROP or an immature retina? **(Fig. 4)**
- If there is an ROP then identify the following:
  - Zone
  - Stage
  - Plus +/–
- Mark the zone and stage the disease **(Figs. 5 to 9)**.

PLUS DISEASE (FIGS. 10A TO C)

Definition: Presence of at least two of the following signs at the posterior pole:

- Venous dilatation
- Arteriolar tortuosity
- Poor pupillary dilatation
- Vascular engorgement of iris
- Vitreous haze

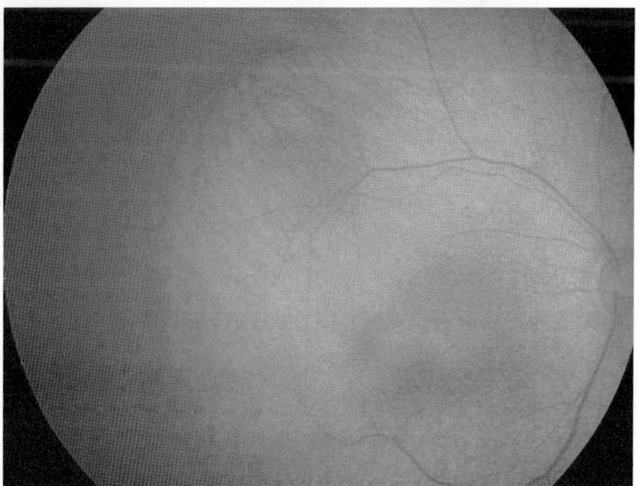

Fig. 4: Immature vascularization with peripheral avascular retina. *(For color version, see Plate 17)*

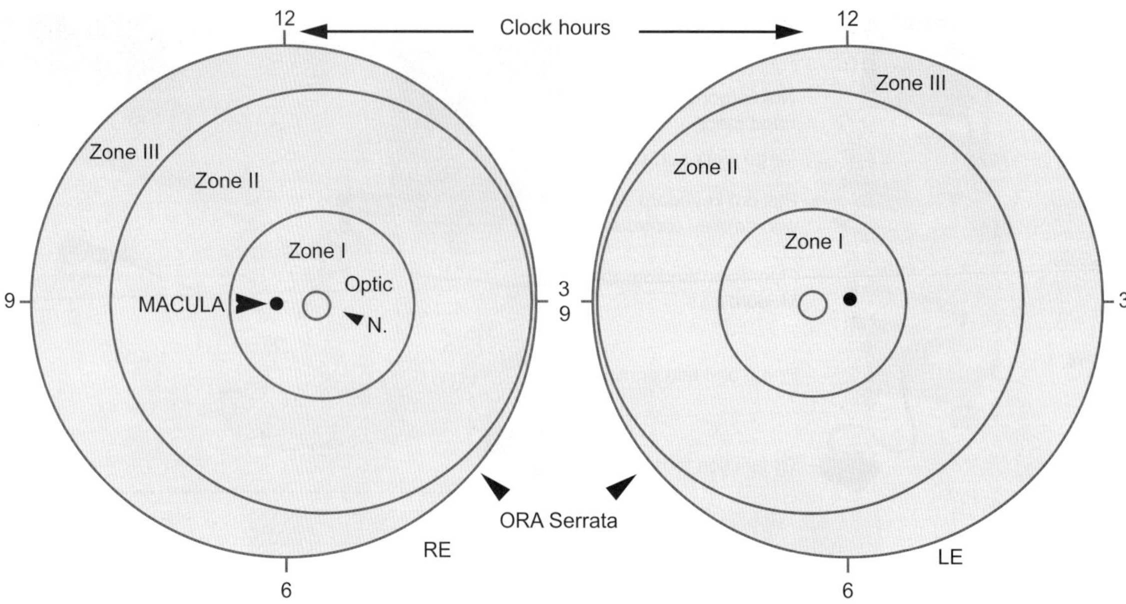

Fig. 5: ROP can be classified into three Zones I, II, III—Zone I-central most area of Retina, around the optic disc extending to a circle with radius twice the distance between disc and macula; Zone II-Ring around the inner circle extending upto the nasal ora; Zone III- includes the remaining temporal crescent of Retina outside zone II.

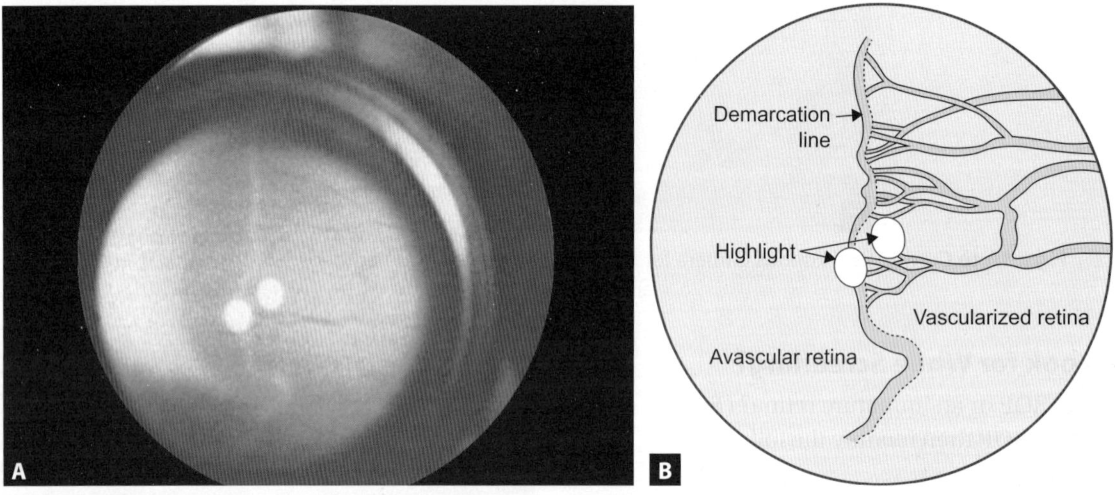

Figs. 6A and B: A thin flat line separates vascular from avascular retina with abnormal branching of vessels posteriorly (indicates earliest sign of abnormal vessel development). *[For color version (Fig. A), see Plate 18]*

AGGRESSIVE POSTERIOR RETINOPATHY OF PREMATURITY (FIG. 11)

This is characterized by the following:

- Rapidly evolving severe plus disease.
- Flat subtle neovascularization in zone 1 or posterior zone 2.
- Intraretinal shunting, hemorrhages.
- Rapid progression to stage 4 or 5 without passing through stage 2 or 3 leading to retinal detachment.
- Requires repeated laser treatment.

Is Retinopathy of Prematurity Treatable/ What are the Available Treatment Options?

Now that we have understood that abnormal vessels come from avascular retina, ablating the peripheral avascular

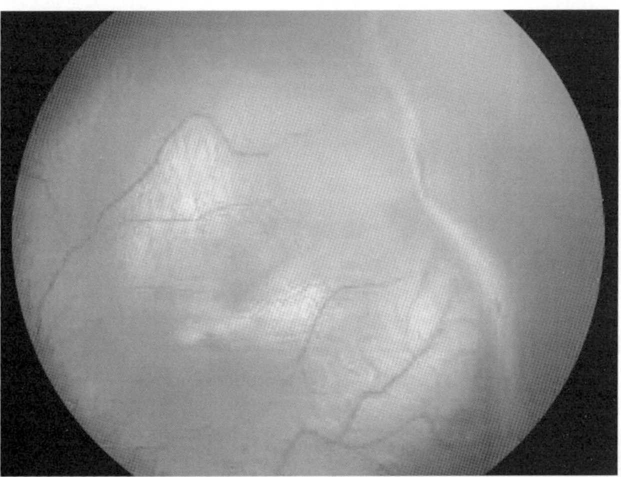

Fig. 7: *Stage II:* The Ridge—this is the hallmark of the stage 2 disease. It arises from the demarcation line and has length and width. It extends above the plane of the retina. *(For color version, see Plate 18)*

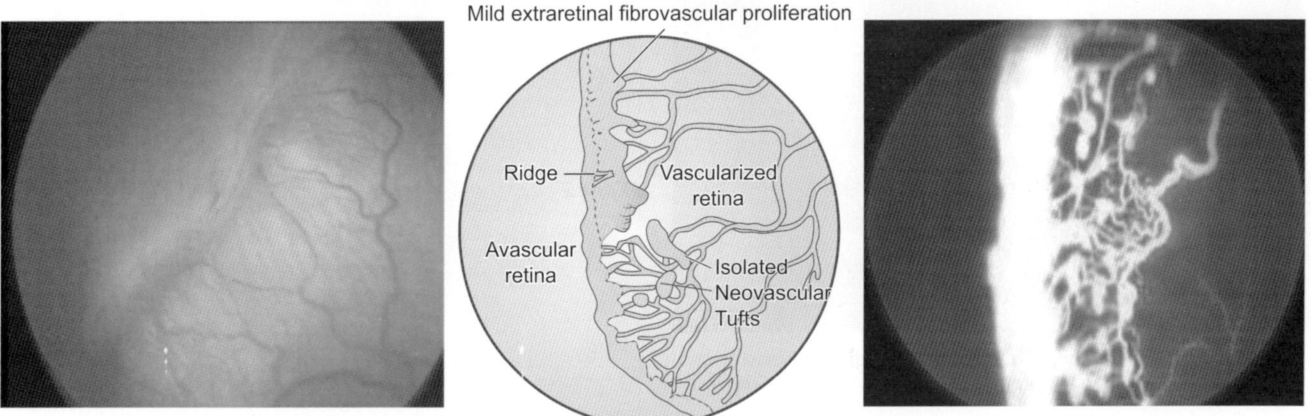

Fig. 8: Stage III: Extraretinal fibrovascular proliferation–new vessels grow beyond the ridge into the vitreous (this may lead to retinal detachment).

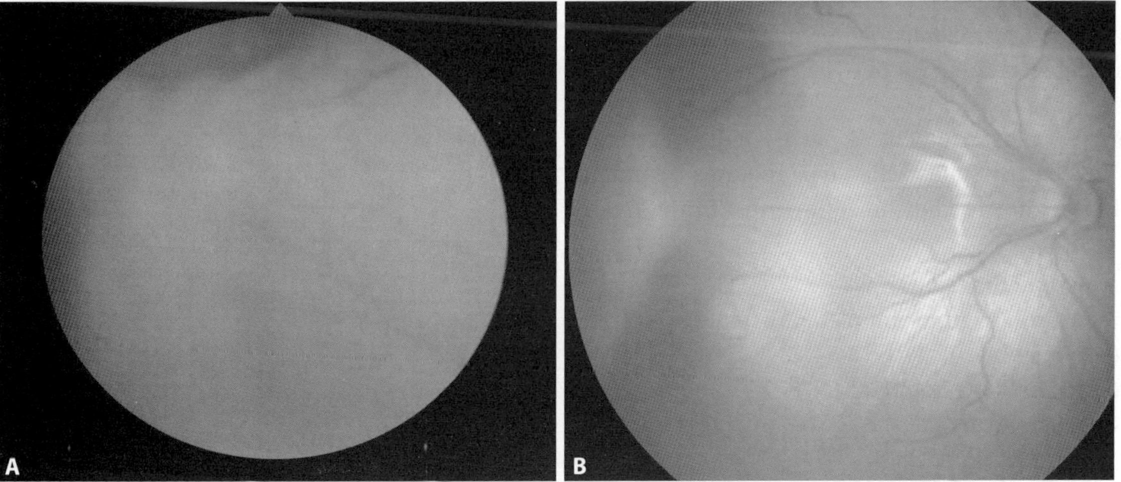

Figs. 9A and B: Partial retinal detachment (A) Stage IVa: Macula not involved; (B) Stage IVb: Macula involved. *(For color version, see Plate 18)*

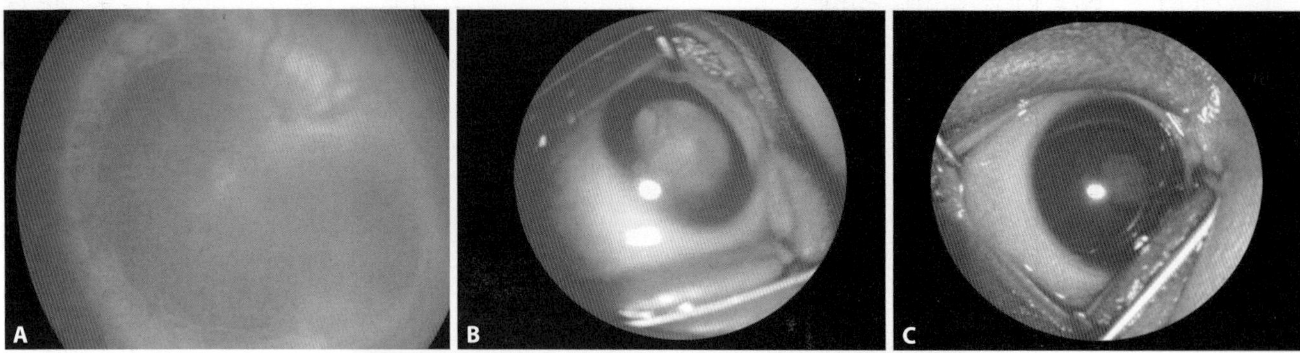

Figs. 10A to C: Plus disease. *(For color version, see Plate 18)*

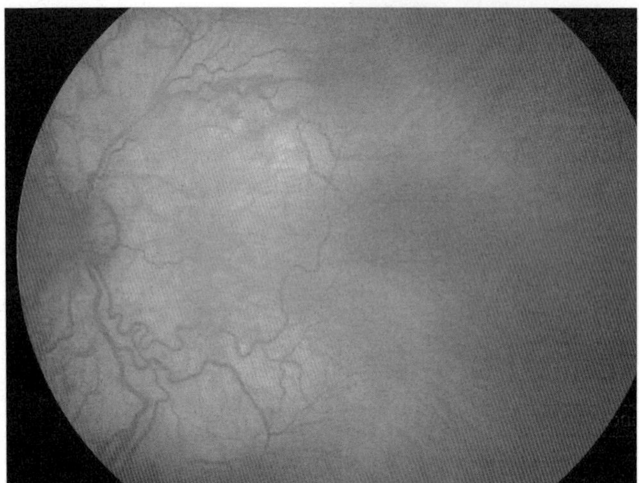

Fig. 11: Left eye of a preterm infant with aggressive posterior retinopathy of prematurity (APROP). *(For color version, see Plate 19)*

retina can lead to regression of the ROP. Earlier CRYO-ROP Study treatment guidelines were followed, but with ETROP Study, there has been a paradigm shift from cryotherapy to laser treatment. Laser therapy is more precise and reduces the unfavorable side effects of CRYO with >90% success rate.

Laser treatment protocol as per ETROP study is as follows. This clearly states which type requires treatment and which are to be kept on follow-up **(Table 1 and Boxes 1 and 2)**.

When can we end the follow up:

- Retinal vascularization completed (usually by 40th or 45 weeks of PMA).
- Regression of ROP noted.
- ROP advances to the stage where treatment is indicated.

Treatment Options (Figs. 12 and 13)

- Laser
- Antivascular endothelial growth factor injections (Anti-VEGFs)
  - Primary therapy in aggressive posterior retinopathy of prematurity (APROP) as it improves the media haze prior to laser.
- Surgery
  - Vitrectomy
  - Scleral buckle

TABLE 1: Zone-wise follow ups and treatment.

Zone 1		
No Plus	Stage 1	Follow
	Stage 2	Follow
	Stage 3	Treat
Plus	Stage 1	Treat
	Stage 2	Treat
	Stage 3	Treat
Zone 2		
No Plus	Stage 1	Follow
	Stage 2	Follow
	Stage 3	Follow
Plus	Stage 1	Follow
	Stage 2	Treat
	Stage 3	Treat

BOX 1: Type 1: Requires treatment.

- *Zone 1*: Any stage with plus disease, stage 3 with or without plus disease.
- *Zone 2:* Stage 2 or 3 with plus disease.

BOX 2: Type 2: Requires observation.

- *Zone 1:* Stage 1 or stage 2 without plus disease.
- *Zone 2:* Stage 3 without plus disease.

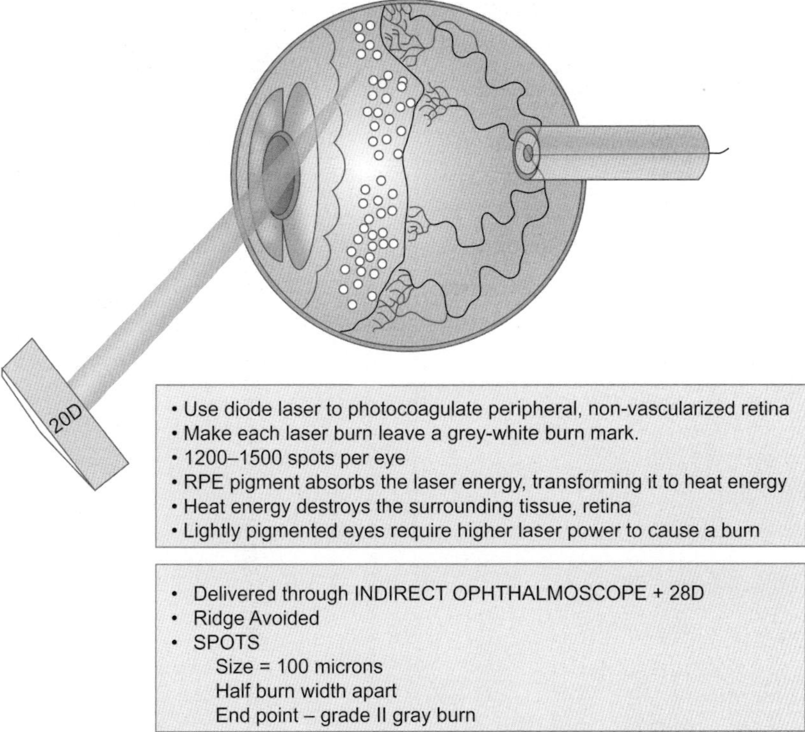

Fig. 12: Laser.

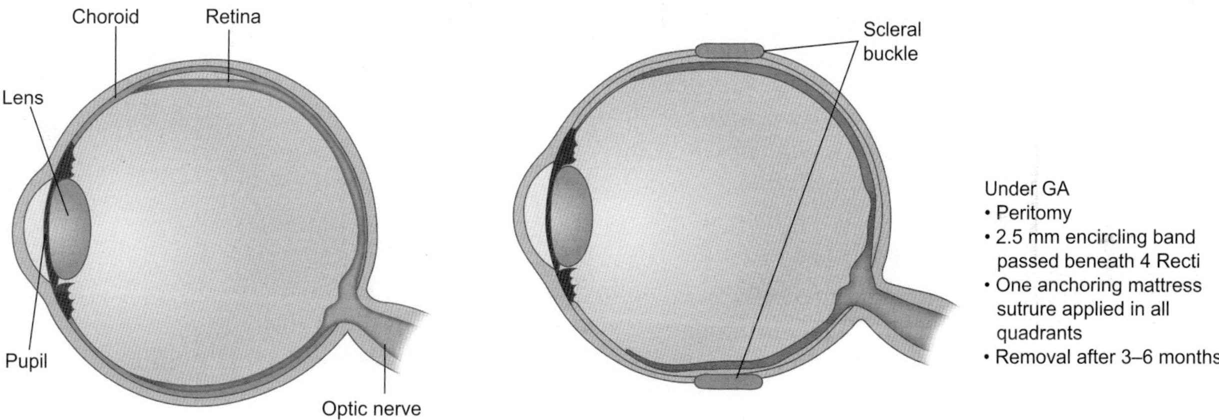

Fig. 13: Scleral buckle.

SUGGESTED READING

1. Cryotherapy for retinopathy of prematurity cooperative group. Multicentric trial of retinopathy of prematurity: 3 months outcome. Arch Ophthalmol. 1990;108:195-204.
2. Early Treatment of Retinopathy of Prematurity Cooperative Group. Revised indications for treatment of retinopathy of prematurity: results of early treatment of retinopathy of prematurity randomized trial. Arch Ophthalmol. 2003;121:1684-96.
3. Fierson WM. Screening examination of premature infants for retinopathy of prematurity. Pediatrics. 2013;131:189-95
4. Jalali S, Anand R, Kumar H, Dogra MR, Azad R, Gopal L. Programme planning and screening strategy in retinopathy of prematurity. Indian J Ophthalmol. 2003;51(1):89-99.
5. Pejawar R, Vinekar A, Bilagi A. National Neonatology Foundation's Evidence-based Clinical Practise Guidelines (2010). India, New Delhi: Retinopathy of Prematurity, NNF; 2010. pp. 253-62.
6. Terry TL. Extreme prematurity and fibroblastic overgrowth of persistent vascular sheath behind each crystalline lens. I. Preliminary report. Am J Ophthalmol. 1942;25:203-4.

SECTION 18

Ear, Nose, and Throat

Section Editor: *Ameet Kishore*

Newborn Hearing Screening and Management

Neevita Narayan

INTRODUCTION

Hearing impairment in children across the world contributes to a serious obstacle to their development and education, including language acquisition. According to a range of studies and surveys conducted in different countries, around 2–5 in every 1,000 neonates and infants have congenital or early childhood onset sensorineural deafness or severe-to-profound hearing impairment. The prevalence of hearing impairment is much more common than other common congenital anomalies that are screened for **(Table 1)**.

Deaf and hearing-impaired children often experience delayed development of speech, language, and cognitive skills, which may result in slow learning and difficulty progressing in school.

Congenital and early childhood onset of severe-to-profound hearing impairment may affect the auditory neural pathway of children at a later developmental stage if appropriate and optimal interventions are not provided within the critical period of central auditory pathway development. Therefore, early detection is extremely important aspect in providing appropriate support for hearing-impaired babies that will help them enjoy equal opportunities in society alongside all other children.

TABLE 1: Comparison of the incidence of common congenital anomalies.

Disorder	*Rate per 100,000*
Adrenal hyperplasia	2
Galactosemia	2
Phenylketonuria	3
Sickle cell disease	47
Hypothyroidism	28
Down's syndrome	100–125
Hearing impairment	200–400

Universal screening is preferable, since about 50% of infants with hearing loss are not discovered if neonatal hearing screening is restricted to only high-risk groups **(Box 1)**.

CLINICAL PEARLS

- Almost 50% children born with hearing impairment have no known risk factors.
- Therefore, high risk register is not good enough.
- Hearing screening should be applied universally to all babies.

BOX 1: The high risk register.

List of situations where a hearing impairment can be expected:

- Family history of permanent childhood sensorineural hearing loss
- In utero infection such as *Cytomegalovirus*, *Rubella* toxoplasmosis, or *Herpes*
- Craniofacial anomalies, including those with morphological abnormalities of the pinna and ear canal
- Neonatal indicators, specifically hyperbilirubinemia at a serum level requiring exchange transfusion, persistent pulmonary hypertension of the newborn (PPHN) associated with mechanical ventilation, and conditions requiring the use of extracorporeal membrane oxygenation (ECMO)
- Postnatal infections associated with sensorineural hearing loss, including bacterial meningitis
- Stigmata or other findings associated with a syndrome known to include a sensorineural or conductive hearing loss or eustachian tube dysfunction
- Syndromes associated with progressive hearing loss such as neurofibromatosis, osteopetrosis, and Usher syndrome
- Neurodegenerative disorders, such as Hunter syndrome, or sensory motor neuropathies, such as Charcot-Marie-Tooth syndrome
- Parental or caregiver concern regarding hearing, speech, language, and/or developmental delay
- Head trauma
- Recurrent or persistent otitis media with effusion lasting for at least 3 months

The Joint Committee on Infant Hearing (JCIH), position statement 2019, endorses early detection and early intervention for all infants who are, or who are at risk of being or becoming, hard of hearing. The goals *of early hearing detection and intervention (EHDI)* are to maximize language and communication competence, literacy development, and psychosocial well-being for children who are hard of hearing. Without appropriate language exposure and access, these children will fall behind their hearing peers in communication, language, speech, cognition, reading, and social-emotional development, and delays may continue to affect the child's life into adulthood. With early detection and appropriate, targeted intervention, developmental milestones for an infant who is hard of hearing can be expected to be achieved, more accurately reflecting the child's true potential. Focusing on the importance of prompt diagnosis and timely, high-quality early intervention for such infants, EHDI systems should facilitate seamless transitions for infants and their families through the processes of screening, audiologic and medical diagnosis, and intervention.

Universal newborn hearing screening (UNHS) has resulted in significantly lowering the average age of identification. Screening is a necessary first step, but does not ensure the next critical steps of timely identification and diagnosis of children who are hard of hearing, amplification, and referral to early intervention, all with the goal of promoting language development.

The goal of EHDI is to assure that all infants are identified as early as possible, and appropriate intervention initiated, no later than 3–6 months of age. There is a body of literature which demonstrates that children and families experience optimal outcomes when these benchmarks are met. Additionally, communication and linguistic competence (in spoken language, signed language, or both) are achievable when timelines are met, and when optimal audiologic and early intervention services are accessible.

UNIVERSAL NEWBORN HEARING SCREENING/EARLY HEARING DETECTION AND INTERVENTION 1-3-6 GOALS

- All infants should undergo hearing screening prior to discharge from the birth hospital and no later than 1 month of age, using physiologic measures with objective determination of outcome.
- All infants whose initial birth-screen and any subsequent rescreening warrant additional testing should have appropriate audiologic evaluation to confirm the infant's hearing status no later than 3 months of age.
- A concurrent or immediate comprehensive otologic evaluation should occur for infants who are confirmed to be hard of hearing.
- All infants who are hard of hearing in one or both ears should be referred immediately to early intervention in order to receive targeted and appropriate services.
- A simplified, coordinated point of entry into an intervention system appropriate for identified children is optimal.
- Early intervention services should be offered through an approach that reflects the family's preferences and goals for their child, and should begin as soon as possible after diagnosis but no later than 6 months of age.
- The child and family should have immediate access, through their audiologist, to high-quality, well-fitted, and optimized hearing aid technology. Access should also be assured, depending on the child's needs, to cochlear implants (CI), hearing assistive technologies, and visual alerting and informational devices.

NEWBORN HEARING SCREENING PROGRAMS AND SCREENING TECHNIQUES

Multidisciplinary teams of professionals including audiologists, physicians, and nursing personnel are needed to establish the UNHS component of EHDI programs. An audiologist with experience in evaluating newborns and young children should be involved in the development and oversight of each component of the hearing screening program, whenever possible, at the individual or at hospital level. Hospitals and agencies should also designate a physician to oversee the medical aspects of the EHDI program. Reporting and communication protocols must be well-defined, and such protocols must include the content of reports to physicians and to families, documentation of results in medical records, flow of screening result information from hospital-based medical records to outpatient records. Hospitals should identify and define the referral pathway and systems for ensuring that each baby who does not pass in-patient screening has access to a pediatric audiologist who can complete the outpatient rescreening, and when indicated, complete a diagnostic audiologic evaluation according to the EHDI 1-3-6 goals.

OBJECTIVE PHYSIOLOGIC SCREENING MEASURES

Objectively-determined physiologic measures must be used to screen newborns and young infants to identify those who may be hard of hearing.

Currently such measures include automated otoacoustic emission (OAE) and auditory brainstem response (ABR). Automated OAE protocols use either transient-evoked OAEs (TEOAE) or distortion-product OAEs (DPOAE). Both automated OAE and ABR technologies provide noninvasive recordings of physiologic activity underlying normal auditory function. Both are easily performed in neonates and infants, and both have been successfully used for UNHS programs.

There are, however, important differences between the two measures. OAE measures a physiologic response from the cochlear outer hair cells, while ABR measurements reflect both cochlear status, as well as auditory neural function extending beyond the cochlea into the brainstem. Thus, the ABR response reflects activity from a greater portion of the auditory pathway than does the OAE.

For this reason, ABR will result in a failed outcome when screening infants with auditory neuropathy, whereas screening with OAEs will result in a pass for the baby with *auditory neuropathy*.

Both OAE and ABR screening technologies can be used to detect whether the child has a sensory hearing loss. However, the results obtained using either technology are affected by outer ear or middle ear dysfunction that might be present. Therefore, conditions of the outer ear and/or middle ear would result in a failed hearing screening in the presence of normal cochlear and/or neural function.

Use of OAE as a screening tool is likely to result in a higher fail rate in the immediate postbirth period as compared with automated auditory brainstem response (AABR). OAE test is faster and easier than AABR, but with higher false positive rate. The most ideal hearing screening protocol should be tailored according to the center. **Flowcharts 1 and 2** give examples of protocols that can be used for both the well-baby nursery and the neonatal intensive care unit (NICU) graduates.

KEY COMPONENTS OF AN AUDIOLOGIC DIAGNOSTIC EVALUATION IN AN INFANT

Audiologic diagnosis of the infant is the sole purview of the audiologist with specific skills, knowledge, and access

Flowchart 1: Newborn hearing screening protocol: Well-baby nursery.

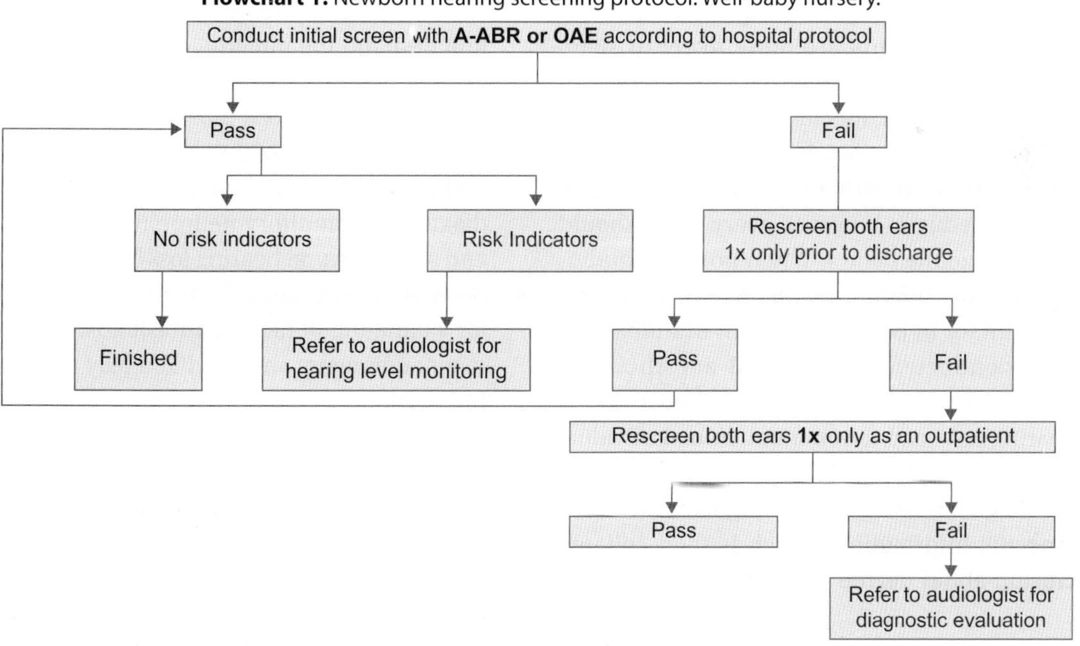

(A-ABR: automated auditory brainstem response; OAE: otoacoustic emission)

Source: Created by ASHA with information adapted from "Year 2019 Position Statement: Principles and Guidelines for Early Hearing Detection and Intervention Programs," by The Joint Committee on Infant Hearing. The Journal of Early Hearing Detection and Intervention. 2019;4(2):1-44.

Flowchart 2: Newborn Hearing Screening Protocol: NICU.

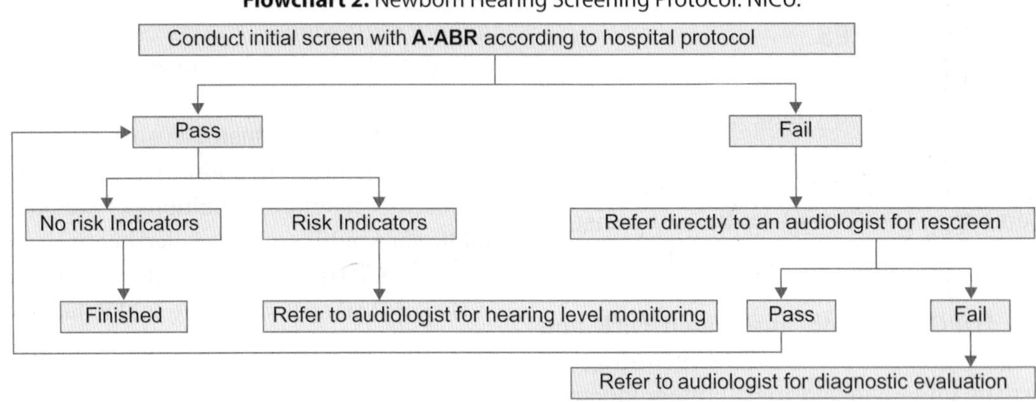

(A-ABR: automated auditory brainstem response; OAE: otoacoustic emission)
Source: Created by ASHA with information adapted from "Year 2019 Position Statement: Principles and Guidelines for Early Hearing Detection and Intervention Programs," by The Joint Committee on Infant Hearing. The Journal of Early Hearing Detection and Intervention. 2019;4(2):1-44.

to all necessary equipment for infant and early childhood audiologic diagnostic evaluations. Testing is performed to quantify frequency-specific thresholds for air- and bone-conduction stimuli, and to determine the type and degree of hearing loss in each ear to guide the fitting of hearing aids.

In keeping with the 1-3-6 (or 1-2-3) EHDI goals, audiologic diagnosis should be completed no later than 2–3 months of age. This earlier age facilitates the diagnostic process as infants are more likely to sleep for prolonged periods of time required to complete all measures. In children with special health needs, delay in diagnosis of hearing loss may be unavoidable due to attention paid to other health/time-urgent diagnostic and treatment procedures; however, every effort should be made to minimize the delays. When possible, audiologists can evaluate infants in the NICU, pediatric intensive care unit, or in conjunction with examinations or procedures conducted with general anesthesia or sedation. Infant hearing should be assessed only by battery of hearing tests and never stand-alone individual test. Test battery approach should be followed for correct and accurate diagnosis of infant hearing loss. Each test highlights specific information, which is then collated and a conclusion about degree and type of hearing loss is made.

- *Auditory brainstem response* is the gold standard test for threshold estimation for infants and children who cannot complete behavioral audiologic assessment. ABR provides ear- and frequency-specific threshold estimates that are necessary for the diagnosis of the type, degree, and configuration of hearing loss and provision of amplification.
- *Measures of middle ear function* should be completed as part of the diagnostic audiologic process for infants and young children. Either tympanometry or wideband reflectance can be used to characterize middle ear function.
- *Acoustic reflexes* are an important test of middle ear function and the integrity of auditory brainstem path ways.
- *Otoacoustic emissions* provide important information about the integrity of the outer hair cells of the cochlea and provide critical information about the differential diagnosis of auditory neuropathy spectrum disorder and sensorineural hearing loss (SNHL).
- *Behavioral assessment* of hearing is the gold standard for estimation of hearing thresholds. Visual reinforcement audiometry and condition play audiometry (CPA; for toddlers 24+ months) are established methods based on conditioned responses to sound.

OTOACOUSTIC EMISSIONS

Otoacoustic emissions (OAE) are sounds generated from the outer hair cells of the cochlea transmitted across the middle ear to the external ear canal, where they can be recorded. The production of an OAE is a marker for inner ear health and a simple way to screen for hearing loss. There are two types of OAE: spontaneous OAE (SOAE), which occur continuously without external stimuli, and evoked OAE (EOAE), which requires an acoustic stimulus prior to its measurement.

The ease of performing OAE is permitted now with automated units that include an aural probe that contains a speaker to deliver the acoustic stimulus and a microphone to detect the emissions **(Fig. 1)**. These systems provide an easily reproducible, noninvasive method to assess hearing in newborns, young children, and adults who are unable to cooperate for conventional hearing tests. The all-or-nothing response from OAE makes OAE an excellent screening test for hearing loss. The UNHS has widely been adopted in most of developed countries.

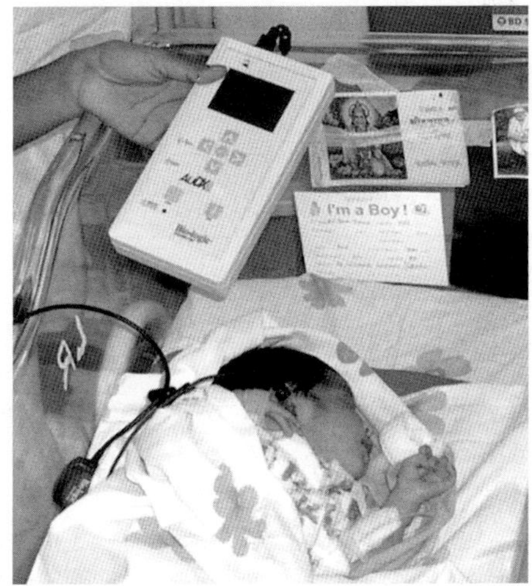

Fig. 1: Otoacoustic emissions being tested in the nursery.

AUDITORY BRAINSTEM RESPONSE

Evoked potentials are electrical potentials that occur in a group of neurons in response to stimulation of a sensory organ which can be recorded by surface electrodes. Testing evoked potentials is useful in assessing the integrity of neuronal pathways both at sensory and motor levels of neural control. Early auditory evoked potentials include cochlear and brainstem auditory-evoked potentials, popularly known as electrocochleogram, and auditory brainstem response. Evoked potential audiometry is a neurotheological test to assess auditory pathway function in response to auditory stimuli.

Auditory brainstem response mainly assesses brainstem functions and integrity. These evoked potentials are widely used for assessment of the cochlear functions, auditory nerve, and the brainstem. Most common indications for auditory evoked potentials include routine newborn hearing screening for auditory pathway deficits, detecting retro cochlear pathologies, intraoperative and intensive care monitoring, frequency-related measurement of auditory sensitivity, and for diagnosing some demyelinating disorders in initial stages **(Figs. 2 and 3)**.

AUTOMATED AUDITORY BRAINSTEM AUDIOMETRY

The AABR screener is a dedicated hearing screening device which provides information not only about the

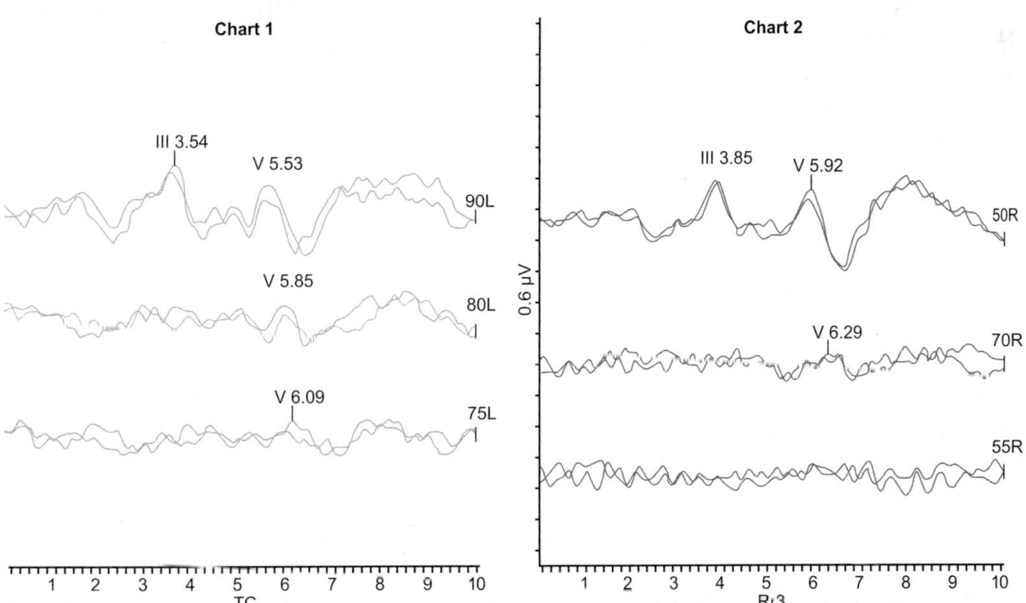

Fig. 2: Typical normal auditory brainstem response (ABR) response in left (Chart 1) and right (Chart 2) ears with wave III and V marked.

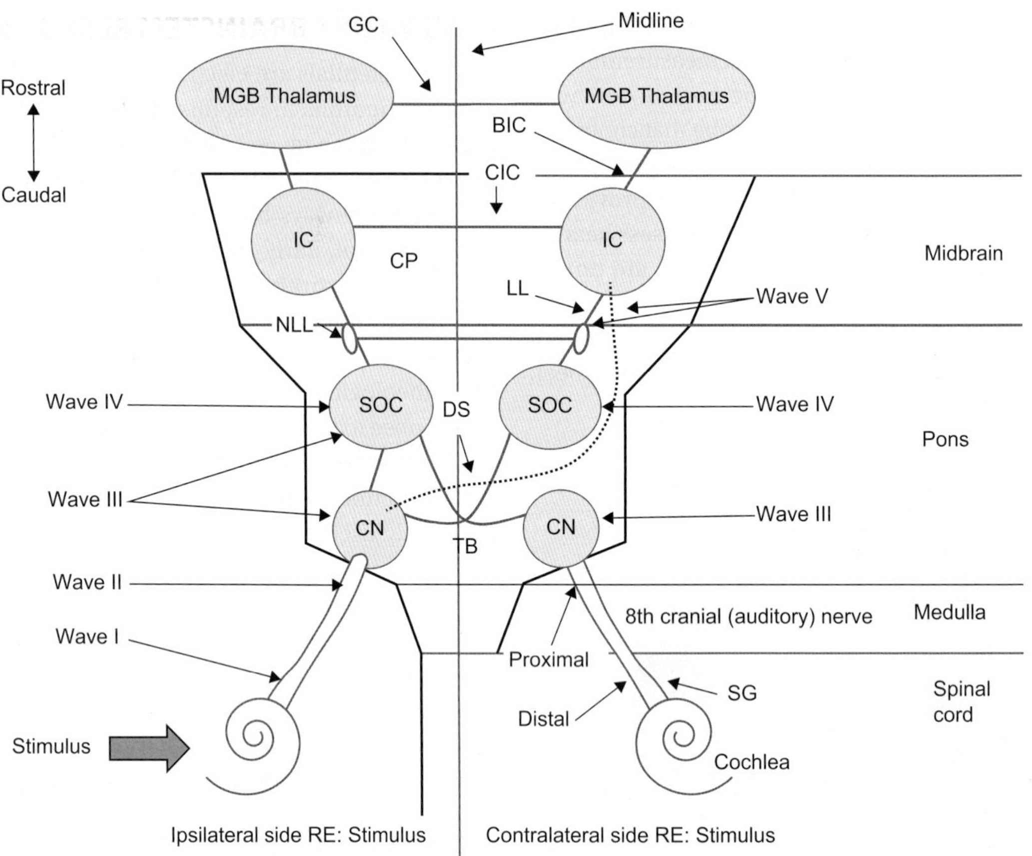

Fig. 3: Generators of the auditory brainstem response (ABR) response.

outer/middle ear and cochlea but also about the auditory pathway up to the brainstem. AABR has an agreement with conventional auditory brainstem response up to 98%. It uses a 35 dB near hearing level click. No operator interpretation is needed and it can be used on the ward and during oxygen therapy without disturbance from ambient noise. The time necessary for screening varies with the setting, but ranges from 4 to 15 minutes.

TYMPANOMETRY

The tympanometry is an objective measure of middle ear effusion or eustachian tube dysfunction. It provides information about the compliance or mobility of the tympanic membrane, the pressure within the middle ear and the volume of the external ear canal. Tympanograms are classified as type A (normal), type B (indicating fluid behind the tympanic membrane), or type C (indicating eustachian tube dysfunction). The objective data obtained by tympanometry are a useful adjunct in the diagnosis and follow-up of middle ear disease.

ASSESSING INFANT/TODDLER WITH AUDITORY NEUROPATHY SPECTRUM DISORDER

Auditory neuropathy spectrum disorder (ANSD) may occur in association with specific conditions (i.e., extreme prematurity, hyperbilirubinemia, and hydrocephalus), or it may present in infants where no obvious causative factor is identified.

Audiological characteristics include the presence of OAEs and/or cochlear microphonics accompanied by poor morphology of the ABR and absent or elevated middle ear muscle reflexes. Pure-tone audiometry, when the infant is developmentally able to participate in behavioral testing, is typically characterized by bilateral or unilateral fluctuating or stable thresholds which may range from mild to profound. Some of these children may have severe neurological involvement and may not ever be able to participate in behavioral evaluation. Until such time that reliable behavioral thresholds can be determined and hearing status appears to be stable, infants with auditory neuropathy may require frequent audiological monitoring to assess progression, improvement, or fluctuation in electrophysiological threshold estimates. ABR monitoring, however, cannot be used to determine or to demonstrate change in hearing sensitivity, as the hallmark Wave V is not present in ABR recordings of infants or children with auditory neuropathy.

Additional Testing Considerations

Additional laboratory testing to be considered in the process of evaluating a newborn or infant diagnosed with SNHL and to rule out the most common etiologies that impact intervention plans include (1) connexin gene, (2) electrocardiogram, and (3) urine and saliva swabs for congenital cytomegalovirus (cCMV).

Connexin 26 and Connexin 30 Genes

Mutations in this gene account for a significant number of nonsyndromic cases. As the inheritance is autosomal recessive, these children frequently have a negative family history for other family members who are deaf or hard of hearing. In the absence of other risk factors, these children may or may not pass the birth screen. Developmental surveillance and parental concern play an important role in monitoring infants who are unknowingly at risk for progressive hearing changes due to this genetic condition.

Electrocardiogram

An electrocardiogram is carried out among children who are profoundly deaf to identify a long QT interval—Jervell and Lange-Nielsen syndrome. This rare autosomal recessive inherited condition can result in sudden death if undetected and therefore, the benefit far outweighs the cost of what may seem an unnecessary medical procedure.

Congenital Cytomegalovirus

The cCMV infection is a leading cause of congenital infection, occurring in 0.2–2% of live births worldwide and is a leading cause of nongenetic unilateral or bilateral SNHL. Since children with cCMV can develop late onset SNHL, all infants who test positive on a neonatal screen for cCMV require periodic monitoring by audiology to identify changes in hearing thresholds, with the provision of appropriate amplification and early intervention as indicated.

Incidence of Genetic Disorders

In large population studies, around 50% of the etiologies related to being deaf or hard of hearing are designated as hereditary; hundreds of syndromes and many different individual genes have been identified. The evaluation, therefore, should include a review of family history of specific genetic disorders or syndromes, genetic testing for gene mutations such as GJB2 (connexin-26), and syndromes commonly associated with early-onset hearing loss (see Risk Factors, **Table 2**).

Surveillance and Rescreening for Children with Risk Factors

The majority of all infants identified as hard of hearing will be followed closely by an audiologist and otolaryngologist and receive indicated intervention and support services. However, a significant number of children will pass the newborn screen or rescreen who are at risk for later-onset hearing loss.

Table 2 shows a revised list of risk factors since the 2007 JCIH statement. The recommendations for follow-up and evaluation on this list of risk factors pertain to infants who pass the newborn screen or rescreen. These recommendations for follow-up are based on the fact that standard newborn screening procedures and protocols do not identify all children who are deaf or hard of hearing due to missed mild or neural hearing loss, progressive hearing loss, and delayed-onset hearing loss.

As shown in **Table 2**, the prior 11 risk factors listed in JCIH 2007 are now listed as 12 separate factors and divided into subgroups of predominantly perinatal (risk factors 1–9) and perinatal or postnatal (risk factors 10–12). In addition, the recommendations for follow-up and monitoring have been modified and are described in greater detail, and the age of audiologic diagnostic follow-up for children with risk factors who passed newborn hearing screening has been lowered for most risk factors to by 9 months of age. Supporting evidence for the revised JCIH risk factor recommendations is provided in the following sections.

Perinatal Risk Factors

The first nine risk factors occur solely in the perinatal period.

1. *Risk factor 1:* A history of family members being hard of hearing with onset in childhood, has consistently been shown to be predictive that the diagnosis is secondary

TABLE 2: Risk factors for early childhood hearing loss: guidelines for infants who pass the newborn hearing screen. Need for follow-up.

	Risk factor classification	*Recommended diagnostic follow-up*	*Monitoring frequency*
	Perinatal		
1.	Family history* of early, progressive, or delayed onset permanent childhood hearing loss	by 9 months	Based on etiology of family hearing toss and caregiver concern
2.	Neonatal intensive care of >5 days	by 9 months	
3.	Hyperbilirubinemia with exchange transfusion regardless of length of stay	by 9 months	As per concerns of on-going surveillance of hearing skills and speech milestones
4.	Aminoglycoside administration for >5 days**	by 9 months	
5.	Asphyxia or hypoxic Ischemic Encephalopathy	by 9 months	
6.	Extracorporeal membrane oxygenation (ECMO)*	No later than 3 months after occurrence	Every 12 months to school age or at shorter intervals based on concerns of parent or provider
7.	In utero infections, such as herpes, rubella, syphilis, and toxoplasmosis	by 9 months	As per concerns of on-going surveillance
	In utero infection with cytomegalovirus (CMV)*	No later than 3 months after occurrence	Every 12 months to age 3 or at shorter intervals based on parent/provider concerns
	Mother + Zika and infant with no laboratory evidence and no clinical findings	Standard	As per AAP (2017) Periodicity schedule
	• Mother + Zika and infant with laboratory evidence of Zika + clinical findings • Mother + Zika and infant with laboratory evidence of Zika—clinical findings	• A-ABR by 1 month • A-ABR by 1 month	• ABR by 4–6 months or VRA by 9 months • ABR by 4–6 months: Monitor as per AAP (2017) Periodicity schedule (Adebanjo et al., 2017)
8.	Certain birth conditions or findings: • Craniofacial malformations including microtia/atresia, ear dysplasia, oral facial clefting, white forelock, and microphthalmia • Congenital microcephaly. Congenital or acquired hydrocephalus • Temporal bone abnormalities	by 9 months	As per concerns of on going surveillance of hearing skills and speech milestones
9.	Over 400 syndromes have been identified with atypical hearing thresholds.*** For more information, visit the Hereditary Hearing Loss website (Van Camp & Smith, 2016)	by 9 months	According to natural history of syndrome or concerns
	Perinatal or postnatal		
10.	Culture-positive infections associated with sensorineural hearing loss,*** including confirmed bacterial and viral (especially herpes viruses and varicella) meningitis or encephalitis	No later than 3 months after occurrence	Every 12 months to school age or at shorter intervals based on concerns of parent or provider
11.	Events associated with hearing loss: • Significant head trauma especially basal skull/temporal bone fractures • Chemotherapy	No later than 3 months after occurrence	According to findings and or continued concerns
12.	Caregiver concern**** regarding hearing, speech, language, developmental delay and/or developmental regression	Immediate referral	According to findings and or continued concerns

*Infants at increased risk of delayed onset or progressive hearing loss
**Infants with toxic levels or with a known genetic susceptibility remain at risk
***Syndromes (Van Camp & Smith, 2016)
****Parental/caregiver concern should always prompt further evaluation.
(A-ABR: automated auditory brainstem response; AAP = American Academy of Pediatrics; VRA = visual reinforcement audiometry)

to a spectrum of genetic causes, and therefore stands alone as a particularly concerning risk factor.

2. *Risk factor 2:* Infants who require care in the NICU or special care nursery for >5 days is used as an indicator of illness severity.
3. *Risk factor 3:* Hyperbilirubinemia as a risk factor for hearing loss is impacted by multiple factors including illness severity, birth weight, rate of rise of bilirubin, clinical findings, postnatal age of the infant, and gestational age, as all premature infants have some degree of hyperbilirubinemia. Management of these infants should be based on established protocols. Hyperbilirubinemia requiring exchange transfusion is the only risk factor for which close follow-up is recommended regardless of length of stay in the NICU.
4. *Risk factor 4:* Aminoglycoside administration of >5 days is reaffirmed; administration of aminoglycoside antibiotics for <5 days is considered a risk factor only if toxic blood levels are identified or if there is a family history of a mitochondrial genetic mutation associated with aminoglycoside sensitivity for SNHL. Several mitochondrial deoxyribonucleic acid (DNA) mutations of the 12S ribosomal ribonucleic acid (rRNA) gene are known to be associated with an increased risk of aminoglycoside-induced hearing loss. However, aminoglycosides are one of the most common medications administered in the NICU. Studies have examined the frequency of the mitochondrial gene mutations in NICU populations and identified a rate of approximately 1–1.8%.
5. *Risk factor 5:* Perinatal asphyxia, also termed hypoxic ischemic encephalopathy, particularly if requiring hypothermia treatment, is noted, because of the illness severity of this subgroup of infants and the significant increase in permanently elevated hearing thresholds.
6. *Risk factor 6:* Extracorporeal membrane oxygenation (ECMO) is specifically noted because of the increased risk of delayed-onset hearing loss.
7. *Risk factor 7:* In utero infections (i.e., herpes, rubella, syphilis, and toxoplasmosis) pose a risk and require follow-up by 9 months of age. cCMV infection is a leading cause of congenital infection occurring in 0.2–2% of live births worldwide and is a leading cause of nongenetic unilateral or bilateral early, progressive, and delayed onset SNHL. Therefore, the recommendation for follow-up audiologic assessment of infants with cCMV is no later than 3 months of age. Zika virus has been added to the list of in utero infections associated with hearing loss.
8. *Risk factor 8:* All craniofacial conditions and physical conditions associated with hearing loss are now included as the 8th risk factor (formerly risk factors 5 and 6).
9. *Risk factor 9:* More than 400 syndromes and genetic disorders associated with atypical hearing thresholds (formerly risk factors 7 and 8) are now included as the 9th risk factor.
10. *Risk factor 10:* Perinatal and postnatal confirmed bacterial and/or viral meningitis or encephalitis (especially herpes viruses and varicella and hemophilus influenza and pneumococcal meningitis are included in the 10th risk factor.
11. *Risk factor 11:* Predominantly postnatal events of significant head trauma particularly injury to the mastoid and chemotherapy comprise the 11th risk factor category.
12. *Risk factor 12:* Family/caregiver concern regarding hearing, speech, language, or development requires attention. The recommendation is immediate referral after discussion with family. When a caregiver expresses concern that the baby is not responsive to sound in the home environment, or about speech and/or language delays, it is recommended that the primary care provider obtain additional medical and language history and evaluate the child carefully for middle ear effusion.

MANAGEMENT OF HEARING LOSS FOLLOWING DIAGNOSIS OF HEARING LOSS

Mild-moderate conductive hearing loss: Conductive hearing losses in infants can be due to various reasons. Most common would be otitis media which can be treated by otolaryngologist by oral medication or ventilation tubes. Few may be due to craniofacial deformity or microtia-atresia, which may require bone conduction device use for early speech and language development.

Mild-severe sensory hearing loss: Infants diagnosed with this type of hearing loss require immediate referral to pediatric audiologists for early intervention program, which requires timely fitting of hearing aids before 3 months of age and enrolment in speech and language intervention with timely monitoring of its development.

Severe-profound sensory hearing loss: Infants diagnosed with hearing loss in this severity would require early intervention similar to mild-severe SNHL, with very strict surveillance of speech and language development. Many infants with this type of hearing loss would probably require a further intervention with Cochlear Implants for complete auditory access and speech and language development, as hearing aids do not provide adequate auditory access to sound for proper speech and language development equivalent to their hearing peers.

Neural or retro cochlear hearing loss: Infants having hearing loss due to auditory nerve deficiency, would probably get limited benefits from Cochlear Implants as well. Families are however provided options to avail either the limited benefit from Cochlear Implants or can have auditory access with auditory brainstem implants, or can choose an option away from mainstream to sign language. Families must be provided with all these options for the child as early as possible so that there is no ambiguity about which way to proceed.

SUGGESTED READING

1. Cannon MJ, Griffiths PD, Aston V, Rawlinson WD. Universal newborn screening for congenital CMV infection: what is the evidence of potential benefit? Rev Med Virol. 2014;24(5):291-307.
2. Cone-Wesson B, Vohr BR, Sininger YS, Widen JE, Folsom RC, Gorga MP, et al. Identification of neonatal hearing impairment: infants with hearing loss. Ear Hear. 2000;21(5):488-507.
3. de Lyra-Silva KA, Sanches SG, Neves-Lobo IF, Ibidi SM, Carvallo RM, et al. Middle ear muscle reflex measurement in neonates: Comparison between 1000Hz and 226Hz probe tones. Int J Pediatr Otorhinolaryngol. 2015; 79(9):1510-5.
4. Doutre SM, Barrett TS, Greenlee J, White KR. Losing Ground: Awareness of Congenital Cytomegalovirus in the United States. J Early Hear Detect Intervent. 2016;9(1):1-53.
5. Gorga MP, Johnson TA, Kaminski JR, Beauchaine KL, Garner CA, Neely ST. Using a combination of click- and tone burst-evoked auditory brain stem response measurements to estimate pure-tone thresholds. Ear Hear. 2006;27(1):60-74.
6. Gravel J, Berg A, Bradley M, Cacace A, Campbell D, Dalzell L, et al. New York State universal newborn hearing screening demonstration project: effects of screening protocol on inpatient outcome measures. Ear Hear. 2000;21(2):131-40.
7. Hood LJ. Auditory neuropathy/dys-synchrony disorder: diagnosis and management. Otolaryngol Clin North Am. 2015;48(6):1027-40.
8. Johnson JL, White KR, Widen JE, Gravel JS, James M, Kennalley T, et al. A multicenter evaluation of how many infants with permanent hearing loss pass a two-stage otoacoustic emissions/automated auditory brainstem response newborn hearing screening protocol. Pediatrics. 2005;116(3):663-72.
9. Kim SH, Choi HS, Han YE, Choi BY. Diverse etiologies manifesting auditory neuropathy characteristics from infants with profound hearing loss and clinical implications. Int J Pediatr Otorhinolaryngol. 2016;86:63-7.
10. Moeller MP, Carr G, Seaver L, Stredler-Brown A, Holzinger D. Best Practices in family-centered early intervention for children who are deaf or hard of hearing: an international consensus statement. J Deaf Stud Deaf Educ. 2013;18(4):429-45.
11. Morton CC, Nance WE. Newborn hearing screening-a silent revolution. N Engl J Med. 2006;354(20):2151-64.
12. Nance WE. The genetics of deafness. Ment Retard Dev Disabil Res Rev. 2003;9(2):109-19.
13. Norrix LW. Hearing thresholds, minimum response levels, and cross-check measures in pediatric audiology. Am J Audiol. 2015;24(2):137-44.
14. Norton SJ, Gorga MP, Widen JE, Folsom RC, Sininger Y, Cone-Wesson B, et al. Identification of neonatal hearing impairment: evaluation of transient evoked otoacoustic emission, distortion product otoacoustic emission, and auditory brain stem response test performance. Ear Hear. 2000;21(5):508-28.
15. Orzan E, Murgia A. Connexin 26 deafness is not always congenital. Int J Pediatr Otorhinolaryngol. 2007;71(3): 501-7.
16. Raveh E, Buller N, Badrana O, Attias J. Auditory neuropathy: clinical characteristics and therapeutic approach. Am J Otolaryngol. 2007;28(5):302-8.
17. Ross SA, Ahmed A, Palmer AL, Michaels MG, Sánchez PJ, Bernstein DI, et al.; National Institute on Deafness and Other Communication Disorders CHIMES Study. Detection of congenital cytomegalovirus infection by real-time polymerase chain reaction analysis of saliva or urine specimens. J Infect Dis. 2014;210(9):1415-8.
18. Sanford CA, Hunter LL, Feeney MP, Nakajima HH. Wideband Acoustic Immittance: Tympanometric Measures. Ear Hear. 2013;34:65s-71s.
19. Santos RL, Aulchenko YS, Huygen PL, van der Donk KP, de Wijs IJ, Kemperman MH, et al. Hearing impairment in Dutch patients with connexin 26 (GJB2) and connexin 30 (GJB6) mutations. International Journal of Pediatric Otorhinolaryngology. 2005;69(2):165-74.
20. Tarkan Ö, Sari P, Demirhan O, Kiroğlu M, Tuncer Ü, Sürmelioğlu Ö, et al. Connexin 26 and 30 mutations in paediatric patients with congenital, non-syndromic hearing loss treated with cochlear implantation in Mediterranean Turkey. J Laryngol Otol. 2013;127(1): 33-7.

21. The Journal of Early Hearing Detection and Intervention. Volume 4 Issue 3 pages 1-118. Journal of Early Hearing Detection and Intervention: Volume 9 Issue 1, pages 1-53, 4(3). (2019). Available from https://doi.org/10.26077/1aag-nc88 [Last accessed March, 2025].
22. Tomblin JB, Oleson JJ, Ambrose SE, Walker E, Moeller MP. The influence of hearing aids on the speech and language development of children with hearing loss. JAMA Otolaryngol Head Neck Surg. 2014;140(5):403-9.
23. Uhler K, Heringer A, Thompson N, Yoshinaga-Itano C. A tutorial on auditory neuropathy/dyssynchrony for the speech-language pathologist and audiologist. Semin Speech Lang. 2012;33(4):354-66.
24. Van Camp G, Smith R (2017). Hereditary Hearing Loss Homepage. Retrieved from http://hereditaryhearingloss.org/.
25. van Dyk M, Swanepoel de W, Hall JW 3rd. Outcomes with OAE and AABR screening in the first 48 h-Implications for newborn hearing screening in developing countries. Int J Pediatr Otorhinolaryngol. 2015;79(7):1034-40.
26. Walker EA, Holte L, Spratford M, Oleson J, Welhaven A, Harrison M. Timeliness of service delivery for children with later-identified mild-to-severe hearing loss. Am J Audiol. 2014;23(1):116-28.
27. Yamamoto AY, Mussi-Pinhata MM, Isaac Mde L, Amaral FR, Carvalheiro CG, Aragon DC, et al. Congenital cytomegalovirus infection as a cause of sensorineural hearing loss in a highly immune population. Pediatr Infect Dis J. 2011;30(12):1043-6.
28. Yoshinaga-Itano C, Baca RL, Sedey AL. Describing the trajectory of language development in the presence of severe-to-profound hearing loss: a closer look at children with cochlear implants versus hearing aids. Otol Neurotol. 2010;31(8):1268-74.
29. Yoshinaga-Itano C, Sedey AL, Coulter DK, Mehl AL. Language of early- and later-identified children with hearing loss. Pediatrics. 1998;102(5):1161-71.

Hoarseness in Pediatric Age Group

Sharad Nair, Ameet Kishore

INTRODUCTION

Communication or speech of children plays a key role in everyday life. Dysphonia and hoarseness are the terminology used for altered voice quality. Dysphonia is a commonly encountered clinical problem in pediatric practice. "Hoarseness" and "dysphonia" are terms used to describe changes in voice quality. In the pediatric population, the prevalence of hoarseness ranges from 6 to 23% of 4–12 years old children. The etiology of hoarseness can be classified as infectious, inflammatory, iatrogenic, traumatic, congenital, and functional.

Hoarseness can negatively affect the lives of children physically, socially, and emotionally. In contrast to the commonly held belief that children do not appear aware or concerned about the sound of their voices, children as young as 6 years express concerns about dysphonia.

The characteristic head and neck anatomy in children has an impact on voice production and dysphonia. The new born baby has a small mandible, smallmouth, large head, more fat pads at the cheeks, and tongue filling the entire oral cavity. All these anatomical characteristics have an impact on the speech of the child.

Behaviors of the male child are more impulsive and aggressive than a female child and are allied to anxiety, spirit of leadership, and excessive hyperactivity. These profiles of male child directly reflect in phonatory mechanisms leading to vocal abuse and thus making them more prone to pediatric hoarseness. As age increases in childhood, the larynx undergoes structural changes due to masculine hormones in adolescence, leading to enlargement of laryngeal dimension. In male adolescent, the new glottic configuration is characterized by longer vocal folds along with the acute angle of thyroid cartilage approximately 90°. During the adolescent period of male child, symptoms of hoarseness tend to decrease.

Such types of changes are not seen in adolescent girls. In adolescent girls, the vocal folds elongate 3–4 mm whereas in boys, it increases by 1 cm. Children in family with siblings are often prone for dysphonia and hoarseness **(Table 1)**.

One study showed that 65% of the children suffering from altered voice quality belonged to large families, i.e., more than two children, 30% of the children had a family history of dysphonia, and 57% of them are male child.

TABLE 1: Etiology.

Acquired lesion	*Congenital lesion*	*Functional*	*Thyroid issues*
• Vocal fold nodule • Vocal fold polyp • Vocal fold cyst • Laryngopharyngeal reflux • Vocal fold hemorrhagic polyp • Vocal cord granuloma • Laryngeal papilloma • Vocal fold sulcus • Vocal cord paralysis • Spasmodic dysphonia	• Anterior commissure synechiae • Laryngeal webs • Glottic stenosis • Vocal fold cyst • Vocal fold sulcus	• Impaired laryngeal mobility • Psychogenic • Adolescent voice disorders	

It is noteworthy that noisy surroundings need excessive demand for loud talking which increases the risk of hoarseness in voice. Phonotrauma in noisy environment is an important risk factor for causing hoarseness among children.

VOCAL NODULES

The most common etiology for hoarseness of voice among children is vocal fold nodules, which have been seen in 38–78% of the pediatric patients evaluated for hoarseness. Vocal abuse is an important factor for the development of vocal fold lesions due to phonotrauma, especially vocal nodules. Vocal nodules develop from repeated trauma to the vocal cords, resulting in an inflammatory reaction and damage to the microscopic layers of the vocal cord. They are often bilateral and commonly located at the junction of the anterior one-third and posterior two-thirds of the vocal fold where pressure of contact between the vocal cords is greatest **(Fig. 1)**.

Vocal Polyps

Vocal cord polyps are rarely seen in children. They are usually unilateral mostly noted in the superficial layer of vocal cord. They are more commonly encountered in a girl child with recent onset hoarseness. The lesion is mostly limited to children who scream sharply and suddenly **(Fig. 2)**.

Vocal Cord Cyst

Classified as epidermiod or mucus retention cyst. The former kind of cyst is diagnosed with dilated vasculature over its surface and have dense keratinized epithelium **(Fig. 3)**. Mucus retention cyst of vocal cord develops with obstructed glandular ducts which can easily rupture **(Fig. 4)**.

Sulcus Vocalis

Sulcus vocalis is a rare lesion affecting one or both of the mucosal surfaces of the vocal folds. It is characterized by a linear groove on the mucosal surface of the vocal fold with varying depths, at times approaching or touching the vocal ligament thus affecting the vibratory function of vocal cords leading to hoarseness of voice **(Fig. 5)**.

Vocal Cord Granuloma and Vocal Cord Hemorrhagic Polyp

These are usually formed as a response to local trauma to the vocal cord during intubation, chemical effect of laryngopharyngeal reflux or acute phonotraumatic effect. These are benign inflammatory lesions in response to trauma **(Figs. 6 and 7)**.

Juvenile Onset Recurrent Respiratory Papillomatosis

An infection of the upper airway by the human papilloma virus (HPV). Viral transmission is usually acquired from birth. Approximately 75% of cases present before 5 years of age and 25% occur between 5 and 12 years of age, which is thought to be caused by latent virus remaining in the laryngeal tissues. The symptoms can progress from mild hoarseness to dyspnea and stridor as the papillomas progress and obstruct the glottic airway **(Fig. 8)**.

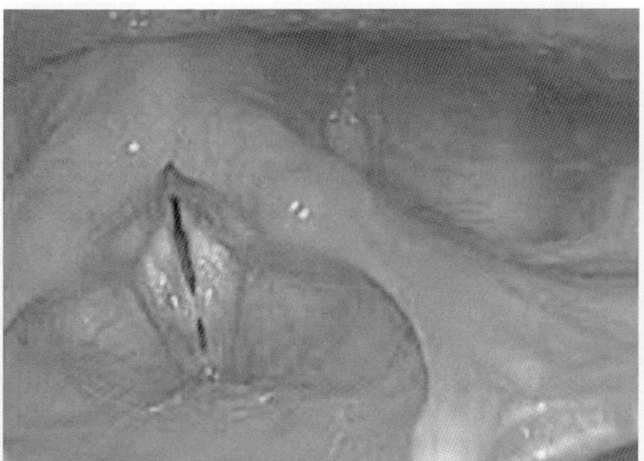
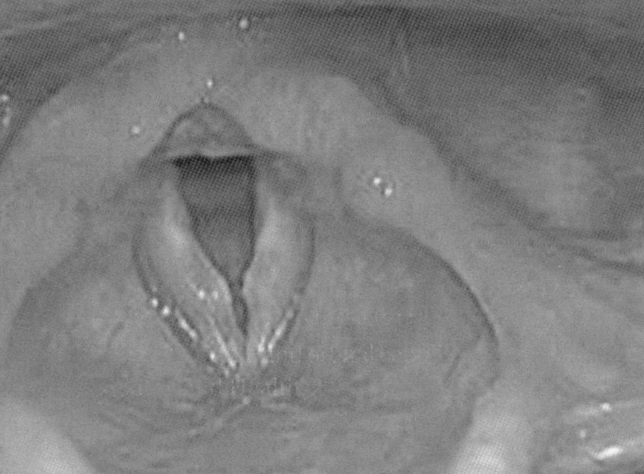

Fig. 1: Laryngoscopic image of a 7-year-old boy with bilateral vocal cord nodule. *(For color version, see Plate 19)*

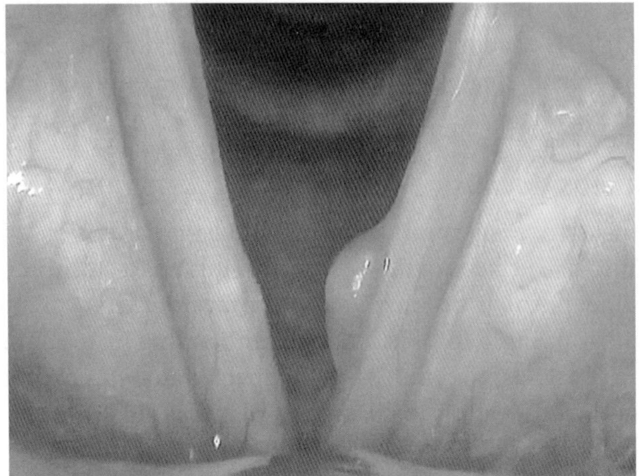

Fig. 2: Laryngoscopic image of 9-year-old girl with left vocal cord polyp. *(For color version, see Plate 19)*

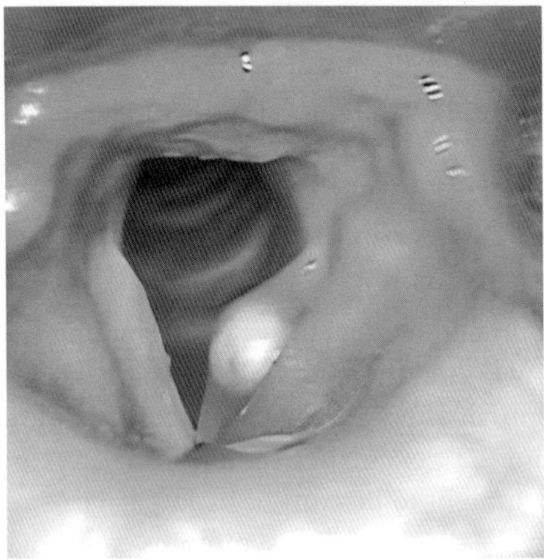

Fig. 3: Laryngoscopic image of left vocal cord epidermoid cyst. *(For color version, see Plate 19)*

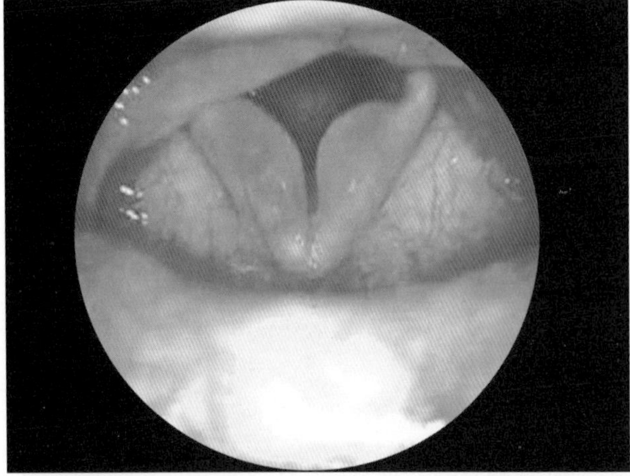

Fig. 4: Laryngoscopic image of bilateral vocal cord mucus retention cyst. *(For color version, see Plate 20)*

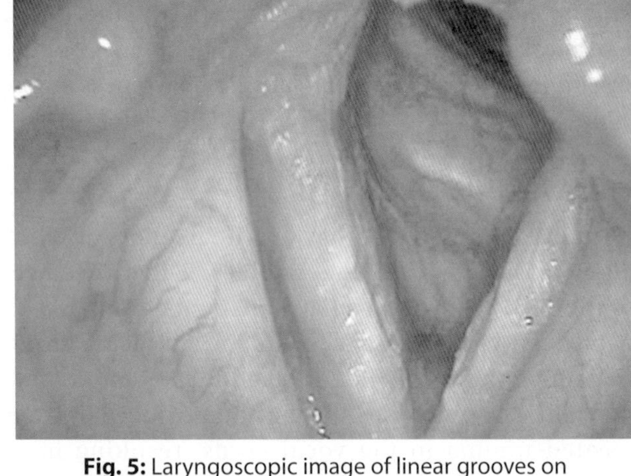

Fig. 5: Laryngoscopic image of linear grooves on bilateral vocal cords. *(For color version, see Plate 20)*

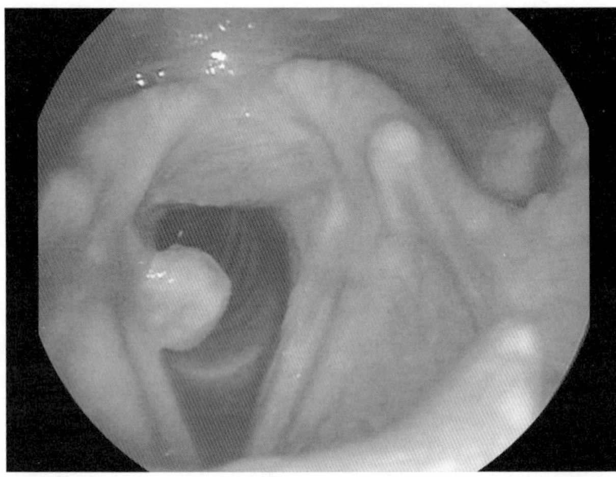

Fig. 6: Laryngoscopic image of right vocal cord granuloma. *(For color version, see Plate 20)*

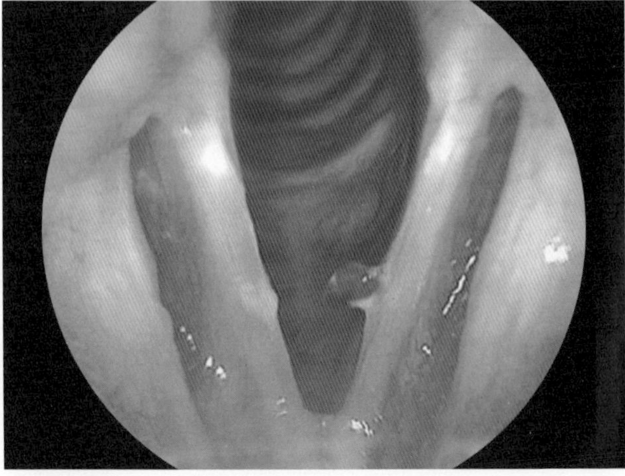

Fig. 7: Laryngoscopic image of hemorrhagic polyp. *(For color version, see Plate 20)*

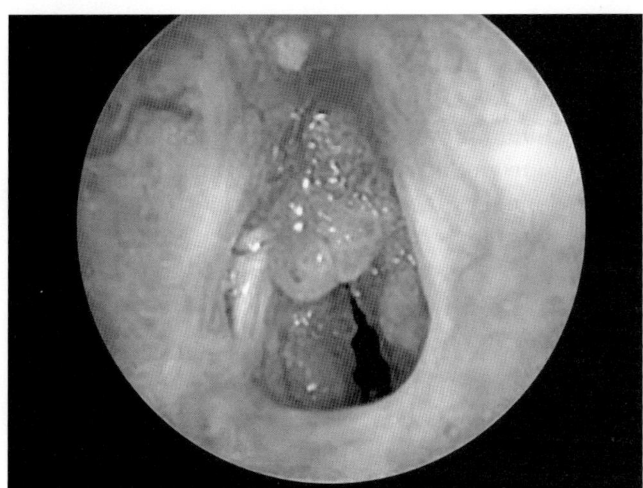

Fig. 8: Laryngoscopic image of juvenile onset juvenile onset recurrent respiratory papillomatosis (JORRP) of larynx. *(For color version, see Plate 20)*

The pediatric form, juvenile onset recurrent respiratory papillomatosis (JORRP), is the more aggressive subtype. Laryngeal mucosal RRP is affected most often by the low-risk subtypes, human papillomavirus (HPV)-6, and HPV-11, which accounts for approximately 90% of JORRP.

The child or the young adult usually presents with hoarseness or weak cry which can worsen into severe respiratory distress that can require an airway stabilization with multiple debulking surgery which is the mainstay of treatment. Children who require more than four surgical procedures have rapid regrowth, or airway compromise should be considered for adjunct medical therapy.

Alpha interferon was the first widely employed of these therapies and now available as pegylated interferon. The cyclooxygenase-2 enzyme is a growth stimulator and overexpressed in RRP, and celecoxib, a nonsteroidal anti-inflammatory drug, may inhibit the papilloma growth.

Cidofovir is an antiviral and the most widely used adjunct therapy for RRP, although there is insufficient evidence from randomized controlled trials to support the efficacy of antiviral agents. Cidofovir reduces the efficiency of deoxyribonucleic acid (DNA) transcription on the growing DNA chain. Dose ranges of 2.5–15 mg/mL have been reported, and a review of the literature recently indicated that higher infiltrated doses result in longer relapse free times. Furthermore, previous concerns of use of cidofovir and increased malignant transformation have been refuted by studies demonstrating no statistical difference in cidofovir and noncidofovir groups.

Bevacizumab is a chemotherapeutic agent used to inhibit growth of papillomas. Bevacizumab is recombinant humanized monoclonal immunoglobulin G1 antibody that binds to and inhibits the biologic activity of human vascular endothelial growth factor *in vitro* and *in vivo*. There is evidence that vascular endothelial growth factor is an important factor in the development of RRP, and there have been some recent reports of promising results achieved with relatively high dosing (45–50 mg) of bevacizumab in all patients treated. The dose approved by the US Food and Drug Administration is 12.5 mg.

The HPV vaccination includes the viral subtypes responsible for laryngeal papillomatosis, and will hopefully decrease transmission and result in future eradication of this disease in children.

The factors that lead to virus activation have not been identified; however, gastroesophageal reflux disease (GERD) and laryngopharyngeal reflux (LPR) have been suggested. When chronically exposed to pepsin and gastric contents, the inflammation induced by chronic acid exposure may result in the expression of HPV in the ciliated respiratory epithelium of the larynx, possibly contributing to more advanced presentations of the disease or a more frequent need for surgical debridement. Some of the concerning findings in disease progression of RRP, such as laryngeal webs, may be diminished or even prevented if these children receive antireflux therapy. This emphasizes the importance of initiating antireflux medication in children who have evidence of RRP.

Laryngitis and Laryngo-pharyngeal Reflux

Children have smaller airways than adults and are more susceptible to inflammation and edema of the subglottic airway. Laryngitis is usually related to viral respiratory tract infections in children but can occur secondary to acute vocal strain and submucosal vocal cord inflammation or hemorrhage. Laryngotracheobronchitis, or croup, is commonly viral in origin and affects children <5 years of age. Management is conservative with steroids reserved for airway compromise. Young infants <6 months old are more likely to have viral infection superimposed on a congenital defect of the airway such as laryngomalacia or subglottic stenosis, especially if noisy breathing is present prior to illness **(Fig. 9)**.

A toxic appearing child is more likely to have bacterial tracheitis, retropharyngeal abscess, or epiglottitis. Chronic laryngitis is less likely to be infectious. If symptoms of

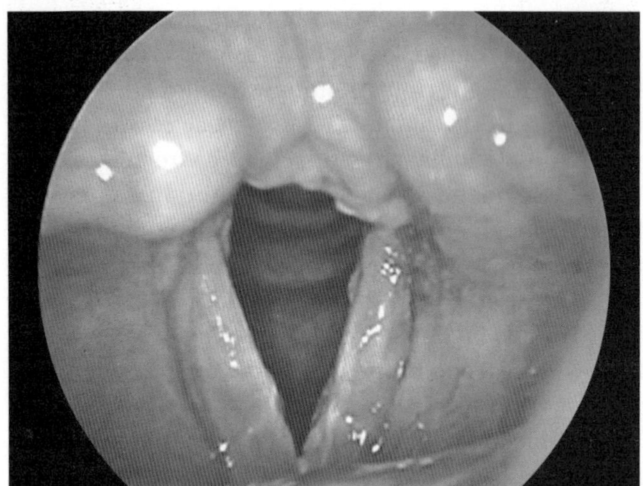

Fig. 9: Laryngoscopic image of chronic laryngitis owing to laryngopharyngeal reflux (LPR) with interarytenoid edema. *(For color version, see Plate 20)*

laryngitis last for >3 months, chronic changes, such as mucosal edema and thickened epithelium, can occur in the larynx. Chronic systemic diseases, medications, dehydration, allergies, and gastroesophageal reflux are common causes of chronic laryngitis. Treatment requires correction of the underlying disorder.

Gastroesophageal reflux disease and LPR disease are common causes of pediatric hoarseness. Laryngopharyngeal reflux is defined as reflux of gastric or duodenal juices beyond the esophagus into the larynx, oropharynx, or nasopharynx.

Recent pediatric literature tends to identify LPR as a distinct disease process, not as an extension of GERD. Chronic cough, vomiting, dysphagia, bitter taste, and laryngospasm are common presentations. Children with radiographic evidence of GERD often demonstrate LPR findings as described earlier. Laryngoscopic changes found in LPR include lingual tonsil hyperplasia (69%), postglottic edema (83%), arytenoid edema and loss of arytenoid architecture (55%), ventricular obliteration (39%), and true vocal cord edema (67%). A total of 66% showed improvement with speech and pharmacotherapy.

Treatment options for LPR include lifestyle modifications, medical therapy, and surgical therapy.

Lifestyle modifications include avoiding diet triggers, postural positioning, and altering food composition with thicker feeds. If lifestyle modifications are insufficient, first-line therapies are proton pump inhibitors (PPIs). Esomeprazole has been shown to provide the greatest benefit, but in children lansoprazole and omeprazole are the only PPIs approved by the Food and Drug Administration. Histamine-2 receptor antagonists are second line, and are helpful for weaning off of PPIs. If symptoms are life threatening or the child has failed maximal medical therapy, Nissen fundoplication may be considered.

PARALYSIS OF VOCAL CORDS

Child with weak cry or hoarseness should be evaluated with a laryngoscope to rule out any vocal cord paralysis. The condition may or may not be associated with symptoms of clinical or subclinical aspiration. Unilateral vocal cord paralysis may present with symptoms of chronic aspiration, weak or absent cry.

In bilateral vocal cord paralysis, the vocal cords assume a midline position, thus protecting the airway from aspiration and permitting a normal cry. Children will often compensate well early in life and may not be symptomatic until they become more active or suffer an acute respiratory infection. Diagnosis relies on laryngoscopy, but other adjuncts such as ultrasound and laryngeal electromyography may also be helpful in making the diagnosis and formulating a treatment plan. Causes include neurologic, iatrogenic, birth-related trauma, or idiopathic.

Damage to the recurrent laryngeal nerve can occur during cardiothoracic surgery, thyroid surgery, or tracheoesophageal fistula repair. The most common surgery that puts the nerve at risk is ligation of patent ductus arteriosus. Neurologic causes include hydrocephalus, Arnold–Chiari malformation, posterior fossa tumors, and meningomyelocele. Children with vocal cord paralysis should have prompt airway and swallow evaluations, as well as imaging of the chest and brain.

Congenital Abnormalities

An infant that presents with an unusual cry or respiratory distress or hoarseness should be evaluated for congenital abnormalities of the larynx, including laryngeal webs and hemangiomas.

Patients with concomitant cardiac anomalies have higher incidence of congenital laryngeal anomalies. Failure of resorption of the epithelial layer that normally obliterates during the development of the glottis results in laryngeal webbing, or incomplete separation of the vocal cords. These can occur anywhere along the vocal cords.

Atresia, or complete webbing of the larynx, is incompatible with life and requires tracheostomy at birth.

Laryngeal webs are commonly associated with other airway abnormalities, DiGeorge and velocardiofacial syndromes. Presentation varies depending on the degree of airway obstruction with altered cry quality, and treatment correlates with the severity. Small anterior webs can be treated with sharp dissection or lasers; larger webs may require laryngeal stents, reconstruction, or tracheostomies.

Functional Voice Disorders

Dysphonia in the absence of an underlying structural or neurologic pathology is known as a functional voice disorder. Abnormal contraction of laryngeal musculature compensating for another abnormality can lead to functional dysphonia. Causes of increased laryngeal tone include vocal misuse, maladaptation following respiratory infection, inflammation, compensation for underlying glottic insufficiency, and psychological causes.

Treatment of functional dysphonia focuses on speech therapy, cognitive behavior therapy (CBT) and rebalancing the laryngeal mechanism (speech therapy) to produce normal voice. Children with psychogenic dysphonia typically have a normal cry, laugh, and cough, and is a diagnosis of exclusion, with treatment targeting the underlying disorder.

EVALUATION AND EXAMINATION

A multidisciplinary approach including a pediatrician, ear-nose-throat (ENT) Surgeon, and speech language pathologist is the key to diagnosis. Etiological diagnosis for pediatric hoarseness is usually done by clinical assessment and flexible nasopharyngolaryngoscopic evaluation. The poor cooperation of the children during fiberoptic video examination is often a hindrance to the diagnosis.

Transnasal flexible endoscope is often useful in all cases of pediatric hoarseness for identifying the morphodynamic alterations. Videolaryngoscopy examination gives large magnification, better angle of visualization, better illumination, and resolution.

Ultrasound is a noninvasive test useful for assessing the upper respiratory anatomy and pathological findings in infants and children. Laryngeal ultrasound is a help to assess the subglottic diameter as well as laryngeal stenosis, subglottic hemangiomas, and vocal fold paralysis.

Computed tomography (CT) and magnetic resonance imaging are usually advised for any neoplastic assessment in the larynx. Any laryngeal stenosis is assessed by CT scan. Virtual endoscopy has been advised and nowadays used as a replacement for classical laryngeal endoscopy during follow-up. It is often helpful for assessing the topography of stenosis and tumors.

Diagnostic biopsy of the tumor or papillomatosis lesions is done to find out the pathological diagnosis.

Perceptual analysis involving a speech language pathologist is another key component of voice evaluation in children, and several tools are currently available for assessing these qualities. Perceptual analysis of voice by the patient, the parent, clinician and speech language pathologist is important in the comprehensive assessment of pediatric hoarseness. Parental questionnaires such as the Pediatric Voice outcome Survey, the Pediatric Voice Related Quality of Life questionnaire, and the Pediatric Voice Handicap Index are available.

TREATMENT

Multidisciplinary approach involving the pediatrician, oto-rhino-laryngologist, speech language therapist, child psychologist, and pediatric neurologist helps mitigating issues of hoarseness in a child comprehensively. There is a significant role of parents and peers in proper rehabilitation in such situations. Their role as home tutors and support can never be underestimated.

The treatment of pediatric hoarseness need individual basis. The therapeutic options available are counseling, voice re-education, medical treatment, psychotherapy, and surgical intervention.

Voice Therapy in Treating a Hoarse Child

The aim of the voice therapy is to return the child's voice from hoarseness to normal or best possible voice of the child within normal physiologic and anatomic capabilities and satisfy the children's social, occupational, and emotional vocal requirements. Voice therapy is usually given by professional speech and language pathologists once or twice per week and each session is approximately 30 minutes. The type of voice therapy and frequency of sessions are planned on basis of requirement of the child. The voice therapy is classified into three types. Hygienic voice therapy is made to enhance the behaviors which protect the vocal folds from injury. Symptomatic voice therapy is designed to treat abnormal voice quality; physiological voice therapy is designed to optimize the voice production.

Medical Treatment

Proton pump inhibitors are the treatment of choice in dysphonia due to LPR. The lifestyle modification in LPR includes avoidance of heavy meals, alcohol, smoking (passive), and late meals. Sleeping with head end elevation of the bed and reduction of the body weight shows benefit to the patient.

In the case of functional dysphonia, the etiology is usually multifactorial such as misuse of voice or strain and laryngeal muscle tension thus requiring psychotherapeutic medications to alleviate the symptoms.

In the case of spasmodic dysphonia, there is focal dystonia affecting the laryngeal muscles during speech. It may be adductor spasmodic dysphonia (common) or abductor one (rare). Child with adductor spasmodic dysphonia often presents with voice breaks and usually treated with botulinum toxin. Vocal fold granuloma is occasionally associated with LPR, voice abuse, intubation, infection, multifactorial, and idiopathic. Treatment of vocal fold granuloma options varies and includes antireflux medication, voice rest, surgical excision, and speech therapy. Botulinum toxin injection is useful in these cases, particularly in recalcitrant granuloma especially in idiopathic case.

Surgical Treatment

Surgical interventions are eventually required if even after proper diagnosis and rehabilitation the child does not improve in terms of the voice quality.

In some specific situations the surgery is offered as the first line if there is clarity that rehabilitative measures would not work as in cases of JORRP or in situations where the airway also has to be secured with adequate control of pathology causing the hoarseness. Micro laryngeal surgery (with operating microscope or endoscopic) cold steel technique or laser assisted modalities help negate some causes of hoarseness while everything else has failed.

The CO_2 laser is quite effective for the treatment of vocal fold polyp and nodules. It will completely excise the polyp without injuring adjacent tissue and bleeding. A combination of vocal hygiene and CO_2 laser is highly effective treatment for vocal fold lesions such as polyp and nodules.

Surgical intervention is also helpful in correcting unilateral vocal cord paralysis that causes hoarseness by means of medialization thyroplasty that is done to close the gap between the paralyzed cord and the normal cord after adequate period for compensation is allowed.

KEY POINTS

- Hoarseness (dysphonia) is defined as a disorder characterized by altered vocal quality, pitch, loudness, or vocal effort that impairs communication or reduces voice-related quality of life.
- Impaired communication is defined as a decreased or limited ability to interact vocally with others.
- Reduced voice-related quality of life is defined as a self-perceived decrement in physical, emotional, social, or economic status as a result of voice-related dysfunction.
- The clinician should not routinely prescribe antibiotics to treat hoarseness in children.
- The clinician and speech language therapist should advocate voice therapy for patients diagnosed with hoarseness that reduces voice-related quality of life.
- The clinician should diagnose hoarseness in children with altered voice quality, pitch, loudness, or vocal effort that impairs communication, or reduces quality of voice in a child.
- The clinician should assess the child with hoarseness by history and/or physical examination for factors that modify management, such as one or more of the following: recent surgical procedures involving the neck or affecting the recurrent laryngeal nerve, recent endotracheal intubation, radiation treatment to the neck, an exposure to tobacco abuse, and over usage of voice.
- The clinician should visualize the child's larynx, or refer the patient to a clinician who can visualize the larynx, when hoarseness fails to resolve by a maximum of three months after onset, or irrespective of duration if a serious underlying cause is suspected.
- The clinician should not obtain computed tomography or magnetic resonance imaging of the child with a primary complaint of hoarseness prior to visualizing the larynx.
- The clinician should not prescribe anti-reflux medications for children with hoarseness without signs or symptoms of gastroesophageal reflux disease or chronic laryngitis.
- The clinician should not routinely prescribe oral corticosteroids to treat hoarseness.
- The clinician should visualize the larynx before prescribing voice therapy and document/communicate the results to the speech-language pathologist.
- The clinician should prescribe, or refer the patient to a clinician who can prescribe, botulinum toxin injections for the treatment of hoarseness caused by adductor spasmodic dysphonia.
- The clinician may perform laryngoscopy at any time in a patient with hoarseness, or may refer the child to a clinician who can visualize the larynx.
- The clinician may prescribe anti-reflux medication for children with hoarseness and signs of chronic laryngitis.
- The clinician may educate/counsel parents of the child with hoarseness about control/preventive measures.

SUGGESTED READING

1. Amir M, Youssef T. Management and anatomical observation in vocal cord paralysis. Clin Respir J. 2010;4(4): 202-7.
2. Aronson AE, Bless DM. Treatment of voice disorders. In: Aronson AE, Bless DM (Eds). Clinical Voice Disorders, 4th edition. NewYork: Thieme; 2009. pp. 231-70.
3. Block BB, Brodsky L. Hoarseness in children: the role of laryngopharyngeal reflux. Int J Pediatr Otorhinolaryngol. 2007;71(9):1361-9.
4. Carifi M, Napolitano D, Morandi M, Dall'Olio D. Recurrent respiratory papillomatosis: current and future perspectives. Ther Clin Risk Manag. 2015;11:731-8.
5. Connelly A, Clement WA, Kubba H. Management of dysphonia in children. J Laryngol Otol. 2009;123(6): 642-7.
6. Jeong WJ, Lee SJ, Lee WY, Chang H, Ahn SH. Conservative management for vocal fold polyps. JAMA Otolaryngol Head Neck Surg. 2014;140(5):448-52.
7. Martins RH, Branco A, Tavares EL, Gramuglia AC. Clinical practice: vocal nodules in dysphonic children. Eur J Pediatr. 2013;172(9):1161-5.
8. Martins RH, Goncalves TM, Neves DS, Fracalossi TA, Tavares EL, Moretti-Ferreira D. Sulcus vocalis: evidence for autosomal dominant inheritance. Genet Mol Res. 2011;10(4):3163-8.
9. Martins RH, Hidalgo Ribeiro CB, Fernandes de Mello BM, Branco A, Tavares EL. Dysphonia in children. J Voice. 2012;26(5):674.e17-674.e20.
10. Martins RH, Santana MF, Tavares EL. Vocal cysts: clinical, endoscopic, and surgical aspects. J Voice. 2011;25(1): 107-10.
11. Morgan JE, Zraick RI, Griffin AW, Bowen TL, Johnson FL. Injection versus medialization laryngoplasty for the treatment of unilateral vocal fold paralysis. Laryngoscope. 2007;117(11):2068-74.
12. Nardone HC, Recko T, Huang L, Nuss RC. A retrospective review of the progression of pediatric vocal fold nodules. JAMA Otolaryngol Head Neck Surg. 2014;140:233-6.
13. Petrocheilou A, Tanou K, Kalampouka E, Malakasioti G, Giannios C, Kaditis AG. Viral croup: diagnosis and a treatment algorithm. Pediatr Pulmonol. 2014;49(5):421-9.
14. Ribeiro LL, Paula KM, Behlau M. Voice-related quality of life in the paediatric population: Validation of the Brazilian version of the pediatric voice-related quality-of life survey. Codas. 2014;26(1):87-95.
15. Smith ME, Roy N, Stoddard K. Unilateral vocal fold paralysis in adolescents and young adults. Int J Pediatr Otorhinolaryngol. 2008;72(9):1311-6.
16. Smith ME. Care of the child's voice: a pediatric otolaryngologist's perspective. Semin Speech Lang. 2013;34(2): 63-70.
17. Tavares EL, Brasolotto A, Santana MF, Padovan CA, Martins RH. Epidemiological study of dysphonia in 4-12 year-old children. Braz J Otorhinolaryngol. 2011; 77(6):736-46.
18. Ulis JM, Yanagisawa E. What's new in differential diagnosis and treatment of hoarseness? Curr Opin Otolaryngol Head Neck Surg. 2009;17(3):209-15.
19. Verduyckt I, Remacle M, Jamart J, Benderitter C, Morsomme D. Voice-related complaints in the pediatric population. J Voice. 2011;25(3):373-80.
20. Wilcox LJ, Hull BP, Baldassari CM, Derkay CS. Diagnosis and management of recurrent respiratory papillomatosis. Pediatr Infect Dis J. 2014;33(12):1283-4.

Otitis Media in Children

Ameet Kishore

INTRODUCTION

Otitis media or infection of middle ear cleft is probably one of the most common infections in childhood. Probably 70% of children would have at least one episode of acute otitis media by 4 years of age and 80–90% of children would have had at least one episode of otitis media with effusion.

ACUTE OTITIS MEDIA

Acute otitis media (AOM) is an acute infection of the middle ear cleft by pus forming organisms. Acute infections of the middle ear in children are common. AOM usually presents between the ages of 3 months–3 years with a peak between the ages of 6 and 9 months.

Etiology and Pathology

The incidence is higher in the colder months, in children attending daycare centers and in those children who are not breastfed.

The following conditions predispose children to recurrent episodes of AOM:

- Cleft palate, immunodeficiency (AIDS, leukemia, and immunosuppressive drugs), and adenoid hypertrophy (this may block the Eustachian tube and also be a source of infection).
- Usually, AOM is a complication of eustachian tube dysfunction that occurred during an acute viral upper respiratory tract infection.
- Bacterial co-infections with viruses are common, whereas isolated viral infections are reported to make up only 20% of AOM infections. Bacteria can be isolated from middle ear fluid cultures in 50–90% of cases of AOM and otitis media with effusion (OME). *Streptococcus pneumoniae, Haemophilus influenzae,* and *Moraxella catarrhalis* are the most common organisms.
- *H. influenzae* has become the most prevalent organism among children with severe or refractory AOM following the introduction of the pneumococcal conjugate vaccine.

Risk factors for AOM are listed in **Box 1**.

Clinical Symptoms and Signs

The older child will complain of severe otalgia and general unwellness, whereas infants and younger children who are less able to communicate may not be able articulate their symptoms. Where possible direct questioning regards fever, disturbed sleep pattern, and hearing loss may direct the clinician to the diagnosis. In the case of these younger children, as their primary and only presenting symptom may be that they are systemically unwell, examination of ears is mandatory. Anecdotally infants with AOM are often reported to rub or bang their ears. In most cases a history of a preceding upper respiratory tract infection will be identified.

An AOM diagnosis requires moderate-to-severe bulging of the tympanic membrane, **(Fig. 1)** new onset of otorrhea not caused by otitis externa, or mild bulging of the tympanic membrane associated with recent onset of ear pain (<48 hours) or erythema.

BOX 1: Risk factors for acute otitis media.

- Age (younger)
- Allergies
- Craniofacial abnormalities
- Exposure to environmental smoke or other
- Respiratory irritants
- Exposure to group day care
- Family history of recurrent acute otitis media
- Gastroesophageal reflux
- Immunodeficiency
- No breastfeeding
- Pacifier use
- Upper respiratory tract infections

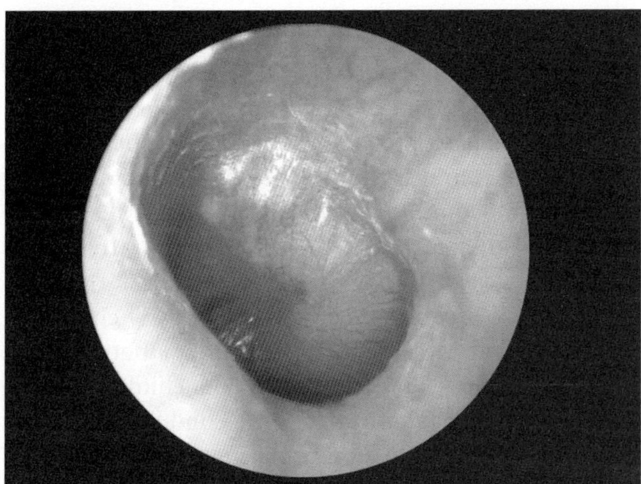

Fig. 1: Acute otitis media—bulging of tympanic membrane. *(For color version, see Plate 21)*

In some cases the tympanic membrane will have already ruptured leading to pus discharge and a rapid improvement in symptoms. Examination of the ear will demonstrate a bulging tympanic membrane with prominent blood vessels on its surface or the tympanic membrane will be obscured by pus in the canal.

Management

For the majority of children AOM is usually a self-resolving condition. First-line treatment for all children with AOM remains adequate analgesia and effective control of fever.

Analgesics are particularly important at bedtime because disrupted sleep is one of the most common symptoms motivating parents to seek care. Ibuprofen is preferred, given its longer duration of action and its lower toxicity in the event of overdose. Topical analgesics, such as benzocaine, can also be helpful.

Antibiotic usage in the management of children with AOM remains debated with most advocating a 24–72 hours period of watch full waiting. Antibiotic treatment has been proven to reduce pain, rate of tympanic membrane perforation, and episodes of contralateral AOM, but this must be considered against the potential adverse events of antibiotic usage such as vomiting, diarrhea, or rash.

The majority of published guidelines for AOM recommend that routine antibiotic prescription should be avoided in mild-to-moderate cases and when there is a diagnostic uncertainty in patients who are 2 years of age or older. Antibiotics are recommended in children of 2 years and younger, most commonly a 5-day course of amoxicillin or a macrolide in patients allergic to penicillin.

BOX 2: Treatment strategy for acute otitis media.

Initial presentation

- Diagnosis established by physical examination findings and presence of symptoms: Treat pain
- Children of 6 months or older with otorrhea or severe signs or symptoms [moderate or severe otalgia, otalgia for at least 48 hours, or temperature of 102.2°F (39°C) or higher]: Antibiotic therapy for 10 days
- Children six to 23 months of age with bilateral acute otitis media without severe signs or symptoms: Antibiotic therapy for 10 days
- Children six to 23 months of age with unilateral acute otitis media without severe signs or symptoms: Observation or antibiotic therapy for 10 days
- Children of 2 years or older without severe signs or symptoms: Observation or antibiotic therapy for five to seven days

Persistent symptoms (48–72 hours)

- Repeat ear examination for signs of otitis media
- If otitis media is present, initiate or change antibiotic therapy
- If symptoms persist despite appropriate antibiotic therapy, consider intramuscular ceftriaxone (Rocephin), clindamycin, or tympanocentesis

A large prospective study of this strategy found that two out of three children will recover without antibiotics. The American Academy of Family Physicians recommended not prescribing antibiotics for otitis media in children two to 12 years of age with nonsevere symptoms if observation is a reasonable option.

High-dose amoxicillin should be the initial treatment (80–90 mg/kg/day). Children who have taken amoxicillin in the past 30 days, who have conjunctivitis, or who need coverage for β-lactamase–positive organisms should be treated with high-dose amoxicillin/clavulanate. Oral cephalosporins, such as cefuroxime, may be used in children who are allergic to penicillin.

Antibiotic therapy for AOM is often associated with diarrhea. Probiotics and yogurts containing active cultures reduce the incidence of diarrhea and should be suggested for children receiving antibiotics for AOM. The strategy for management of AOM is summarized in **Box 2**.

Children with persistent, significant AOM symptoms despite at least 48–72 hours of antibiotic therapy should be re-examined. If a bulging, inflamed tympanic membrane is observed, therapy should be changed to a second-line agent.

Otitis media with effusion (OME) is often seen as a sequel of AOM and must be managed appropriately.

OME can occur during the resolution of AOM once the acute inflammation has resolved. Among children who have had an episode of AOM, as many as 45% have persistent effusion after 1 month, but this number decreases to 10% after 3 months. Management of OME is described in the next section.

Recurrent Acute Otitis Media

Recurrent AOM is defined if the child has 3 or more episodes of AOM in 6 months. It may be managed either expectantly, with a long term course of antibiotics, such as amoxicillin for 6 weeks, or surgically with ventilation tubes. Studies have identified those children that are diagnosed with AOM before the age of 2 years as being at higher risk of recurrence. Various guidelines recommend that any child with four or more episodes of AOM over a period of 6 months or 6 episodes in 12 months may be considered for ventilation tube insertion.

Factors such as frequency, severity, and impact on activities of daily living of the effects of recurrent AOM should be taken into account when considering ongoing management, as should associated factors such as the occurrence of febrile convulsions, mastoiditis, and the presence of ventriculoperitoneal shunts.

Complications of Acute Otitis Media

Rare complications of AOM include mastoiditis, meningitis, and intracranial abscesses. Population-based studies in the Netherlands, where antibiotic usage for AOM is less common have demonstrated an increase in the incidence of mastoiditis. Many of the large trials looking at antibiotic usage for AOM excluded children who were systemically unwell. It should also be noted that the majority of evidence in these reviews is derived from research in first world countries and it is not known whether these management protocols are appropriate for populations out with this group of countries and/or populations from developing countries that have a higher risks of complications.

CLINICAL PEARLS

- Most common between 6–9 months of age.
- Bulging tympanic membrane is the most reliable diagnostic sign.
- Ibuprofen is preferred over paracetamol.
- Watchful waiting (24–72 hrs) is appropriate for mild/moderate symptoms in children >2 years.
- First-line antibiotic: High-dose amoxicillin.
- In recurrent AOM consider ventilation tube insertion.

OTITIS MEDIA WITH EFFUSION

Otitis media with effusion (OME) is a chronic middle ear effusion due to nonpurulent inflammation of the mucosa of the middle ear cleft. It is also defined as the presence of middle ear fluid without the symptoms and signs of acute ear infection. It is also called serous otitis media, secretory otitis media (SOM), nonsuppurative otitis media, or glue ear.

The OME is commonly a disease of early childhood with an overall prevalence of about 33% between the ages of 2 and 6 years. With up to 80% children having OME before the age of 10 years. The condition fluctuates with relapses and remission being common. Over 50% of the episodes resolve within 3 months.

Etiology

The OME often follows an initial upper respiratory tract infection. It may also be preceded by episode of AOM. Obstruction of the Eustachian, particularly at the nasopharyngeal end has a role to play in the development of OME. This is probably due to the fact that an obstructed tube prevents adequate drainage of the effusion.

Risk Factors

Screening surveys of healthy children between infancy and age 5 years show 15–40% point prevalence in OME. Furthermore, among children examined at regular intervals for 1 year, 50–60% of child care attendees and 25% of school-aged children were found to have an OME at some point during the examination period, with peak incidence during the winter months. The prevalence of OME is highest in those aged 2 years or younger, and it sharply declines in children older than 6 years.

List of risk factors:

- Boys are affected more than girls.
- Siblings with OME.
- Repeated upper respiratory tract infections.
- Children attending daycare and thus prone to repeated upper respiratory tract infection (URTI)
- Bottle fed babies
- Use of pacifier
- Allergic rhinitis or atopy
- Adenoid hypertrophy
- Trisomy 21
- Primary ciliary dyskinesia or Kartagener's syndrome resulting in abnormal mucociliary function
- Palatal abnormalities such as cleft palate

- Craniofacial anomalies
- Parental smoking
- Barotrauma

Pathology

A variety of changes have been identified in SOM:

- *Inflammatory:* Most infections are caused by viruses, the most common of which is respiratory syncytial virus. Others are adenovirus and influenza. Bacterial infection is secondary with *S. pneumoniae, H. influenzae,* and *M. catarrhalis* being the common pathogens. Mediators of inflammation and inflammatory cells are found in the effusion.
- *Mucosal:* Goblet cell proliferation with mucus production. Alteration in mucosal clearance mechanism.
- *Allergy:* An IgE mediated response does not appear to be the primary causal factor, but may be associated.
- *Changes in middle ear cleft:* Reduced mastoid pneumatization is associated with history of ear infections and appears to be a risk factor for SOM. It is unclear whether this is genetic or environmental.
- *Middle ear gas composition:* Middle ear gas is deficient in patients with SOM. It is felt that this may be related more to excessive diffusion of gas through blood rather than Eustachian tube dysfunction.

Clinical Features

The most common presentation is a hearing loss. This may either be identified by parents or often by teachers at school. This may sometimes result in impairment of speech and language development or may give rise to behavioral abnormalities. Fever and other constitutional symptoms are absent. Occasionally children with OME present with ear pain due to secondary acute infection that often follows a cold.

Diagnosis

Diagnosis is based on otoscopic examination. The tympanic membrane appears dull, retracted and demonstrates reduced mobility on pneumatic otoscopy or Valsalva maneuver. If there is an effusion in the middle ear, this appears as an amber colored fluid **(Fig. 2)**. Occasionally, an air fluid level or bubbles may be visible **(Fig. 3)**.

American clinical practice guidelines have strongly advocated the use of pneumatic otoscopy as the primary diagnostic method for OME. The sensitivity of pneumatic otoscopy is 85–93% and its specificity from 71 to 89%. This can be carried out with a closed system in a handheld otoscope or with a Siegel's pneumatic speculum, viewed with headlight illumination or microscope.

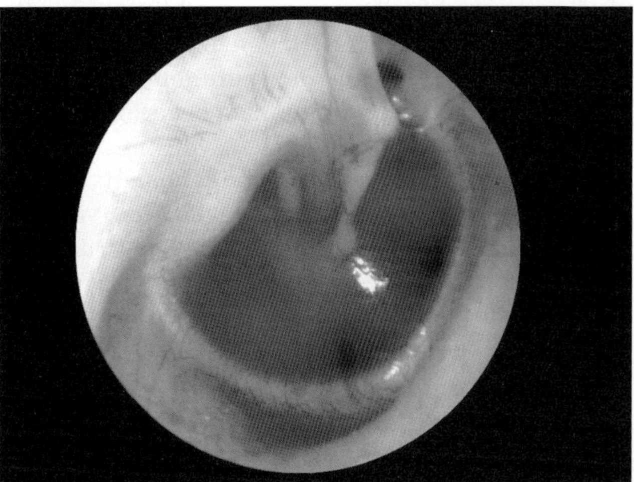

Fig. 2: Otitis media with effusion (OME)—Amber colored fluid in middle ear. *(For color version, see Plate 21)*

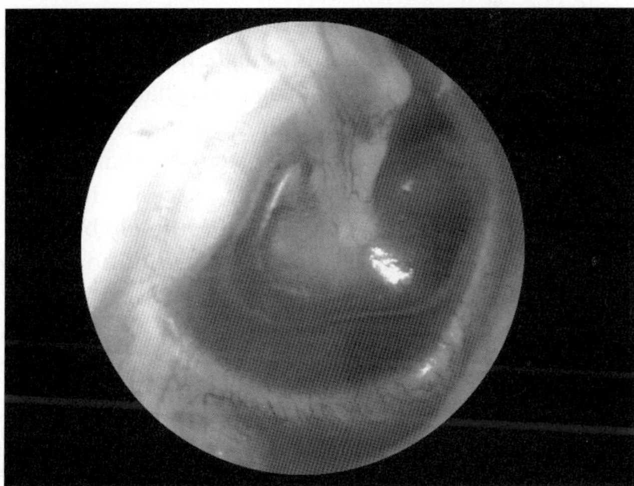

Fig. 3: Otitis media with effusion (OME)—Air fluid level. *(For color version, see Plate 21)*

Investigation

The patient's hearing must be assessed. According to American Academy of Family Physicians (AAFP), the American Academy of Otolaryngology–Head and Neck Surgery (AAO-HNS), and the American Academy of Pediatrics (AAP) subcommittee on OME, audiology is a necessary component of the evaluation of certain patients with this condition.

This is useful for the assessment of disease severity and to monitor progress. In an older child or an adult this is done by way of a pure tone audiogram. In a younger child, age appropriate behavioral tests of hearing are carried out.

Impedance audiogram or tympanometry is also performed to assess middle ear compliance. Tympanometry has a sensitivity and specificity of 70–90% for the detection of middle ear fluid. The presence of a flat tympanogram (type B) is highly suggestive of the presence of middle ear effusion.

Management

Any treatment instituted is aimed to relieve the symptoms caused by the condition, i.e., hearing loss (and its effect on speech and behavior) or secondary infections. It should also be tailored to prevent recurrence **(Box 3)**.

In half of the children with otitis media with effusion, this will resolve spontaneously within 3 months. It is therefore prudent to reassess the child's hearing 3 months after initial presentation. In the remaining half who do not resolve spontaneously, further intervention is required.

Decongestants, antihistamines, steroids, or antibiotics do not significantly improve the outcome in otitis media with effusion and should not routinely be used. Myringotomy with insertion of a ventilation tube (grommet) is currently the treatment of choice for persistent middle ear effusion. In children above the age of 4 with enlarged adenoids, an adenoidectomy reduces the chance of recurrent effusion.

Antibiotics are useful only in a minority of patients with chronic OME or recurrent AOM and any benefit is only short term. The antibiotic of choice is amoxicillin with clavulanic acid.

BOX 3: Diagnosis and treatment of otitis media with effusion.

- Evaluate tympanic membranes at every well-child and sick visit if feasible; perform pneumatic otoscopy or tympanometry when possible (consider removing cerumen)
- If transient effusion is likely, reevaluate at 3-month intervals, including screening for language delay; if there is no anatomic damage or evidence of developmental or behavioral complications, continue to observe at 3–6-month intervals; if complications are suspected, refer to an otolaryngologist
- For effusion that appears to be associated with anatomic damage, such as adhesive otitis media or retraction pockets, reevaluate in 4–6 weeks; if abnormality persists, refer to an otolaryngologist
- Antibiotics, decongestants, and nasal steroids are not indicated

Most guidelines recommend that if the effusion has been present for greater than 3 months and there is an associated disability in the form of a hearing loss of greater than 25–30 dB on average through speech frequencies, proven on audiogram, then either surgery in the form of myringotomy and ventilation tube insertion with or without adjuvant adenoidectomy or a trial of hearing aids is appropriate. In the interim the use of devices to encourage autoinflation (ear popping) have been advocated.

Myringotomy is a procedure where an incision is made in the tympanic membrane and any middle ear fluid is aspirated. Myringotomy alone has only short-term benefit. Myringotomy with insertion of a ventilation tube (grommet) is currently the treatment of choice for persistent middle ear effusion **(Fig. 4)**. The myringotomy is performed under general anesthesia. A radial incision is made in the antero-inferior quadrant of the tympanic membrane. Grommets may be made of silicone or metal and are inserted so as to keep the incision patent and allow ventilation of the middle ear. The grommet usually extrudes spontaneously in 9–12 months.

In children above the age of 4 with enlarged adenoids, an adenoidectomy reduces the chance of recurrent effusion. Various studies have shown that adenoidectomy in this age group leads to reduced failure rates, fewer days with OME, and a reduced rate of future tympanostomy tube insertion. In children younger than 4, adenoidectomy is not recommended in this age group because the benefits are limited and of questionable clinical significance.

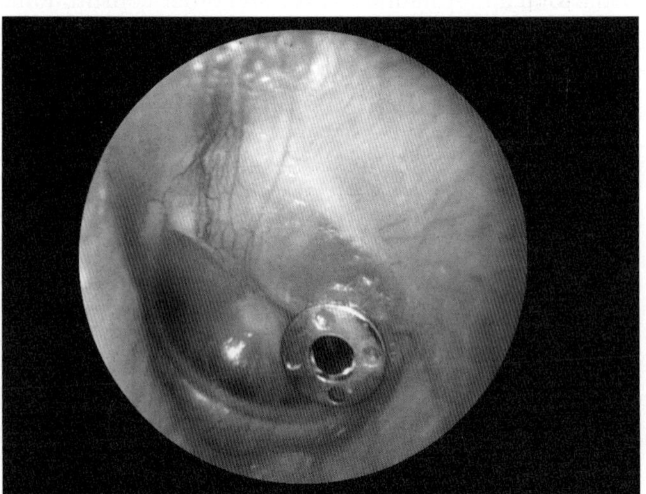

Fig. 4: Grommet in place. *(For color version, see Plate 21)*

Sequelae

In most children OME subsides spontaneously or following intervention. However, the condition itself or its treatment may result in long term structural or functional changes to the middle ear.

The above changes may lead to a degree of conductive hearing loss. Persistence of effusion would also cause prolonged hearing loss. It has been shown that prolonged hearing loss at early age has an effect on speech, language, and may lead to behavioral changes.

Two rare complications of OME are transient hearing loss potentially associated with language delay, and chronic anatomic injury to the tympanic membrane requiring reconstructive surgery. Children should be screened for speech delay at all visits.

In a minority of children the Eustachian tube dysfunction persists into adulthood. This may lead to permanent changes in the middle ear such as atelectasis of the tympanic membrane, adhesive otitis media, tympanic membrane perforation, or cholesteatoma. Most of these will result in a degree of conductive hearing loss in that ear. Such permanent changes to the middle ear structure are broadly classed as chronic otitis media.

CLINICAL **PEARLS**

- Most common cause of hearing loss in young children.
- Pneumatic otoscopy is more accurate than standard otoscopy.
- Tympanogram Type B (flat curve) strongly suggests OME.
- No fever or acute illness.
- Decongestants, antihistamines, and steroids are not helpful.
- Spontaneous resolution in ~50% within 3 months—repeat hearing assessment before deciding on intervention.
- Indications for grommets: Effusion >3 months + hearing loss ≥25–30 dB or developmental concerns.
- Adenoidectomy helps in children >4 yrs with enlarged adenoids and persistent OME.

CHRONIC SUPPURATIVE OTITIS MEDIA

For most tympanic membrane perforations associated with AOM the discharge will settle spontaneously and the underlying perforation will heal without any intervention being required. However in a small number of children the perforation will not heal and they can end up with a chronically or intermittently discharging ear. Chronic otorrhea can also occur following ventilation tube insertion. The management for both remains the same with treatment with either topical or oral antibiotics. Recent Cochrane reviews show the use of topical quinolone eardrops to be superior to oral antibiotics in clearing the discharge. In cases where topical aminoglycosides are used these should be used for no longer than 2 weeks. Chronically discharging ears put patients at greater of risk of developing intracranial infections and abscesses. Where the discharge fails to respond to appropriate antibiotic therapy onward referral to exclude an underlying cholesteatoma or for surgery to repair the perforation or remove the ventilation tube is advised. In the case of an asymptomatic tympanic membrane perforation no treatment is required.

CLINICAL **PEARLS**

- Persistent otorrhoea through a perforated tympanic membrane lasting ≥6 weeks.
- Topical quinolones are more effective than oral antibiotics.
- Refer non-healing perforations or persistent discharge—especially if cholesteatoma is suspected.
- No treatment needed for dry, asymptomatic perforations—but monitor.

Mastoiditis

Mastoiditis is infection in the air cells in the mastoid process of the temporal bone. The infection is preceded by AOM and caused by the same organisms. Swelling will be identified in the postauricular sulcus due to the occurrence of a cellulitis or subperiosteal abscess. Urgent referral is required for intravenous antibiotics and possible surgery to drain the pus. Associated complications include facial palsy, sigmoid sinus thrombosis, meningitis and extradural, temporal lobe, and posterior fossa abscesses.

CLINICAL **PEARLS**

- Suspect mastoiditis in any child with AOM and postauricular swelling, tenderness, or protruding pinna.
- Requires urgent ENT referral for IV antibiotics ± surgical drainage.
- Facial palsy or neurological symptoms = potential intracranial spread—emergency!

Cholesteatoma

Cholesteatoma is a process whereby squamous epithelium that would normally migrate out via the external auditory canal fails to do so and is caught in the middle ear cleft. This may be either a congenital process where a keratin pearl has become entrapped behind the tympanic membrane during development or an acquired process where the middle ear respiratory epithelium changes to become squamous epithelium or a retraction pocket develops in the tympanic membrane that is unable to effectively clear itself. The mechanisms of the development of acquired cholesteatomas are poorly understood and probably multifactorial. Clinically, cholesteatomas present with recurrent intermittent or chronic foul smelling otorrhea with or without hearing loss. There is an associated risk of developing permanent hearing loss due to damage to the ossicles as well as intracranial complications as discussed earlier. Any patient with a suspected cholesteatoma should be referred and will need surgical intervention.

CLINICAL PEARLS

- Chronic, foul-smelling, painless otorrhea.
- Conductive hearing loss often accompanies discharge.
- Any suspicion = prompt ENT referral; the definitive treatment is surgical.

KEY POINTS

- Otitis media is one of the most common childhood infections and a leading cause of hearing loss in young children.
- *Acute otitis media (AOM):* Most common between 6 and 9 months; diagnosis relies on a bulging tympanic membrane.
- *Management of AOM:* Analgesia (ibuprofen preferred) is essential; antibiotics reserved for younger children, severe disease, or persistent symptoms; high-dose amoxicillin is first-line.
- Watchful waiting (24–72 hours) is appropriate in mild/moderate cases in children >2 years.
- Recurrent AOM may require ventilation tube insertion, particularly with ≥4 episodes in 6 months or ≥6 in 12 months.
- *Otitis media with effusion (OME):* Common after AOM; half resolve within 3 months. Diagnosis is best made with pneumatic otoscopy and tympanometry (Type B curve).
- No role for decongestants, antihistamines, or steroids in OME.
- *Indications for grommets:* Effusion >3 months with hearing loss ≥25–30 dB or developmental concerns; adenoidectomy helps in children >4 years with enlarged adenoids.
- *Chronic suppurative otitis media (CSOM):* Persistent otorrhea through a perforation; topical quinolones are superior to oral antibiotics.
- Mastoiditis and cholesteatoma are serious complications and require urgent ENT referral.

SUGGESTED READING

1. American Academy of Family Physicians, American Academy of Otolaryngology-Head and Neck Surgery, American Academy of Pediatrics Subcommittee on Otitis Media With Effusion. Otitis media with effusion. Pediatrics. 2004;113(5):1412-29.
2. Arrieta A, Singh J. Management of recurrent and persistent acute otitis media: new options with familiar antibiotics. Pediatr Infect Dis J. 2004;23(2 Suppl):S115-24.
3. El Feghaly RE, Nedved A, Katz SE, Frost HM. New insights into the treatment of acute otitis media. Expert Rev Anti Infect Ther. 2023;21(5):523-34.
4. Harmes KM, Blackwood RA, Burrows HL, Cooke JM, Harrison RV, Passamani PP. Otitis media: diagnosis and treatment. Am Fam Physician. 2013;88(7):435-40.
5. Jacobs MR, Dagan R, Appelbaum PC, Burch DJ. Prevalence of antimicrobial-resistant pathogens in middle ear fluid: multinational study of 917 children with acute otitis media. Antimicrob Agents Chemother. 1998;42(3):589-95.
6. Lambert M. AAO-HNS releases updated guideline on management of otitis media with effusion. Am Fam Physician. 2016;94(9):747-9.
7. Lieberthal AS, Carroll AE, Chonmaitree T, Ganiats TG, Hoberman A, Jackson MA, et al. The diagnosis and management of acute otitis media. Pediatrics. 2013; 131(3):e964-99.
8. Marchetti F, Ronfani L, Nibali SC, Tamburlini G. Delayed prescription may reduce the use of antibiotics for acute otitis media: a prospective observational study in primary care. Arch Pediatr Adolesc Med. 2005;159(7): 679.
9. Rosenfeld RM, Schwartz SR, Pynnonen MA, Tunkel DE, Hussey HM, Fichera JS, et al. Clinical Practice Guideline: Tympanostomy Tubes in Children. Otolaryngol Neck Surg. 2013;149(S1).
10. Rosenfeld RM, Shin JJ, Schwartz SR, Coggins R, Gagnon L, Hackell JM, et al. Clinical Practice Guideline: Otitis Media with Effusion (Update). Otolaryngol Neck Surg. 2016;154(S1).
11. Shekelle PG, Takata G, Newberry SJ, Coker T, Limbos MA, Chan LS, et al. Management of acute otitis media: update. Evid ReportTechnology Assess. 2010;(198):1-426.
12. Suzuki HG, Dewez JE, Nijman RG, Yeung S. Clinical practice guidelines for acute otitis media in children: a systematic review and appraisal of European national guidelines. BMJ Open. 2020;10(5):e035343.
13. Van Den Aardweg MT, Schilder AG, Herkert E, Boonacker CW, Rovers MM. Adenoidectomy for otitis media in children. Cochrane ENT Group (Eds). Cochrane Database Syst Rev. 2010:CD007810.

CHAPTER 158

Pediatric Sinusitis

Devinder Rai

INTRODUCTION

Paranasal sinuses in childhood are difficult to evaluate because of their variability in size, shape, and patterns of development. However, the child's sinuses are affected by a wide spectrum of conditions including congenital abnormalities, inflammatory, traumatic, and neoplastic conditions.

The sinuses are air filled cavities in the mid-face communicating with the nasal cavity through narrow ostia. Type 2 pseudostratified columnar ciliated epithelium lining provide mucociliary activity for its mucous clearance which takes place in a predetermined physiological pathway. There are four sets of sinuses on each side.

Maxillary and Ethmoid sinuses are present at birth but are diminutive in size. As sinus development progresses opacification or mucous membrane thickening continues to be physiological till about 6 years of age. It is likely due to either redundant normal mucosa, or an abundance of tears or an easily occluded ostium. Both these sinuses attain full size by 15 or 16 years of age.

Sphenoid sinus is underdeveloped and nonpneumatized at birth and only starts to aerate at about 3 years of age. The varying degrees of pneumatization of the sphenoid sinus results in three types, i.e., conchal, presellar, and sellar and completing it by about age 15 years.

Frontal sinus is not present at birth. It starts appearing at the age of 6 as a cranial extension of an ethmoidal cell completing its aeration by the age of 15. Depending upon the extent of aeration of the frontal recess, it forms a narrow hourglass shaped doorway leading to the frontal sinus.

In 2016 the International Frontal Sinus Anatomy Classification (IFAC) classified the frontal recess cells based on their anatomic origin into three groups determining their frontal sinus drainage pathways.

Anterior frontal cells push the drainage pathway medially, posteriorly or posteromedial, include the agger nasi cell (ANC), supra agger cell (SAC), and supra agger frontal cell (SAFC).

Posterior frontal cells push the drainage pathway anteriorly, include supra bulla cell (SBC), supra bulla frontal cell (SBFC), and supra orbital ethmoid cell (SOEC).

Medial cells push the drainage pathway laterally, include the frontal septal cell (FSC).

RHINOSINUSITIS

European position paper on rhinosinusitis and nasal polyposis (EPOS) defines pediatric rhinosinusitis clinically as an inflammation of the nose and paranasal sinuses characterized by two or more symptoms, one of which should be either:

- Nasal blockage/obstruction/congestion or
- Nasal discharge (anterior or posterior nasal drip
- +/– facial pain/pressure
- +/– cough as opposed to reduction
- +/– loss of smell

And/or

- Endoscopic signs of:
  - Nasal polyps, and/or mucopurulent discharge primarily from the middle meatus, and/or
  - Edema/mucosal obstruction primarily in the middle meatus
  - Adenoid hypertrophy
- Computerized tomography of paranasal sinus changes mucosal changes within the osteo-meatal complex and the sinuses

The common predisposing events that set the stage for acute bacterial sinusitis are acute viral upper respiratory infections that result in a viral rhinosinusitis (a diffuse mucositis that predisposes to approximately 80% of bacterial sinus infections) and allergic inflammation (that predisposes to 20% of bacterial sinus infections). Children have 6–8 viral upper respiratory infections each year; it is estimated that 5–13% of these infections may be complicated by a secondary bacterial infection of the paranasal sinuses.

Due to viral rhinitis, there is increased nasal discharge or rhinorrhea along with nasal congestion and edema of the nasal mucosa. Another effect of viral infection is that there is ciliary dysfunction leading to impaired clearance of secretions particularly in the sinuses. This leads to stasis, which over a period undergoes secondary infection leading to bacterial sinusitis along with all its signs and symptoms.

Sinusitis in children is also associated with an increased risk of complications. The complications of sinusitis may be divided into orbital, intracranial, and local complications. The increased risk may be attributed to the low immunity of the children as well as the low bone density of the lamina and the fovea ethmoidalis.

CLASSIFICATION

According to duration of sinusitis:

- Acute sinusitis (7 days–4 weeks)
- Subacute sinusitis (4–12 weeks)
- Chronic sinusitis (persistence of symptoms beyond 3 months)

According to etiology or the causative factors:

- Viral
- *Bacterial:* The usual bacteria implicated in sinusitis are *Streptococcus pneumoniae*, *Haemophilus influenzae*, and *Moraxella catarrhalis*. Other lesser common bacteria isolated were *Staphylococcus aureus*, *Bacteroides*, *Peptostreptococcus*, *Fusobacterium*, and *Prevotella*.
- *Fungal:* In immunocompetent children the usual fungal species responsible are *Aspergillus* and *Candida*. However, in immunocompromised individuals, there is a greater incidence of invasive fungal sinusitis with *Rhizopus* and *Mucor spp*. Thus, the cause of immunocompromised if any should be searched for in any child suffering from fungal sinusitis. The cause could be uncontrolled type 1 diabetes, children undergoing steroid therapy, human immunodeficiency virus (HIV) infection, or those suffering from neoplastic conditions of the blood cell.

According to phenotype:

- *Chronic rhinosinusitis without polyposis—CRSsNP:* Children are inherently prone to allergies, viral, and bacterial infections, which is manifested as nasal discharge and nasal obstruction.
- *Chronic rhinosinusitis with nasal polyposis—CRSwNP:* Relatively common in adults but, is rarely seen in children. Any child with polyposis should be further examined to rule out ciliary dyskinesia syndromes, cystic fibrosis, and other similar diseases.

SYMPTOMOLOGY

The typical symptoms of nasal obstruction, nasal discharge, and headache as seen in the adult population are rarely seen among young children. Thus, indirect signs are considered as pointers to a possible sinusitis in infants and young children.

The diagnosis of pediatric rhinosinusitis is usually based on a combination of history and physical examination, laboratory investigation, and radiological findings.

The first and perhaps most common clinical indicator of sinusitis in children is similar to that of a viral upper respiratory tract infection which is refractory to supportive therapy. According to Lusk, it is virtually impossible to differentiate between an upper respiratory tract infection and rhinosinusitis during the first 7–10 days of symptomatology. Symptoms may include:

- Rhinorrhea which may be serous or mucopurulent
- Nasal congestion
- Cough—which is more common in children rather than adults
- Low grade fever, malaise, and irritability
- Dental pain

However, in more advanced cases, there may be high-grade fever and a profuse purulent nasal discharge. Always this should also raise the suspicion of a nasal foreign body in infants. Once excluded, this may be the sign of acute sinusitis. Several warning signs point to an impending complication of acute sinusitis like: periorbital pain and swelling.

Double vision in more advanced cases leading to loss of vision in extreme cases.

Signs indicating intracranial involvement such as meningismus and altered sensorium.

DIAGNOSIS

A high clinical suspicion and rapid diagnosis is a must for pediatric sinusitis due to rapid progression of infection.

A detailed history and clinical examination including anterior rhinoscopy is a must in every case.

Flexible fiberoptic nasoendoscopy is an invaluable tool to better assess the nasal cavity, the sinus prechambers, and the nasopharynx for adenoids.

Laboratory investigations include nasal smears for bacteriology, blood work for leukocytosis, culture, and for diagnosis of sepsis. The gold standard for the diagnosis of acute bacterial sinusitis is the recovery of bacteria in high density ($\geq 10^4$ colony-forming units/mL) from the cavity of a paranasal sinus. Blood investigations may also rule out immunodeficiency conditions and ciliary dyskinesia.

In children below 6 years of age with uncomplicated sinusitis radiography is generally not indicated. However, the American College of Radiology has taken the position that the diagnosis of acute uncomplicated sinusitis should be made on clinical grounds alone. They support this position by noting that plain radiographs of the paranasal sinuses are technically difficult to perform, particularly in very young children. Correct positioning may be difficult to achieve and therefore the radiographic images may overestimate and underestimate the presence of abnormalities within the paranasal sinuses.

The CT scans of the paranasal sinuses should be reserved for patients in whom surgery is being considered as a management strategy (strong recommendation based on good evidence and strong panel consensus).

In complicated cases, radiography is invaluable in assessing the extent of disease as well as differentiating the type of complications present.

In case of a suspected intracranial complication magnetic resonance imaging (MRI) may be considered as it has greater sensitivity and specificity as compared to a computed tomography (CT) scan.

Lumbar puncture maybe considered to confirm the presence of meningitis; however, an ophthalmology consult must be sought prior to this invasive procedure to rule out raised intracranial tension (ICT), as it may be fatal in such cases.

TREATMENT

For the sake of discussion, treatment of pediatric sinusitis can be divided into uncomplicated cases and cases with complications. However, treatment strategies are aimed to be aggressive due to the fulminant and rapid progression of infection in children.

The mainstay of treatment of acute uncomplicated bacterial sinusitis is antibiotics, which may be parenteral or oral depending upon variables such as severity, general condition of the child. In all suspected cases of complications hospital admission and intravenous (IV) antibiotics are a must.

Supportive therapy including systemic and topical decongestants is controversial once sinusitis has set in.

Saline nasal wash/rinse sprays are indicated as it lowers the viral/allergen load. It also removes the discharge allowing the topical intranasal corticosteroid therapy to reach the middle meatus.

Intranasal corticosteroids (INCS) can be instituted in children >2 years of age. Mometasone is preferred due to its lesser systemic absorption.

A short burst of systemic corticosteroids may be given in atopic children to manage the symptoms but should be used with caution in fungal sinusitis. The following treatment algorithm has been recommended by the Subcommittee on Management of Sinusitis and Committee on Quality Improvement Pediatrics in 2001.

In complicated cases of sinusitis, the treatment is more aggressive as compared and involves prompt radiography to diagnose the complication. The treatment is as has been described earlier.

Adenoids have been implicated in contributing to recurrent rhinosinusitis due to bio-film formation and lowered local immunity. Hypertrophy of the adenoids further causes lack of nasal breathing and resultant nasal secretion stasis along with sleep disordered breathing. The bacterial biofilms is usually present in the furrows of the adenoidal tissue and tends to be polymicrobial and antibiotic resistant. Therefore, in recurrent pediatric chronic rhinosinusitis (CRS) not responding to medical treatment, removal of adenoid tissue has been recommended as a first line surgical management by the EPOS and American Academy of Otolaryngology-Head and Neck Surgery (AAO-HNS).

Functional endoscopic sinus surgery (FESS) is indicated where adenoid removal and medical management have not been successful or in those who have cystic fibrosis (CF), nasal polyps, antro-choanal polyps, or allergic fungal sinusitis.

ADJUNCTIVE THERAPY

Biologics Treatment of type II inflammatory disease by biologics which target key cytokines interleukin (IL)-4, IL-5, and IL-13 as well as immunoglobulin (Ig)E have emerged in recent times. Omalizumab which targets IgE is a monoclonal antibody has been shown to exhibit significant improvement in polyp size and nasal symptoms as well as in concurrent asthma.

This can be given to children who are 6 years or older. Another monoclonal antibody Dupilumab which targets IL-4 and IL-13 receptors has been approved by the Federal Drug Administration (FDA) for children and adults, 12 years or older.

European Forum for Research and Education in Allergy and Airway Disease (EUFOREA) have laid down five criteria for administering biologics adjunct therapy in CRSwNP:

- Evidence of type II inflammation
- Need for two or more courses of systemic corticosteroids in the past year
- Significant impairment of quality of life (QOL)
- Significant loss of smell
- Diagnosis of asthma

COMPLICATIONS

There is an increased incidence of complications in pediatric sinusitis due to the following reasons:

- Thinner bony septa and sinus walls
- Greater porosity of bones
- Larger vascular foramina
- Open suture lines

The complications occurring in sinusitis can be divided into local, orbital, and intracranial complications.

Local Complications

The basic premise of sinusitis is that it is always rhinologic in origin. The ideology being that rhinitis causes the nasal mucosa to undergo inflammation leading to edema and blockage of the sinus prechambers leading to accumulation of secretions in them which undergo secondary infections leading to sinusitis. The local complications of sinusitis are particularly more common in children as compared to adults due to the immature bony skeleton and incompletely closed foramina.

In an acute case there is an incidence of frontal bone osteomyelitis, which is termed as Potts Puffy Tumor. This is a misnomer as there is no actual tumor but a subperiosteal collection of pus in the frontal bone usually secondary to frontal sinusitis.

The other local complications of sinusitis in children are mucoceles and pyoceles. A pyocele is a collection of pus within a walled cavity usually present in the ethmoid or the sphenoid sinus leading to a myriad of symptoms depending on the sinus involved and its surrounding structures. A similar presentation but when the walled cavity contains sterile fluid it is termed as a mucocele.

Sphenoidal mucoceles are considered more dangerous due to the proximity of the optic nerve, in the posterolateral wall of the sphenoid sinus, which invariably gets compressed leading to visual deficits. According to various studies once the optic nerve gets involved or compressed, the surgeon has about 60 minutes to decompress the nerve to save its function before irreversible functional deficits occur. The "golden hour" concept.

Orbital Complications

The incidence of orbital complications is higher with about 75% of pediatric sinusitis cases presenting with an orbital complication. This greater incidence of orbital complications can be attributed to the close relationship between the sinuses and the orbit, which are separated only by a thin bone, the lamina papyracea, which has congenital dehiscences.

Chandler et al., divided orbital complications into five stages:

1. Stage of preseptal cellulitis
2. Stage of orbital cellulitis
3. Stage of subperiosteal abscess
4. Stage of orbital abscess
5. Stage of cavernous sinus thrombosis

Preseptal Cellulitis

This is the first stage of orbital complications of sinusitis. About 30% of children with sinusitis have preseptal cellulitis as the initial presentation. The signs include eyelid edema and erythema. There is normal extraocular muscle movement and normal vision. Radiologic findings include diffuse thickening of the lids and conjunctiva.

Medical therapy is usually sufficient in preseptal cellulitis which consists of IV antibiotics, head end elevation, and warm compresses. Decongestant therapy consisting of mucolytics, topical, and systemic decongestants should be instituted to facilitate drainage of sinuses.

Orbital Cellulitis

This stage consists of postseptal infection, which is characterized by eyelid edema and erythema. On external examination, chemosis and proptosis may be present. Extraocular muscle movement may or may not affect in this stage. Vision is normal though blurring may be present due to proptosis. There is no discrete abscess however localized inflammation signs are positive. Radiologically there is a low attenuation next to lamina papyracea.

Orbital cellulitis stage may be managed the same as the stage of preseptal cellulitis. However, due to advanced stage frequent visual acuity testing and extraocular movement testing is warranted. Surgical drainage is indicated if no improvement or worsening of symptoms is seen after 48 hours of medical therapy.

Subperiosteal Abscess

This is characterized by pus formation between the periorbita and the lamina papyracea. This displaces the orbital contents downward and laterally. On local examination there is proptosis, chemosis, and total ophthalmoplegia. There is thus an increased risk of residual visual sequelae. The pus may rupture through the septum and present in the eyelids. On computed tomography (CT) scanning there is a rim enhancing hypodensity with mass effect adjacent to lamina.

Treatment consists of combined medical and surgical approaches. Only medical therapy has a success rate of about 50–67%. Combined approach is successful in 95–100% of the cases. Due to the morbidity associated with loss of eye function, an aggressive approach is required comprising surgical drainage with medical therapy consisting of IV antibiotics, systemic and topical decongestants, and supportive therapy **(Flowcharts 1 and 2)**.

Flowchart 1: Algorithm for management of persistent or severe upper respiratory tract infection.

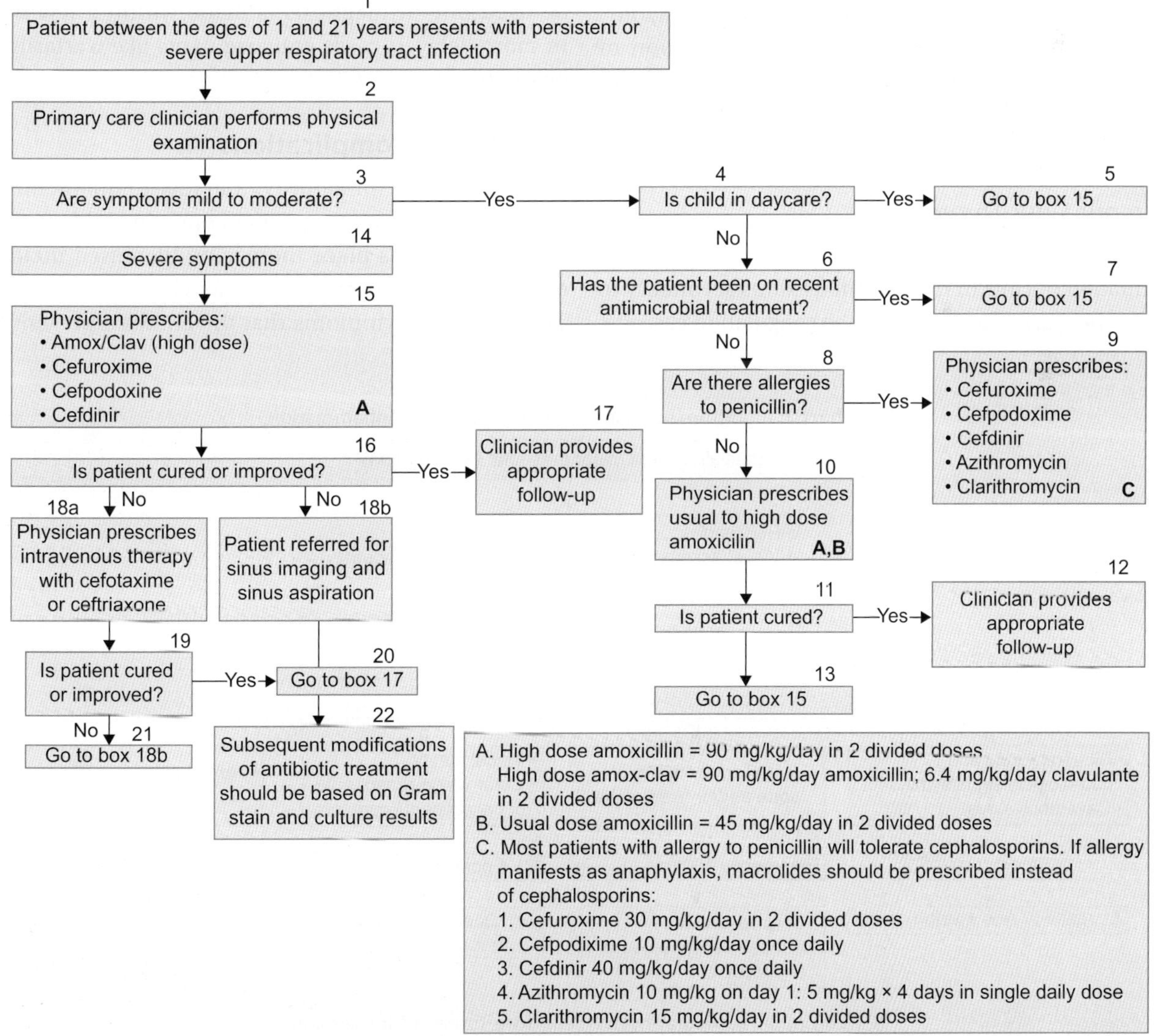

The surgical approach depends upon the location and extent of the abscess in question. In case of medial abscesses an endoscopic orbital decompression is preferred. However, in case of lateral abscesses an external ethmoidectomy via lynch incision or a transcaruncular approach is considered best.

Orbital Abscess

This is characterized by pus formation within orbital tissues. On local examination there is exaggeration of signs seen in subperiosteal abscess. There is visual impairment, which may range from blurring of vision to total visual loss. Vision loss constitutes an emergency and according to studies, the surgeon has about 100 minutes to save the vision before the loss becomes irreversible. On CT scanning there is a rim enhancing hypodensity within the orbital tissue, which may extend to the intraconal region.

Orbital abscess with its ominous complication of irreversible vision loss must be treated aggressively with surgical drainage the primary modality of treatment in addition to medical therapy.

Cavernous Sinus Thrombosis

This dreaded complication of sinusitis is characterized by formation of clots in the cavernous sinus secondary to infection because of activation of the coagulation cascade. This condition is associated with chemosis, exophthalmos, decrease or loss of vision, headaches or paralysis of the cranial nerves 3, 4, 5, and 6. Other common signs include signs of raised ICT and sepsis. Infection can spread to contralateral sinus within 24–48 hours.

Clinical acuity and testing is paramount to diagnosis as the signs and symptoms of cavernous sinus thrombosis are characteristic. However, imaging used in confirming diagnosis consists of MRI venogram in addition to CT scan. Cerebral angiography is invasive and not very sensitive to the diagnosis of cavernous sinus thrombosis.

Treatment includes early diagnosis and prompt medical therapy consisting of IV antibiotics. Drainage of sinuses to remove the source of infection is a must and should be done as soon as possible. The role of anticoagulants like heparin is controversial. Heparin should be used only if diagnosis is made within a few hours. In more delayed cases anticoagulants like warfarin may be tried.

Intracranial Complications

Due to the bony immaturity, thin fovea ethmoidalis and numerous foramina that remain open in children till full ossification takes place there is an increased incidence of intracranial complications as compared to adults. The signs and symptoms that the children present with

Flowchart 2: Algorithm for management of persistent inflammation.

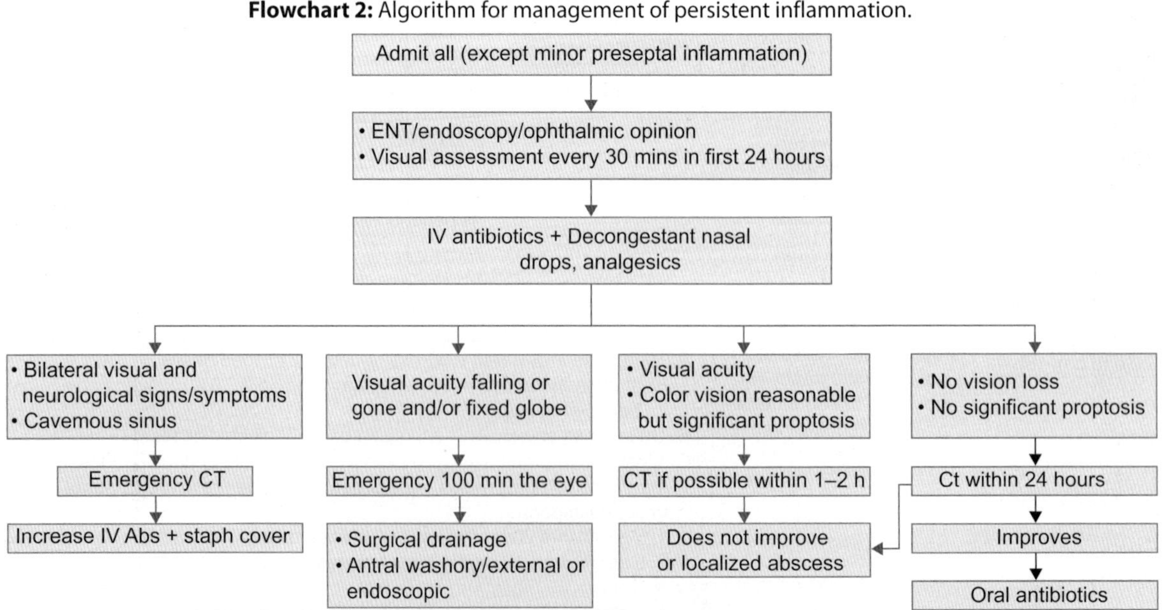

(CT: computed tomography; ENT: ear-nose-throat; IV: intravenous)

are also subtle, thus a high degree of suspicion is needed to diagnose the intracranial complications.

There are five types of intracranial complications of sinusitis in children:

1. Meningitis
2. Epidural abscess
3. Subdural abscess
4. Brain abscess
5. Cavernous sinus thrombophlebitis

These complications can also be considered as a spectrum of progression of disease. Thus, the symptoms can be quite overlapping with confusion to the surgeon. However, the final diagnosis is often made radiologically. The common symptoms include general symptoms such as fever, irritability, vomiting, seizures, and altered sensorium. Specific symptoms include hemiparesis, visual disturbances, and other neurological deficits. Thus ruling out sinusitis is an important part of working up a child with such symptoms even with no preceding complaints of nasal discharge or obstruction.

The most common microorganisms isolated in children include *S. pneumoniae*, *S. aureus*, Gram-negative rods, and anaerobes.

Meningitis

Acute bacterial meningitis follows sinusitis and presents with all the general malaise symptoms in the child. Additionally, the child may have neck rigidity on examination and photophobia, and may also present with cranial nerve palsies. Upon examination, the various tests done are the Kernig's sign and Brudzinki's sign. Radiologically, there may be enhancement along the meninges but with no abscess formation.

Epidural and Subdural Abscess

Due to the usual ambiguity between the two types of abscesses, which are close to one another, they may be considered together. They present with fever with chills and rigors, headache, and vomiting. Due to raised ICT there may be features of papilledema upon fundoscopic examination. Epidural and subdural abscess are differentiated from one another radiologically. Epidural abscess presents with a rim shaped enhancement on CT scanning, whereas subdural abscess presents with biconvex or crescentic enhancing lesions. Subdural abscess also have a higher rate of residual neurological sequelae, which are present in 35–55% of the cases.

Intracerebral Abscess

In the present antibiotic era, brain abscesses have become extremely rare. However, if present they present the surgeon as an emergency with symptoms of altered sensorium, focal neurological deficits, seizures, and papilledema. There is also a grave prognosis as there is a 20–30% risk of mortality associated with it. On CT scanning there is hypodense lesion in the brain, usually in the frontal or temporoparietal lobe with peripheral rim enhancement.

CLINICAL PEARLS

- Antibiotics in all cases of sinusitis in children <2 years of age or in those who have had a complication in the past.
- Early recognition of warning signs a must for successful treatment and prevention of complications.
- Limited role of antihistaminics and systemic decongestants, IV antibiotics is the mainstay of treatment.
- Multidisciplinary team to successfully diagnose and treat sinusitis and its complications.
- Early radiography may remove doubt in most cases.
- Adenoidectomy is the first line of surgical management in uncomplicated cases.
- Prompt surgical intervention is a must in case of visual deficit and threatening complications.

KEY POINTS

- Bacterial sinusitis in children is usually preceded by viral rhinitis, which is one of the most common diseases in children.
- Usual bacteria implicated are *S. pneumoniae, H. influenzae,* and *M. catarrhalis*.
- The symptoms include runny nose, nasal obstruction, fever, and cough.
- High index of suspicion, anterior rhinoscopy and nasoendoscopy is a must to diagnose pediatric sinusitis.
- Increased rate of complications of sinusitis in children, which may be local, orbital, or intracranial.
- In case of complications IV antibiotics, prompt management, and imaging is a must.
- Surgery may be needed on an emergent basis to prevent vision loss in advanced orbital complications.

SUGGESTED READING

1. American Academy of Pediatrics. Subcommittee on Management of Sinusitis and Committee on Quality Improvement. Clinical practice guideline: management of sinusitis. Pediatrics. 2001;108(3):798-808.
2. Chandler JR, Langerbrunner DJ, Stevens ER. The pathogenesis of orbital complications in acute rhinosinusitis. Laryngoscope. 1970;80(9):1414-28.

3. Dalgorf DM, Harvey RJ. Anatomy of the nose and paranasal sinuses. In: Watkinson JC, Raymond CW (Eds). Scott Brown's Otorhinolaryngology Head and Neck Surgery, 8th edition. Boca Raton: CRC press; 2019. pp. 961-76.
4. Fokkens WS, Viskers AS, Backer V, Conti D, Corso ED, Gevaert P, et al. EPOS/EUFOREA update on indications and evaluation of biologics in chronic rhinosinusitis with nasal polyps. Rhinology. 2023;61(3):194-202.
5. Lusk RP, Stankiewicz JA. Pediatric rhinosinusitis. Otolaryngology—Head and Neck Surgery. 1997;117(3): S53-7.
6. Miller AJ, Amedee RG. Sinus anatomy and function. In: Bailey BJ et al. (Eds). Otolaryngology—Head and Neck Surgery. Philadelphia: Lippincott Williams & Wilkins; 2006. pp. 413-21.
7. Ott NL, O'Connell EJ, Hoffman AD, Beatty CW, Sachs MI. Childhood Sinusitis. Mayo Clin Proc. 1991;66:1238-47.
8. Philpott C. Rhinosinusitis: Definitions and diagnosis. In: Watkinson JC, Raymond CW (Eds). Scott Brown's Otorhinolaryngology Head and Neck Surgery, 8th Edition, Vol 1. Boca Raton: CRC press; 2019: pp 1025-36.
9. Tweedie DJ. Paediatric Rhinosinusitis and its complications. In: Watkinson JC, Raymond CW (Eds). Scott Brown's Otorhinolaryngology Head and Neck Surgery, 8th Edition. Boca Raton: CRC press; 2019: pp. 261-78.
10. Wormald PJ, Hoseman W, Callejas C, Weber RK, Kennedy DW, Citardi MJ, et al. The International Frontal Sinus Anatomy Classification (IFAC) and classification of the extent of endoscopic frontal sinus surger (EFSS). Int Forum Allergy Rhinol. 2016.;6(7):677-96.

Stridor in Children

Arvind S Bais

INTRODUCTION

Stridor means noisy-breathing. It is loud noise <10% of the new born babies have some kind of noisy breathing but all of them do not fit into the category of congenital laryngeal stridor. Which comprises of group of conditions present since birth.

CLINICAL PEARLS

- It is important to know that no clinical entity as congenital laryngeal stridor exists.
- Upper airway evaluation is the basic need in every case.

In clinical practice, a variety of terms are frequently used to describe the noisy breathing which are given in **Table 1**.

It is essential to know that there are some basic differences between the larynx of an infant and adult larynx. A proper understanding of which helps in treatment planning.

Infant larynx:

- Situated higher up in the neck close to the base of the tongue
- The size is small
- Epiglottis is infolded
- The aryepiglottic folds are large
- The internal diameter of the larynx is small
- The mucous membrane of the larynx is loosely attached, especially in the subglottic region
- The entire cartilaginous framework of the larynx is soft

TABLE 1: Terms frequently need to describe noisy breathing.

	Site of origin
Wheeze	Intrathoracic airways
Stridor	Extrathoracic airways
Rattle	Either of the above or both
Biphasic sound	Trachea

CLINICAL PEARL

- As the internal diameter of the infant larynx is small even 1 mm of edema in the subglottic area narrows the airway to approximately 50% as compared to adults in whom no significant change occurs.

The causes of stridor can be divided into: (A) Congenital and (B) Acquired.

CONGENITAL CAUSES

- Laryngotracheal stenosis
- Laryngeal atresia
- Laryngomalacia
- Tracheomalacia or
- Laryngeal webs
- Laryngeal cysts
- Vascular abnormalities such as:
  - Aberrant left subclavian artery
  - Innominate artery compression
  - Double aortic arch
- Vocal cord palsy

ACQUIRED CAUSES

- Laryngeal trauma
- Epiglottitis
- Croup
- Acquired causes prefix Multiple Laryngeal Papilloma
- Retropharyngeal abscess
- Bilateral abductor palsy of the vocal cords
- Cystic hygroma
- Large tonsils and adenoids may cause stridor during sleep
- Hemangioma may be congenital or acquired
- Foreign bodies in the airway, i.e., larynx, trachea, and the bronchus
- Reflux laryngitis
- Inhalation of toxic fumes/gases

Laryngotracheal Stenosis

- Narrowing of the larynx wait and watch if the symptoms are mild.
- If severe stridor is present do tracheostomy.
- Laryngotracheal reconstruction can be done at a later date. Procedure is known as laryngotracheoplasty

Laryngeal Atresia

It is usually incompatible with life.

Laryngomalacia

- Causes stridor while crying feeding there is inward collapse of the cartilaginous framework of the larynx leading to inspiratory stridor.
- Stridor is more when the baby is lying on his back and is a common condition.

DIAGNOSIS

Use flexible endoscope to assess the status of the larynx in spontaneous respiration. It is a self-limiting disease.

Symptoms usually subside by 2–3 years of age.

> **CLINICAL PEARL**
>
> Reassure the parents regarding clinical improvement over a period of time. No surgery is required. Small frequent feeds and burping is required.

Tracheomalacia

- The incidence ranges between 1 in 1,500 and 1 in 2,000 children. Diagnosis is by computed tomography (CT) and magnetic resonance imaging (MRI).
- Bronchoscopy reveals flattening of the trachea anteriorly or at the junction of middle and lower third of the trachea use of antibiotics is recommended to prevent bronchitis.
- In severe cases surgery is indicated.

> **CLINICAL PEARL**
>
> The parents should be advised to bring their child for regular check-up in order to minimize unnecessary usage of antibiotics and overcome anxiety amongst family members.

Laryngeal Webs

In the third month of gestation if the larynx fails to get canalized web forms. In majority of cases webs are located anteriorly, thickness may vary:

- Patient presents with severe stridor.
- Immediate measure requires tracheostomy following endoscopy.
- Ablation of the web by CO_2 laser.

Laryngeal Cysts

True congenital cysts of the larynx are extremely rare. There is severe stridor endoscopy reveals cystic swilling completely distorting the view of the larynx, originating from the aryepiglottic folds. Manage by Aspiration of fluid from the cyst, allow it to collapse, and then followed by complete excision of the cyst wall. The procedure is known as deroofing and excision.

ACQUIRED CAUSES

Epiglottitis

Inflammation of the supraglottic larynx caused by *Haemophilus influenzae* type B and rarely by streptococci and pneumococci. Assess by:

- Postural inspiratory stridor
- Drooling and sudden onset of severe sore throat
- Thick mucus secretion
- High temperature
- Lack of cough

Recommended:

- Pulse oximetry
- Monitor arterial blood gas (ABGS)
- Humidification
- Oxygenation

> **CLINICAL PEARL**
>
> There is no evidence to show that the systemic corticosteroid is useful, but can be given the use of HIB vaccine has reduced the incidence.

Croup

Most common between 6 months and 5 years of age. Commonly occurs in winter and is viral in origin.

Symptoms

- Inspiratory stridor
- Fever
- Barking cough
- Hoarse voice

Diagnosis

Lateral X-ray of the neck in extended position will reveal enlarged edematous epiglottis, called as Thumb sign or a tapered subglottic area called "steeple sign" is seen.

Management

Always admit the child. Humidification does not give much relief. Administer nebulized adrenaline. For moderate-to-severe cases systemic or nebulized corticosteroids is recommended. Avoid beta agonist.

CLINICAL PEARL

- Some children with COVID-19 may also present like croup. Though very rare but has to be kept in mind.
- Repeated clinical examination is most desired intervention as the clinical condition may worsen.

FOREIGN BODIES IN AIRWAYS

History of aspiration of foreign bodies in most of the cases occasionally no history of aspiration yet the child may have violent cough, breathing difficulty, difficulty in swallowing, and inspiratory stridor.

Management:

- Ensure adequate airway
- Oxygenation in severe stridor
- Prophylactic antibiotics and systemic corticosteroids to be given on need based cases.
- Plan for quick intervention in form of pan endoscopy, i.e., laryngoscopy, bronchoscopy, and in few cases esophagoscopy is required because foreign bodies in the upper end of esophagus is a common cause of unsuspected partial airways obstruction.
- Endoscopic procedure requires good team work between pediatrician, otolaryngologist and anesthetist.
- Premedication is always by atropine injection.
- Spontaneous anesthesia by use of nitrous oxide, oxygen, and halothane.
- Rarely muscle relaxant may be given.

Instruments:

- All types of rigid pediatric laryngoscopes including anterior commissure laryngoscope rigid bronchoscopes with internal diameter of 2.5 mm, 3 mm, 4 mm, or 6 mm with facility for ventilation telescopes with an angle of 0°, 30°, and 70° and all types of foreign body removal forceps and powerful suction apparatus is a must.
- Tracheostomy tray should be kept ready one may need it at times.

CLINICAL PEARLS

- Bronchoscopy needed.
- Always prefer to use rigid endoscopes as a flexible bronchoscope fails to give the depth of the field.

SUBGLOTTIC HEMANGIOMA

- May be congenital or acquired.
- Large hemangioma produces inspiratory stridor.
- Removal by CO_2 laser.
- Radiotherapy is contraindicated.
- Always look for cutaneous hemangioma.
- May spontaneously resolve if small.

In all cases of stridor the essential broad principles of approach is as follows:

- Proper history taking and clinical observation followed by auscultation.
- Note the type of stridor.
- Any relationship with change of posture. Note does it gets aggravated or stops by change of posture or while feeding.
- Note the duration of stridor.
- Is it continuous, regular, or intermittent?
- Any change in the pattern of stridor while crying.
- Is there any aspiration while taking feeds?

CLINICAL PEARLS

- Do not classify stridor as wheeze as one may miss upper airway obstructive pathology.
- Always look for respiratory distress, at times even slow respiratory rate. There may be evidence of hypoxia, hypercarbia, and even cyanosis.

ABNORMALITIES OF THE CRY

- In unilateral vocal cord palsy weak cry.
- In bilateral vocal cord palsy the cry is weak but clear.
- Absent or Muffled cry is noted in laryngeal web.
- Hoarse cry due to excessive crying or inflammation.

CLINICAL PEARLS

- Hunger.
- Emotion.
- Pain all can also cause cry in babies
- Rule them out

Flowchart 1: Workup of a child with stridor.

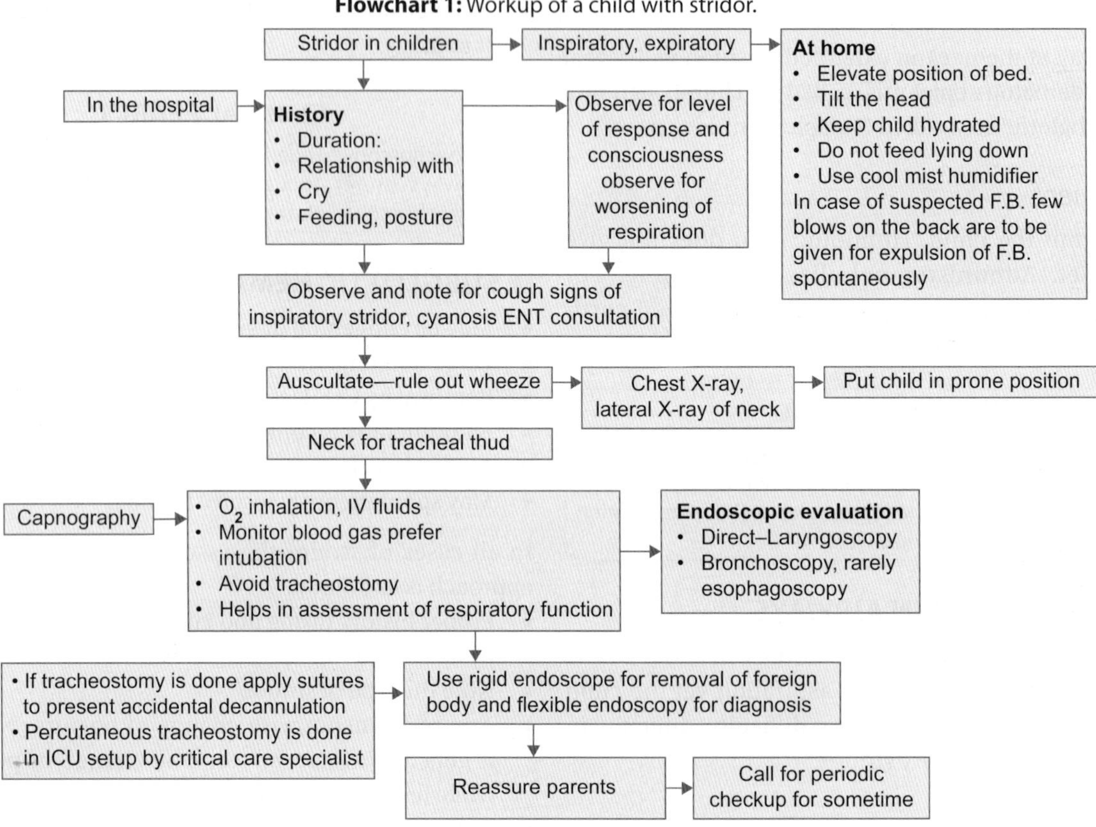

PHYSICAL SIGNS

Inspiratory stridor:

- Breathing is rapid.
- Recession of the suprasternal and intercostal spaces.
- In drawing of the epigastric region.
- Flaring of the nostrils.

NASAL PATENCY TEST

Put a small piece of cotton in front of the baby's nostril and observe for to and fro movement of cotton. Less movement on one or both sides gives an idea of nasal block. Also pass soft rubber catheter from the nose to the nasopharynx, it checks the patency and breaks the membranous choanal atresia if any.

RADIOLOGY

- Lateral skiagram of neck in extended position is a must. Take care of occipital protuberance in children.
- CT and MRI is very helpful in cases of stenosis and tracheomalacia.
- Contrast radiography in cases of suspected vascular abnormalities.
- Chest X-ray PA (Postero Anterior) and lateral view should always be done.

KEY POINTS

- Supraglottic lesion causes inspiratory stridor while subglottic pathology may cause biphasic stridor
- Clinical evaluation, it is a must
- Follow the principle of observation, palpation, and auscultation of the chest, neck, and also for any tracheal Thud (loud tracheal sound).
- Never hesitate to consult anesthetist and ear-nose-throat (ENT) surgeon for proper management of airway, i.e., intubation, oxygenation tracheostomy, and for endoscopy.
- Monitor oxygen saturation and arterial blood gas estimation.
- Ultrasonography may be needed in vocal cord palsy.
- Prefer laryngeal intubation than tracheostomy as much as possible.
- In severe cases of stridor shift the patient to operation theater (OT) where all facilities for anesthesia, ventilator support, tracheostomy, and endoscopy are available.
- Flexible endoscopy is helpful for screening, but for removal of foreign bodies from the airway, rigid endoscopy is preferred.
- Never use jet ventilation anesthesia in cases of surgery of multiple papilloma of the larynx because of seedling and recurrence.

- If there is delay in setting up OT trolley always intubate the child and oxygenate.
- For laryngoscopic evaluation with a rigid laryngoscope in infants never try to lift the epiglottis with the tip of laryngoscope as severe laryngeal spasm may occur. Just wait for few seconds spontaneous visualization is possible because in infants the larynx is very close to the base of the tongue.
- If foreign body such as seed of any such object has been removed piecemeal then always do a check bronchoscopy before discharging the patient from the hospital as a small foreign bodies if left in the bronchus may cause serious complications later on.
- Be careful in bronchoscopy as one may override a foreign body and nothing may be found.
- Carina is the thinnest part of tracheobronchial tree respect it while doing the endoscopy. A small tear may lead to spontaneous pneumothorax.
- Never waste time in removing a foreign body especially in demonstrating its location as it may slip deeper down and make the whole procedure difficult and time consuming.
- Gastroesophageal reflux may play a major role in acquired abnormalities in older children.

SUGGESTED READING

1. Cummings CW, Richardson MA, Haughey BH, Thomas JR, Harker LA, Robbins KT, et al. Stridor and airway management. In: David Albert, Susanna Leighton (Eds). Otolaryngology Head and Neck surgery, 3rd edition. Mosby: Elsevier; 2017. pp. 285-8.
2. Cummings CW. Congenital disorders of the larynx. Otolaryngology Head and Neck surgery. Philadelphia: Elsevier; 2017. pp. 262-84.
3. Seiden AM, Gluckman JL, Padhya JA, Wilson KM et al. Congenital disorders. Otolaryngology the Essentials. pp. 247-51.
4. Sigler BA, Schuring LT. Ear Nose and Throat Disorders. Mosby Clinical Nursing Series. US: Mosby; 1993. pp. 190-5.

Upper Airway Obstruction and Sleep-related Breathing Disorder

Ashwani Kumar, Ameet Kishore

INTRODUCTION

Upper airway obstruction refers to the partial or complete blockage of the upper airway. Obstructive sleep-disordered breathing describes a spectrum of abnormal breathing patterns during sleep characterized by snoring and increased respiratory effort. Habitual snoring during sleep, the hallmark indicator of increased upper airway resistance, is an extremely frequent occurrence during childhood, with a median incidence of about 10% among preschool and school-aged children, with subsequent declines in frequency after 12 years of age. Sleep-disordered breathing in children is a timely public health concern, given the increasing rates of obesity and hyperactivity in this population. This activity highlights the role of the interprofessional team in the diagnosis and treatment of this condition.

The estimated prevalence of snoring in children is 3–12%, while obstructive sleep apnea (OSA) affects 1–10%. The majority of these children have mild symptoms, and many outgrow the condition. The OSA often results from adenotonsillar hypertrophy, neuromuscular disease, and craniofacial abnormalities.

Sleep-disordered breathing refers to a pathophysiologic spectrum that includes snoring, upper airway resistance syndrome (UARS), obstructive hypopnea syndrome, and OSA. The mildest form of OSA in children is UARS. Affected children have symptoms of OSA but lack the accompanying polysomnographic findings. While many children demonstrate intermittent snoring and mouth breathing, severe form OSA results in worst clinical sequelae such as failure to thrive, behavior problems, enuresis, and cor pulmonale.

The exact polysomnographic criteria that differentiate between innocent snoring and snoring that is associated with adverse consequences, have yet to be defined. Nevertheless, a consensus statement has been generated, and defines a set of empiric criteria, on the basis of which we currently estimate that of the many children with habitual snoring; approximately 2–3% will have clinically relevant disease. Therefore, the ratio between symptomatic habitual snoring and OSA is usually between 3:1 and 5:1.

As demonstrated in one study a large percentage of children with hyperactivity or inattentive behaviors had underlying sleep disordered breathing. These children would be cared for more effectively with appropriate recognition and treatment of sleep-disordered breathing than with the use of stimulant medications **(Flowchart 1)**.

PATHOPHYSIOLOGY

Physical examination reveals adenotonsillar hypertrophy in most children with OSA. Whenever lymphoid tissue in a child occupies a disproportionate amount of space in the oropharyngeal region, it causes a compromise airway.

Flowchart 1: Sleep related breathing disorders.

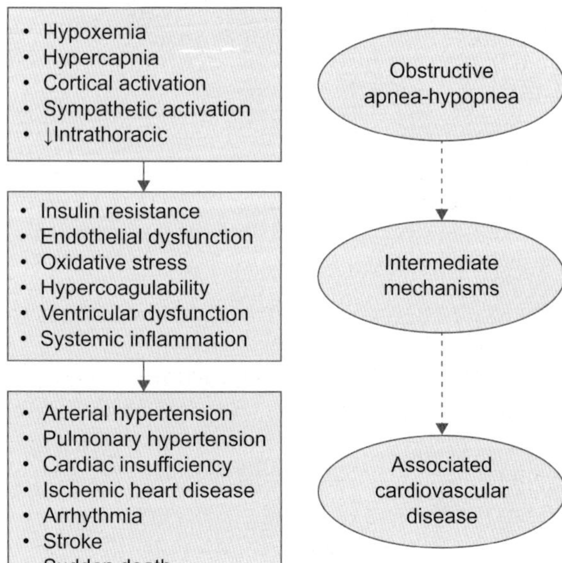

Children with craniofacial syndromes have fixed anatomic variations that predispose them to airway obstruction, while in children with neuromuscular disease, obstruction is caused by hypotonia. The problem can be made more intense by associated anatomic conditions such as craniofacial abnormalities, obesity, laryngomalacia, and conditions with diminished neuromuscular tone as in Down syndrome and cerebral palsy.

It is however during sleep they exhibit signs of the full spectrum of airway obstruction. This is due to the relaxation of the oropharyngeal muscle leading to further obstruction. These children may usually snore loudly with cessation of breathing for short intervals with sternal retraction and paradoxical movement of the chest. The negative physiological outcome includes hypoxemia, hypercapnia, and acidosis which lead to arousals, awakenings, and a poor quality sleep. These children demonstrate a variety of behavioral problems including hyperactivity, lack of stamina, poor attention spans and daytime sleepiness or tiredness.

These disturbances in sleep are collectively called sleep related breathing disorders (SRBD). One such syndrome is called UARS where a child with a significantly obstructive nose causes snoring, mouth breathing without significant apneas but a significant increase in respiratory effort related arousal giving rise to daytime fatigue and poor performance.

CLINICAL PRESENTATION

The most common presentation in children younger than 5 years is snoring. Other night time symptoms frequently reported by parents include mouth breathing, increased respiratory effort, supra-sternal and intercostal retraction, nocturnal sweating, abnormal sleep posture (hyper-extension of the neck), restless nocturnal sleep, frequent awakenings during night, and observed respiratory pauses.

Poor growth and failure to thrive are more common in children with sleep-disordered breathing. Growth velocity increases after adenotonsillectomy. The hypothesized etiology for failure to thrive is increased work of breathing, with subsequent increase in baseline caloric expenditure. Decreased production of growth hormone during fragmented sleep may contribute further to poor growth **(Box 1)**.

Children with significant OSA if not treated may land up with cor pulmonale, right ventricular hypertrophy, congestive heart failure, pulmonary hypertension and edema, failure to thrive, and are at a definitive risk for permanent neurologic damage and even death.

BOX 1: Symptoms and signs of obstructive sleep apnea syndrome.

Symptoms:

- Snoring
- Labored breathing during sleep
- Gasping for air/snorting noises/observed episodes of apnea
- Sleeping in a seated position or with the neck hyperextended
- Cyanosis
- Cor pulmonale
- Sleep enuresis (especially secondary enuresis)*
- Excessive daytime sleepiness
- Attention-deficit/hyperactivity disorder
- Learning problems/poor academic performance
- Unusual daytime behavior

Physical examination:

- Adenotonsillar hypertrophy
- Lingual tonsils
- Craniofacial abnormalities
- Growth disturbances
- Failure to thrive
- Underweight or overweight
- Laryngeal pathology

*Enuresis after at least 6 months of continence.

Enuresis associated with OSA often resolves after successful treatment of sleep-disordered breathing. Increased urine production results from hormonal dysregulation. These alterations are accompanied by increased levels of catecholamines and frequent arousal that further contribute to enuresis.

The prevalence of OSA in children is 1–4% and surprisingly up to 10% of children may present with primary snoring. Physical examination should include the patient's weight, height, and body mass index. Detailed physical examination of a child suspected of having OSA must include evaluation of the child's general appearance, with special emphasis to craniofacial characteristics such as midface hypoplasia, micrognathia, and occlusal relationships. Adenoid facies is perhaps the most common observation. Evaluation for nasal obstruction depends on the child's age. Septal deviation, choanal atresia, nasolacrimal cysts, and nasal aperture stenosis must be considered in infants. In older children, nasal polyps and turbinate hypertrophy must be ruled out.

Tonsil size should ideally be scaled from 1–4. Scale 1 being mild hypertrophy and scale 4 would compromise

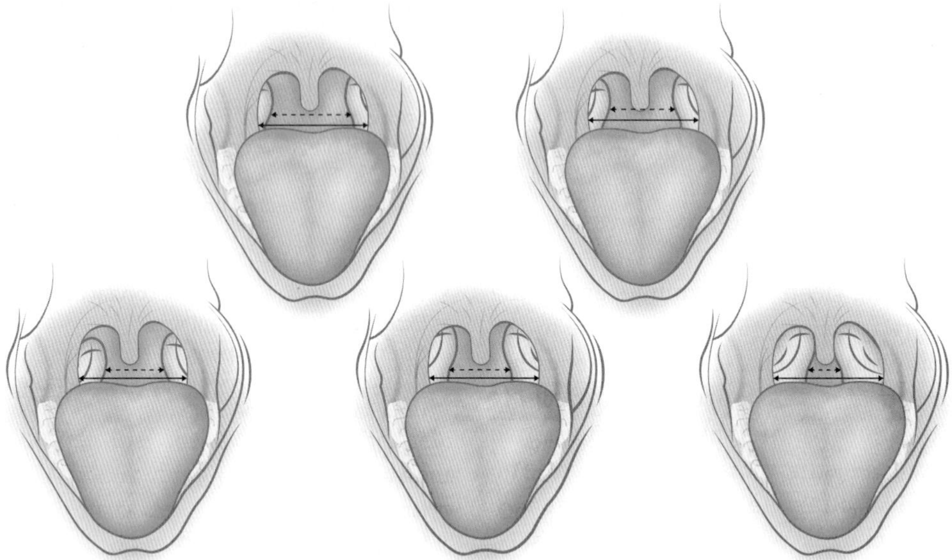

Fig. 1: Standardized tonsillar hypertrophy grading scale. *(0)* Tonsils are entirely within the tonsillar fossa. *(1+)* Tonsils occupy <25% of the lateral dimension of the oropharynx as measured between the anterior tonsillar pillars. *(2+)* Tonsils occupy <50% of the lateral dimension of the oropharynx. *(3+)* Tonsils occupy <75% of the lateral dimension of the oropharynx. *(4+)* Tonsils occupy 75% or more of the lateral dimension of the oropharynx.

>75% of the oropharyngeal airway. The adenoid size is best evaluated with a soft tissue lateral neck radiograph to assess the anteroposterior dimension of the nasopharynx. However, the correlation to the clinical symptoms is still effected by subjectivity **(Figs. 1 and 2)**.

POLYSOMNOGRAPHY

Polysomnography is necessary for diagnosis and treatment of patients with multiple medical comorbidities, children with craniofacial syndromes, and patients with an unclear etiology (which includes patient with modest physical findings or examination findings inconsistent with severity of apnea), and to determine the degree of apnea.

Polysomnography is the gold standard for the diagnosis of OSA and disordered breathing however, the lack of reliable sleep laboratories for children, excess cost, and lack of consensus on interpretation of polysomnograms as reasons it is not required for diagnosis. Children may have sleep disruption because of an increased effort to breathe but show no evidence of apnea on polysomnography. This condition is called UARS.

In a large majority the clinical decision-making is shown to be accurate. However, it may benefit a child with severe problems to consult with a pulmonologist and a cardiologist to rule out the other significant and dangerous complications of OSA.

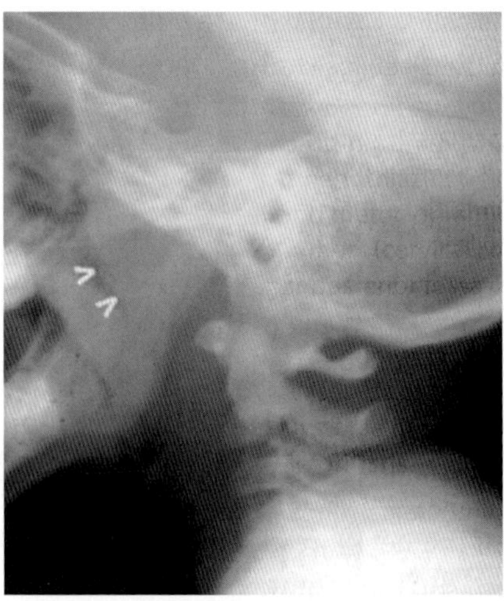

Fig. 2: Lateral neck radiograph. Arrows indicate prominent adenoidal tissue in the posterior nasopharynx, resulting in upper airway narrowing.

OTHER DIAGNOSTIC EXAMINATIONS

Pulse oximetry, often recommended as screening tool but is not an accurate predictor of OSA because large numbers of children have sleep disturbance without desaturations.

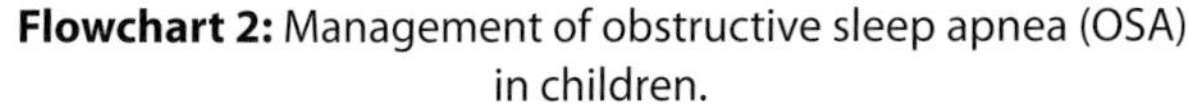

Flowchart 2: Management of obstructive sleep apnea (OSA) in children.

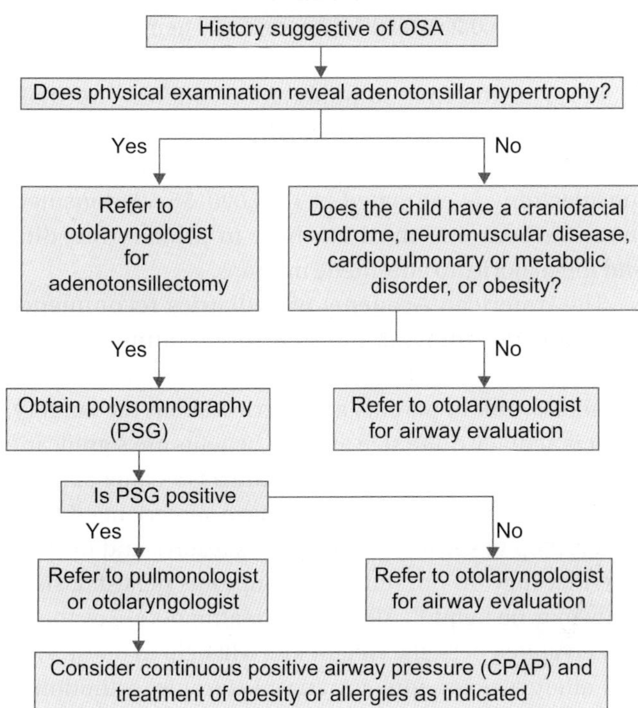

In addition, subgroups of children who have night time desaturations do not have OSA **(Flowchart 2)**.

The use of video photography to record apneic events and night time arousals in children has shown mixed results and poor predictive accuracy. Airway fluoroscopy provides information on the degree of obstruction and the dynamics of the child's airway. However, this procedure rarely is used because flexible fiberoptic nasopharyngoscopy is more reliable with no radiation exposure and can be performed as office procedure.

Cervical computed tomography and magnetic resonance imaging also demonstrate pharyngeal lymphoid hyperplasia. When nasopharyngoscopy is unavailable, lateral neck radiography should be considered as a reliable alternative for detecting adenoid hypertrophy. There is some suggestion that behavioral patterns may also be associated with reduced verbal abilities and language scores possibly a result of hypoxemia induced dysfunction of the frontal lobe. However, this supposition needs to be substantiated with research in future.

MANAGEMENT

Antibiotics therapy helps in the treatment of recurrent tonsillitis and adenoiditis. Reduction of postinfectious lymphoid hyperplasia relieves the obstruction. Even small reductions in adenotonsillar size can eliminate snoring and OSA. An established pattern of recurrent infections accompanied by sleep disturbance may warrant consideration of adenotonsillectomy.

Weight loss is an excellent therapeutic measure in obese children, but it can be a difficult process. Allergy testing and treatment of allergic rhinitis are important in children with OSA secondary to nasal obstruction. There is a temporary benefit in use of intranasal corticosteroid but is unlikely to provide definitive therapy.

Unfortunately there are few randomized studies in the efficacy of the tonsillectomy and adenoidectomy for children with OSA. Adenotonsillectomy should be considered first line of therapy for OSA provided adenotonsillar hyperplasia is present. Outcomes appear to improve regardless of the measure used and show a definite improvement in snoring, OSA, enuresis, behavior, and growth following adenotonsillectomy.

Uvulopalatopharyngoplasty is indicated when a thick soft palate and a long uvula are present.

Tracheotomy is reserved for use in children with severe OSA, who have failed to improve with other medical and surgical treatments and in special cases in which these modalities are contraindicated or not tolerated. Tracheotomy must be considered in children for whom traditional surgery is unlikely to be of benefit, such as those with Pierre Robin syndrome.

Children with craniofacial syndromes presents more commonly with OSA. Children who have syndromes with craniosynostosis, such as Apert's syndrome, Crouzon's disease, Pfeiffer's syndrome, and Saethre-Chotzen syndrome; abnormalities of the skull base; and accompanying maxillary hypoplasia may have nasopharyngeal obstruction.

Children with syndromes that involve micrognathia, such as Treacher Collins syndrome, Pierre Robin syndrome, and Goldenhar' syndrome, become obstructed at the hypopharyngeal level. In children with trisomy 21, narrow upper airway combined with macroglossia and hypotonic musculature predisposes them to OSA.

The surgical management of craniofacial syndromes and OSA in children frequently requires more than standard adenotonsillectomy which involves tracheotomy.

In children with midfacial hypoplasia, craniofacial advancement may be indicated. Glossopexy, mandibular distraction or advancement, or tongue suspension should be considered in patients with micrognathia.

> **CLINICAL PEARLS**
>
> - Tonsil size does not always correlate with severity of obstructive sleep apnea as determined by polysomnography.
> - Primary care physician can assess adenoid size by ordering a soft tissue lateral radiograph of the nasopharynx from a good center.

Children with other comorbidities such as craniofacial, neuromuscular, genetic, and allergic abnormalities are at a higher risk for persistent postoperative OSA and also at a higher risk of postoperative complication such as respiratory embarrassment and residual airway obstruction.

Long-term follow-up shows a dramatic improvement in the quality of life scores after adenotonsillectomy with reduction in the number of upper respiratory episodes, and hospital visit and admissions. A reduction in problem behaviors and cognitive impairment was seen after adenotonsillectomy. Studies suggested that in a majority of children enuresis resolves or improves after the surgery.

> **CLINICAL PEARLS**
>
> - Adenotonsillectomy is effective in reducing physiological, behavioral, and cognitive sequelae in patients with adenotonsillar hypertrophy, and obstructive sleep apnea.
> - Some patients with obesity develop recurrent obstructive sleep apnea after adenotonsillectomy. The primary care physician must emphasize weight reduction and continue to monitor the signs and symptoms of obstructive sleep apnea after surgery.

ADENOTONSILLECTOMY

Adenoidectomy and adenotonsillectomy remain the most commonly performed operations in children. However, they are also the most discussed, appreciated, denounced, and least studied procedures in the history of ear-nose-throat (ENT) surgery. While the indications have changed over the decades. The essential surgery remains the same with the advent of laser, coblation, high frequency diathermy, etc. The intraoperative bleeding has reduced dramatically; however, the traditional surgery with blunt dissection and snare still seems to have a large number of favorable references.

Adenoidectomy however has become more effective and definitive with the introduction of nasal endoscopy coupled with powered instrumentation like shavers made by Medtronics. The operative and postoperative complications are dehydration, velopharyngeal insufficiency, and hemorrhage. Hemorrhage remains the most common serious problems of the surgery. The incidence is reported from 0.2 to 0.22% from primary hemorrhage and from 0.1 to 3% for secondary hemorrhage.

Fever in the first 36 hours is considered "normal." It is important to maintain hydration in hospital and immediate postoperative period. Mortality from tonsillectomy is estimated at 1/16,000–35,000 tonsillectomies. About one-third attribute to primary bleeding and the majority to anesthetic mishaps.

The American Academy of Pediatrics recommends adenotonsillectomy as the first line treatment in any child with OSA and enlargement of the tonsils and adenoids. A lot of parents are worried about the surgery, but it is actually quite safe and the benefits are significant. In some kids, however, there is residual OSA after surgery. Thus, all children with OSA who have surgery need to be followed up to see if there symptoms resolve and to make sure that they do not return. If symptoms persist, a sleep study may be helpful. Alternative treatments are available if sleep apnea persists. Weight loss will help in obese kids, and allergy treatments, intranasal steroids, orthodontic work, and continuous positive airway pressure (CPAP) can benefit some kids.

> **CLINICAL PEARL**
>
> - There are no studies to date that demonstrate significant negative clinical effect of tonsillectomy on the immune system.

RED FLAG SIGNS AND SYMPTOMS OF OBSTRUCTIVE SLEEP APNEA

- Loud or noisy breathing, snoring, or mouth breathing during sleep.
- Brief pauses in breathing during sleep or difficulty breathing during sleep.
- Restless sleep (i.e., lots of tossing and turning)
- Sweating heavily during sleep.
- Bedwetting
- Sleeping in odd positions (e.g., neck hyperextended).
- Inattentiveness and lack of focus at school.
- Excessive daytime sleepiness (e.g., child regularly falls asleep in school).
- Poor academic performance
- Irritable mood, aggressiveness, other behavioral problems.
- Morning headaches

KEY POINTS

- Screening for snoring should be part of routine health maintenance visits in all children; if snoring is present, a more detailed evaluation should follow (good evidence; strong recommendation). *Note:* Obstructive sleep apnea syndrome is unlikely in children who do not have habitual snoring.
- Complex, high-risk patients should be referred to a subspecialist (good evidence for increased surgical risk in these patients and consequent need for more complex management; strong recommendation).
- Patients who have cardiorespiratory failure cannot wait for elective evaluation. These patients are not covered in the AAP guideline because it is expected that they will be in an intensive care setting and managed by a subspecialist.
- The diagnostic evaluation should be thorough. The history and physical examination have been shown to be poor in differentiating between primary snoring and obstructive sleep apnea syndrome (strong evidence). Polysomnography is the diagnostic method of choice; it is the only test that quantifies sleep and ventilatory abnormalities. Other screening techniques, such as videotaping, audiotaping, nocturnal pulse oximetry, and daytime nap polysomnography, may be helpful if the results are positive. However, these tests have high false-negative rates, and they do not assess the severity of the syndrome (disease severity is useful in determining treatment and follow-up). When the results of other diagnostic tests are negative, polysomnography should be performed; additional audiotaping is necessary (strong evidence; strong recommendation).
- In most children, adenotonsillectomy is a first line treatment for obstructive sleep apnea syndrome; continuous positive airway pressure is an option in patients who are not surgical candidates or do not respond to surgical treatment (strong evidence; strong recommendation). *Note:* Potential complications of adenotonsillectomy include anesthetic-related medical problems, pain, and poor oral intake in the immediate postoperative period, and hemorrhage. Patients with obstructive sleep apnea syndrome may have respiratory complications (e.g., worsening of the syndrome, pulmonary edema); death attributable to severe respiratory complications has been reported in patients with severe obstructive sleep apnea syndrome. Risk factors for complications after adenotonsillectomy in children with obstructive sleep apnea syndrome include age younger than 3 years, cardiac complications of the syndrome (e.g., right ventricular hypertrophy), severe obstructive sleep apnea syndrome determined by polysomnography, failure to thrive, obesity, prematurity, recent respiratory infection, craniofacial anomalies, and neuromuscular disorders (the last two risk factors are not discussed in the AAP Guideline).

SUGGESTED READING

1. AAO-HNS Position Statement—Treatment of Obstructive Sleep Apnea. [online] Available from https://www.entnet.org/resource/position-statement-treatment-ofobstructive-sleep-apnea/ [Last accessed March, 2025].
2. American Thoracic Society. Standards and indications for cardiopulmonary sleep studies in children. Am J Respir Crit Care Med. 1996;153(2):866-78.
3. Beebe DW. Neurobehavioral morbidity associated with disordered breathing during sleep in children: a comprehensive review. Sleep. 2006;29(9):1115-34.
4. Bhattacharjee R, Kheirandish-Gozal L, Spruyt K, Mitchell RB, Promchiarak J, Simakajornboon N, et al. Adenotonsillectomy Outcomes in Treatment of obstructive sleep apnea in children. Am J Respir Crit Care Med. 2010;182(5):676-83.
5. Brietzke SE, Gallagher D. Brieztke 2006—The effectiveness of tonsillectomy and adenoidectomy in the treatment of pediatric obstructive sleep apnea/hypopnea syndrome: A meta- analysis. Epstein 2009—Clinical Guidelines for Evaluation, Management and long-term care of obstructive sleep apnea in adults. Otolaryngol Head Neck Surg. 2006;134(6):979-84.
6. Brietzke SE, Katz ES, Roberson DW. Can history and physical examination reliably diagnose pediatric obstructive sleep apnea/hypopnea syndrome? A systematic review of the literature. Otolaryngol Head Neck Surg. 2004;131(6):827-32.
7. Brietzkes SE, Gallagher D. The effectiveness of tonsillectomy and adenoidectomy in the treatment of pediatric obstructive sleep apnea/hypopnea syndrome: a meta-analysis. Otolaryngol Head Neck Surg. 2006;134(6):979-84.
8. Brown KA, Laferriere A, Lakheeram I, Moss IR. Recurrent hypoxemia in children is associated with increased analgesic sensitivity to opiates. Anesthesiology. 2006;105(4):665-9
9. Carroll JL, McColley SA, Marcus CL, Curtis S, Loughlin GM. Inability of clinical history to distinguish primary snoring from obstructive sleep apnea syndrome in children. Chest. 1995;108(3):610-8.
10. Chervin RD, Archbold KH, Dillon JE, Panahi P, Pituch KJ, Dahl RE, et al. Inattention, hyperactivity, and symptoms of sleep-disordered breathing. Pediatrics. 2002;109(3):449-56.
11. Chervin RD, Ruzicka DL, Giordani BJ, Weatherly RA, Dillon JE, Hodges EK, et al. Sleep-disordered breathing, behavior, and cognition in children before and after adenotonsillectomy. Pediatrics. 2006;117(4):e769-78.
12. Cohen SR, Simms C, Burstein FD, Thomsen J. Alternatives to tracheostomy in infants and children with obstructive sleep apnea. J Pediatr Surg. 1999;34(1):182-6.

13. De Serres LM, Derkay C, Sie K, Biavati M, Jones J, Tunkel D, et al. Impact of adenotonsillectomy on quality of life in children with obstructive sleep disorders. Arch Otolaryngol Head Neck Surg. 2002;128(5):489-96.
14. Farber JM. Clinical practice guideline: diagnosis and management of childhood obstructive sleep apnea syndrome. Pediatrics. 2002;110(6):1255-7.
15. Gozal D, Crabtree VM, Sans CO, Witcher LA, Kheirandish-Gozal L. C-reactive protein, obstructive sleep apnea, and cognitive dysfunction in school-aged children. Am J Respir Crit Care Med. 2007;176(2):188-93.
16. Gozal D, Kheirandish-Gozal L. Sleep apnea in children—treatment considerations. Paediatr Respir Rev. 2006; 7(Suppl 1):S58-61.
17. Gozal D. Sleep-disordered breathing and school performance in children. Pediatrics. 1998;102(3 Pt 1): 616-20.
18. Kheirandish L, Goldbart AD, Gozal D. Intranasal steroids and oral leukotriene modifier therapy in residual sleep-disordered breathing after tonsillectomy and adenoidectomy in children. Pediatrics. 2006;117:e61-6.
19. Kribbs NB, Pack AI, Kline LR, Smith PL, Schwartz AR, Schubert NM, et al. Kribbs 1993—Objective Measurement of Patterns of Nasal CPAP Use by Patients with obstructive sleep apnea. Am Rev Respir Dis. 1993;147(4):887-95.
20. Marcus CL, Ward SL, Mallory GB, Rosen CL, Beckerman RC, Weese-Mayer DE, et al. Use of nasal continuous positive airway pressure as treatment of childhood obstructive sleep apnea. J Pediatr. 1995;127(1):88-94.
21. Marcus CL. Pathophysiology of childhood obstructive sleep apnea: current concepts. Respir Physiol. 2000; 119(2-3):143-54.
22. McColley SA, April MM, Carroll JL, Naclerio RM, Loughlin GM. Respiratory compromise after adenotonsillectomy in children with obstructive sleep apnea. Arch Otolaryngol Head Neck Surg. 1992;118(9):940-3.
23. Monasterio FO, Drucker M, Molina F, Ysunza A. Distraction osteogenesis in Pierre Robin sequence and related respiratory problems in children. J Craniofac Surg. 2002; 13(1):79-83.
24. Richards W, Ferdman RM. Prolonged morbidity due to delays in the diagnosis and treatment of obstructive sleep apnea in children. Clin Pediatr (Phila). 2000;39(2):103-8.
25. Rosen CL, D'Andrea L, Haddad GG. Adult criteria for obstructive sleep apnea do not identify children with serious obstruction. Am Rev Respir Dis. 1992;146(5 Pt 1): 1231-4.
26. Rosen GM, Muckle RP, Mahowald MW, Goding GS, Ullevig C. Postoperative respiratory compromise in children with obstructive sleep apnea syndrome: can it be anticipated? Pediatrics. 1994;93(5):784-8.
27. Tauman R, Gulliver TE, Krishna J, Montgomery-Downs HE, O'Brien LM, Ivanenko A, et al. Persistence of obstructive sleep apnea syndrome in children after adenotonsillectomy. J Pediatr. 2006;149(6):803-8.
28. Waters KA, Everett FM, Bruderer JW, Sullivan CE. Obstructive sleep apnea: the use of nasal CPAP in 80 children. Am J Respir Crit Care Med. 1995;152(2):780-5.
29. Weaver EM, Maynard C, Yueh B. Weaver 2004—Survival of Veterans with Sleep Apnea—CPAP vs Surgery. Otolaryngol Head Neck Surg. 2004;130(6):659-65.
30. Weaver TE, Grunstein RR. Weaver 2008—Adherence to CPAP Therapy—The Challenge to Effective Treatment. Proc Am Thorac Soc. 2008;5(2):173-8.

SECTION 19

Orthopedics

Section Editor: *Rujuta Mehta*

CHAPTER 161

Septic Arthritis

Viraj Shingade, Mandar Agashe

INTRODUCTION

Septic arthritis continues to be one of the major causes of orthopedic disability in pediatric population. Although the management is not very difficult, it usually needs a multidisciplinary approach. Most of the neonates are either missed in diagnosis in early stages or they are managed by a medical person single-handed and they lead to outcomes like deformity and limb shortening. If diagnosis is made timely and management is done by the team including neonatologist, pediatrician, pediatric orthopedic surgeon, microbiologist, and radiologist, most of these cases can be cured completely without any remnant deformity or disability. This chapter gives useful information about how to diagnose it at the earliest and what should be the approach for the treatment.

HOW COMMON IS THE PROBLEM?

Septic arthritis refers to bacterial invasion of the joint space and the subsequent inflammatory response.

The incidence of septic arthritis in India is approximately 1 in 1,500 live births. Although bone and joint infections are quite common, the diagnosis of septic arthritis is not always straightforward.

MECHANISM/PATHOPHYSIOLOGY OF THE PROBLEM

Septic arthritis usually is of hematogenous origin, but can arise through direct inoculation. It can occur from the primary seeding of the synovial membrane, secondarily from infection in the adjacent metaphyseal bone or directly from infection in the adjoining epiphysis.

When septic arthritis occurs, bacteria rapidly gain access to the joint cavity and within a matter of hours cause synovitis and formation of fibrinous exudates followed by areas of synovial necrosis. Endotoxins are released. This leads to destruction of the synovium and cartilage matrix. Proteases, peptidases, and collagenases are released from the leukocytes and synovial cells. These enzymes breakdown the cellular and extracellular structures of the cartilage. The loss of glycosaminoglycans is the first measurable change in articular cartilage, occurring as early as 8 hours after bacteria are introduced into the joint. Loss of glycosaminoglycans softens the cartilage and may cause it to be susceptible to increased wear. Collagen destruction follows and is responsible for visible change in cartilage appearance. Elevation of the intracapsular pressure, thrombosis causes impairment of the intracapsular vascular supply which causes articular destruction. Destruction of the joint space leads to long-term sequelae in a significant percentage of patients. In certain joints like hip, infection distends and softens joints capsule and may cause joint subluxation or dislocation.

WHICH ARE THE SUSCEPTIBLE GROUPS IN NEONATES?

Septic arthritis in the neonates is seen in two distinct groups. One is the neonate, who is sick, premature, and needs intensive care. The other group is healthy neonate, who has been discharged from the hospital and then presents 2–3 weeks later with bone and joint infection.

When to Suspect (Flowchart 1)?

Clinically, septic arthritis usually presents with obvious swelling of one or more joints. Symptoms include edema, erythema, joint effusion, and tenderness. Patients tend to keep the affected joint in a position that maximizes intracapsular volume and comfort. Refusal to move an affected joint is referred to as pseudoparalysis and even passive movement may be painful. Systemic symptoms, such as fever, malaise, and poor appetite, are also seen in most patients. If the infection involves a lower extremity,

Flowchart 1: How to diagnose and treat a baby with septic arthritis.

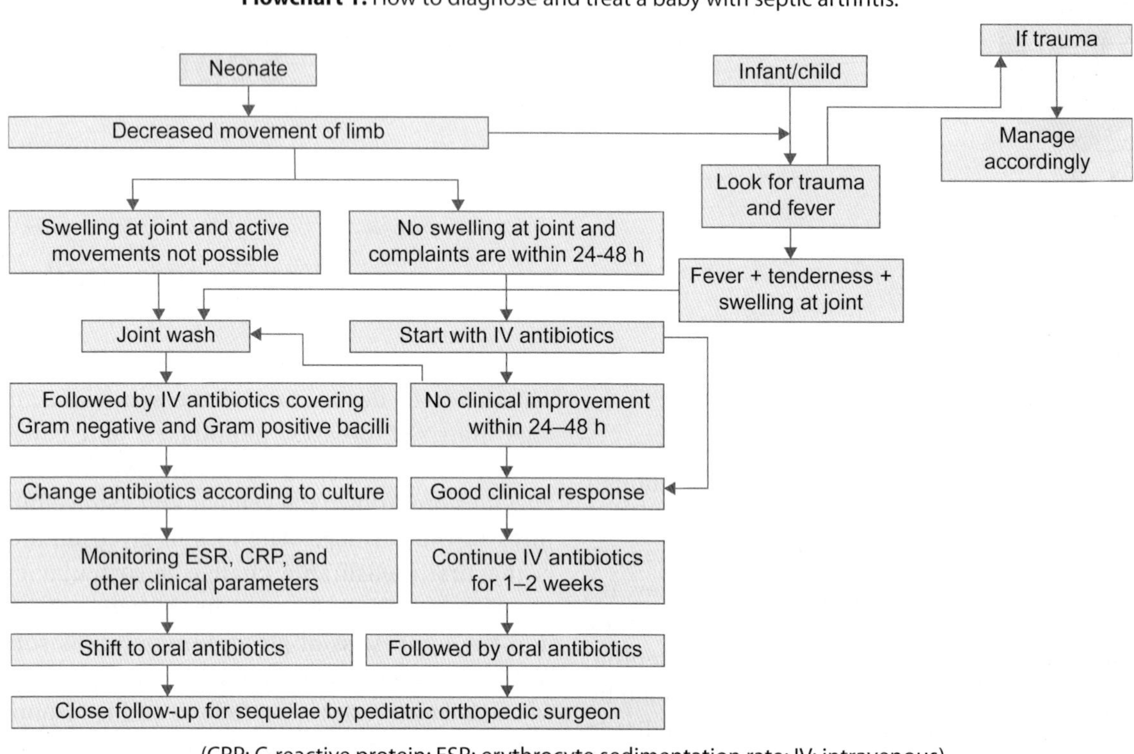

(CRP: C-reactive protein; ESR: erythrocyte sedimentation rate; IV: intravenous)

the child will often have a limp or will be unable to bear weight on the limb. A history of antecedent trauma is quite common. Trauma rarely results in a delayed limp. The clinician should elicit specific details regarding any traumatic event. Did the child cry and limp or refuse to bear weight immediately after the trauma? If the answers to these questions are no and there was a period of time between the injury and time symptoms appeared, the suspicion of infection should increase.

WHICH ARE THE MOST COMMON JOINTS INVOLVED?

Knees and the hips being most commonly affected (80%), other commonly affected joints include the ankles, wrists, elbows, and shoulders.

What are Clinical Clues for Diagnosis in Neonate?

The initial presentation is with swelling of a limb or joint and reluctance to move the limb. There may be irritability on handling, e.g., when changing the nappies. Sometimes, the reluctance to move a limb is so severe as to cause a pseudoparalysis. Septic arthritis of the hip may cause the baby to hold the leg flexed, abducted, and externally rotated.

In the fulminant form of septic arthritis, signs of bone and joint involvement may occur at the time of, or some times after the signs of, sepsis. The babies are lethargic with or without fever, do not tolerate feeds, and may have abdominal distension and jaundice. Multiple bones or joints may be involved.

What are Clinical Clues in Infants and Older Children?

Typical symptoms like high grade fever, and warmth or hot extremity may not be present. Limping, refusal to walk, and refusal to bear weight may be the earliest symptom.

CHALLENGES IN DIAGNOSING SEPTIC ARTHRITIS

Many immunocompromised children fail to have fever and may show lowered white blood cell count. X-rays may be reported as normal in early phase of the disease. Ultrasound, bone scan, or magnetic resonance imaging (MRI) suggest a process of inflammation and effusion, but cannot diagnose septic arthritis confirmatively in the early stage of disease. The damage to the cartilage, growth plate, and bone due to avascularity and enzymatic destruction sets in very early. The cartilage destruction starts as early as 8 hours following the onset of infection. The avascularity sets in within 24–48 hours of the tamponade. The biggest challenge is, therefore, to control the infection and drain the joint before the damage takes place. Understanding the limitations of investigations for confirmation of diagnosis, it is important that physician should have high index of suspicion and should start treatment as earliest as possible.

WHICH ARE OTHER DIFFERENTIAL DIAGNOSES?

It includes hemarthrosis, traumatic effusion, transient synovitis, reactive arthritis, Lyme arthritis, juvenile rheumatoid arthritis, arthritis of acute rheumatic fever, and slipped capital femoral epiphysis.

WHICH ARE THE MOST COMMON CAUSATIVE ORGANISMS?

In the neonatal period, *Staphylococcus aureus* remains a common organism, but Group B β-hemolytic streptococcus and gram-negative enteric bacilli are also frequently identified. No bacteria are grown from the blood or joint fluid of 50% cases of typical septic arthritis.

Other contributing organisms could be methicillin-resistant *S. aureus* (MRSA), gram-negative organisms (Enterobacteriaceae) fungal species like *Aspergillus* and *Candida*. Tuberculosis and syphilis must be considered in atypical case contexts.

WHAT INVESTIGATIONS ARE SUPPORTIVE TO CONFIRM THE DIAGNOSIS?

The most important diagnostic test is clinical acumen. Positive changes on X-ray suggest that the disease is already in its advanced stage. Hence to diagnose the condition in its early stage, optimum use of investigations like ultrasound and MRI can be done.

Radiographs

The role of plain X-ray film in the diagnosis of early bone and joint sepsis is often undervalued. It is because the most sought after change is osteopenia or bone lysis, which takes 7–10 days to develop. Actually, deep soft tissue swelling with obliteration of fat plane is the earliest radiographic evidence of infection. Unlike older children, radiographic changes appear early in neonatal age group. The thin periosteum ruptures easily, and osteolytic lesions, soft tissue swelling, and periosteal elevation are often seen within 7 days of onset of infection. Erosion of the cortex, cavitation in the metaphysic or epiphysis can be seen as early as 3 days of onset of infection.

Ultrasonography

Ultrasonography (USG) is very useful to detect any joint effusion and subperiosteal edema. Although USG cannot clearly differentiate between pus and synovial fluid, in experienced hands USG-guided aspiration may be very useful to confirm the diagnosis.

Bone Scan

Bone scans are both sensitive and specific. They are often abnormal within 2–3 days of onset of symptoms.

Magnetic Resonance Imaging

In selected cases, an MRI is the most sensitive. It shows changes of marrow edema and helps to differentiate between transient synovitis, inflammatory arthritis, and septic arthritis by virtue of changes in marrow edema and synovial lining.

Hematological Investigations

A routine hemogram (complete blood count) with erythrocyte sedimentation rate (ESR) and C-reactive protein (CRP) are usually required and helpful to diagnose and monitor the course of treatment. In the community setting, CRP is useful parameter and is highly sensitive for infection. In an immunocompromised child, it may not be very reliable. Rather than a single value, changing trend in a CRP is more informative.

Erythrocyte sedimentation rate is not very useful in neonates, but with chronicity of infection, a decreasing trend in ESR usually indicates subsidence of infection.

Blood culture must be routinely performed and sometimes it can identify the pathogen. However, the blood sample must be promptly analyzed after collection and any contamination must be prevented.

Organism identification is extremely important for both confirmation of the diagnosis and guiding antimicrobial selection. Needle aspiration is likely to grow an organism in almost 50–60% of cases whereas blood cultures yield positive results in one-third to little more than half of specimens.

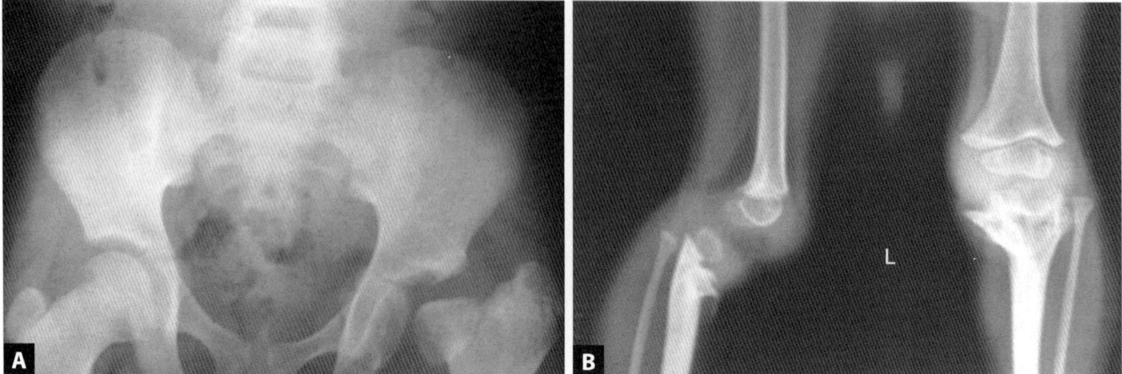

Figs. 1A and B: (A) An X-ray pelvis in an 8-year-old child who suffered septic arthritis of left hip in neonatal age group. Left femoral head shows growth arrest and gross collapse and incongruity; (B) An X-ray of knee in a 5-year-old child who suffered septic arthritis in neonatal period. There is gross deformity and growth arrest of proximal tibia. Child had gross shortening of limb and deformity.

HOW TO PROCEED FOR THE MANAGEMENT ONCE DIAGNOSIS IS MADE (FLOWCHART 1)?

Early diagnosis and treatment of septic arthritis is usually highly effective and usually achieves a clinically normal joint. Consequently, it is essential that children with septic arthritis are urgently referred to treatment centers and it is essential that the latter centers commence treatment as soon as possible. Prompt diagnosis and treatment of septic arthritis is not only rewarding, but also saves the child from a lifelong disability.

The treatment is a team approach which involves pediatrician, pediatric orthopedic surgeon, pediatric intensivist (particularly in sick neonates), microbiologist, and radiologist.

Treatment is directed towards obtaining a rapid cure as the sequelae of septic arthritis can be quite devastating **(Figs. 1 and 2)**. Any suspicion of the infection in a neonate should initiate prompt investigation to identify the site and source of the infection. Ideally, a joint or bone aspirate or positive blood culture must be obtained before commencing antimicrobial therapy. However, often this is not the case, and many neonates have received oral or intravenous antibiotics before they reach the definitive treatment center. In any case, if there is no improvement in clinical parameters within 48–72 hours of antimicrobial administration, then surgical intervention is mandatory.

Prompt surgical drainage and thorough wash of the joint is necessary. Open surgical drainage of the certain joints is essential to prevent necrosis (e.g., head of the femur or humerus). The current trend is towards mini-invasive surgeries **(Figs. 3 and 4)**, particularly in neonates; or arthroscopic joint lavage rather than big incisions. Smaller joints can usually be effectively treated by regular aspiration and rarely need open surgical drainage.

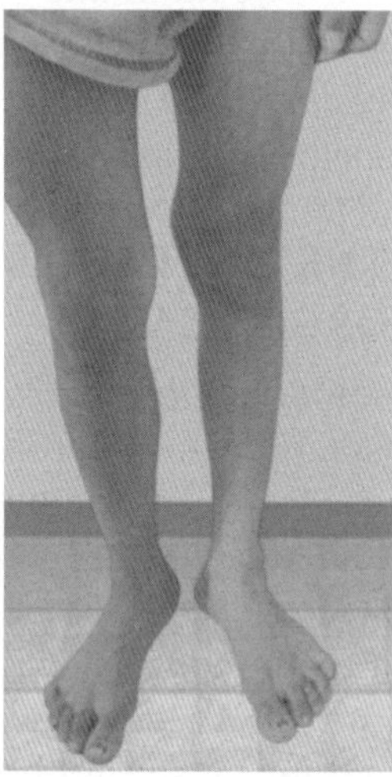

Fig. 2: Clinical photograph of the same child whose X-ray is shown in Figure 1A suggesting gross shortening of left lower limb. *(For color version, see Plate 21)*

Drainage of pus by a pediatric orthopedic surgeon decompresses the joint with drainage of pus leading to increased vascularity and healing. The antibiotics which were not able to reach the local site due to tight compartment like pressure are able to reach the infection site after drainage of pus. This ultimately results in rapid healing of bone and joint due to clearance of tissue-destroying fluid and also due to decrease in the tamponade effect on the delicate circulation around the growth plate.

Pus or fluid obtained during surgery must be sent for Gram staining and appropriate culture which helps in selection of proper antibiotics. Involvement of pediatric orthopedic surgeon at the onset of treatment itself is

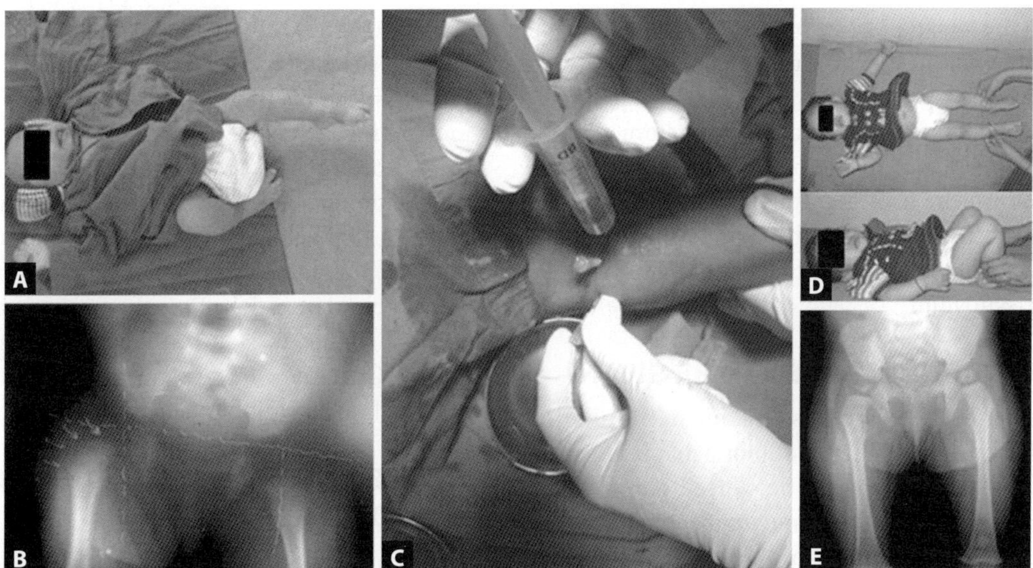

Figs. 3A to E: (A) Clinical photograph of a 25-day-old neonate with septic arthritis right hip. There is fixed flexion deformity at right hip and baby refuses to move the right lower limb; (B) An X-ray shows right hip dislocation, which is due to inflamed synovium pushing the head outside the acetabulum; (C) Joint wash of the right hip was done by mini-invasive technique using 16 G needles through multiple ports. This was followed by course of intravenous and then oral antibiotics; (D) Clinical photographs showing one and half year follow-up with full range of movement at right hip joint and no limb length discrepancy; (E) X-ray done at 15 months suggests growth is getting affected and small-sized epiphysis of right hip.

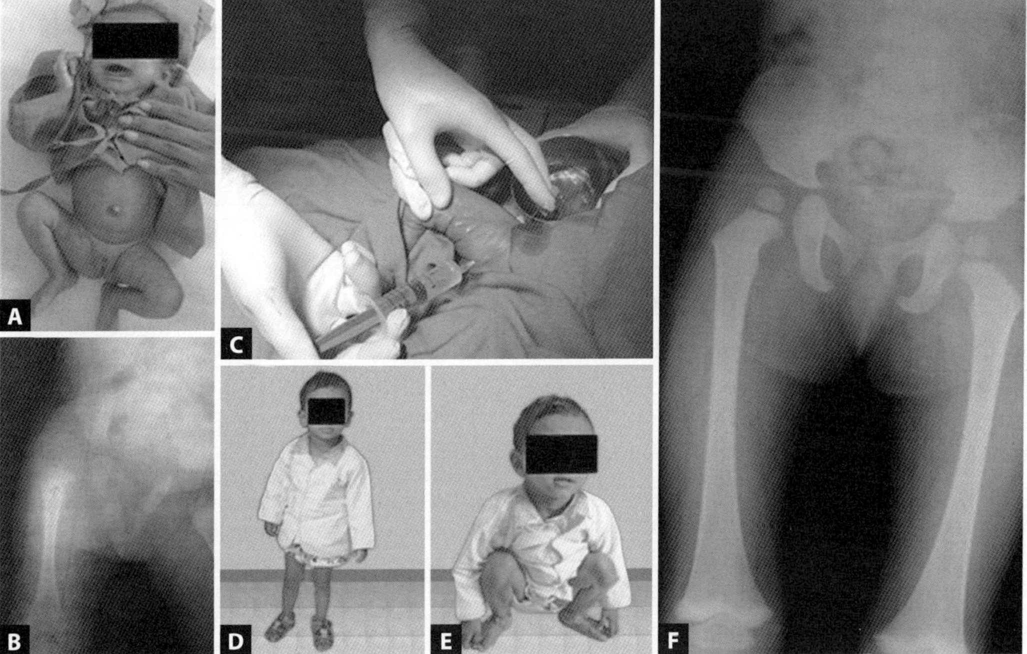

Figs. 4A to F: (A) Clinical photograph of a 28-day-old neonate with septic arthritis right hip. There is fixed flexion deformity at right hip and painful movements of right lower limb; (B) X-ray shows right hip dislocation as well as lytic changes in proximal femur; (C) Joint wash of the right hip was done by mini-invasive technique using 16 G needles through multiple ports. This was followed by course of intravenous and then oral antibiotics; (D and E) Clinical photographs showing two and half year follow-up with full range of movement at right hip joint and no limb length discrepancy; (F) X-ray done at two and half years suggests normal recovery; no growth arrest, no limb length discrepancy.

important as he or she is the person who is going to manage the sequelae in future. These children need long-term follow-up.

Antimicrobial therapy should commence immediately after drainage of pus. Antimicrobial therapy is guided by Gram stain on the aspirated pus. Up to 50% of joint aspirates are sterile in septic arthritis, possibly because joint fluid is bacteriostatic or because the organisms are limited to the synovium.

WHICH ANTIBIOTICS NEED TO BE GIVEN?

Since gram-positive organisms are most frequently responsible for the infection, an antibiotic that is effective against these organisms should be started empirically. In infants and children, a third-generation cephalosporins (e.g., cefotaxime, ceftriaxone) are the drug of choice combined with amikacin or gentamicin which provide coverage against many *S. aureus* (methicillin-sensitive *S. aureus*), most streptococci, *Haemophilus influenzae,* and *Kingella kingae.*

Linezolid, vancomycin, teicoplanin, and tobramycin are reserved until there is a positive report to support their use. Once an organism has been identified, coverage can be narrowed based on results of susceptibility testing.

WHICH IS THE PREFERRED ROUTE OF ANTIBIOTICS?

The initiation of treatment should be with intravenous antibiotics only. The oral route is preferred for maintenance phase.

HOW LONG ANTIBIOTICS NEED TO BE GIVEN?

The duration of parenteral antimicrobial therapy is a matter of debate. While the final choice is decided by the prevalent pathogen in the bacteriological and culture report, the duration of intravenous treatment varies from 7 days to 5 weeks.

There are many studies which has proven efficacy of minimum 3 weeks of intravenous antibiotics followed by 2–3 weeks of oral therapy (total 4–6 weeks). The author follows the regimen of 2–3 weeks of intravenous antibiotics followed by oral antibiotics for 2–3 weeks at our center. Few studies have indicated a shortened course of appropriate antibiotics for 3 weeks is as efficacious as 6 weeks of parenteral therapy.

Close monitoring of the clinical, blood, and radiological parameters is required to ensure that the treatment is effective and the outcome satisfactory. Antibiotics can usually be stopped by 6 weeks if the child has improved. Radiographs must be taken 6 monthly to see for any sequelae which develop in future.

Based on the latest review of literature, use of intravenous antibiotics till child improves clinically and starts weight bearing, followed by oral antibiotics for 4–6 weeks seems to be a standard regimen. The duration of antibiotics depends on the clinical recovery rather than a fixed time frame. To start with, an intravenous route is preferred. Once the clinical signs improve and CRP levels touch baseline, the antibiotic may be given orally.

WHERE AND WHO SHOULD PERFORM THE JOINT ASPIRATION?

Although older literature mentions about drainage in the emergency room, recent guidelines suggest to be done under aseptic atmosphere like operation theater or sterile neonatal intensive care unit/pediatric intensive care unit room. It should be done by a person well worse with anatomy of particular joint (preferably by pediatric orthopedic surgeon).

Is Simple Joint Aspiration Sufficient or a Joint Wash Need to be done?

Joint wash gives an additional advantage of reducing the bacterial load and thereby better chances of healing.

CLINICAL PEARLS

- Suspect septic arthritis in all neonates with decreased movements of limb or painful movements of limb.
- Suspect septic arthritis in all toddlers or children having gait disturbance with history of fever.
- Give joint lavage as earliest as possible.
- Joint lavage should be given in aseptic conditions preferably in operation theater or sterile neonatal intensive care unit/pediatric intensive care unit room (preferably by pediatric orthopedic surgeon who will keep follow-up of the case managing sequelae in long term).
- Send joint fluid for microbiological evaluation.
- X-rays and ultrasonography are helpful in diagnosis.
- Empirical antibiotics should be commenced after prompt drainage of joint collections.
- Start antibiotics with intravenous route only.
- Further choice of antibiotics will depend on culture report and clinical course
- Once clinical course is better shift to oral route of antibiotics.
- Keep patient in long-term follow-up for observation of sequelae and their subsequent management.

Hence, whenever a pediatric orthopedic surgeon is available he should be involved in the management and a thorough joint wash should be done rather than simple aspiration.

What is the Role of Plaster Cast/Splints/ Traction?

Plaster cast/splints help in immobilization of the joint and better healing particularly initial 1–2 weeks of treatment. Hip spica is needed in cases of septic hip dislocations to achieve the containment. Joint should not be immobilized for prolonged time to avoid stiffness. In children, traction helps in reducing the pain as well as correcting the deformity. On traction, movements need to be started as earliest as possible.

KEY POINTS

- Septic arthritis is a surgical as well as medical emergency.
- Prevention of sequelae by starting treatment urgently is the key to success.
- The treatment needs a team approach by pediatrician, pediatric orthopedic surgeon, neonatologist, microbiologist, and radiologist.
- Small setups where facilities are not available should refer the patient urgently to tertiary center where treatment needs to be started by the team on emergency basis.
- Septic arthritis if untreated will cause growth plate disturbances or damage, subsequent shortening of affected limb and lifelong deformity. Hence, the need for urgent diagnosis and treatment.

SUGGESTED READING

1. Curtiss PH, Klein L. Destruction of articular cartilage in septic arthritis. II. In vivo studies. J Bone Joint Surg Am. 1965;47(8):1595-604.
2. Fox L, Sprunt K. Neonatal osteomyelitis. Pediatrics. 1978; 62(4):535-42.
3. Narang A, Kumar PK. Bone and joint infection in neonates. Indian J Pediatr. 1988;62:535-42.
4. Pääkkönen M, Kallio MJ, Kallio PE, Peltola H. Sensitivity of erythrocyte sedimentation rate and C-reactive protein in childhood bone and joint infections. Clin Orthop Relat Res. 2014;468(3):861-6.
5. Rutz E, Brunner R. Septic arthritis of the hip-current concepts. Hip Int. 2009;19(Suppl 6):S9-12.
6. Sultan J, Hughes PJ. Septic arthritis or transient synovitis of the hip in children: the value of clinical prediction algorithms. J Bone Joint Surg Br. 2010;92(9):1289-93.
7. Syriopoulou VP, Smith AL. Osteomyelitis and septic arthritis. In: Feigin RD, Cherry JD, Demmler GJ, Kaplan SD, editors Textbook of Pediatric Infectious Diseases, 2nd edition. Philadelphia, PA: WB Saunders; 1987. pp. 759-79.

CHAPTER 162

Angular and Rotational Deformities in Children

Taral V Nagda, Venkatadass K

INTRODUCTION

Any deviation from the normal alignment of the limb in coronal plane is termed as angular deformity and that in transverse or axial plane is termed as rotational (torsional) deformity. While angular deformities are obviously seen as outward or inward deviation of legs, children with rotational deformities often present with either in-toeing or out-toeing walking. This chapter discusses in brief the common causes of these abnormalities and an algorithmic approach to each of this clinical scenario.

ANGULAR DEFORMITIES IN CHILDREN

Genu varum (bow legs) and genu valgum (knock knees) are the most common angular deformities for which the child is brought to the pediatric orthopedic clinic.

Normal Variation During Growth

Before going to the pathological genu varum and valgum, it is important to know the normal variation during growth. Most newborns have bow legs, with 10–15° of varus angulation. This gradually corrects until 18–24 months of age. After 2 years, there is valgus angulation with maximum valgus occurring around 4 years of age. The limb usually reaches normal adult alignment of 6–7° of valgus by around 11 years of age.

Clinical Assessment

Clinical evaluation of a child with an angular deformity includes looking at gait of the child, table examination for joint range of movements and rotational profile. In addition, special examination points are:

- *Alignment:* A line joining center of the hip joint and center of ankle passes through center of knee normally. In genu valgum, the line passes on lateral side of the center of knee and in genu valgum it passes medial to the center of knee.
- *Measurements:* Include measuring intercondylar distance (ICD) in case of genu varum and intermalleolar distance (IMD) in case of genu valgum. These are measured in standing or supine position. To minimize the error, measurement should be done in a standard fashion with patella facing forward. Fat thighs and internal femoral torsion can exaggerate the clinical appearance of genu valgum and internal tibial torsion can clinically exaggerate clinical appearance of genu varum.

Radiological Assessment of Alignment of Lower Limb

Although standing anteroposterior and lateral X-rays of the knee will be useful for diagnosis in most cases of angular deformities the detailed analysis of the deformities in children who need correction need complete analysis with full length standing radiograph of both lower limbs covering from both the hip joints to ankle joints with patellae facing anteriorly. This should be standardized as management decisions are made based on this radiograph. Mechanical axis is drawn by the line joining the center of the femoral head to the center of tibial plafond. Usually, it passes through the center of the knee joint. Medial deviation of mechanical axis is seen in genu varum and lateral deviation is seen in genu valgum. The measure of the deviation of mechanical axis of lower limb from the center of knee joint is called as "mechanical axis deviation (MAD)". The other angles which needs to be routinely measured are mechanical lateral distal femoral angle, medial proximal tibial angle, modified tibiofemoral angle (TFA), and joint line convergence angle **(Fig. 1)**.

Genu Varum (Flowchart 1)

Causes of genu varum are given in **Box 1**.

Physiological Genu Varum

Bow legs usually become prominent when the child starts walking and the parents get concerned about the deformity. Physiological genu varum is common in early walkers and in obese children. In physiologic genu varum, there may be associated tibial intorsion. There are no other significant positive findings on clinical examination.

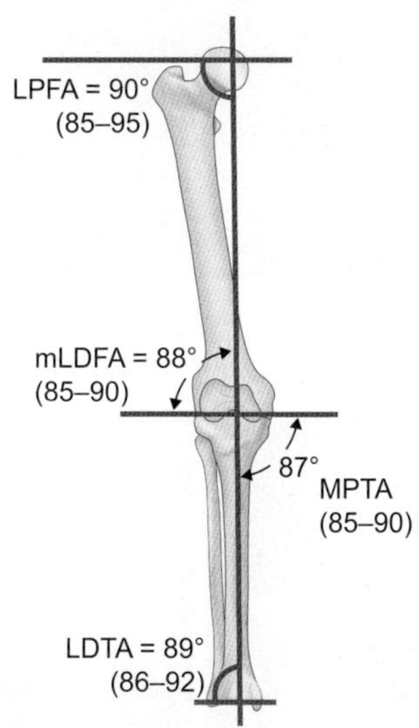

Fig. 1: Mechanical axis of lower limb. (LDTA: lateral distal tibial angle; LPFA: lateral proximal femoral angle; mLDFA: mechanical lateral distal femoral angle; MPTA: medial proximal tibial angle)

X-rays of the knees may show an apparent delay in the ossification of the medial side of the distal femoral and proximal tibial epiphyses or flaring of the medial distal femoral metaphysis. The physes are normal. Majority of children <2 years of age have physiological genu varum, which needs reassurance to parents and follow-up evaluation. The genu varum that persists after 2 years of age is considered to be pathological and needs to be investigated further.

Nutritional Rickets

Nutritional rickets is one of the most common causes for bowed legs in developing countries. The typical clinical scenario would be a child presenting with bowed legs and on clinical examination will have other signs of active rickets. The X-rays show cupping and flaring of the metaphysis with widening of the physis. Active rickets will have to be treated with vitamin D supplements and the deformity needs to be observed. The children with active rickets who are not responding to vitamin D supplements are likely to have vitamin D resistant rickets and they need to be investigated preferably by a pediatric endocrinologist and managed accordingly.

It is not uncommon to see children presenting with bowlegs after the active rickets has healed. The persistent deformity needs to be corrected to get the mechanical axis of the lower limb to normal. Guided growth in the form

Flowchart 1: Approach to a child with genu varum (bow legs).

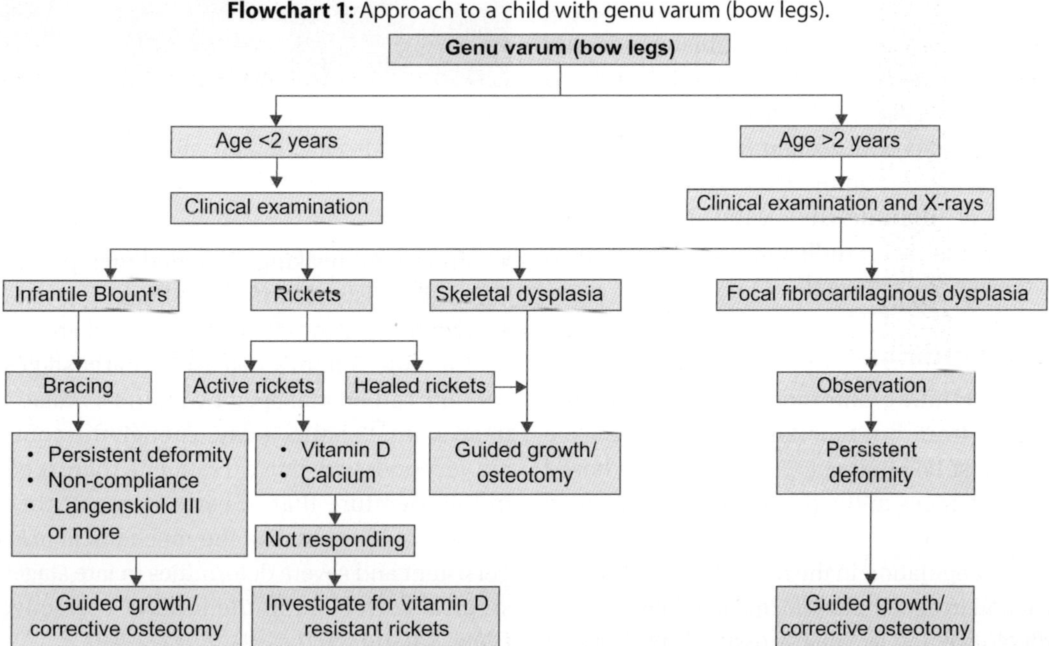

BOX 1: Causes of genu varum.
- Physiological genu varum
- Infantile Blount's disease
- Metabolic disorders
- Skeletal dysplasias
- Focal fibrocartilaginous dysplasia

of temporary hemiepiphysiodesis with a tension band plate (8-plate) applied on the lateral side is the preferred form of treatment when the physes remains open. The parents must be counseled well about the need for regular follow-up X-rays at 3–4 monthly intervals and the need for 8-plate removal once the deformity is corrected. In children for whom the physes are closed or those with sick physis not responding to guided growth, the deformity is corrected by osteotomy.

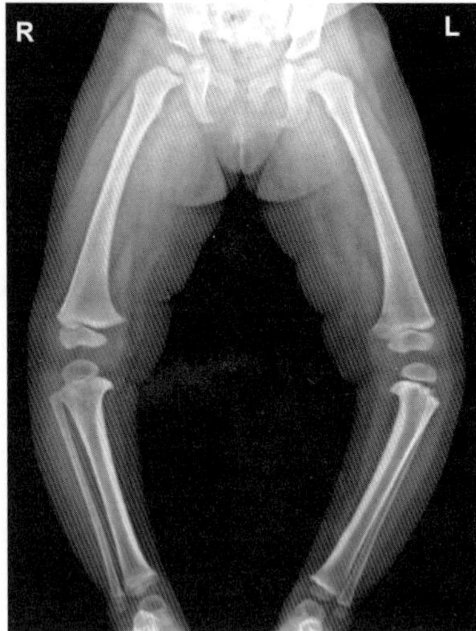

Fig. 2: An X-ray of a child with bilateral Blount's disease.

Blount's Disease

Blount's disease also called as tibia vara is classified into three types based on the age of onset of the deformity.
- *Infantile tibia vara:* <3 years
- *Juvenile tibia vara:* 4–10 years
- *Adolescent tibia vara:* >10 years

Infantile Blount's disease is considered to be a disorder on the other end of the spectrum of physiological bowing.

Clinical Features

The two major features which helps in differentiating physiologic genu varum from infantile tibia vara is that the child is usually obese (>95th percentile) and the presence of lateral thrust while walking. This sudden lateral knee movement with weight bearing is caused by varus instability at the joint. This sign, though not pathognomonic of infantile tibia vara, increases the level of suspicion and is an indication for radiography, regardless of the age of the patient.

Radiographic Findings

A standardized standing anteroposterior view of the lower extremities from hip to ankle with both patellae facing forward must be obtained. The diagnosis is based on radiographic changes in the proximal end of the tibia as follows **(Fig. 2)**:
- A sharp varus angulation in the metaphysis
- A widened and irregular physeal line medially
- A medially sloped and irregularly ossified epiphysis

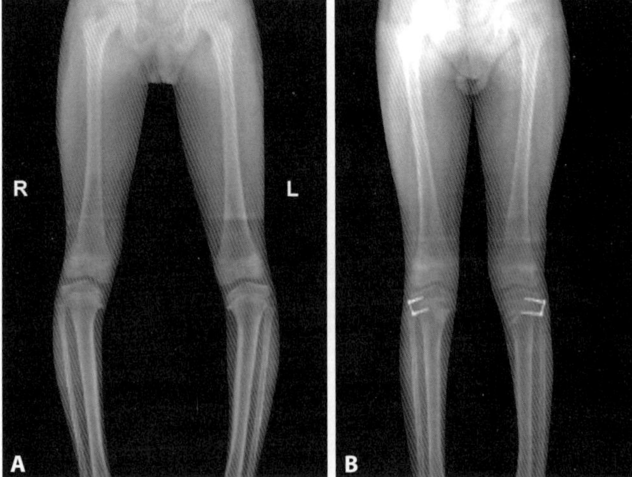

Figs. 3A and B: (A) Preoperative X-ray of a 7-year-old boy with bilateral Blount's disease; (B) 2 years follow-up X-ray after osteotomy showing normal alignment of the lower limbs.

- Prominent beaking of medial metaphysis with lucent cartilage islands within the beak
- Lateral subluxation of the proximal end of the tibia

Infantile Blount's disease in early stages and young patients can be managed by Blount's brace, which needs to be worn 23 hours a day. Though the compliance rates are very poor with brace treatment, there is good evidence in the literature that in early stages of the disease just braces could normalize the mechanical axis of the limb. Persistent and severe deformities in late stages will require surgical correction in the form of corrective osteotomy **(Figs. 3A and B)**.

Skeletal Dysplasia

Children with genu varum secondary to skeletal dysplasia usually have associated short stature. The dysplasia could be either at the epiphysis, metaphysis, or the diaphysis. The common dysplasias which present with genu varum are achondroplasia, pseudoachondroplasia and metaphyseal chondrodysplasia (Schmid/McKusick) and hereditary multiple exostosis. Genu varum in these children will need surgical correction to restore the mechanical axis. It is worthwhile considering growth modulation or guided growth in these patients while the physes are open. Those children who are not ideal for growth modulation will need corrective osteotomy.

Focal Fibrocartilaginous Dysplasia

Focal fibrocartilaginous dysplasia is a rare cause of unilateral genu varum in an infant or toddler. Careful clinical examination reveals that the deformity is slightly more distal than the knee joint. On weight bearing and walking, the child may have a lateral thrust along with associated hyperextension of the knee which is not a feature of Blount's disease.

Radiographic Findings

X-rays show a characteristic abrupt varus at the metaphyseal-diaphyseal junction of the tibia, clearly not involving the physis. There is cortical sclerosis in and around the area of the abrupt varus on the medial cortex. A radiolucent lesion may be seen just proximal to the area of cortical sclerosis, which probably corresponds to the fibrocartilaginous tissue. The etiology of this defect and the pathogenesis of the deformity are unknown.

The importance of recognizing this variation of infantile tibia vara is that the deformity can resolve without surgery. Surgical treatment may be necessary if the deformity progresses or fails to resolve during a period of observation or orthotic management.

> **CLINICAL PEARLS**
>
> *Pointers to pathological genu varum:*
> - Age >2 years
> - Lateral thrust on walking
> - Hyperextension while standing
> - Acute bowing in the tibia
> - Unilateral bowing

Genu Valgum (Flowchart 2)

Causes of genu valgum are given in **Box 2**.

Valgus alignment of the lower extremities is normal in a child between 2 years and 6 years of age. The maximum amount of physiologic valgus occurs between the ages of 2 years and 4 years, after which the alignment of the lower extremity assumes a mild valgus femoral-tibial angle, the normal alignment in an adult.

In a younger child, X-rays are not routinely indicated.

Alignment X-rays are indicated in the following situations:

- Presence of short stature
- History of trauma or infection
- Features suggestive of metabolic bone disease
- Asymmetrical genu valgum

Flowchart 2: Approach to a child with genu valgum (knock knees).

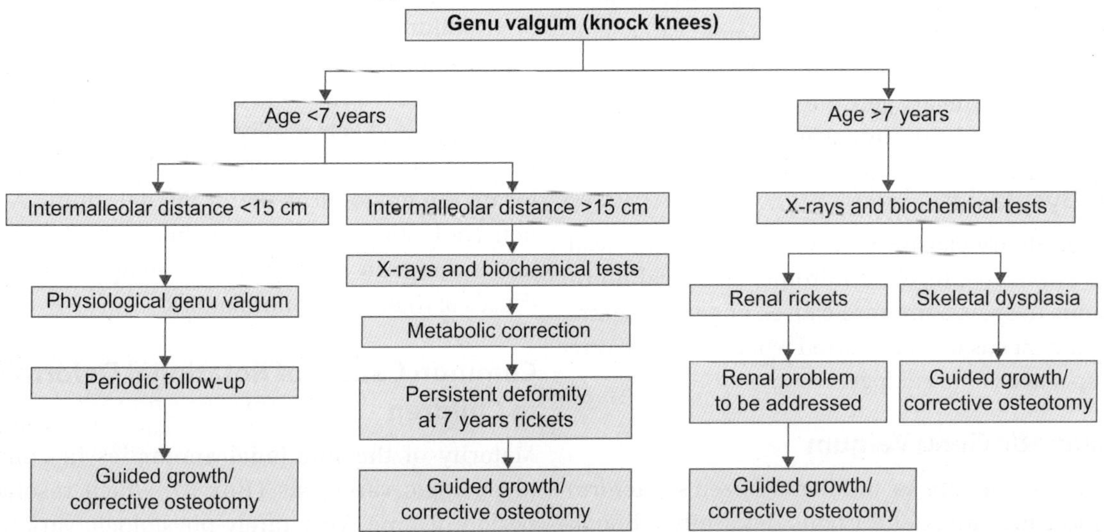

BOX 2: Causes of genu valgum.

- Physiological genu valgum
- Metabolic
- Post-traumatic
- Skeletal dysplasias
- Hereditary multiple exostosis

The rotational profile of the extremity must be evaluated carefully because an apparent increase in valgus may result from increased femoral anteversion.

Idiopathic Genu Valgum

Significant genu valgum that persists after 7 years of age without any identifiable underlying cause is usually labeled as idiopathic genu valgum. Surgical correction is indicated when there is significant MAD (the mechanical axis passing lateral to the lateral-tibial plateau). If untreated this may lead to gait disturbance, difficulty in running, knee discomfort, patellar malalignment, and evidence of ligamentous instability. Growth modulation with medial hemiepiphysiodesis using a tension band plate or a percutaneous epiphysiodesis screw is currently the preferred method of achieving correction while the physis is open **(Figs. 4A and B)**. However, one must be aware that in genu valgum, correction is rapid and 3-monthly monitoring with X-rays is mandatory to avoid over correction and development of opposite deformity. In children who present late where the physis is fused, corrective osteotomy is indicated.

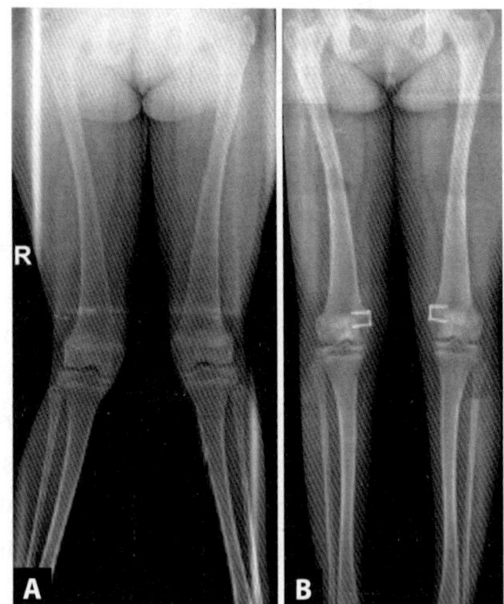

Figs. 4A and B: (A) A 12-year-old girl with idiopathic genu valgum; (B) A 1-year follow-up X-ray after bilateral hemiepiphysiodesis showing complete correction of deformity.

Metabolic Disorders

Genu valgum may be presenting feature of a child with chronic renal failure. Apart from nutritional rickets, renal rickets must be ruled out in all children presenting with genu valgum by doing renal function tests. Correcting the metabolic abnormality gets the first priority in these children followed by deformity correction later on.

Skeletal Dysplasia

Multiple hereditary exostosis, spondyloepimetaphyseal dysplasia, Ellis–Van Creveld syndrome, and focal fibrocartilaginous dysplasia are rare causes of genu valgum. The deformity needs to be corrected when there is severe MAD irrespective of the etiology.

Post-traumatic Genu Valgum

Proximal tibial fracture in toddlers (Cozen's fracture) is known to cause unilateral valgus deformity. Though the etiology of this condition remains undetermined, there is strong evidence in the literature that most of these deformities would correct spontaneously and hence need to be observed periodically for improvement of the deformity.

CLINICAL PEARL

- Beware of unilateral deformity; it is most likely to be pathological.

ROTATIONAL DEFORMITIES IN CHILDREN

Rotational deformities in children manifest as either in-toeing or out-toeing while walking. Parents bring their children seeking opinion for abnormal inward or outward positioning of the feet while walking. Though majority of the rotational deformities in early childhood are benign and gets resolved spontaneously with growth, it is important to do a thorough clinical examination to locate the anatomical site of the deformity. A comprehensive history along with a thorough physical examination helps in differentiating benign from pathologic causes of rotational abnormalities.

Common Causes of Rotational Deformities in Children

Majority of the rotational anomalies in children are physiologic variations **(Box 3)**, which resolve over a period of time. Very rarely physiologic variations may persist or become rigid deformities, which then would warrant a surgical intervention. Pathologic causes of rotational deformities need to be identified and managed appropriately.

Pathologic Causes for Rotational Deformities

Pathological causes for rotational deformities are given in **Box 4**.

Evaluation of Child with Rotational Deformity

A good history with systematic clinical examination is recommended in all children presenting with in-toeing or out-toeing while walking. The following findings would point towards a pathologic cause of rotational deformity:

- A hypoxic or infective event in neonatal period
- Delayed developmental milestones
- A family history of hip dysplasia or a neurologic disorder
- Spasticity, a neurologic deficit, or signs of muscular dystrophy
- Limping or another abnormality of gait of sudden onset
- Deformities of the foot

BOX 3: Physiologic causes for rotational deformities.

In-toeing

- *Foot:*
  - Metatarsus adductus
  - Skew foot
- Leg: Internal tibial torsion
- Hip: Increased femoral anteversion

Out-toeing

- *Foot:*
  - Pes calcaneovalgus
  - Pes planovalgus
- *Leg:* External tibial torsion
- *Hip:*
  - External rotation contracture
  - Femoral retroversion

BOX 4: Pathological causes of rotational deformities.

- Cerebral palsy
- Hereditary neurologic disorders—Charcot–Marie–Tooth disease and Friedrich ataxia
- Mild tibial deficiencies
- Blount's disease
- Metabolic disorders
- Skeletal dysplasia
- Rigid pes planus with or without tarsal coalition
- Slipped capital femoral epiphysis

The Three-step Rotational Profile (Flowchart 3)

- *Step 1 [foot progression angle (FPA)]:* Make the child walk in a straight line and look for the FPA. FPA is the angle between the longitudinal axis of the foot and an imaginary line of progression of the body through space **(Fig. 5)**. A positive or external FPA of 0–20° is considered normal, but the angle varies with age and may necessitate observation over time and correlation with the remainder of the physical examination. A negative FPA indicates that the child is walking with in toeing. FPA is also an important indicator of dynamic causes of in- toeing such as tibialis anterior overactivity.
- *Step 2 [external rotation and internal rotation (IR) at both hip joints]:* Femoral anteversion is diagnosed clinically when a child has more IR than external rotation of the hip. In infants, IR of the hip averages 40°, with a range of 10–60°, and external rotation averages 65° with a range of 45–90°
- *Step 3 [thigh foot angle (TFA)]:* It is determined in the prone position as the angle between the longitudinal axis of the foot (usually along the second ray) and the longitudinal axis of the thigh, with the knee flexed to 90° and the ankle in neutral position **(Fig. 6)**. Factors influencing the TFA include tibial torsion and any hind foot or forefoot deformities. The average TFA is negative or internal by 5° in infants, and becomes positive or external by 10° by approximately 8 years of age.

Investigations

As benign variations in the rotational profile of the lower extremities are quite common in children, imaging is not routinely required in the assessment of an in-toeing or out-toeing gait unless indicated by a clinically suspected pathology. It is also important to know that deformities in the rotational or axial plane are difficult to interpret on standard two-dimensional radiographs. Indications for supplemental radiographic imaging include the presence of leg-length discrepancy, asymmetric findings, limp, pain, spasticity, recent changes in gait, persistence of a deformity into adolescence, and cosmetic concerns. Children older than 6 months who present with a leg-length discrepancy, an asymmetric rotational profile, or both should have an anteroposterior radiograph of the

Flowchart 3: Approach to a child with rotational profile.

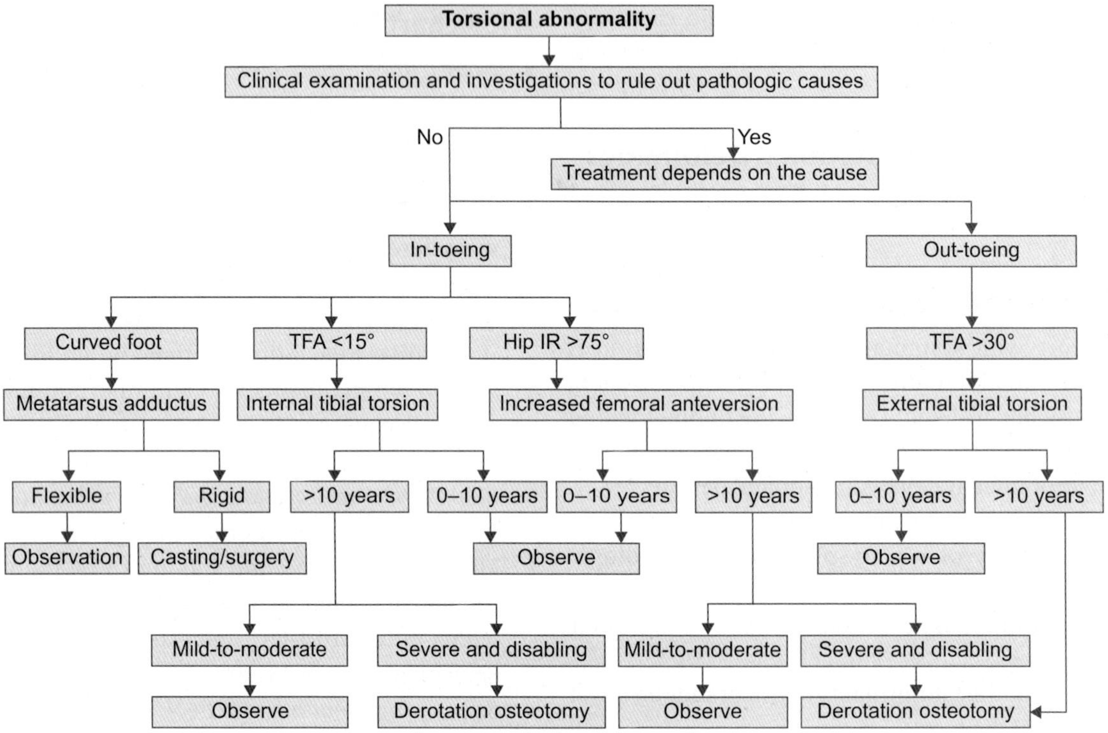

- **Torsional abnormality**
  - Clinical examination and investigations to rule out pathologic causes
    - Yes → Treatment depends on the cause
    - No (and after treatment) →
      - In-toeing
        - Curved foot → Metatarsus adductus
          - Flexible → Observation
          - Rigid → Casting/surgery
        - TFA <15° → Internal tibial torsion
          - 0–10 years → Observe
          - >10 years
            - Mild-to-moderate → Observe
            - Severe and disabling → Derotation osteotomy
        - Hip IR >75° → Increased femoral anteversion
          - 0–10 years → Observe
          - >10 years
            - Mild-to-moderate → Observe
            - Severe and disabling → Derotation osteotomy
      - Out-toeing
        - TFA >30° → External tibial torsion
          - 0–10 years → Observe
          - >10 years → Derotation osteotomy

(IR: internal rotation; TFA: tibiofemoral angle)

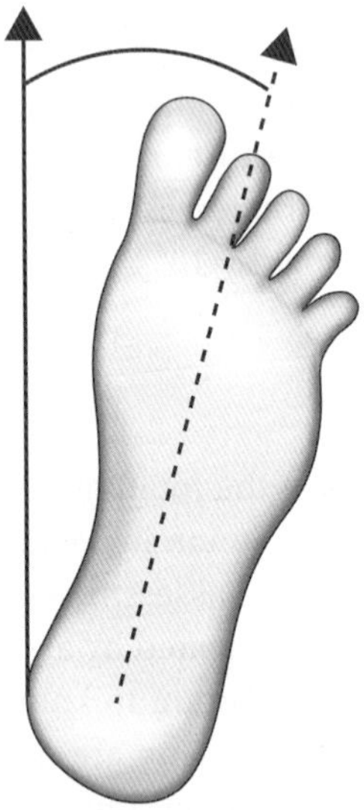

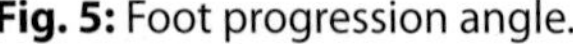

Fig. 5: Foot progression angle.

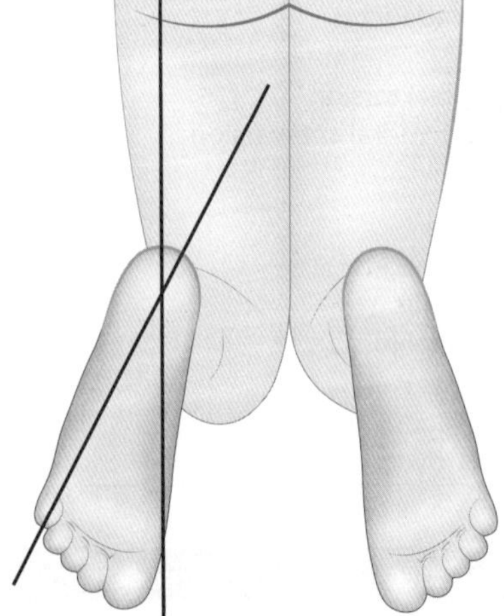

Fig. 6: Thigh foot angle.

pelvis to rule out hip dysplasia or other abnormalities of the hip. In children with symptomatic rotational anomaly, 3D instrumented gait analysis and rotational profile of lower limbs using CT scan can help to qualify and quantify the site and magnitude of the deformity.

In-toeing

The three most common causes of in-toeing are persistent femoral anteversion, internal tibial torsion, and metatarsus adductus. In-toeing is usually the result of metatarsus adductus in an infant, of internal tibial torsion in a toddler, and of femoral anteversion both in children older than 2.5 years and in adolescents.

Among causes for out-toeing, which is less common, are diminished femoral anteversion and, less frequently, femoral retroversion, external tibial torsion, pes calcaneovalgus, and external rotational contracture of the hip. Out-toeing, when seen in newborns, is often a consequence of intrauterine positioning of the foot in dorsiflexion against the shin, or calcaneovalgus. In infants and toddlers, it is often the result of external capsular contracture of the hip, and in older children the consequence of true bone torsion or pes planovalgus.

A comprehensive recording of the patient's history combined with a thorough physical examination are essential for differentiating benign from pathologic causes of rotational abnormalities. Studies present various conclusions in terms of the age beyond which the persistence of in-toeing is abnormal. However, the general consensus is that no natural correction of a rotational malalignment should be expected beyond the age of 10 years, although exceptions to this do occur.

Metatarsus Adductus

In metatarsus adductus, there is inward deviation of the forefoot relative to the hind foot. Metatarsus adductus is the most common congenital foot deformity and it resolves spontaneously in >90% of children. A rigid forefoot adduction deformity with a prominent plantar crease, which often requires surgical management, is termed as "metatarsus varus" by some authors. For simplicity, these deformities are now classified as actively correctable, passively correctable or rigid.

The clinical hallmark of the condition is medial deviation of the forefoot relative to the hind foot. When the foot is viewed from the plantar surface, the sole of the foot appears bean shaped.

It is important to establish the degree of flexibility of the deformity. In mild cases, the foot will correct actively when the lateral border of the foot is stimulated. In less flexible cases, the foot will not correct actively but can easily be corrected passively. A rigid deformity has a medial soft-tissue crease at the tarsometatarsal level and a medial soft-tissue contracture that prevents passive correction of the foot.

If the metatarsus adductus is flexible and spontaneously corrects as the foot is stimulated into active eversion, it does not warrant any treatment. These mild deformities will resolve gradually. Parents should be reassured and shown how to gently stretch the foot and how to stimulate it to achieve active correction. Passively correctable deformities can either be casted or be maintained on a splint. Majority of the rigid deformities will be corrected by serial casting. Surgical intervention is indicated very rarely for those patients with persistent deformity or those presenting late with rigid deformities and in older patients with recurrence of the deformities.

Tibial Torsion

Tibial torsion is defined by the angular difference between the transmalleolar axis and the bicondylar axis of the knee. Medial tibial torsion is most apparent when infants first begin to walk. This contributes to physiologic genu varum, which often presents in toddlers younger than 2.5 years. A slightly externally rotated hip combined with an internally rotated tibia will give the appearance of genu varum even if the knee is normal in the coronal plane. This "apparent genu varum" is frequently confused with true infantile tibia vara (Blount's disease), but can usually be differentiated from the latter by serial physical examinations done over a period of a few months. If torsion alone is present, the knee with the patella facing forward has an orientation that ranges from neutral to slight valgus. Classic tibial torsion usually improves spontaneously, whereas true Blount disease tends to progress to greater varus deformity. External tibial torsion, which is less common than classic tibial torsion, has a greater potential for persistence into adolescence.

Physical examination of the lower extremities is normal or may show physiologic genu varum and negative TFA. Medial tibial torsion resolves spontaneously and hence does not need any treatment. Efforts aimed at changing the torsional profile of a long bone with an orthosis or other splint is generally ineffective. It is better to avoid such devices as there is a possibility of creating a second deformity through the joints.

Due to the benign natural history of the condition and the generally unattractive and ineffective nature of orthotic management, observation and parental education are the main forms of treatment of tibial torsion. A small segment of the population with severe (>2 standard deviation above the mean) medial tibial torsion that does not resolve spontaneously may need treatment. On the other hand, excessive external tibial torsion might not resolve and, therefore, might need treatment at a later age.

In either case, moderate-to-severe deformities that fail to resolve should alert the orthopedist to the possibility of an underlying neurologic problem, such as cerebral palsy.

Surgical management by rotational osteotomy may therefore be necessary in the rare situation in which the child has persistent functional or cosmetic problems after 8 years of age. Rotational tibial osteotomies should probably be performed only in a child with a persistent deformity exceeding 15° internal FPA or 30° external FPA at age 8 years or older, thereby ensuring that no other rotational change or gait accommodation is likely to occur, and in whom definite functional and psychological disturbances appear to be present.

FEMORAL ANTEVERSION

Femoral version is defined as the angular difference between the axis of the femoral neck and the transcondylar axis of the knee. Medial femoral torsion is a common clinical problem during early childhood. It is twice as common in girls as in boys. Normally, children are born with an average femoral anteversion of 40°, which diminishes to approximately 12–16° at skeletal maturity, resolving at a rate of approximately 1.5° per year. This "normalization" with growth is usually achieved by approximately 8–10 years of age.

The child sits with the limbs in the W position, walks with an in-toeing gait with the patella medially rotated and runs in an awkward pattern. The appearance while running is described as egg-beater pattern and the walking is described as pigeon-toed gait. Tripping as a result of crossing the feet may occur in some children.

Clinical examination reveals increased IR and decreased external rotation. Imaging is not routinely indicated, unless there is asymmetrical version. A computed tomography scan or magnetic resonance imaging is needed to exactly measure the amount of version and this is only indicated for surgical planning rather than as a diagnostic aid.

Majority of the children resolve spontaneously and the parents need to be reassured and also counseled to encourage their child sit cross-legged and avoid "W sitting". In a select group of children with persistent increased femoral anteversion (IR > 80°) with severe cosmetic and functional limitation derotation osteotomy of the proximal femur is indicated to correct the deformity.

CLINICAL PEARLS

- In-toeing is more common than out-toeing
- Majority of rotational anomalies resolve with growth
- No role for orthotics
- Corrective osteotomy only after 10 years of age

KEY POINTS

- Many children with angular and rotational deformities can have physiological malpositions which correct over time.
- Angular deformities in a child who has at least 2 years of growth left are treated with guided growth using growth modulation plate.
- Corrective osteotomies may be needed for angular deformities where <2 years of growth is remaining or guided growth is contraindicated and for correction of pathological rotational deformities.

SUGGESTED READING

1. Herring JA. Tachdjian's Pediatric Orthopaedics: From the Texas Scottish Rite Hospital for Children, 5th edition. Philadelphia, PA: Saunders-Elsevier; 2013.
2. Joseph B, Nayagam S, Loder RT, Torode I. Paediatric Orthopaedics: A System of Decision-Making. London, United Kingdom: CRC Press, Taylor & Francis Group; 2009.
3. Lovell WW, Winter RB, Morrissy RT, Weinstein SL. Lovell and Winter's Pediatric Orthopaedics, 6th edition. Philadelphia, PA, USA: Lippincott Williams & Wilkins; 2006.
4. Staheli LT. Rotational problems in children. J Bone Joint Surg Am. 1993;75:939-49.

Approach to a Child with a Limp

Sandeep A Patwardhan, Anirban Chatterjee, Arjun A Dhawale

INTRODUCTION

A limp is any deviation from the normal gait pattern. The incidence of limping in children is unknown. A child walking with an abnormal gait pattern is a cause of concern for parents and the attending pediatrician. As a number of conditions may be the cause of a limp, a systematic approach is needed for appropriate treatment to be initiated.

DIAGNOSIS

Abnormal gait can be antalgic **(Flowchart 1)** or nonantalgic. Common abnormal gait patterns are shown in **Box 1** and common causes of limp in different age groups are shown in **Box 2**. A detailed history, physical examination, laboratory tests, and imaging are necessary for making a diagnosis. Common tests are shown in **Table 1**.

HISTORY

The importance of obtaining a detailed history from the child or parents cannot be overemphasized. Some of the important questions to be answered are: is the onset acute, insidious, or chronic? Is the limp persistent or periodic, static or progressive and if there are any systemic symptoms like fever or weight loss. If there is pain,

Flowchart 1: Algorithm for antalgic gait.

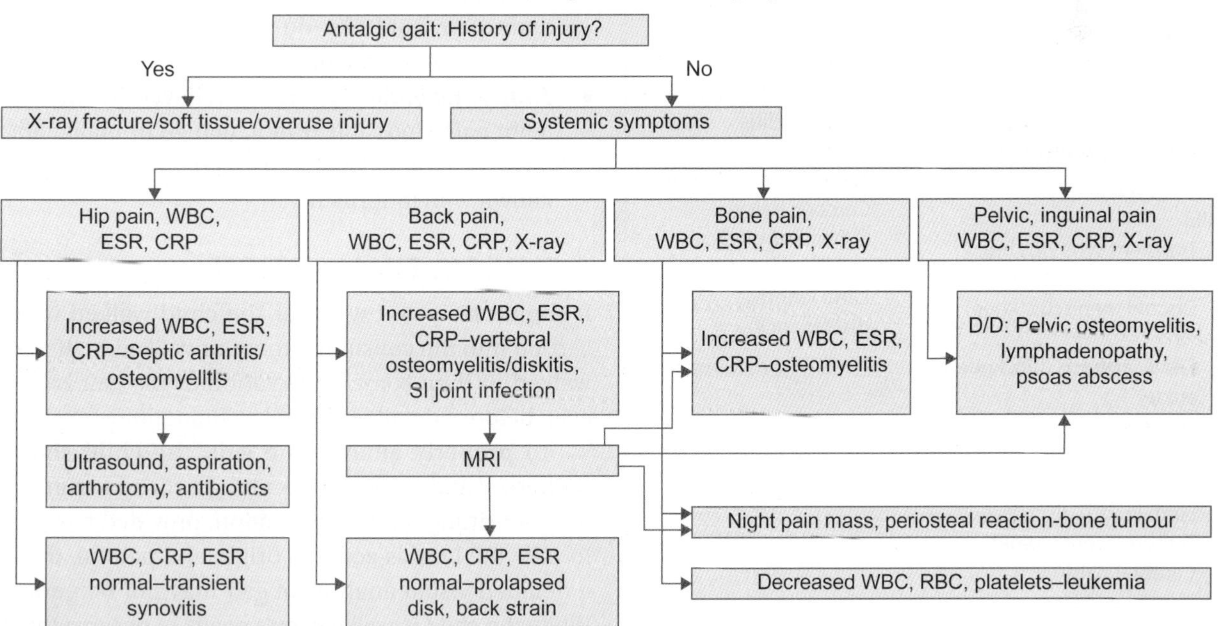

(CRP: C-reactive protein; DD: differential diagnosis; ESR: erythrocyte sedimentation rate; MRI: magnetic resonance imaging; RBC: red blood cell; WBC: white blood cell)

BOX 1: Common abnormal gait patterns.

Short limb gait:
- When limb length discrepancy (LLD) >5%
- Toe walk/shoulder drops on same side
- Compensatory knee bend on contralateral side

Trendelenburg gait:
- Weak abductors, abnormal fulcrum
- Pelvis drops on opposite side
- Compensatory leaning on affected side

Antalgic gait:
- Short stepping
- Reduced stance time on affected side
- Spine pain
- Slow stiff gradual movement to avoid jarring

BOX 2: Common causes of limp in different age groups.

Toddlers 1–3 years
- Mild pain
  - Transient synovitis (hip)
  - Toddlers fracture
  - Seronegative spondyloarthropathy
- Severe and night pains
  - Septic arthritis (hip, knee, ankle)
  - Tumors
- Painless
  - Cerebral palsy
  - Muscular dystrophy
  - Coxa vara (hip)
  - Developmental dysplasia of the hip
  - Torsional problems

Child 4–10 years
- Mild
  - Transient synovitis hip
  - Legg-Calvé-Perthes
  - Discoid meniscus (knee)
- Severe
  - Septic arthritis (hip, knee, ankle)
  - Leukemias
  - Tumors
- Painless
  - Limb length discrepancy
  - Tethered cord (spine)
  - Cerebral palsy
  - Muscular dystrophy
  - Coxa vara (hip)
  - Developmental dysplasia of the hip
  - Torsional problems

Adolescents 11–15 years
- Mild to moderate
  - Slipped capital femoral epiphysis
  - Residual hip dysplasia
  - Chondrolysis (hip)
  - Overuse syndromes
  - Osteochondritis dissecans
  - Tarsal coalitions
  - Seronegative spondyloarthropathy
- Severe
  - Sickling crisis
  - Malignant tumors
  - Osteomyelitis
- Painless
  - Tethered cord (spine)
  - Cerebral palsy
  - Other neurological conditions
  - Limb length discrepancy

TABLE 1: Tests for diagnosis.

Test	*Condition*
Complete blood count	Polymorphs increased in infective or inflammatory pathologies
C-reactive protein	Level increased in infective or inflammatory pathologies
Erythrocyte sedimentation rate	Level increased in infective or inflammatory pathologies
Synovial fluid analysis	Septic arthritis: leukocyte count increased (>50,000/cmm), turbid synovial fluid; transient synovitis: leukocyte count increased (<15,000/cmm), clear synovial fluid
Synovial fluid culture	Septic arthritis: Growth; transient synovitis: no growth
Throat culture	Acute rheumatic fever: group A streptococci
Blood culture	Positive in infective pathologies

is it localized and what its aggravating and relieving factors are. Some examples are:

- *Mechanical:* Pain on loading, relieved by rest
- *Inflammatory:* Continuous pain but relieved by nonsteroidal anti-inflammatory medicines (NSAIDs)
- *Infective:* Continuous pain, not relieved by NSAIDs, night pain could be due to chronic granulomatous diseases like tuberculosis
- *Tumor:* Relentless pain, not relieved by medication; night pain—possible tumor, benign or malignant with the exception of osteoid osteoma, where pain relief is known with ibuprofen.

CLINICAL EXAMINATION

It should be noted whether the child walked in or was carried into the consulting room or walked in. If the child walked in then some observation of the gait is possible even before a detailed clinical examination.

To properly analyze the gait, the child should be undressed and made to walk along a corridor, run, and get up from sitting/squatting position, provided it is painless. In case the limp is acute in origin and painful, then such a detailed visual analysis of gait may not be performed. While the child is walking, one needs to observe the trunk, the pelvis, hips, knees, and the ankle foot complex individually. One also needs to observe the shoes, especially the wear characteristics of the heel and sole.

Local Examination

At the end of the history and examination of the gait, one should have narrowed down the differential diagnosis (DD) and also mentally decide which limb, which bone or which joint needs to be examined in more detail. To avoid missing out any subtle signs, examination should include the spine and lower extremities including hip joints, knee joints, and ankle-foot complex with the child suitably undressed. A useful dictum to follow for local examination of a part is look, feel, move, measure, and perform (special tests).

Focal examination should be done if infection or trauma is suspected.

CLINICAL PEARLS

- Onset, duration, and progress of limp and associated or absence of pain must be elicited clearly.
- Origin of pathology in a limping child may be from the foot to the spine.
- Think of the most common conditions first according to age.

DIFFERENTIAL DIAGNOSIS

Transient Synovitis

Transient synovitis is commonly seen in children aged 3–8 years with acute onset of hip pain and limping with a decreased range of movements. Often, there is a history of a preceding viral illness. Ultrasound findings of joint effusion with no elevation of C-reactive protein and erythrocyte sedimentation rate (ESR) with a normal or slight elevation in white blood cell count help corroborate the diagnosis. Treatment is observation, rest, and analgesics.

Septic Arthritis

Septic arthritis can occur at any age from the neonatal period. There is an acute onset of pain, limping, and fever with restricted hip range of movements. Differentiation from transient synovitis is based on history of fever, inability to bear weight, elevated ESR, and leukocytosis (>12,000 cells/mL). The probability of a diagnosis of septic arthritis increases with the number of criteria present; ultrasound to assess joint effusion and synovial thickening. Radiographs, although not helpful in the early stages, identifies associated osteomyelitis, soft-tissue swelling, or hip subluxation. Early intervention with hip arthrotomy and 6 weeks of antibiotic coverage as per the culture sensitivity is the standard of care.

Osteomyelitis

Osteomyelitis in children usually occurs as a result of hematogenous spread of bacteria. The most common organism is *Staphylococcus aureus*, with incidence of methicillin-resistant *S. aureus* (MRSA) increasing. The child will present with fever, limping, localized swelling, and tenderness. Although metaphyseal involvement is more common, the diaphysis may be involved less often. In acute osteomyelitis, early radiographs may only show soft-tissue swelling and radiographs after a few weeks will show periosteal reaction **(Figs. 1A and B)** and bone destruction. A 6-week course of appropriate antibiotics is initiated after obtaining blood cultures and local cultures after surgical drainage.

Fracture

Children with trauma to the lower extremity may present with a limp. These could commonly occur while playing or due to motor vehicle accidents. Fractures of the femur and tibia are common injuries and are diagnosed with appropriate radiographs. Treatment depends on the location and type of fracture and the age of the patient. Closed treatment of long bone fractures with casting or elastic nailing is usually the norm. Epiphyseal injuries and joint injuries should be identified with a thorough local examination and if suspected then an magnetic resonance imaging is useful.

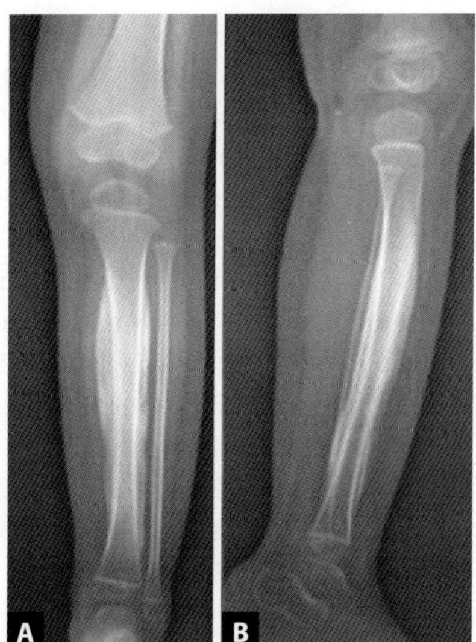

Figs. 1A and B: Periosteal reaction of the tibia, the differential diagnosis could be osteomyelitis, healing fracture, or Caffey's disease.

Limb Length Discrepancy

Children with a limb length discrepancy (LLD) will toe walk on the shorter side. The shortening may be due to developmental dysplasia of the hip (DDH), congenital short femur, postinfective physeal growth arrest, or hemimelia **(Fig. 2)**. Apart from treatment of the primary pathology, a lower extremity scanogram will document the LLD. Treatment is usually a shoe raise and observation for a difference of up to 2 cm. For a greater LLD, lengthening of the short limb with an external fixator or an epiphysiodesis of the contralateral extremity are options after serial documentation of the discrepancy.

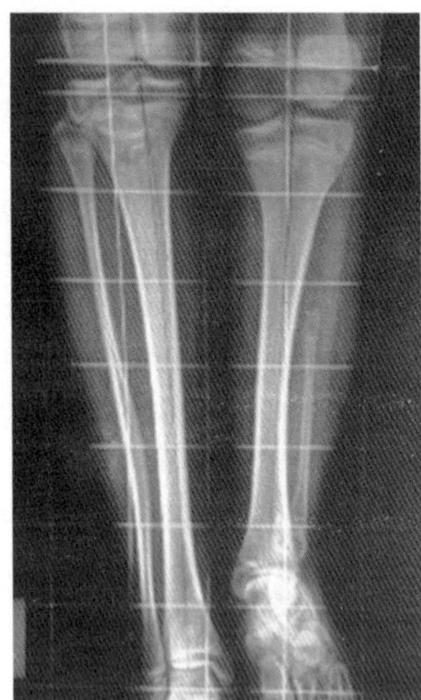

Fig. 2: Limb length discrepancy in a child with fibular hemimelia.

Developmental Dysplasia of Hip

Incidence of neglected DDH is higher in India and other developing countries due to the absence of screening programs and unequal distribution of healthcare facilities and personnel in urban and rural areas. This often results in a missed diagnosis of DDH and children present with a limp **(Fig. 3)**. Diagnosis of DDH in a child of walking age can be made clinically on hip examination by eliciting a telescopy sign and restricted abduction with LLD. The pelvis anteroposterior radiograph will confirm the diagnosis of DDH. Treatment depends on the age of the child. After walking age, open reduction is necessary and may be combined with a femoral and acetabular osteotomy to relocate the head into the acetabulum.

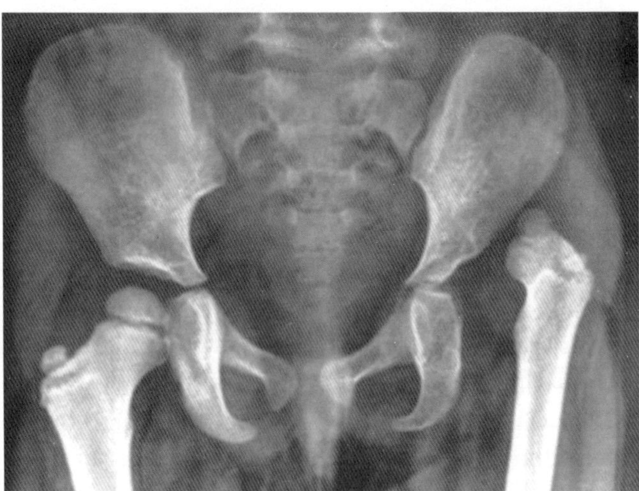

Fig. 3: Developmental dysplasia of the hip.

Slipped Capital Femoral Epiphysis

Slipped capital femoral epiphysis is more common in overweight adolescent boys. Onset of limp and pain could be insidious in stable slips or acute with inability to bear weight in unstable slips. Some patients may complain of knee pain (due to referred pain). Patients will have restricted range of hip movements, with obligatory external rotation on flexion and restricted internal rotation. Anteroposterior and lateral hip X-rays are diagnostic of the slip. Bilateral involvement could occur. An endocrinology workup should be completed. Treatment is dependent on the degree of slip and usually involves surgery with *in-situ* pinning for mild-to-moderate slips and management of any underlying endocrinological condition, if present.

Perthes Disease

Legg-Calvé-Perthes disease usually presents with a painful limp with restricted internal rotation of the hip in children between 6 and 11 years. The prognosis is better in younger children due to the better remodeling potential of the capital femoral epiphysis. Although many theories have been postulated, the etiology is not well defined. The pelvis radiograph will show collapse or extrusion depending on the stage of the disease **(Fig. 4)**. Treatment depends on the age of the patient and stage of the disease, the principle being to contain the hip with an abduction cast, femoral varus osteotomy, or an acetabular shelf procedure.

Osteoid Osteoma

The child will present with boring pain in the extremity with worsening at night and typically NSAIDs will relieve the pain. A computed tomography scan can confirm the diagnosis with a sclerotic ring surrounding a nidus being

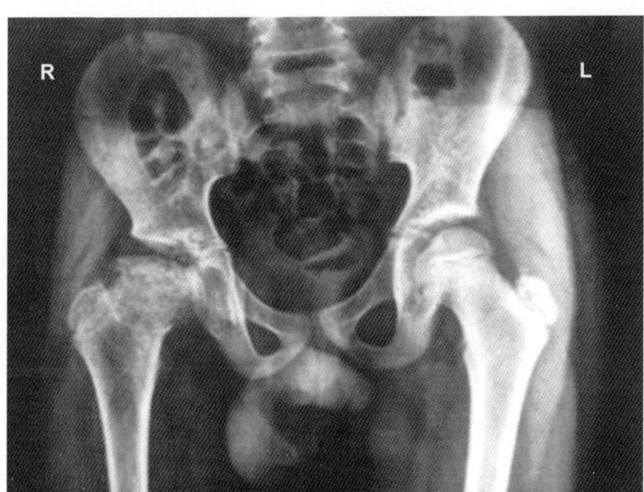

Fig. 4: Perthes disease of the right hip in an 11-year-old male with extrusion and flattening of the head.

the classical radiographic appearance. Treatment is image-guided radiofrequency ablation or surgical excision.

Juvenile Arthritis

Juvenile arthritis is an important DD in a child with a limp who presents with pain in the knee, ankle, or subtalar joints. Swelling with some restriction of movement will be present along with an elevated ESR and antinuclear antibody positive titer, although this may often be negative. Orthopedic intervention is rarely needed.

CLINICAL PEARLS

What to tell the parents?

- A limp is often the tip of the iceberg.
- Investigations are necessary to prove diagnosis or rule out sinister pathology.
- Surgical intervention is very often required, especially in painless limps to prevent future problems.

CONCLUSION

A referral to a pediatric orthopedic specialist is warranted if there is a mild painful limp, not responsive to conservative therapy for more than 10 days; if the limp is associated with severe pain, especially at night; if there is a persistent limp with all basic investigations normal, and if an obvious orthopedic abnormality is diagnosed on investigations.

KEY POINTS

- Onset, duration, progress, and associated symptoms and age of a limping child are your most valuable diagnostic criteria.
- Supportive and relevant investigations will lead to accuracy in management.
- Early and timely referral significantly affect outcome.
- Unilateral painless limp should never be ignored.
- Bilateral limp usually indicative of as generalized or systemic involvement or bilateral pathology which requires correct prioritization of problems.

SUGGESTED READING

1. Aronsson DD, Loder RT, Breur G, Weinstein SL. Slipped capital femoral epiphysis: current concepts. J Am Acad Orthop Surg. 2006;14(12):666-79.
2. Boscainos PJ, Cousins GR, Kulshreshtha R, Oliver TB, Papagelopoulos PJ. Osteoid osteoma. Orthopedics. 2013;36(10):792-800.
3. Flynn JM, Widmann RF. The limping child: evaluation and diagnosis. J Am Acad Orthop Surg. 2001;9(2):89-98.
4. Gill KG. Pediatric hip: pearls and pitfalls. Semin Musculoskelet Radiol. 2013;17(3):328-38.
5. Herring JA. Tachdjian's Pediatric Orthopaedics: From the Texas Scottish Rite Hospital for Children, 5th edition. Philadelphia: Saunders-Elsevier; 2013.
6. Kocher MS, Mandiga R, Zurakowski D, Barnewolt C, Kasser JR. Validation of a clinical prediction rule for the differentiation between septic arthritis and transient synovitis of the hip in children. J Bone Joint Surg Am. 2004; 86-A(8):1629-35.
7. Sawyer JR, Kapoor M. The limping child: a systematic approach to diagnosis. Am Fam Physician. 2009;79(3): 215-24.
8. Shah H. Perthes disease: evaluation and management. Orthop Clin North Am. 2014;45(1):87-97.
9. Sultan J, Hughes PJ. Septic arthritis or transient synovitis of the hip in children: the value of clinical prediction algorithms. J Bone Joint Surg Br. 2010;92(9):1289-93.
10. Weinstein SL, Mubarak SJ, Wenger DR. Developmental hip dysplasia and dislocation: Part II. Instr Course Lect. 2004;53:531-42.

Pulled Elbow, Growing Pains, and Flatfoot

Premal Naik, Hitesh B Chauhan

PULLED ELBOW

Pulled elbow is a common injury in children under the age of 5 years. It is a minor soft-tissue injury of the radio-humeral joint caused by sudden traction on the hand, wrist, or forearm.

Incidence

Five percent of all upper limb injuries less than 10 years age:

- Boys more than girls
- Left more than right.

Mechanism of Injury

Forcible traction applied to the child's pronated hand or wrist with the elbow extended; common circumstances, which leads to such traction injury, are:

- Child's forearm or hand is held firmly by a parent as the child attempts to run away
- Child is lifted by an adult from the ground by his/her hands
- Child may be lifted by the hand from a lying or sitting position or may be swung around by the hands/wrist while playing.

Pathology

Traction on pronated forearm with extended elbow → partial escape of radial head from annular ligament → pulled elbow.

Clinical Features (Flowchart 1)

Child presents with painful dangling arm (infant will present with pseudoparalysis), child does not use the affected limb for holding objects, keeps the elbow extended and forearm pronated, and resists supination of forearm. There is no obvious tenderness, edema, or deformity at elbow.

Flowchart 1: Algorithm for pulled elbow patient.

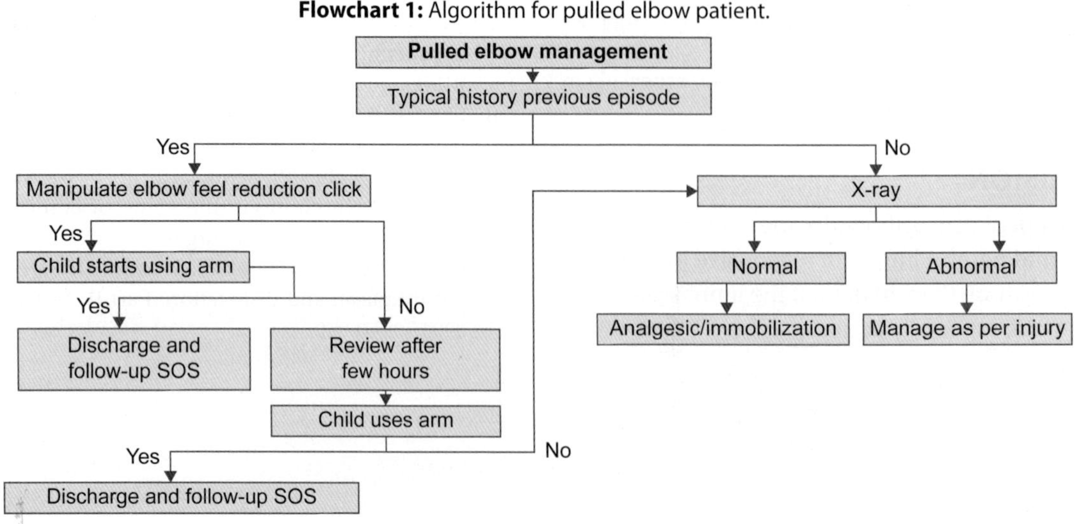

Investigations

Pulled elbow is a clinical diagnosis, but when the mode of trauma and history are not corroborative, X-ray is indicated.

Treatment

Reduction Maneuver

- Hold the child's wrist with one hand and with other hand support the elbow and palpate the radial head → supinate the forearm with upward push on the radial head → click is felt with radial head reduction
- Sometimes pronation and flexion of elbow is also required for reduction
- Click signals successful reduction, the child will be playful and will use the arm after sometime
- If the child is not using arm immediately, should be sent home with analgesics and should be called the next day.

Precautions

An important aspect in the management of pulled elbow is to advise the parents to avoid traction on the child's arm. They should not pull child from hands or wrists. Parents should be advised to discuss this with neighbors and relatives who are expected to handle the child any time.

> **CLINICAL PEARL**
>
> Look for mode of trauma or mechanism of injury, age of the child, absence edema or deformity at elbow, pronation attitude of forearm, and presence of previous history of similar complaints → clinically pulled elbow → reduction maneuver → feel click → dramatic improvement in movements → no immobilization required.

GROWING PAINS (FLOWCHART 2)

These are idiopathic benign pains or discomfort in children.

Incidence

- Fifteen to thirty percent of all children
- More common in girls.

Etiology

Idiopathic in nature, no documented cause has been discovered.

Flowchart 2: Algorithm for growing pains.

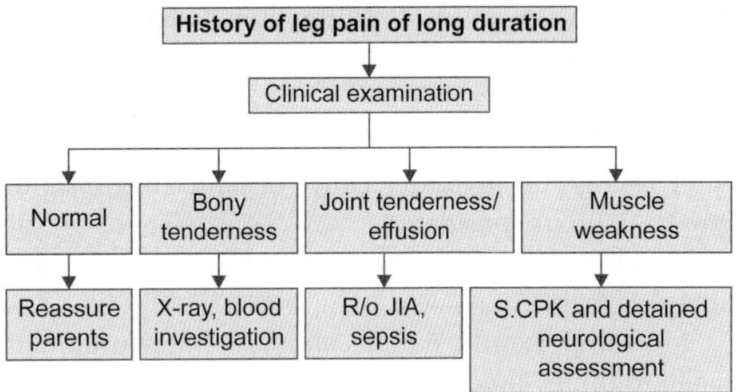

(JIA: juvenile idiopathic arthritis; S. CPK: serum creatine phosphokinase)

Clinical Features

Growing pain is a diagnosis of exclusion. All other causes of leg aches are to be excluded before stamping it as growing pain.

- History is typically vague and of long duration
- Not associated with any functional disability
- Usually occurs at night (just before going to sleep). Occasionally child may get up from sleep due to pain
- Pain is most commonly in calf and ankle region and sometimes is so severe that child cries with pain
- Few children demand massaging for relief of pain
- Primarily involves lower extremities and is mostly bilateral
- Typically child resumes normal activity next day.

On Examination

- Normal walking pattern without limp
- No local tenderness or swelling in joints and muscles
- No muscular spasticity or restriction of joints movements
- No wasting or neurological deficit. Gower test will be negative
- No limb length discrepancy or limb wasting.

Investigations

If history is not corroborative, any other condition should be ruled out with X-rays and blood investigations.

Differential Diagnosis

If there is history of trauma and excessive exertion with local bony tenderness, rule out stress fracture with X-ray. Tumor-like osteoid osteoma, osteogenic sarcomas, or

Ewing's give rise to night pain, but are more aggressive and associated with localized swelling, tenderness and limb wasting.

Management

After ruling out any other cause of pain, diagnosis of growing pains is considered.

No specific treatment, hot fomentation, massage, and analgesic may help.

Most importantly, parents should be reassured and made to understand that growing pain are self-limiting and will subside in due course of time. One can be made to understand relation of pain with sudden increase in height of their child (growth spurt) in last few months.

Relapse may occur in next growth spurt. If any other symptoms like swelling, wasting, and fever develop on follow-up, child should be subjected to further investigation.

> **CLINICAL PEARL**
>
> Long and vague history, bilateral lower extremity, night pain, mainly calf and ankle, normal activities next day, no clinical findings → no radiological findings → diagnosis of exclusion → reassurance, diversion of mind, relapses may occur → look for warning signals.

FLATFOOT

Absence of medial longitudinal arch of foot is known as flatfoot **(Flowchart 3)**.

Incidence

It occurs approximately 20–30% of general population.

Flowchart 3: Algorithm for flatfoot patient.

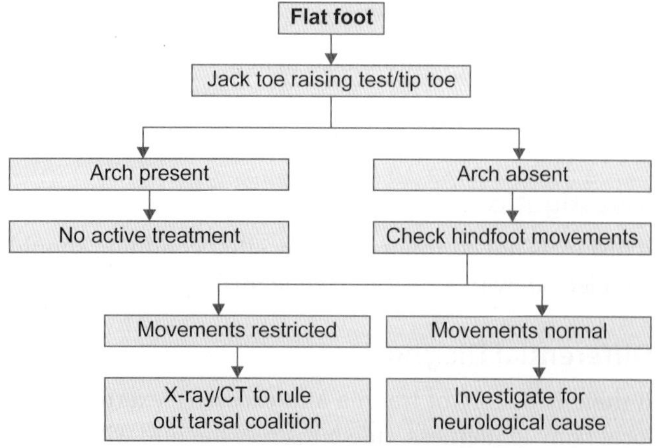

(CT: computed tomography)

Classification

- *Flexible flatfoot:* Arch is absent when patient bears weight but appears off weight. It is be due to hyperlaxity of ligaments **(Fig. 1)**
- *Rigid flatfoot:* Arch is absent all the time, whether child is bearing weight or not. It may be due to:
  - Tarsal coalition
  - Juvenile chronic arthritis
- *Neuromuscular flatfoot:* Flatfoot secondary to muscular imbalance, weakness or spasticity. Common causes are:
  - Cerebral palsy
  - Spina bifida.

Differential Diagnosis

Other conditions which give similar appearance as of flatfoot are:

- Congenital vertical talus
- Accessory navicular.

Clinical Features

- Primarily parents complaint of awkward appearance of foot, uneven shoe ware, or sometimes pain
- Family history may be positive: parents tend to have joint laxity and sometimes flatfeet as well. Tarsal coalitions can be autosomal dominant or recessive
- Many parents are bothered about future participation in sports and army recruitment.

Examination

- *In flexible flatfeet:* Arch disappears on standing, and reappears on taking weight off. Arch also reappears when patient stands on toes **(Fig. 2)**

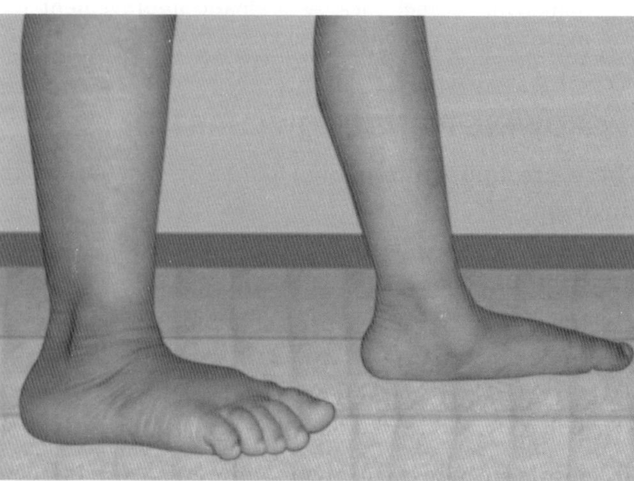

Fig. 1: Patient with flexible flatfoot.

- *Wind up test or Jack toe raising test:* In flexible flatfoot, arch can be reproduced by extending great toe at metatarsophalangeal joint **(Fig. 3)**
- General assessment of signs of hyperlaxity should be looked for hyperextension of elbows, thumb touching to forearm, knee hyperextension
- In rigid flatfeet, arch is always absent, on or off weight. Extension of great toe or standing on toes does not form arch
- Movements of the hindfoot are restricted in rigid flatfeet and free in flexible flatfeet
- Heel is in valgus and corrects on tiptoeing in flexible feet
- Tendo achilles tightness should be looked for
- Detailed neurological examination if any suggestive findings are present.

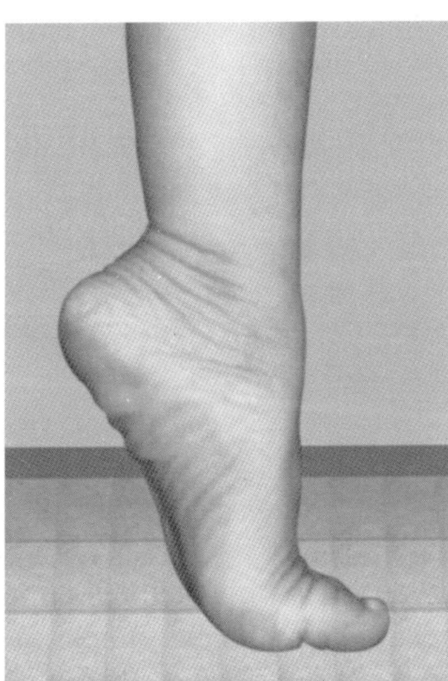

Fig. 2: Same patient showing good arch on tip toe.

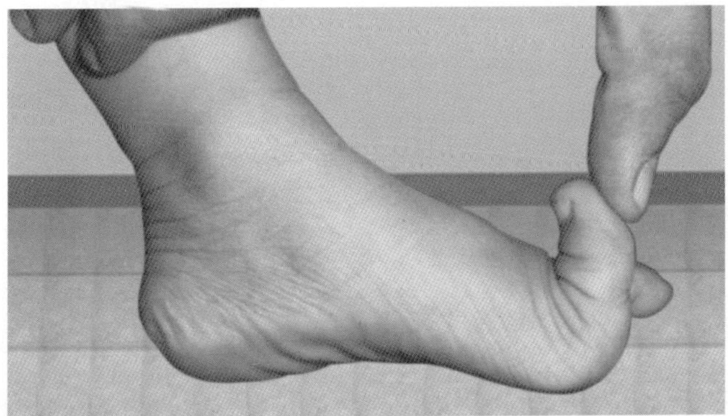

Fig. 3: Same patient showing good arch on extension of great toe.

Investigations

- In flexible flatfeet, no investigations are required, clinical diagnosis is adequate
- In rigid flatfeet, X-rays and computed tomography scan are helpful to rule out tarsal coalitions.

Management

- *In flexible flatfeet:*
  - Parents are reassured regarding benign nature of deformity
  - Promote bare feet walking in sand and garden
  - Special shoes have no role in management of flexible flatfeet (in fact early shoe wearing in city kids is found to have high incidence of flatfeet compared to rural children walking bare feet)
  - Arch support only if severe shoe wear and feet pain
  - Rarely surgery is advised for failed conservative treatment
- *In tarsal coalitions:* Initially, conservative treatment in form of cast followed by splints and arch support is given. If it fails then bar excision surgery is required
- *In neuromuscular flatfeet:* Initial conservative treatment is orthosis. If it fails than surgery in form of muscle balancing or arthrodesis is required.

CLINICAL PEARL

Absence of medial longitudinal arch, complaining of awkward feet and gait pattern, uneven shoe wear and tear, sometimes pain → Look for hyperlaxity, hindfoot movements, presence of arch off weight, jack toe raising test, neurological examination → Absence of radiological signs → Reassurance, barefoot walking, rigid arch support for pain.

KEY POINTS

- Commonly loss of medial longitudinal arch.
- Changes in the hindfoot movement.
- Associated with hyperlaxity.
- Differentiate from tarsal coalition and neurological flatfeet.
- Forcible traction in pronation is the common mechanism.
- Painful nonusage of arm results.
- Reduce on outpatient department (OPD) basis two gentle attempts.
- Reduction click gives dramatic relief.
- Cause is idiopathic.
- Commonly calf pain at night.
- Stretching exercises and hydration maximum relief.

SUGGESTED READING

1. Evans AM. Growing pains: contemporary knowledge and recommended practice. J Foot Ankle Res. 2008;1(1):4.
2. Fabry G. Clinical practice. Static, axial, and rotational deformities of the lower extremities in children. Eur J Pediatr. 2010;169(5):529-34.
3. Harris EJ, Vanore JV, Thomas JL, Kravitz SR, Mendelson SA, Mendicino RW, et al. Diagnosis and treatment of pediatric flatfoot. J Foot Ankle Surg. 2004;43(6):341-73.
4. Irie T, Sono T, Hayama Y, Matsumoto T, Matsushita M. Investigation on 2331 cases of pulled elbow over the last 10 years. Pediatr Rep. 2014;6(2):5090.
5. Krul M, van der Wouden JC, van Suijlekom-Smit LW, Koes BW. Manipulative interventions for reducing pulled elbow in young children. Cochrane Database Syst Rev. 2009;(4):CD007759.
6. Mohanta MP. Growing pains: practitioners' dilemma. Indian Pediatr. 2014;51(5): 379-83.
7. Mosca VS. Flexible flatfoot in children and adolescents. J Child Orthop. 2010;4(2):107-21.
8. Petersen H. Growing pains. Pediatr Clin North Am. 1986; 33(6):1365-72.
9. Weiser P. Approach to the patient with noninflammatory musculoskeletal pain. Pediatr Clin North Am. 2012;59(2): 471-92.

CHAPTER 165

Clubfoot Treatment: Current Concepts

Rujuta Mehta, Alaric J Aroojis, Rupesh Wod

INTRODUCTION

Clubfoot is the one of the most frequent congenital musculoskeletal deformities seen by a pediatrician and referred to a pediatric orthopedic surgeon. With an incidence of 1.2 per 1,000 live livebirths, it is estimated that over 35,000 children are born with clubfoot in India every year. Significant advances have been made over the last few decades regarding the treatment of clubfoot, with a paradigm shift toward more conservative methods of management. This chapter will give the reader an overview of diagnosis and management in concurrence with the changing scenario.

DEFINITION

The term congenital talipes equino varus (CTEV) aptly describes the complex amalgamation of the following deformities of the entire foot: congenital, from birth; talipes, tali = talus and ankle bone, pes = foot; equino, (equinus like a horse's heel) foot fixed in excessive plantar flexion at ankle joint complex; and varus, hindfoot turned inward with subluxation of talonavicular joint. Clubfoot is defined as a congenital foot deformity characterized by equinus of the ankle joint complex, varus through the hindfoot subtalar joint complex, cavus of the midfoot, and adduction of the forefoot **(Fig. 1)**.

CLINICAL PEARL

- Deformity in CTEV is CAVE; Cavus, Adductus, Varus and Equinus.

ETIOLOGY

Multifactorial inheritance system due to intrauterine environment factor leads to idiopathic CTEV and the associated underlying causes lead to secondary/non-idiopathic CTEV **(Box 1)**.

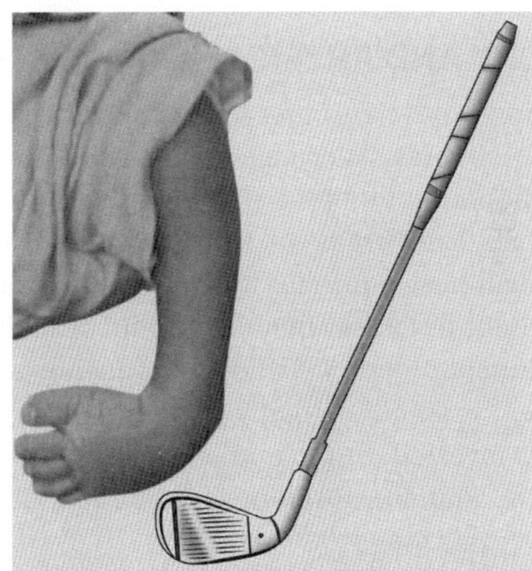

Fig. 1: Clubfoot resembling Golf Club

BOX 1: Etiology.

Most common etiology
- Idiopathic (various theories)
- Neuromuscular etiology, e.g.,
  - Spinal dysraphism/spina bifida
- *Syndromic/genetic etiology, e.g.,:*
  - Arthrogryposis multiplex congenita (AMC)
  - Streeter's dysplasia (constriction band syndrome)
  - Secondary to decrease of size of the uterus resulting from early rupture of amnion with chorion remaining intact

Rarer syndromic etiology
- *Autosomal dominant:* Whistling face/Freeman–Sheldon syndrome (cranio-carpo-tarsal syndrome)
- *Autosomal recessive:*
  - Diastrophic dwarfism (micromelia)
  - Larsen syndrome
  - Down's syndrome
  - Mobius syndrome

PATHOLOGY

Bony and soft-tissue pathology coexist in clubfeet. It is a deformation occurring during the second trimester of pregnancy and not an embryonic malformation except in the teratologic variety. Congenital clubfoot is a complex three-dimensional deformity. The tarsal bones, which are mostly made up of cartilage, are in the most extreme positions of flexion, adduction, and inversion at birth. The talus is in severe plantar flexion, its neck is deflected medially, plantar ward and its head is dislocated out of its socket. The navicular, cuboid, and calcaneus are medially rotated. The ligaments of the posterior-medial aspects of the ankle and the capsules of tarsal joints are very thick, taut, and contracted.

HISTORY AND PHYSICAL EXAMINATION

The treating physician must have a sensitive and kind approach to babies. After a general examination to rule out nonidiopathic clubfeet, parents must be reassured that their baby's deformity will be corrected in a few weeks. The baby will have a normal-looking and functional foot throughout life as long as they are faithful to all the details of the treatment program. Radiographs are not necessary.

The heel is small, medially rotated, and in equinus. The foot is inverted on the end of the tibia. The midfoot is in cavus, and the forefoot is adducted. There is a deep crease on the medial and posterior borders of the foot. The lateral border of the foot is curved. There may be calf muscle atrophy. There is a varying degree of resistance to dorsiflexion and eversion in the foot, i.e., fixed deformity.

It should be differentiated from positional deformity of the foot, which is not fixed, and the foot can be dorsiflexed; the metatarsus adductus, which has only forefoot adduction deformity; and the calcaneo-valgus deformity of the foot, which has excessive dorsiflexion of the foot, in which the toes usually touch the shin.

There are multiple systems to classify clubfoot based on physical examination but commonly used are Pirani, Dimeglio, and PAVER scoring system. The Pirani score is a simple, easy tool for assessing the severity of each of the components of clubfoot. It consists of six different physical examination findings; hindfoot contracture score and midfoot contracture score **(Fig. 2)**, each scored 0 for no abnormality, 0.5 for moderate abnormality, or 1 for severe abnormality. Each foot is assigned a total score, the maximum being 6 points, with a higher score indicating a more severe deformity and 0 point being corrected clubfoot or normal foot. Routine clinical use of one or

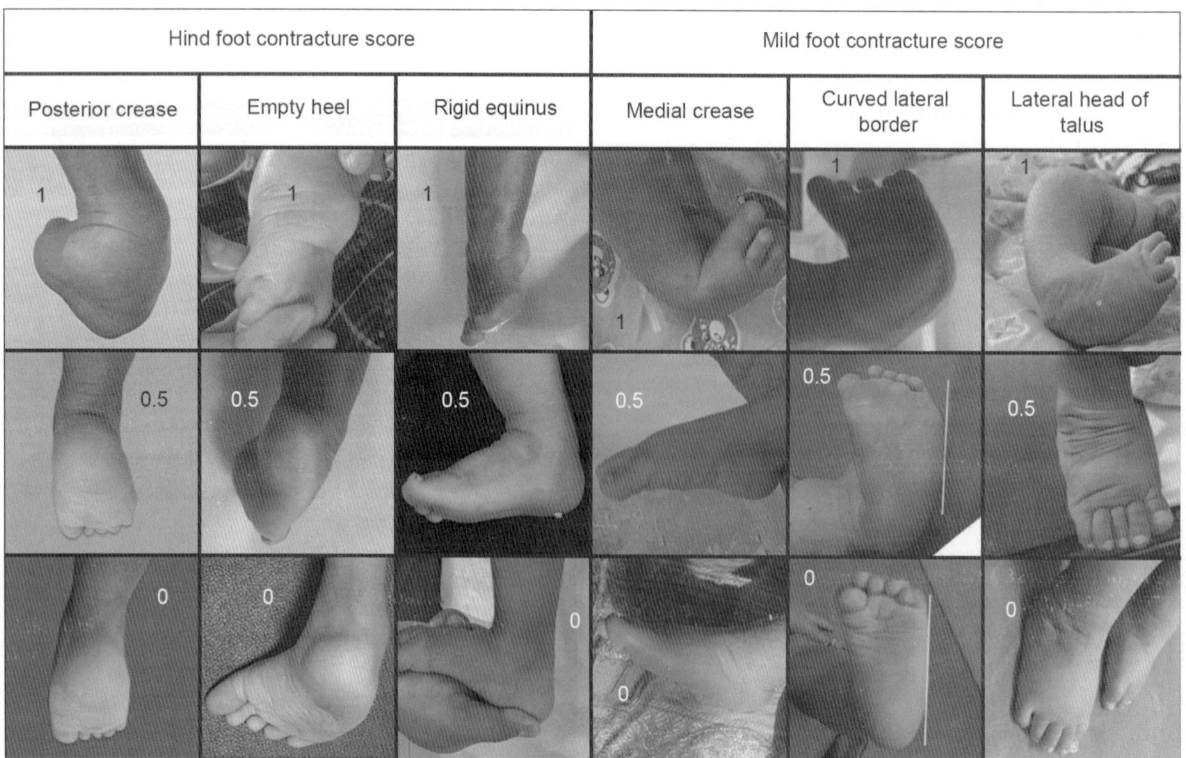

Fig. 2: Pirani score.

both of these classification systems can be helpful in determining prognosis and documenting maintenance of correction or recurrence over time.

ROLE OF PRENATAL DETECTION

Clubfoot can be diagnosed prenatally, commonly by ultrasound in the second trimester and by other techniques such as magnetic resonance imaging (MRI) or karyotyping. But the diagnosis will finally be confirmed only after delivery. As it is difficult to determine on ultrasound whether the feet are actually clubfoot or whether it is a positional defect, whether they are "standard" or atypical, prenatal diagnosis has some limitations.

MANAGEMENT

Treatment of clubfoot as a generic term cannot be clubbed together. It is therefore subdivided as follows:

- Treatment in the prewalking age.
- Treatment after independent walking is achieved.

Treatment in the Prewalking Age

The most widely practiced current standard of care for treatment of clubfeet in the first 6 months of life is the Ponseti method of treatment **(Figs. 3A to E)**. This is a combination of weekly plastering and a semi-invasive procedure of percutaneous tenotomy of the Achilles tendon at the final step of correction. This technique of manipulation and casting is based on anatomical studies and a biomechanical understanding of the "kinematic coupling" of the subtalar joint. It corrects all elements of the deformity, resulting in a functional, pain-free, plantigrade foot with good mobility, without calluses, and without the need for wearing special or modified shoes. Foot examination and corrective manipulations are best done with the baby resting on the mother's lap. When applying the plaster cast, the baby is placed at one end of the table to provide room for the mother and assistant on either side. It is best if the baby is breastfed through the treatment.

Results of the Ponseti Method of Clubfoot Treatment

The Ponseti method is a safe and effective treatment for congenital idiopathic clubfoot and radically decreases the need for extensive corrective surgery. It is the most effective method for children <1 or 2 years of age **(Figs. 4A to D)**.

CLINICAL PEARLS: TREATMENT PROTOCOL

- Treatment can begin as early as first week of life.
- Complex deformity yields better under influence of relaxin with serial casts.
- Deformity is corrected within few weeks with weekly serial casts.
- Achilles tenotomy after correction usually within 5–6 weeks and final cast for 3 weeks.
- After cast removal, foot abduction brace to be worn for 23 hours per day for first 3 months.
- After 3 months worn brace at night time and nap time in afternoon till age of 4 years.
- Adherence to protocol is a must.

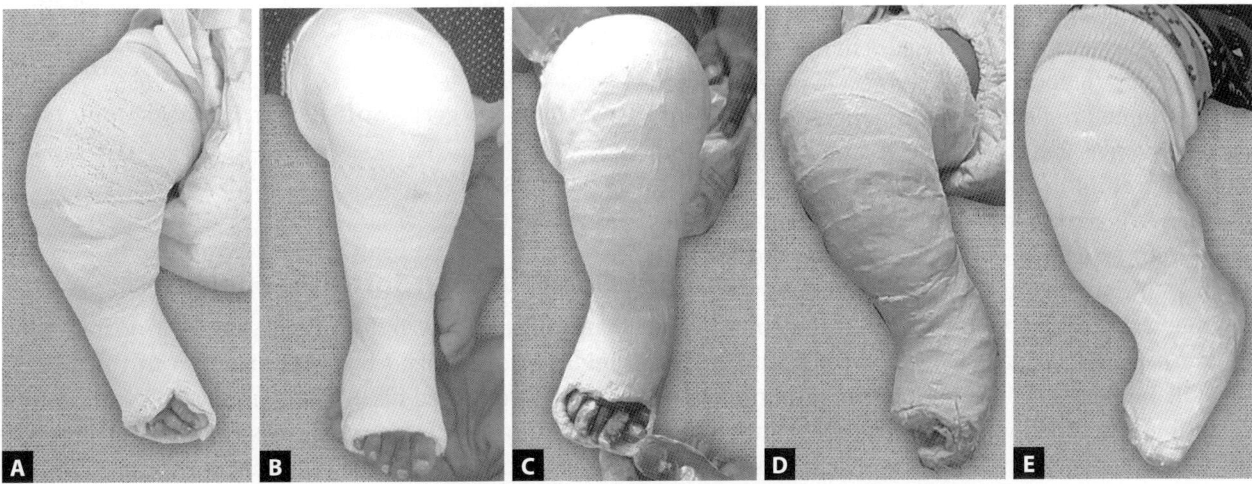

Figs. 3A to E: Technique of Ponseti cast.

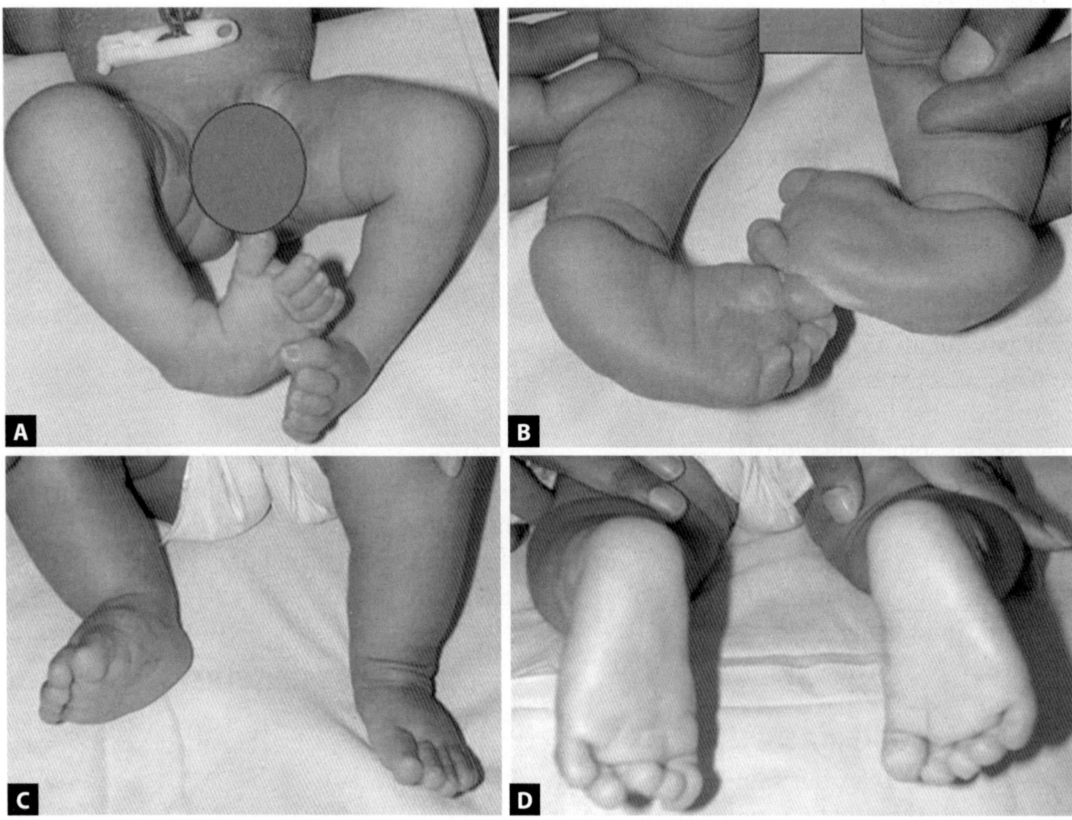

Figs. 4A to D: Result of Ponseti method of treating clubfoot in a 1-week-old neonate. The deformity is fully corrected after five serial manipulations and casting followed by a percutaneous tendo-Achilles tenotomy.

Treatment after Independent Walking is Achieved

Children with clubfoot often present after the walking age, especially in low- and middle-income countries where approximately 80% of children with clubfoot are born. With advancing age, there is increased stiffness of the soft tissue structures and decreased remodeling potential of the bones of the foot. Not all clubfeet in older children are rigid—some are flexible and amenable to stretching and conservative treatment. The treatment of clubfoot in the older child is challenging and was traditionally performed using complex soft tissue and bony surgeries ranging from extensive soft-tissue releases and external fixation with the Ilizarov apparatus to bony osteotomies and triple arthrodesis, often with poor outcomes in the long term. Now it has been changed to conservative treatment utilizing Ponseti principles of serial manipulation and casting, combined with limited surgery such as soft tissue release, tendon transfer, or lateral column shortening osteotomy.

However, the number of casts required are more in comparison with younger children, and a modification in the bracing protocol is required to improve compliance in older children. There is a real and high risk of relapse in approximately one-third of these children but is amenable to re-casting and minor surgical procedures.

Surgical options:

- *Open surgery:* Soft-tissue releases and tendon transfer
- Bony surgery
- Fixators

Open Surgery: Soft-tissue Releases

The most widely followed surgery is a posteromedial release popularized by Vincent Turco in the 1960–70s after he published his original monograph with a 16-year follow-up. This surgery addresses almost all the deforming pathoanatomical structures on the anterior medial and posterior aspects of the foot and their abnormal

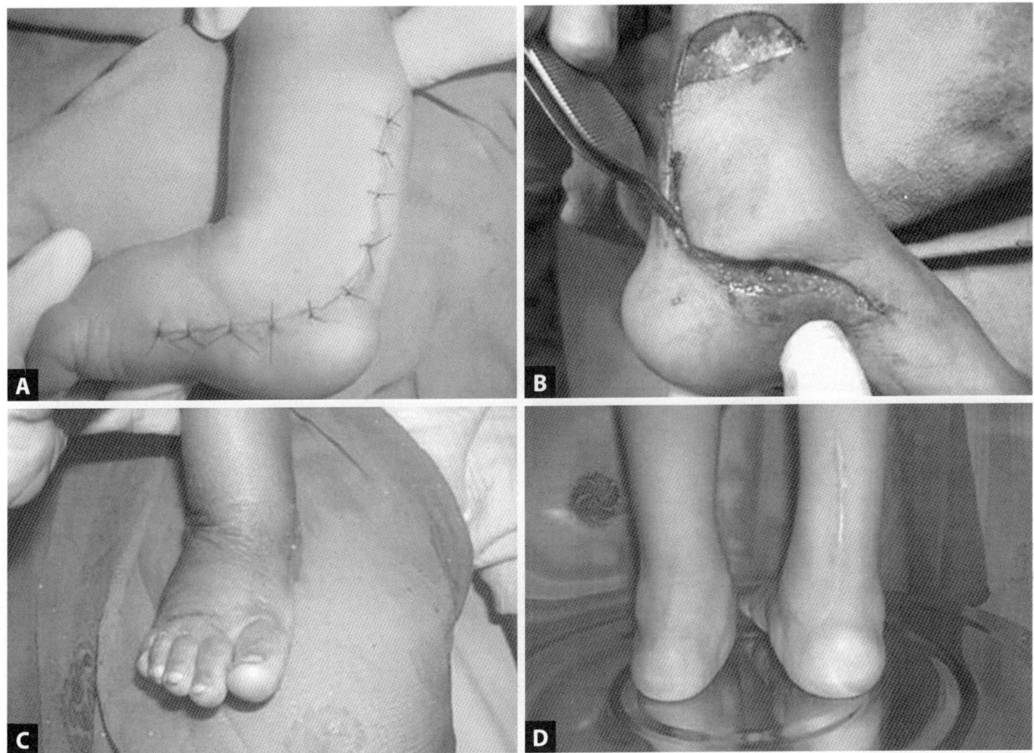

Figs. 5A to D: Steps and result of posteromedial release surgical open release for a 17-month-old boy.
(For color version, see Plate 22)

interrelationships. Results of this surgery are highly gratifying and long-lasting **(Figs. 5A to D)**, but not without their share of complications and morbidity.

Open Surgery: Tendon Transfer

Tendon transfers are indicated for age groups above 3–5 years mainly for residual uncorrected components of clubfoot deformities. Tibialis transfer to the medial cuneiform bone is indicated for dynamic supination and persistent metatarsus adductus deformity, which particularly occurs with relapses of the conservative or Ponseti method of plastering.

Bony Surgery

The incidence of bony surgeries has plummeted in recent years, particularly with the success of conservative techniques; however, it deserves mention.

- *Osteotomies:* Particularly for hind- and midfoot correction above the age of 5 years, after majority of the tarsal bones have ossified.
- *Talectomy/naviculectomy:* This is a surgery with a very select place for the treatment of severe arthrogrypotic feet where the deformity is so severe and no other operation can work so as to prevent plantigrade shoe wear.
- *Triple arthrodesis:* This is a salvage procedure done at or around skeletal maturity for very severe or recalcitrant clubfeet, for the purpose of relieving pain or to facilitate normal shoe wear.

Fixators

In 1989, Dr BB Joshi from Mumbai, India, started using an indigenous external fixation system for gradual distraction of multiplanar deformities of clubfoot. The process has been analogous to an external version of Ponseti principles which gradually unlocks the talus and brings about a complete correction of all components of clubfoot, however, complex the deformity. Fixators are invaluable for neglected and relapsed and rigid clubfeet, particularly 3–14 years **(Figs. 6A to D)**.

Clubfoot is referred at any age and treatment can be instituted irrespective of age of referral. A simple flowchart on treatment of clubfoot treatment is depicted in **Flowchart 1**.

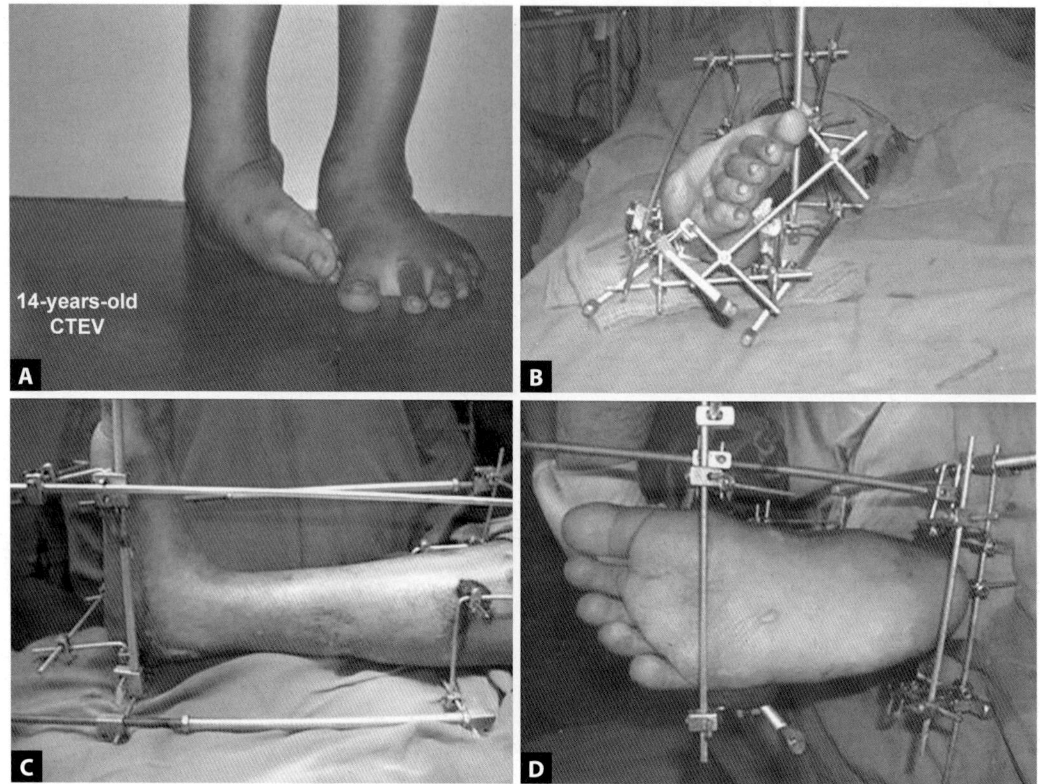

Figs. 6A to D: Deformity, frame, and result of external fixation system for neglected clubfoot.

Flowchart 1: Treatment of clubfoot.

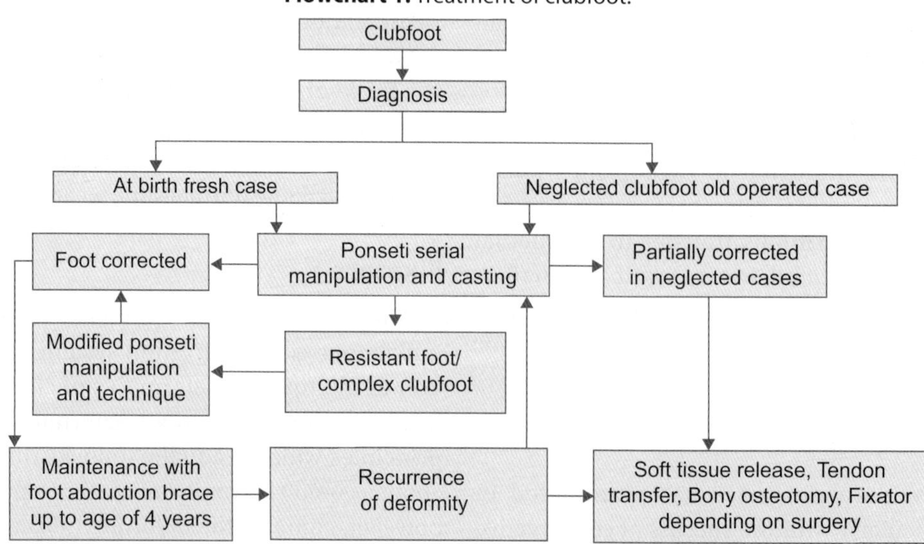

ROLE OF EXERCISES AND SPLINTS

Any method of CTEV correction requires maintenance of correction and sustaining the same till skeletal maturity. This is achieved by using special footwear in the form of ankle-foot orthosis or stiff medial border shoes mounted on an abduction bar with external rotation correction. These are essentially static devices and need to be supplemented with active and assisted active exercises and stimulation of the muscles of the lateral aspect of the foot regularly several times a day over a number of years.

The importance of a regular follow-up and prevention of relapse thus cannot be overemphasized.

CLINICAL PEARLS: COUNSELING TO THE PARENTS

- Treat early.
- Maintain serial casting and bracing protocol.
- Correct treatment will ensure full correction of deformity and good function.
- Surgery when indicated can give good results.
- Postoperative bracing and rehabilitation has a vital role.

KEY POINTS

- Clubfeet vary in severity and presentation.
- Early conservative treatment in the form of serial Ponseti casts is highly successful.
- Recurrences are amenable to successful treatment too.
- Now neglected or resistant feet regardless of age can be treated with Ponseti principles of serial manipulation and casting, combined with limited surgery.

SUGGESTED READING

1. Cooper DM, Dietz FR. Treatment of idiopathic clubfoot. A thirty-year follow-up note. J Bone Joint Surg Am. 1995;77(10):1477-89.
2. Faldini C, Fenga D, Sanzarello I, Nanni M, Traina F, Rosa MAA. Prenatal Diagnosis of Clubfoot: A Review of Current Available Methodology. Folia Med (Plovdiv). 2017;59(3):247-53.
3. Kite JH. The Clubfoot. New York, NY, USA: Grune & Stratton; 1964.
4. Laaveg SJ, Ponseti IV. Long-term results of treatment of congenital club foot. J Bone Joint Surg Am. 1980;62(1):23-31.
5. Morcuende JA, Weinstein SL, Dietz FR, Ponseti IV. Plaster cast treatment of clubfoot: the Ponseti method of manipulation and casting. J Pediatr Orthop B. 1994; B(3):161-7.
6. Penny N, Aroojis A, Mehtani A, Banskota B. Clubfoot Correction in Walking Age Children: A Review. J Foot Ankle Surg (Asia Pacific). 2021;XX(X):1-8.
7. Pirani S, Outerbridge HK, Sawatzky B, Stothers K. A reliable method of clinically evaluating a virgin clubfoot evaluation. In 21st SICOT congress. 1999;29:2-30.
8. Ponseti IV, Zhivkov M, Davis N, Sinclair M, Dobbs MB, Morcuende JA. Treatment of the complex idiopathic clubfoot. Clin Orthop Relat Res. 2006;451:171-6.
9. Ponseti IV. Congenital Clubfoot. Fundamentals of Treatment. Oxford, United Kingdom: Oxford University Press; 1996.
10. Ruzzini L, De Salvatore S, Longo UG, Marino M, Greco A, Piergentili I, et al. Prenatal Diagnosis of Clubfoot: Where are we now? Systemic Review and Meta-Analysis. Diagnostics (Basel). 2021;11(12):2235.
11. Shah A, Mehta R, Aroojis A. The Ponseti method of clubfoot treatment in walking age children: is it effective? A study of 56 children from 1 to 10 years of age. J Pediatr Orthop B. 2019;28(2):159-66.
12. Turco VJ. Surgical correction of the resistant club foot. One-stage posteromedial release with internal fixation: a preliminary report. J Bone Joint Surg Am. 1971;53(3): 477-97.
13. Joshi B, Prabhoo R, Kanaji B, Kaushik S. Correction of CTEV by Controlled Differential Fractional Distraction Using JESS. In: Management of Clubfoot by Joshi's External Stabilization System (JESS) [Internet]. 1st ed. Jaypee Brothers Medical Publishers (P) Ltd.; 2010. p. 38. Available from: https://www.jaypeedigital.com/book/9788184488876/chapter/ch3.

Developmental Dysplasia of the Hip

Rujuta Mehta, Rupesh Wod, Jayanth S Sampath

INTRODUCTION

Hip instability is the most common abnormality in newborn infants. It ranges from mild looseness to complete hip dislocation. Developmental dysplasia of the hip (DDH) is benign as a "silent" condition, so pain is uncommon until later stages, which makes it harder to detect and more difficult to treat unless detected. So screening and early detection of DDH are most important to prevent morbidity and long-term complications. Mild infantile hip instability resolves naturally in most infants during the first few weeks of life, but some infants need evaluation or treatment depending on persistent hip instability, or hip dislocation. If detected early successfully treated with a Pavlik harness and, lately, with closed or open reduction with or without femoral or pelvic osteotomy and hip spica application. This chapter gives a complete overview of DDH and its guidelines.

SPECTRUM OF DEVELOPMENTAL DYSPLASIA OF HIP

Developmental dysplasia of the hip or developmental dysplasia of the hip (DDH) is a term used to describe a spectrum of conditions, from hip subluxation and dislocation to acetabular dysplasia, where the hip joint fails to develop normally during childhood. In the past, descriptions such as congenital hip dislocation or CDH were used, but it is not congenital as it is not always present at birth. So now the preferred term is developmental dysplasia of the hip, which includes the embryonic, fetal, and infantile periods. All of the aforementioned terms refer to the same condition.

INCIDENCE OF DEVELOPMENTAL DYSPLASIA OF HIP

The widely quoted figure of 1–2 cases of dislocation per 1,000 live births is an approximation. The reported incidence of DDH in the literature is influenced by genetic and racial factors, cultural practices (tight swaddling of neonates among Native Americans), experience and training of the examiner, diagnostic criteria applied, and age of the child at presentation. The incidence of neonatal hip instability may be as high as 1 in 100. Since the vast majority of unstable hips in neonates resolve spontaneously, this is termed *physiological instability.*

CLINICAL PEARL

- A significant number of clinically unstable hips resolve spontaneously in the first few weeks of life. This is termed physiological instability. Hip ultrasound scan should be done as early screening tool in such cases.

CAUSES AND RISK FACTORS

Teratologic dislocations are caused by neuromuscular conditions such as Arthrogryposis Multiplex Congenita (AMC), spina bifida, Larsen syndrome, and diastrophic dysplasia. A specific cause may not be readily identifiable in typical dislocations. Genetic and ethnic factors play a key role. A positive family history in 1st degree relatives increases the risk of DDH. Wynne Davies reported a risk of 6% with 1 affected sibling, 12% risk with an affected parent, and 36% when a parent and a sibling are affected.

Other risk factors for DDH, relative risk, and the presumed pathogenetic mechanisms are summarized in **Table 1**.

DIAGNOSING DEVELOPMENTAL DYSPLASIA OF THE HIP

Clinical Examination

There are no pathognomonic physical findings in DDH which will help the clinician make a reliable diagnosis at any age and in every child. Considerable skill, experience, and patience are therefore essential if an accurate

TABLE 1: Risk factors for developmental dysplasia of the hip (DDH), relative risk, and the presumed pathogenetic mechanisms.

Risk factor	***Relative risk***	***Mechanism***
Breech presentation (See note later)	5–6 times (greater risk if frank breech with hip flexion and knee extension)	Intrauterine compression, though preterm breech babies also at risk
"Clicky" hips at birth	8 times compared to normal hip examination at birth	
Birth order	>50% of DDH in 1st born	Tight uterus
Girls	3–6 times greater than boys	Greater susceptibility in girl babies to the maternal hormone relaxin causes ligamentous laxity
Side affected	*Left:* Right ratio of 3:1	Left occipitoanterior position causes the left hip to rest against the mother's spinal column
Oligohydramnios	Higher risk if clinically significant, low risk if diagnosis made on sonography	Intrauterine compression
Postural foot deformity	Risk varies from 1 in 27 for postural Talipes to 1 in 5 for calcaneovalgus feet	Extraneous compression of the hip on the affected side
Improper swaddling practice during first year of life **(Fig. 1)**	Risk up to 2 times	Attempts to forcibly correct the hip and knee physiological flexion contractures result in abnormal joint reaction forces across the hip joint

Note: Successful external cephalic version for breech presentation reduces but does not abolish DDH risk. Ultrasound screening of the hips for babies in this category is recommended.

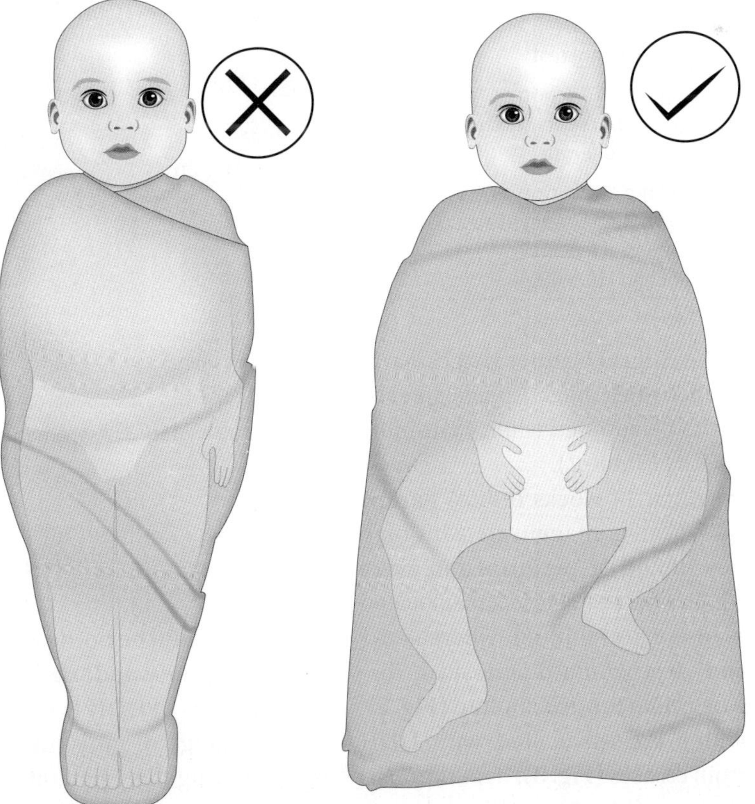

Fig. 1: Traditional improper swaddling (X) and safe swaddling (√).

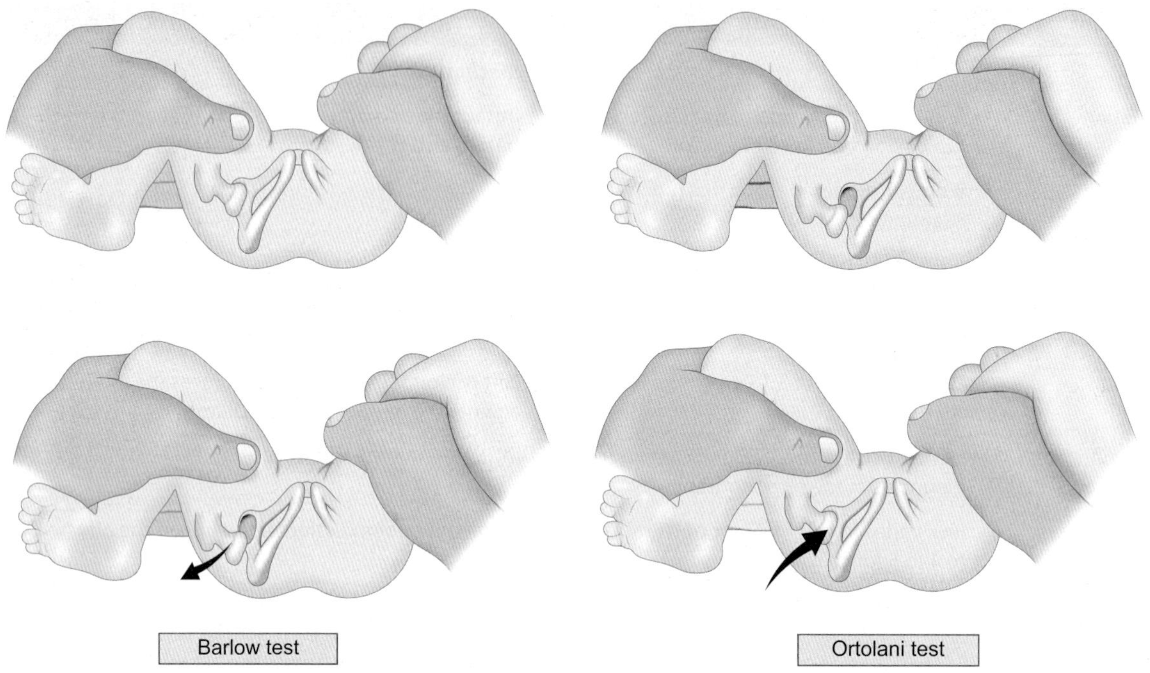

Fig. 2: Barlow test and Ortolani test.

TABLE 2: Clinical test important for screening of developmental dysplasia of the hip (DDH) according to age.	
Age	***Clinical test***
0–14 weeks	Barlow and Ortolani test
14 weeks–6 months	• Reduced hip abduction • Leg length discrepancy/Galeazzi Test (short affected femur)
6 months and above	• Reduced hip abduction • Leg length discrepancy/Galeazzi Test (short affected femur) • Limp (if child is walking)

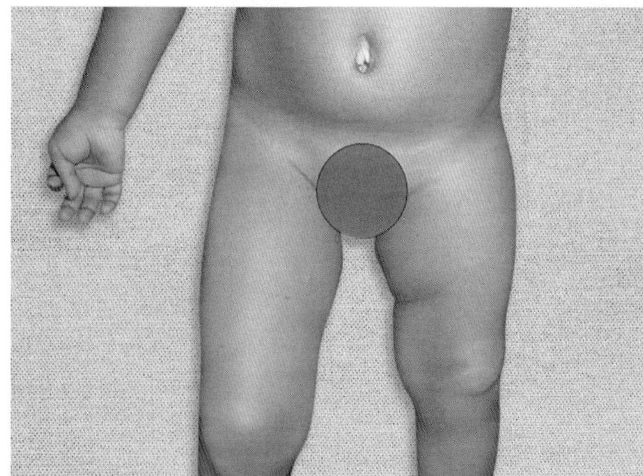

Fig. 3: Asymmetry of groin creases.

diagnosis is to be made. The clinical features suggestive of DDH change as the child becomes older. An age-specific approach therefore needs to be adopted when examining the child with suspected DDH **(Table 2)**.

At or soon after birth (first 14 weeks of life) Barlow and Ortolani tests are provocative maneuvers with high specificity for DDH. They should be performed in every child at or soon after birth. Barlow test detects an enlocated hip which dislocates from the acetabulum, whereas the Ortolani is a "relocation" test which diagnoses a dislocated hip as it reduces back into the acetabulum **(Fig. 2)**. Other clinical signs which are associated with DDH include asymmetrical groin creases **(Fig. 3)**, hyperlordosis **(Fig. 4)**, positive Galeazzi test **(Fig. 5)**, and limb length discrepancy. Reduced hip abduction (<60°) is a sensitive clinical indicator of DDH in children over the age of 3 months.

DDH should be borne in mind when examining a child with a limp or waddling gait. An important principle in the diagnosis of DDH is to detect asymmetry in the limbs (length, range of movement, etc.). However, it is worth remembering that bilateral DDH is frequently missed due to lack of asymmetry.

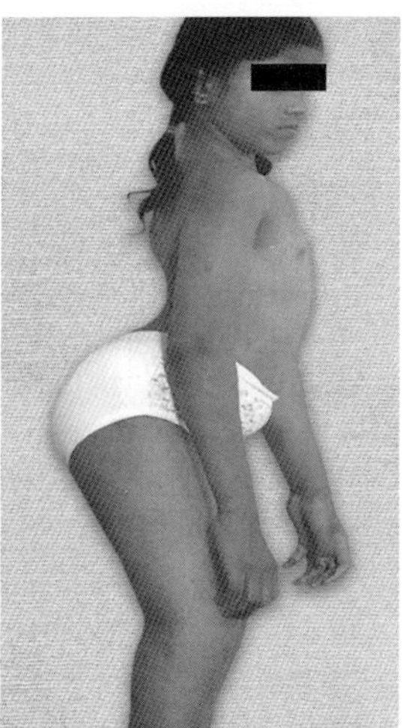

Fig. 4: Hyperlordosis.

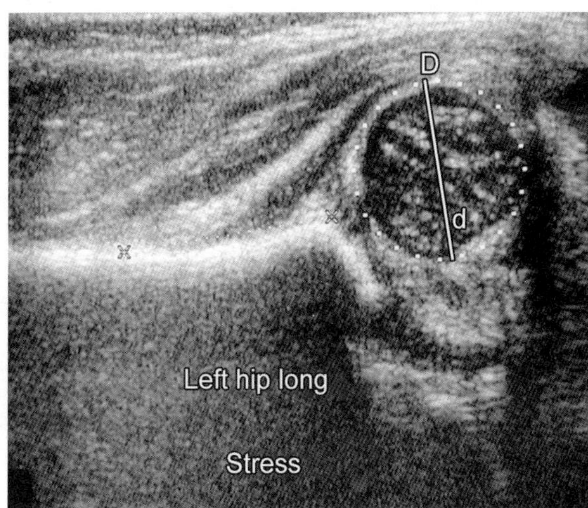

Fig. 6: Ultrasound image of left hip dislocated on stress.

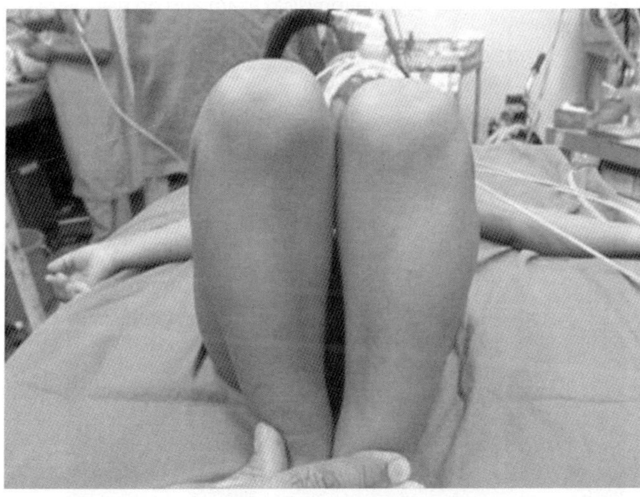

Fig. 5: Positive Galeazzi test.

CLINICAL PEARL

- All newborns, irrespective of risk factors, should undergo a careful examination of the hip by a pediatrician at or soon after birth. Barlow and Ortolani tests should be performed and the results clearly documented.

INVESTIGATIONS

Though clinical tests for DDH have high specificity (>90%), they lack sensitivity particularly in neonates and infants (around 60% only). By no means does a normal clinical examination rule out DDH. The clinician should therefore select an investigation which will conclusively confirm or rule out DDH. The choice of test again depends on the age of the child.

0–14 weeks of age: Ultrasound scanning of the hips using the Graf (Static) and Harcke (Dynamic) methods is recommended in children younger than 14 weeks.

In the Graf method, α and β angles are calculated and these angles guide treatment. The α angle is an indicator of the extent of development of the bony acetabulum ("Bony Roof"). The β angle is an indicator of development of the cartilaginous roof **(Fig. 6)**.

The Graf method is precise and has been standardized to a high degree. Specific training in ultrasound scanning for hip dysplasia is necessary in order to obtain good quality ultrasound scans.

Ideally, all new-born babies should undergo a hip ultrasound scan. Though practiced in certain parts of Europe, Universal Neonatal Ultrasound Hip Screening cannot be justified due to cost, logistical hurdles, and the relatively low incidence of abnormal hips requiring treatment. As mentioned earlier, many physiologically immature hips will resolve spontaneously by 6 weeks of age. Universal screening may result in overtreatment of immature hips and the possibility of iatrogenic complications such as avascular necrosis of the femoral head.

Selective Ultrasound Hip Screening based on risk factors for DDH has been implemented more widely in the UK, US, and other developed nations, as well as our country **(Table 3)**.

Children older than 14 weeks: A good quality antero-posterior X-ray of the pelvis will clearly demonstrate the problem in the vast majority of cases. Various lines are

TABLE 3: Guidelines for screening for developmental dysplasia of the hip. (As per National DDH Expert Group)

Clinical workup	***Imaging recommendations***	***Timing for referral to orthopedics***
Risk factors: • Breech presentation • Family history of DDH • Improper swaddling practices • History of hip instability in any previous clinical exam *Clinical tests:* • Ortolani test (<14 weeks) Barlow test (<14 weeks) • Limited hip abduction (>14 weeks) • Galeazzi test/leg length discrepancy (>14 weeks) Sign of limp (walking age)	*Indications for imaging:* • One or more risk factor(s) present • Positive Barlow in baby <6 weeks • Inconclusive/uncertain clinical exam *Age-dependent imaging recommendations:* • Ultrasound at 6 weeks if babies <6 weeks of age • Immediate ultrasound for babies 6–14 weeks of age • Immediate ultrasound or AP pelvis X-ray for babies between 14 weeks–6 months of age • Immediate AP pelvis X-ray for babies >6 months of age *Imaging alternatives:* Ultrasound before 6 weeks of age if baby is at risk for loss to follow-up anteroposterior (AP) pelvis X-ray not earlier than 14 weeks of age if quality ultrasound is not available	*Urgent:* Abnormal imaging findings *Abnormal clinical exam:* • Positive Ortolani • Positive Barlow in baby >6 weeks • Limited hip abduction • Positive Galeazzi test/leg length discrepancy • Limp in walking age child. *Not urgent:* Positive Barlow in baby <6 weeks *(May spontaneously resolve. Only refer if first imaging is abnormal)* *Referral not required:* • Normal physical exam and no risk factors present • Normal imaging findings

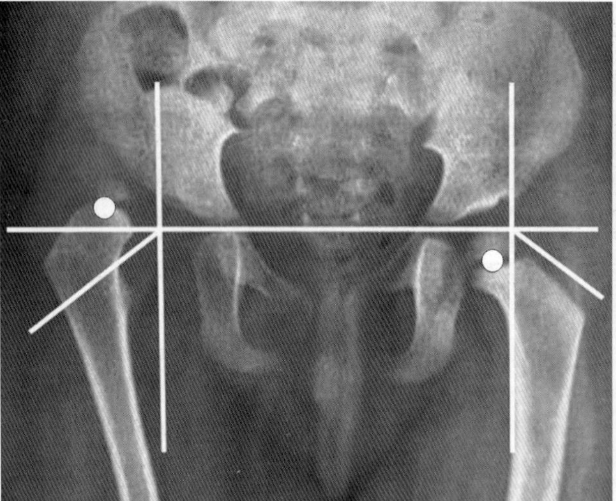
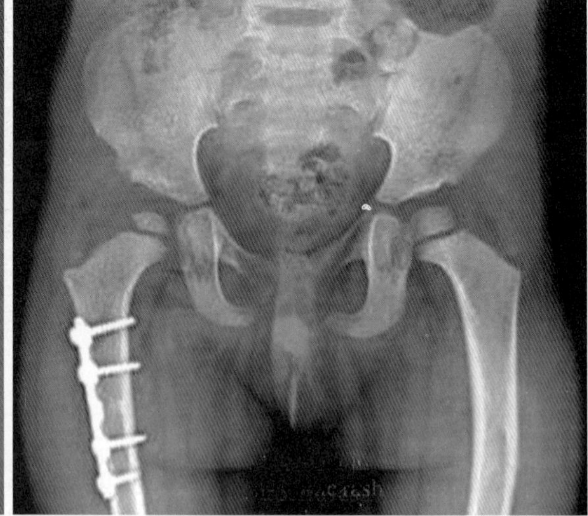

Fig. 7: X-ray image of right developmental dysplasia of the hip (DDH) with marking of lines and relocated same hip after operation.

drawn on the X-ray by orthopedic surgeons as illustrated but these are probably of little interest to pediatricians. Briefly, in pelvis radiograph the Hilgenreiner's (horizontal) line and Perkin's (perpendicular) line divides it in four quadrants as shown in **Figure 7**. The normal hip lies in the inner-lower quadrant (left hip of **Fig. 7**) and outside of this quadrant is suggestive of DDH (right hip of first image of **Fig. 7**).

DEVELOPMENTAL DYSPLASIA OF THE HIP SCREENING AND CARE PATHWAY

The Paediatric Orthopaedic Society of India (POSI) took the lead in setting up a high-level DDH Expert Group comprising of members of various national organizations such as, the Indian Academy of Pediatrics (IAP), National Neonatology Forum of India (NNFI),

Flowchart 1: Algorithm for developmental dysplasia of the hip (DDH) screening in India.

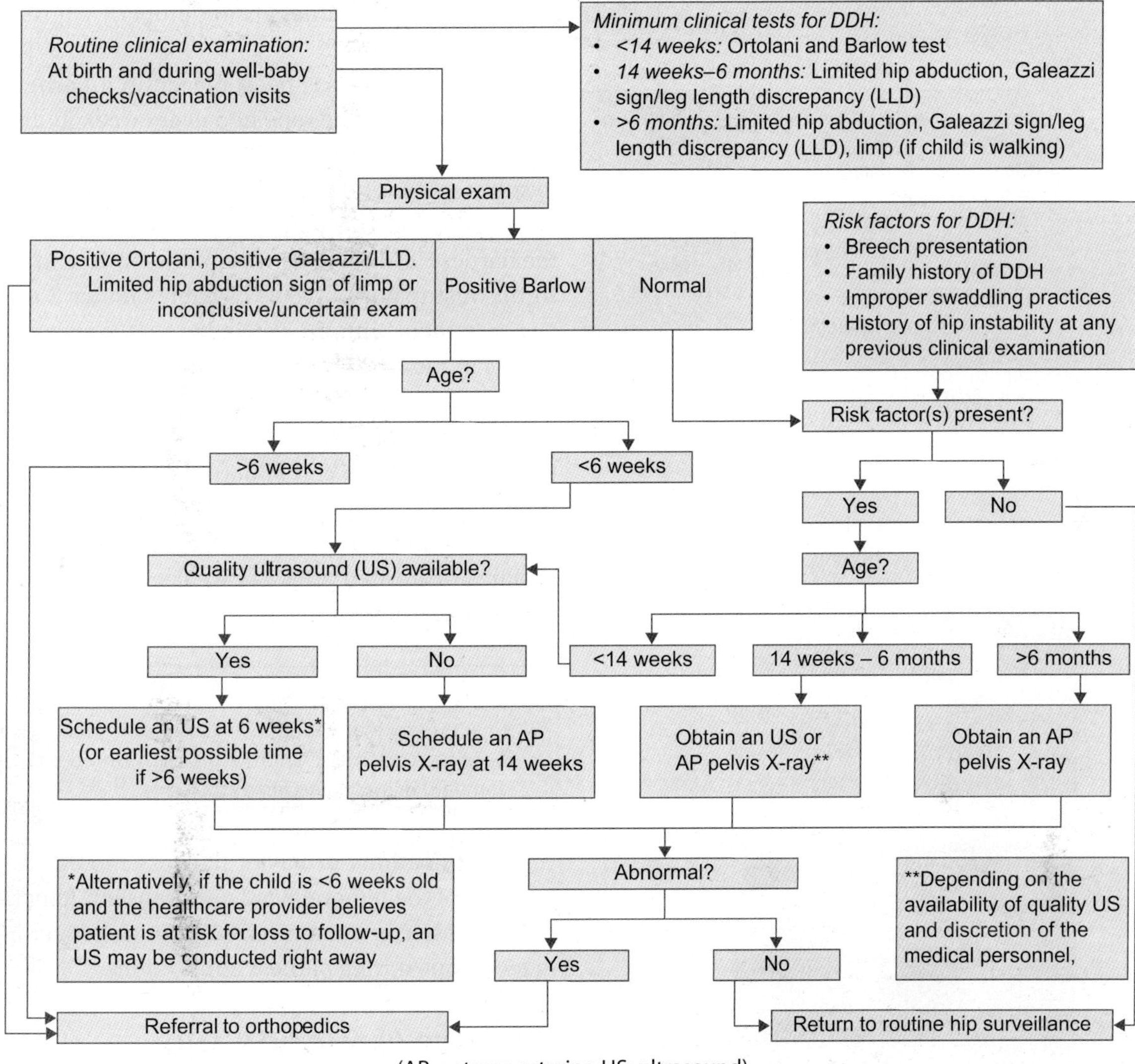

(AP: anteroposterior; US: ultrasound)

Indian Radiological and Imaging Association (IRIA), Indian Federation for Ultrasound in Medicine and Biology (IFUMB), Indian Orthopaedic Association (IOA), and the Federation of Obstetric and Gynaecological Societies of India (FOGSI); with each organization nominating a few representatives involved in pediatric care, in order to establish contextually-relevant screening guidelines for DDH in India **(Flowchart 1)**. The goal is to develop practice guidelines that is feasible to be implemented across the country's diverse healthcare settings. This pathway has the potential to standardize diagnosis and management decisions and decrease the prevalence of walking-age DDH on a national scale.

WHAT ARE THE TREATMENT OPTIONS?

Treatment of DDH is entirely dependent on the age of the child. The younger the child at diagnosis, less the intervention required. *It is therefore important that the diagnosis is made as soon after birth as possible.*

Figure 8 summarizes the treatment options for DDH at different ages. Note that the treatment becomes progressively more invasive with increasing age at treatment.

PAVLIK HARNESS

Pavlik harness is one of the most common nonoperative treatment methods because it is simple, easy to use,

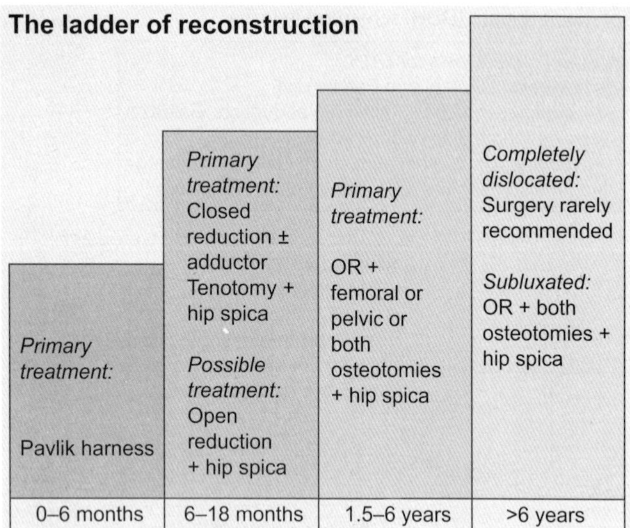

Fig. 8: Treatment options for developmental dysplasia of the hip (DDH) at different ages.

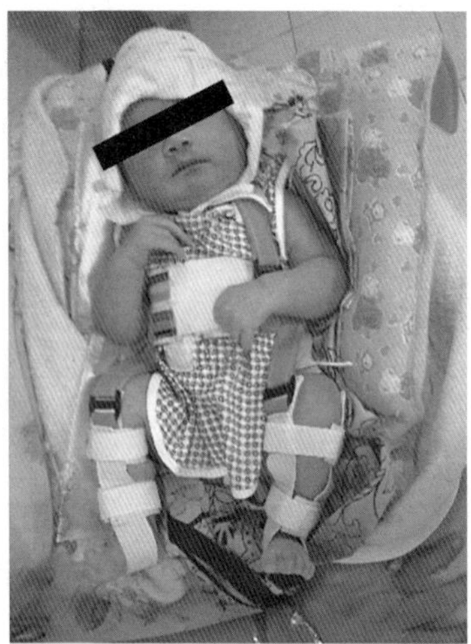

Fig. 9: Baby wearing Pavlik harness.

baby friendly, and have excellent results. The Pavlik harness can be used to correct stable dysplasia, unstable dysplasia, or hips that are dislocated at rest. The baby can kick both legs freely within the harness and it does not interfere with normal growth of the baby **(Fig. 9)**. The Pavlik harness is applied by first placing the chest strap just below the nipple line. The child's feet are placed in the stirrups, the hips are placed in 90–120° of flexion, and the anteromedial flexion straps are secured. The posterior abduction straps are fastened loosely to allow for the abduction of the hips to occur by gravity alone (<70°). Abduction should never be forced by the straps on the harness. Excessive flexion must be avoided; it will occur if the harness is not properly adjusted as the child grows.

Once the baby has been placed in a harness, ultrasound scans must be repeated every week in dislocated, 2–4 weekly in dislocatable, and 4–6 weekly in stable dysplastic hip until the hip is anatomically located back in the hip joint. This may take 2–4 weeks. Average time in the harness is likely to be worn between 10 and 12 weeks. In the vast majority (95%) of babies under 3 months of age, treatment with the Pavlik harness is successful, and results in radiographically normal hips when assessed at 5 years of age.

Red flag for Pavlik Harness is irreducibility and teratologic hip. The end of harness is instituted when hip is normal on ultrasonography (USG) or radiograph (IHDI grade I) directly or after night-time weaning. If the hip remains dislocated after 3–4 weeks of harness wear, the use of the harness should be discontinued.

CLINICAL PEARL

- In summary, early diagnosis (soon after birth) and Pavlik harness treatment should be considered as the gold standard in managing hip dysplasia.

Complications of Pavlik harness include avascular necrosis of the femoral head and transient femoral nerve palsy. These can be minimized through proper attention to technique during harness application.

CLOSED REDUCTION AND HIP SPICA APPLICATION

If the child is older than 6 months at diagnosis, Pavlik harness is not appropriate. In this group (6 months–12 months), an arthrogram will be necessary. A short general anesthetic is given. A radio-opaque dye is also instilled into the hip joint to provide contrast. If the hip can be reduced without undue force, a hip spica is applied. The total period in the Hip spica ranges from 2 to 6 months followed by hip abduction brace from 4 to 6 months.

The term *closed* reduction refers to reducing a dislocated joint without the need for an incision. This is in contrast to an *open* reduction where an incision is necessary.

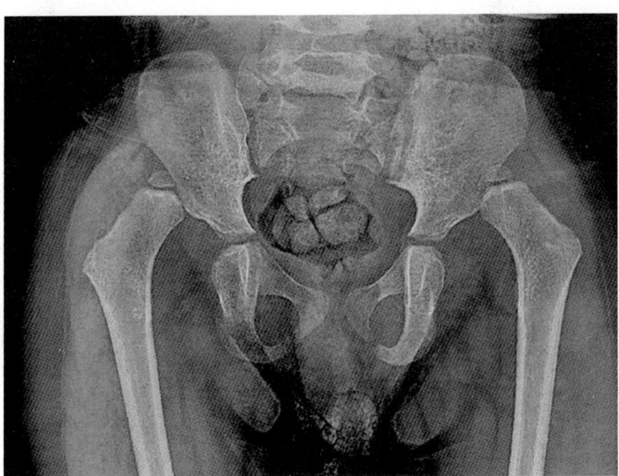

Fig. 10: Neglected bilateral developmental dysplasia of the hip (DDH) in the older child.

SURGICAL TREATMENT

Open Reduction

Indicated when unable to relocate in closed reduction or re-dislocation of hip. Open reduction in generally done with medial hip approach in <1 year age and anterior or anterolateral approach in child >1 years of age.

Open Reduction with Femoral and Pelvic Osteotomy

In a dislocated hip, concomitant acetabular dysplasia (shallow acetabulum) is almost always present. Children <18 months of age possess considerable remodeling capacity and early reduction of the hip typically results in spontaneous resolution of the acetabular dysplasia. In children older than 18 months at presentation, an additional procedure in the form of a pelvic osteotomy is usually required. In addition to the pelvic osteotomy, a femoral osteotomy is also sometimes required.

Unilateral neglected DDH can be treated safely up to the age of 8 years. The upper limit of age for treatment of *bilateral* neglected DDH **(Fig. 10)** is approximately 5 years. In children older than these age thresholds, there is unacceptably high incidence of iatrogenic complications which compromises the eventual outcome.

CLINICAL PEARL

- The key to successful management of DDH is to identify risk factors for DDH in the newborn, confirm the diagnosis by hip ultrasound scan, and institute early appropriate treatment.

KEY POINTS

- First screening for DDH clinically in neonatal intensive care unit (NICU)—Barlow's and Ortolani test
- Hips with persistent instability at 6 weeks need to be treated.
- Prewalking DDH treatment is more successful than post-walking. A painless unilateral limp or a bilateral waddle in a child must always be investigated for DDH.
- Surgical treatment is indicated postwalking and can have a successful outcome.
- Various options are available for the neglected DDH, surgically.
- All varieties of DDH should be treated to eliminate the lurch and prevent secondary osteoarthritis, and problems with the lumbar spine which may occur if left untreated.

SUGGESTED READING

1. Aroojis A, Anne RP, Li J, Schaeffer E, Kesavan TMA, Shah S, et al. Surveillance for Developmental Dysplasia of the Hip in India: Consensus Guidelines From the Pediatric Orthopaedic Society of India, Indian Academy of Pediatrics, National Neonatology Forum of India, Indian Radiological and Imaging Association, Indian Federation of Ultrasound in Medicine and Biology, Federation of Obstetric and Gynaecological Societies of India, and Indian Orthopaedic Association. Indian Pediatr. 2022;59(8):626-35.
2. Barlow T. Early diagnosis and treatment of congenital dislocation of the hip. J Bone Joint Surg. 1962;44-B: 292.
3. Biedermann R, Eastwood DM. Universal or selective ultrasound screening for developmental dysplasia of the hip? A discussion of the key issues. J Child Orthop. 2018;12(4):296-301.
4. Dunn P. The anatomy and pathology of congenital dislocation of the hip. Clin Orthop Relat Res. 976;119: 23-7.
5. Gage J, Winter R. Avascular necrosis of the capital femoral epiphysis as a complication of closed reduction of congenital dislocation of the hip. J Bone Joint Surg. 1972; 74-A:624.
6. Graf R. Classification of hip joint dysplasia by means of sonography. Arch Orthop Trauma Surg. 1984;102(4): 248-55.
7. Harcke H, Kumar J. The role of ultrasound in the diagnosis and management of congenital dislocation and dysplasia of the hip. J Bone Joint Surg. 1991;73-A(4): 622-8.
8. International Hip Dysplasia Institute. Hip dysplasia brochures. [online] Available from https://hipdysplasia.

org/get-involved/hip-dysplasia-brochures/ [Last assessed March, 2025].
9. Kelley SP, Feeney MM, Maddock CL, Murnaghan ML, Bradley CS. Expert-Based Consensus on the Principles of Pavlik Harness Management of Developmental Dysplasia of the Hip [published correction appears in JB JS Open Access. 2019;4(4):e0054.
10. Klisic PJ. Congenital dislocation of the hip: a misleading term. J Bone Joint Surg. 1989;71(1):136.
11. Laurenson R. The acetabular index: a critical review. J Bone Joint Surg. 1959;41-B(4):702-10.
12. Ortolani M. Congenital hip dysplasia in the light of early and very early diagnosis. Clin Orthop Relat Res. 1976;119: 6-10.
13. POSI. Development of DDH Screening Guidelines and DDH Care Pathway. [online] Available from https://www.posi.in/DDH-screening-guideline-for-India.html [Last accessed March, 2025].
14. Severin E. Contribution to the knowledge of congenital dislocation of the hip joint. Acta Chir Scand. 1941; 84:1.
15. Strayer L. Embryology of the human hip joint. Clin Orthop Relat Res. 1971;74:221-40.
16. Suzuki S, Yamamuro T. Correlation of fetal posture and congenital dislocation of the hip. Acta Orthop Scand. 1986;57(1):81-4.
17. Vaidya S, Aroojis A, Mehta R. Developmental Dysplasia of Hip and Post-natal Positioning: Role of Swaddling and Baby-Wearing. Indian J Orthop. 2021;55(6):1410-6.
18. Wenger DR. Congenital hip dislocation: Techniques for primary open reduction including femoral shortening. Instr Course Lect. 1989;38:343.

Index

Page numbers followed by *b* refer to box, *f* refer to figure, *fc* refer to flowchart, and *t* refer to table.

A

B

C

D

E

F

G

H

I

J

K

M

N

O

P

Q

R

S

U

V